AF305921

Orthopedic Surgical Pathology

Dedication

To my wife, Danielle Myriam, with love
Michel Forest

Technical note

Unless otherwise specified, histological staining used for
all figures is hematoxylin-erythrosin-saffron.

Editorial note

References given in the text in the Harvard (name–date)
system are listed in the Library for the Pathologist on
page 773.

For Churchill Livingstone

Commissioning Editor: Sheila Khullar, Gavin Smith
Copy Editor: Holly Regan-Jones
Project Manager: Nora Naughton
Design Direction: Jeanette Jacobs

Orthopedic Surgical Pathology:
Diagnosis of Tumors and Pseudotumoral Lesions of Bone and Joints

Edited by

Michel Forest MD

Professor of Pathology, Head of the Department of Pathology, Hospital Cochin, Paris, France

Associate Editors

Bernard Tomeno MD

Professor of Orthopedic Surgery, Head of the Department of Orthopedic Surgery, Hospital Cochin, Paris, France

Daniel Vanel MD

Head of Department of Radiology, Institute Gustave Roussy, Villejuif, France

Foreword by

Peter G. Bullough MD

Director of Laboratory Medicine, Hospital for Special Surgery, Professor of Pathology,
Cornell University Medical College, New York, USA

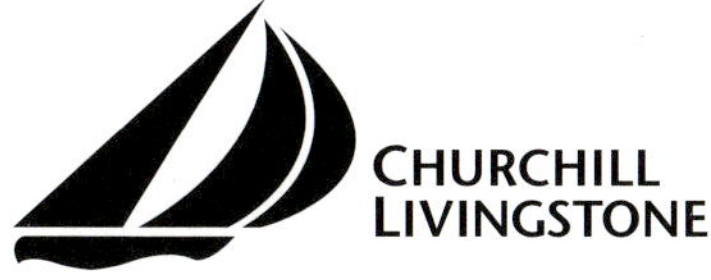

EDINBURGH LONDON NEW YORK PHILADELPHIA SAN FRANCISCO SYDNEY TORONTO 1988

CHURCHILL LIVINGSTONE
A Division of Harcourt Brace and Company Limited

Robert Stevenson House, 1–3 Baxter's Place, Leith Walk
Edinburgh, EH1 3AF.

© Harcourt Brace and Company Limited

 is a registered trademark of Harcourt Brace and Company Limited

ISBN 0 443 05540 8

British Library Cataloguing in Publication Data
A catalogue record for this book is available from the British Library.

Library of Congress Cataloging in Publication Data
A catalog record for this book is available from the Library of Congress.

Medical knowledge is constantly changing. As new information becomes available, changes in treatment, procedures, equipment and the use of drugs become necessary. The editors/authors/contributors and the publishers have, as far as it is possible, taken care to ensure that the information given in the text is accurate and up to date. However, readers are strongly advised to confirm that the information, especially with regard to drug usage, complies with latest legislation and standards of practice.

The
publisher's
policy is to use
**paper manufactured
from sustainable forests**

Printed in Hong Kong

Contents

Contributors

Claire Alapetite MD
Assistant, Department of Radiotherapy. Institut Curie, Paris

Jacques Amouroux MD
Professor of Pathology, Department of Pathology, Hôpital Avicenne, Bobigny

Philippe Anract MD
Assistant Professor, Department of Orthopedic Surgery, Hôpital Cochin, Paris

Anne-Marie Bergemer MD
Assistant Professor, Department of Pathology, Hôpital Bretonneau, Tours

Henri Carlioz MD
Professor of Orthopedic Surgery, Department of Pediatric Orthopedics, Hôpital Armand Trousseau, Paris

Jean Michel Coindre MD
Professor of Pathology, Department of Pathology, Cancer Center Fondation Bergonié, Bordeaux

Jean Marc Cosset MD
Professor and Head of the Department of Radiotherapy, Institut Curie, Paris

Jerome Couturier MD
Cytogenetican, Laboratory of Cytogenetics, Institut Curie, Paris

Jacques Diebold MD
Professor of Pathology, Department of Pathology, Hôpital Hôtel Dieu, Paris

Michel Forest MD
Professor of Pathology, Department of Pathology, Hôpital Cochin, Paris

Brigitte Laguerre MD
Department of Medical Oncology, Institut Curie, Paris

Veronique Pacault-Legendre MD
Psychiatrist, Department of Orthopedic Surgery, Hôpital Cochin, Paris

Pierre Pouillart MD
Professor of Oncology, Department of Oncology, Institut Curie, Paris

Suzy Scholl MD
Department of Medical Oncology, Institut Curie, Paris

Lorraine G. Shapeero MD
Department of Radiology, USUHS Bethesda, USA

Bernard Tomeno MD
Professor of Orthopedic Surgery, Department of Orthopedic Surgery, Hôpital Cochin, Paris

Marie Cecile Vacher-Lavenu MD
Professor of Pathology, Department of Pathology, Hôpital Cochin, Paris

Daniel Vanel MD
Head of the Department of Radiology, Institut Gustave Roussy, Villejuif

Philippe Vielh MD
Cytologist, Laboratory of Cytology, Institut Curie, Paris

Foreword

On November 2nd 1993, the New York Bone Pathology Club, of which I have the honor to be secretary, held their regular monthly meeting as they had for the previous 15 years. Normally, the meeting would have been held at one of the New York hospitals in which the various members work; this particular meeting was held in Paris, France, at the Groupe Hôspitalier Cochin.

This special event had been planned many months before by one of our club members, Dr Lauren Ackerman, who was to have spent a sabbatical that autumn at l'hôpital Cochin in the department of Professor Michel Forest. He had met Professor Forest in `1991 during the course of another visit to Paris and discovered that he was not only a passionate student of skeletal diseases but had amassed a large volume of material which he had very thoroughly documented. Each was delighted to have met the other. Dr Ackerman came back to New York excited at the prospect of working with Professor Forest at l'Hôpital Cochin in 1993. Unfortunately, just a month or so before he was to leave for Paris with his wife, Lauren died after a very short illness. He was 88 years old.

Dr Ackerman was not only one of the great surgical pathologists of the United States but because of his writings as well as his truly charismatic personality, his influence was felt worldwide. He reminded me of that great Russian impresario who left such a lasting impression in both London and Paris during the second decade of this century, Sergei Diaghilev. Both of them were larger than life, full of restless energy, with an encyclopedic knowledge. They also shared, and enjoyed, that rare ability to recognize talent and, most importantly, to nurture it.

On November 3rd 1993, Lauren's friends from the New York Bone Club, together with Professor Forest's department and colleagues, held a seminar in his honor. I am sure Lauren would have been delighted by this conjunction of the Gallic and Anglo-Saxon world of bone pathology, by the quality of the papers presented and perhaps, most of all, by the grand dinner held later that evening at that great Parisian landmark, le restaurant Mercure Galant. He would have been especially pleased by the New Yorkers' surprise and delight at the wonderful museum of skeletal material collected by the great Baron Dupuytren during the early 19th century in the legendary times of Bichat, Bayle and Laennec when the new pathology of the Paris school was the envy of the world. However, I think what made the greatest impression on all of us was the meticulous documentation of the cases which had come under Professor Forest's review.

Some years before our visit, Professor Forest and his surgical colleague Professor Bernard Tomeno had published a two-volume loose-leaf book entitled Les tumeurs osseuses de l'appareil locomoteur. The aphorisms which preface the book should be writ large in every department where tumors are diagnosed and treated.

JAMAIS

de traitement sans diagnostic (ce qui 9 fois sur 10, au moins, signifie pas de traitement sans biopsie).

JAMAIS

de prélèvements opératoires envoyés moitié à Paul, moitié à Pierre (fussent-ils des anatomo-pathologistes de grand renom).

NE PAS ENTREPRENDRE

de traitement sans la certitude de pouvoir assurer la suite (techniquement, intellectuellement, psychologiquement) quelle que soit l'évolution. (I believe only a book emanating from France would have an introductory section entitled Psychopathology and bone tumor diagnosis.

NE PAS CONSIDÉRER

l'anatomo-pathologie comme une science devinatoirè: donner des renseignements cliniques, joindre une radiographie au prélèvement.

NE PAS ASSIMILER

la réponse du pathologiste à un oracle incontestable: la

confronter au contexte, la discuter avec son auteur, recommencer la biopsie si nécessaire.

The illustrations in that book were very fine but limited in number because of the restrictions of the publication. The text was in French, unfortunately limiting the potential audience for the work.

I urged Professor Forest to consider writing a text in English so that the large English-speaking medical community, unfortunately ignorant of Professor Forest's native French, should have the opportunity of sharing in both his wide experience and his passionate involvement with skeletal pathology.

The resultant exquisitely illustrated and scholarly volume is now in your hands. It will surely be at the forefront of the emerging internationalism of French medicine. Professor Forest and his colleagues deserve both our admiration and thanks for having undertaken this great work.

Peter G Bullough MD
Director of Laboratory Medicine
Hospital for Special Surgery
Professor of Pathology
Cornell University Medical College
New York, USA

Preface

In the field of Bone pathology and especially in that of bone tumors, the surgical pathologist not only has to deal with technical problems, but must also have knowledge of rare and often difficult lesions. Most pitfalls encountered are due to lack of knowledge of the imaging features or the inability to distinguish tumors from reactive processes.

A lot of information has recently been provided in several excellent texts dealing with all aspects of bone and joint diseases and bone tumors, presented as reviews of current concepts, personal experiences or medical atlases. We have tried not to duplicate our predecessors but to stress first of all, the radiological and pathological links.

The approach of this work is twofold. It has to reflect the fact that a pathological report presents all the imaging information and enhances particular points in relation to the needs of the orthopedic surgeon or the oncologist. Each chapter, conceived as a review, therefore deals not only with pathology, but also with imaging, special techniques such as flow cytometry or cytogenetics and recent trends in treatment. Furthermore the main part of the book, on pathology, is complemented by general chapters on methods of diagnosis and treatment which should be very useful as overviews, even if there is some unavoidable overlap.

The second point is that the key to pathological diagnosis often relies more on illustrations than on text. We have tried, whenever possible, to give simultaneous illustrations of the gross and imaging findings. Clinical X-rays are complemented by some high-resolution radiographs of specimen slabs. The characteristic histological features are shown on several figures, frequently with the use of polarized light. Cytological features are demonstrated on imprint material. On the other hand, illustrations of immunohistochemistry are limited, to save space, but this technique is thoroughly discussed, when necessary. The illustrations cover usual features, rare cases and some misdiagnoses made by ourselves or our colleagues, on pathology or imaging.

Current knowledge is documented by references, most of them oriented to pathology and imaging. To avoid some repetition, major textbooks are given in the text using the Harvard System and grouped at the end of the book.

This work deals only with diagnosis of orthopedic material; cranial and facial lesions are excluded. Moreover, it should be stressed that the choice of pseudotumoral lesions is unavoidably selective, being guided by the available material and not by the frequency of the lesion.

Special acknowledgements are due to the staff of Churchill Livingstone; including Geoffrey Nuttall, former Editorial Director, who gave the initial impetus to the work, and Gavin Smith, former Medical Editor, who coordinated the project with the greatest skill and patience, followed by Sheila Khullar, Medical Commissioning Editor.

Nora Naughton, Projects Manager, did a tremendous technical job dealing with many intricate printing problems, and we are greatly indebted to her for that.

We extend our thanks and appreciation to M.F. Garreau, Head of the Library of Pathology of the Pierre et Marie Curie University, Paris for checking and providing many of the countless references and to Dr Allan J Darby, Consultant Pathologist at the Robert Gordon and Agnes Hunt Orthopaedic Hospital, UK for his corrections to the English terminology used in bone pathology.

Michel Forest
Bernard Tomeno
Daniel Vanel

Paris, October, 1997.

Psychopathology and bone tumor pathology

V. Pacault-Legendre

The biopsy of a bone tumor allows a name to be given to the illness from which the patient suffers. Making a diagnosis, however, does not result from an encounter between the patient and the person returning the verdict: the patient and the pathologist neither see nor speak to each other and they almost never meet. The pathologist possesses a few facts concerning the patient (sex, age, location of the tumor...) and the patient knows that the rest of his life will depend on what the pathologist sees and says.

Notification of diagnosis, established by the pathologist, will be passed onto the patient and it is at this very particular and critical moment, when the verdict is issued, that the second role of the pathologist becomes manifest, i.e. the role of a third person between the patient and the surgeon.

The preceding remarks, although apparently obvious, are nonetheless important in helping to understand that the pathologist is vitally important to the patient suffering from a bone tumor. This position of a third person, physically absent but present through the written word (articulated by the surgeon), is extremely important, particularly at the time when the diagnosis is given by the surgeon to the patient. This third person will have considerable influence and effect on any psychopathological reactions related to bone tumor casess.

Bone tumors occur at any age and can be either benign or malignant. These simple remarks throw some light on the range and variety of psychical reactions which may be observed before and after biopsy is carried out on patients suffering from bone tumors. In spite of rapid evolution of therapeutic protocols and the excellent prognosis of some bone tumors, some aspects of human behavior are unchanging: anguish in the face of death and the specter induced by occurrence of a tumor.

BEFORE THE BIOPSY

As mentioned above, bone tumors are sometimes benign, often malignant and can affect children, adults or elderly persons. They sometimes occur and develop quickly; often revealing themselves through pain, or the appearance of a 'palpable mass', which can be seen on a part of the body. At this early stage, before the patient has even taken medical advice, psychological reactions help protect the subject; feelings of anguish and the shadow cast by the possible existence of a tumor do not last long. From this early stage and with an, as yet, undiagnosed tumor, feelings of despondency and anxiety begin to grow.

At this point, the patient is reminded of his mortality and resents the brutal interruption into his activities, passions and, indeed, life. He may dwell upon death in the hope of averting it, to bide time.

The patient then makes the decision to discuss this with his immediate circle and his doctor, eventually seeking surgical advice. Now, he needs to feel reassured, at a time of great physical and mental suffering. Instead, however, the patient is being told that his anxiety *is* well founded, a biopsy *is* necessary and this biopsy will make a diagnosis possible. His worst fears are realised and a third party enters the picture: the pathologist. The latter's involvement will spare the surgeon from having to fight a duel with the patient.

When the patient is an adult, he is naturally afraid of premature death; his mortality is made dramatically plain, even although he knows that malignancy has not yet been established. His hope is tinged with fear. At this stage, nightmares often appear. For instance, the patient dreams that he is working in a factory, merrily making coffins. The patient fears death or mutilation and wonders what the cost of his survival will be. Sometimes, to allay this fear, he invents scenarios, as though rationalizing his illness can help him get the upper hand over the unknown. Some patients ask many questions, hoping that medical, scientific and objective information will reassure them. Their aim is to avoid having to face their overwhelming fears alone.

Children, on the other hand, live very much in the present; when their body suffers, they wish only to be relieved from this suffering so that they can continue with games, school and everyday life unhindered. In these cases, it is the parents who are often extremely distressed. They are overcome by a fear of the death of their child and by the suffering their children may have to endure. Eventually, they may communicate their anguish to the child instead of helping them continue with daily life as normal.

DURING BIOPSY AND ANALYSIS

The biopsy is usually a straightforward surgical operation but it is very emotionally loaded for the patient. The gap between the ease of operation and psychological burden of the patient at the time of the operation is immense.

During the short period of time spent in hospital for tumor biopsy, the patient is very often alone. His physical condition does not usually entail special treatment: nurses and doctors rarely see him.

For the patient's immediate family, this is a very emotional moment as they do not yet have a name for the disease. Each person fights against their own anxieties, which are dependent on their individual relationship with the patient. Often, during the period of uncertainty when the diagnosis is still unknown, family members put themselves in the position of the patient; in the position of the person who may have a tumor. They are all worried and may avoid talking about what worries them.

The waiting period whilst the pathologist carefully carries out his work is often problematic for the patient. This time is very difficult to bear, with little to do and the patient may be entirely absorbed in his own anxiety. Away from his daily occupation, family and professional world, he may begin to question the meaning of his life and its future.

He is waiting for the verdict; for the few words from the pathologist which, relayed to him by the surgeon will, at last, separate fact from fantasy, and hopefully pave the way out of uncertainty.

This period of waiting is often a time when the subconscious is at work, preparing the patient to face a grave diagnosis. Many dreams reported by patients throw a light on this process: dreams of endless running in the case of a tumor located in the leg, or dreams of amputation. In most cases, the part of the body suffering from the tumor is at the core of the dream and is the focus of the patient's attention and anxiety. Often, the patient speaks of himself as though he were reduced to the affected part of his body. He will react to this but only at a later stage, when he realizes he has not shrunk to the sick part of his body, and will accept the idea of losing a limb in order to stay alive. He will realize that he, as a person, remains undamaged.

This time of uncertainty, between the biopsy and the diagnosis, cannot be shortened. The pathologist needs a few days to perform his work on the biopsy sample and the patient also needs this period of waiting, during which he will develop psychological reactions to the possible advent of the tumor.

Usually the surgeon simply tells the patient they must wait for the diagnosis, but he may already be in a position to answer some questions, especially when clinical examination points to the likelihood of a malignant tumor. Nothing precise can be said until the pathologist has made his diagnosis known. At this point, a third party enters the picture, a mediator so to speak, embodied in the pathologist. Thanks to this third party, patient and surgeon can avoid direct conflict. At the time of disclosure of diagnosis, there will be three persons 'present': the patient, the surgeon and the pathologist. Even though only the patient and surgeon actually meet, the pathologist's diagnosis will serve to support their discussion.

AFTER THE BIOPSY: DISCLOSING THE RESULT

The pathologist sends the biopsy report, via the surgeon,

to an addressee whom he does not know and will never meet: the patient. With the help of a few clinical facts given to him, he can only imagine the patient. He will not see him and will not talk to him. The pathologist can only wonder how the patient will react to the diagnosis. How will his findings affect those concerned? Most of the time, such questions remain unanswered.

Occasionally, after a week or so, the examination of a biopsy specimen may provide a few more clues to the patient's life. However, even though the role played by the pathologist is chiefly technical, it is also a very humane one and, more often than not, the pathologist himself is unaware of this. Indeed, it is the pathologist who presides, in absentia, over the moment when the surgeon announces the diagnosis of the tumor to the patient.

When the result is negative, i.e. when the tumor is benign, everyone is relieved. Even in this favorable circumstance, however, the patient needs time to digest this result. Anguish and anxiety do not vanish at once; the patient can harbor doubts. Is the diagnosis unquestionable? Are errors impossible? These are just a few of the questions a patient may ask. Many will have nightmares in the nights following the announcement of the diagnosis, even if it is negative. Anxiety *will* reduce gradually, but the patient may feel that he has had a 'close shave with death'. At this point, the patient has obviously already undergone a long process of self-assessment; he has been able to frame this event in the context of his life as a whole. He has taken note of how precarious and valuable each day of life is.

When the result is positive and in accordance with clinical facts i.e. when the tumor is established, diagnosed and confirmed in the report of the pathologist, it is the surgeon's responsibility to give the results to the patient, with the help and the support of this report.

The initial gut reaction of the patient being told they have a malignant tumor is usually one of astonishment. The specter of death becomes real. Even if statistics are favorable or new therapeutic protocols improve the prognosis, the patient has heard the worst possible diagnosis: his life is in danger. Psychological reactions to this event can differ according to the past life of each person, but they cannot be avoided and are, in the patient's eyes, scarcely affected by progress in therapeutic techniques. The patient once again needs time in order to accept this reality. Very often, the patient neither hears nor remembers the medical explanations supporting the diagnosis.

An uncertainty has been lifted but other questions now arise. After the verdict comes offers of treatment or discussions of possible surgical intervention. A prognosis may also be suggested to the patient. It is the living part of the patient that must be addressed: the patient will often rebel and behave aggressively towards the surgeon, the pathologist or other persons. Sometimes, he will express guilt over his tumor and occasionally he will simply not accept the diagnosis. The surgeon must then remain with the patient, listen to him and support him in order to help him accept often radical treatment which will potentially mutilate him. In doing so, the surgeon will have the support of the pathologist and his report from the biopsy. Indeed, as already mentioned, the surgeon is not the only person accountable for the diagnosis imposed on the patient. Thanks to the mediation of a third party, the pathologist, whose diagnosis is trusted and respected, the patient will invariably accept the proposal for treatment made by the surgeon, even in the most severe and difficult of cases. The patient can then direct his energy towards continuing life under conditions which remain acceptable to him, instead of towards a fruitless conflict with the therapist.

CONCLUSION

The role played by the pathologist is a dual one. Firstly, the pathologist performs the very precise technical work necessary to establish a diagnosis. The latter role may be unseen, but is as necessary as the former in the field of bone tumors. It is the humane role of intervening between the surgeon and the patient as a vital third party.

The pathologist studies tissue sections but he must bear in mind that behind these sections stands a human being to whom his words will not only convey information, but also have a profound impact on the patient's physical and mental well-being.

Methods of Diagnosis

1

Imaging

D. Vanel   L.G. Shapeero

INTRODUCTION

Bone imaging techniques have undergone significant changes during the last decade. Ultrasound, computed tomography (CT) and recently magnetic resonance imaging (MRI) have been added to arteriography, bone scanning and conventional X-ray, which remains the primary examination. At the same time, survival in malignant primary bone tumors has improved with chemotherapy.[1,2] Conservative surgery continues to give improved results but imaging plays a major role in diagnosis, local and distant staging, monitoring of the effectiveness of treatment and detection of recurrences.

IMAGING TECHNIQUES

Plain films

These remain the mandatory first step and are often the diagnostic key, allowing the diagnosis of the 'don't touch' lesions. They use X-rays and visualize on a film the attenuation of the X-ray beam by the structure studied. This attenuation depends on the density of the organs studied and their thickness. Multiple projections, magnification and soft tissue techniques improve the diagnostic capabilities and allow a global view of the whole lesion, with good spatial resolution. The main limitations are:

- the superimposition of all the structures;
- a partial destruction of the cortex can be overlooked unless studied in a tangential way and a small lytic lesion can disappear when surrounded by dense bone;
- deeply located bones are poorly studied, because of soft tissue superimposition; plain films are therefore more useful to study peripheral than central bones;
- the poor detection of soft tissue involvement, as muscles and non-calcified masses have the same density.

Ultrasonography

This has a limited role in bone imaging as it cannot image through cortical bone. It is limited to the soft tissues, where it can differentiate solid from cystic masses and

guide a needle biopsy. Color flow Doppler sonography allows the visualization and measurement of the flow in a mass.

Computed tomography (CT)

CT also uses X-rays and the image looks like a plain X-ray. The image is, however, obtained in a completely different way. The CT image is the indirect image of a slice of the body. Instead of the X-ray film, there are detectors, which are much more sensitive. They allow a high number of measurements of the attenuation of the object. An algorithm reconstructs the matricial image of the slice, which appears on a television screen. A selected part of the information is then reproduced on film. The size of the matrix (usually 512×512) defines the spatial resolution of the image. Different areas of the results can be reproduced on the films (for example, bone or soft tissue windows). The complete information can be kept on disks, but is partially lost on the films.

The X-ray tube rotates around the patient during the

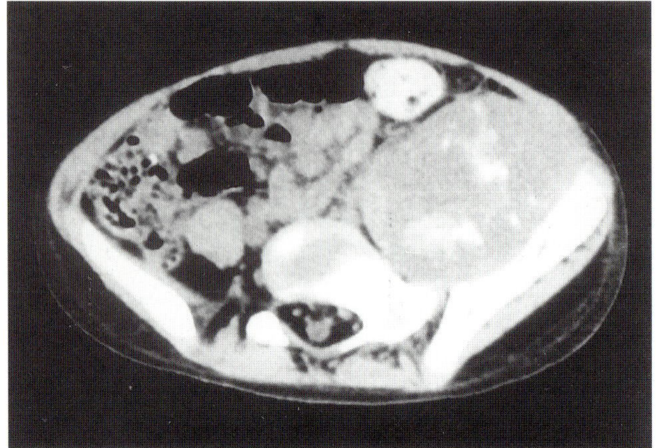

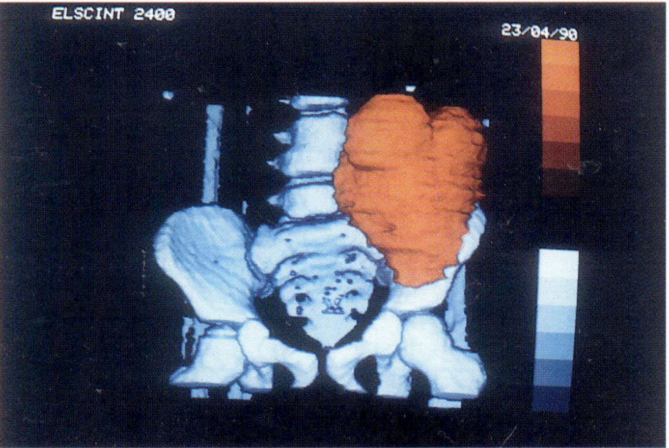

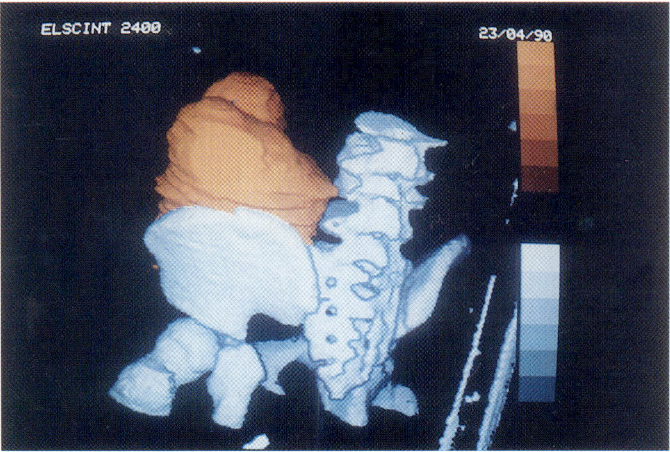

Fig. 1.1 Ewing's sarcoma of the left iliac wing. Involvement of soft tissue is well evaluated on CT (a). Three-D reconstructions (b: anterior and c: posterior views) allow a better understanding of the volume and relations between tumor and tissue (in red) before radiation therapy or surgery.

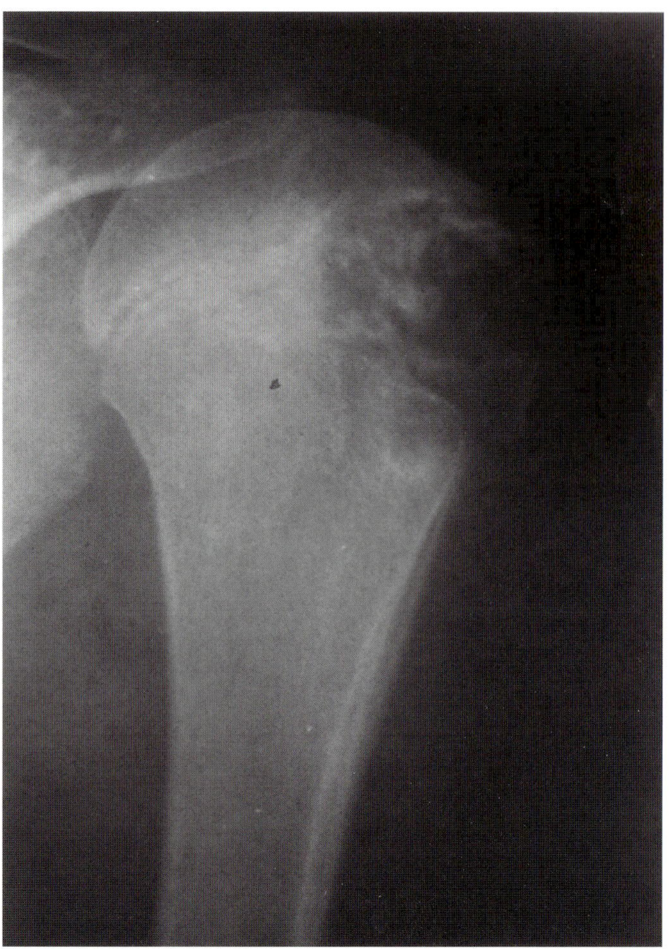

Fig. 1.2 Mineralised and lytic tumor of the proximal epiphysis of the humerus, before closure of the epiphyseal plate: chondroblastoma.

X-ray emission. The detectors usually turn at the same time (third-generation CT). On fourth-generation CT a static array of detectors receives the information, then the table moves and another slice is studied. On the new helical CTs, the table moves during the operation, allowing a continuous flow of images. The attenuation depends on the slice studied. At the end of the rotation, multiple measurements have been acquired. The computer then allots to each elementary part of the image (called a pixel) a numerical value. The Hounsfield scale uses different densities: air density is −1000, fat −100, water 0, dense bone +1000. Each pixel is reproduced on a gray scale (lowest densities are black, highest white). Different parameters include the slice thickness (from 0.1 to 10 mm), gap between the slices, matrix, field of view, acquisition time (usually around 1 s per slice). Contrast injection increases the density of vascularized lesions. As it is a computer image, measurements such as distances or density can easily be taken. Multiple contiguous slices allow reconstruction in different planes (coronal, sagittal or oblique) or in volume (Fig. 1.1).

The main advantages of CT are a greater contrast resolution than plain films and cross-sectional sections, helping study of central bones. It is also a convenient way of guiding interventional radiology, such as biopsies or intratumoral injections. Its sensitivity is much lower than MRI.

Magnetic resonance imaging (MRI)

MRI has emerged as the most significant advance for imaging musculoskeletal tumors because of its excellent

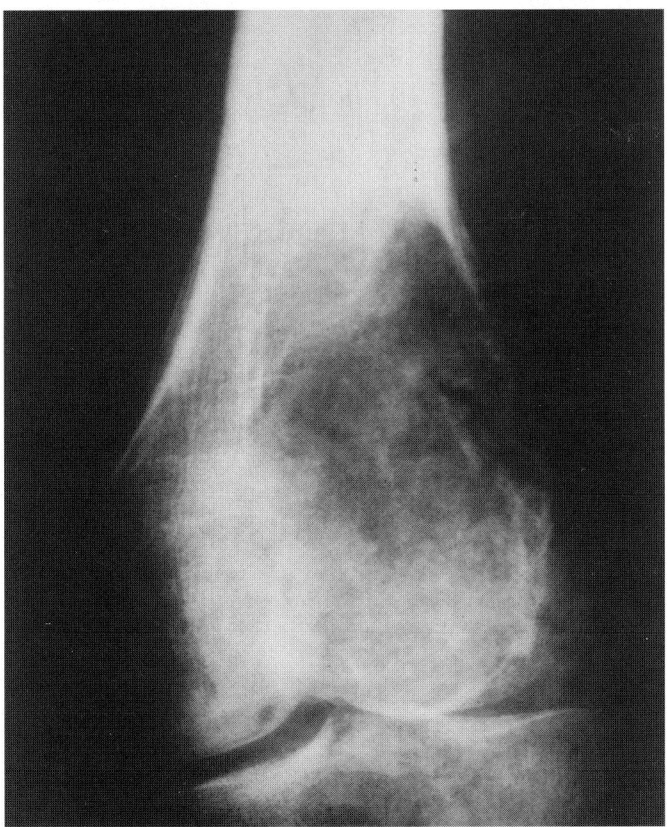

Fig. 1.3 Epiphysiometaphyseal tumor of the distal femur, after closure of the epiphyseal plate: giant cell tumor.

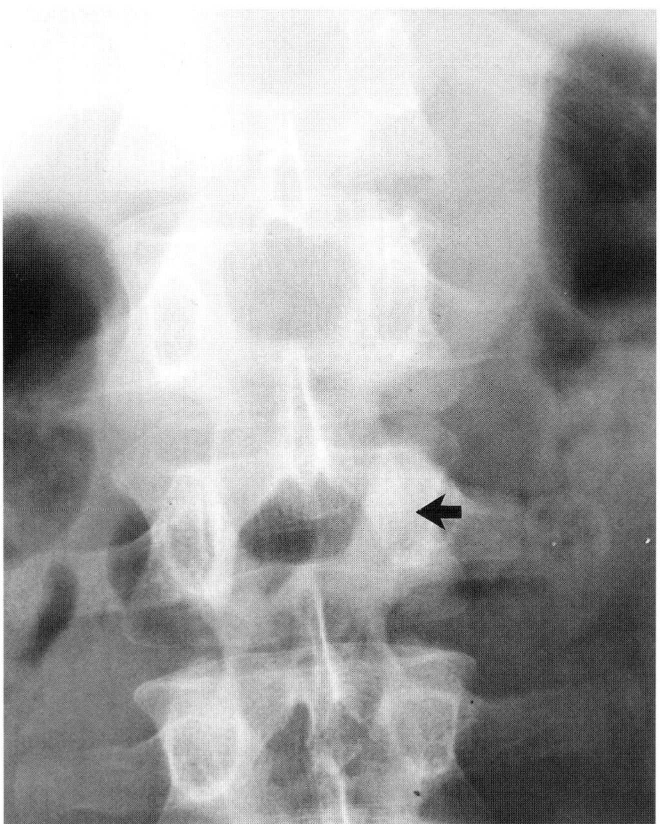

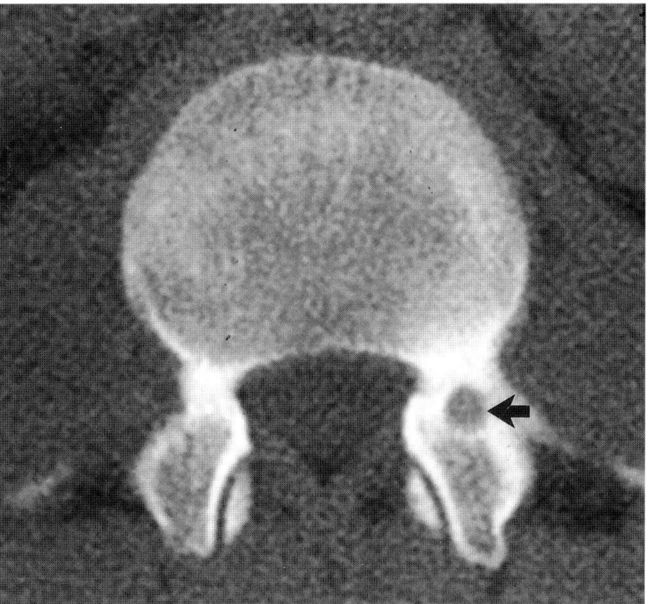

Fig. 1.4 Back pain. On plain film (a) hardly visible sclerosis of the right pedicle of L2 (arrow). On CT (b), the nidus is well depicted, surrounded by a sclerotic reaction: osteoid osteoma.

soft tissue contrast and multiplanar imaging capability.[3-10]

The human body is mainly made of water (H_2O). The protons (H+) are elementary charged spinning particles so they behave like small magnets. All these magnets are randomly oriented, so there is no global magnetization. If the body is placed in a strong homogeneous magnetic field, the magnets align in only two possible directions: in the same direction or opposite to the main field. Slightly more align with the main field, so the body becomes magnetized. If a radiofrequency wave is sent at the same frequency as the rotation speed of the protons, part of its energy can be transferred to the protons, which become excited. The return to the initial state at the end of the stimulation characterizes the tissue and is used on the MR image. In particular, the interactions between the protons and the network correspond to the T1 value of the tissue and the interactions between the different protons to the T2 value. Other useful parameters are the number of mobile protons and the flow. For example, air contains no protons, so its signal is zero whatever the acquisition sequence selected (thus air appears black). Cortical bone or calcifications contain no mobile protons and are also black. Fat, containing slowly moving

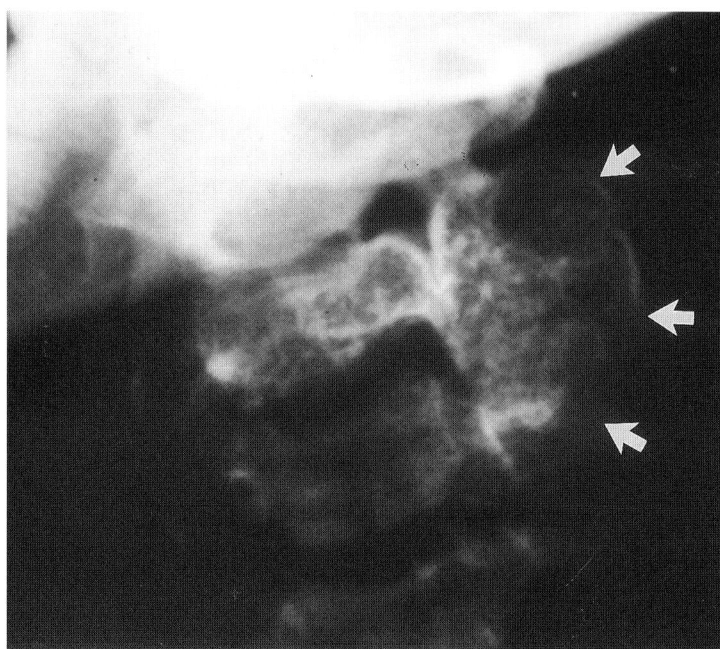

Fig. 1.5 Expansile, well-limited (arrows), partially ossified tumor of the posterior arch of C3 in a child: osteoblastoma.

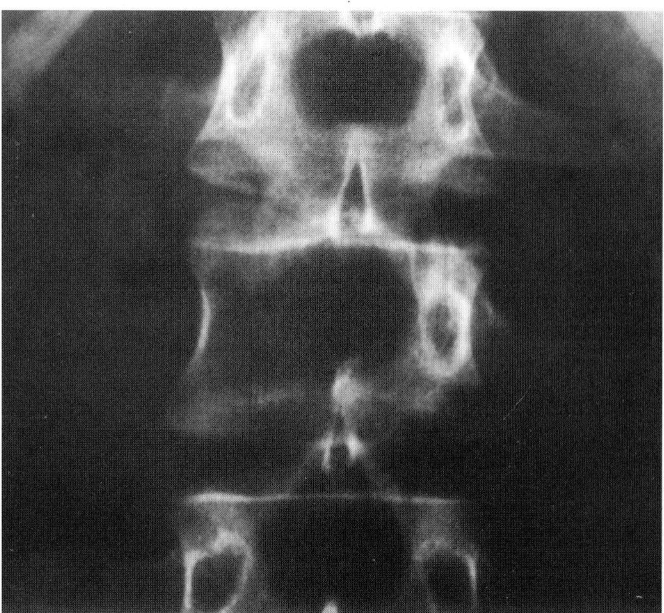

Fig. 1.6 Large, purely lytic tumor of the posterior arch of L2 in a child: aneurysmal bone cyst.

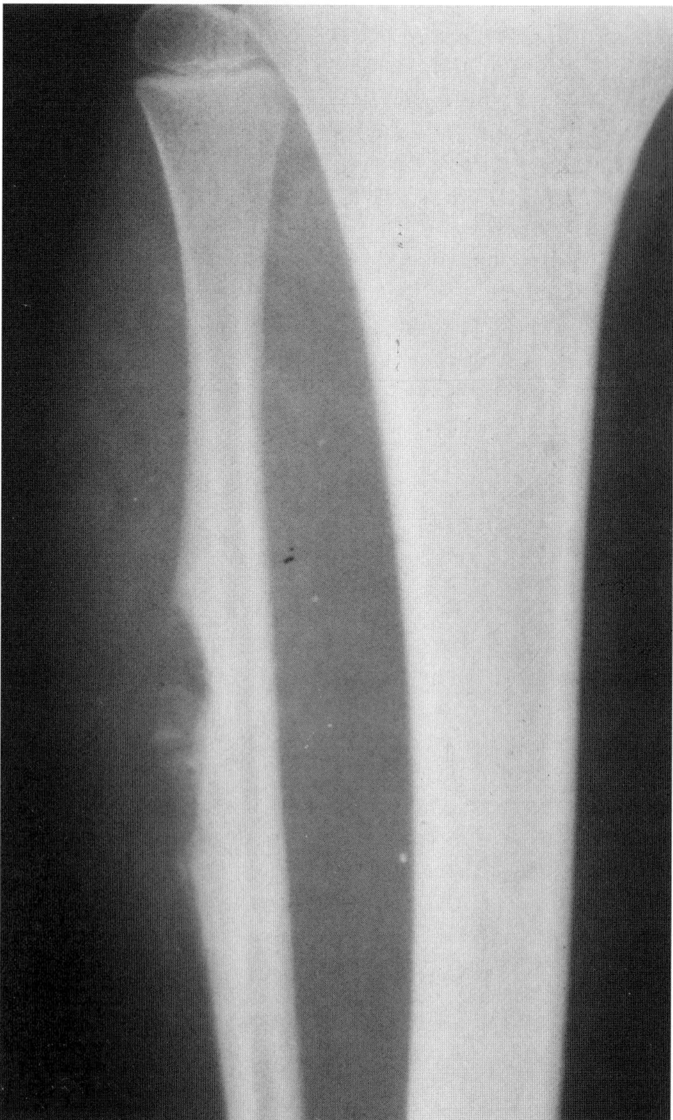

Fig. 1.7 Periosteal Ewing's sarcoma of the shaft of the fibula. The 'saucerization' is typical, with perpendicular periosteal bone formations.

protons, returns its energy to the network on T1-weighted sequences (sequences emphasizing the T1 values) and will have a high signal (that is, will appear white) on T1-weighted sequences. Water, made of homogeneous fast-moving protons, will give a high signal on T2-weighted images.

Contrast medium allows the tissues to return their energy faster and so to produce a high signal on T1-weighted sequences.

The initial MRI should be performed before the initial biopsy. A surface coil, which improves the spatial resolution, should be used whenever possible to improve the signal-to-noise ratio.

New sequences are being developed to decrease the examination time or improve the specificity. Conventional T1 and T2-weighted spin-echo sequences are still very useful, as they allow a reproducible evaluation.

Fast spin-echo T2-weighted sequences retain a strong T2-weighting but save time (by a factor of 4–16). Their main drawback is the high signal intensity of fat, similar to that of water, which is inconvenient for evaluation of bone tumors. A fat presaturation method (a technique saturating all the fat protons before the sequence starts and so obliterating the signal of fat) must be used.[11,12] It requires a very homogeneous field, which is not available in every MR unit.

STIR (short tau inversion recovery) sequences can also be used to cancel the fat signal, but the acquisition time is long and the number of slices that can be acquired is usually too limited for studying musculoskeletal tumors.

Angiographic MRI techniques are now reliable enough to be of practical use.[13] They permit visualization of vessels without injection of contrast medium.

Dynamic MR studies after injection of contrast medium are a major improvement in the detection of tumor versus inflammation. They study the changes in the MR signal after injection within the time limit. Different dynamic gadolinium-enhanced MR techniques have been developed: the region of interest (ROI) technique uses a preselected part of the image and obtains curves to evaluate contrast uptake in the selected region after injection.[14] However, only the selected region is studied, so only an average of the whole ROI is obtained. To overcome this limitation several non-operator-dependent techniques have been developed that display the physiologic information in one single image.

Factor analysis of medical imaging sequences allows a pixel-by-pixel evaluation of contrast uptake in the entire image.[15] This very sophisticated software is not currently available.

First-pass techniques show the maximum enhancement rate during the first pass of the contrast agent by calculating the 'first-pass' slope value on a pixel-by-pixel basis.[16–18] The display of the steepest slope of each pixel on the entire image with a gray scale identical to the maximum enhancement rate provides an easily read parametric image.

Gadolinium-enhanced MRI subtraction imaging[19] is the simple dynamic technique which we currently use. Precontrast spin-echo T1-weighted images (matrix 128 × 256, 1aq, TR/TE: 300/17) are required for an acquisition time of 45 s. After a rapid bolus injection of contrast medium, fast spin-echo sequences are obtained at 45 s, 1.5 min and 5 min. The postcontrast scans are subtracted from precontrast scans on an MR work station console. Malignant viable tissue takes up contrast medium early (before 2 min) and inflammatory changes later (after

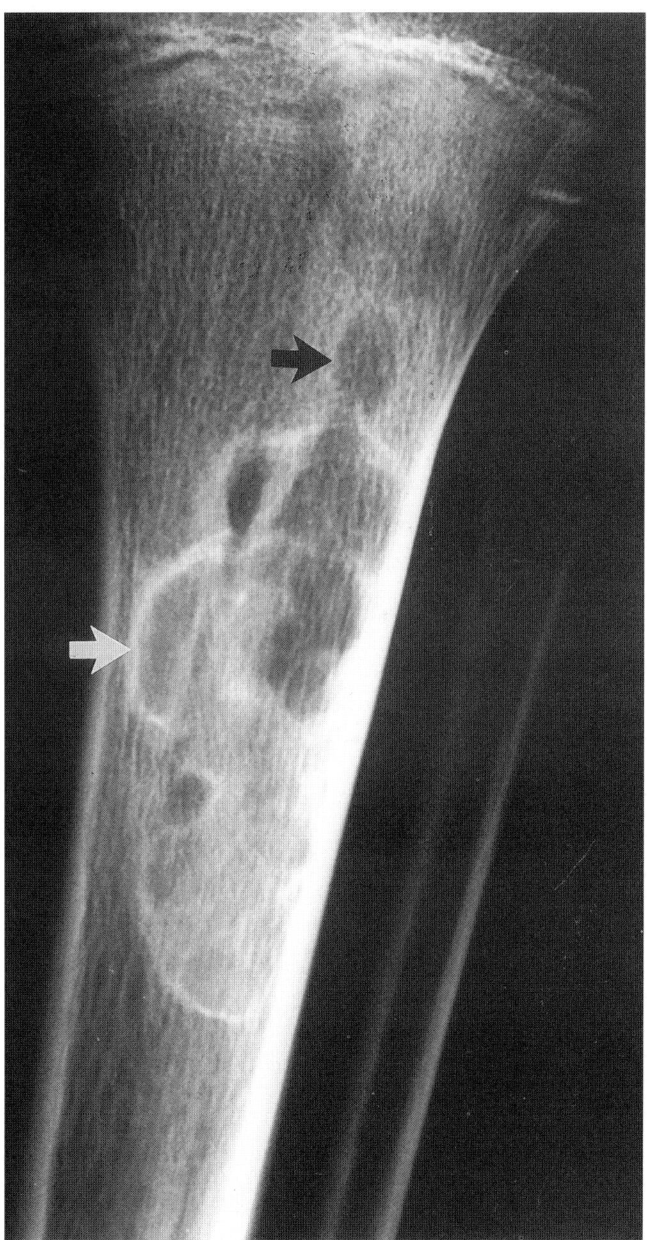

Fig. 1.8 Painless tumor of the shaft of the proximal tibia in a child: the lesion is centered on the cortex and well limited. The margins are of type 1A (white arrow) and 1B (black arrow): non-ossifying fibroma. The lesion has started to ossify in its oldest part (the furthest from the epiphyseal plate), which is a normal way to heal.

2 min). For differentiating the tissues, an acquisition less than 2 min is thus mandatory, but faster acquisition times may improve the results. Ultrafast MRI sequences allow both good spatial (128 × 128 matrix) and temporal (3 s per image) resolution. Coverage of the whole volume of the tumor is not yet possible.

The patient lies in the unit, at the center of a strong magnetic field. Contraindications to the use of this strong field are: cardiac pacemakers, ocular magnetic particles, recent surgical vascular clips, which could move, and claustrophobia. The operator selects the sequences and so the 'weighting' of the image, the axis, slice thickness, gap and field of view. Several levels are acquired in the same time. The patient does not have to move in order to obtain different orientations or levels. Contrast medium can be injected intravenously.

Bone scan

Bone scanning uses the intravenous injection of technetium 99 m diphosphonates. The radionuclide uptake of the lesion depends on the reactive or reparative response to the tumor and not on the tumor itself. The main advantages are the ability to study the whole body and a high sensitivity, but it has poor specificity and a poor spatial resolution. The negative diagnostic value of bone scan is high: a negative examination usually rules out an active lesion. The exceptions are lesions growing very fast and

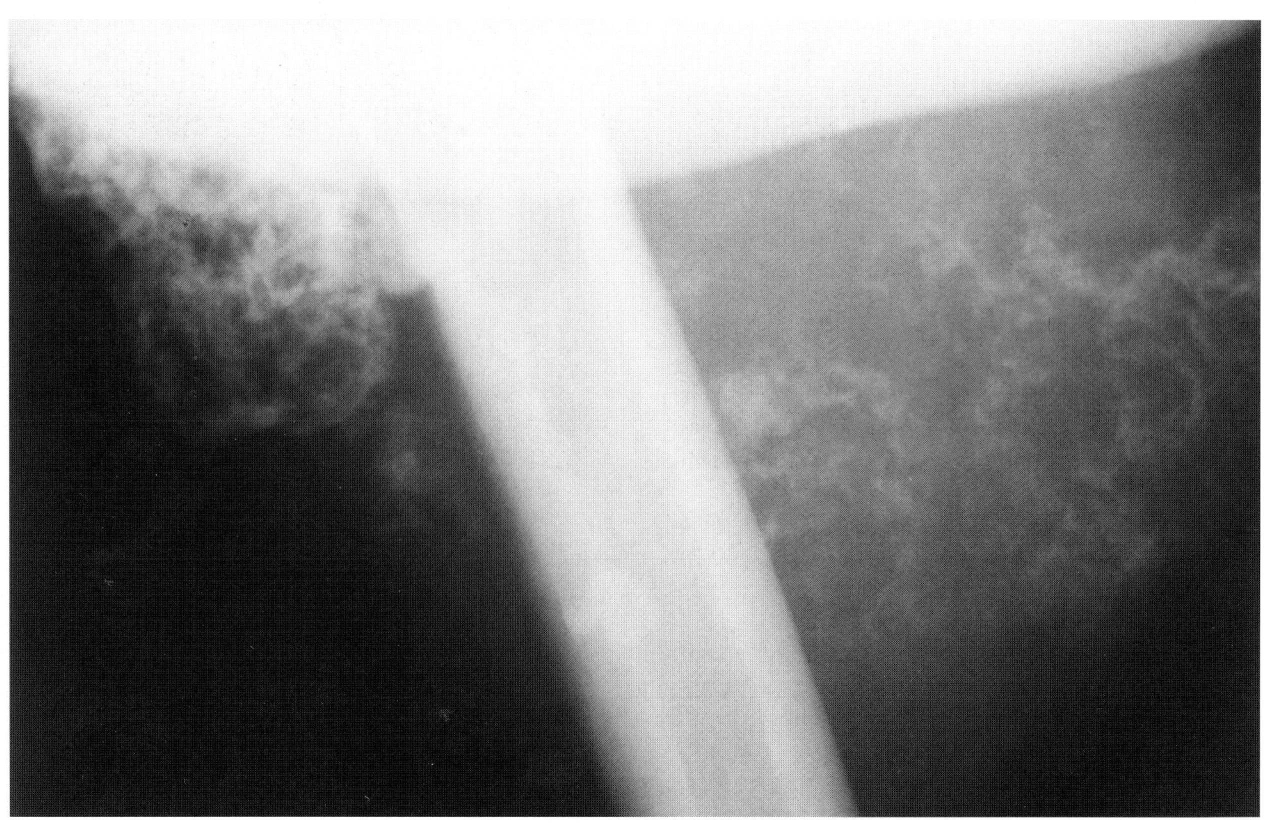

Fig. 1.9 (a and b) Typical arcuate cartilaginous calcifications in a chondrosarcoma of the proximal femur.

those which are purely lytic, which may remain undetected. Triple-phase imaging brings additional information. Serial images are taken after injection. The first phase corresponds to arterial flow, the second, after 1 or 2 min, to blood pool and the third, after 2 h, to bone uptake.

Arteriography

The role of arteriography in the diagnosis and staging of bone tumors has almost completely disappeared. It remains a useful technique for interventional radiology, such as embolization before biopsy to prevent bleeding or chemoembolization of some malignant tumors, still mainly in research protocols.

DIAGNOSIS

Diagnostic criteria

The diagnostic approach is statistical[20,21] and consists of evaluating various clinical and imaging data in order to select the most probable diagnosis. The radiologist can

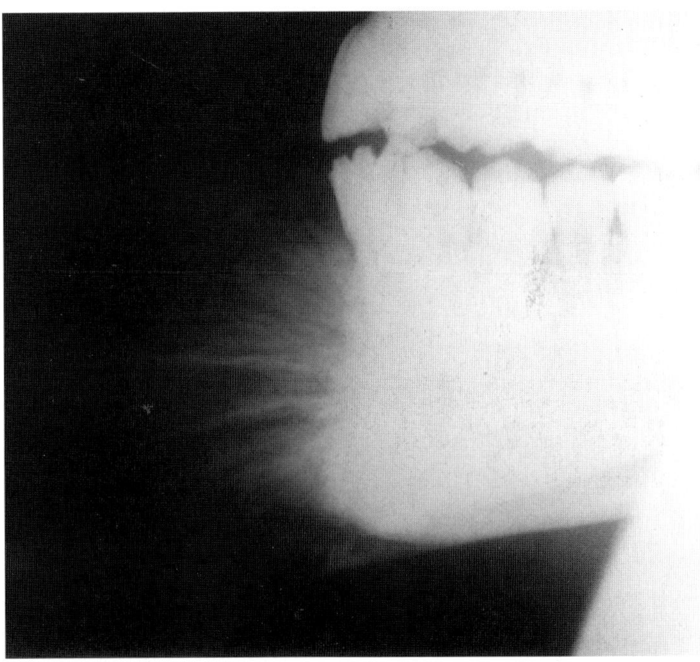

Fig. 1.11 Ewing's sarcoma of the mandible, with typical perpendicular periosteal bone formations.

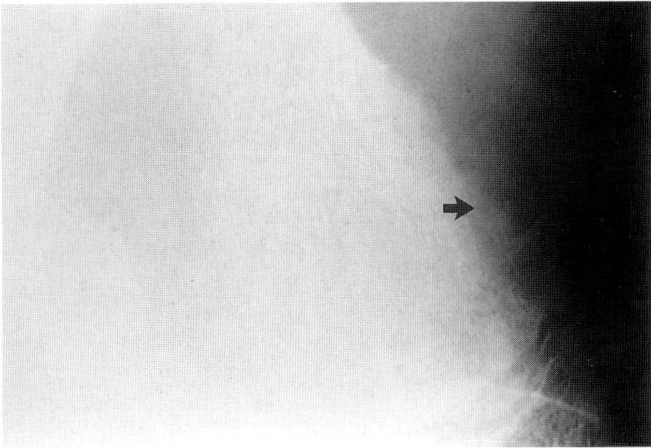

Fig. 1.10 Aggressive lytic and sclerotic lesion of the distal femoral shaft and metaphysis in a child. Although the lesion is poorly limited, the thick, regular periosteal bone formation (arrow) suggests a benign process: staphylococcal osteomyelitis.

Fig. 1.12 Periosteal desmoid tumor. Plain film. The pattern is aggressive: osteolysis of the cortex and periosteal bone formation (arrow). The location (posterior aspect of the medial condyle of the femur) allows the correct diagnosis. No biopsy is necessary.

study the whole specimen and the pathologist a more limited part of the lesion, but in greater detail. Combining both radiological and histological criteria is the most accurate way.

Age is important: before 5 years old, a malignant tumor is almost always metastatic neuroblastoma; between 5 and 15, it is often osteosarcoma or Ewing's sarcoma; after 40, it tends to be metastasis or myeloma.

Clinical symptoms vary little and are most often pain and swelling. Although fever suggests infection, it may also be found in Ewing's sarcoma or, more rarely, in osteoblastoma. Laboratory examination is usually normal.

The location of the tumor is also very helpful. Some tumors are more common in particular bones. Adamantinoma, usually found in the adult, selectively involves the tibia. Epiphyseal tumors are few: chondroblastoma in childhood (Fig. 1.2), giant cell tumor (Fig. 1.3) and the rare calcified clear cell chondrosarcoma in the young adult. The only three benign tumors involving the posterior arch of the vertebrae of children are the osteoid osteoma with its small nidus (Fig. 1.4), the larger calcified

osteoblastoma (Fig. 1.5) and the non-ossified aneurysmal bone cyst (Fig. 1.6). In these special locations, the radiological range is very limited and, moreover, composed of tumors with very different patterns. Many lesions involve the metaphyses or shafts of bones.

In addition, the aggressiveness of some tumors may relate to their location in the axial or appendicular skeleton: for example, in the hand, cartilaginous tumors are almost always benign whereas, in the pelvis, they are often malignant, whatever the radiological and histological pattern.

Tumor size is useful and easy to use. Statistically, when

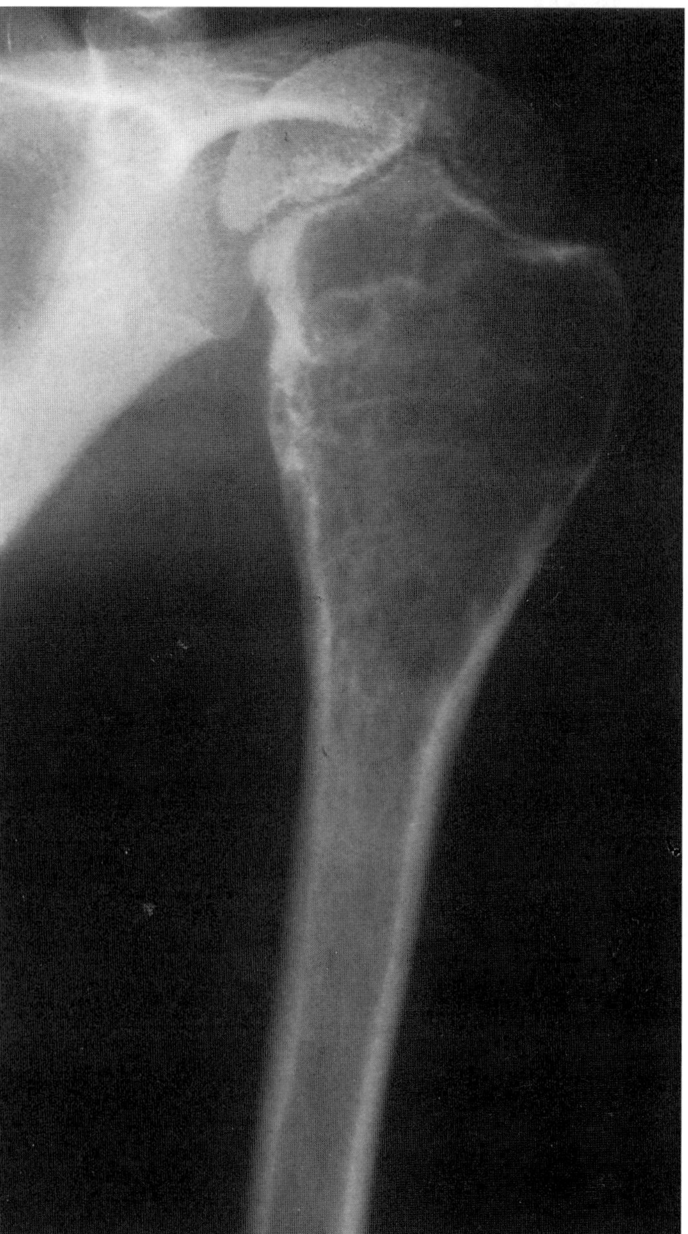

Fig. 1.14 Focal well-demarkated lytic lesion of the proximal metaphysis of the humerus in a child: simple bone cyst.

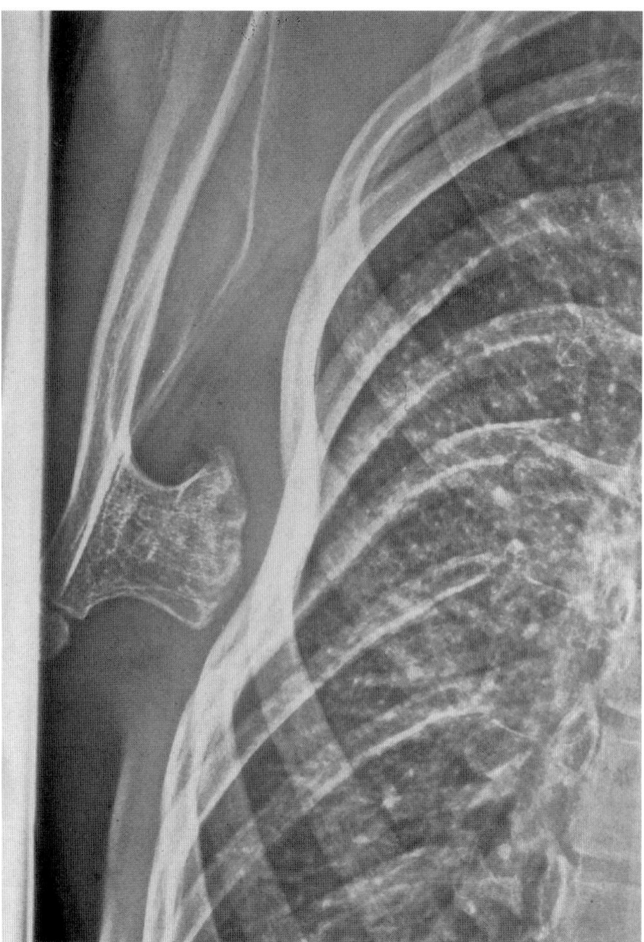

Fig. 1.13 Exostosis of the scapula. The cortex of the lesion is in continuity with the cortex of the normal bone, allowing the diagnosis.

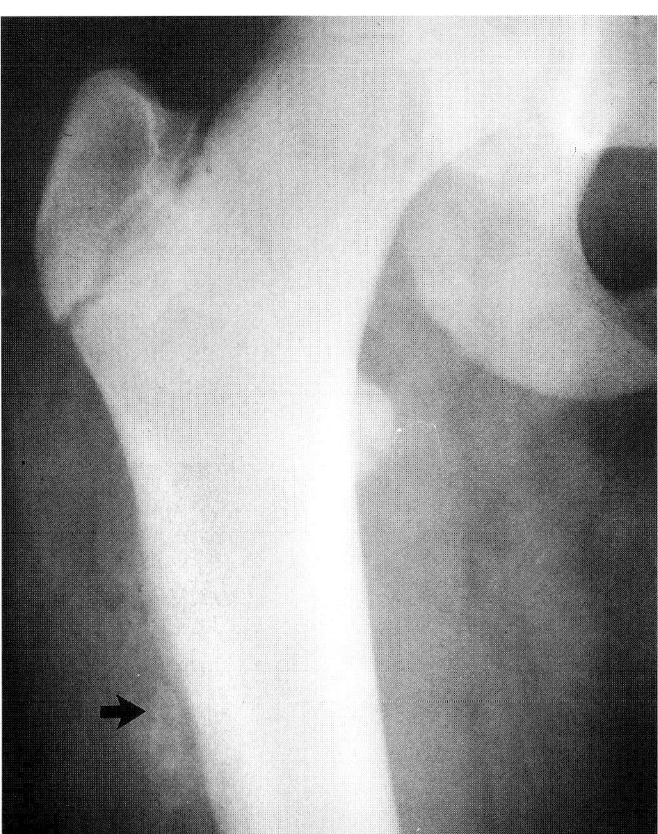

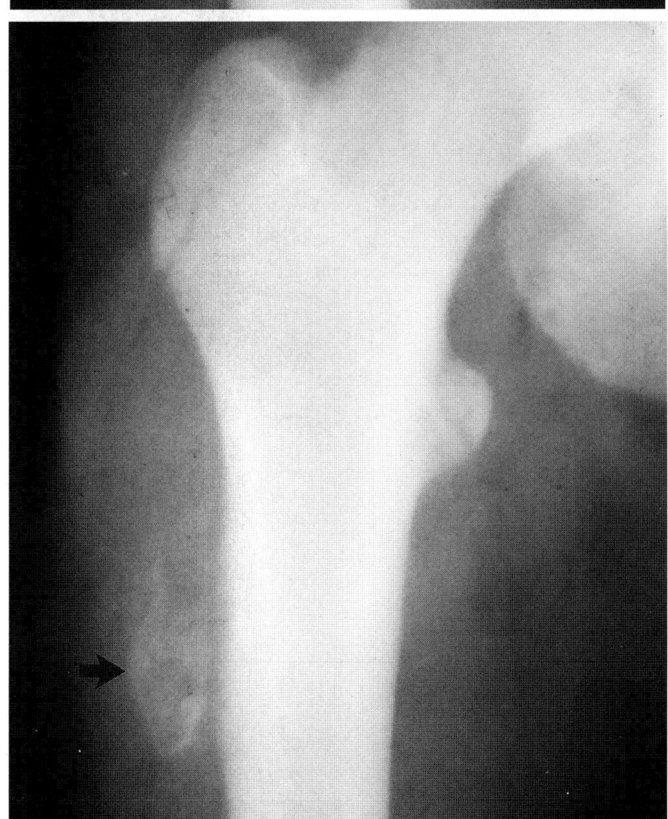

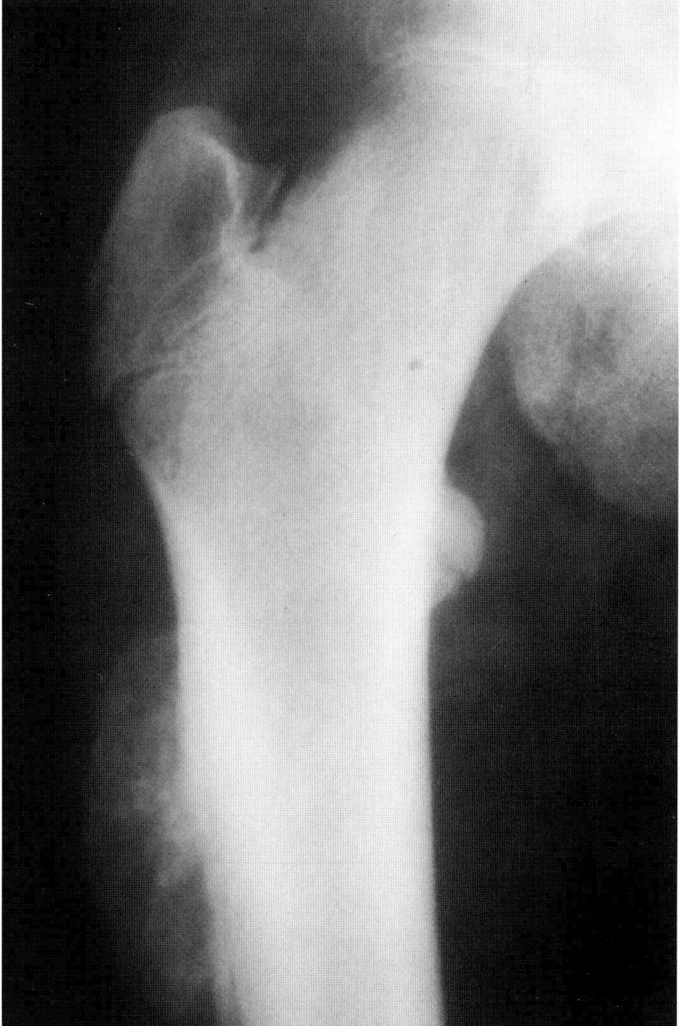

discovered, a tumor less than 6 cm diameter is benign, but may be either benign or malignant when bigger than 6 cm.

The axis of the lesion is also useful to determine. Tumors are rarely centrally located, as in a simple bone cyst. They are most often eccentric, more developed on one side of the bone. For example, a cortical location, centered on the cortex, is necessary to diagnose a non-ossifying fibroma. Finally, the tumor may be a surface lesion: periosteal tumors[22,23] produce 'saucerization' of the cortex on radiographs (Fig. 1.7). Parosteal lesions are masses attached in a sessile fashion to the cortex. The non-involvement of the medullary cavity must be evaluated (on MRI) and seems a reliable sign of local disease, without metastases, in osteosarcomas.[24]

The first step in the radiological evaluation of a bone tumor is to determine its limits by conventional radiology. The patterns of bone destruction indicate the aggressiveness of the lesion (Fig. 1.8). Type 1 is the geographic

Fig. 1.15 Plain films. Pain. Three weeks later (a), calcified soft tissue mass at the periphery (arrow) with a clear center, suggestive of myositis ossificans. One month later (b), the lesion is far more calcified, with a typical pattern (arrow). Two months later (c), the lesion is more ossified. It disappeared slowly and spontaneously.

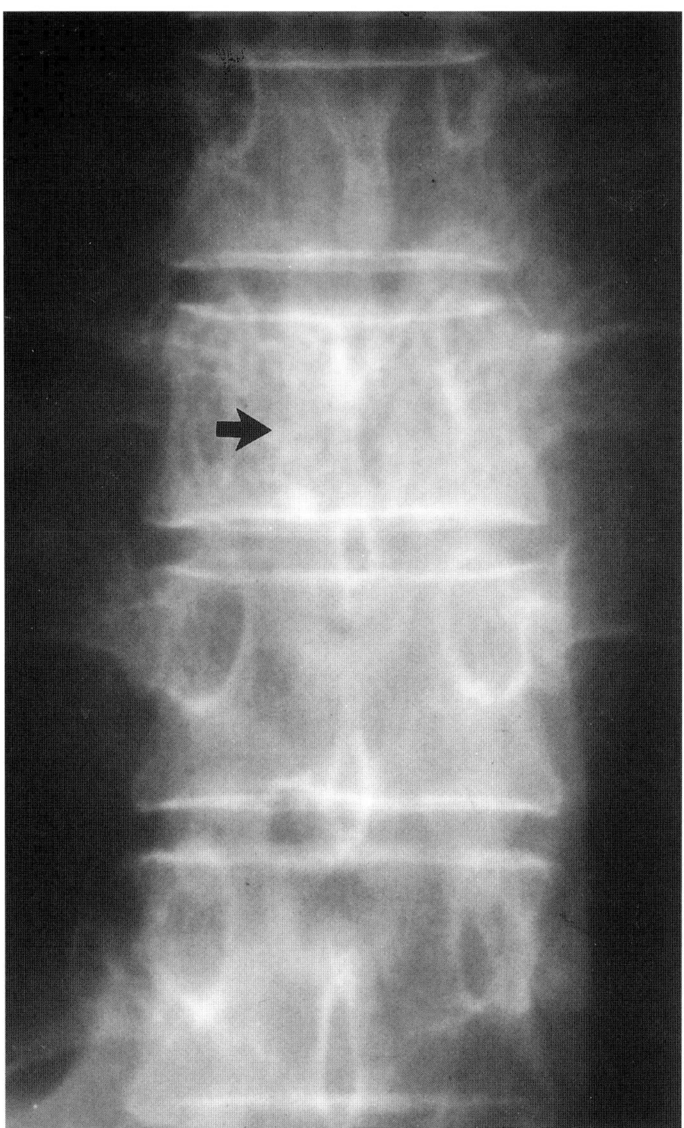

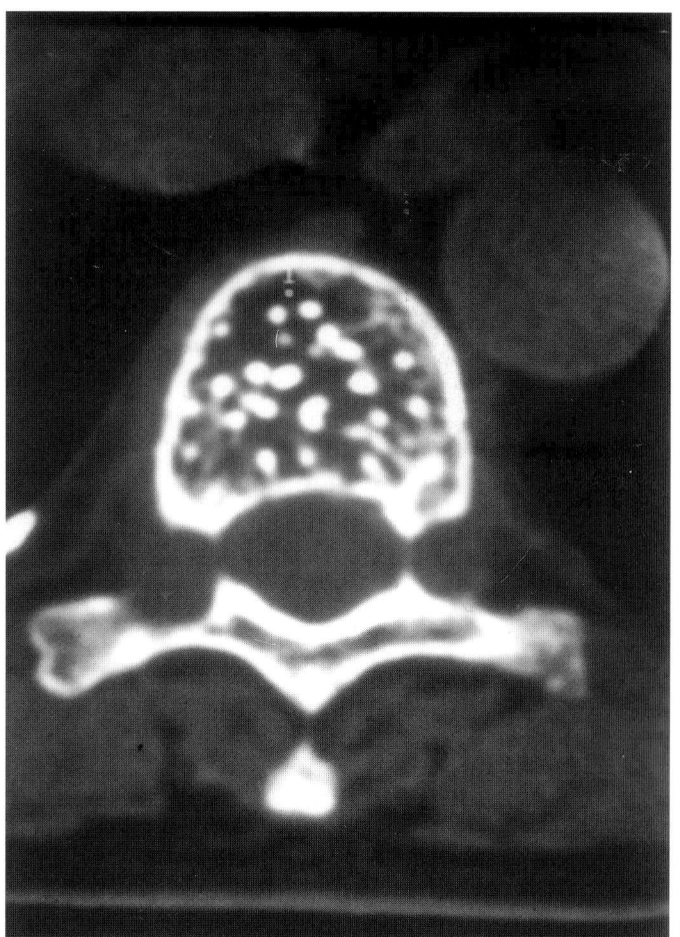

Fig. 1.16 Plain film. (a) Typical striated vertebra suggesting an angioma. This pattern can also be seen in metastases of thyroid or kidney cancers. In this context, CT (b) confirms the diagnosis of benign angioma, by revealing the fatty density of the lesion (here 60).

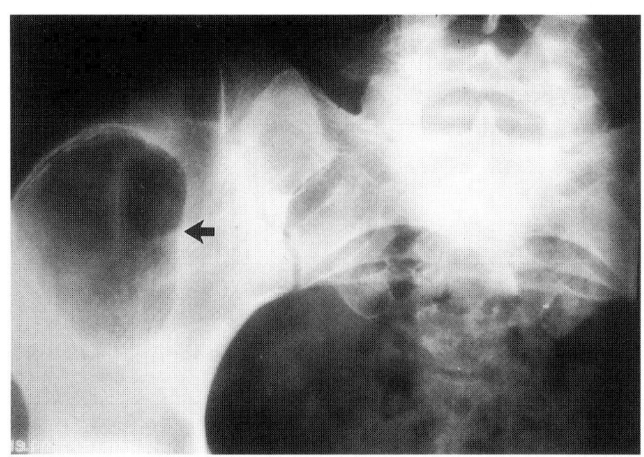

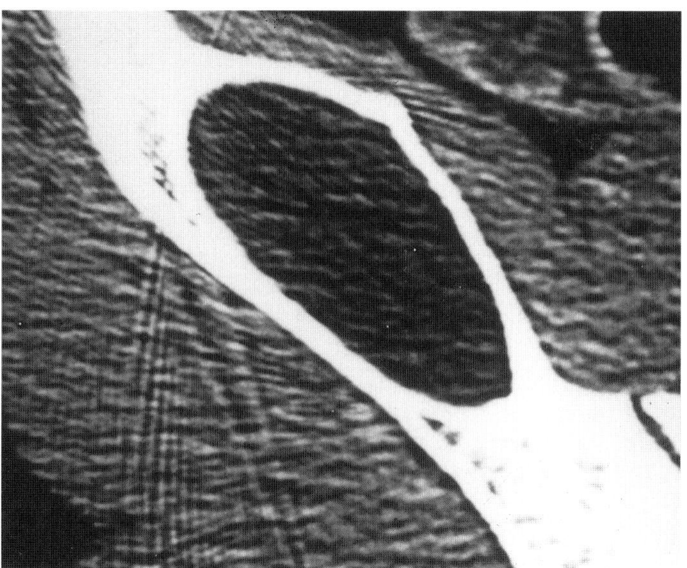

Fig. 1.17 Well-limited lytic painless lesion of the iliac wing in a child. (a) Plain film. On CT (b), the zero density allows the diagnosis of water and thus of a simple bone cyst in an atypical location.

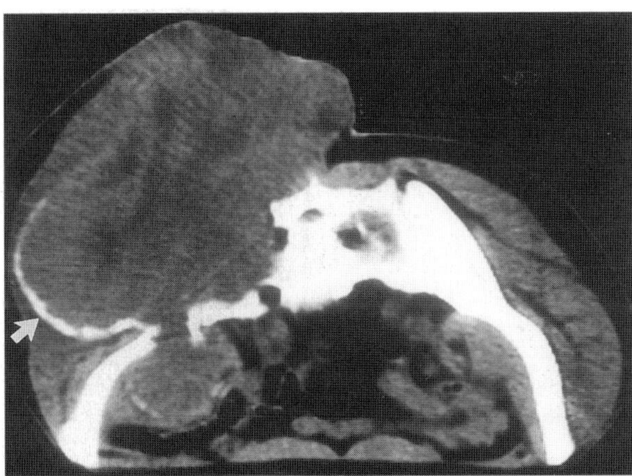

Fig. 1.18 Large tumor of the sacrum and iliac bone in a young adult. CT with the patient in a prone position reveals a thin periosteal bone formation at the periphery of the lesion (arrow), allowing the diagnosis, in spite of the size, of a slowly growing lesion: benign giant cell tumor.

pattern. 1A is characterized by a rim of sclerosis between the normal and lytic areas. The lesion grows so slowly that not only are all trabeculae inside it destroyed, but also there is enough time to build a sclerotic reaction at the periphery of the lesion. 1B indicates a very well-differentiated lesion, with sharp separation from normal bone, but no sclerosis. The lesion grows slowly enough to allow the osteoclasts to destroy all normal trabeculae inside, thus making the difference from normal bone radiologically obvious, but too fast to allow a sclerotic reaction to appear. 1C shows a less sharp margin, indicating that some trabeculae have not yet disappeared inside the lesion. Type 2 is the moth-eaten pattern, made of multiple holes separated by as yet undestroyed bone, and indicates a more aggressive growth. Type 3 is the permeative pattern in which the transition between normal and involved bone is impossible to determine. This indicates a very rapid progression of the lesion. The pattern of the tumor margin only relates to the speed of progression of the lesion and not directly to its malignancy. For example, acute osteomyelitis or eosinophilic granuloma at the beginning may display a permeative pattern and low-grade chondrosarcoma a type 1B margin. Type 1A margins are only seen in non-malignant lesions.

The type of matrix must be studied. Most lesions appear radiolucent on the radiographs. To be detected, a lytic lesion must involve the cortex of the bone, or the matrix must be sufficiently calcified. That may be because the tumor itself is forming bone (osteosarcoma) or is calcified or because of reactive bone formation (Ewing's sarcoma). The typical arcuate or ring calcifications of cartilaginous tumors are explained by the calcification of the fibrous tissue surrounding the round, non-calcified nodules of cartilage (Fig. 1.9). The difference between active and reactive bone formation may be impossible to determine on radiographs.

Periosteal bone formation is the normal way in which the periosteum reacts to any aggression. The pattern of the layer of periosteal formation reacting to the tumor crossing the cortex depends on the speed of tumor progression. When the tumor grows slowly, the periosteum has enough time to build a thick layer of bone (Fig. 1.10). When multiple layers of periosteal formation are present, there is probably a succession of fast and slow growth phases. The periosteal formations are built during the slow phases. This pattern is classic in Ewing tumors, but non-pathognomonic. Spiculated periosteal formations are a very useful radiological sign, strongly suggesting malignancy (Fig. 1.11). They are also seen, rarely, in avulsion injuries, angiomas and infections. Perpendicular spicules are usually seen in extensive lesions of the medullary cavity, such as Ewing's sarcoma. The sunburst pattern is made of spicules diverging from the tumor center, more frequent in osteosarcoma. The Codman's triangle indicates an elevated periosteal reaction, broken by the growth of the tumor. It can be seen in both benign and malignant processes.

Cortical disruption and soft tissue involvement usually indicate aggressiveness. A thin layer of new bone formation ossified around the tumor suggests a slow evolution and therefore a benign process, even if the cortex is destroyed. On the other hand, tumor on both sides of existing cortex indicates a very aggressive lesion.

Multiple lesions change the picture. Metastases are by far the most frequent multiple lesions.

The first necessary step is to diagnose benign lesions definitively based on clinical and radiologic signs, for which biopsy is not necessary.

Fibrous cortical defect

Fibrous cortical defect is a benign bone lesion often found in children, most frequently between the ages of 6 and 11 years. It is always an accidental finding. When painful, other lesions should be considered. The posteromedial side of the distal femoral metaphysis, superior portion of the tibia, fibula and, more rarely, of the humerus, ribs and iliac bone are the sites most often involved. Radiographs should be evaluated in multiple projections and the following findings are typical. A metaphyseal lesion is centered on the cortex of a long bone in contact with the cartilaginous growth plate. The lesion usually measures less than 3 cm, is oriented along the bone axis, oval in shape and lytic and has well-defined margins, sometimes with a thin sclerotic border. Fibrous cortical defect may expand but not disrupt the outer margin of the cortex. There is neither periosteal reaction nor soft tissue mass and no problems with bone growth. The radiologic findings and absence of pain are so typical that they are diagnostic. Often fibrous cortical defect resolves spontaneously. Rarely, it becomes a non-ossifying fibroma with involvement of the medullary cavity.

Non-ossifying fibroma (Fig. 1.8)

Non-ossifying fibroma may spontaneously appear or may develop from the transformation of a fibrous cortical defect. Children with this lesion are usually older than 8 years. The lesion is usually asymptomatic but produces pain when fractured (one-third of cases, particularly in the distal

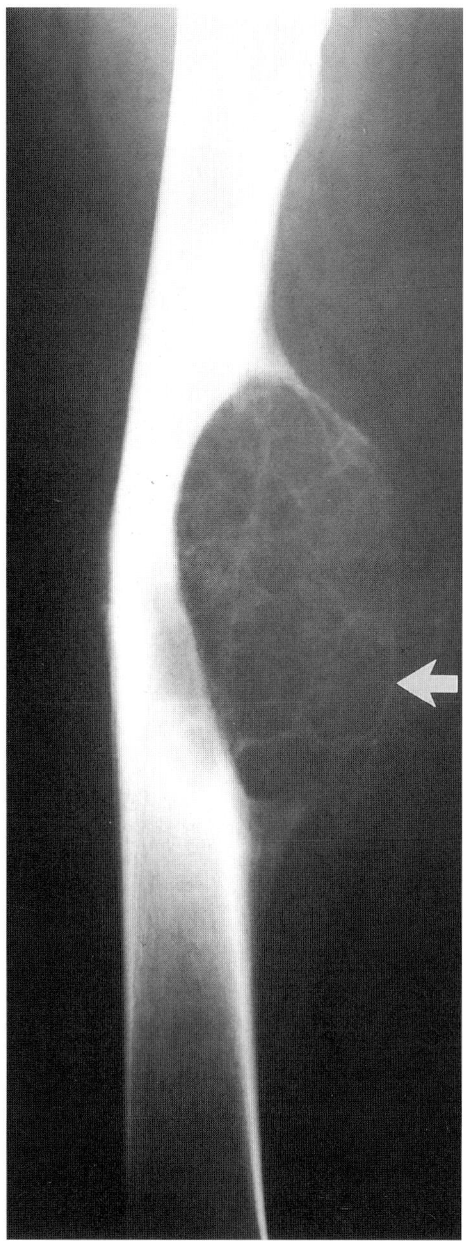

A

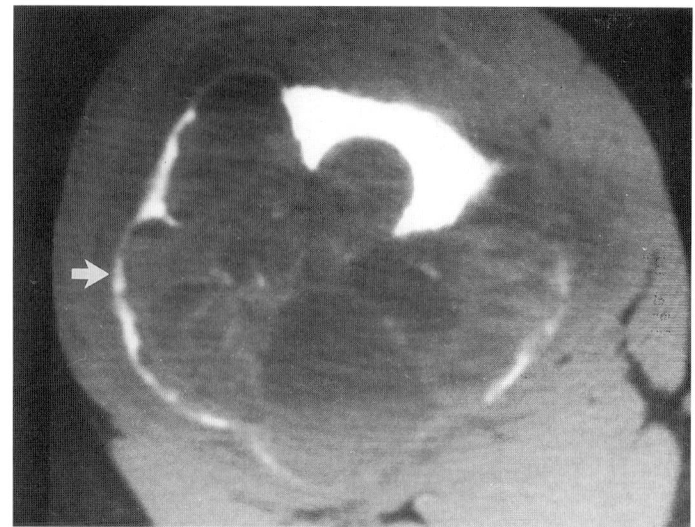

B

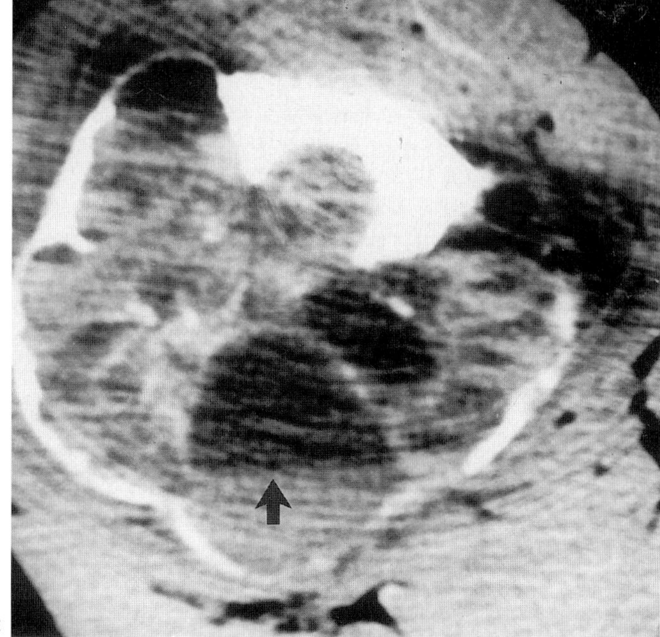

C

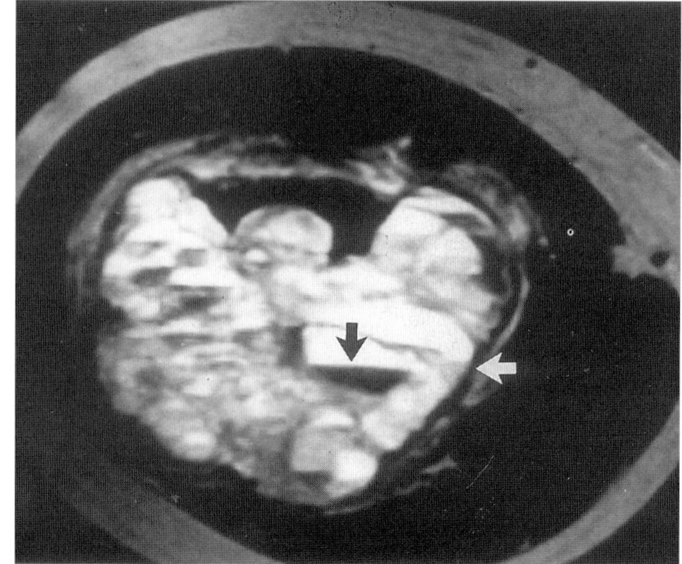

D

Fig. 1.19 Well-demarkated lytic periosteal tumor of the femoral shaft. The thin periosteal formation at the periphery of the tumor (arrow) is visible on plain film (a), but better on CT (bone (b) and soft tissue (c) windows). It is less visible on MRI ((d) T2-weighted axial image), but the fluid–fluid levels (black arrows) are better depicted.

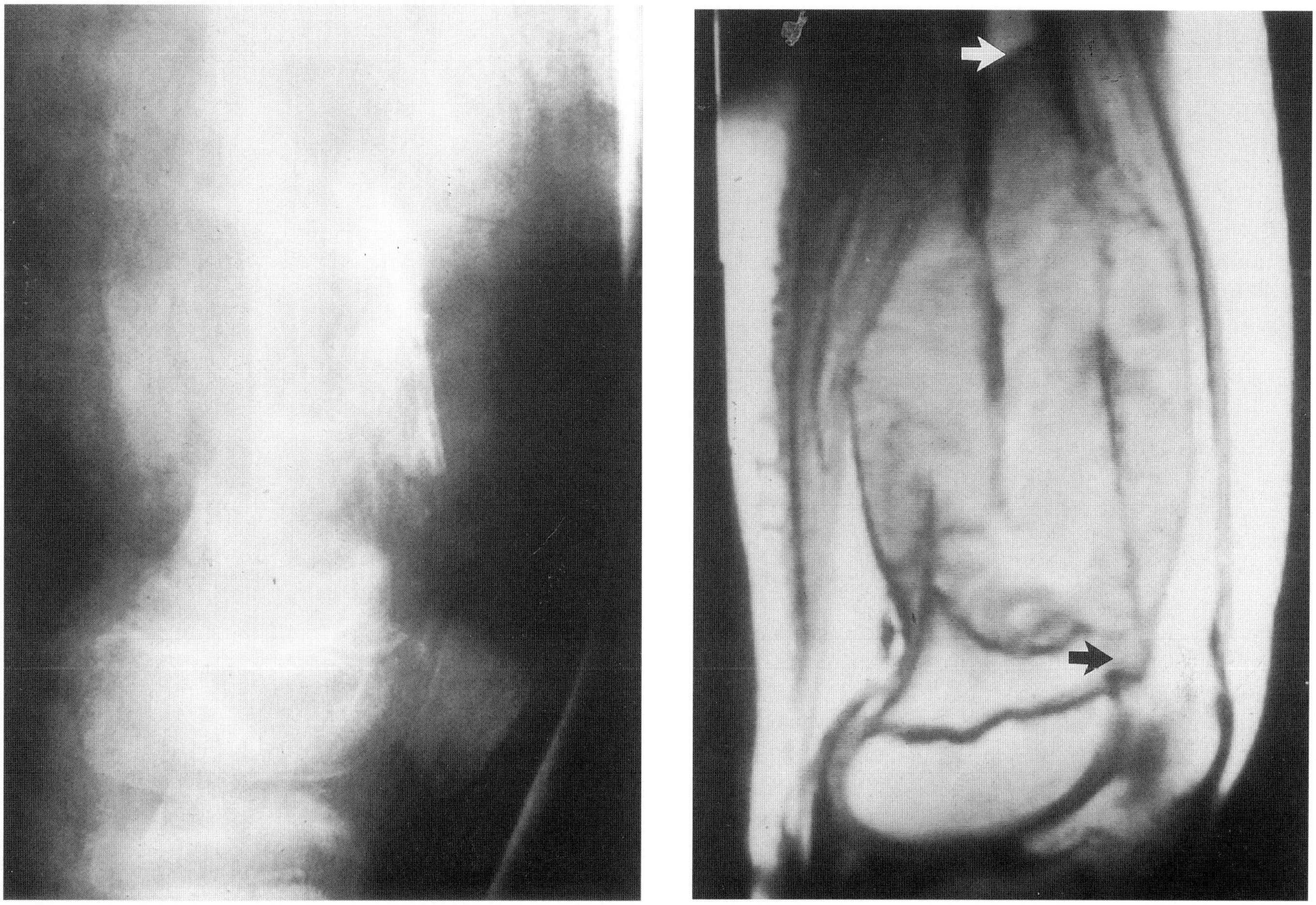

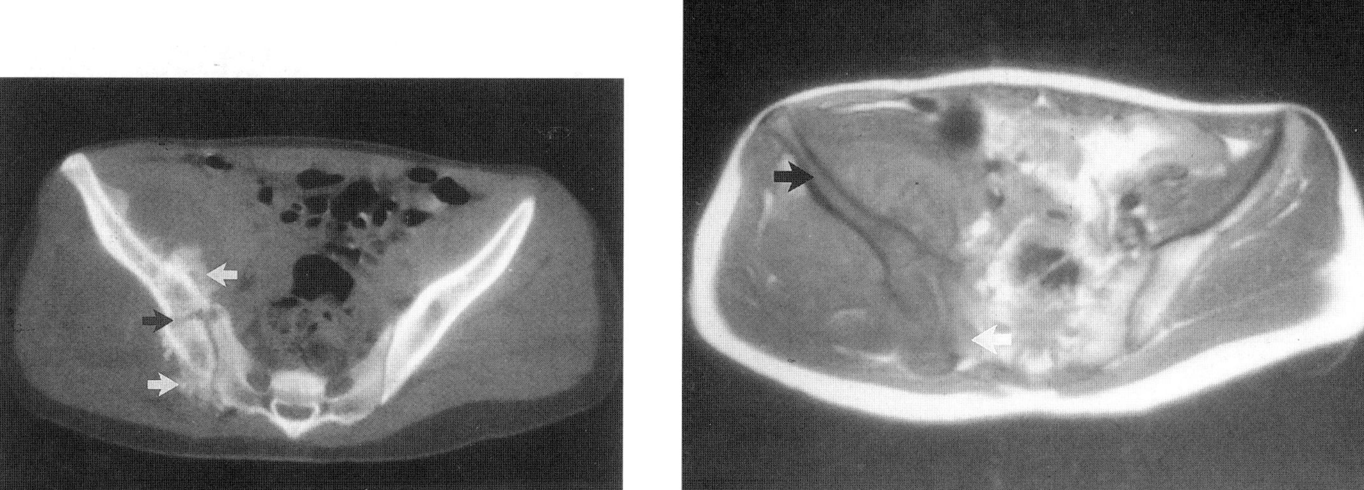

Fig. 1.20 Osteosarcoma of the distal femur in a 9-year-old girl. There is a fracture and a cast. The extension of the tumor is poorly detected on plain film (a). On MRI ((b) T1-weighted sagittal image), its extension into the medullary cavity (white arrow) and the metaphysis is well visualized. The lesion does not involve the epiphyseal plate but the anterior extension into soft tissues (black arrow) makes it impossible to save the epiphysis.

Fig. 1.21 Osteosarcoma of the right iliac wing in a 17-year-old girl. On CT (a), the fracture (black arrow) and the ossifications (white arrows) are easily detected. On MRI ((b) T1-weighted axial image), they are hardly visible, but their extension into the whole iliac wing and the lateral part of the sacrum is impeccably rendered.

tibia). On radiographs, non-ossifying fibroma is usually larger than the fibrous cortical defect and measures 2–7 cm in size. It is metaphyseal in location, adjacent to cartilaginous growth plates. Non-ossifying fibroma appears as a well-defined cortical lesion, centered on the cortex and oriented along the long axis of the bone. The internal border is well defined while the external border expands the cortex, which is thin and often intact. The lesion is lytic, but sometimes dense bone formation occurs in the older portion of the lesion which is the segment farthest from the cartilaginous growth plate. The prognosis is usually favorable, with spontaneous disappearance; there is no malignant degeneration. Here, too, radiologic findings and absence of symptoms are diagnostic.

Periosteal desmoid (Fig. 1.12)

Periosteal desmoid is a common benign tumor in children, particularly in boys aged between 10 and 15 years. Although usually asymptomatic, it is frequently discovered after trauma. Radiographically, its location is typical: the posterior part of the medial femoral condyle just beneath the adductor tubercle. One third of cases are bilateral. The lesion is similar to the fibrous cortical defect, with erosion of the cortex and peripheral sclerosis. When the outer part of the lesion is lytic with perpendicular periosteal reaction and soft tissue masses, differentiation from periosteal sarcoma may be difficult. Its typical location is suggestive. If there is any doubt, close follow-up is needed to confirm the benign nature and to prevent more aggressive treatment.

Fibrous dysplasia

This lesion is frequently found in children and adolescents. The monostotic form is more frequent and is often asymptomatic unless deformity or focal symptoms develop. The radiologic appearance depends on the degree of ossification of the lesions and on their expansile nature. Typically, fibrous dysplasia is a homogeneous, slightly opaque medullary lesion which obscures the trabeculation and extends to the cortex. It sometimes expands bone and shows a 'ground glass' appearance, contrasting with adjacent normal bone. Lesions may also be purely radiolucent or very dense with disappearance of the border between the cortex and medullary cavity. They also can be inhomogeneous with multiple calcifications. Various appearances can be combined. There is no periosteal reaction or soft tissue mass without coexistent fracture.

Osteochondroma or exostoses

Osteochondromas or exostoses are frequent in children and teenagers. Patients usually present with an asympto-

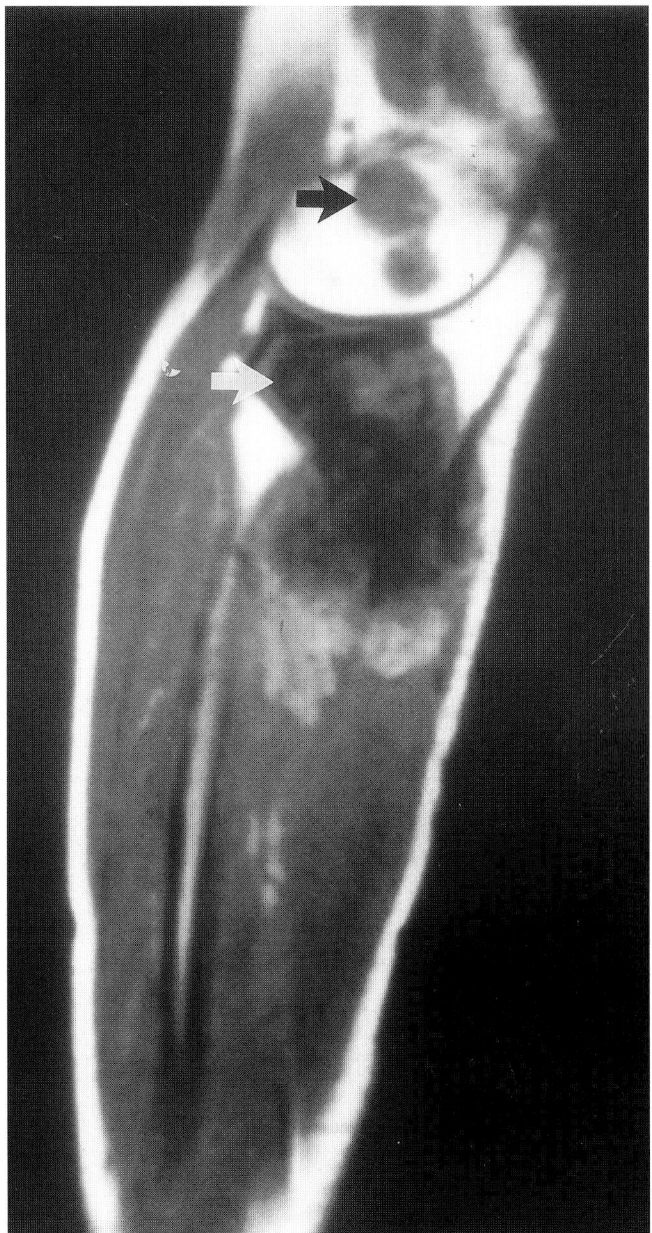

Fig. 1.22 Osteosarcoma of the proximal tibia. Sagittal T1-weighted spin-echo image. The tumor, as well as the two skip metastases of the distal femur (arrow), exhibit a low signal.

matic firm mass that develops in bone with enchondral growth. It is generally revealed by palpation of an asymptomatic firm mass. On radiographs, the findings are typical. The lesion is metaphyseal in location but points to the end of the long bones (most commonly the distal femur and the proximal humerus). Several projections are needed to evaluate the base of the lesion. The key to diagnosis is to show continuity of the cortex of the normal bone with that of the osteochondroma (Fig. 1.13).

Chondroma

Chondroma is also a frequent lesion and is found in the

hand in half of the cases. It is fortuitously discovered; pain and swelling only appear after fracture. On radiographs, although it is usually centered on the bone, it is occasionally eccentric or periosteal in location. It is round or oval, lytic and contains cartilaginous calcifications. Borders are well defined and the cortex can be thinned and expansile. There is no periosteal reaction or lesion in the soft tissues without fracture.

Simple bone cyst (Fig. 1.14)

This is the most frequent of the benign lesions of the peripheral skeleton. Eighty to 90% of the patients are aged between 3 and 19 years and boys are more often involved than girls. Simple bone cyst is asymptomatic until fractured. Fifty percent of the lesions are located in the proximal humerus and 25% in the femur. Radiographically, bone cysts develop in the metaphysis and do not cross the cartilaginous growth plate. They occupy the medullary cavity in the long axis of the bone, being widest in the metaphysis and becoming narrower as they approach the diaphysis. It is lytic and well defined and sometimes has localized dense bone when found in the extremities, especially on the diaphyseal side. The cortex is expansile and thinned, but not destroyed. While growing, the cyst migrates into the diaphysis and is separated from the cartilaginous growth plate by normal bone. When growth ceases, it becomes ovoid. Fracture occurs in two-thirds of patients with bone cysts and presents a typical radiographic appearance with a bone fragment within the cyst cavity.

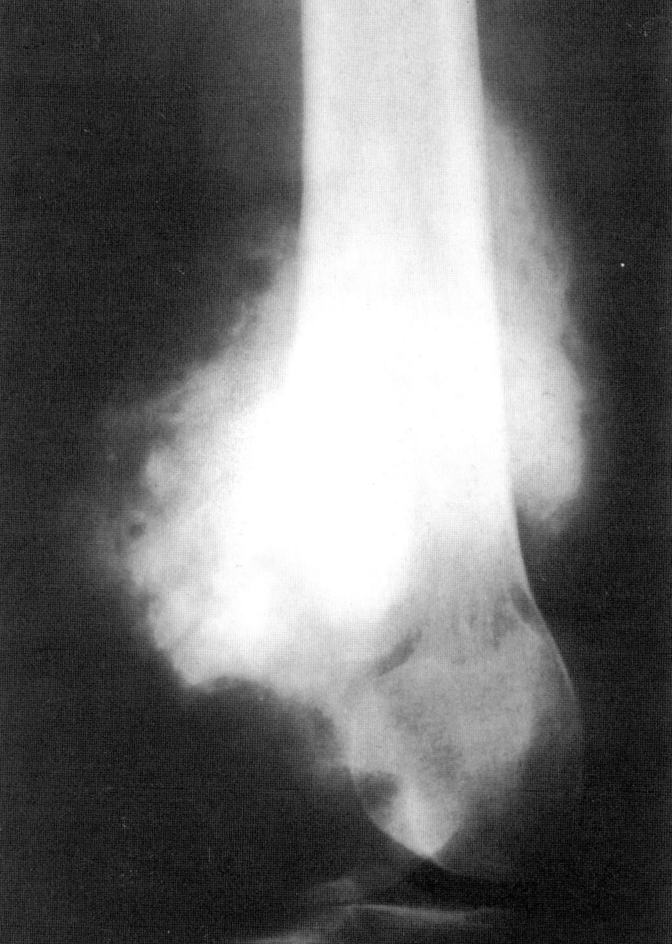

A

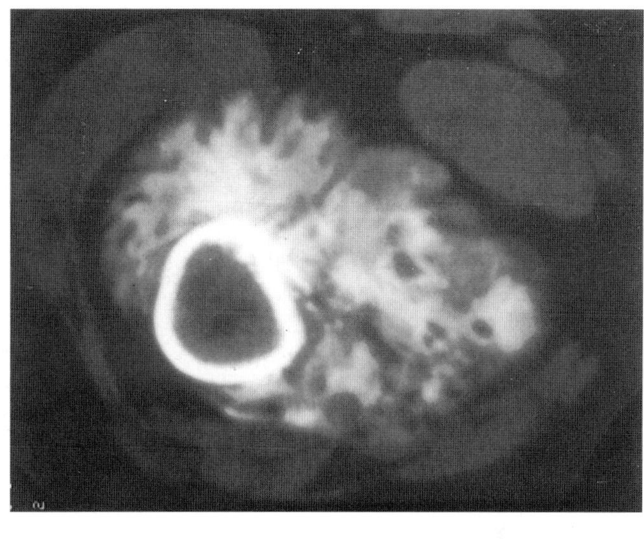

B

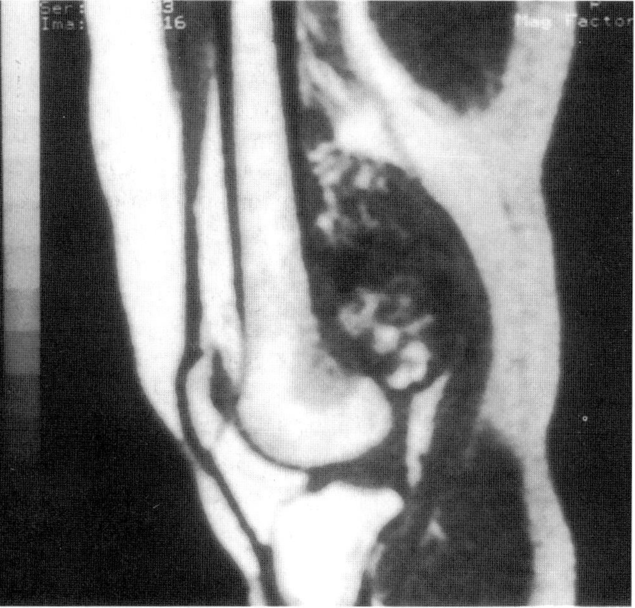

C

Fig. 1.23 Parosteal osteosarcoma. Ossified mass has developed mainly outside the shaft of the femur. (a) Plain film; (b) CT with a bone window; (c) MRI T1-weighted sagittal image. Ossifications are better depicted on plain film and CT while the non-involvement of the medullary cavity, visible on CT, is much better conveyed on MRI.

Vertebral angiomas

Vertebral angiomas can occur in any age group. Radiographically they enlarge vertebrae and cause striations within the vertebral body.

Myositis ossificans (Fig. 1.15)

This lesion must be recognized, as biopsy is not necessary and can be harmful because histologic diagnosis can be very difficult. Patients are usually aged under 30 years and trauma is found in two-thirds of the cases. Swelling of the soft tissues appears with maximal pain during the second and third weeks, redness of skin, limitation of movement, fever and increase of the sedimentation rate. The lesion is most commonly located in the arm, thigh, pelvis or the

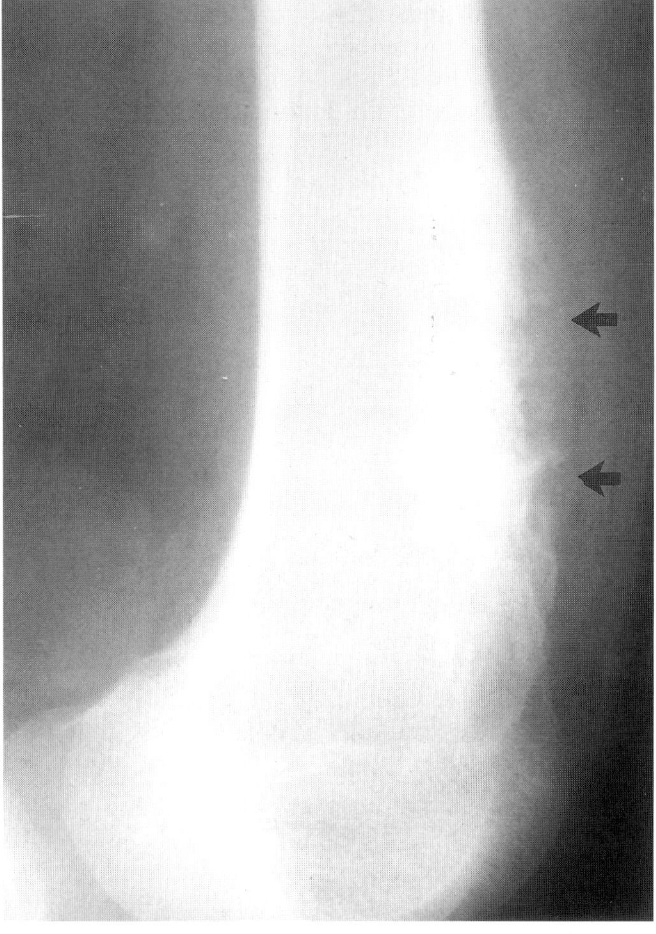

A

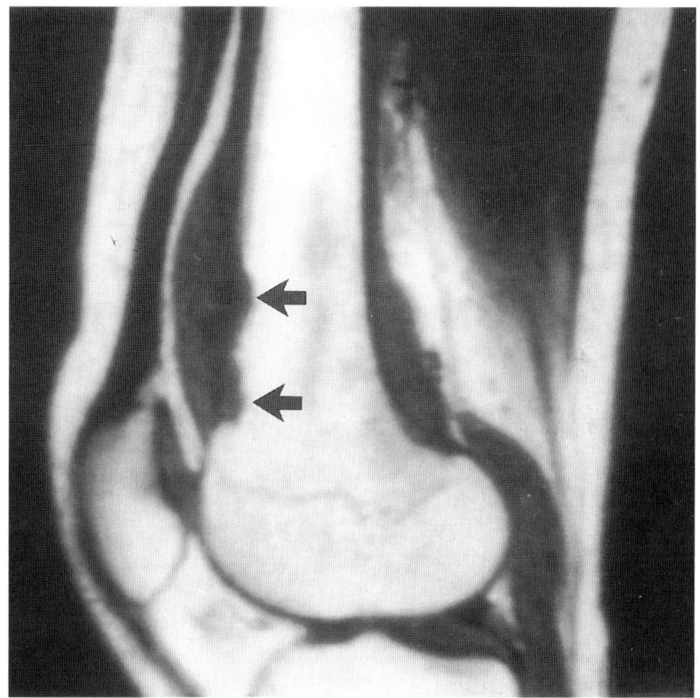

C

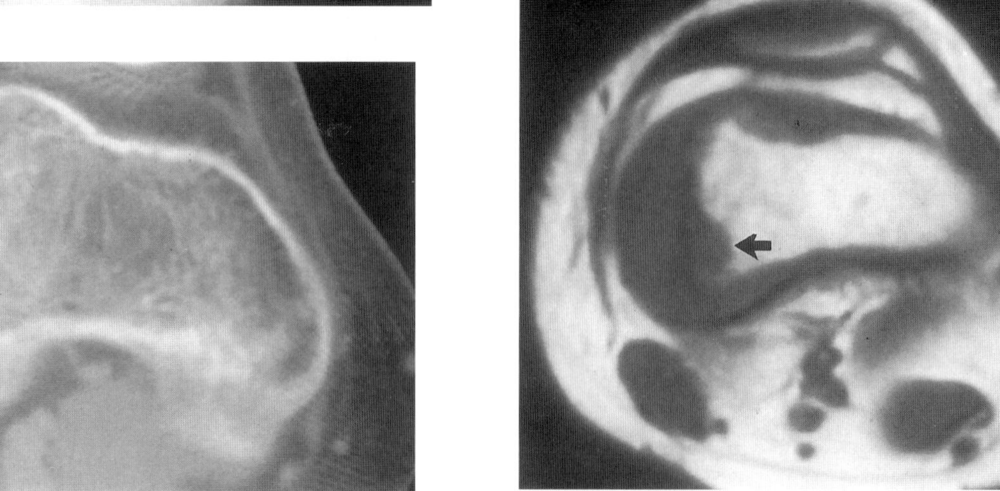

B

D

Fig. 1.24 Periosteal osteosarcoma of the shaft of the femur. Plain film. (a) Saucerization of the cortex; ossified tumor has developed in the soft tissue. The ossification of the tumor is readily detected on CT ((b) arrow) and not on MRI ((c and d) axial and sagittal T1-weighted images), but the involvement of the medullary cavity is only visible on MRI (arrows).

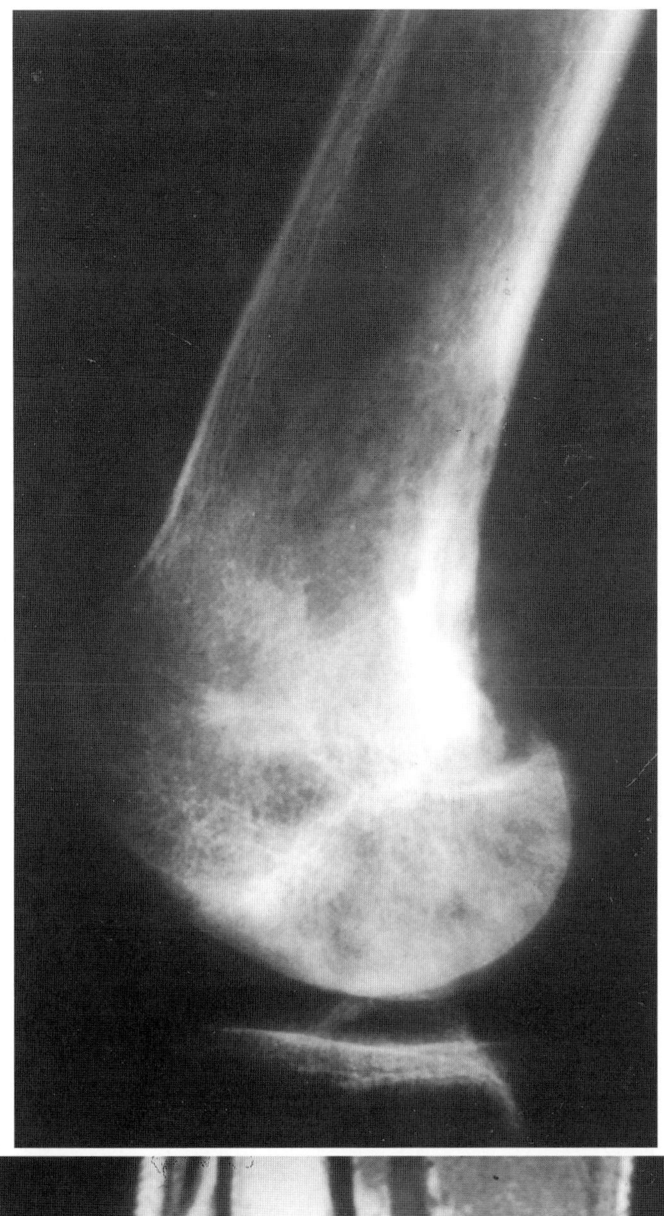

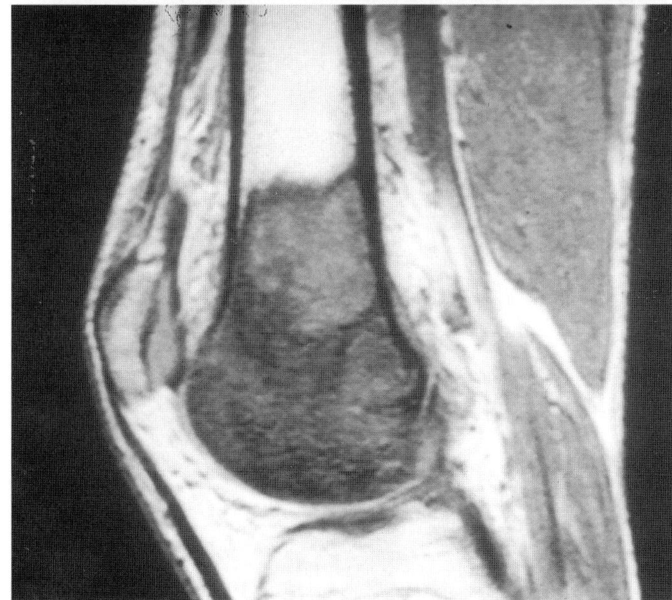

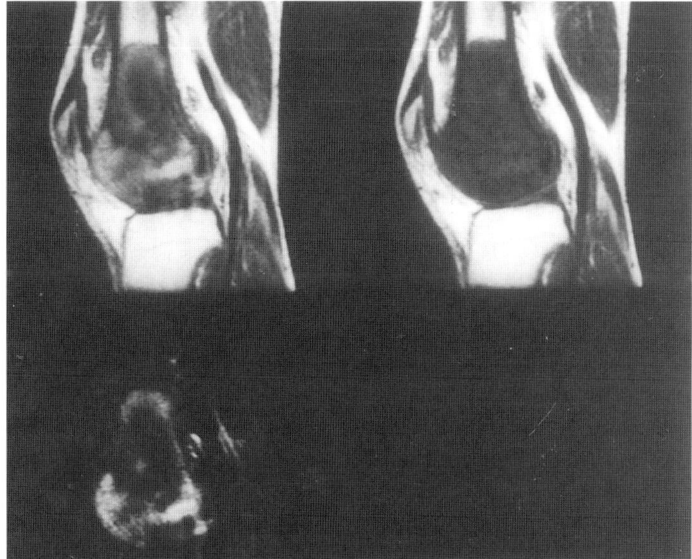

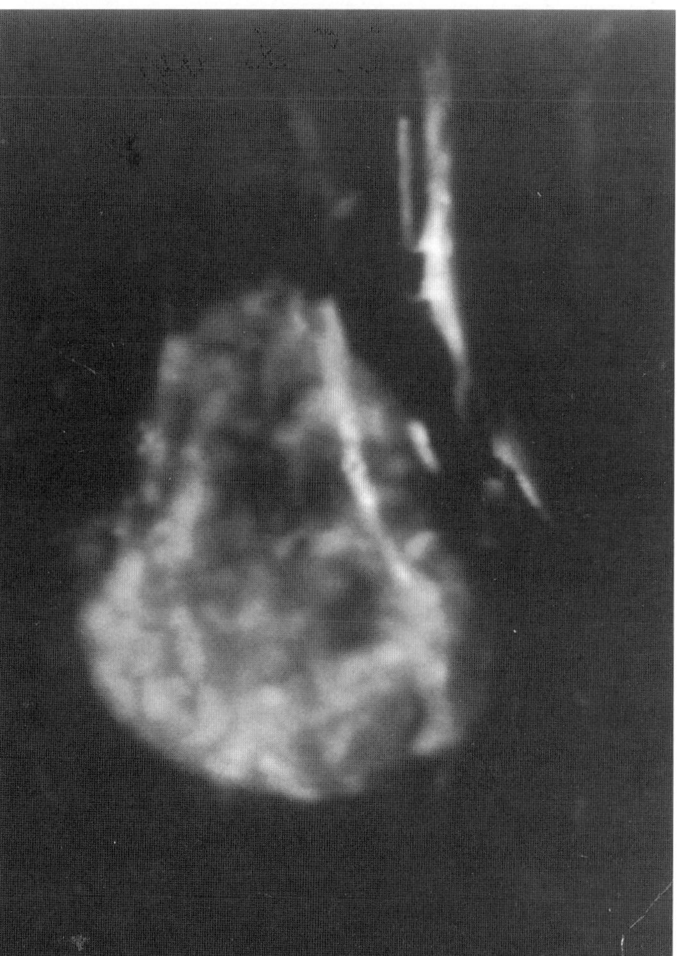

Fig. 1.25 Osteosarcoma of the distal femur. Faintly delineated lytic lesion on plain films (a). On MR images (sagittal T1-weighted spin-echo), the tumor abuts on the extremity of the bone: the involvement of the joint cannot be reliably evaluated (in this case it was free at surgery). (b). T1-weighted sagittal images before (top right), 45 s after injection (top left) and subtraction (bottom), displaying the viable part of the tumor (c). This can also be visualized on a 3-D reconstruction (d).

first and second metacarpals. Initial radiographs are normal but within 3–4 weeks ossification appears in the soft tissues. Thus myositis ossificans, when first radiographically apparent, resembles a soft tissue mass. The lesion progressively ossifies and appears as a mass with a lucent center and calcified periphery which is diagnostic, particularly when previous images are available. The lesion evolves progressively to spontaneous regression.

In other cases, evidence favors a malignant lesion. Examination for metastases and MRI examination before biopsy must be performed.

Finally, some diagnoses are difficult. In these cases, the next step is CT. Problems can result from bone locations which are difficult to evaluate on conventional X-ray (short, flat bones, especially the pelvis, sacrum, sternum and vertebrae). Sometimes, the study of the tumor matrix can provide features necessary for the diagnosis. There may be small calcifications allowing diagnosis of cartilaginous tumor or osteoid matrix. Measurement of the density can help characterize fat (Fig. 1.16), fluid (Fig. 1.17), fibrous or calcified tissue. Axial study and high contrast provide basic diagnostic principles: small lytic regions of the cortex, localized involvement of the soft tissues and thin peripheral periosteal reactions can be seen better than on plain films. Lesions with slow evolution which displace and expand the cortex peripherally (Fig. 1.18) can be distinguished from more aggressive lesions which cross the cortex. CT can show the tumor on both sides of the cortex before it is destroyed. This is the case for Ewing's sarcoma and osteosarcomas. If a tumor of this type is not ossified, it is probably a Ewing's sarcoma; if the tumor is ossified, it is probably an osteosarcoma.[26] CT allows measurement of the thickness of the non-calcified cap of an osteochondroma tumor: the cap is thin in benign lesions and thick (more than 3 cm) in chondrosarcomas.[27,28] The cap can also be evaluated by ultrasonography.[29] CT is the examination of

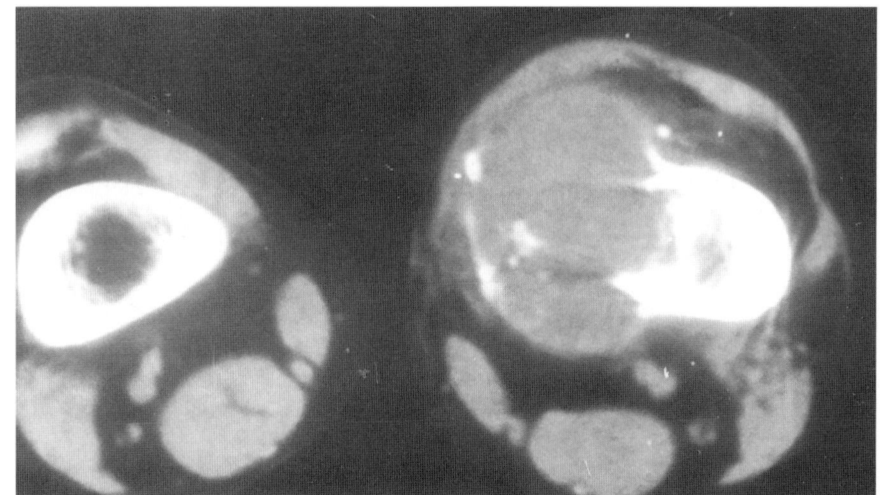

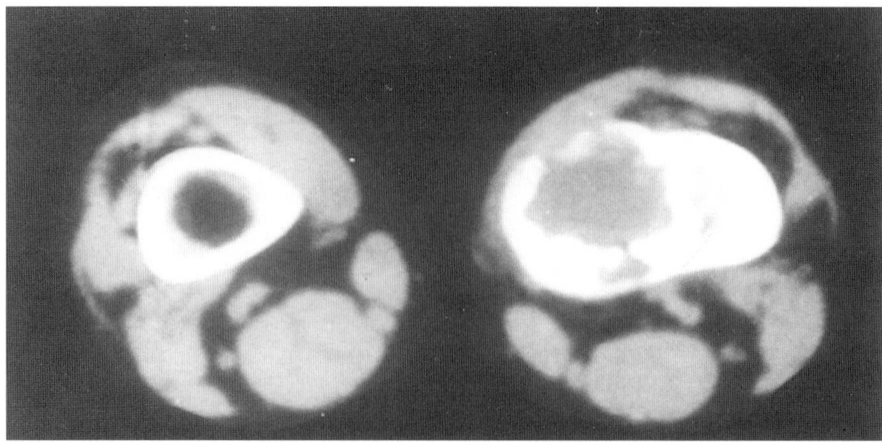

Fig. 1.26 CT images of an osteosarcoma of the distal left femur, before (a) and after (b) chemotherapy. All signs of treatment efficacy are visible: the tumor is smaller, better limited and more ossified.

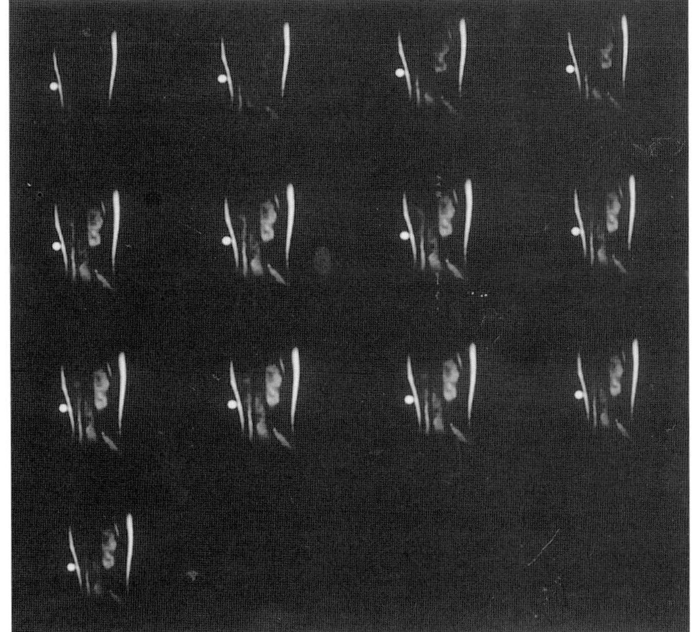

A

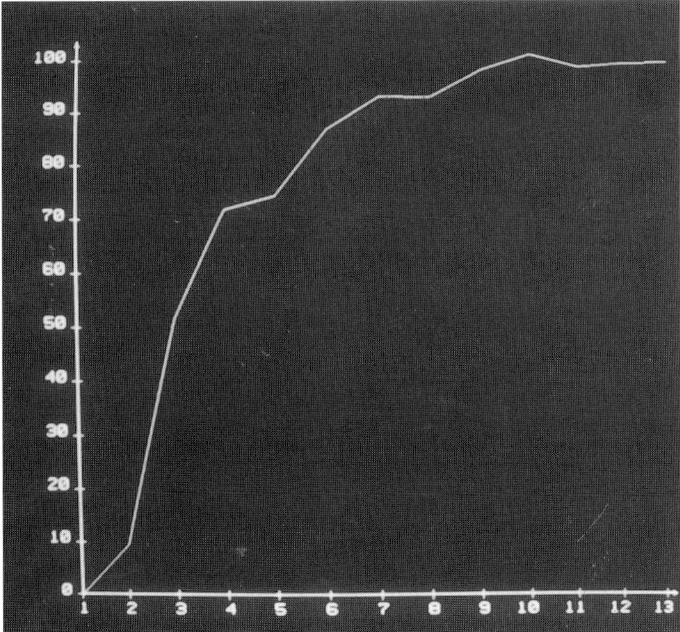

C

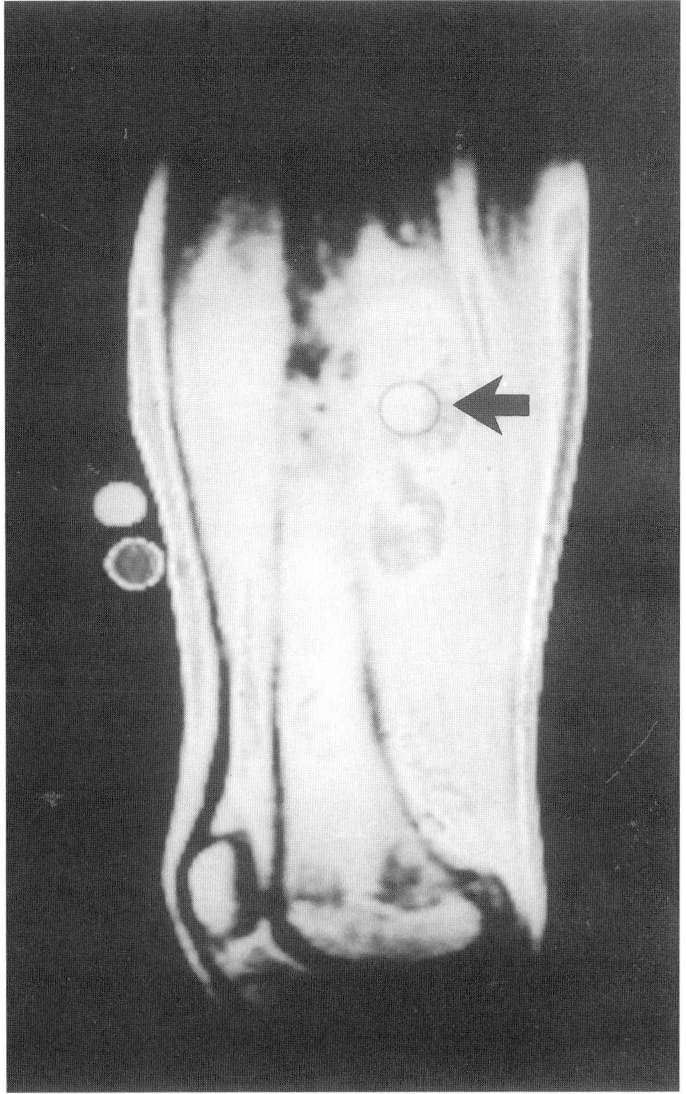

B

Fig. 1.27 Osteosarcoma of the femoral shaft. Region of interest (ROI) technique. (a) Multiple acquisitions are realized at regular intervals here every 45 s. (b) The ROI is selected (arrow). (c) The curve indicates the uptake of contrast medium.

choice for the demonstration of the nidus of an osteoid osteoma in dense bone. Although the nidus is better evaluated and detected on CT than on MRI, the inflammatory reaction is more obvious on MRI.[30]

Usually MRI is not useful for characterization of bone tumors.[31,32] Calcifications are poorly detected and T1 and T2 measurements are not reliable and reproducible because most large tumors are heterogeneous. Moreover, there is a significant overlap between T1 and T2 values of benign and malignant tissues. MRI can define fluid levels in blood-filled cavities, especially in aneurysmal bone cysts[33] (Fig. 1.19). The levels are also detected on CT, but the contrast is far superior on MRI. This sign is non-pathognomonic and indicates only layering phenomenon with supernatant and deposit in some cystic cavities. Spin-echo sequences combined with contrast images help differentiate cartilaginous lesions.[34–36] If there is no enhancement after injection of contrast medium, the lesion is benign. Septal ring and arc enhancement is seen in some enchondromas and intense, usually heterogeneous non-septal enhancement in high-grade chondrosarcomas. The use of dynamic sequences seems reliable in adults if very fast acquisitions are performed. An uptake less than 6 s after visualization of the arteries suggests malignancy.

STAGING

Local extent

Local extent and staging is based on magnetic resonance imaging.[3–10] The main advantages are high contrast and the possibility of choosing the plane of examination without moving the patient.

Intramedullary extension

MRI, with its inherently superior tissue contrast resolution, allows accurate depiction of medullary bone (high signal) as opposed to cortical bone (low signal) on T1 spin echo sequences. Diaphyseal and metaphyseal intermedullary extension, as well as spread across the growth plate in the child, are best observed in the longitudinal (Figs. 1.20, 1.21). Although CT can also evaluate extension, it is limited to the axial plane.[37–39] MRI has a few limitations such as the inability to detect very small lesions and the overestimation of the tumor volume on T2-weighted sequences because of peritumoral edema. The latter can be solved by the use of dynamic sequences.[40] With accurate evaluation of tumor extent, the surgeon can determine the level of bone resection and the size of the prosthesis. The growth plate in children and the joints in adults can sometimes be preserved when uninvolved. Skip lesions (small metastases separated from the primary tumor by healthy tissue) are easily detected on MR scans parallel to the long axis of the bone (Fig. 1.22). In periosteal tumors, MRI demonstrates the location and its extension into cortex and the medullary cavity[23] (Figs 1.23, 1.24). CT can also define the extent of diaphyseal periosteal lesions but not of metaphyseal periosteal tumors, as the normal cancellous bone of the metaphysis is heterogeneous.

MRI also very adequately depicts soft tissues, vessels and their relationship to the tumor. The extension into the soft tissues can be overevaluated on MRI, because of peritumoral edema. Dynamic sequences are helpful to define the difference. Both CT and MRI can show skin and subcutaneous extension. Intraarticular extension remains a very difficult problem[41] (Fig. 1.25). When the lesion is far from the joint or obviously within the joint, the cases are

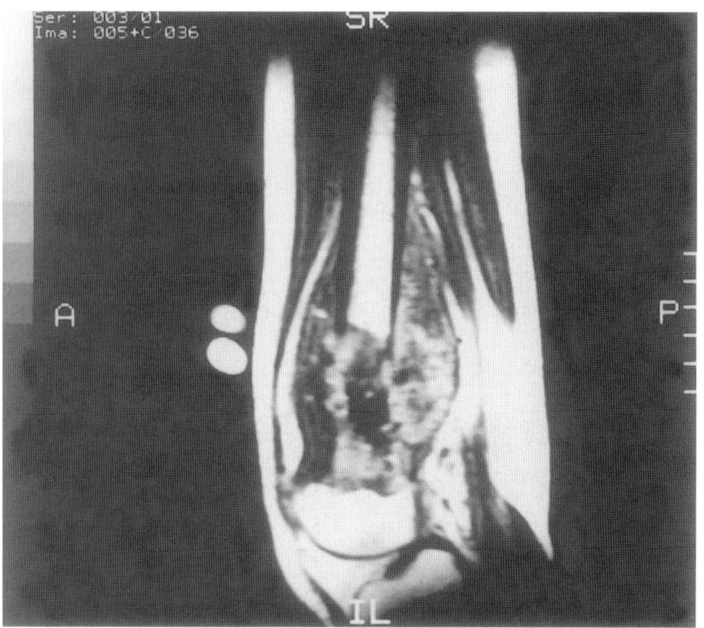

A

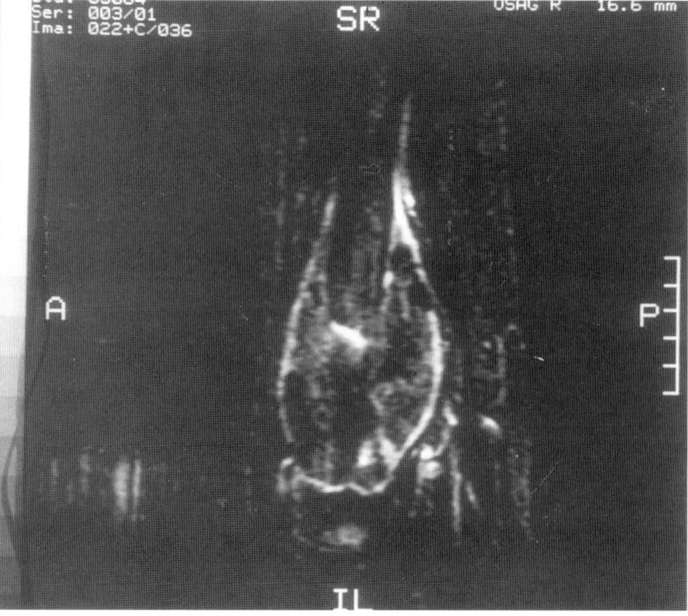

B

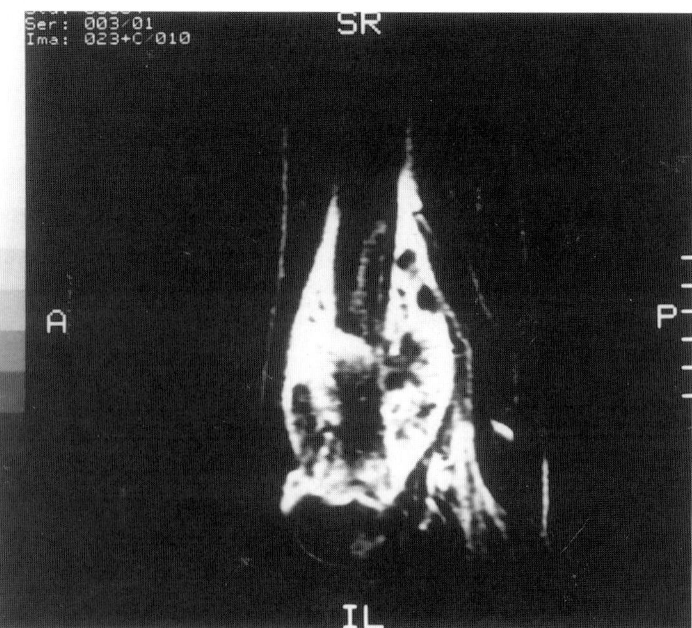

C

Fig. 1.28 Osteosarcoma of the distal femur. T1-weighted sagittal images, after injection (a) and subtraction of the images obtained 45 s (b) and 5 min after injection (c) from the native images. In this good responder, only small foci of viable tumor are visible at 45 s. At 5 min, both the viable tumor and the granulation tissue have increased their signal.

easily solved. When the tumor abuts on the joint, a frequent situation, involvement of the joint is often overevaluated. Joint effusion does not mean involvement. Adequate assessment of tumor extension has practical consequences. A malignant tumor should never be opened during surgery but a non-involved joint can be opened, allowing preservation of muscles and good function with a prosthesis. Conversely, an involved joint should be removed en bloc to prevent spillage of tumor. The real question we cannot answer is: if the surgeon excises the involved bone, will there be tumor cells remaining in the joint?

In summary, MRI should be used as the principal test for evaluating extension of malignant tumors.

EXAMINATION OF DISTANT SPREAD

Bone metastases and multiple lesions are best detected on radionuclide bone scans. Pulmonary metastases are evaluated on conventional chest radiographs and chest CT.[42]

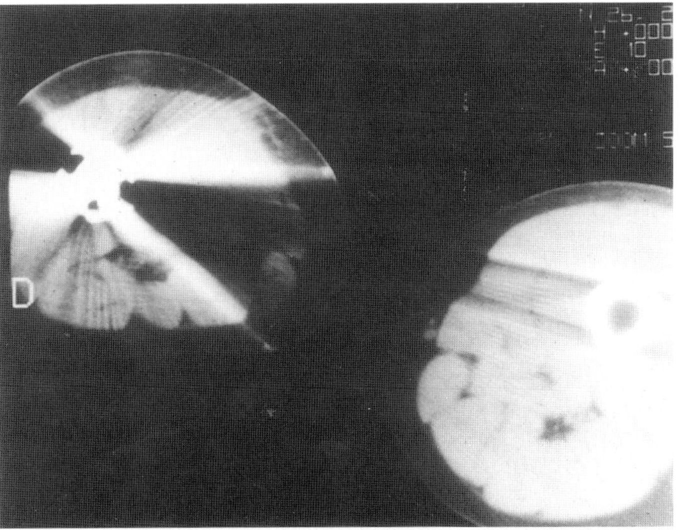
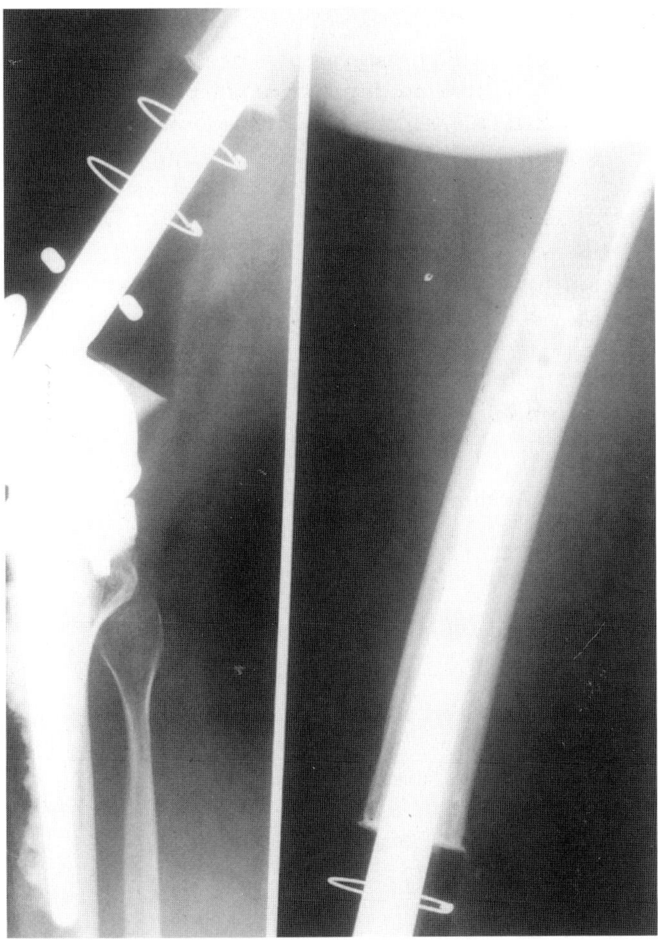
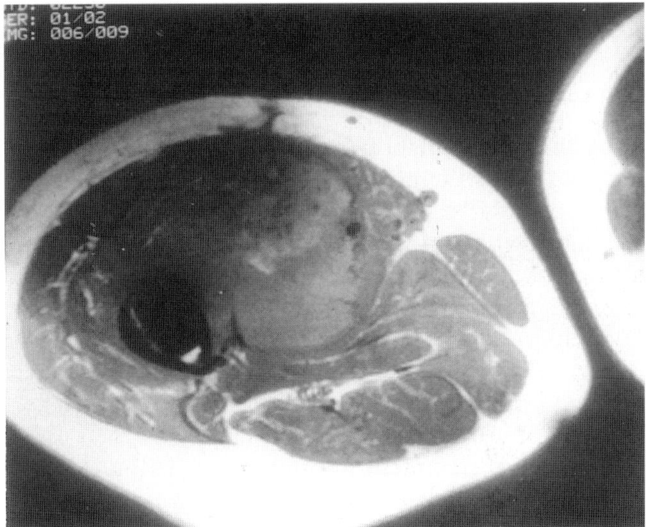
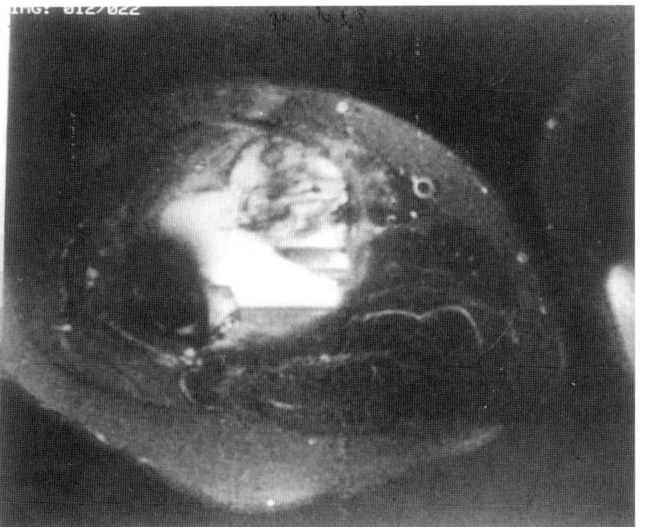

Fig. 1.29 Prosthesis of the right femur in an osteosarcoma. On the plain films (a), requested because of further pain, nothing is visible. On CT (b), there are too many artifacts. On MRI (axial T1 and T2 images), the recurrence is obvious. Fluid–fluid levels are easily detected. There are almost no artifacts from the titanium prosthesis.

Table 1.1 The choice of the imaging technique

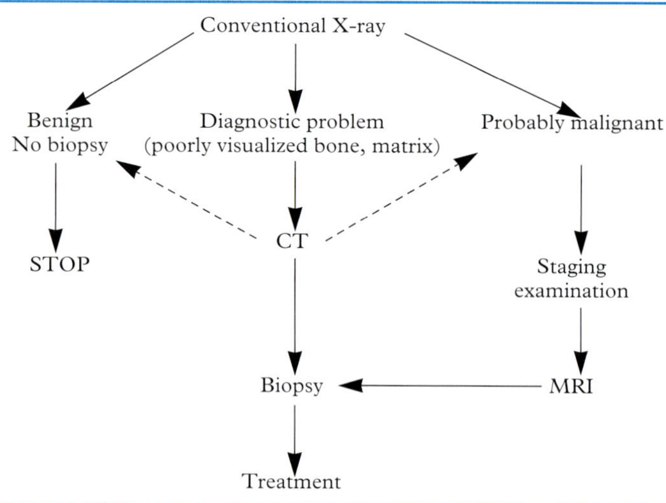

EVALUATION OF EFFECTIVENESS AND FOLLOW-UP OF TREATMENT

Most primary malignant bone tumors are treated with preoperative chemotherapy before removal. After surgery, histologic study of the tumor can be carried out to estimate effectiveness of the treatment. If effective, the same treatment will be continued postoperatively; if not, treatment should be changed.

Plain films and CT can provide information on the size of the tumor, its margins and presence of calcified or ossified matrix. Decrease in tumor size, better demarcation and ossification have been considered as good indicators of effective treatment in osteosarcoma (Fig. 1.26). In fact, even with increased tumor size, there are still 20% good responders (the increase in size is usually secondary to bleeding in these cases) and when it decreases, there are only two-thirds of good responses, so size is not completely reliable as a marker.[43]

Sonography with color flow Doppler is an easy to use and efficient technique to evaluate the effectiveness of preoperative chemotherapy in malignant tumors (osteosarcomas), but only when the cortical bone is destroyed by the tumor.[44]

MRI provides a more accurate study of the tumoral volume than other imaging techniques and the clinical examination, but with the same limitations. Signal decrease on T2-weighted sequences in the tumor involving the soft tissues suggests increased ossification or presence of more fibrous tissue in the tumor. Increase of the tumor volume and persistence of high signal intensity of the tumor and peritumoral edema on T2-weighted sequences are reliable indicators of a poor response, even after only one cycle of chemotherapy.[45] On T1-weighted spin echo sequences there are no reliable indicators of a good response on non-contrasted MRI. The signal of normal tissues does not change during chemotherapy.[46] MR imaging with dynamic contrast-enhanced images is useful for differentiating postchemotherapeutic change from viable tumor, for viable tumor enhances rapidly and the postchemotherapeutic inflammatory changes enhance slowly[14–19] (Figs 1.27, 1.28). This allows a precise mapping of the active tumor and a study of the whole tumor volume. Detection of residual viable tumor is more accurate in osteosarcomas, with usually massive nests of tumor, than in Ewing's sarcoma because, with this tumor, isolated viable tumor cells, which are too small to detect, may remain after treatment.[47,48] Problems may arise when growth factors are associated with chemotherapy, as they stimulate yellow to red marrow reconversion.[49] New islands of red marrow, when abutting on the tumor, may mimic tumor growth.

Bone scintigraphy can also be used to monitor the effectiveness of treatment, in both static and dynamic ways. The results are reliable, but the spatial resolution is inferior to MRI.

DETECTION OF LOCAL RECURRENCES

After placement of a prosthesis, if a local recurrence is suspected MRI can be used, provided the prosthesis is non-paramagnetic, e.g. titanium. Titanium is increasingly used, making MRI very efficient (Fig. 1.29).

CONCLUSION

Plain films must be used first to study a bone tumor, followed by CT in the case of diagnostic problems (Table 1.1). MRI is the modality of choice for local staging, evaluating response to preoperative chemotherapy and long-term follow-up (Table 1.2).

Table 1.2 Role of the imaging modalities in the local evaluation of a bone tumor

	Plain films	Bone scan	CT	MRI
Diagnosis Calcifications,	+++ (long bones)	+	++++	+
ossifications	+++	0	++++	0
Periosteum, cortex	+++	0	++++	+
Tissue characterization	+	0	+++	+
Extension	+	++	++	++++
Soft tissues	+	0	+++	++++
Medullary cavity	+	++	++	++++
Skip lesions	0	+++	+	+++
Joint	+	+	++	+++
Skin, vessels	0	0	+++	++++
Follow-up under and after treatment	+	++	++	++++

REFERENCES

1. Kalifa C, Mlika N, Dubousset J, Contesso G, Vanel D, Lumbroso J. Expérience du protocole T10 dans le Service de Pédiatrie de l'Institut Gustave-Roussy. Bull Cancer 1988: 75: 207–211

2. Rosen G, Caparros B, Huvos A G et al. Preoperative chemotherapy for osteogenic sarcoma: selection of postoperative adjuvant chemotherapy based on the response of the primary tumor to preoperative chemotherapy. Cancer 1982: 49: 1221–1230

3. Aisen A M, Martel W, Braunstein E M, McMilin K I, Philips W A, Kling T F. MRI and CT evaluation of primary bone and soft tissue tumors. AJR 1986: 146: 749–756

4. Bloem J L, Taminiau A H M, Eulderink F, Hermans J, Pauwels E K J. Radiologic staging of primary bone sarcoma. MRI, scintigraphy, angiography and CT correlated with pathologic examination. Radiology 1988: 169: 805–810

5. Bohndorf K, Reiser M, Lochner B, Feaux de Lacroix W, Steinbrich W. Magnetic resonance imaging of primary tumors and tumor like lesions of bone. Skeletal Radiol 1986: 15: 511–517

6. Boyko O B, Cory D A, Cohen M D, Provisor A, Mirkin D, De Rosa G P. MR imaging of osteogenic and Ewing's sarcoma. AJR 1987: 148: 317–322

7. Hudson T M, Hamlin D J, Enneking W F, Petterson H. MRI of bone and soft tissue tumors. Early experience in 31 patients compared with CT. Skeletal Radiol 1985: 13: 134–146

8. Reiser M, Rupp N, Biehl T, Allgoyer B, Heller H J, Lukas P, Fink U. MRI in the diagnosis of bone tumors. Eur J Radiol 1985: 5: 1–7

9. Sundaram M, McGuire M H, Herbold D R, Wolverson M K, Heiberg E. Magnetic resonance imaging in planning limb-salvage surgery for primary malignant tumors of bone. J Bone Joint Surg (Am) 1986: 68: 809–819

10. Vanel D, Di Paola R, Contesso G. Magnetic resonance imaging in musculoskeletal primary malignant tumors. In: Kressel HY Ed Magnetic resonance annual. New York: Raven Press, 1987: 237–261

11. Mirowitz S A, Apicella P, Reinus W R et al. MR imaging of bone marrow lesions: relative conspicuousness on T1-weighted, fat-suppressed T2-weighted, and STIR images. AJR 1994: 162: 215–221

12. Pui M H, Chang S K. Comparison of inversion recovery fast spin-echo (FSE) with T2-weighted fat-saturated FSE and T1-weighted MR imaging in bone marrow lesion detection. Skeletal Radiol 1996: 25: 149–152

13. Swan J S, Grist T M, Sproat I A et al. Musculoskeletal neoplasms: preoperative evaluation with MR angiography. Radiology 1995: 194: 519–524

14. Erleman R, Reiser M, Peters P E. Musculo-skeletal neoplasms: static and dynamic Gd-DTPA-enhanced MR imaging. Radiology 1989: 171: 767–77

15. Bonnerot V, Charpentier A, Frouin F, Kalifa C, Vanel D, Di Paola R. The use of factor analysis of dynamic MR imaging in predicting the response of osteosarcoma to chemotherapy. Invest Radiol 1992: 27: 847–855

16. Verstraete K L, De Deene Y, Roels H et al. Benign and malignant musculoskeletal lesions: dynamic contrast-enhanced MR imaging parametric 'first-pass' images depict tissue vascularization and perfusion. Radiology 1994: 192: 835–843

17. Verstraete K L, Dierick A, De Deene Y et al. First-pass images of musculoskeletal lesions: a new and useful diagnostic application of dynamic contrast-enhanced MRI. Magn Reson Imaging 1994: 12: 687–702

18. Verstraete K L, Vanzieleghem B, De Deene Y et al. Static, dynamic and first-pass MR imaging of musculoskeletal lesions using gadodiamide injection. Acta Radiol 1995: 36: 27–36

19. De Baere T, Vanel D, Shapeero L G, Charpentier A, Terrier P, Di Paola M. Contrast enhanced subtraction MRI for evaluating osteosarcoma after chemotherapy. Radiology 1992; 185: 587–592

20. Lodwick G S, Wilson A J, Farrel C, Virtama P, Smeltzer F M, Ditrich F. Estimating rate of growth in bone lesions: observer performance and error. Radiology 1980: 134: 585–590

21. Madewell J E, Ragsdale B D, Sweet D E. Radiology and pathology analysis of solitary bone lesions. Radiol Clin North Am 1981: 19: 715–748

22. Unni K K, Dahlin D C, Beabout J W. Periosteal osteogenic sarcoma. Cancer 1976: 37: 2476–2486

23. Shapeero L G, Vanel D, Sundaram M et al. Periosteal Ewing sarcoma. Radiology 1994: 191: 825–831

24. Campanacci M, Middi P, Gherlinzoni F, Guerra A, Bertoni F, Neff J R. Parosteal osteosarcoma. J Bone Joint Surg (Br) 1984: 66: 313–321

25. Regent D, Tamisier J N, Fery A, Bernard C, Delagoutte J P, Pourel J P, Gaucher A. Intérêt du traitement de l'information dans l'exploration scanographique des lésions focales bénignes de l'os. Rev Rhum Mal Osteoartic 1986: 53: 77–82

26. Brown K T, Kattapuram S S V, Rosentahl D I. Computed tomography analysis of bone tumors: patterns of cortical destruction and soft tissue extension. Skeletal Radiol 1986: 15: 448–451

27. Hudson T M, Springfield D S, Spanier S S, Enneking W F, Hamlin D J. Benign exostoses and exostosis chondrosarcomas: evaluation of cartilage thickness by CT. Radiology 1984: 153: 595–599

28. Kenney P J, Gilula L A, Murphy W A. The use of CT to distinguish osteochondroma and chondrosarcoma. Radiology 1981: 138: 129–137

29. Malghem J, Van De Berg B, Noel H, Maldague B. Benign osteochondromas: evaluation of cartilage cap thickness by ultrasound. Skeletal Radiol 1992: 21: 33–37

30. Assoun J, Richardi G, Railhac J J et al. Osteoid osteoma: MR imaging versus CT. Radiology 1994: 191: 217–223

31. Ma L D, Frassica F J, Scott W W et al. Differentiation of benign and malignant musculoskeletal tumors: potential pitfalls with MR imaging. Radiographics 1995: 15: 349–366

32. Petterson H, Slone R M, Spanier S, Gillepsy T III, Fitzsimmons J R, Scott K N. Musculoskeletal tumors: T1 and T2 relaxation times. Radiology 1988: 167: 783–785

33. Hudson T M, Hamlin D J, Fitzsimmons J R. MRI of fluid levels in aneurysmal bone cysts and in anticoagulated human blood. Skeletal Radiol 1985: 13: 267–270

34. De Beuckeleer L H L, De Schepper A M A, Ramon F. Magnetic resonance imaging of cartilaginous tumors: is it useful or necessary? Skeletal Radiol 1996: 25: 137–141

35. Geirnaerdt M J A, Bloem J L, Eulderink F et al. Cartilaginous tumors: correlation of gadolinium-enhanced MR imaging and histopathologic findings. Radiology 1993: 186: 813–817

36. Janzen D L, Logan P M, O'Connell J X et al. MR imaging of intramedullary chondroid tumors of bone: correlation of abnormal peritumoral marrow and soft-tissue signal intensity with tumor type. Radiology 1995: 197(P): 194

37. Azouz E M, Esseltine D W, Chevalier L, Gledhill R B. Radiologic evaluation of osteosarcoma. J Can Assoc Radiol 1982: 33: 167–171

38. Hudson T M, Schieber L M, Springfield D S, Hawkins I F, Enneking W F, Spanier S S. Radiologic imaging of osteosarcoma. Role in planning surgical treatment. Skeletal Radiol 1983: 10: 137–146

39. Vanel D, Contesso G, Couanet D, Piekarski J D, Sarrazin D, Masselot J. CT in evaluation of 41 Ewing's sarcomas. Skeletal Radiol 1982: 9: 8–13

40. Lang P, Honda G, Roberts T et al. Musculoskeletal neoplasms: perineoplastic edema versus tumor on dynamic postcontrast MR images with spatial mapping of instantaneous enhancement rates. Radiology 1995: 197: 831–839

41. Schima W, Amann G, Stiglbauer R et al. Preoperative staging of osteosarcoma: efficacy of MR imaging in detecting joint involvement. AJR 1994: 163: 1171–1175

42. Vanel D, Henri-Amar M, Lumbroso J et al. Pulmonary evaluation of patients with osteosarcoma: roles of standard radiography, tomography, CT, scintigraphy and tomoscintigraphy. AJR 1984: 143: 519–523

43. Holscher H C, Bloem J L, Vanel D, Hermans J, Nooy M A, Taminiau A H M, Henry-Amar M. Osteosarcoma: chemotherapy-induced changes at MR imaging. Radiology 1992: 182: 839–844

44. Van der Woude H J, Bloem J L, Schipper J et al. Changes in tumor perfusion induced by chemotherapy in bone sarcomas: color Doppler flow imaging compared with contrast-enhanced MR imaging and three phase bone scintigraphy. Radiology 1994: 12: 687–702

45. Holscher H C, Bloem J L, Van Der Woude H J et al. Can MRI predict the histopathological response in patients with osteosarcoma after the first cycle of chemotherapy? Clin Radiol 1995: 50: 384–390

46. Holscher H C, Van Der Woude H J et al. Magnetic resonance relaxation times of normal tissue in the course of chemotherapy: a study in patients with bone sarcoma. Skeletal Radiol 1994: 23: 181–185

47. Kauffman W M, Fletcher B D, Hanna S L et al. MR imaging findings in recurrent primary osseous Ewing sarcoma. Magn Reson Imaging 1994: 12: 1147–1153

48. Van Der Woude H J, Bloem J L, Holscher H C et al. Monitoring the effect of chemotherapy in Ewing's sarcoma of bone with MR imaging. Skeletal Radiol 1994: 23: 493–500

49. Ryan S P, Weinberger E, White K S et al. M R imaging of bone marrow in children with osteosarcoma: effect of granulocyte colony-stimulating factor. AJR 1995: 165: 915–920

2

Biopsy

P. Anract   B. Tomeno

INTRODUCTION

Bone biopsy is a surgical procedure whose aim is to supply the pathologist with sufficient material, together with the clinical and radiologic data, to enable him to make as reliable a diagnosis as possible.

This procedure must be a routine preliminary to the total treatment of a tumoral lesion of the locomotor system. The absence of a biopsy before the treatment of a lesion that is tumoral in principle must be an exception duly supported by the clinical and radiologic features and by the length of experience of the clinician responsible for such a decision.[1]

While the maximum clinical, radiologic and biochemical data must be assembled to guide and plan the biopsy, this must not be delayed by arrangements for complementary investigations which can easily be made while awaiting the results of the biopsy.

INDICATIONS FOR BIOPSY

Every lesion of tumoral appearance in which the diagnosis of a frankly benign and non-progressive nature is not evident must be biopsied before definitive treatment. In practice, many malignant tumors of the locomotor system have seen their prognosis largely modified by the use of neoadjuvant chemotherapy before surgical resection.[2,3] Moreover, surgical treatment is often facilitated by the reduction in tumoral volume resulting from chemotherapy treatment.[3]

Images of tumoral appearance may be infections whose clinical background is sometimes obscure, multiple lesions without a known primary cancer and especially solitary lesions which may correspond to an infection, a dystrophy or a tumor of the locomotor system. The biopsy is intended to establish a firm diagnosis of the causal lesion: infective, dystrophic or tumoral.

If there is a tumor, the biopsy must allow definition of

the histologic type, its malignant or benign nature, the histologic grade, the possible presence of dedifferentiated zones and the performance of more specific studies by means of immunohistochemistry, ultrastructural examination, flow cytometry and identification of the karyotype if this is necessary.

In the near future, study of markers on the biopsy material may have prognostic and predictive value for the sensitivity of the tumor to chemotherapy (e.g. P glycoprotein for multidrug resistance).[4]

In some asymptomatic lesions of tumoral appearance where the diagnosis is obvious from the clinical and radiologic findings, biopsy may be dispensed with. This is the case with some fibrous dysplasias, osteochondromas and non-ossifying fibromas, which often do not require treatment and simply need surveillance.

For other tumors whose benign nature is certain, such as a chondroma of the extremities or a typical osteoid osteoma, treatment will consist of an initial excisional biopsy.[5] For obviously metastatic lesions which would benefit from osteosynthesis or prosthetic surgery, biopsy can also be performed during the definitive procedure.

In the special case of tumors that are probably benign and not cartilaginous or ossified, an immediate frozen section will confirm the benign nature and allow treatment at the same time. This is the case with benign giant cell tumors. In all other cases, biopsy must be a preliminary to the definitive treatment of the lesion.

BIOPSY TECHNIQUE

Choice of technique

The biopsy must be performed in a center specializing in the surgery of tumors of the locomotor system and preferably by the surgeon who will assume responsibility for the patient treated by resection.[1] Mankin clearly showed in 1982[6] and confirmed in a study in 1992[7] that biopsy performed by unspecialized teams is burdened with complications and diagnostic errors to an extent that may compromise conservative surgery or even the prognosis of the patient.

Once a decision to perform a biopsy has been taken, a choice must be made between an open technique or a percutaneous method (using an aspiration needle or a drill). While these two last techniques are cost effective (six times cheaper according to Skrzynski[8]) and while they can be performed without general anesthesia or even under outpatient conditions and with a lower incidence of complications, their success level of 54–84%[8–12] remains lower than that of surgical biopsy.[8]

In Skrzynski's series of 62 patients,[8] percutaneous biopsies gave 84% correct results as against 96% for open biopsies performed by the same surgeon and studied by the same pathologist. In this study, 13% of needle biopsies

yielded no pathologic tissue, in 35 of the cases the pathologist was unable to determine the benign or malignant nature of the lesion and 6% led to errors of histologic grading.

In a prospective study made by Kreicbergs,[11] based on 300 patients, fine-needle aspiration gave a positive and correct diagnosis in 84% of cases. In 8% of cases the material obtained was inadequate and in 8% the pathologist was unable to reach a conclusion even though the sample was tumoral. Most of these diagnostic difficulties concerned benign tumors and chondrosarcomas. Ewing's sarcoma never posed any diagnostic difficulties.

It seems that in the best series, with a rigorous selection of patients, the success rate of percutaneous biopsies is around 80%. Moreover, with a small amount of material, the type and histologic grade are difficult to assess[11,13] and complementary investigations (immunohistochemical, microelectronic) are sometimes impossible.

Most authors report excellent reliability of this technique for secondary tumors, lymphomas, myelomas and cases of recurrence of a previously identified tumor.[8,11] It is more reliable when performed by the surgical oncologist in overall charge of the patient, in close collaboration with the pathologist, and when it is strictly planned.[1]

To improve the yield, the biopsy should be performed after using imaging assessment, guided by CT and using a trocar system (rather than an aspiration needle) and should yield at least three fragments, one of which should be examined by frozen section to insure the presence of pathologic tissue.[8] These conditions are restrictive and seem to us difficult to apply in current practice. Ahlström and Aström[14] propose a drill system with a coaxial blade, making it possible to obtain a larger amount of tissue from different zones and facilitating perforation of the cortices.

The surgical biopsy has the advantage of greater reliability, with 96% of positive and correct results in specialized centers.[8,15] The diagnosis is more certain and the amount of tissue removed allows precise histologic diagnosis, grading and supplementary investigations (immunohistochemistry, ultrastructure). For tumors secondary to an unidentified cancer, an adequate amount of tissue may help in the search for the primary lesion. However, there are some special cases:

- tumors of the pelvis or spine where access is difficult: a needle biopsy may be attempted and if this fails it does not compromise the performance of an open biopsy[16,17]; Fig. 2.1a,b
- recurrences of a malignant tumor: a cytologic diagnosis is often sufficient;
- probable secondary tumors, hematologic tumors and Ewing's sarcomas, in which diagnosis by needle aspiration has a reliability approaching 100%.[8,11]

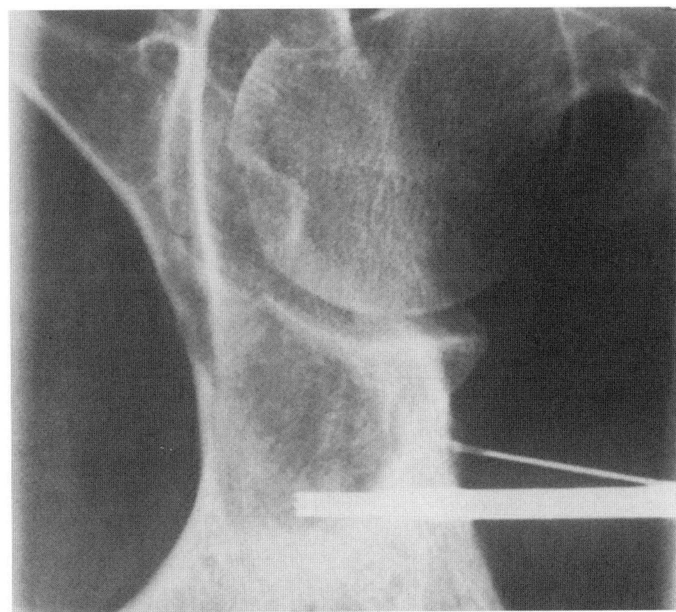

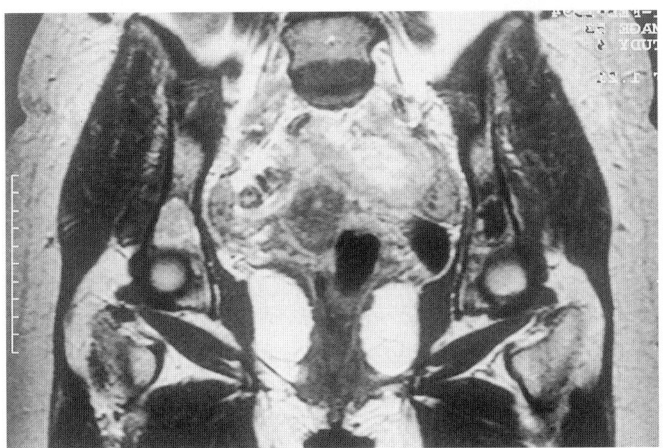

Fig. 2.1 (a) Percutaneous biopsy for tumor of the acetabulum area. The diagnosis was chondrosarcoma and a resection was performed. The final diagnosis based on the resection was dedifferentiated chondrosarcoma. The anaplastic component was missed at percutaneous biopsy. (b) MRI of the tumor.

Surgical biopsy

Preoperative planning

This is essential. The clinical examination should assess extension into the soft parts and relationship with the neurovascular axes. Assessment by radiology and by MRI should define:

- the precise site of the lesion in relation to reliable landmarks (such as joint-line, great trochanter, etc);
- any possible articular extension;
- invasion of the soft parts.

Use of a tourniquet

A tourniquet is not contraindicated and greatly facilitates

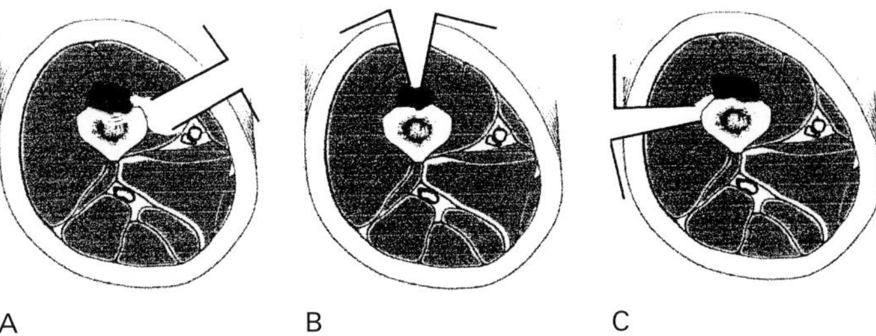

Fig. 2.2 For malignant tumors it is more appropriate to use the most direct surgical approach without exposing the neurovascular bundles. (a) The surgical approach of this femoral tumor is not adequate: the neurovascular bundles exposure constrains the surgeon to sacrifice them during the resection or to perform a contamined resection. Surgical approach of the femur (b) passing through the muscular fibers is adequate. Incision for the biopsy (c) along the same incision that will be used for surgery is the best choice. In these two cases, the scar could be removed together with the tumor and the neurovascular bundles could be preserved during the resection.

the surgical procedure. However, the limb must not be exsanguinated by a compression bandage to avoid the migration of tumoral cells into the circulation.[16,18]

Route of access

If the tumor is benign, the classic surgical approaches to the limbs are used. If there is any doubt as to the malignancy of the lesion, it is preferable to use the shortest and most direct route of approach, in the path of the future route of access for surgical resection, without aponeurotic stripping and without exposing the neurovascular bundles.[5] Indeed, the biopsy scar must be removed together with the tumor during the resection so as to prevent local recurrence (Fig. 2.2). Moreover, it is necessary to preserve and not to traverse any muscular flaps which may be used to cover major losses of substance subsequent to excisional surgery; this is the case with the muscle flap of the gluteus maximus during disarticulation of the hip.[5]

When resection of a tumor is to be undertaken it is always necessary to plan the access route to avoid compromising the performance of conservative surgery. In the multicenter study of Mankin[6,7] resectional surgery had to be modified in 20% of cases because of a complication or faulty technique during the biopsy.

Removal of the sample

This must be adequate and not fragmented. If it is a tumor of the soft parts, the removal is made with the scalpel in the shape of a 1–2 cm cube. For intraosseous tumors and if the cortex has been weakened, the removal may sometimes be made with a curette. It is often necessary to cautiously trephine the cortex using circular or ovoid orifices so as not to weaken the bone. A curette or trephine, as proposed by Akerman[19] and Tomeno[5] (Fig. 2.3a,b), will remove enough tissue if the tumor is firm.

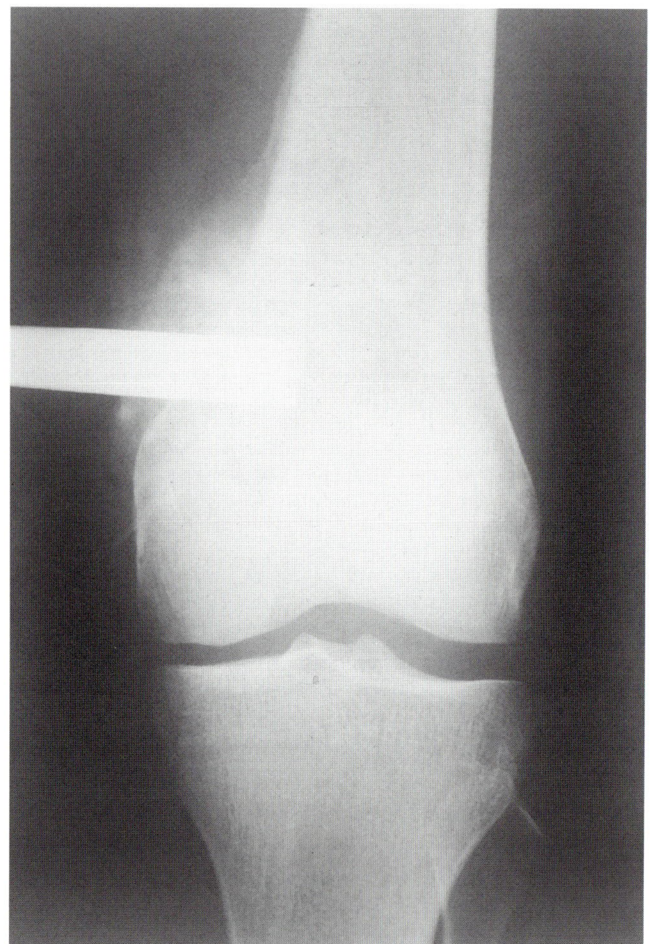

A

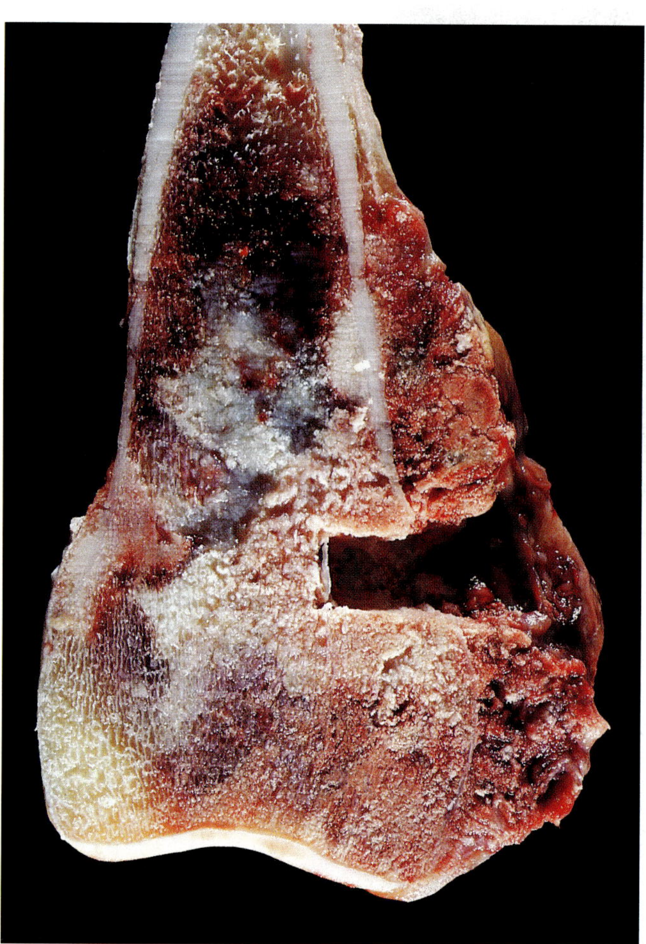

B

Fig. 2.3 (a) Trephine biopsy of osteosarcoma of distal femur. (b) Same case: resected specimen after chemotherapy, demonstrating the track of the biopsy. (Courtesy of M Forest MD.)

It is never acceptable to be satisfied with sampling a peripheral periosteal reaction to the tumor, since in most cases this is non-tumoral. It is essential to biopsy the osteolytic regions, which are the most significant zones for the pathologist (Fig. 2.4).

In case of doubt, radiologic monitoring during the procedure can confirm the correct localization of the sampling.

Ideally, an immediate frozen section of one of the biopsy fragments should be made before closure of the operation site to confirm the presence of tumoral tissue, thus allowing repetition of the sampling if necessary.

The cortical windows can be blocked with a plug of methylmethacrylate; losses of substance after biopsy of the soft parts can be filled with local hemostatic agents.

Closure must be made in layers using sutures which do not grasp the margins widely and, if drainage is needed, this should have its exit orifice close to the scar and in its long axis, since this too must be excised with the tumor in one piece. In all cases, drainage is preferable to the development of a hematoma, which is a source of tumoral dissemination.

Informing the pathologist

The pathologist is unable to make a diagnosis if he is not supplied with the clinical findings, a radiograph and a report of the operation. The clinical data must specify the age, sex and previous history and give a clinical account of the current episode. The pathologist must be supplied with the radiographs of the lesion. The operative report gives the gross findings and helps to orientate the specimen.

Handling of the sample

Ideally, the sample is sent immediately to the pathologist, without fixation and without opening or dissecting the specimen. An immediate frozen section may confirm the presence of tumoral tissue. The pathologist may then retain the unfixed fragments for ultrastructural, immunohistochemical and possibly cytogenetic study. It may be useful to make imprints.

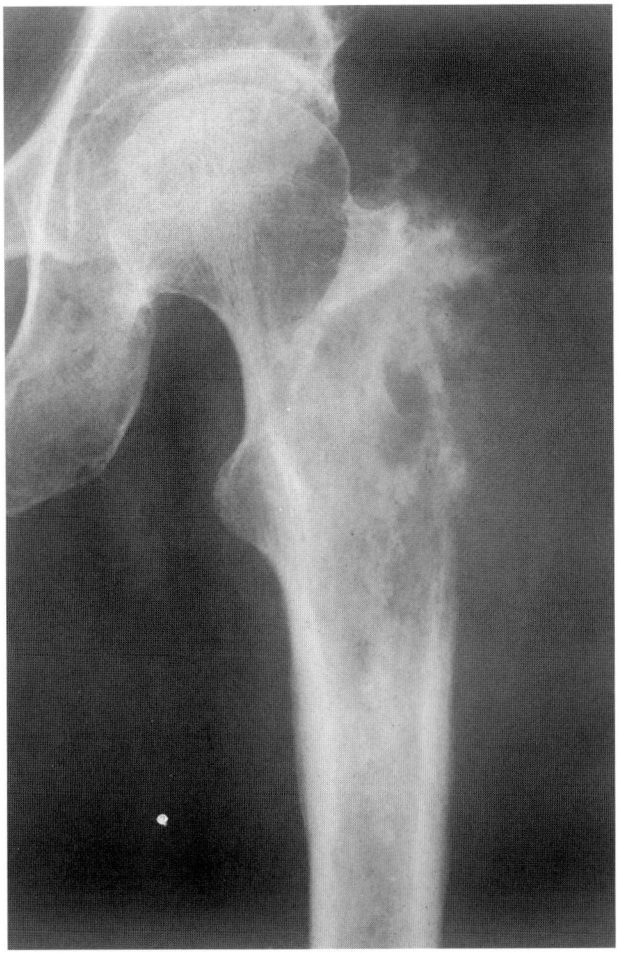

Special cases

In a case where the sample is negative or the result inconsistent with the clinical context and radiologic findings, it is preferable to repeat the biopsy rather than to miss a malignant tumor or to treat a benign tumor in an unnecessarily aggressive manner.

An illustrative case, often encountered, is that of a request for an opinion on a tumoral pathology in a patient cared for in another department and posing a diagnostic problem. A glance at the sections or a simple viewing of the radiographs is quite unsatisfactory. In such cases it is essential to review the entire clinical history from the beginning and to have available all the complementary investigations and sections before the pathologist can give a useful opinion.

CONCLUSION

The biopsy of a lesion of tumoral appearance of the locomotor system is a surgical procedure which must be conducted in a specialized department. The biopsy forms an integral part of the treatment of a tumor and must be scrupulously planned, with an eye to any possible subsequent treatment. The biopsy can be made by a percutaneous route or as an open procedure; this latter technique is still more reliable for primary tumors of the locomotor system.

Finally, it should be borne in mind that the diagnosis of a tumor is based on a synthesis of the clinical, radiologic and pathologic findings, calling for close collaboration between the surgeon, radiologist and pathologist.

Fig. 2.4 X-ray of a dedifferentiated chondrosarcoma of proximal femur. The calcified regions correspond to the chondrosarcomatous component and the zones of osteolysis to the anaplastic component. It is essential to biopsy both zones to obtain a correct and complete diagnosis.

REFERENCES

1. Springfield D S, Rosenberg A. Editorial. Biopsy: complicated and risky. J Bone Joint Surg (Am) 1996: 78: 639–643
2. Rosen G, Marcove R C, Caparros B, Nirenberg A, Kosloff C, Huvos A G. Primary osteogenic sarcoma. The rationale for preoperative chemotherapy and delayed surgery. Cancer 1979: 43: 2163–2177
3. Jaffe N. Chemotherapy for malignant bone tumors. Orthop Clin North Am 1989: 20: 487–503
4. Wunder J S, Bell R S, Wold L, Andrulis I L. Expression of the multidrug resistance genes in osteosarcoma: a pilot study. J Orthop Res 1993: 11: 396–403
5. Tomeno B. La biopsie dans les tumeurs des os. Chirurgie 1982: 108: 353–355
6. Mankin H J, Lange T A, Spanier S S. The hazards of biopsy in patients with malignant primary bone and soft tissue tumors. J Bone Joint Surg (Am) 1982: 64: 1121–1127
7. Mankin H J, Mankin C J, Simon M A. The hazards of the biopsy, revisited. J Bone Joint Surg (Am) 1996: 78: 656–663
8. Skrynski M C, Biermann J S, Montag A, Simon M A. Diagnostic accuracy and charge-savings of outpatient core needle biopsy compared with open biopsy of musculoskeletal tumors. J Bone Joint Surg (Am) 1996: 78: 644–649
9. De Santos L A, Murray J A, Ayala A G. The value of percutaneous needle biopsy in the management of primary bone tumors. Cancer 1979: 43: 735–744
10. El Khoury G Y, Terepka R H, Mickelson M R, Rainville K L, Zaleski C T. Fine needle aspiration biopsy of bone. J Bone Joint Surg (Am) 1983: 64: 522–525
11. Kreicbergs A, Bauer H C, Brosjö O, Lindholm J, Skoog L, Söderlund V. Cytological diagnosis of bone tumours. J Bone Joint Surg (Br) 1996: 78: 258–263
12. Moore T M, Meyers M H, Patzakis M J, Terry R, Harvey J P. Closed biopsy of musculoskeletal lesions. J Bone Joint Surg (Am) 1979: 61: 375–380
13. Walaas L, Kindblom L G. Fine-needle aspiration biopsy in preoperative diagnosis of chordoma: a study of 17 cases with application of electron microscopic, histochemical and immunocytochemical examination. Hum Pathol 1991: 22: 22–28
14. Alhström K H, Aström K G. CT guided biopsy performed by means of coaxial biopsy system with an eccentric drill. Radiology 1993: 188: 549–552
15. Bröstrom L A, Harris M A, Simon M A, Cooperman D R, Nilsonne U. The effect of biopsy on survival of patients with osteosarcoma. J Bone Joint Surg (Br) 1979: 61: 209–212
16. Stoker D J, Kissin C M. Percutaneous vertebral biopsy: a review of 135 cases. Clin Radiol 1985: 36: 569–577

17. Roy Camille R, Saillant G, Mamoudy P, Leonard P. Biopsie du corps vertébral par voie postérieure transpédiculaire. Rev Chir Orthop 1983: 69: 147–149

18. Engell H C. Cancer cells in the blood. A five to nine year follow up study. Ann Surg 1959: 149: 457–461

19. Ackerman W. Application of the trephine for bone biopsy. JAMA 1963: 184: 133–139

3

Flow cytometry

P. Vielh

INTRODUCTION

Flow cytometry is a technique offering a rapid, reproducible and quantitative measurement of a large number of physical and fluorescence-associated parameters.

Pioneering works are those of Moldavan[1] who developed an apparatus in which red blood cells in suspension were forced through a capillary on a microscope stage, the passage of each cell being registered by a photodetector attached to the microscope eyepiece. Crosland-Taylor[2] introduced the principle of laminar flow for flow cytometry, named hydrodynamic focusing, and showed that a suspension of red blood cells injected slowly in the center of a faster flowing stream permitted focusing of the cells within the core of the wider stream. Coulter[3] also showed that the electric conductance of the fluid stream containing the cells was locally modified proportionally to the volume of each cell and could be used to identify it and to measure its volume.

Finally, the use of fluorescence was introduced by Kamentsky[4] and was applied to the so-called orthogonal flow systems by Van Dilla[5]; the development of these latter flow cytometers allowed the construction of the first fluidic systems to sort selected cells according to the principle first described by Fulwyler.[6]

Further developments of flow cytometry included the blending of physics, optics, electronics and computer science.

Today, the availability of numerous monoclonal antibodies, the synthesis of a large number of fluorochromes excited by a single wavelength, the stabilization and optimization of the optical and mechanical parts of the flow systems and their high degree of automation allow the use of flow cytometers as user-friendly tools for routine clinical applications such as immunophenotyping of cell surface markers and quantitation of DNA content and cell proliferation.

PRINCIPLES OF FLOW CYTOMETRY

The principle of flow cytometry is based on the analysis of parameters on a cell-by-cell basis performed on a monodispersed suspension of cells (Fig. 3.1). A single-file flow of cells is passed through a sensing region where optical and electrical signals are generated and measured. This flow is generated by introducing the monodispersed suspension of cells through a narrow tube immersed in a flowing sheath of fluid (Fig. 3.1) whose hydrodynamic properties generate a laminar flow and reduce the diameter of the stream to the size of the cells to be analyzed.

Except for volume, the measurement of cell parameters requires illumination by a light source (Fig. 3.1) which more generally consists of a laser since, in contrast to an arc lamp which provides a continuous spectrum of excitation wavelengths, it delivers a highly stable, coherent, plane polarized, intense and monochromatic beam of light.

Generally, cells to be analyzed are prelabeled with one or more fluorescent dyes depending on the parameter(s) studied, i.e. cellular antigens and/or DNA content. Cellular antigens may be studied by direct or indirect fluorescent methods using specific antibodies generated against membrane, intracytoplasmic or nuclear antigens.

The fluorochromes most commonly linked to antibodies are fluorescein isothiocyanate, phycoerythrin, Texas red and allophycocyanin. DNA content analysis requires the use of intercalating or non-intercalating fluorochromes. Intercalating fluorochromes such as propidium iodide and ethidium bromide form complexes with double-stranded DNA, whereas non-intercalating fluorochromes are specific for regions of the DNA rich in either adenine and thymine or guanine and cytosine; examples of non-intercalating fluorochromes specific for the adenine and thymine regions are diamidinophenylindole and the different Hoechsts.

Light focused on to the stream physically interacts with each cell and excites the fluorochrome with which the cell has been stained, leading to light scattering and fluorescence respectively (Fig. 3.1).

The intensity and the spatial distribution of the scattered light is related to the size, shape and electric properties of the cells analyzed. Light scattering can be measured at small (forward) angle for cell size estimation and/or at wide (right or orthogonal) angle for cell asymmetry, cell surface roughness and internal granular structure of the cell.

Excitation by the incident light beam consists of the absorption of photons of given wavelengths; this excitation is followed by the isotropic emission of photons of lower energy and higher wavelengths, namely fluorescence. Since the fluorescent light is much less intense than the incident light, the detection system consists of properly selected dichroic filters and sensitive photomultiplier tubes. Each photomultiplier tube converts light into electrical signals which are analog impulses with varying intensities and durations. These signals are electronically amplified (Fig. 3.1) by linear or logarithmic amplifiers and digitized by an analog-to-digital converter. The digital signals are then processed by the computer (Fig. 3.1) using powerful software programs in order to display interpretable and relevant condensed information in the form of parameter lists, cytograms or histograms.

ANALYSIS OF DNA CONTENT AND CELL PROLIFERATION

The DNA content of any quiescent normal human cell is a constant and is characterized by 23 pairs of chromosomes. Cells leave the quiescent state to undergo a series of sequential steps, named the cell cycle. Based on total DNA content, the cell cycle can be divided into three

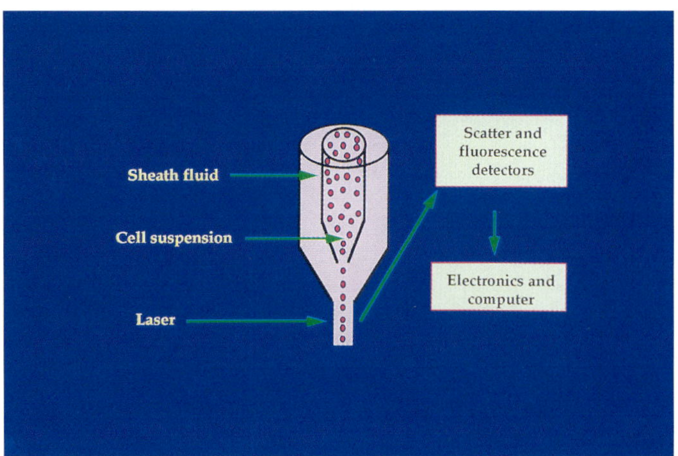

Fig. 3.1 Schematic representation of a flow cytometer.

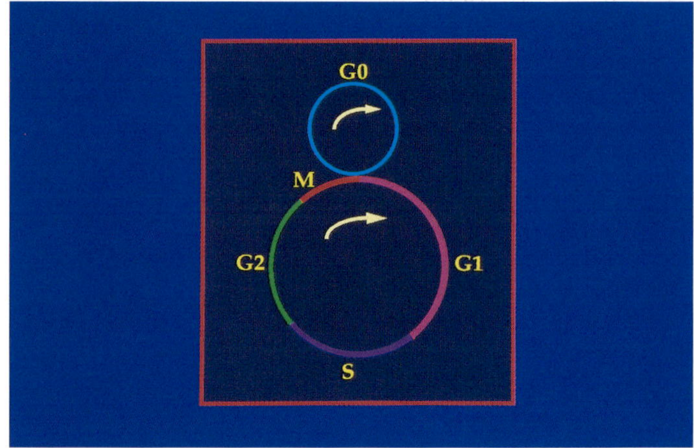

Fig. 3.2 The components of the cell cycle.

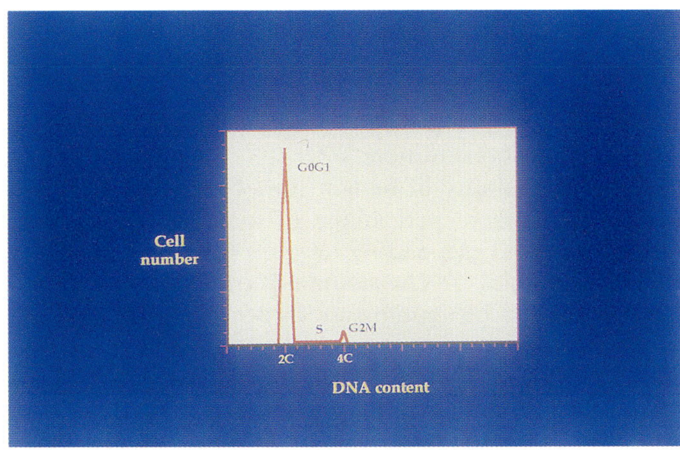

Fig. 3.3 The flow cytometric histogram represents cell number versus fluorescence DNA content of a DNA-diploid cell population.

components (Fig. 3.2): cells in G0 (gap 0 or quiescent phase) and G1 (gap 1) phase have a 2C DNA content which corresponds to two haploid (2 × 23) sets of chromosomes; cells in G2 (gap 2) and M (mitosis) phase have a 4C DNA content which corresponds to four haploid (4 × 23) sets of chromosomes; and cells in S (synthesis) phase have a DNA content of any value between 2C and 4C corresponding to the asynchronous duplication of DNA of heterogeneous cell populations. A typical corresponding flow cytometric histogram of DNA content is illustrated in Figure 3.3.

By contrast with normal tissues, malignant cells are characterized by genetic instability leading to chromosomal abnormalities. These chromosome aberrations are qualitative (translocations, inversions) or quantitative (deletions, losses, duplications). The latter may alter the total DNA content and flow cytometry is therefore a straightforward technique for detecting the presence of cells with abnormal DNA content.

While ploidy refers to the number of chromosomes seen at metaphases in a karyotype, DNA ploidy represents measurement of total DNA content by cytometry but not its organization or disorganization. DNA ploidy of a cell is proportional to the fluorescence intensity of specific dyes which have a stoichiometric interaction with DNA and is expressed by its DNA index. DNA index is the ratio of the mode of the relative DNA content of the G0G1 cells of the sample divided by the mode of the relative measurements of the DNA-diploid G0G1 reference cells. Therefore, by definition, DNA index of a DNA-diploid cell population is 1.0, whereas DNA index of a DNA-aneuploid cell population is different from 1.0; for example, DNA index of a DNA-triploid or DNA-tetraploid tumor is 1.5 or 2.0, respectively. A tumor with more than one DNA-aneuploid peak is defined as DNA multiploid and has at least two DNA indices.

Some problems may be encountered in the interpretation of DNA histograms. The first is that differences in quantitative fluorescence intensity between normal and malignant cells of equivalent DNA content may be observed. Indeed, DNA conformation is often critical for the interaction of the fluorescent dye and a staining procedure adapted for a given tumor type is not always applicable to another type of lesion.

The second problem arises when the coefficient of variation, which is the ratio of the width at midheight to the height of the peak, is too broad. A wide coefficient of variation may result from poor alignment of the flow cytometer, from partially degraded material or from malignant cells because of their inherent genetic variability. Therefore a single peak with a broad coefficient of variation or an asymmetry of G0G1 peak may mask a malignant DNA near-diploid cell population. The third problem is the detection of a true DNA-tetraploid stemline in the presence of a DNA-diploid cell population. Beside the fact that normal cells contain double the normal amount of DNA during the G2 phase of their cycle, a peak at twice the normal diploid amount of DNA may result from clumping of nuclei. This may be eliminated by seeking the presence of other peaks at the hexaploid position resulting from aggregation of three nuclei and by using software including doublet discrimination and pulse processing.

This emphasizes the necessity for permanent quality control as recommended by the guidelines proposed at the 1993 DNA Cytometry Consensus Conference for the implementation of clinical DNA cytometry.[7]

Cell cycle analysis also includes measurement of S-phase fraction. The presence of cellular debris often leads to a background signal which has to be subtracted exponentially. After background correction, appropriate algorithms must be applied to the DNA histograms to derive the percentage of cells in S phase. Mathematical procedures for approximating the S-phase fraction include the so-called peak reflect method,[8] consisting of subtraction of twice the left portion of the G0G1 peak and twice the right portion of the G2 M peak, as well as more sophisticated models using a polynomial equation[9] or a series of broadened gaussian distributions[10] and the rectangular approximation method[11] with its variant named the trapezoidal procedure[12] in which the S-phase fraction is approximated by a trapezoid truncated at the G0G1 and G2 M means.

S-phase fraction measurement can be obscured by a high background composed of cellular debris. It may also be overestimated by the contribution of a large number of normal cycling cells such as lymphocytes or by the presence of doublets due to nuclear clumping. Lymphocytes will be discriminated and gated using the leukocyte common antigen, whereas doublets can be efficiently excluded by pulse processing analyzing the duration of the fluorescence pulse which is longer for doublets than for single nuclei.

Finally, the overlapping of peaks in DNA-multiploid tumors often precludes an accurate calculation of the S-phase fraction. In such cases, tumor cell proliferation can be measured by flow cytometry after incorporation of 5-bromodeoxyuridine, an analog of thymidine, by using specific monoclonal antibodies.[13]

PROCEDURES AND APPLICATIONS

A monodispersed suspension of cells is mandatory for flow cytometric analysis. Such a suspension is not hard to obtain with cells that normally lack intercellular junctions, such as red blood cells or lymphocytes from nodes, but is difficult to prepare from benign or malignant solid tumors.

Preparation of cells from fresh or frozen tissue usually requires mechanical disaggregation and/or enzymatic digestion. Mechanical disaggregation may consist of scraping cells from a piece of tissue or mincing it with razor blades followed by fine-needle syringing of the suspension which is then filtered through nylon mesh.

Enzymatic methods employ enzymes such as trypsin, pepsin, pronase and hyaluronidase in order to degrade selective components of the connective tissue and the final separation of nuclei from other cellular components may be achieved by the use of non-ionic detergents.

A very convenient method, including procedures for long-term storage of fresh or frozen samples, preparation and staining of nuclei using a detergent-trypsin protocol and propidium iodide, as well as standardization of the results, has been described by Vindelöv.[14–16] By contrast, Hedley[17,18] first published a technique for preparation and staining of formalin-fixed, paraffin-embedded archival material. Briefly, thick (30–60 μm) sections are prepared from paraffin blocks, dewaxed in xylene, rehydrated in decreasing concentrations of ethanol and soaked in distilled water. Cells and bare nuclei are isolated by treatment

with 0.5% pepsin at pH 1.5 and stained with a DNA-specific dye after neutralization, washing and treatment with RNase.

Few works concern flow cytometric analysis of DNA in miscellaneous bone tumors.[19–22]

The vast majority of benign tumors are DNA diploid, whereas a variable percentage of malignant tumors are DNA aneuploid, depending on their histology. Examples of DNA-diploid, DNA-aneuploid and DNA-multiploid flow cytometric histograms are shown in Figures 3.4, 3.5 and 3.6 respectively. Osteosarcomas[23–25] and chondrosarcomas[26–28] are predominantly DNA aneuploid, while Ewing's sarcomas,[29] as well as chordomas[30,31] and adamantinomas,[32] are more frequently DNA diploid.

It is also interesting to note that DNA aneuploidy has

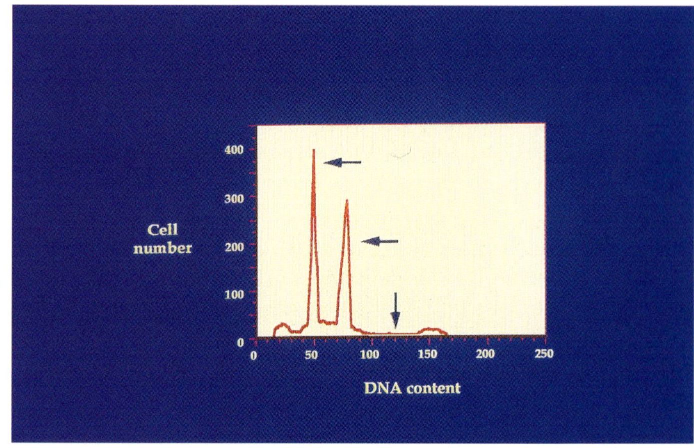

Fig. 3.5 DNA-aneuploid osteosarcoma. DNA index = 1.56 (lower horizontal arrow). S-phase fraction = 10% (vertical arrow). The upper horizontal arrow corresponds to the DNA-diploid peak.

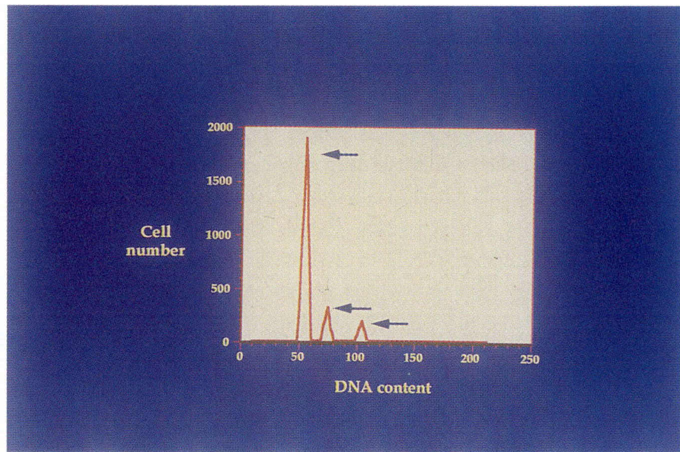

Fig. 3.6 DNA-multiploid chondrosarcoma. The first horizontal arrow corresponds to the DNA-diploid peak. The two other horizontal arrows define two peaks with DNA indices = 1.39 (DNA-hyperdiploid) and 2.02 (DNA-tetraploid). The overlap of the different peaks precludes the calculation of S-phase fraction.

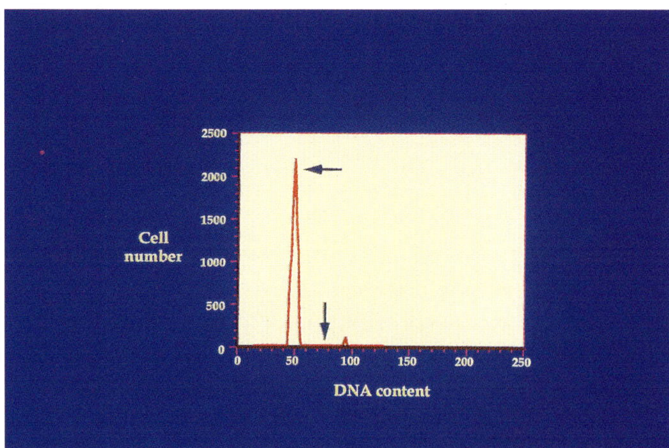

Fig. 3.4 DNA-diploid giant cell tumor. DNA index = 1 (horizontal arrow). S-phase fraction = 2.3% (vertical arrow).

been associated with a shorter overall survival in osteo-sarcomas,[24] chondrosarcomas[28] and Ewing's sarcomas.[29] However, these series are retrospective studies performed on paraffin-embedded blocks. Therefore, long-term prospective studies with larger series of patients are now needed to confirm these interesting results and to ascertain the clinical value of flow cytometric analysis of bone tumors.

REFERENCES

1. Moldavan A. Photo-electric technique for the counting of microscopical cells. Science 1934: 80: 188–189
2. Crosland-Taylor P J. A device for counting small particles suspended in a fluid through a tube. Nature 1953: 171: 37–38
3. Coulter W H. High speed automatic blood cell counter and cell size analyzer. Proc Natl Electronics Conf 1956: 12: 1034–1042
4. Kamentsky L A, Melamed M R, Derman H. Spectrophotometer: new instrument for ultrarapid cell analysis. Science 1965: 150: 630–631
5. Van Dilla M A, Trujillo T T, Mullaney P F, Coulter J R. Cell microfluorimetry: a method for rapid fluorescence measurement. Science 1969: 163: 1213–1214
6. Fulwyler M J. Electronic separation of biological cells by volume. Science 1965: 150: 910–911
7. Shankey T V, Rabinovitch P S, Bagwell B et al. Guidelines for the implementation of clinical DNA cytometry. Cytometry 1993: 28: 61–68
8. Barlogie B, Spitzer G, Hart J et al. DNA-histogram of human hematopoietic cells. Blood 1976: 48: 245–258
9. Dean P, Jett J. Mathematical analysis of DNA distributions derived from flow microfluorometry. J Cell Biol 1974: 60: 523–527
10. Fried J. Method for the quantitative evaluation of data from flow microfluorometry. Comp Biomed Res 1976: 9: 263–276
11. Baisch H, Gohde W, Linden W. Analysis of PCP-data to determine the fraction of cells in the various phases of the cell cycle. Radiat Environ Biophys 1975: 12: 31–39
12. Baisch H, Beck H, Christensen I et al. A comparison of mathematical models for the analysis of DNA histograms by flow cytometry. Cell Tissue Kinet 1982: 15: 235–249
13. Gratzner H G. Monoclonal antibodies to 5-bromo and 5-iododeoxyuridine: a new reagent for detection of DNA replication. Science 1982: 218: 474–475
14. Vindelöv L L, Christensen I J, Keiding N, Spang-Thomsen M, Nissen N I. Long-term storage of samples for flow cytometric DNA analysis. Cytometry 1983: 3: 317–322
15. Vindelöv L L, Christensen I J, Nissen N I. A detergent-trypsin method for the preparation of nuclei for flow cytometric DNA analysis. Cytometry 1983: 3: 323–327
16. Vindelöv L L, Christensen I J, Nissen N I. Standardization of high-resolution flow cytometric DNA analysis by the simultaneous use of chicken and trout red blood cells as internal reference cells. Cytometry 1983: 3: 328–331
17. Hedley D W, Friedlander M L, Taylor I W, Rugg C A, Musgrove E A. Method for analysis of cellular DNA content of paraffin-embedded pathological material using flow cytometry. J Histochem Cytochem 1983: 31: 1333–1335
18. Hedley D W. Flow cytometry using paraffin-embedded tissue: five years on. Cytometry 1989: 10: 229–241
19. Kreicbergs A, Silfverswärd C, Tribukait B. Flow DNA analysis of primary bone tumors. Relationship between cellular DNA content and histopathologic classification. Cancer 1984: 53: 129–136
20. Heliö H, Karaharju E, Nordling S. Flow cytometric determination of DNA content in malignant and benign bone tumors. Cytometry 1985: 6: 165–171
21. Mankin H J, Connor J F, Schiller A L, Perlmutter N, Alho A, McGuire M. Grading of bone tumors by analysis of nuclear DNA content using flow cytometry. J Bone Joint Surg (Am) 1985: 67: 404–413
22. Xiang J, Spanier S S, Benson N A, Braylan R C. Flow cytometric analysis of DNA in bone and soft-tissue tumors using nuclear suspensions. Cancer 1987: 59: 1951–1958
23. Hiddeman W, Roessner A, Wörman B et al. Tumor heterogeneity in osteosarcoma as identified by flow cytometry. Cancer 1987: 59: 324–328
24. Bauer H C F, Kreicbergs A, Silfverswärd C, Tribukait B. DNA analysis in the differential diagnosis of osteosarcoma. Cancer 1988: 61: 2532–2540
25. Look A T, Douglass E C, Meyer W H. Clinical importance of near-diploid stemlines in patients with osteosarcoma of an extremity. N Engl J Med 1988: 318: 1567–1572
26. Alho A, Connor J F, Mankin H J, Schiller A L, Campbell C J. Assessment of malignancy of cartilage tumors using flow cytometry. J Bone Joint Surg (Am) 1983: 65: 779–785
27. Coughlan B, Feliz A, Ishida T, Czerniak B, Dorfman H D. p53 expression and DNA ploidy of cartilage lesions. Hum Pathol 1995: 26: 620–624
28. Adler C P, Herget G W, Neuburger M. Cartilaginous tumors. Prognostic applications of cytophotometric DNA analysis. Cancer 1995: 76: 1176–1180
29. Dierick A M, Langlois M, Van Oostveldt P, Roels H. The prognostic significance of the DNA content in Ewing's sarcoma: a retrospective cytophotometric and flow cytometric study. Histopathology 1993: 23: 333–339
30. Hruban R H, Traganos F, Reuter V E, Huvos A G. Chordomas with malignant spindle cell components. A DNA flow cytometric and immunohistochemical study with histogenetic implications. Am J Pathol 1990: 137: 435–447
31. Naka T, Fukuda T, Chuman H et al. Proliferative activities in conventional chordoma: a clinicopathologic, DNA flow cytometric, and immunohistochemical analysis of 17 specimens with special reference to anaplastic chordoma showing a diffuse proliferation and nuclear atypia. Hum Pathol 1996: 27: 381–388
32. Hazelbag H M, Fleuren G J, Cornelisse C J, Van Den Broek L J C M, Taminiau A H M, Hogendoorn P C W. DNA aberrations in the epithelial cell component of adamantinoma of long bones. Am J Pathol 1995: 147: 1770–1779

4

Cytogenetics

J. Couturier

It has been known for a number of years that cancer cells show chromosome aberrations. However, it is only in the last decade that cytogenetics has made a significant and often decisive contribution to the diagnosis (and sometimes to the prognosis) of certain solid tumors, particularly in sarcomas (for review, see[1] and Sandberg & Bridge 1995).

This has been made possible by progress in tumor cell culture and in karyotype analysis, which has improved the reliability and power of cytogenetic studies. Specific chromosome changes have been identified in more than 20 tumor types. These characteristic rearrangements can not only aid the diagnosis in tumors of confusing origin, but also the classification of neoplasia[1,2] (Sandberg & Bridge 1995). Specific chromosome changes can actually allow the recognition of tumor subtypes within a given histologic type (in lipoma, for example) or establish a connection between tumors of diverse histological type (as between Ewing's sarcoma and peripheral neuroectodermal tumors (Sandberg & Bridge 1995).[1]

Lastly, identification of chromosome rearrangements directs molecular approaches toward the search for genes involved in tumor pathogenicity.[3] These studies have led to the discovery of characteristic fusion genes in a number of tumor types. The identification of specific chimeric RNAs provides the possibility of detection of tumor cells by polymerase chain reaction (PCR) and enables a reliable diagnosis to be made from very small samples. Recently, new approaches to the detection of chromosome changes, based on in situ hybridization, have been developed.[4,5]

These techniques, which have led to the development of a 'molecular cytogenetics', are of interest to the pathologist because they help to fill the gap between molecular biology and morphology.

In this chapter, we shall examine bone and soft tissue tumors in which cytogenetic analysis can be of help for the pathologist.

CHROMOSOME REARRANGEMENTS IN TUMORS

Chromosome abnormalities observed in tumors are usually clonal: all tumor cells possess the same rearrangement. Surprisingly, even certain benign tumors such as lipoma, show clonal and recurrent chromosomal changes.

A tumor often exhibits several, sometimes many, rearrangements. A hierarchy exists among these changes. First, there is an initial rearrangement of high specificity. Then, the tumor cell accumulates additional abnormalities, of lower specificity but generally not random. Furthermore, in the course of tumor progression, a doubling of the chromosome set, leading to a tetraploidy, may occur. All these secondary events help to determine the degree of genetic evolution of the tumor. In certain tumor types, for example in osteosarcomas, changes observed at the time of diagnosis are already so complex that the recognition of an initial rearrangement is impossible.

Several types of rearrangement are observed in solid tumors: the most frequent are translocations, inversions, deletions and amplifications.

Translocations are exchanges of chromosome segments between non-homologous chromosomes. Inversions are intrachromosomal rearrangements. These karyotypic abnormalities are described according to an international nomenclature.[6] For example, translocations are designated by the letter t, followed by the numbers of both chromosomes involved, then by the numbers identifying bands in which the breakpoints occur, preceded by p for the short arm and q for the long arm. The translocation of Ewing's sarcoma is thus expressed as: t(11;22)(q24;q12).

Translocations and inversions may cause breaks within genes located at the breakpoints, forming a fusion gene.[3] The genes involved often encode transcription factors and fusion gene products may have oncogenic effects, leading to deregulation of cell proliferation.

Deletions of chromosome segments result in loss of tumor suppressor genes. Amplifications of chromosome regions, which often lead to the duplication of genes involved in cell proliferation, can take the form of homogeneously staining regions (hsr) or double-minute chromosomes.

COLLECTION OF SAMPLES FOR CYTOGENETIC ANALYSIS

The essential condition for the success of cytogenetic analysis is good viability of tumor cells. Thus, tumor samples should be obtained and placed in culture medium as soon as possible after surgical excision. A tumor fragment, about $0.5-1$ cm^3, should be taken as aseptically as possible in a non-necrotic area and placed in containers filled with culture medium. Media maintaining stable pH, such as L15 or HEPES-buffered media, are recommended.

Tumor specimens should be taken immediately to the cytogenetic lab, at room temperature. If necessary, it is possible to keep the sample in culture medium overnight at room temperature.

CYTOGENETIC METHODOLOGIES

Karyotypic analysis

This is the conventional cytogenetic approach. Tumor samples are mechanically or enzymatically disaggregated and processed with colchicine incubation, hypotonic treatment and fixation, either immediately or after a variable culture time. This depends on the tumor type under study. Metaphase chromosomes are analyzed, after banding techniques, by microscope examination.

Karyotypic analysis provides a precise identification (if the karyotype is not too complex) of all numerical and structural abnormalities present in the tumor. A knowledge of the expected rearrangement is theoretically not required. It is by this method that all known specific rearrangements of solid tumors have been identified and it remains the routine technique in tumor cytogenetics.

Limitations of this approach are related to the fact that it is a time-consuming technique, not easily standardizable and requiring highly specialized personnel. In addition, certain types of tumors show a relatively low mitotic index and do not proliferate in culture. Furthermore, karyotypes observed in solid tumors may be very complex, preventing a complete identification of the rearrangements. These limitations have prompted great interest in in-situ hybridization techniques.

Fluorescent in situ hybridization (FISH)

This technique allows the detection of specific DNA sequences of known chromosome localization (probe) on tumor nuclei or metaphases.[4] Briefly, the probe, chosen to correspond with the chromosome regions expected to be rearranged in the tumor studied, is labeled, generally with biotin or digoxygenin, and hybridized to nuclei and metaphase preparations. The probe binds to the corresponding region of the DNA in nuclei or chromosomes. The labeled hybrids are recognized by fluorescent immunodetection and appear as spots in the nuclei or on chromosomes.

Various types of probes can be used according to the suspected diagnosis. Alphoid probes recognize the centromere of specific chromosomes (Fig. 4.1), enabling detection of numerical abnormalities in interphase nuclei. Double hybridization and detection of double color in cosmid probes located on both sides of the breakpoint make it possible to recognize translocations in nuclei or metaphases (Fig. 4.2). Translocations can also be recognized on metaphases using double hybridization with chromosome

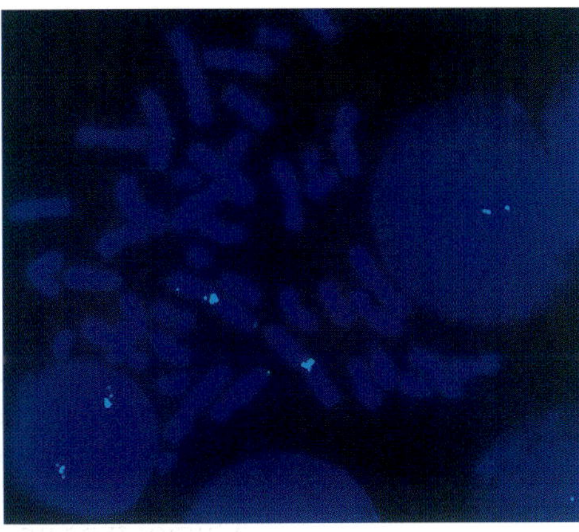

Fig. 4.1 Fluorescent in situ hybridization (FISH) of an alpha satellite probe specific for chromosome 1, on a preparation of normal metaphases and nuclei. The probe recognizes the centromeric region of chromosome 1. Spots corresponding to the two copies of chromosome 1 are also visible in interphase nuclei.

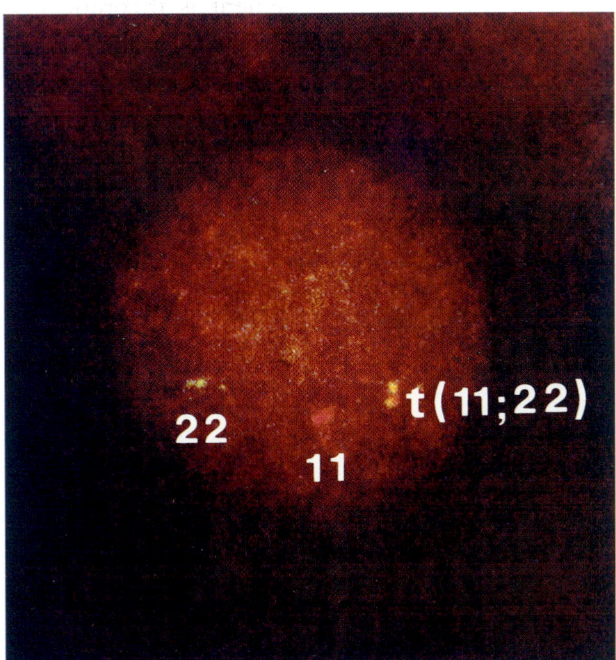

Fig. 4.2 Detection of translocation t(11;22) by FISH on interphase nucleus in Ewing's sarcoma. The preparation has been cohybridized with two cosmid probes corresponding to gene FLI1, located on chromosome 11 (red signal), and to gene EWS, on chromosome 22 (green signal). Signals of both probes are fused on the translocated element. (Courtesy of A. Aurias MD.)

'painting' probes specific for both chromosomes involved in the rearrangement. These 'painting' probes recognize whole chromosomes, so their interphasic domain is too large and ill defined for use on nuclei.

FISH is a very sensitive technique which has the advantage, using suitable probes, of being applicable to interphase nuclei, thus allowing the study of tumors lacking analyzable mitoses with conventional cytogenetic technique. In pathology, it is also applicable on paraffin-embedded tissue sections, although with some difficulties related to the effectiveness of hybridization and to the sectioning of nuclei. A limitation of the technique is that it requires information about the putative chromosome regions involved for the selection of appropriate probes.

Comparative genomic hybridization (CGH)

This particular technique of FISH is the most recently developed approach.[4–7] It allows an overview of quantitative abnormalities, gains and losses, of chromosome segments in a tumor. Roughly, tumor DNA plays the role of the probe. It is labeled with a green fluorochrome and mixed with normal DNA labeled with a red one and hybridized to normal metaphase preparations.

Green and red labeled DNAs hybridize competitively to the metaphases and the green-to-red fluorescence ratio along the chromosomes reflects the over- or under-representation of defined chromosome regions in the tumor. The fluorescent image is captured, digitized and processed. Amplified or duplicated regions appear with a relative excess of green fluorescence, whereas deleted regions show an excess of red. With the aid of adapted software, ratio profiles can be obtained for each chromosome pair.

As a conventional cytogenetic technique, CGH has the advantage of exploring the whole chromosome material of the tumor, but without requiring the presence of mitoses. However, it has several limitations. It yields information on imbalanced changes, gains and losses, only. Ploidy abnormalities and structural rearrangements, such as translocations, which often are of diagnostic value, escape the method. Moreover, its sensitivity is seriously hampered by contamination of tumor with normal cells (stroma and inflammatory cells).

In spite of these shortcomings, CGH may be a useful tool for screening a high number of tumors to identify gains and losses of chromosome segments which could be associated with tumor progression and have prognostic implications.

CHARACTERISTIC CHROMOSOME ABNORMALITIES IN BONE AND SOFT TISSUE TUMORS

We discuss below the tumor types for which the chromosome rearrangements are specific or consistent enough to be of diagnostic relevance for the pathologist. Characteristic translocations are reported in Table 4.1.

Lipoma

These benign tumors may present clonal chromosome abnormalities, especially involving chromosome 12

Table 4.1 Characteristic translocations and gene fusions in bone and soft tissue tumors

Tumor type	Translocation	Fusion gene	References
Liposarcoma	t(12;16)(q13;p11)	CHOP/FUS-TLS	8
Ewing's sarcoma	t(11;22)(q24;q12)	FLI1/EWS	15
" "	t(21;22)(q22;q12)	ERG/EWS	16
" "	t(7;22)(p22;q12)	ETV1/EWS	17
Melanoma of soft parts	t(12;22)(q13;q12)	ATF-1/EWS	18
Myxoid chondrosarcoma	t(9;22)(q22;q12)	TEC/EWS	19
Synovial sarcoma	t(X;18)(p11.2;q11.2)	SSX/SYT	22

(Sandberg & Bridge 1995),[1] but surprisingly, they form a cytogenetically heterogeneous group. Rearrangements of 12q13–15 are seen in 55% of tumors with a clonal abnormality. They are due to translocations with 3q27–28, 1p32–34, 2p21–23, 21q21–q22 and other less frequent chromosome bands. Other cytogenetic types of tumor lack translocations of chromosome 12 and show rearrangements of 6p21–23 or rearrangement or loss of 13q14. Future molecular studies will certainly shed light on the genetic process underlying the cellular proliferation in this group of tumors.

Liposarcoma

Among the various histological types, the myxoid liposarcoma is cytogenetically the best characterized. A t(12;16)(q13;p11) is consistently found in this tumor (Sandberg & Bridge 1995),[1] as the sole abnormality or associated with a trisomy 8 as a non-random additional abnormality (Fig. 4.3). The molecular breakpoint in chromosome 12 is different from that of lipoma. It involves the transcription factor gene CHOP. This gene is rearranged with the gene TLS/FUS, located on chromosome 16[3,8] (Table 4.1), which has similarities with the EWS gene involved in Ewing's sarcoma. The translocation results in a TLS/FUS-CHOP fusion transcript,[9] detectable by PCR, leading to a chimeric protein with oncogenic properties. This translocation is a useful marker for the differential diagnosis of myxoid liposarcoma, especially in cases of poorly differentiated tumor.

Well-differentiated liposarcomas are characterized by the presence of ring chromosomes, large marker chromosomes which may contain hsr and telomeric associations. These supernumerary rings and giant marker chromosomes have been shown, by chromosome 'painting' and CGH, to be composed of chromosome 12 material, with coamplification of genes SAS and MDM2.[10]

Giant cell tumor

This tumor does not show specific translocation but in 75% of the cases presents non-clonal telomeric associations,[11] end-to-end fusions of apparently whole chromo-

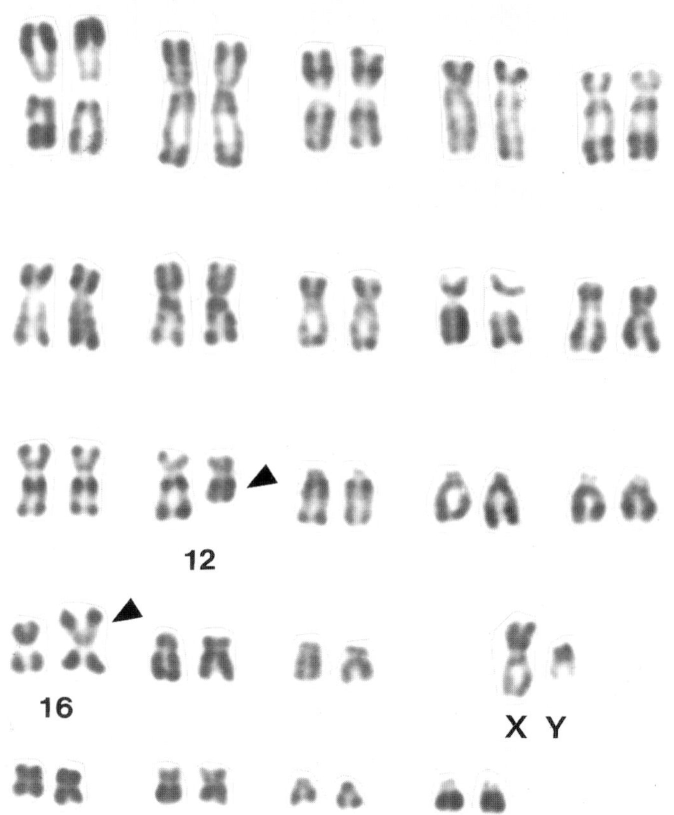

Fig. 4.3 Karyotype of a myxoid liposarcoma (R-banding) showing the characteristic translocation t(12;16)(q13;p11).

somes (Fig. 4.4), an abnormality observed in other tumors of fibrohistiocytic or fibroblastic origin.[1] Telomeres most commonly involved include 11p and 19q. Clonal rearrangements are sometimes observed (Fig. 4.4). Attempts have been made to correlate the presence of clonal abnormalities with prognosis.[12] Although the number of studies is still scarce, available data suggest the possibility of an association between the presence of clonal aberrations and risk of recurrence.

Ewing's sarcoma and peripheral primitive neuroectodermal tumors

About 90% of Ewing's sarcomas (skeletal and extraskeletal) and peripheral primitive neuroectodermal tumors show a specific translocation (Figs 4.2, 4.5):t(11;22)(q24;q12).[13] This rearrangement shared by both tumor types provides evidence for their histogenetic relationship and is an important marker for the diagnosis of small round cell tumors.[14] The translocation results in a fusion of the EWS gene, on chromosome 22, with the transcription factor gene FLI1, on chromosome 11,[15] leading to a hybrid transcript and an oncogenic chimeric protein. In about 5% of the cases, the EWS gene is fused with genes other than FLI1,[15–17] but with similar properties (Table 4.1).

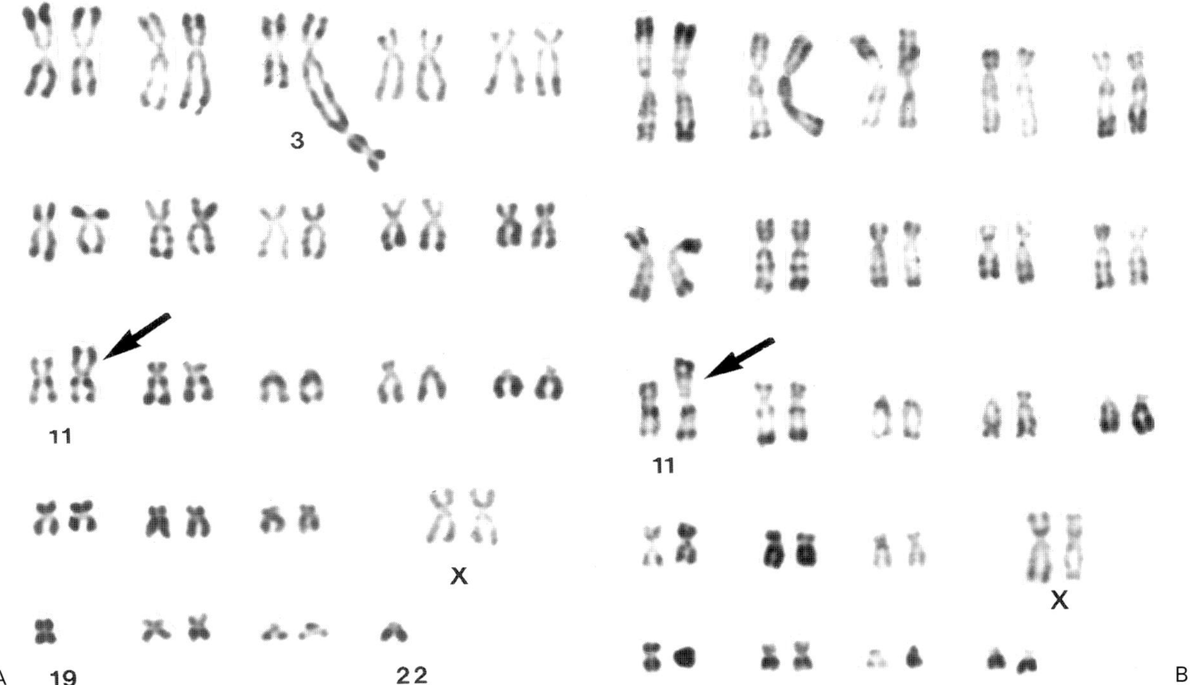

Fig. 4.4 Karyotypes of two cells from a giant cell tumor of bone (R-banding). (a) Characteristic terminal associations, in this cell between chromosomes 3, 19 and 22. In addition, presence of an unbalanced translocation t(11;14) (arrow). (b) Presence of the t(11;14) in another cell of the tumor, showing that this abnormality was clonal.

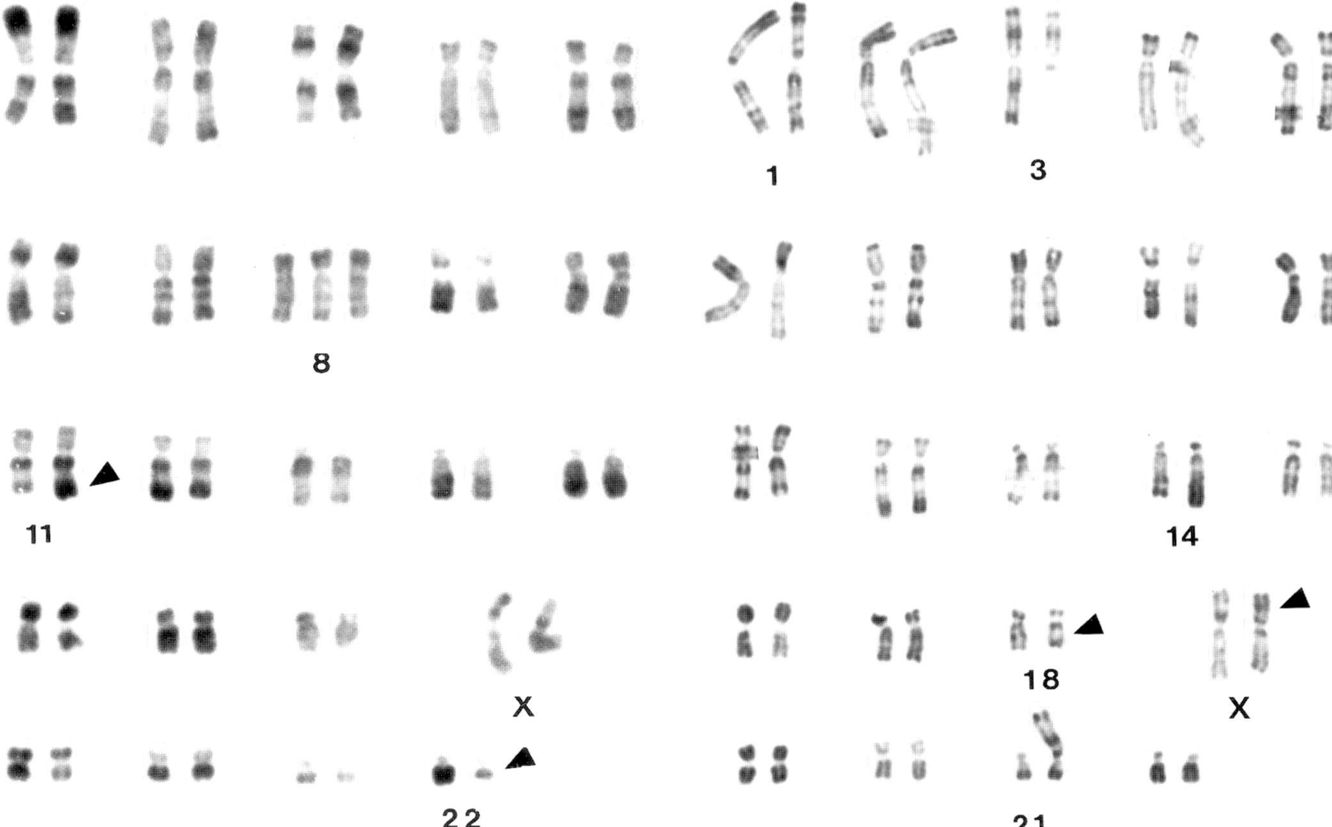

Fig. 4.5 Karyotype of a Ewing's sarcoma (R-banding) showing the characteristic translocation t(11;22)(q24;q12). Presence of trisomy 8 as additional abnormality.

Fig. 4.6 Karyotype of a synovial sarcoma (R-banding) showing the characteristic translocation t(X;18)(p11.2;q11.2). Presence of two other translocations, t(1;14) and t(3;21), as additional rearrangements.

Thus, cytogenetics and PCR appear to be particularly useful in this group of tumors which is often challenging for the pathologist. Interestingly, the EWS gene is involved in other tumor types (Table 4.1). In the clear cell sarcoma (malignant melanoma of soft parts), a translocation t(12;22)(q13;q12) exists which fuses the EWS gene with the ATF-1 gene.[18] In extraskeletal myxoid chondrosarcomas, a recurrent t(9;22)(q22;q12) has been found in which the EWS gene is fused to the TEC gene.[19]

Synovial sarcoma

More than 90% of synovial sarcomas are characterized by a translocation t(X;18)(p11.2;q11.2)[20] (Fig. 4.6), which results in a fusion of the SYT gene on chromosome 18 to one of two genes sharing large homology, SSX1 and SSX2, on chromosome X.[21] No correlation seems to exist between the two breakpoints on chromosome X and the histological subtypes, mono- or biphasic. Conventional karyotypic analysis or FISH[22] has proved useful in this tumour which can raise difficult problems of differential diagnosis.

CONCLUSION

The identification of characteristic rearrangements of diagnostic value has made cytogenetics (and molecular biology) an important adjunct to conventional histological analysis, particularly in soft tissue tumors which often present difficult challenges to the pathologist.

Karyotypic analysis of solid tumors was hampered by the frequent difficulty in obtaining a sufficient number of metaphases of good morphology. This obstacle is now potentially circumvented by the development of new approaches based on FISH on nuclei from fresh and paraffin-embedded material.

Such approaches are currently being popularized by the availability of an increasing number of commercial probes. However, in spite of the vital information chromosome analysis can provide, it must be emphasized that such studies, which remain at the border between diagnostic routine and research, are delicate and can be reliably performed only by a cytogenetic laboratory trained in the study of solid tumors.

REFERENCES

1. Sreekantaiah C, Ladanyi M, Rodriguez E, Chaganti R S K. Chromosomal aberrations in soft tissue tumors. Relevance to diagnosis, classification, and molecular mechanisms. Am J Pathol 1994: 144: 1121–1134
2. Fletcher J A, Kozakewitch H P, Hoffer F A et al. Diagnostic relevance of clonal cytogenetic aberrations in malignant soft tissue tumors. N Engl J Med 1991: 324: 436–442
3. Rabbits T H C. Chromosomal translocations in human cancers. Nature 1994: 372: 143–149
4. Waldman F M, Sauter G, Sudar D, Thompson C T. Molecular cytometry of cancer. Hum Pathol 1996: 27: 441–449
5. Hermsen M A J A, Meijer G A, Baak J P A, Joenje H, Walboomers J J M. Comparative genomic hybridization: a new tool in cancer pathology. Hum Pathol 1996: 27: 342–349
6. ISCN. An international system for human cytogenetic nomenclature. Basel: Karger, 1995
7. Kallioniemi A, Kallioniemi O, Sudar D et al. Comparative genomic hybridization: a powerful new method for cytogenetic analysis of solid tumors. Science 1992: 258: 818–821
8. Rabbits T H, Forster A, Larson R, Nathan P. Fusion of the dominant negative transcription regulator CHOP with a novel gene FUS by translocation t(12;16) in malignant liposarcoma. Nature Genet 1993: 4: 175–180
9. Kuroda M, Ishida T, Horiuchi H et al. Chimeric TLS/FUS-CHOP gene expression and heterogeneity of its junction in human myxoid and round cell sarcoma. Am J Pathol 1995: 147: 1221–1227
10. Pedeutour F, Suijkerbuijk R F, Forus A et al. Complex composition and co-amplification of SAS and MDM2 in ring and giant rod marker chromosomes in well-differentiated liposarcoma. Genes Chromosomes Cancer 1994: 10: 85–94
11. Bridge J A, Neff J R, Mouron B J. Giant cell tumor of bone: chromosomal analysis of 48 specimens and review of the literature. Cancer Genet Cytogenet 1992: 58: 2–13
12. McComb E N, Johansson S L, Neff J R, Nelson M, Bridge J A. Chromosomal anomalies exclusive of telomeric associations in giant cell tumor of bone. Cancer Genet Cytogenet 1996: 88: 163–166
13. Turc-Carel C, Aurias A, Mugneret F et al. Chromosomes in Ewing's sarcoma. I. An evaluation of 85 cases and remarkable consistency of t(11;22)(q24;q12). Cancer Genet Cytogenet 1988: 32: 229–238
14. Delattre O, Zucman J, Plougastel B et al. The Ewing family of tumors: a sub-group of small round-cell tumors defined by specific chimeric transcripts. N Engl J Med 1994: 331: 294–299
15. Delattre O, Zucman J, Plougastel B et al. Gene fusion with an ETS DNA-binding domain caused by chromosome translocation in human tumours. Nature 1992: 359: 162–165
16. Sorensen P H B, Lessnick S L, Lopez-Terrada D, Liu X F, Triche T J, Denny C T. A second Ewing's sarcoma translocation, t(21;22), fuses the EWS gene to another ETS-family transcription factor, ERG. Nature Genet 1994: 6: 146–151
17. Jeon I-S, Davis J N, Braun B S et al. A variant Ewing's sarcoma translocation (7;22) fuses the EWS gene to the ETS gene ETV1. Oncogene 1995: 10: 1229–1234
18. Zucman J, Delattre O, Desmaze C et al. EWS and ATF-1 gene fusion induced by the t(12;22) translocation in malignant melanoma of soft parts. Nature Genet 1993: 4: 341–345
19. Labelle Y, Zucman J, Stenman G et al. Oncogenic conversion of a novel orphan nuclear receptor by chromosome translocation. Hum Molec Genet 1995: 4: 2219–2226
20. Limon J, Mrozek K, Mandahl N et al. Cytogenetics of synovial sarcoma: presentation of ten new cases and review of the literature. Genes Chromosomes Cancer 1991: 3: 338–345
21. Crew A J, Clark J, Fischer C et al. Fusion of two genes SSX1 and SSX2, encoding proteins with homology to the Kruppel-associated box in human synovial sarcoma. EMBO J 1995: 14: 2333–2340
22. Shipley J, Crew J, Birdsall S et al. Interphase fluorescence in situ hybridization and reverse transcription polymerase chain reaction as a diagnostic aid for synovial sarcoma. Am J Pathol 1996: 148: 559–567

5

Electron microscopy

M.C. Vacher-Lavenu

GENERAL CONSIDERATIONS

In spite of technical difficulties, sometimes due to the hardness of the tissues, electron microscopy has been used to describe the different ultrastructural patterns of bone lesions and has contributed to a better understanding of the pathogenesis of disease.

The purpose of a conventional ultrastructural study is not to discover new images or hypothetical specific markers but to contribute to diagnosis and electron microscopy retains some practical value today.[1] In orthopedic surgical pathology, it is used for the localization of Birbeck granules and detection of features of differentiation which cannot be be detected at the optical level. However its place is less important than before the advent of immunochemistry and cytogenetics.

Recent studies have focused on immunoelectron microscopic techniques. Although there are relatively few diagnostic applications, these techniques offer considerable potential for resolving issues in tumor pathology and provide clues as to the origins of metastatic tumors of unknown primary sites, for example. These techniques are not yet routinely available but this powerful tool exists and allows the localization of proteins (antigens) at the subcellular level.

The aim of this chapter is not to be exhaustive but to analyze some contributions of electron microscopy.

Some procedural recommendations must be borne in mind. To be effective, electron microscopy necessitates good fixation in a well-preserved specimen, careful selection of the study area, wide sampling, an experienced pathologist and correlation with optical findings. The diagnosis can be further supported by ultrastructural studies of embedded aspirated material.

Fine-needle biopsy is now increasingly used and ultrastructural study may be a useful complementary technique.[2] Cytologic features in smears are correlated with light and electron microscopic findings and immunocytochemistry of embedded aspirated material in the preoperative diagnostic investigation of cartilaginous, osteogenic and other tumors.[3,4]

When examining an electron micrograph, one should bear in mind a set of questions to be answered. To identify the nature of a proliferation it is necessary to study the morphological information methodically, first by the analysis of the elements used for optical study and second by the analysis of the different cell structures: cytoplasm, nucleus, cellular membrane, relationship with other cells. Finally, the extracellular matrix should be analyzed.

It is necessary to keep in mind that the small size of an electron microscopic sample makes the findings of deposits, inclusions or other infrequent details a matter of chance.

As for the ultrastructural features, only a few salient points concerning bone neoplasms are listed here. For further details, see the sections on specific lesions.

In the nucleus, two elements are studied: the fibrous lamina and nuclear inclusions. The fibrous lamina is interposed between the inner nuclear membrane and the peripheral chromatin or nucleoplasm (nuclear matrix). A thickened fibrous lamina is peculiar to chondroblastoma and chondromyxoid fibroma but is also reported in non-tumor cells such as myofibroblasts and synovial intimal cells.[5]

According to Ghadially,[5] intranuclear inclusions are interesting but their significance remains unclear or controversial. The following aspects are of interest. Bundles of densely packed 10 nm intermediate filaments are seen in

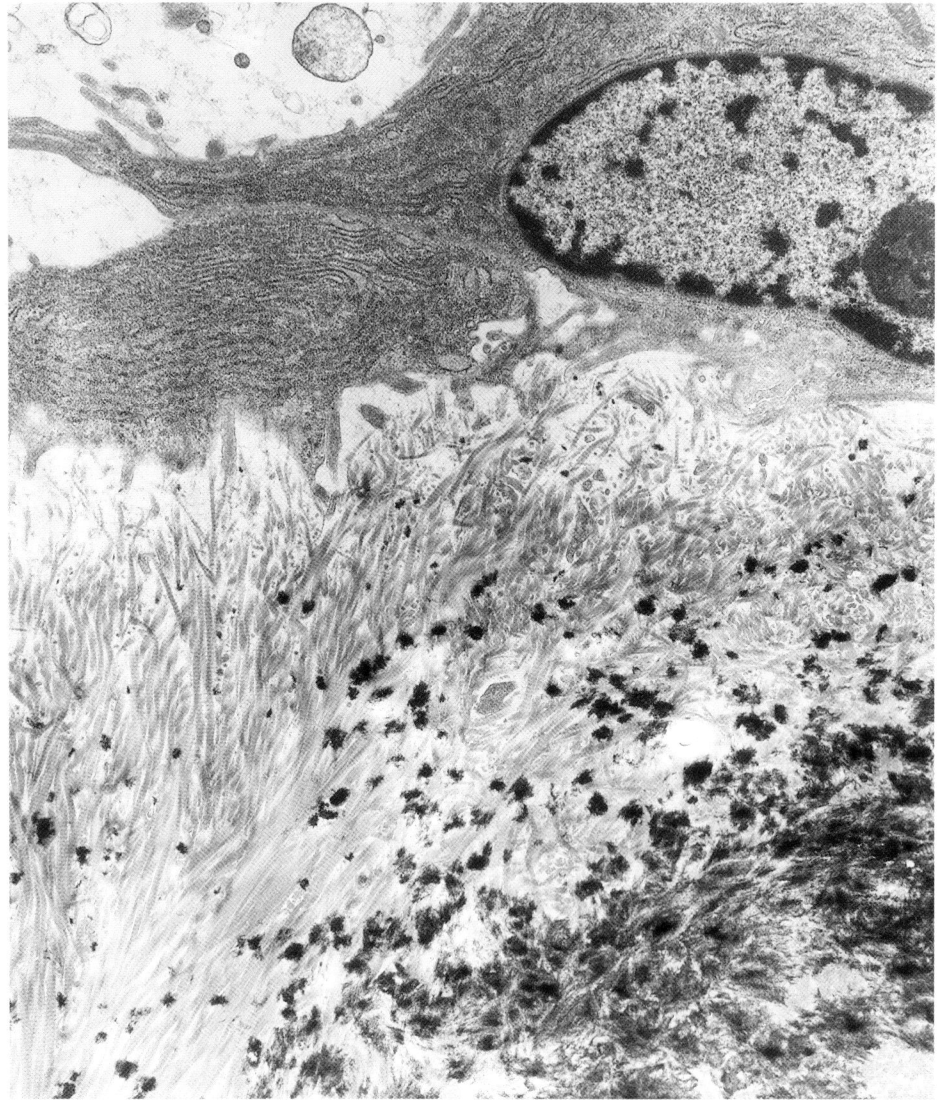

Fig. 5.1 Calcified bone matrix. (Top) An osteoblast contains prominent rough endoplasmic reticulum. (Bottom) Electron-dense hydroxyapatite crystal deposits on (probable type I) collagen fibers with banding periodicity constitutes the calcified bone matrix. Some matrix vesicles are seen. (Uranyl acetate and lead citrate ×21 000)

soft tissue sarcomas and chondroblastomas. Paracrystalline undulating membranous structures[5] are reported in parosteal osteosarcoma[6] and tubular honeycomb intranuclear inclusions may be found. The latter are usually seen in the cytoplasm, often joined directly to the endoplasmic reticulum, and are considered to be a special area of the microtubuloreticular complex. They are also observed in both the cytoplasm and nucleus of osteosarcoma cells[7] and vermicellar nuclear inclusions are also possible.[8] Paramyxovirus-like inclusions of Paget's disease are discussed on page 63.

The extracellular matrix is significant for a proper diagnosis. Bone and cartilage tumors present two types of matrix, generally well delineated.

The osteoid matrix is defined as an unmineralized precursor matrix of bone. Figure 5.1 shows a typical area of bone-forming activity.[9] Clusters of calcium crystals are randomly distributed on or along type I collagen bundles and become more densely packed near the calcified matrix. These hydroxyapatite deposits (Fig. 5.2) are often associated with matrix vesicles.[10] They are seen, for example, in human osteogenic tumors[11] and seem to be common in both normal and pathologic calcification processes.

In mature cartilage, compartments appear in the intercellular matrix.

The pericellular matrix, in intimate contact with the plasma membrane, is free of fibrillar collagen and rich in proteoglycans. The territorial matrix is made of collagen fibrils in a network-like distribution in the inner part but are more parallel in the outer part. Proteoglycan granules are also present. In the interterritorial compartment, fibrils

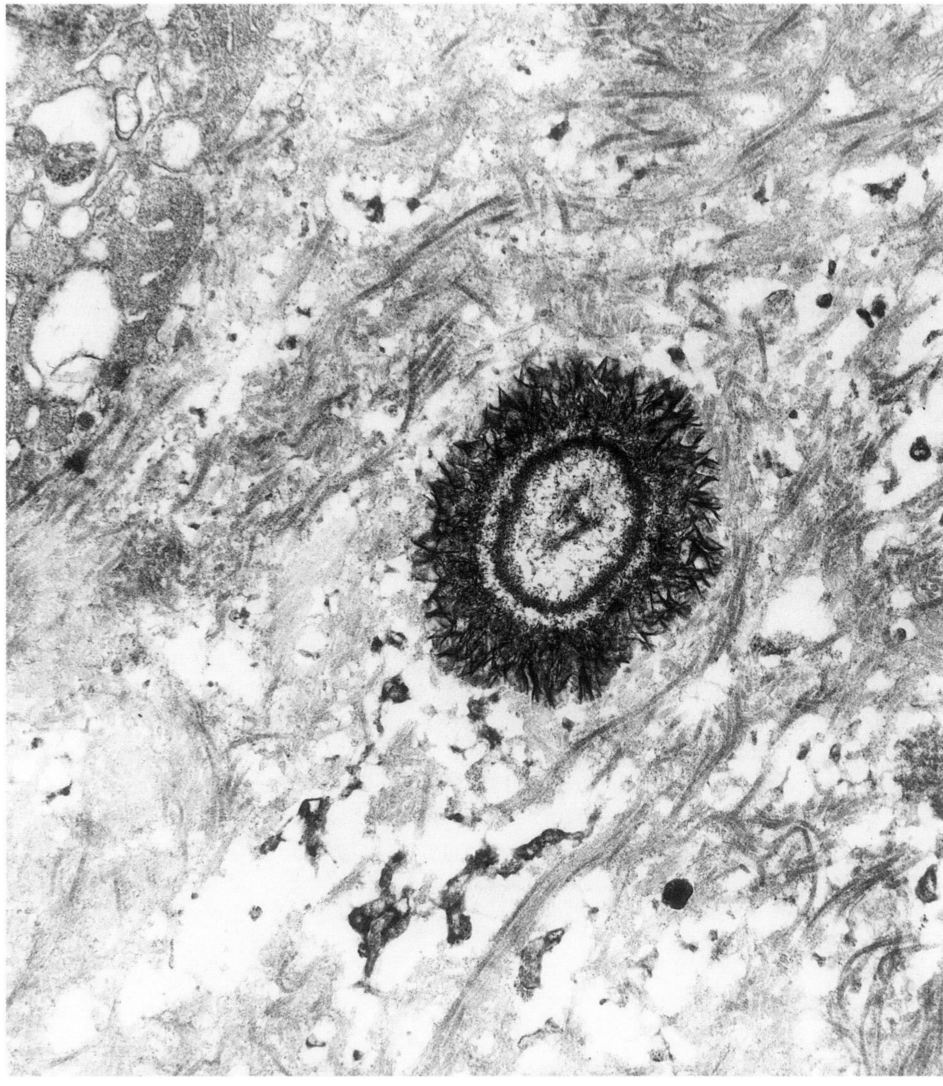

Fig. 5.2 Osteoid extracellular matrix. Hydroxyapatite crystals are seen at the center within randomly dispersed collagen fibrils and matrix vesicles. (Uranyl acetate and lead citrate ×25 000)

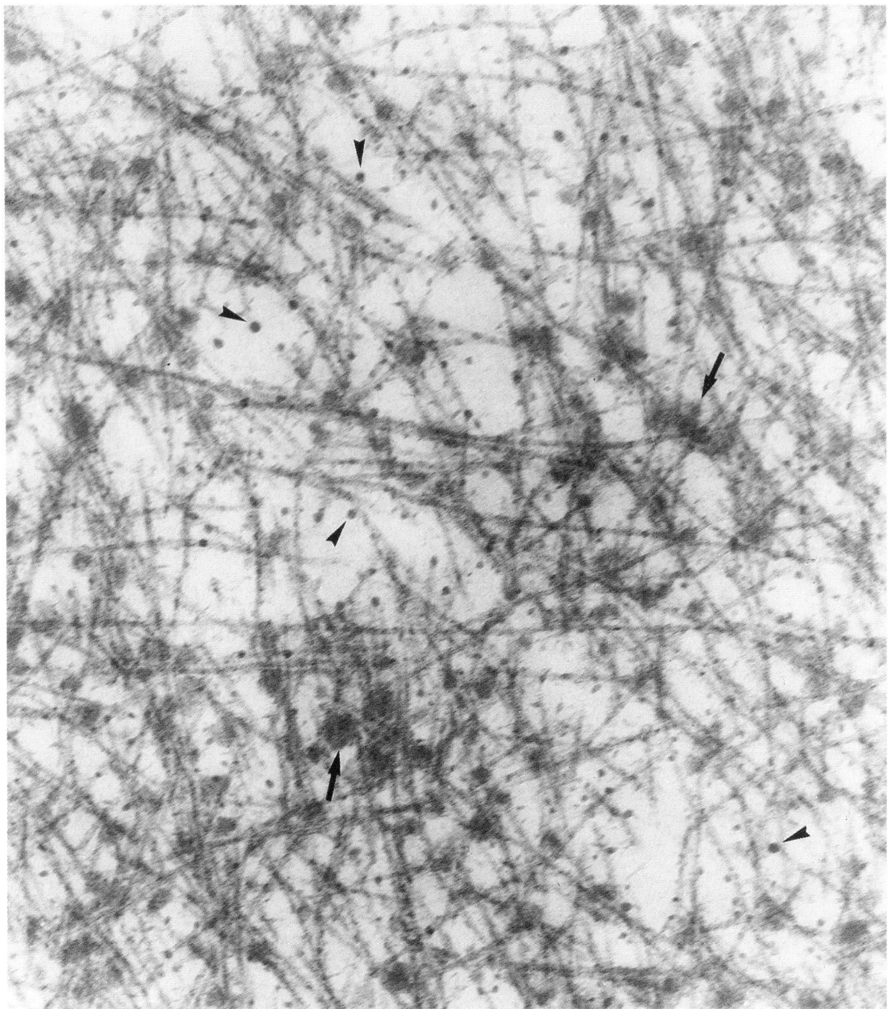

Fig. 5.3 Cartilaginous extracellular matrix. Proteoglycan (core protein and chondroitin sulfates) granules (arrowheads) in a loose meshwork of banded (probable type II) collagen fibrils with electron-dense matrix vesicles (arrows). (Uranyl acetate and lead citrate ×39 000)

are parallel and the density of proteoglycans is lower. In this last compartment, the process of mineralization is associated with matrix vesicles.[12]

Immature cartilage exhibits the same aspect without zones. The cartilaginous extracellular matrix is made up almost exclusively of a loose meshwork of striated, type II collagen fibrils,[13] punctuated by proteoglycan granules (Fig. 5.3)[12] and other macromolecules.

The ultrastructural aids to diagnosis for each disease entity are mentioned briefly below, with stress on specific features or points of interest.

BONE-FORMING TUMORS

Osteoblastoma

At the ultrastructural level, osteoid osteoma and osteo-

blastoma reveal the same features.[13,14,15,16] Neoplastic osteoblasts resemble normal osteoblasts[17] and possess eccentric, irregular and indented nuclei, well-developed, sometimes markedly dilated, rough endoplasmic reticulum with the Golgi apparatus in a juxtanuclear creation (Fig. 5.4). Multinucleated giant cells appear to be similar to other osteoclast-like cells (Fig. 5.5) with numerous cytoplasmic mitochondria, Golgi cisternae and vesicles and lysosomes. The presence of a ruffled border[14,18] depends on the contact with the bone surface. These giant cells, as with most osteoclast-like cells, may exhibit centriole away from the nuclei.[14,19]

The stroma is collagenous and consists of densely packed calcified collagen fibers with matrix vesicles.[20,21] Normal osteocytes are embedded in the osteoid matrix.

Electron microscopy is not a great help in the differential diagnosis of osteoblastoma and osteosarcoma.

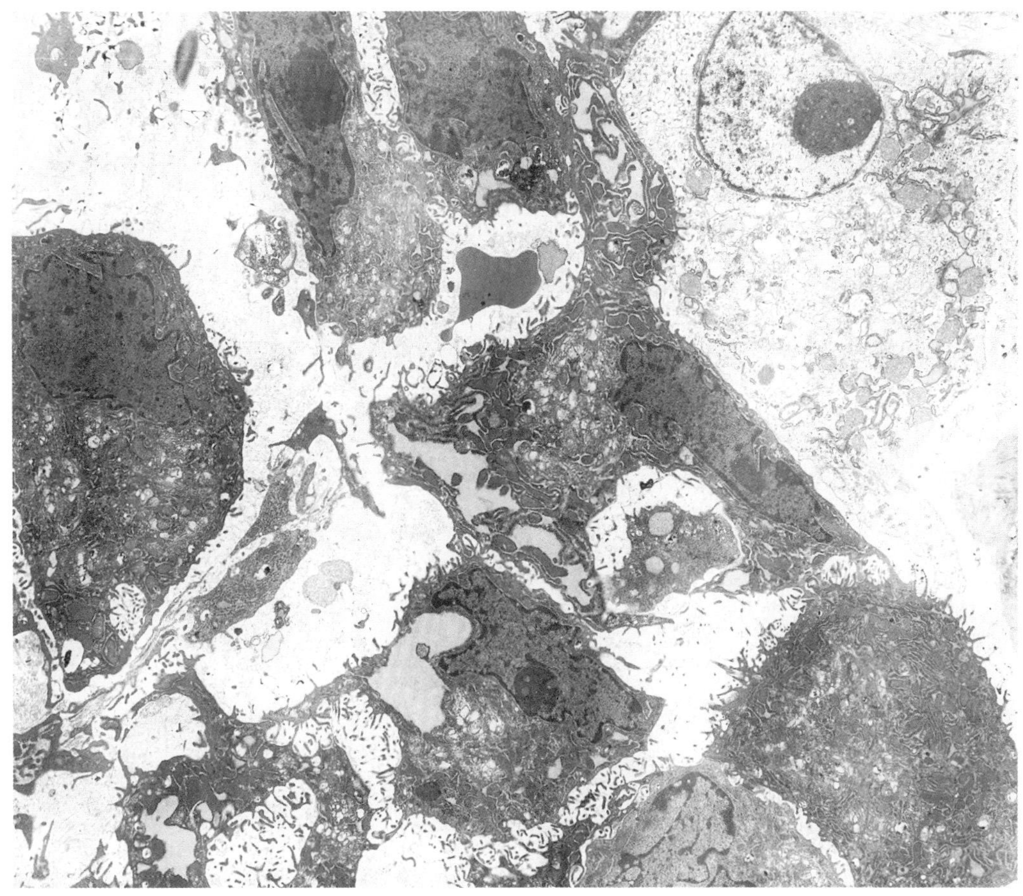

Fig. 5.4 Osteoblastoma. Osteoblasts show eccentric irregular nuclei with abundant rough endoplasmic reticulum and microvilli. No osteoid is present in this field. (Uranyl acetate and lead citrate ×12 000)

Osteosarcoma may show areas that are indistinguishable from benign or aggressive forms of osteoblastoma; however, lipid droplets are not seen in most osteoblastoma cells.[16]

Osteosarcoma

Basic well-differentiated osteoblasts (Fig. 5.6a) are typified by the following features:[17,22–28] polygonal to oval shape, an eccentric large nucleus with marginated heterochromatin and irregular contours, prominent nucleolus, well-developed rough endoplasmic reticulum, an often dilated Golgi apparatus distant from the nucleus, few mitochondria, free ribosomes, microfilaments, and a scalloped membrane or florid microvilli at the cell surface. Occasional lipid droplets, lysosomes and glycogen pockets are observed (Fig. 5.6b) as well as primitive cell junctions and mitochondria containing microcrystal deposits. Abundant 7 nm microfilaments have also been described.[29,30]

Tumor cells are embedded in a more or less dense and mineralized type I collagen extracellular matrix. Osteoid substance contains electron-dense deposits of hydroxyap-

atite crystals on irregularly disposed bundles of collagen fibers in close relationship to matrix vesicles[31] which are also present in chondrosarcoma and osteoblastoma.[21] These extracellular matrix vesicles are located between cells and the calcifying front. The aggregation of crystals into nodules and minicalcospherites leads to membrane rupture. The spherical nodules contribute to the formation of the calcifying front.[21]

Foci of cartilaginous differentiation show chondroblastic cells characterized by the usual features of cartilaginous cells (scalloped membrane, abundant amounts of glycogen, dilated cisternae of rough reticulum). Some authors describe four subtypes of chondroblast cells but this is of little practical interest.[32]

Fibroblastic differentiation[33] is characterized by elongated, spindle-shaped cells with central nuclei, fairly well-developed rough endoplasmic reticulum, more frequent lysosomes and numerous microfilaments. Myofibroblastic cells are numerous in the fibroblastic type of osteosarcomas.

Transitional stages between the different types of cell are seen, as well as undifferentiated cells[13,25,34] with reduced cytoplasm and organelles. Eventually, the scanty

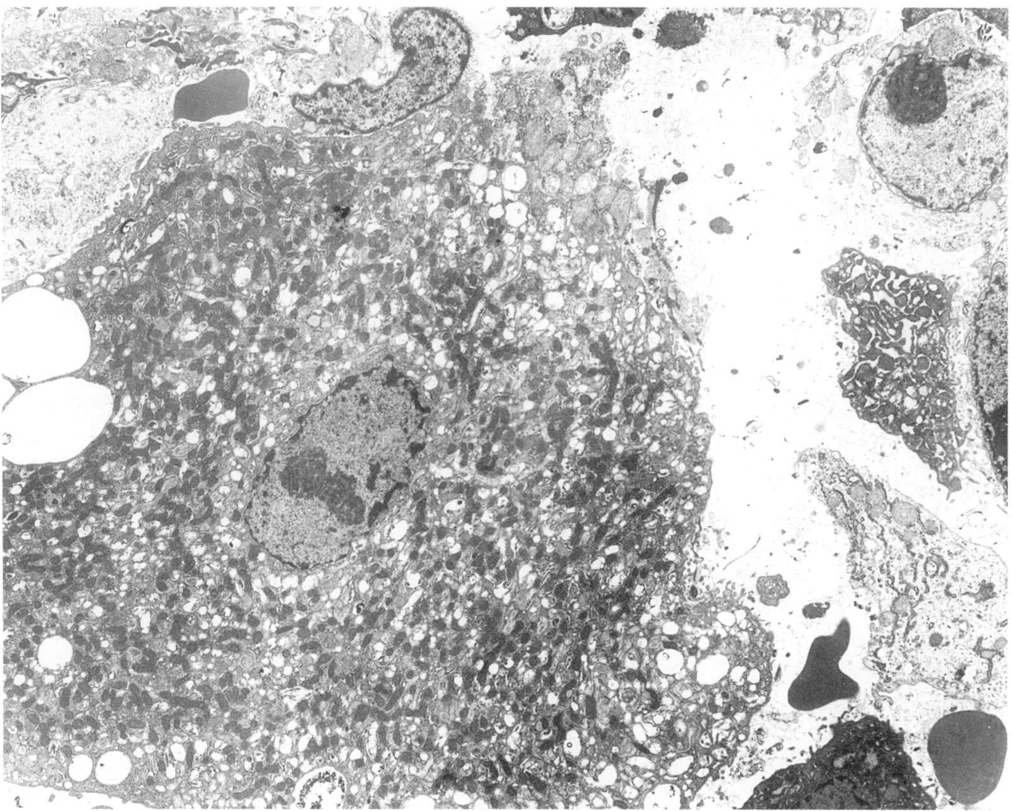

Fig. 5.5 Osteoblastoma. Part of an osteoclast-like cell in a benign osteoblastoma. Numerous mitochondria are associated with copious cytoplasmic vacuoles. (Uranyl acetate and lead citrate ×12 500)

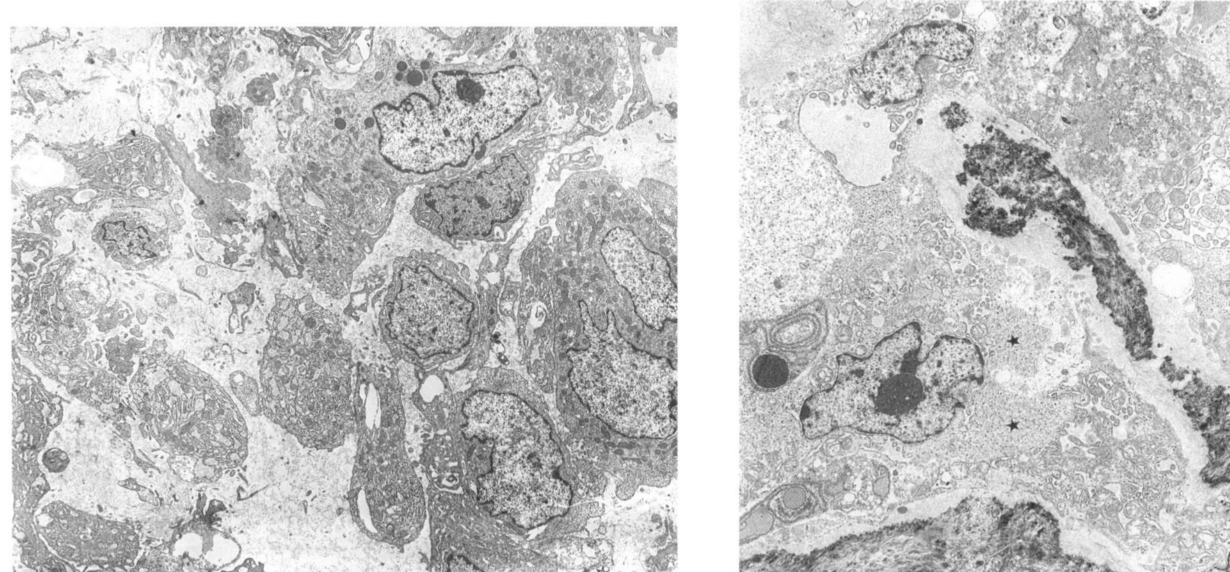

A

B

Fig. 5.6 (a) Osteosarcoma. Tumor cells show pleomorphic nuclei with prominent nucleoli, well-developed, moderately dilated rough endoplasmic reticulum and rounded mitochondria. Lipid droplets are seen in the upper cell. A multinucleated osteoclast-like cell is present at the right edge of the electron micrograph. No osteoid is identified in the extracellular matrix of this field. (Uranyl acetate and lead citrate ×11 000) (b) Osteosarcoma. Electron-dense high areas correspond to calcified (mineralized) osteoid matrix. A few lipid droplets are seen at the lower left corner of the field. Dilated rough endoplasmic reticulum filled with medium-dense finely granular material is observed at the upper left. Clusters of glycogen patches (*) are visible. (Uranyl acetate and lead citrate ×13 000)

rough endoplasmic reticulum adopts an annular or lamellar configuration.[30]

Curious unexplained images are occasionally encountered in the nucleus and cytoplasm of osteosarcomatous cells. Intracellular tubuloreticular complexes[6,23,35,36] associated with the rough and smooth reticulum have been observed in osteosarcomas, in both the cytoplasm and the nucleus, in a great variety of mammalian tissues.

Another type of intracisternal microtubular complex has been reported in the cytoplasm of osteosarcoma cells.[7] Coated parallel tubules are situated within the dilated rough endoplasmic reticulum cisternae of mononuclear cells. In cross-section, the appearance is that of hexagonal crystalline arrays. These structures, of unknown significance, have also been seen in melanoma and in the chondrocytes of one case of mucopolysaccharidosis type IV.[7]

Nuclear inclusions ultrastructurally similar to papovavirus[23,30] consisting of round electron-dense bodies adjacent to nucleoli have been described. They are observed in both neoplastic osteoblasts and osteoclast-like cells.

Finally, one case of osteosarcoma exhibited well-formed desmosomes and perinuclear tonofilaments in all four surgically resected specimens.[37]

Some osteosarcomas are *giant cell rich*. The ultrastructure of most of the multinucleated cells show the characteristic features of normal osteoclasts: many small vesicles and rounded mitochondria, narrow rough endoplasmic cisternae and a villous cell surface.[22,23,30] When they are mixed with osteoblasts, size and multinucleation are the principal arguments in favor of their osteoclastic nature.

The ultrastructural information about *small cell osteosarcomas* is restricted to about 10 published cases.[38–41] The nucleocytoplasmic ratio is high with euchromatic nuclei. The spindle, oval or polygonal tumor cells are larger than those of Ewing's sarcoma, form solid aggregates and produce frequent desmosome-like junctions. Organelles, particularly rough endoplasmic reticulum, although some are

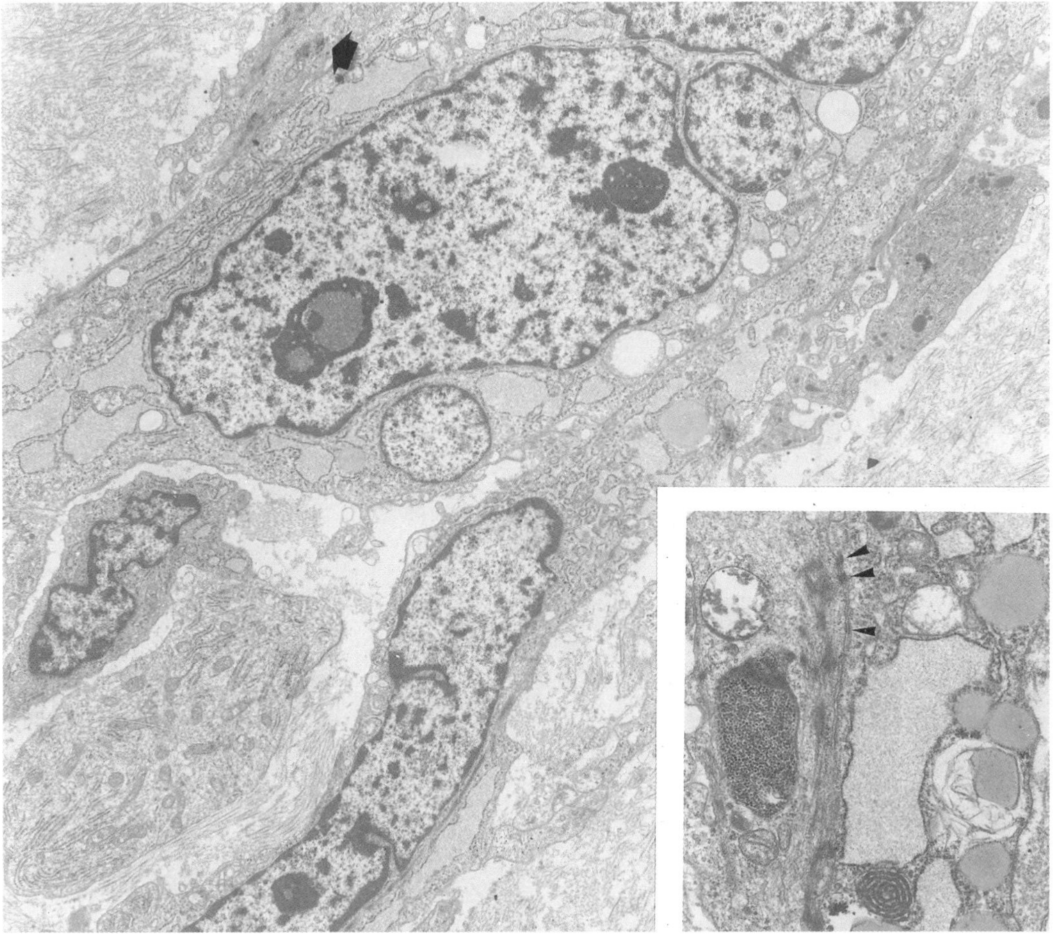

Fig. 5.7 Parosteal osteosarcoma. Spindle cell with large nucleus and well-developed rough endoplasmic reticulum. Microfilaments with dense bodies (arrow) are visible along the cell membrane. (Uranyl acetate and lead citrate ×7500) (Inset) Parosteal osteosarcoma. A group of membrane-bound glycogen particles near myofilaments, dilated rough endoplasmic cisternae and lipid droplet can be seen. Tiny primitive junctions (arrowhead) are present. A fortuitous pseudospiral of rough endoplasmic reticulum cisternae is observed. (Uranyl acetate and lead citrate ×14 500)

still more numerous than in Ewing's sarcoma. Glycogen, however, is less plentiful in small cell osteosarcoma. If present, foci of osseous matrix contribute to the right diagnosis. Electron microscopy can therefore help in the differential diagnosis between this entity and classic Ewing's sarcoma or lymphoma but is not useful for atypical Ewing's sarcoma or the undifferentiated component of mesenchymal chondrosarcoma.[39–41]

Myofibroblasts[27,42,43] are described in *parosteal osteosarcomas* and conventional osteosarcomas, characterized by bundles of actin microfilaments with dense bodies situated under the cell membrane or around the nucleus (Fig. 5.7). Foci of fragmented basement membrane are seen. Fibroblasts and myofibroblasts are more numerous in parosteal osteosarcomas and rudimentary cell junctions may be seen (Fig. 5.7 inset). Paracrystalline undulating membranous structures[5] may be observed in the nuclei of dense cells in human parosteal osteosarcoma[6] as well as tubular honeycomb intranuclear inclusions. They are associated with nuclear vermicellar bodies, large numbers of interchromatin granules and prominent perichromatin granules.

No information is available about the ultrastructural aspects of *central well-differentiated osteosarcomas*. Three cases have been studied in our department. The predominant cells show the features of fibroblastic cells (Fig. 5.8), with a central nucleus, an occasionally dilated well-developed rough endoplasmic reticulum, intermediate microfilaments, lipid droplets and glycogen particles. Intracytoplasmic collagen fibers are observed.

These fibroblastic cells are mixed with myofibroblastic cells and a smaller number of osteoblastic elements. The nucleus of osteoblastic cells is eccentric with a prominent nucleolus. Organelles are the same as fibroblastic ones but the rough endoplasmic reticulum cisternae are very developed with glycogen, primitive cell junctions and an electron-dense core within the mitochondria.

Myofibroblastic cells contain peripheral bundles of myofilaments with dense bodies (Fig. 5.8). A thickened fibrous lamina is rarely noted in myofibroblastic-like cells. Giant multinucleated cells are inconspicuous and resemble osteoclasts. Intermediate types of cells are often noted.

The extracellular matrix is composed of osteoid without significant differences from the classic tumoral form.

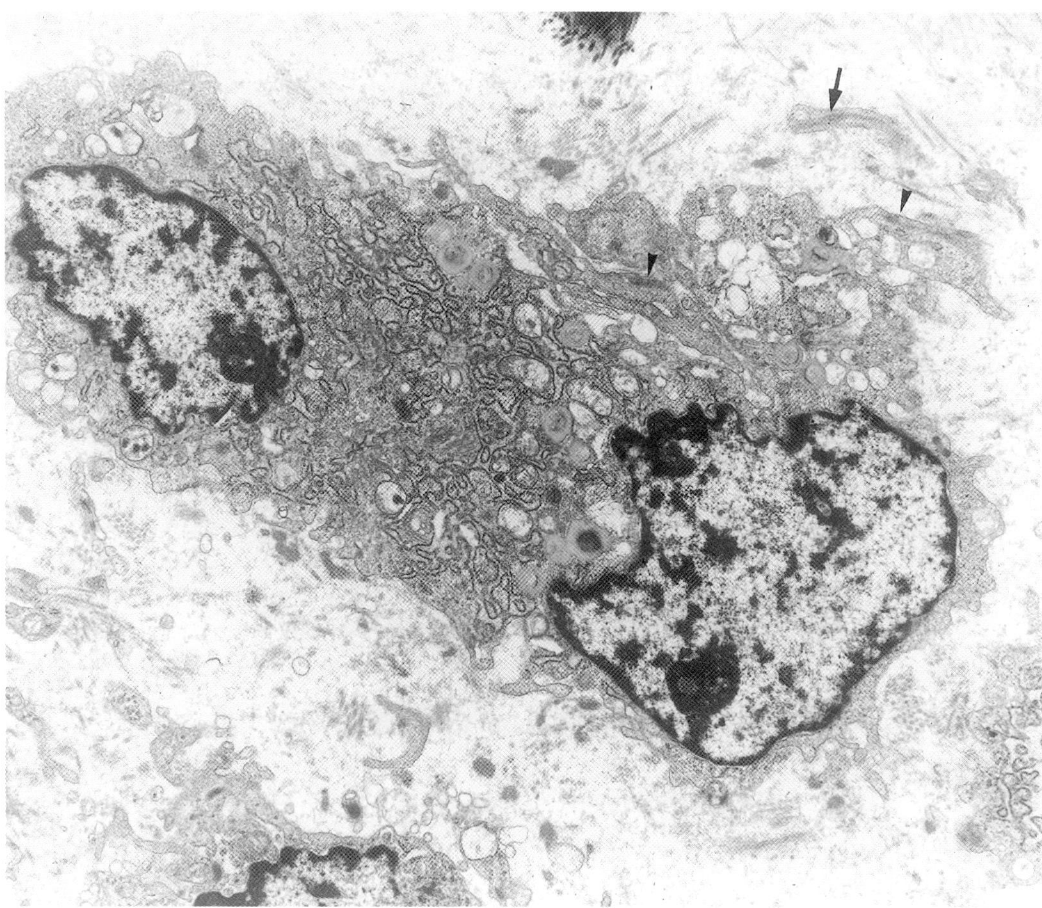

Fig. 5.8 Intraosseous well-differentiated osteosarcoma. Binucleated cells showing well-developed rough endoplasmic reticulum, lipid droplets, bundles of microfilaments under the cell membrane (arrowheads), intramitochondrial dense bodies and a collagen fiber in a cytoplasmic process (arrow). Dark mineralized osteoid matrix is visible in the middle upper part of the electron micrograph. (Uranyl acetate and lead citrate ×17 000)

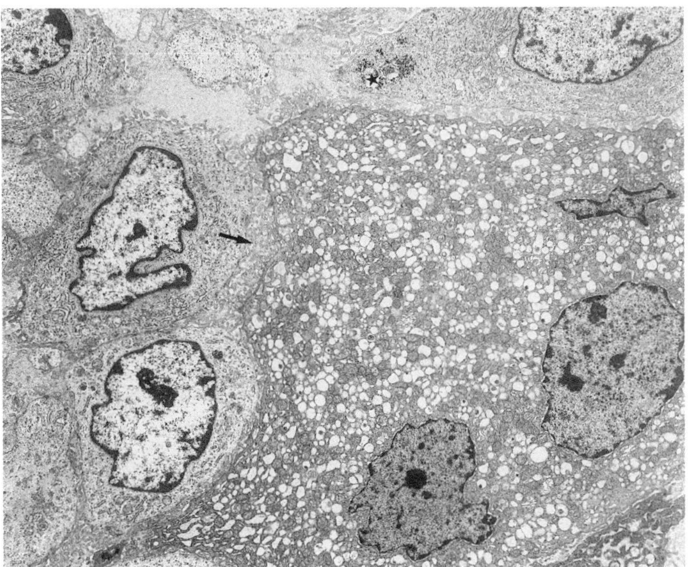

A

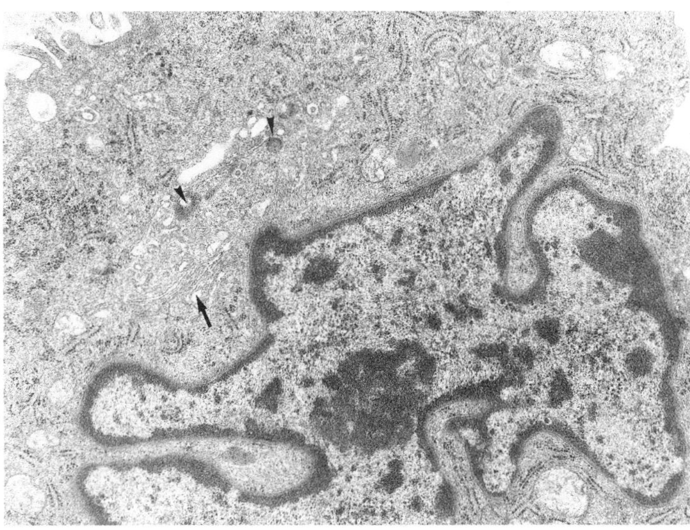

B

Fig. 5.9 (a) Chondroblastoma. Electron microscopy shows a multinucleated giant cell, with its cytoplasm crowded with organelles and surrounded by round mononuclear cells. Microvilli are seen between the giant cell and the mononuclear ones (arrow). In the upper center field can be seen an occasional cluster of glycogen particles (*). The intercellular substance of low electron density is scanty. (Uranyl acetate and lead citrate × 6500) (b) Chondroblastoma. Ultrastructural detail of a tumor cell showing irregular-shaped nucleus with a prominent nuclear fibrous lamina and cytoplasmic organelles such as Golgi apparatus (arrow), isolated lipid droplets (arrowhead) and branching rough endoplasmic reticulum. A few surface microvilli are seen in the upper left cornor. (Uranyl acetate and lead citrate ×23 000)

CARTILAGINOUS TUMORS

Chondroblastoma

This tumor is composed of mononuclear cells intermixed with variable numbers of multinucleated osteoclast-like giant cells without unusual features (Fig. 5.9a).[13,16,44–53] Some of the mononuclear cells are round or polygonal poorly differentiated cells, usually with a high nuclear–cytoplasmic ratio and few cytoplasmic organelles. The others are more or less well-differentiated chondroid cells that show an amount of glycogen particles varying from cell to cell, lipid inclusions, numerous mitochondria, well-developed rough endoplasmic reticulum and Golgi apparatus and surface microvilli (Fig. 5.9b). Diffuse intermediate filaments are often seen in the cytoplasm.

The nucleus, frequently indented and lined by heterochromatin, possesses a fibrous lamina of 30–60 nm thickness interposed between the inner nuclear membrane and the peripheral chromatin of the nuclear matrix. This feature, of unknown significance, is fairly specific for chondroblastoma and chondromyxoid fibroma (Fig. 5.10c).

The pericellular matrix is sparse and of various kinds: granular and fibrillar or chondroid with clusters of crystals or calcified globules in close contact with the collagen fibers. Ultrastructural cytochemical demonstration of proteoglycans and calcium in the extracellular matrix of chondroblastoma supports the theory that chondroblastomas are of chondrogenic origin[52] although some other observations support a histiocytic origin.[53] The absence of lacunae under scanning[51] or conventional transmission electron microscopy around the tumor cells can be explained by the immaturity of the cartilage.

It is necessary to emphasize the common ultrastructural features (not only a thick fibrous lamina) between chondroblastoma and chondromyxoid fibroma, although the presence of undifferentiated cells may help to distinguish chondroblastoma at the ultrastructural level.[51]

Chondromyxoid fibroma

The tumor cells are stellate myofibroblasts and fibroblastic cells intermixed with chondroblasts. The cells are more pleomorphic and elongated than those of chondroblastoma[16,44] but many of the tumor cells are similar in ultrastructure.

Characteristic tumor cells[16,44,54–56] contain a Golgi apparatus, a rough endoplasmic reticulum, glycogen particles and microfilaments. Some elements are myofibroblasts; their cytoplasm contains peripheral bundles of myofilaments in parallel arrays oriented to the long axis of the cell, with scattered fusiform dense bodies (Fig. 5.10a,b). Cytoplasmic projections and pinocytotic vesicles are seen at the cell periphery. Sometimes, zonula adherens or desmosome-like attachments are observed.[44,55]

The nucleus shows deep indentations and a thick fibrous lamina along the inner nuclear membrane, as seen

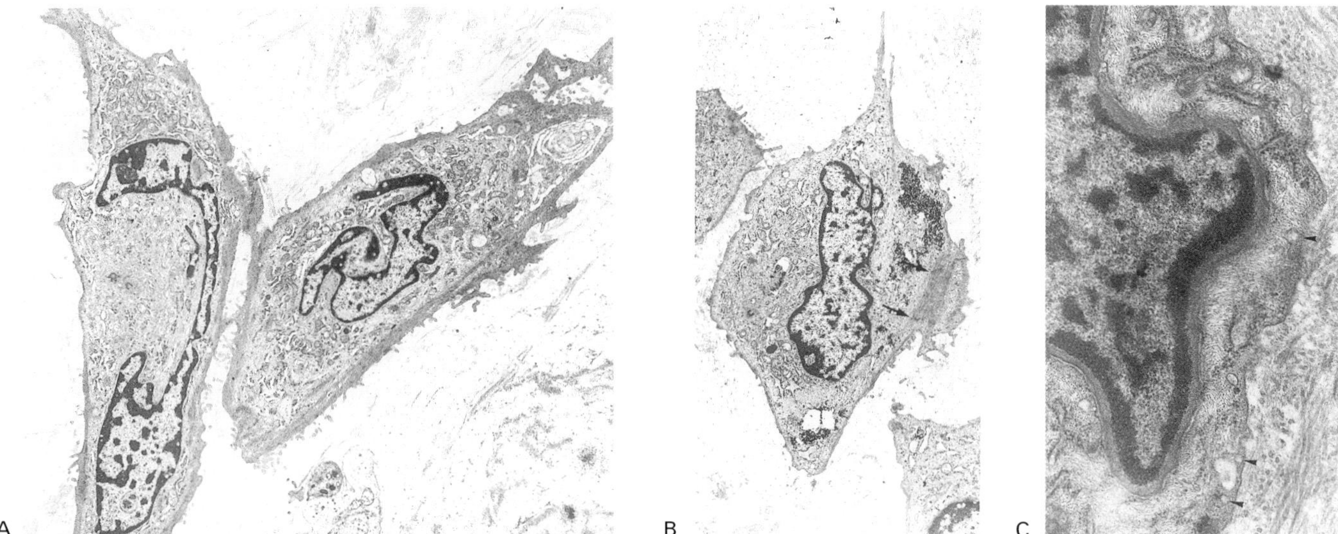

Fig. 5.10 (a) Chondromyxoid fibroma. Two tumor cells show an irregular indented nucleus with marginated heterochromatin. Centrioles are visible in the cytoplasmic area situated in the concavity of the nucleus. Note the subplasmalemmal bundles of actin microfilaments with interspersed fusiform dense bodies. Immature short microvilli are seen on the free cell surface. The abundant loose matrix is chondroid with fine fibrils. (Uranyl acetate and lead citrate ×9000) (b) Chondromyxoid fibroma. This tumor cell exhibits large amounts of glycogen, a pronounced elongated projection, spicular cytoplasmal membrane processes and an area of microfilaments with electron-dense focal aggregates (fusiform bodies), with evidence of periodic banding (arrow). (Uranyl acetate and lead citrate ×9000) (c) Chondromyxoid fibroma. Detail of a conspicuous thick nuclear fibrous lamina. Collagen fibers are seen in the vicinity of the tumor cell. Intracytoplasmic intermediate filaments and pinocytotic vesicles (arrowheads) are noticed under the cell membrane. (Uranyl acetate and lead citrate ×22 000)

in chondroblastoma (Fig. 5.10c). The nuclear irregularities are marked in the aggressive atypical form of chondromyxoid fibroma cells.[44]

Nuclear inclusions consisting of densely packed parallel bundles of 10 nm microfilaments may be observed, as we have noticed in some cases of malignant fibrohistiocytoma (personal observations). Lipid droplets are less numerous than in enchondroma.[16]

The multinucleated giant cells are similar to osteoclast-like cells of other bone lesions. The matrix is made of fine immature fibrils, electron-dense granules of proteoglycans with prominent myxoid zones and eventually mature collagen fibers and long spacing collagen.

Chondrosarcoma

The ultrastructural features of the cartilaginous cells depend on the degree of differentiation. The light criteria correlate well with the ultrastructural findings.

The basic features are common to all.[13,44,57–60] The cell membrane is scalloped with short, spicular, footlike processes, forming peaked ends on the surface depressions. The rough endoplasmic reticulum is well developed and occasionally dilated and the cisternae contain flocculant material of moderate electron density. Mitochondria are usually surrounded by rough endoplasmic cisternae. Lipid droplets and clusters of glycogen particles are frequently observed. The Golgi complex is conspicuous. Intermediate filaments are widely dispersed in the cytoplasm.

The nucleus is round to oval in shape, sometimes indented and filled with euchromatin with a single dense homogeneous nucleolus.

The immediate pericellular matrix is sparse with fine amorphous proteoglycan granules delimiting lacunae and becoming more fibrillar. A clear zone is seen between the cell and the matrix. The fibrils are mixed with matrix vesicles and electron-dense granules. Collagen fibers with 64 nm periodicity are scarce (Fig. 5.11a,b).

In myxoid chondrosarcomas, the tumor cells are widely distributed in an abundant loose matrix and show a dilated rough endoplasmic reticulum.[60]

Osteoblasts may resemble chondroblasts so the finding of hydroxyapatite crystals deposits is important for the differential diagnosis. However, primary mineralization with matrix vesicles and calcifying nodules has been observed in chondrosarcoma.[11]

The fine structure reveals no specific differences between well-differentiated chondrosarcoma and benign cartilaginous lesions such as enchondromas, chondromyxoid fibromas and even non-neoplastic chondrocytes.[16,44,60] In high-grade chondrosarcomas, the tumor cells contain abundant vimentin filaments, an increased number of lipid droplets and fewer cytoplasmic organelles.[13,57,60] Of course, the shape of the cells also varies and many adopt a spindly fibroblastic appearance with a high nuclear–cytoplasmic ratio. The nuclear pleomorphism is conspicuous.

Ultrastructural curiosities have been reported in chon-

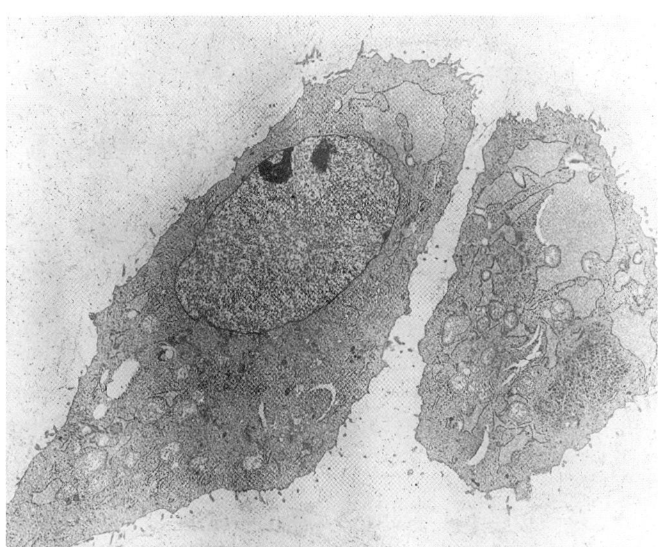
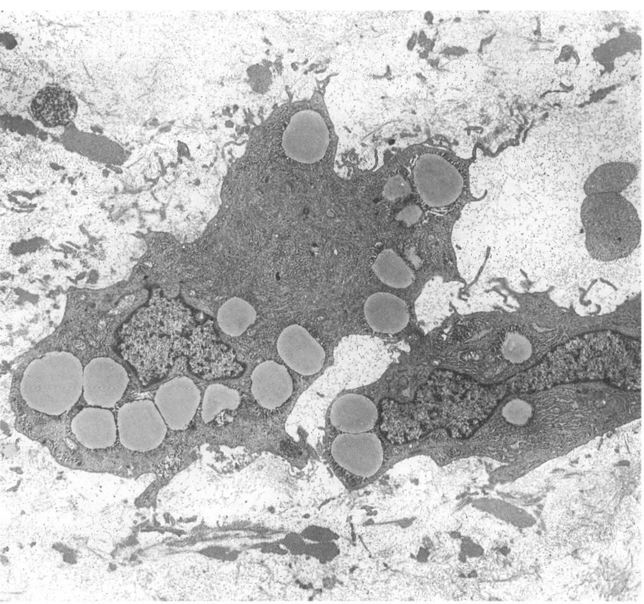

Fig. 5.11 (a) Grade II chondrosarcoma. Two tumor cells show ergastoplasmic dilated cisternae which contain a fine flocculent substance, short processes of the cytoplasmic membrane and some glycogen rosettes ($\star$). The granular amorphous matrix of lacuna consists of proteoglycan granules. (Uranyl acetate and lead citrate ×12 500) (b) Chondrosarcoma. Spindle-shaped grade III tumor cells with scalloped cell surface. Lipid droplets are apparent and associated with clusters of glycogen particles. Note the pleomorphic nuclei with margin heterochromatin. The rough endoplasmic reticulum cisternae are well developed. In the extracellular matrix, small dense granules of proteoglycans are enmeshed in fine fibrils with electron-dense vesicles. (Uranyl acetate and lead citrate ×14 500)

drosarcomas, such as the amianthoid fibers described by Ghadially[61] in a case of chondrosarcoma. This seems to be a degenerative change caused by coalescence of collagen fibers.

Intracytoplasmic eosinophilic hyaline globules in cartilaginous neoplasms have been studied by scanning and transmission electron microscopy, as well as electron probe X-ray microanalysis.[62] About 70% of chondrosarcomas were found to contain spherical, non-membrane-bound bodies localized within the profiles of dilated cisterns of the rough endoplasmic reticulum. These hyaline globules are secretory products of a glycoprotein nature admixed with peroxidized lipids, calcium and sulfur.

Intramitochondrial paracrystalline inclusions 50 nm in diameter and of unknown significance have been reported in three cases of chondrosarcoma.[63] These structures may be artifacts or degenerative changes.

Intracisternal bundles of tubules have been observed in *myxoid chondrosarcoma*[64–66] but, more often, in extraskeletal myxoid chondrosarcomas.[67] Their nature is undetermined, but they are probably not related to paramyxovirus. No diagnostic import is attributed to these structures and they have also been reported in a case of osteosarcoma.[7]

Most of the morphologic features described above are more or less associated with spindle-shaped cells resembling fibroblasts. The ultrastructure of different degrees of cartilaginous differentiation, according to the grading of chondrosarcomas, exhibits a wide spectrum of morphological associations. The more differentiated the neoplasm, the more likely it is that its cells will contain characteristic findings. However, the same lesion may often contain ultrastructural differences with foci of different stages of differentiation or maturation.

The chondroblasts of *clear cell chondrosarcomas* show large clusters of glycogen particles, sometimes lost during the chemical processing of the tissue, and few organelles similar to those of classic chondrosarcoma[13,68–72] (Fig. 5.12b). The cytoplasm contains a well-developed Golgi complex and a dilated rough endoplasmic reticulum, often closely associated with rounded mitochondria. Bundles of microfilaments are occasionally observed. The cell membrane is scalloped with many microvillous processes. The nucleus is regular or indented with an occasionally prominent nucleolus (Fig. 5.12a).

When multinucleated giant cells are present, they exhibit the characteristic features of osteoclasts. The appearance of the intercellular substance is loose with sparse dense glycosaminoglycan granules, thin fibrils and matrix vesicles as in immature cartilage, with[70,71] or without mature collagen fibers,[68,69] depending on the stage of differentiation.[71] At the ultrastructural level, clear cell chondrosarcoma closely resembles chondroblasts and chondroblastoma.

The ultrastructural features of the chondrosarcomatous component of *dedifferentiated chondrosarcomas* are similar to those of conventional chondrosarcoma (Fig. 5.13). The dedifferentiated sarcoma component shows the ultrastruc-

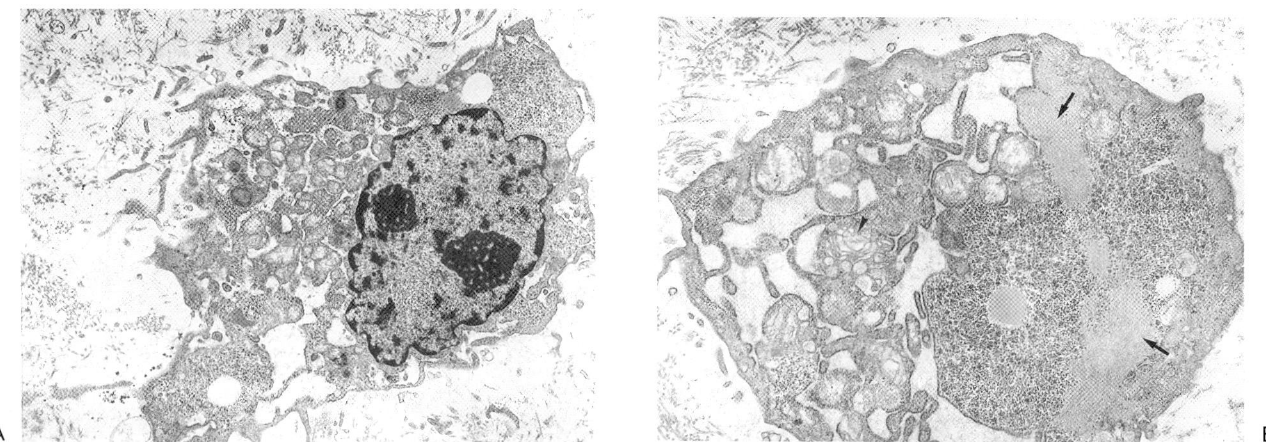

Fig. 5.12 (a) Clear cell chondrosarcoma. The nucleus contains two prominent nucleoli (nucleolonema). Note numerous microvillous processes and no obvious pericellular clear zone. Collagen fibers are seen within the intercellular matrix. (Uranyl acetate and lead citrate ×20 000) (b) Clear cell chondrosarcoma. Detail of the cytoplasm. Note large amount of glycogen rosettes, round mitochondria protruding into dilated rough endoplasmic reticulum, Golgi apparatus (arrowhead) and intermediate type 10 nm filaments (arrow). (Uranyl acetate and lead citrate ×25 000)

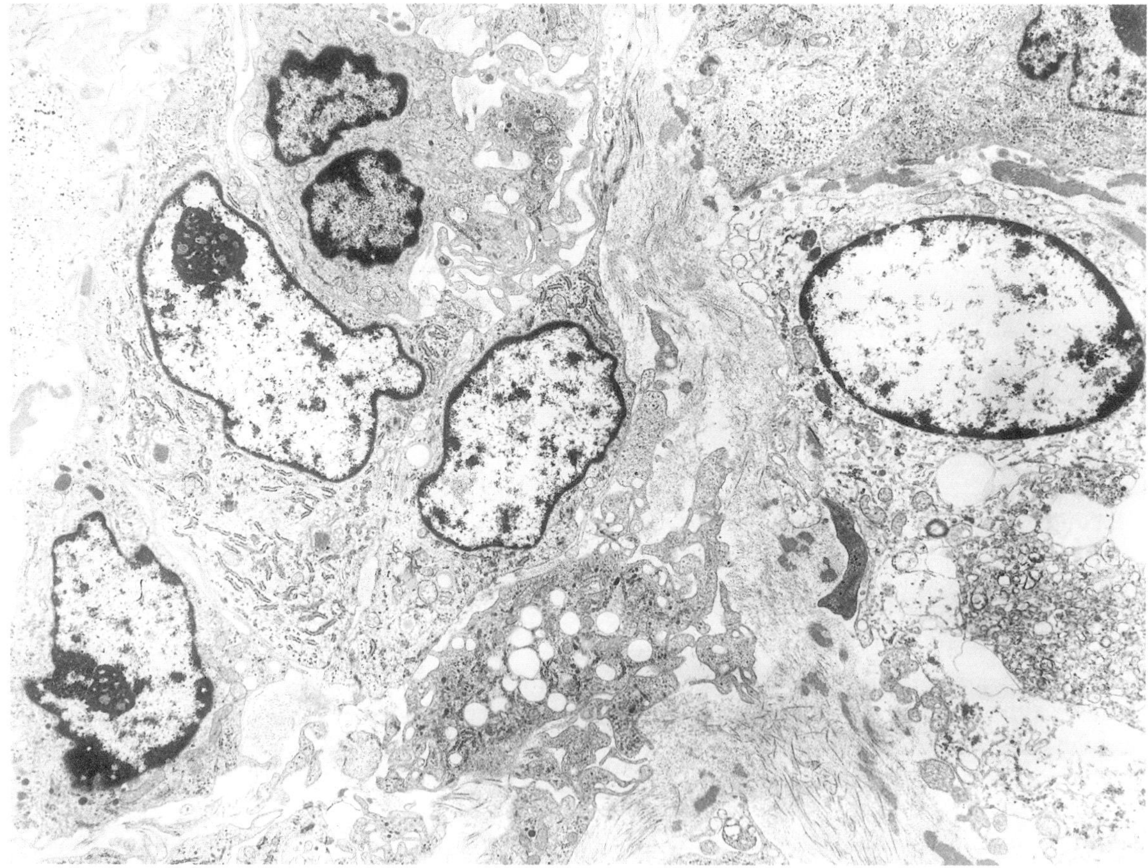

Fig. 5.13 Dedifferentiated chondrosarcoma. High-grade sarcomatous tumor cells in the non-chondroid component such as the one with the round nucleus on the right, are interpreted as poorly differentiated elements, or as in the middle left part of the electron micrograph as fibroblastic. (Uranyl acetate and lead citrate ×14 000)

tural characteristics of fibrosarcoma,[73] malignant fibrous histiocytoma[73,74] (the most frequent), rhabdomyosarcoma,[73,75] osteosarcoma or undifferentiated sarcoma.[13,76,77]

Mesenchymal chondrosarcoma exhibits two components: poorly differentiated cells mixed with differentiated cartilaginous cells. The ultrastructural features are similar in

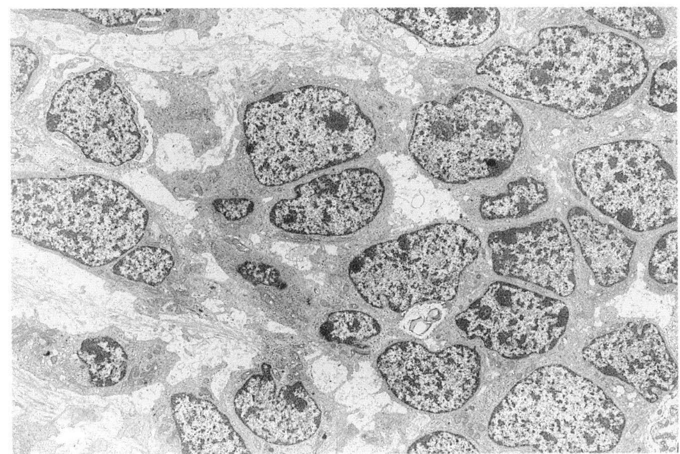

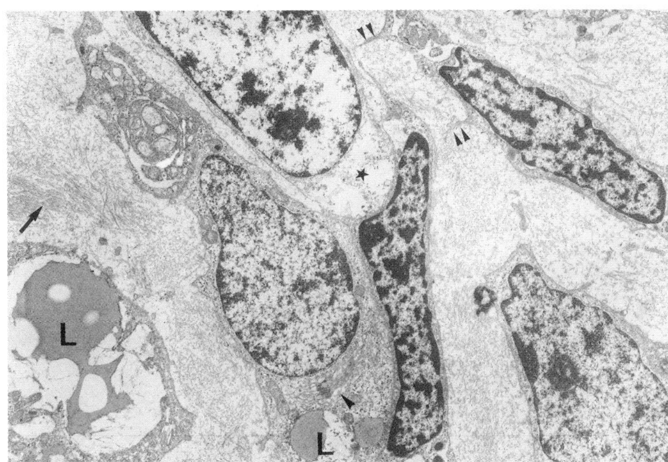

Fig. 5.14 (a) Mesenchymal chondrosarcoma. Low power view of clusters of round or spindle-shaped, poorly differentiated tumor cells showing large nuclei and paucity of cytoplasmic organelles. The matrix is sparse. (Uranyl acetate and lead citrate ×12 000) (b) Mesenchymal chondrosarcoma. High nuclear–cytoplasmic ratio. The scanty cytoplasm contains few organelles: lipid droplets (L), Golgi apparatus (arrowhead) and rough endoplasmic reticulum. Cytoplasmic glycogen granules were extracted and distorted during processing (★). In the intercellular spaces, finely granular or amorphous material contains randomly oriented collagen fibrils (arrow). The cell membrane exhibits indented edges (double arrowheads). (Uranyl acetate and lead citrate ×18 500)

both bone and soft tissue mesenchymal chondrosarcomas.[13,16,56,60,78–82]

The poorly differentiated mesenchymal cells are round or spindle shaped and contain sparse cytoplasmic organelles, little or no glycogen and rare lipid droplets (Fig. 5.14b). The size and shape of the cells and the number of organelles are similar to those of the small cell osteosarcomas,[40] but nuclei have smooth profiles and hydroxyapatite crystals are not seen. They also resemble Ewing's sarcoma cells. The cytoplasmic membranes are cohesive and cytoplasmic projections are infrequent (Fig. 5.14a). Desmosome-like or primitive junctions are occasionally observed.

The extracellular matrix is very scant and contains col-lagen fibers (Fig. 5.14b). These features are comparable with the cartilage formation in the primitive mesenchyme in embryo.

The cartilaginous areas show the fine structure of typical chondrosarcomas previously described, but some subtle differences are noticed.[16] In ordinary chondrosarcomas the cells are usually larger and more irregular, with prominent dilated rough endoplasmic reticulum. The cells of the cartilaginous component show a well-developed Golgi complex, glycogen particles, more or less dilated rough endoplasmic reticulum and irregular cell processes with scalloping. Matrix vesicles with calcium crystal deposits may be present.

ROUND CELL TUMORS OF BONE

Ultrastructural study remains very useful in cases of round cell sarcomas of bone and for the diagnosis of *Ewing's sarcoma of bone*, even if its role is not the same as in the past. Cytogenetic studies are necessary to support the diagnosis but are not always available.

The abundant literature describes an essentially identical ultrastructure for classic Ewing's sarcoma of bone,[13,83–95] even in vitro and in true cases of extraskeletal Ewing's sarcoma. The cytoplasm has more or less large aggregates of glycogen granules and a paucity of cytoplasmic organelles consisting of free ribosomes, small round mitochondria, scarce rough endoplasmic reticulum, small Golgi apparatus and eventually lipid vacuoles (Fig. 5.15a,b).

Glycogen is always found in Ewing's tumor but may be present in small quantities. α glycogen, rosette-like aggregates, are particularly prominent in Ewing's sarcoma. Intermediate 10 nm filaments are sometimes found.[96]

The nucleus is round or ovoid, rarely deeply indented with diffusely distributed euchromatin. The nucleolus is small and single. The cell membrane is smooth or with occasional short processes.

There is debate about the reality of neurosecretory granules in true Ewing's sarcoma.[13,97] Lysosomes are also seen in tumor cells and they may mimic neurosecretory granules. The extraskeletal form contains less glycogen and more cytoplasmic processes.[98]

Intercellular connections, such as small desmosome-like or, more frequently, rudimentary cell junctions, are detected but are not a consistent finding. Small desmosomes were noted in 20% of 71 cases reported by Erlandson.[13]

Some tumor cells show differentiating features of endothelial cells, such as basement membrane-like deposits.[99]

As well as the principal tumor cells, darker, intermediate, irregularly shaped cells are usually observed. They are of different electron density and less numerous than the principal cells. The cell contours are irregular and the nucleus is indented with clumps of heterochromatin. Cytoplasmic organelles are more numerous.

Atypical Ewing's sarcoma[13,87,90,93] is reported to show

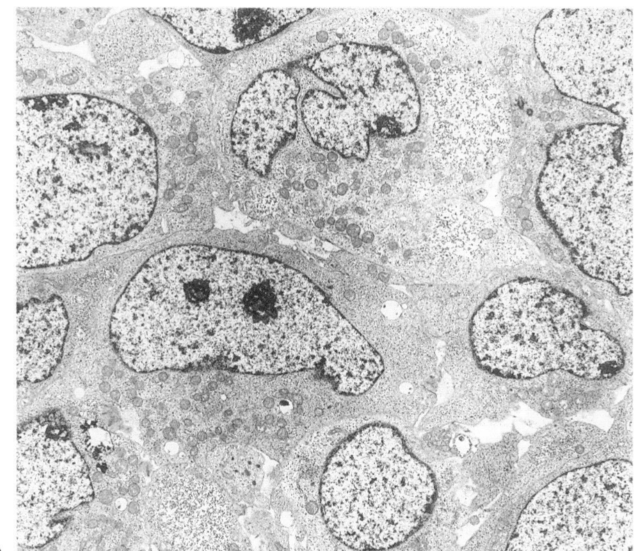

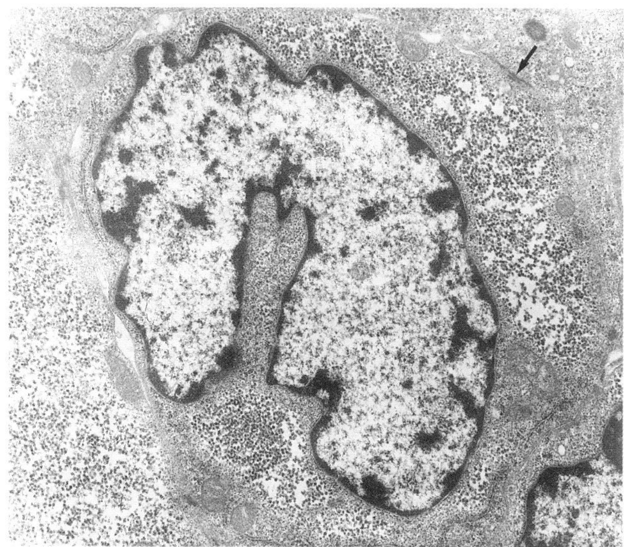

Fig. 5.15 (a) Ewing's sarcoma. Nest of round to polygonal monomorphic tumor cells containing focal deposits of cytoplasmic glycogen particles and few cytoplasmic organelles, uniform nuclei with finely dispersed chromatin (euchromatin) and mostly inconspicuous nucleoli. No junctions or cell processes. (Uranyl acetate and lead citrate ×13 000) (b) Ewing's sarcoma. Detail of a tumor cell showing sparse organelles, such as mitochondria and free ribosomes, and large pools of cytoplasmic glycogen rosettes. A primitive intercellular junction is seen (arrow) as a discrete density of the cell membrane. Note a prominent nuclear cleft. (Uranyl acetate and lead citrate ×23 000)

a greater variation in size and contour with a prominent heterochromatic nucleus with a large nucleolus and more conspicuous intermediate filaments and cell junctions.

Peculiar ultrastructural features have been reported in Ewing's sarcoma, such as nuclear filamentous paramyxovirus-like inclusions,[100] bundles of tonofilaments with keratin positivity[101] and banded structures with a periodicity of 250 nm[102] (perhaps a new form of long-spacing collagen).

Two points are interesting from an ultrastructural point of view. First is the problem of neuroectodermal differentiation as dentritic processes containing dense-core granules and longitudinally aligned microtubules, considered to be neuroblastoma-like features have been described.[97,103] Ultrastructural studies of 71 cases of typical Ewing's sarcoma revealed no evidence of neuroectodermal differentiation[13] but in atypical forms, electron microscopy can reveal the evidence of neuroblastic features[92] fuelling the debate about the reality of peripheral PNET and the real place of Ewing's sarcoma.

At the ultrastructural level, the tumor cells of *peripheral neuroectodermal tumors of bone* closely resemble Ewing's sarcoma, but from the ultrastructural point of view, some authors find it difficult to believe that Ewing's sarcoma is a peripheral PNET.[13,97] The cells are characterized by a few bounded dense-core granules interpreted as neurosecretion, neuromicrotubules and more dendritic-like cell processes.[92,104,105] Electron microscopy is one of the important ways to identify this entity. The ultrastructural features resemble peripheral neuroepithelioma and neuroectodermal tumors.[97,105]

Second, ultrastructural study is still of interest for the differential diagnosis of small round cell tumors of bone.[106,107] Small cell osteosarcoma shows more organelles and forms osteoid but mesenchymal chondrosarcoma cells can be indistinguishable from those of Ewing's sarcoma.[95] Neuroblastoma contains synaptic junctions and interdigitating cytoplasmic processes with production of neurites containing microtubules, neurotubules and a few dense-core mitochondria and secretory granules, usually without glycogen.[108,109] A lymphoma may be possible when glycogen is sparse or absent and tiny junctions are present but immunohistochemistry makes the distinction between lymphoma and other neoplasms. In most cells of embryonal rhabdomyosarcoma, there is early formation of myofibrils with single thick (myosin) filaments and adjacent thin (actin) filaments. Irregular electron-dense bodies (Z lines) may be seen along the fibrils.

SPECIAL PROBLEMS

The contribution of electron microscopy to improving diagnosis and explaining pathogenesis is discussed in the following three entities: chordoma, adamantinoma and fibrous dysplasia.

Chordoma

The following ultrastructural features characterize the conventional form of chordoma in which physaliferous cells are prominent.[13,110–119]

The cytoplasm contains some glycogen granules and occasionally lipid droplets, scattered ribosomes and well-developed Golgi apparatus. Also present are scattered cytoplasmic vacuoles of various size. Some appear as intra-cytoplasmic lumens studded by sparse microvilli.

The vacuoles of the physaliferous cells are important. Some may represent sequestered extracellular space, while others are dilated intercellular spaces lined by microvilli. There are also small membrane-bound, glycogen-containing vacuoles, in addition to free cytoplasmic glycogen.[110,119]

Another ultrastructural characteristic of chordoma is a close relationship between mitochondria and rough endoplasmic reticulum profiles in the cytoplasm. Their significance is unknown. These mitochondria–RER complexes are considered to be typical of chordomas where they are seen frequently but not in all cases.[112,122–124] The mitochondrial membranes are compressed with a thinner middle compartment, as seen in Figure 5.16a and b. The aspect is that of dumb-bell-shaped mitochondria with bulbous ends alternating with profiles of rough endoplasmic reticulum in a regular fashion. Sometimes circular rings are seen when mitochondria are partially or completely surrounded by a strand of rough endoplasmic reticulum.

The dilated rough endoplasmic reticulum may be filled with a proteinaceous material such as collagen, glycoaminoglycans and glycoproteins or is left empty by degenerative changes.[59]

Nuclei are irregular with marked indentations and single prominent nucleoli or mostly rounded with smooth outlines. Some physaliferous cells are multinucleated.

Intercellular junctions, such as zonula adherens or desmosomes with associated cytokeratin filaments, are fairly frequent and support the epithelial nature of this tumor.

Chordoma is a well-known example of a tumor in which the formation of both tonofilaments and bundles of intermediate-type filaments and desmosomes (or desmosome-like cell junctions) are observed,[13, 118, 123, 125] as well as cytoplasmic processes and pinocytotic vesicles.

Basement membrane material[118,123] or a discontinous basal lamina is occasionally seen.

The extracellular matrix is often abundant and myxoid similar to myxoid chondrosarcoma or it may have a finely granular appearance with proteoglycan particles.[123,127]

Using electron microscopy, five stages of evolution have been described for the tumor cells[127] with a progressive increase of glycogen particles. Spindle cells, stellate cells and physaliferous cells appear to belong to the spectrum of a single cell type[110,113,114,117,128] rather than being distinct cells.[111,117]

Although usually absent in classic chordoma, the presence of microtubular inclusions within the endoplasmic reticulum seems to be of diagnostic importance. Even though they are not specific (for example, they are observed in myxoid chondrosarcoma[66]), these inclusions are considered to be an important feature in support of the concept of 'chondroid chordoma'.[128] These crystalline, tubular structures in the rough endoplasmic reticulum,

arranged in parallel arrays, were first described by Valderrama et al[129] in two cases of so-called chondroid chordoma. The ultrastructural detection of these images thus seems to constitute a helpful differential marker for this unusual form of chordoma. However these microtubular inclusions are not specific as they are reported, although rarely detected, in conventional chordoma.[124,130] Compared to classic chordomas, relatively few desmosomes and intermediate filaments are noticed in chondroid chordomas.[131] As stated by Erlandson, 'It is possible that chondroid chordomas may be a heterogeneous group of neoplasms'.[13]

Electron microscopy can be helpful in identifying the

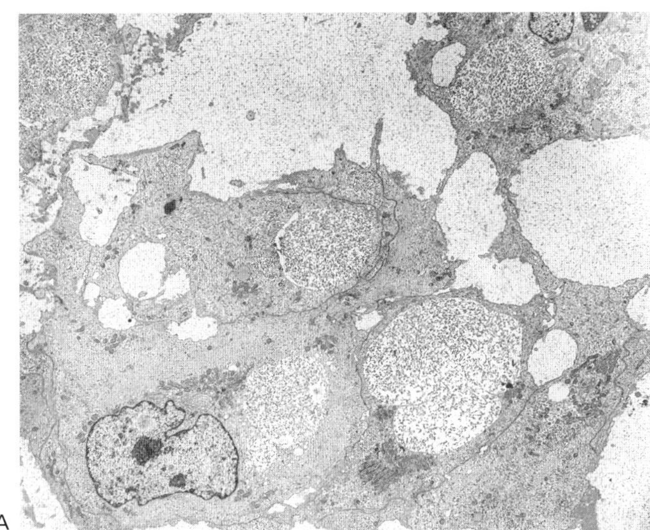

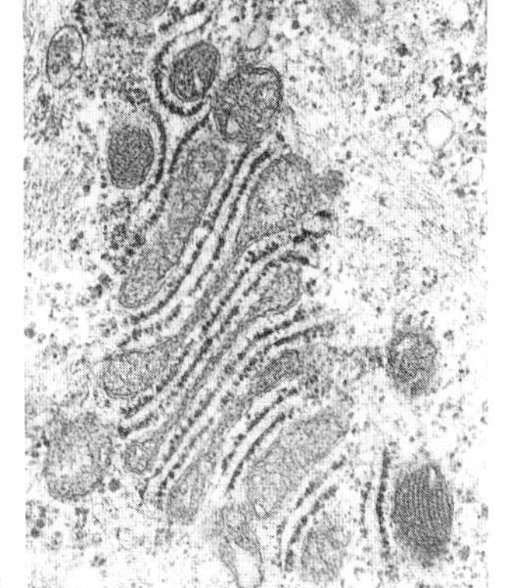

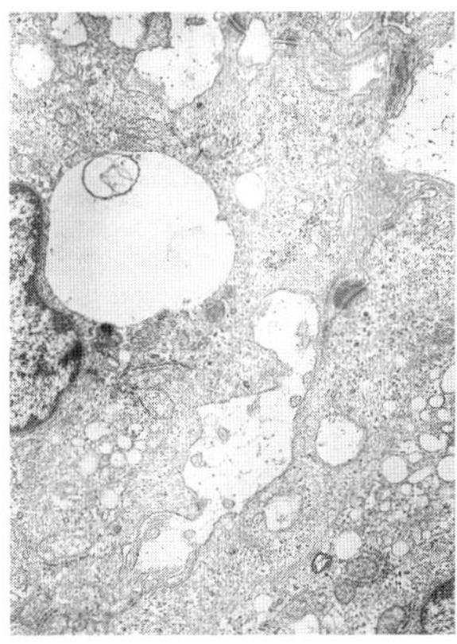

Fig. 5.16 (a) Chordoma. Electron micrograph of cluster of physaliferous tumor cells showing abundant membrane-bound glycogen deposits. In the lower left corner, intracytoplasmic fibrils occupy most of the cell cytoplasm. An abundant granular loose matrix contains proteoglycan particles. Intercellular cystic space and intracytoplasmic lumen are bordered by low microvillous projections. (Uranyl acetate and lead citrate ×11 500) (b) Chordoma. Detail of mitochondria–RER complexes. Note that the mitochondria are attenuated in the central regions and bulbous at their ends. In the lower left area, intermediate filaments are seen. (Uranyl acetate and lead citrate ×29 000) (c) Chordoma. Detail. Cytoplasmic clear vacuoles of various sizes and several desmosome-like junctions are visible. In the center, immature microvillous processes are seen in a dilated intercellular space. (Uranyl acetate and lead citrate ×22 000)

components of a *dedifferentiated chordoma*[13,117,132] and also for differential diagnosis, as in the case of a chordoma presenting as a soft tissue tumor unrelated to bone. Ultrastructural study provides elements for the differential diagnosis in cases of extraskeletal myxoid chondrosarcomas and parachordomas. The cells of an extraskeletal myxoid chondrosarcoma show no evidence of tonofilaments, desmosomal junctions or mitochondria–RER complexes. These organized complexes have however been described in grade I chondrosarcomas.[13] Ultrastructural features of chordomas are similar to those observed in the entity called parachordoma, especially the primitive cell junctions, discontinuous basal lamina, surface projections, small lumina with microvillous-like projections, bundles of intermediate filaments, glycogen particles and cytoplasmic vacuoles.[59,115,121,125,133] These are also seen in chordoma-like soft tissue sarcomas,[134] the differences being very subtle. The clustering of the cells within a largely structureless stroma is also comparable, but much greater variations in the size and cytoplasmic contents of cells are observed in

chordomas and the large vacuolated physaliferous cells do not have a close parallel in parachordomas.

The characteristics of the matrix may help to differentiate these tumors. In chondrosarcoma, fine fibrils, vesicles and granules are observed. In chordoma, the matrix is scarce and finely granular or may appear amorphous. In chordoid sarcoma, as well as in extraskeletal myxoid chondrosarcoma, the stromal component is a fibrillary and/or granular amorphous material.[116] The matrix also differs from metastatic adenocarcinoma but the findings of desmosomes and intracytoplasmic lumina bordered by microvilli may be similar.[125]

Adamantinoma

This tumor shows similar pleomorphism at the ultrastructural and histological levels. Desmosomes, basal lamina and cytoplasmic bundles of tonofilaments characterize this lesion.[135–141] The cells look like keratinocytes. The cytoplasm contains the usual organelles: mitochondria, endoplasmic reticulum, Golgi apparatus and a few glycogen

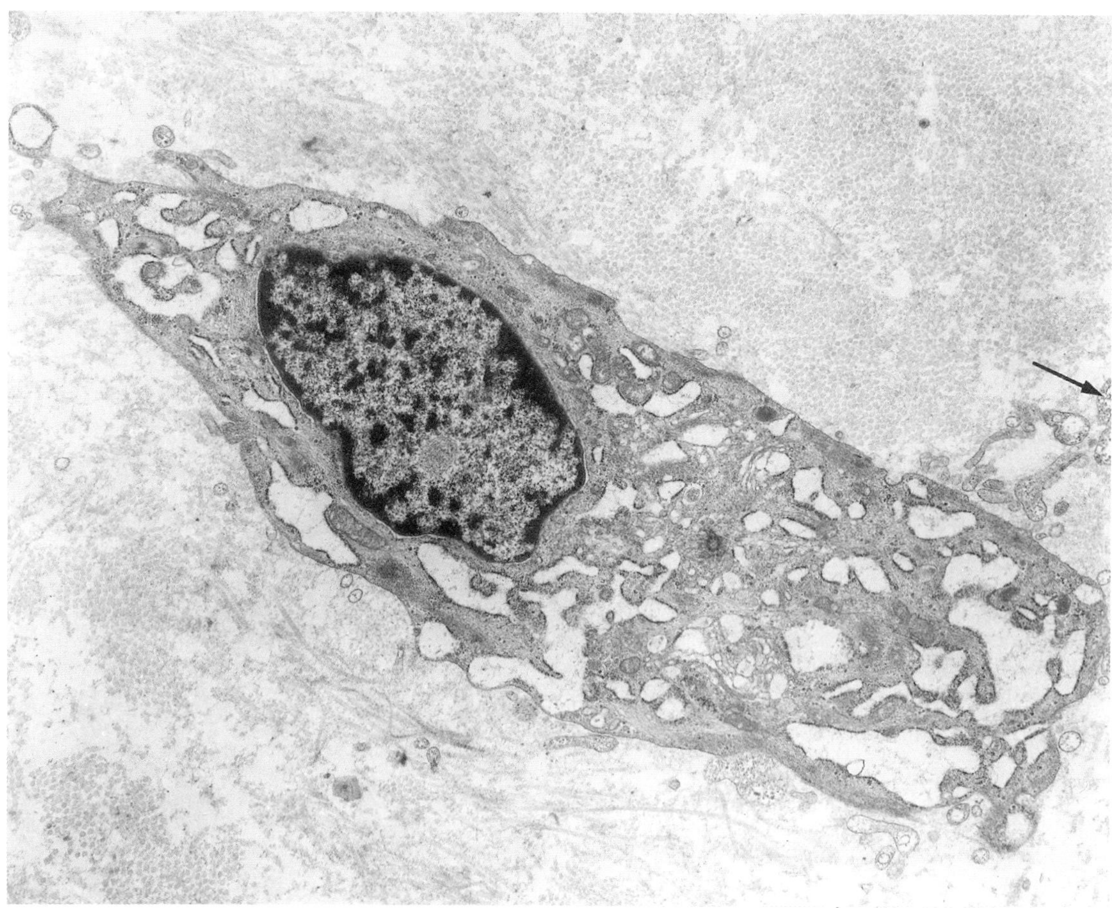

Fig. 5.17 Fibrous dysplasia. Spindle-shaped myofibroblastic cell with dilated well-developed rough endoplasmic reticulum and microfilaments in the peripheral area of the cytoplasm. Scanty glycogen particles are seen in short cell processes (arrow). The centriole is not far from the Golgi apparatus. The extracellular matrix is collagen. (Uranyl acetate and lead citrate ×13 500)

granules. These epithelial cells exhibit cytoplasmic extensions and, often, microvilli. Actin myofilaments have been reported,[139,141] and, as in our experience, rudimentary cilia.[141] More interesting are the ultrastructural features of endothelial differentiation, including rod-shaped structures interpreted as Weibel–Palade bodies:[142, 143] although published illustrations are not very convincing.

The intercellular matrix is composed of collagen fibers with capillaries. Spindle-shaped fibroblasts and rare myofibroblasts are observed and constitute the mesenchymal component. An amorphous granular proteoglycan-like material occupies the intercellular spaces.[144]

Fibrous dysplasia

In the fibrous component, the cells are fibroblasts, myofibroblasts and many intermediate types. In the cytoplasm of most of the cells, the rough endoplasmic reticulum and Golgi complexes are well developed. Lipid droplets and glycogen may be present.[13,16,145,146] Other elongated cells resemble myofibroblasts (Fig. 5.16) with the typical myofilaments at the periphery of the cytoplasm and dense bodies along these filaments. An incomplete basal lamina is not infrequent.

The central nucleus shows a condensation of heterochromatin against the nuclear membrane[146] and a prominent nucleolus with an irregular contour. Sometimes a prominent fibrous lamina[147,148] is reported.

Usually, the spindle-shaped cells are arranged in parallel with the collagen bundles. In the osseous component, the osteoblast-like cells have a fibroblastic appearance. The matrix consists of osteoid and immature woven bone trabeculae. The presence of well-defined matrix vesicles is reported.[146,148,149] The ultrastructural aspects seem to be related to an abnormal osteoblastic maturation of the bone-forming mesenchyme.

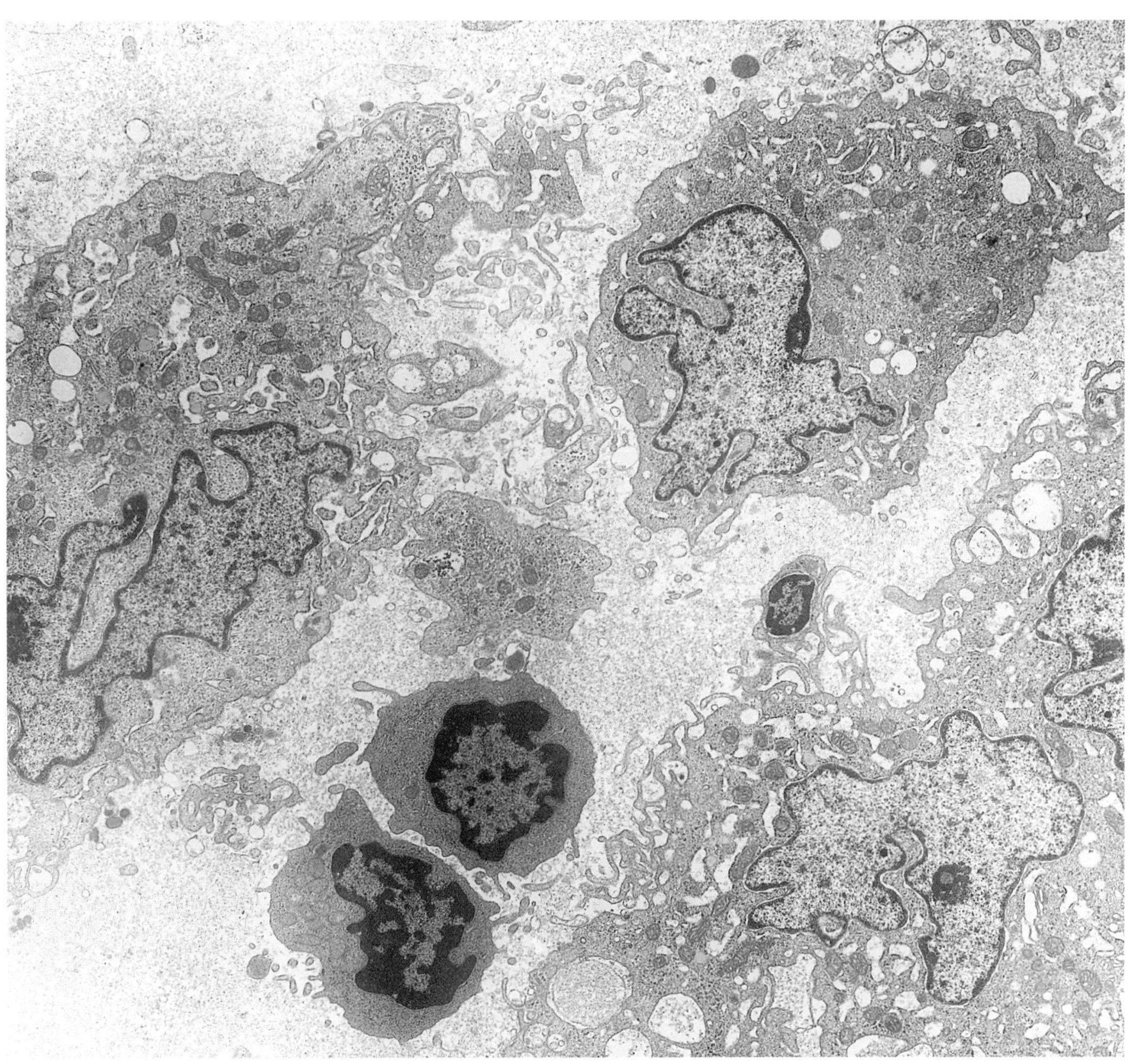

Fig. 5.18 Eosinophilic granuloma. Electron micrograph showing mononuclear histiocytic cells with irregular, deeply cleaved nuclei and two eosinophils. (Uranyl acetate and lead citrate ×15 000)

ULTRASTRUCTURAL MARKERS

The search for specific ultrastructural markers is one of the aims of electron microscopy. In some instances such as paramyxovirus-like inclusions and Birbeck bodies, the findings are often regarded as specific but are not truly pathognomonic.

Eosinophilic granuloma

Histiocytosis X is thought to be a proliferative disease of Langerhans cells characterized by the presence of a highly specific marker, Birbeck bodies or granules. The widespread distribution of Langerhans cells in pathologic tissues has been shown by electron microscopy and immunohistochemistry[150] and thus Birbeck bodies are not pathognomonic of histiocytosis X. The ultrastructural appearances are similar to those of other histiocytes and to Langerhans cells of the skin.

In bone lesions,[13,151–155] the cytoplasm of Langerhans-like cells contain various types of rod-shaped, flask-shaped or tennis racket-shaped Birbeck granules which are most commonly found at or near the cell membrane (Figs 5.18, 5.19).

The abundant cytoplasm presents the usual well-developed organelles: ribosomes, mitochondria, rough ER and prominent Golgi complex with a variable number of cytoplasmic vacuoles and primary and secondary lysosomes.

The cell surface is raised into filopodia. Moderate to extreme convolution of the cell membranes can be observed. Cell junctions and basal lamina are absent. The nucleus is irregular and indented.

Birbeck bodies, the hallmark of these histiocytes (Fig. 5.19), have the two-dimensional appearance of pentalaminar structures of about 34 nm in width[13,156] and various profile lengths (between 190 and 360 nm); a few are in continuity with the cell surface membrane.

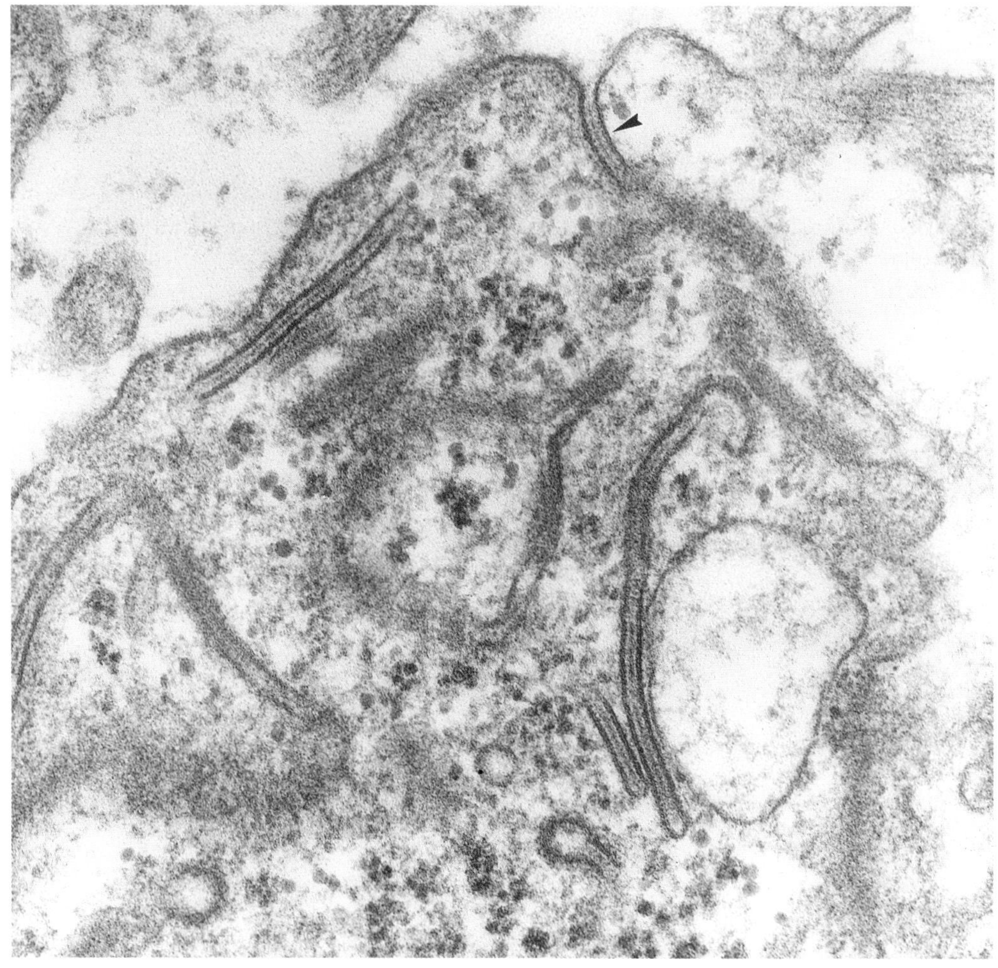

Fig. 5.19 Eosinophilic granuloma. High power view showing cytoplasmic detail of a histiocyte containing multiple Birbeck bodies of various shapes. One is closely associated with the cell membrane (arrowhead) as an invagination. Another opens on a vesicle (distended into a sac). The pentalaminar zipper-like core and rod-shaped structure is apparent. The parallel membranes with a central axial line are visible. (Uranyl acetate and lead citrate ×40 000)

Invaginations of the plasmalemmal membrane are supposed to be the origin of this zipper-like structure. The dense central line with a periodicity of about 9–12 nm between the opposing membranes of the granules probably represents a cellular surface coating similar to a glycocalyx. Its three-dimensional shape is a cup or a disk or a combination of the two.

Birbeck bodies have been reported in mitotically active cells.[15]

Some intercellular membranes, under special conditions, can look like Birbeck granules, even in epithelial cells (enterocytes).[157] These images have to be compared with those of peculiar intercellular attachments. Where neighboring cells are in contact, rare intercellular Birbeck-like pentalaminar structures, with membranes belonging to opposing cells, can be seen. Some of these complexes show distinct periodicity of the central lamina (the sandwiched lattice layer) and are morphologically indistinguishable from the pentalaminar component of nearby Birbeck granules; the term 'lattice junction' is proposed for this supposed specific junctional structure of monohistiocytic cells[155] which can occur in a variety of circumstances.[156]

Trilaminar membranous loops[154,156,158] are often unusual but non-specific cytoplasmic membranous complexes most commonly observed in the Langerhans-like cell. Also called worm-like particles, cored tubules, octopus-like images and comma-shaped bodies, they are tortuous and do not show central lamellae.

Lysosomal granules with lamellar internal membranes are also described as potentially useful diagnostic features.[154]

The presence of Langerhans cell granules seems to be a constant feature in histiocytosis X, but is without pronostic significance.[154]

Paget's disease and paramyxovirus-like inclusions in bone diseases not associated with Paget's disease

In Paget's disease, ultrastructural examination of the osteoclasts reveals cytoplasmic and nuclear inclusions[159–164] that resemble the nucleocapsids of the *Paramyxoviridae* virus.[165–169] They are located in one or more nuclei in the same field. Inclusions are present in 85% of the osteoclasts and involve 15–75% of the nuclear cross-sectioned area.[165] They are much more numerous in the cytoplasm than in the nuclei.

Cytoplasmic inclusions are seen in 30–40% of pagetic biopsies[165] and appear randomly dispersed. One case of osteosarcoma in Paget's disease[166] has been reported with nuclear inclusions in the osteosarcomatous component.

Inclusions with the same ultrastructural features, are found in the nuclei of some other pathologic conditions, such as giant cell tumor of bone (Fig. 5.20a). They appear as bundles of parallel tubulofilamentous structures more or less randomly oriented, dispersed or in stacked parallel rows or forming a thumbprint, with paracristalline arrangement (Fig. 5.20b). The filamentous structures are 12–15 nm in diameter and 100–300 µm long[163] with a

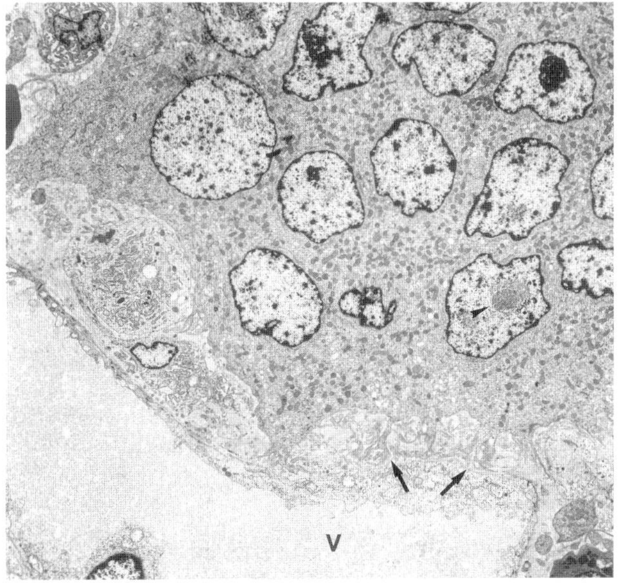

A

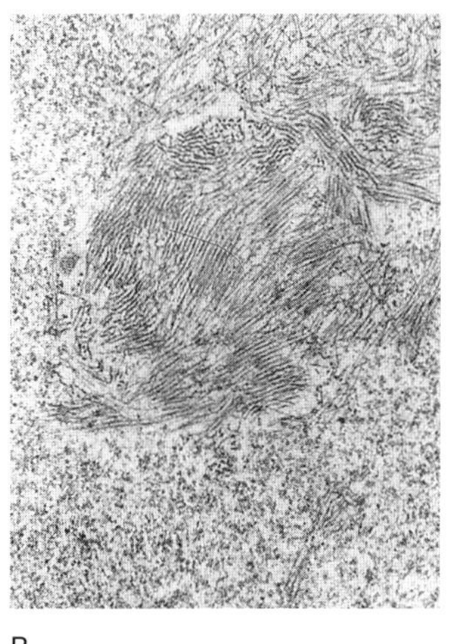

B

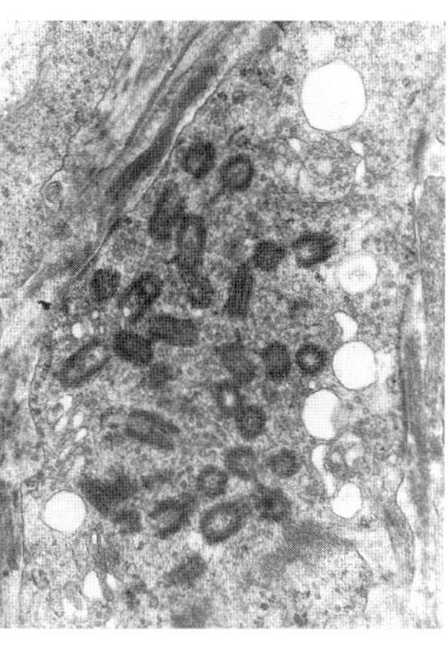

C

Fig. 5.20 (a) Giant cell tumor of bone. Osteoclast-like cell showing multiple nuclei. One of them contains a filamentous inclusion (arrowhead). Numerous round or oval mitochondria and vesicles are seen in the cytoplasm. At the bottom, a ruffled border (arrows) is observed near the lumen of a vessel (V). (Uranyl acetate and lead citrate ×9000) (b) Giant cell tumor of bone. Detail of a tubulofilamentous intranuclear inclusion in tissue culture. (Uranyl acetate and lead citrate ×21 000) (c) Giant cell tumor of bone. Giant centrosphere made of diplosomes observed in a cytoplasmic extension of a multinucleated giant cell. (Uranyl acetate and lead citrate ×20 500)

clear central core and peripheral densities of about 5–7 nm in diameter. A distance of 20 nm regularly separates the filaments. A light and dark periodicity of about 5 nm[160,172] or 10–12 nm[164] according to the literature, gives the filaments a striated appearance, probably due to a helical formation.[161,164,168]

A goniometric study has shown a group of parallel microtubules with a triangular arrangement and a center-to-center distance of 30 nm. Some inclusions appeared to be composed of two sets of tubules at an angle of about 60°. The measurement cannot be considered valid however, unless the sections are not truly longitudinal.[169] The size of the inclusion area is not constant; sometimes two or more clusters are observed, not membrane bound and not attached to the nucleolus. These findings show similarities to measles virus infection[170] and to the virus of subacute sclerosing panencephalitis.[171]

Osteoclasts of Paget's disease are involved in active bone resorption and present a well-developed, deeply folded ruffled border and a high number of nuclei with varying sizes and shapes in the same cell.[164] Cell membrane interdigitations between mononuclear cells and osteoclasts occur frequently and seem to indicate an increased tendency to cell fusion.[162] No mitoses are found in any of the giant cells. The cytoplasmic organelles are those usually encountered in osteoclast-like cells (Figs 5.5, 5.20a). The centrioles are either near a nucleus or grouped in a giant centrosphere near the cell membrane in a cell process[19] (Fig. 5.20c).

As previously indicated, nuclear inclusions in giant cell tumors of bone are identical to those found in Paget's disease[164, 172–176] but less frequent. Forty-nine percent of 43 cases of giant cell tumors of bone, either fresh or cultured, have shown these ultrastructural inclusions.[176] In our series of 73 giant cell tumors studied ultrastructurally, a meticulous search for nuclear inclusions showed the same percentage of inclusions. These inclusions have also been described in giant cell tumors associated with Paget's disease[177] and in other skeletal disorders: two brothers with pycnodysostosis,[178] one case of oxalosis,[179] one case of Ewing's sarcoma[100] and three cases of osteopetrosis.[180,181] It is surprising that the inclusions are seen in reduced bone resorption – osteopetrosis – and in increased osteoclastic activity – Paget's disease.[182] Very similar paramyxovirus-like inclusions are also observed in polymyositis[183–185] where they appear in the nucleus and/or the cytoplasm. The real significance of these inclusions in bone pathology is still uncertain.

REFERENCES

1. Erlandson R A, Rosaï J. A realistic approach to the use of electron microscopy and other ancillary diagnostic techniques in surgical pathology. Am J Surg Pathol 1995: 19: 247–250
2. Kindblom L G. Light and electron microscopic examination of embedded fine-needle aspiration biopsy specimens in the preoperative diagnosis of soft tissue and bone tumors. Cancer 1983: 51: 2264–2277
3. Walaas L, Kindblom L G, Gunterberg B, Bergh P. Light and electron microscopic examination of fine needle aspirates in the preoperative diagnosis of osteogenic tumors. A study of 21 osteosarcomas and two osteoblastomas. Diagn Cytopathol 1990: 6: 27–38
4. Walaas L, Kindblom L G, Gunterberg B, Bergh P. Light and electron microscopic examination of fine needle aspirates in the preoperative diagnosis of cartilaginous tumors. Diagn Cytopathol 1990: 6: 396–408
5. Ghadially F N. Ultrastructure of the cell and matrix. 3rd ed. London: Butterworth, 1988
6. Murray A B, Buscher H, Erfle V, Biehl T, Gossner W. Intranuclear undulating membranous structures in cells of a human parosteal osteosarcoma. Ultrastruct Pathol 1983: 5: 163–170
7. Marquart K H. Intracisternal crystalline arrays of coated parallel tubules in cells of a human osteosarcoma. Virchows Arch Pathol Anat Pathol Anat Histol 1981: 391: 309–313
8. Murray A B, Becke H, Marquart K H. Vermicellar bodies on osteosarcoma cell nuclei. Ultrastruct Pathol 1984: 6: 363
9. Fornasier V L. Osteoid: an ultrastructural study. Hum Pathol 1977: 8: 243–254
10. Sela J. Bone remodeling in pathologic conditions. A scanning electron microscopic study. Calcif Tissue Res 1977: 23: 229–234
11. Sela J, Bab I A, Muhlrad A, Stein H. Extracellular matrix vesicles in human osteogenic neoplasm: an ultrastructural and enzymatic study. Cancer 1981: 48: 1602–1610
12. Hunziker E, Herrmann W. Ultrastructure of cartilage. In: Bonucci E, Motta P M, Eds. Ultrastructure of skeletal tissues. Boston: Kluwer, 1990, pp 79–99
13. Erlandson R A. Diagnostic transmission electron microscopy of tumors. New York: Raven Press, 1994
14. Steiner G C. Ultrastructure of osteoblastoma. Cancer 1977: 39: 2127–2136
15. Aparisi T, Arborgh B, Ericsson J L E. Studies on the fine structure of osteoblastoma with notes on the localization of nonspecific acid and alkaline phosphatase. Cancer 1978: 41: 1811–1822
16. Johannessen J V. Soft tissues, bones and joints. In: Johannessen J V, Ed. Electron microscopy in human medicine, vol 4. New York: McGraw-Hill, 1981
17. Scherft J P, Groot C G. The electron microscopic structure of the osteoblast. In: Bonucci E, Motta P M, Eds. Ultrastructure of skeletal tissues. Boston: Kluwer, 1990, pp 209–222
18. Steiner G C. The ultrastructure of bone tumors. In: Bonucci E, Motta P M, Eds. Ultrastructure of skeletal tissues. Boston: Kluwer, 1990, pp 271–291
19. Vacher-Lavenu M C, Louvel A, Daudet-Monsac M, Abelanet R. Configuration et position des centrioles des cellules mono et multinucléées des tumeurs à cellules géantes des os longs. Ann Anat Pathol (Paris) 1981: 25: 331–339
20. Bonucci E, De Santis E. Ultrastructure of osteoblastoma with particular reference to calcification and matrix vesicles. In: Donath A, Courvoisier B, Eds. Bone and tumors. Berne: Hans Huber, 1980, pp 232–236
21. Sela J, Bab I A, Muhlrad A, Stein H. Extracellular matrix vesicles in human osteogenic neoplasm: an ultrastructural and enzymatic study. Cancer 1981: 48: 1602–1610
22. Ghadially F N, Metha P N. Ultrastructure of osteogenic sarcoma. Cancer 1970: 25: 1457–1467
23. Ferguson R J, Yunis E J. The ultrastructure of human osteosarcoma: a study of nine cases. Clin Orthop 1978: 131: 234–246
24. Garbe L, Monges G, Pellegrin E, Payan H. Ultrastructural study of osteosarcomas. Hum Pathol 1981: 12: 891–896

25. Grundmann E, Roessner A, Immenkamp M. Tumor cells in osteosarcoma as revealed by electron microscopy. Implications for histogenesis and subclassification. Virchows Arch B Cell Pathol Incl Mol Pathol 1981: 36: 257–273

26. Aparisi T, Stark A, Ericsson J L. Human osteogenic sarcoma. Study of the ultrastructure with special notes on the localization of alkaline and acid phosphatase. Int Orthop 1982: 6: 171–179

27. Martinez-Tello F J, Navas-Palacios J J. The ultrastructure of conventional, parosteal, and periosteal osteosarcomas. Cancer 1982: 50: 949–961

28. Ballance W A, Mendelsohn G, Carter J R, Abdul-Karim F W, Jacobs G, Majley J T. Osteogenic sarcoma. Malignant fibrous histiocytoma subtype. Cancer 1988: 62: 763–771

29. Reddick R L, Michelitch H J, Levine A M, Triche T J. Osteogenic sarcoma: a study of the ultrastructure. Cancer 1980: 45: 64–71

30. Shapiro F. Ultrastructural observations on osteosarcoma tissue: a study of 10 cases. Ultrastruct Pathol 1983: 4: 151–161

31. Williams A H, Schwinn C P, Parker J W. The ultrastructure of osteosarcoma: a review of twenty cases. Cancer 1967: 37: 1293–1301

32. Stark A, Aparisi T, Ericsson J L. Human osteogenic sarcoma. Fine structure of the chondroblastic type. Ultrastruct Pathol 1984: 6: 51–67

33. Stark A, Aparisi T, Ericsson J L. Human osteogenic sarcoma. Fine structure of the fibroblastic type. Ultrastruct Pathol 1984: 7: 301–319

34. Aho A J, Aho H J. Ultrastructure of human osteosarcoma. Malignant transformation of a multipotential connective tissue cell. Pathol Res Pract 1982: 174: 53–67

35. Jenson A B, Spjut H J, Smith M N, Rapp F. Intracellular branched tubular structures in osteosarcoma. Cancer 1971: 27: 1440–1448

36. Paschall H A, Paschall M M. Electron microscopic observations of 20 human osteosarcomas. Clin Orthop 1975: 111: 42–56

37. Dardick I, Schatz J, Colgan T. Osteogenic sarcoma with epithelial differentiation. Ultrastruct Pathol 1992: 16: 463–474

38. Ringus J C, Riddell R H. Small cell osteosarcoma: ultrastructural description and differentiation from atypical Ewing's sarcoma. Lab Invest 1981: 44: 55A (abstract)

39. Dickersin G R, Rosenberg A E. The ultrastructure of small-cell osteosarcoma, with a review of the light microscopy and differential diagnosis. Hum Pathol 1991: 22: 267–275

40. Mawad J, Mackay B, Raymond A K, Ayala A G. Electron microscopy in the diagnosis of small cell tumors of bone. Ultrastruct Pathol 1994: 18: 263–268

41. Mawad J, Mackay B, Raymond A K. An ultrastructural study of small cell osteosarcoma. Mod Pathol 1988: 364: 61A (abstract)

42. Vuletin J C. Myofibroblasts in paraosteal osteogenic sarcoma. Arch Pathol Lab Med 1977: 101: 272

43. Reddick R L, Popovsky M A, Fantome J C, Michelitch H J. Paraosteal osteogenic osteosarcomas: ultrastructural observations in three cases. Hum Pathol 1980: 11: 373–380

44. Steiner G C. Ultrastructure of benign cartilaginous tumors of intraosseous origin. Hum Pathol 1979: 10: 71–86

45. Welsh R A, Mayer A T. A histogenetic study of chondroblastoma. Cancer 1964: 17: 578–589

46. Wellmann K F. Chondroblastoma of the scapula. A case report with ultrastructural observations. Cancer 1969: 24: 408–416

47. Huvos A G, Marcove R C, Erlandson R A, Mike V. Chondroblastoma of bone. A clinicopathologic and electron microscopic study. Cancer 1972: 29: 760–771

48. Levine G L, Bensch K G. Chondroblastoma – the nature of the basic cell. A study by means of histochemistry, tissue culture, electron microscopy and autoradiography. Cancer 1972: 29: 1546–1562

49. Meary R, Abelanet R, Forest M. Les chondroblastomes bénins des os. Etude anatomoclinique et ultrastructurale à propos de 11 observations. Rev Chir Orthop Reparatrice App Mot 1975: 61: 717–734

50. Ushigome S, Takakuwa T, Shinagawa T et al. Ultrastructure of cartilaginous tumors and S-100 protein in the tumors with reference to the chondroblastoma, chondromyxoid fibroma and mesenchymal chondrosarcoma. Acta Pathol Jpn 1984: 34: 1285–1300

51. Fadda M, Manunta A, Rinonapoli G, Zirattu G, De Santis E. Ultrastructural appearance of chondroblastoma. Int Orthop 1994: 18: 389–392

52. Mii Y, Miyauchi Y, Miura S et al. Ultrastructural cytochemical demonstration of proteoglycans and calcium in the extracellular matrix of chondroblastomas. Hum Pathol 1994: 25: 1290–1294

53. Morimoto K, Okada S. Electron microscopic and immunohistochemical studies on chondroblastoma (in Japanese). Nippon Seikeigeka Gakkai Zasshi 1992: 66: 668–674

54. Tornberg D N, Rice R W, Johnston A D. The ultrastructure of chondromyxoid fibroma. Its biologic and diagnosis implications. Clin Orthop 1973: 95: 295–299

55. Ushigome S, Sodemoto Y, Shinagawa T, Kishida H, Yamazaki M. Chondromyxoid fibroma of bone, an electron microscopic observation. Acta Pathol Jpn 1982: 32: 113–122

56. Ushigome S, Takakuwa T, Shinagawa T et al. Ultrastructure of cartilaginous tumors and S-100 protein in the tumors with reference to the chondroblastoma, chondromyxoid fibroma and mesenchymal chondrosarcoma. Acta Pathol Jpn 1984: 34: 1285–1300

57. Erlandson R A, Huvos A G. Chondrosarcoma: a light and electron microscopic study. Cancer 1974: 34: 1642–1652

58. Pardo-Mindan F J, Guillen F J, Villas C, Vasquez J J. A comparative ultrastructural study of chondrosarcoma, chordoid sarcoma, and chordoma. Cancer 1981: 47: 2611–2619

59. Povysil C, Matejovsky Z. A comparative ultrastructural study of chondrosarcoma, chordoid sarcoma, chordoma and chordoma periphericum. Pathol Res Pract 1985: 179: 546–559

60. Martinez-Tello F J, Navas-Palacios J J. Ultrastructural study of conventional chondrosarcomas and myxoid and mesenchymal chondrosarcomas. Virchows Arch A Pathol Anat Histol 1982: 396: 197–211

61. Ghadially F N, Lalonde J M A, Yong N K. Amianthoid fibres in a chondrosarcoma. J Pathol 1980: 130: 147–151

62. Del Rosario A D, Bui H X, Singh J, Ginsburg R, Ross J S. Intracytoplasmic eosinophilic hyaline globules in cartilaginous neoplasms: a surgical, pathological, ultrastructural, and electron probe X-ray microanalytic study. Hum Pathol 1994: 25: 1283–1289

63. Jaworski R C. Intramitochondrial paracrystalline inclusion in chondrosarcoma. Pathology 1984: 16: 172–173

64. Vernick S H, Kay S, Escobar M, Sperber E, Rosato F. Intracisternal tubules in myxoid chondrosarcoma. Arch Pathol Lab Med 1977: 101: 566

65. Wetzel W J, Reuhl K R. Microtubular aggregates in the rough endoplasmic reticulum of a myxoid chondrosarcoma. Ultrastruct Pathol 1980: 1: 519–525

66. Wolford J F, Bedetti C D. Skeletal myxoid chondrosarcoma with microtubular aggregates within endoplasmic reticulum. Arch Pathol Lab Med 1988: 112: 77–81

67. Payne C, Dardick I, Mackay B. Extraskeletal myxoid chondrosarcoma with intracisternal microtubules. Ultrastruct Pathol 1994: 18: 257–261

68. Forest M, Le Charpentier Y, Postel M et al. Une nouvelle variété de chondrosarcome: les sarcomes dits 'chondroblastiques' ou chondrosarcomes 'à cellules claires'. Etude anatomo-clinique et ultrastructurale de 5 observations. Arch Anat Cytol Pathol 1978: 26: 5–11

69. Le Charpentier Y, Forest M, Postel M, Tomeno B, Abelanet R. Clear-cell chondrosarcoma. A report of five cases including ultrastructural study. Cancer 1979: 44: 622–629

70. Angervall L, Kinblom L G. Clear cell chondrosarcoma. A light- and electron microscopic and histochemical study of two cases. Virchows Arch Pathol Anat Histol 1980: 389: 27–41

71. Faraggiana T, Sender B, Glicksman P. Light- and electron-microscopic study of clear cell chondrosarcoma. Am J Clin Pathol 1981: 75: 117–121

72. Ohno T, Park P, Oguro K et al. Ultrastructural study of a clear cell chondrosarcoma. Ultrastruct Pathol 1986: 10: 321–330

73. Têtu B, Ordonez N G, Ayala A G, Mackay B. Chondrosarcoma with additional mesenchymal component (dedifferentiated chondrosarcoma) II. An immunohistochemical and electron microscopic study. Cancer 1986: 58: 287–298

74. Abenoza P, Neumann P M, Manivel C, Wick M R. Dedifferentiated chondrosarcoma: an ultrastructural study of two cases, with immunocytochemical correlations. Ultrastruct Pathol 1986: 10: 529–538

75. Astorino R N, Tesluk H. Dedifferentiated chondrosarcoma with a rhabdomyosarcomatous component. Hum Pathol 1985: 16: 318–320

76. Kahn L B. Chondrosarcoma with dedifferentiated foci. A comparative and ultrastructural study. Cancer 1976: 37: 1365–1375

77. Jaworski R C. Dedifferentiated chondrosarcoma. An ultrastructural study. Cancer 1984: 53: 2674–2678

78. Steiner G C, Mirra J M, Bullough P G. Mesenchymal chondrosarcoma. A study of the ultrastructure. Cancer 1973: 32: 929–939

79. Fu Y S, Kay S. A comparative ultrastructural study of mesenchymal chondrosarcoma and myxoid chondrosarcoma. Cancer 1974: 33: 1531–1542

80. Bertoni F, Picci P, Bacchini P et al. Mesenchymal chondrosarcoma of bone and soft tissues. Cancer 1983: 52: 533–541

81. Mikata A, Iri H, Inuyama Y. Mesenchymal chondrosarcoma: a case report with an ultrastructural study and review of Japanese literature. Acta Pathol Jpn 1977: 27: 93–109

82. Dobin S M, Donner L R, Speights V O Jr. Mesenchymal chondrosarcoma. A cytogenetic, immunohistochemical and ultrastructural study. Cancer Genet Cytogenet 1995: 83: 56–60

83. Friedman B, Gold H. Ultrastructure of Ewing's sarcoma of bone. Cancer 1968: 22: 307–322

84. Hou-Jensen K, Priori E, Dmochowski L. Studies on ultrastructure of Ewing's sarcoma of bone. Cancer 1972: 29: 280–286

85. Povysil C, Hatejovsky Z. Ultrastructure of Ewing's tumor. Virchows Arch A Pathol Anat Histol 1977: 374: 303–316

86. Mahoney J P, Alexander R W. Ewing's sarcoma. A light- and electron-microscopic study of 21 cases. Am J Surg Pathol 1978: 2: 283–298

87. Llombart-Bosch A, Blanche R, Peydro Olaya A. Ultrastructural study of 28 cases of Ewing's sarcoma: typical and atypical forms. Cancer 1978: 41: 1362–1378

88. Llombart-Bosch A, Peydro Olaya A, Gomar A. Ultrastructure of one Ewing's sarcoma of bone with endothelial character and a comparative review of the vessels in 27 cases of typical Ewing's sarcoma. Pathol Res Pract 1980: 167: 71–87

89. Llombart-Bosch A, Blache R, Peydro-Olaya A. Round-cell sarcoma of bone and their differential diagnosis (with particular emphasis on Ewing's sarcoma and reticulosarcoma). A study of 233 tumors with optical and electron microscopic techniques. Pathol Annu 1982: 17: 113–145

90. Llombart-Bosch A, Peydro-Olaya A. Scanning and transmission electron microscopy of Ewing's sarcoma of bone (typical and atypical variants). An analysis of nine cases. Virchows Arch A Pathol Anat Histopathol 1983: 398: 329–346

91. Llombart-Bosch A, Lacombe M J, Contesso G, Peydro-Olaya A. Small round blue cell sarcoma of bone mimicking atypical Ewing's sarcoma with neuroectodermal features. An analysis of five cases with immunohistochemical and electron microscopic support. Cancer 1987: 60: 1570–1582

92. Llombart-Bosch A, Lacombe M J, Peydro-Olaya A, Perez-Bacete M, Contesso G. Malignant peripheral neuroectodermal tumours of bone other than Askin's neoplasm: characterization of 14 new cases with immunohistochemistry and electron microscopy. Virchows Arch A Pathol Anat Histopathol 1988: 412: 421–430

93. Navas-Palacios J J, Aparicio-Duque R, Valdes M D. On the histogenesis of Ewing's sarcoma. An ultrastructural, immunohistochemical, and cytochemical study. Cancer 1984: 53: 1882–1901

94. Akhtar M, Ali M A, Sabbah R. Aspiration cytology of Ewing's sarcoma. Light and electron microscopic correlations. Cancer 1985: 56: 2051–2060

95. Mackay B, Donner L, Ordonez N G. Small round cell tumor. In: Russo J, Sommers SC, Eds. Tumor diagnosis by electron microscopy, vol 3. New York: Field & Wood, 1990, pp 281–313

96. Erlandson R A. Ewing's sarcoma with intermediate filaments (case 8). Ultrastruct Pathol 1983: 5: 323–328

97. Ushigome S, Shimoda T, Takaki K et al. Immunocytochemical and ultrastructural studies of the histogenesis of Ewing's sarcoma and putatively related tumors. Cancer 1989: 64: 52–62

98. Mierau G W. Extraskeletal Ewing's sarcoma (peripheral neuroepithelioma). Ultrastruct Pathol 1985: 9: 91–98

99. Roessner A, Voss B, Rauterberg J, Immenkamp M, Grundman E. Biologic characterization of human bone tumors. I. Ewing's sarcoma. A comparative electron and immunofluorescence microscopic study. J Cancer Res Clin Oncol 1982: 104: 171–180

100. Vacher-Lavenu M C, Carlioz A, Forest M, Tomeno B. Inclusions nucléaires dans un sarcome d'Ewing. Ann Pathol 1991: 11: 54–55

101. Greco M A, Steiner G C, Fazzini E. Ewing's sarcoma with epithelial differentiation: fine structural and immunohistochemical study. Ultrastruct Pathol 1988: 12: 317–325

102. Ghadially F N, Mierau G W. An unusual banded structure in Ewing's sarcomas. J Submicrosc Cytol 1985: 17: 645–650

103. Schmidt D, Mackay B, Ayala A G. Ewing's sarcoma with neuroblastoma-like features. Ultrastruct Pathol 1982: 3: 143–151

104. Jaffe R, Santamaria M, Yunis E J et al. The neuroectodermal tumor of bone. Am J Surg Pathol 1984: 8: 885–894

105. Steiner G C, Graham S, Lewis M M. Malignant round cell tumour of bone with neural differentiation (neuroectodermal tumour). Ultrastruct Pathol 1988: 12: 505–512

106. Mierau G W, Berry P J, Orsini E N. Small round cell neoplasm: can electron microscopy and immunohistochemical studies accurately classify them? Ultrastruct Pathol 1985: 9: 99–111

107. Mawad J K, Mackay B, Raymond A K, Ayala A G. Electron microscopy in the diagnosis of small round cell tumors of bone. Ultrastruct Pathol 1994: 18: 263–268

108. Triche T J, Ross W E. Glycogen containing neuroblastoma with clinical and histopathologic features of Ewing's sarcoma. Cancer 1978: 41: 1425–1432

109. Mackay B, Ordonez N G. Adult neuroblastoma of bone: a case report. Ultrastruct Pathol 1987: 11: 455–464

110. Friedmann I, Harrison D F N, Bird E S. The fine structure of chordoma with particular reference to the physaliferous cell. J Clin Pathol 1962: 15: 116–125

111. Spjut H J, Luse S A. Chordoma: an electron microscopic study. Cancer 1964: 17: 643–656

112. Erlandson R A, Tandler B, Lieberman P H, Higinbotham N L. Ultrastructure of human chordoma. Cancer Res 1968: 28: 2115–2125

113. Murad T M, Murthy M S N. Ultrastructure of chordoma. Cancer 1970: 25: 1204–1215

114. Pena C E, Horvat B L, Fisher E R. The ultrastructure of chordoma. Am J Clin Pathol 1970: 53: 544–551

115. Kay S, Schatzki P F. Ultrastructural observations of a chordoma arising in the clivus. Hum Pathol 1972: 3: 403–413

116. Pardo-Mindan F J, Guillen F J, Villas C, Vasquez J J. A comparative ultrastructural study of chondrosarcoma, chordoid chordoma and chordoma. Cancer 1981: 47: 2611–2619

117. Miettinen M, Lehto V P, Virtanen I. Malignant fibrous histiocytoma within a recurrent chordoma: a light microscopic, electron microscopic and immunohistochemical study. Am J Clin Pathol 1984: 82: 738–743

118. Persson S, Kindblom L G, Angervall L. Classical and chondroid chordoma. A light-microscopic, histochemical, ultrastructural and immunohistochemical analysis of the various cell types. Pathol Res Pract 1991: 187: 828–838

119. Kubota T, Sato K, Kabuto H et al. Immunohistochemical and ultrastructural study of skull base chordomas. Noshuyo Byori 1994: 11: 23–28

120. Wick M R, Burgess J H, Manivel J C. A reassessment of 'chordoid sarcoma'. Ultrastructural and immunohistochemical comparison with chordoma and skeletal myxoid chondrosarcoma. Mod Pathol 1988: 1: 433–443

121. Carstens P H B. Chordoid tumor: a light, electron microscopic, and immunohistochemical study. Ultrastruct Pathol 1995: 19: 291–295

122. Moss T H. Chordomas. In: Tumours of the nervous system. An ultrastructural atlas. Berlin: Springer-Verlag, 1986, pp 129–135

123. Rutherfoord G S, Davies A G. Chordoma – ultrastructure and immunohistochemistry: a report based on the examination of six cases. Histopathology 1987: 11: 775–787
124. Ueda Y, Nakanishi I. Microtubular aggregates in the rough endoplasmic reticulum of sacrococcygeal chordoma. Ultrastruct Pathol 1991: 15: 77–82
125. Ghadially F N. Diagnostic electron microscopy of tumours. 2nd ed. London: Butterworth, 1985
126. Walaas L, Kindblom L G. Fine-needle aspiration biopsy in the preoperative diagnosis of chordoma: a study of 17 cases with application of electron microscopic, histochemical, and immunocytochemical examination. Hum Pathol 1991: 22: 22–28
127. Thiery J P, Mazabraud A, Mognot J, Durigon M. Etude au microscope électronique d'un chordome sacré. Caractérisation de diverses étapes évolutives des cellules tumorales. Ann Anat Pathol 1977: 22: 193–204
128. Mierau G W, Weeks D A. Chondroid chordoma. Ultrastruct Pathol 1987: 11: 731–737
129. Valderrama E, Lipper S, Kahn L B, Marc J. Chondroid chordoma: electron-microscopic study of two cases. Am J Surg Pathol 1983: 7: 625–632
130. Begin L R. Intracisternal microtubular aggregates in classic (non chondroid) chordoma. J Submicrosc Cytol Pathol 1995: 27: 295–301
131. Niwa J, Hashi K, Minase T. Immunohistochemical and electron microscopic studies on intracranial chordomas: difference between typical chordomas and chondroid chordomas. Noshuyo Byori 1994: 11: 15–21
132. Miettinen M, Karaharju E, Järvinen H. Chordoma with a massive spindle-cell sarcomatous transformation. A light- and electron-microscopic and immunohistochemical study. Am J Surg Pathol 1987: 11: 563–570
133. Shin H J, Mackay B, Ichinose H, Ayala A G, Romsdahl M M. Parachordoma. Ultrastruct Pathol 1994: 18: 249–256
134. Miettinen M, Gannon F H, Lackman R. Chordomalike soft tissue sarcoma in the leg: a light and electron microscopic and immunohistochemical study. Ultrastruct Pathol 1992: 16: 577–586
135. Rosai J. Adamantinoma of the tibia. Electron microscopic evidence of its epithelial origin. Am J Clin Pathol 1969: 51: 786–792
136. Unni K K, Dahlin D C, Beabout J W, Ivins J C. Adamantinoma of long bones. Cancer 1974: 64: 1796–1805
137. Yoneyama T, Winter W G, Milsow L. Tibial adamantinoma: its histogenesis from ultrastructural studies. Cancer 1977: 40: 1138–1142
138. Knapp R H, Wick M R, Scheithauer B W, Unni K K. Adamantinoma of bone: an electron microscopic and immunohistochemical study. Virchows Arch A Pathol Anat Histopathol 1982: 398: 75–86
139. Pieterse A S, Smith P S, McClure J. Adamantinoma of long bones: clinical, pathological and ultrastructural features. J Clin Pathol 1982: 35: 780–786
140. Perez-Atayde A R, Kozakewich H P W, Vawter G F. Adamantinoma of the tibia. An ultrastructural and immunohistochemical study. Cancer 1985: 55: 1015–1023
141. Mori H, Yamamoto S, Hiramatsu K, Miura T, Moon N F. Adamantinoma of the tibia. Ultrastructural and immunohistochemical study with reference to histogenesis. Clin Orthop 1984: 190: 299–310
142. Llombart-Bosch A, Ortuno-Pacheco G. Ultrastructural findings supporting the angioblastic nature of the so-called adamantinoma of the tibia. Histopathology 1978: 2: 189–200
143. Povysil C, Matejovsky Z. Ultrastructure of adamantinoma of long bones. Virchows Arch A Pathol Anat Histol 1981: 393: 233–244
144. Eisenstein K, Pitcock J A. Adamantinoma of the tibia. Arch Pathol Lab Med 1984: 108: 246–250
145. Greco M A, Steiner G C. Ultrastructure of fibrous dysplasia of bone: a study of its fibrous, osseous, and cartilaginous components. Ultrastruct Pathol 1986: 10: 55–66
146. Bertrand G, Minard M F, Simard C, Rebel A. Etude ultrastructurale d'un cas de dysplasie fibreuse monostotique. Ann Anat Pathol 1978: 23: 81–90
147. Nunez E A, Horwith M, Krook L, Whalen J P. An electron microscopic investigation of human familial bone dysplasia. Am J Pathol 1979: 94: 1–18
148. Ohira O. Electron microscopic studies of fibrous dysplasia. J Jpn Orthop Assoc 1981: 55: 497–507
149. Hirohata K, Morimoto K, Kimura H. Ultrastructure of bone and joint diseases. 2nd ed. Tokyo: Igaku-Shoin, 1981
150. Hammar S, Bockus D, Remington F, Bartha M. The widespread distribution of Langerhans cell in pathologic tissue: an ultrastructural and immunohistochemical study. Hum Pathol 1986: 17: 894–905
151. Basset F, Nezelof C, Mallet R, Turiaf J. Nouvelle mise en évidence, par la microscopie électronique, de particules d'allure virale dans une seconde forme clinique de l'histiocytose X, le granulome éosinophile de l'os. Cr Acad Sci Paris 1965: 261: 5719–5720
152. Friedman B, Hanaoka H. Langerhans cell granules in eosinophilic granuloma of bone. J Bone Joint Surg (Am) 1969: 51: 367–374
153. Katz R L, Silva E G, De Santos L A, Lukeman J M. Diagnosis of eosinophilic granuloma of bone by cytology, histology and electron microscopy of transcutaneous bone-aspiration biopsy. J Bone Joint Surg (Am) 1980: 62: 1284–1290
154. Mierau G W, Favara B E, Brenman J M. Electron microscopy in histiocytosis X. Ultrastruct Pathol 1982: 3: 137–142
155. Robb I A, Jimenez C L, Carpenter B F. Birbeck granules or Birbeck junctions? Intercellular 'zipperlike' lattice junctions in eosinophilic granuloma of bone. Ultrastruct Pathol 1992: 16: 423–428
156. Favara B E, McCarthy R C, Mierau G W. Histiocytosis X. Hum Pathol 1983: 14: 663–676
157. Martinez Gonzalez M A, Ortega Serrano M P. Birbeck-like granules in an epithelial cell. Ultrastruct Pathol 1994: 18: 457–458
158. Basset F, Escaig J, Le Crom M. A cytoplasmic membranous complex in histiocytosis X. Cancer 1972: 29: 1380–1386
159. Rebel A, Malkani K, Basle M. Anomalies nucléaires des ostéoclastes de la maladie osseuse de Paget. Nouv Presse Med 1974: 20: 1299–1301
160. Rebel A, Malkani K, Basle M, Bregeon C. Osteoclast ultrastructure in Paget's disease. Calcif Tissue Res 1976: 20: 187–199
161. Mills B G, Singer F R. Nuclear inclusions in Paget's disease of bone. Science 1976: 194: 201–202
162. Schulz A, Delling G, Ringe J D, Ziegler R. Morbus Paget des Knochens. Untersuchungen zur Ultrastruktur der Osteclasten und ihrer Cytopathogenese. Virchows Arch A Pathol Anat Histol 1977: 376: 309–328
163. Gherardi G, Lo Cascio V, Bonucci E. Fine structure of nuclei and cytoplasm in Paget's disease of bone. Histopathology 1980: 4: 63–74
164. Mills B G. Comparison of the ultrastructure of a malignant tumor of the mandible containing malignant cells with Paget's disease of bone. J Oral Pathol 1981: 10: 203–215
165. Harvey L, Gray T, Beneton M N et al. Ultrastructural features of the osteoclasts from Paget's disease of bone in relation to a viral aetiology. J Clin Pathol 1982: 35: 771–779
166. Viola M V, Eilon G, Lazarus M. Virus-like inclusions in osteosarcoma cells arising in Paget's disease. Lancet 1982: 1: 848
167. Singer F R, Mills B G. Evidence for a viral etiology of Paget's disease. Clin Orthop 1983: 178: 245–251
168. Rebel A, Malkani K, Basle M, Bregeon C. Osteoclast ultrastructure in Paget's disease. Clin Orthop 1987: 217: 4–8
169. Malkani K, Basle M, Rebel A. Goniometric observations of nuclear inclusions in osteoclasts in Paget's bone disease. J Submicrosc Cytol 1976: 8: 229–236
170. Kallman F, Admas J M, Williams R L, Imagawa D T. Fine structure of cellular inclusions in measles virus infections. J Biophys Biochem Cytol 1959: 6: 379–392
171. Oyanagi S, Meulen V, Katz M, Koprowski H. Comparison of subacute sclerosing panencephalitis and measles viruses. J Virol 1971: 7: 176–187

172. Welsh R A, Mayer A T. Nuclear fragmentation and associated fibrils in giant cell tumour of bone. Lab Invest 1970: 22: 63–72

173. Le Charpentier Y, Le Charpentier M, Forest M et al. Inclusions intranucléaires dans une tumeur osseuse à cellules géantes. Mise en évidence au microscope électronique. Nouve Presse Med 1977: 6: 259–262

174. Vacher-Lavenu M C, Louvel A, Daudet-Monsac M, Le Charpentier Y, Abelanet R. Inclusions tubulo-filamenteuses intranucléaires dans les cellules multinucléées des tumeurs cellules géantes des os. Etude ultrastructurale d'une série de 31 tumeurs. Cr Acad Sci Paris 1981: 293: 639–644

175. Schajowicz F, Ubios A M, Santini Araujo E, Cabrini L. Virus like intranuclear inclusions in giant cell tumor of bone. Clin Orthop 1985: 201: 247–250

176. Abelanet R, Daudet-Monsac M, Laoussadi S, Forest M, Vacher-Lavenu M C. Frequency and diagnostic value of the virus-like filamentous intranuclear inclusion in giant cell tumor of bone, not associated with Paget's disease. A study of 43 cases. Virchows Arch A Pathol Anat Histopathol 1986: 410: 65–68

177. Mirra J M, Bauer F C, Grant T T. Giant cell tumor with viral-like intranuclear inclusions associated with Paget's disease. Clin Orthop 1981: 158: 243–251

178. Beneton M N, Harris S, Kanis J A. Paramyxovirus-like inclusions in two cases of pycnodysostosis. Bone 1987: 8: 211–217

179. Bianco P, Silvestrini G, Ballanti P, Bonucci E. Paramyxovirus-like nuclear inclusions identical to those of Paget's disease of bone detected in giant cells of primary oxalosis. Virchows Arch A Pathol Anat Histopathol 1992: 421: 427–433

180. Mills G B, Yabe H, Singer F R. Osteoclasts in human osteopetrosis contain viral-nucleocapsid-like nuclear inclusions. J Bone Miner Res 1988: 3: 101–106

181. Yabe H, Singer F R, Tucker W S, Mills B G. Paget-like inclusion in osteopetrosis and hereditary neuromuscular and skeletal disease. J Bone Miner Res 1986: 1 (suppl 1): 221

182. Marks S C, Popoff S N. Ultrastructural biology and pathology of the osteoclast. In: Bonucci E, Motta P M, Eds. Ultrastructure of skeletal tissues. Boston: Kluwer, 1990, pp 240–252

183. Chou S M. Myxovirus-like structures in a case of human chronic polymyositis. Science 1967: 158: 1453–1455

184. Chou S M. Myxovirus-like structures and accompanying nuclear changes in chronic polymyositis. Arch Pathol 1968: 86: 649–658

185. Yunis E J, Smaha F J. Inclusion body myositis. Lab Invest 1971: 25: 240–248

Pathology of tumors

6

Osteoma and bone island

M. Forest

OSTEOMA

Introduction, clinical data and skeletal distribution

Osteomas are protruding lesions developing on the surface of bone and most commonly found in the skull and facial bones. They can be single or multiple in association with the Gardner syndrome; in this autosomal-dominant disorder, osteomatosis or wavy thickening of the cortex may precede the clinical finding of polyposis.[1,2]

Isolated extracranial osteomas of the long and flat bones are exceedingly rare, as is location in the soft tissues.[3] They are usually found in adults and are more frequent in males (Schajowicz 1994).

The lesion is slow growing[4] and usually asymptomatic, but pain has been recorded in some cases.[5,6]

Various locations have been reported: pelvis,[5,7] clavicle,[6] tubular bones of the extremities,[8] femur (Figs 6.1–6.6), humerus, ulna, tibia, ribs (Unni 1996), but most of the lesions occur in the lower extremities.[9]

Imaging

On plain films, the lesion appears as a very dense, round or ovoid sclerotic mass with sharply demarcated borders.[2] It adheres to the cortex with a wide implant base, protruding towards the soft tissues. The surface is smooth or lobulated. No periosteal reaction and bone destruction are found, but in some cases, the lesion can extend through the cortex into the medullary fat[4,10] (Fig. 6.2).

On conventional and computed tomography, lytic areas are not seen in the homogeneous mass, which appears very dense and well defined. The underlying cortex is normal or thickened.[9] Some lesions show an increased uptake on bone scans.[4,5]

Pathology

On gross examination, the elongated or lobular mass is very dense, ivory-like and covered by a fine fibrous

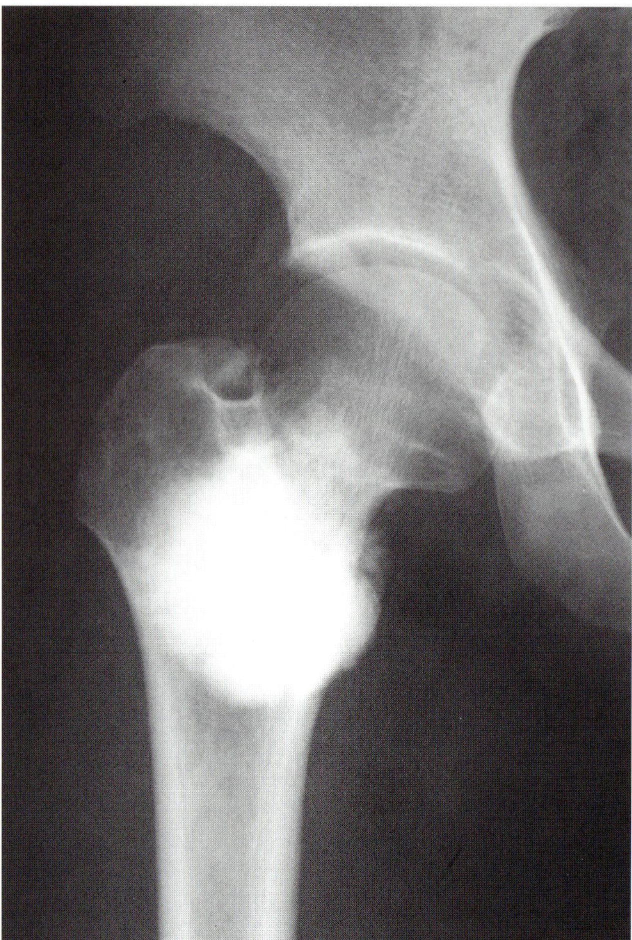

Fig. 6.1 Osteoma appearing as a dense sclerotic mass in front of the metaphysis of the femur.

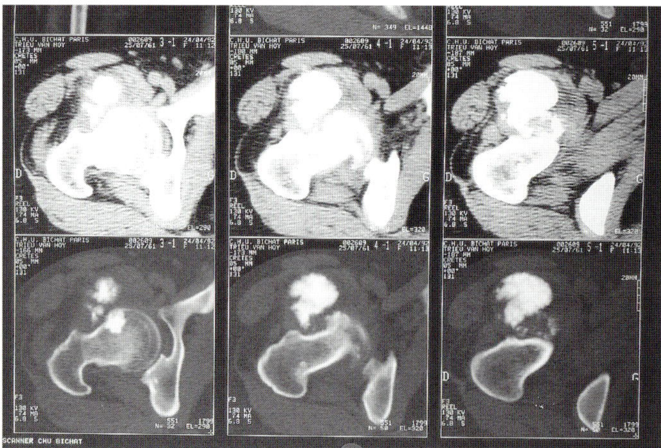

Fig. 6.2 Same case as Fig. 6.1. On CT scan, the lesion is extending into the cervical neck of the femur.

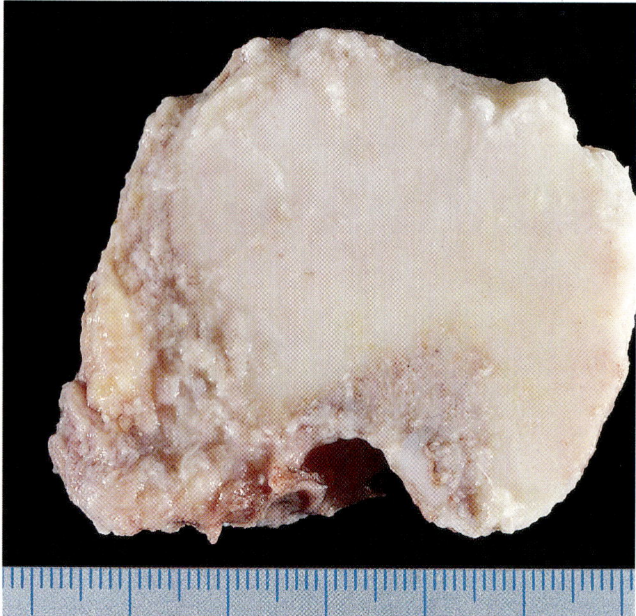

Fig. 6.3 Same case as Fig. 6.1. Gross appearance of the well-circumscribed mass.

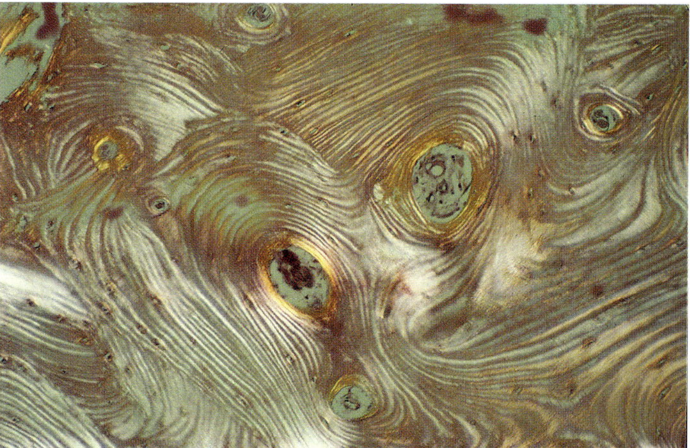

Fig. 6.4 Same case as Fig. 6.1. Lamellar bone exhibiting a cortical architecture (polarized light).

periosteal membrane (Fig. 6.3). Some are described as giant parosteal osteomas in the pelvis[7] or metacarpals;[8] their size can vary from 2.5 to 20 cm,[9] though usually it does not exceed 5–6 cm.

On histological study, in long and flat bone locations, rare cases show some trabecular structure with medullary tissue and fat (spongious form[11]). Most are composed of dense lamellar or compact cortical bone, with Haversian systems and even, sometimes, a pagetoid architecture or accretion lines in the peripheral part (Mirra 1989, Schajowicz 1994) (Figs 6.4, 6.5). There is no cartilaginous component. The lesion is covered by a thin layer of spindle cells.[9]

An ultrastructural study has shown an undisturbed cellular maturation of osteoblasts, producing an osteoid matrix with a mineralizing front and matrix vesicles (Schulz 1980).

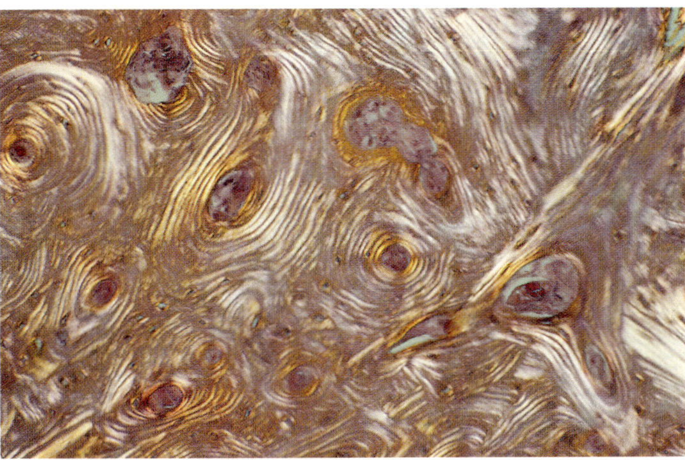

Fig. 6.5 Same case as Fig. 6.1. Histology is similar in the intramedullary component (polarized light).

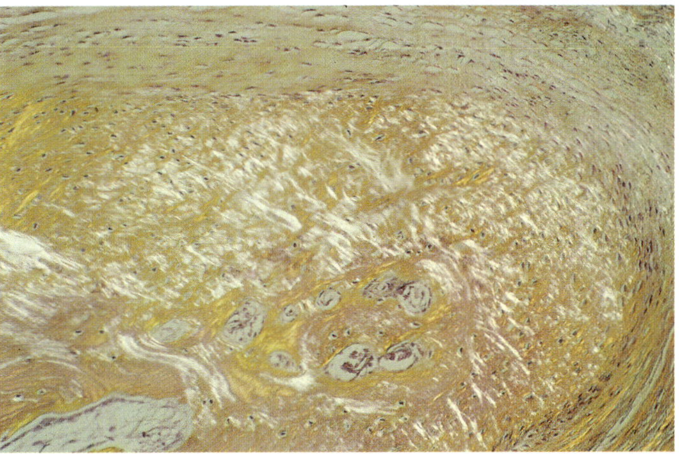

Fig. 6.6 Same case as Fig. 6.1. A few areas of woven bone in the outer margin (polarized light).

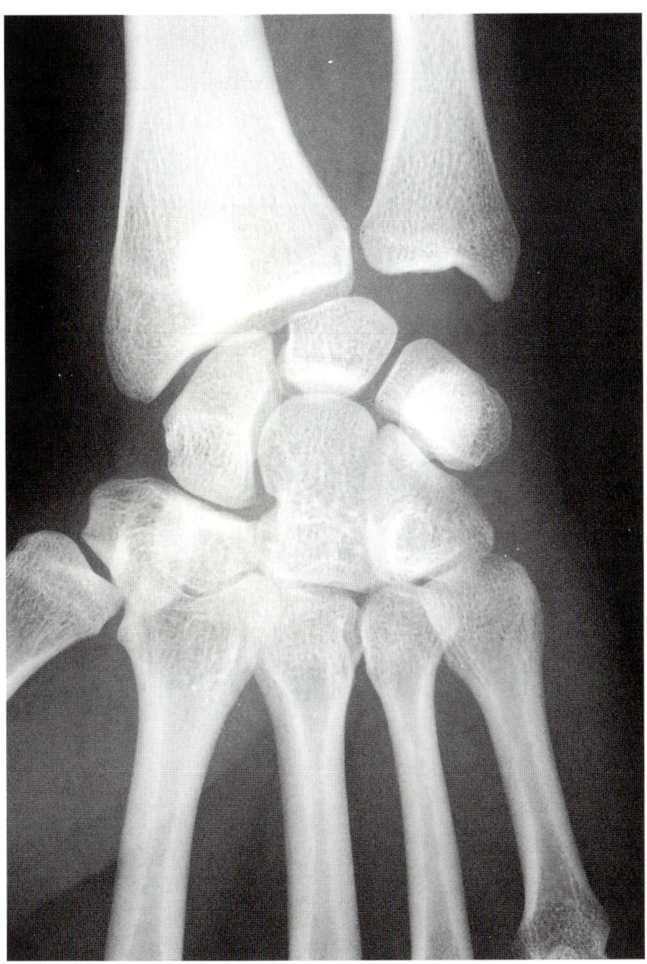

Fig. 6.7 Bone island in the lower epiphysis of the radius.

Fig. 6.8 Bone island in the acetabular area.

Treatment

Treatment is by excision of the mass with the underlying cortex. There is no recurrence or malignant transformation.

Differential diagnosis

Some differential diagnoses on imaging are easily ruled out by gross or histological examination: myositis ossificans,

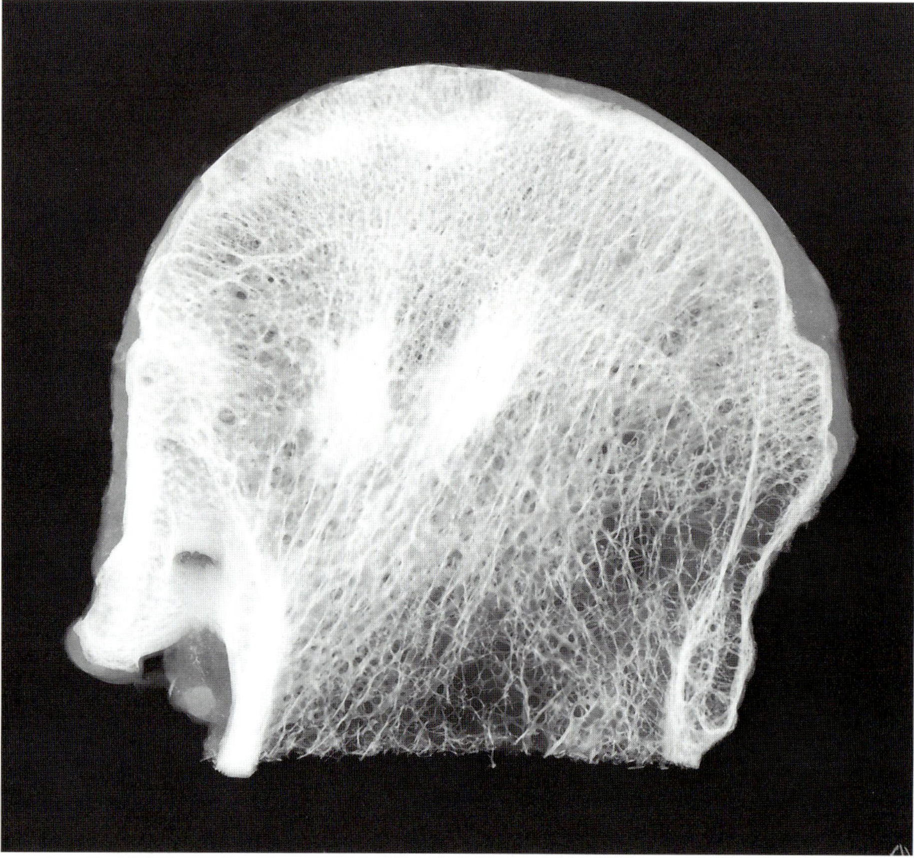

Fig. 6.9 Bone islands as an incidental finding in an osteoarthritic femoral head.

periosteal osteoblastomas or lipomas, osteochondromas with involuted cartilaginous caps or simple periosteal reactions.

A major problem arises in excluding a parosteal osteosarcoma; imaging may be quite similar even if, in most cases, homogeneous density and smooth borders are lacking in the sarcoma. Histology may also be quite similar, with 'normalization' of a part of the sarcoma, that is, cortical bone which appears normal. The most important point is to exclude a spindle cell proliferation, even without cytological atypia, in the periphery of the osteoma,[7] or in the Haversian systems, a subtle but decisive element leading to the diagnosis of sarcoma.[9]

Comments for the surgical pathologist

Parosteal osteoma is definitely not a semimalignant lesion.[12] It has to be differentiated from parosteal osteosarcoma, not by biopsy but by a thorough histological examination of the completely resected tumor.[13] Any report on this very rare lesion should refer, on imaging, to the absence of areas of lucency and on histology, to the absence of spindle cell proliferation.[9]

BONE ISLAND

Introduction, clinical data and skeletal distribution

Bone islands or enostoses are single or infrequent areas of mature compact bone located in cancellous bone.[14,15]

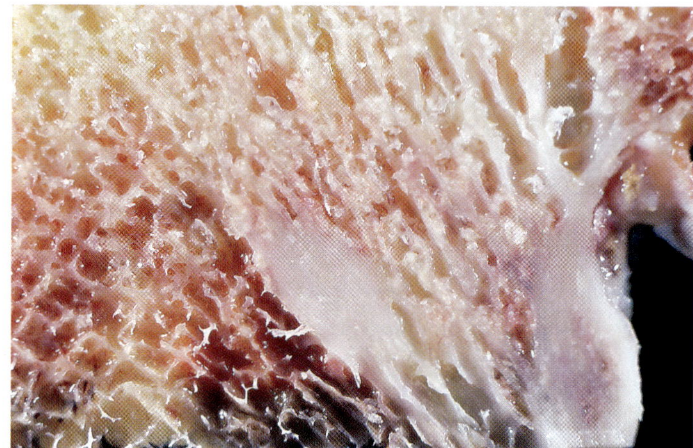

Fig. 6.10 Bone island in a femoral head, in continuity with the trabeculae of cancellous bone.

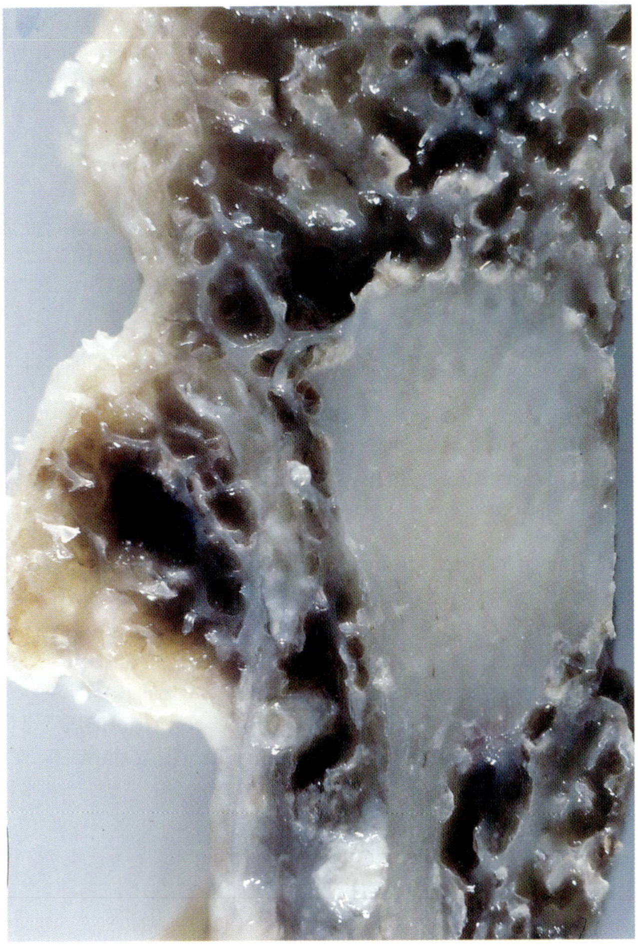

Fig. 6.11

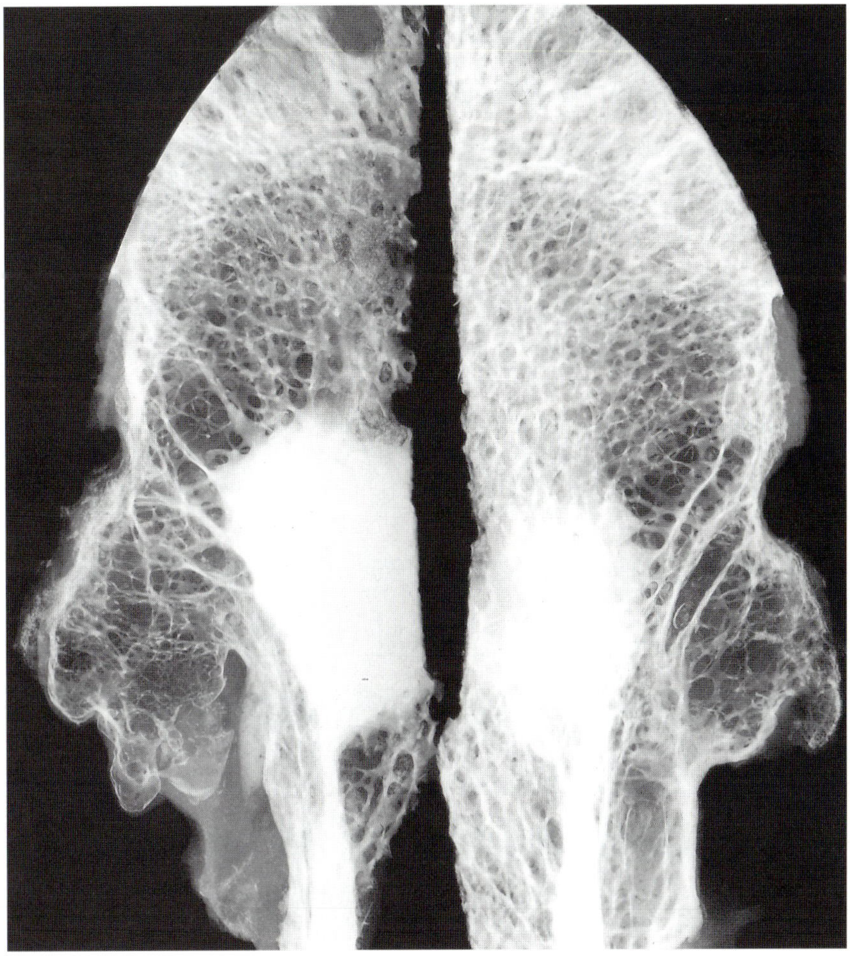

Fig. 6.12

Figs 6.11, 6.12 Bone island closely linked to the cortex, in an osteoarthritic femoral head.

They are found predominantly in the bones of adults and rarely in children, in approximately 1% of the population, with no sexual predilection. Usual sites are the pelvis, the proximal end of the femur, the humerus and ribs.[14,16] Bone islands can be found anywhere, but they are rare in the spine (thoracic and lumbar spine[17,18]) and extremely rare in the skull. In long tubular bones, they are located in the epiphysis or metaphysis.

They are presumed to be developmental abnormalities: focal failure of bone resorption occurring during the process of skeletal maturation and modeling.[19,20]

Imaging

On plain films, bone islands appear as round or ovoid well-delineated areas of cortical density within cancellous bone, on the long axis of the trabecular architecture and with sizes ranging from 1 mm to 15 mm (Figs 6.7, 6.8).

Peripheral spiculations merge with the surrounding

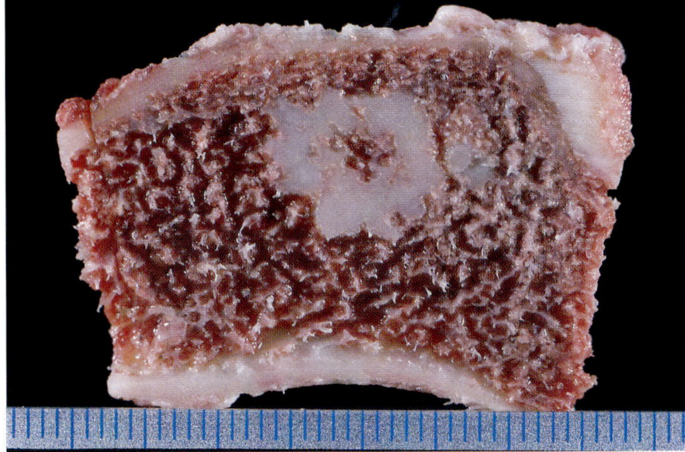

Fig. 6.13 Unusual bone island in the iliopubic ramus with serrated contours.

bone trabeculae in a 'brush-like' fashion.[21] Some may be partly connected with the endosteal surface of the cortex.[15,22] Lesions of more than 2 cm are described as

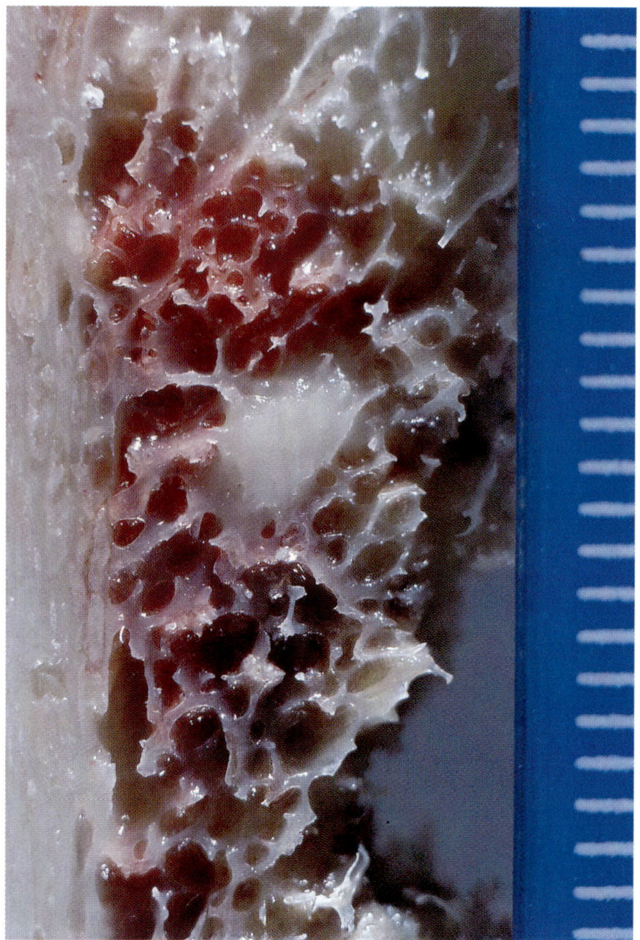

Fig. 6.14 Bone island located in the lower metaphysis of the femur.

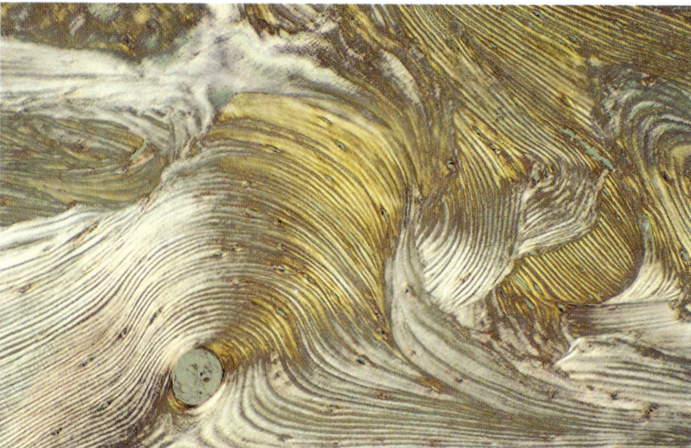

Fig. 6.15 Cortical architecture of a bone island (polarized light).

'giant bone islands' in various locations: tibia,[23] ilium,[24] femur[25–28] or even spine and sacrum (Mirra 1989).

On CT scans, the contour of bone is unaltered; on T1- and T2-weighted MRI sequences, they present a low signal intensity as cortical bone.[21] Most lesions do not change in size but some may increase or decrease or even disappear.[30–34]

On radionuclide bone scan, bone islands usually show no activity, but increased uptake has been reported,[23,28,35–37] sometimes in relation to growing activity,[36] or the size of the lesion,[28] though an enlarging lesion may show a normal bone scan.[37,38]

Pathology

On gross examination, bone islands are small, white-yellow, circular or oblong masses (Figs 6.9–6.14). On histology, they show compact, mature lamellar bone with Haversian systems (Fig. 6.15). Occasionally, some woven bone may be found[20,23] or a central mild bone remodeling.[22,29] Various factors have been suggested for a positive bone scan: size,[26] rate of growth,[21,28] bone remodeling,[20] or increased metabolic activity in the surrounding cancellous bone.[23]

Differential diagnosis

Differential diagnosis can only be seen clearly on imaging: calcified nidus of an osteoid osteoma, osteoblastoma, osteoblastic metastases or even sclerotic osteosarcoma for rare giant bone islands. A significant increase in size in repeated radiographs may suggest that biopsy is necessary.[20]

Bone islands are similar to the lesions of osteopoikilosis. There is, perhaps, also some link with a localized form of osteosclerosis involving a segment of the vertebral bodies (chiefly L3–L4), without alteration of the vertebral contour or disk space, in adults,[39,40] even if the lesions are segmental, less sharply defined and continuous with the cortex.

Comments for the surgical pathologist

A bone island is a 'leave alone' lesion; one has only to search histologically for a mild bone remodeling in cases of growing or hot lesions on bone scans.

REFERENCES

1. Chang C H, Piatt E D, Thomas K E, Watne A L. Bone abnormalities in Gardner's syndrome. Am J Roentgenol Radium Ther Nucl Med 1968: 103: 645–652
2. Greenspan A. Benign bone-forming lesions: osteoma, osteoid osteoma, and osteoblastoma. Clinical, imaging, pathologic, and differential considerations. Skeletal Radiol 1993: 22: 485–500
3. Schweitzer M E, Greenway G, Resnick D, Haghighi P, Snoots W E. Osteoma of soft parts. Skeletal Radiol 1992: 21: 177–180

4. Baum P A, Nelson M C, Lack E E, Bogumill G P. Case report of 560 parosteal osteoma of the tibia. Skeletal Radiol 1989: 18: 406–409

5. Cervilla V, Haghighi P, Resnick D, Sartoris D J. Case report of 596 parosteal osteoma of the acetabulum. Skeletal Radiol 1990: 19: 135–137

6. Meltzer C C, Scott W W Jr, McCarthy E F. Case report of 698 osteomas of the clavicle. Skeletal Radiol 1991: 20: 555–557

7. Mirra J M, Gold R H, Pignatti G, Remotti F. Case report of 497 compact osteomas of iliac bone. Skeletal Radiol 1988: 17: 437–442

8. Stern P J, Lim E V A, Krieg J K. Giant metacarpal osteoma. A case report. J Bone Joint Surg (Am) 1985: 67: 487–489

9. Bertoni F, Unni K K, Beabout J W, Sim F H. Parosteal osteoma of bones other than of the skull and face. Cancer 1995: 75: 2466–2473

10. Houghton M J, Heiner J P, De Smet A A. Osteoma of the innominate bone with intraosseous and parosteal involvement. Skeletal Radiol 1995: 24: 455–457

11. Alfonso C, Laus M, Ferrari D, Pignatti G. Osteoma of the proximal femur. Chir Organi Mov 1994: 79: 339–343

12. Tamarit L V, Pardo J. Parosteal osteoma: clinicopathologic approach. Pathol Annu 1977: 12: 373–387

13. O'Connel J X, Rosenthal D I, Mankin H J, Rosenberg A E. Solitary osteoma of a long bone. A case report. J Bone Joint Surg (Am) 1993: 75: 1830–1834

14. Kim S K, Barry W F Jr. Bone island. Am J Roentgenol Radium Ther Nucl Med 1964: 92: 1301–1306

15. Kim S K, Barry W F Jr. Bone islands. Radiology 1968: 90: 77–78

16. Onitsuka H. Roentgenologic aspects of bone islands. Radiology 1977: 123: 607–612

17. Resnick D, Nemcek A A Jr, Haghighi P. Spinal enostoses (bone islands). Radiology 1983: 147: 373–376

18. Broderick T W, Resnick D, Goergen T G, Alazraki N. Enostosis of the spine. Spine 1978: 3: 167–170

19. Greenspan A. Sclerosing bone dysplasias – a target-site approach. Skeletal Radiol 1991: 20: 561–583

20. Greenspan A, Steiner G, Knutzon R. Bone island (enostosis): clinical significance and radiologic and pathologic correlations. Skeletal Radiol 1991: 20: 85–90

21. Greenspan A. Bone island (enostosis): current concepts – a review. Skeletal Radiol 1995: 24: 111–115

22. Lagier R, Nussle D. Anatomy and radiology of a bone island. RÖFO 1978: 128: 261–264

23. Gold R H, Mirra J M, Remotti F, Pignatti G. Case report of 527 giant bone islands of tibia. Skeletal Radiol 1989: 18: 129–132

24. Smith J. Giant bone islands. Radiology 1973: 107: 35–36

25. Greenspan A, Klein M J. Giant bone island. Skeletal Radiol 1996: 25: 67–69

26. Brien E W, Mirra J M, Latanza L, Fedenko A, Luck J Jr. Giant bone island of femur. Case report, literature review, and its distinction from low grade osteosarcoma. Skeletal Radiol 1995: 24: 546–550

27. Ehara S, Kattapuram S V, Rosenberg A E. Giant bone island. Computed tomography findings. Clin Imaging 1989: 13: 231–233

28. Sickles E A, Genant H K, Hoffer P B. Increased localization of 99mTc pyrophosphate in a bone island: case report. J Nucl Med 1976: 17: 113–115

29. Avery G R, Wilsdon J B, Malcom A J. Giant bone island with some central resorption. Skeletal Radiol 1995: 24: 59–60

30. Blank N, Lieber A. The significance of growing bone islands. Radiology 1965: 85: 508–511

31. Ngan H. Growing bone islands. Clin Radiol 1972: 23: 199–201

32. Hoffman R R Jr, Campbell R E. Roentgenologic bone-island instability in hyperparathyroidism. Case report. Radiology 1972: 103: 307–308

33. Simon K, Mulligan M E. Growing bone islands revisited. A case report. J Bone Joint Surg (Am) 1985: 67: 809–811

34. Gower D J, Tytle T, Brumback R. Enlarging endostoma (bone island) of the spinous process. Neurosurgery 1992: 30: 608–609

35. Greenspan A, Stadalnik R C. Bone island: scintigraphic findings and their clinical application. Can Assoc Radiol J 1995: 46: 368–379

36. Davies J A K, Hall F M, Goldberg R P, Kasdon E J. Positive bone scan in a bone island. Case report. J Bone Joint Surg (Am) 1979: 61: 943–945

37. Hall F M, Goldberg R P, Davies J A, Fainsinger M H. Scintigraphic assessment of a bone island. Radiology 1980: 135: 737–742

38. Go R T, El Khoury G Y, Wehbe M A. Radionuclide bone image in growing and stable bone island. Skeletal Radiol 1980: 5: 15–18

39. Ackermann W, Schwarz G S. Non-neoplastic sclerosis in vertebral bodies. Cancer 1958: 11: 703–708

40. McCarthy E F, Dorfman H D. Idiopathic segmental sclerosis of vertebral bodies. Skeletal Radiol 1982: 9: 88–91

7

Osteoid osteoma and osteoblastoma

M. Forest

OSTEOID OSTEOMA

Introduction and clinical data

An osteoid osteoma is a benign osteoblastic lesion of limited growth, frequently inducing a huge reactive bone formation. It was first described as a clinicopathological entity by Jaffe in 1935;[1] the small round or oval pathologic process was called a nidus.[2]

Osteoid osteoma accounts for 10–12% of all benign bone tumors. It can be found at any age, but most cases occur in the first three decades with an average age at presentation of 19 years.[3] It is rarely found in very young children[4] and may be difficult to diagnose in children.[5] It is also uncommon in the elderly.[6] There is a definite male prevalence with a mean ratio of male to female patients of 2.2:1.[7]

A dull, aching pain is the main clinical symptom. This is worse at night and in more than 70% of patients is relieved by salicylates.[8] Pain of a few weeks' or even years' duration may precede any radiological finding or may be referred to an adjacent bone or joint.[9,10] Some osteoid osteomas are painless,[11,12] with an incidence of 1.6%[7] to 5% of cases;[3] most of these have been reported in the fingers.[13]

Clinical symptoms may be tenderness and swelling,[6] a mass or a limp with muscle atrophy in the lower extremities.[9] In the spine, osteoid osteoma is frequently associated with a spinal deformity due to spasm; this painful scoliosis of rapid onset may also precede radiographic changes.[14,15]

Intraarticular osteoid osteomas are associated with many symptoms, which can mask the true diagnosis: limitation of joint motion, synovitis, joint effusion, capsular contracture, advanced epiphyseal development, subluxation or even osteoarthritis.[16–20]

Patients frequently connect symptoms with local trauma, but this is disputable.

Skeletal distribution

Osteoid osteomas can be found anywhere in the skeleton;

"

in about 50% of cases, the femur (Fig. 7.1) and the tibia are involved. In the femur, the proximal end, the neck and intertrochanteric regions are generally affected. In long bones, the location is metaphyseal or diaphyseal and rarely epiphyseal.

Approximately 10% occur in the spine (Fig. 7.2), chiefly in the lumbar and cervical vertebrae involving the posterior elements, and rarely in the vertebral body.[14,21] Osteoid osteomas are unusual in the pelvis, the coccyx and the sacrum.[22,23]

In the hand (Figs 7.3, 7.4), lesions occur predominantly in the proximal or distal phalanx, sometimes with segmental digital hypertrophy, pseudoclubbing and, on X-ray, a cortical hypertrophy with a poorly visible nidus.

In the foot, the metatarsals and the calcaneus may be involved, and in the talus it is almost always in a subperiosteal location[24] (Figs 7.5–7.8).

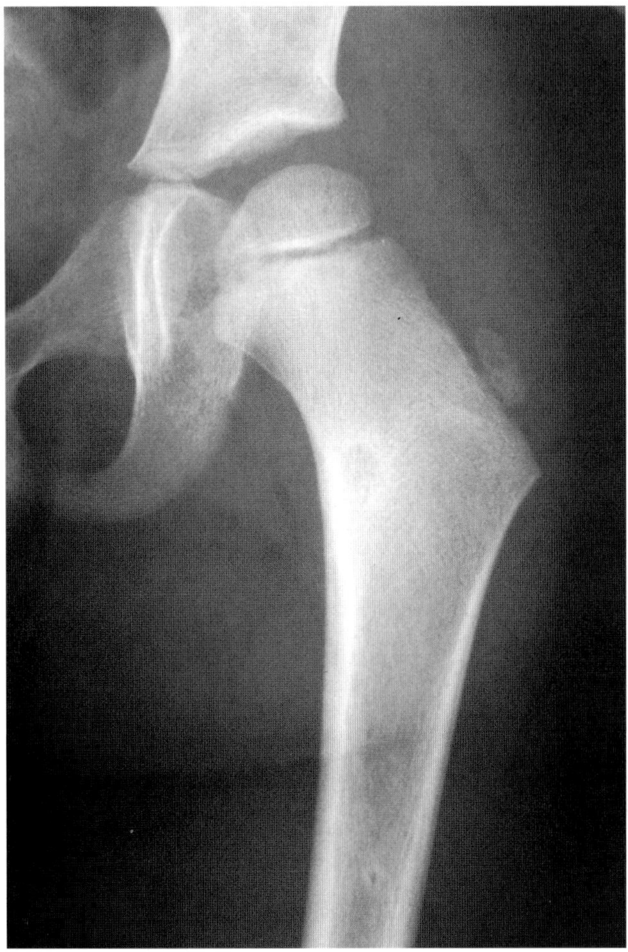

Fig. 7.1 Osteoid osteoma in the metaphysis of the femur.

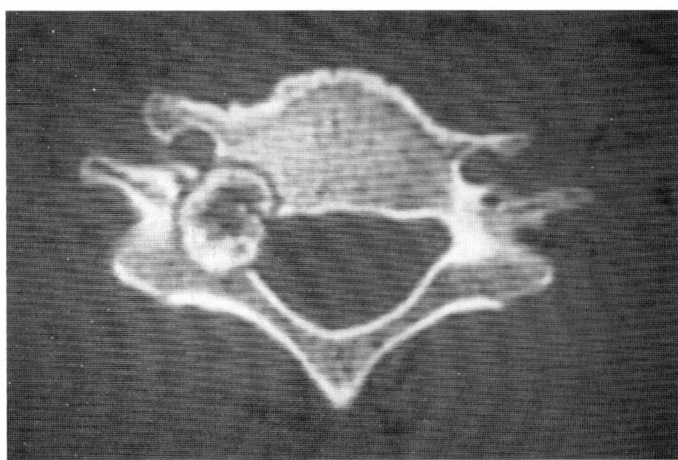

Fig. 7.2 Osteoid osteoma at the C6 vertebral level.

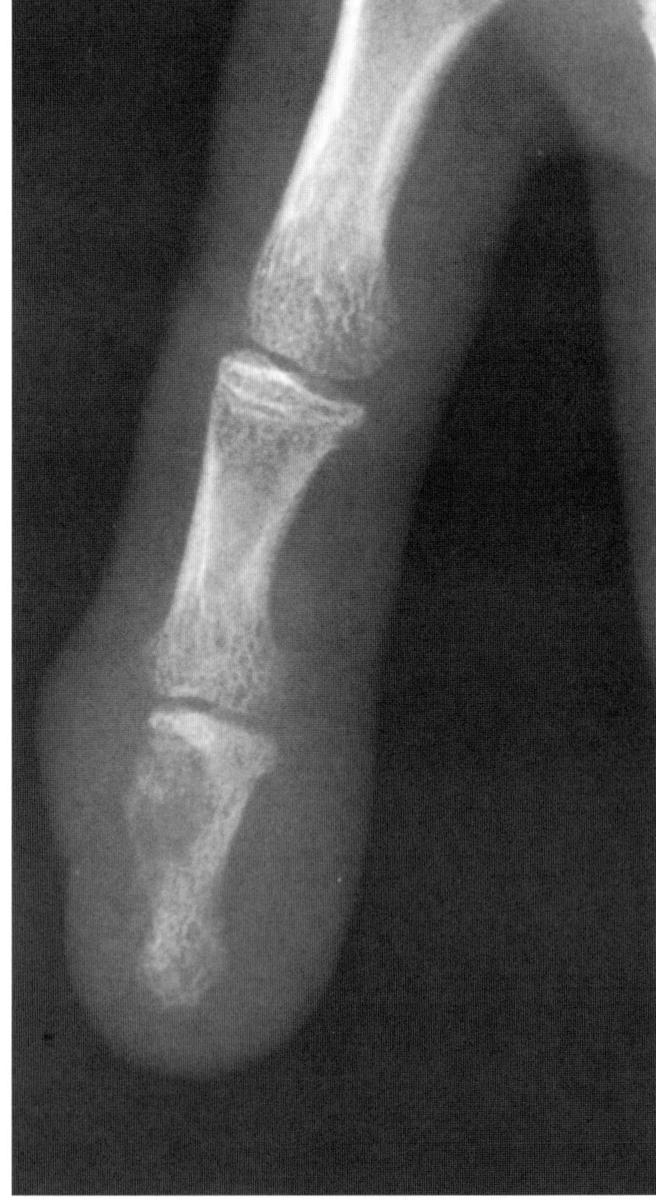

Fig. 7.3

Fig. 7.3, 7.4 Osteoid osteomas in phalangeal locations.

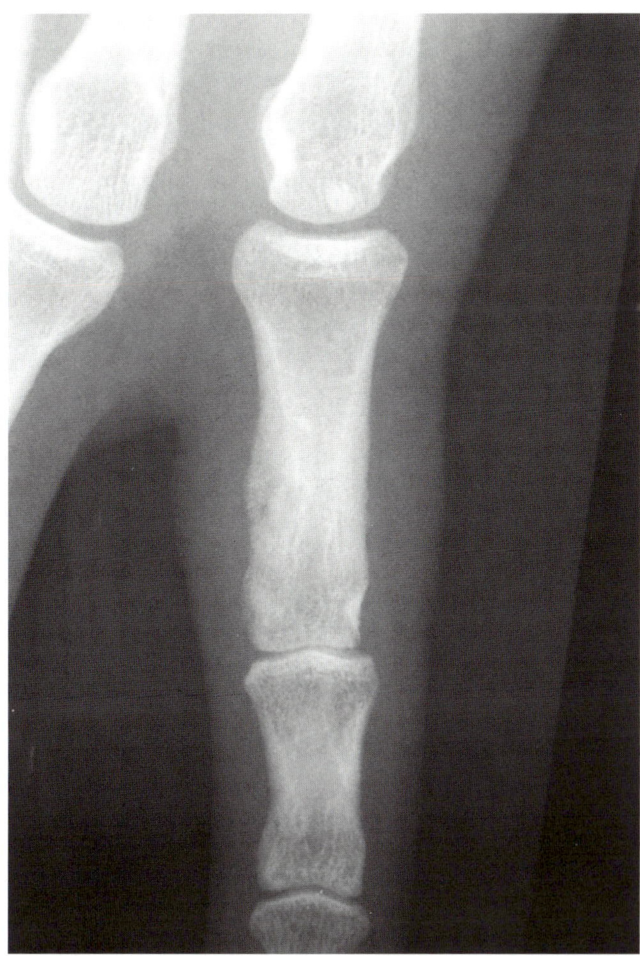

Fig. 7.4

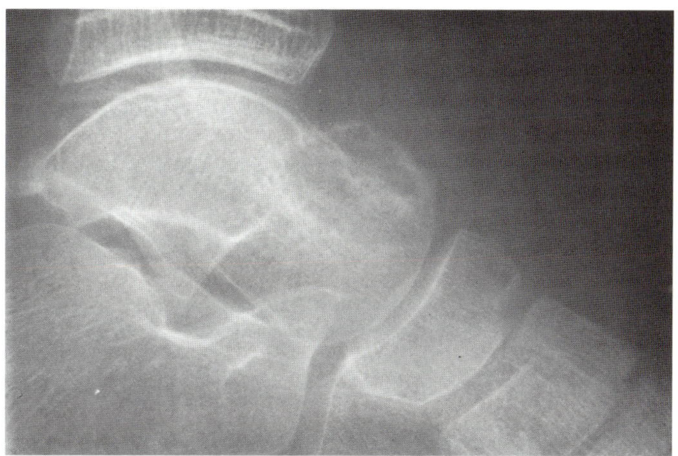

Fig. 7.5

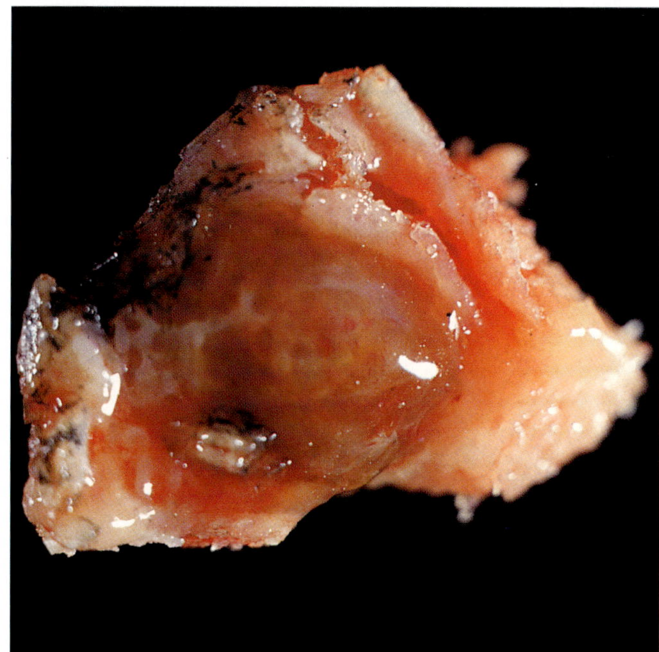

Fig. 7.6
Figs 7.5, 7.6 Subperiosteal osteoid osteoma of the talus.

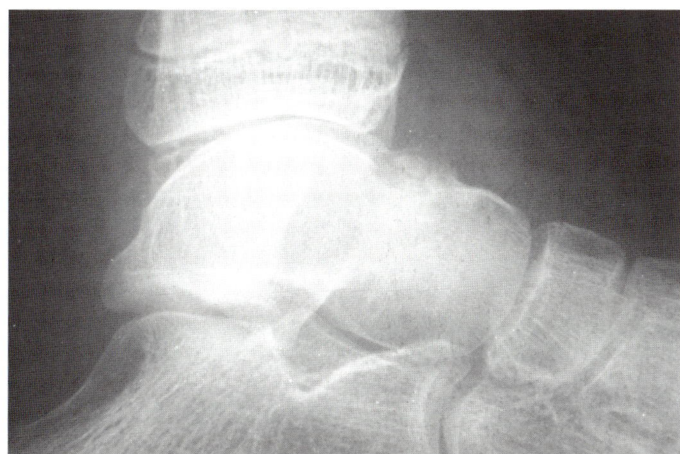

Fig. 7.7

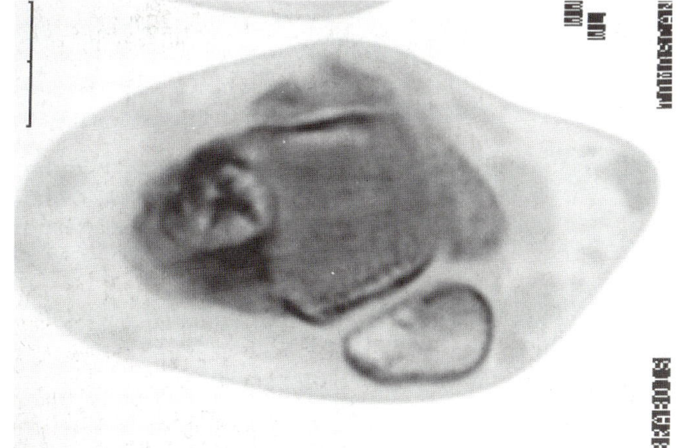

Fig. 7.8

Figs 7.7, 7.8 Subperiosteal osteoid osteoma of the talus with a 15-year clinical course (Fig. 7.8: MRI).

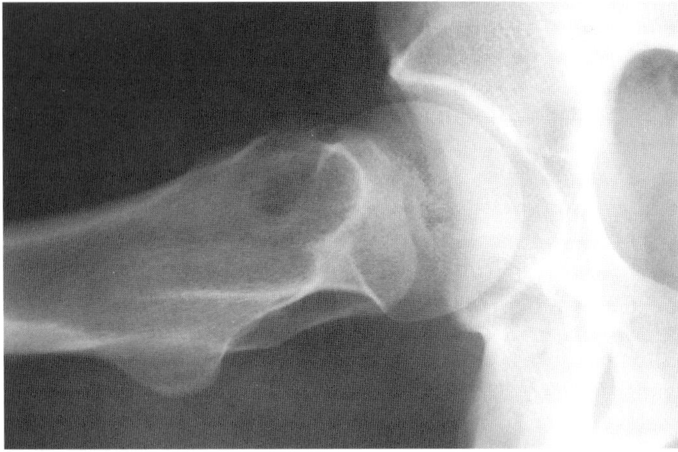

Fig. 7.9 Radiolucent nidus in a femoral location.

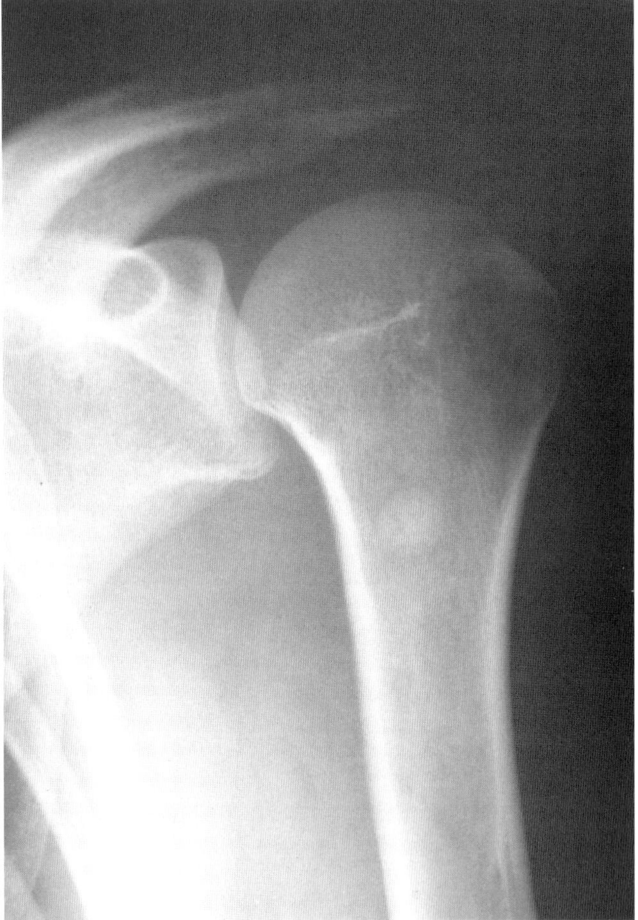

Fig. 7.10 Radiopaque nidus in a humeral location.

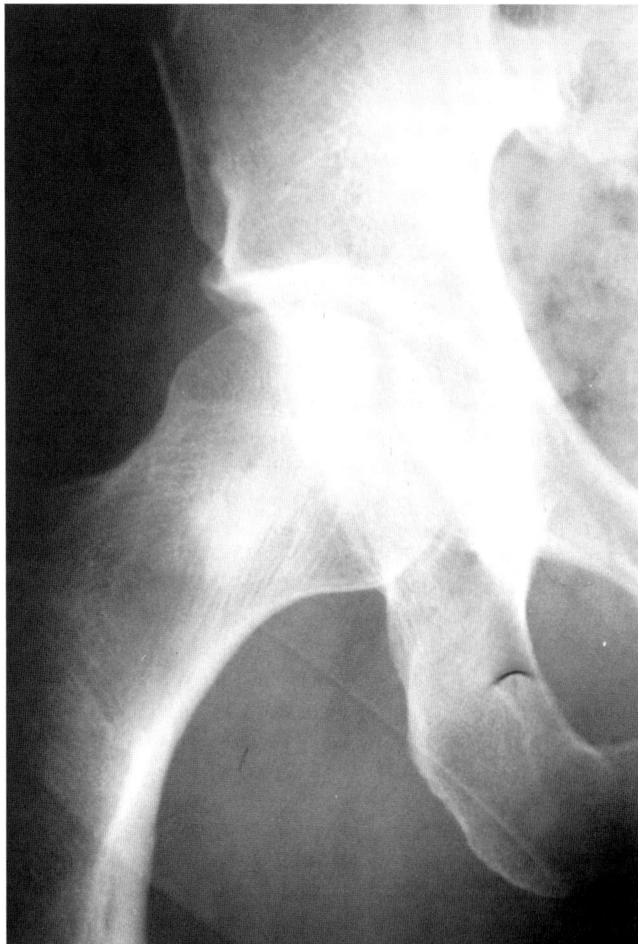

Fig. 7.11 Radiopaque nidus in a femoral location.

Imaging

On plain films, the nidus appears as a well-delineated area of radiolucency (Fig. 7.9) or as a more radiopaque lesion with maturation and calcification (Figs 7.10, 7.11).

Ossification may predominate in the center, leading to the appearance of a ring or annular sequestrum (Figs 7.12, 7.13). There is no correlation between the degree of mineralization and the duration of symptoms.

Reactive bone formation is often asymmetrical with respect to the long axis of the shaft and the location of the nidus (Wilner 1982). It is quite marked in children and may mimic the lamellated periosteal reaction of a Ewing's sarcoma (Unni 1996). The perifocal zone of reactive bone may extend a considerable distance beyond the nidus and may obscure it (Figs 7.14, 7.15).

Radiographic localization of the nidus and the different degrees of osteosclerosis have led to a radiological classification still used today.[9,25]

The most common lesion is the cortical osteoid osteoma, with a fusiform sclerotic thickening on the shaft and a radiolucent nidus centrally positioned (femur, tibia). A cancellous or medullary osteoid osteoma is mostly found in the femoral neck, the small bones of hand and foot and the vertebrae. Reactive osteosclerosis is less marked and may be some distance from the nidus. Subperiosteal osteoid osteoma is the least common, the

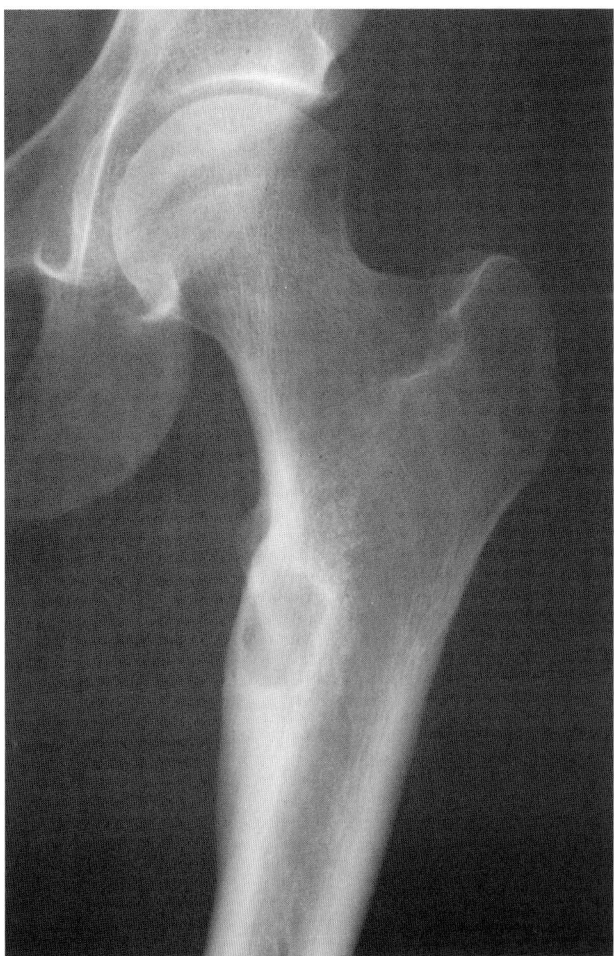

Fig. 7.12

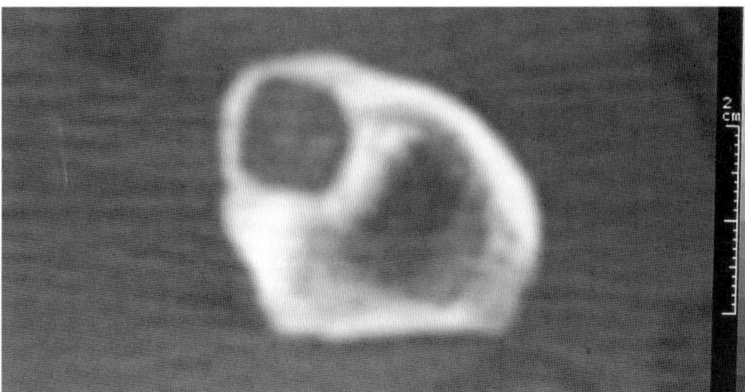

Fig. 7.13

Figs 7.12, 7.13 Cortical osteoid osteoma of the femur; the nidus is also well demonstrated on CT scan.

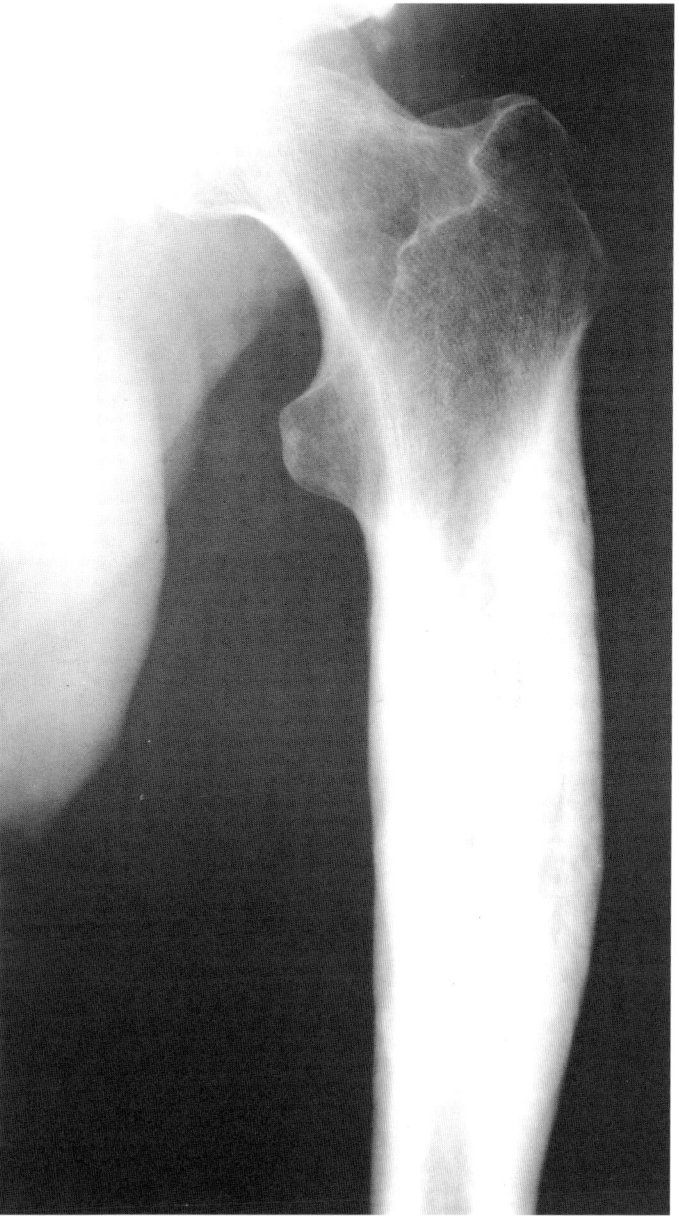

Fig. 7.14 Osteoid osteoma of the femur: massive osteosclerosis obscuring the nidus.

juxtacortical mass excavating the cortex, usually without sclerosis.

Intraarticular osteoid osteomas are of the cancellous and subperiosteal types. There is usually a lack of extensive sclerosis due to the relative position of the periosteum. In the experience of the Armed Forces Institute of Pathology (AFIP), reactive changes may be found in the adjacent cancellous bone,[3] particularly in the elbow,[16] as well as periosteal reactions on both sides of the joint.[26] The most commonly reported sites are the femoral neck, the elbow and the neck of the talus (Figs 7.16, 7.17). An associated disuse osteoporosis has been reported in various locations[27–29] (Fig. 7.18).

The osteoblastic activity and increased blood flow both support isotope uptake in the region. Bone scan is extremely sensitive,[30–33] with false results being extremely rare.[34] A classic double density sign has been described, with a focal intense isotope uptake within a more diffuse area of increased activity.[35,36]

Angiography is now rarely performed. It reveals an intense and circumscribed blush persisting late in the

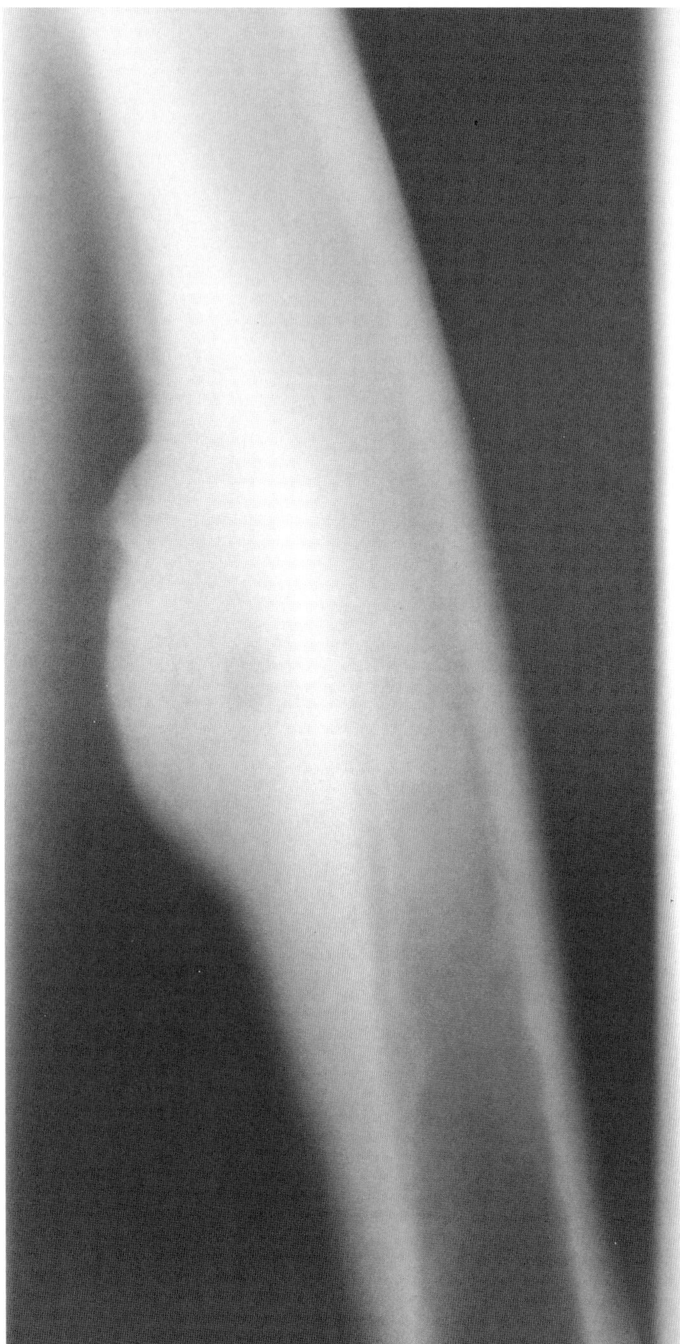

Fig. 7.15 Osteoid osteoma of the femur: nidus centrally located in the reactive bone.

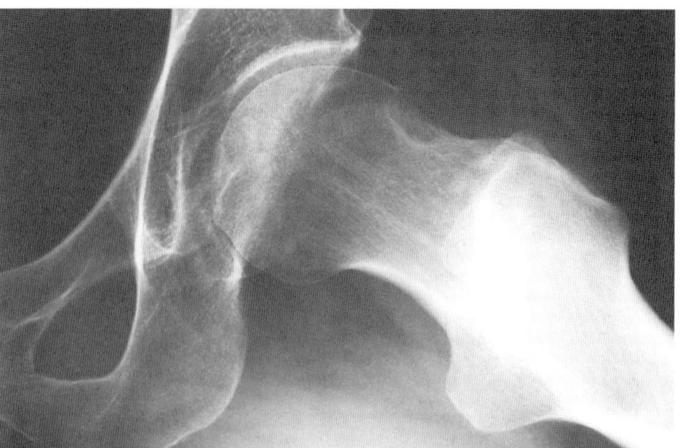

Fig. 7.16 Subperiosteal and intracapsular osteoid osteoma of the femoral neck.

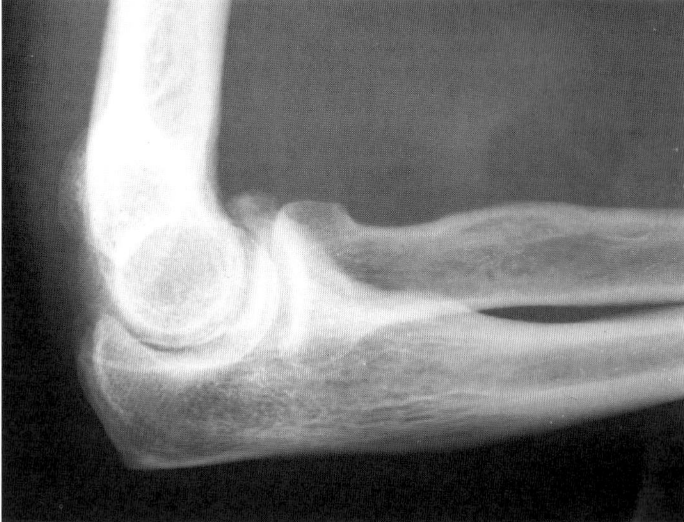

Fig. 7.17 Unusual nidus developed from the olecranon and protruding into the articular cavity of the elbow.

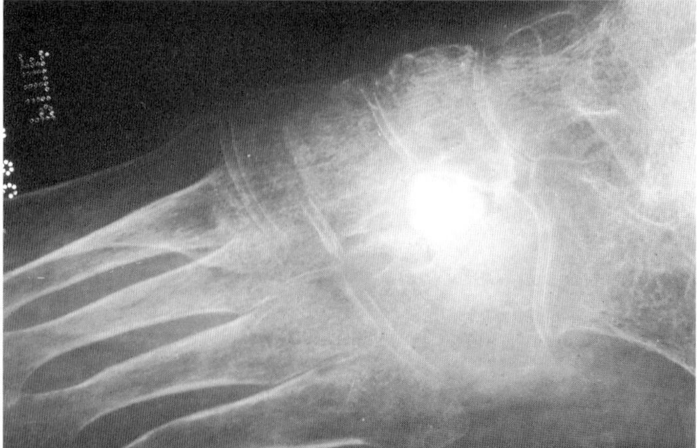

Fig. 7.18 Osteoid osteoma in tarsal location inducing a disuse osteoporosis.

venous phase and responding to the dilated capillary network of the nidus.[37–39]

Plain tomography[40] has been replaced by CT which is now regarded as the definitive technique in the study of the extent, size and location in bone of an osteoid osteoma, with the ability to locate the lesion in both the transverse and sagittal planes.[41–44] The nidus appears as a well-defined, low-density area with smooth borders which

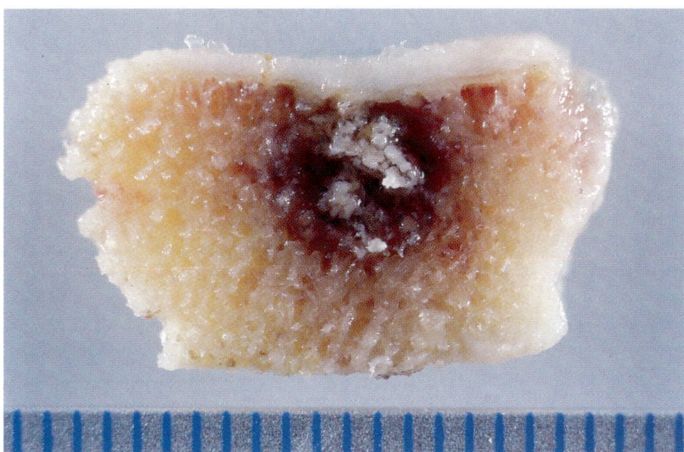

Fig. 7.19 Highly vascularized nidus in a cuneiform bone.

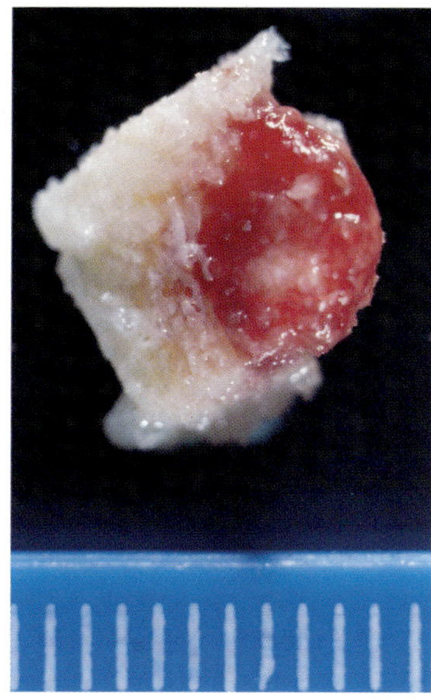

Fig. 7.20 Highly vascularized nidus in the phalanx of a great toe.

differ from those seen in osteomyelitis; variable amounts of punctate, amorphous or dense central mineralization may be found.[3] CT is particularly useful in the examination of vertebral lesions.[42]

Identification of the nidus using MRI produces variable results;[41,43,45] there is a decreased signal intensity on both T1- and T2-weighted images and an increased signal intensity in the surrounding area on T2 correlating with diffuse marrow abnormalities.[3,46–48] A calcified nidus appears as a low-intensity signal. For some authors, MRI findings are uncharacteristic, showing a reactive soft tissue mass, edema[45,47,49,50] or synovitis and joint effusion,[51] even if the nidus may occasionally be clearly visualized.[48]

Gross pathology

The nidus appears as a reddish-brown granular or gritty mass, sharply demarcated and ranging in size from a few millimeters to 10–15 millimeters maximum. More calcified lesions are yellow–white (Figs 7.19–7.26).

Subperiosteal osteoid osteomas protude from the surface of bone and can be easily shelled out from the skeletal bed; they may be encapsulated by the periosteum.[52]

In cortical osteoid osteomas, the nidus is usually situated at the junction of the new and old cortex (Lichtenstein 1975).

The term 'giant osteoid osteoma' has been suggested for osteoblastomas, but genuine giant osteoid osteomas do themselves exist according to the cases reported by Lichtenstein in the humerus, femur and lumbar vertebra.

Histopathology

The histological structure of a nidus is that of a highly vascularized stroma with hyperemic capillaries associated with interlacing trabeculae of osteoid or woven bone (Figs 7.27–7.34). Osteoblasts are the main cellular com-

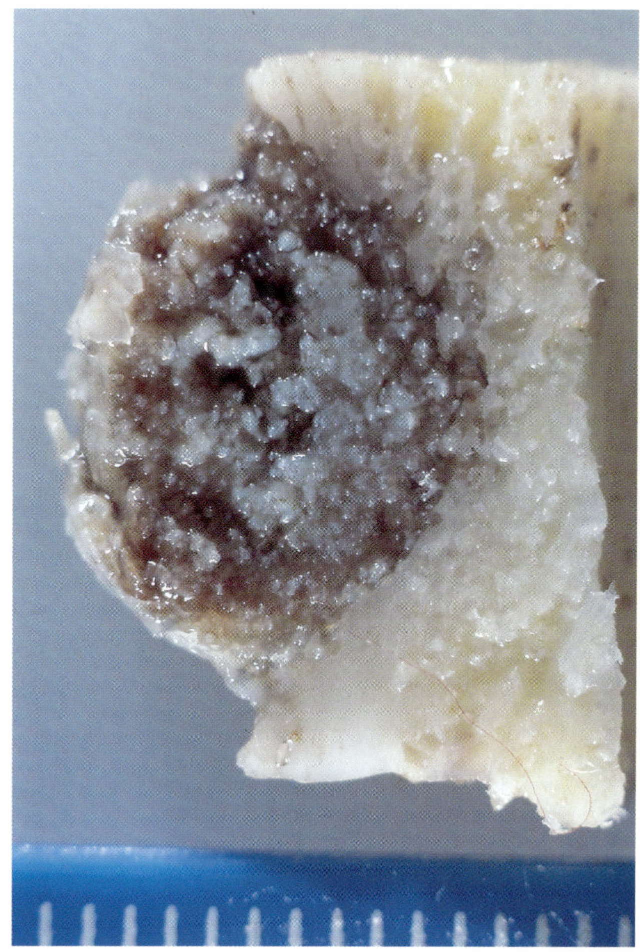

Fig. 7.21 Highly vascularized subperiosteal nidus of the femoral neck.

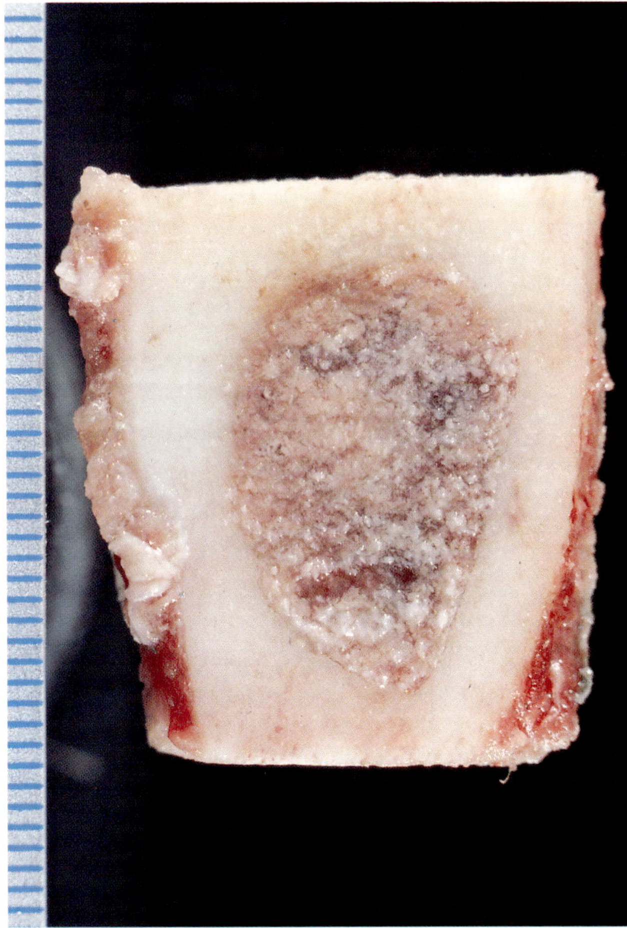

Fig. 7.22

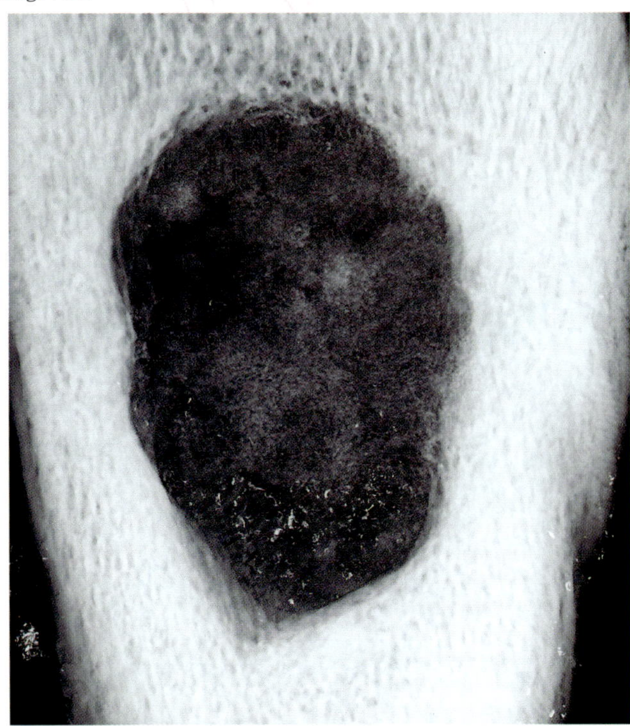

Fig. 7.23

Figs 7.22, 7.23 Osteoid osteoma of the femur with faint calcifications.

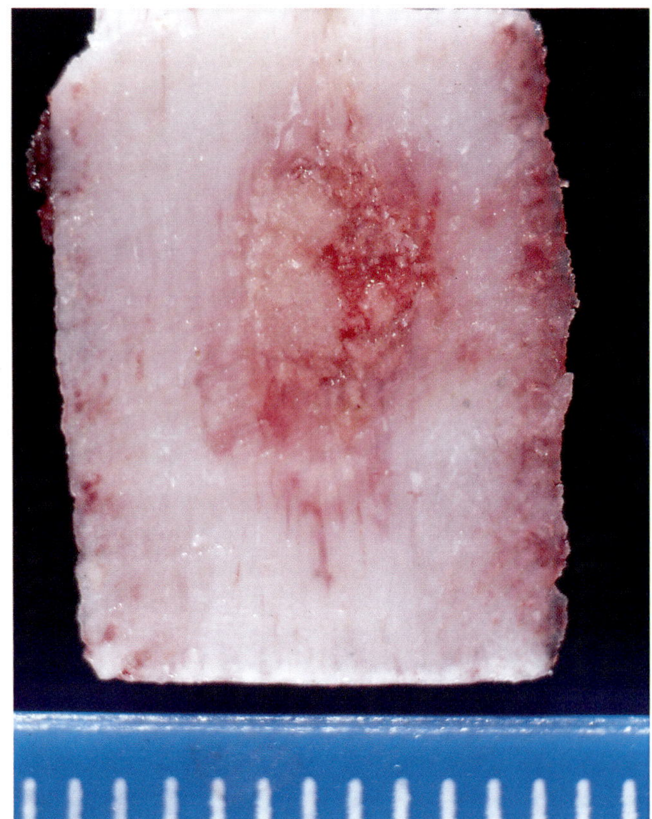

Fig. 7.24

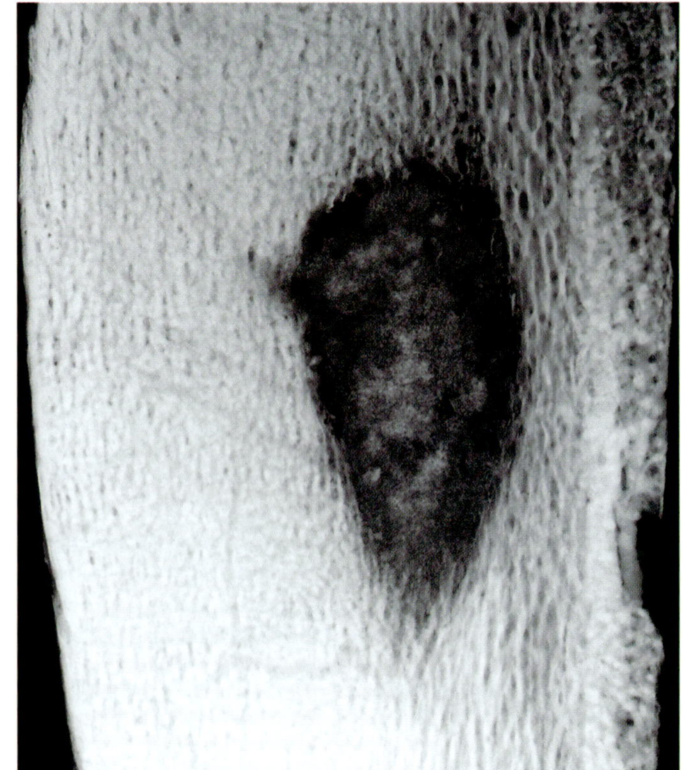

Fig. 7.25

Figs 7.24, 7.25 Osteoid osteoma of the femur with moderate calcifications.

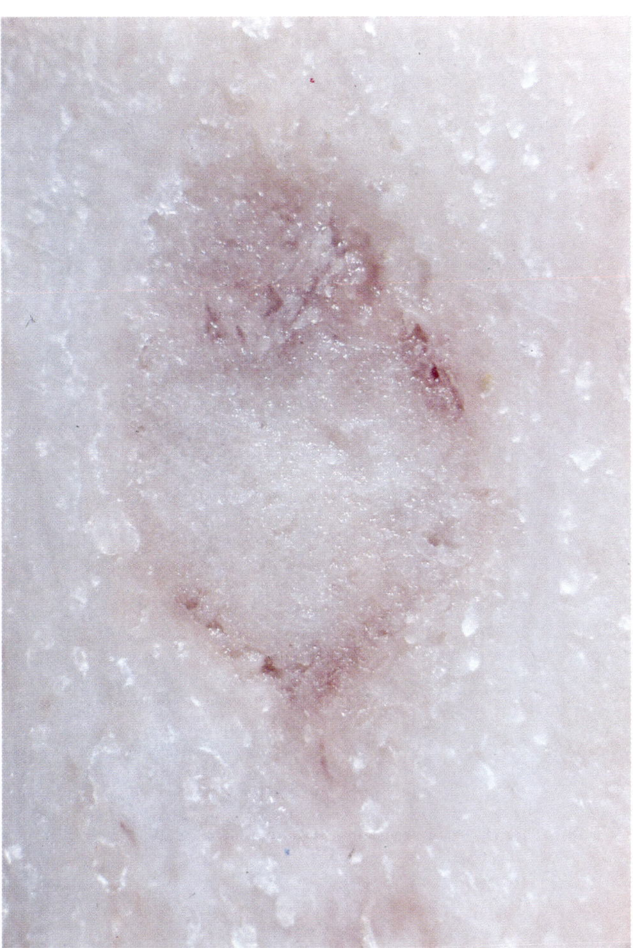

Fig. 7.26 Highly calcified intracortical osteoid osteoma of the femur.

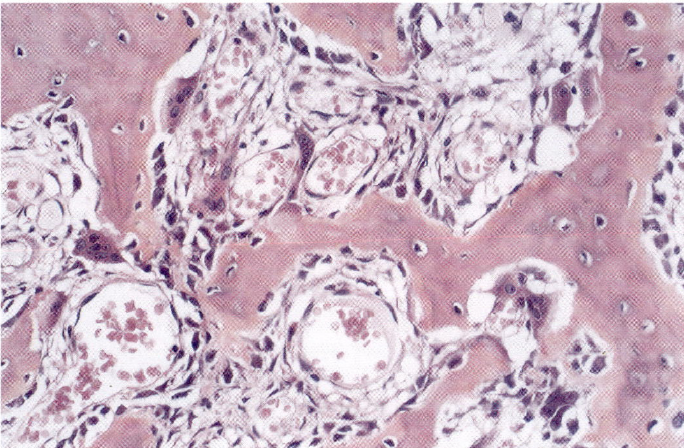

Fig. 7.27

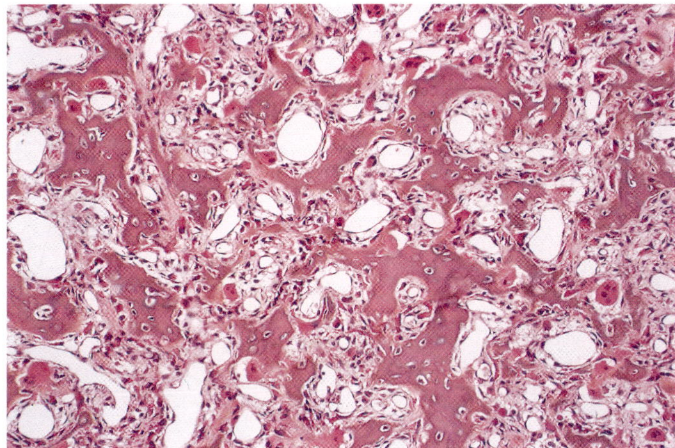

Fig. 7.28

Figs 7.27, 7.28 Usual histology of a nidus: osteoblastic and osteoclastic cells, meshwork of new bone and prominent vascularization.

ponent, with plump nuclei, an occasional normal mitotic figure and in particular, a normally prominent osteoblastic narrowing of the surfaces. Osteoclasts may be numerous but are rarely in apposition to the mineralized osteoid.[53] Some scattered lymphocytes and plasma cells may be found.

Calcification is usually central; some osteoid osteomas may show compact osteoid (Lichtenstein 1975). In sclerotic lesions with broad trabeculae a prominent mosaic pattern of cement lines which mimics that seen in Paget's disease may be found. At the periphery, a loose fibrovascular band is located between the nidus and the surrounding bone.

Remodeling of bone and hypervascularization are found in periosteal thickening or diffuse cancellous bone sclerosis.

Three evolutionary disease stages have been delineated by Huvos (1991): a first stage of active proliferative osteoblasts in a highly vascularized stroma and minimal bone production, an intermediate stage with osteoid and a mature or so-called 'osteoma' stage with well-calcified compact trabeculae of atypical bone. Even if the nidus can be considered a dynamic process of bone formation, mineralization and resorption,[53] the histologic stages do not correlate with the clinical symptoms.[8]

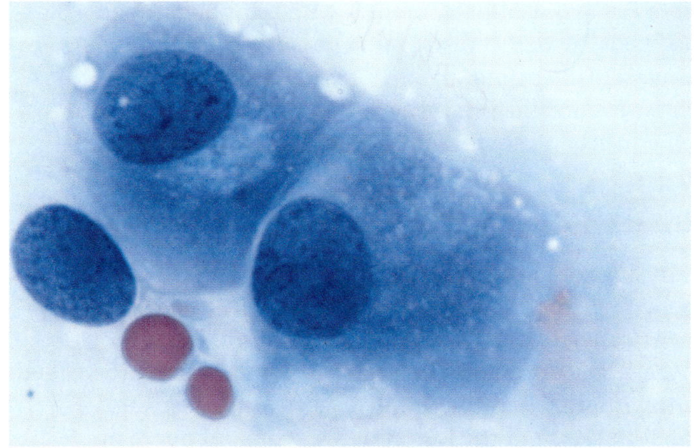

Fig. 7.29 Imprint cytology of a nidus: osteoblasts exhibiting a peripheral located nucleus.

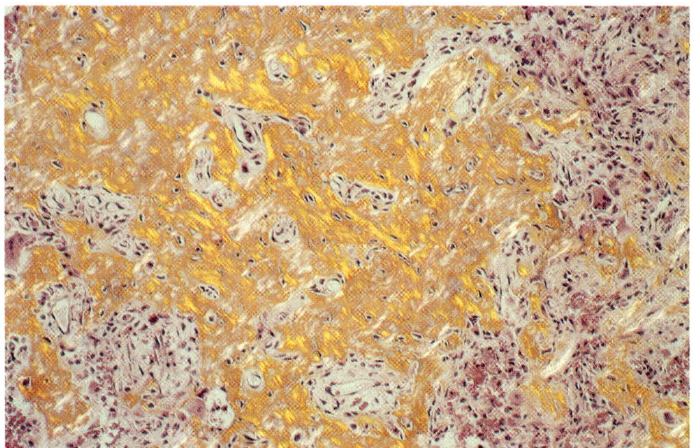

Fig. 7.30 Woven bone formation in an osteoid osteoma of the humerus (polarized light).

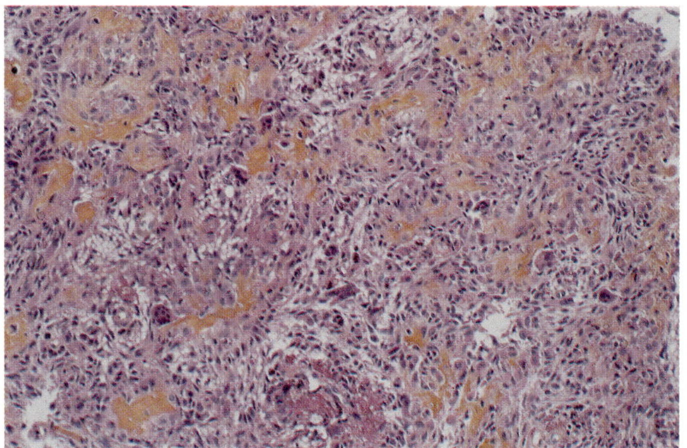

Fig. 7.31 Unusual more cellular area with closely packed cells and giant cells, in an otherwise classic osteoid osteoma.

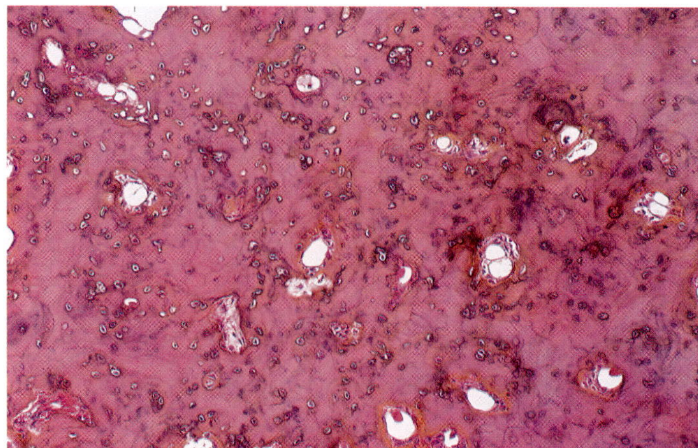

Fig. 7.32

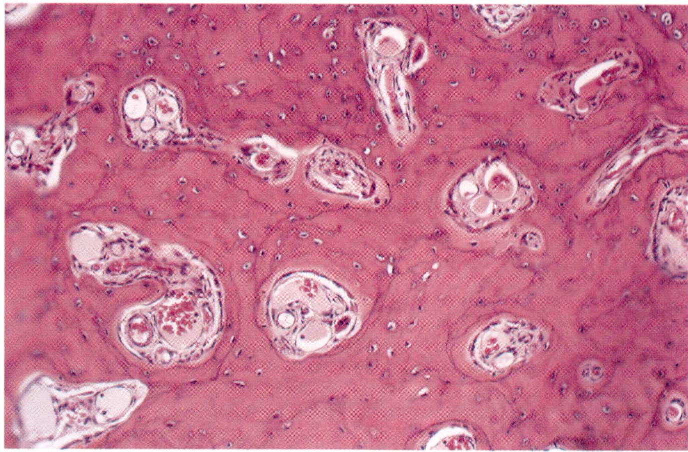

Fig. 7.33

Figs 7.32, 7.33 Osteosclerotic nidus with prominent cement lines.

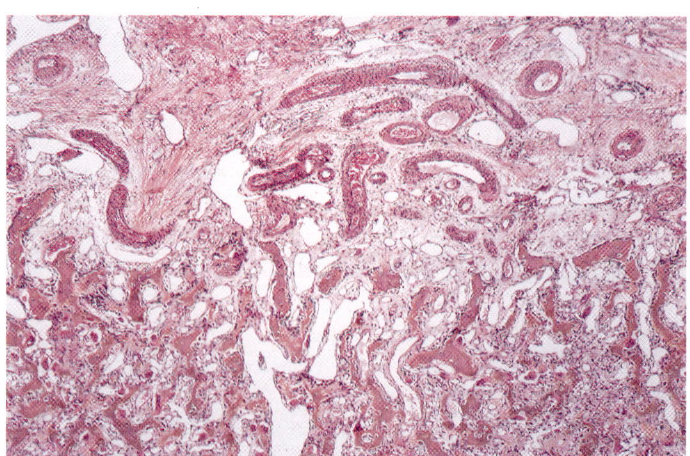

Fig. 7.34 Peripheral vascularization of a nidus.

In intraarticular lesions, synovial changes have been described as a lymphofollicular synovitis[54–58] (Fig. 7.35); there is a synovial proliferation with lymphocytes and plasma cells usually distributed in lymphoid clusters or perivascular cuffing, mimicking an early rheumatoid synovitis. Joint fluid is typical of mechanical disease with low cell counts and increased protein levels.

Histochemistry and immunohistochemistry

Pain in osteoid osteoma has been studied in several reports, histochemically and more recently immunohistochemically, as well as at an ultrastructural level.

On silver impregnation staining, axons can be identified ramifying through the nidus or appearing as groups entering at the edge of the lesion. Unmyelinated nerve fibers are close to the abundant nutrient arteries and it is presumed that pain is generated by vascular pressure[59] and transmitted by sensitive autonomic nerves.[60–65] S-100 protein positivity, as well as positivity for PGP9.5, has confirmed the existence of fine nerve fibers, usually close to the blood

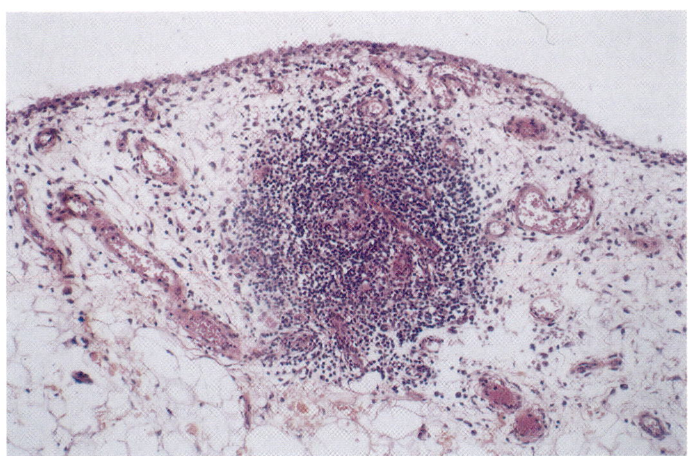

Fig. 7.35 Intraarticular osteoid osteoma of the femoral neck: lymphofollicular synovitis.

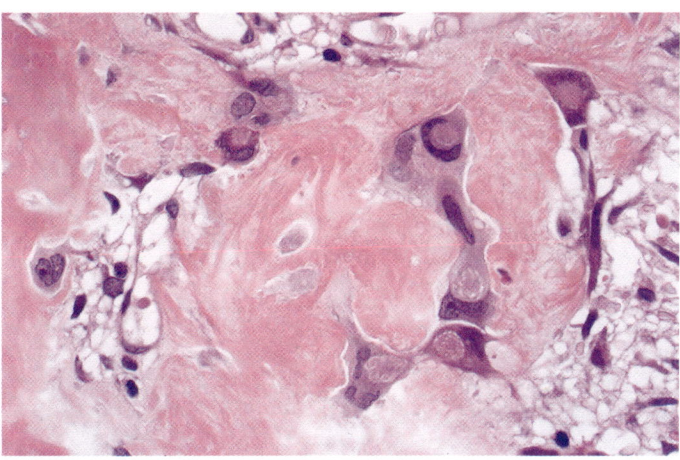

Fig. 7.36 Osteoid osteoma with a 15-year clinical course (see Figs 7.7, 7.8): smudged osteoblasts close to a non-calcified osteoid matrix.

vessels (PGP9,5 demonstrating the terminal regions of fine nerve fibers[66]).

Myelinated fibers have recently been found on electron microscopy.[67]

Radioimmunoassays have demonstrated an increased synthesis of prostaglandins, especially prostaglandin E2.[68–70] The role of prostaglandin E2 and prostacyclin (PGI2) is to stimulate nerve endings by vasodilatation and to reduce the threshold for stimulation of pain receptors.[71] This very high prostaglandin biosynthetic activity is reversible upon removal of the nidus.[71] PGE2 immunoreactivity has been found in the cytoplasm of the osteoblasts.[66] The role of prostaglandins has even been suggested in the development of the nidus itself.[8,68]

Other immunohistochemical studies are of limited value in the diagnosis of osteoid osteoma, i.e. positive staining of the osteoblasts with osteonectin[72,73] or immunoreactivity with osteocalcin.[74]

Immunological characteristics of the joint fluid have been studied, suggesting a local T cell-mediated activation of the immune system induced by a presumed antigen or release of PGE2 or cytokines;[75] cells bearing IL-2R have been demonstrated in the synovial tissue and lymphoid follicles are composed of B and T cells, T lymphocytes being mainly of the CD4 phenotype.[75]

Electron microscopy

Several ultrastructural reports have shown similarities in the cellular component of the nidus with normal osteoblasts, with the exception of some irregular or indented nuclei. Osteogenic cell differentiation with a mineralization process involving matrix vesicles is seen.[76–79]

Osteoid osteoma has been also studied using scanning electron microscopy[80–82] which reveals a spongy structure of bone, calcifying globules and, paradoxically, the greatest degree of immaturity in the central zone.[82]

Course, treatment and prognosis

The natural course of osteoid osteoma is variable. The nidus can persist for several years without any indication of involution (Lichtenstein 1975) (Fig. 7.36). Spontaneous healing with gradual loss of symptoms has been reported, leaving some sclerosis or cortical thickening, but only evidenced by clinical and radiological findings.[9,59,83–86] There is no true malignant transformation, only disputable diagnoses.[87]

Removal of the nidus cures the disease with prompt relief of pain. Thickened reactive bone may resolve after successful surgery (Unni 1996). In some cases, removal of reactive bone may only relieve symptoms.[86] Patients can be cured even when the nidus is not found.

Surgical localization may be facilitated by CT-guided wire placement, thin section CT scans and successively burring through the reactive bone, or CT-guided drill needle excision.[88–90] Intraoperative or postoperative bone scintigraphy is also used.[91–93] Tetracycline labeling gives a golden-yellow fluorescence under UV light,[94] but the results are inconsistent in some reports.[11] Intraoperative radiography of the specimen is normal practice.

Recently, long-term administration of non-steroidal antiinflammatory medication has also been advocated.[95]

Recurrence, sometimes with a very long asymptomatic interval, is due to the persistence of the nidus or to its incomplete removal.[96–99] Rarely, recurrence may be related to multiple lesions. Multicentric lesions can occur synchronously or metachronously in the same bone or in two adjacent bones.[100–102] Multiple lesions have been reported in periosteal locations (Lichtenstein 1975, Schajowicz 1994, Unni 1996),[103] in vertebrae,[104–106] in the hand[107–109] and also in children.[110]

Differential diagnosis

On imaging, many lesions are included: stress fractures,

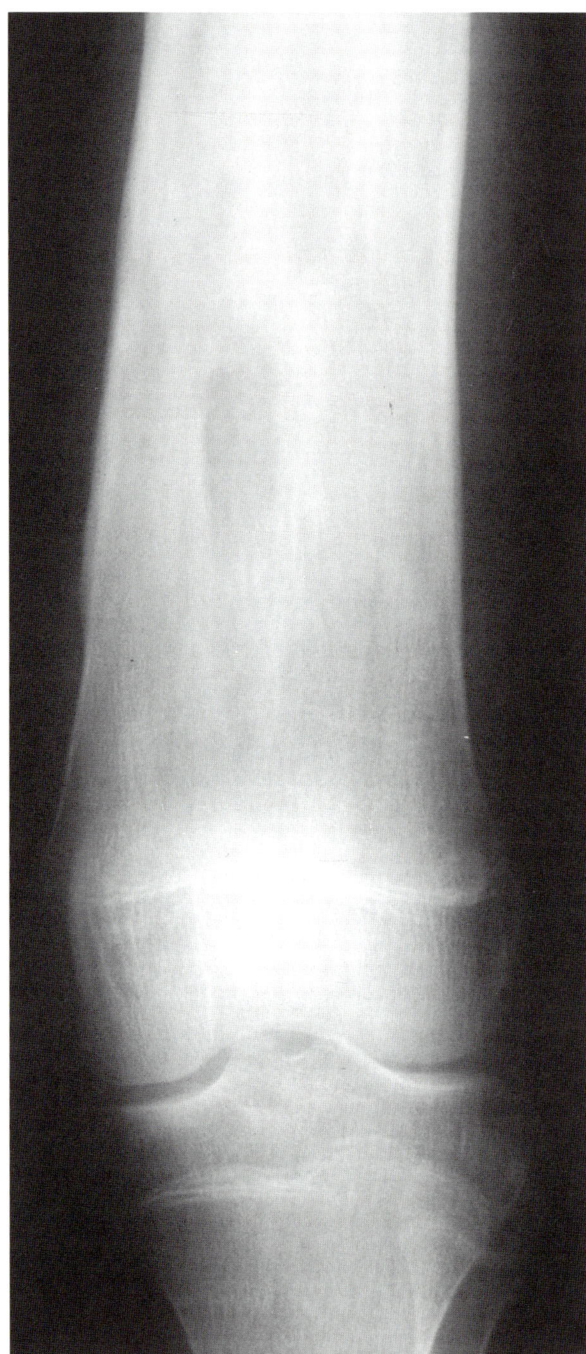

Fig. 7.37

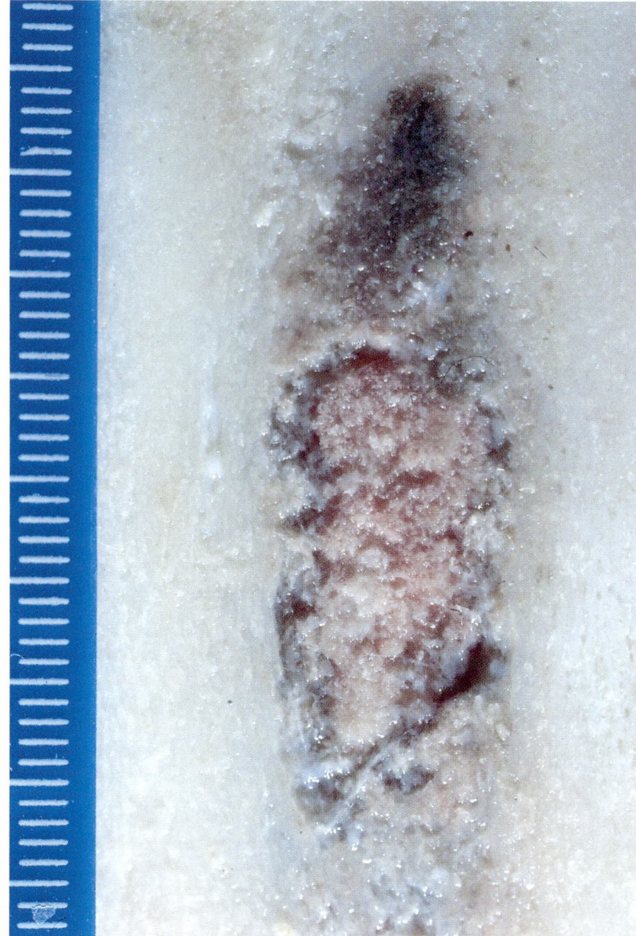

Fig. 7.38

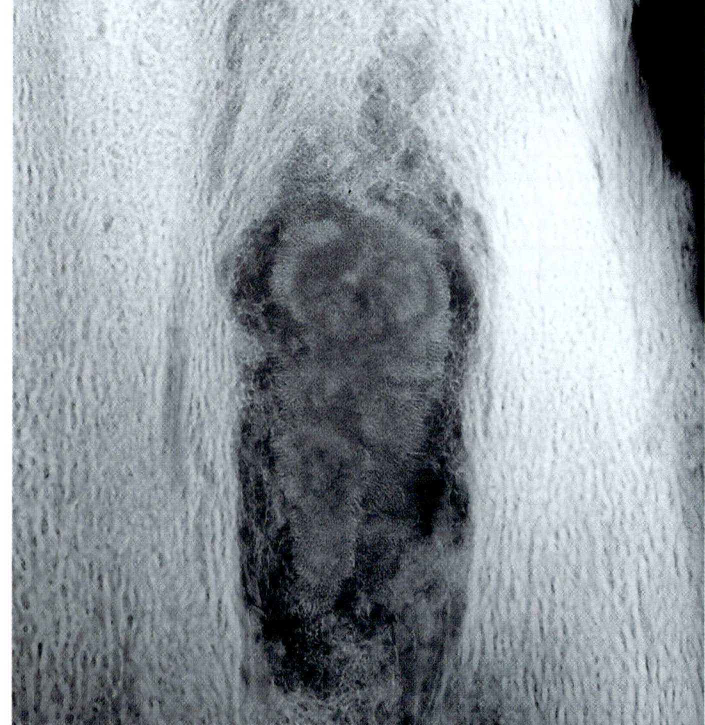

Fig. 7.39

Figs 7.37–7.39 Osteoblastoma of the femur with associated osteomalacia.

intracortical abscess, sclerosing osteomyelitis,[8] bone islands, osteoblastic metastasis,[12,111] or even hemangiomas.[112]

For the pathologist, the main differential diagnosis is osteoblastoma and there are some reports of 'transformation' of an osteoid osteoma into osteoblastoma.[113–116]

For some authors, both lesions are benign osteoblastic tumors with closely similar histologic aspects.[7,116–120] They can be separated by their size[60] or by their location in bone. Using the two criteria, Schajowicz & Lemos[117] have proposed a new classification: circumscribed osteoblastoma with a nidus of less than 2 cm and cortical, medullary and periosteal location, and genuine osteoblastoma with a nidus larger than 2 cm and multifocal osteoblastomas (medullary or periosteal). If we refer to Lichtenstein, 'Size as a criterion is arbitrary and unrealistic . . . it should be clear that resemblance at times does not establish identity'.

For a diagnosis of osteoblastoma, one has to rely on a brisk osteoblastic proliferation, a more disordered architecture, an expanding lesion with growth potential and differences in pain and reactive bone formation.

Asymptomatic lesions, found as solitary hotspots on bone scans, have been reported in ribs and can mimic osteoid osteoma.[121] Histologically, they presumably represent a reactive or reparative process with a moderately fibrous stroma, remodeling of bone and new bone formation without prominent osteoblastic rimming. A similar case has been studied on the scapula, following trauma, with a zonal architectural pattern; Mirra suggested the term 'fibroosseous reparative pseudotumor' (FORP) for this asymptomatic lesion.[122]

Comments for the surgical pathologist

Even the skilled bone pathologist is faced with some difficult problems: fragmentation or crumbling of the nidus by thorough curettage, a crushed nidus in one or several cores of bone obtained using interventional radiological techniques, a piece of bone with absence of any nidus despite meticulous serial slices, reembedding of the tissue and numerous sections, histological similarities between osteoid osteoma and osteoblastoma and a reliance on imaging and on the clinical course, particularly in spinal locations.

OSTEOBLASTOMA

Introduction and clinical data

An osteoblastoma is a benign osteoblastic tumor of progressive growth, with a potential for local bone destruction and aggressiveness. The name 'osteoblastoma' was proposed simultaneously, but separately, by Lichtenstein and Jaffe.[123–125]

It accounts for 1% of all bone tumors and approximately 3% of all benign tumors, with a male:female prevalence ratio of 2–3:1.

Peak incidence appears to be between 7 and 20 years of age.[126] In the experience of the Mayo Clinic, the mean age is 20 years;[127] 70% of cases occur in the second and third decade of life.

Clinical symptoms, lasting in duration for between a few weeks and 2 years, are boring pain, local tenderness or swelling. Amelioration of pain by salicylates is, at best, intermittent.

In vertebral cases, scoliosis appears in one-third to half of the cases,[128,129] due to muscle spasm[21,129,130] and neurologic symptoms may be related to cord compression. A single case has been reported with systemic toxicity, cachexia, clubbing and periosteal reactions.[131,132]

Osteoblastoma is one of the causes of tumor-induced osteomalacia;[133–138] metabolic disturbances improve or completely disappear on removal of the tumor (Figs 7.37–7.39).

Skeletal distribution

Virtually any bone can be affected, but the most common sites are the vertebral column including the sacrum

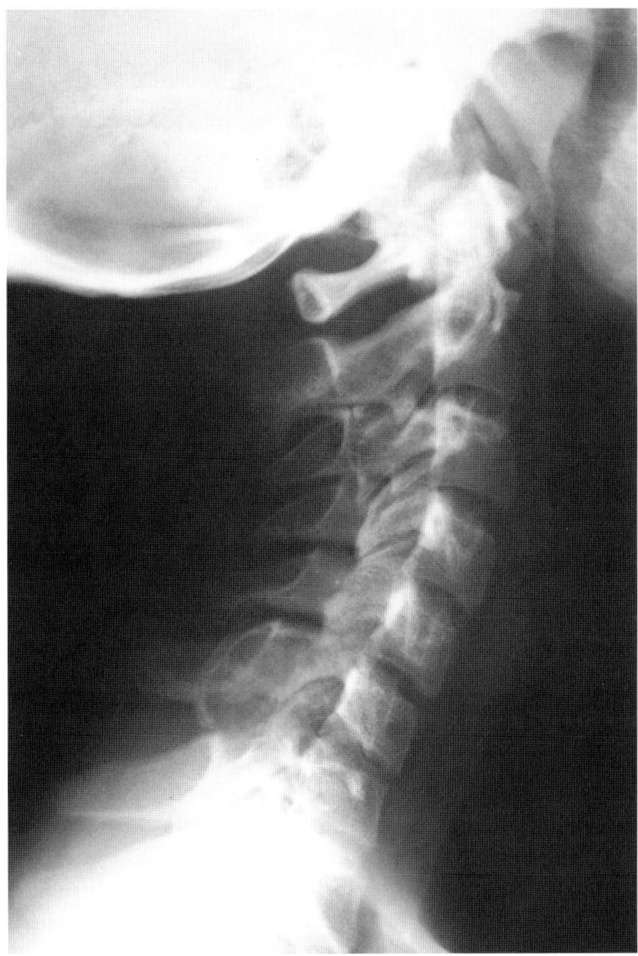

Fig. 7.40 Osteoblastoma of the sixth cervical vertebra.

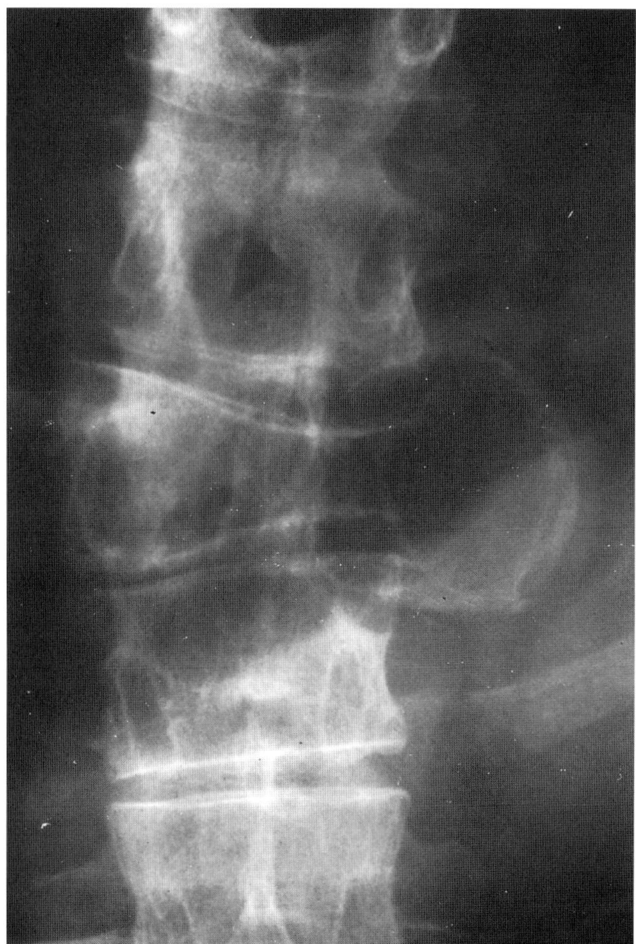

Fig. 7.41 Osteoblastoma at the T12 level.

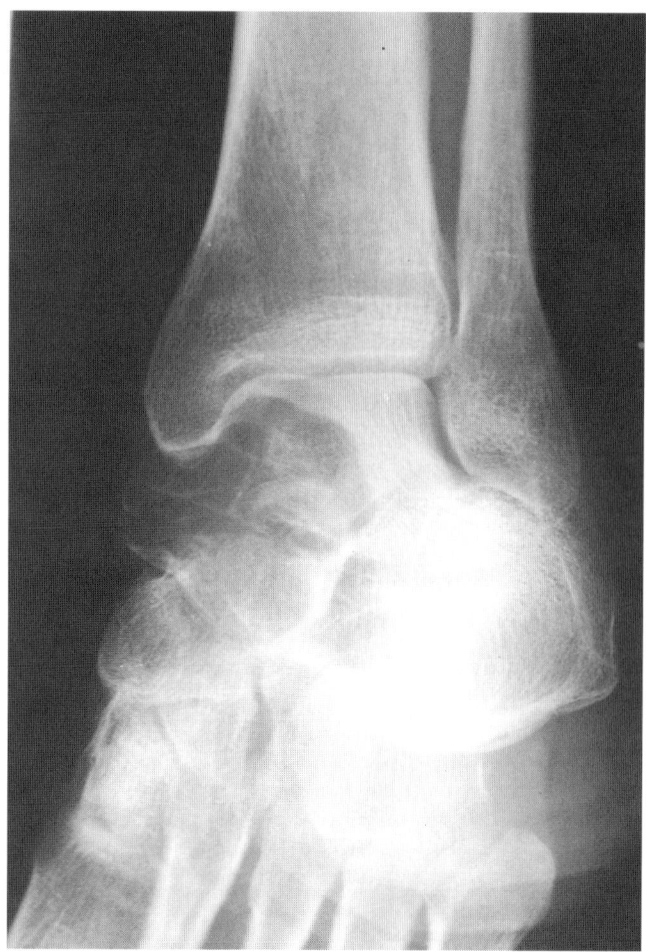

Fig. 7.42 Osteoblastoma of the talus with a secondary aneurysmal bone cyst component.

(Figs 7.40, 7.41), the femur and tibia[139,140] and the bones of the foot, chiefly the dorsal part of the neck of the talus[24] (Fig. 7.42).

Imaging

There is a broad spectrum of radiographic findings and about 12% of cases are suggestive of malignancy, showing cortical expansion and destruction.[127]

On plain films, osteoblastoma may be identical to osteoid osteoma, but with less reactive sclerosis[41] (Fig. 7.43). Usually, it is a well-circumscribed, expansile, radiolucent lesion, with a thin shell of peripheral new bone and eventually a periosteal reaction of solid type. Flecks of calcification or irregular calcified deposits may be found; mottled calcifications can mimic the ground glass appearance of fibrous dysplasia (Campanacci 1990) (Fig. 7.44).

Attenuation of the cortex and expansion of bone may also resemble an aneurysmal bone cyst, especially in the small tubular bones.[139,141,142] In long bones, the lesion is metaphyseal or diaphyseal (proximal part of the shaft);

epiphyseal involvement is unusual.[142–144] The lesion is often eccentric.

In the spine, the thoracic and lumbar vertebrae are the most common sites; the tumor originates from the posterior elements (pedicle and lamina) and involvement of the vertebral body only is rare.[21,127,130,145] Two adjacent vertebrae may be involved[146] and pathologic fractures can occur. In long-standing cases, tumors become heavily ossified,[147] leaving only a calcified shell. A blow-out expansile lesion is also common in the spine. Tumors can extend into the epidural space and paraspinal tissues.

Juxtacortical or periosteal locations have been reported, the tumor being limited by a thin shell of periosteal bone[148,149] (Fig. 7.45).

Multifocal lesions are rare[41,117,150] though a most unusual case has been reported, involving several bones of the lower extremity.[151]

On bone scans, there is an intense focal accumulation of radionuclides;[139] scintigraphy may be useful in the spine.[130]

Angiography is seldom performed, but shows a pro-

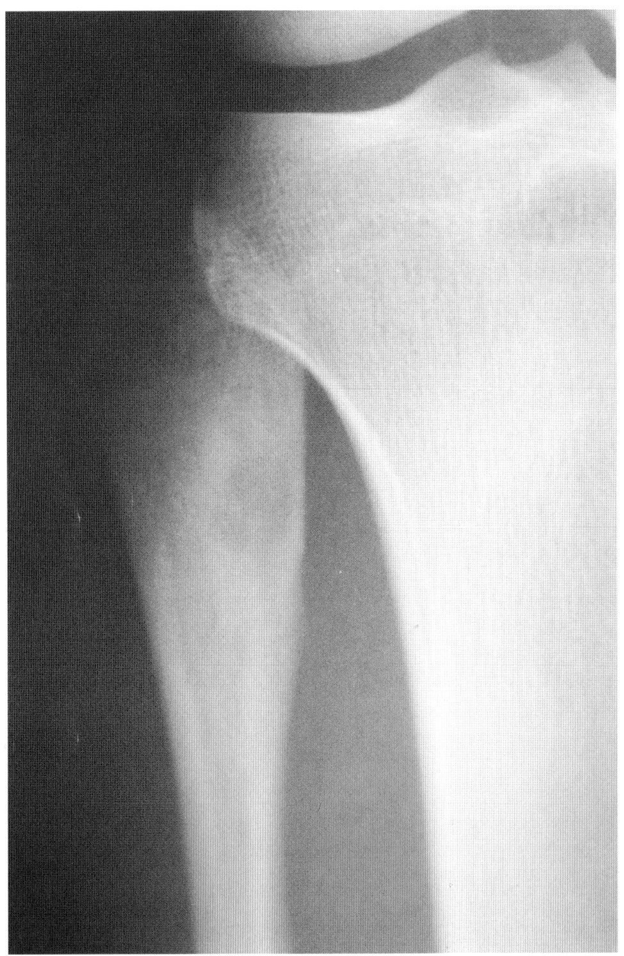

Fig. 7.43 Well-circumscribed lytic osteoblastoma of the fibula.

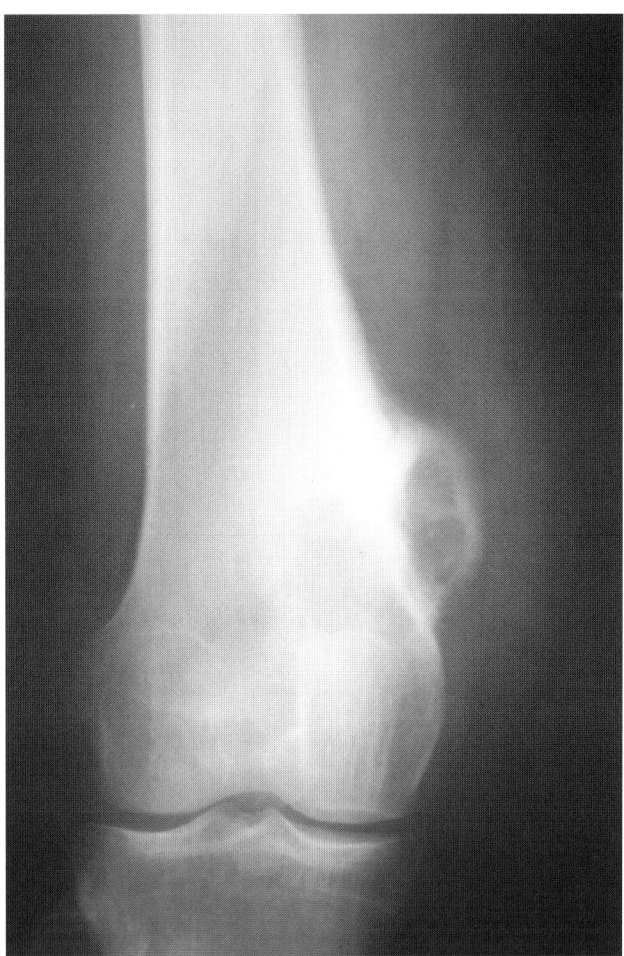

Fig. 7.45 Periosteal osteoblastoma of the femur.

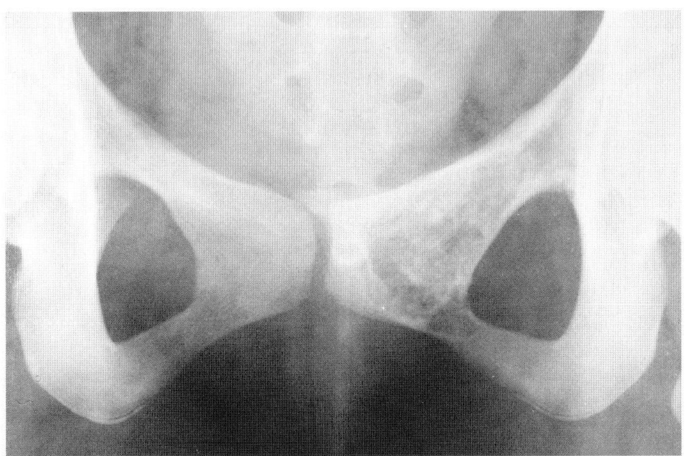

Fig. 7.44 Mottled calcifications in an osteoblastoma of the pubis.

nounced tumor blush at the capillary phase that persists into the venous phase. Some tumors are avascular.[152]

Computed tomography is by far the best imaging procedure, particularly in the spine[130,153] and pelvis,[139] delineating the location of the tumor and its size and revealing calcifications or ossifications, cortical destruction and any associated soft tissue extension.

MRI shows a low and intermediate signal intensity on T1-weighted images and a high signal on T2, reflecting the changes in the bone marrow and soft tissues.[139] In vertebral locations, it can delineate the degree of extension into the spinal canal; in the same site, an unusual flare phenomenon has been described, simulating a malignant tumor and corresponding to a widespread inflammatory response to the lesion.[154]

MRI can also detect multiple aneurysmal bone cyst components with fluid–fluid levels.[155]

Gross pathology

Osteoblastomas range in size from approximately 2 to 12 cm. They appear as highly vascular tissue, reddish-brown or chalky white and grayish in color[126] and with a granular or gritty texture.

The tumor interface is sharp, sometimes with scalloped margins.[126] The soft tissue extension may be limited by a thin calcified periosteal shell.

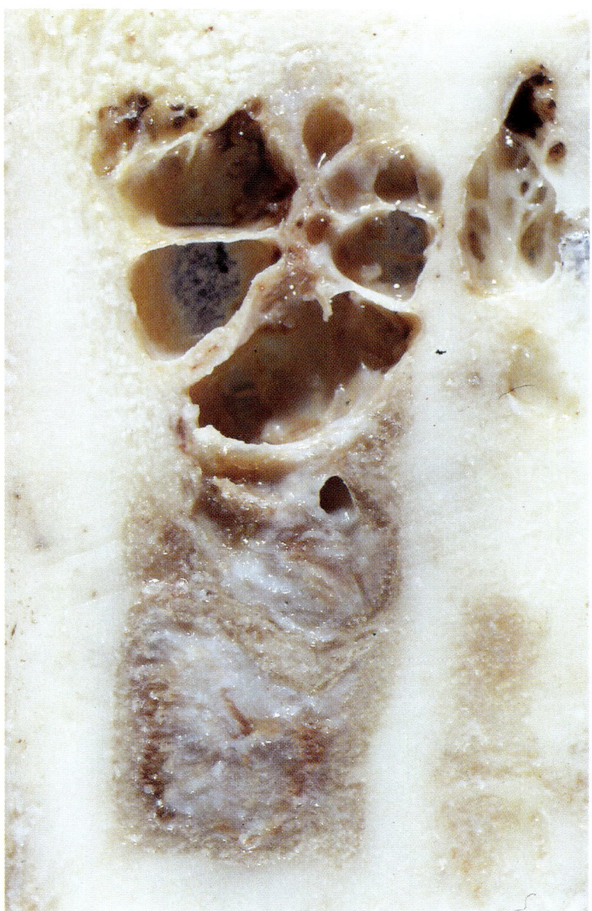

Fig. 7.46

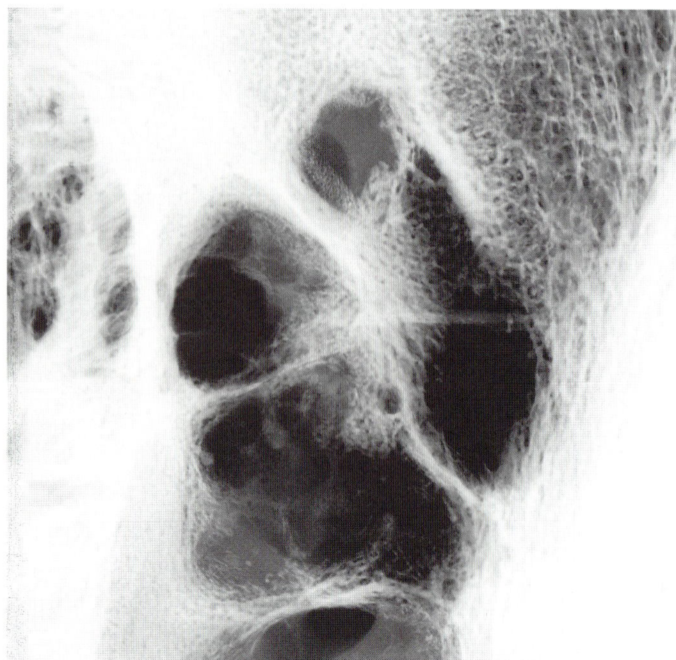

Fig. 7.47

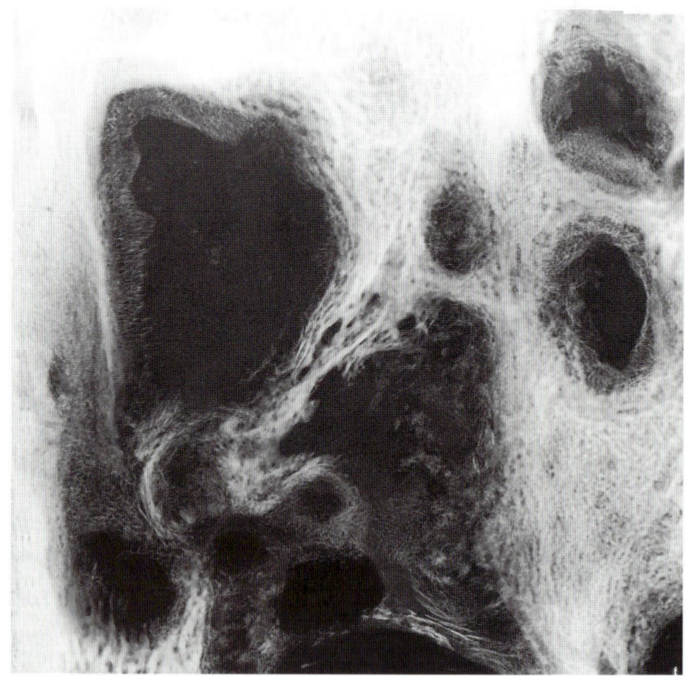

Fig. 7.48

Figs 7.46–7.48 Secondary aneurysmal bone cyst-like changes in a recurrence of a femoral osteoblastoma.

Hemorrhages or, more often, cystic degeneration can be found, but expansile lesions usually correspond to a secondary aneurysmal bone cyst component (Figs 7.46–7.48).

Histopathology

Osteoblastoma, unlike osteoid osteoma, shows variations in its histologic pattern[127] (Figs 7.49–7.54). The stroma comprises a loosely fibrovascular tissue, with many thin-walled capillaries; some spindly cells may be found (Huvos 1991), but the main cell component is made up of local aggregates of osteoblasts in different stages of differentiation (Lichtenstein 1975). Osteoblasts look plump and active, but the few mitotic figures are normal. The nucleus has regular contours with a single prominent nucleolus.[127] There appears, eventually, a focal rimming of osteoblasts around the bone component. Multinucleated giant cells may be found in moderate numbers.

Osteoid and immature bone trabeculae of variable thickness can lead to heavily calcified areas or large bony masses.[156] In some cases, dense sheets of osteoid are associated with little intervening connective tissue stroma (Lichtenstein 1975) or bone develops a pagetoid pattern with irregular cement lines.[127] The amount of osteoid and bone can vary in a single tumor, as can the degree of calcification.

The tumor does not infiltrate or permeate the surrounding normal bone trabeculae; a multifocal growth should not, therefore, be confused with permeation.[127,140]

In a few cases, bizarre osteoblasts with smudged chro-

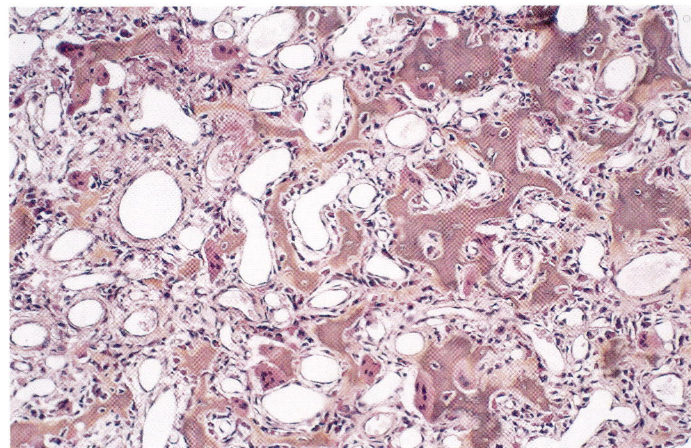

Fig. 7.49 Osteoblastoma of a femur.

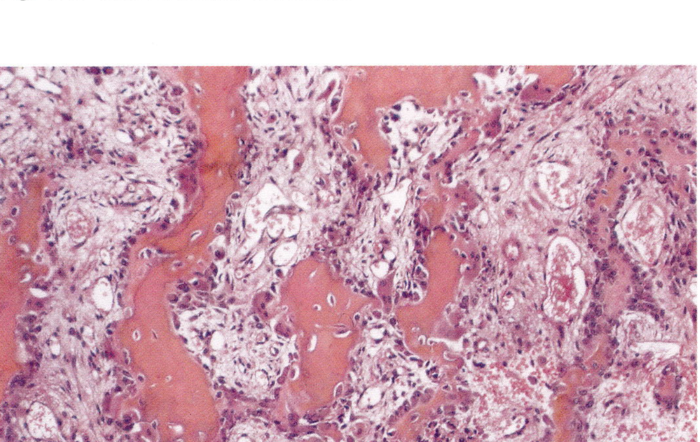

Fig. 7.50 Osteoblastoma of an atlas.

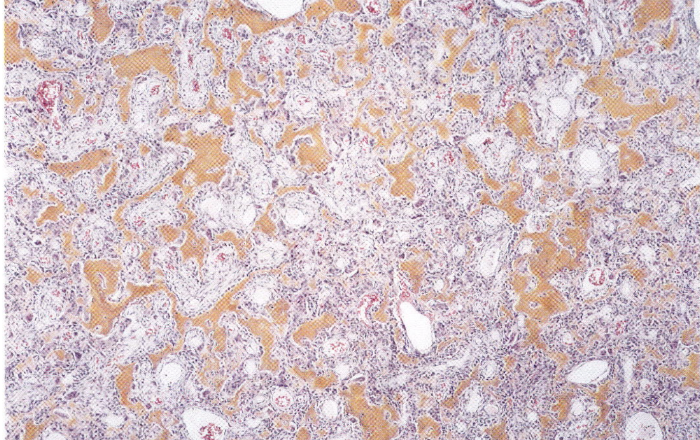

Fig. 7.51 Osteoblastoma of a rib.

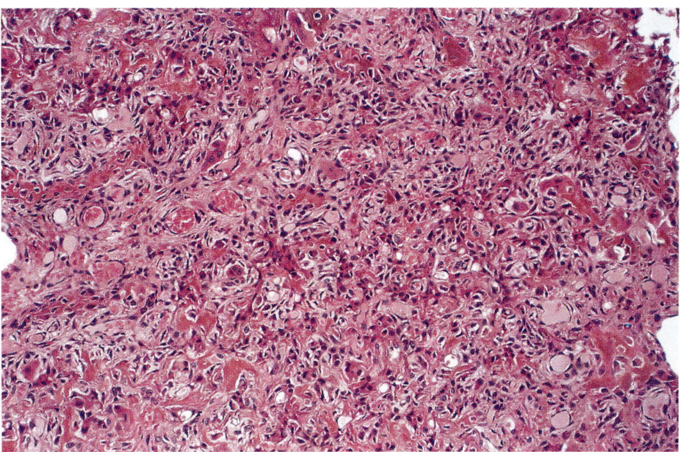

Fig. 7.52 Limited bone formation in an osteoblastoma.

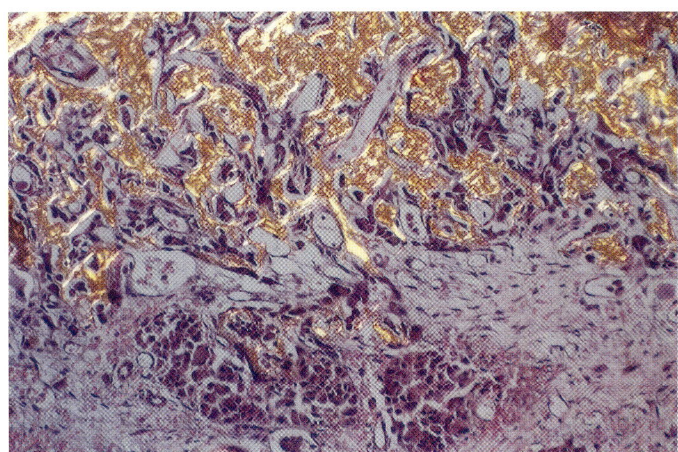

Fig. 7.53 Immature bone formation in an osteoblastoma (polarized light).

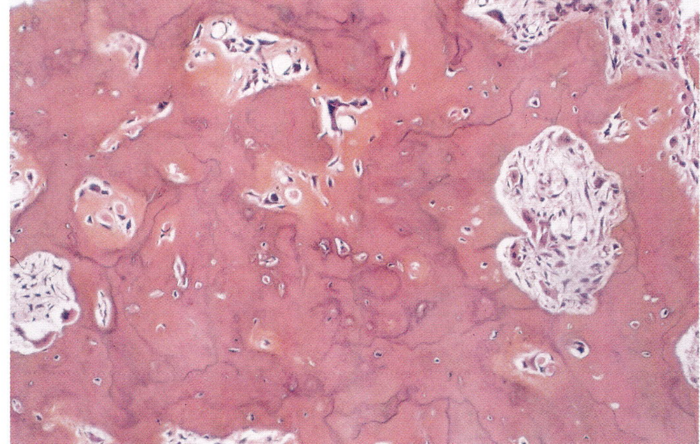

Fig. 7.54 Heavily calcified areas in an osteoblastoma.

matin and multinucleated forms can be found, but these show no mitotic activity, and correspond to degenerative changes.[127,157,158]

A secondary aneurysmal bone cyst component is responsible for a rapid destructive growth with an incidence of 10–16% of cases.[127,140–142,155,159]

Some metaplastic hyaline cartilage is not unusual after recurrence, corresponding presumably to microfractures.[140] A chondroosteoid material or even hyaline cartilage has been found in some cases, merging with the osteoblastoma component, with no evidence of fracture.[160,161] A peripheral chondroid component has also comprised part of a very unusual rib osteoblastoma.[162]

Aggressive osteoblastomas have been described as a distinct clinicopathologic entity by Dorfman & Weiss.[163] They seem to be quite similar to the cases described by Schajowicz as malignant osteoblastomas.[164] Occurring in older patients, they are osteolytic and expanding tumors which destroy the cortex and invade the adjacent bones and soft tissues; they may even cross the joint space.[163] They often recur, but do not metastasize. Since first being described, many cases have been reported.[165–171]

Histologically, osseous trabeculae are broad and irregular, sometimes with a lace-like osteoid. Characteristically, cytology is unusual: besides some spindle stromal cells, osteoblasts are larger, with eosinophilic cytoplasm and prominent, plump, hyperchromatic and vesicular nuclei with one or more nucleoli, resulting in an epithelioid appearance. These cytoplasmic findings have been related to a wide Golgi system and a rich rough endoplasmic reticulum.[140] Osteoblasts are distributed in sheets or scattered. Mitotic rate is low, with no atypical figures (Figs 7.55–7.60).

It should be stressed that the relationship between this aggressive behavior and the unusual histology has been disputed in recent reports from the Mayo Clinic and the Memorial Sloan-Kettering Cancer Center of New York. Epithelioid cells are frequently found in osteoblastomas, often with a multifocal pattern,[127,140] and most tumors do not pursue an aggressive clinical course; there does not seem to be any histological predictor of aggressive behavior.[127,140] Conversely, Mirra & Bertoni[172] regard aggressive osteoblastomas as genuine low-grade osteosarcomas.

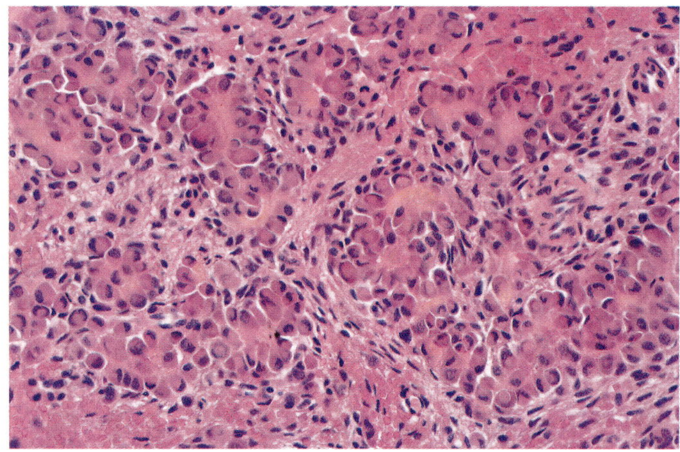

Fig. 7.55 Epithelioid osteoblasts in a vertebral osteoblastoma.

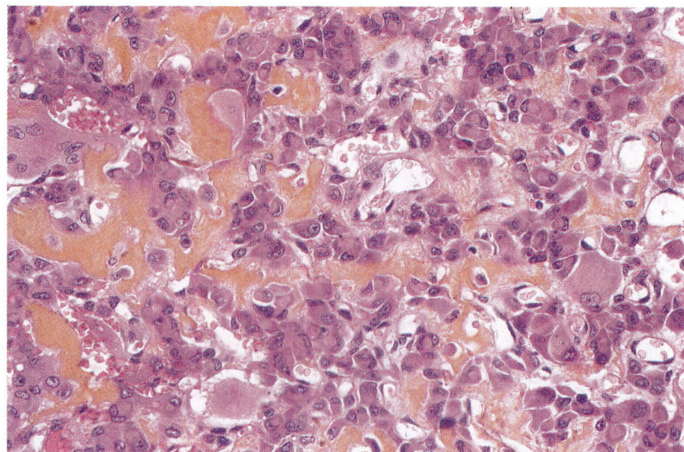

Fig. 7.56 Epithelioid osteoblasts in an osteoblastoma of a rib.

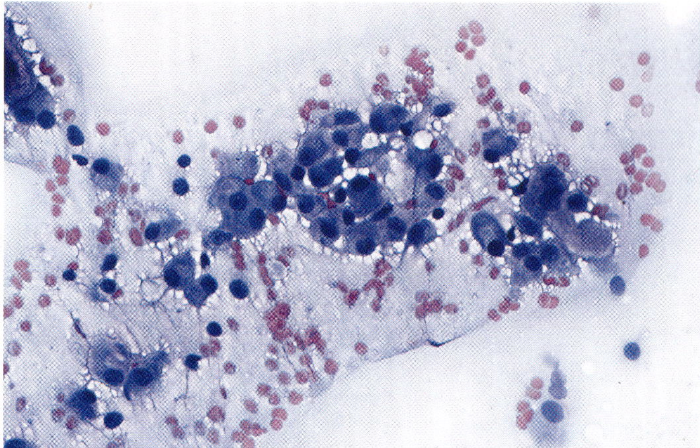

Fig. 7.57

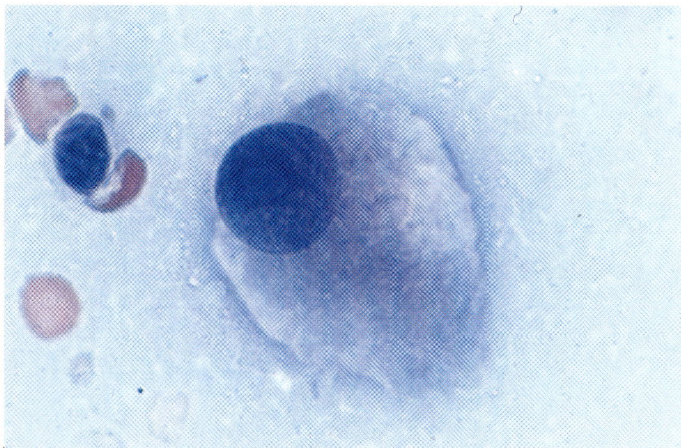

Fig. 7.58

Figs 7.57, 7.58 Imprint cytology of an osteoblastoma demonstrating the osteoblastic cell component.

Cytopathology

On smears, osteoblasts usually appear as mononucleated or occasionally binucleated cells, with an eccentric nucleus

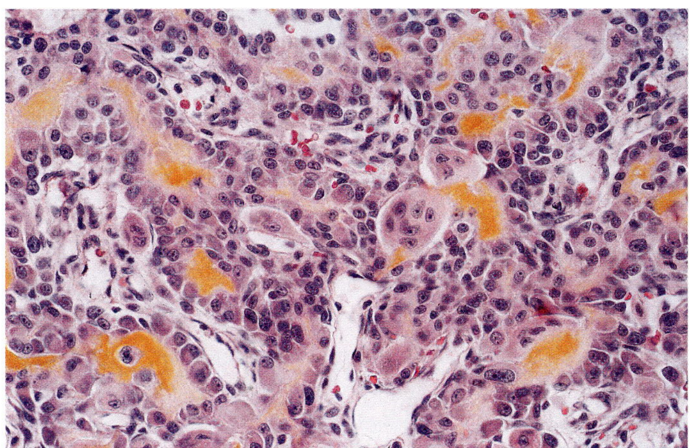

Fig. 7.59

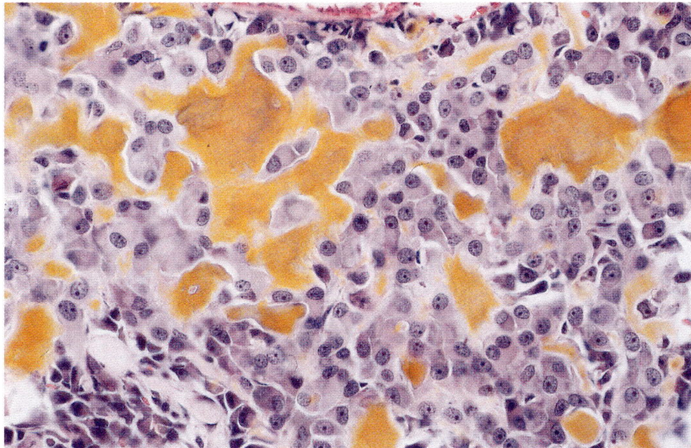

Fig. 7.60

Figs 7.59, 7.60 Osteoblastoma of a rib mimicking an osteoblastoma-like osteosarcoma, but without any infiltrating pattern and with a benign clinical course.

and an abundant, well-demarcated cytoplasm.[173] They are associated with osteoclast-like giant cells of varying size. Osteoid resembles a pinkish fibrillar material.[173]

Immunohistochemistry

A positive staining has been found with osteonectin, a glycoprotein recognized as a differentiation marker of normal osteogenic cells.[174] S-100 protein-positive cells have been found in cases of aggressive osteoblastomas, in the vicinity of calcifying osteoid.[175]

Flow cytometry

Osteoblastoma may show a normal DNA content on flow DNA analysis[176] or on DNA cytophotometry.[144] Aggressive osteoblastomas can be diploid or aneuploid[177] (Schajowicz 1994). A DNA aneuploidy has been found without histological change and with a favorable clinical course[177] but aneuploid peaks have been detected in osteoblastomas transforming to osteosarcomas[178] and hyperploidy detected by microspectrophotometric analysis.[179] This tumor progression to osteosarcoma has shown an aneuploid pattern *before* the detection of histological malignancy, but the very short clinical course may suggest an osteosarcoma from the onset.[180]

Cytogenetics

A three-way unbalanced translocation has been described in a vertebral osteoblastoma, involving chromosomes 15, 17 and 20, with a loss of the chromosome 17 short arm, the latter also being frequently seen in osteosarcomas.[181]

Electron microscopy

Osteoblasts resemble their normal counterparts, but with some irregular indented nuclei,[182–184] large and prominent perinuclear Golgi zones[173,185] and a dilated rough endoplasmic reticulum.[186] Some cells are spindle shaped with abundant intermediate cytofilaments. Multinucleated giant cells are osteoclasts with ruffled borders.[173] The process of mineralization appears to be similar to that of normal bone, with production of matrix vesicles.[80,185,187]

Scanning electron microscopy shows an irregular pattern of bone formation and a spongy structure (Hirohata et al 1981). The localization of alkaline phosphatase activity is similar to that of normal osteoblasts and is increased in aggressive osteoblastomas.[184,188]

In two cases of osteoblastomas with tumor-induced osteomalacia, no secretory granules or other specific features have been found.[134]

The osteoblasts of aggressive osteoblastomas have a similar morphology, but with more immature cells and poorly developed organelles.[182,188]

Course, treatment and prognosis

Rare cases of spontaneous or radiation-induced transformation to osteosarcomas have been reported.[115,127,157,159,170,189–199] Some of them may, however, have been osteosarcomas from the very onset (Huvos 1991).[127,172]

Treatment consists of thorough curettage or a complete resection, which appears to be curative.[157] The role of radiation therapy is disputable,[130] with a risk of radiation-induced sarcoma.[142] Chemotherapy may be useful for recurrent aggressive tumors or those in surgically inaccessible locations.[200]

Recurrences after many years sometimes occur if removal is incomplete,[139,142,201–203] with a rate of 10–21%;[127,142] they are more frequent in the spine and the pelvis.[129] The histologic appearance of recurrences is usually similar to that of the original tumor, but it may be more aggressive.[165]

Differential diagnosis

An aneurysmal bone cyst may be confused with an osteoblastoma, particularly in the spine, if the underlying tumor is not adequately sampled on biopsy.

Differential diagnosis with osteoid osteoma is often quite difficult and small incipient tumors may appear similar. To address this, quantitative histological analysis has been performed, which shows a greater amount of stromal tissue in osteoblastoma.[204] Osteoblastoma also has a less organized pattern, with more irregular distribution of osteoid and calcification, thicker woven bone, more vascularization and, most characteristically, an active proliferation of osteoblasts (Lichtenstein 1975, Schajowicz 1994). Areas resembling aneurysmal bone cysts are not found in osteoid osteomas.

Osteoblastomas must be differentiated from osteosarcomas,[192] the latter showing cells arranged in a compact pattern with a greater nuclear pleomorphism and atypical mitotic activity. Osteoblastomas should also be differentiated from osteoblastoma-like osteosarcoma[172] which shows a permeation of the surrounding tissue, with entrapped host bone and, in some cases, areas of usual osteosarcoma with spindle cells. The interface between the tumor and surrounding bone is the most useful diagnostic feature.[205]

Comments for the surgical pathologist

The brisk cellular osteoblastic activity of osteoblastomas may, in some cases, lead to a false diagnosis of osteosarcoma: one has to rely for diagnosis on the cytology and the loose vascular stroma. Conversely, osteoblastoma-like osteosarcomas may be misdiagnosed and study of the peripheral growth pattern of the tumor on sufficient material from the lesional borders is essential.

REFERENCES

1. Jaffe H L. Osteoid osteoma. A benign osteoblastic tumor composed of osteoid and atypical bone. Arch Surg 1935: 31: 709–728
2. Jaffe H L, Lichtenstein L. Osteoid osteoma. J Bone Joint Surg (Am) 1940: 22: 645–682
3. Kransdorf M J, Stull M A, Gilkey F W, Moser R P Jr. Osteoid osteoma. Radiographics 1991: 11: 671–696
4. Orlowski J P, Mercer R D. Osteoid osteoma in children and young adults. Pediatrics 1977: 59: 526–532
5. Kaweblum M, Lehman W B, Bash J, Strongwater A, Grant A D. Osteoid osteoma under the age of five years. The difficulty of diagnosis. Clin Orthop 1993: 296: 218–224
6. Cohen M D, Harrington T M, Ginsburg W W. Osteoid osteoma: 95 cases and a review of literature. Semin Arthritis Rheum 1983: 12: 265–281
7. Jackson R P, Reckling F W, Mants F A. Osteoid osteoma and osteoblastoma. Similar histologic lesions with different natural histories. Clin Orthop 1977: 128: 303–313
8. Healey J H, Ghelman B. Osteoid osteoma and osteoblastoma. Current concepts and recent advances. Clin Orthop 1986: 204: 76–85
9. Freiberger R H, Loitman B S, Herpern M, Thompson T C. Osteoid osteoma, a report on 80 cases. Am J Roentgenol Radium Ther Nucl Med 1959: 82: 194–205
10. Kattapuram S V, Kushner D C, Philips W C, Rosenthal D I. Osteoid osteoma: an unusual cause of articular pain. Radiology 1983: 147: 383–387
11. Klein M H, Shankman S. Osteoid osteoma: radiologic and pathologic correlation. Skeletal Radiol 1992: 21: 23–31
12. McDermott M B, Kyriakos M, McEnery K. Painless osteoid osteoma of the rib in an adult. Cancer 1996: 77: 1442–1449
13. Wiss D A, Reid B S. Painless osteoid osteoma of the fingers – report of three cases. J Hand Surg (Am) 1983: 8: 914–917
14. Pettine K A, Klassen R A. Osteoid osteoma and osteoblastoma of the spine. J Bone Joint Surg (Am) 1986: 68: 354–361
15. Azouz E M, Kozlowski K, Marton D, Sprague P, Zerhouni A, Asselah F. Osteoid osteoma and osteoblastoma of the spine in children. Report of 22 cases with brief literature review. Pediatr Radiol 1986: 16: 25–31
16. Bauer T W, Zehr R J, Belhobek G H, Marks K E. Juxtaarticular osteoid osteoma. Am J Surg Pathol 1991: 15: 381–387
17. Moser R P Jr, Kransdorf M J, Brower A C et al. Osteoid osteoma of the elbow. A review of six cases. Skeletal Radiol 1990: 19: 181–186
18. Norman A, Dorfman H D. Osteoid osteoma inducing pronounced overgrowth and deformity of bone. Clin Orthop 1975: 110: 233–238
19. Norman A, Abdelwahab I F, Buyon J, Matzkin E. Osteoid osteoma of the hip simulating an early onset of osteoarthritis. Radiology 1986: 158: 417–420
20. Clark C R, Ozonoff M B, Drennan J C. Case report 157. Osteoid osteoma of the femoral neck with localized synovitis. Skeletal Radiol 1981: 6: 286–289
21. Kirwan E O, Hutton P A N, Pozo J L, Ransford A O. Osteoid osteoma and benign osteoblastoma of the spine. Clinical presentation and treatment. J Bone Joint Surg (Br) 1984: 66: 21–26
22. Bettelli G, Capanna R, Van Horn J R, Ruggieri P, Biagini R, Campanacci M. Osteoid osteoma and osteoblastoma of the pelvis. Clin Orthop 1989: 247: 261–271
23. Capanna R, Ayala A, Bertoni F et al. Sacral osteoid osteoma and osteoblastoma: a report of 13 cases. Arch Orthop Trauma Surg 1986: 105: 205–210
24. Capanna R, Van Horn J R, Ayala A, Picci P, Bettelli G. Osteoid osteoma and osteoblastoma of the talus: a report of 40 cases. Skeletal Radiol 1986: 15: 360–364
25. Edeiken J, DePalma A F, Hodes P J. Osteoid osteoma (roentgenographic emphasis). Clin Orthop 1966: 49: 201–206
26. Schlesinger A E, Hernandez R J. Intracapsular osteoid osteoma of the proximal femur: findings on plain film and CT. AJR 1990: 154: 1241–1244
27. Spence A J, Lloyd-Roberts G S. Regional osteoporosis in osteoid osteoma. J Bone Joint Surg (Br) 1961: 43: 501–507
28. Wiener S N, Kirschenbaum D. Osteoid osteoma presenting as regional osteoporosis. Clin Nucl Med 1980: 5: 68–69
29. Bergeron P, Beauregard C G, Gagnon S, McKay Y. Case report 831. Juxtaarticular osteoid osteoma. Skeletal Radiol 1994: 23: 161–163
30. Smith F W, Gilday D L. Scintigraphic appearances of osteoid osteoma. Radiology 1980: 137: 191–195
31. Winter P F, Johnson P M, Hilal S K, Feldman F. Scintigraphic detection of osteoid osteoma. Radiology 1977: 122: 177–178
32. Lisbona R, Rosenthall L. Role of radionuclide imaging in osteoid osteoma. AJR 1979: 132: 77–80
33. Bilchik T, Heyman S, Siegel A, Alavi A. Osteoid osteoma: the role of radionuclide bone imaging, conventional radiography, and computed tomography in its management. J Nucl Med 1992: 33: 269–271
34. Fehring T K, Green N E. Negative radionuclide scan in osteoid osteoma. A case report. Clin Orthop 1984: 185: 245–249
35. Helms C A, Hattner R S, Vogler J B 3rd. Osteoid osteoma: radionuclide diagnosis. Radiology 1984: 151: 779–784
36. Helms C A. Osteoid osteoma: the double density sign. Clin Orthop 1987: 222: 167–173

37. Lindbom A, Lindvall N, Soderberg G, Spjut H. Angiography in osteoid osteoma. Acta Radiol (Stockh) 1960: 54: 327–333

38. O'Hara J P 3rd, Tegtmeyer C, Sweet D E, McCue F C. Angiography in the diagnosis of osteoid osteoma of the hand. J Bone Joint Surg (Am) 1975: 57: 163–166

39. Lateur L, Baert A L. Localisation and diagnosis of the osteoid osteoma of the carpal area by angiography. Skeletal Radiol 1977: 2: 75–79

40. Swee R G, McLeod R A, Beabout J W. Osteoid osteoma: detection, diagnosis, and localization. Radiology 1979: 130: 117–123

41. Greenspan A. Benign bone-forming lesions: osteoma, osteoid osteoma and osteoblastoma. Clinical, imaging, pathologic, and differential considerations. Skeletal Radiol 1993: 22: 485–500

42. Gamba J L, Martinez S, Apple J, Harrelson J M, Nunley J A. Computed tomography of axial skeletal osteoid osteomas. AJR 1984: 142: 769–772

43. Goldman A B, Schneider R, Pavlov H. Osteoid osteoma of the femoral neck: report of four cases evaluated with isotopic bone scanning, CT and MR imaging. Radiology 1993: 186: 227–232

44. Herrlin K, Ekelund L, Lövdahl R, Persson B. Computed tomography in suspected osteoid osteomas of tubular bones. Skeletal Radiol 1982: 9: 92–97

45. Yeager B A, Schiebler M L, Wertheim S B et al. MR imaging of osteoid osteoma of the talus. J Comput Assist Tomogr 1987: 11: 916–917

46. Glass R B, Poznanski A K, Fisher M R, Shkolnik A, Dias L. MR imaging of osteoid osteoma. J Comput Assist Tomogr 1986: 10: 1065–1067

47. Thompson G H, Wong K M, Konsens R M, Vibhakar S. Magnetic resonance imaging of an osteoid osteoma of the proximal femur: a potentially confusing appearance. J Pediatr Orthop 1990: 10: 800–804

48. Yamamura S, Sato K, Sugiura H, Asano M, Takahashi M, Iwata H. Magnetic resonance imaging of inflammatory reaction in osteoid osteoma. Arch Orthop Trauma Surg 1994: 114: 8–13

49. Woods E R, Martel W, Mandell S H, Crabbe J P. Reactive soft-tissue mass associated with osteoid osteoma: correlation of MR imaging features with pathologic findings. Radiology 1993: 186: 221–225

50. Biebuyck J C, Katz L D, McCauley T. Soft tissue edema in osteoid osteoma. Skeletal Radiol 1993: 22: 37–41

51. Assoun J, Richard G, Railhac J J et al. Osteoid osteoma: MR imaging versus CT. Radiology 1994: 191: 217–223

52. Tanaka C, Fujiwara Y, Yamamuro T, Nakashima Y, Haebara H. Intraperiosteal osteoid osteoma. A case report. Clin Orthop 1983: 175: 190–192

53. Johnston A D. Clinical problems in osteoid osteoma. Evidence of osteoclastic aversion to osteoid. Bull Hosp Jt Dis 1962: 23: 80–94

54. Snarr J W, Abell M R, Martel W. Lymphofollicular synovitis with osteoid osteoma. Radiology 1973: 106: 557–560

55. Corbett J M, Wilde A H, McCormack L J, Evarts C M. Intra-articular osteoid osteoma, a diagnostic problem. Clin Orthop 1974: 98: 225–230

56. Alani W O, Bartal E. Osteoid osteoma of the femoral neck simulating an inflammatory synovitis. Clin Orthop 1987: 223: 308–312

57. Cronemeyer R L, Kirchmer N A, De Smet A A, Neff J R. Intraarticular osteoid osteoma of the humerus simulating synovitis of the elbow: a case report. J Bone Joint Surg (Am) 1981: 63: 1172–1174

58. Ruggieri P, Biagini R, Ferraro A, Picci P, Capanna R. Osteoid osteoma of the elbow. A study of twelve cases. Ital J Orthop Traumatol 1989: 15: 154–163

59. Golding J S R. The natural history of osteoid osteoma. J Bone Joint Surg (Br) 1954: 36: 218–229

60. Byers P D. Solitary benign osteoblastic lesions of bone. Osteoid osteoma and benign osteoblastoma. Cancer 1968: 22: 43–57

61. Sherman M S, McFarland G. Mechanism of pain in osteoid osteoma. South Med J 1965: 58: 163–166

62. Schulman L, Dorfman H D. Nerve fibers in osteoid osteoma. J Bone Joint Surg (Am) 1970: 52: 1351–1356

63. Halperin N, Gadoth N, Reif R, Axer A. Osteoid osteoma of the proximal femur simulating spinal root compression. Clin Orthop 1982: 162: 191–194

64. Esquerdo J, Fernandez C F, Gomar F. Pain in osteoid osteoma: histological facts. Acta Orthop Scand 1976: 47: 520–524

65. Ippolito E, Postacchini R. Osteoid osteoma of the neck of the femur simulating the lumboradicular syndrome (2 cases report). Ital J Orthop Traumatol 1983: 9: 497–500

66. Hasegawa T, Hirose T, Sakamoto R, Seki K, Ikata T, Hizawa K. Mechanism of pain in osteoid osteomas: an immunohistochemical study. Histopathology 1993: 22: 487–491

67. Greco F, Tamburrelli F, Laudati A, La Cara A, Di Trapani G. Nerve fibres in osteoid osteoma. Ital J Orthop Traumatol 1988: 14: 91–94

68. Makley J T, Dunn M J. Prostaglandin synthesis by osteoid osteoma. Lancet 1982: 2: 42

69. Wold L E, Pritchard D J, Bergert J, Wilson D M. Prostaglandin synthesis by osteoid osteoma and osteoblastoma. Mod Pathol 1988: 1: 129–131

70. Greco F, Tamburrelli F, Ciabattoni G. Prostaglandins in osteoid osteoma. Int Orthop 1991: 15: 35–37

71. Ciabattoni G, Tamburrelli F, Greco F. Increased prostacyclin biosynthesis in patients with osteoid osteoma. Eicosanoids 1991: 4: 165–167

72. Jundt G, Schulz A, Berghäuser K H, Fisher L W, Gehron-Robey P, Termine J D. Immunocytochemical identification of osteogenic bone tumors by osteonectin antibodies. Virchows Arch A Pathol Anat Histopathol 1989: 414: 345–353

73. Dreyer T, Welkerling H, Delling G. Morphologische Charakteristika und Besonderheiten des Osteoidosteoms. Pathologe 1990: 11: 290–294

74. Vermeulen A H, Vermeer C, Bosman F T. Histochemical detection of osteocalcin in normal and pathological human bone. J Histochem Cytochem 1989: 37: 1503–1508

75. Lafforgue P, Senbel E, Boucraut J et al. Elbow synovitis related to an intraarticular osteoid osteoma of the humerus, with immunologic and histochemical studies. J Rheumatol 1992: 19: 633–636

76. De Giuli C, Frontino G. Rilievo al microscopico electronico di particolari strutture endocellulari in un caso di osteoma osteoide. Arch Ital Pat Clin Tumori 1968: 11: 35–51

77. Marotti F. Osservazioni preliminari sull'ultrastruttura dell'osteoma-osteoide. Clin Ortop 1975–76: 26: 109–118

78. Steiner G C. Ultrastructure of osteoid osteoma. Hum Pathol 1976: 7: 309–325

79. Tamburrelli F, Greco F, Laudati A, Bucca C. L'osteoma osteoide: aspetti ultrastrutturali. Arch Putti Chir Organi Mov 1989: 37: 199–207

80. Sela J. Bone remodeling in pathologic conditions. A scanning electron microscopic study. Calcif Tissue Res 1977: 23: 229–234

81. Fadda M, Delrio A N, Zirattu G. L'osteoma osteoide. Studio al microscopio elettronico a scansione. Arch Putti Chir Organi Mov 1990: 38: 105–111

82. Fadda M, Zirattu G, Laneri P, De Santis E. Scanning electron microscopy of osteoid osteoma. Int Orthop 1994: 18: 72–76

83. Sabanas A O, Bickel W H, Moe J H. Natural history of osteoid osteoma of the spine. Am J Surg 1970: 91: 880–889

84. Vickers C, Pugh D C, Ivins J C. Osteoid osteoma. A fifteen year follow up of an untreated patient. J Bone Joint Surg (Am) 1959: 41: 357–358

85. Moberg E. The natural course of osteoid osteoma. J Bone Joint Surg (Am) 1951: 33: 166–170

86. Sim F H, Dahlin D C, Beabout J W. Osteoid osteoma: diagnostic problems. J Bone Joint Surg (Am) 1975: 57: 154–159

87. Wahl H, Dominok G W. Osteoid-Osteom und maligne Entartung. Zentralbl Chir 1978: 103: 1490–1492

88. Voto S J, Cook A J, Weiner D S, Ewing J W, Arrington L E. Treatment of osteoid osteoma by computed tomography guided excision in the pediatric patient. J Pediatr Orthop 1990: 10: 510–513

89. Doyle T, King K. Percutaneous removal of osteoid osteoma using CT control. Clin Radiol 1989: 40: 514–517

90. Ward W G, Eckardt J J, Shayestehfar S, Mirra J, Grogan T,

Oppenheim W. Osteoid osteoma diagnosis and management with low morbidity. Clin Orthop 1993: 291: 229–235

91. Ghelman B, Thompson F M, Arnold W D. Intraoperative radioactive localization of an osteoid osteoma. Case report. J Bone Joint Surg (Am) 1981: 63: 826–827

92. Ghelman B, Vigorita V J. Postoperative radionuclide evaluation of osteoid osteomas. Radiology 1983: 146: 509–512

93. Vigorita V J, Ghelman B. Localization of osteoid osteoma – use of radionuclide scanning and autoimaging in identifying the nidus. Am J Clin Pathol 1983: 79: 223–225

94. Ayala A G, Murray J A, Erling M A, Raymond A K. Osteoid osteoma. Intraoperative tetracycline fluorescence demonstration of the nidus. J Bone Joint Surg (Am) 1986: 68: 747–751

95. Kneisl J S, Simon M A. Medical management compared with operative treatment for osteoid-osteoma. J Bone Joint Surg (Am) 1992: 74: 179–185

96. Dunlop J A, Morton K S, Eliott G B. Recurrent osteoid osteoma. Report of a case with a review of the literature. J Bone Joint Surg (Br) 1970: 52: 128–130

97. Worland R L, Ryder C T, Johnston A D. Recurrent osteoid osteoma. Report of a case. J Bone Joint Surg (Am) 1975: 57: 277–278

98. Norman A. Persistence or recurrence of pain: a sign of surgical failure in osteoid osteoma. Clin Orthop 1978: 130: 263–266

99. Regan M W, Galey J P, Oakeshott R D. Recurrent osteoid osteoma. Case report with a ten-year asymptomatic interval. Clin Orthop 1990: 253: 221–224

100. Glynn J J, Lichtenstein L. Osteoid osteoma with multicentric nidus. A report of two cases. J Bone Joint Surg (Am) 1973: 55: 855–858

101. Greenspan A, Elguezabel A, Bryk D. Multifocal osteoid osteoma. A case report and review of the literature. Am J Roentgenol Radium Ther Nucl Med 1974: 121: 103–106

102. Larsen L J, Mall J C, Ichtertz D F. Metachronous osteoid-osteomas. Report of a case. J Bone Joint Surg (Am) 1991: 73: 612–614

103. Kenan S, Abdelwahab I F, Klein M J, Hermann G, Lewis M M. Case report 864. Elliptical, multicentric periosteal osteoid osteoma. Skeletal Radiol 1994: 23: 565–568

104. Lundeen M A, Herring J A. Osteoid-osteoma of the spine: sclerosis in two levels. A case report. J Bone Joint Surg (Am) 1980: 62: 476–478

105. Calderoni P, Gusella A, Martucci E. Multiple osteoid osteoma in the 7th dorsal vertebra. Ital J Orthop Traumatol 1984: 10: 257–260

106. Keret D, Harcke H T, McEwen G D, Bowen J R. Multiple osteoid osteomas of the fifth lumbar vertebra. A case report. Clin Orthop 1989: 248: 163–168

107. Alcalay M, Clarac J P, Bontoux D. Double osteoid osteoma in adjacent carpal bone. A case report. J Bone Joint Surg (Am) 1982: 64: 779–780

108. Resnick D. Double osteoid osteoma in adjacent carpal bones. J Bone Joint Surg (Am) 1982: 64: 1399

109. Allieu Y, Lussiez B, Benichou M, Cenac P. A double nidus osteoid osteoma in a finger. J Hand Surg (Am) 1989: 14: 538–541

110. Nelson M C, Lack E E, Freedman M T. Case report 856. Multifocal osteoid osteoma in a 2.5-year-old child. Skeletal Radiol 1994: 23: 465–467

111. Abdelwahab I F, Norman A. Osteoblastic metastasis of lymphoepithelioma simulating osteoid osteoma. A case history. Bull Hosp Jt Dis Orthop Inst 1981: 41: 63–68

112. Schajowicz F, Rebecchini A C, Bosch-Mayol G. Intracortical haemangioma simulating osteoid osteoma. J Bone Joint Surg (Br) 1979: 61: 94–95

113. Sung H W, Liu C C. Can osteoid osteoma become osteoblastoma? A case report. Arch Orthop Trauma Surg 1979: 95: 217–219

114. Bettelli G, Tigani D, Picci P. Recurring osteoblastoma initially presenting as a typical osteoid osteoma. Report of two cases. Skeletal Radiol 1991: 20: 1–4

115. Pieterse A S, Vernon-Roberts B, Paterson D C, Cornish B L, Lewis P R. Osteoid osteoma transforming to aggressive (low grade malignant) osteoblastoma: a case report and literature review. Histopathology 1983: 7: 789–800

116. Morton K S, Quenville N F, Beauchamp C P. Aggressive osteoblastoma. A case previously reported as recurrent osteoid osteoma. J Bone Joint Surg (Br) 1989: 71: 428–431

117. Schajowicz F, Lemos C. Osteoid osteoma and osteoblastoma. Closely related entities of osteoblastic derivation. Acta Orthop Scand 1970: 41: 272–291

118. De Santis E, Priolo F. Neoplasie osteoblastiche benigne dell'ossa: correlazioni cliniche ed anatomo-radiografiche fra osteoma osteoide ed osteoblastoma. Radiol Med (Torino) 1980: 66: 289–296

119. Morton K S, Vassar P S, Krikerbocker W J. Osteoid osteoma and osteoblastoma: reclassification of 43 cases using Schajowicz's classification. Can J Surg 1975: 18: 148–152

120. De Souza Diaz L, Frost H M. Osteoid osteoma-osteoblastoma. Cancer 1974: 33: 1075–1081

121. McCarthy E F, Moses D C, Zibreg J W, Dorfmann H D. Painless fibro-osseous lesion of the rib resembling osteoid osteoma: a report of six cases. Skeletal Radiol 1985: 13: 263–266

122. Kessler S, Mirra J M, Gordon P. Case report 823. Fibro-osseous pseudotumor of the scapula. Skeletal Radiol 1994: 23: 73–77

123. Jaffe H L. Benign osteoblastoma. Bull Hosp Jt Dis 1956: 17: 141–151

124. Lichtenstein L. Benign osteoblastoma. A category of osteoid and bone-forming tumors other than classical osteoid osteoma, which may be mistaken for giant-cell tumor or osteogenic sarcoma. Cancer 1956: 9: 1044–1052

125. Lichtenstein L, Sawyer W R. Benign osteoblastoma. J Bone Joint Surg (Am) 1964: 46: 755–765

126. Gitelis S, Schajowicz F. Osteoid osteoma and osteoblastoma. Orthop Clin North Am 1989: 20: 313–325

127. Lucas D R, Unni K K, McLeod R A, O'Connor M I, Sim F H. Osteoblastoma: clinicopathologic study of 306 cases. Hum Pathol 1994: 25: 117–134

128. Mehta M H, Murray R O. Scoliosis provoked by painful vertebral lesions. Skeletal Radiol 1977: 1: 223–230

129. Akbarnia B A, Rooholamini S A. Scoliosis caused by benign osteoblastoma of the thoracic or lumbar spine. J Bone Joint Surg (Am) 1981: 63: 1146–1155

130. Janin Y, Epstein J A, Carras R, Khan A. Osteoid osteomas and osteoblastomas of the spine. Neurosurgery 1981: 8: 31–38

131. Mirra J M, Cove K, Theros E, Paladugu R, Smasson J. A case of osteoblastoma associated with severe systemic toxicity. Am J Surg Pathol 1979: 3: 463–471

132. Theros E G, Mirra J M, Smasson J, Cove K, Paladugu R. Osteoblastoma of the left femur associated with toxic manifestations. Skeletal Radiol 1979: 4: 157–162

133. Weidner N, Santa Cruz D. Phosphaturic mesenchymal tumors. A polymorphous group causing osteomalacia or rickets. Cancer 1987: 59: 1442–1454

134. Yoshikawa S, Nakamura T, Takagi M, Imamura T, Okano K, Sasaki S. Benign osteoblastoma as a cause of osteomalacia. J Bone Joint Surg (Br) 1977: 59: 279–286

135. Boriani S, Campanacci M. Osteoblastoma associated with osteomalacia (presentation of a case and review of the literature). Ital J Orthop Traumatol 1978: 4: 379–382

136. Nuovo M A, Dorfman H D, Sun C C, Chalew S A. Tumor-induced osteomalacia and rickets. Am J Surg Pathol 1989: 13: 588–599

137. Lee D Y, Choi I H, Lee C K, Ching C Y, Cho K H. Acquired vitamin D-resistant rickets caused by aggressive osteoblastoma of the pelvis: a case report with ten years follow-up and review of the literature. J Pediatr Orthop 1994: 14: 793–798

138. Fukumoto Y, Tarui S, Tsukiyama K et al. Tumor-induced vitamin D resistant hypophosphatemic osteomalacia associated with proximal renal tubular dysfunction and 1,25-dihydroxyvitamin D deficiency. J Clin Endocrinol Metab 1979: 49: 873–878

139. Kroon H M, Schurmans J. Osteoblastoma: clinical and radiological findings in 98 new cases. Radiology 1990: 175: 783–790

140. Della Rocca C, Huvos A G. Osteoblastoma: varied histological presentations with a benign clinical course. An analysis of 55 cases. Am J Surg Pathol 1996: 20: 841–850

141. Tonai M, Campbell C J, Ahn G H, Schiller A L, Mankin H J. Osteoblastoma: classification and report of 16 patients. Clin Orthop 1982: 167: 222–235

142. Marsh B W, Bonfiglio M, Brady L P, Enneking W F. Benign osteoblastoma: range of manifestations. J Bone Joint Surg (Am) 1975: 57: 1–9

143. Raymond A K, Raymond P G, Edeiken J. Case report 531. Epiphyseal osteoblastoma distal end of femur. Skeletal Radiol 1989: 18: 143–146

144. Adler C P. Case report 255. Osteoblastoma of the lesser trochanter of the left femur. Skeletal Radiol 1984: 11: 65–68

145. Boriani S, Capanna R, Donati D, Levine A, Picci P, Savini R. Osteoblastoma of the spine. Clin Orthop 1973: 91: 141–151

146. Paige M L, Michael A S, Brodin A. Case report 647. Benign osteoblastoma causing spinal cord compression and spastic paresis. Skeletal Radiol 1991: 20: 54–57

147. Abdelwahab I F, Frankel V H, Klein M J. Case report 351. Aggressive osteoblastoma of the third lumbar vertebra. Skeletal Radiol 1986: 15: 164–169

148. Goldman R L. The periosteal counterpart of benign osteoblastoma. Am J Clin Pathol 1971: 56: 73–78

149. Gentry J F, Schechter J J, Mirra J M. Case report 574. Periosteal osteoblastoma of rib. Skeletal Radiol 1989: 18: 551–555

150. Michelacci M, Vasina P G. Considerazioni su un caso di osteoblastoma multifocale a sede insolita. Arch Putti Chir Organi Mov 1986: 36: 275–284

151. O'Connell J X, Rosenthal D I, Mankin H J et al. A unique multifocal osteoblastoma-like tumor of the bones of a single lower extremity. Report of a case. J Bone Joint Surg (Am) 1993: 75: 597–602

152. Laurin S. Angiography of benign bone tumors. Acta Radiol Diagn (Stockh) 1981: 22: 601–607

153. Azouz E M, Kozlowski K, Marton D, Sprague P, Zerhouni A, Asselah F. Osteoid osteoma and osteoblastoma of the spine in children: report of 22 cases with brief literature review. Pediatr Radiol 1986: 16: 25–31

154. Crim J R, Mirra J M, Eckardt J J, Seeger L L. Widespread inflammatory response to osteoblastoma: the flare phenomenon. Radiology 1990: 177: 835–836

155. Vade A, Wilbur A, Pudlowski R, Ghosh L. Case report 566. Osteoblastoma of sacrum with secondary aneurysmal bone cyst. Skeletal Radiol 1989: 18: 475–480

156. Marcove R C, Alpert M. A pathologic study of benign osteoblastoma. Clin Orthop 1963: 30: 175–181

157. McLeod R A, Dahlin D C, Beabout J W. The spectrum of osteoblastoma. AJR 1976: 126: 321–325

158. Mirra J M, Kendrick R A, Kendrick R E. Pseudomalignant osteoblastoma versus arrested osteosarcoma: a case report. Cancer 1976: 37: 2005–2014

159. Dorfman H D, Rosenthal D L, Mankin H J, Fosburg M J, Schiller A. Aggressive osteoblastoma, ilium, with secondary aneurysmal bone cyst. N Engl J Med 1980: 303: 866–873

160. Bertoni F, Unni K K, Lucas D R, McLeod R A. Osteoblastoma with cartilaginous matrix. An unusual morphologic presentation in 18 cases. Am J Surg Pathol 1993: 17: 69–74

161. Eisenbrey A B, Huber P J, Rachmaninoff N. Benign osteoblastoma of the spine with multiple recurrences: case report. J Neurosurg 1969: 31: 468–473

162. Zabski Z A, Cutler S S, Yermakov V. Unclassified benign tumor of the rib. Osteochondroblastoma. Cancer 1975: 36: 1009–1015

163. Dorfman H D, Weiss S W. Borderline osteoblastic tumors. Problems in the differential diagnosis of aggressive osteoblastoma and low grade osteosarcoma. Semin Diagn Pathol 1984: 1: 215–234

164. Schajowicz F, Lemos C. Malignant osteoblastoma. J Bone Joint Surg (Br) 1976: 58: 202–211

165. Kenan S, Floman Y, Robin G C, Laufer A. Aggressive osteoblastoma. A case report and review of the literature. Clin Orthop 1985: 195: 294–298

166. Miyayama H, Sakamoto K, Ide M et al. Aggressive osteoblastoma of the calcaneus. Cancer 1993: 71: 346–353

167. Morton K S, Quenville N F, Beauchamp C P. Aggressive osteoblastoma: a case previously reported as a recurrent osteoid osteoma. J Bone Joint Surg (Br) 1989: 71B: 428–431

168. Roessner A, Metze K, Heymer B. Aggressive osteoblastoma. Pathol Res Pract 1985: 179: 433–438

169. Revell P A, Scholtz C L. Aggressive osteoblastoma. J Pathol 1979: 127: 195–198

170. Mitchell M L, Ackerman L V. Metastatic and pseudomalignant osteoblastoma: a report of two unusual cases. Skeletal Radiol 1986: 15: 213–218

171. Unni K K, Dahlin D C. Premalignant tumors and conditions of bone. Am J Surg Pathol 1979: 3: 47–60

172. Bertoni F, Unni K K, McLeod R A, Dahlin D C. Osteosarcoma resembling osteoblastoma. Cancer 1985: 55: 416–426

173. Walaas L, Kindblom L S. Light and electron microscopic examination of fine-needle aspirates in the preoperative diagnosis of osteogenic tumors: a study of 21 osteosarcomas and two osteoblastomas. Diagn Cytopathol 1990: 6: 27–38

174. Serra M, Morini M C, Scotlandi K et al. Evaluation of osteonectin as a diagnostic marker of osteogenic bone tumors. Hum Pathol 1992: 23: 1326–1331

175. Ishida T, Dorfman H D. S-100 protein in osteogenic tumors (letter). Am J Surg Pathol 1994: 18: 857–858

176. Kreicbergs A, Silfversward C, Tribukait B. Flow DNA analysis of primary bone tumors. Relationship between cellular DNA content and histopathologic classification. Cancer 1984: 53: 129–136

177. Mellin W, Dierschauer W, Hiddemann W et al. Flow cytometric DNA analysis of bone tumors. Curr Top Pathol 1989: 80: 122–123

178. Heliö H, Karaharju E, Nordling S. Flow cytometric determination of DNA content in malignant and benign bone tumours. Cytometry 1985: 6: 165–171

179. Bauer H C, Kreicbergs A, Silfversward C, Tribukait B. DNA analysis in the differential diagnosis of osteosarcoma. Cancer 1988: 61: 1430–1436

180. Grace J, McCarthy S, Stankovic R, Marsden W. Malignant transformation of osteoblastoma: study using image analysis microdensitometry. J Clin Pathol 1993: 46: 1024–1029

181. Mascarello J T, Krous H F, Carpenter P M. Unbalanced translocation resulting in the loss of the chromosome 17 short arm in an osteoblastoma. Cancer Genet Cytogenet 1993: 69: 65–67

182. Steiner G C. Ultrastructure of osteoblastoma. Cancer 1977: 39: 2127–2136

183. Steiner G C. The ultrastructure of bone tumors. In: Bonucci E, Motta P M, Eds. Ultrastructure of skeletal tissues. Boston: Kluwer, 1990, pp 271–273

184. Aparisi T, Arborgh B, Ericsson J L. Studies on the fine structure of osteoblastoma with notes on the localization of nonspecific acid and alkaline phosphatase. Cancer 1978: 41: 1811–1822

185. Bonucci E, De Santis E. Ultrastructure of osteoblastoma with particular reference to calcification and matrix vesicles. In: Donath A, Courvoisier B, Eds. Bone and tumors. Berne: Hans Huber, 1980, pp 232–236

186. Brown G A, Cooper R R, Maynard J A, Bonfiglio M. Endoplasmic reticulum size and morphology in bone disorders. Relationship to protein synthesis and malignancy. Clin Orthop 1974: 101: 278–285

187. Yoshida H, Miyazaki S, Yumoto T. Matrix vesicles in bone tumors. Ultrastructural analysis and their significance in neoplastic bone formation. Acta Pathol Jpn 1991: 41: 610–617

188. Hachisuka Y, Ogino M, Asai H, Segawa M, Maeda I, Zyougiku H, Shinndo N. An electron microscopic study on osteoblastoma. Ultrastructure and fine localization of alkaline phosphatase (in Japanese). Nippon Seikeigeka Gakkai Zasshi 1992: 66: 1221–1231

189. Loizaga J M, Calvo M, Lopez Barea F, Martinez Tello F J, Perez Villanueva J. Osteoblastoma and osteoid osteoma. Clinical and morphological features on 162 cases. Pathol Res Pract 1993: 189: 33–41

190. Beyer W F, Kûhn H. Can an osteoblastoma become malignant? Virchows Arch A Pathol Anat Histopathol 1985: 408: 297–305

191. Seki T, Fukuda H, Ishii Y, Hanaoka H, Yatabe S. Malignant transformation of benign osteoblastoma. J Bone Joint Surg (Am) 1975: 57: 424–426

192. Marsh H O, Choi C B. Primary osteogenic sarcoma of the cervical spine originally mistaken for benign osteoblastoma. A case report. J Bone Joint Surg (Am) 1970: 52A: 1467–1471

193. Schulze K J. Maligne Entartung eines benignen Osteoblastoms (Jaffe–Lichtenstein). Beitr Orthop Traumatol 1968: 15: 136–137

194. Schuhr E U, Bader G. Maligne Entartung eines Osteoblastoms-gleichzeitig ein Beitrag zu Doppeltumoren des Knochens. Zentralbl Chir 1978: 103: 177–181

195. Stutch R. Osteoblastoma – a benign entity? Orthop Rev 1975: 4: 27–33

196. Grundmann E, Hobik H P, Immenkamp M, Roessner A. Histo-diagnostic remarks of bone tumors, a review of 3026 cases registered in 'Knochengeschwulstregister Westfalen'. Pathol Res Pract 1979: 166: 5–24

197. Merryweather R, Middlemiss J H, Sanerkin N G. Malignant transformation of osteoblastoma. J Bone Joint Surg (Br) 1980: 62: 381–384

198. Mayer L. Malignant degeneration of so called benign osteoblastoma. Bull Hosp Jt Dis 1967: 28: 4–13

199. Dalinka M K, Chunn S P. Osteoblastoma – benign or malignant precursor? Report of a case. J Can Assoc Radiol 1972: 23: 214–216

200. Camitta B, Wells R, Segura A, Unni K K, Murray K, Dunn D. Osteoblastoma response to chemotherapy. Cancer 1991: 68: 999–1003

201. Jackson R P. Recurrent osteoblastoma: a review. Clin Orthop 1978: 131: 229–233

202. Gertzbein S D, Cruickshank B, Hoffman H, Taylor G A, Cooper P W. Recurrent benign osteoblastoma of the second thoracic vertebra. J Bone Joint Surg (Br) 1973: 55: 841–847

203. Bisset G S, Kaufman R A, Towbin R, Bove K E. Case report 452. Recurrent sacral osteoblastoma. Skeletal Radiol 1987: 16: 666–669

204. Aszodi K. Benign osteoblastoma: quantitative histological distinction from osteoid osteoma. Arch Orthop Unfallchir 1977: 88: 359–368

205. Nojima T, Yamaguchi H, Nagashima K, Nagai Y, Kanda M. Osteosarcoma resembling osteoblastoma and its heterotransplantation into nude mice. Acta Pathol Jpn 1992: 42: 75–81

8

Osteosarcoma

M. Forest

CHAPTER CONTENTS

INTRODUCTION AND CLINICAL DATA

Osteosarcoma is a tumor in which the osteoblastic cell component directly produces tumoral bone, at least focally. It is the most frequent malignant bone tumor, if one excludes myeloma (25% Unni), and is twice as common as chondrosarcoma.[1]

Males are affected more frequently, with a ratio of 1.5–2:1.[2] More than 50% of patients are between 10 and 20 years old (Huvos 1991) and about 60% develop the tumor in the second decade.

Osteosarcoma is rare in young children but the clinical presentation, radiographic and pathologic features are similar to those of older children and adolescents.[3–5] Osteosarcoma is even rarer in infants.[6–11]

Some tumors may be part of the Li–Fraumeni syndrome, an autosomal-dominant condition including leukemia, soft tissue sarcomas, brain, breast and adrenocortical carcinomas.[12] Rare cases have been reported with the Rothmund–Thompson syndrome.[13–17]

About 10% occur in patients older than 60 years[18], with a higher incidence in flat bones; more than half are secondary to a preexisting bone disease.[18]

Clinical symptoms are pain, swelling, a palpable mass and sometimes a limitation of joint motion. Local inflammatory signs and venous stasis are found in advanced tumors.

Pathological fracture is uncommon (chiefly in osteolytic forms) and is not an indicator of poor prognosis (Figs 8.1, 8.2). Chemotherapy is the usual treatment.[19,20]

Abnormal carbohydrate metabolism, elevation of growth hormone and high somatomedin levels have been seen as a 'panneoplastic syndrome' in some cases.[21,22] High β human gonadotrophin ectopic production has been reported in one case.[23] Osteosarcoma may respond to a broad spectrum of steroids, glucocorticoid types being the most useful.[24] The only suggestive laboratory finding is an elevation of alkaline phosphatases related to the reactive or tumoral new bone formation.

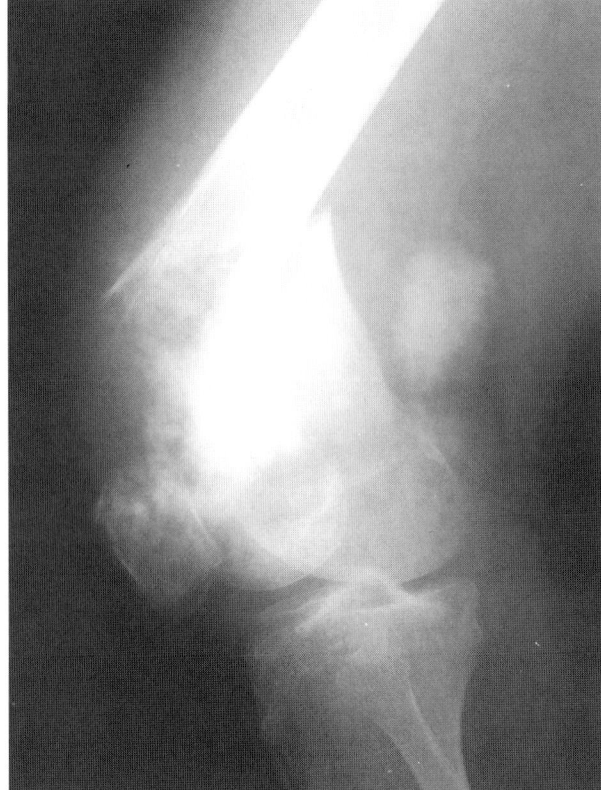

Fig. 8.1

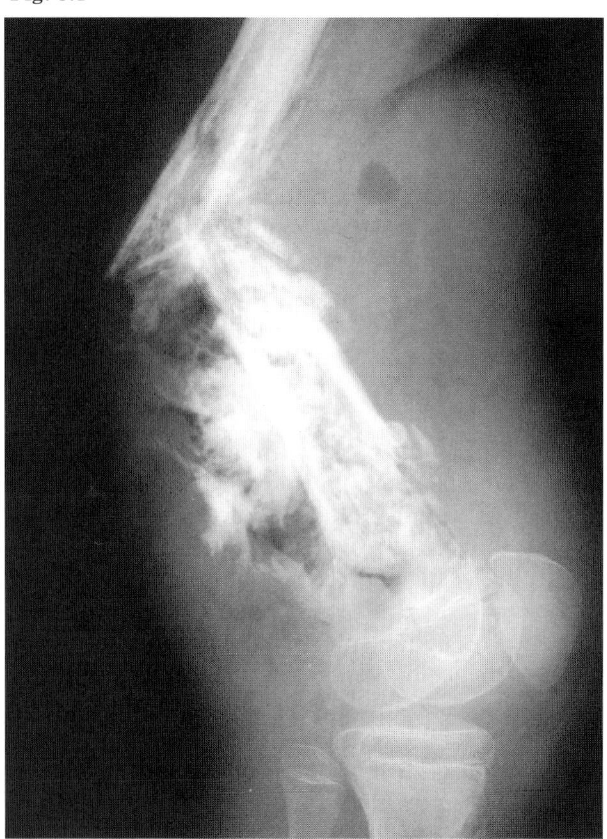

Fig. 8.2

Figs 8.1, 8.2 Osteosarcoma: pathological fractures in femoral locations.

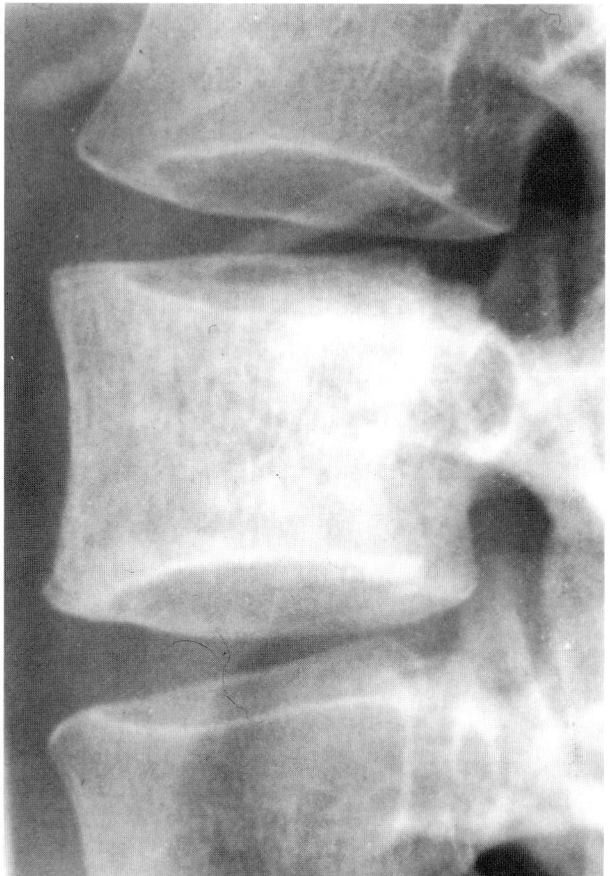

Fig. 8.3 Osteosarcoma involving the body of L3.

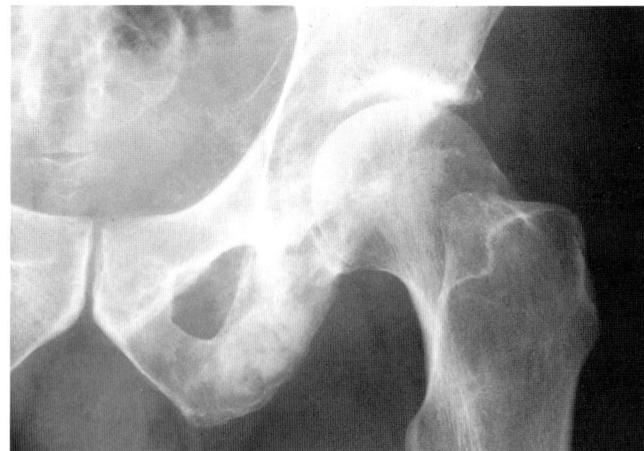

Fig. 8.4 Osteosarcoma in pelvic location.

Osteosarcoma is rarely a cause of oncogenic osteomalacia.[25–28]

SKELETAL DISTRIBUTION

Almost any bone in the body can be affected. Typical locations are the lower end of the femur (40%), the upper end

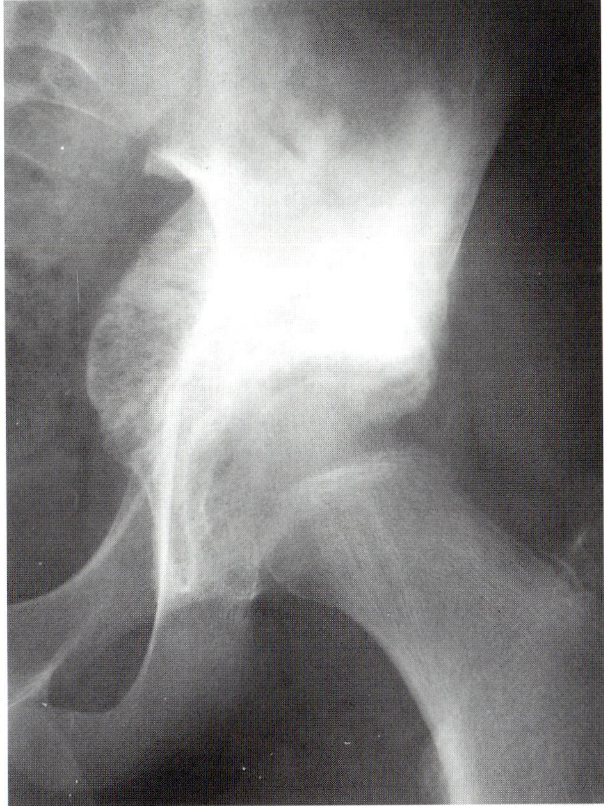

Fig. 8.5

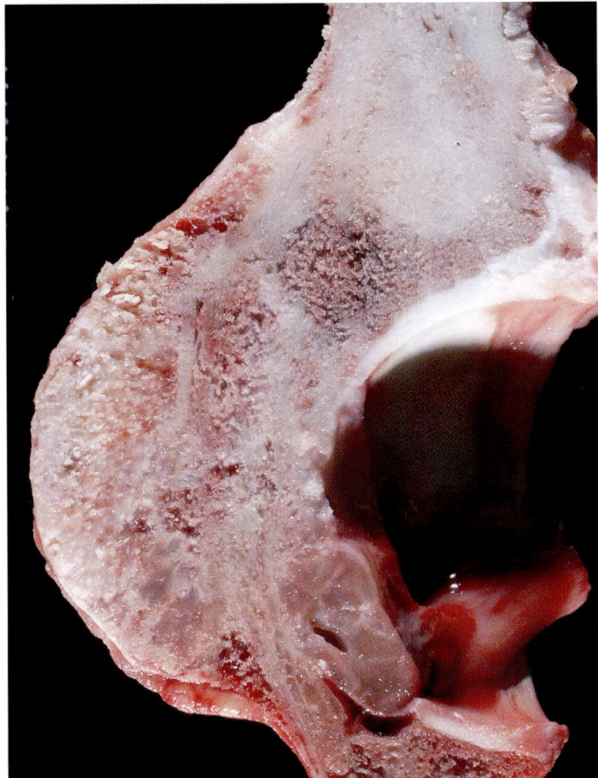

Fig. 8.6

Figs 8.5, 8.6 Osteosarcoma of the iliac bone invading the joint space of the hip.

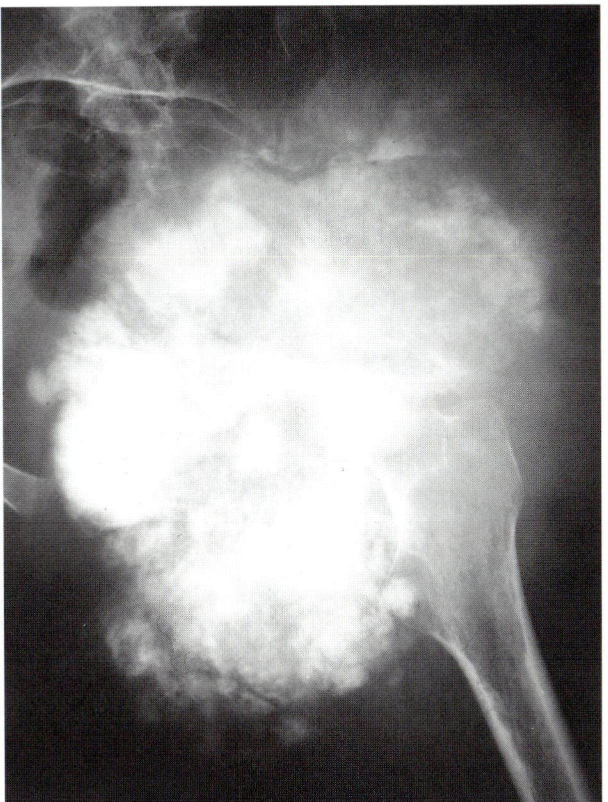

Fig. 8.7

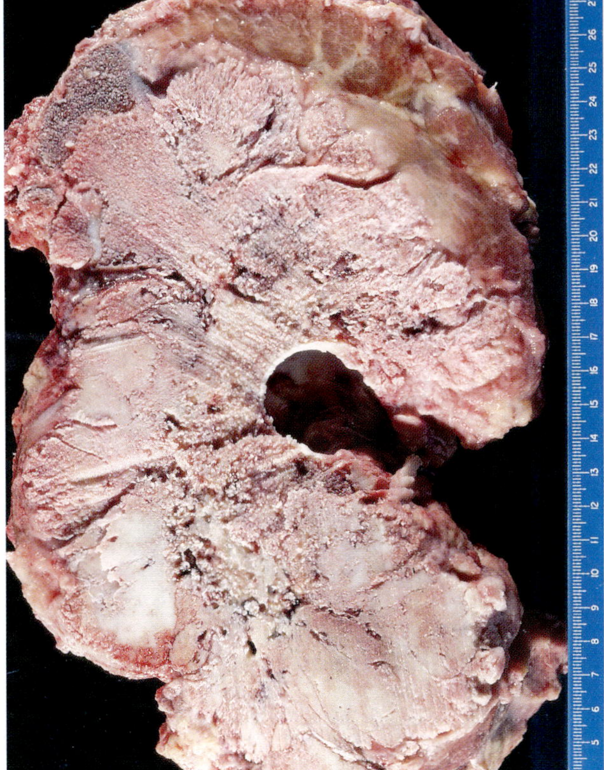

Fig. 8.8

Figs 8.7, 8.8 Huge osteoblastic osteosarcoma of the iliac bone around the acetabulum.

of the tibia (16%) and, less frequently, the upper end of the humerus (15%). Osteosarcomas are rare in the spine, with an incidence ranging from 1% to 3%[29–34] (Fig. 8.3). About half of the spinal cases are secondary to other conditions. Pain and neurologic deficits are related to epidural extension. They predominate in the lower portion of the vertebral column, involving the vertebral body and extending to the neural arch and the spinal canal.

Less than 9% occur in the pelvis[35] (Figs 8.4–8.8); usually, these are large tumors, with extension across the joints and into large veins; most of them are of chondroblastic histologic form and many are radiation induced or secondary to Paget's disease.

Osteosarcomas in the hands account for 0.18% of all cases in the Mayo Clinic files.[36] Men and women are affected equally in the older age group; many of these lesions are of surface origin.

Primary tumors in the foot are equally rare.[37,38] Most of them are also secondary to radiation or Paget's disease.[37]

IMAGING

Diagnosis has to be made on plain films[39] (Figs 8.9–8.24).

The earliest changes are mottled radiolucent or radiopaque areas with minimal periosteal bone formation[40] (Huvos 1991). Mineralization of the matrix may give a ground glass, cloud-like or ivory pattern.[41] So-called sclerosing osteosarcomas exhibit increased density due to the mineralized bone forming between intact residual normal bone trabeculae[41] and any sclerotic intramedullary lesion looking like a cumulus cloud is an osteosarcoma.[42] Small flocculent or ring-like calcifications are calcium deposits or enchondral ossification in the cartilage part of the sarcoma.[42]

Some tumors are purely lytic. Osteolytic forms account for 30%, osteosclerotic ones for 45% and mixed forms for 25% of tumors. Internal margins usually show a moth-eaten appearance or permeative destruction.[43]

Periosteal reactions can mineralize in a period of 10 days to 3 weeks, varying with the age of the patient.[44] They can be lamellated or spiculated. The Codman trian-

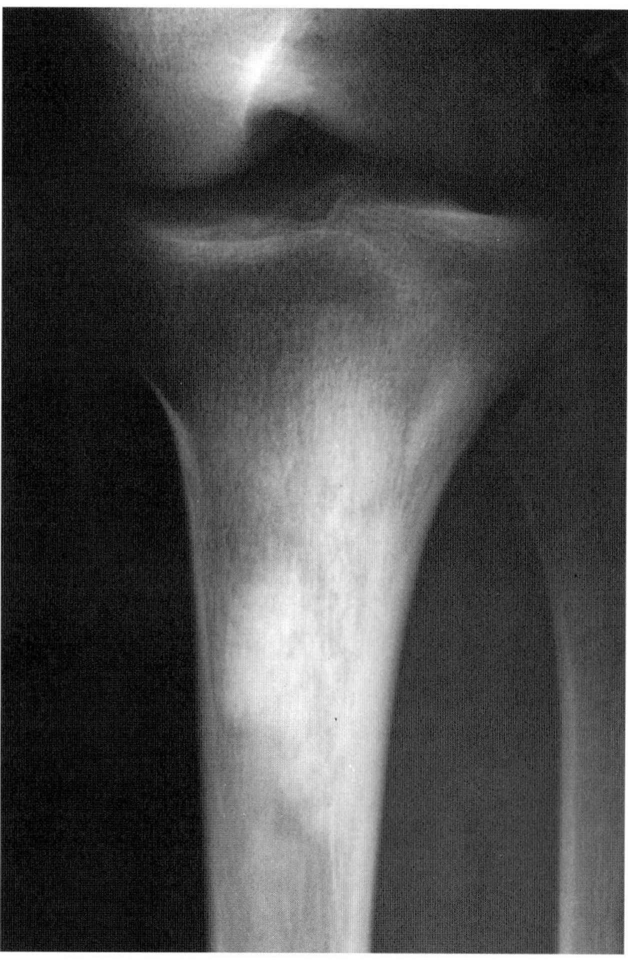

Fig. 8.9 Cumulus cloud appearance of an osteosarcoma of the tibia.

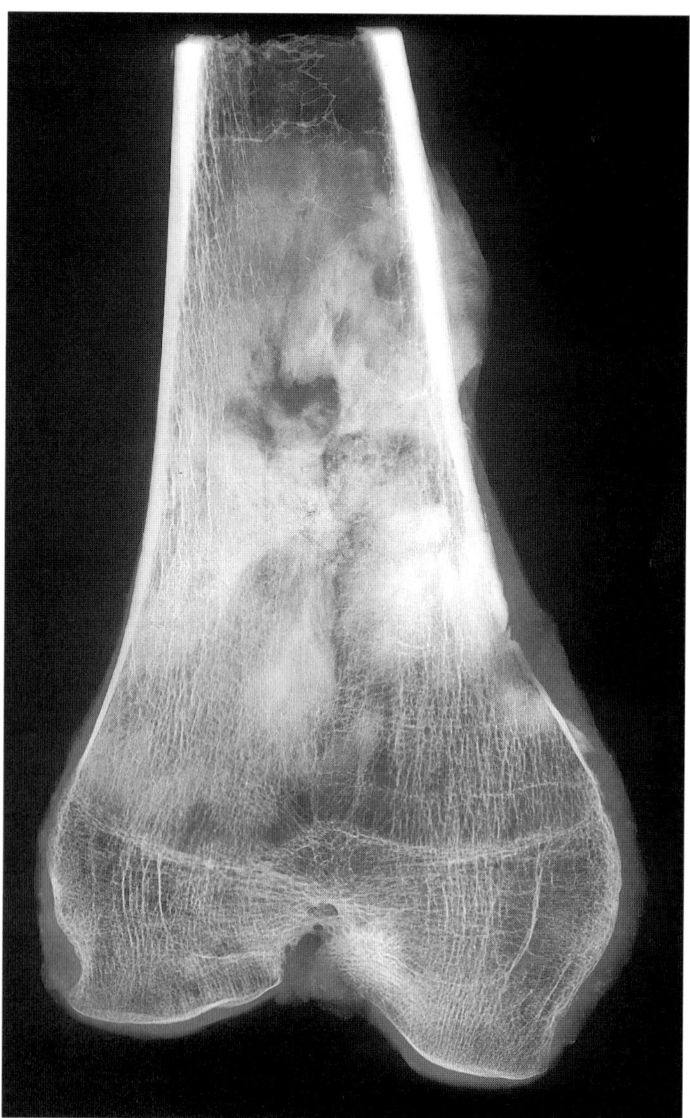

Fig. 8.10 Mottled calcifications of an osteosarcoma of the femur.

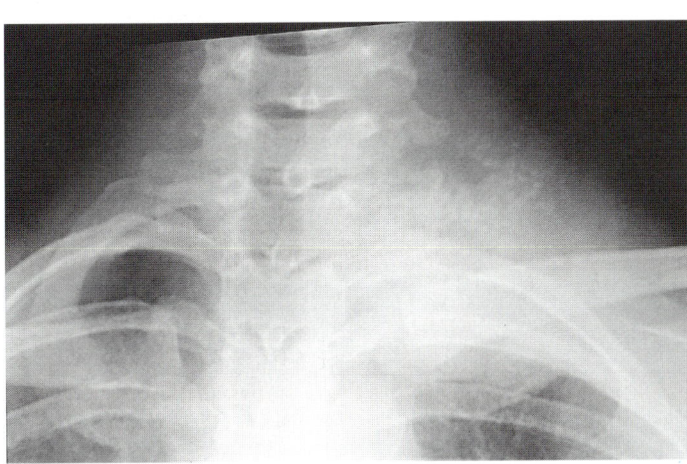

Fig. 8.11

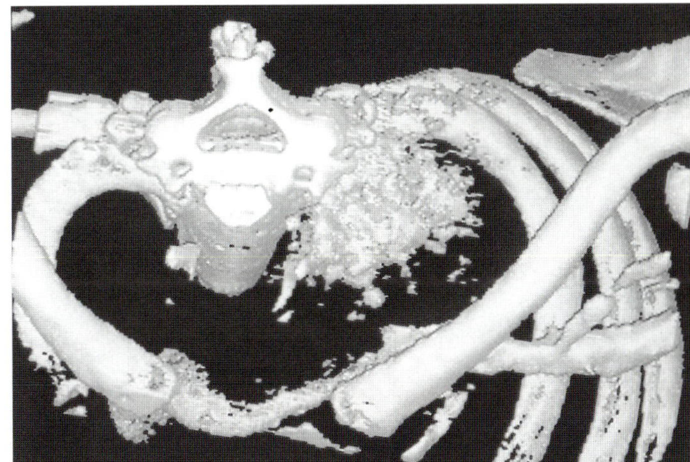

Fig. 8.12

Figs 8.11, 8.12 Osteosarcoma of the first rib: bone production well demonstrated on 3-D CT.

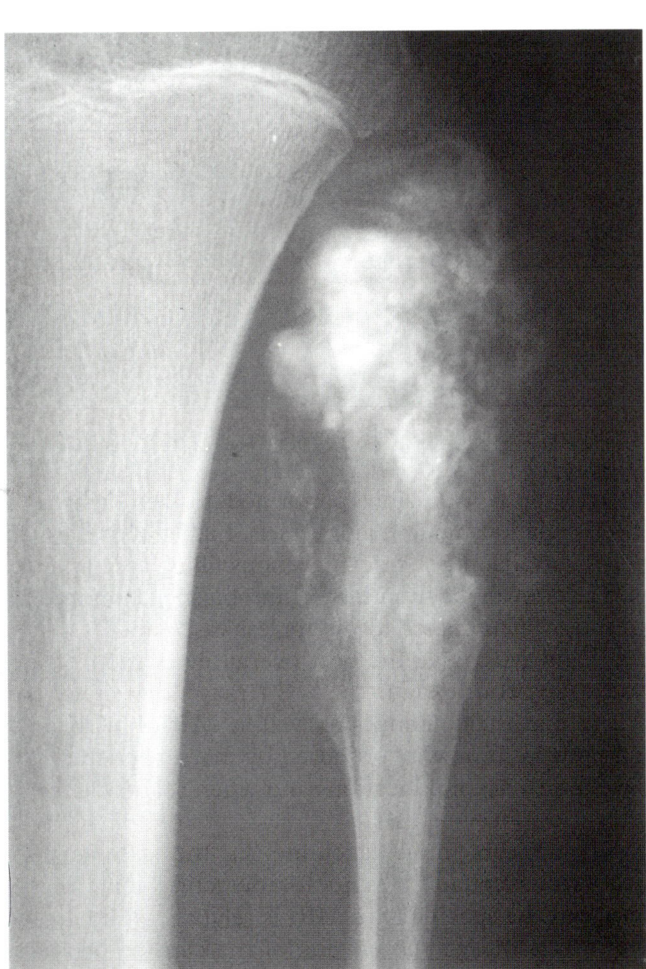

Fig. 8.13

Figs 8.13, 8.14 Some calcified areas in a predominantly lytic osteosarcoma of the fibula (chondroblastic osteosarcoma).

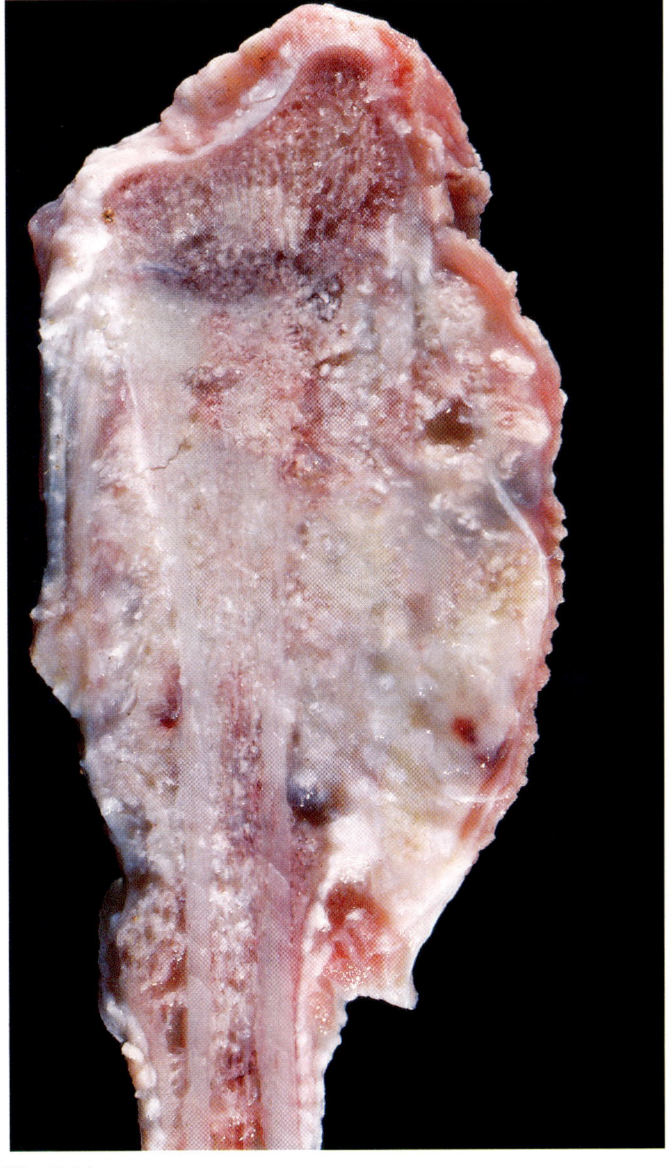

Fig. 8.14

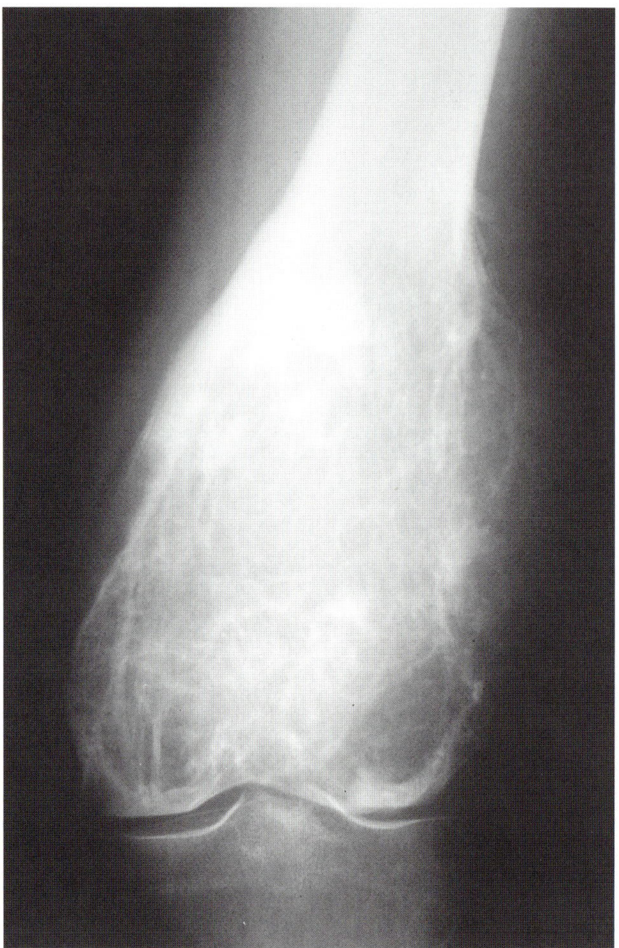

Fig. 8.15

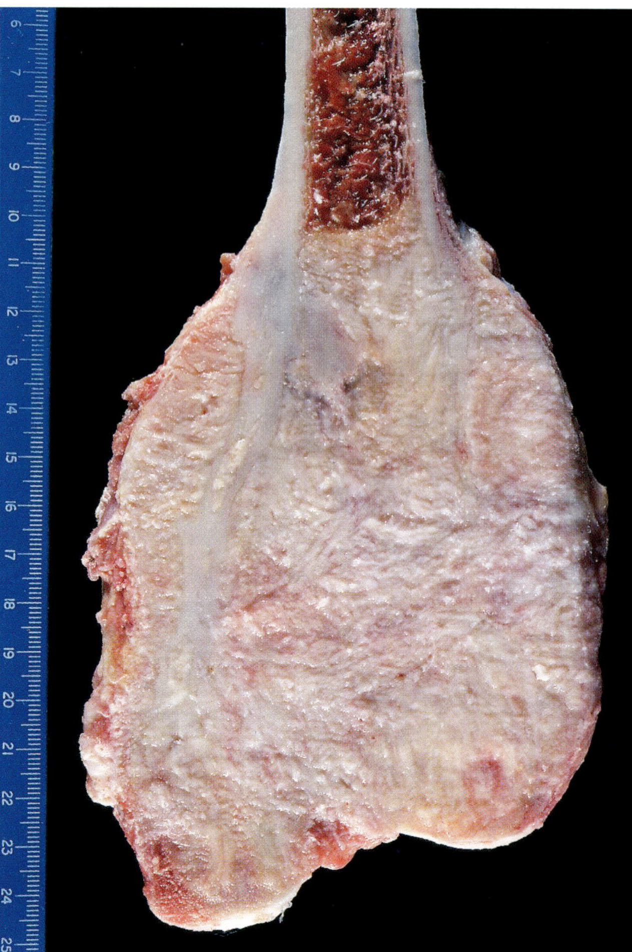

Fig. 8.16

Figs 8.15–8.17 Very few calcifications in a femoral osteosarcoma (fibroblastic osteosarcoma).

gle, an elevation of intact periosteum caused by reactive bone, may be unilateral[44] and secondarily infiltrated by the sarcoma (Figs 8.25, 8.26). Long, thin and divergent spicules create the sunburst pattern composed of reactive and tumoral bone production.[44] Periosteal bone production may be entirely lacking (Huvos 1991).

In long tubular bones, metaphyseal involvement is usually eccentric with secondary epiphyseal extent in 80% of cases. Diaphyseal or epiphyseal locations are unusual (see Ch. 9). Articular cartilage acts as a barrier but tumor may invade the joint cavity. The growth plate is a relative barrier and massive epiphyseal involvement is common. The extraosseous tumoral component may present extensive calcification and mimic a parosteal osteosarcoma (Schajowicz 1994) (Figs 8.27–8.30).

Radionuclide bone scans show an abnormal uptake. Misleadingly extensive responses are related to marrow hyperemia, periosteal new bone or synovial fluid (Greenfield & Arrington 1995) but, in some reports, isotope scan does not demonstrate a greater intramedullary extension when correlated with gross specimens.[45]

Distant spread is usually assessed by scintigraphy and CT scans.[39]

Angiography is mainly performed to demonstrate the tumor's relationship to major vessels. Filling of the vessels at an early arterial phase or early venous filling corresponds to rapid arteriovenous shunting.[46] Fibroblastic, chondroblastic and most differentiated forms are less vascular.[46]

CT and MRI give the best overall evaluation of intra- and extraosseous extent.[39,42,47] CT may show subtle cortical and periosteal changes as well as MRI, but this latter technique is somewhat obscured by marrow edema.[48] CT is useful in vertebral locations and when searching for skip metastases.[49]

MRI appears more accurate in the assessment of intraosseous extent[47,50] and for detecting joint involvement, but the specificity of MRI is relative, with false-positive results due to the bowing of the capsule or reactive synovial changes.[51] Epiphyseal involvement with an open growth plate is a common finding. MRI is superior to plain films in detecting transphyseal spread which recurs in 70–80% of cases.[52,53]

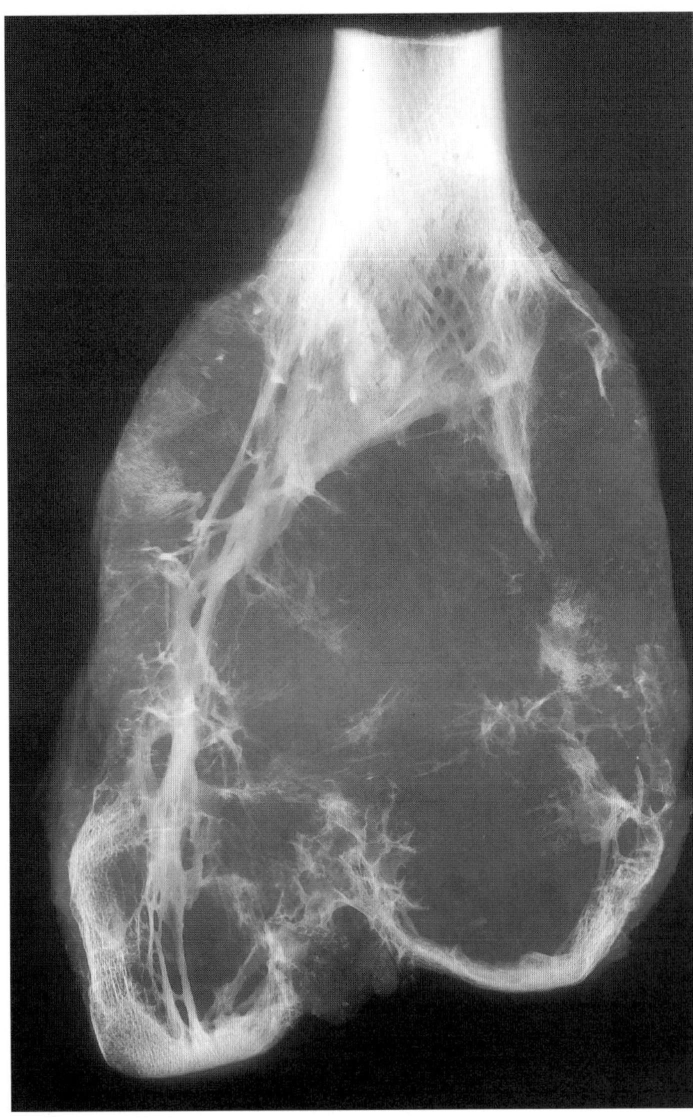

Fig. 8.17

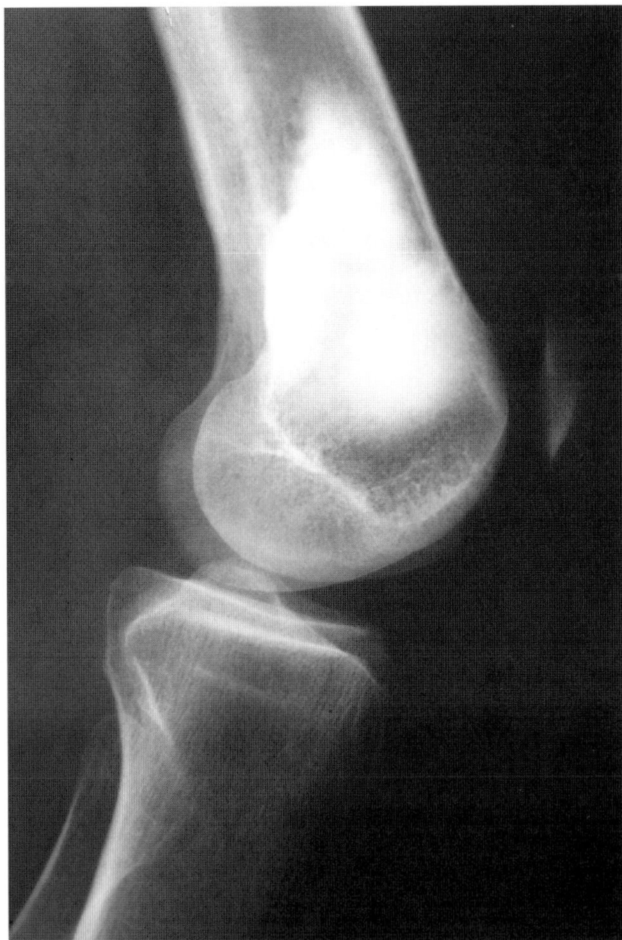

Fig. 8.18 Sclerosing osteosarcoma of the femur.

GROSS PATHOLOGY

Osteosarcoma can appear as a yellow-white dense, sclerotic and calcified mass; the fibrous component is gray-white and the tumoral cartilage is blue-gray. Undifferentiated tumors are soft and fleshy. Hemorrhages, necrosis or cystic degeneration are usual. Medullary extension can be of a considerable length, especially in osteoblastic osteosarcomas (Huvos 1991).

Skip metastases[54–57] are solitary separate tumoral foci occurring synchronously without pulmonary metastases, with an incidence of up to 19% in one series[54] (Figs 8.31–8.33). They may be intraosseous or transarticular. In other series, the clinical incidence is much lower, from 0.7%[55] to 1%,[56] or even absent.[57]

In skeletally immature patients, the physis cannot restrain the tumor invasion in most cases and epiphyseal extension is massive in more than half of the cases,

the plate being partially or completely crossed and the tumor abutting against the articular cartilage[58,59] (Figs 8.34–8.37). Invasion of joints may occur in 19–24% of cases[51] and does not correlate with tumor size, except for very large tumors[60] (Figs 8.38–8.43).

In the knee, tumor invasion is prevalent in the intercondylar region with extension to the cruciate ligaments. It has been recently postulated that, in the knee joint, fatty connective tissue and the superficial synovial layer may be detached and elevated by the tumor, preventing extension into the joint space.[61]

In the joints of the pelvis, there may be a direct relationship between transarticular tumor spread and lack of joint mobility.[62]

HISTOPATHOLOGY

The histologic classification established by Dahlin,[63,64] separating osteoblastic, chondroblastic and fibroblastic types, is still widely used. In osteoblastic forms (Figs 8.44–8.54), tumoral osteoid appears as a fine lace-like network, as streamers, sheets, interlacing trabeculae

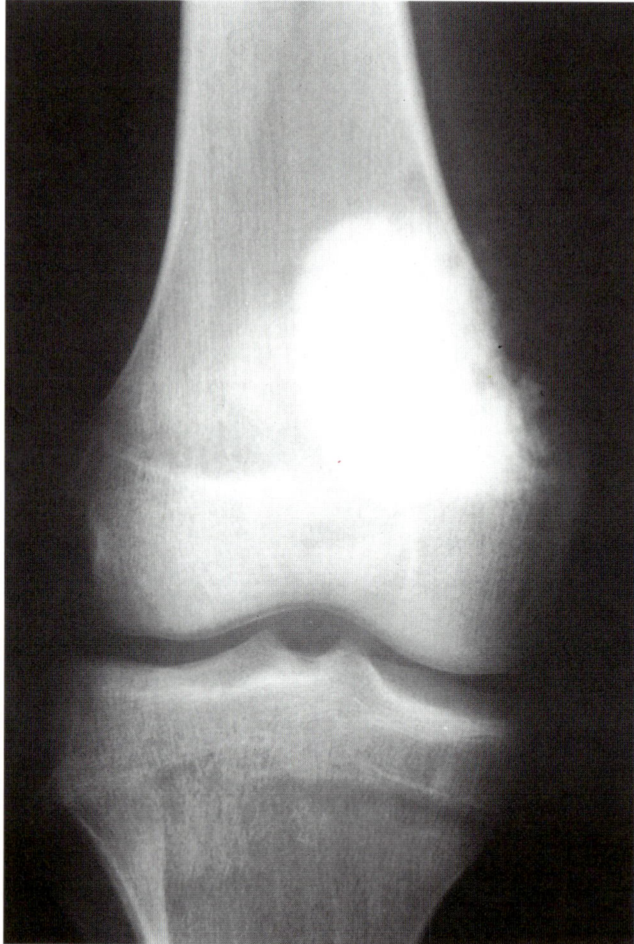

Fig. 8.19

Figs 8.19–8.21 Sclerosing osteosarcoma of the femur.

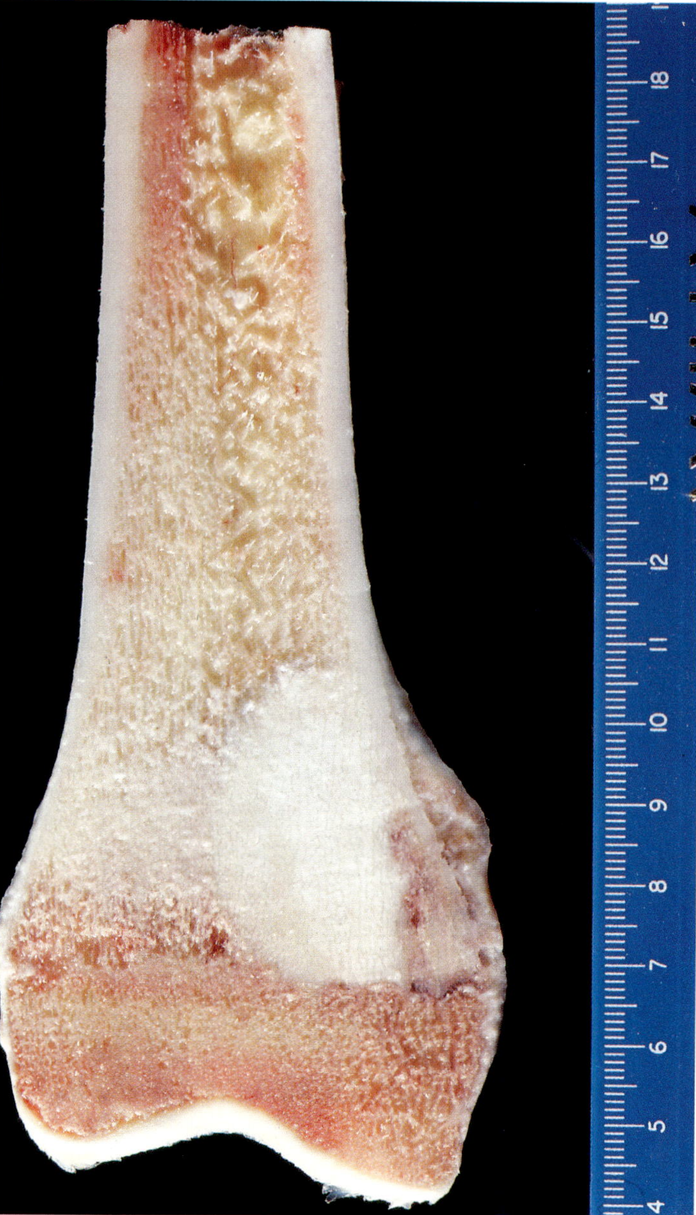

Fig. 8.20

or massive deposits. The sclerosing type of osteosarcoma involves osteoid or immature tumoral woven bone surrounding or deposited on the remnants of normal cancellous bone. In rare cases, tumor cells are not seen in the newly formed bone and diagnosis has to be made on the permeative pattern. Heavily ossified areas may be due to the 'normalization pattern' established by Phemister in 1926: osteoblasts are smaller, darker and more regular and look like embedded osteocytes in the ossified tumor areas.

The osteoid-forming activity has been studied as an index to demonstrate the degree of differentiation of the tumor.[65–67] Osteoid is frequently difficult to differentiate from hyalinized collagen although some methods of testing have been reported, including picrosirius staining with polarization[68] or fixation in cyanuric chloride.[69] However, they are not widely used.

The chondroid component of chondroblastic osteosarcomas may appear as scattered foci or as a predominantly cartilaginous matrix with a malignant appearance (Figs 8.55–8.58). Cartilage lobules with a myxoid or hyaline matrix merge with the stroma of spindle cells. Metaplastic bone formation and enchondral ossification are common.

Fibroblastic osteosarcomas may mimic fibrosarcomas, with a herringbone pattern and limited collagen matrix (Fig. 8.59).

In all forms, cellular pleomorphism, hyperchromatic nuclei with prominent nucleoli, typical or atypical mitoses, hemorrhages and spontaneous necrosis of up to 70% of the tumor (Schajowicz 1994) are common findings (Figs 8.60–8.62).

The Broders method of grading[70,71] is controversial as there is wide variation in the tumor. For many authors, results are not reproducible and most tumors are of grade 3 or 4.[72,73]

Resistance of cartilage to tumor invasion has been studied in vitro and in vivo;[74] enzyme activity of osteosarcoma and endothelial cells seems to be inhibited by a cartilage-derived, low molecular weight collagenase inhibitor. Other

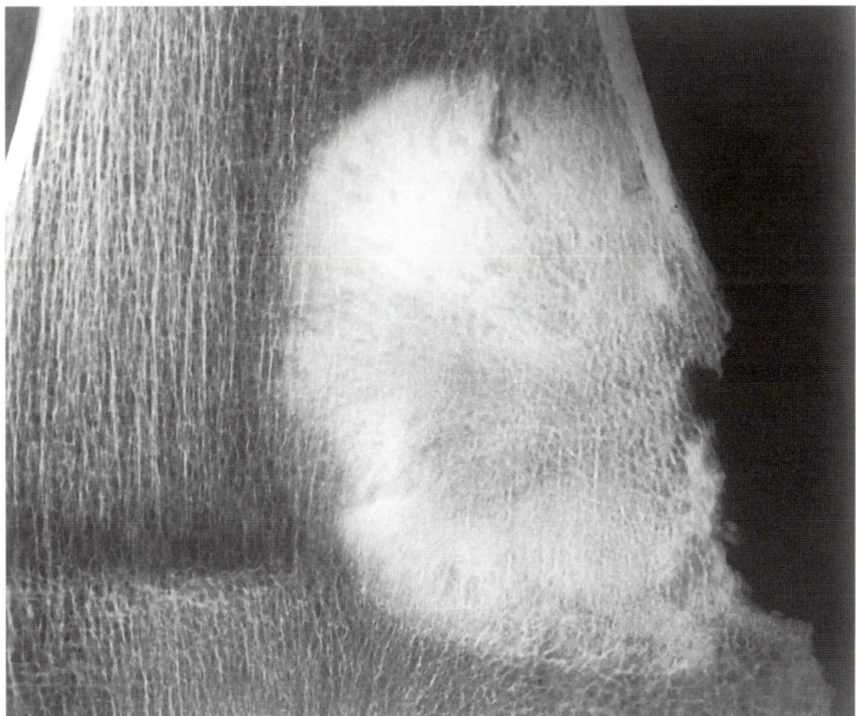

Fig. 8.21

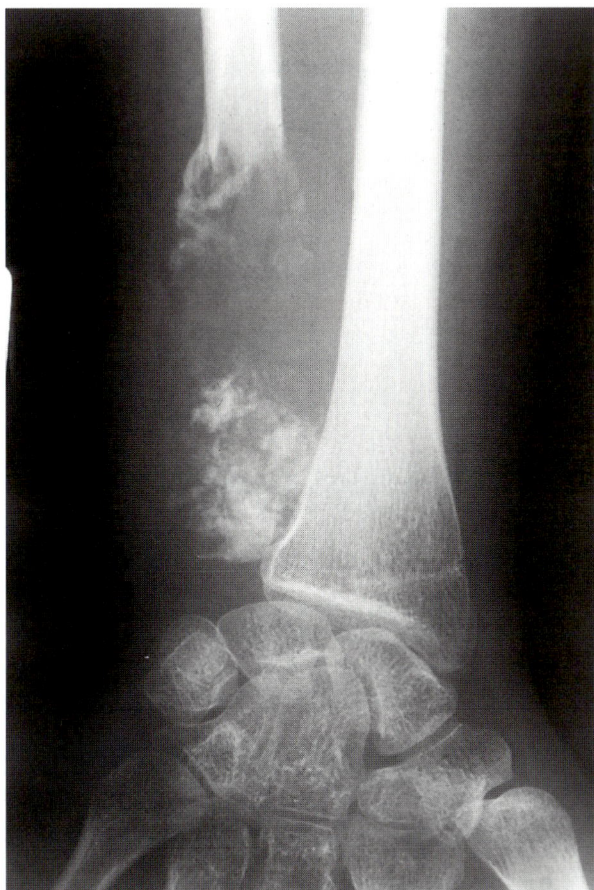

Fig. 8.22

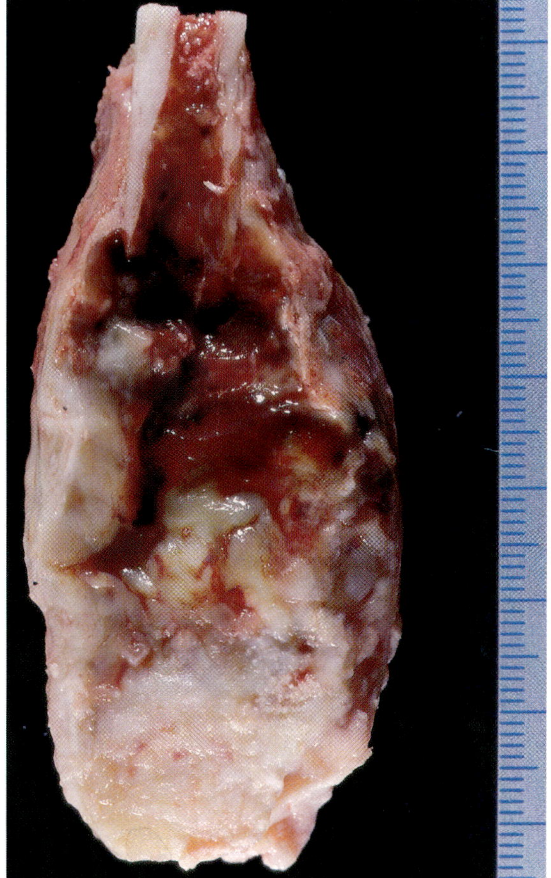

Fig. 8.23

Figs 8.22, 8.23 Predominantly lytic osteosarcoma of the ulna.

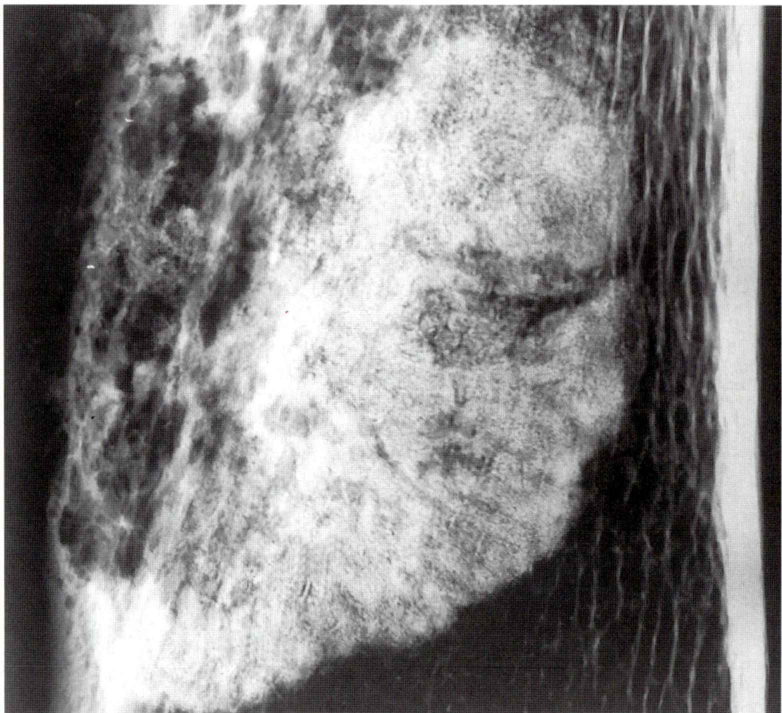

Fig. 8.24 Osteosarcoma of the femur: permeative destruction of the cortex.

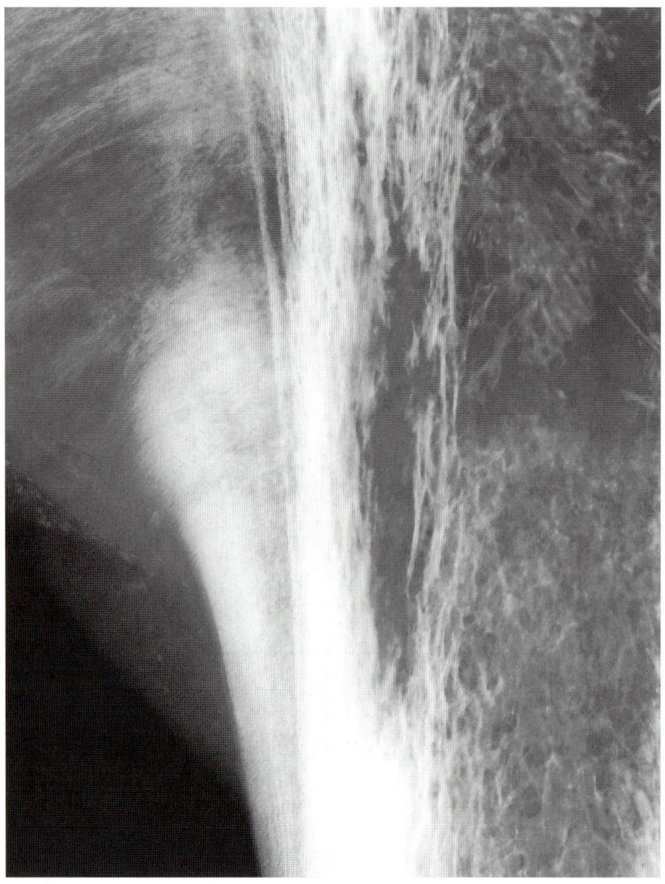

Fig. 8.25

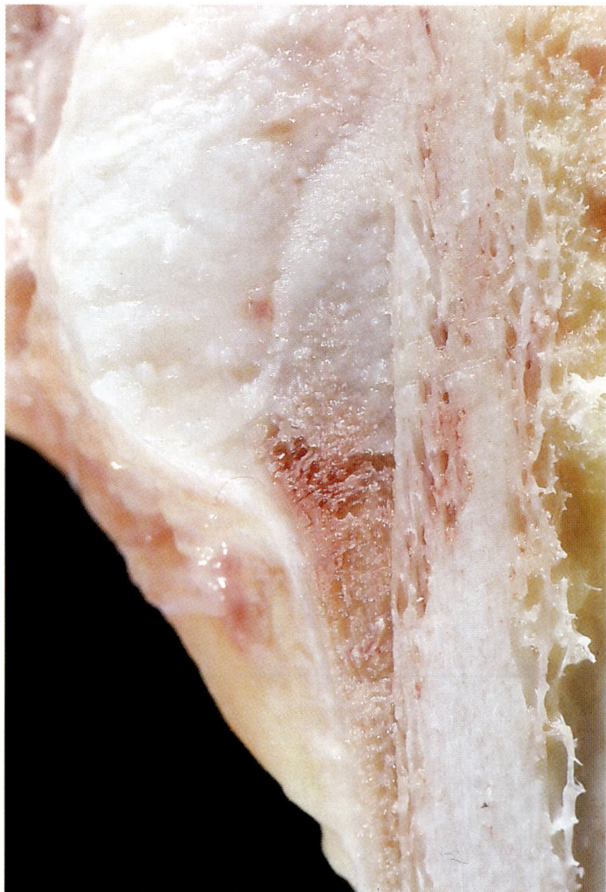

Fig. 8.26

Figs 8.25, 8.26 Codman triangle in a femoral osteosarcoma.

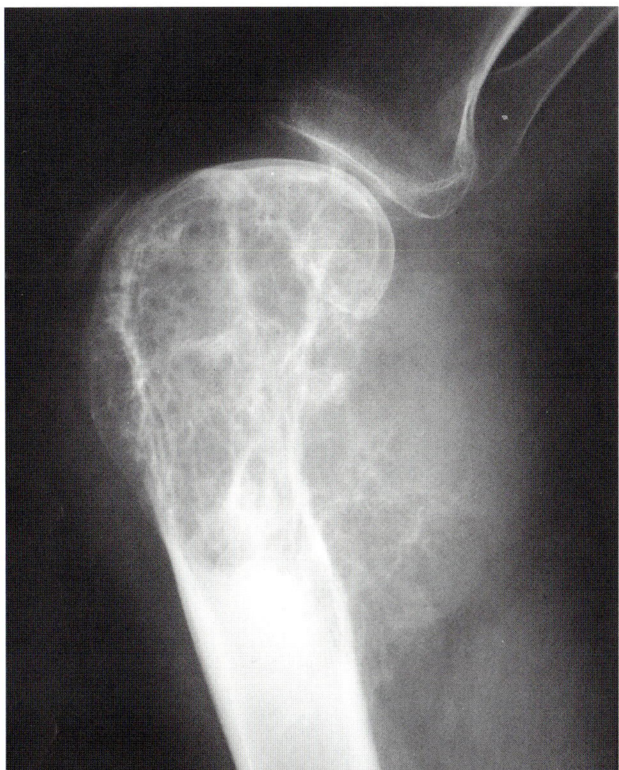

Fig. 8.27

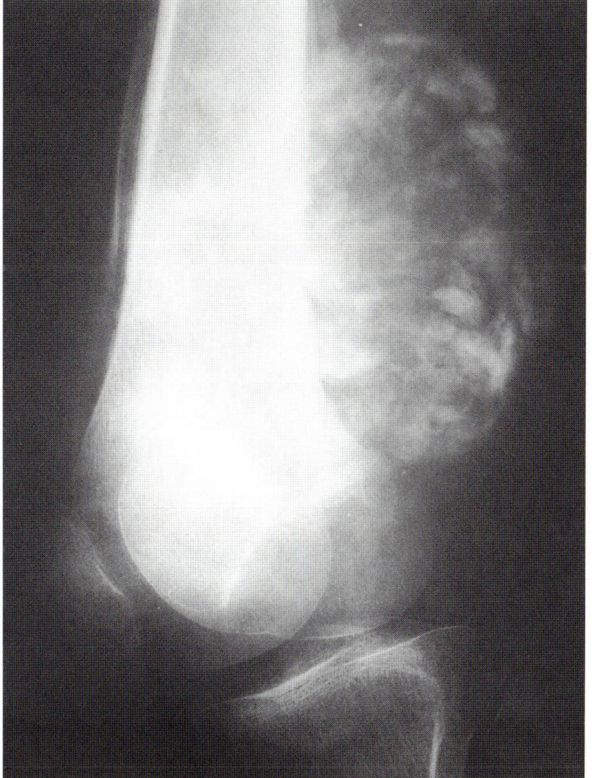

Fig. 8.29

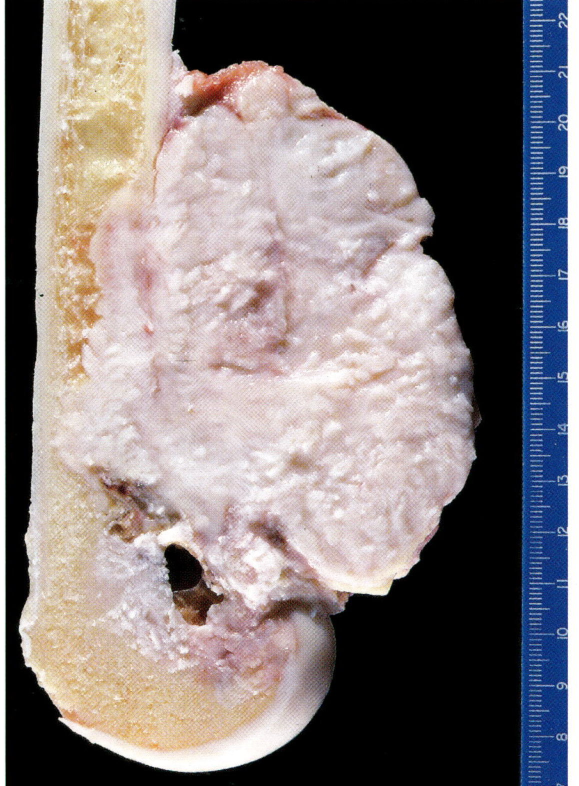

Fig. 8.28

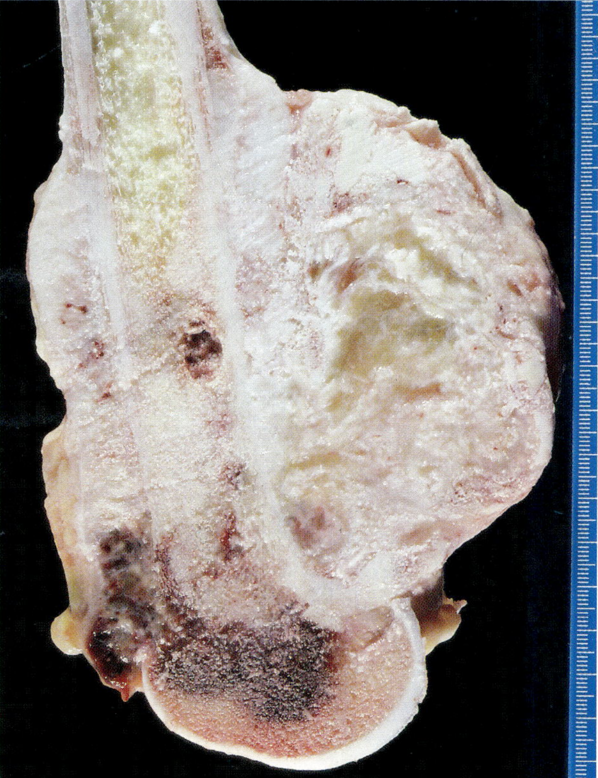

Fig. 8.30

Figs 8.27, 8.28 Soft tissue extension of a fibroblastic osteosarcoma of the femur.

Figs 8.29, 8.30 Soft tissue extension of a chondroblastic osteosarcoma of the femur.

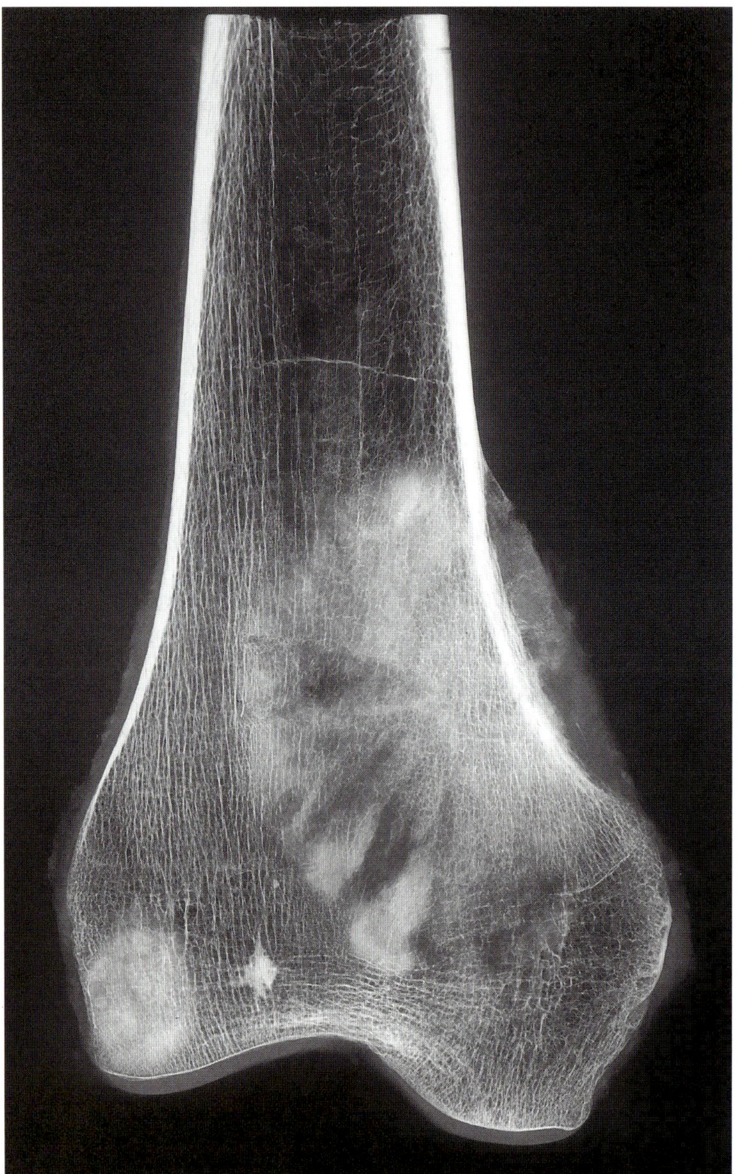

Fig. 8.31 Osteosarcoma of the femur with satellite tumoral foci at initial presentation.

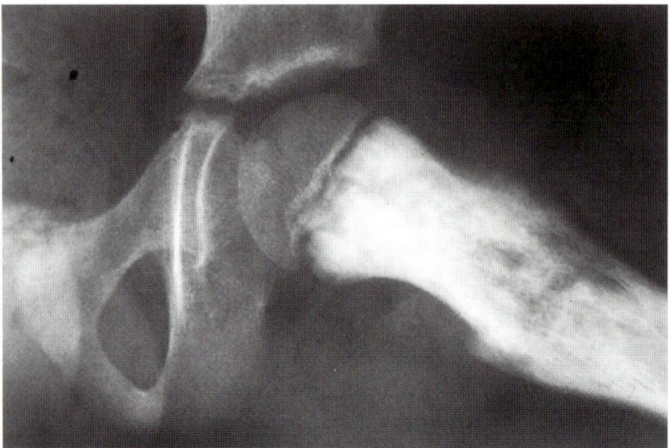

Fig. 8.34 Osteosarcoma of the femur abutting the growth plate.

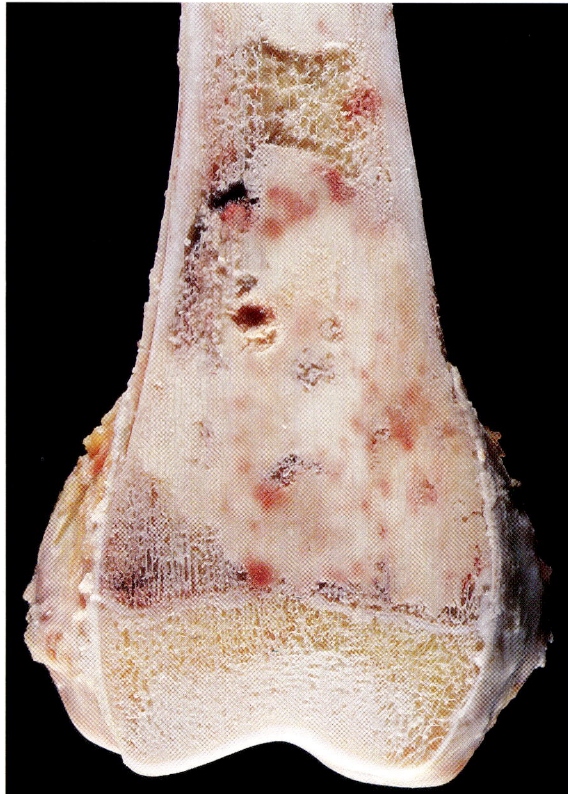

Fig. 8.32

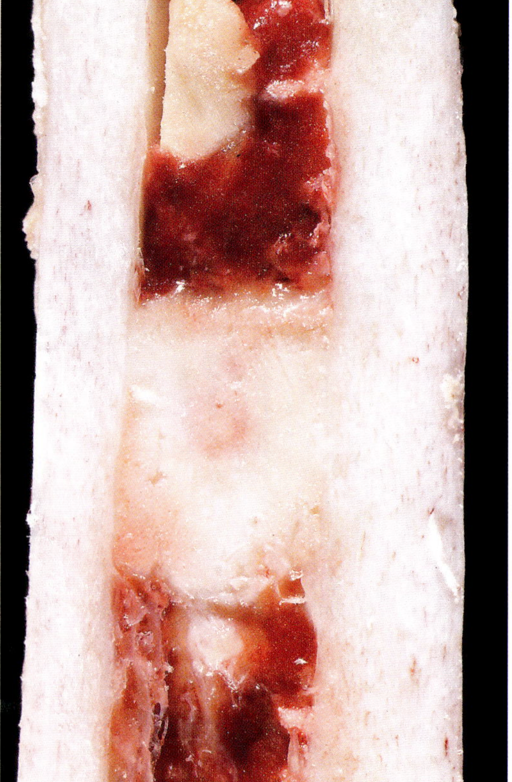

Fig. 8.33

Figs 8.32, 8.33 Osteosarcoma of the femur with skip lesions in the upper diaphysis.

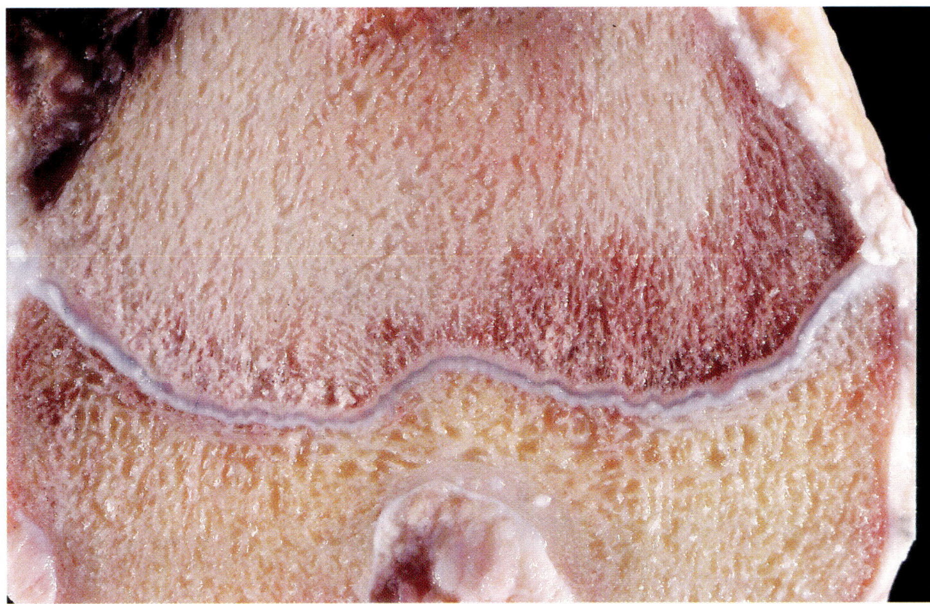

Fig. 8.35 Osteosarcoma of the femur abutting the growth plate.

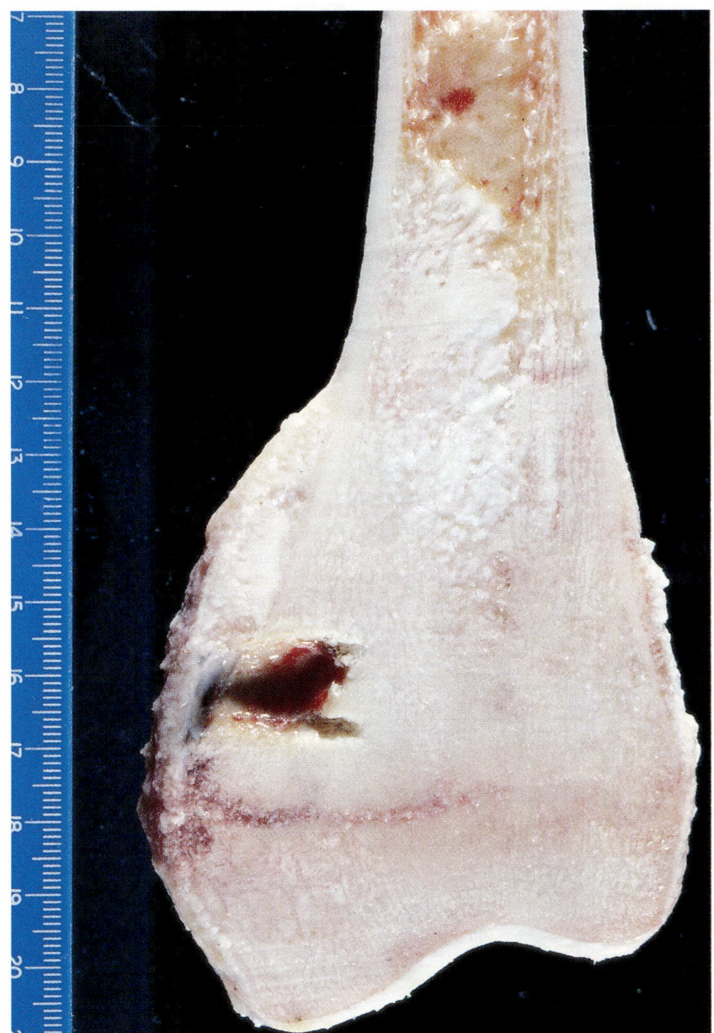

Fig. 8.36 Sclerosing osteosarcoma of the femur abutting the growth plate remnant.

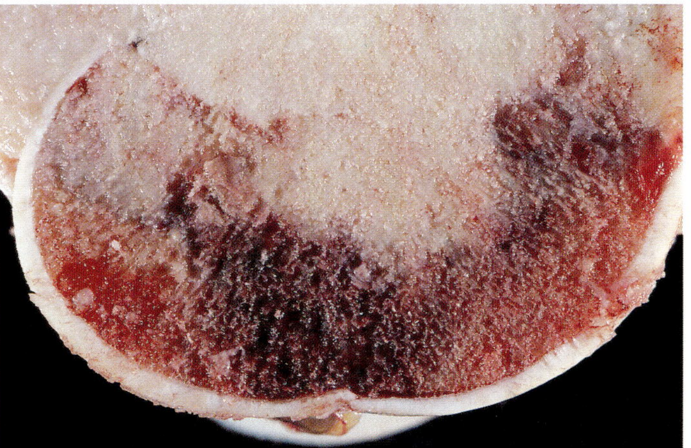

Fig. 8.37 Metaphyseal osteosarcoma of the femur with epiphyseal extension.

studies have shown that part of the epiphyseal plate may be destroyed by spread of the tumor along vascular channels or in epiphyseal vessels in the perichondral ring.[75] The same vascular budding and chondroblastic resorption occur in the articular cartilage.[59]

The soft tissue tumoral component may be covered by the periosteum or by a pseudocapsule comprising an inner compressed rim of normal tissue (compression zone) and an outer rim of inflammation and neovascularization (reactive zone).[76] Macrophages are found in the compressive zone and mast cells, macrophages, fibroblasts and lymphocytes in the reactive zone. Identification of a compression zone has been correlated with a better 5-year survival.[76]

Periosteal reactions are due to various stimuli; implicated physical and chemical changes are tension, pressure

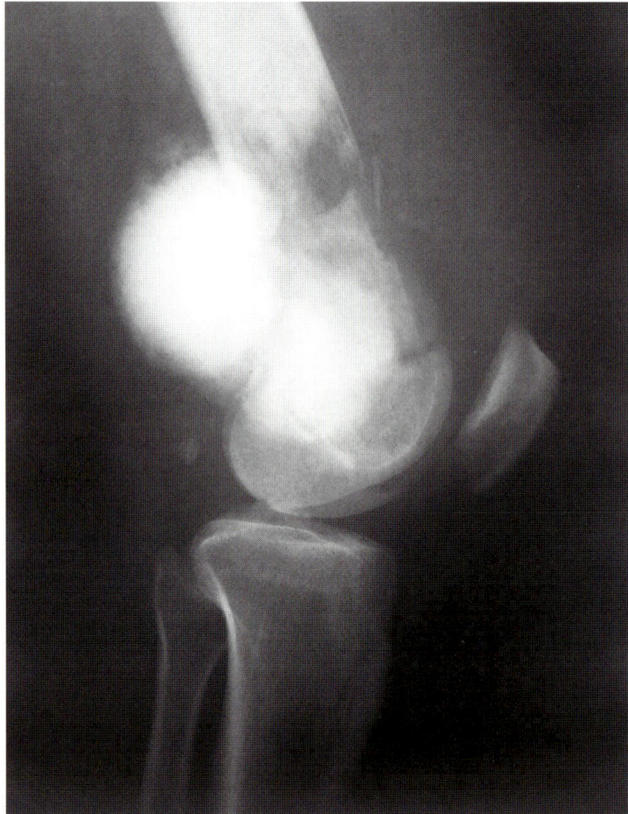

Fig. 8.38

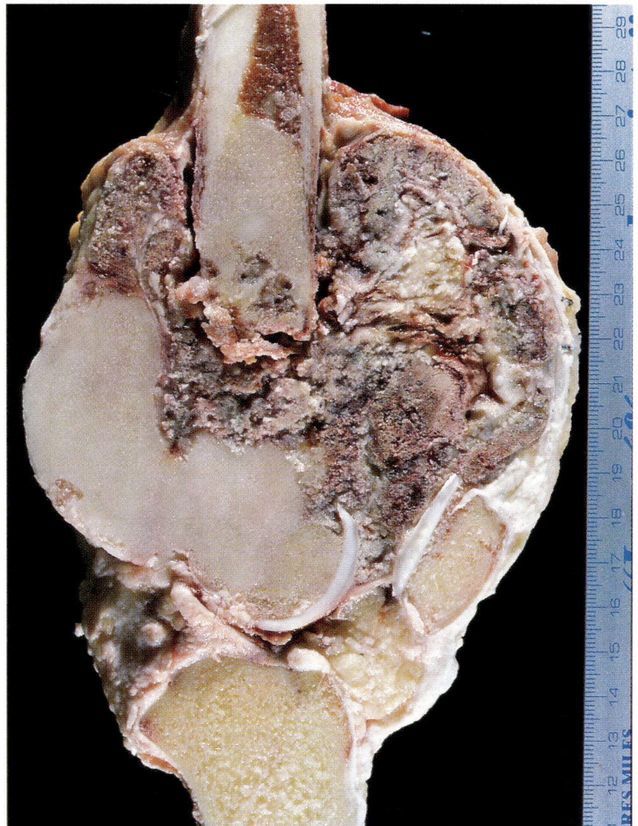

Fig. 8.39

Figs 8.38, 8.39 Involvement of the knee joint by a femoral osteosarcoma.

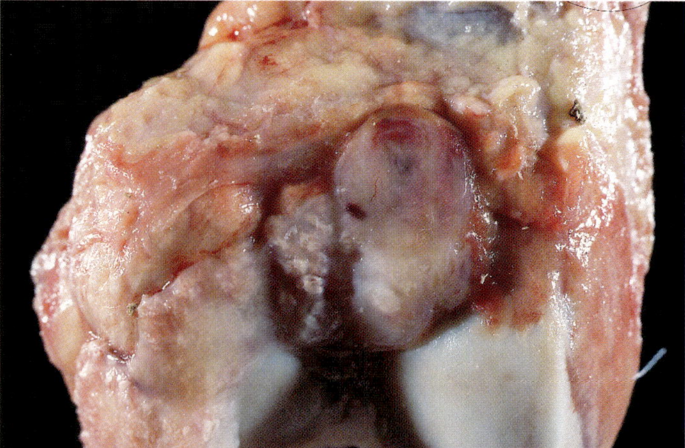

Fig. 8.40

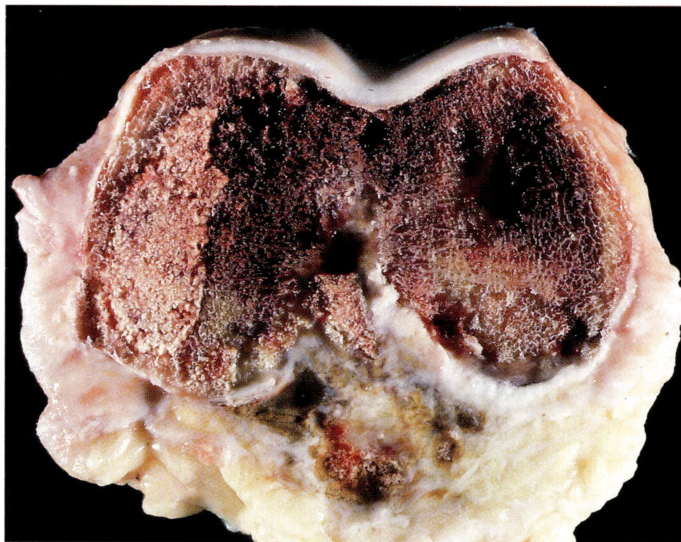

Fig. 8.41

Figs 8.40, 8.41 High-grade osteosarcoma of the femur: intercondylar involvement of the knee joint.

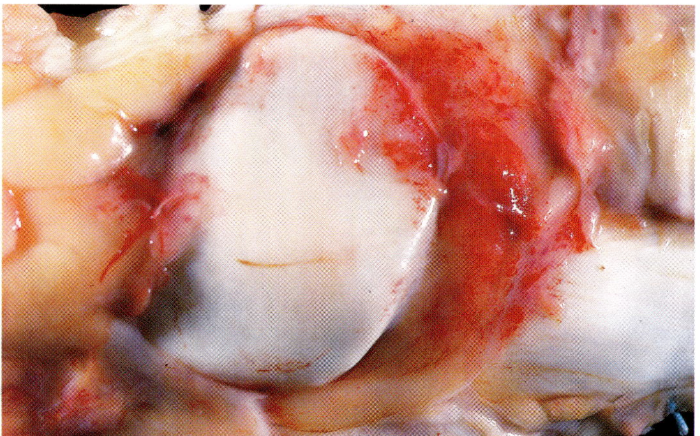

Fig. 8.42 Femoral osteosarcoma: reactive hyperemia of the synovium of the knee joint, without tumoral extension.

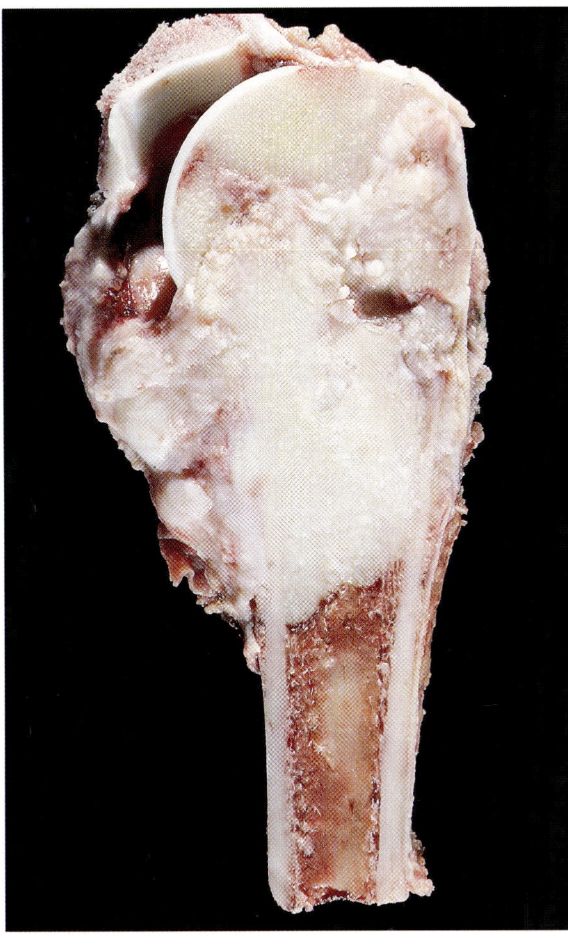

Fig. 8.43 Humeral osteosarcoma with involvement of the joint capsule.

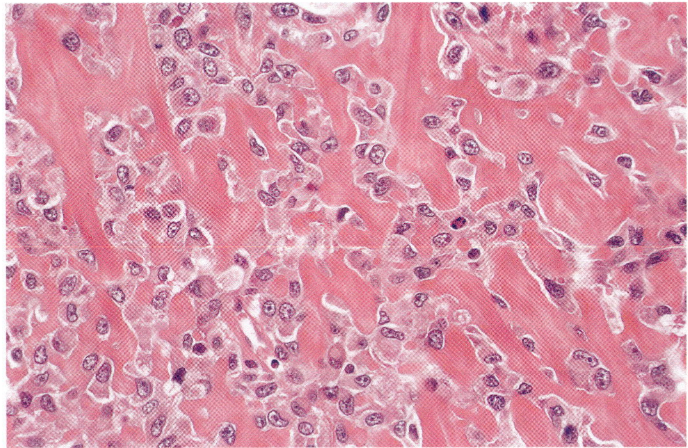

Fig. 8.44

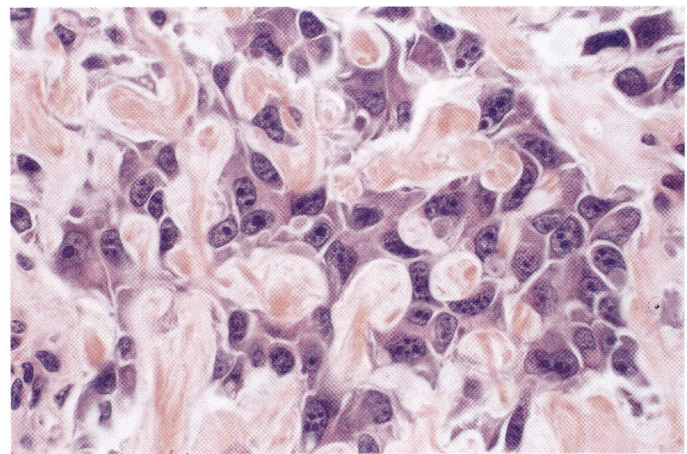

Fig. 8.46

Figs 8.44–8.46 Osteoblastic osteosarcomas with osteoid production.

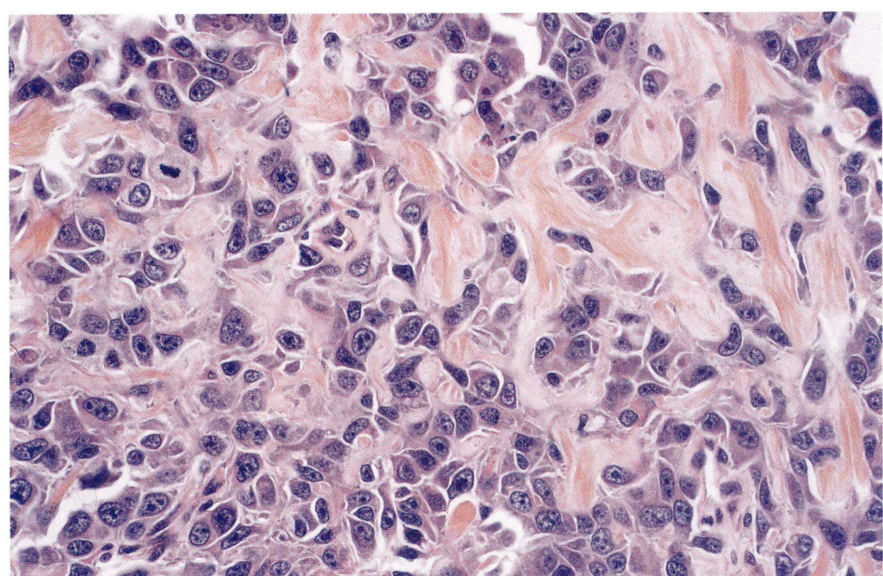

Fig. 8.45

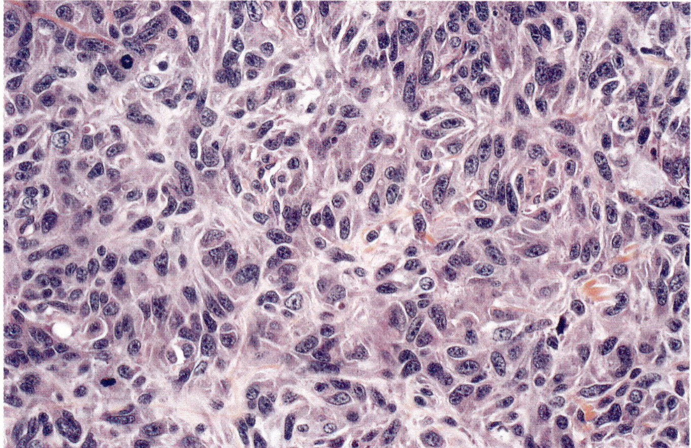

Fig. 8.47

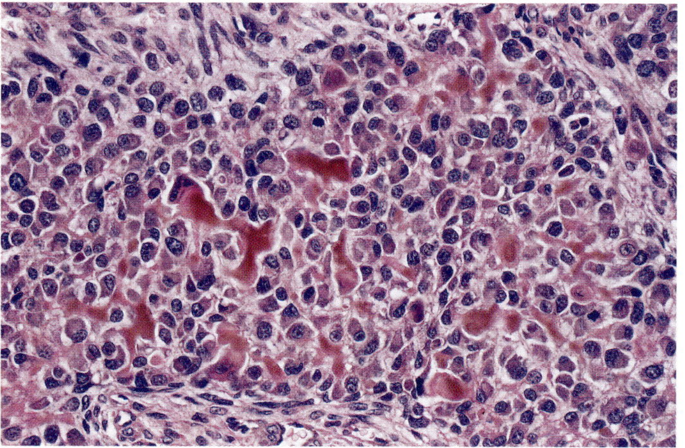

Fig. 8.48

Figs 8.47, 8.48 Osteoblastic osteosarcomas: minute flecks of bone formation.

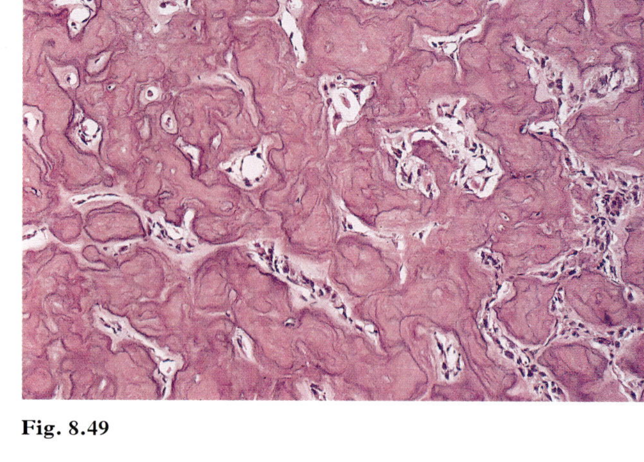

Fig. 8.49

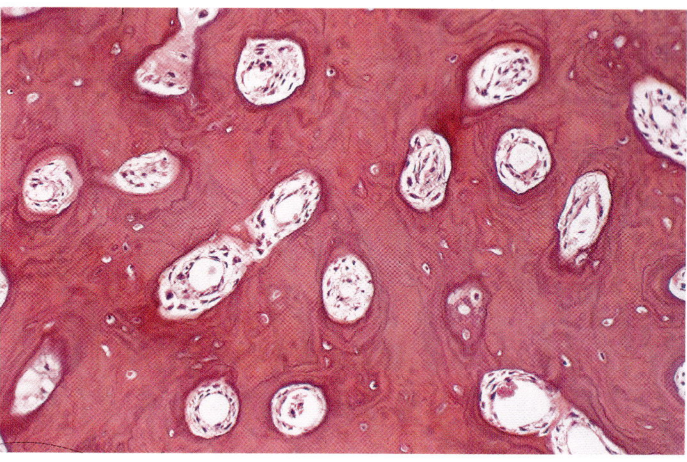

Fig. 8.50

Figs 8.49, 8.50 Osteoblastic osteosarcomas: massive bone formation with irregular cement lines.

disturbances affecting the intercellular fluid (exudates, hemorrhages) and differences in electric potential influencing the blood circulation and the proliferation of reactive osteoblasts, as well as fibroblasts.[77]

CYTOPATHOLOGY

Some reports show cytological examination as having (Figs 8.63–8.69) a high accuracy rate, ranging from 67% to 94%.[78,79] In other reports about 30% of aspirates are insufficient for diagnosis and only 40% give a correct diagnosis.[80,81] Distinction from malignant fibrous histiocytoma, high-grade chondrosarcoma or osteoblastoma may be quite difficult.

Apart from reactive giant cells, osteoblasts are the predominant cells. They are large, round or polygonal shaped cells with a pink cytoplasm. There is an increased nucleocy-

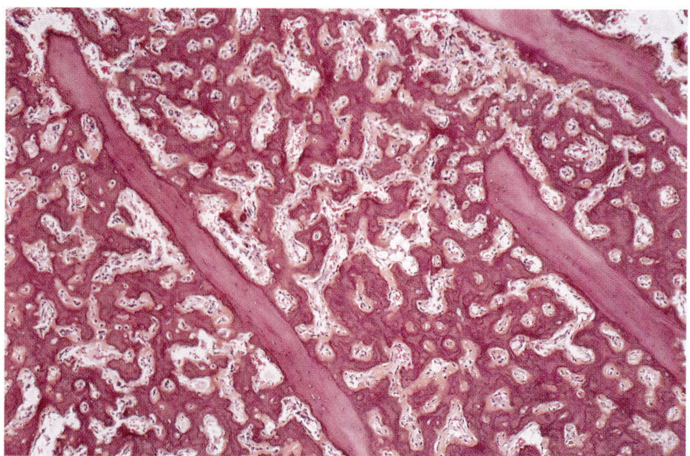

Fig. 8.51 Osteoblastic osteosarcoma: tumoral bone abutting the trabeculae of cancellous bone.

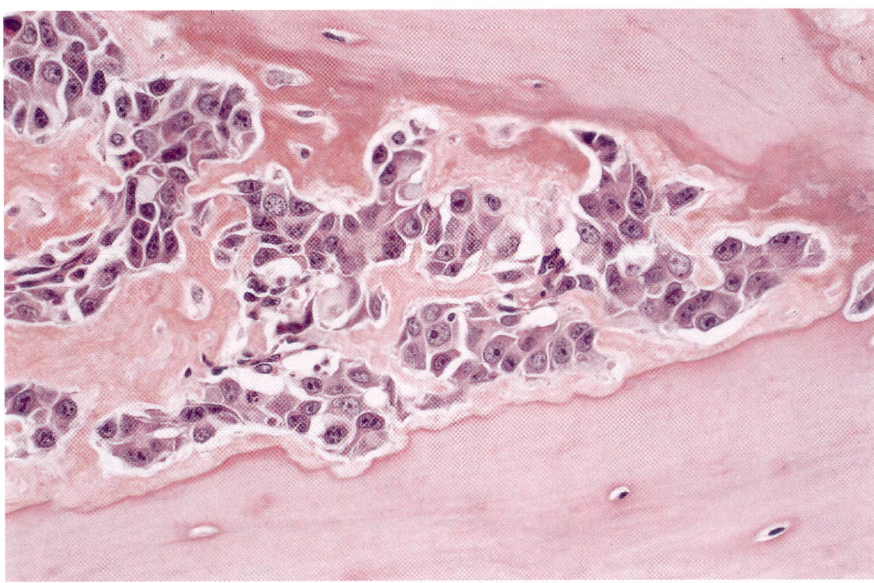

Fig. 8.52 Osteoblastic osteosarcoma: permeation of the cortex and tumoral bone production.

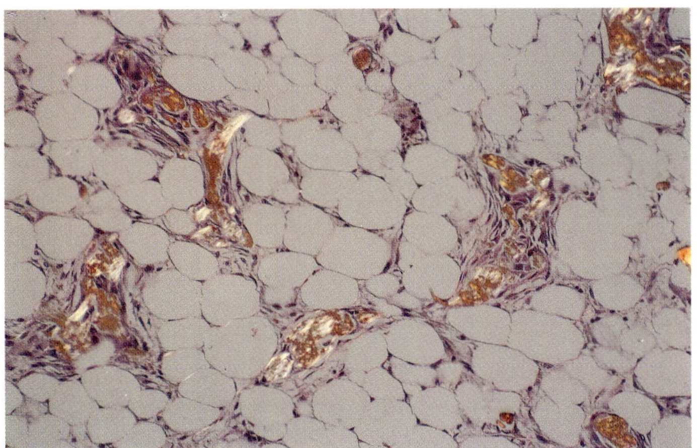

Fig. 8.53 Osteoblastic osteosarcoma: unusual infiltrative pattern of the marrow (polarized light).

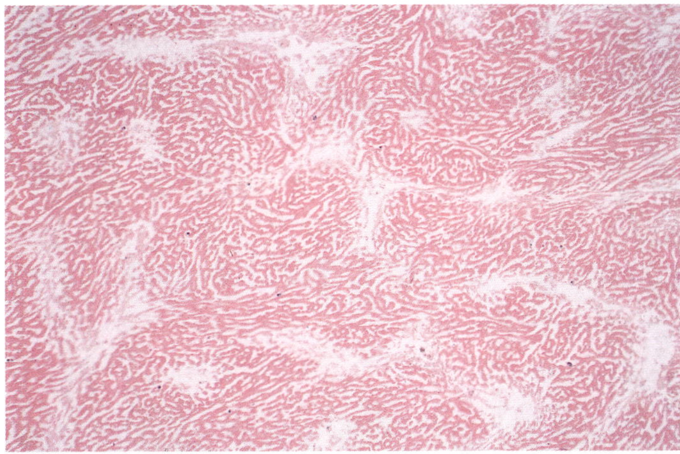

Fig. 8.54 Osteoblastic osteosarcoma: massive drop-out of tumor cells.

toplasmic ratio and increased nuclear size; nuclei are irregular with prominent nucleoli and coarse chromatin with clumping. Abnormal mitoses and large tumoral multinucleated cells are common. Differentiated osteoblasts have a plasmacytoid or epithelioid appearance with an eccentric nucleus[80,82] but the perinuclear cytoplasmic clear one is lacking. The osteoid matrix appears as an amorphous pink fibrillar material on May-Grunwald-Giemsa staining.[82]

A gelatinous chondroid matrix is found in chondroblastic osteosarcomas.[79] Fibroblastic osteosarcomas, obviously, have spindle-shaped cells.

Imprint techniques are valuable adjuncts not only to frozen but also to permanent sections.[83–85] Cytology also has a role in the expanding field of percutaneous bone biopsy. Aspirated osseous blood in stained smears or paraffin-embedded blood clot can include a significant cytological tumoral component.[86]

IMMUNOHISTOCHEMISTRY

Monoclonal antibodies against osteosarcoma-associated antigens have been developed but unfortunately they have a broad reactivity. A unique monoclonal antibody (TmMR-2) appears to be specific for mesenchymal cells of osseous differentiation;[87,88] it does not react with normal chondroblasts or chondrocytes but may give positive results in malignant fibrous histiocytomas, synovial sarcomas and even chondrosarcomas.

Reactivities of osteosarcomas with monoclonal and polyclonal antibodies against filamentous proteins and

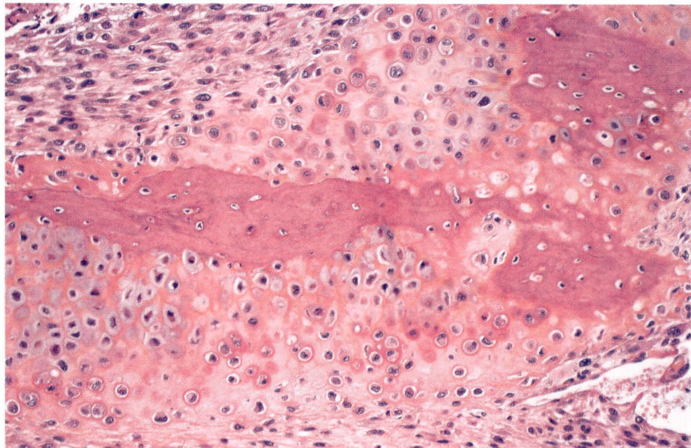

Fig. 8.55

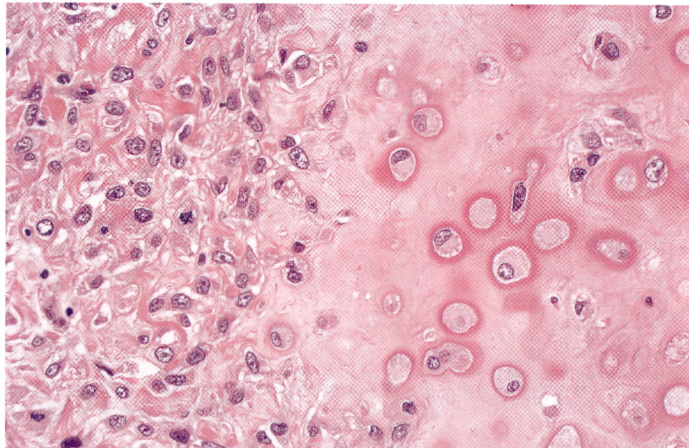

Fig. 8.57

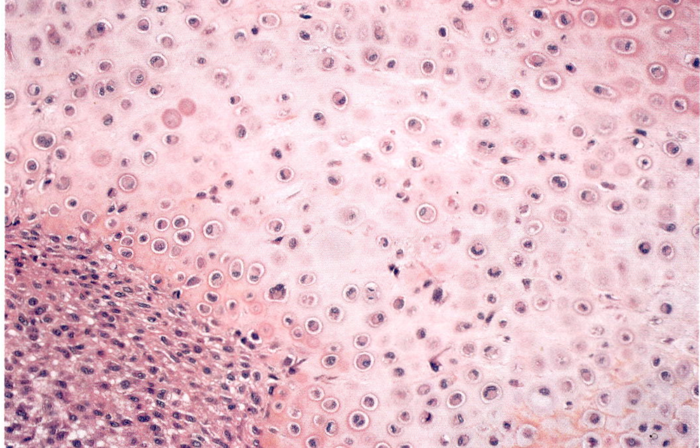

Fig. 8.56

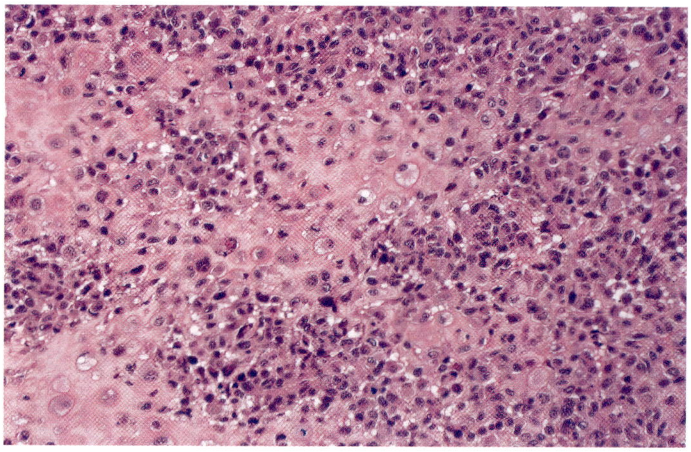

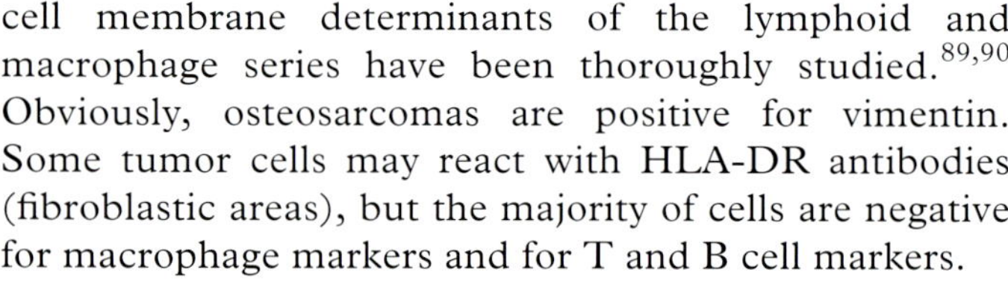

Fig. 8.58

Figs 8.55–8.58 Cartilaginous fields of chondroblastic osteosarcomas.

cell membrane determinants of the lymphoid and macrophage series have been thoroughly studied.[89,90] Obviously, osteosarcomas are positive for vimentin. Some tumor cells may react with HLA-DR antibodies (fibroblastic areas), but the majority of cells are negative for macrophage markers and for T and B cell markers.

Osteosarcomas may occasionally express some immunologic features of histiocytic differentiation (factor XIIIa) or myofibroblastic differentiation (α smooth muscle actin and desmin); some cells can even show an epithelial immunophenotype.[90]

S-100 protein has been demonstrated not only in the chondroblastic areas but also in some osteoblastic areas, positivity being related to the calcification of osteoid tissue.[90–92] Immunohistochemical studies as well as ultrastructural examination show a significant degree of ALPase activity, irrespective of the cytological diversity.[93,94]

Several non-collagenous proteins (osteonectin, osteocalcin, bone morphogenetic protein) have been investigat-

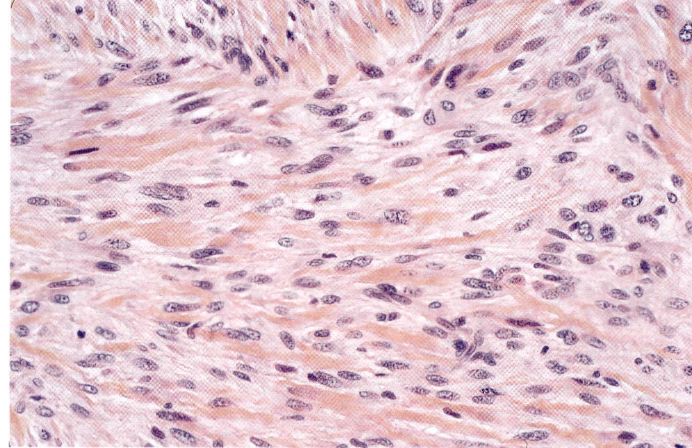

Fig. 8.59 Fibroblastic osteosarcoma.

ed in osteosarcomas. Osteonectin is a phosphorylated glycoprotein produced by osteoblasts showing binding properties for collagen type I as well as for hydroxyapatite; it

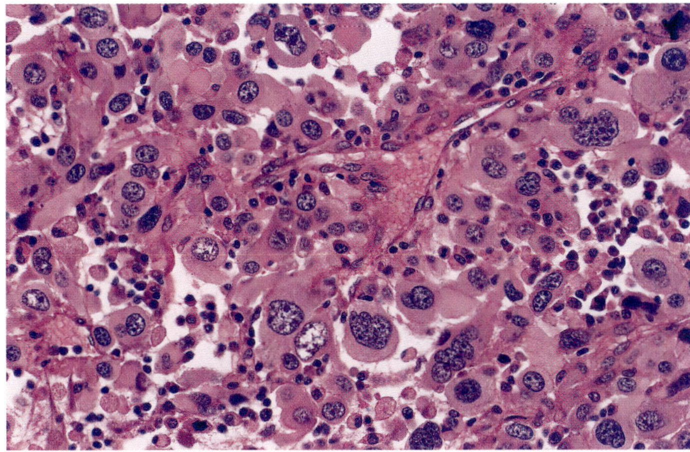

Fig. 8.60

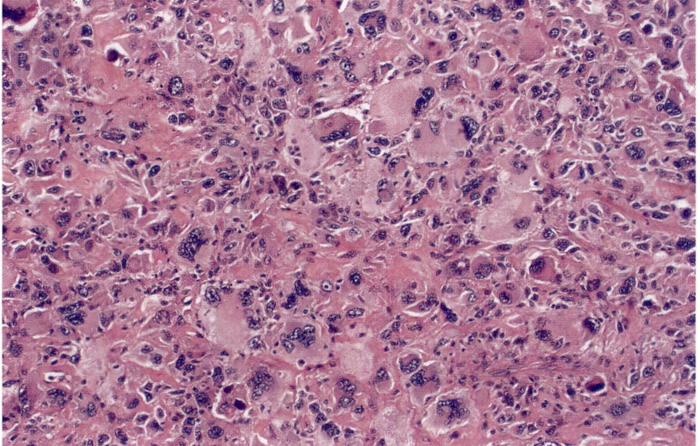

Fig. 8.61

Figs 8.60, 8.61 Marked cytological pleomorphism in high-grade osteosarcomas.

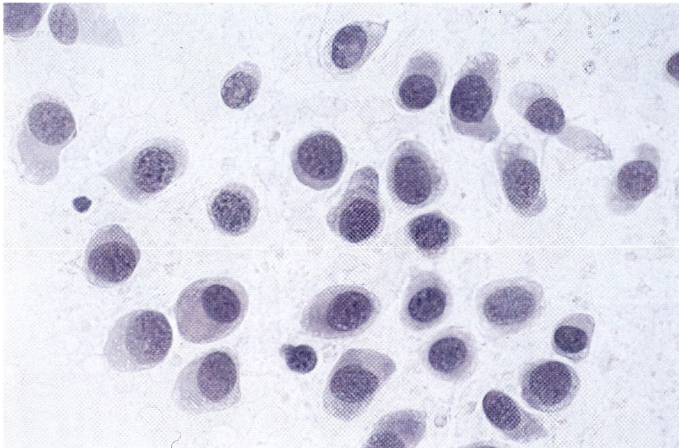

Fig. 8.63

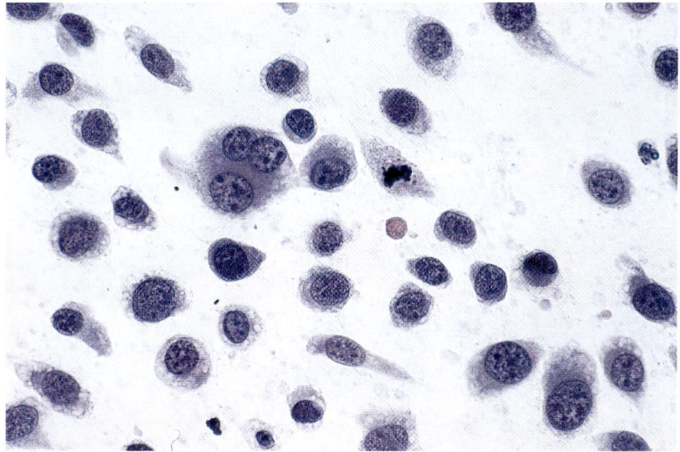

Fig. 8.64

Figs 8.63, 8.64 Imprint cytology of osteoblastic osteosarcomas.

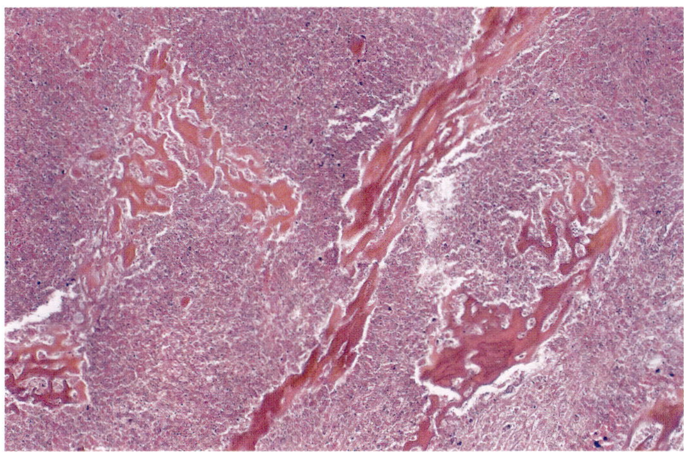

Fig. 8.62 Spontaneous necrosis in a femoral osteosarcoma.

occurs in bone cells if active matrix synthesis takes place.[95] Immunostaining has been reported in osteogenic lesions[95,96] but it appears that osteonectin cannot be regarded as a bone-specific protein, as it is found in some fibrosarcomas and chondrosarcomas.[97,98] However, in situ hybridization of osteonectin mRNA might be useful in differentiating osteosarcomas from non-osteogenic bone tumors.[99]

Osteocalcin (bone γ-carboxyglutamic acid-containing protein, BGP) is the most abundant non-collagenous protein in bones and may participate in the process of mineralization.[100] Immunolocalization of osteocalcin in osteosarcomas may be intra- and extracellular[101,102] or solely intracellular.[90,103,104] Osteocalcin, a cell marker of osteoblastic differentiation, may be useful in the differential diagnosis with malignant fibrous histiocytoma,[105] even if some positivity has been reported with the latter tumor and also with chondrosarcomas.

Bone morphogenetic proteins (BMPs) are potent inducers of bone formation in heterotopic sites by host mesenchymal cells. These regulatory peptides belong to the transforming growth factor β superfamily.[106] Immunolocalization has been found in osteosarcomas, but also in

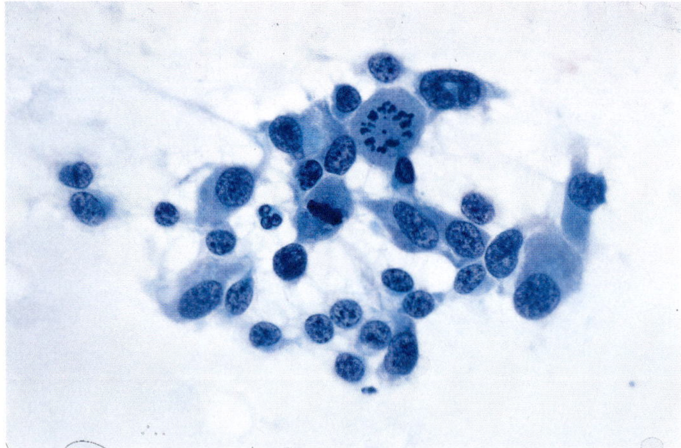

Fig. 8.65

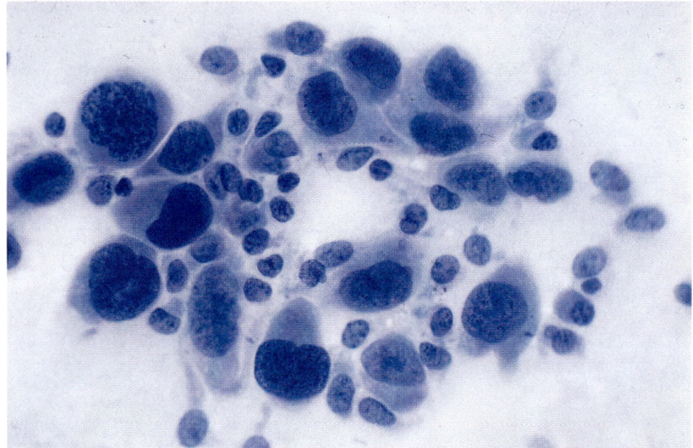

Fig. 8.66

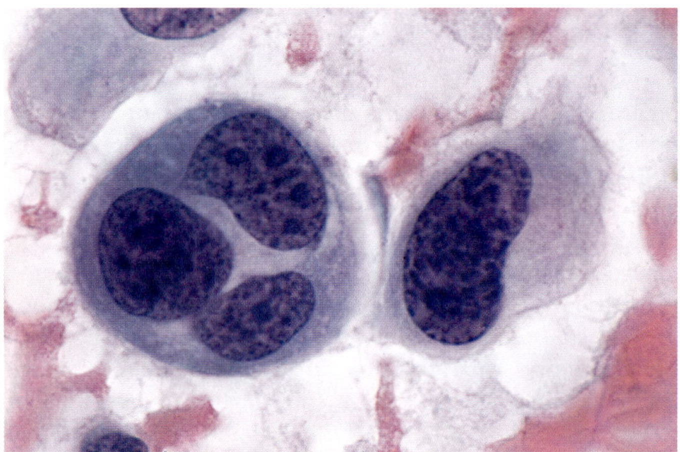

Fig. 8.67

Figs 8.65–8.67 Imprint cytology of high-grade osteoblastic osteosarcomas.

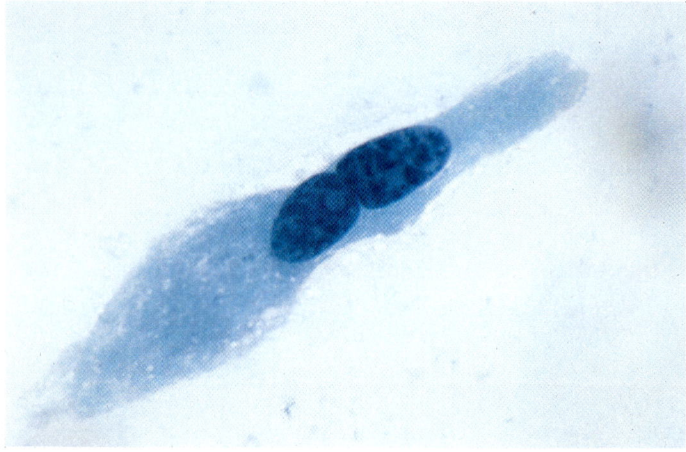

Fig. 8.68 Imprint cytology of a fibroblastic osteosarcoma.

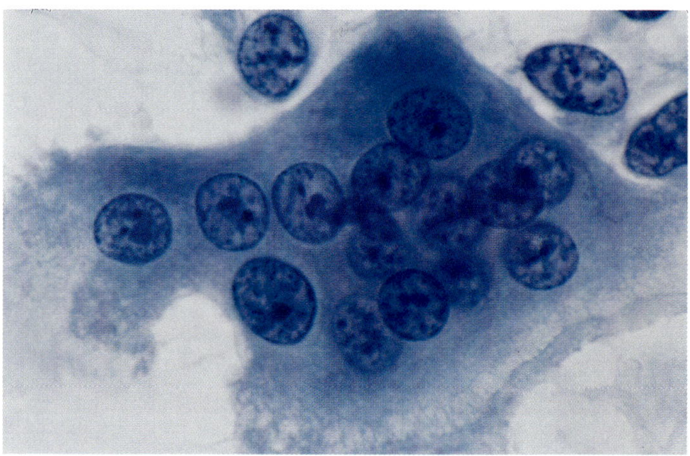

Fig. 8.69 Imprint cytology of osteosarcoma: osteoclast-like reactive giant cell.

typical or dedifferentiated chondrosarcomas and malignant fibrous histiocytomas.[107,108] Bone morphogenetic activity of osteosarcomas appears to be correlated with a worse prognosis.[109,110]

Different collagen types have been studied by biochemistry, chromatography, immunohistochemistry and immunoelectron microscopy.[111–114] Osteoblastic areas show exclusively collagen type I, chondroblastic areas collagen type II and eventually I, V and VI, fibroblastic areas collagen type I–III and VI and anaplastic fields collagen type III with a very low collagen synthesis.[115,116] Type IV collagen is found in the stroma of fibroblastic, well-differentiated and telangiectatic osteosarcomas, maybe in relation to a myofibroblastic or angioblastic differentiation of tumor cells.[116] Identification of collagen types II and VI may be useful in the differential diagnosis with chondrosarcomas.[116]

Molecular genetic research in osteosarcoma has some implications for immunohistochemical techniques. The development of osteosarcoma is partly the result of mutations of two tumor suppressor genes: the retinoblastoma susceptibility (Rb-1) gene and the p53 gene.[117–122] Inactivation of the p53 suppressor gene located on chromosome 17 has been extensively studied in osteosarcoma. Development of a monoclonal antibody clone PAb 240 recognizing a mutant p53 protein and a monoclonal antibody PAb 421 recognizing both wild-type and mutant forms[119,122] has shown an expression in 29–75% of tumors[123] but without correlation with histological subtypes, DNA ploidy patterns or response to preoperative chemotherapy.[124,125]

Some osteosarcomas may also exhibit overexpression of the MYC protooncogene due to gene amplification[126] but the clinical and biological significance is not finally established.

Expression of the members of the β1 integrin family and extracellular matrix ligands has been studied in osteosarcoma tissues. α4 and α5 fibronectin receptors predominate, correlating with the strong expression of fibronectin in the stroma. Adhesive interaction of tumor cells with the extracellular matrix has a role in the metastatic process.[127] Expression of the protooncogene bcl–2 is related to the inhibition of apoptosis and in osteosarcoma, immunohistochemistry shows negative to strong results.[128] This reaction may have an important future role as a predictive factor for prognosis, as well as the expression of receptor-type protein tyrosine kinase ErbB-2 evaluated with monoclonal antibody or by immunoblotting.[129]

Proliferation behavior of osteosarcoma may be assessed by the monoclonal antibody Ki-67 directed against a nuclear antigen present in all the active phases of the cell cycle;[130] immunohistological results are comparable to flow cytometry.[130] In a recent study, there was a good correlation between Ki-67 expression and the level of malignancy; biological aggressiveness with high levels of Ki-67 labeling reflects a worse prognosis, despite a good response to chemotherapy.[131]

FLOW CYTOMETRY

DNA analysis can be performed by microspectrophotometry of tissue sections or flow cytometry of cell suspensions from fresh tissue. Most high-grade osteosarcomas are hyperploid[132–135] and hyperploidy and aneuploidy are the same in the areas of osteoblastic, chondroblastic and fibroblastic differentiation.[136–138]

The metastasis-free survival rate appears to be related to the percentage of cells in S phase.[135,138] However, there may be a high degree of heterogeneity in the same tumor;[139] near diploid variants in one report showed a better response to adjuvant chemotherapy.[140] After chemotherapy, mean S-phase value is lower and the number of tumors without DNA aneuploidy is higher.[141] There is a distinct relationship between DNA content and the grade of tumor regression[142] but in one report, ploidy determination did not prove useful in predicting the histologic response.[143]

CYTOGENETICS

Cytogenetic changes in osteosarcomas appear very complex with a great variety of both numerical and structural abnormalities.[144–147] Most common structural changes are unbalanced translocations, deletions, double-minute or ring chromosomes. In many cases, deletions are at 13q14 and 17p13 (corresponding to the Rb and p53 tumor suppressor genes).[144,147]

ELECTRON MICROSCOPY

The diagnostic value of ultrastructural study is currently somewhat restricted. The most significant finding may be the demonstration of hydroxyapatite crystals deposited on or along collagen fibers, in very anaplastic tumors.

Osteosarcoma presents the differentiation of a pluripotent mesenchymal cell toward osteoblastic, fibroblastic, chondroblastic or even myofibroblastic and angioblastic cell lines.[148–151] Osteoblasts have an eccentric nucleus, an abundant cytoplasm with a marked development of the rough endoplasmic reticulum and a large perinuclear Golgi zone. The nucleus may be quite irregular and indented with prominent chromatin aggregates and one or more huge nucleoli. Primary mineralization comprises matrix vesicles and calcifying nodules between the cells and the calcifying fronts; it is one of the ultrastructural parameters for osteoblastic bone tumors.[152,153]

OTHER TECHNIQUES

Enzyme histochemical investigations show that all tumor cells in osteosarcomas contain abundant alkaline phosphatase[154,155] but some anaplastic tumors may not show any increase.[156] Plastic embedding has been used for a quantitative analysis of cytology, bone formation and mineralization.[157] The process of differentiation has also been studied by biochemical and topological analysis.[158,159]

Loops of DNA within the nucleolus in the cellular interphase are nucleolar organizer regions. Associated proteins can be located by a silver staining technique (AgNORs). In osteosarcomas, there is a positive correlation between the number of AgNORs and the proliferation potential[160] but the predictive value for metastatic disease is unclear.[161]

In cell cultures, one can study the mechanism of mineralization[162] or the resorption of the collagenous bone matrix.[163,164] It should be remembered that osteosarcoma cell lines have been extensively used to define the normal osteoblast phenotype.

Morphology and biology of osteosarcoma may be investigated by nude mice xenografts[165] and combined studies on bone formation by human osteosarcoma cells in vitro and in nude mice have shown the respective roles of collagen, alkaline phosphatase and BMP in tumoral bone formation.[166]

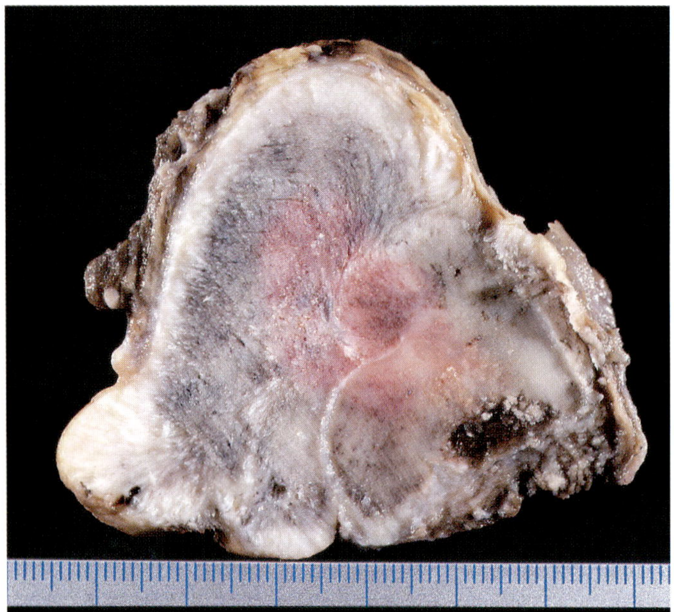

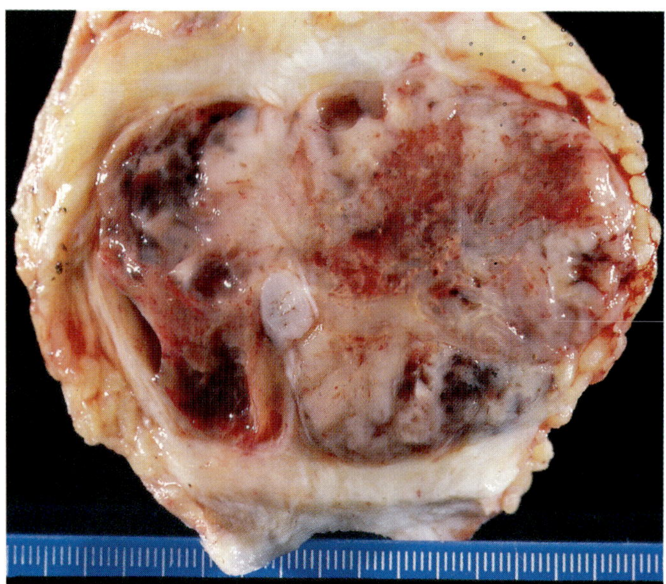

Fig. 8.71 Recurrence of a resected femoral osteosarcoma in the thigh.

Fig. 8.70 Lung metastasis of an osteoblastic osteosarcoma with massive bone formation.

Experimental bone tumors have been produced by radiation, viruses and chemical carcinogens, especially beryllium.[167]

COURSE, TREATMENT AND PROGNOSIS

In more than 90% of cases, the usual site of metastasis is the lung[168] (Fig. 8.70), occurring in most cases in the first 2 years (Campanacci 1990). Patients with tumors responding to chemotherapy may develop pulmonary metastases,[169] with a histology and degree of differentiation equal to the primary tumor in more than 60% of cases.[170] However, adjuvant chemotherapy seems to affect the development of pulmonary metastases, delaying their appearance and reducing their numbers.[171,172] Very rarely, some pulmonary metastases may temporarily regress.[173] The ratio of extent of the involved marrow segment to the total length of long bone has been correlated with the finding of pulmonary metastases.[174]

At post mortem examination, metastases spreading by the hematogenous route are found in 50% of cases, chiefly in the lung, bones, pleura and heart.[175] Incidence of extrapulmonary sites is higher among patients treated by adjuvant chemotherapy, with these patients living longer.[176]

Lymphatic metastases may occur with an incidence of about 10% for large tumors.[177,178] The incidence is higher in autopsy material.[179,180] Lymph nodes can show sinus histiocytosis only[181,182] or may calcify and ossify.[183,184]

Skeletal metastases are metaphyseal or diaphyseal lesions in long bones, but they occur more frequently in the spine, the pelvis, the skull and ribs (Wilner 1982). They can precede the lung lesions.[185]

Treatment is surgical (limb-sparing procedures in long

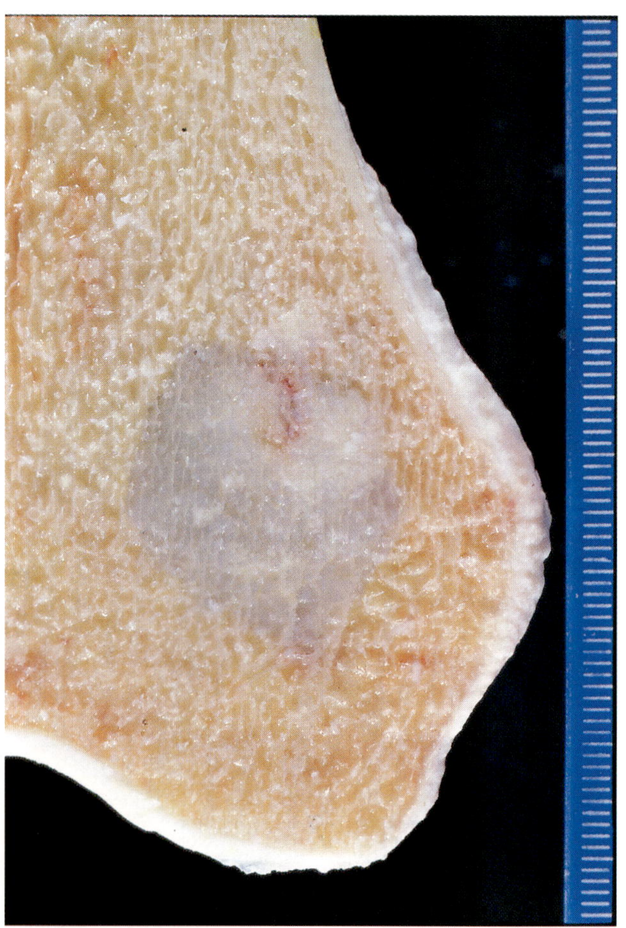

Fig. 8.72 Smallest high-grade osteoblastic osteosarcoma in our series (femoral location).

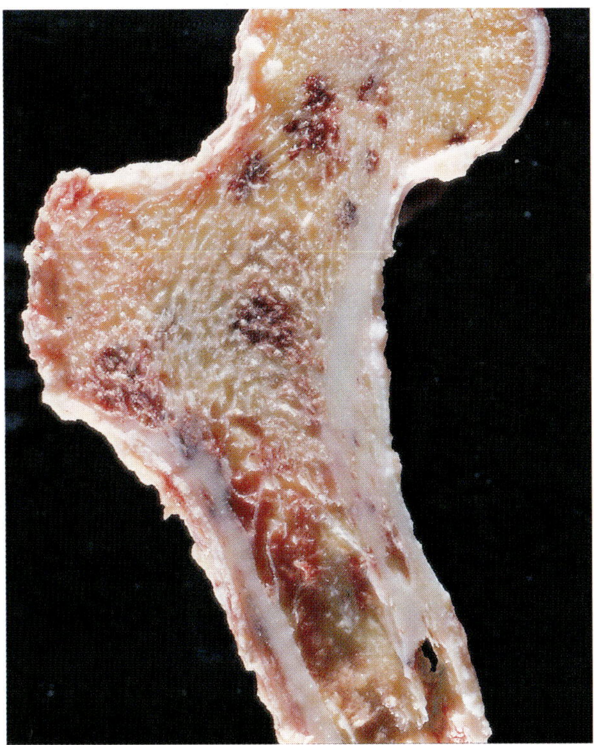

Fig. 8.73

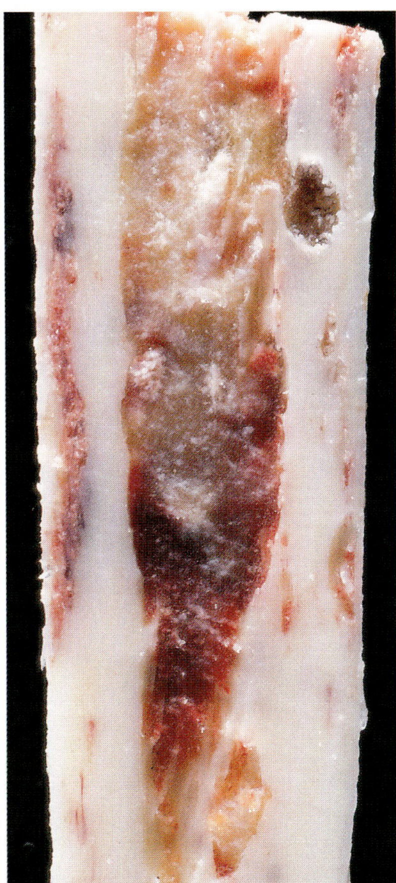

Fig. 8.74

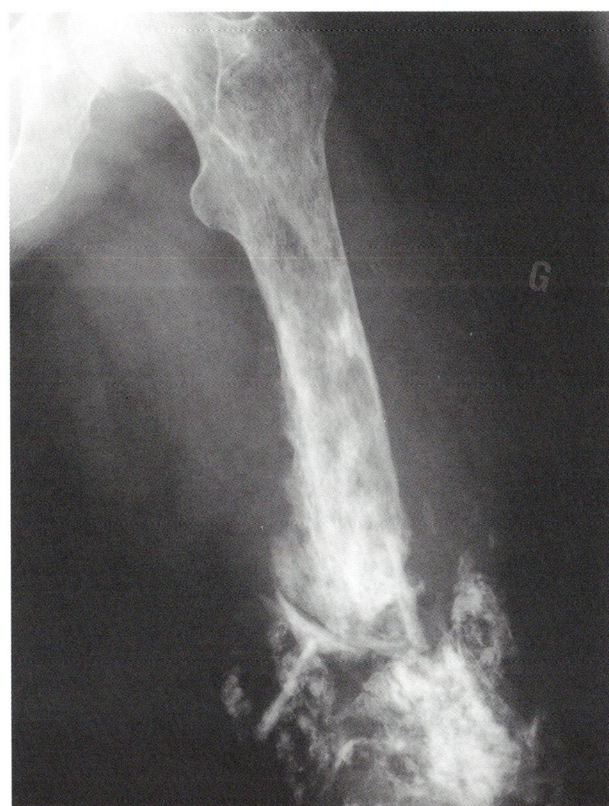

Fig. 8.75

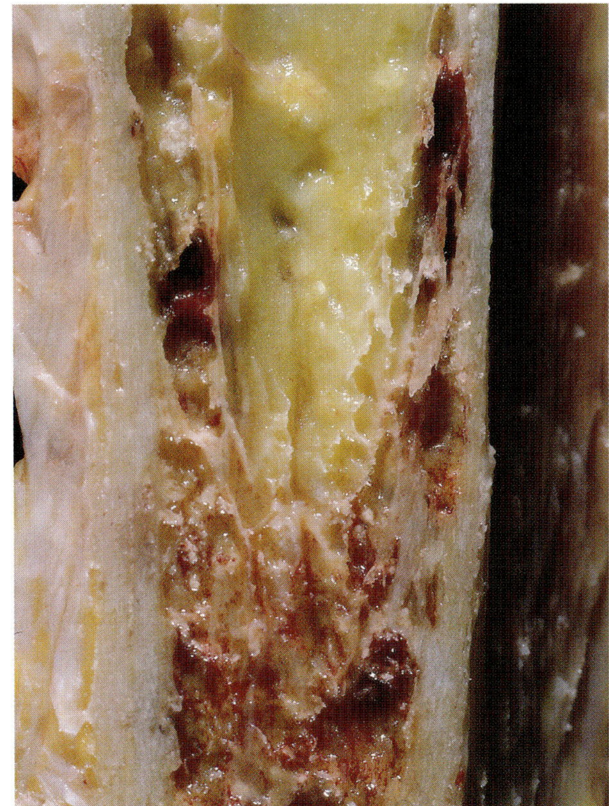

Fig. 8.76

Figs 8.73–8.76 Two cases of radiation osteitis of the femur, with lytic and sclerotic changes.

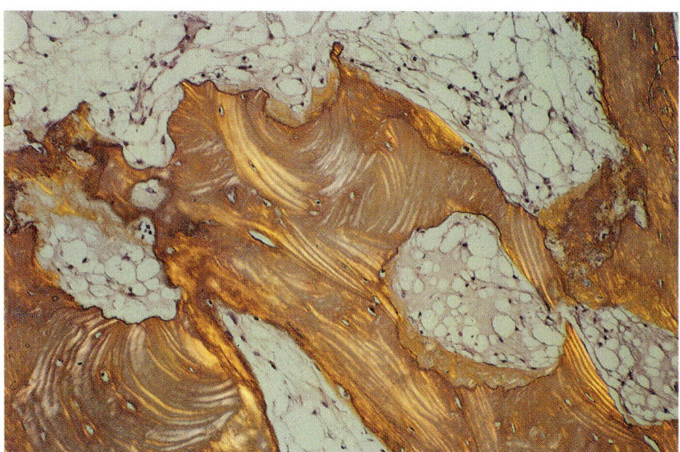

Fig. 8.77 Radiation osteitis: osteolysis associated with new bone formation (polarized light).

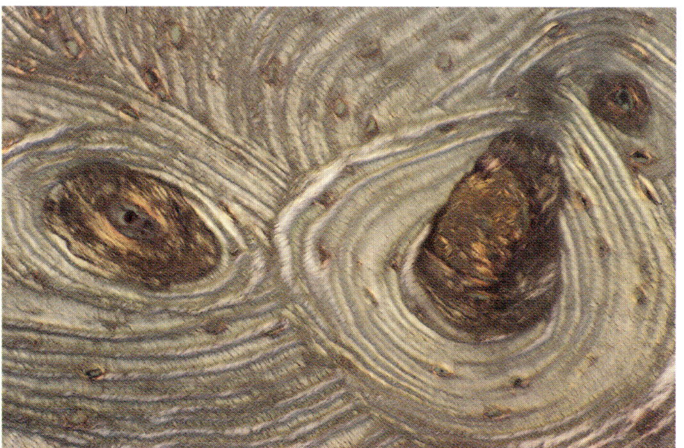

Fig. 8.78 Radiation osteitis: Haversian canals being filled by new bone (polarized light).

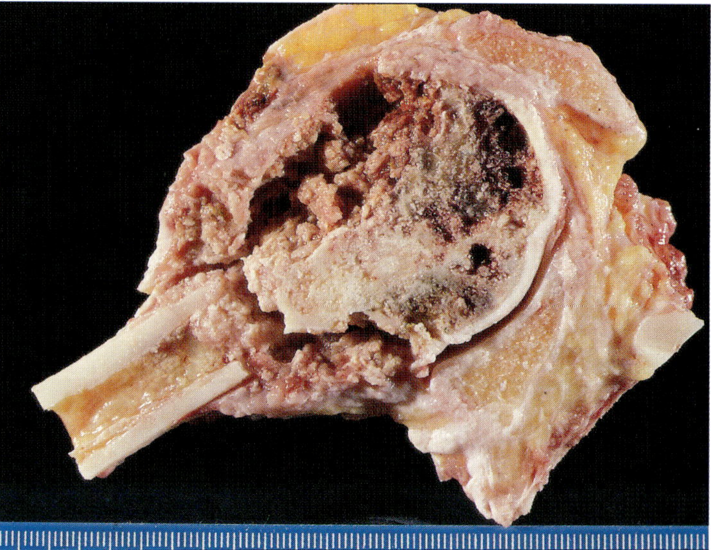

Fig. 8.79 Humeral osteosarcoma with no response to intraarterial chemotherapy: pathological fracture.

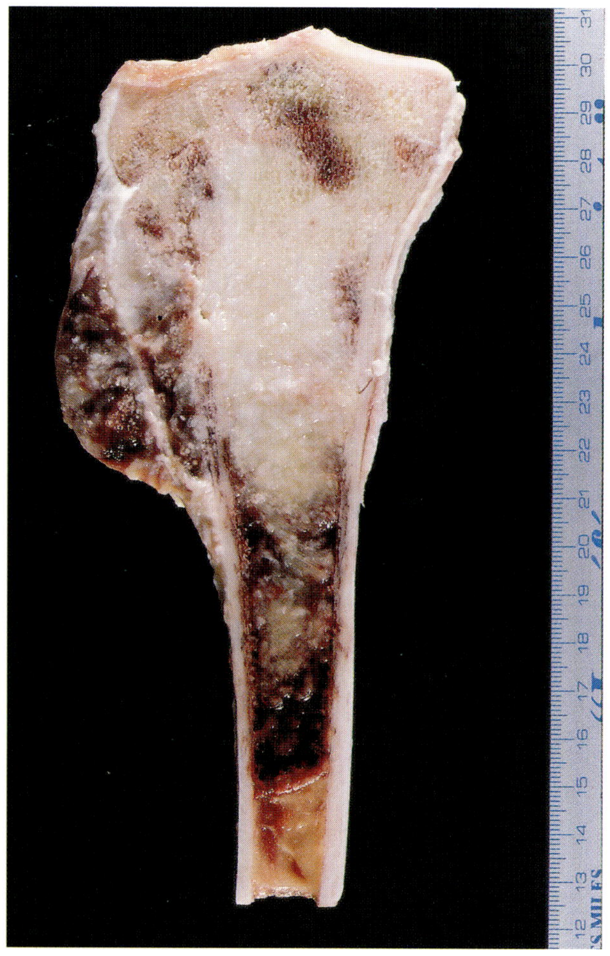

Fig. 8.80 Chondroblastic osteosarcoma of the tibia with poor response to intraarterial chemotherapy.

bones), associated in the usual form of osteosarcoma with pre- and postoperative chemotherapy. Survival at 5 years is between 60% and 80%. Radiation therapy is of more restricted value.

Incidence of local recurrence after limb-sparing surgery is about the same as after transmedullary amputation and is low, from 2% to 5% of cases[186] (Fig. 8.71).

There is a lack of correlation between radiological appearance, histological grading and prognosis.[187,188] Tumors of the proximal femur, trunk and pelvis have a worse prognosis,[189,190] as do tumors of more than 10 cm diameter[191,192] or more than 150 cm^3 absolute tumor volume[193] (the size being unrelated to the histological grading; Fig. 8.72) or tumors with local invasion of two ore more adjacent structures.[191,194] The extent of spontaneous necrosis (independent of tumor size) may indicate a rapid clinical course.[195]

Osteosarcomas with skip metastases have the same risk

of death as osteosarcomas metastasizing to distant organs[196] but this finding is somewhat disputed.[190]

Pretreatment levels of serum alkaline phosphatase or levels measured in the tumor and metastases are strongly related to the prognosis.[197–199] Pretreatment LDH enzyme levels also have a definite prognostic value.[200]

PATHOLOGICAL STUDIES AFTER RADIATION THERAPY AND CHEMOTHERAPY

Few studies have examined *morphological changes after radiation therapy*. In some osteosarcomas, the central part is not the most radioresistant: in studying the proliferation capacity of tumor cells on cultures, the central core appears as sensitive as the peripheral, well-oxygenated areas.[201]

Associated bone changes are known as radiation osteitis (Ewing) (Figs 8.73–8.78) and include well-circumscribed lytic areas in the cortex or cortical thickening in long bones and diffuse areas of sclerosis made of coarsened trabecular structures in the pelvis.[202] Percutaneous needle biopsy has been used to differentiate radiation necrosis from tumor extension.[203]

In a multivariate analysis, the strongest predictor of a

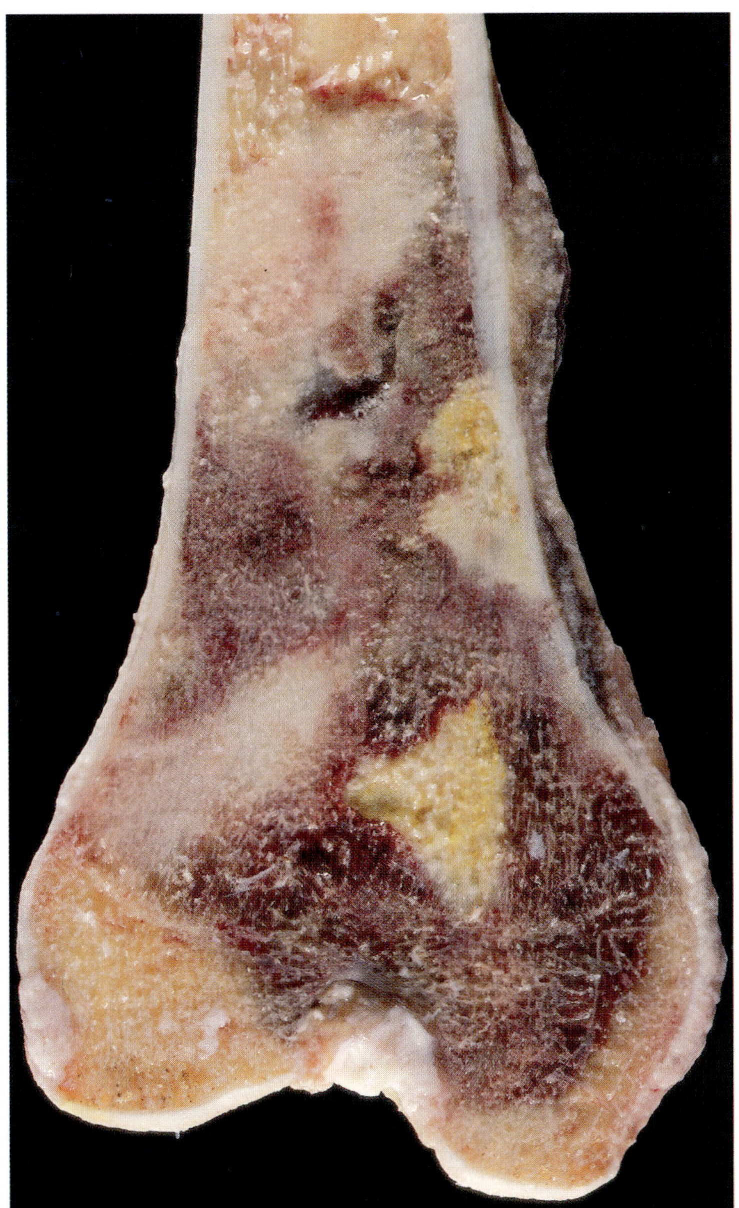

Fig. 8.81

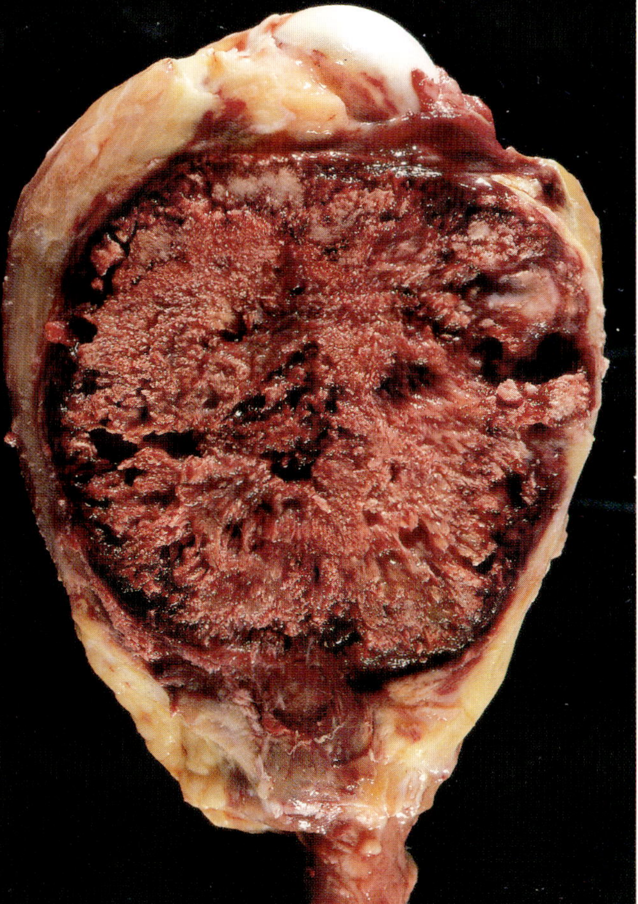

Fig. 8.82

Figs 8.81, 8.82 Necrotic and hemorrhagic changes induced by chemotherapy in femoral osteosarcomas.

disease-free outcome is the *degree of histologic response to preoperative chemotherapy.*[190,204]

In some series, fibroblastic osteosarcomas seem to have a better prognosis[205] and a high degree of chondroblastic differentiation is associated with a poor response to chemotherapy. In a quantitative study of nuclear size, the grade of differentiation of osteosarcomas has been found to be a significant factor[206] but usually, the morphological phenotype is of limited value in predicting the response to chemotherapy.[207]

Since the first reports of Huvos,[208–210] the work-up of surgical specimens has been thoroughly delineated. The plane of section is chosen to demonstrate the maximal areas of tumor growth;[211] on an entire slab specimen, after X-ray, mapped sections are made along with a study of the two remaining hemispheres.[212] The regional mapping of bone destruction may be guided by preoperative arteriograms.[212]

Needle biopsy[213] is marked by a lack of diagnostic sensitivity, but imprint cytology on gross specimens is very useful for a rapid evaluation of the effect of therapy.[214]

Gross examination is not reliable[212] (Figs 8.79–8.87), showing a shrinkage of the tumor size, well-defined margins and fibrotic or sclerotic bone.[211] The degree of capsule formation may be related to the adjuvant treatment: a thick hyaline stratified membrane is found, continuous with the periosteum.[215,216] In pediatric patients, there is a slowing of growth plate activity, with subsequent recovery.[217]

Induced necrosis is shown by cell 'drop out' or 'ghost cells' with no residual nucleocytoplasmic details[212] (Fig. 8.88). Ultrastructural findings are fatty deposits, irregular dilatations of rough endoplasmic reticulum and shrinkage of nuclear chromatin.[218]

'Bizarre' cells are usually found (Figs 8.89, 8.90). These are large and irregular; hyperchromatic and multiple nuclei show clumping and smudging of the chromatin;[212] the cytoplasm may be vacuolated with eosinophilic globules.[212,219] These changes may be lethal or sublethal, but the cells are considered viable for practical purposes.[212,220]

Lace-like osteoid and tumor bone remain intact (Figs 8.91, 8.92). Reparative changes are a regenerative loose or hyaline fibrovascular stroma with reactive fibroblasts and osteoblasts[211,212] and new bone deposition around necrotic trabeculae.[219] Some lymphocytes, plasma cells and hemosiderin-laden macrophages may be found (Fig. 8.93), along with blood-filled sinusoidal spaces and hemorrhages.

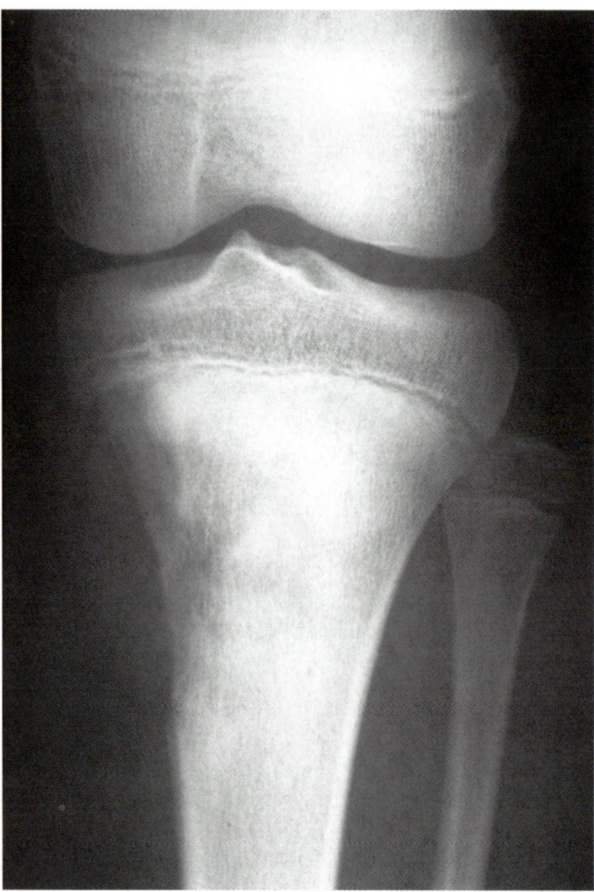

Fig. 8.83

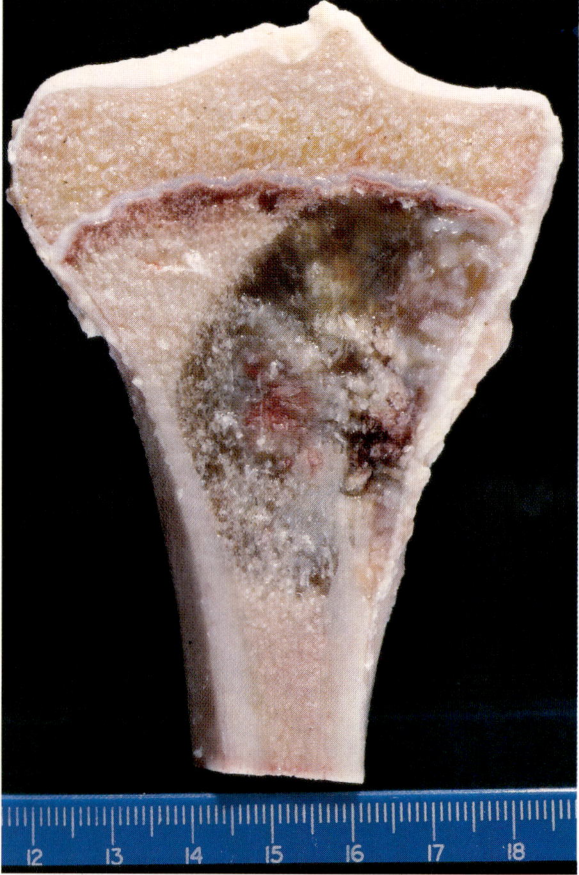

Fig. 8.84

Figs 8.83–8.85 Osteoblastic osteosarcoma of the tibia with complete necrosis induced by intraarterial chemotherapy.

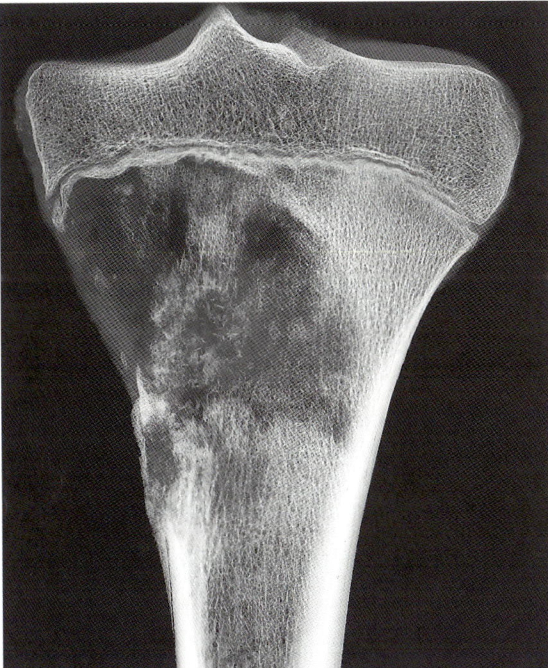

Fig. 8.85

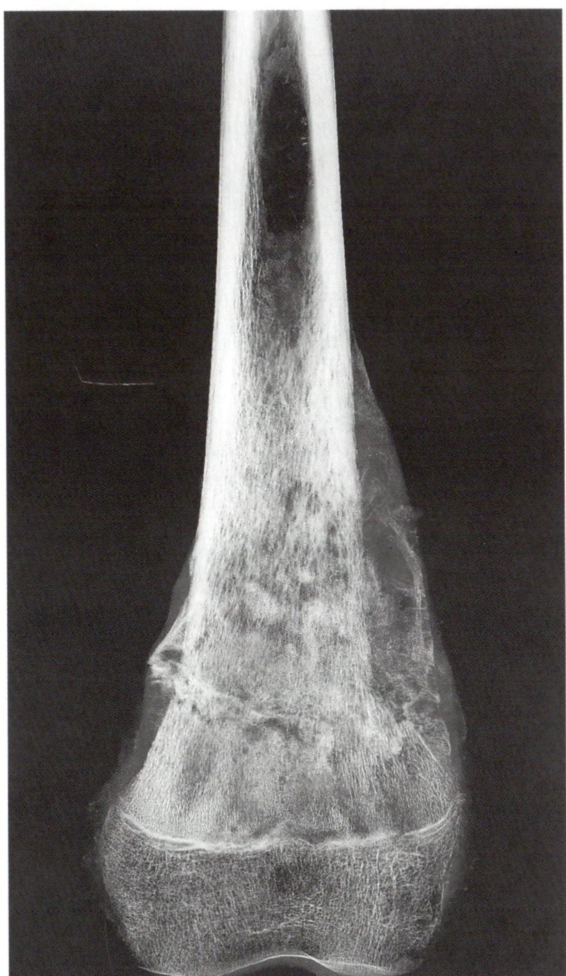

Fig. 8.86 Pathologic fracture during the course of chemotherapy.

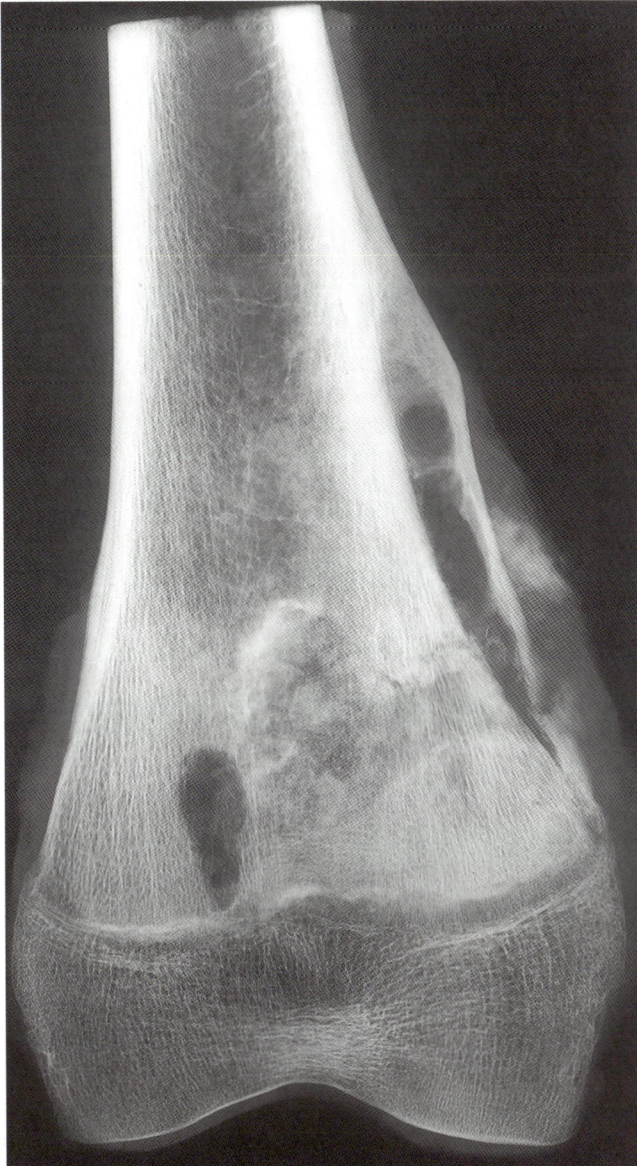

Fig. 8.87 Solid periosteal reaction developing during the course of chemotherapy.

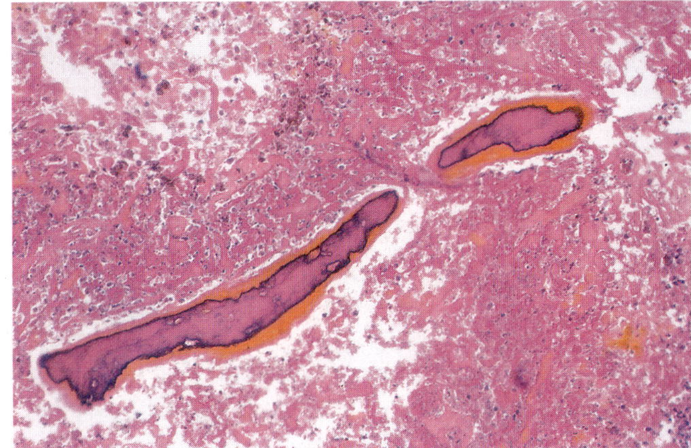

Fig. 8.88 Total drop-out of tumor cells induced by chemotherapy.

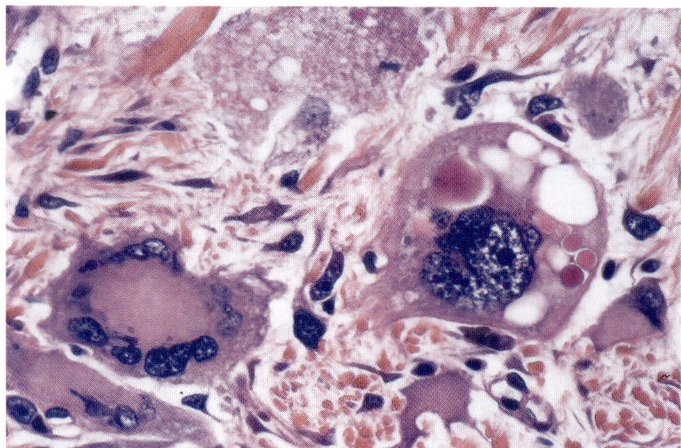

Fig. 8.89 'Bizarre cells' after intraarterial chemotherapy, with vacuolated cytoplasm and eosinophilic globules.

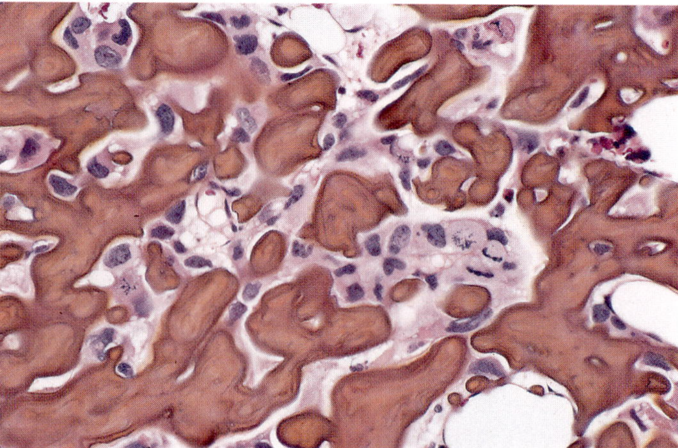

Fig. 8.92 Few residual tumor cells after intraarterial chemotherapy.

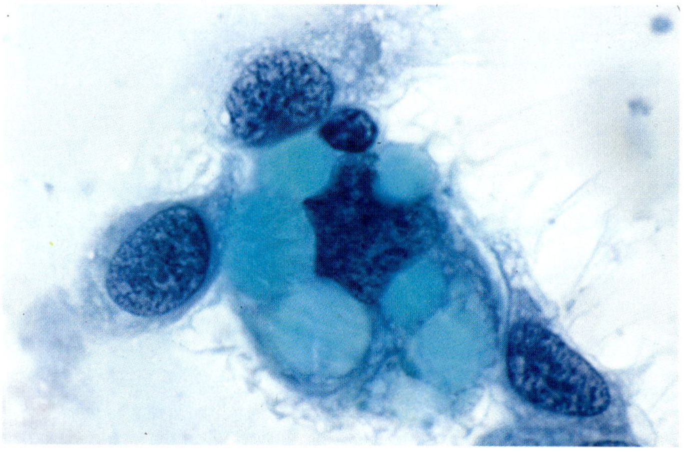

Fig. 8.90 Imprint cytology of 'bizarre cells' after chemotherapy.

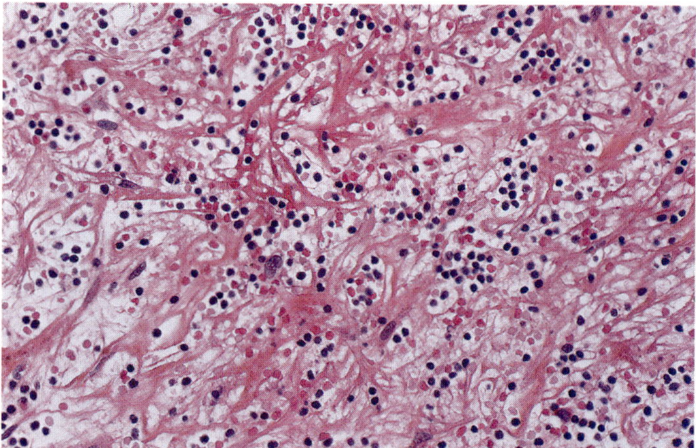

Fig. 8.93 Lymphocytic infiltrates after intraarterial chemotherapy.

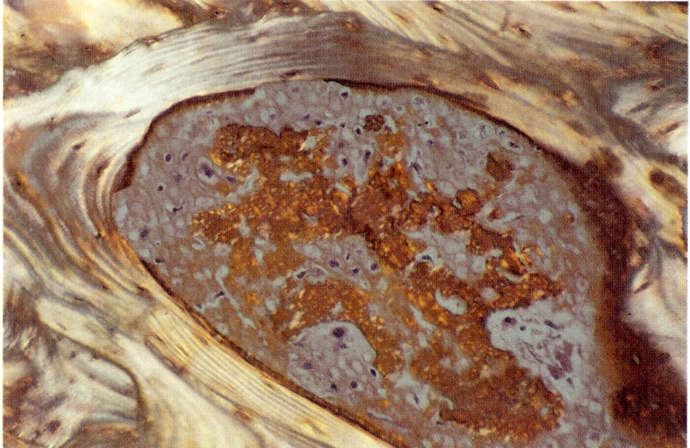

Fig. 8.91 Persistence of tumor bone after intraarterial chemotherapy (polarized light).

Collagen analysis after chemotherapy has shown a higher collagen production in vitro and a differentiation of residual bone tumor.[221] Residual viable tumor is located at the interface of tumor and normal bone structures ('sanctuary sites')[212,222] or may be centrally located.[223]

Histologic response to preoperative chemotherapy is assessed by the percentage of tumor necrosis. Usually, four stages are used: stage 1 (little or no effect), stage 2 (areas of 40–60% of viable tumor), stage 3 (more than 90% of tumor necrosis), stage 4 (no viable tumor).[224] A more intricate six-stage regression scale has also been advocated.[225] In the experience of the Instituto Rizzoli and in our own daily practice, standardization of grading seems unrealistic and only a rough estimate of a good, fair or poor response may be possible.

One has to remember that the changes are the sum of spontaneous and chemotherapy-induced necrosis. Spontaneous hemorrhagic or coagulative necrosis may involve 20–50% of the tumor and is more pronounced in the central intramedullary area.[219,226–228] Spontaneous necrosis is found in more than half of cases of high-grade osteosarcoma[227] and it has been stated that it is impossible for that reason to discern intermediate grades of necrosis; the response is either manifest (up to 90% of necrosis) or not.[226]

Patients with a poor histologic response in the primary tumor may have good histologic response in pulmonary metastases.[229]

Cross-resistance to drugs is termed 'multidrug resistance' (MDR). MDR results from the overexpression of a multidrug resistance gene (mdr 1) mRNA; the protein product, P-glycoprotein, works as a drug efflux pump, decreasing the intracellular concentration of cytostatic agents. P-glycoprotein is located at the cell surface and in the Golgi apparatus of resistant cells;[230,231] ultrastructural studies demonstrate membrane vesicles and cytoplasmic vacuoles containing cytostatic drugs.[231]

Expression of the mdr gene can be detected by point mutations on PCR analysis[232] or by immunohistochemistry using antibodies to P-glycoprotein with a specific membrane staining. High levels of mdr 1 expression have been found by PCR in up to 90% of osteosarcomas[233,234] but the interpretation of the results is unclear: there may be poor response to treatment[235,236] or no ability to predict the outcome of therapy. Furthermore, a recent study has shown that there is no correlation between the levels of mdr 1 expression measured by reverse transcription and PCR and the P-glycoprotein staining.[237] It is possible that alternative biochemical pathways independent of P-glycoprotein contribute to MDR.[231]

Nevertheless, for some authors, P-glycoprotein status is related to the clinical outcome and appears as an independent predictor for the extent of tumor necrosis after chemotherapy.[234,238] However, in a recent study, experimental observations and clinical data have shown that the poor outcome of tumors with P-glycoprotein overexpression is more related to their lack of response to chemotherapy than to their metastatic dissemination.[239] In any case, the prognostic significance of the P-glycoprotein level has to be correlated with a long-term follow-up.[234]

DIFFERENTIAL DIAGNOSIS

Typical osteosarcoma will not be confused with other bone lesions, if two major histological problems are resolved:

1. finding areas of tumoral bone formation in chondroblastic and fibroblastic osteosarcomas;
2. differentiating osteoid or tumoral bone from reactive bone formation: one has to rely on the regular structure of bone, the osteoblastic rimming, the surrounding cells or the loose and vascular stroma found in reactive lesions (see Ch. 49).

COMMENTS FOR THE SURGICAL PATHOLOGIST

Despite many studies dealing with the most complex sarcoma of bone, daily diagnosis is generally made with plain films and well-processed histological sections. Frozen sections may be used to show the adequacy of the biopsy specimen[240] but we, and others,[241] do not use them as a guide for an immediate and irreversible surgical procedure.

In spite of some positive results, we are reluctant to rely solely on fine-needle aspiration for a definite diagnosis. Needle biopsies have to be interpreted in close relationship with the radiological findings[242,243] and they give poor results in blastic, cystic or hemorrhagic osteosarcomas.[242]

REFERENCES

1. Dorfman H D, Czerniak B. Bone cancers. Cancer 1995: 75: 203–210
2. Campanacci M, Bacci G, Bertoni F, Picci P, Minutillo A, Franceschi C. The treatment of osteosarcoma of the extremities: twenty years' experience at the Istituto Ortopedico Rizzoli. Cancer 1981: 48: 1569–1581
3. Carter J R, Abdul-Karim F W. Pathology of childhood osteosarcoma. Perspect Pediatr Pathol 1987: 9: 133–170
4. Kellie S J, Pratt C B, Parham D M, Fleming I D, Meyer W H, Rao B N. Sarcomas (other than Ewing's) of flat bones in children and adolescents. A clinicopathologic study. Cancer 1990: 65: 1011–1016
5. Kazakewich H, Perez-Atayde A R, Goorin A M, Wilkinson R H, Gebhardt M C, Vawter G F. Osteosarcoma in young children. Cancer 1991: 67: 638–642
6. Siegal G P, Dahlin D C, Sim F H. Osteoblastic osteogenic sarcoma in a 35 month old girl. Report of a case. Am J Clin Pathol 1975: 63: 886–890
7. Atik O S, Caglar M, Bolukbasi S, Gogus S, Gogus M T. Osteogenic sarcoma of the distal femur in a young child. Hum Pathol 1982: 13: 766

8. Levy M L, Jaffe N. Osteosarcoma in early childhood. Pediatrics 1982: 70: 302–303
9. Luiz C P, Al Kharusi W, Sethu A U, Buhl L, Al Lamki Z. Osteosarcoma in a 26-month-old girl. Cancer 1992: 70: 894–896
10. Sanchis-Alfonso V, Fernandez-Fernandez C I, Donat J, Llombart-Bosch A. Osteoblastic osteogenic sarcoma in a 13-month-old girl. Pathol Res Pract 1994: 190: 207–210, 211
11. Graham N J, Cairns R A, Anderson R A. Osteosarcoma in a 19-month-old girl. Can Assoc Radiol J 1996: 47: 33–45
12. Porter D E, Holden S T, Steel C M, Cohen B B, Wallace M R, Reid R. A significant proportion of patients with osteosarcoma may belong to Li-Fraumeni cancer families. J Bone Joint Surg (Br) 1992: 74: 883–886
13. Baro P R, Bastart F M, Bartrina J R, Mateo J M, Vidal M T. Case report 529. Osteosarcoma of calcaneus with Rothmund–Thompson syndrome. Skeletal Radiol 1989: 18: 136–139
14. Sim F H, DeVries E M, Miser J S, Unni K K. Case report 760. Osteoblastic osteosarcoma (grade 4) with Rothmund–Thompson syndrome. Skeletal Radiol 1992: 21: 543–545
15. Molina M I, Santolaya J M, Delgado A et al. Syndrome de

Rothmund–Thomson et ostéosarcome. Arch Pediatr 1995: 2: 865–870

16. Cumin I, Cohen J Y, David A, Mechinaud F, Avet-Loiseau H, Harousseau J L. Rothmund–Thomson syndrome and osteosarcoma. Med Pediatr Oncol 1996: 26: 414–416

17. Leonard A, Craft A W, Moss C, Malcom A J. Osteogenic sarcoma in the Rothmund–Thomson syndrome. Med Pediatr Oncol 1996: 26: 249–253

18. Huvos A G. Osteogenic sarcoma of bones and soft tissues in older persons. A clinicopathologic analysis of 117 patients older than 60 years. Cancer 1986: 57: 1442–1449

19. Verhaven E, De Boeck H, Opdecam P. Osteosarcoma appearing as a pathologic fracture. Acta Orthop Belg 1991: 57: 437–441

20. Jaffe N, Spears R, Eftekhari F et al. Pathologic fracture in osteosarcoma. Impact of chemotherapy on primary tumor and survival. Cancer 1987: 59: 701–709

21. McMaster J H. Carbohydrate metabolism in osteosarcoma. Int Orthop 1977: 1: 19–21

22. Goodman M A, McMaster J H, Drash A L, Diamond P E, Kappakas G S, Scranton P E Jr. Metabolic and endocrine alterations in osteosarcoma patients. Cancer 1978: 42: 603–610

23. Kalra J K, Mir R, Kahn L B, Wessely Z, Shah A B. Osteogenic sarcoma producing human chorionic gonadotrophin. Case report with immunohistochemical studies. Cancer 1984: 53: 2125–2128

24. Walker M J, Chaudhuri P K, Beattie C W, Das Gupta T K. Steroid receptors in malignant skeletal tumors. Cancer 1980: 45: 3004–3007

25. Wyman A L, Paradinas F J, Daly J R. Hypophosphataemic osteomalacia associated with a malignant tumour of the tibia: report of a case. J Clin Pathol 1977: 30: 328–335

26. Kruse H P, Kuhlencord T F, Ringe J D. Osteosarcoma in vitamin D-resistant hypophosphatemic osteomalacia. In: Donath A, Courvoisier B, Eds. Bone and tumors. Berne: Hans Huber, 1980, pp 210–217

27. Cheng C L, Ma J, Wu P C, Mason R S, Posen S. Osteomalacia secondary to osteosarcoma. A case report. J Bone Joint Surg (Am) 1989: 71: 288–292

28. Park Y K, Unni K K, Beabout J W, Hodgson S F. Oncogenic osteomalacia: a clinicopathologic study of 17 bone lesions. J Korean Med Sci 1994: 9: 289–298

29. Barwick K W, Huvos A G, Smith J. Primary osteogenic sarcoma of the vertebral column: a clinicopathologic correlation of ten patients. Cancer 1980: 46: 595–604

30. Patel D V, Hammer R A, Levin B, Fisher M A. Primary osteogenic sarcoma of the spine. Skeletal Radiol 1984: 12: 276–279

31. Shives T C, Dahlin D C, Sim F H, Pritchard D J, Earle J D. Osteosarcoma of the spine. J Bone Joint Surg (Am) 1986: 68: 660–668

32. Tigani D, Pignatti G, Picci P, Savini R, Campanacci M. Vertebral osteosarcoma. Ital J Orthop Traumatol 1988: 14: 5–13

33. Sundaresan N, Schiller A L, Rosenthal D I. Osteosarcoma of the spine. In: Sundaresan N, Schmidek H H, Schiller A L, Rosenthal D I, Eds. Tumors of the spine. Philadelphia: W B Saunders, 1990, pp 128–145

34. Miller T T, Abdelwahab I F, Hermann G, Morgello S. Case report 735. Vertebral osteosarcoma. Skeletal Radiol 1992: 21: 277–279

35. Fahey M, Spanier S S, Van Der Griend R A. Osteosarcoma of the pelvis. A clinical and histopathological study of twenty-five patients. J Bone Joint Surg (Am) 1992: 74: 321–330

36. Okada K, Wold L E, Beabout J W, Shives T C. Osteosarcoma of the hand, a clinicopathologic study of 12 cases. Cancer 1993: 72: 719–725

37. Mirra J M, Kameda N, Rosen G, Eckardt J. Primary osteosarcoma of toe phalanx: first documented case. Review of osteosarcoma of short tubular bones. Am J Surg Pathol 1988: 12: 300–307

38. Chan Y F, Llewellyn H. Sclerosing osteosarcoma of the great toe phalanx in an 11-year-old girl. Histopathology 1995: 26: 281–284

39. Murphy W A Jr. Imaging bone tumors in the 1990s. Cancer 1991: 67: 1169–1176

40. De Santos L A, Edeiken B S. Subtle early osteosarcoma. Skeletal Radiol 1985: 13: 44–48

41. Sweet D E, Madewell J E, Ragsdale B D. Radiologic and pathologic analysis of solitary bone lesions. Part III: matrix patterns. Radiol Clin North Am 1981: 19: 785–814

42. Hudson T M, Schiebler M, Springfield D S, Hawkins I F Jr, Enneking W F, Spanier S S. Radiologic imaging of osteosarcoma: role in planning surgical treatment. Skeletal Radiol 1983: 10: 137–146

43. Madewell J E, Ragsdale B D, Sweet D E. Radiologic and pathologic analysis of solitary bone lesions. Part I: internal margins. Radiol Clin North Am 1981: 19: 715–748

44. Ragsdale B D, Madewell J E, Sweet D E. Radiologic and pathologic analysis of solitary bone lesions. Part II: periosteal reactions. Radiol Clin North Am 1981: 19: 749–783

45. Goldman A B, Becker M H, Braunstein P, Francis K C, Genierser N B, Firooznia H. Bone scanning – osteogenic sarcoma. Correlation with surgical pathology. AJR 1975: 124: 83–90

46. Yaghmai I. Angiographic features of osteosarcoma. Am J Roentgenol Radium Ther Nucl Med 1977: 129: 1073–1081

47. Gillespy T 3rd, Manfrini M, Ruggieri P, Spanier S S, Pettersson H, Springfield D S. Staging of intraosseous extent of osteosarcoma: correlation of preoperative CT and MR imaging with pathologic macrolides. Radiology 1988: 167: 765–767

48. Greenfield G B, Warren D L, Clark R A. MR imaging of periosteal and cortical changes of bone. Radiographics 1991: 11: 611–623

49. Schreiman J S, Crass J R, Wick M R, Maile C W, Thompson R C Jr. Osteosarcoma: role of CT in limb-sparing treatment. Radiology 1986: 161: 485–488

50. O'Flanagan S J, Stack J P, McGee H M, Dervan P, Hurson B. Imaging of intramedullary tumor spread in osteosarcoma. A comparison of techniques. J Bone Joint Surg (Br) 1991: 73: 998–1001

51. Schima W, Amann G, Stigbauer R et al. Preoperative staging of osteosarcomas: efficacy of MR imaging in detecting joint involvement. AJR 1994: 163: 1171–1175

52. Norton K I, Hermann G, Abdelwahab I F, Klein M J, Granowetter L F, Rabinowitz J G. Epiphyseal involvement in osteosarcoma. Radiology 1991: 180: 813–816

53. Panuel M, Gentet J C, Scheiner C et al. Physeal and epiphyseal extent of primary malignant bone tumors in childhood. Correlation of preoperative MRI and the pathologic examination. Pediatr Radiol 1993: 23: 421–424

54. Enneking W F, Kagan A. 'Skip' metastases in osteosarcoma. Cancer 1975: 36: 2192–2205

55. Malawer M M, Dunham W K. Skip metastases in osteosarcoma: recent experience. J Surg Oncol 1983: 22: 236–245

56. Anani A P, Costa J, Remagen W. L'échappement métastatique dans la moelle osseuse (skip métastase) de l'ostéosarcome. Fréquence et implications cliniques. Ann Pathol 1987: 7: 193–197

57. Lewis R J, Lotz M J. Medullary extension of osteosarcoma. Implications for rational therapy. Cancer 1974: 33: 371–375

58. Simon M A, Bos G D. Epiphyseal extension of metaphyseal osteosarcoma in skeletally immature individuals. J Bone Joint Surg (Am) 1980: 62: 195–204

59. Ghandur-Mnaymneh L, Mnaymneh W A, Puls S. The incidence and mechanism of transphyseal spread of osteosarcoma of long bones. Clin Orthop 1983: 177: 210–215

60. Simon M A, Hecht J D. Invasion of joints by primary bone sarcomas in adults. Cancer 1982: 50: 1649–1655

61. Sato K, Miura T, Nakanishi K, Sugiura H. Specific mechanism of the knee joint preventing tumor invasion. Acta Orthop Scand 1993: 64: 320–322

62. Abdelwahab I F, Miller T T, Hermann G, Klein M J, Kenan S, Lewis M M. Transarticular invasion of joints by bone tumors: hypothesis. Skeletal Radiol 1991: 20: 279–283

63. Dahlin D C. Pathology of osteosarcoma. Clin Orthop 1975: 111: 23–32

64. Dahlin D C, Unni K K. Osteosarcoma of bone and its important recognizable varieties. Am J Surg Pathol 1977: 1: 61–72

65. Ishii S, Yamawaki S, Sasaki T et al. Analysis of osteoid-forming activity of human osteosarcoma implanted into nude mice. Int Orthop 1982: 6: 215–223

66. Usui M, Sasaki T, Yagi T, Kobayashi M, Matsuno T. A

histological study on osteosarcoma. Part I: relationship between modes of osteoid formation and differentiation of tumor cells (in Japanese). Nippon Seikeigeka Gakkai Zasshi 1984: 58: 793–801

67. Wang D, Gao F X. Prognosis based on stereological study of neoplastic osteoid classification in osteosarcoma (in Chinese). Chung-Hua, Ping Li-Hsueh Tsa Tsih 1990: 19: 268–270

68. Junqueira L C, Assis Figueiredo M T, Torloni H, Montes G S. Differential histologic diagnosis of osteoid. J Pathol 1986: 148: 189–196

69. Yoshiki S. A simple histological method for identification of osteoid matrix in decalcified bone. Stain Technol 1973: 48: 233–238

70. Unni K K, Dahlin D C. Grading of bone tumors. Semin Diagn Pathol 1984: 1: 165–172

71. Meister P, Konrad E, Lob G, Janka G, Keyl W, Stûrz H. Osteosarcoma. Histological evaluation and grading. Arch Orthop Trauma Surg 1979: 94: 91–98

72. Huvos A G. Clinicopathologic spectrum of osteogenic sarcoma. Recent observations. Pathol Annu 1979: 14: 123–144

73. Yunis E J, Barnes L. The histologic diversity of osteosarcoma. Pathol Annu 1986: 21: 121–141

74. Kuettner K E, Pauli B U, Soble L. Morphological studies on the resistance of cartilage to invasion by osteosarcoma cells in vitro and in vivo. Cancer Res 1978: 38: 277–287

75. Enneking W F, Kagan A 2nd. Transepiphyseal extension of osteosarcoma: incidence, mechanism, and implications. Cancer 1978: 41: 1526–1537

76. Miura Y, Suda A, Watanabe Y, Yamakawa M, Imai Y. Inflammatory cells in the pseudocapsule of osteosarcoma. A clinicopathologic analysis. Clin Orthop 1994: 300: 225–232

77. Vermeij J. The periosteal reaction in bone tumours. In: Price C H G, Ross F G M, Eds. Bone – certain aspects of neoplasia. London: Butterworth, 1973, pp 113–122

78. Kumar R V, Rao C R, Hazarika D, Mukherjee G, Gowda B M. Aspiration biopsy cytology of primary bone lesions. Acta Cytol 1993: 37: 83–89

79. White V A, Fanning C V, Ayala A G, Raymond A K, Carrasco C H, Murray J A. Osteosarcoma and the role of fine-needle aspiration. A study of 51 cases. Cancer 1988: 62: 1238–1246

80. Layfield L J, Glasgow B J, Anders K H, Mirra J M. Fine needle aspiration cytology of primary bone lesions. Acta Cytol 1987: 31: 177–184

81. Layfield L J, Armstrong K, Zaleski S, Eckardt J. Diagnostic accuracy and clinical utility of fine-needle aspiration cytology in the diagnosis of clinically primary bone lesions. Diagn Cytopathol 1993: 9: 168–173

82. Walaas L, Kindblom L G. Light and electron microscopic examination of fine-needle aspirates in the preoperative diagnosis of osteogenic tumors: a study of 21 osteosarcomas and two osteoblastomas. Diagn Cytopathol 1990: 6: 27–38

83. Bloustein P A, Silverberg S G. Rapid cytologic examination of surgical specimens. Pathol Annu 1977: 12: 251–278

84. Owings R M. Rapid cytologic examination of surgical specimens: a valuable technique in the surgical pathology laboratory. Hum Pathol 1984: 15: 605–614

85. Wilkerson J A, Crowell W T. Intraoperative cytology of osseous lesions. Diagn Cytopathol 1986: 2: 5–12

86. Hewes R C, Vigorita V J, Freiberger R H. Percutaneous bone biopsy: the importance of aspirated osseous blood. Radiology 1983: 148: 69–72

87. Tsai C C, McGuire M H, Mellitt R J et al. Monoclonal antibody to human osteosarcoma: a novel Mr26,000 protein recognized by murine hybridoma TMMR-2. Cancer Res 1990: 50: 152–158

88. Farrands P A, Perkins A, Sully L, Hopkins J S et al. Localisation of human osteosarcoma by antitumour monoclonal antibody. J Bone Joint Surg (Br) 1983: 65: 638–640

89. Lôning T, Liebsch J, Delling G. Osteosarcoma and Ewing's sarcomas. Comparative immunocytochemical investigation of filamentous proteins and cell membrane determinants. Virchows Arch A Pathol Anat Histopathol 1985: 407: 323–336

90. Hasegawa T, Hirose T, Kudo E, Hizawa K, Usui M, Ishii S. Immunophenotypic heterogeneity in osteosarcomas. Hum Pathol 1991: 22: 583–590

91. Okajima K, Honda I, Kitakawa T. Immunohistochemical distribution of S-100 protein in tumors and tumor-like lesions of bone and cartilage. Cancer 1988: 61: 792–799

92. Nakamura Y, Becker L E, Marks A. S-100 protein in tumors of cartilage and bone. An immunohistochemical study. Cancer 1983: 52: 1820–1824

93. Yoshida H, Adachi H, Hamada Y et al. Osteosarcoma: ultrastructural and immunohistochemical studies on alkaline phosphatase-positive tumor cells constituting a variety of histologic types. Acta Pathol Jpn 1988: 38: 325–338

94. Minamizaki T, Yoshida H, Yumoto T. Alkaline phosphatase-positive and negative bone tumors. Ultrastructural and immunohistochemical studies of fibroblast-like tumor cells. Pathol Res Pract 1990: 186: 633–641

95. Schulz A, Jundt G, Berghäuser K H, Gehron-Robey P, Termine J D. Immunohistochemical study of osteonectin in various types of osteosarcoma. Am J Pathol 1988: 132: 233–238

96. Serra M, Morini M C, Scotlandi K et al. Evaluation of osteonectin as a diagnostic marker of osteogenic bone tumors. Hum Pathol 1992: 23: 1326–1331

97. Bosse A, Vollmer E, Bôcker W et al. The impact of osteonectin for differential diagnosis of bone tumors. An immunohistochemical approach. Pathol Res Pract 1990: 186: 651–657

98. Jundt G, Schulz A, Berghäuser K H, Fisher L W, Gehron-Robey P, Termine J D. Immunocytochemical identification of osteogenic bone tumors by osteonectin antibodies. Virchows Arch A Pathol Anat Histopathol 1989: 414: 345–353

99. Park Y K, Yang M H, Park H R. The impact of osteonectin for differential diagnosis of osteogenic bone tumors: an immunohistochemical and in situ hybridization approach. Skeletal Radiol 1996: 25: 13–17

100. Ohta T, Mori M, Ogawa K, Matsuyama T, Ishii T. Immunocytochemical localization of BGP in human bones in various developmental stages and pathological conditions. Virchows Arch A Pathol Anat Histopathol 1989: 415: 459–466

101. Iwasaki R, Yamamuro T, Kotoura Y, Okumura H, Kasai R, Nakashima Y. Immunohistochemical study of bone GLA protein in primary bone tumors. Cancer 1992: 70: 619–624

102. Park Y K, Yang M H, Kim Y N, Park H R. Osteocalcin expression in primary bone tumors. In situ hybridization and immunohistochemical study. J Korean Med Sci 1995: 10: 263–268

103. Takada J, Ishii S, Ohta T et al. Usefulness of a novel monoclonal antibody against human osteocalcin in immunohistochemical diagnosis. Virchows Arch A Pathol Anat Histopathol 1992: 420: 507–511

104. Vermeulen A H, Vermeer C E, Bosman F T. Histochemical detection of osteocalcin in normal and pathological human bone. J Histochem Cytochem 1989: 37: 1503–1508

105. Ushigome S, Shimoda T, Fukunaga M, Takakuwa T, Nakajima H. Immunocytochemical aspects of the differential diagnosis of osteosarcoma and malignant fibrous histiocytoma. Surg Pathol 1988: 1: 347–357

106. Yoshikawa H, Rettig W J, Lane J M et al. Immunohistochemical detection of bone morphogenetic proteins in bone and soft-tissue sarcomas. Cancer 1994: 74: 842–847

107. Yoshikawa H, Rettig W J, Takaoka K et al. Expression of bone morphogenetic proteins in human osteosarcoma. Immunohistochemical detection with monoclonal antibody. Cancer 1994: 73: 85–91

108. Jin Y, Yang L J. The relationship between bone morphogenetic protein and neoplastic bone diseases. Clin Orthop 1990: 259: 233–238

109. Yoshikawa H, Takaoka K, Hamada H, Ono K. Clinical significance of bone morphogenetic activity in osteosarcoma. A study of 20 cases. Cancer 1985: 56: 1682–1687

110. Yoshikawa H, Takaoka K, Masuhara K, Ono K, Sakamoto Y. Prognostic significance of bone morphogenetic activity in osteosarcoma tissue. Cancer 1988: 61: 569–573

111. Remberger K, Gay S. Immunohistochemical demonstration of different collagen types in the normal epiphyseal plate and in

benign and malignant tumors of bone and cartilage. Z Krebsforsch Klin Onkol 1977: 90: 95–106

112. Stern R, Wilczek J, Thorpe W P, Rosenberg S A, Cannon G. Procollagens as markers of the cell of origin of human bone tumors. Cancer Res 1980: 40: 325–328

113. Lanzer W L, Liotta L A, Yee C, Arar H A, Costa J. Synthesis of procollagen type II by a xenotransplanted human chondroblastic osteosarcoma. Am J Pathol 1981: 104: 217–226

114. Shapiro F D, Eyre D R. Collagen polymorphism in extracellular matrix of human osteosarcoma. J Natl Cancer Inst 1982: 69: 1009–1016

115. Roessner A, Voss B, Rauterberg J, Immenkamp M, Grundmann E. Biologic characterization of human bone tumors. II Distribution of different collagen types in osteosarcoma – a combined histologic, immunofluorescence and electron microscopic study. J Cancer Res Clin Oncol 1983: 106: 234–239

116. Ueda Y, Nakanishi I. Immunohistochemical and biochemical studies on the collagenous proteins of human osteosarcomas. Virchows Arch B Cell Pathol 1989: 58: 79–88

117. Benedict W F, Fung Y K, Murphree A L. The gene responsible for the development of retinoblastoma and osteosarcoma. Cancer 1988: 62: 1691–1694

118. Hansen M F. Molecular genetic considerations in osteosarcoma. Clin Orthop 1991: 270: 237–246

119. Araki N, Uchida A, Kimura T et al. Involvement of the retinoblastoma gene in primary osteosarcomas and other bone and soft-tissue tumors. Clin Orthop 1991: 270: 271–277

120. Scholz R B, Kabisch H, Weber B, Roser K, Delling G, Winkler K. Studies of the RBI gene and the p53 gene in human osteosarcomas. Pediatr Hematol Oncol 1992: 9: 125–137

121. Wadayama B, Toguchida J, Shimizu T et al. Mutation spectrum of the retinoblastoma gene in osteosarcomas. Cancer Res 1994: 54: 3042–3048

122. Wadayama B, Toguchida J, Yamaguchi T, Sasaki M S, Kotoura Y, Yamamuro T. p53 expression and its relationship to DNA alterations in bone and soft tissue sarcomas. Br J Cancer 1993: 68: 1134–1139

123. Nishikawa T, Yamamoto T, Mizuno K, Fujimori T, Maeda S, Ugai K. Expression of the p53 protein in human osteosarcoma (in Japanese). Nippon Seikeigeka Gakkai Zasshi 1994: 68: 400–406

124. Ueda Y, Dockhorn-Dworniczak B, Blasius S et al. Analysis of mutant p53 protein in osteosarcomas and other malignant and benign lesions of bone. J Cancer Res Clin Oncol 1993: 119: 172–178

125. Grundmann E, Roessner A, Ueda Y, Schneider-Stock R, Radig K. Current aspects of the pathology of osteosarcoma. Anticancer Res 1995: 15: 1023–1032

126. Ladanyi M, Park C K, Lewis R, Jhanwar S C, Healey J H, Huvos A G. Sporadic amplification of the MYC gene in human osteosarcomas. Diagn Mol Pathol 1993: 2: 163–167

127. Kawaguchi S, Uede T. Distribution of integrins and their matrix ligands in osteogenic sarcomas. J Orthop Res 1993: 11: 386–395

128. Posl M, Amling M, Werner M et al. Osteosarkom-Apoptose und Proliferation. Untersuchung zur bcl-2-Expression. Pathologe 1994: 15: 337–344

129. Onda M, Matsuda S, Higaki S et al. ErbB-2 expression is correlated with poor prognosis for patients with osteosarcoma. Cancer 1996: 77: 71–78

130. Vollmer E, Roessner A, Wuisman P, Hârle A, Grundmann E. The proliferation behavior of bone tumors investigated with the monoclonal antibody Ki-67. Curr Top Pathol 1989: 80: 91–114

131. Scotlandi K, Serra M, Manara M C et al. Clinical relevance of Ki-67 expression in bone tumors. Cancer 1995: 75: 806–814

132. Mankin H J, Gebhardt M C, Springfield D S, Litwak G J, Kusazaki K, Rosenberg E. Flow cytometric studies of human osteosarcoma. Clin Orthop 1991: 270: 169–180

133. Kreicbergs A, Broström L A, Cewrien G, Einhorn S. Cellular DNA content in human osteosarcoma. Aspects of diagnosis and prognosis. Cancer 1982: 50: 2476–2481

134. Bauer H C F, Kreicbergs A, Silfersward C, Tribukait B. DNA analysis in the differential diagnosis of osteosarcoma. Cancer 1988: 61: 1430–1436

135. Bauer H C. DNA cytometry of osteosarcoma. Acta Orthop Scand 1988: S228 (suppl): 1–39

136. Kreicbergs A, Silfersward C, Tribukait B. Flow DNA analysis of primary bone tumors. Relationship between DNA content and histopathologic classification. Cancer 1984: 53: 129–136

137. Bauer H C F, Kreicbergs A, Silfersward C, Tribukait B. Ploidy and morphology in osteosarcoma. Anal Quant Cytol Histol 1989: 11: 96–103

138. Bauer H C F, Kreicbergs A, Silfersward C. Prognostication including DNA analysis in osteosarcoma. Acta Orthop Scand 1989: 60: 353–360

139. Hiddemann W, Roessner A, Wôrmann B et al. Tumor heterogeneity in osteosarcoma as identified by flow cytometry. Cancer 1987: 59: 324–328

140. Look A T, Douglass E C, Meyer W H. Clinical importance of near diploid tumor stem lines in patients with osteosarcoma of an extremity. N Engl J Med 1988: 318: 1567–1572

141. Vollmer E, Mellin W, Roessner A, Bôcker W. Proliferation kinetics of bone tumors. Acta Histochem (Iena) 1990: 39 (suppl): 163–174

142. Bôsing T, Roessner A, Hiddemann W, Mellin W, Grundmann E. Cytostatic effects in osteosarcomas as detected by flow cytometric DNA analysis after preoperative chemotherapy according to the COSS80/82 protocol. J Cancer Res Clin Oncol 1987: 113: 369–375

143. Baldini N, Manara M C, Scotlandi K, Sangiorgi L, Serra M. Analysis of DNA content in high-grade osteosarcoma. In: Novak J F, McMaster J H, Eds. Frontiers of osteosarcoma research. Seattle: Hogrefe & Huber, 1993, pp 243–244

144. Biegel J A, Womer R B, Emanuel B S. Complex karyotypes in a series of pediatric osteosarcomas. Cancer Genet Cytogenet 1989: 38: 89–100

145. Mertens F, Mandahl N, Örndal C et al. Cytogenetic findings in 33 osteosarcomas. Int J Cancer 1993: 55: 44–50

146. Ozisik Y Y, Meloni A M, Peier A et al. Cytogenetic findings in 19 malignant bone tumors. Cancer 1994: 74: 2268–2275

147. Fletcher J A, Gebhardt M C, Kozakewich H P. Cytogenetic aberrations in osteosarcomas. Nonrandom deletions, rings and double-minute chromosomes. Cancer Genet Cytogenet 1994: 77: 81–88

148. Reddick R L, Michelitch H J, Levine A M, Triche T J. Osteogenic sarcoma: a study of the ultrastructure. Cancer 1980: 45: 64–71

149. Grundmann E, Roessner A, Immenkamp M. Tumor cell types in osteosarcoma as revealed by electron microscopy. Implications for histogenesis and subclassification. Virchows Arch B Cell Pathol Incl Mol Pathol 1981: 36: 257–273

150. Martinez-Tello F J, Navas-Palacios J J. The ultrastructure of conventional, parosteal, and periosteal osteosarcomas. Cancer 1982: 50: 949–961

151. Stark A, Aparisi T, Ericsson J L. Human osteogenic sarcoma; fine structure of the osteogenic type. Ultrastruct Pathol 1983: 4: 311–329

152. Sela J, Bab I A, Muhlrad A, Stein H. Extracellular matrix vesicles in human osteogenic neoplasms: an ultrastructural and enzymatic study. Cancer 1981: 48: 1602–1610

153. Yoshida H, Miyazaki S, Yumoto T. Matrix vesicles in bone tumors. Ultrastructural analysis and their significance in neoplastic bone formation. Acta Pathol Jpn 1991: 41: 610–617

154. Sanerkin N G. Definitions of osteosarcoma, chondrosarcoma, and fibrosarcoma of bone. Cancer 1980: 46: 178–185

155. Bendix-Hansen K, Myhre-Jensen O. Enzyme histochemical investigations on bone and soft tissue tumours. Acta Pathol Microbiol Immunol Scand (A) 1985: 93: 73–80

156. Roessner A, Mellin W, Hiddemann W, Voss B, Vollmer E, Grundmann E. New cytomorphologic methods in the diagnosis of bone tumors: possibilities and limitations. Semin Diagn Pathol 1984: 1: 199–214

157. Delling G, Schulz A, Seifert G. Morphology of osteosarcoma: new qualitative and quantitative investigations. Pathol Res Pract 1978: 162: 166–177

158. Althoff J, Quint P, Hôhling H J, Roessner A, Grundmann E. Biological characterization of human bone tumors. IV Combined biochemical and histological analyses of different osteosarcomas. Pathol Res Pract 1985: 180: 383–391

159. Althoff J, Quint P, Hôhling H J, Roessner A, Grundmann E. Biological characterization of human bone tumors. V Zonal characterization of osteosarcoma: topological biochemical analysis correlated with morphology. Pathol Res Pract 1985: 180: 392–399

160. Ohno T, Tanaka T, Takeuchi S, Matsunaga T, Mori H. Nucleolar organizer regions in bone tumors. Clin Orthop 1991: 272: 287–291

161. Clohisy J C, Schajowicz F, Vaziri D M et al. Assessment of argyrophilic nucleolar organizer region quantification in benign and malignant bone tumors. Clin Orthop 1995: 310: 229–236

162. Fedde K N. Human osteosarcoma cells spontaneously release matrix-vesicle-like structures with the capacity to mineralize. Bone Miner 1992: 17: 145–151

163. Fukushima H, Novak J F, McMaster J H, Asanuma K, Yong M C. Bone resorption in osteogenic sarcoma. I. Release of calcium by tumor cells, normal fibroblasts, and macrophages. Clin Orthop 1983: 180: 268–277

164. Novak J F, Fukushima H, McMaster J H, Asanuma K, Simpson K A. Bone resorption in osteogenic sarcoma. II Resorption of the bone collagenous matrix by tumor cells, normal fibroblasts and macrophages. Eur J Cancer Clin Oncol 1984: 20: 939–946

165. Llombart-Bosch A, Carda C, Boix J, Pellin A, Peydro-Olaya A. Value of nude mice xenografts in the expression of cell heterogeneity of human sarcomas of bone and soft tissue. Pathol Res Pract 1988: 183: 683–692

166. Ogose A, Motoyama T, Hotta T, Watanabe H, Takahashi H E. Bone formation in vitro and in nude mice by human osteosarcoma cells. Virchows Arch 1995: 426: 117–125

167. Komitowski D. Experimental bone tumors as models of human bone tumors. Pathol Res Pract 1979: 166: 72–79

168. Meyer W H, Schell M J, Kumar M et al. Thoracotomy for pulmonary metastasis osteosarcoma: an analysis of prognostic indications of survival. Cancer 1987: 59: 374–379

169. Derstappen T, Roessner A, Mûller K M, Grundmann E. Morphology of pulmonary metastases from osteosarcoma during chemotherapy. J Cancer Res Clin Oncol 1987: 113: 241–248

170. Dunn D, Dehner L P. Metastatic osteosarcoma to lung. A clinicopathologic study of surgical biopsies and resections. Cancer 1977: 40: 3054–3064

171. Bacci G, Avella M, Picci P, Briccoli A, Dallari D, Campanacci M. Metastatic patterns in osteosarcoma. Tumori 1988: 74: 421–427

172. Jaffe N, Smith E, Abelson H T, Frei E 3rd. Osteogenic sarcoma: alterations in the pattern of pulmonary metastasis with adjuvant chemotherapy. J Clin Oncol 1983: 1: 251–254

173. Ogihara Y, Takeda K, Yanagawa T, Hirasawa Y. Spontaneous regression of lung metastases from osteosarcoma. Cancer 1994: 74: 2798–2803

174. Hermann G, Leviton M, Mendelson D et al. Osteosarcoma: relation between extent of marrow infiltration on CT and frequency of lung metastases. AJR 1987: 149: 1203–1206

175. Uribe-Botero G, Russell W O, Sutow W W, Martin R G. Primary osteosarcoma of bone. A clinicopathologic investigation of 243 cases, with necropsy studies in 54. Am J Clin Pathol 1977: 67: 427–435

176. Giuliano A E, Feig S, Eilber F R. Changing metastatic patterns of osteosarcoma. Cancer 1984: 54: 2160–2164

177. Forsted D H, Dalinka M K, Kaplan F, Ochs R H. Case report 48. Osteosarcoma originating in tibia, with metastases in soft tissue, lymph node and possibly in the skeleton. Skeletal Radiol 1978: 2: 179–180

178. English R, Dicks-Mireaux C, Malone M, Scott R. Osteosarcoma – presumed lymph node metastases in two cases. Skeletal Radiol 1989: 18: 289–293

179. Caceres E, Zaharia M, Tantalean E. Lymph node metastasis in osteogenic sarcoma. Surgery 1969: 65: 421–422

180. Caceres E, Zaharia M, Calderon R. Incidence of regional lymph node metastasis in operable osteogenic sarcoma. Semin Surg Oncol 1990: 6: 231–233

181. Shrikhande S S, Rao R S. Histopathological study of regional lymph nodes in osteosarcoma. J Surg Oncol 1977: 9: 371–377

182. Rao R S, Rao D N. Prognostic significance of the regional lymph nodes in osteosarcoma. J Surg Oncol 1977: 9: 123–130

183. Weitzner S. Osteosarcoma of humerus with axillary lymph node metastases. Clin Orthop 1973: 90: 233–235

184. Madsen E H. Lymph node metastases from osteoblastic osteogenic sarcoma visible on plain films. Skeletal Radiol 1979: 4: 216–218

185. Thayer L, Rogers L F. Unicentric osteosarcoma of bone with subsequent skeletal metastases. Skeletal Radiol 1979: 4: 148–153

186. Campanacci M, Laus M. Local recurrence after amputation for osteosarcoma. J Bone Joint Surg (Br) 1980: 62: 201–207

187. Lockshin M D, Higgins I T. Prognosis in osteogenic sarcoma. Clin Orthop 1968: 58: 85–103

188. Gravanis M B, Whitesides T E Jr. The unreliability of prognostic criteria in osteosarcoma. Am J Clin Pathol 1970: 53: 15–20

189. Bentzen S M, Poulsen H S, Kaae S et al. Prognostic factors in osteosarcomas. A regression analysis. Cancer 1988: 62: 194–202

190. Glasser D B, Lane J M, Huvos A G, Marcove R C, Rosen G. Survival, prognosis and therapeutic response in osteogenic sarcoma. The Memorial Hospital experience. Cancer 1992: 69: 698–708

191. Spanier S S, Shuster J J, Van Der Griend R A. The effect of local extent of the tumor on prognosis in osteosarcoma. J Bone Joint Surg (Am) 1990: 72: 643–653

192. Petrilli A S, Gentil F C, Epelman S et al. Increased survival, limb preservation, and prognostic factors for osteosarcoma. Cancer 1991: 68: 733–737

193. Bieling P, Rehan N, Winkler P et al. Tumor size and prognosis in aggressively treated osteosarcoma. J Clin Oncol 1996: 14: 848–858

194. Wuisman P, Enneking W F, Roessner A. Local growth and the prognosis of osteosarcoma. Int Orthop 1992: 16: 55–58

195. Bjôrnsson J, Inwards C Y, Wold L E, Sim F H, Taylor W F. Prognostic significance of spontaneous tumor necrosis in osteosarcoma. Virchows Arch A Pathol Anat Histopathol 1993: 423: 195–199

196. Wuisman P, Enneking F. Prognosis for patients who have osteosarcoma with skip metastasis. J Bone Joint Surg (Am) 1990: 72: 60–68

197. Thorpe W P, Reilly J J, Rosenberg S A. Prognostic significance of alkaline phosphate measurements in patients with osteogenic sarcoma receiving chemotherapy. Cancer 1979: 43: 2178–2181

198. Levine A M, Rosenberg S A. Alkaline phosphatase levels in osteosarcoma tissue are related to prognosis. Cancer 1979: 44: 2291–2293

199. Bacci G, Picci P, Ferrari S et al. Prognostic significance of serum alkaline phosphatase measurements in patients with osteosarcoma treated with adjuvant or neoadjuvant chemotherapy. Cancer 1993: 71: 1224–1230

200. Bacci G, Ferrari S, Sangiorgi L et al. Prognostic significance of serum lactate dehydrogenase in patients with osteosarcoma of the extremities. J Chemother 1994: 6: 204–210

201. Urtasun R C, McConnachie P, Merz T. Radiation damage to the periphery and center of human osteogenic sarcoma. Histologic and tissue culture studies. Cancer 1973: 31: 1354–1358

202. Paling M R, Herdt J R. Radiation osteitis: a problem of recognition. Radiology 1980: 137: 339–342

203. Edeiken B, De Santos L A. Percutaneous needle biopsy of the irradiated skeleton. Radiology 1983: 146: 653–655

204. Davis A M, Bell R S, Goodwin P J. Prognostic factors in osteosarcoma: a critical review. J Clin Oncol 1994: 12: 423–431

205. Taylor W F, Ivins J C, Pritchard D J, Dahlin D C, Gilchrist G S, Edmonson J H. Trends and variability in survival among patients with osteosarcoma: a 7-year update. Mayo Clin Proc 1985: 60: 91–104

206. Apel R, Delling G, Krumme H, Winkler K, Salzer-Kuntschik M. Nuclear polymorphism in osteosarcoma as a prognostic factor for the effect of chemotherapy. A quantitative study. Virchows Arch A Pathol Anat Histopathol 1985: 405: 215–223

207. Schulz A, Fischer H P, Breithaupt H, Pralle H. Therapie-Response verschiedener histologischer Subtypen des Osteosarkoms unter hochdosierter Methotrexat-Behandlung. Onkologie 1983: 6: 296–304

208. Huvos A G, Rosen G, Marcove R C. Primary osteogenic sarcoma. Pathologic aspects in 20 patients after treatment with

chemotherapy en bloc resection and prosthetic bone replacement. Arch Pathol Lab Med 1977: 101: 14–18

209. Marroum M C, Huvos A G, Rosen G. Pathologic aspects of chemotherapy response in the treatment of osteogenic sarcoma. An analysis of two cases. Oncology 1977: 34: 273–280

210. Jaffe N, Knapp J, Chuang V P et al. Osteosarcoma: intra-arterial treatment of the primary tumor with cis-diammine-dichloroplatinum II (CDP). Angiographic, pathologic and pharmacologic studies. Cancer 1983: 51: 402–407

211. Ayala A G, Raymond A K, Jaffe N. The pathologist's role in the diagnosis and treatment of osteosarcoma in children. Hum Pathol 1984: 15: 258–266

212. Raymond A K, Chawla S P, Carrasco C H et al. Osteosarcoma chemotherapy effect: a prognostic factor. Semin Diagn Pathol 1987: 4: 212–236

213. Ayala A G, Zornoza J. Primary bone tumors: percutaneous needle biopsy. Radiologic-pathologic study of 222 biopsies. Radiology 1983: 149: 675–679

214. Delling G, Krumme H, Salzer-Kuntschik M. Morphological changes in osteosarcoma after chemotherapy-COSS 80. J Cancer Res Clin Oncol 1983: 106 (suppl): 32–37

215. Hirano T, Iwasaki K, Kumashiro T, Sadamatsu T. Encapsulation around malignant bone tumors after preoperative adjuvant treatment. Nippon Seikeigeka Gakkai Zasshi 1992: 66: 31–37

216. Picci P, Sangiorgi L, Rougraff B T, Neff J R, Casadei R, Campanacci M. Relationship of chemotherapy-induced necrosis and surgical margins to local recurrence in osteosarcoma. J Clin Oncol 1994: 12: 2699–2705

217. Bar-On E, Beckwith J B, Odom L F, Eilert R E. Effects of chemotherapy on human growth plate. J Pediatr Orthop 1993: 13: 220–224

218. Grundmann E, Roessner A, Schlake W et al. Combined ultrastructural, histochemical, and autoradiographic study of osteosarcoma after preoperative chemotherapy according to the COSS80 protocol. J Cancer Res Clin Oncol 1983: 106 (suppl): 25–31

219. Misdorp W, Hart G, Delemarre J F, Voûte P A, Van Der Eijken J W. An analysis of spontaneous and chemotherapy-associated changes in skeletal osteosarcomas. J Pathol 1988: 156: 119–128

220. Klein M J, Kenan S, Lewis M M. Osteosarcoma. Clinical and pathological considerations. Orthop Clin North Am 1989: 20: 327–345

221. Tsuchiya H, Ueda Y, Tomita K, Nakanishi I, Roessner A. Chemotherapeutic effect on osteosarcoma on basis of collagen analysis: a proposal of the induction of osteosarcoma differentiation. J Cancer Res Clin Oncol 1993: 119: 702–706

222. Picci P, Bacci G, Campanacci M et al. Histologic evaluation of necrosis in osteosarcoma induced by chemotherapy. Regional mapping of viable and nonviable tumor. Cancer 1985: 56: 1515–1521

223. Delling G, Pompesius-Kempa M, Welkerling H et al. Morphological investigation of tumor growth and distribution of viable tumour areas in osteosarcomas after chemotherapy. Chir Organi Mov 1990: 75 (S1): 45–47

224. Rosen G, Caparros B, Huvos A G et al. Preoperative chemotherapy for osteogenic sarcoma: selection of postoperative adjuvant chemotherapy based on the response of the primary tumor to preoperative chemotherapy. Cancer 1982: 49: 1221–1230

225. Salzer-Kuntschik M, Brand G, Delling G. Bestimmung des morphologischen Regressionsgrades nach Chemotherapie bei malignen Knochentumoren. Pathologe 1983: 4: 135–141

226. Von Hochstetter A R. Spontaneous necrosis in osteosarcomas. Virchows Arch A Pathol Anat Histopathol 1990: 417: 5–8

227. Springfield D S, Schakel M E Jr, Spanier S S. Spontaneous necrosis in osteosarcoma. Clin Orthop 1991: 263: 233–237

228. Hayashi K. Histopathological study of the effect of preoperative chemotherapy on osteosarcoma (in Japanese). Nippon Seikeigeka Gakkai Zasshi 1994: 68: 151–161

229. Nachman J, Simon M A, Dean L, Shermeta D, Dawson P, Vogelzang N J. Disparate histologic responses in simultaneously resected primary and metastatic osteosarcoma following intravenous neoadjuvant chemotherapy. J Clin Oncol 1987: 5: 1185–1190

230. Molinari A, Cianfriglia M, Meschini S, Calcabrini A, Arancia G. P-glycoprotein expression in the Golgi apparatus of multidrug-resistant cells. Int J Cancer 1994: 59: 789–795

231. Dietel M. What's new in cytostatic drug resistance and pathology. Pathol Res Pract 1991: 187: 892–905

232. Stein U, Walther W, Wunderlich V. Point mutations in the mdr1 promoter of human osteosarcomas are associated with in vitro responsiveness to multidrug resistance relevant drugs. Eur J Cancer 1994: 30A: 1541–1545

233. Stein U, Wunderlich V, Haensch W, Schmidt-Peter P. Expression of the mdr1 gene in bone and soft tissue sarcomas in adult patients. Eur J Cancer 1993: 29A: 1979–1981

234. Baldini N, Scotlandi K, Barbanti-Brodano G et al. Expression of P-glycoprotein in high-grade osteosarcomas in relation to clinical outcome. N Engl J Med 1995: 333: 1380–1385

235. Wunder J S, Bell R S, Wold L, Andrulis I L. Expression of the multidrug resistance gene in osteosarcoma: a pilot study. J Orthop Res 1993: 11: 396–403

236. Imanishi T, Abe Y, Suto R et al. Expression of the human multidrug resistance gene (MDR 1) and prognostic correlation in human osteogenic sarcoma. Tokai J Exp Clin Med 1994: 19: 39–46

237. Kandel R A, Campbell S, Noble-Topham S, Bell R, Andrulis I L. Correlation of p-glycoprotein detection by immunohistochemistry with mdr-1 mRNA levels in osteosarcomas. Pilot study. Diagn Mol Pathol 1995: 4: 59–65

238. Serra M, Scotlandi K, Manara M C. Analysis of P-glycoprotein expression in osteosarcoma. Eur J Cancer 1995: 31A: 1998–2002

239. Scotlandi K, Serra M, Nicoletti G et al. Multidrug resistance and malignancy in human osteosarcoma. Cancer Res 1996: 56: 2434–2439

240. Weatherby R P, Unni K K. Practical aspects of handling orthopedic specimens in the surgical pathology laboratory. Pathol Annu 1982: 17: 1–31

241. Fechner R E, Huvos A G, Mirra J M, Spjut H J, Unni K K. A symposium on the pathology of bone tumors. Pathol Annu 1984: 19: 125–194

242. Ayala A G, Raymond A K, Ro J Y, Carrasco C H, Fanning C V, Murray J A. Needle biopsy of primary bone lesions M.D. Anderson experience. Pathol Annu 1989: 24: 219–251

243. Kindblom L G. Light and electron microscopic examination of embedded fine-needle aspiration biopsy specimens in the preoperative diagnosis of soft tissue and bone tumors. Cancer 1983: 51: 2264–2277

Osteosarcoma: variants

M. Forest

CYTOLOGICAL VARIANTS

Osteosarcoma has been reported with the appearance of a *chondroblastoma*, showing broad areas of rounded, oval or polyhedral cells with an eosinophilic cytoplasm and round, reniform or indented nuclei.[1]

Osteosarcoma may mimic a *clear cell chondrosarcoma* (Fig. 9.1), but without S-100 positivity; neoplastic cells have a clear or finely granular eosinophilic cytoplasm.[2] Ultrastructurally, the water-clear cytoplasm corresponds to an accumulation of glycogen or a vacuolar degeneration.[3]

Osteosarcoma has shown focal *rhabdomyosarcomatous features*[4] and a myofibroblastic differentiation.[5]

Reactive giant cells may be a major component, with sparse osteoid production, leading to a misdiagnosis of giant cell tumor (Mirra 1989, Fechner & Mills 1993) (Figs 9.2, 9.3). In order to diagnose osteosarcoma, one has to study the background of mononuclear cells showing pleomorphism and atypical mitoses (Fechner & Mills 1993).

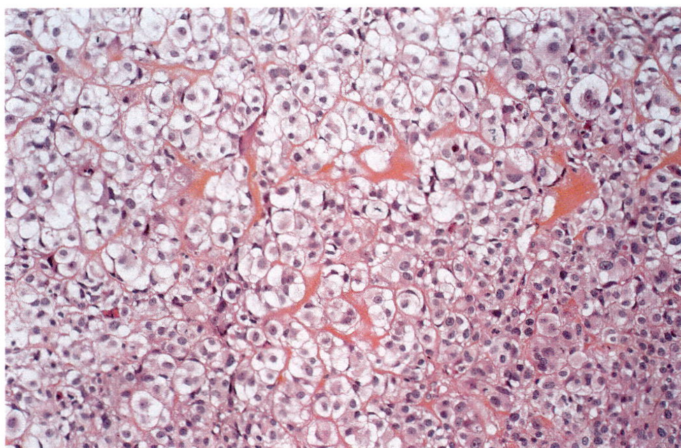

Fig. 9.1 Clear cell component of a typical osteoblastic osteosarcoma of the femur.

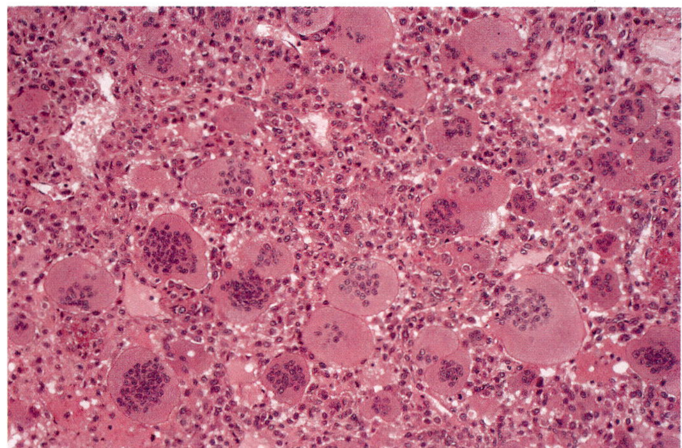

Fig. 9.2

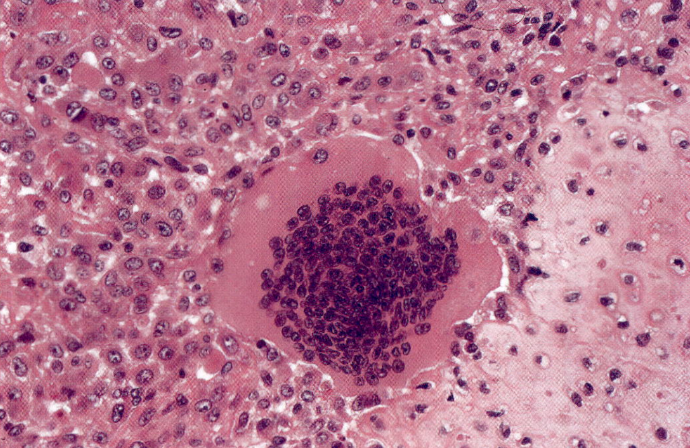

Fig. 9.3

Figs 9.2, 9.3 Cellular fields, close to the soft tissue extension of a femoral osteosarcoma mimicking a genuine giant cell tumor.

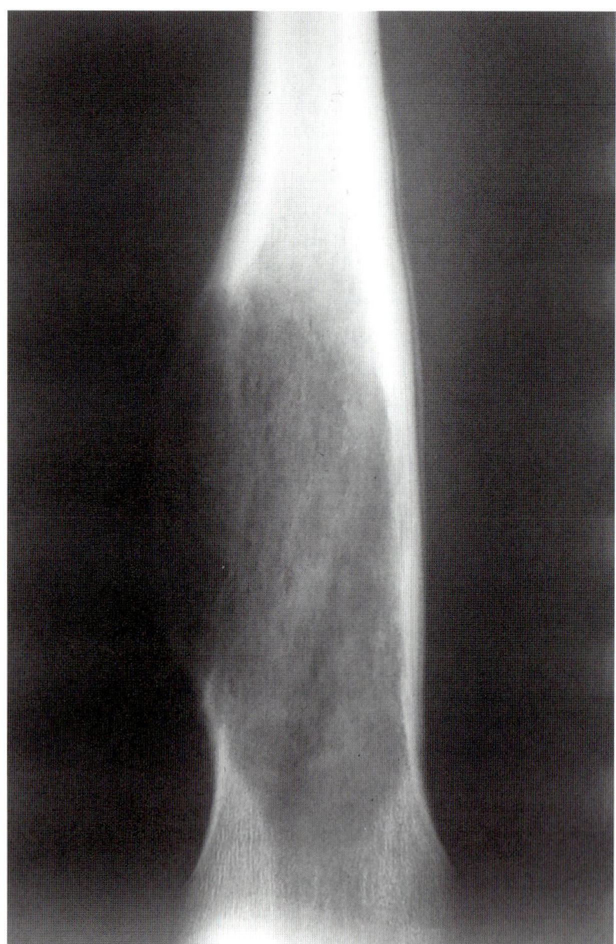

Fig. 9.4 Small cell osteosarcoma of the femur.

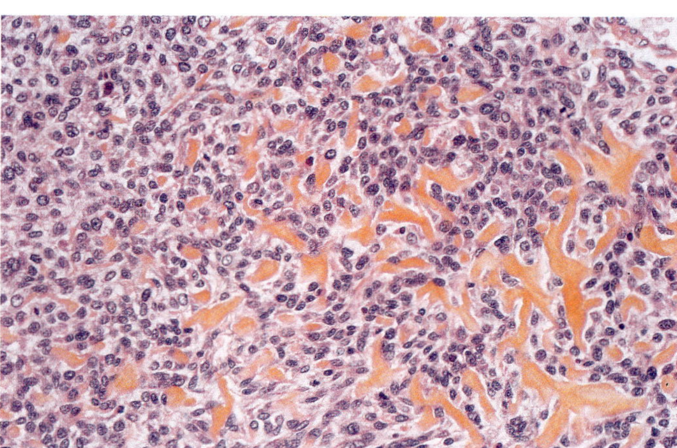

Fig. 9.5 Osteoid formation in a small cell osteosarcoma.

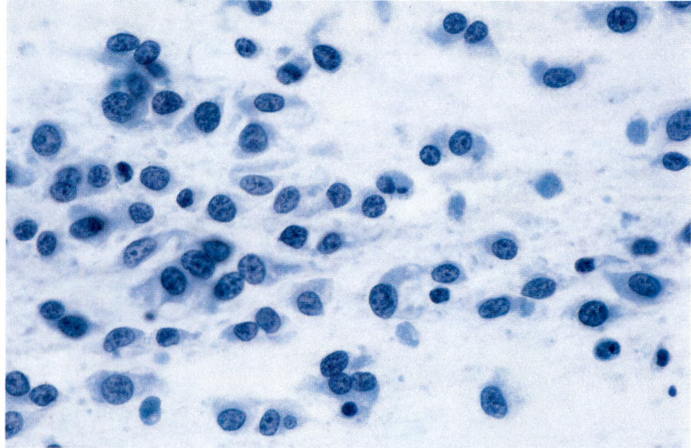

Fig. 9.6 Imprint cytology of a small cell osteosarcoma.

Most osteosarcomas have focal clusters of benign multinucleated giant cells. Incidence of so-called giant cell-rich osteosarcomas is about 3% in the Bristol Bone Tumor registry,[6] appearing as metaphyseal or diaphyseal lesions, predominantly lytic and with ill-defined margins. Osteosarcoma may be juxtaposed with a preexisting benign giant cell tumor[8] or identified in the clinical course of this latter condition.[7] Tumoral giant cells are mostly found in anaplastic tumors, malignant fibrous histiocytoma-like osteosarcomas or tumors secondary to Paget's disease.

Osteoid production can demonstrate a striking pattern, creating *rosettoid structures* composed of bundles of collagen, sometimes in continuity with the usual lace-like pattern.[9]

Small cell osteosarcoma is a rare variant (4% of all osteosarcomas[10]), being more frequent in the metaphyseal region of long bones, distal femur, tibia and proximal humerus[11,12] (Figs 9.4–9.6). There is wide variation in the radiographic appearance, ranging from lytic to osteosclerotic lesions with permeative destruction of the shaft.[11,13,14] Sheets of round cells produce an osteoid matrix. The cells have minimal cytoplasm; the nucleus is round or oval with finely dispersed chromatin similar to Ewing's sarcoma. Others may resemble the cells of large cell lymphomas or may be spindle shaped.[12] Intracytoplasmic glycogen can be found, as well as foci of tumoral cartilage. Reticulin production is absent or scanty.

Small cell osteosarcomas exhibit immunoreactivity for vimentin, osteonectin, osteocalcin and alkaline phosphatase. A minority of cells may react with muscle-specific actin, Leu-7, S-100 protein and cytokeratin.[15] On electron microscopy, an abundant rough endoplasmic reticulum and well-developed collagen fibers have been related to the osteoblastic differentiation but in most cases, the

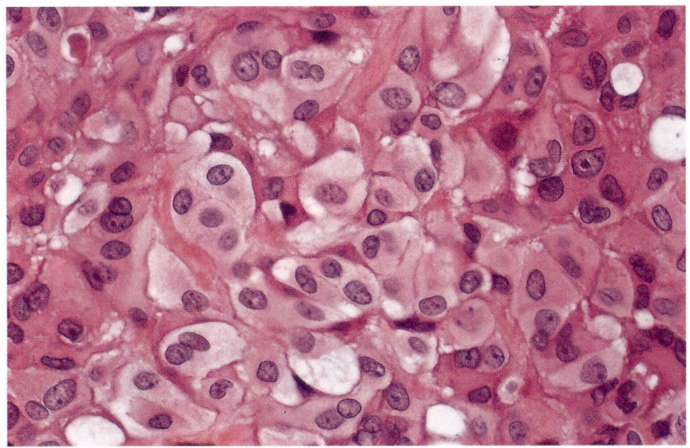

Fig. 9.7 Epithelioid cells in a femoral osteoblastic osteosarcoma.

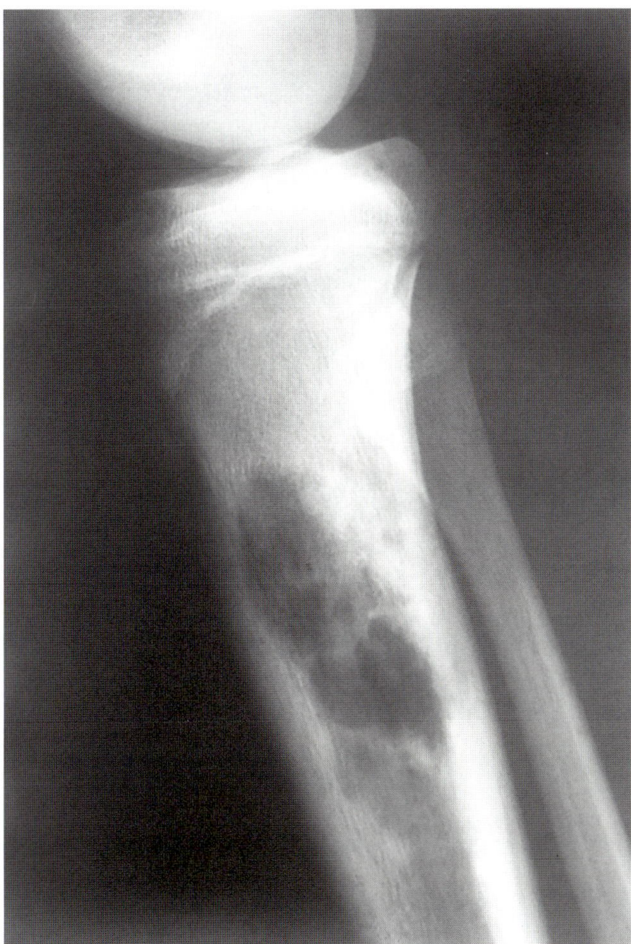

Fig. 9.8

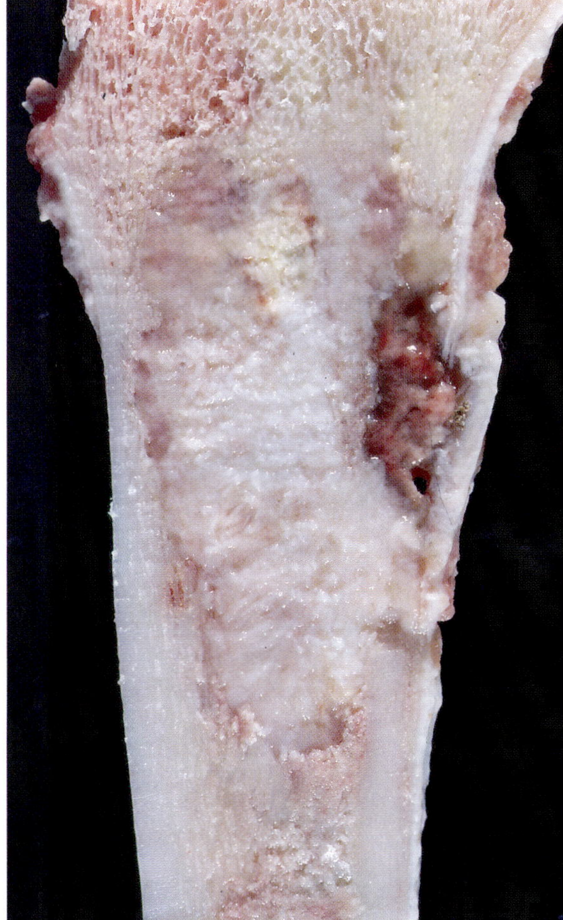

Fig. 9.9

Figs 9.8, 9.9 MFH-like osteosarcoma of the tibia.

cytoplasm is poorly differentiated; there is a high nuclear cytoplasmic ratio and overlap with Ewing's sarcoma cells.[14,15–17] Variable amounts of glycogen are found,[14,15,18] as well as deposits of hydroxyapatite crystals[19] or prominent flocculent deposits in the matrix.[20]

A chromosomal translocation involving chromosomes 11 and 22, similar to that found in Ewing's sarcoma, has been described[21] but not confirmed in another study.[22] Furthermore, the cells of a small cell osteosarcoma of the soft tissues have shown strong immunoreactivity to a monoclonal antibody recognizing the glycoprotein p30/32 MIC2, as in Ewing's sarcoma and PNET of bone.[23]

Small cell osteosarcomas may be viewed as tumors in which Ewing's cells proceed towards an osteoblastic or chondroblastic differentiation[24] or as a more primitive intermediate stage between Ewing's sarcoma and osteosarcoma.[25] Metastases are found in the lungs, the bones and the central nervous system.[14,26] The treatment is surgery and chemotherapy;[12] there seems to be a lack of correlation between the response to preoperative chemotherapy and the prognosis.[12,27] Local control may be achieved by irradiation[28] but the prognosis is worse than that of classical osteosarcomas.[27]

The definitive criterion for the differential diagnosis is the finding of osteoid[19] but with immunohistochemistry, one can exclude Ewing's sarcomas, neuroectodermal tumors, lymphomas or metastases from neuroblastomas or rhabdomyosarcoma. For mesenchymal chondrosarcomas, only the finding of low-grade tumoral cartilage is definitive.

VARIATIONS IN PATTERN

In otherwise typical osteosarcomas, some cells may show a *coexpression of cytokeratins* and *epithelial membrane antigen*; *epithelioid-like* cells with a pale or eosinophilic cytoplasm

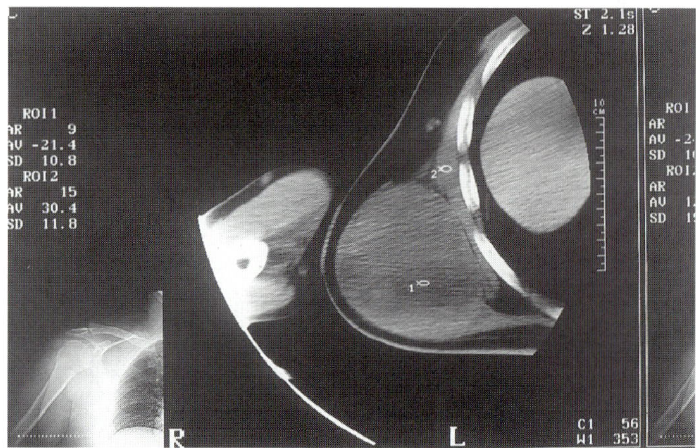

Fig. 9.12

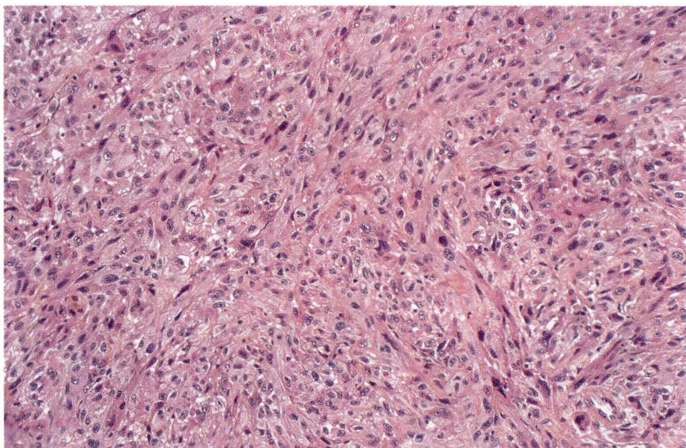

Fig. 9.10   Same case. MFH-like areas on the biopsy.

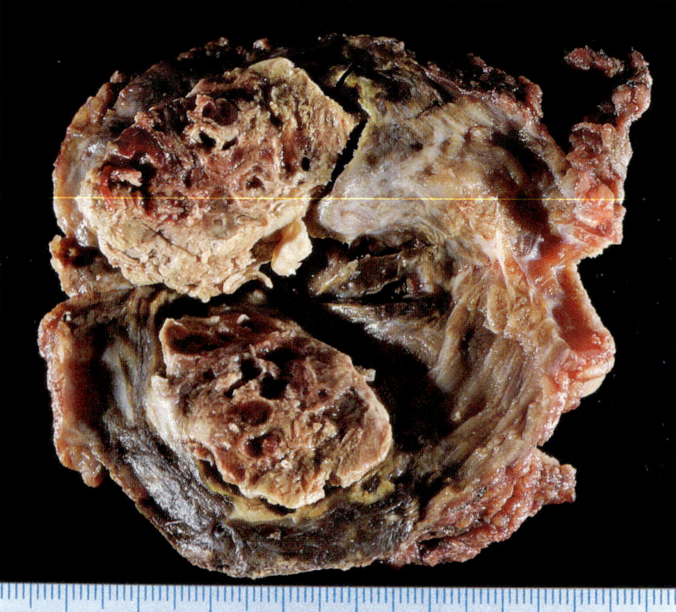

Fig. 9.13

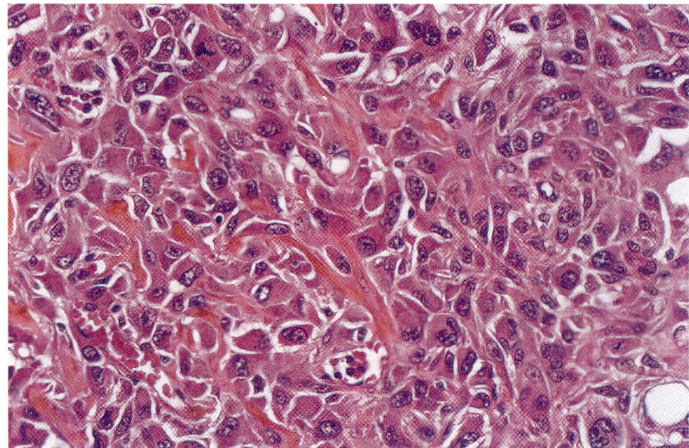

Fig. 9.11   Same case. Osteoblastic osteosarcoma in the study of the resection specimen.

Figs 9.12, 9.13   Unusual telangiectatic osteosarcoma of the soft tissues located in the axilla. Shrinkage of the tumor after intraarterial chemotherapy.

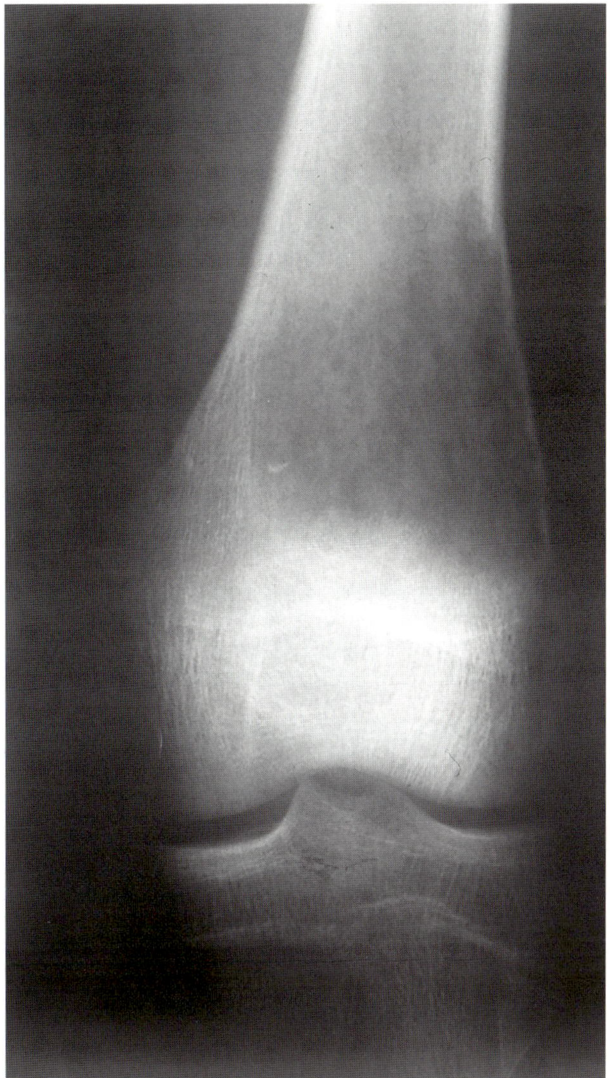

Fig. 9.14

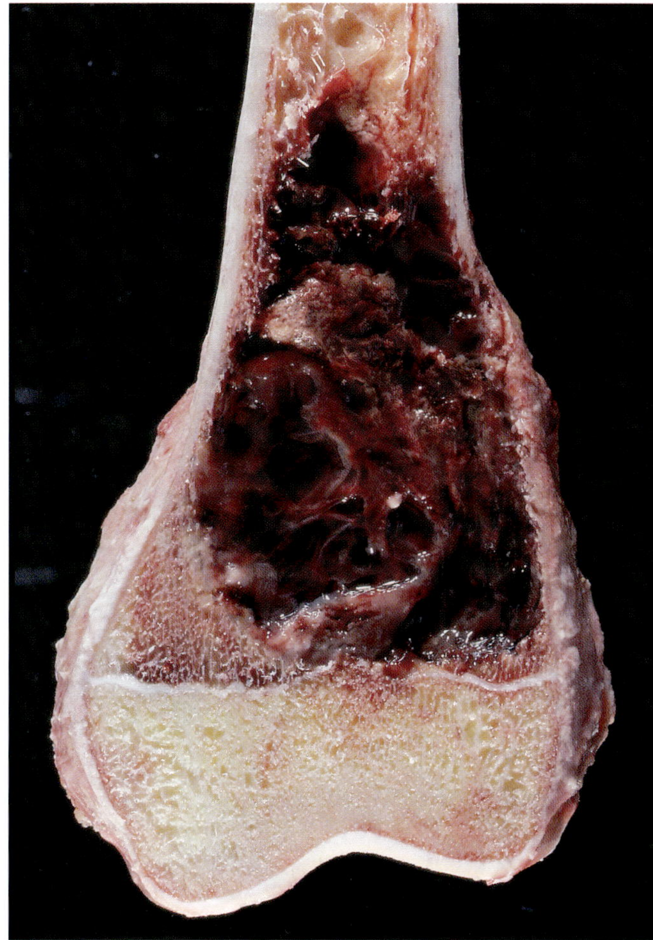

Fig. 9.15

Figs 9.14, 9.15 Purely lytic telangiectatic osteosarcoma of the femur.

are distributed in an alveolar or trabecular pattern[29–32] (Fig. 9.7). Some tumors contain fully developed epithelial structures with glandular, tubular and squamous differentiation.[29,33–35]

On electron microscopy, well-formed desmosomes and tonofilaments are found;[36] similar features have been reported in a chondrosarcoma.[37] For some authors, these unusual variants may represent true carcinosarcomas of bone.[33,38]

Frequently, a diagnosis of malignant fibrous histiocytoma is made from the biopsy of the soft tissue extension of an osteosarcoma and osteoid or bone formation is found in the central part of the resection specimen[39,40] (Figs 9.8–9.11).

MFH-like osteosarcomas are mostly found in patients older than 60 years of age (Huvos 1991)[41] with an incidence ranging from 8% to 30% of all osteosarcomas. The cellular component comprises spindle-shaped cells in short irregular fascicles and storiform pattern, histiocytic-

like and pleomorphic cells or large multinucleated tumor cells with prominent phagocytosis and eosinophilic bodies.[39] Osteoclast-like reactive giant cells may be present.

The ALPase activity or immunoreactivity with osteocalcin and collagen type I is more useful for the differential diagnosis than the usual histiocytic markers[40–42] or positivity for vimentin. In xenografts of athymic mice, the spindle-shaped cell proliferation is intensely positive for alkaline phosphatase.[40] Ultrastructural examination shows a fibroblastic, histiocytic or osteoblastic differentiation of tumoral cells.[39,40]

The Ki-67 labeling index has been found to be significantly lower than that of malignant fibrous histiocytomas of bone and the p53 overexpression is detected less frequently.[41] Malignant fibrous histiocytoma-like areas in osteosarcomas do not correlate with a poorer prognosis.[41]

Rare osteosarcomas (1%) have to be differentiated from

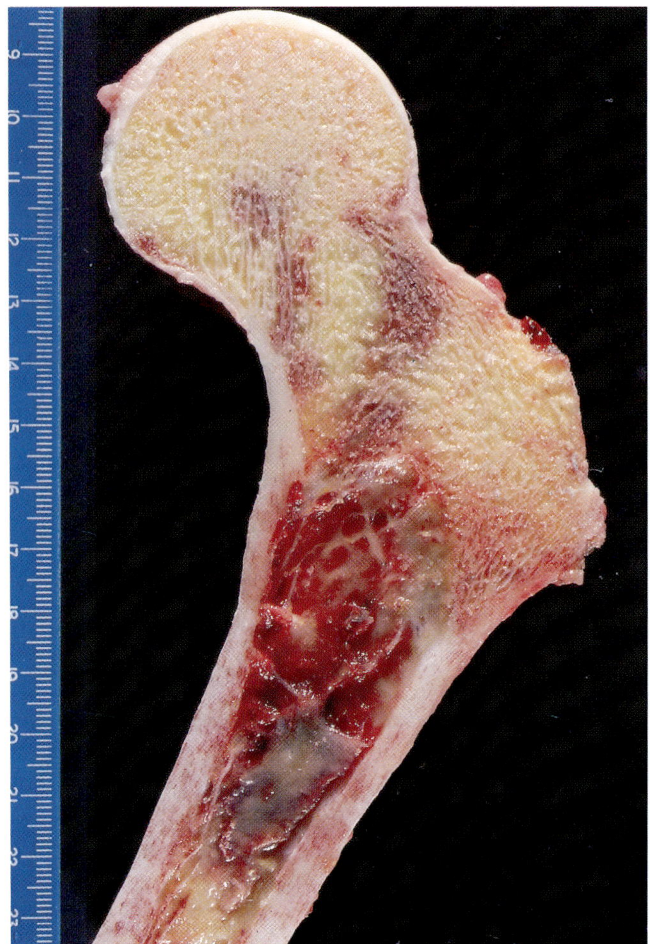

Fig. 9.16

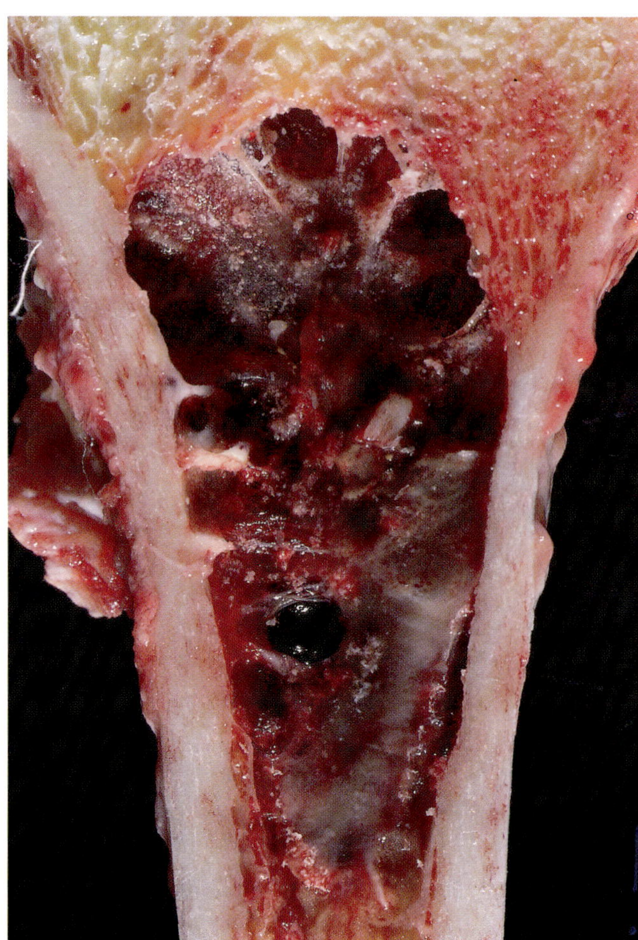

Fig. 9.17

Figs 9.16, 9.17 Metaphyseal telangiectatic osteosarcoma of the femur appearing as a blood-filled cavity.

osteoblastomas, especially in vertebral lesions involving the sacrum.[43] For some authors, they are similar to the so-called aggressive osteoblastomas.[43]

Histologically, the trabeculae of tumoral bone are rimmed by plump osteoblasts with an eosinophilic cytoplasm and a round nucleus with prominent nucleolus.[43] Occasionally mitotic activity is found. Spindle cells with a lace-like osteoid or a heavily ossified matrix are important findings. On ultrastructural examination, the tumoral cells have an eccentrically placed, irregular and indented nucleus; the rough endoplasmic reticulum is dilated.[44]

The diagnosis may be quite difficult on small biopsies[43] and one has also to exclude osteoblastomas with a multifocal growth without destruction of bone or pseudomalignant osteoblastomas with bizarre cells.[45] One has to search for a permeating pattern of growth, with entrapment of normal host trabeculae, and confirm the absence of the loose, vascular intertrabecular tissue or maturation towards the edges usually found in osteoblastomas.[43,44] A more esoteric method is successful transplantation into nude mice, suggesting malignancy.[44]

Telangiectatic osteosarcoma was first described by Paget in 1854 and termed malignant bone aneurysm by Ewing in 1922. It accounts for 2% of all osteosarcomas if the radiographic criterion is a purely lytic lesion[46] and for 11% if one allows a minimal sclerosis corresponding to tumoral bone formation.[47,48] Pathological fractures occur in about a quarter of cases.[46,48,49] It can be found secondary to fibrous dysplasia or Paget's disease or may be induced by irradiation.[48] Telangiectatic osteosarcomas in the soft tissues are rare, but the diagnostic difficulties are the same[52,53] (Figs 9.12, 9.13).

Sites of occurrence are the same as those of typical osteosarcomas[50] but in some series, there is a prevalence in the distal end of the femur and femoral diaphysis[48] or the femoral diaphysis and fibular metaphysis.[47] On imaging, they usually appear as purely metaphyseal lytic lesions (Fig. 9.14), with infiltrative margins, cortical destruction, soft tissue extension and periosteal reactions;[49] some may have limited areas of sclerosis. They extend into the epiphysis up to the articular cartilage and may involve the joint capsule.[49] Some tumors simulate an

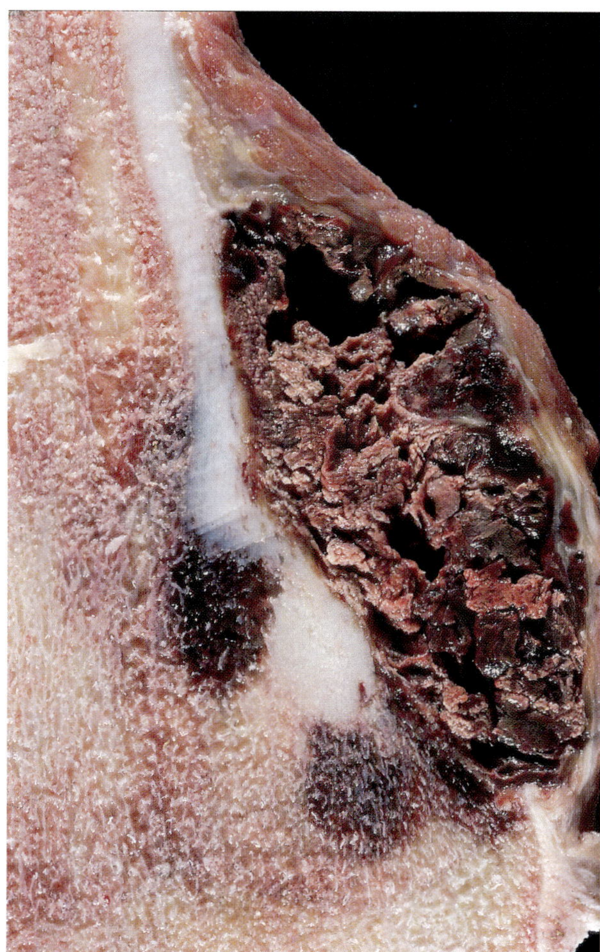

Fig. 9.18 Peripheral telangiectatic osteosarcoma of the lower femoral metaphysis.

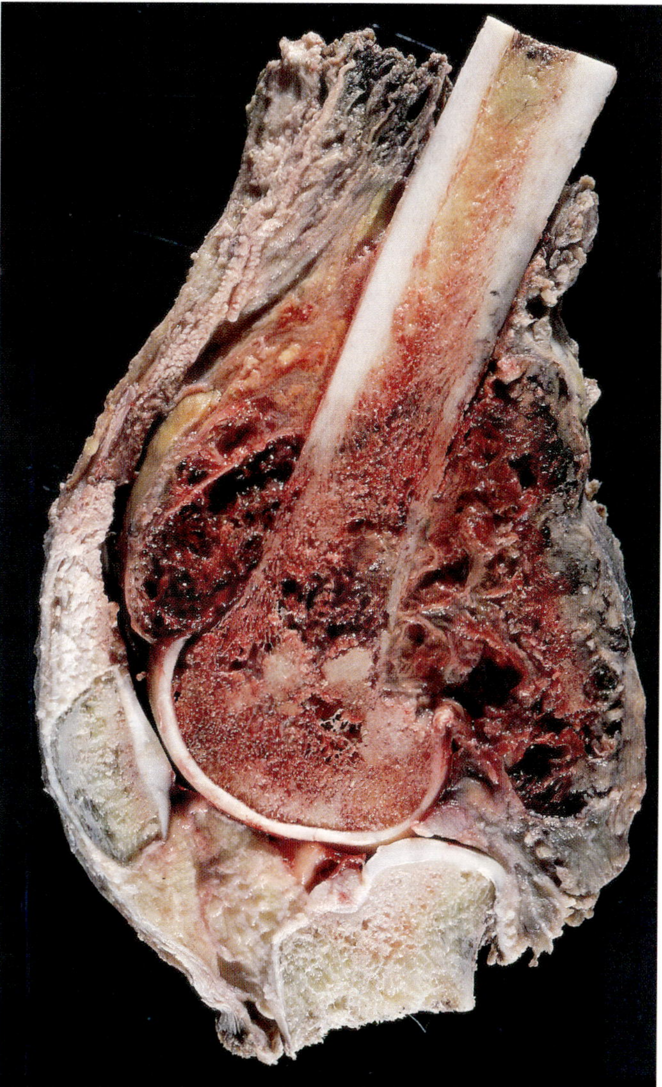

Fig. 9.19 Femoral telangiectatic osteosarcoma with extensive soft tissue involvement and pathologic fracture.

aneurysmal bone cyst[54] while others have the radiographic appearance of a blow-out or expansile pseudocystic lesion.[46,48] CT can demonstrate fluid levels similar to an aneurysmal bone cyst; on MRI, there is a rather specific high signal intensity.[55]

Gross examination (Figs 9.15–9.25) may reveal a cavity filled with hemorrhagic and necrotic tissue looking like a 'bag of blood'[48] or a multicystic mass resembling an aneurysmal bone cyst.

Histologically (Figs 9.26–9.30), malignant cells and slight osteoid production are detected in the blood and necrotic debris, along with numerous reactive giant cells; cytospins or tumor imprints are very useful for the diagnosis. When the pattern is similar to an aneurysmal bone cyst, the cyst walls and the lining are formed by anaplastic tumor cells, usually associated with reactive giant cells or hemosiderin-laden macrophages; there is a brisk mitotic activity with atypical forms. Osteoid matrix appears as a thin lace-like pattern.

Cells lining the blood-filled spaces do not react with the antifactor VIII antigen, but ALPase activity is highly posi-

tive.[56] On ultrastructural examination, the finding of an incomplete endothelial lining[57] has not been confirmed in another study,[56] which showed osteoblast-like cells, macrophages and reactive multinucleated cells on the lining.

The distribution of metastases is the same as with typical osteosarcomas; lung metastases have been reported with the classic structure of an aneurysmal bone cyst.[58]

With surgical treatment alone, telangiectatic osteosarcomas are almost always lethal.[46,59,60] There has been a recent improvement in prognosis, however, maybe due to the good response to chemotherapy, as the widespread vascularity may allow a better perfusion by chemotherapeutic drugs (Huvos 1991:[61,62]). Now, more than 80% of patients remain disease free. Pulmonary metastases may also regress after chemotherapy.[63]

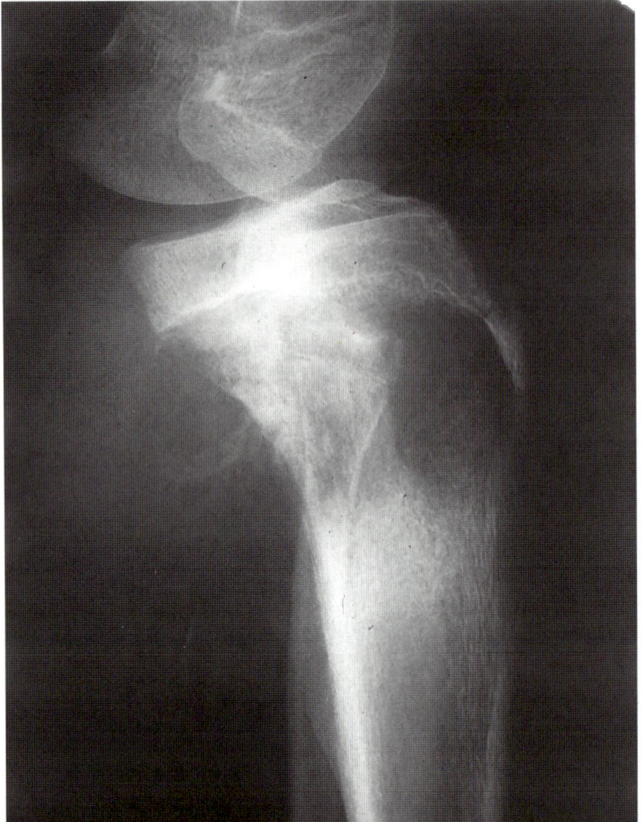

Fig. 9.20

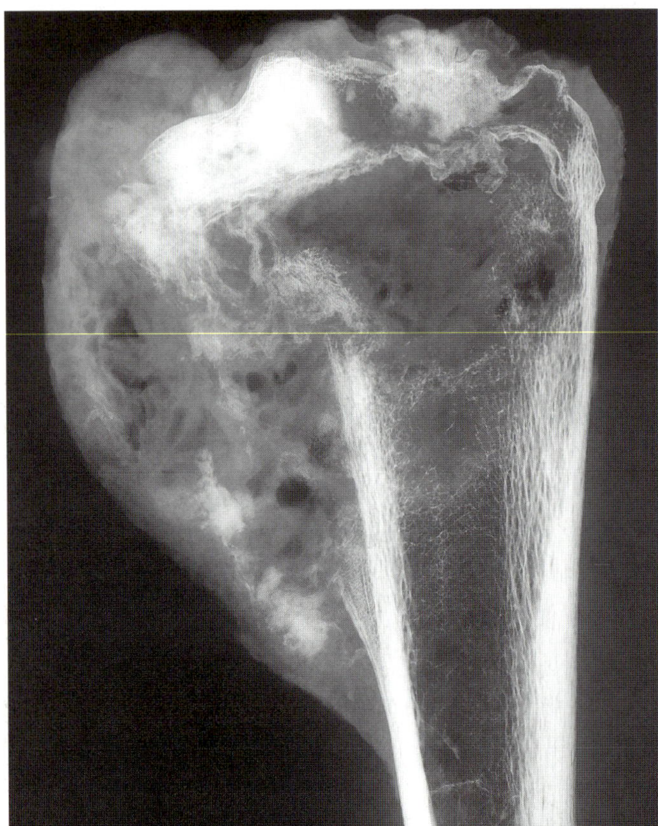

Fig. 9.22

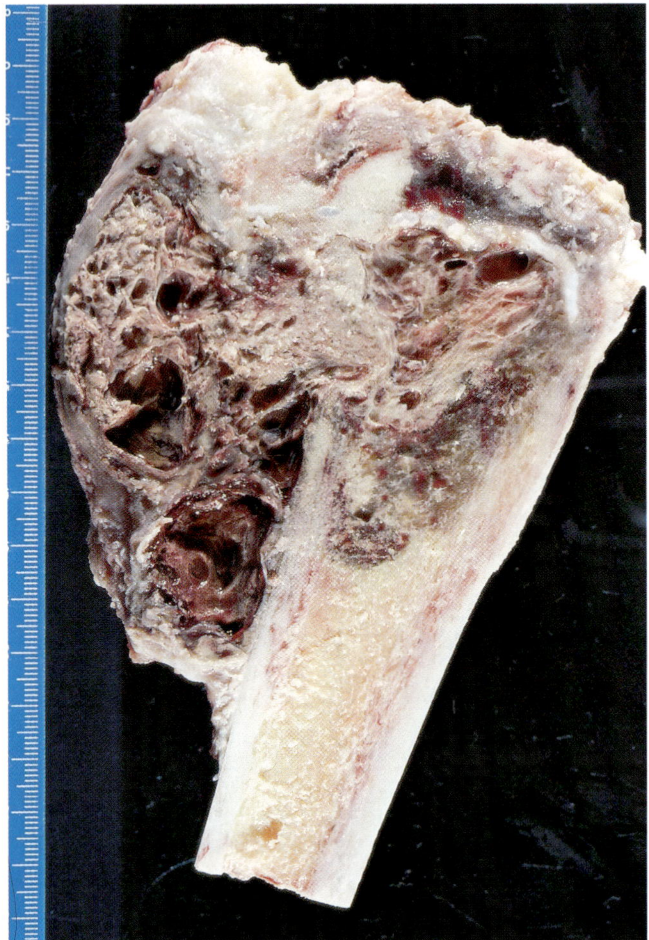

Fig. 9.21

Figs 9.20–9.22 Osteoblastic osteosarcoma of the tibia with a telangiectatic component.

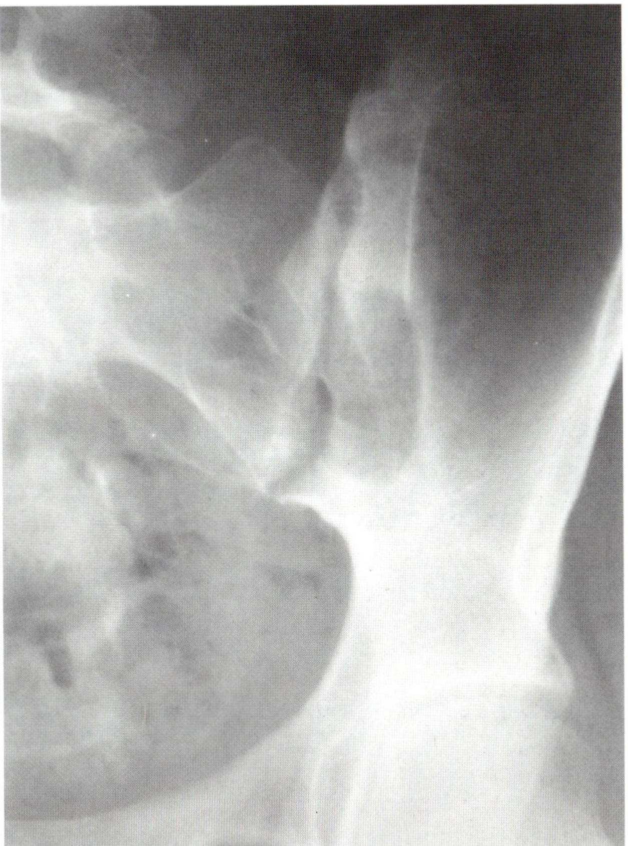

Fig. 9.23

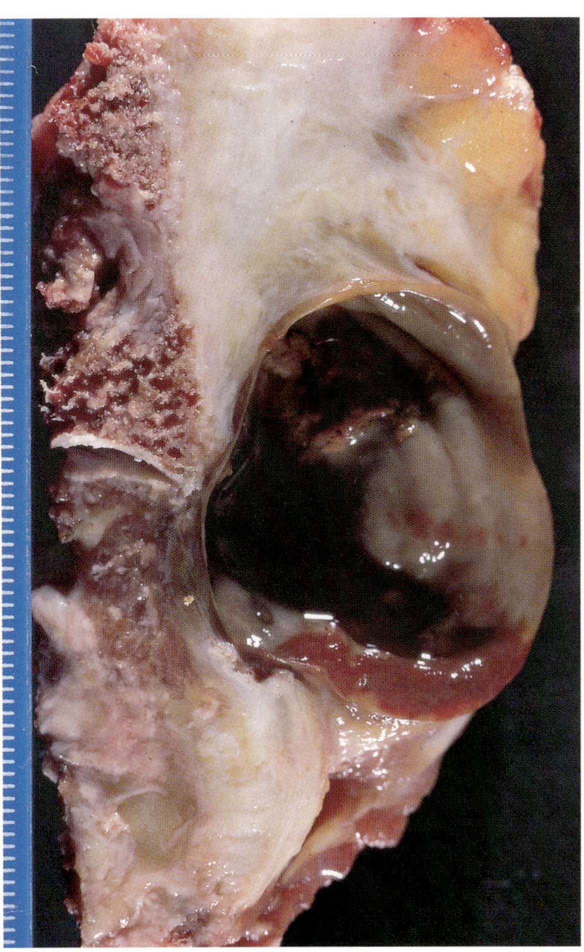

Fig. 9.24

Figs 9.23, 9.24 Telangiectatic osteosarcoma involving the sacroiliac joint.

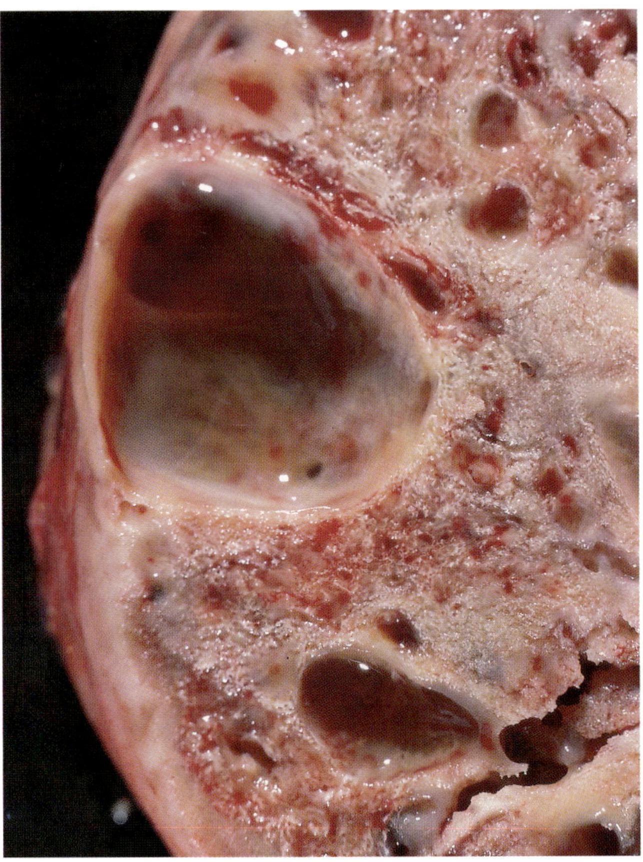

Fig. 9.25 Cystic changes in a femoral osteoblastic osteosarcoma with no telangiectatic pattern.

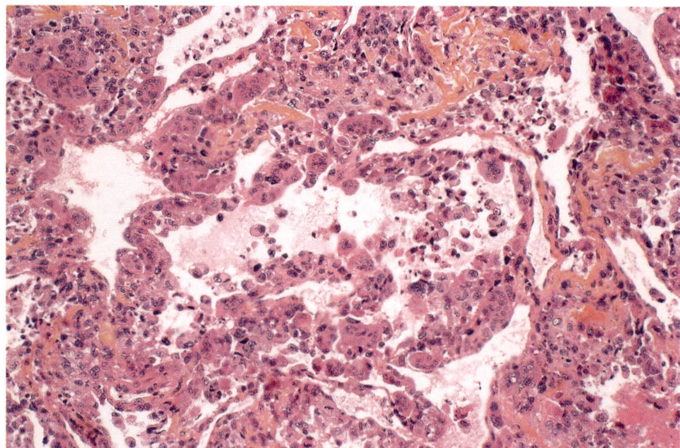

Fig. 9.26

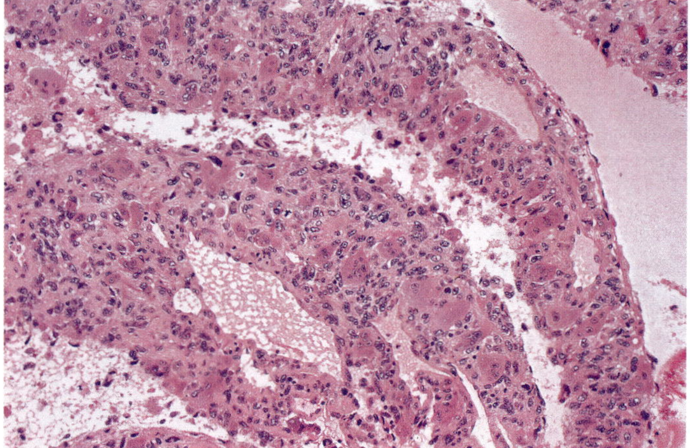

Fig. 9.27

Figs 9.26, 9.27 Telangiectatic osteosarcomas: cyst walls with a sarcomatous cell component.

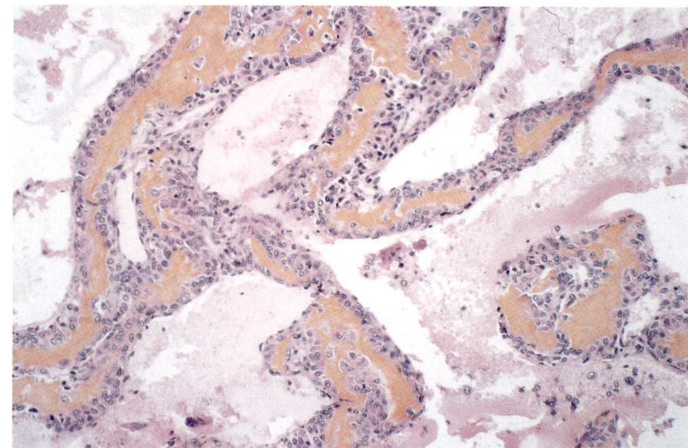

Fig. 9.28

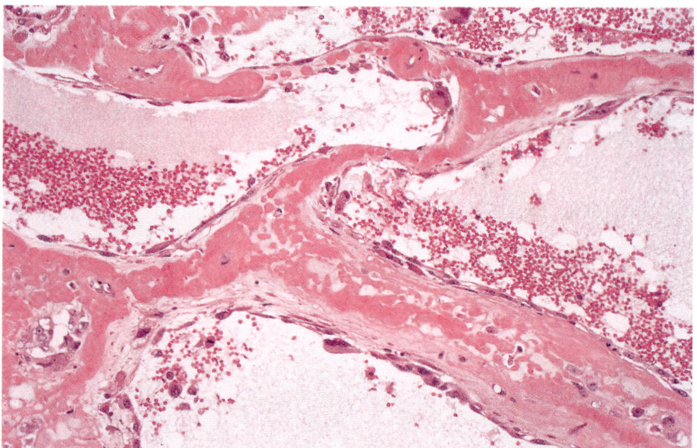

Fig. 9.29

Figs 9.28, 9.29 Telangiectatic osteosarcomas: osteoid production in the cyst walls.

The main differential diagnosis is an aneurysmal bone cyst. Imaging may be quite similar,[64] with a rapidly spreading destruction in aneurysmal bone cysts, sharply defined margins and 'eggshell' periosteal new bone appearing later. For a diagnosis of sarcoma, one has to search for anaplastic cells, atypical mitoses and a lace-like pattern of osteoid. Histomorphometric techniques have been applied to this lesion:[65] in 77% of cases, discrimination from an aneurysmal bone cyst was established on the basis of quantitative nuclear characteristics (nuclear surface areas and mitotic index).

Most of the clinicopathologic findings on *central low-grade osteosarcomas* (1–2% of osteosarcomas) have been issued from the Mayo Clinic files[66–68] but shorter series[69–71] or single case reports[72–80] also provide unusual features (Figs 9.31–9.43). Patients are, on average, one decade older than those presenting with the usual forms; there is no sex predominance. Main symptoms are pain and swelling, often with a very protracted course. Some

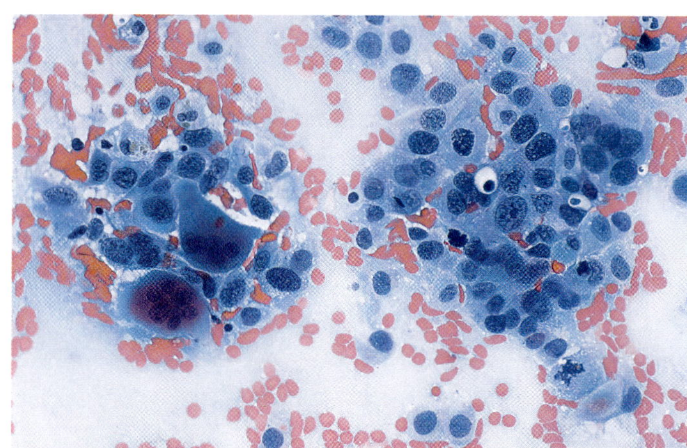

Fig. 9.30 Telangiectatic osteosarcoma: cytology of the blood in the cystic spaces: tumoral osteoblasts and numerous reactive giant cells.

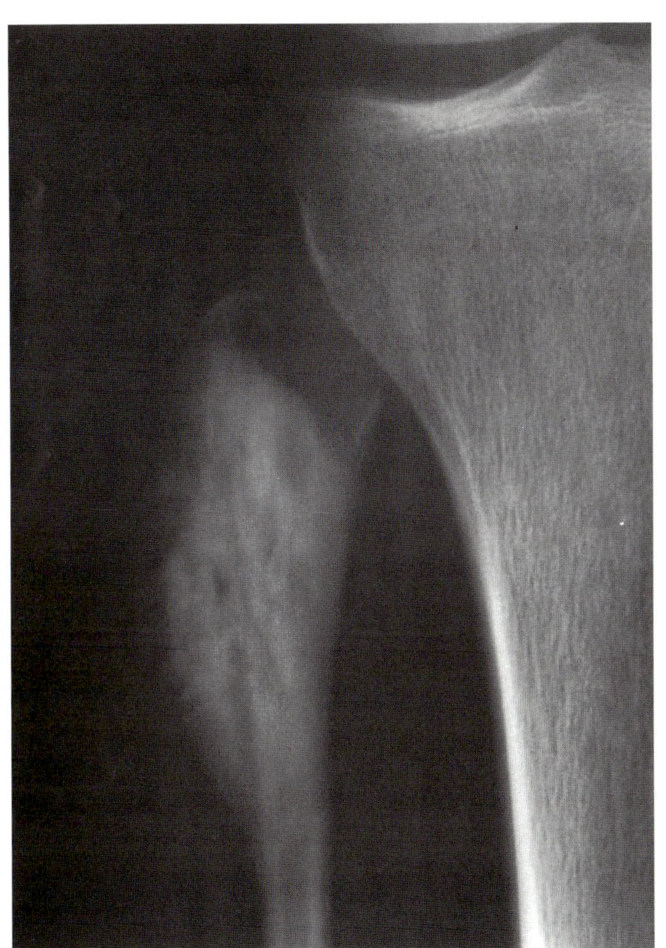

Fig. 9.31

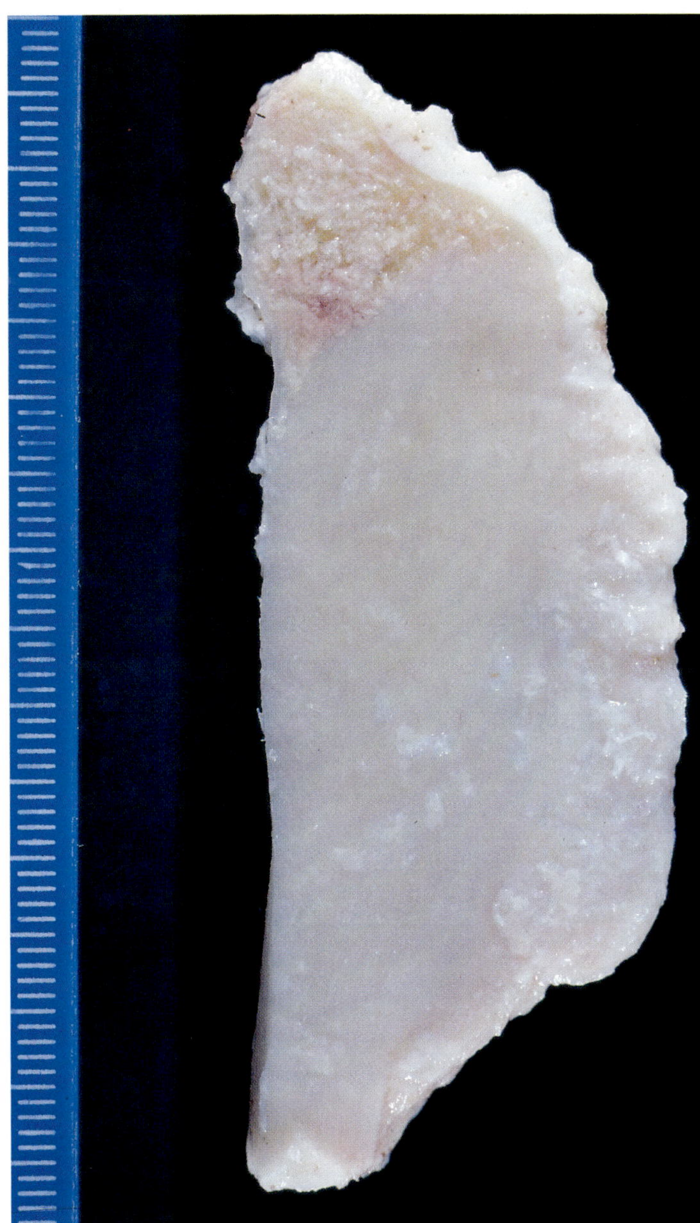

Fig. 9.32

Figs 9.31, 9.32 Well-differentiated osteosarcoma of the upper end of the fibula.

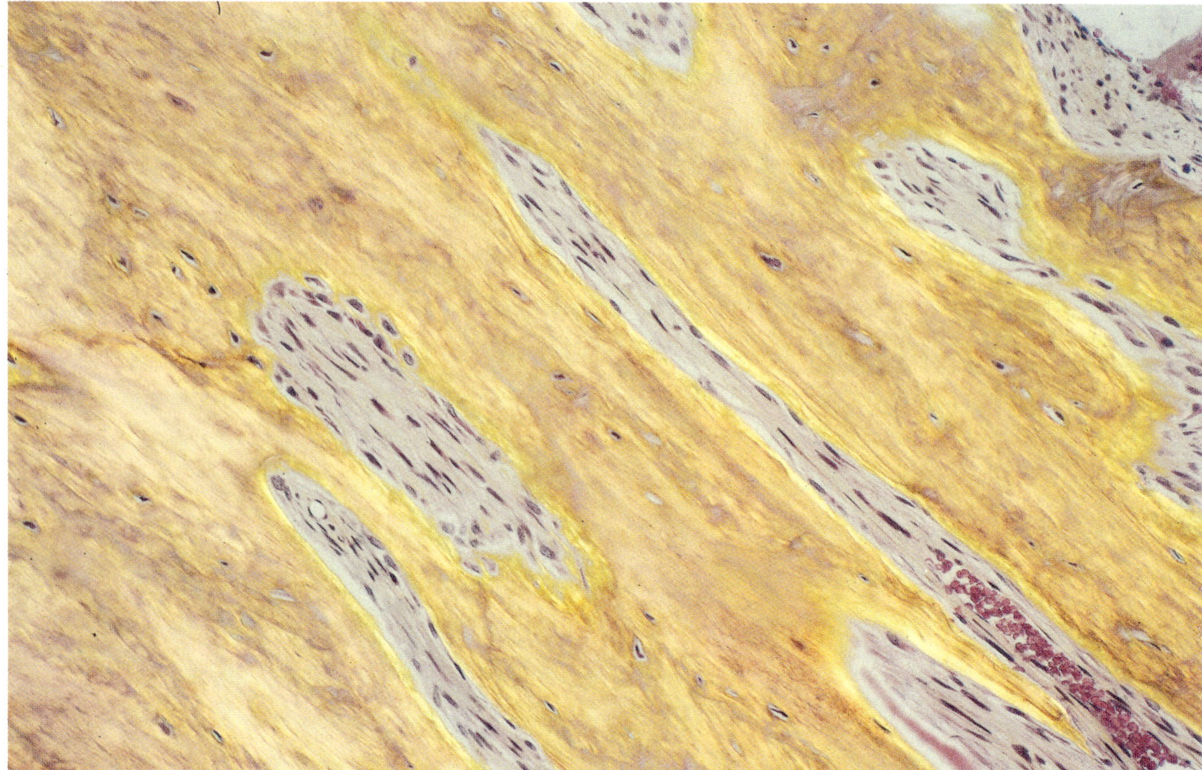

Fig. 9.33

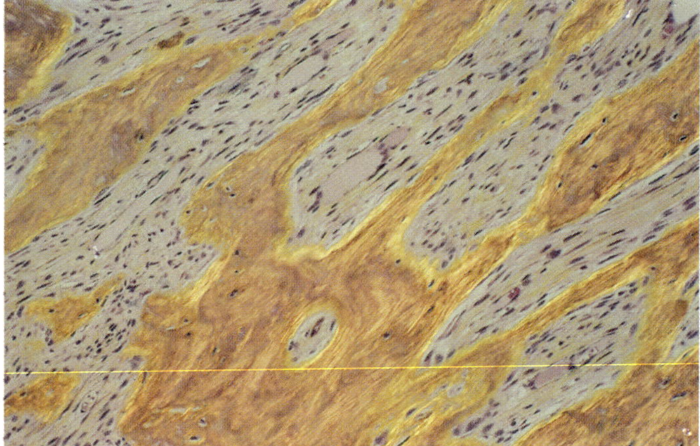

Fig. 9.34

Figs 9.33, 9.34 Same case. Massive formation of large trabeculae of tumoral bone with minimal cytological atypia (polarized light).

patients may be asymptomatic. The most common sites are in the long bones in a metaphyseal location, but also the diaphysis or epiphysis if the growth plate is closed. A diaphyseal site has been reported.[66] The femur (chiefly the distal part) and tibia are most affected, other locations being the flat bones (15%) or the bones of the hand and foot (4%).

On imaging, some cases in long bones appear to develop in the cortical region, but most involve the medullary area over 5–10 cm. In about half of the cases, the lesion is expansive, with or without trabeculations. It may be entirely radiolucent, densely blastic or have some matrix mineralization. Tumoral borders show poor margination or a sclerotic rim. It should be stressed that the X-ray findings change with the evolution of the lesion.[70] Definite cortical destruction, soft tissue mass, cumulus cloud mineralization and periosteal reactions are found in advanced tumors as well as pathologic fractures, aneurysmal bone cyst aspects or even simple cyst formation. In about 50% of cases, early lesions may simulate a benign process, chiefly fibrous dysplasia.

CT scans, MRI and xerography may be useful to detect cortical destruction, even if it is limited.[70] Gross aspects depend on the amount of mineralized tumoral bone, which varies from a firm, whitish, gritty tissue to highly sclerotic tumors.

Histologically, the fibrous tumoral tissue is predominant, with bundles of spindle-shaped elongated cells in fairly uniform arrangement; overall anaplasia is very subtle and mitoses are rare, without abnormal forms. Collagen production may be important, with focal hyalinization and overall hypocellularity. Large seams of irregular calcified osteoid without prominent osteoblastic rimming can be quite similar to that of a parosteal

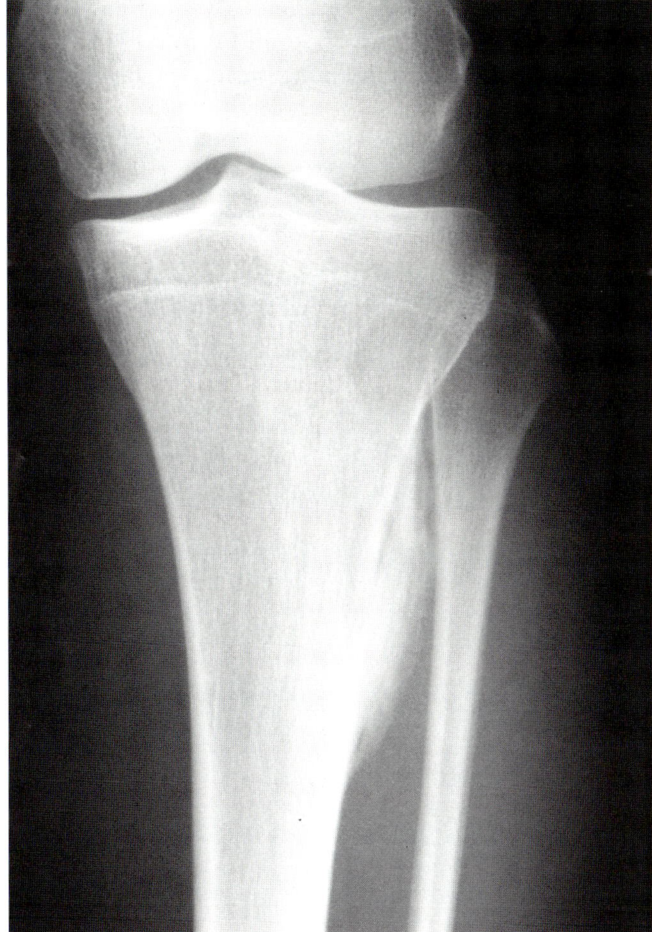

Fig. 9.35

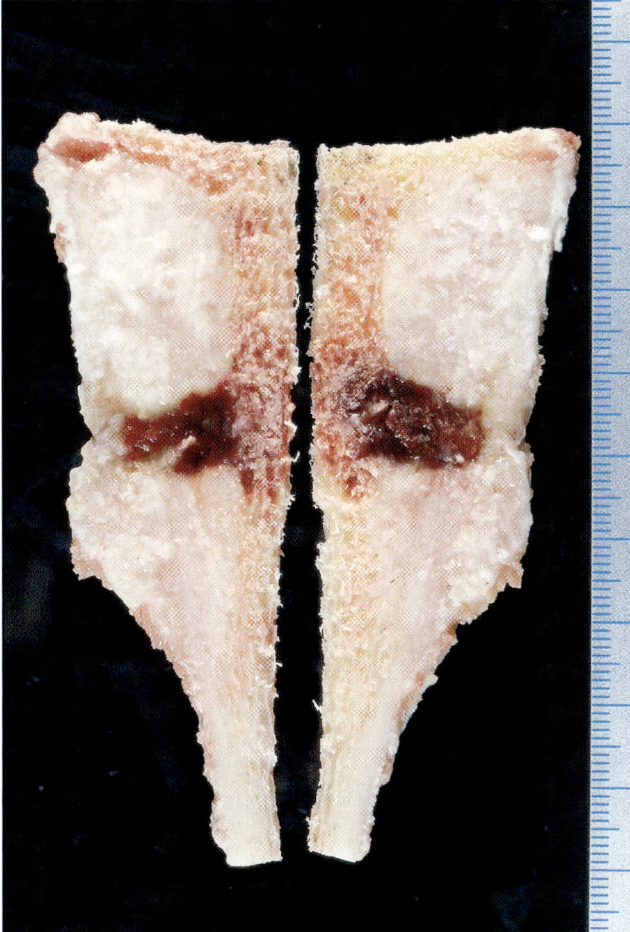

Fig. 9.36

Figs 9.35, 9.36 Well-differentiated osteosarcoma of the upper end of the tibia.

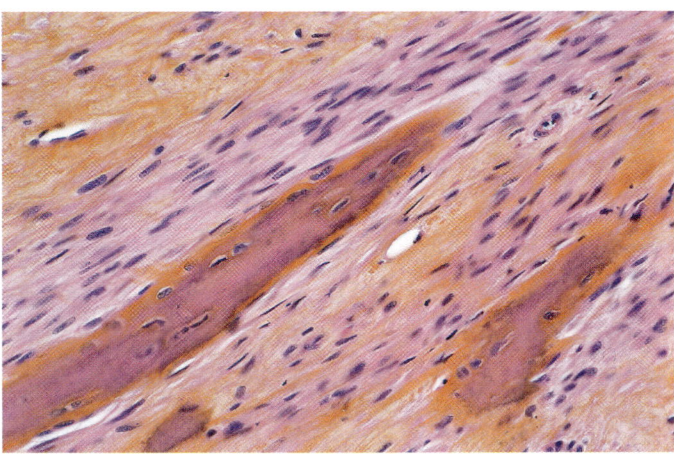

Fig. 9.37

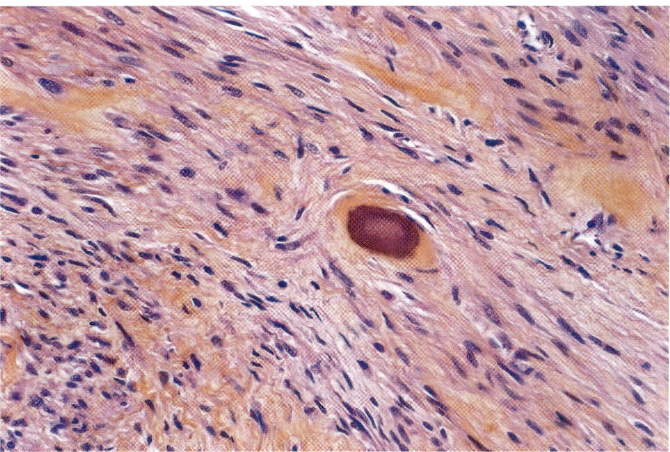

Fig. 9.38

Figs 9.37, 9.38 Same case. Long slivers of tumoral bone, small islands of bone resembling fibrous dysplasia and some atypia of the elongated cells.

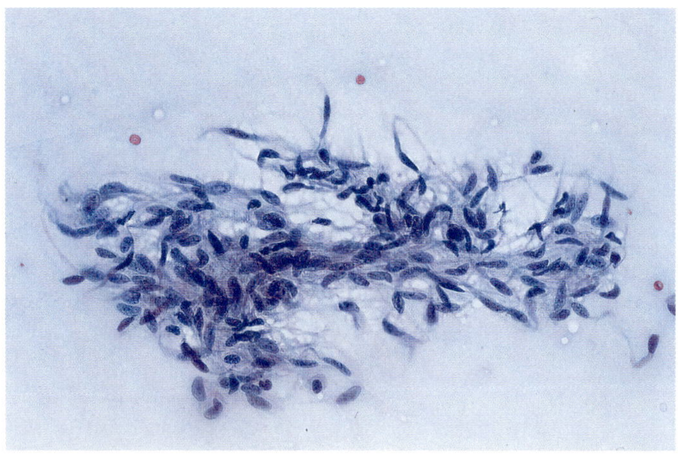

Fig. 9.39 Same case. Imprint cytology: fibroblast-like tumoral cells.

osteosarcoma. Some tumors have only scanty bone production, with small flecks of osteoid sometimes mimicking the 'Chinese characters' of fibrous dysplasia. On the other hand, massive bone production may lead to a 'normalization' of tumoral trabecular bone. Small foci of tumoral cartilage can be detected with only slight nuclear atypia.

On ultrastructural examination, osteoblastic, fibroblastic and chondroblast-like cells are found, but the most frequent cell type is myofibroblast-like, as in parosteal osteosarcomas.

The prognosis compared with typical forms is good, with a metastatic rate of about 10%, if adequate treatment is performed, that is, wide tumor resection. Chemotherapy is ineffective when the tumor is generally well differentiated. If initial treatment is a limited local excision,

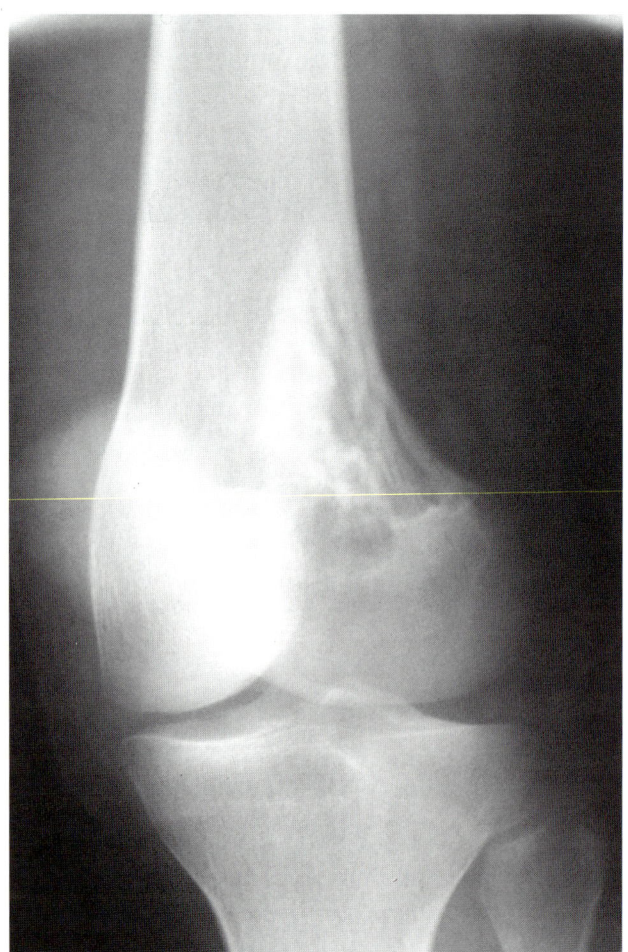

Fig. 9.40

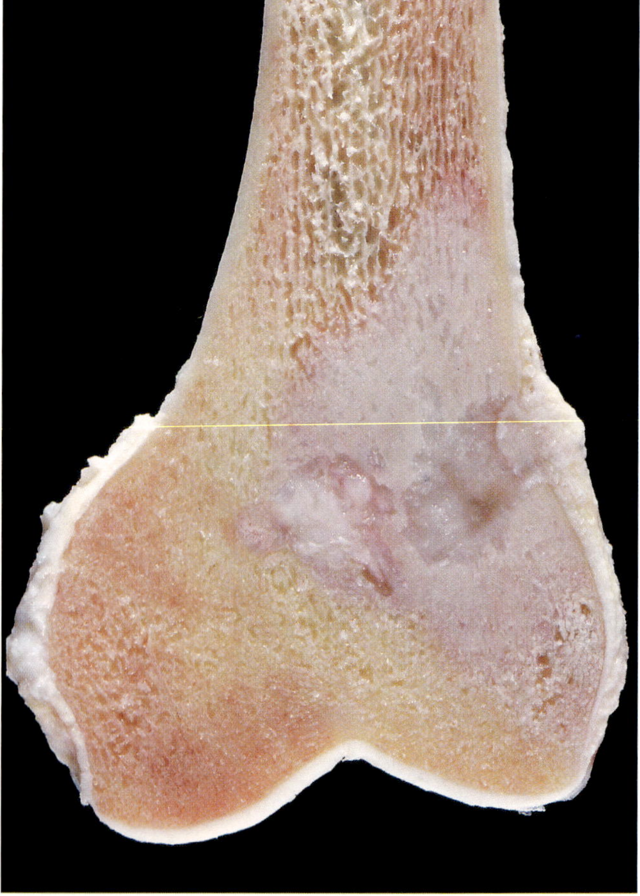

Fig. 9.41

Figs 9.40, 9.41 Well-differentiated osteosarcoma of the lower metaphysis of the femur.

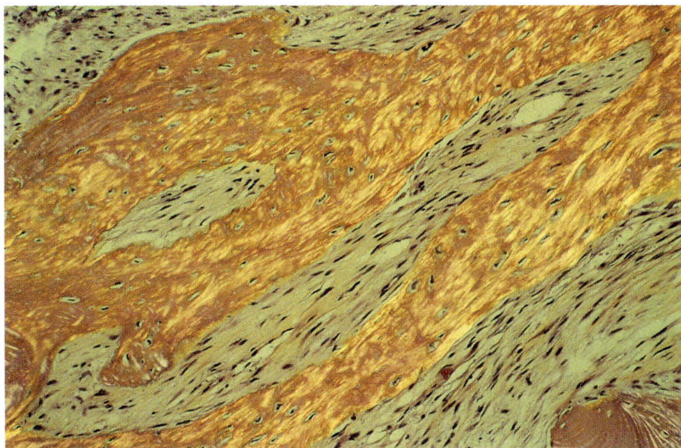

Fig. 9.42

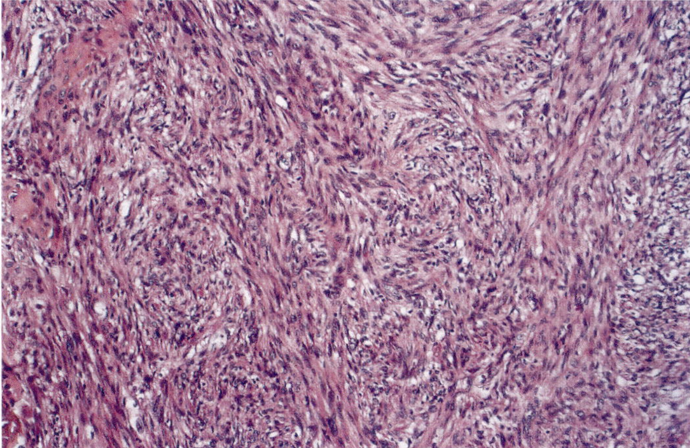

Fig. 9.43

Figs 9.42, 9.43 Same case. Most of the tumor is well differentiated (polarized light) while the central part is dedifferentiated.

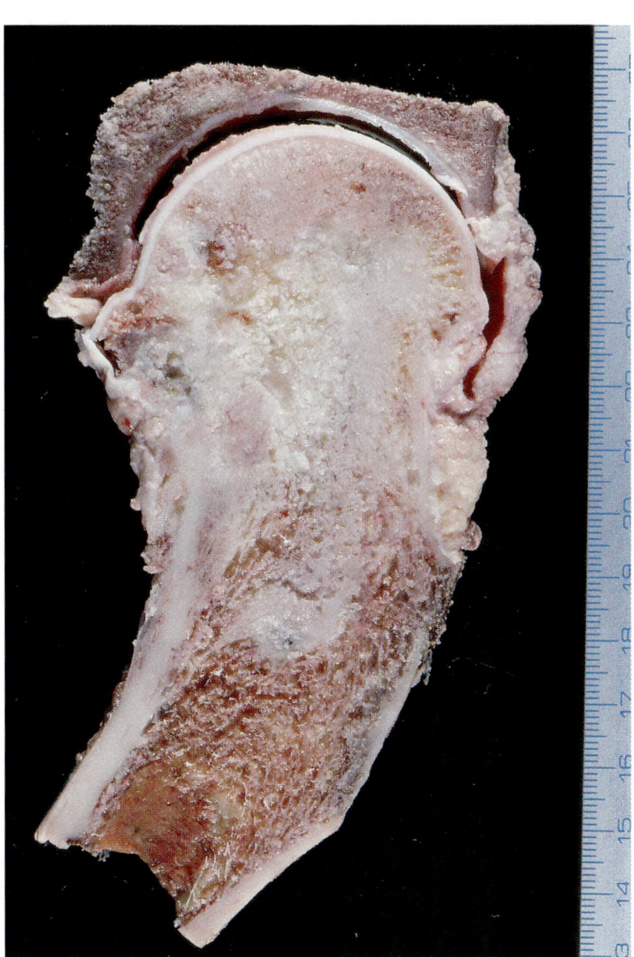

Fig. 9.44 Osteosarcoma of the femur centered on the epiphysis with extension to the joint capsule.

one or multiple recurrences may occur, sometimes after a fairly long period of time, and in 15% of cases, transformation to a typical high-grade tumor.[68,71] This progression or so-called 'dedifferentiation' is also known in parosteal osteosarcomas. The recognition of low- and high-grade tumoral components at the time of initial surgery is a rare event.[68,79]

The main diagnostic difficulty is not parosteal osteosarcoma, if the pathologist knows the tumor location, but fibrous dysplasia. The search for plump or elongated nuclei and chromatin clumping is important but the pattern of lesional bone, and particularly long slivers of bone running in parallel, is one of the most useful clues to the diagnosis (Mirra 1989), with the finding of tumoral infiltration, destruction of the cortex and extension through the periosteum.[67,68]

VARIATIONS IN BONE LOCATION

Epiphyseal location in long bones is rare[81–85] (Fig. 9.44); most of the tumors are predominantly lytic lesions. They may disrupt the cortex with joint involvement.[85] The main diagnostic problems occur on imaging, which presents some radiologic features of clear cell chondrosarcomas, chondroblastomas and enchondromas.[85]

Diaphyseal osteosarcomas occur in 7% of cases in the Mayo Clinic files,[86] involving mostly the femur, tibia and humerus (Figs 9.45, 9.46). The duration of symptoms is greater than for patients with metaphyseal tumors, but the prognosis is similar.[86] On X-ray, they appear as a dense cortical sclerosis, a purely lytic lesion with a pathological fracture or with the classic features of osteosarcomas.[87–89] Small tumors have been reported[90] and sclerotic medullary spread into the shaft.[87] In 20% of cases, they can mimic a Ewing's sarcoma.[86]

Intracortical osteosarcomas are the rarest form.[91–98] They

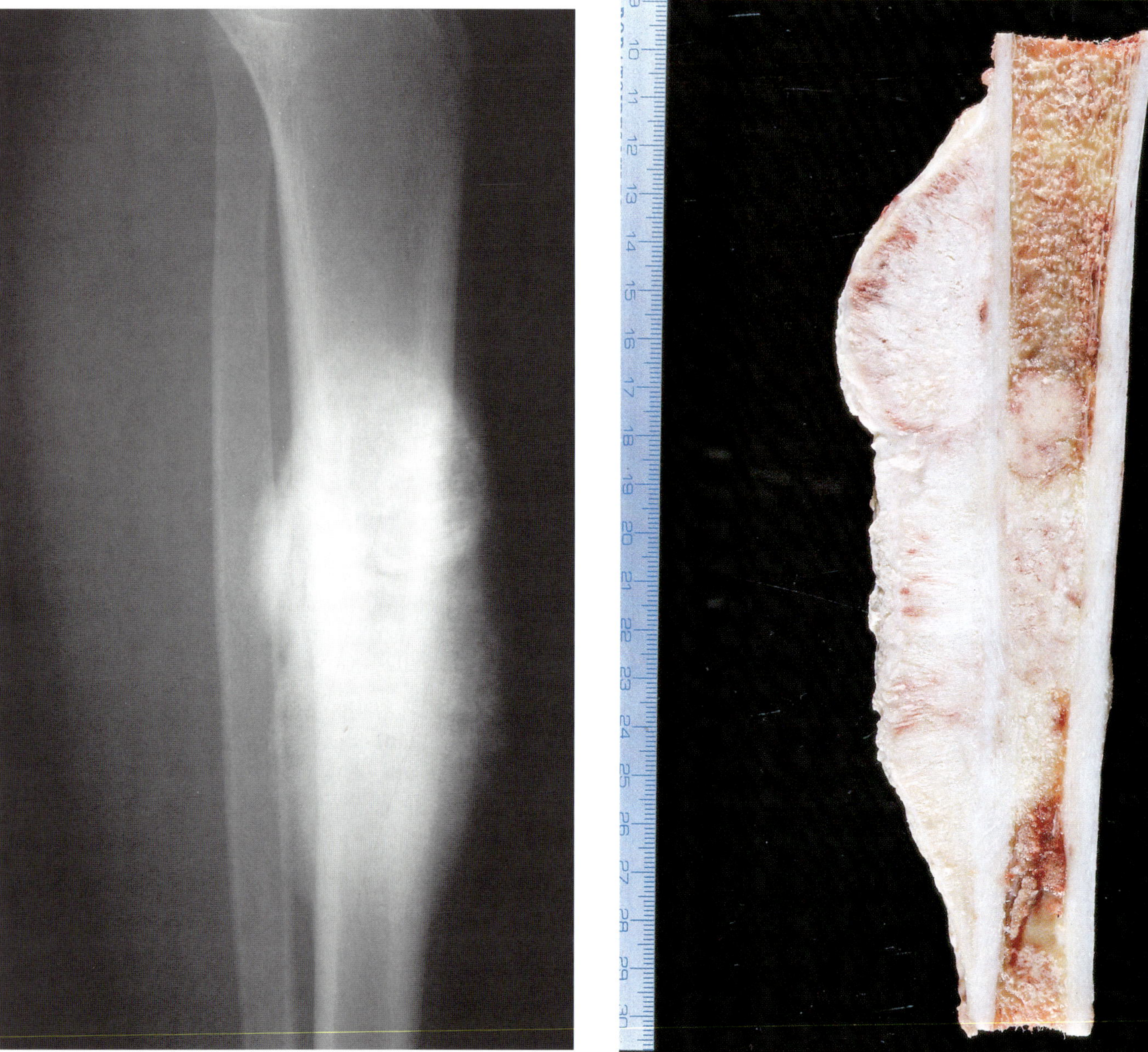

Fig. 9.45

Fig. 9.46

Figs 9.45, 9.46 Diaphyseal osteosarcoma of the tibia shaft with massive soft tissue involvement.

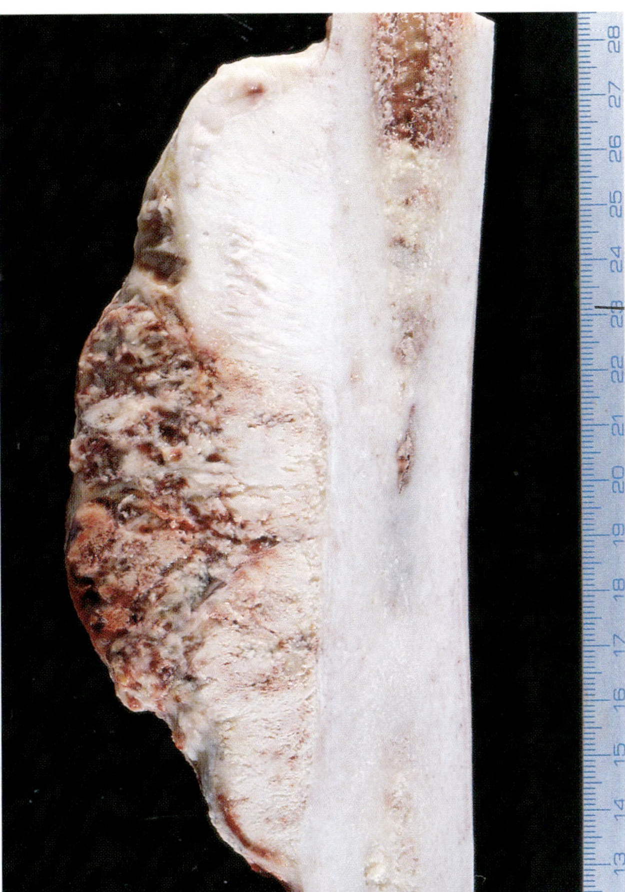

Fig. 9.47

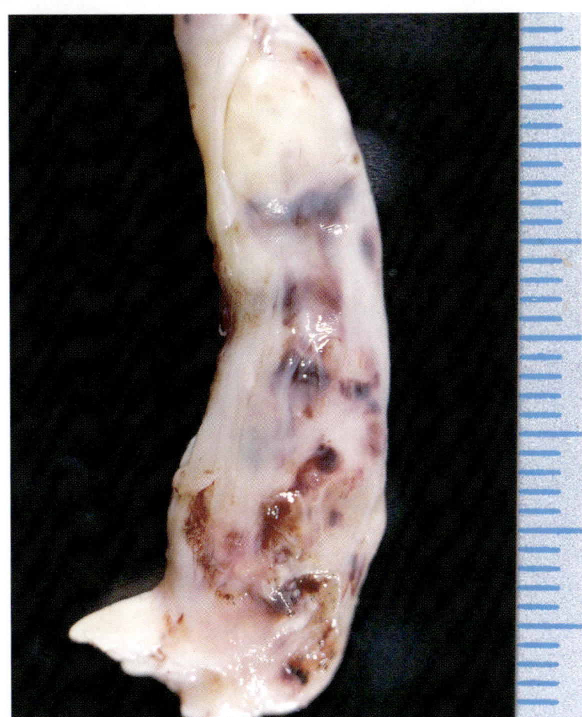

Fig. 9.48

Figs 9.47, 9.48 High-grade surface osteosarcoma of the femur, with tumoral extension into the deep femoral vein.

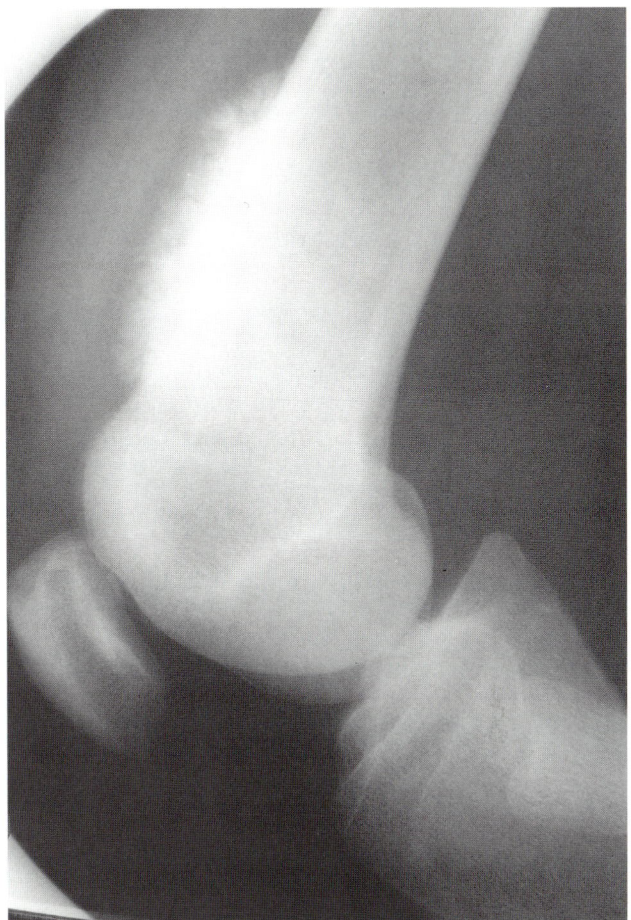

Fig. 9.49

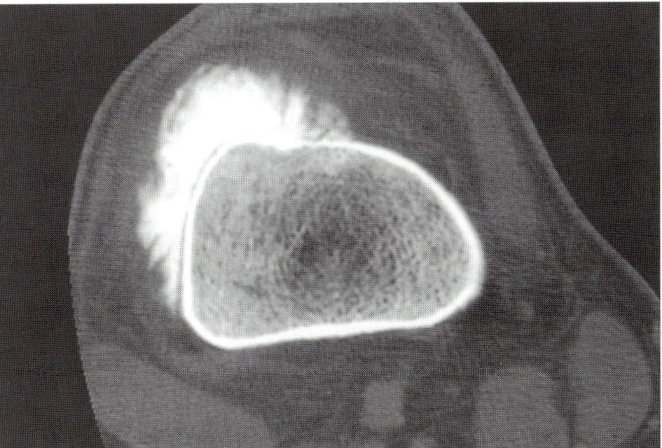

Fig. 9.50

Figs 9.49–9.54 High-grade surface osteosarcoma of the femur. On CT scan, the medullary cavity is uninvolved. A 3-D CT was performed. Gross examination and high-definition radiography show a surface tumor. Histology exhibits an osteoblastic cellular component, ruling out a parosteal osteosarcoma (polarized light).

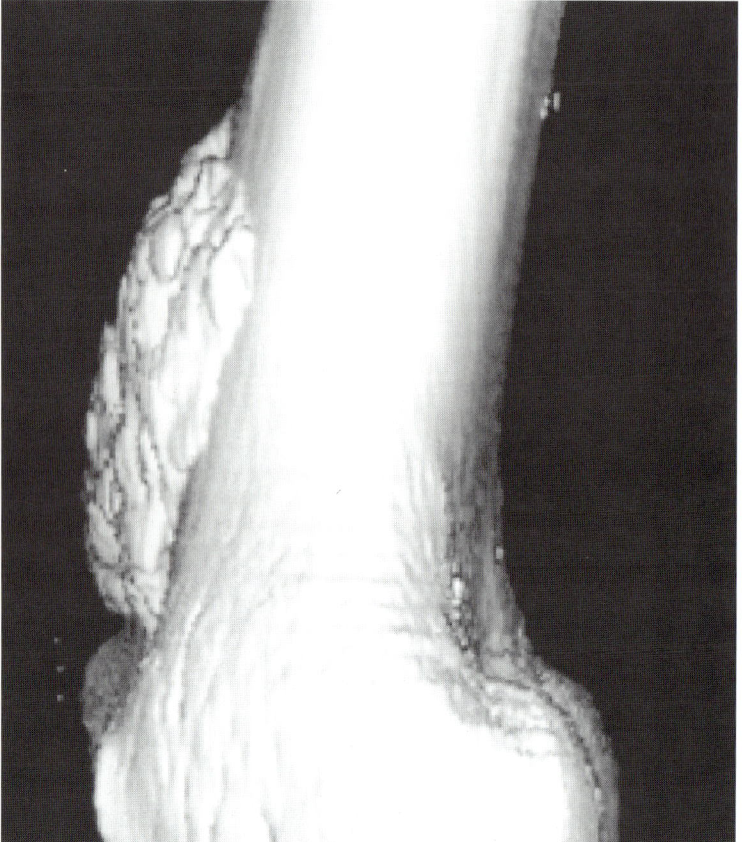

Fig. 9.51

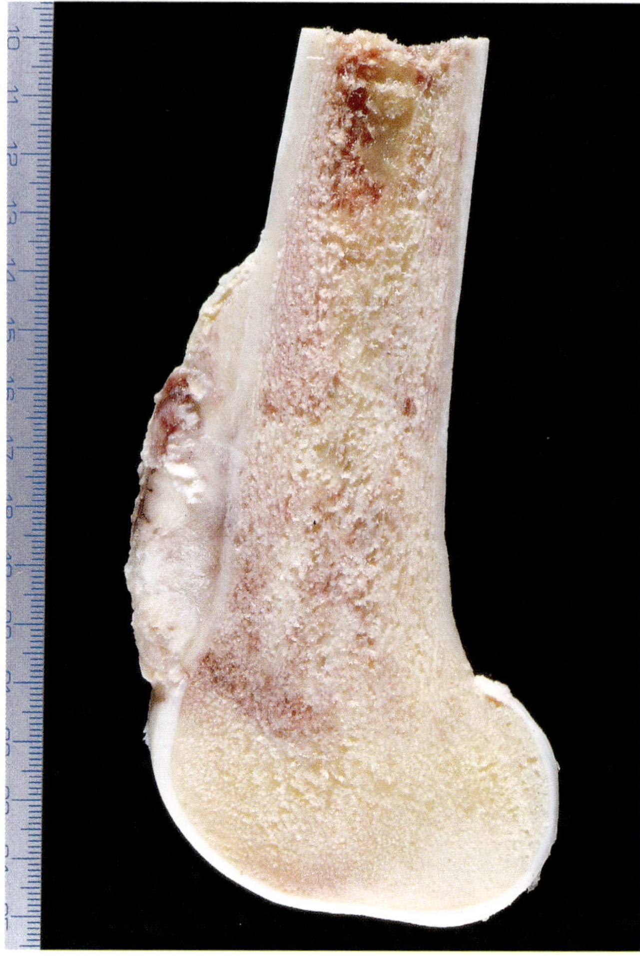

Fig. 9.52

are confined to the cortex with no involvement of the medullary canal or the soft tissues. They are predominantly located in the diaphysis of long bones of the lower extremities (femur, tibia). On X-ray, they appear as an intracortical lucency of 1–7 cm surrounded by thickened bone[91,95] and may be confused with an osteoid osteoma, an osteoblastoma, a non-ossifying fibroma or even a Brodie abscess (Fechner & Mills 1993). The progression to typical osteosarcoma may be rapid,[92] with extension to the soft tissues and the medullary cavity.[97] An intracortical small cell osteosarcoma has been described.[98]

Surface osteosarcomas[99,100] comprise periosteal lesions, originating from the deep layer of the periosteum, and parosteal lesions arising from the outer fibrous layer.[101]

The rarest variety is a high-grade osteosarcoma (0.6% of all osteosarcomas,[102]) (Figs 9.47–9.54). In long bones, common locations are diaphyseal or diaphyseal-metaphyseal, involving mostly the distal femur[103] followed by the humerus.[104] They appear as a partially mineralized mass, more dense close to the cortex, with variable periosteal reactions. MRI shows the lack of marrow involvement and CT the matrix calcifications and periosteal new bone formation.[105]

Grossly, they are bulky, multilobulated tumors attached to the outer cortical surface by a broad base, with superficial or absent cortical destruction.[102]

Histologically, the tumors exhibit microscopic involvement of the medullary cavity in more than one-third of cases.[104]

One has to exclude dedifferentiated parosteal osteosarcomas, periosteal osteosarcomas or even extraosseous osteosarcomas.[106] The spread, metastases and treatment are the same as for typical osteosarcomas. An unusual case has been reported at the site of a previously treated aneurysmal bone cyst.[107]

Periosteal osteosarcoma has been established as a distinct clinicopathologic entity by Unni et al[108] after the description of Lichtenstein in 1955[109] (Figs 9.55–9.58). It accounts for 1.5–2% of all osteosarcomas, in patients with a mean age of 21 years and no sex predominance. Symptoms are pain, swelling, tenderness or a limb mass. The proximal diaphysis of long bones is involved,[110] with a predilection for the proximal tibia and femur.[111–114] Involvement of the flat bones is rare.[115–117] A bilateral metachronous periosteal osteosarcoma has been reported, involving the femur.[118]

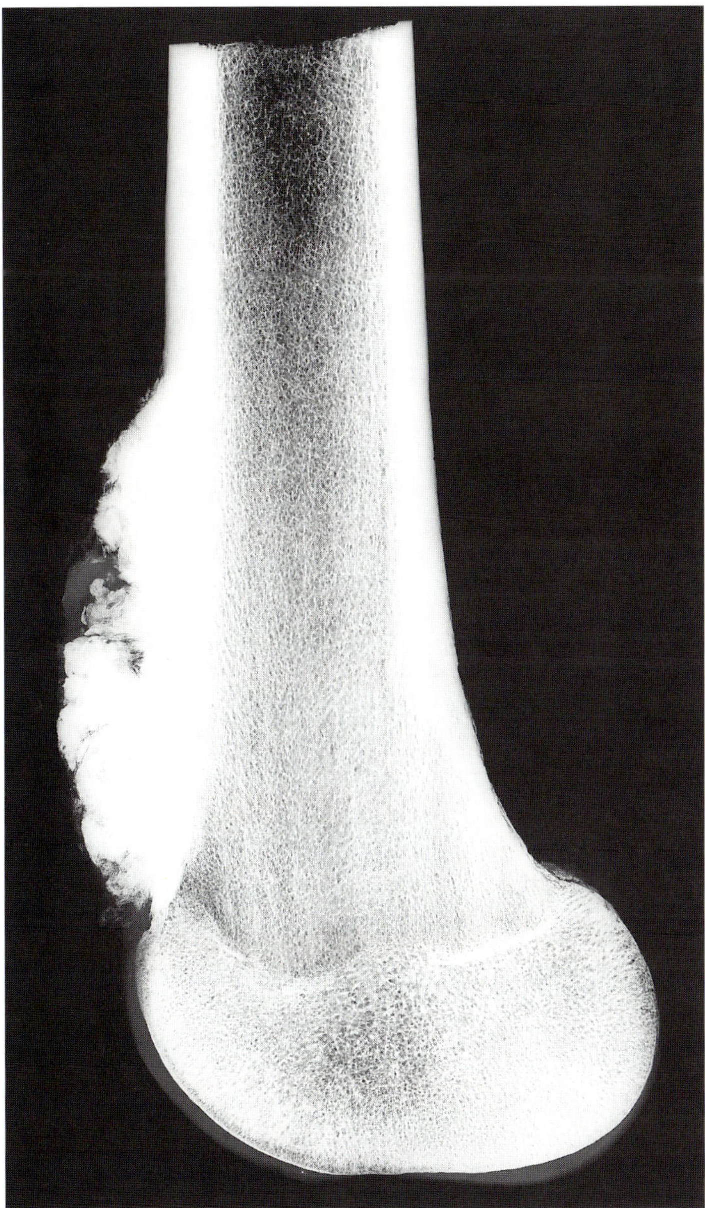

Fig. 9.53

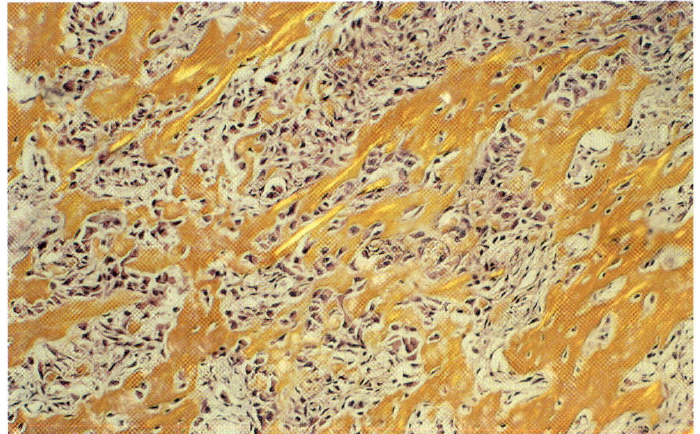

Fig. 9.54

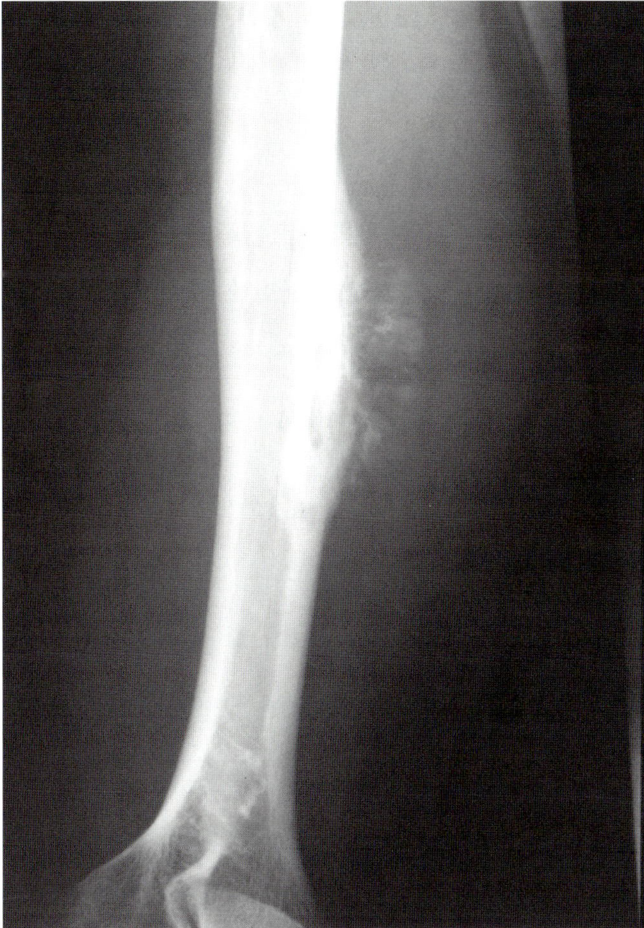

Fig. 9.55 Periosteal osteosarcoma of the humerus.

On X-ray, it appears as a radiolucent peripheral lesion with a more mineralized portion at the base. A spiculated pattern of calcifications is found, perpendicular to the long axis of bone,[110] or in some cases, stippled calcifications.[112] The underlying cortex is eroded or thickened with saucerization.[110] Codman triangles are not unusual.

On gross examination, a rounded or fusiform mass with a mean diameter of 10 cm is well demarcated by a fibrous capsule. Lobulated cartilage and spicules of bone are obvious.

Histologically, lace-like osteoid production is often very reduced. Chondroid areas are predominant, showing anaplastic peripheral spindle cells[108] and in the center, some areas of enchondral ossification. The periphery of the tumor is covered by the periosteum, with a proliferation of immature cells. Reactive periosteal bone produces broad spicules. Infiltration of the Haversian canals may occur, as well as bone marrow involvement.[111,112,119]

On ultrastructural examination, the tumor comprises most types of osteosarcoma cells[120] or mostly chondroblast-like cells.[121]

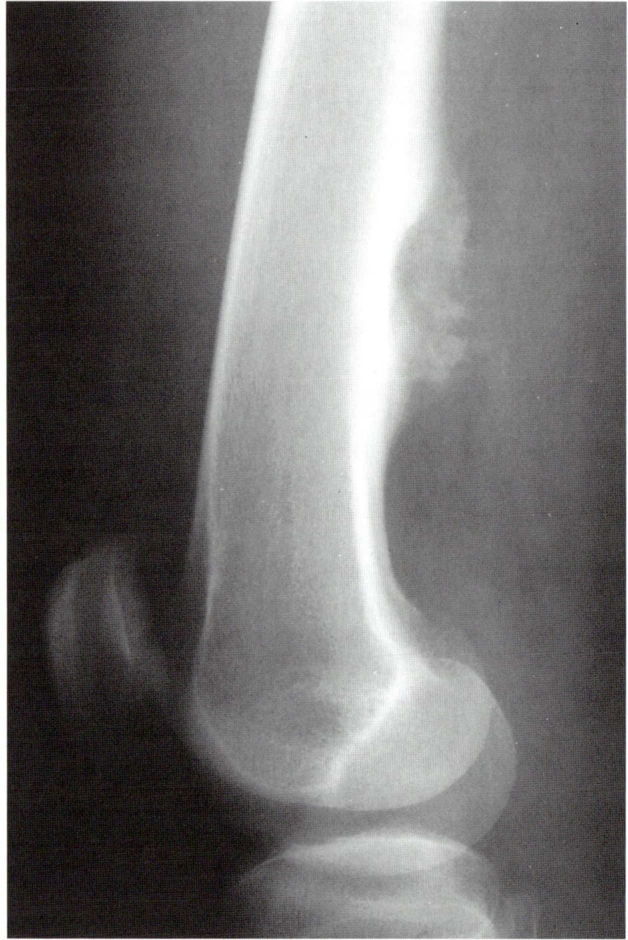

Fig. 9.56

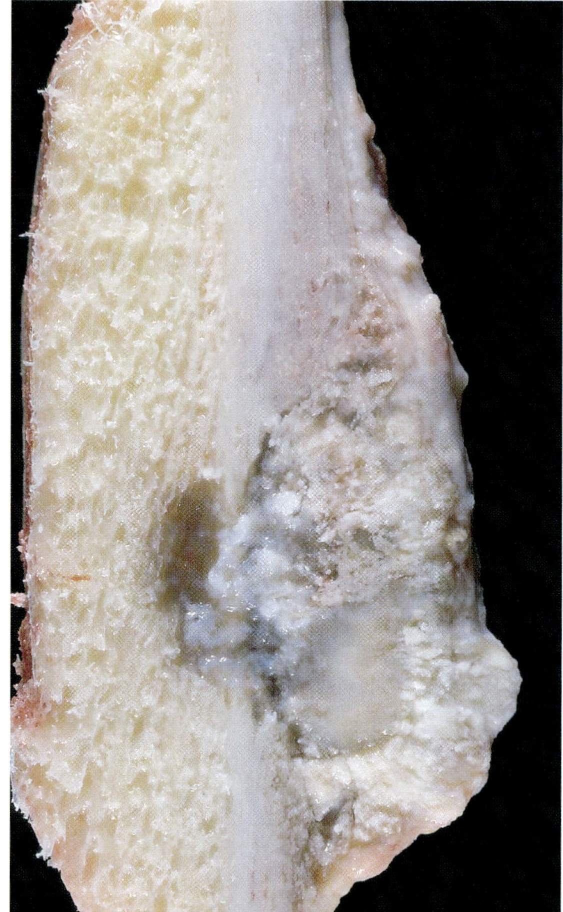

Fig. 9.57

Figs 9.56, 9.57 Periosteal osteosarcoma of the femur.

The treatment is wide surgical resection. There is a relatively high rate of recurrences (13%) and metastases (15–20%), chiefly involving the lungs. Medullary extension does not seem to herald a poor prognosis.[112]

The main differential diagnosis is from periosteal chondrosarcoma. This is found in older patients, in a metaphyseal location; it is less painful with a slower clinical course.[122] There is neither osteoid production nor brush-like reactive spicules, but granular or popcorn opacities may be seen on X-ray. They are larger, more rounded tumors and the lobular, well-differentiated cartilage is of grade I–II.[122] With a double immunostaining method, using proliferative cell nuclear antigen (PCNA) and S-100 protein, it has been shown very clearly that a periosteal osteosarcoma is a proliferation of osteoblastic cells while periosteal chondrosarcoma is composed of chondroblastic cells.[123]

Parosteal or juxtacortical osteosarcomas occur mostly in the second to fourth decades of life,[124] with an incidence of 5% of all osteosarcomas[125] and a slight female preponder-

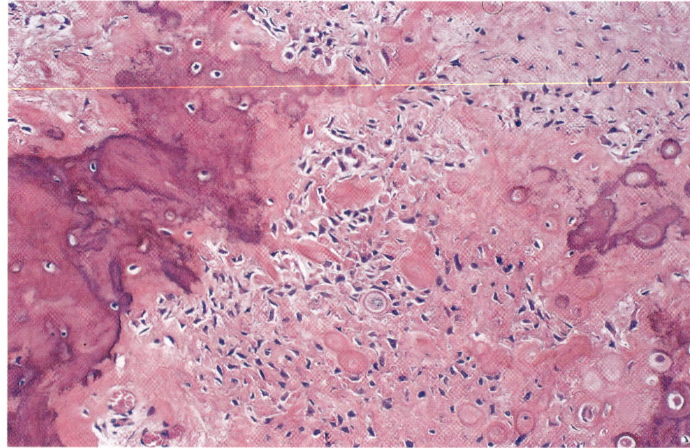

Fig. 9.58 Periosteal osteosarcoma: calcification of the cartilaginous component and spindle tumoral cells.

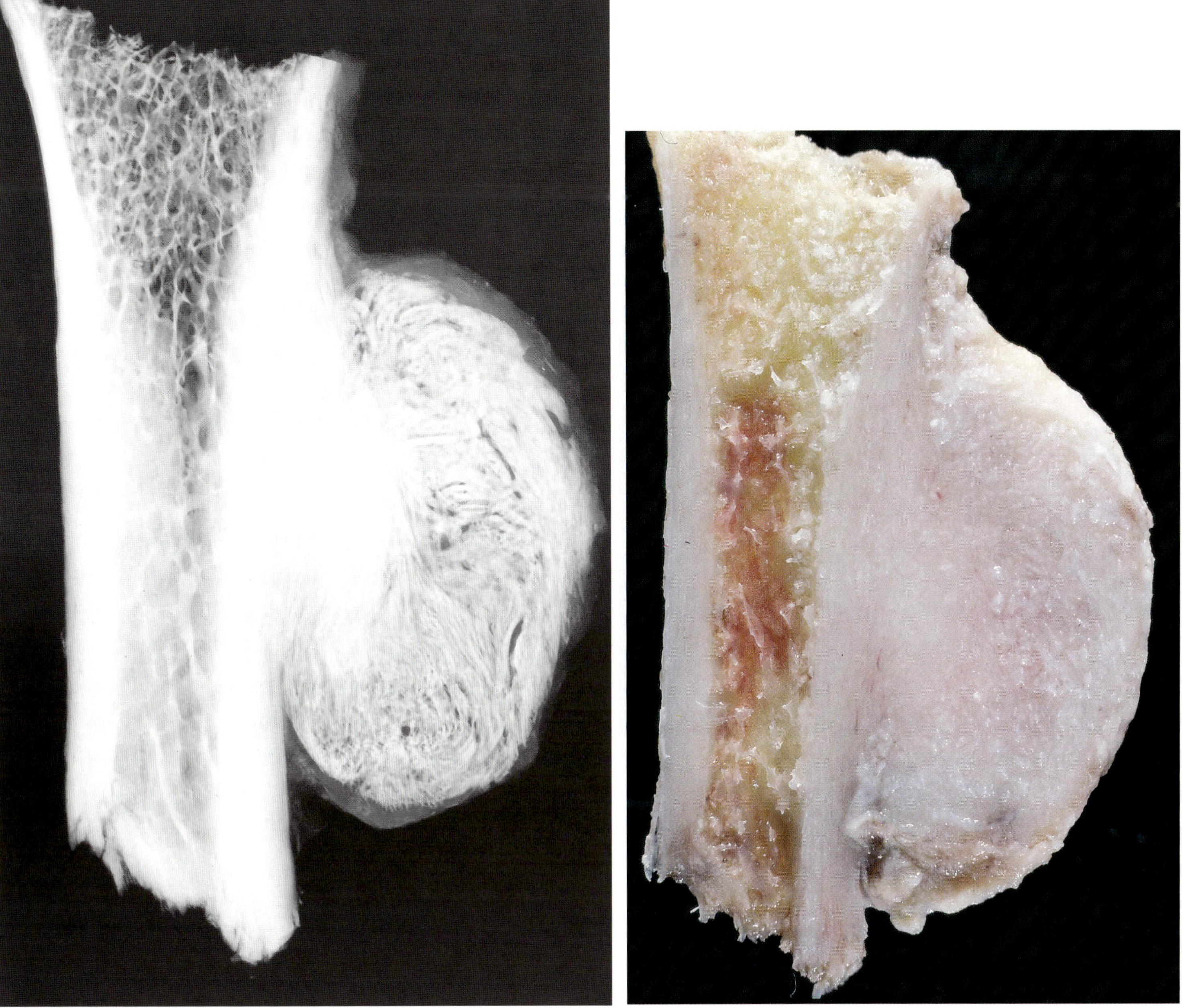

Fig. 9.59

Fig. 9.60

Figs 9.59, 9.60 Small parosteal osteosarcoma of the fibula exhibiting a steel-wool appearance of bone production, as described by Mirra.

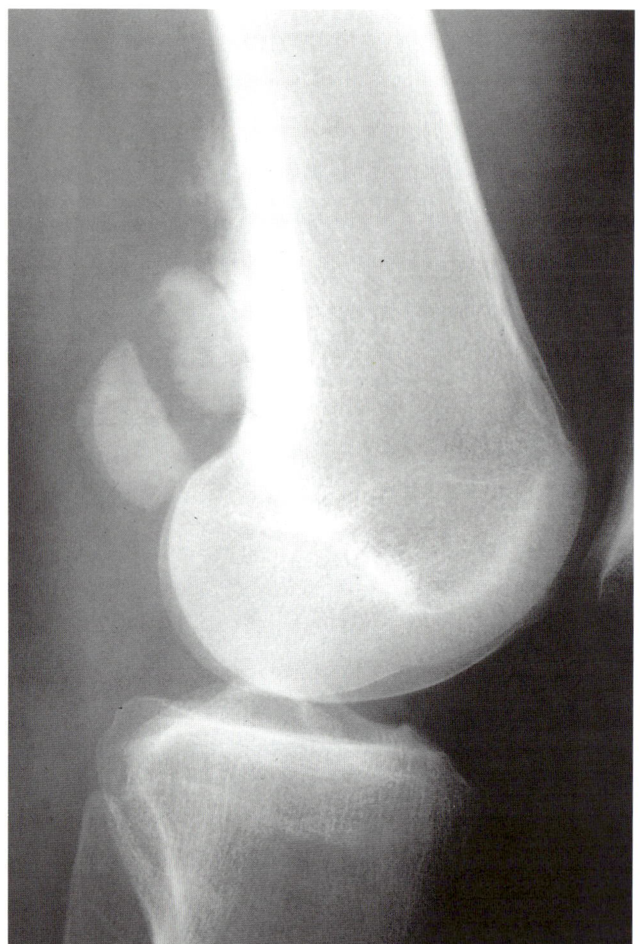

Fig. 9.61

Fig. 9.62

Figs 9.61, 9.62 Small parosteal osteosarcoma of the lower metaphysis of the femur.

ance.[124,126] The clinical course may take several years with pain, swelling, a palpable mass or some stiffness of the adjacent joint. Some cases are completely painless.[127] Parosteal osteosarcoma may be secondary to irradiation.[128]

In more than 70% of cases, the posterior aspect of the lower femoral shaft is involved.[124,129–131] In other long bones, the tumor is metaphyseal (proximal part of the tibia or humerus), rarely diaphyseal. Rare cases have been reported in the hand,[132,133] the foot[134] or in unusual locations such as the pubis.[135] A case has been described in soft tissue.[136]

On imaging, the tumor appears as an oval or spherical, dense, lobulated mass with a broad base (Figs 9.59–9.70); it is denser at the base and may exhibit some prominent sclerosis of the cortex.[137] There is no periosteal reaction. In more than half of the cases, a periosteal lucency or cleavage plane 1–3 mm wide is found between the tumor and the cortex, representing a periosteal thickening.[125] The lucency, best detected on CT, may become totally obliterated by the tumor.[137–139] The outer margins may be smooth or irregular and the tumor tends to grow circumferentially, with encirclement of the shaft in large lesions.[140]

Radiolucencies may be found in the mass in half of the cases:[141] radiolucent separation between lobules, peripheral radiolucencies corresponding to low-grade malignant tissue or fibrous tissue mixed with fat, deep radiolucencies corresponding to high-grade dedifferentiated areas.

Satellite lesions can be located in the soft tissues at initial presentation or in recurrences.[124,130]

On gross examination, parosteal osteosarcomas are large, sessile or, rarely, pedunculated with a mean length of 10 cm; they can reach massive proportions.[137] The ossified, hard, gritty, white tumors may have fibrous areas or a peripheral thin cartilaginous cap.[124,140] Rare tumors are cystic.[142,143]

Histologically (Figs 9.71–9.82), a hypocellular spindle cell stroma with minimal cytological atypia and rare mitoses is associated with long trabeculae of osteoid and woven bone. Streamers of disorganized woven bone may

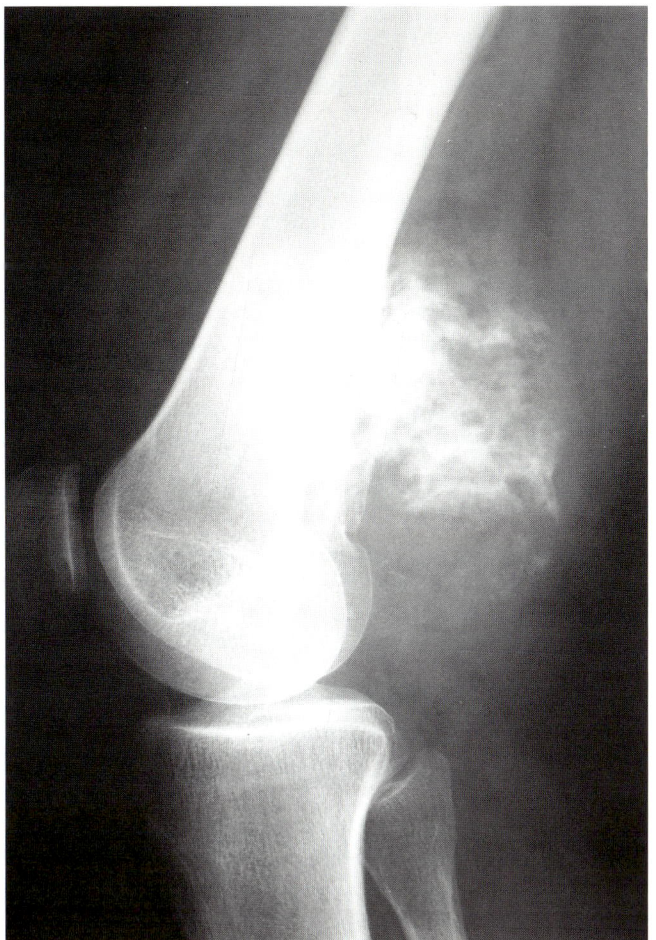

Fig. 9.63

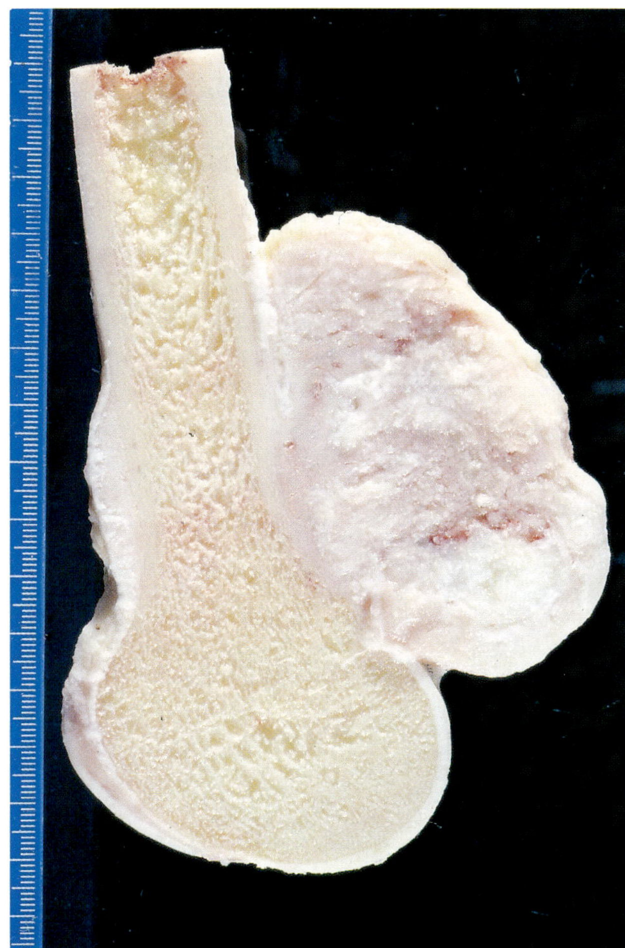

Fig. 9.64

Figs 9.63–9.65 Typical size of a parosteal osteosarcoma at initial presentation (lower end of femur).

merge with well-formed trabeculae with an occasional osteoblastic rimming, by a process of normalization,[100] and sometimes with a peculiar steel-wool appearance on X-ray (Mirra 1989). The calcified tissue with a lamellar structure may present cement lines, simulating Paget's disease.[125] Islands of low-grade tumoral cartilage are found in more than half of the cases, sometimes forming peripheral cartilaginous caps.

Rare cases may show nodular clusters of osteoclast-like giant cells not associated with areas of hemorrhage.[144] Some areas have a more pronounced cytological pleomorphism but anaplasia may only be found in the more cellular peripheral areas.[125] Near to the cortex, the well-differentiated tumoral bone is difficult to separate from reactive bone, on imaging[138] as well as on histology.[125]

A histological grading is given in some series, based either on cellularity, anaplasia and mitotic activity of the fibrous, osseous and cartilaginous components or on the fibrous and cartilaginous areas alone;[130,140,145–147] howev-

er, the system separating well-differentiated tumors, high-grade surface tumors and dedifferentiated areas is the most widely used.

A morphometric analysis of silver-stained nucleolar organizer regions (AgNOR) has shown a decrease in total AgNOR volume per nucleus and in the number of AgNOR per nucleus and an increase in single AgNOR volume compared with central osteosarcomas.[148]

Ultrastructurally, fibroblast-like cells and myofibroblasts are the main cell types.[121,149,150] A prominent fibrous lamina may be related to the slower progression of the tumor.[121] Large numbers of paracrystalline, undulating membranous structures in the nuclei have been reported.[151]

The cytogenetic findings show unusual supernumerary ring chromosomes[152,153] or telomeric association or fusion, also reported in a giant cell tumor with osteosarcomatous transformation, a giant cell variant of osteosarcoma and in giant cell tumors of bone.

The treatment is wide segmental resection and the sur-

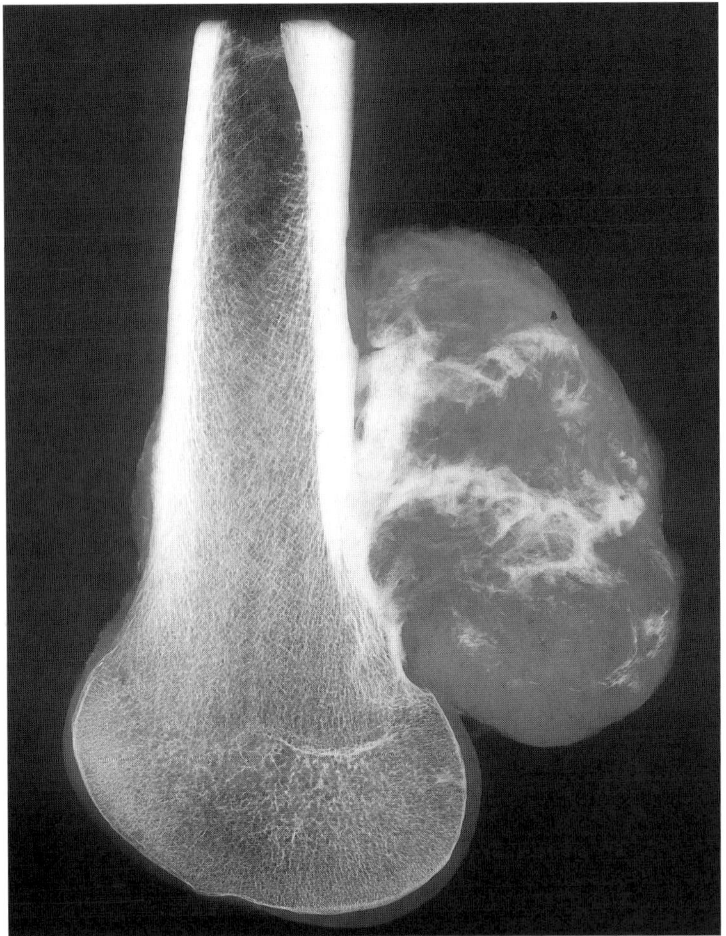

Fig. 9.65

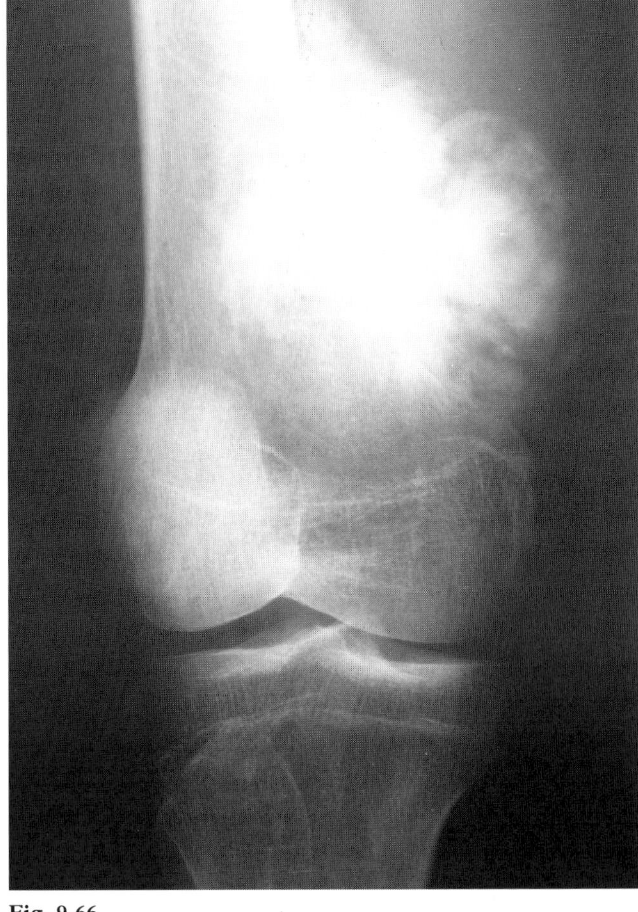

Fig. 9.66

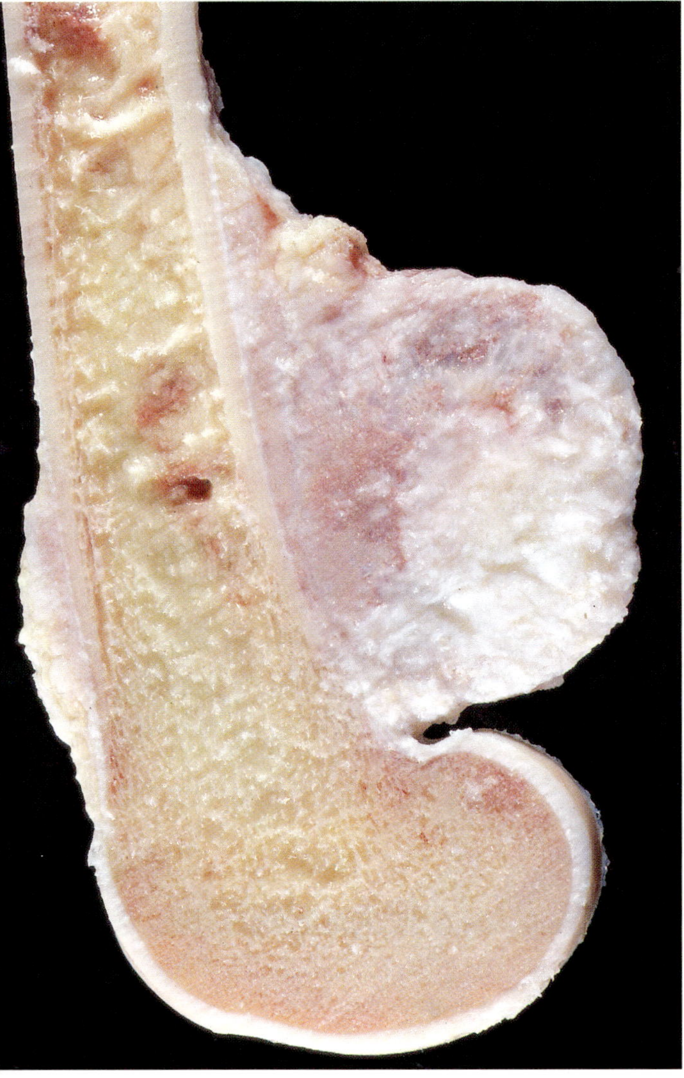

Fig. 9.67

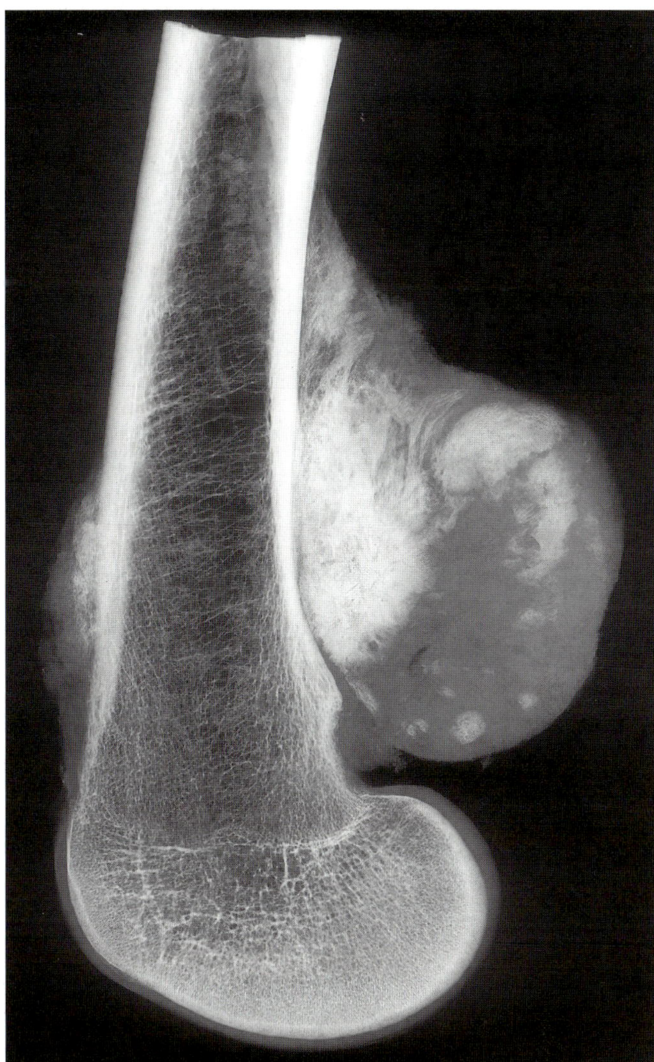

Fig. 9.68

Figs 9.66–9.68 Parosteal osteosarcoma of the femur encircling the femoral shaft.

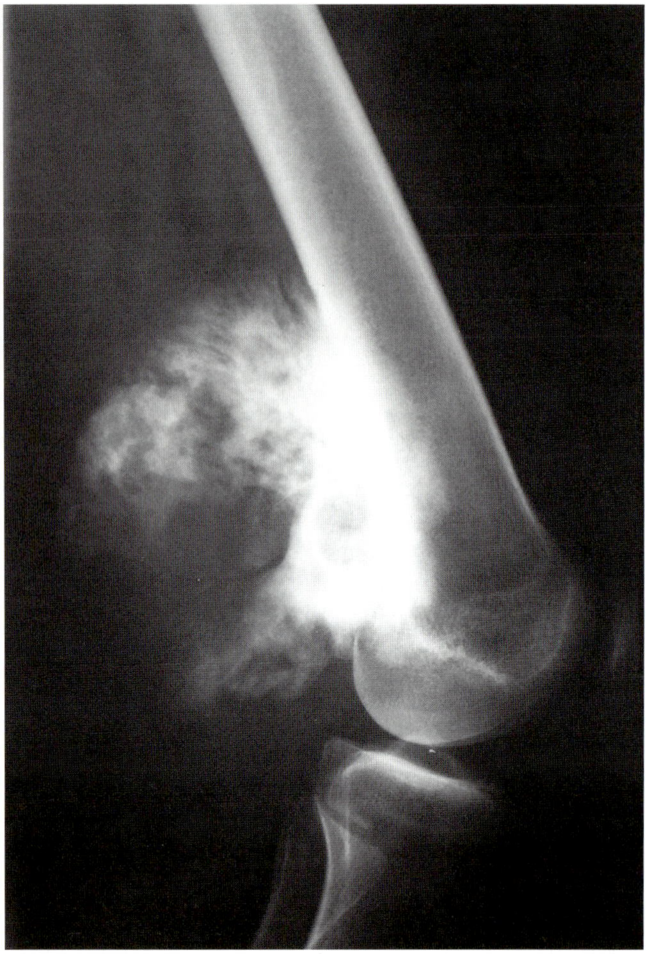

Fig. 9.69

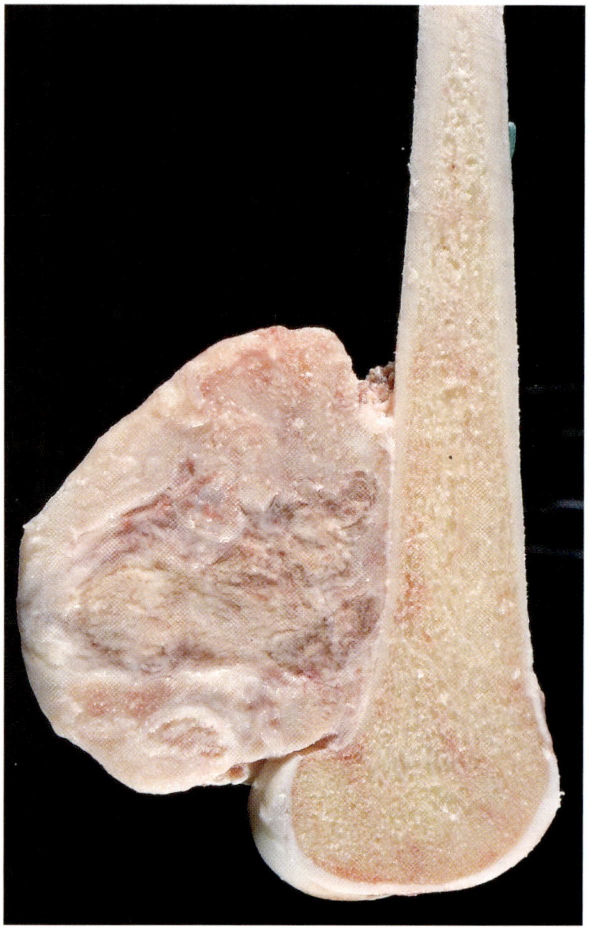

Fig. 9.70

Figs 9.69, 9.70 Large parosteal osteosarcoma of the femur exhibiting lucent areas (fibroblastic tumoral component).

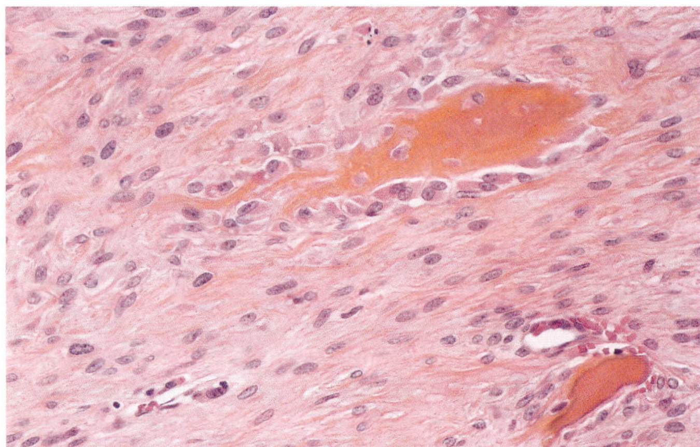

Fig. 9.71 Parosteal osteosarcoma: limited tumoral bone formation in a fibrous stroma mimicking fibrous dysplasia.

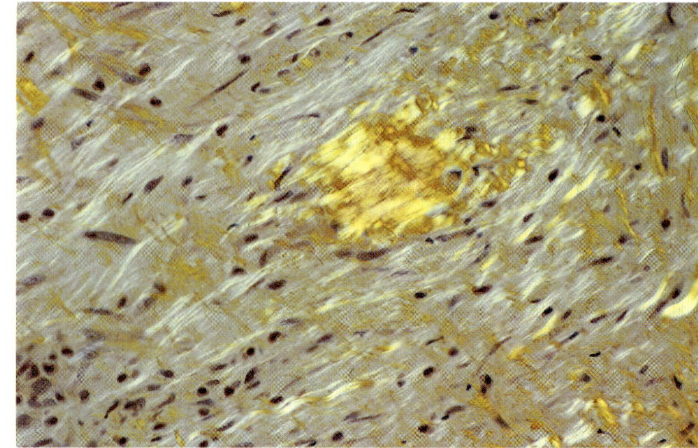

Fig. 9.72 Parosteal osteosarcoma: minute area of calcification of the collagen fibers in the fibrous stroma (polarized light).

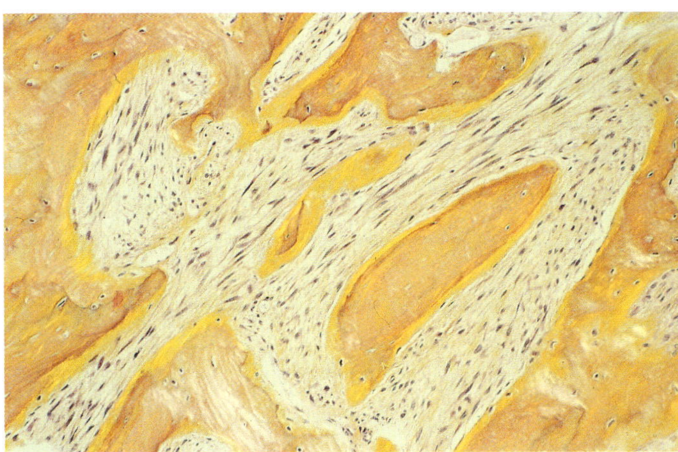

Fig. 9.73

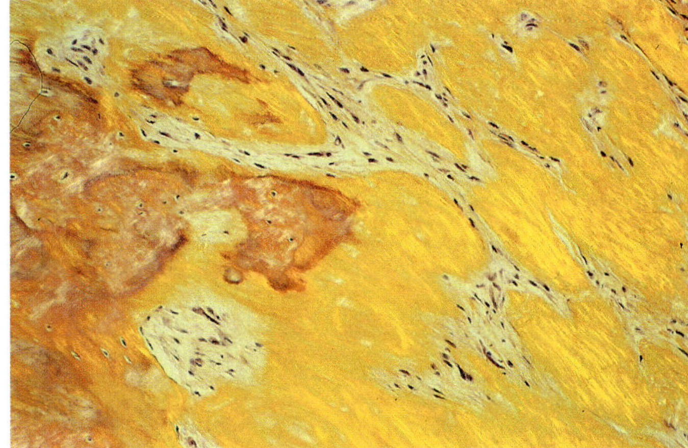

Fig. 9.74

Figs 9.73, 9.74 Woven bone formation in parosteal osteosarcoma (polarized light).

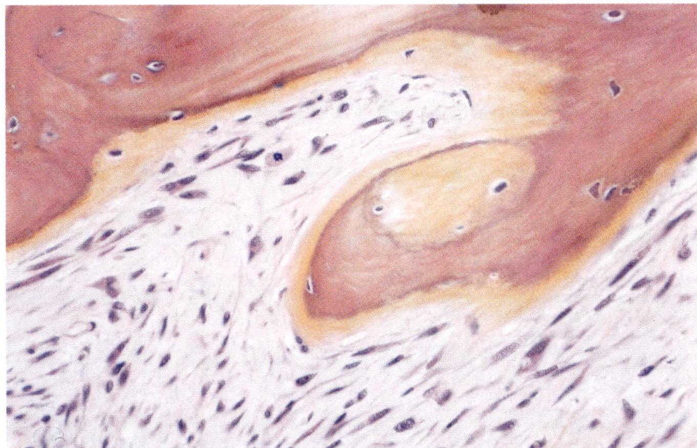

Fig. 9.75 Parosteal osteosarcoma: slight nuclear pleomorphism of the cellular component and rare normal mitotic figures.

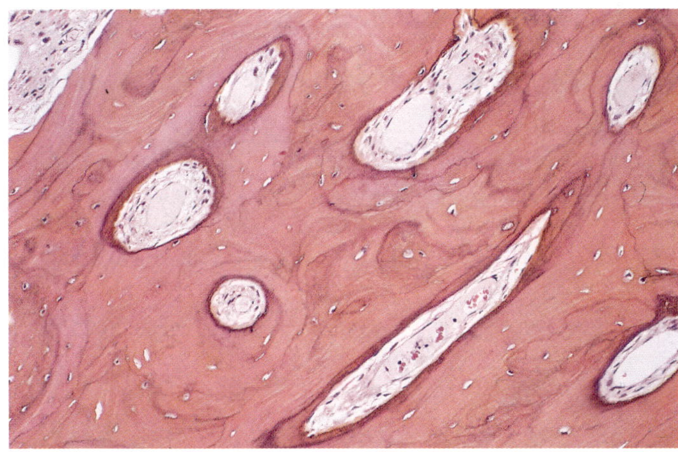

Fig. 9.76 Massive well-differentiated bone formation in a parosteal osteosarcoma.

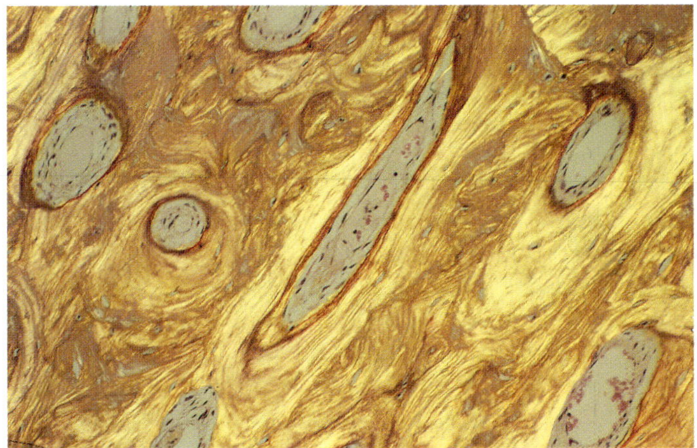

Fig. 9.77

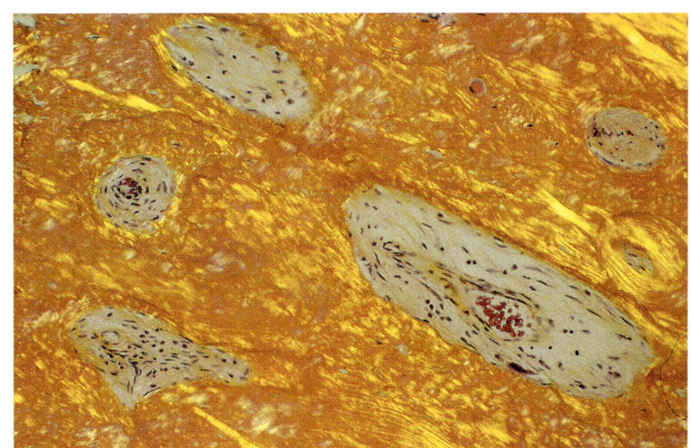

Fig. 9.78

Figs 9.77, 9.78 Parostal osteosarcoma: fields of tumoral bone on polarization study.

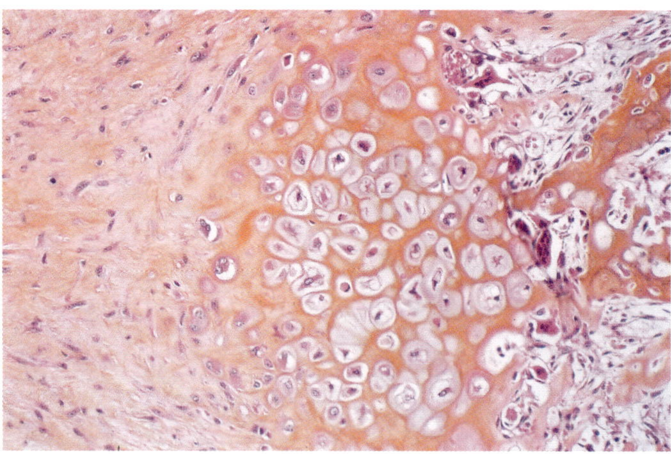

Fig. 9.79

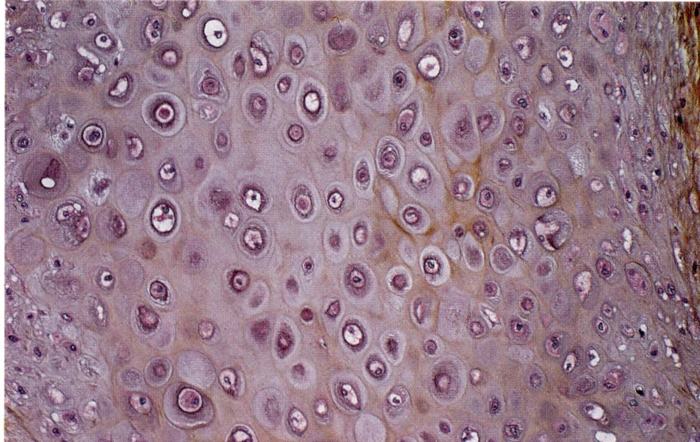

Fig. 9.80

Figs 9.79, 9.80 Peripheral cartilaginous component of parosteal osteosarcomas.

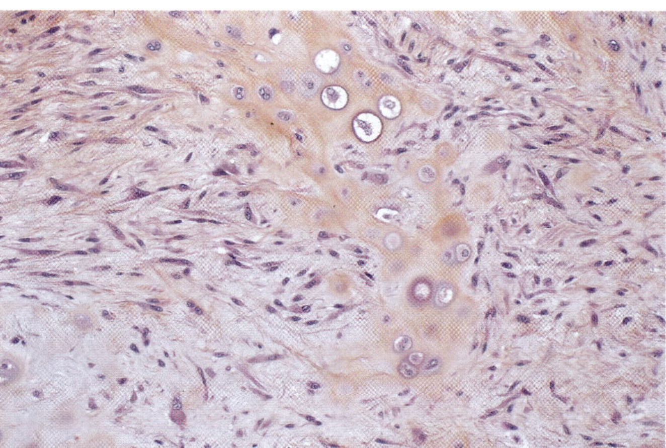

Fig. 9.81

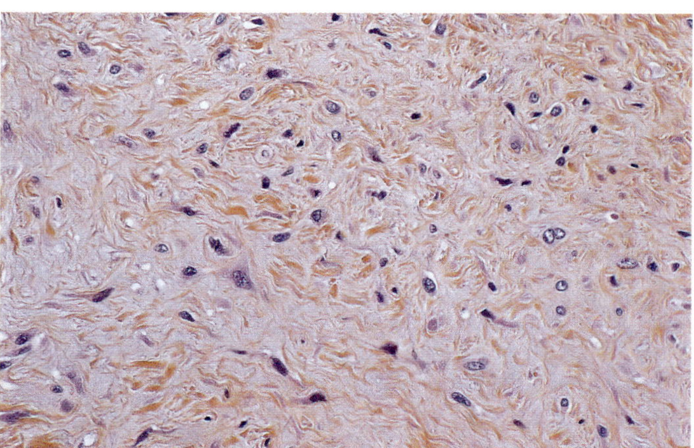

Fig. 9.82

Figs 9.81, 9.82 Peripheral areas of parosteal osteosarcomas: cartilaginous and spindle cell proliferation.

vival rate is 80% of cases at 10 years.[125] Metastases are found, usually in the lungs, with either low-grade or low- and high-grade components.[100,154] Medullary involvement, found in 28% of cases at the Mayo Clinic, is not correlated with local recurrences or metastases if the tumor is well differentiated.[124–126,139,155,156]

The risk of metastasis is linked to the dedifferentiation of the tumor, occurring in 20–33% of cases as a primary manifestation or on recurrences of dedifferentiation.[157–161] Clinical symptoms are severe pain and rapid growth.[158] On X-ray, the dedifferentiated areas correspond to deep lytic defects or amorphous and irregular calcifications; CT is useful for detecting these,[138,139] as well as the more frequent medullary involvement (43%,[125]), but there may be some false-positive results.[162] The dedifferentiated areas are hypervascularized on arteriograms.[100] Aneuploidy has been demonstrated.[163] The treatment is preoperative chemotherapy followed by surgery and adjuvant chemotherapy, but there is no change in the low-grade component.[139]

The main differential diagnosis of a parosteal osteosarcoma is an intraosseous well-differentiated osteosarcoma (Figs 9.83, 9.84), but this usually has a major medullary component. Extension into the medullary cavity, if it is less than 25%,[125] does not rule out a diagnosis of parosteal osteosarcoma.[156] The spindle cell stroma is the clue to excluding very rare osteomas or the more common reactive periosteal bone formations.

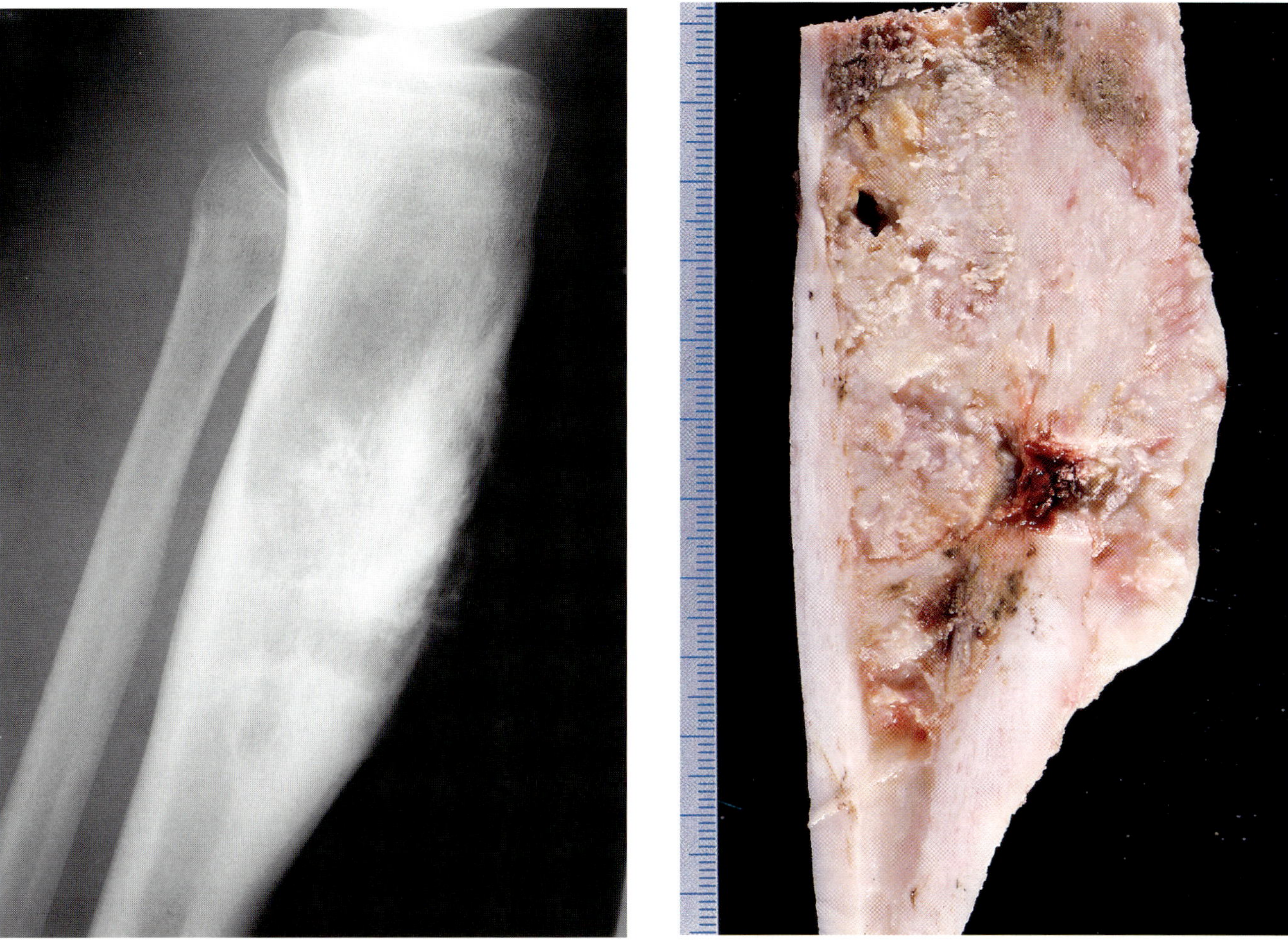

Fig. 9.83   **Fig. 9.84**

Figs 9.83, 9.84 Well-differentiated osteosarcoma of the tibia: imaging, gross pathology and histology do not resolve whether this is a surface tumor or an intramedullary sarcoma with prominent soft tissue extension.

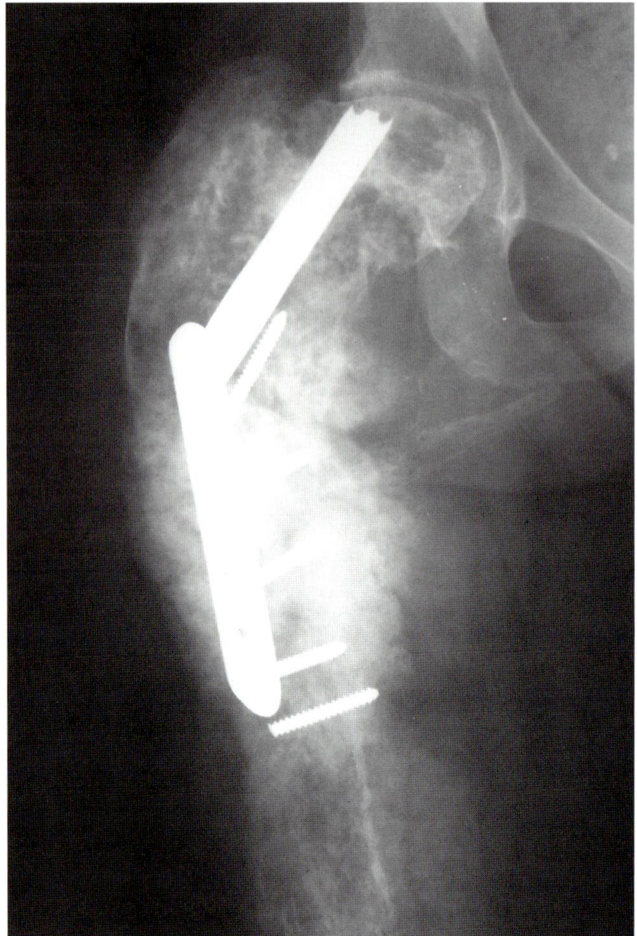

Fig. 9.85

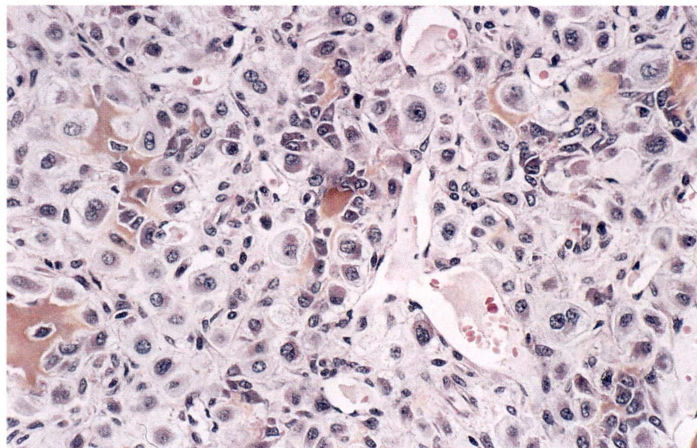

Fig. 9.86

Figs 9.85, 9.86 Osteosarcoma occurring in fibrous dysplasia of the femur.

OSTEOSARCOMATOSIS

An uncommon entity is the rapid, simultaneous and usually symmetrical appearance of osteosarcomas of histologically analogous stage[164] (1.5% of all osteosarcomas), first described by Silverman.[165] Various attempts have been made to classify the clinical patterns,[166–168] synchronous and asynchronous types having markedly different clinical courses.

Young patients with rapidly appearing sclerotic synchronous lesions have a poor prognosis, as do tumors in adults. Early or late lytic or blastic metachronous lesions in adults have a longer survival,[169,170] representing late metastases or possible new primary sarcomas.[168,171]

A possible mechanism for multiple osteosarcomas with no evidence of pulmonary metastases may be spread via the vertebral venous plexus system.[172–177] For many authors, osteosarcomatosis is a manifestation of a metastatic disease; most patients present a dominant skeletal tumor[176–180] with skeletal metastases occurring prior to pulmonary metastases[172] or being detected concurrently or earlier in the course of the disease.[181]

An unusual miliary osteosarcomatosis has been described.[175]

SECONDARY OSTEOSARCOMAS

Osteosarcomas have been reported as a secondary lesion in many conditions, but chiefly in the course of fibrous dysplasia, Paget's disease and radiation therapy.

Osteosarcomas in fibrous dysplasia occur in monostotic and polyostotic forms,[182,183] with a frequency of 0.5%[184] to 2.5%[185] (Figs 9.85, 9.86). Some tumors are radiation induced. Without radiation, the interval between the diagnosis of fibrous dysplasia and that of a sarcoma ranges from 2 to 30 years.[185,186] The prognosis is poor.

Osteosarcomas in Paget's disease (Figs 9.87–9.92) are slightly more frequent in men than in women; the mean age at diagnosis is 64 years,[187] with an incidence of 1%.[188] In most cases, they are found in polyostotic dis-

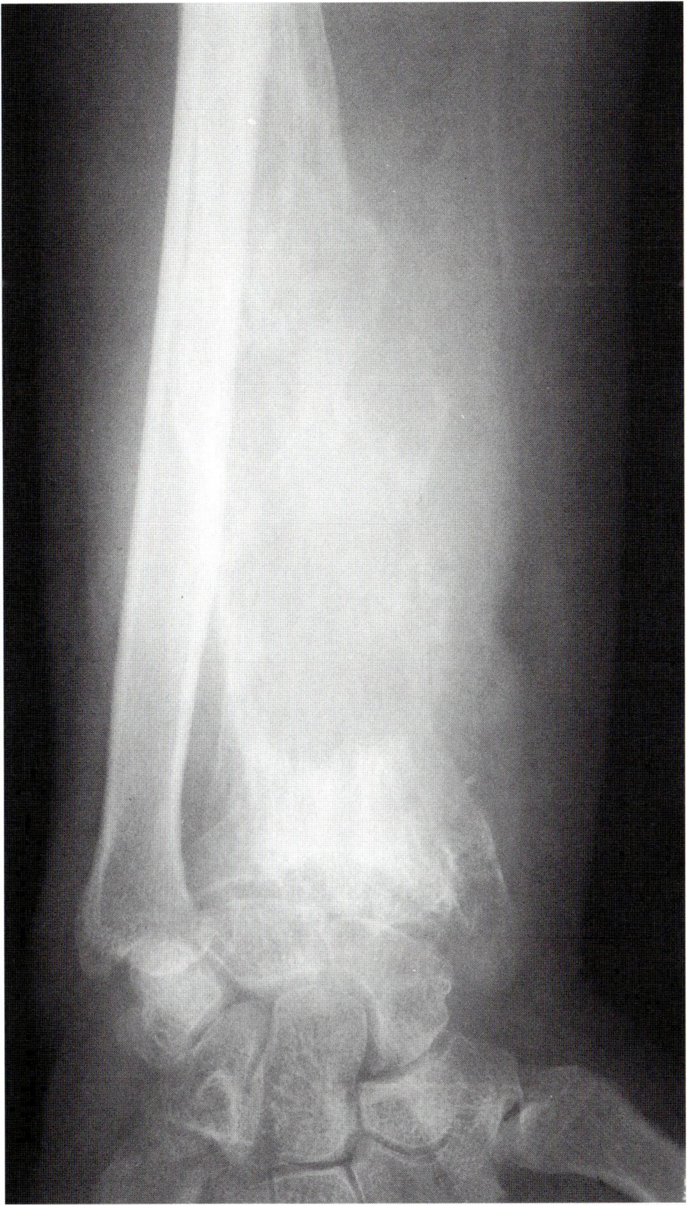

Fig. 9.87

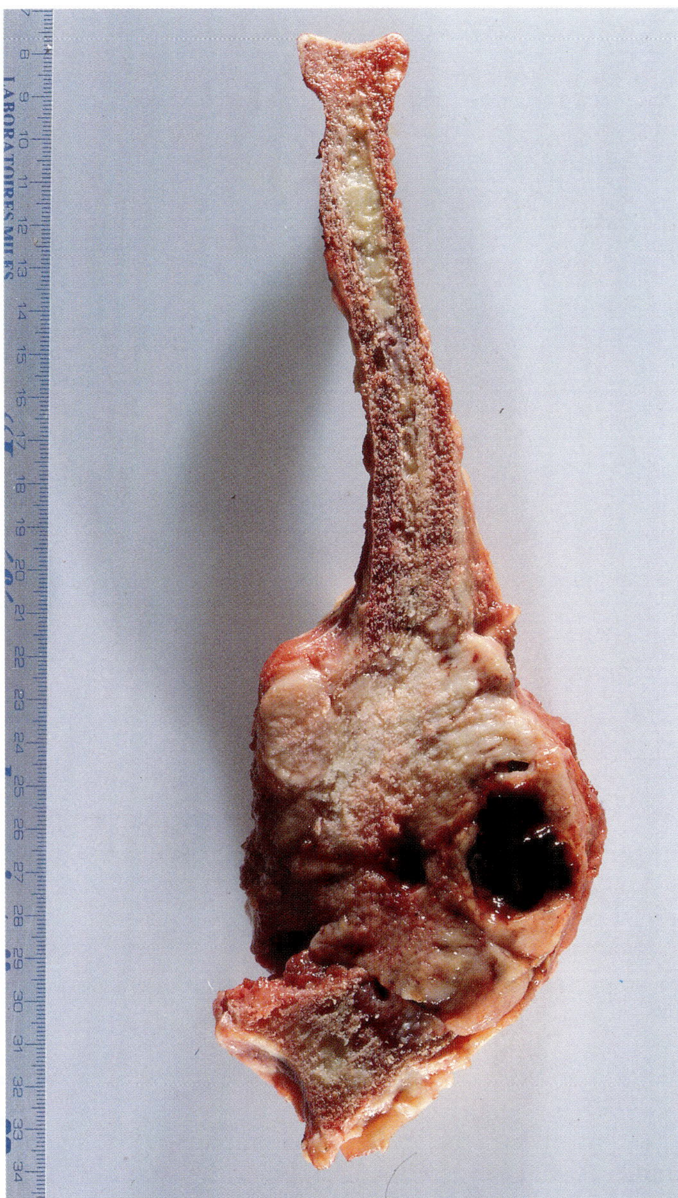

Fig. 9.88

Figs 9.87, 9.88 Osteosarcoma occurring in Paget's disease of the radius.

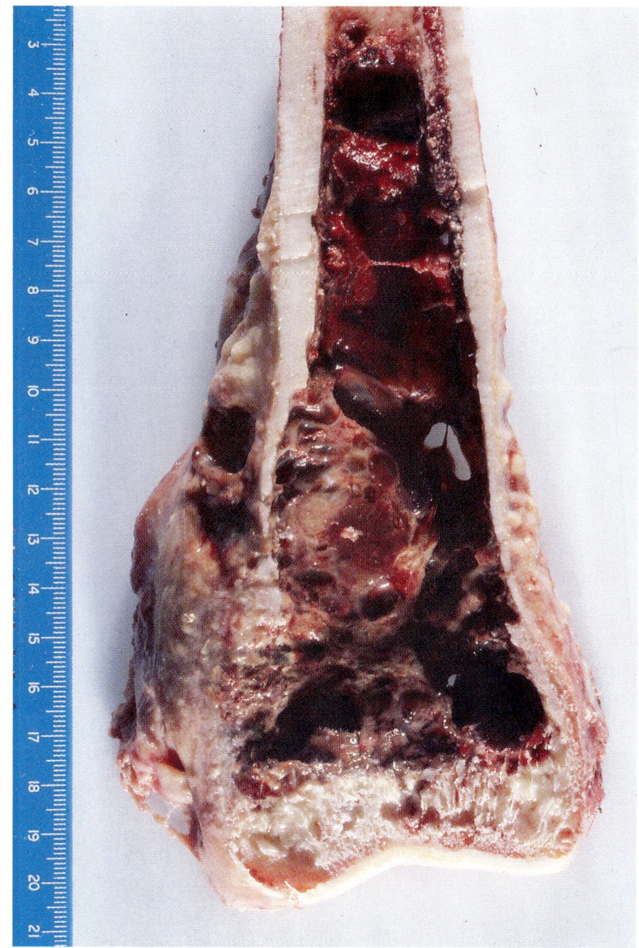

Fig. 9.89 Telangiectatic osteosarcoma occurring in Paget's disease of the femur.

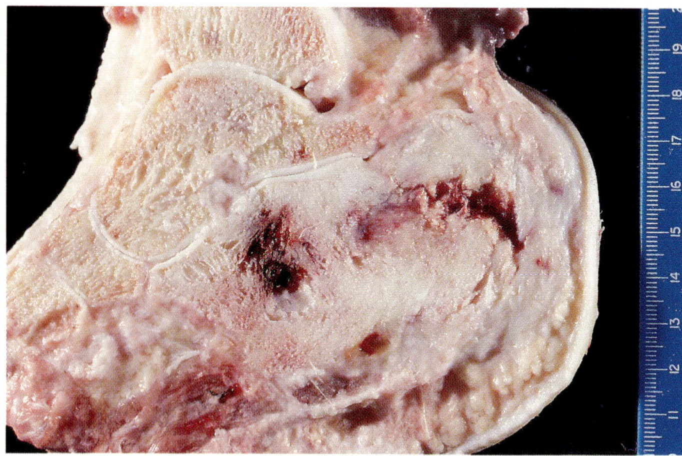

Fig. 9.90 Osteosarcoma occurring in Paget's disease of the calcaneus.

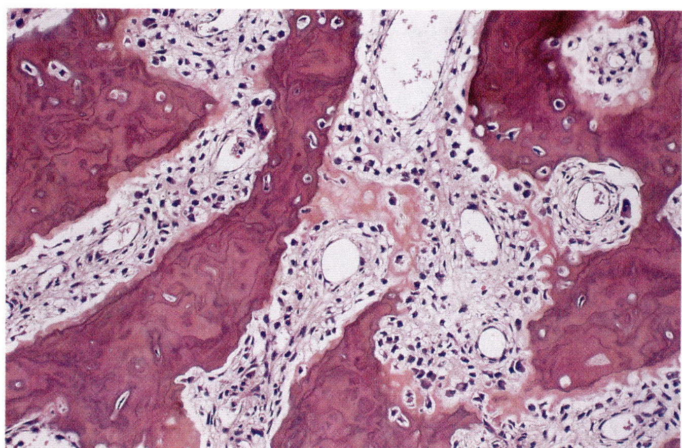

Fig. 9.91 Osteosarcoma invading pagetic bone.

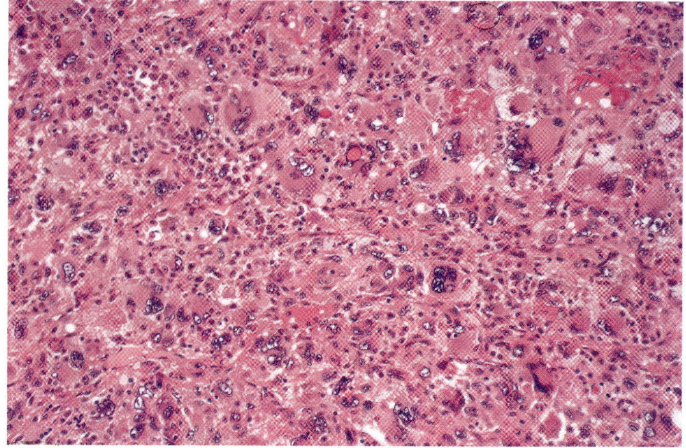

Fig. 9.92 Giant cell-rich osteosarcoma in Paget's disease.

ease, involving the pelvis and sacrum, the femur, humerus, tibia and craniofacial bones.[187,189] The 5-year survival is only 10% in the experience of the Mayo Clinic.

The risk of induction of an *osteosarcoma by radiation* is very low (0.02–0.8%,[190]), with an absorbed dose ranging from 4000 to 7000 rads,[191] but it is the second most common secondary bone sarcoma, following Paget's sarcoma,[192] and mostly found in the sixth decade of life (Figs 9.93–9.96).

Irradiation is usually given for malignant entities: carcinomas of the breast, uterus, cervix,[193] lymphomas[189] or, in children, Ewing's sarcomas, retinoblastomas or Hodgkin's disease.[194–196] Typical locations are the pelvis and shoulder regions.[192,195,197]

Criteria for a radiation-induced sarcoma have been defined by Cahan et al[198] and modified by Arlen et al:[199] tumors occurring in an irradiated field, histologic or radiologic evidence of the preexisting condition of bone, latent period of 3–4 years, histological proof of the osteosarcoma

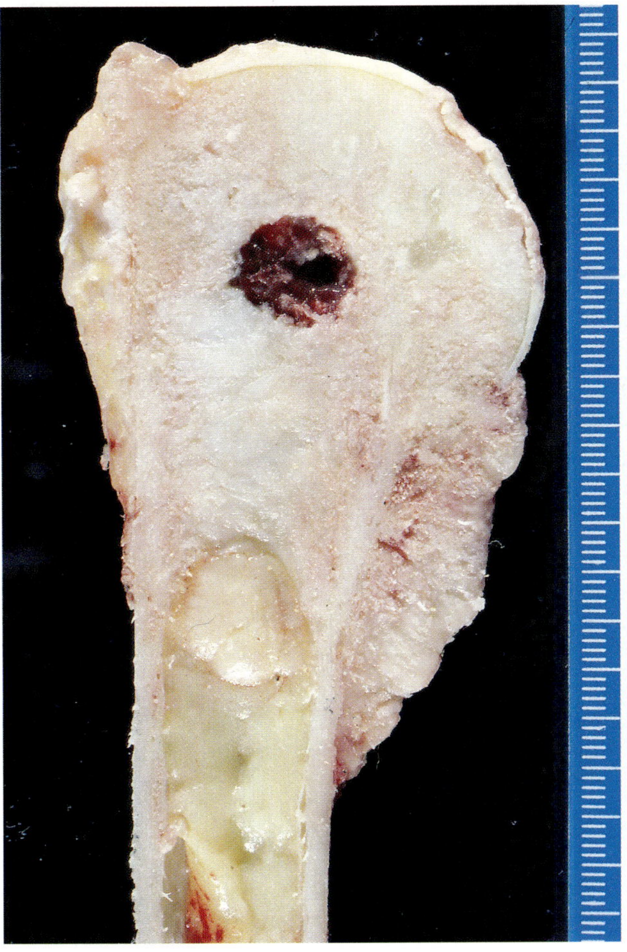

Fig. 9.93 Radiation-induced humeral osteosarcoma (irradiation of a breast carcinoma).

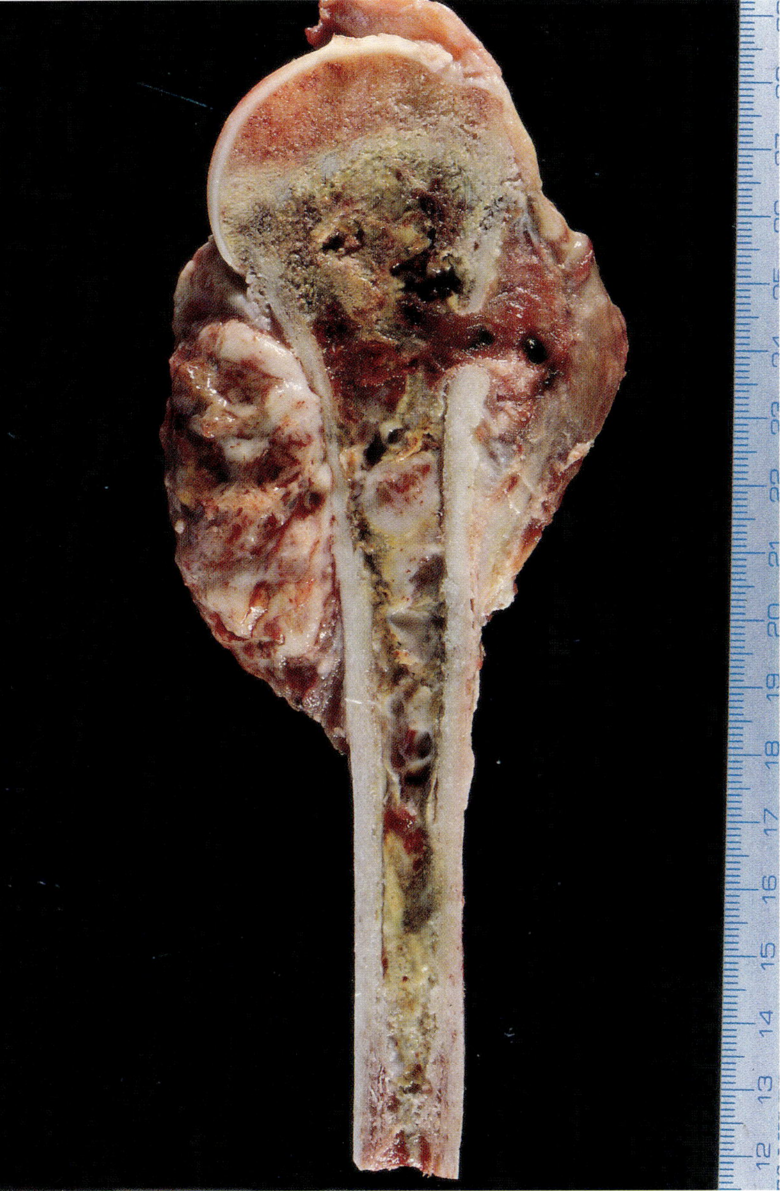

Fig. 9.94 Radiation-induced humeral osteosarcoma (irradiation of a breast carcinoma, with a latent period of 20 years).

and preexisting osteitis. The median latent period is 11 years. A radiation osteitis is demonstrated in 50–60% of cases,[200,201] but may be impossible to identify,[195] especially on histology, as it is destroyed by the expanding tumor.

A multicentric radiation-induced osteosarcoma has been reported.[202] A cytogenetic analysis has shown complex karyotypic changes including deletion of chromosome 13.[203]

The prognosis is poor, with an overall survival rate of 10–30%.[204] Locations in the vertebral column, pelvis and shoulder girdle have the worst prognosis.[205] Osteosarcomas may be induced by *Thorotrast administration*, with a mean latent period of 26 years.[206] Thorotrast particles within the immediate area of the tumor are demonstrated by autoradiography, scanning and transmission electron microscopy, but chiefly by X-ray spectrometry.[207]

Osteosarcomas in *constitutional diseases* such as: osteogenesis imperfecta,[208–212] osteopetrosis,[213] melorrheostosis[214] and osteopoikilosis are presumably unrelated lesions.[215]

Osteosarcomas and *non-ossifying fibromas* are also inde-

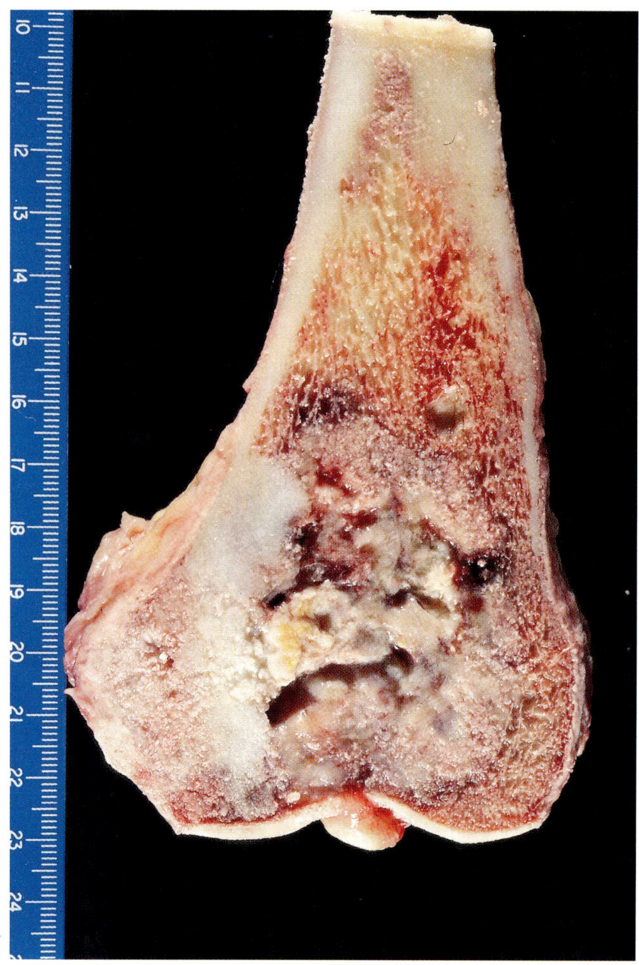

Fig. 9.95 Radiation-induced femoral osteosarcoma after irradiation of an osteoid osteoma.

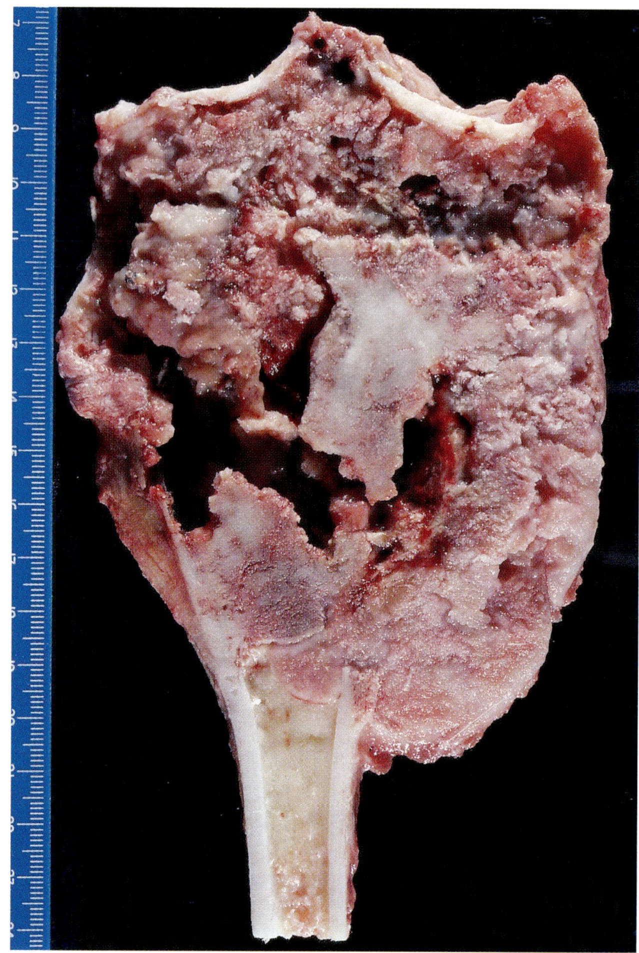

Fig. 9.96 Radiation-induced tibial osteosarcoma after irradiation of an aneurysmal bone cyst.

pendent lesions.[216] Osteosarcomas have been reported in enchondromas,[217] enchondromatosis, osteochondromas[218,219] and osteochondromatosis.[220]

Osteosarcomas developing on *bone infarcts* are rare[221–224] and survival is poor, with more than 70% succumbing.[222]

In *children*, some malignancies (retinoblastoma and Wilms' tumor) predispose to osteosarcoma without radiation therapy,[190] but radiation shortens the interval to second malignant tumor.[225] Osteosarcoma is the most frequent secondary malignant tumor in children[226] and the prevalence is increasing with longer survival times. Chemotherapy may also have some effect on the induction of a secondary bone sarcoma.[193,227]

REFERENCES

1. Schajowicz F, De Prospero J D, Cosentino E. Case report 641. Chondroblastoma-like osteosarcoma. Skeletal Radiol 1990: 19: 603–606
2. Raymond A K, Murphy G F, Rosenthal D I. Case report 425. Chondroblastic osteosarcoma: clear cell variant of femur. Skeletal Radiol 1987: 16: 336–341
3. Povysil C, Matejowski Z, Zidkova H. Osteosarcoma with a clear-cell component. Virchows Arch A Pathol Anat Histopathol 1988: 412: 273–279
4. Otsuka T, Matsui N, Ohta H, Hattori M, Nakamura T. Osteosarcoma with deeply eosinophilic rhabdomyoblast cells in a lung metastatic focus. A case report. Clin Orthop 1993: 293: 307–309
5. Hasegawa T, Shibata T, Hirose T, Seki K, Hizawa K. Osteosarcoma with epithelioid features. An immunohistochemical study. Arch Pathol Lab Med 1993: 117: 295–298
6. Bathurst N, Sanerkin N, Watt I. Osteoclast-rich osteosarcoma. Br J Radiol 1986: 59: 667–673
7. Sundaram M, Martin A S, Tayob A A. Case report 182. Osteosarcoma arising in giant cell tumor of tibia. Skeletal Radiol 1982: 7: 282–285
8. Kenan S, Abdelwahab I F, Klein M J, Lewis M M. Case report 863. Osteosarcoma associated with giant cell tumor. Skeletal Radiol 1995: 24: 55–58
9. Kim H, Park C, Lee Y B, Jin S Y, Ro J Y, Ayala A G. Case report 643. Osteosarcoma of ribs with giant rosettoid structures. Skeletal Radiol 1990: 19: 609–612
10. Sim F H, Unni K K, Beabout J W, Dahlin D C. Osteosarcoma

with small cells simulating Ewing's tumor. J Bone Joint Surg (Am) 1979: 61: 207–215

11. Edeiken J, Raymond A K, Ayala A G, Benjamin R S, Murray J A, Carrasco HC. Small-cell osteosarcoma. Skeletal Radiol 1987: 16: 621–628

12. Ayala A G, Ro J Y, Raymond A K et al. Small cell osteosarcoma. A clinicopathologic study of 27 cases. Cancer 1989: 64: 2162–2173

13. Martin S E, Dwyer A, Kissane J M, Costa J. Small-cell osteosarcoma. Cancer 1982: 50: 990–996

14. Roessner A, Immenkamp M, Hiddemann W, Althoff J, Miebs T, Grundmann E. Case report 331. Small cell osteosarcoma of the tibia with diffuse metastatic disease. Skeletal Radiol 1985: 14: 216–225

15. Devaney K, Vinh T N, Sweet D E. Small cell osteosarcoma of bone: an immunohistochemical study with differential diagnostic considerations. Hum Pathol 1993: 24: 1211–1225

16. Dickersin G R, Rosenberg A E. The ultrastructure of small-cell osteosarcoma, with a review of the light microscopy and differential diagnosis. Hum Pathol 1991: 22: 267–275

17. Navas-Palacios J J, Aparicio-Duque R, Valdes M D. On the histogenesis of Ewing's sarcoma. An ultrastructural, immunohistochemical and cytochemical study. Cancer 1984: 53: 1882–1901

18. Park Y K, Ryu K N, Ahn J H, Yang M H. A small cell osteosarcoma on the calcaneus. J Korean Med Sci 1995: 10: 147–151

19. Mawad J K, Makay B, Raymond A K, Ayala A G. Electron microscopy in the diagnosis of small round cell tumors of bone. Ultrastruct Pathol 1994: 18: 263–268

20. Papadimitriou J C, Drachenberg C B. Ultrastructural features of the matrix of small cell osteosarcoma (letter). Hum Pathol 1994: 25: 430–431

21. Noguera R, Navarro S, Triche T J. Translocation (11;22) in small cell osteosarcoma. Cancer Genet Cytogenet 1990: 45: 121–124

22. Giovannini M, Selleri L, Biegel J A, Scotlandi K, Emanuel B S, Evans G A. Interphase cytogenetics for the detection of the t(11;22)(q24;q12) in small round cell tumors. J Clin Invest 1992: 90: 1911–1918

23. Robinson L H, Pitt M J, Jaffe K A, Siegal G P. Small cell osteosarcoma of the soft tissue. Skeletal Radiol 1995: 24: 462–465

24. Roessner A, Jürgens H. Round cell tumors of bone. Pathol Res Pract 1993: 189: 111–136

25. Schajowicz F, McGuire M H. Diagnostic difficulties in skeletal pathology. Clin Orthop 1989: 240: 281–310

26. Sanjay B, Raj G A, Vishwakarma G. A small-cell osteosarcoma with multiple skeletal metastases. Arch Orthop Trauma Surg 1988: 107: 58–60

27. Bertoni F, Present D, Bacchini P, Pignatti G, Picci P, Campanacci M. The Istituto Rizzoli experience with small cell osteosarcoma. Cancer 1989: 64: 2591–2599

28. Stea B, Cavazzana A, Kinsella T J. Small-cell osteosarcoma: correlation of in vitro and clinical radiation response. Int J Radiat Oncol Biol Phys 1988: 15: 1233–1238

29. Hasegawa T, Hirose T, Kudo E, Hizawa K, Usui M, Ishii S. Immunophenotypic heterogeneity in osteosarcomas. Hum Pathol 1991: 22: 583–590

30. Yoshida H, Yumoto T, Adachi H, Minamizaki T, Maeda N, Furuse K. Osteosarcoma with prominent epithelioid features. Acta Pathol Jpn 1989: 39: 439–445

31. Yunis E J, Barnes L. The histologic diversity of osteosarcoma. Pathol Annu 1986: 21: 121–141

32. Richter D, Bosse A, Weber A, Müller K M, Muhr G. Das epithelioide Osteosarkom. Langensbecks Arch Chir 1995: 380: 354–358

33. Kramer K, Hicks D G, Palis J et al. Epithelioid osteosarcoma of bone. Immunocytochemical evidence suggesting divergent epithelial and mesenchymal differentiation in a primary osseous neoplasm. Cancer 1993: 71: 2977–2982

34. Adler C P. Osteosarkom der distalen Radius-Epi-Metaphyse mit pseudoepithelialen Ausdifferenzierungen. Verh Dtsch Ges Pathol 1974: 58: 272–274

35. Meister P, Konrad E A, Wallmuller-Strycker A. Metastasiertes Osteosarkom mit undifferenzierten karzinomähnlichen Anteilen. Arch Orthop Trauma Surg 1980: 96: 75–78

36. Dardick I, Schatz J E, Colgan T J. Osteogenic sarcoma with epithelial differentiation. Ultrastruct Pathol 1992: 16: 463–474

37. Ling L L, Steiner G C. Primary multipotential malignant neoplasm of bone: chondrosarcoma associated with squamous cell carcinoma. Hum Pathol 1986: 17: 317–320

38. Hutter R V, Foote F W Jr, Francis K C, Sherman R S. Primitive multipotential primary sarcoma of bone. Cancer 1966: 19: 1–25

39. Ballance W A Jr, Mendelsohn G, Carter J R, Abdul-Karim F W, Jacobs G, Makley J T. Osteogenic sarcoma. Malignant fibrous histiocytoma subtype. Cancer 1988: 62: 763–771

40. Yoshida H, Yumoto T, Minamizaki T. Osteosarcoma with features mimicking malignant fibrous histiocytoma. Virchows Arch A Pathol Anat Histopathol 1992: 421: 229–238

41. Naka T, Fukuda T, Shinohara N, Iwamoto Y, Sugioka Y, Tsuneyoshi M. Osteosarcoma versus malignant fibrous histiocytoma of bone in patients older than 40 years. Cancer 1995: 76: 972–984

42. Ushigome S, Shimoda T, Fukunaga M, Takakuwa T, Nakajima H. Immunocytochemical aspects of the differential diagnosis of osteosarcoma and malignant fibrous histiocytoma. Surg Pathol 1988: 1: 347–357

43. Bertoni F, Unni K K, McLeod R A, Dahlin D C. Osteosarcoma resembling osteoblastoma. Cancer 1985: 55: 416–426

44. Nojima T, Yamaguchi H, Nagashima K, Nagai Y, Kanda M. Osteosarcoma resembling osteoblastoma and its heterotransplantation into nude mice. Acta Pathol Jpn 1992: 42: 75–81

45. Mirra J M, Kendrick R A, Kendrick R E. Pseudomalignant osteoblastoma versus arrested osteosarcoma. Cancer 1976: 37: 2005–2014

46. Matsuno T, Unni K K, McLeod R A, Dahlin D C. Telangiectatic osteogenic sarcoma. Cancer 1976: 38: 2538–2547

47. Bertoni F, Bacchini P, Donati D, Martini A, Picci P, Campanacci M. Osteoblastoma-like osteosarcoma. The Rizzoli Institute experience. Mod Pathol 1993: 6: 707–716

48. Huvos A G, Rosen G, Bretsky S S, Butler A. Telangiectatic osteogenic sarcoma: a clinicopathologic study of 124 patients. Cancer 1982: 49: 1679–1689

49. Mervak T R, Unni K K, Pritchard D J, McLeod R A. Telangiectatic osteosarcoma. Clin Orthop 1991: 270: 135–139

50. Farr G H, Huvos A G, Marcove R C, Higinbotham N L, Foote F W Jr. Telangiectatic osteogenic sarcoma. A review of twenty-eight cases. Cancer 1974: 34: 1150–1158

51. Bertoni F, Pignatti G, Bacchini P, Picci P, Bacci G, Campanacci M. Telangiectatic or hemorrhagic osteosarcoma of bone: a clinicopathologic study of 41 patients at the Rizzoli Institute. Prog Surg Pathol 1989: 10: 63–82

52. Chung E B, Enzinger F M. Extraskeletal osteosarcoma. Cancer 1987: 60: 1132–1142

53. Mirra J M, Fain J S, Ward W G, Eckardt J J, Eilber F, Rosen G. Extraskeletal telangiectatic osteosarcoma. Cancer 1993: 71: 3014–3019

54. Kaufman R A, Towbin R B. Telangiectatic osteosarcoma simulating the appearance of an aneurysmal bone cyst. Pediatr Radiol 1981: 11: 102–104

55. Vanel D, Tcheng S, Contesso G et al. The radiological appearances of telangiectatic osteosarcoma. A study of 14 cases. Skeletal Radiol 1987: 16: 196–200

56. Yoshida H, Adachi H, Naniwa S, Yumoto T, Morimoto K, Furuse K. High alkaline phosphatase activity of telangiectatic osteosarcoma (TOS) and its diagnostic significance. Acta Pathol Jpn 1987: 37: 305–313

57. Roessner A, Hobik H P, Immenkamp M, Grundmann E. Ultrastructure of telangiectatic osteosarcoma. J Cancer Res Clin Oncol 1979: 95: 197–207

58. Adler C P. Case report 111. Telangiectatic osteosarcoma of the femur with features of an aggressive aneurysmal bone cyst. Skeletal Radiol 1980: 5: 56–60

59. Campanacci M, Pizzoferrato A. Osteosarcoma emorragico. Chir Organi Mov 1972: 60: 409–421

60. Larsson S E, Lorentzon R, Boquist L. Telangiectatic osteosarcoma. Acta Orthop Scand 1978: 49: 589–594

61. Bacci G, Picci P, Ferrari S, Sangiorgi L, Zanone A, Brach del Prever A. Primary chemotherapy and delayed surgery for non-metastatic telangiectatic osteosarcoma of the extremities. Results in 28 patients. Eur J Cancer 1994: 30A: 620–626

62. Pignatti G, Bacci G, Picci P et al. Telangiectatic osteogenic sarcoma of the extremities. Results in 17 patients treated with neoadjuvant chemotherapy. Clin Orthop 1991: 270: 99–106

63. Chawla S P, Benjamin R S. Effectiveness of chemotherapy in the management of metastatic telangiectatic osteosarcoma. Am J Clin Oncol 1988: 11: 177–180

64. Gomes H, Menanteau B, Gaillard D, Behar C. Telangiectatic osteosarcoma. Pediatr Radiol 1986: 16: 140–143

65. Ruiter D J, Cornelisse C J, Van Rijssel T G, Van der Velde E A. Aneurysmal bone cyst and telangiectatic osteosarcoma. A histopathological and morphometric study. Virchows Arch A Path Anat Histol 1977: 373: 311–325

66. Unni K K, Dahlin D C, McLeod R A, Pritchard D J. Intraosseous well-differentiated osteosarcoma. Cancer 1977: 40: 1337–1347

67. Kurt A M, Unni K K, McLeod R A, Pritchard D J. Low-grade intraosseous osteosarcoma. Cancer 1990: 65: 1418–1428

68. Choong P F, Pritchard D J, Rock M G, Sim F H, McLeod R A, Unni K K. Low grade central osteogenic sarcoma. Clin Orthop 1996: 322: 198–206

69. Campanacci M, Bertoni F, Capanna R, Cervellati C. Central osteosarcoma of low grade malignancy. Ital J Orthop Traumatol 1981: 7: 71–78

70. Ellis J H, Siegel C L, Martel W, Weatherbee L, Dorfman H. Radiologic features of well-differentiated osteosarcoma. AJR 1988: 151: 739–742

71. Bertoni F, Bacchini P, Fabbri N et al. Osteosarcoma. Low-grade intraosseous-type osteosarcoma, histologically resembling parosteal osteosarcoma, fibrous dysplasia and desmoplastic fibroma. Cancer 1993: 71: 338–345

72. Unni K K. Case report 136. Central low-grade osteosarcoma of tibia. Skeletal Radiol 1981: 6: 65–67

73. Lodwick G S. Case report 169. Low grade osteosarcoma of the tibia. Skeletal Radiol 1981: 7: 139–141

74. Vriens J P, Vosmer A M, Vos A K. Oorspronkelijke stukken. Het goed gediferentieerde intra-ossale osteosarcoom (the well-differentiated intraosseous osteosarcoma). Ned Tijdschr Geneeskd 1984: 128: 2210–2213

75. Petrovichev N N, Khmelev O N, Lukyanchenko A B, Karapetyan R M. Intraosteal well differentiated osteogenic sarcoma (Russian). Arkh Patol 1988: 50(8): 71–74

76. Xipell J M, Rush J. Case report 340. Well differentiated intraosseous osteosarcoma of the left femur. Skeletal Radiol 1985: 14: 312–316

77. Sundaram M, Herbold D R, McGuire M H. Case report 370. Low grade (well-differentiated) intramedullary osteosarcoma. Skeletal Radiol 1986: 15: 338–342

78. Sim F H, Kurt A M, McLeod R A, Unni K K. Case report 628. Low-grade central osteosarcoma. Skeletal Radiol 1990: 19: 457–460

79. Iemoto Y, Ushigome S, Fukunaga M, Nikaido T, Asanuma K. Case report 679. Central low-grade osteosarcoma with foci of dedifferentiation. Skeletal Radiol 1991: 20: 379–382

80. Tokito T, Ushijima M, Hara N, Oda Y, Tsuneyoshi M. Case report 812. Well-differentiated osteosarcoma arising in the right third rib. Skeletal Radiol 1993: 22: 549–551

81. Mink J H, Gold R H, Mirra J M, Grant T T, Eilber F R. Case report 65. Highly anaplastic epiphyseal osteolytic osteosarcoma. Skeletal Radiol 1978: 3: 69–72

82. Unni K K. Case report 214. Osteosarcoma (high grade) of the upper end of the tibia. Skeletal Radiol 1982: 9: 129–131

83. Raymond A K, Murphy G F, Rosenthal D I. Case report 425. Chondroblastic osteosarcoma: clear-cell variant of femur. Skeletal Radiol 1987: 16: 336–341

84. Paltiel H J, Wilkinson R H, Kozakewich H P. Case report 507. Osteosarcoma of the distal femoral epiphysis. Skeletal Radiol 1988: 17: 527–530

85. Tsuneyoshi M, Dorfman H D. Epiphyseal osteosarcoma: distinguishing features from clear cell chondrosarcoma, chondroblastoma, and epiphyseal enchondroma. Hum Pathol 1987: 18: 644–651

86. Sim F H, Frassica F J, Unni K K. Osteosarcoma of the diaphysis of long bones: clinicopathologic features and treatment of 51 cases. Orthopedics 1995: 18: 19–23

87. Haworth J M, McCall I W, Park W M, Watt I. Sclerotic medullary spread in diaphyseal osteosarcoma. Skeletal Radiol 1979: 4: 212–215

88. Haworth J M, Watt I, Park W M, Roylance J. Diaphyseal osteosarcoma. Br J Radiol 1981: 54: 932–938

89. Ellman H, Gold R H, Mirra J M. Roentgenographically 'benign' but rapidly lethal diaphyseal osteosarcoma: a case report. J Bone Joint Surg (Am) 1974: 56: 1267–1269

90. Gold R H, Ellman H, Mirra J M. Case report 23. Intramedullary osteosarcoma of the femur. Skeletal Radiol 1977: 1: 235–236

91. Kyriakos M. Intracortical osteosarcoma. Cancer 1980: 46: 2525–2533

92. Picci P, Gherlinzoni F, Guerra A. Intracortical osteosarcoma: rare entity or early manifestation of classical osteosarcoma? Skeletal Radiol 1983: 9: 255–258

93. Vigorita V J, Jones J K, Ghelman B, Marcove R C. Intracortical osteosarcoma. Am J Surg Pathol 1984: 8: 65–71

94. Anderson R B, McAlister J A Jr, Wrenn R N. Case report 585. Intracortical osteosarcoma of tibia. Skeletal Radiol 1989: 18: 627–630

95. Mirra J M, Dodd L, Johnston W, Frost D B, Barton D. Case report 700. Primary intracortical osteosarcoma of femur, sclerosing variant, grade 1 to 2 anaplasia. Skeletal Radiol 1991: 20: 613–616

96. Lopez-Barea F, Rodriguez-Peralto J L, Gonzalez-Lopez J, Sanchez-Herrera S, Sanchez del Charco M. Intracortical osteosarcoma. A case report. Clin Orthop 1991: 268: 218–222

97. Greenspan A, Wold L. Cortical osteosarcoma involving the medullary cavity and soft tissue. A case report. J Bone Joint Surg (Am) 1994: 76: 1399–1404

98. Kyriakos M, Gilula L A, Becich M J, Schoenecker P L. Intracortical small cell osteosarcoma. Clin Orthop 1992: 279: 269–280

99. Schajowicz F, McGuire M H, Santini Araujo E, Muscolo D L, Gitelis S. Osteosarcomas arising on the surfaces of long bones. J Bone Joint Surg (Am) 1988: 70: 555–564

100. Raymond A K. Surface osteosarcoma. Clin Orthop 1991: 270: 140–148

101. Kenan S, Abdelwahab I F, Klein M J, Hermann G, Lewis M M. Lesions of juxtacortical origin (surface lesions of bone). Skeletal Radiol 1993: 22: 337–357

102. Wold L E, Unni K K, Beabout J W, Pritchard D J. High-grade surface osteosarcomas. Am J Surg Pathol 1984: 8: 181–186

103. Sonneland P R, Unni K K. Case report 258. High-grade 'surface' osteosarcoma arising from the femoral shaft. Skeletal Radiol 1984: 11: 77–80

104. Okada K, Kubota H, Ebina T, Kobayashi T, Abe E, Sato K. High-grade surface osteosarcoma of the humerus. Skeletal Radiol 1995: 24: 531–534

105. Cheung H, Lau R L, Hsu S Y. Case report. Primary high grade surface osteosarcoma. Clin Radiol 1995: 50: 194–197

106. Yamaguchi H, Nojima T, Yagi T, Masuda T, Sasaki T. High grade surface osteosarcoma of the left ilium. A case report and review of the literature. Acta Pathol Jpn 1988: 38: 235–240

107. Wuisman P, Roessner A, Blasius S, Grünert J, Vestering T, Winkelmann W. High malignant surface osteosarcoma arising at the site of a previously treated aneurysmal bone cyst. J Cancer Res Clin Oncol 1993: 119: 375–378

108. Unni K K, Dahlin D C, Beabout J W. Periosteal osteogenic sarcoma. Cancer 1976: 37: 2476–2485

109. Lichtenstein L. Tumours of periosteal origin. Cancer 1955: 8: 1060–1069

110. De Santos L A, Murray J A, Finklestein J B, Spjut H J, Ayala A G. The radiographic spectrum of periosteal osteosarcoma. Radiology 1978: 127: 123–129

111. Spjut H J, Ayala A G, De Santos L A, Murray J A. Periosteal

osteosarcoma. In: Management of primary bone and soft tissue tumors. Chicago: Year Book Medical, 1977, pp 79–95

112. Hall R B, Robinson L H, Malawar M M, Dunham W K. Periosteal osteosarcoma. Cancer 1985: 55: 165–171

113. Ritts G D, Pritchard D J, Unni K K, Beabout J W, Eckardt J J. Periosteal osteosarcoma. Clin Orthop 1987: 219: 299–307

114. Dahlin D C. Case report 27. Periosteal osteosarcoma of the right femur. Skeletal Radiol 1977: 1: 249–252

115. Chan M M, McGuire L J. Test and Teach Number 59. Diagnosis. Periosteal osteogenic sarcoma. Pathology 1989: 21: 17–18, 65–66

116. Lawson J P, Barwick K W. Case report 162. Periosteal osteosarcoma of rib. Skeletal Radiol 1981: 7: 63–65

117. Oda Y, Hashimoto H, Tsuneyoshi M, Masuda S. Case report 793. Periosteal osteosarcoma of the clavicle. Skeletal Radiol 1993: 22: 375–377

118. Howat A J, Dickens D R, Boldt D W, Waters K D, Campbell P E. Bilateral metachronous periosteal osteosarcoma. Cancer 1986: 58: 1139–1143

119. Sonobe H, Iwata J, Furihata M, Ohtsuki Y, Mizobuchi H, Yamamoto H. Periosteal osteosarcoma of the femur with bone marrow involvement: a case report. Pathol Int 1994: 44: 407–411

120. Saito N, Fujioka F, Uchiyama S, Ono S. Periosteal osteosarcoma of the femur: a pathological and ultrastructural study (in Japanese). Nippon Seikeigeka Gakkai Zasshi 1991: 65: 1028–1034

121. Martinez-Tello F J, Navas-Palacios J J. The ultrastructure of conventional, parosteal and periosteal osteosarcomas. Cancer 1982: 50: 949–961

122. Bertoni F, Boriani S, Laus M, Campanacci M. Periosteal chondrosarcoma and periosteal osteosarcoma Two distinct entities. J Bone Joint Surg (Br) 1982: 64: 370–376

123. Chano T, Matsumoto K, Ishizawa M, Morimoto S, Hukuda S, Okabe H. Periosteal osteosarcoma and parosteal chondrosarcoma evaluated by double immunohistochemical staining. Report of 2 cases. Acta Orthop Scand 1994: 65: 355–358

124. Unni K K, Dahlin D C, Beabout J W, Ivins J C. Parosteal osteogenic sarcoma. Cancer 1976: 37: 2644–2675

125. Okada K, Frassica F J, Sim F H, Beabout J W, Bond J R, Unni K K. Parosteal osteosarcoma. A clinicopathological study. J Bone Joint Surg (Am) 1994: 76: 366–378

126. Van Der Heul R O, Von Ronnen J R. Juxtacortical osteosarcoma. J Bone Joint Surg (Am) 1967: 49: 415–439

127. Lorentzon R, Larsson S E, Boquist L. Parosteal (juxtacortical) osteosarcoma. A clinical and histopathological study of 11 cases and a review of the literature. J Bone Joint Surg (Br) 1980: 62: 86–92

128. Masuda S, Murakawa Y. Post-irradiation parosteal osteosarcoma. A case report. Clin Orthop 1984: 184: 204–207

129. Campanacci M, Giunti A. Periosteal osteosarcoma. Review of 41 cases, 22 with long-term follow-up. Ital J Orthop Traumatol 1976: 2: 23–35

130. Campanacci M, Picci P, Gherlinzoni F, Guerra A, Bertoni F, Neff J R. Parosteal osteosarcoma. J Bone Joint Surg (Br) 1984: 66: 313–321

131. Adler C P. Parosteal (juxtacortical) osteosarcoma of the distal femur. Pathol Res Pract 1980: 169: 388–395

132. Stark H H, Jones F E, Jernstrom P. Parosteal osteogenic sarcoma of a metacarpal bone. J Bone Joint Surg (Am) 1971: 53: 47–53

133. Van der Walt J D, Ryan J F. Parosteal osteogenic sarcoma of the hand. Histopathology 1990: 16: 75–78

134. Kersjes W, Grebe P, Runkel M, Stôrkel S, Schild H. Parosteal osteosarcoma of the talus. Skeletal Radiol 1995: 24: 217–219

135. Green P W, Ilardi C F, Bitter J J, Dee R D. Case report 260. Parosteal osteosarcoma of the pubis. Skeletal Radiol 1984: 11: 141–143

136. Yi E S, Shmookler B M, Malawer M M, Sweet D E. Well-differentiated extraskeletal osteosarcoma. A soft-tissue homologue of parosteal osteosarcoma. Arch Pathol Lab Med 1991: 115: 906–909

137. Smith J, Ahuja S C, Huvos A G, Bullough P G. Parosteal (juxtacortical) osteogenic sarcoma. A roentgenological study of 30 patients. J Can Assoc Radiol 1978: 29: 167–174

138. Levine E, De Smet A A, Huntrakoon M. Juxtacortical osteosarcoma: a radiologic and histologic spectrum. Skeletal Radiol 1985: 14: 38–46

139. Lindell M M Jr, Shirkhoda A, Raymond A K, Murray J A, Harle T S. Parosteal osteosarcoma: radiologic-pathologic correlation with emphasis on CT. AJR 1987: 148: 323–328

140. Farr G H, Huvos A G. Juxtacortical osteogenic sarcoma. An analysis of fourteen cases. J Bone Joint Surg (Am) 1972: 54: 1205–1216

141. Bertoni F, Present D, Hudson T, Enneking W F. The meaning of radiolucencies in parosteal osteosarcoma. J Bone Joint Surg (Am) 1985: 67: 901–910

142. Kricun M E, Stead J. Case report 289. 'Cystic' parosteal osteosarcoma. Skeletal Radiol 1984: 12: 227–231

143. Wuisman P, Harle A, Bosse A, Roessner A. 'Cystic' parosteal osteosarcoma. A case treated by resection. Fr J Orthop Surg 1988: 2: 487–490

144. Sciot R, Samson I, Dal Cin P et al. Giant cell rich parosteal osteosarcoma. Histopathology 1995: 27: 51–55

145. Ahuja S C, Villacin A B, Smith J, Bullough P G, Huvos A G, Marcove R C. Juxtacortical (parosteal) osteogenic sarcoma. Histological grading and prognosis. J Bone Joint Surg (Am) 1977: 59: 632–647

146. Ritschl P, Wurnig C, Lechner G, Roessner A. Parosteal osteosarcoma. 2–23-year follow-up of 33 patients. Acta Orthop Scand 1991: 62: 195–200

147. Mellin W, Roessner A, Immenkamp M, Boeddinghaus D, Grundmann E. Klassifikation und Differentialdiagnose der juxtakortikalen Osteosarkome. Pathologe 1986: 7: 94–100

148. Schwint A E, Araujo E S, Cole A, Itoiz M E, Cabrini R L. Nucleolar organizer regions in parosteal and central osteosarcomas. Clin Orthop 1996: 327: 253–258

149. Reddick R L, Popovsky M A, Fantone J C 3rd, Michelitch H J. Parosteal osteogenic sarcoma. Ultrastructural observations in three cases. Hum Pathol 1980: 11: 373–380

150. Vuletin J C. Myofibroblasts in parosteal osteogenic sarcoma. Arch Pathol Lab Med 1977: 101: 272

151. Murray A B, Bûscher H, Erfle V, Biehl T, Gössner W. Intranuclear undulating membranous structures in cells of a human parosteal osteosarcoma. Ultrastruct Pathol 1983: 5: 163–170

152. Orndal C, Mandahl N, Rydholm A et al. Supernumerary ring chromosomes in five bone and soft tissue tumours of low or borderline malignancy. Cancer Genet Cytogenet 1992: 60: 170–175

153. Sinovic J F, Bridge J A, Neff J R. Ring chromosomes in parosteal osteosarcoma. Clinical and diagnostic significance. Cancer Genet Cytogenet 1992: 62: 50–52

154. Hermann G, Abdelwahab I F, Klein M J, Kenan S, Lewis M M. Case report 711. Parosteal osteosarcoma of left femur. Skeletal Radiol 1992: 21: 69–71

155. Wolfel D A, Carter P R. Parosteal osteosarcoma. Am J Roentgenol Radium Ther Nucl Med 1969: 105: 142–146

156. Picci P, Campanacci M, Bacci G, Capanna R, Ayala A. Medullary involvement in parosteal osteosarcoma. J Bone Joint Surg (Am) 1987: 69: 131–136

157. Dunham W K, Wilborn W H, Zarzour R J. A large parosteal osteosarcoma with transformation to high-grade osteosarcoma: a case report. Cancer 1979: 44: 1495–1500

158. Wold L E, Unni K K, Beabout J W, Sim F H, Dahlin D C. Dedifferentiated parosteal osteosarcoma. J Bone Joint Surg (Am) 1984: 66: 53–59

159. Sauer D D, Chase D R. Case report 461. Dedifferentiated parosteal osteosarcoma. Skeletal Radiol 1988: 17: 72–76

160. Pintado S O, Lane J, Huvos A G. Parosteal osteogenic sarcoma of bone with coexistent low and high-grade sarcomatous components. Hum Pathol 1989: 20: 488–491

161. Partovi S, Logan P M, Janzen D L, O'Connell J X, O'Connell D G. Low-grade parosteal osteosarcoma of the ulna with dedifferentiation into high-grade osteosarcoma. Skeletal Radiol 1996: 25: 497–500

162. Orcutt J, Ragsdale B D, Curtis D J, Levine M I. Misleading CT in parosteal osteosarcoma. AJR 1981: 136: 1233–1235

163. Van Oven M W, Molenaar W M, Freling N J et al.

Dedifferentiated parosteal osteosarcoma of the femur with aneuploidy and lung metastases. Cancer 1989: 63: 807–811

164. Biagini R, Ruggieri P, De Cristofaro R, Torricelli P, Picci P, Bacci G. Multicentric osteosarcoma. Report of 5 cases. Chir Organi Mov 1991: 76: 113–122

165. Silverman G. Multiple osteogenic sarcoma. Arch Pathol 1936: 21: 88–95

166. Lowber L. Multifocal osteosarcomatosis, a rare entity. Bull Pathol 1968: 9: 52–53

167. Amstutz H C. Multiple osteogenic sarcomata – metastatic or multicentric? Report of two cases and review of literature. Cancer 1969: 24: 923–931

168. Mahoney J P, Spanier S S, Morris J L. Multifocal osteosarcoma: a case report with review of the literature. Cancer 1979: 44: 1897–1907

169. McCarthy E F, Tolo V T, Dorfman H D. Case report 446. Multicentric, metachronous, low grade, sclerosing osteogenic sarcoma. Skeletal Radiol 1987: 16: 592–596

170. Simodynes E E, Jardon O M, Connolly J F. Multiple metachronous osteosarcoma with eleven year survival. A case report. J Bone Joint Surg 1981: 63: 317–322

171. Fitzgerald R H Jr, Dahlin D C, Sim F H. Multiple metachronous osteogenic sarcoma. Report of twelve cases with two long term survivors. J Bone Joint Surg (Am) 1973: 55: 595–605

172. Thayer C, Rogers L F. Unicentric osteosarcoma of bone with subsequent skeletal metastases. Skeletal Radiol 1979: 4: 148–153

173. Pho R W, Lim S M, Satku K. Late metastases from osteogenic sarcoma. A case report. J Bone Joint Surg (Am) 1985: 67: 147–150

174. Olson P N, Prewitt L, Griffiths H J, Cherkna B. Case report 703. Multifocal osteosarcoma. Skeletal Radiol 1991: 20: 624–627

175. Ippolito V, Mirra J M, Fedenko A, Brien E W, Rosen P, Chap L. Case report 827. Miliary osteosarcomatosis. Skeletal Radiol 1994: 23: 143–147

176. Hopper K D, Moser R P Jr, Haseman D B, Sweet D E, Madewell J E, Kransdorf M J. Osteosarcomatosis. Radiology 1990: 175: 233–239

177. Hopper K D, Haseman D B, Moser R P Jr, Sweet D E, Madewell J E. Case report 634. Osteosarcomatosis. Skeletal Radiol 1990: 19: 535–537

178. Parham D M, Pratt C B, Parvey L S, Webber B L, Champion J. Childhood multifocal osteosarcoma. Clinicopathologic and radiologic correlates. Cancer 1985: 55: 2653–2658

179. Cremin B J, Heselson N G, Webber B L. The multiple sclerotic osteogenic sarcoma of early childhood. Br J Radiol 1976: 49: 416–419

180. Gherlinzoni F, Antoci B, Canale V. Case report 250. Multicentric osteosarcomata (osteosarcomatosis). Skeletal Radiol 1983: 10: 281–285

181. Bowerman J W, Crawford B. Case report 21. Multicentric osteosarcoma of skeleton with pulmonary and pleural metastases. Skeletal Radiol 1977: 1: 185–186

182. Schwartz D T, Alpert M. The malignant transformation of fibrous dysplasia. Am J Med Sci 1964: 247: 1–20

183. Huvos A G, Higinbotham N L, Miller T R. Bone sarcomas arising in fibrous dysplasia. J Bone Joint Surg (Am) 1972: 54: 1047–1056

184. Taconis W K. Osteosarcoma in fibrous dysplasia. Skeletal Radiol 1988: 17: 163–170

185. Ruggieri P, Sim F H, Bond J R, Unni K K. Malignancies in fibrous dysplasia. Cancer 1994: 73: 1411–1424

186. Ishida T, Machinami R, Kojima T, Kikuchi F. Malignant fibrous histiocytoma and osteosarcoma in association with fibrous dysplasia of bone. Report of three cases. Pathol Res Pract 1992: 188: 757–763

187. Huvos A G, Butler A, Bretsky S S. Osteogenic sarcoma associated with Paget's disease of bone. A clinicopathologic study of 65 patients. Cancer 1983: 52: 1489–1495

188. Wick M R, Siegal G P, Unni K K, McLeod R A, Greditzer H G 3rd. Sarcomas of bone complicating osteitis deformans (Paget's disease): fifty years' experience. Am J Surg Pathol 1981: 5: 47–59

189. Frassica F J, Sim F H, Frassica D A, Wold L E. Survival and management considerations in postirradiation osteosarcoma and Paget's osteosarcoma. Clin Orthop 1991: 270: 120–127

190. Mark R J, Poen J, Tran L M, Fu Y S, Selch M T, Parker R G. Postirradiation sarcomas. A single-institution study and review of literature. Cancer 1994: 73: 2653–2662

191. Tountas A A, Fornasier V L, Harwood A R, Leung P M. Postirradiation sarcoma of bone. A perspective. Cancer 1979: 43: 182–187

192. Huvos A G, Woodard H Q, Cahan W G et al. Postradiation osteogenic sarcoma of bone and soft tissues. A clinicopathologic study of 66 patients. Cancer 1985: 55: 1244–1255

193. Wiklund T A, Blomqvist C P, Räty J, Elomaa I, Rissanen P, Miettinen M. Postirradiation sarcoma. Analysis of a nationwide cancer registry material. Cancer 1991: 68: 524–531

194. Niebrugge D, Monzon C, Perry M C, Hakami N. Osteogenic sarcoma following Hodgkin's disease. Cancer 1981: 48: 416–418

195. Smith J. Postradiation sarcoma of bone in Hodgkin disease. Skeletal Radiol 1987: 16: 524–532

196. Boivin J F, O'Brien K. Solid cancer risk after treatment of Hodgkin's disease. Cancer 1988: 61: 2541–2546

197. Logan P M, Munk P L, O'Connell J X, Connell D G, Janzen D L. Post-radiation osteosarcoma of the scapula. Skeletal Radiol 1996: 25: 596–601

198. Cahan W C, Woodard H Q, Higinbotham N L et al. Sarcoma arising in irradiated bone. Cancer 1948: 1: 3–29

199. Arlen M, Higinbotham N L, Huvos A G, Marcove R C, Miller T, Shah I C. Radiation-induced sarcoma of bone. Cancer 1971: 28: 1087–1099

200. Bragg D G, Shidnia H, Chu F C, Higinbotham N L. The clinical and radiologic aspects of radiation osteitis. Radiology 1970: 97: 103–111

201. Brady L W. Radiation-induced sarcomas of bone. Skeletal Radiol 1979: 4: 72–78

202. Tillotson C, Rosenberg A, Gebhardt M, Rosenthal D I. Postradiation multicentric osteisarcoma. Cancer 1988: 62: 67–71

203. Ozisik Y Y, Meloni A M, Zalupski M M, Ryan J R, Qureshi F, Sandberg A A. Deletion of chromosome 13 in osteosarcoma secondary to irradiation. Cancer Genet Cytogenet 1993: 69: 35–37

204. Sim F H, Cupps R E, Dahlin D C, Ivins J C. Post radiation sarcoma of bone. J Bone Joint Surg (Am) 1972: 54: 1479–1489

205. Weatherby R P, Dahlin D C, Ivins J C. Post radiation sarcoma of bone: review of 78 Mayo Clinic cases. Mayo Clin Proc 1981: 56: 294–306

206. Harrist T J, Schiller A L, Trelstad R L, Mankin H J, Mays C W. Thorotrast-associated sarcoma of bone. A case report and review of the literature. Cancer 1979: 44: 2049–2058

207. Sindelar W F, Costa J, Ketcham A S. Osteosarcoma associated with Thorotrast administration: report of two cases and literature review. Cancer 1978: 42: 2604–2609

208. Klenerman L, Ockenden B G, Townsend A C. Osteosarcoma occurring in osteogenesis imperfecta. Report of two cases. J Bone Joint Surg (Br) 1967: 49: 314–323

209. Lasson U, Harms D, Wiedemann H R. Osteogenic sarcoma complicating osteogenesis imperfecta tarda. Eur J Pediatr 1978: 129: 215–218

210. Reid B S, Hubbard J D. Osteosarcoma arising in osteogenesis imperfecta. Pediatr Radiol 1979: 8: 110–112

211. Rutkowski R, Resnick P, McMaster J H. Osteosarcoma occurring in osteogenesis imperfecta. A case report. J Bone Joint Surg (Am) 1979: 61: 606–608

212. Gagliardi J A, Evans E M, Chandnani V P, Myers J B, Pacheco C M. Osteogenesis imperfecta complicated by osteosarcoma. Skeletal Radiol 1995: 24: 308–310

213. Kerr H D. A case of osteopetrosis (marble bones) complicated by osteogenic sarcoma. AJR 1936: 35: 212–214

214. Bostman O M, Holmstrom T, Riska E B. Osteosarcoma arising in a melorrheostotic femur. A case report. J Bone Joint Surg (Am) 1987: 69: 1232–1237

215. Mindell E R, Northup C S, Douglass H O Jr. Osteosarcoma associated with osteopoikilosis. Case report. J Bone Joint Surg (Am) 1978: 60: 406–408

216. Kyriakos M, Murphy W A. Concurrence of metaphyseal fibrous defect and osteosarcoma. Report of a case and review of the literature. Skeletal Radiol 1981: 6: 179–186
217. Smith G D, Chalmers J, McQueen M M. Osteosarcoma arising in relation to an enchondroma. A report of three cases. J Bone Joint Surg (Br) 1986: 68: 315–319
218. Van Lerberghe E, Van Damme B, Van Holsbeek M, Burssens A, Hoogmartens M. Case report 626. Osteosarcoma arising in a solitary osteochondroma of the femur. Skeletal Radiol 1990: 19: 594–597
219. Nojima T, Yamashiro K, Fujita M, Isu K, Ubayama Y, Yamawaki S. A case of osteosarcoma arising in a solitary osteochondroma. Acta Orthop Scand 1991: 62: 290–292
220. Tsuchiya H, Morikawa S, Tomita K. Osteosarcoma arising from multiple exostoses lesions: case report. Jpn J Clin Oncol 1990: 20: 296–298
221. Mirra J M, Bullough P G, Marcove R C, Jacobs B, Huvos A G. Malignant fibrous histiocytoma and osteosarcoma in association with bone infarcts; report of four cases, two in caisson workers. J Bone Joint Surg (Am) 1974: 56: 932–940
222. Torres F X, Kyriakos M. Bone infarct-associated osteosarcoma. Cancer 1992: 70: 2418–2430
223. Resnik C S, Aisner S C, Young J W, Levine A. Case report 767. Osteosarcoma arising in bone infarction. Skeletal Radiol 1993: 22: 58–61
224. Desai P, Perino G, Present D, Steiner G C. Sarcoma in association with bone infarcts. Report of five cases. Arch Pathol Lab Med 1996: 120: 482–489
225. Meadows A T, Strong L C, Li F P et al. Bone sarcoma as a second malignant neoplasm in children: influence of radiation and genetic predisposition. Cancer 1980: 46: 2603–2606
226. Bechler J R, Robertson W W, Meadows A T, Womer R B. Osteosarcoma as a second malignant neoplasm in children. J Bone Joint Surg (Am) 1992: 74: 1079–1083
227. Kriss V M, Stelling C B. Osteosarcoma after chemotherapy for neuroblastoma. Skeletal Radiol 1995: 24: 633–635

10

Osteochondroma

M. Forest

INTRODUCTION AND CLINICAL DATA

Osteochondroma or exostosis is a bony outgrowth, capped by cartilage, on the surface of bone (Figs 10.1, 10.2). It is the most common benign bone tumor, usually discovered between 10 and 15 years of age.[1] It usually stops growing when the epiphyseal plate closes. A male-to-female ratio of 1.7–2:1 has been reported but for many authors there is no sex predominance.

Many lesions are asymptomatic; clinical symptoms may be a palpable mass, pain, a fracture through the stalk,[2] infarction in the deeper portion[3] (Fig. 10.3), spinal cord compression,[4] popliteal pseudoaneurysm or popliteal vein thrombosis[5] or a painful overlying bursa.[6–12]

Virchow's 1891 hypothesis has been confirmed by Milgram:[13] displaced epiphyseal cartilage herniaties through a developmental defect in the plate. This mechanism has been reproduced experimentally in rabbits by transplantation of cartilage[14] or periosteal defects.[15]

After irradiation in childhood, 10–12% of patients may develop one or more osteochondromas by damage or disorganization of the growth plate;[16–18] they may occur even in the pelvis and vertebrae.[19]

SKELETAL DISTRIBUTION

Forty to 50% of lesions are found in the lower end of the femur and the upper ends of the tibia and humerus, but any bone may be involved (Figs 10.4–10.17). The scapula and ilium are common sites and those in the pelvis are often large (Wilner 1982). They are uncommon in the spine (3%[20,21]) and rare in the extremities.

IMAGING

The lesion appears large and sessile, more rarely pedunculated. The thin cortex of the osteochondroma merges with the cortex of the bone it is exiting from and its medullary

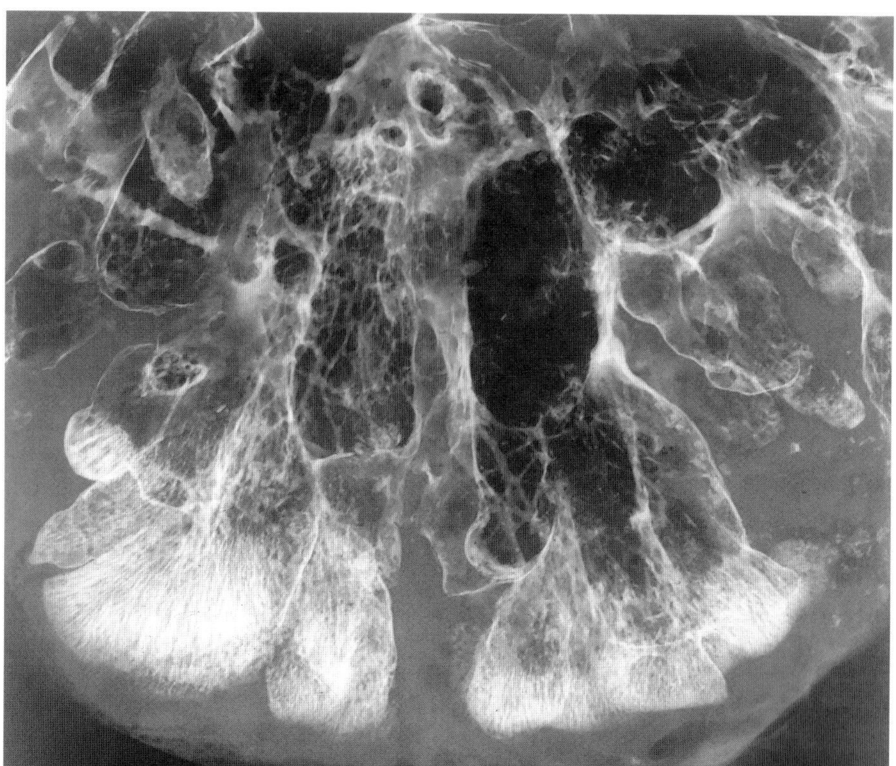

Fig. 10.1 Osteochondroma of the first rib: X-ray of a slab demonstrating the cartilage-capped bony outgrowth.

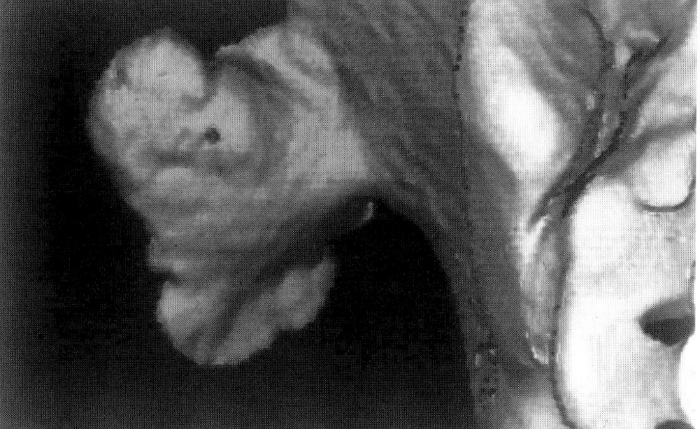

Fig. 10.2 Bony outgrowth of an iliac osteochondroma demonstrated by 3-D CT scan.

cavity is continuous with that of the affected bone. Osteochondromas are oriented towards the diaphysis by the pull of the nearby tendons. The central core may have flocculent densities representing calcified lobules of cartilage.

There may be an associated metaphyseal widening or flaring. Pressure defects may be found on the adjacent bone (more often the tibia), with the development of a synostosis (Wilner 1982) (Figs 10.18, 10.19).

The thickness of the cartilage cap can be evaluated by MRI[22] or ultrasonography,[23] less accurately by CT.[24,25]

Hot bone scans correspond to active enchondral ossification.[26,27]

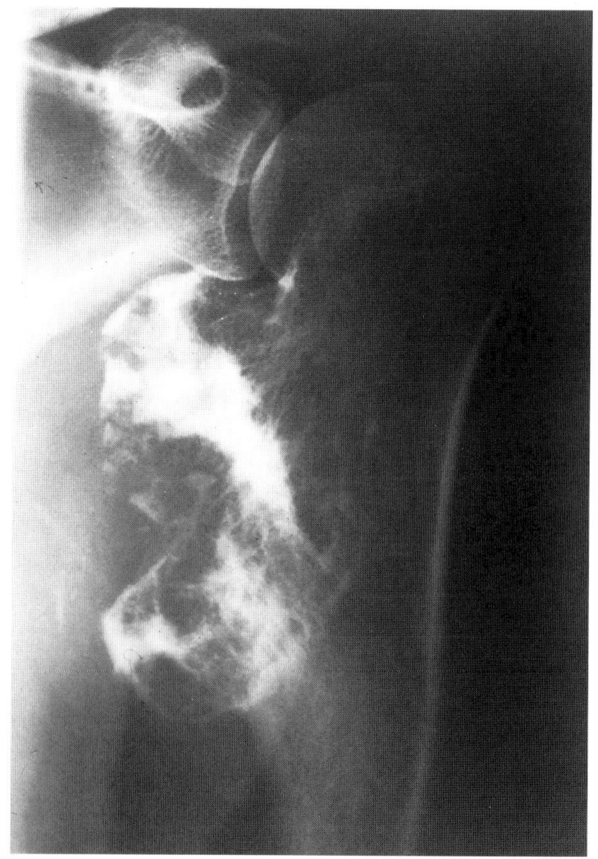

Fig. 10.3 Infarction in the stalk of a humeral osteochondroma, with a clinical course of 30 years.

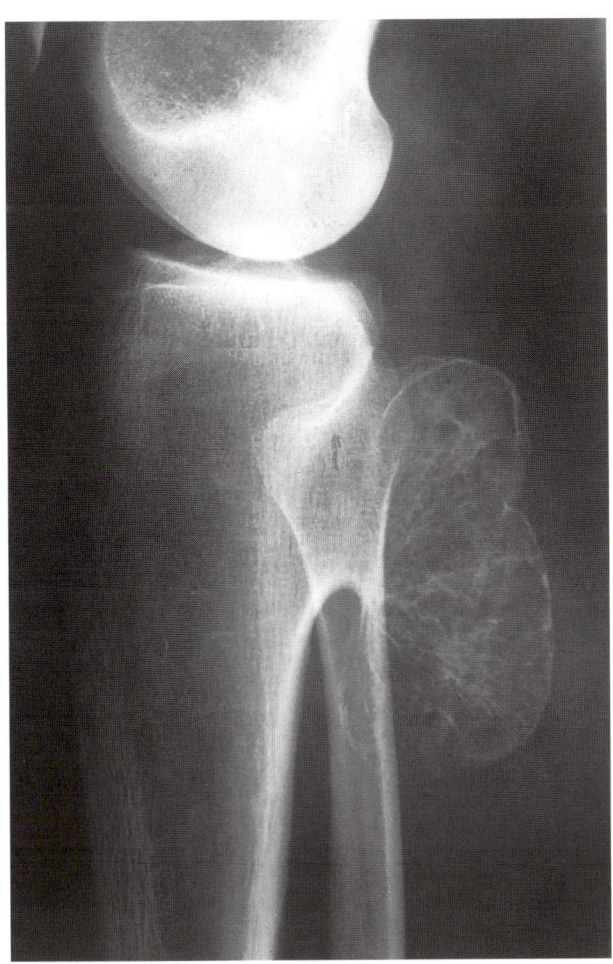

Fig. 10.4

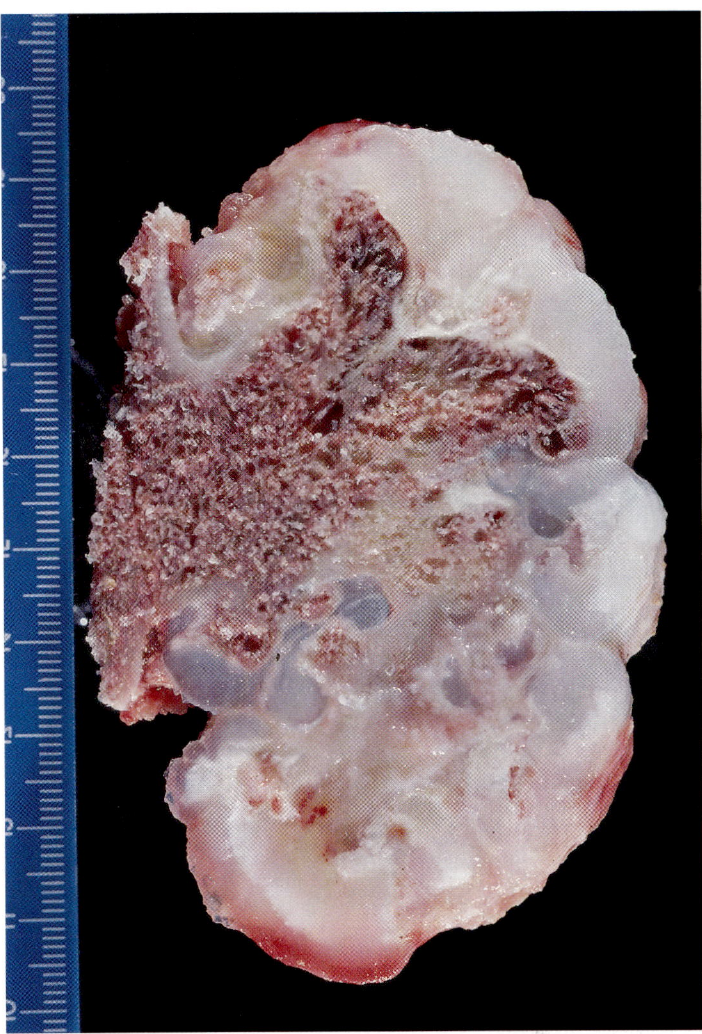

Fig. 10.5

Figs 10.4, 10.5 Osteochondroma of the upper end of the tibia.

GROSS PATHOLOGY

The size is between 1 and 10 cm. The surface may be smooth or lobulated, covered by a thin fibrous layer. The thickness of the cartilage cap is O,1–3 cm in young patients (Figs 10.20, 10.21). In adults it is only a few millimeters thick or it may be entirely absent leaving a surface made of eburnated bone. The central portion is medullary bone with often chalky and gritty calcified areas of cartilage.

HISTOPATHOLOGY

The cartilage cap, covered by the periosteum, looks like a growth plate with columns or clusters of chondrocytes evenly distributed (Figs 10.22–10.24). In the young, some chondrocytes may be binucleated.

PAS-positive cytoplasmic inclusions up to 15 microns have been reported, as in osteochondromatosis.[28]

The process of enchondral ossification leads to medullary bone, with a fatty or hematopoietic marrow and large calcified cartilage areas or calcific debris (Figs 10.25–10.27).

Overlying bursae are chiefly found in large osteochondromas (subscapular region and popliteal fossa) and are attached around the base, with a lining resembling synovium and a synovial-type transudate. Fibrinous rice bodies and secondary synovial chondrometaplasia have been reported.[8,12]

CYTOGENETICS

In some cases, cytogenetic study has shown structural aberrations in the long arm of chromosome 8.[29]

ELECTRON MICROSCOPY

Proliferating mature and degenerating chondrocytes are

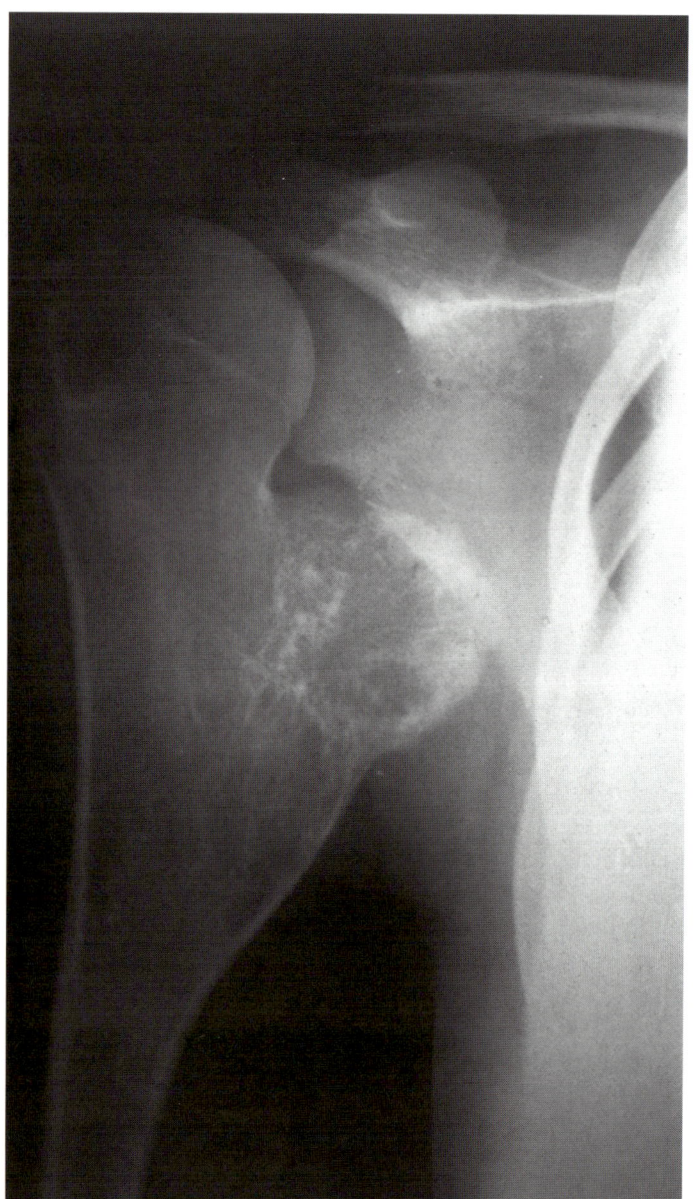

Fig. 10.6

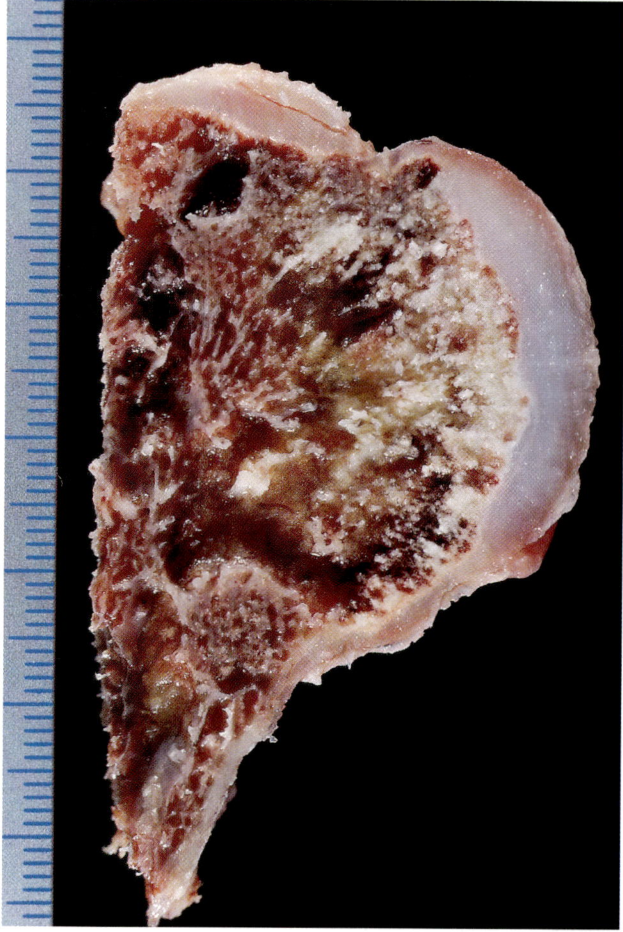

Fig. 10.7

Figs 10.6, 10.7 Osteochondroma of the upper end of the humerus.

indistinguishable from normal chondrocytes.[28,30] The process of mineralization has been studied on SEM.[31]

COURSE, TREATMENT AND PROGNOSIS

The treatment is surgical removal including the periosteum, with recurrences in 2% of cases (Unni 1996). Spontaneous disappearance, a rare event, has been reported.[32–35]

The risk of malignant transformation is about 1–2% of cases (Figs 10.28–10.33); there is no correlation between tumor size or thickness of the cartilage cap[36] and malignancy (Schajowicz 1994). A thick cartilage cap corresponds to a growing cartilage.[37]

Most of the tumors are low-grade chondrosarcomas with clinical symptoms of pain or increased growth of the osteochondroma in an adult.[1] The most frequent sites are the pelvis and the proximal femur (Wilner 1982). The large, irregular, calcified masses appear on X-ray with abnormal dispersed calcifications or an indistinct surface of the cap with lucent zones.[36] Rare secondary osteosarcomas have been reported.[38–41]

DIFFERENTIAL DIAGNOSIS

Concurrent osteochondromas and enchondromas within the same bone[42] have to be differentiated from the familial

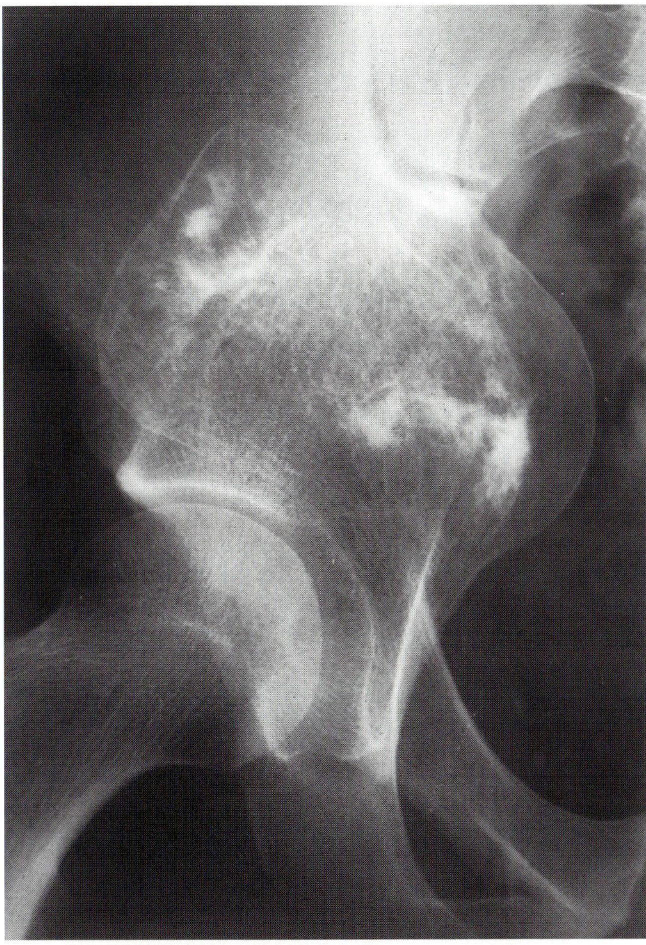

Fig. 10.8

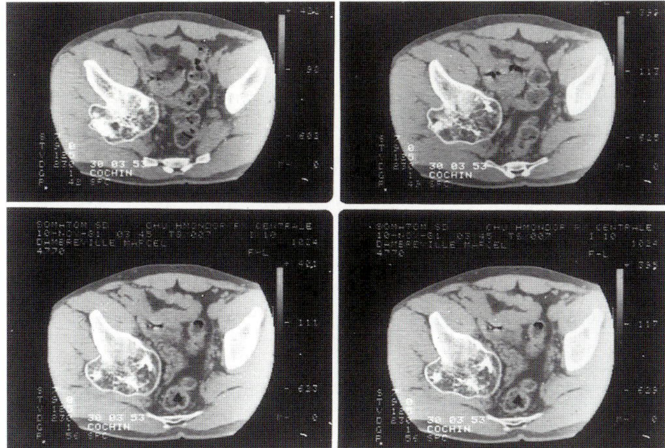

Fig. 10.9

Figs 10.8, 10.9 Unusual osteochondroma of the pelvis involving all the iliac wing.

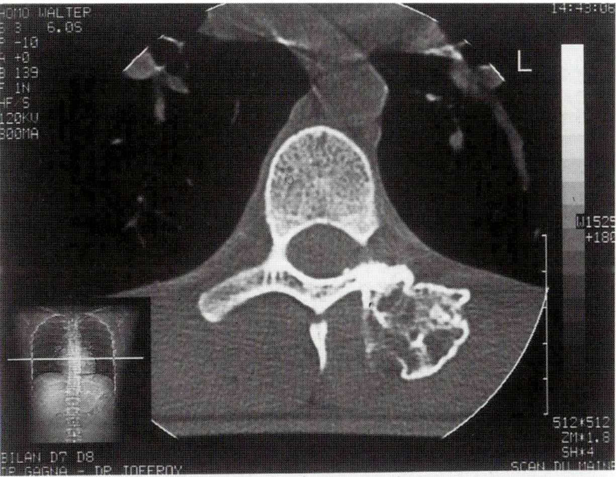

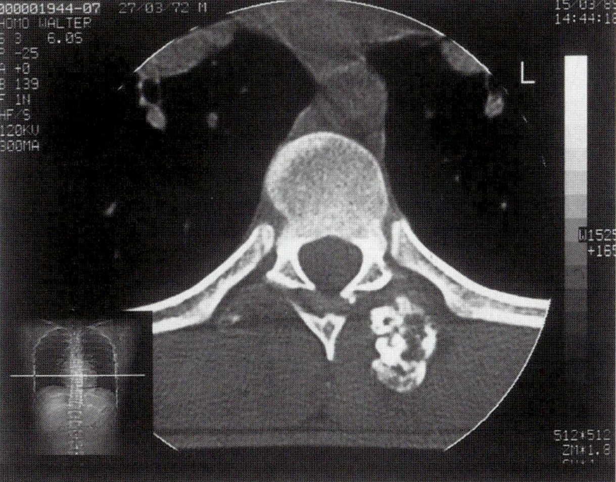

Fig. 10.10

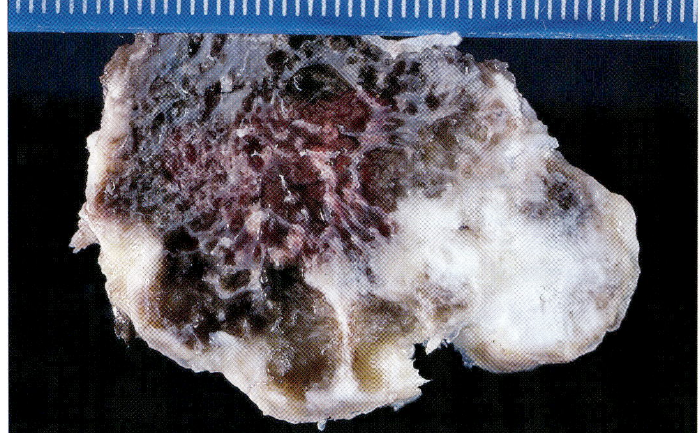

Fig. 10.11

Figs 10.10, 10.11 Osteochondroma of the spine (T7 level).

syndrome of metachondromatosis,[43,44] which displays metaphyseal cartilaginous lesions, periarticular ossifications and calcifications and multiple osteochondromas in the hands and feet.

Turret exostoses are found in the dorsum of the proximal and middle phalanges, after a history of a puncture wound; these lesions are dome-shaped masses of reactive subperiosteal bone caused by a hematoma.[45,46]

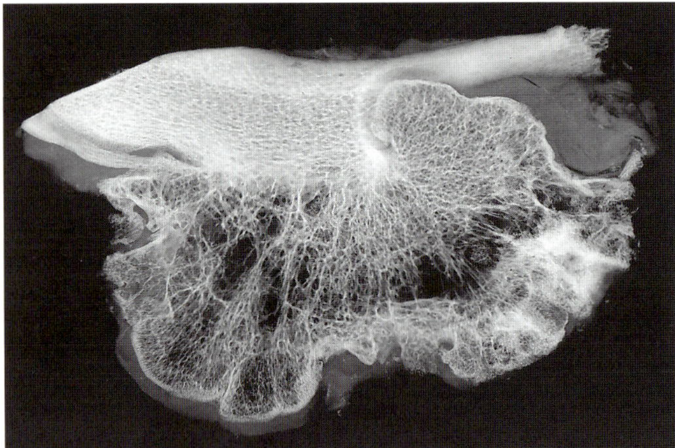

Fig. 10.12

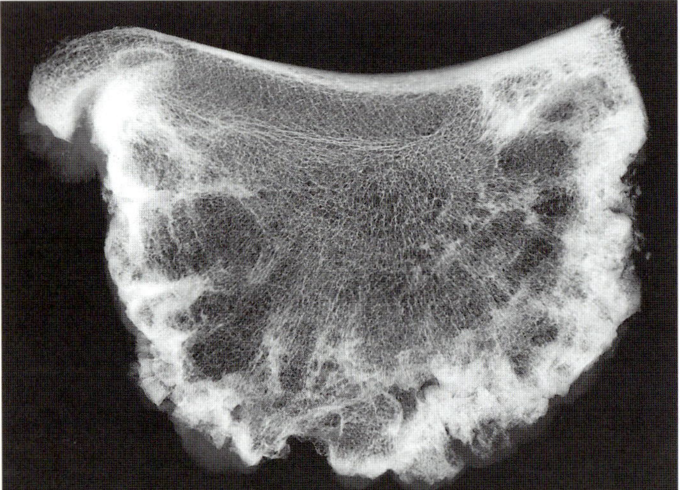

Fig. 10.13

Figs 10.12, 10.13 Osteochondromas of the iliac wing exhibiting one of the hallmarks of the disease: a continuity of the cancellous bone of the lesion with that of normal bone.

Subungual exostoses are found usually on the dorsal and medial aspect of the great toe, frequently after a history of trauma or infection[47,48] (Figs 10.34–10.36). These painful and sometimes ulcerated lesions are the reactive growth of a very cellular fibrocartilaginous tissue merging into mature trabecular bone by intramembranous or enchondral ossification.[48–50]

Bizarre osteochondromatous proliferations involve the small bones of the hands and feet and even the long bones.[51] Gross appearance is that of small osteochondromas, but the underlying cortex is intact. A hypercellular cartilage with irregular calcification, forming lobules or caps, is associated with a spindle cell component and areas of bone formation. There is a high frequency of recurrences, but no metastases (see Ch. 49).

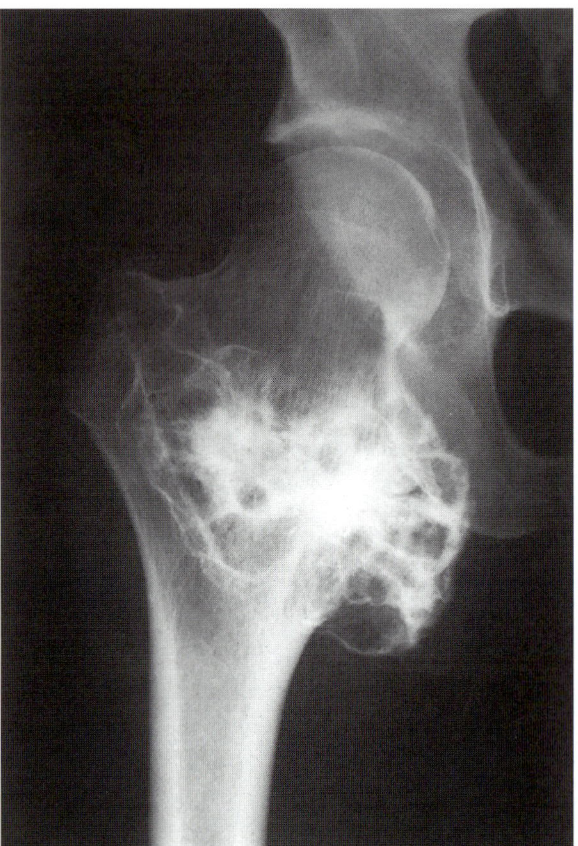

Fig. 10.14

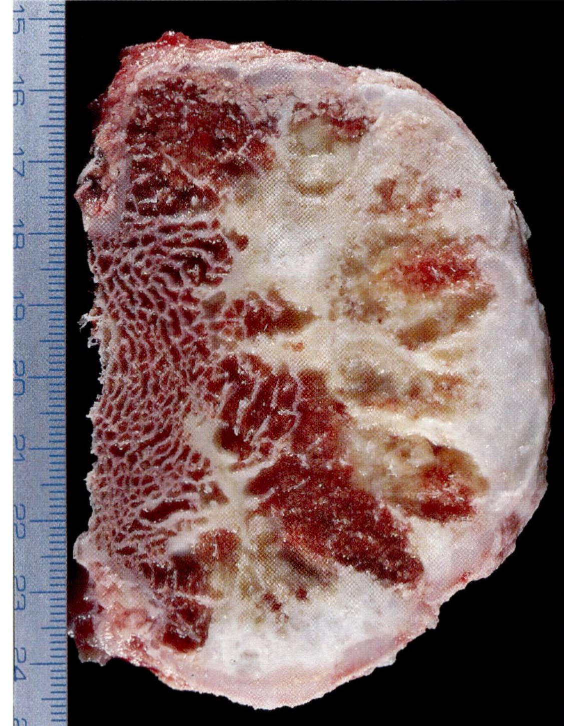

Fig. 10.15

Figs 10.14, 10.15 Large and sessile osteochondroma of the upper end of the femur.

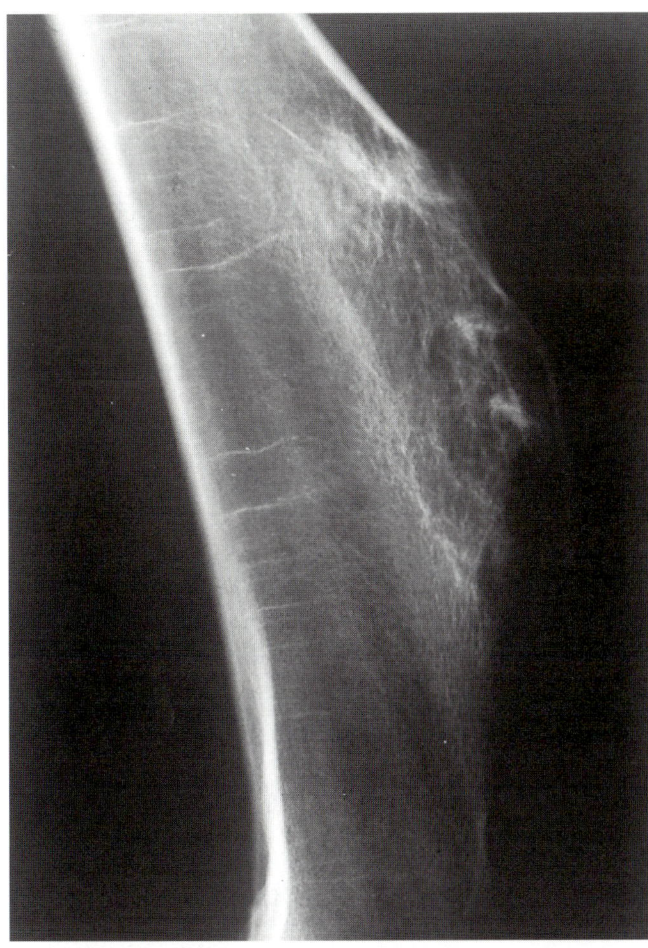

Fig. 10.16 Sessile osteochondroma of the lower femoral metaphysis.

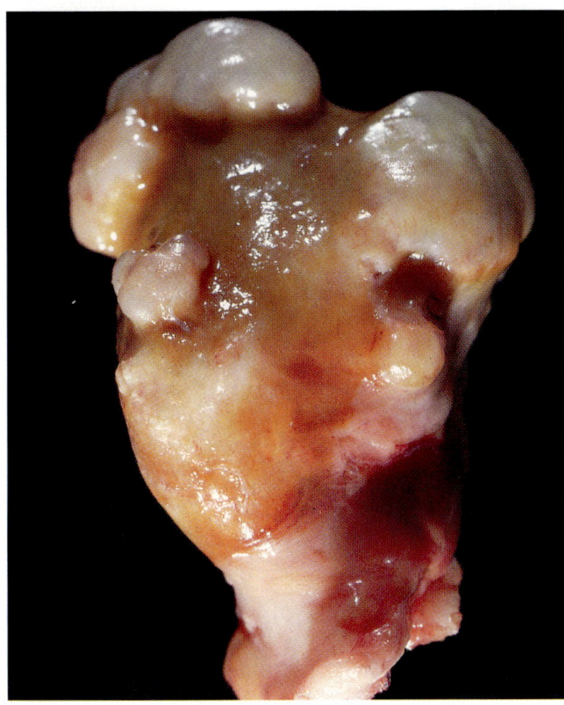

Fig. 10.17 Pedunculated osteochondroma of the lower femoral metaphysis.

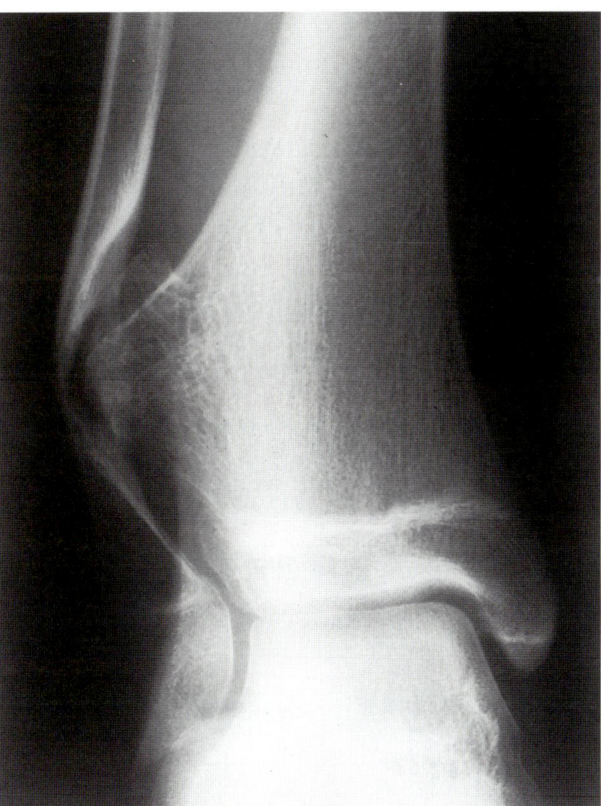

Fig. 10.18 Pressure deformity of the fibula by an osteochondroma of the tibia.

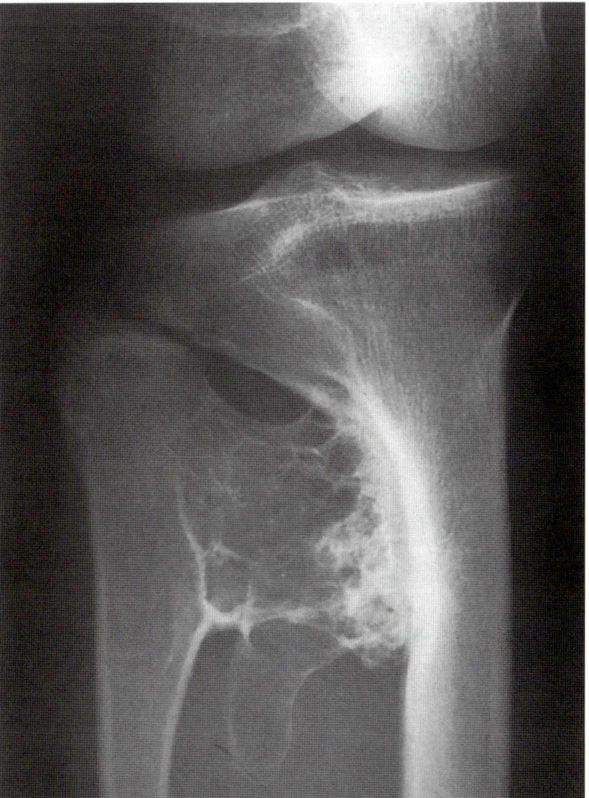

Fig. 10.19 Osteochondroma: synostosis between the tibia and the fibula.

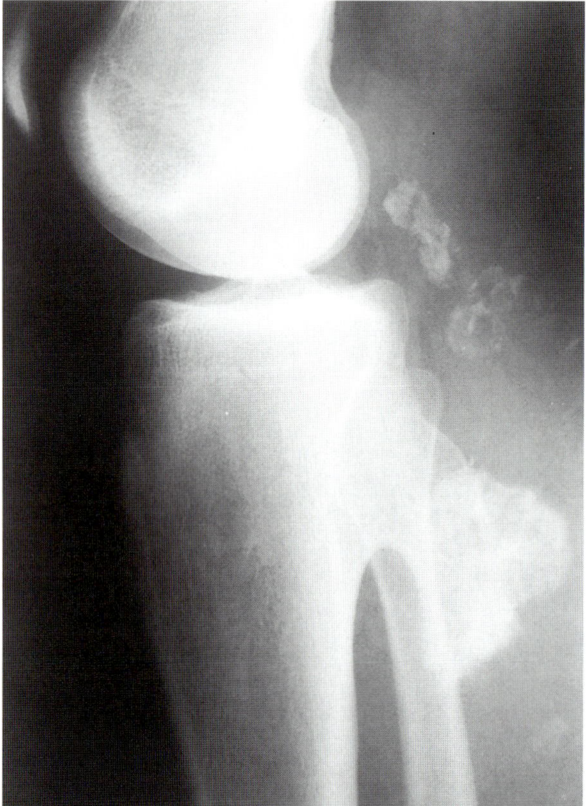

Fig. 10.20

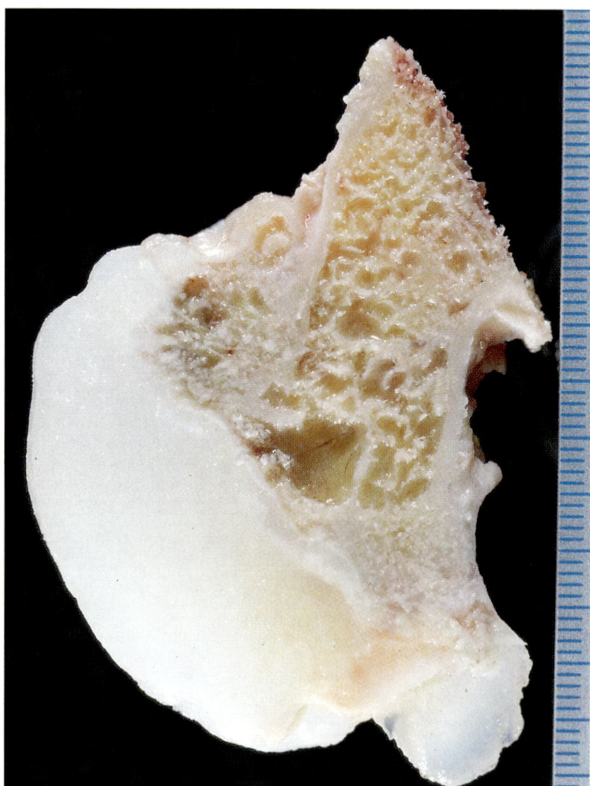

Fig. 10.21

Figs 10.20, 10.21 Thickened cap in a solitary osteochondroma with no cytological anormalities.

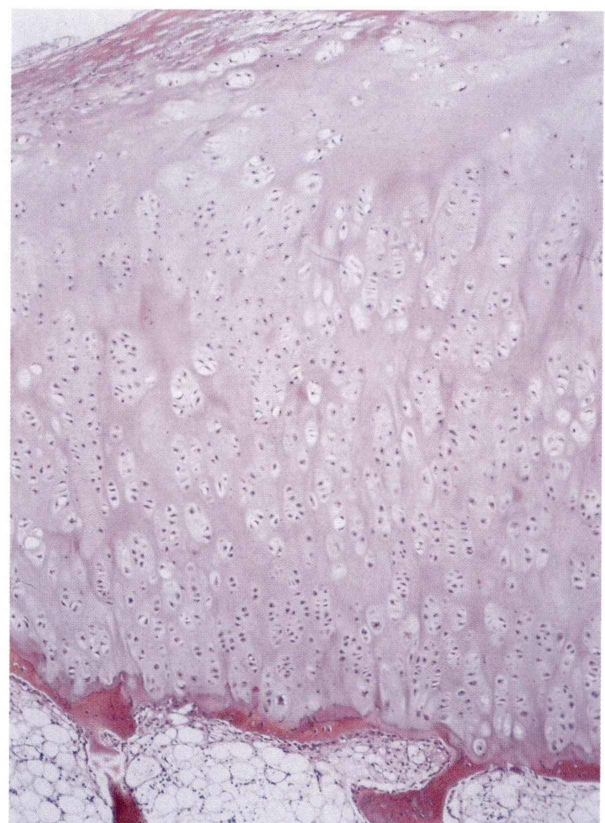

Fig. 10.22

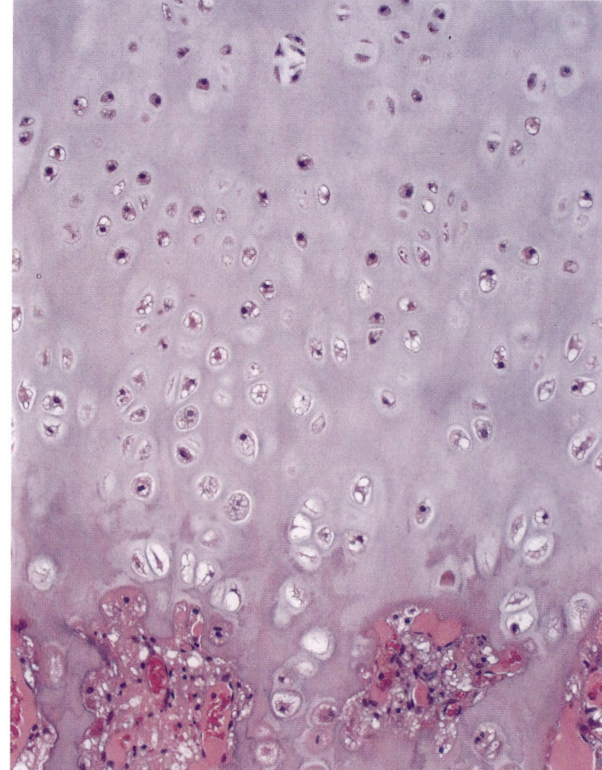

Fig. 10.23

Figs 10.22, 10.23 Cartilage caps of osteochondromas histologically similar to a growth plate.

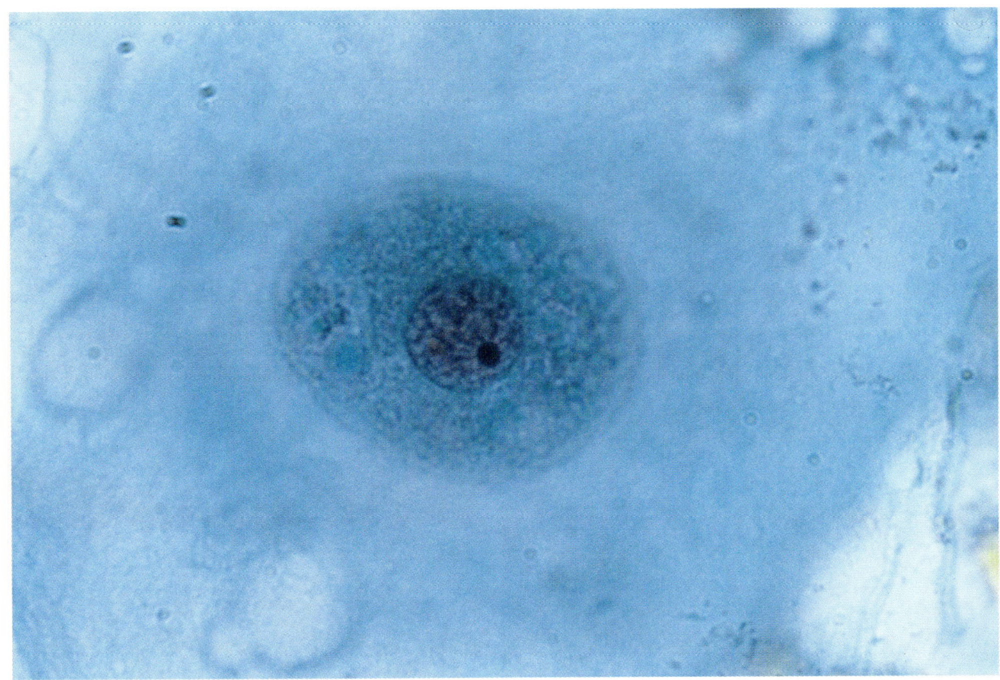

Fig. 10.24 Imprint cytology of the cartilaginous cap on an osteochondroma.

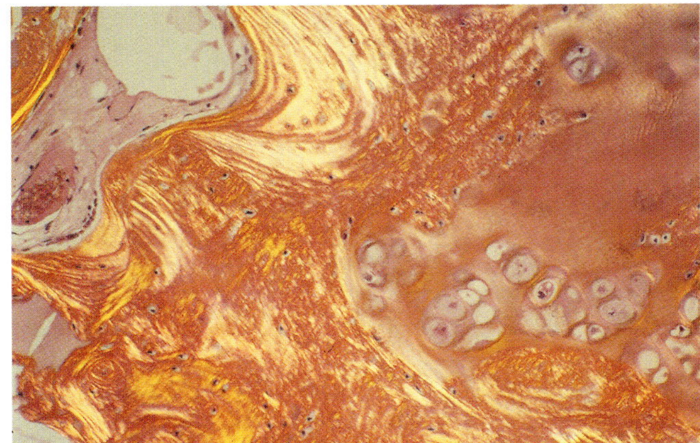

Fig. 10.25 Enchondral ossification of a cartilaginous cap.

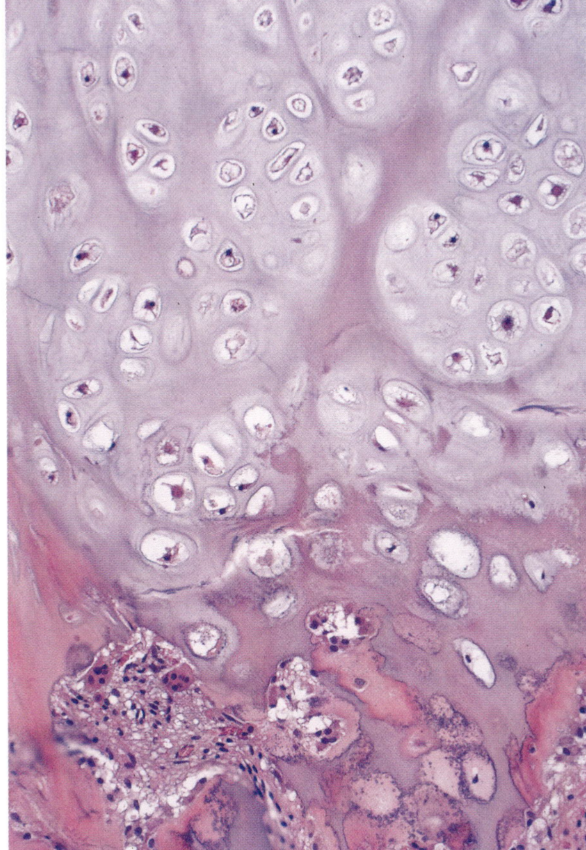

Fig. 10.26

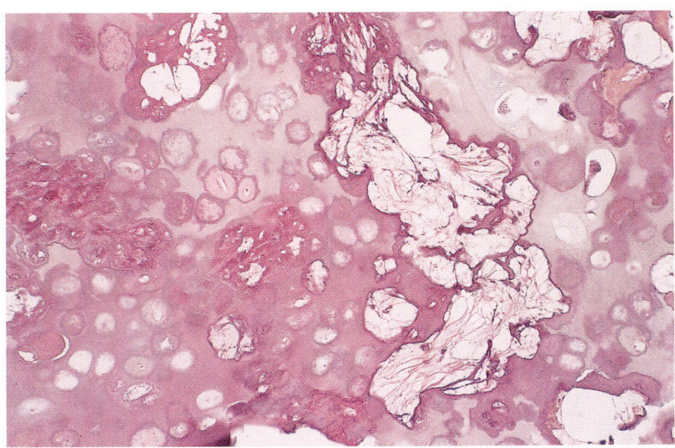

Fig. 10.27

Figs 10.26, 10.27 Osteochondromas: large areas of calcified, ossified or necrotic cartilage in the stalk.

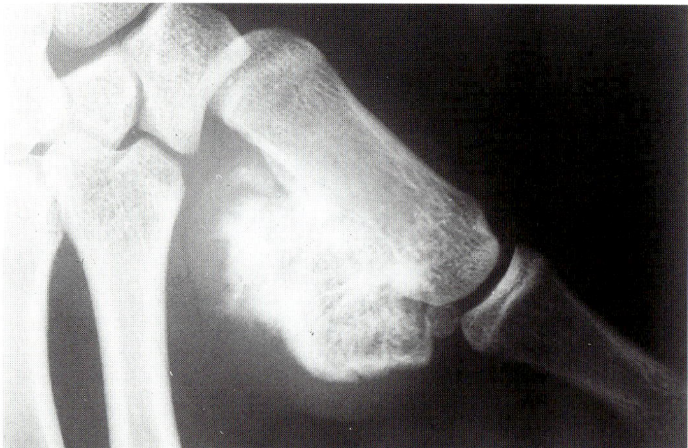

Fig. 10.28

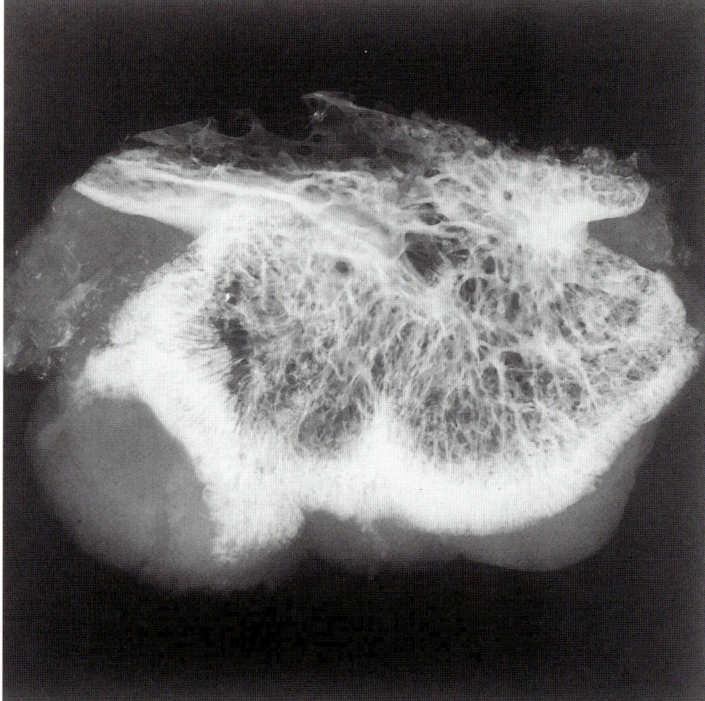

Fig. 10.30

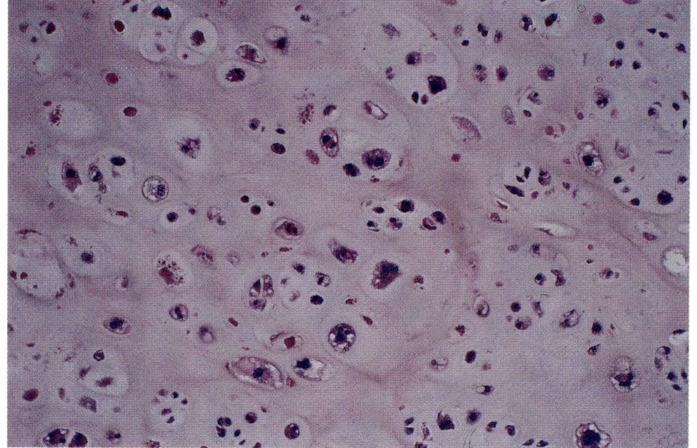

Fig. 10.32

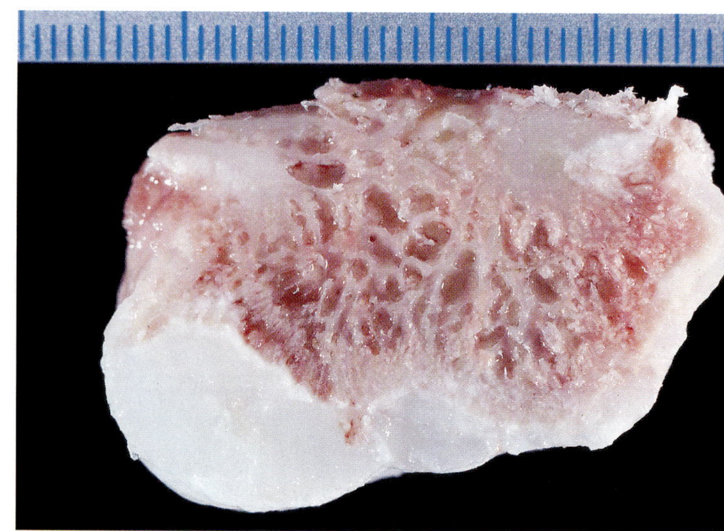

Fig. 10.29

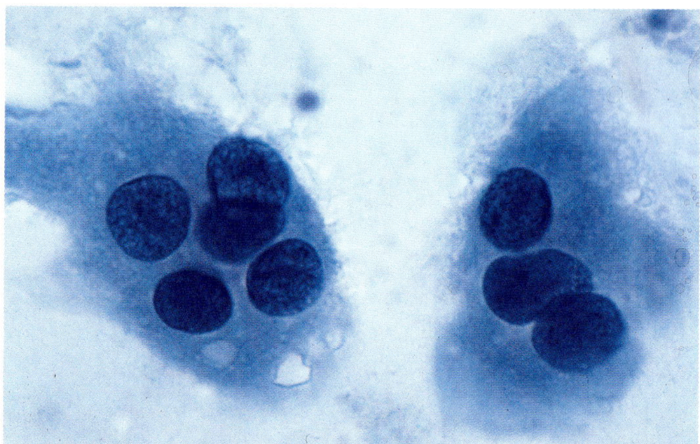

Fig. 10.31

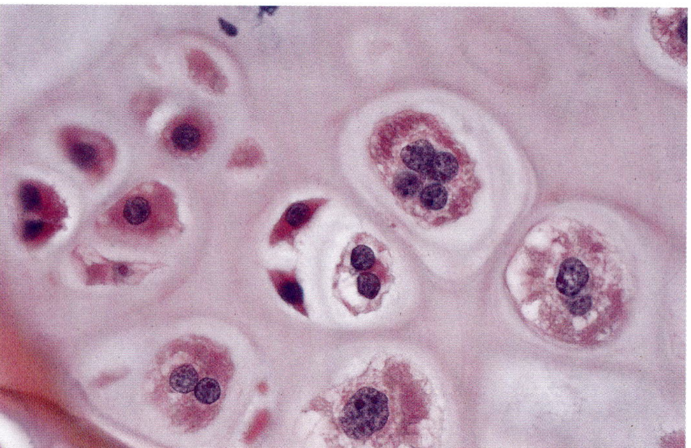

Fig. 10.33

10.28–10.33 Most unusual case of a solitary osteochondroma of a metacarpal, with a limited area of malignant transformation demonstrated by obvious cytological abnormalities.

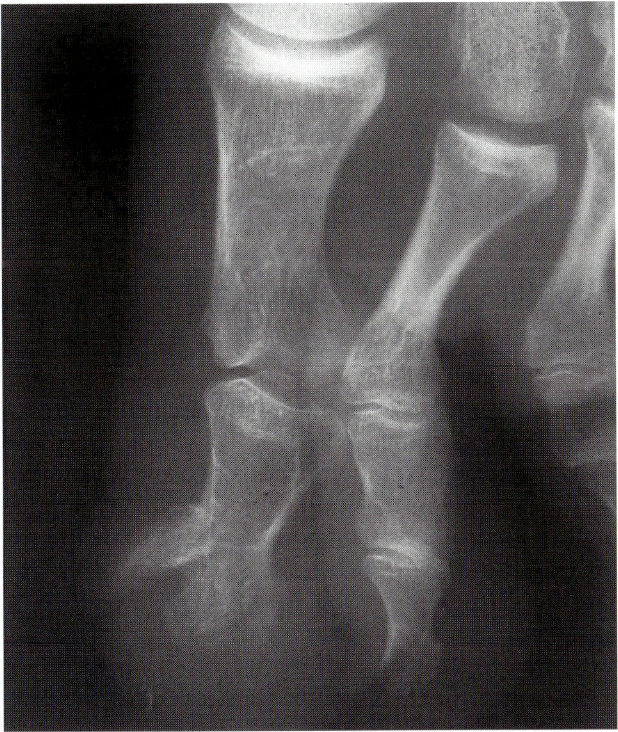

Fig. 10.34

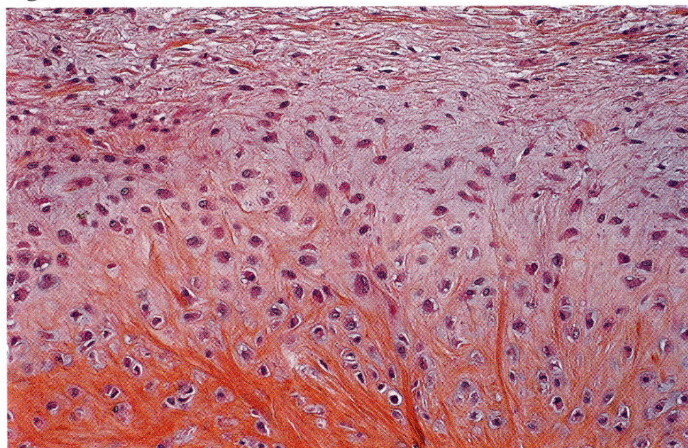

Fig. 10.35

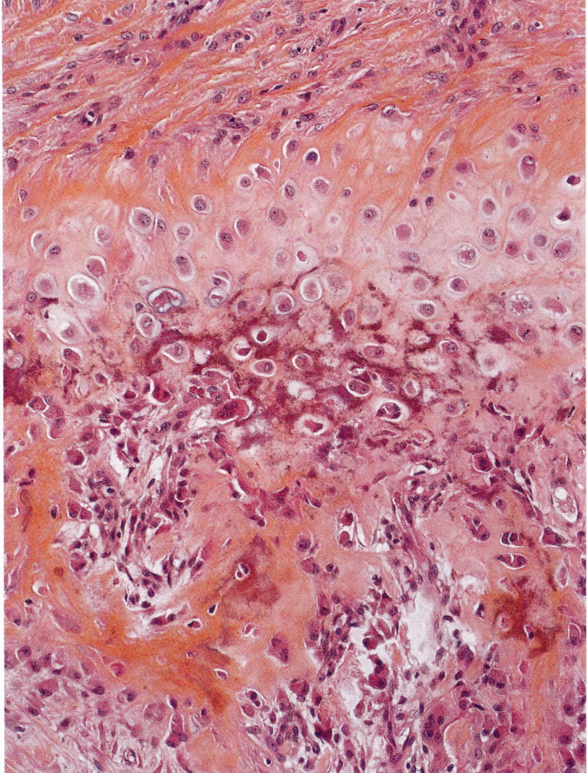

Fig. 10.36

Figs 10.34–10.36 Subungual exostosis of the big toe with periosteal activity and a cellular fibrocartilaginous tissue.

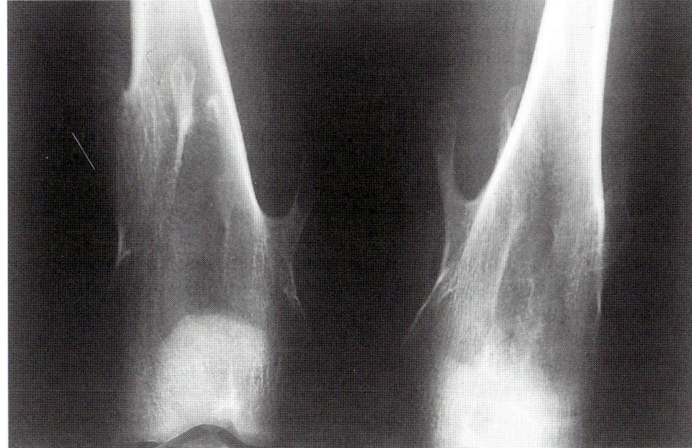

Fig. 10.37

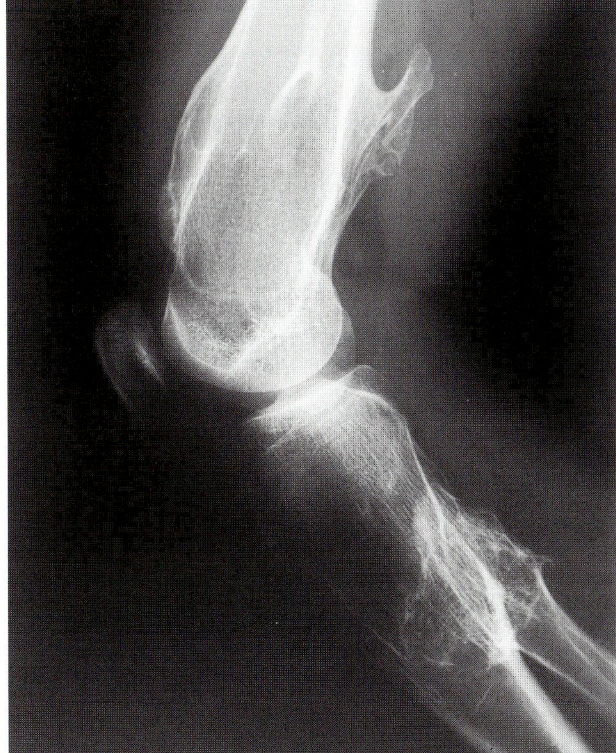

Fig. 10.38

Figs 10.37, 10.38 Cases of osteochondromatosis demonstrating bilateral and symmetrical lesions and flaring of the metaphyses.

OSTEOCHONDROMATOSIS

This is an inherited autosomal-dominant disorder usually discovered before the age of 5[1] (Figs 10.37, 10.38). In some series, there is a male predominance, but this is debated.[52] About 10% of patients have no family history of multiple exostoses.[52]

Osteochondromas are bilateral and symmetrical, but often with a unilateral predilection. They are associated with a defective metaphyseal remodeling: wide flaring of the metaphysis, discrepancies in the growth rate of long bones and in 60% of cases, severe deformities of the forearm.[53,54]

Reactive bursa formation has been reported,[9,12,55] as well as synostoses between adjacent bones.

Constitutional deletions or structural rearrangements of the long arm of chromosome 8[56] and a second locus mapped to the short arm of chromosome 19[57] have been identified.

Malignant degeneration appears to be less frequent than previously stated,[1] ranging from 1.3%[58,59] to 6%[52] and involving chiefly the flat bones.[36] It is very rare in the hand.[60]

Most tumors are well-differentiated chondrosarcomas showing a high uptake on bone scans.[61] Osteosarcomas or malignant fibrous histiocytomas may well represent dedifferentiated chondrosarcomas.[62–65]

COMMENTS FOR THE SURGICAL PATHOLOGIST

Histological sampling of osteochondromas is concentrated on the cartilage cap as the huge central calcified areas are of much less importance.

Malignant transformation, in most cases, is obvious on clinical and radiological findings; focal cytological abnormalities in a normal cartilaginous cap have to be interpreted with caution.

REFERENCES

1. Canella P, Gardini F, Boriani S. Exostosis: development, evolution and relationship to malignant degeneration. Ital J Orthop Traumatol 1981: 7: 293–298
2. Davids J R, Glancy G L, Eilert R E. Fracture through the stalk of pedunculated osteochondromas. A report of three cases. Clin Orthop 1991: 271: 258–264
3. Unger E C, Gilula L A, Kyriakos M. Case report 430. Ischaemic necrosis of osteochondroma of tibia. Skeletal Radiol 1987: 16: 416–421
4. Tajima K, Nishida J, Yamazaki K, Shimamura T, Abe M. Case report 545. Osteochondroma (osteocartilaginous exostosis) of cervical spine with spinal cord compression. Skeletal Radiol 1989: 18: 306–309
5. Gomez-Reino J J, Radin A, Goveric P D. Pseudoaneurysm of the popliteal artery as a complication of an osteochondroma. Skeletal Radiol 1979: 4: 26–28
6. Smithius T. Exostosis bursata. J Bone Joint Surg (Br) 1964: 46: 544–545
7. El Khoury G Y, Bassett G S. Symptomatic bursa formation with osteochondromas. AJR 1979: 133: 895–898
8. Borges A M, Huvos A G, Smith J. Bursa formation and synovial chondrometaplasia associated with osteochondromas. Am J Clin Pathol 1981: 75: 648–653
9. Shogry M E, Armstrong P. Case report 630. Reactive bursa formation surrounding an osteochondroma. Skeletal Radiol 1990: 19: 465–467
10. Griffiths H J, Thompson R C Jr, Galloway H R, Everson L I, Suh J S. Bursitis in association with solitary osteochondromas presenting as mass lesions. Skeletal Radiol 1991: 20: 513–516
11. Cuomo F, Blank K, Zuckerman J D, Present D A. Scapular osteochondroma presenting with exostosis bursata. Bull Hosp Jt Dis 1993: 52: 55–58
12. Schofield T D, Pitcher J D, Youngberg R. Synovial chondromatosis simulating neoplastic degeneration of osteochondroma: findings on MRI and CT. Skeletal Radiol 1994: 21: 99–102
13. Milgram J W. The origins of osteochondromas and enchondromas. A histopathologic study. Clin Orthop 1983: 174: 264–284
14. D'Ambrosia R, Ferguson A B Jr. The formation of osteochondroma by epiphyseal cartilage transplantation. Clin Orthop 1968: 61: 103–115
15. Hwang S K, Park B M. Induction of osteochondromas by periosteal resection. Orthopedics 1991: 14: 809–812
16. Murphy F D, Blount W B. Cartilaginous exostoses following irradiation. J Bone Joint Surg (Am) 1962: 44: 662–668
17. Libshitz H I, Cohen M A. Radiation-induced osteochondromas. Radiology 1982: 142: 643–647
18. DeSimone D P, Abdelwahab I F, Kenan S, Klein M J, Lewis M M. Case report 773. Radiation-induced osteochondroma of the ilium. Skeletal Radiol 1993: 22: 135–137
19. Herman T E, McAlister W H, Rosenthal D, Dehner L P. Case report 691. Radiation-induced osteochondromas (RIO) arising from the neural arch and producing compression of the spinal cord. Skeletal Radiol 1991: 20: 472–476
20. Novick G S, Pavlov H, Bullough P G. Osteochondroma of the cervical spine: report of two cases in preadolescent males. Skeletal Radiol 1982: 8: 13–15
21. Fanney D, Tehranzadeh J, Quencer R M, Nadji M. Case report 415. Osteochondroma of the cervical spine. Skeletal Radiol 1987: 16: 170–174
22. Lee J K, Yao L, Wirth C R. MR imaging of solitary osteochondromas: report of eight cases. AJR 1987: 149: 557–560
23. Malghem J, Vande Berg B, Noel H, Maldague B. Benign osteochondromas and exostotic chondrosarcomas: evaluation of cartilage cap thickness by ultrasound. Skeletal Radiol 1992: 21: 33–37
24. Kenney P J, Gilula L A, Murphy W A. The use of computed tomography to distinguish osteochondroma and chondrosarcoma. Radiology 1981: 139: 129–137
25. Hudson T M, Springfield D S, Spanier S S, Enneking W F, Hamlin D J. Benign exostoses and exostotic chondrosarcomas: evaluation of cartilage thickness by CT. Radiology 1984: 152: 595–599
26. Hudson T M, Chew F S, Manaster B J. Scintigraphy of benign exostoses and exostotic chondrosarcomas. AJR 1983: 140: 581–586
27. Lange R H, Lange T A, Rao B K. Correlative radiographic, scintigraphic and histological evaluation of exostoses. J Bone Joint Surg (Am) 1984: 66: 1454–1459
28. Hwang W S, McQueen D, Monson R C, Reed M H. The significance of cytoplasmic chondrocyte inclusions in multiple osteochondromatosis, solitary osteochondromas, and chondrodysplasias. Am J Clin Pathol 1982: 78: 89–91
29. Mertens F, Rydholm A, Kreicbergs A et al. Loss of chromosome band 8q24 in sporadic osteocartilaginous exostoses. Genes Chromosomes Cancer 1994: 9: 8–12
30. Martinez-Tello F J, Martinez-Gonzalez M A. The ultrastructure of the cartilaginous tumors. In: Bonucci E, Motta P M, Eds. The ultrastructure of skeletal tissues. Boston: Kluwer, 1990, pp 189–190
31. Fadda M, Zirattu G. Il processo di mineralizzazione

nell'osteocondroma. Studio al microscopio ellettronico a scansione. Arch Putti Chir Organi Mov 1991: 39: 289–296

32. Paling M R. The 'disappearing' osteochondroma. Skeletal Radiol 1983: 10: 40–42

33. Copeland R L, Meehan P L, Morrissy R T. Spontaneous regression of osteochondromas. Two case reports. J Bone Joint Surg (Am) 1985: 67: 971–973

34. Montgomery D M, LaMont R L. Resolving solitary osteochondromas. A report of two cases and literature review. Orthopedics 1989: 12: 861–863

35. Castriota-Scanderberg A, Bonetti M G, Cammisa M, Dallapiccola B. Spontaneous regression of exostoses: two case reports. Pediatr Radiol 1995: 25: 544–548

36. Garrison R C, Unni K K, McLeod R A, Pritchard D J, Dahlin D C. Chondrosarcoma arising in osteochondroma. Cancer 1982: 49: 1890–1897

37. Schiller A L. Diagnosis of borderline cartilage lesions of bone. Semin Diagn Pathol 1985: 2: 42–62

38. Schweitzer G, Pirie D. Osteosarcoma arising in a solitary osteochondroma. S Afr J Med 1971: 45: 810–811

39. Slullitel J A, Schajowicz F, Slullitel J. Osteochondrome solitaire avec dégénerescence maligne vers un sarcome osteogénique. Rev Chir Orthop Reparatrice Appar Mot 1971: 57: 471–478

40. Van Lerberghe E, Van Damme B, Van Holsbeeck M, Burssens A, Hoogmartens M. Case report 626. Osteosarcoma arising in a solitary osteochondroma of the femur. Skeletal Radiol 1990: 19: 594–597

41. Nojima T, Yamashiro K, Fujita M, Isu K, Ubayama Y, Yamawaki S. A case of osteosarcoma arising in a solitary osteochondroma. Acta Orthop Scand 1991: 62: 290–292

42. Resnik C S, Levine A M, Aisner S C, Young J W R, Dorfman H D. Case report 522. Concurrent adjacent osteochondroma and enchondroma. Skeletal Radiol 1989: 18: 66–69

43. Maroteaux P. La métachondromatose. Z Kinderheilkd 1971: 109: 246–261

44. Bassett G S, Cowell H R. Metachondromatosis. Report of four cases. J Bone Joint Surg (Am) 1985: 67: 811–814

45. Wissinger H A, McClain E J, Boyes J H. Turret exostosis. Ossifying hematoma of the phalanges. J Bone Joint Surg (Am) 1966: 48: 105–110

46. Lee B S, Kaplan R. Turret exostosis of the phalanges. Clin Orthop 1974: 100: 186–189

47. Landon G C, Johnson K A, Dahlin D C. Subungual exostoses. J Bone Joint Surg (Am) 1979: 61: 256–259

48. Miller-Breslow A, Dorfman H D. Dupuytren's (subungual) exostosis. Am J Surg Pathol 1988: 12: 368–378

49. Ippolito E, Falez F, Tudisco C, Balus L, Fazio M, Morrone A. Subungual exostosis: histological and clinical considerations on 30 cases. Ital J Orthop Traumatol 1987: 13: 81–87

50. Kato H, Nakagawa K, Tsuji t, Hamada T. Subungual exostoses. Clinicopathological and ultrastructural studies of three cases. Clin Exp Dermatol 1990: 15: 429–432

51. Nora F E, Dahlin D C, Beabout J W. Bizarre parosteal osteochondromatous proliferations of the hands and feet. Am J Surg Pathol 1983: 7: 245–250

52. Schmale G A, Conrad E U 3rd, Raskind W H. The natural history of hereditary multiple exostoses. J Bone Joint Surg (Am) 1994: 76: 986–992

53. Shapiro F, Simon S, Glimcher M J. Hereditary multiple exostoses. Anthropometric, roentgenographic, and clinical aspects. J Bone Joint Surg (Am) 1979: 61: 815–824

54. Bock G W, Reed M H. Forearm deformities in multiple cartilaginous exostoses. Skeletal Radiol 1991: 20: 483–486

55. Voegeli E, Laissue J, Kaiser A, Hofer B. Case report 143. Multiple hereditary osteocartilaginous exostoses affecting right femur with an overlying giant cystic bursa (exostosis bursata). Skeletal Radiol 1981: 6: 134–137

56. Yoshiura K, Inazawa J, Koyama K, Nakamura Y, Niikawa N. Mapping of the 8q23 translocation breakpoint of t(8;13) observed in a patient with multiple exostoses. Genes Chromosomes Cancer 1994: 9: 57–61

57. Le Merrer M, Legeai-Mallet L, Jeannin PM et al. A gene for hereditary multiple exostoses maps to chromosome 19p. Hum Mol Genet 1994: 3: 717–722

58. Peterson H A. Multiple hereditary osteochondromata. Clin Orthop 1989: 239: 222–230

59. Voutsinas S, Wynne-Davies R. The infrequency of malignant disease in diaphyseal aclasis and neurofibromatosis. J Med Genet 1983: 20: 345–349

60. Ostlere S J, Gold R H, Mirra J M, Perlman R D. Case report 658. Chondrosarcoma of the proximal phalanx of right fourth finger secondary to multiple hereditary exostoses (MHE). Skeletal Radiol 1991: 20: 145–148

61. Bouvier J F, Chassard J L, Brunat-Mentigny M et al Radionucleide bone imaging in diaphyseal aclasis with malignant change. Cancer 1986: 57: 2280–2284

62. Matsuno T, Ichioka Y, Yagi T, Ishii S. Spindle-cell sarcoma in patients who have osteochondromatosis. A report of two cases. J Bone Joint Surg (Am) 1988: 70: 137–141

63. Tsuchiya H, Morikawa S, Tomita K. Osteosarcoma arising from a multiple exostoses lesion: case report. Jpn J Clin Oncol 1990: 20: 296–298

64. Pucci P, Stilli S. Istiocitoma fibroso maligno su esostosi in paziente affetto da esostosi multiple. Giorn Ital Ortop Traum 1982: 207–209

65. Frassica F J, Unni K K, Beabout J W, Sim F H. Dedifferentiated chondrosarcoma. Report of the clinicopathological features and treatment of seventy-eight cases. J Bone Joint Surg (Am) 1986: 68: 1197–1205

11

Chondroma

M. Forest

INTRODUCTION AND CLINICAL DATA

Chondromas, composed of hyaline cartilage, are the second most common cartilage tumor of bone after osteochondromas (10% of all benign bone tumors). They may occur in a medullary location (enchondroma) or on the surface of bone (periosteal chondroma). It has been assumed that they are caused by the growth plate cartilage becoming fragmented in the central portion.[1]

They are mostly diagnosed after the second decade and there is no sex predominance. They increase in size only during childhood and adolescence (Mulder et al 1993). Some are asymptomatic while others induce a painless swelling or pain due to infraction of plain fractures (20%).

SKELETAL DISTRIBUTION

In 35–60% of cases, chondromas are found in the tubular bones of the hands and mostly the phalanges (Figs 11.1–11.4), less often in the feet. In long bones (25%) (Figs 11.5–11.8), the location is metaphyseal or metadiaphyseal; extension to the epiphysis is unusual.[2] They rarely occur in flat bones or in the spine.[3]

IMAGING

Chondromas appear as a well-marginated radiolucency, with smooth or lobulated contours. A cartilaginous matrix may be found with a ground glass appearance (Wilner 1982) or with mottled calcifications, stippled, coarse conglomerates or a 'popcorn' pattern. Circular ring and arc-shaped densities correspond to the enchondral ossification of cartilage.[4]

The lesion may be expansile with a thinning of the cortex, which may completely disappear in long-standing cases.

CT accurately shows the extent;[2] MRI demonstrates a

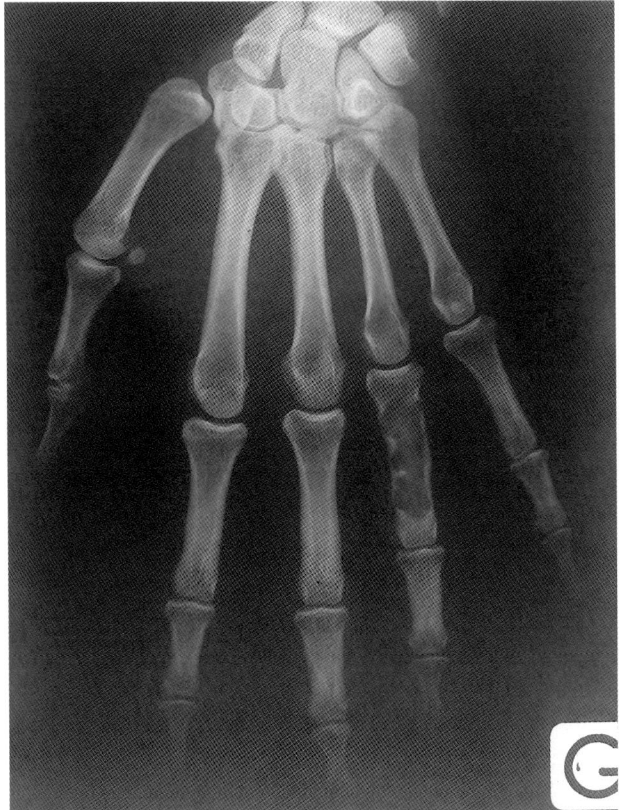

Fig. 11.1

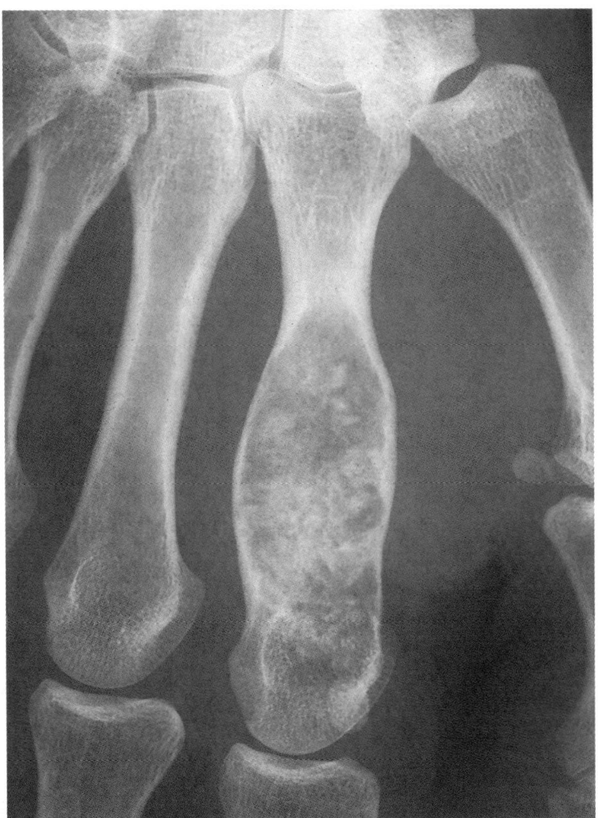

Fig. 11.2

Figs 11.1, 11.2 Enchondromas of short tubular bones of the hand.

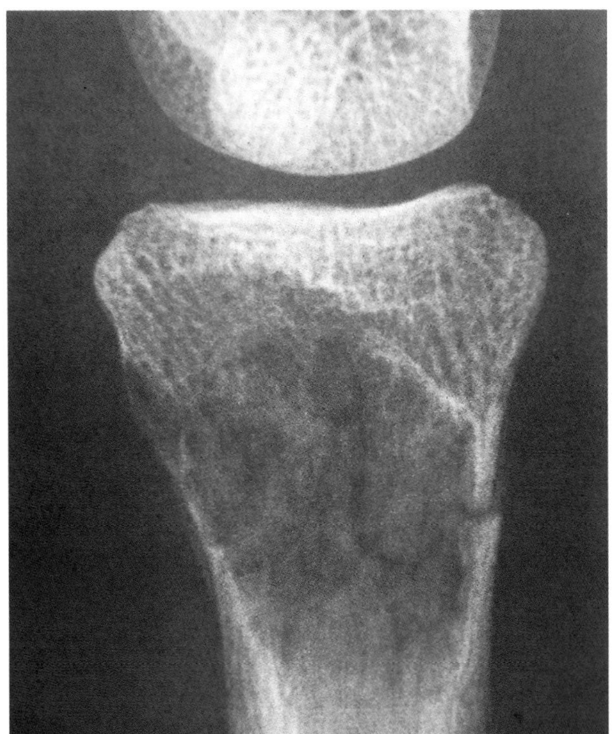

Fig. 11.3

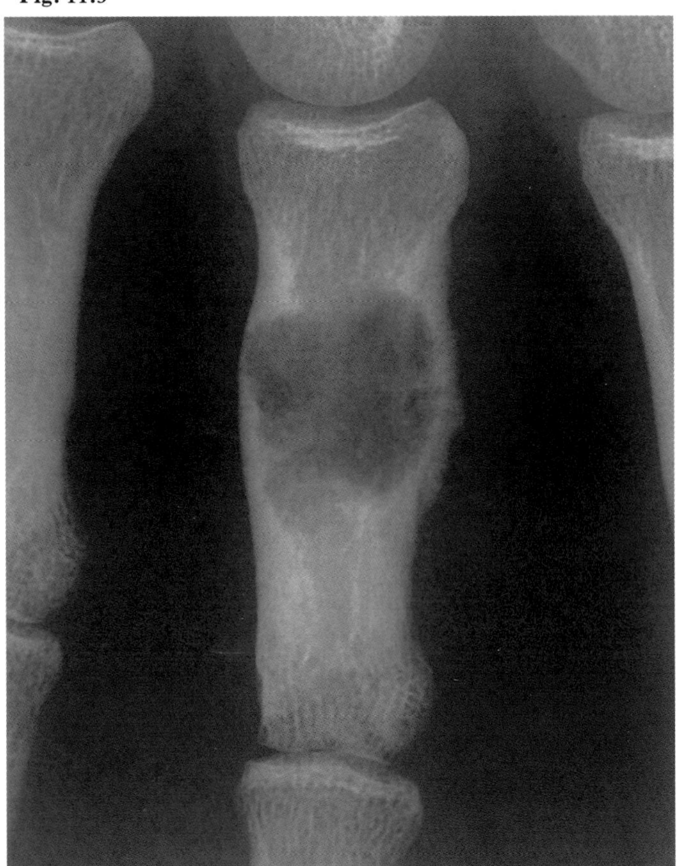

Fig. 11.4

Figs 11.3, 11.4 Enchondromas of the hand: small fracture of the cortex and periosteal reaction.

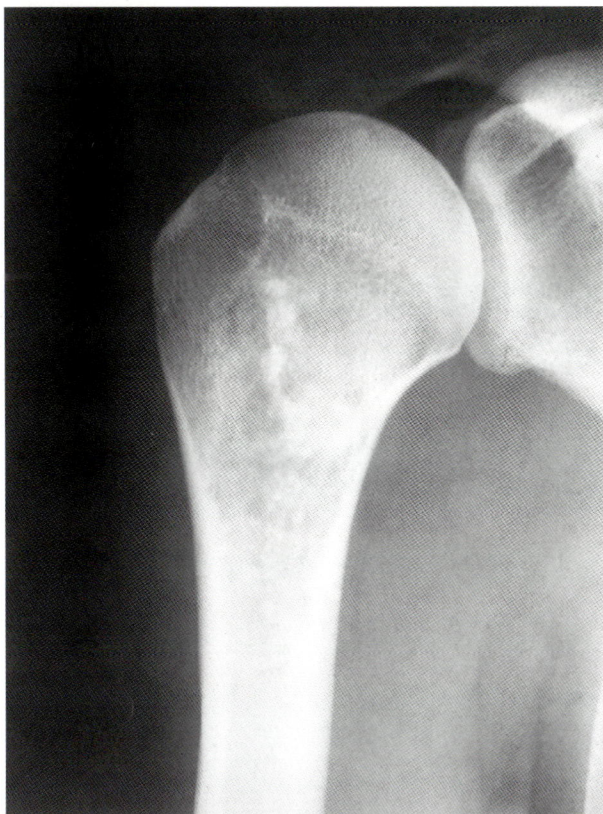

Fig. 11.5

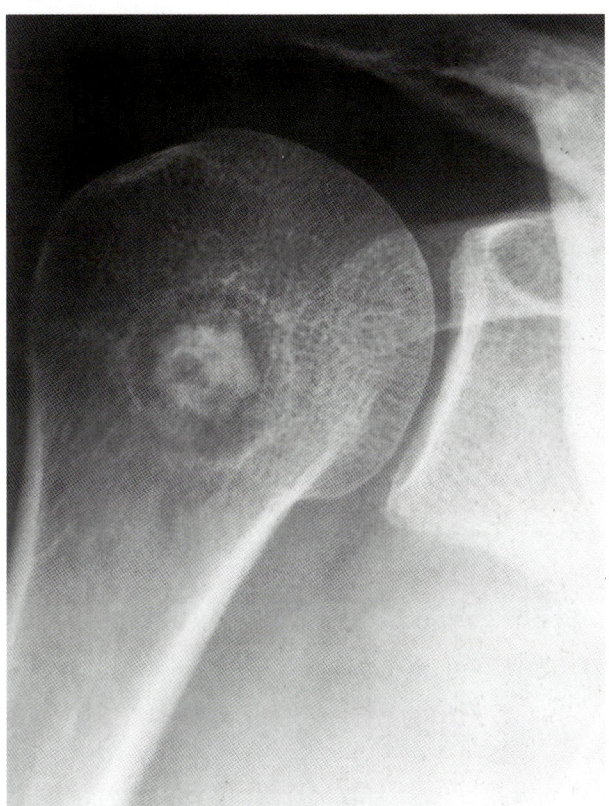

Fig. 11.6

Figs 11.5, 11.6 Enchondromas in the upper end of the humerus.

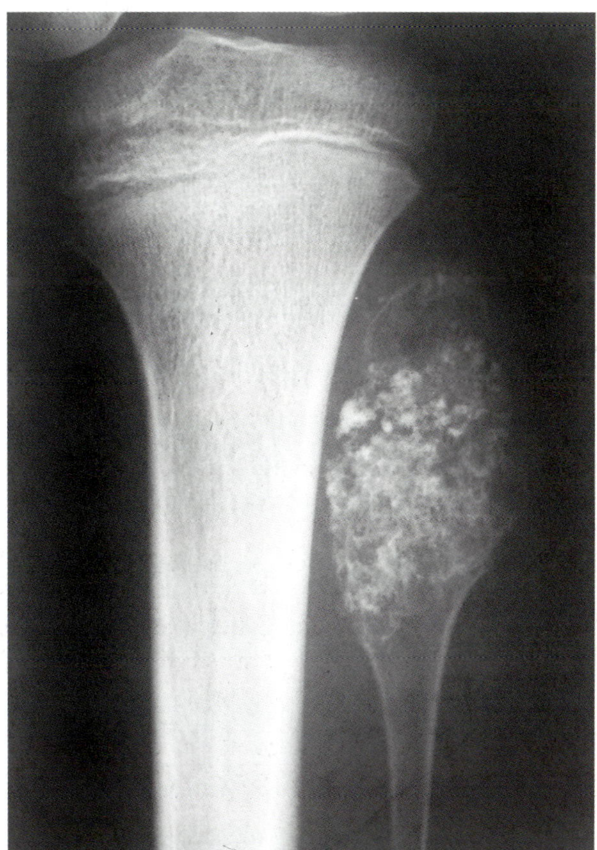

Fig. 11.7

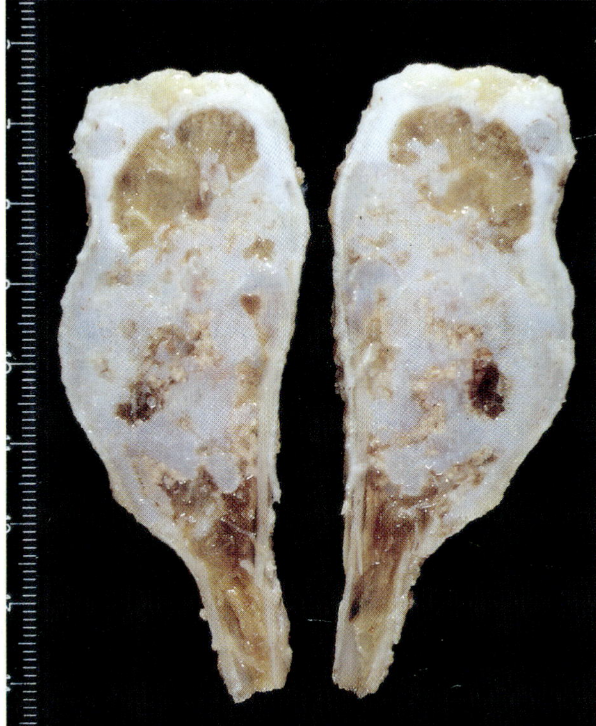

Fig. 11.8

Figs 11.7, 11.8 Enchondroma of the fibula with mottled calcifications and thinning of the cortex.

low signal intensity on T1-weighted images and an increased signal intensity on T2-weighted images (Greenfield & Arrington 1995). Periosteal reactions are due to stress fractures.

GROSS PATHOLOGY

The white or bluish tumoral cartilage is firm and rubbery, sometimes with yellow calcifications. The cortex is thinned or bulging in small tubular bones.

HISTOPATHOLOGY

Lobules of hyaline cartilage are separated by normal marrow and eventually encased by woven or lamellar bone (Mirra 1989), with no permeative growth.

Cartilage cells of uniform size have a small rounded nucleus and in some fields, a vacuolated cytoplasm (Figs 11.9–11.13). In half the cases, hyaline spherical eosinophilic PAS positive, intracytoplasmic globules, averaging 4 microns present. They are secretory products of

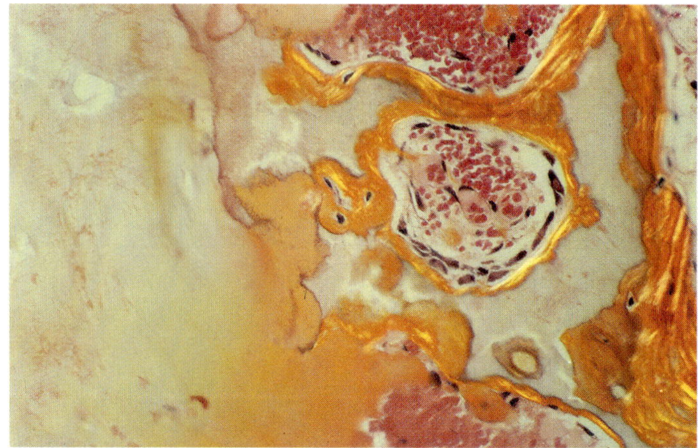

Fig. 11.11 Encasement of cartilage by bone formation in an enchondroma (polarized light).

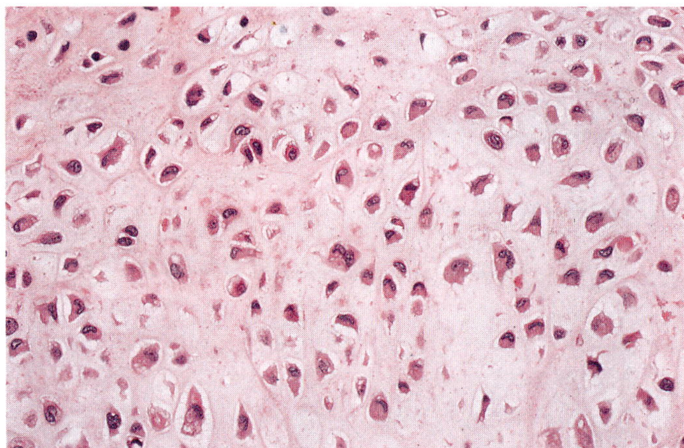

Fig. 11.9

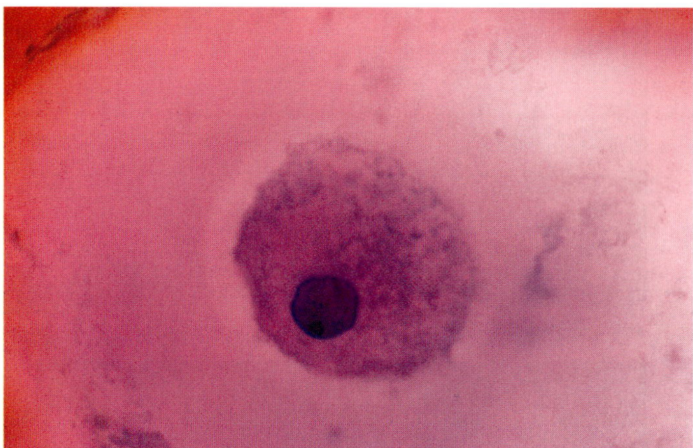

Fig. 11.12

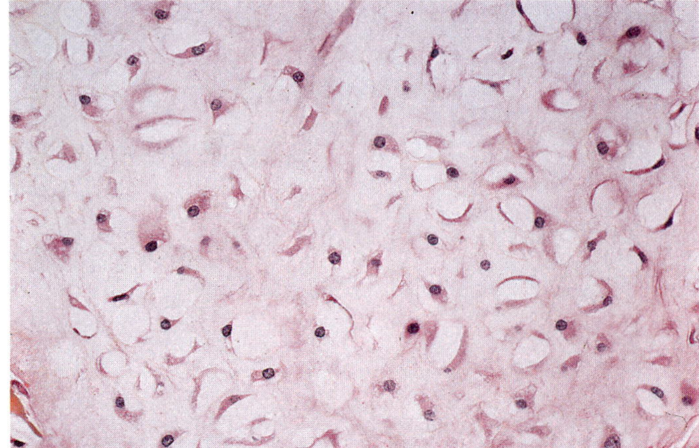

Fig. 11.10

Figs 11.9, 11.10 Normal cellularity in enchondromas of the extremities.

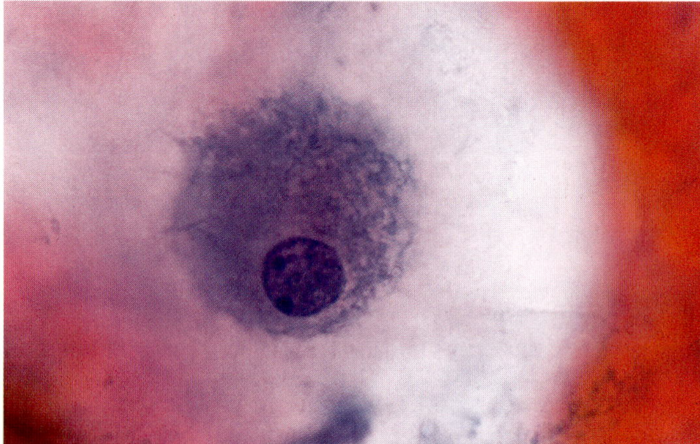

Fig. 11.13

Figs 11.12, 11.13 Imprint cytology of enchondromas demonstrating chondrocytes embedded in the matrix with a low nuclear–cytoplasmic ratio.

probable glycoprotein nature; admixed with lipids, calcium and sulfur.[5]

Mitoses are rare or absent. Chondrocytes may be necrotic or degenerative in calcified regions.[2] Enchondral

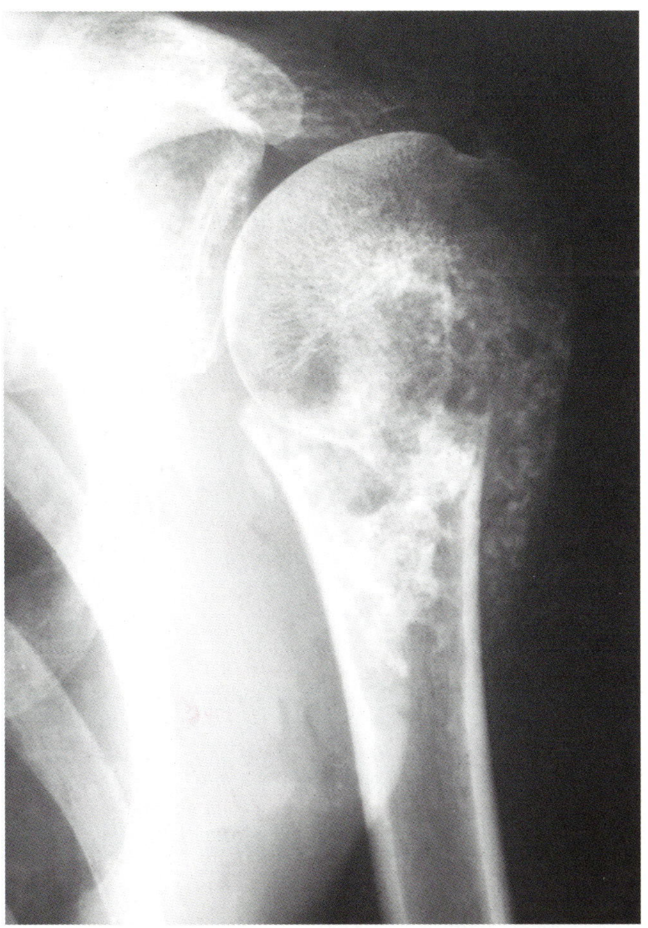

Fig. 11.14

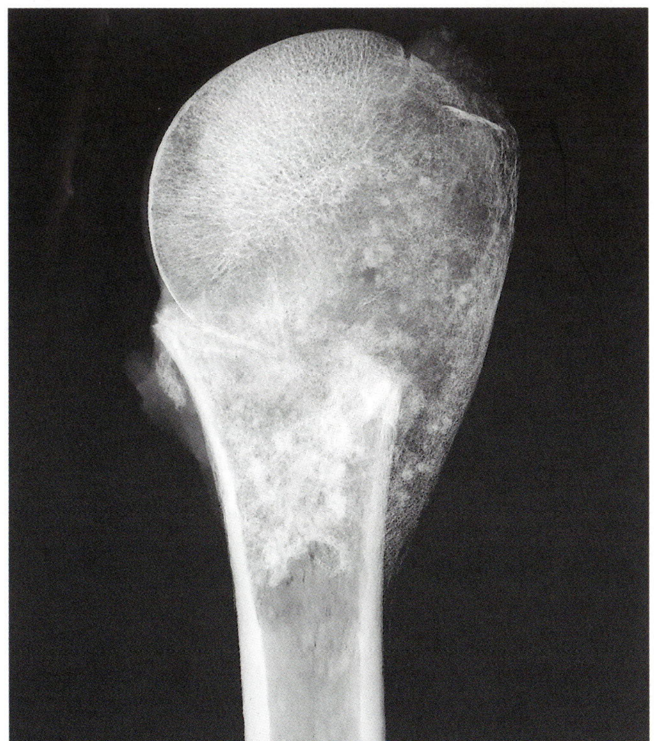

Fig. 11.16

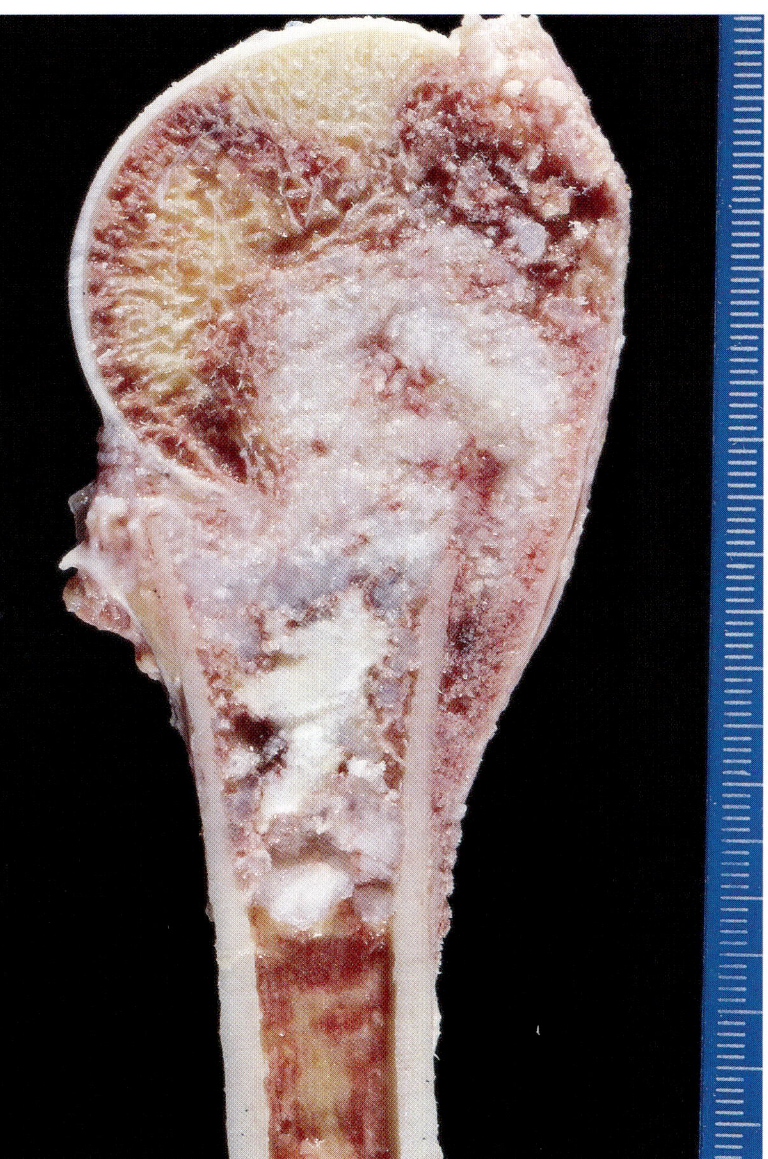

Fig. 11.15

Figs 11.14–11.16 Fracture through an enchondroma of the humerus with a misdiagnosis of chondrosarcoma.

ossification or calcifications are found in variable quantities.

A myxoid aspect is not indicative of malignancy (Schajowicz 1994). It is well known that, in young patients and in the hands and feet, the cellularity and cellular pleomorphism are greater and binucleated chondrocytes are found.

IMMUNOHISTOCHEMISTRY

Immunostaining with S-100 protein is most intense.[6,7] Types II and IX collagens are diffusely distributed in the matrix,[8] with type VI collagen surrounding the cells.[9]

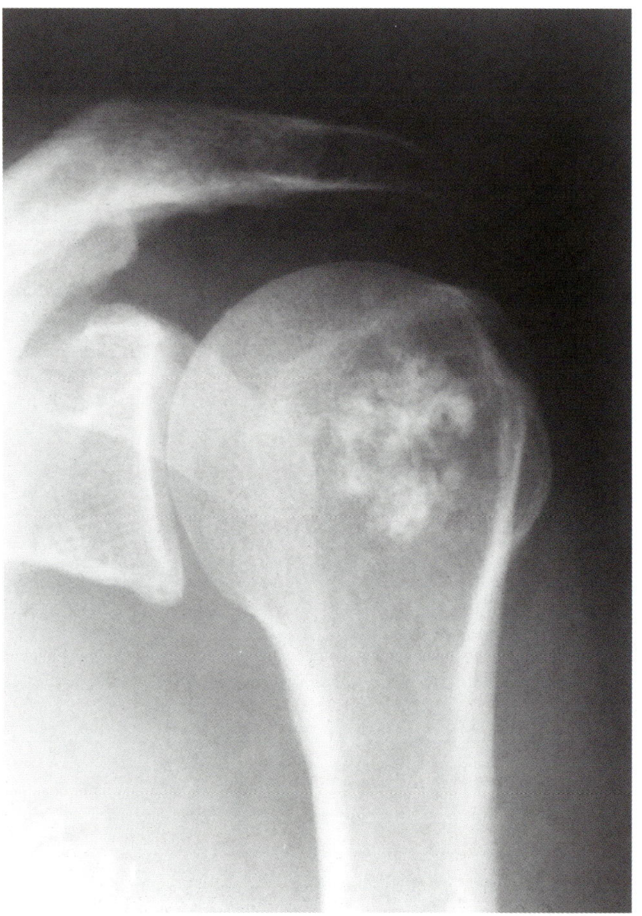

Fig. 11.17

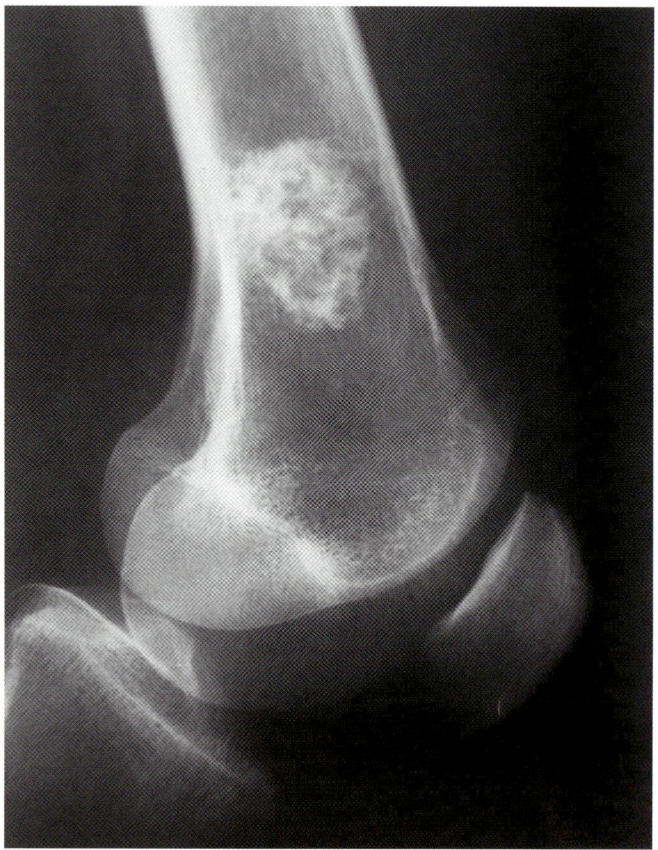

Fig. 11.18

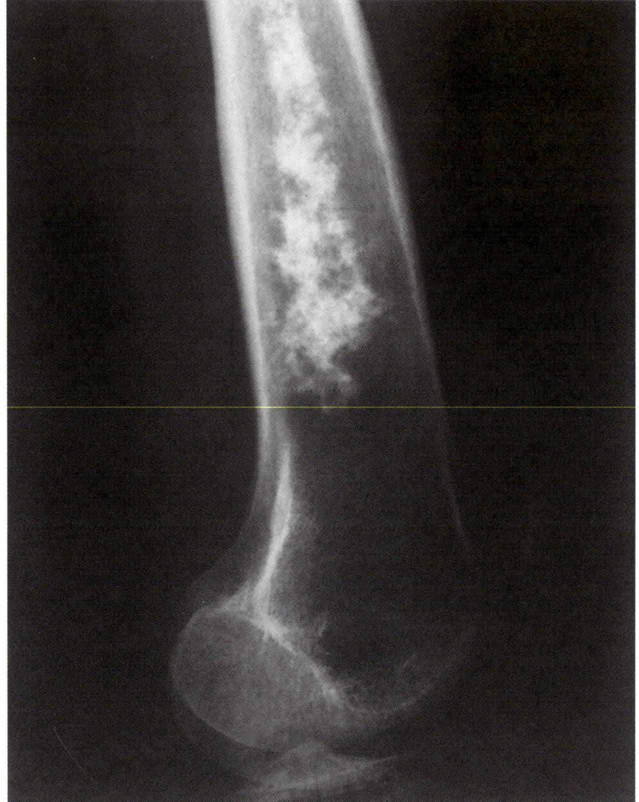

Fig. 11.19

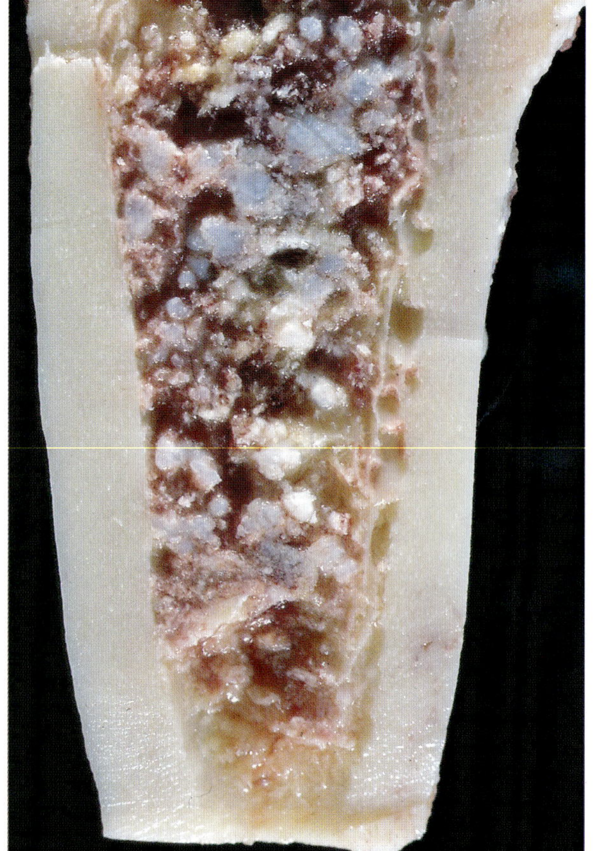

Fig. 11.20

Figs 11.17–11.20 Calcifying enchondromas of the humerus and femur.

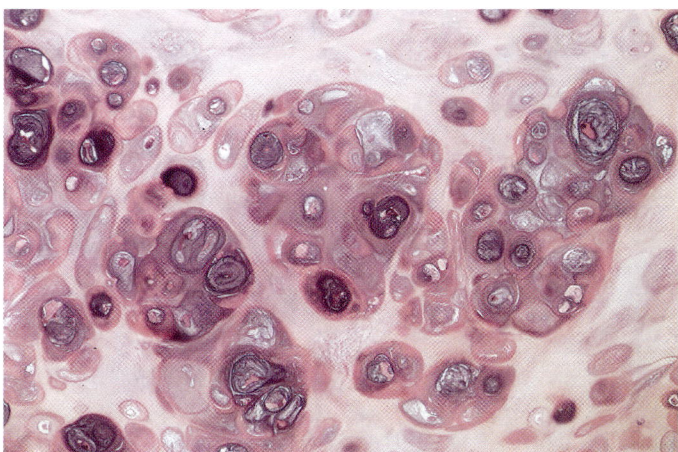

Fig. 11.21

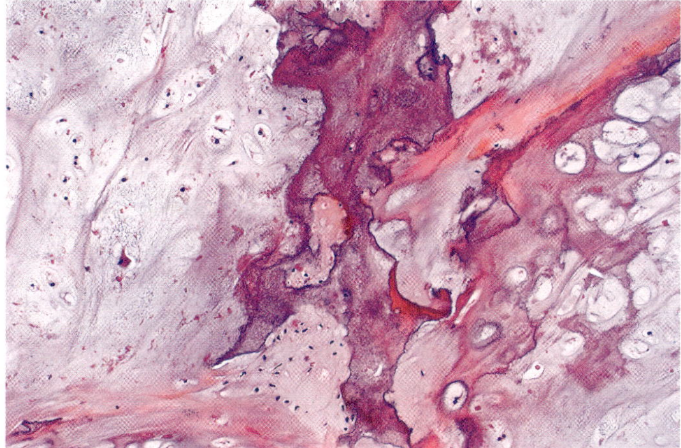

Fig. 11.22

Figs 11.21, 11.22 Calcifying enchondromas of the femur: low cellularity and calcified areas.

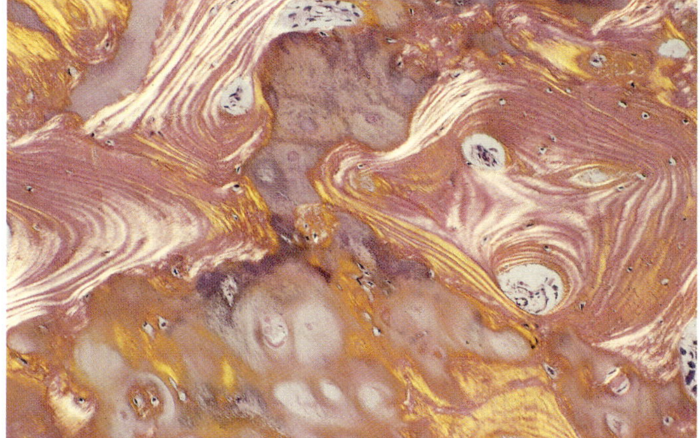

Fig. 11.23 Calcification and ossification in a long-standing case of femoral calcifying enchondroma.

FLOW CYTOMETRY

Usually, the DNA content is diploid,[10] but clear aneuploidy, with separate peaks, has been reported.[11]

ELECTRON MICROSCOPY

Ultrastructurally, the cells may be immature with few

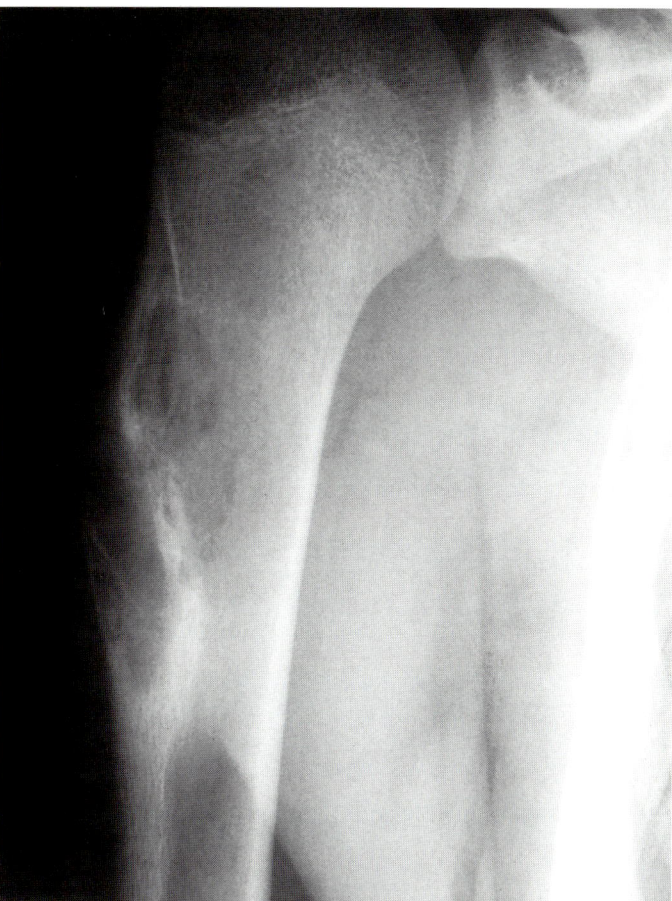

Fig. 11.24

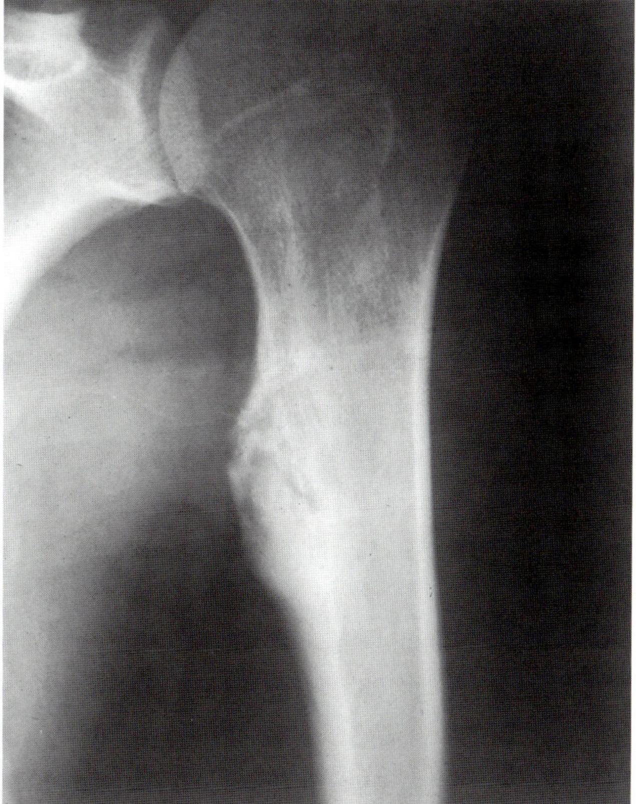

Fig. 11.25

Figs 11.24, 11.25 Enchondroma protuberans of the humerus.

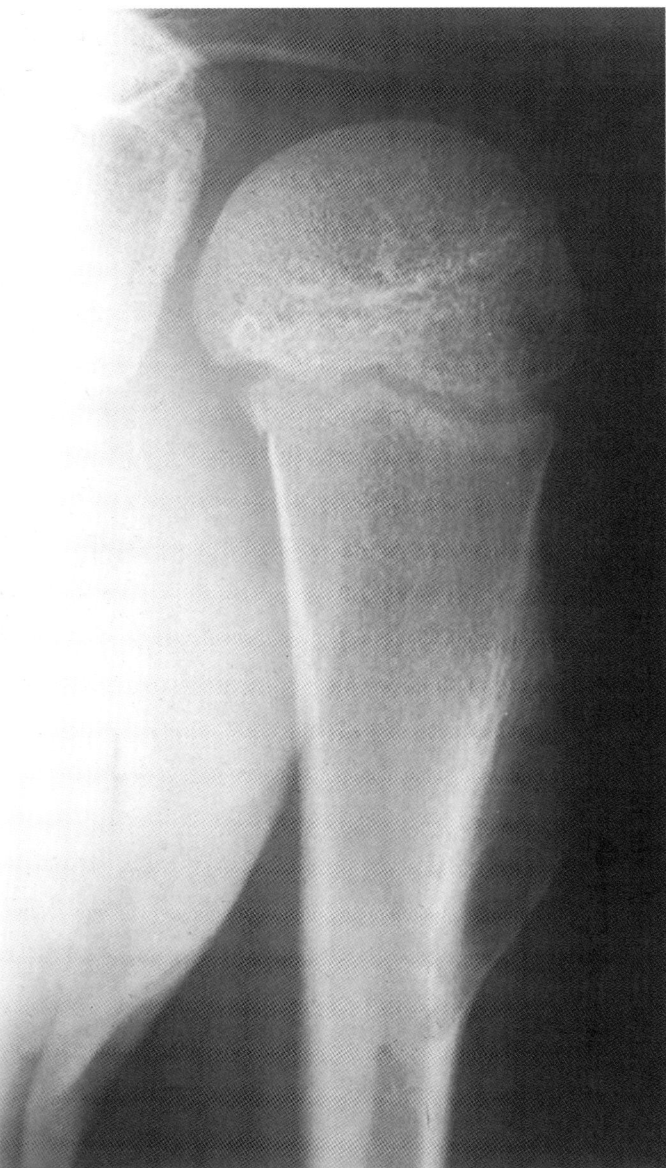

Fig. 11.26 Periosteal chondroma of the humerus.

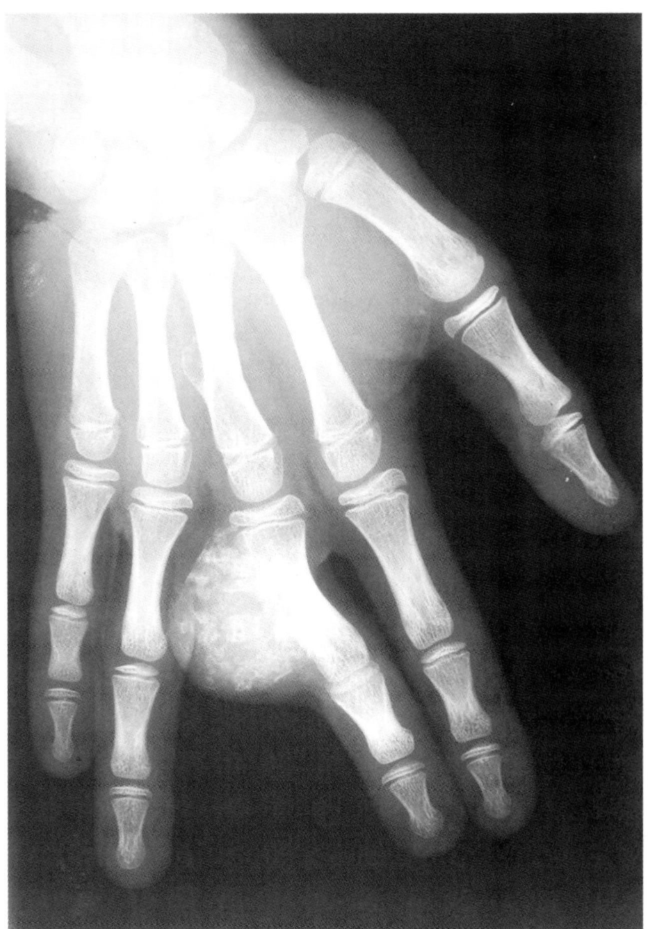

Fig. 11.27 Periosteal chondroma of a phalanx.

cytoplasmic organelles or very developed with a Golgi zone, a dilated rough endoplasmic reticulum, numerous mitochondria, cytoplasmic vacuoles and large amounts of glycogen.[12–15] Some cells are dying or degenerative.[15] Proteoglycan granules are found in the matrix.[14]

COURSE, TREATMENT AND PROGNOSIS

The treatment is thorough curettage; recurrence rates are low (5–10%).[16,17] En bloc resection is performed in small long bones (Schajowicz 1994).

Symptoms of malignant transformation are an increase in size in adults, pain in the absence of trauma and cortical destruction with extraosseous extension.[18] This is a rare event in small bones of the hands and feet.[19,20]

Most tumors are chondrosarcomas involving the long tubular and flat bones, with histological invasion of the intertrabecular spaces and entrapped normal bone (Mirra 1989). The confluent lobules of cartilage are hypercellular, with plump nuclei, binucleate and giant cells and necrosis. Fibrosarcomas, malignant fibrous histiocytomas and osteosarcomas have been reported, most of them presumed to be dedifferentiated chondrosarcomas.[21–25]

Chondrosarcomas should not be confused with a fracture through an enchondroma, with cartilage fragments in the soft tissues and callus showing atypical osteoid and chondroid reactions[4] (Figs 11.14–11.16).

CALCIFYING ENCHONDROMAS

These enchondromas are located in long bones, most often involving the upper humerus, the distal femoral metaphysis and tibia (Schajowicz 1994) (Figs 11.17–11.23). They are long-standing lesions, found in adults. Usually, they are asymptomatic but a pathological fracture can occur.[26]

They may extend down the shaft, with no endosteal cortical erosion or cortical expansion. On X-ray, they appear as centrally located lucencies with sharply defined granular or flocculent deposits or ring-like opacities. An increased uptake on bone scan can differentiate them from bone infarcts.[27]

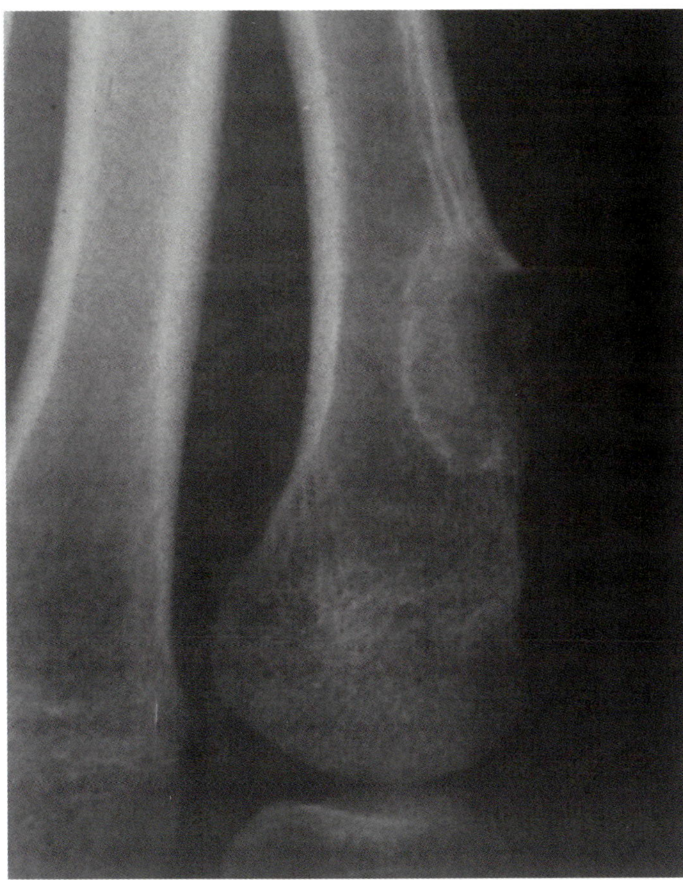

Fig. 11.28

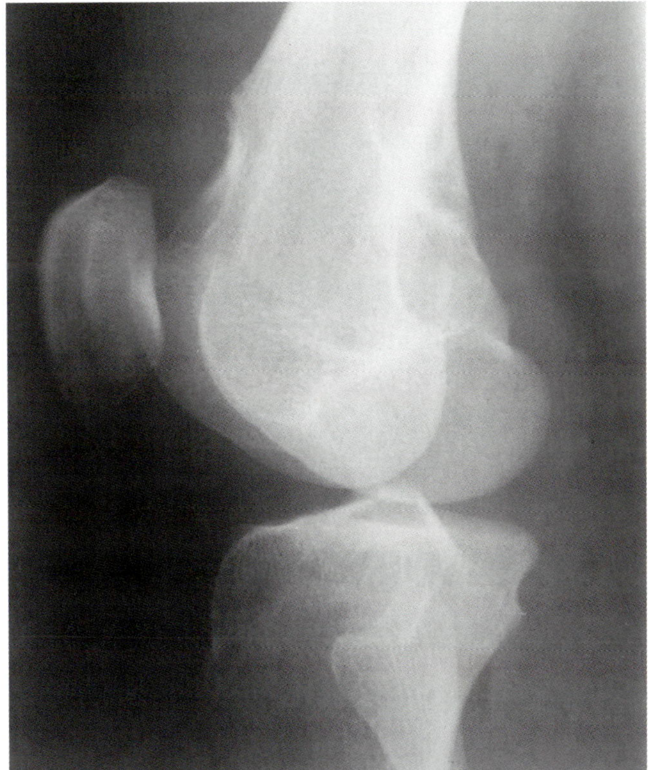

Fig. 11.30

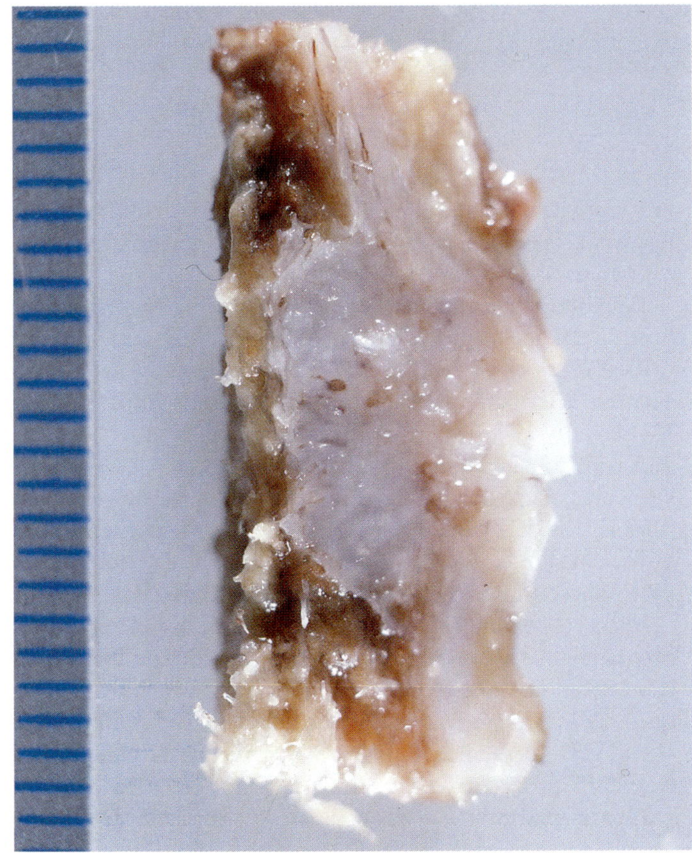

Fig. 11.29

Fig. 11.28, 11.29 Periosteal chondroma of a metacarpal.

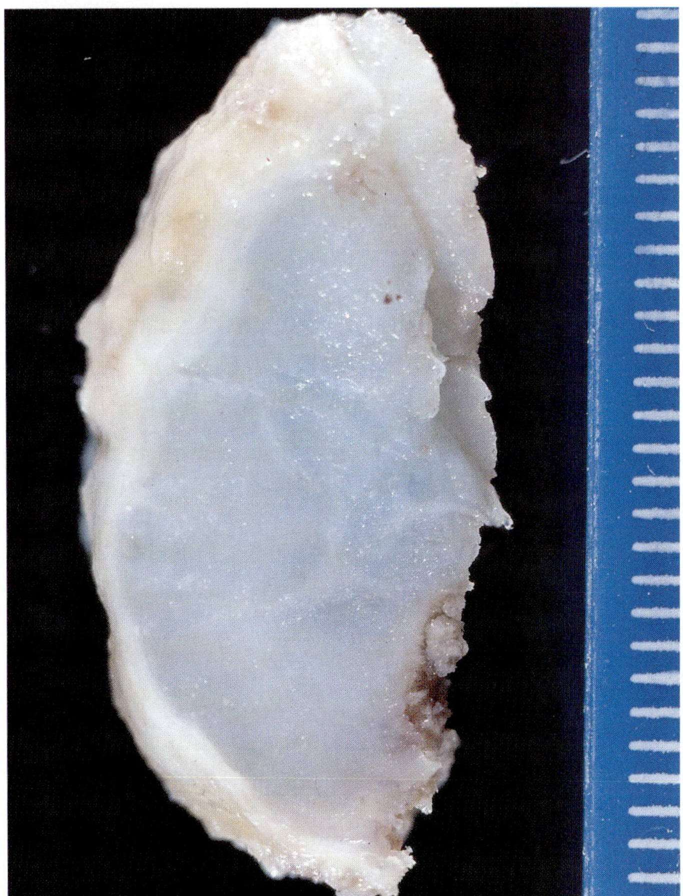

Fig. 11.31

Figs 11.30, 11.31 Periosteal chondroma of the anterior cortex of the femur (associated posterior non-ossifying fibroma).

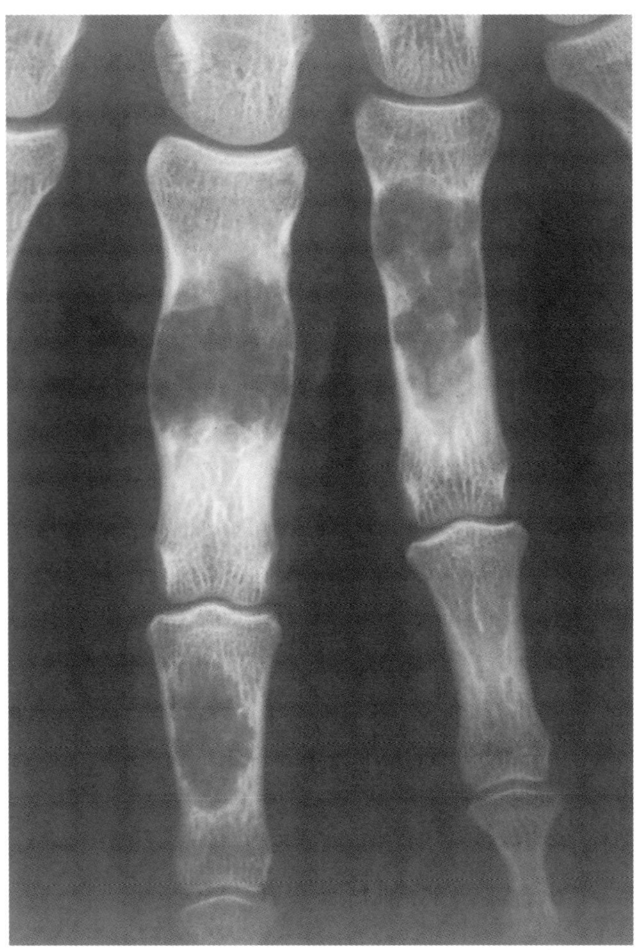

Fig. 11.32

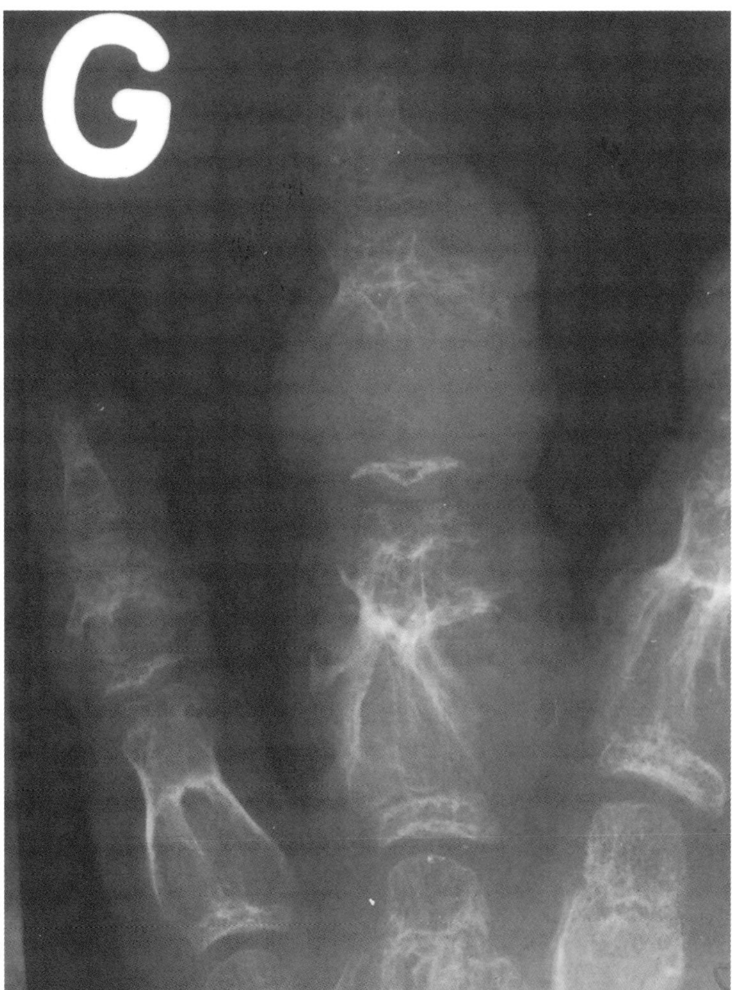

Fig. 11.33

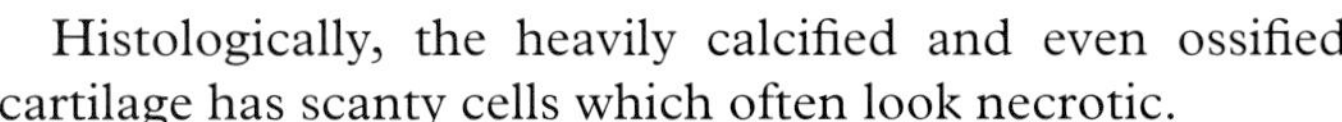

Figs 11.32–11.34 Enchondromatosis in hand and foot locations.

Histologically, the heavily calcified and even ossified cartilage has scanty cells which often look necrotic.

ENCHONDROMA PROTUBERANS

This eccentrically located enchondroma may simulate an osteochondroma, protuding from one side of the bone[28–30] (Figs 11.24, 11.25). Lobulated masses of cartilage are covered by a thin sheath of periosteum, with no cartilage cap.

PERIOSTEAL CHONDROMAS

These account for 20% of chondromas in the Mayo Clinic files[31] but generally they are much rarer (Figs 11.26–11.31). They were defined as a pathological entity by Lichtenstein in 1952[32] and later by Jaffe,[33] under the name of juxtacortical chondroma.

They are usually diagnosed in the second and third decades,[31,34,35] with a male predominance (2:1 ratio). Some

are incidental findings;[36] symptoms of long-standing lesions are pain and swelling. Multiple lesions have been reported.[31,33,36]

Periosteal chondromas are metaphyseal lesions in long bones, chiefly found in the proximal femur and humerus, tibia and bones of the hands.[37–39] Rare locations are the ribs, sacrum, scapula,[40] ilium, spine[41] and pubic symphysis.[31] On X-ray, they appear as a soft tissue mass, slightly lobulated and with focal calcifications in one-third of cases. A saucer-like cortical erosion or scalloping of the cortex with variable sclerosis is associated with buttresses of periosteal new bone[39] and may also be demonstrated by CT.[42] MRI is useful to depict the cartilaginous soft tissue mass.[43]

Some cases may show an absence of cortical erosion or sclerosis,[31,39,44] others may resemble osteochondromas, but the lesion is separated from medullary bone by the cortex.[45] A few cases may exhibit a sclerotic or thin periosteal shell, best seen on CT.[34] Rare cases may be totally intra-cortical[46] or lead to a shortening of the bone.[47]

Gross examination reveals an ovoid chondroid mass

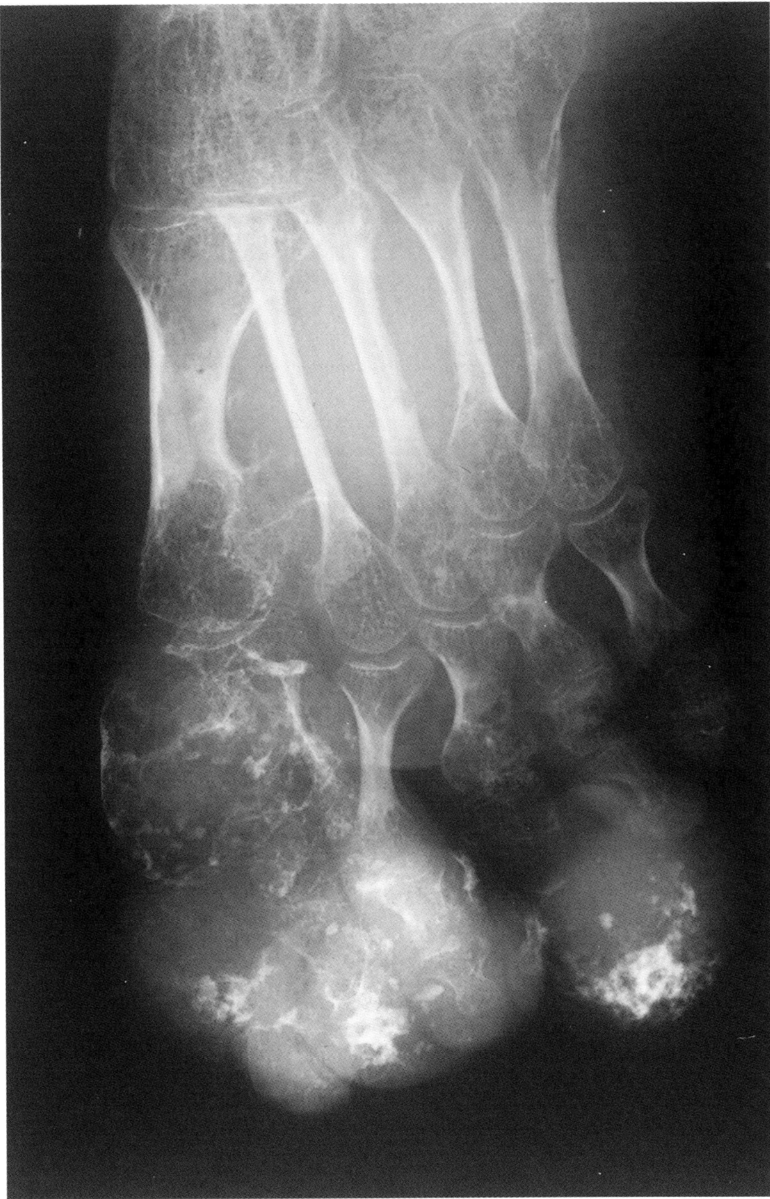

Fig. 11.34

with a prominent lobular pattern,[36] located beneath the periosteum and separated from bone by a thin rim of reactive sclerosis. The mean diameter is 2.5 cm,[36] but large lesions have been reported.[33,48]

Histologically, most tumors are of normal cellularity;[36] some may be hypercellular, with dense and enlarged nuclei, binucleated cells or myxoid changes.[31,49] A cytogenetic study has shown a 12q13–15 rearrangement, also seen in enchondromas.[50]

The treatment is en bloc excision, with no local recurrences[34,36] or a recurrence rate of 3.6%.[51]

These lesions are often misdiagnosed as chondrosarcomas.[38] Periosteal chondrosarcomas are found in older patients,[31] being symptomatic and larger tumors which permeate the underlying bone, with irregular margins.[31] The cellular pleomorphism is greater, but histological differentiation may be difficult. Periosteal chondromas also have to be differentiated from soft tissue chondromas eroding bone.[31]

ENCHONDROMATOSIS

Known also as Ollier's disease, this sporadic condition is usually discovered before 10 years of age.

Enchondromas, often large and eccentric, have a generalized distribution, or are unilateral (Figs 11.32–11.38); they may involve only the hands and feet. Typical locations are the femur and the tibia, less often the flat bones. In the iliac crest, radiating bands of cartilage appear on

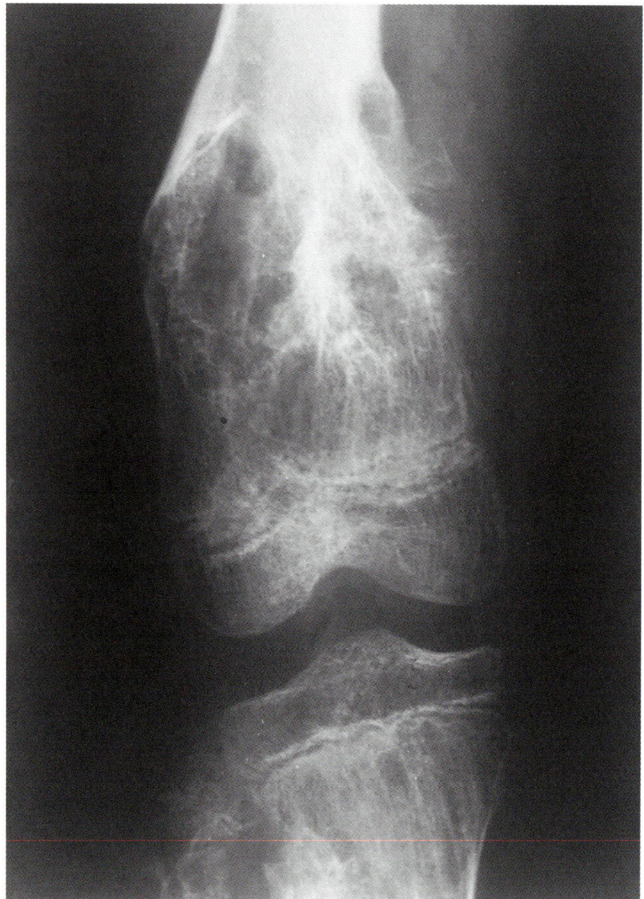

Fig. 11.35

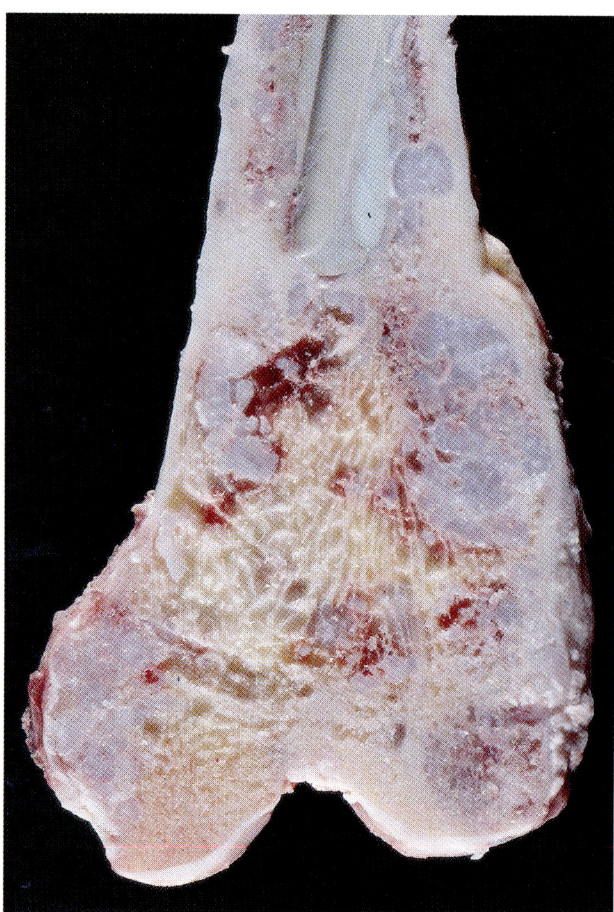

Fig. 11.36

Figs 11.35, 11.36 Enchondromatosis in femoral location.

X-rays as a fan-like pattern. In long bones, they may extend over the whole width of the bone (Wilner 1982), with a streaky texture in the metaphysis. They are often intracortical, periosteal or, rarely, within the articular cartilage.[52] Severe deformities of bone, such as bowing and shortening, may also be seen.

Histologically, a most unusual finding is the report of an association with a giant cell reparative granuloma.[53]

The rate of malignant transformation is about 30%.[17,54] Twenty-five percent of patients present with a sarcoma at the age of 40 years.[55] Osteosarcomas[54,56] and even chordomas[54] have been reported, but the most usual tumors are grade I, II or dedifferentiated chondrosarcomas, which may be multiple.[57–59]

In Ollier's disease, lesions in small bones may have a soft tissue extension or may induce severe deformity in flat bones,[54] so the diagnosis of malignant transformation has to be made on X-ray (huge cortical destruction and soft tissue mass) and on histology (an infiltrative pattern). A morphometric analysis of the nuclear areas of chondrocytes has been performed.[60]

MAFFUCCI'S SYNDROME

This is a congenital, non-hereditary dysplasia, combining enchondromatosis and cavernous or capillary hemangiomas in the skin, subcutaneous tissues or internal organs, appearing sometimes as phleboliths (Fig. 11.39). The sex ratio is equal.[61]

The distribution of nerves and neuropeptides around the chondromas and hemangiomas has been studied by quantitative analysis of immunohistochemical staining, showing a significant increase; Maffuci's syndrome may be a neural abnormality of the neuropeptidergic nervous system.[62]

The incidence of malignant transformation is 15%[61] and MRI may help to identify malignancy, with a higher signal intensity on T2-weighted images compared to enchondromas.[63] Most tumors are chondrosarcomas, sometimes multiple,[64] or, more rarely, fibrosarcomas, vascular sarcomas,[61,65,66] gliomas and carcinomas.[55,67] In some cases, vascular lesions are spindle-cell hemangioendotheliomas, with combined Kaposi-like and cavernous hemangioma-like features; these tumors appear as recur-

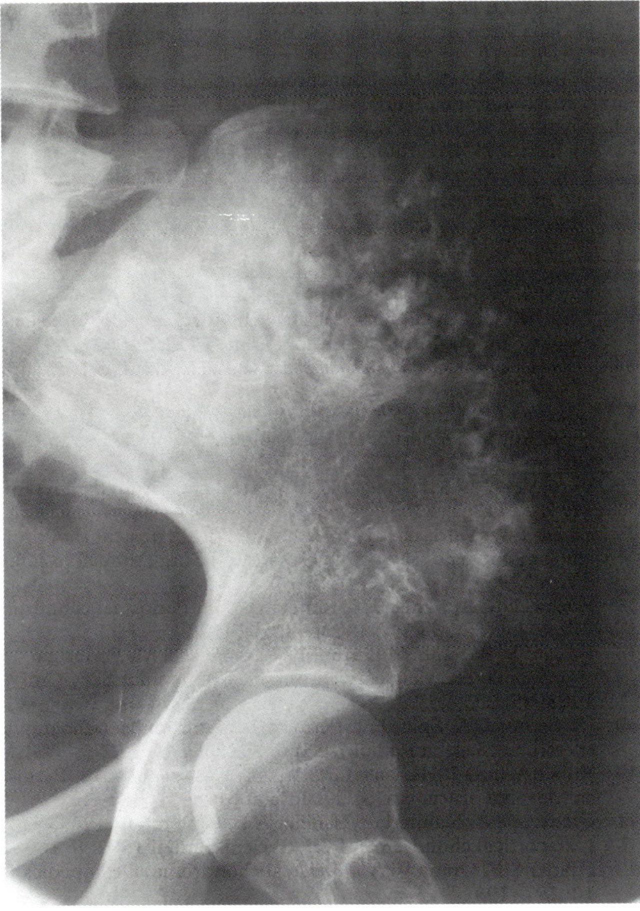

Fig. 11.37

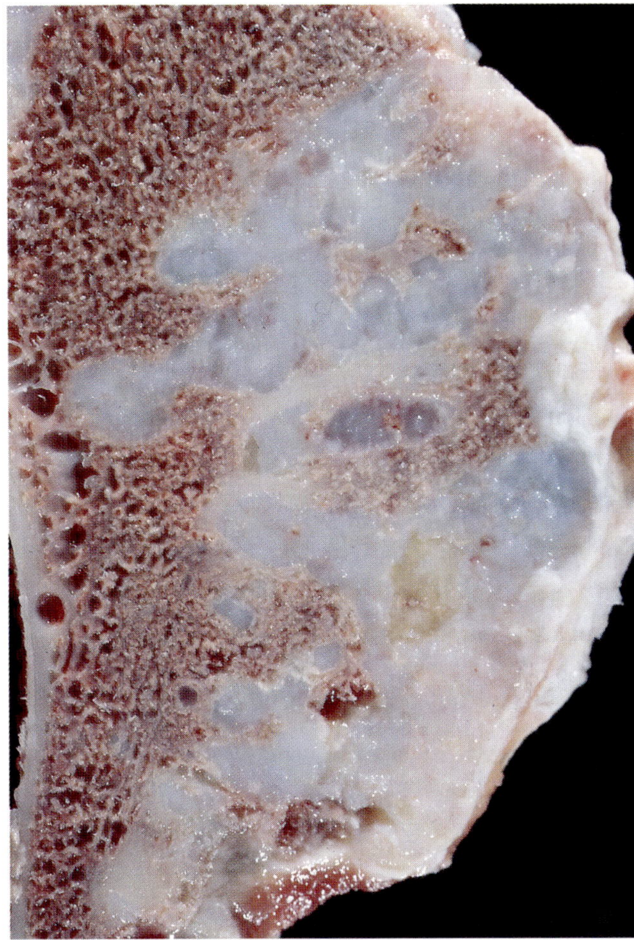

Fig. 11.38

Figs 11.37, 11.38 Enchondromatosis in the iliac wing with a fan-like pattern.

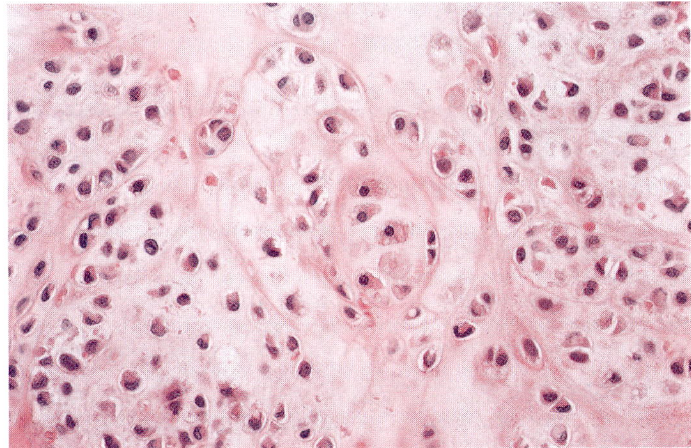

Fig. 11.39 High cellularity in an enchondroma of the hand (Maffucci's syndrome).

rent and multicentric lesions, with proximal spread but no metastasizing potential in the reported cases.[68]

COMMENTS FOR THE SURGICAL PATHOLOGIST

In most cases, the diagnosis of a chondroma is made on radiological findings and the surgical treatment is performed without a biopsy, especially on distal locations.

In cases of a suspected malignant transformation, there is no place for needle aspiration or needle biopsy; an open surgical biopsy is mandatory.

REFERENCES

1. Milgram J W. The origins of osteochondromas and enchondromas. A histopathologic study. Clin Orthop 1983: 174: 264–284
2. Moser R P. Enchondroma. In: Moser R P, Gilkey F W, Madewell J E, Eds. Cartilaginous tumors of the skeleton. AFIP Atlas of radiologic pathologic correlations II. Philadelphia: Hanley & Belfus, 1990, pp 8–34

3. Morard M, De Tribolet N, Janzer R C. Chondromas of the spine: report of two cases and review of the literature. Br J Neurosurg 1993: 7: 551–556

4. Ragsdale B D, Sweet D E, Vinh T N. Radiology as gross pathology in evaluating chondroid lesions. Hum Pathol 1989: 20: 930–951

5. Del Rosario A D, Bui H X, Singh J, Ginsburg R, Ross J S. Intracytoplasmic eosinophilic hyaline globules in cartilaginous neoplasms: a surgical, pathological, ultrastructural, and electron probe X-ray microanalytic study. Hum Pathol 1994: 25: 1283–1289

6. Nakamura Y, Becker L E, Marks A. S-100 protein in tumors of cartilage and bone. An immunohistochemical study. Cancer 1983: 52: 1820–1824

7. Okajima K, Honda I, Kitakawa T. Immunohistochemical distribution of S-100 protein in tumors and tumorlike lesions of bone and cartilage. Cancer 1988: 61: 792–799

8. Kawashima A, Ueda Y, Tsuchiya H, Tomita K, Nagai Y, Nakanishi I. Immunohistochemical localization of collagenous proteins in cartilaginous tumors: characteristic distribution of type IX collagen. J Cancer Res Clin Oncol 1993: 120: 35–40

9. Ueda Y, Oda Y, Tsuchiya H, Tomita K, Nakanishi I. Immunohistological study on collagenous proteins of benign and malignant human cartilaginous tumours of bone. Virchows Arch A Pathol Anat Histopathol 1990: 417: 291–297

10. Cuvelier C A, Roels H J. Cytophotometric studies of the nuclear DNA content in cartilaginous tumors. Cancer 1979: 44: 1363–1374

11. Alho A, Skjeldal S, Pettersen E O, Melvik J E, Larsen T E. Aneuploidy in benign tumors and nonneoplastic lesions of musculoskeletal tissues. Cancer 1994: 73: 1200–1205

12. Winkelmann W, Becker W. Das Chondrom. Ein Beitrage zur feingeweblichen Morphologie. Z Orthop Ihre Grenzgeb 1976: 114: 364–377

13. Walaas L, Kindblom L G, Gunterberg B, Bergh P. Light and electron microscopic examination of fine-needle aspirates in the preoperative diagnosis of cartilaginous tumors. Diagn Cytopathol 1990: 6: 396–408

14. Steiner G C. Ultrastructure of benign cartilaginous tumors of intraosseous origin. Hum Pathol 1979: 10: 71–86

15. Zimny M L, Redler I. Ultrastructure of solitary enchondromas. J Hand Surg (Br) 1984: 9: 95–97

16. Takigawa K. Chondroma of the bones of the hand. A review of 110 cases. J Bone Joint Surg (Am) 1971: 53: 1591–1600

17. Boriani S, Laus M. Chondromas and chondromatosis. A study of 265 cases, 200 with long term follow up. Ital J Orthop Traumatol 1978: 4: 353–357

18. Hamlin J A, Adler L, Greenhaum E I. Central enchondroma – a precursor to chondrosarcoma? J Can Assoc Radiol 1971: 22: 206–209

19. Culver J E Jr, Sweet D E, McCue F C. Chondrosarcoma of the hand arising from a pre-existent benign solitary enchondroma. Clin Orthop 1975: 113: 128–131

20. Wu K K, Frost H M, Guise E E. A chondrosarcoma of the hand arising from an asymptomatic benign solitary enchondroma of 40 years' duration. J Hand Surg (Am) 1983: 8: 317–319

21. Rockwell M A, Enneking W F. Osteosarcoma developing in solitary enchondroma of the tibia. J Bone Joint Surg (Am) 1971: 53: 341–344

22. Slullitel J A, Schajowicz F, Slullitel J. Osteochondrome solitaire avec dégénrescence maligne vers un sarcome osteogénique. Rev Chir Orthop Reparatrice Appar Mot 1971: 57: 471–478

23. Sanerkin N G, Wood C G. Fibrosarcomata and malignant fibrous histiocytomata arising in relation to enchondromata. J Bone Joint Surg (Br) 1979: 61: 366–372

24. Bonfiglio M, Platz C E. Case report 141. Malignant fibrous histiocytoma associated with enchondroma of bone. Skeletal Radiol 1981: 6: 127–130

25. Smith G D, Chalmers J, McQueen M M. Osteosarcoma arising in relation to an enchondroma. A report of three cases. J Bone Joint Surg (Br) 1986: 68: 315–319

26. Lawrance W, Franklin E L. Calcifying enchondroma of long bones. J Bone Joint Surg (Br) 1953: 35: 224–228

27. Telfer C D, Uhthoff H K. Calcifying enchondroma of long bone.

In: Uhthoff H K, Ed. Current concepts of diagnosis and treatment of bone and soft tissue tumors. Berlin: Springer-Verlag, 1984, pp 411–418

28. Caballes R L. Enchondroma protuberans masquerading as osteochondroma. Hum Pathol 1982: 13: 734–739

29. Keating R B, Wright P W, Staple T W. Enchondroma protuberans of the rib. Skeletal Radiol 1985: 13: 55–58

30. Crim J R, Mirra J M. Enchondroma protuberans. Report of a case and its distinction from chondrosarcoma and osteochondroma adjacent to an enchondroma. Skeletal Radiol 1990: 19: 431–434

31. Nojima T, Unni K K, McLeod R A, Pritchard D J. Periosteal chondroma and periosteal chondrosarcoma. Am J Surg Pathol 1985: 9: 666–677

32. Lichtenstein L, Hall J E. Periosteal chondroma: a distinctive benign cartilage tumor. J Bone Joint Surg (Am) 1952: 34: 691–697

33. Jaffe H L. Juxtacortical chondroma. Bull Hosp Jt Dis 1956: 17: 20–29

34. Lewis M M, Kenan S, Yabut S M, Norman A, Steiner G. Periosteal chondroma. A report of ten cases and review of the literature. Clin Orthop 1990: 256: 185–192

35. Fornasier V L, McGonigal D. Periosteal chondroma. Clin Orthop 1977: 124: 233–236

36. Bauer T W, Dorfman H D, Latham J T Jr. Periosteal chondroma. A clinicopathologic study of 23 cases. Am J Surg Pathol 1982: 6: 631–637

37. Rockwell M A, Saiter E T, Enneking W F. Periosteal chondroma. J Bone Joint Surg (Am) 1972: 54: 102–108

38. Boriani S, Bacchini P, Bertoni F, Campanacci M. Periosteal chondroma. A review of twenty cases. J Bone Joint Surg (Am) 1983: 65: 205–212

39. De Santos L A, Spjut H J. Periosteal chondroma: a radiographic spectrum. Skeletal Radiol 1981: 6: 15–20

40. Rubenstein D J, Harkavy L, Glantz L. Case report 518. Periosteal chondroma of scapula. Skeletal Radiol 1989: 18: 47–49

41. Calderone A, Naimark A, Schiller A L. Case report 196. Juxtacortical chondroma of C2. Skeletal Radiol 1982: 8: 160–163

42. Holder S F, Grana W A. Periosteal chondroma. Orthopedics 1987: 10: 197–198

43. Varma D G, Kumar R, Carrasco C H, Guo S Q, Richli W R. MR imaging of periosteal chondroma. J Comput Assist Tomogr 1991: 15: 1008–1010

44. Cooke G M, Pearce J G. Periosteal chondroma. Report of two cases with atypical radiological features. J Can Assoc Radiol 1976: 27: 301–303

45. Greenspan A, Unni K K, Matthews J 2nd. Periosteal chondroma masquerading as osteochondroma. Can Assoc Radiol J 1993: 44: 205–208

46. Abdelwahab I F, Hermann G, Lewis M M, Klein M J. Case report 588. Intracortical chondroma of the left femur. Skeletal Radiol 1990: 19: 59–61

47. Pazzaglia U E, Ceciliani L. Periosteal chondroma of the humerus leading to shortening. A case report. J Bone Joint Surg (Br) 1985: 67: 290–292

48. Jacobson S A. Epichondroma. A supraosseous benign tumor of cartilage. Bull Hosp Jt Dis 1963: 16: 93–101

49. Spjut H J, Nelson P W. Case report 108. Periosteal (parosteal, juxtacortical) chondroma of tibia. Skeletal Radiol 1980: 5: 47–50

50. Mandahl N, Willen H, Rydholm A, Heim S, Mitelman F. Rearrangement of band q13 on both chromosomes 12 in a periosteal chondroma. Genes Chromosomes Cancer 1993: 6: 121–123

51. Nosanchuk J S, Kaufer H. Recurrent periosteal chondroma. Report of two cases and a review of the literature. J Bone Joint Surg (Am) 1969: 51: 375–380

52. Mitchell M L, Ackerman L V. Case report 405. Ollier disease (enchondromatosis). Skeletal Radiol 1987: 16: 61–66

53. Oda Y, Iwamoto Y, Ushijima M, Masuda S, Sugioka Y, Tsuneyoshi M. Case report 877. Giant cell reparative granuloma arising in enchondromatosis. Skeletal Radiol 1994: 23: 669–671

54. Liu J, Hudkins P G, Swee R G, Unni K K. Bone sarcomas associated with Ollier's disease. Cancer 1987: 59: 1376–1385

55. Schwartz H S, Zimmerman N B, Simon M A, Wroble R R, Millar E A, Bonfiglio M. The malignant potential of enchondromatosis. J Bone Joint Surg (Am) 1987: 69: 269–274

56. Braddock G T, Hadlow V D. Osteosarcoma in enchondromatosis (Ollier's disease). Report of a case. J Bone Joint Surg (Br) 1966: 48: 145–149

57. Block R S, Burton R I. Multiple chondrosarcomas in a hand: a case report. J Hand Surg (Am) 1977: 2: 310–313

58. Goodman S B, Bell R S, Fornasier V L, De Demeter D, Bateman J E. Ollier's disease with multiple sarcomatous transformations. Hum Pathol 1984: 15: 91–93

59. Cannon S R, Sweetnam D R. Multiple chondrosarcomas in dyschondroplasia (Ollier's disease). Cancer 1985: 55: 836–840

60. Nakajima H, Ushigome S, Fukuda J. Case report 482. Chondrosarcoma (grade 1) arising from the right second toe in patient with multiple enchondromas. Skeletal Radiol 1988: 17: 289–292

61. Lewis R J, Ketcham A S. Maffucci's syndrome: functional and neoplastic significance. Case report and review of literature. J Bone Joint Surg (Am) 1973: 55: 1465–1479

62. Robinson D, Tieder M, Halperin N, Burshtein D, Nevo Z. Maffucci's syndrome – the result of neural abnormalities? Evidence of mitogenic neurotransmitters present in enchondromas and soft tissue hemangiomas. Cancer 1994: 74: 949–957

63. Unger E C, Kessler H B, Kowalyshyn M J, Lackman R D, Morea G T. MR imaging of Maffucci syndrome. AJR 1988: 150: 351–353

64. Banna M, Parwani G S. Multiple sarcomas in Maffucci's syndrome. Br J Radiol 1969: 42: 304–307

65. Davidson T I, Kissin M W, Bradish C F, Westbury G. Angiosarcoma arising in a patient with Maffucci syndrome. Eur J Surg Oncol 1985: 11: 381–384

66. Lawson J P, Scott G. Case report 602. Spindle cell hemangioendothelioma (SCH) and enchondromatosis (a form of Maffucci syndrome) in a patient with acute myelocytic leukemia (AML). Skeletal Radiol 1990: 19: 158–162

67. Sun T C, Swee R G, Shives T C, Unni K K. Chondrosarcoma in Maffucci's syndrome. J Bone Joint Surg (Am) 1985: 67: 1214–1219

68. Fanburg J C, Meis-Kindblom J M, Rosenberg A E. Multiple enchondromas associated with spindle-cell hemangioendotheliomas. An overlooked variant of Maffucci's syndrome. Am J Surg Pathol 1995: 19: 1029–1038

12

Chondroblastoma

M. Forest

INTRODUCTION AND CLINICAL DATA

Chondroblastoma is a benign cartilage tumor with a chondroblast-like cell component and limited areas of chondroid matrix formation. The term 'benign chondroblastoma' was proposed by Jaffe & Lichtenstein in 1942,[1] following the initial descriptions of Ewing and Codman.[2]

It accounts for 1–3% of all bone tumors, with a male predominance of 2:1.[3] Nearly 90% of patients are in the second and third decades of life. Clinical symptoms are a local swelling or, chiefly, pain, often related to the nearest joint, loss of joint function, joint effusion in 18% of cases[4] or even fractures.[5] The clinical course may be protracted.[6]

SKELETAL DISTRIBUTION

The most frequent sites are the long and short tubular bones (80%[4]), the femur (chiefly in the greater trochanter[7,8]) (Figs 12.1–12.4), the humerus and tibia (Figs 12.5–12.8). Involvement of the flat bones[9] (Figs 12.9–12.10) and the foot, particularly the talus and calcaneus[10,12] (Fig. 12.11) has been reported. Hands[13,14] (Fig. 12.12) or ribs[15–17] are rarely involved. Chondroblastomas in short tubular or flat bones are often found in older patients.[5,18] They are rare in the spine[5,19–21] and the sacrum.[21] In the pelvis, most originate at the site of the triradiate cartilage[22,23] (Fig. 12.13). An unexpected location is the patella.[7,24–26]

Multiple chondroblastomas are unusual[8,27–29] and even rarer are the extraskeletal locations.[30–32]

To sum up, chondroblastomas may develop in any bone formed by endochondral ossification (Mulder et al 1993).

IMAGING

Chondroblastomas nearly always occur in epiphyseal sites

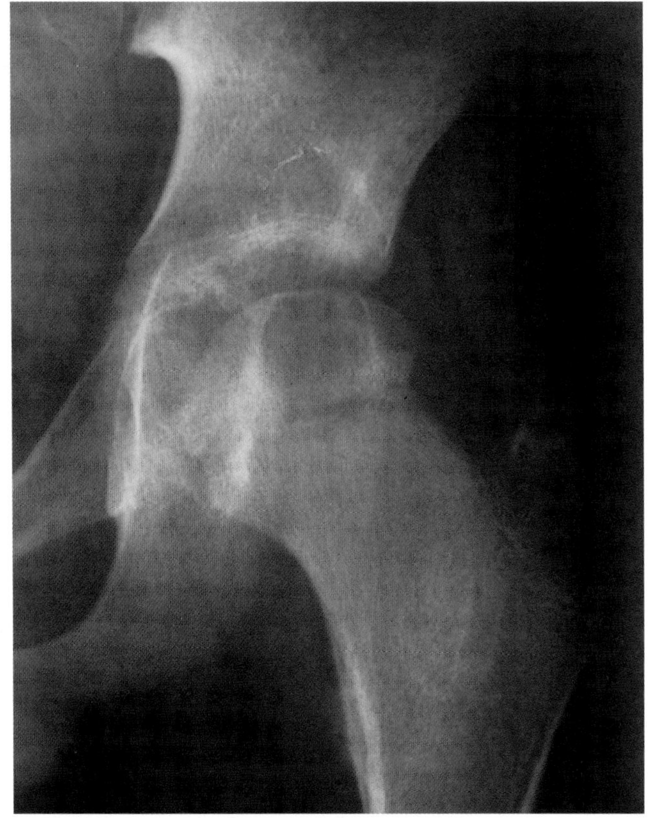

Fig. 12.1

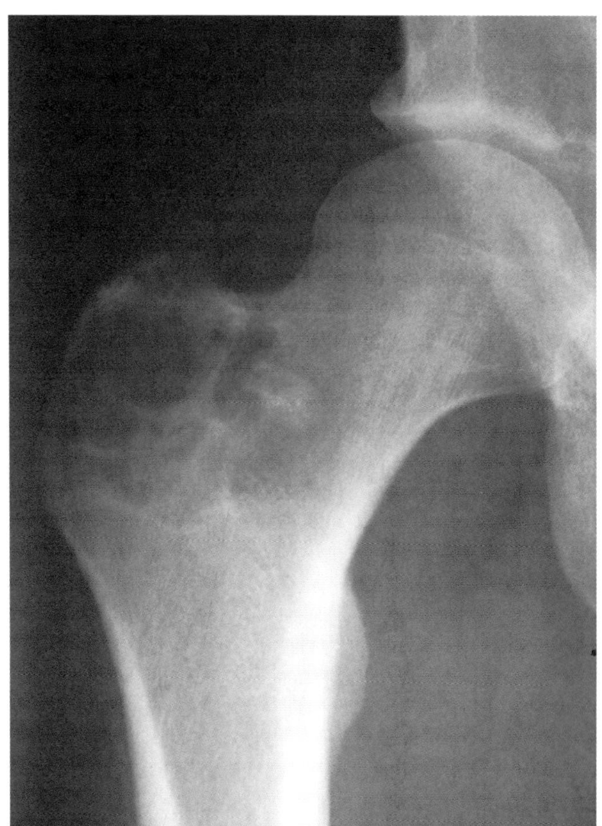

Fig. 12.3

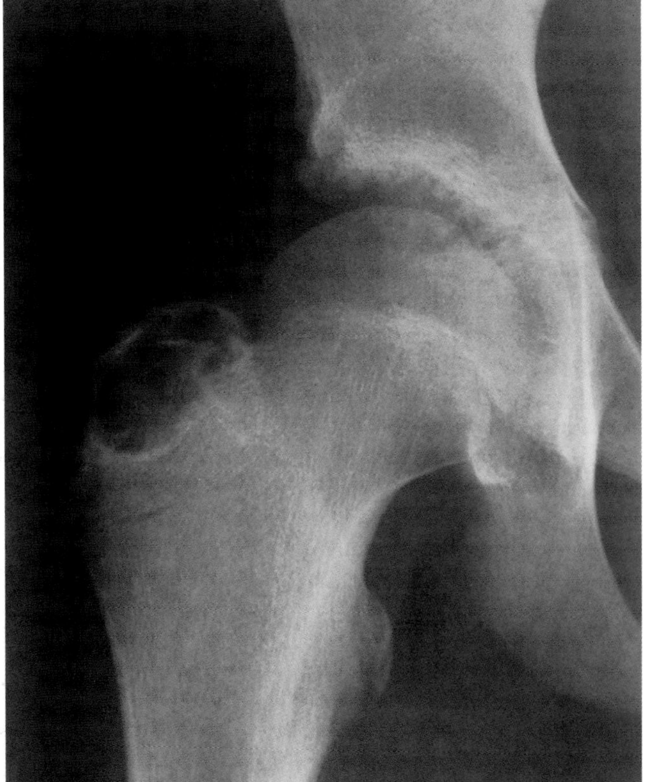

Fig. 12.2

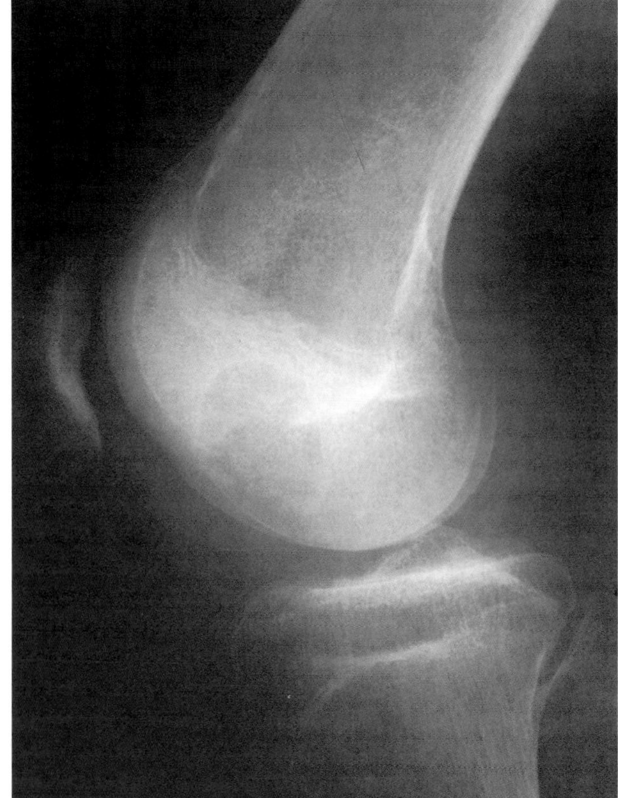

Fig. 12.4

Figs 12.1–12.4 Chondroblastomas in femoral location.

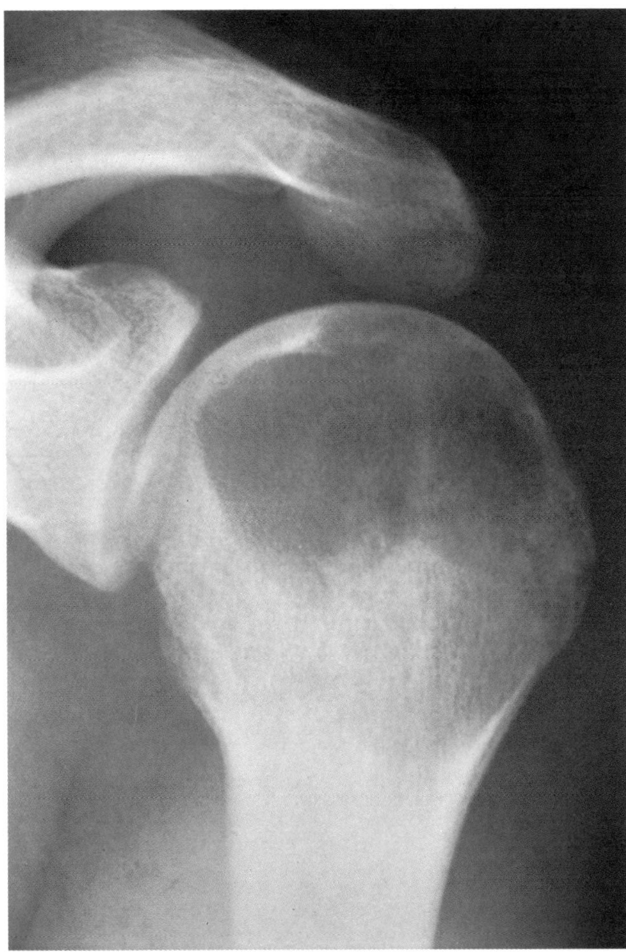

Fig. 12.5 Chondroblastoma of the humerus.

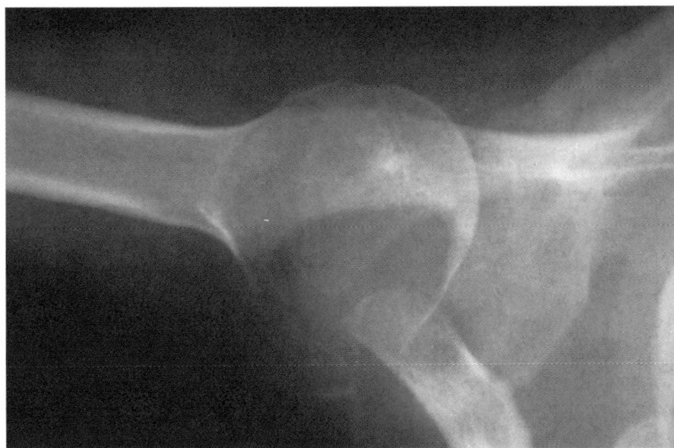

Fig. 12.6 Cystic chondroblastoma of the humerus.

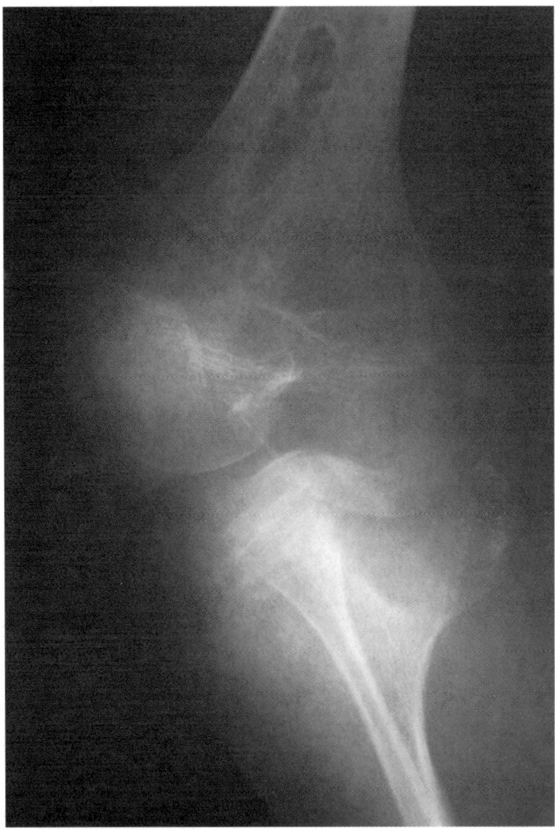

Fig. 12.7 Cystic chondroblastoma of the tibia.

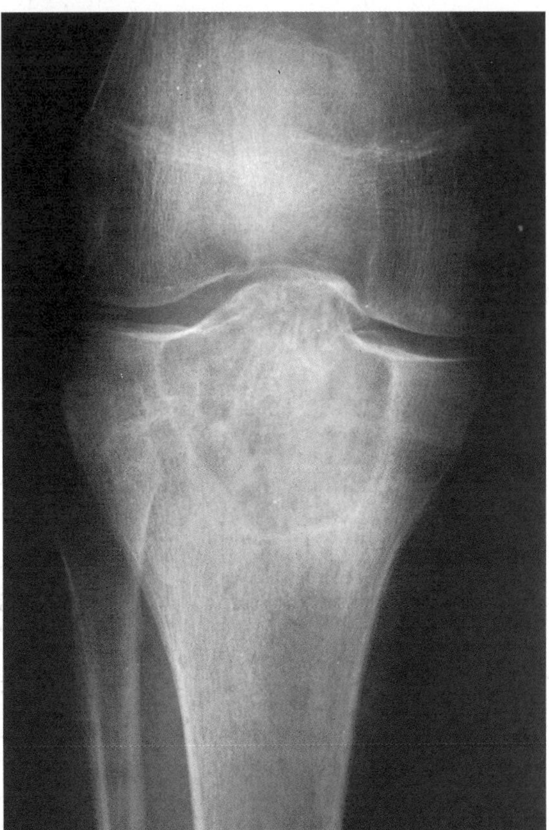

Fig. 12.8 Chondroblastoma of the tibia with faint calcifications.

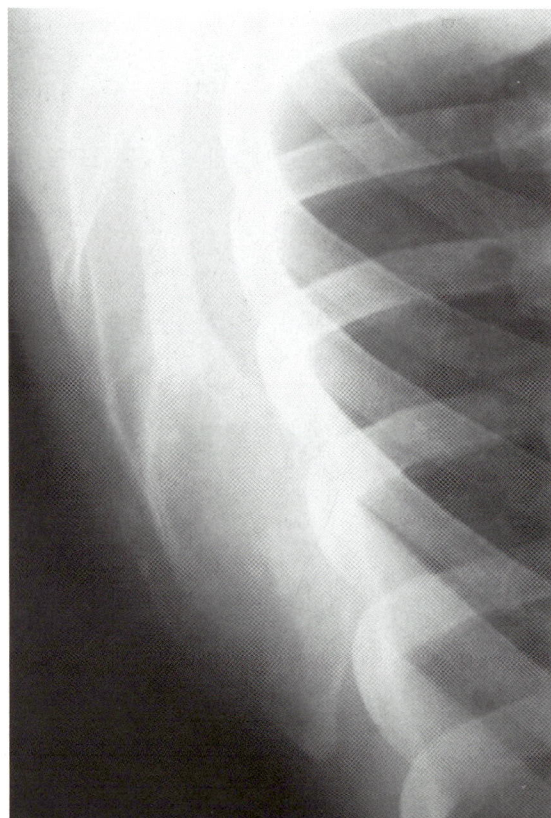

Fig. 12.9

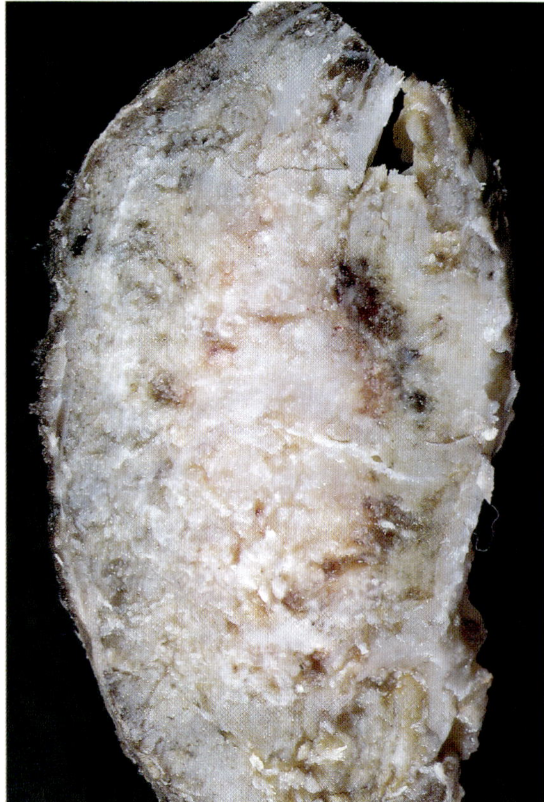

Fig. 12.10

Figs 12.9, 12.10 Chondroblastoma of the scapula.

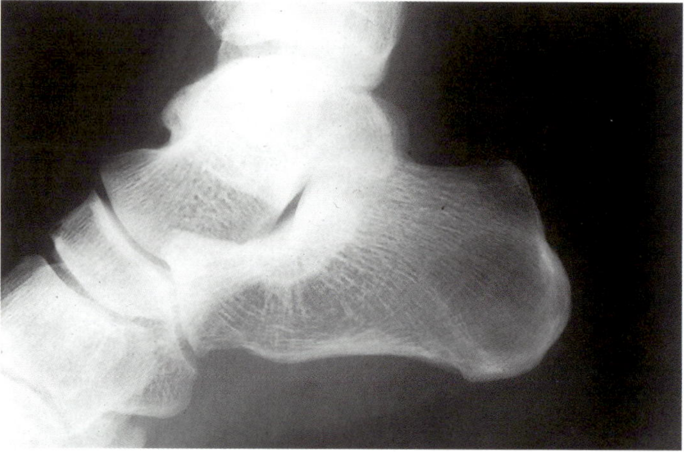

Fig. 12.11 Chondroblastoma of the calcaneus.

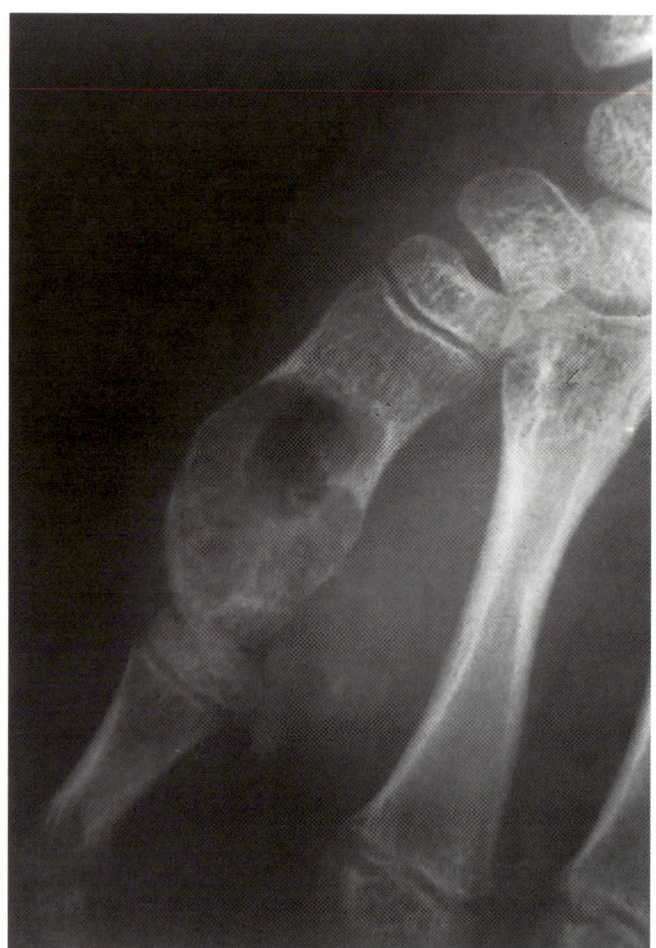

Fig. 12.12 Chondroblastoma of a metacarpal.

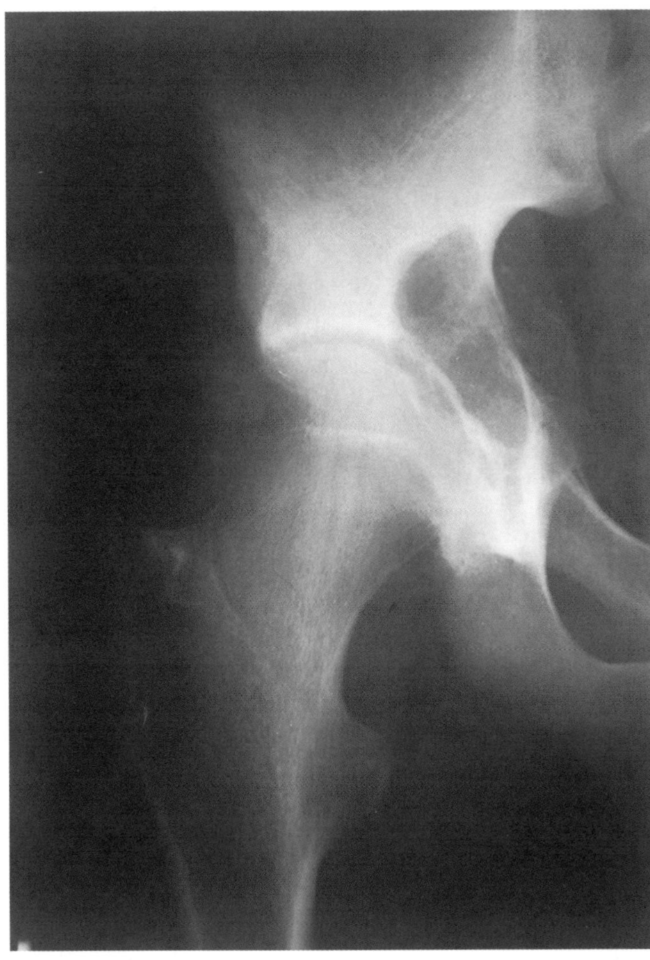

Fig. 12.13 Chondroblastoma in the acetabular area.

related to a primary or secondary center of ossification,[34] usually in eccentric locations and extending into the metaphysis.

Two to 5% of cases are pure metaphyseal, metadiaphyseal or, more rarely, diaphyseal lesions[4,5,8,33,34–44] (Lichtenstein 1977) (Figs 12.14, 12.15). Rare cases are surface or cortical lesions.[8]

The eccentric radiolucency shows a geographic type of destruction with smooth or lobulated margins[5] which are sclerotic in half the cases.[8] This pattern of destruction is the same in long, short or flat bones, but appears more aggressive in flat bones.[45] Trabeculous or ballooning expansion may be found in flat bones with a thin cortex.[5] In a minority of cases (10%[8]), the cortex of long bones shows endosteal erosion or partial destruction.

In the pelvis, chondroblastomas may appear as large osteolytic lesions[24] or heavily calcified tumors.[49] Some have an aggressive growth[5,28,33,35,46–52] with soft tissue involvement, articular implants or even invasion of the adjacent bones.

On plain films, calcifications are found in one-third of cases,[5] appearing as tiny punctate densities[4] or as a more

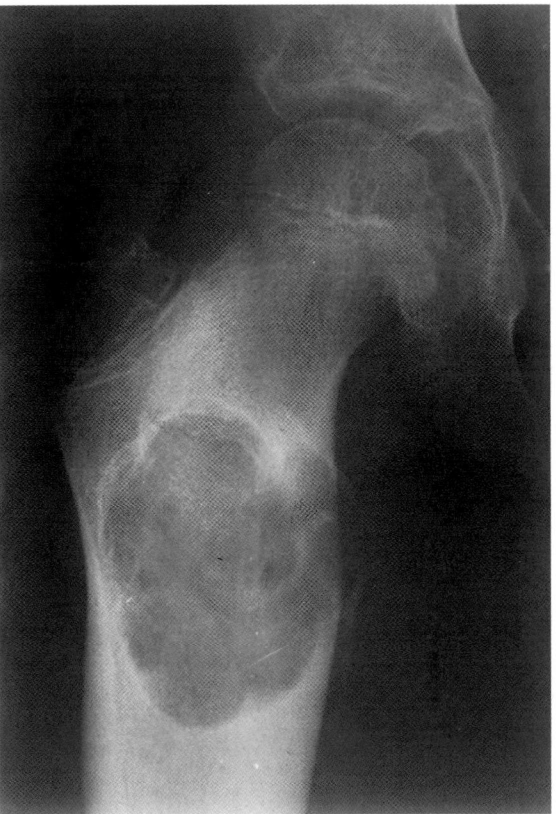

Fig. 12.14

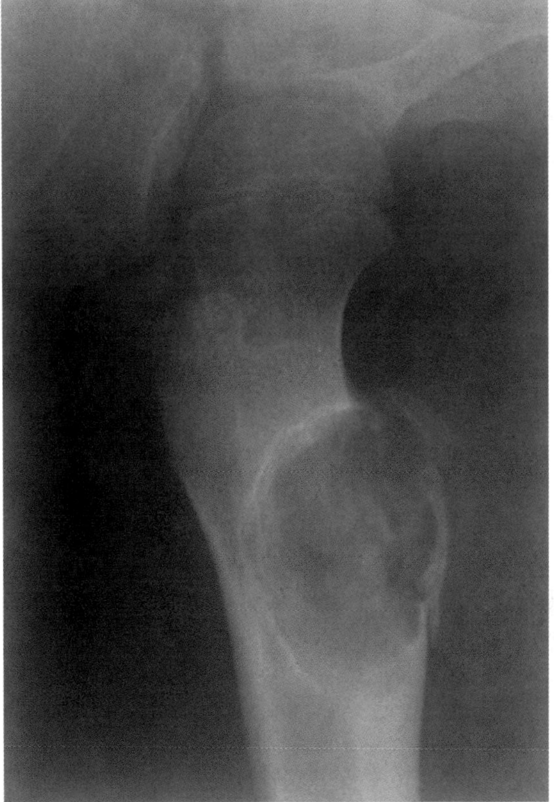

Fig. 12.15

Figs 12.14, 12.15 Metaphyseal chondroblastomas of the femur.

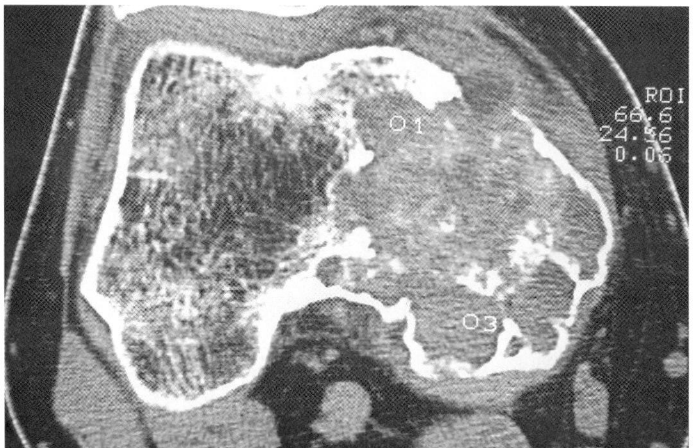

Fig. 12.16 Chondroblastoma of the femur: extent of osteolysis well demonstrated on CT scan.

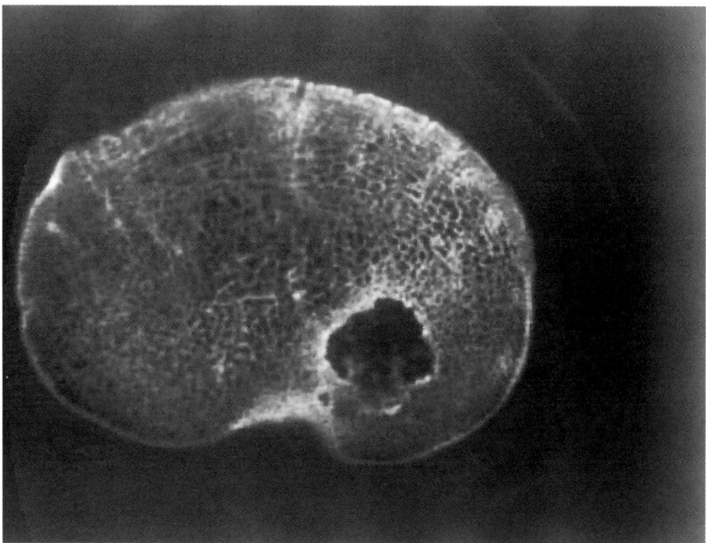

Fig. 12.17 Chondroblastoma of the tibia: sclerotic rim demonstrated on CT scan.

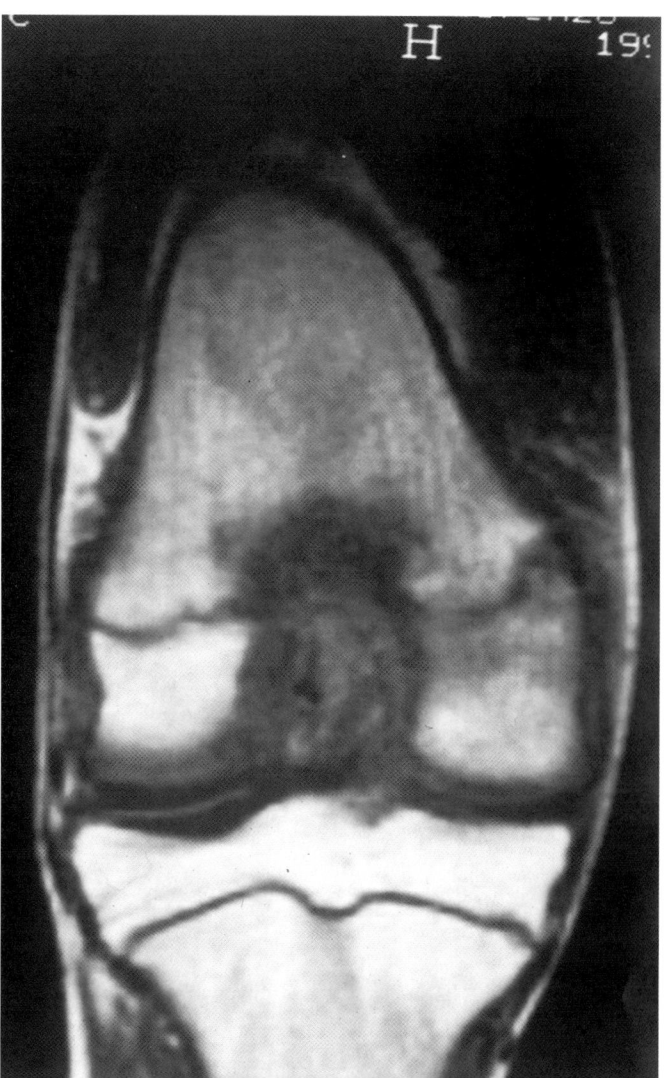

Fig. 12.18 Chondroblastoma of the femur: involvement of the joint cavity demonstrated on MRI.

radiopaque lesion; they are best shown on CT in the majority of patients.[33] In approximately 60% of patients, with tumors in long bones, solid or lamellar periosteal appositional new bone is found.[53,55]

Hot bone scans are related to the increased blood flow and regional hyperemia.[56,57]

CT emphasizes the cortical destruction, the sclerotic rim and the calcifications[58] (Figs 12.16, 12.17).

Chondroblastomas are usually isointense or hypointense compared with muscle on all MR sequences[59] (Fig. 12.18) or there is a low intensity signal in T1-weighted images and a high signal intensity in T2-weighted images related to the bone marrow edema and joint effusion.[60–63] An associated aneurysmal bone cyst may produce a very high signal intensity or even fluid levels. A lobular architecture has been described on MRI.[61]

GROSS PATHOLOGY

The tumor appears as a soft or granular and friable, red-brown or grayish tissue, with yellow calcifications or, less frequently, bluish chondroid islands. This quite vascular and hemorrhagic lesion ranges in size from 1.5 to 7 cm.[5] It may extend to the joint, with involvement of the cruciate ligament attachment or the ligamentum teres.[33] An intact periosteal membrane is found, even when the cortex is thinned or destroyed.

In 10–40% of cases, an aneurysmal bone cyst is present (the so-called 'cystic chondroblastomas'[5,8,22,35,64–68]) and the scarce tumoral tissue is only found in the wall of the

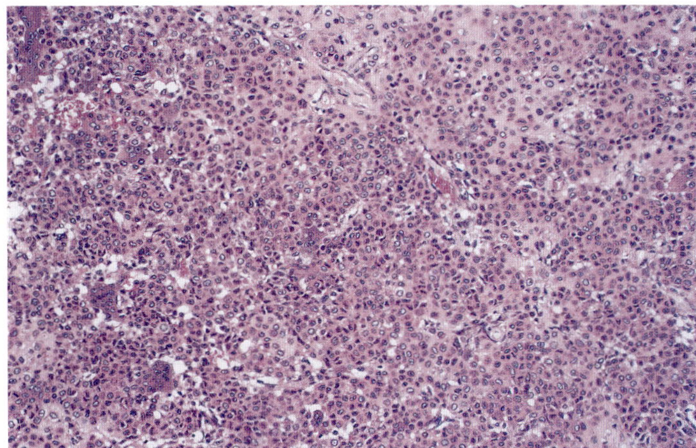

Fig. 12.19

Figs 12.19–12.22 Chondroblastomas: sheets of round or polyhedral cells with indented, grooved or reniform nuclei and little cytoplasm.

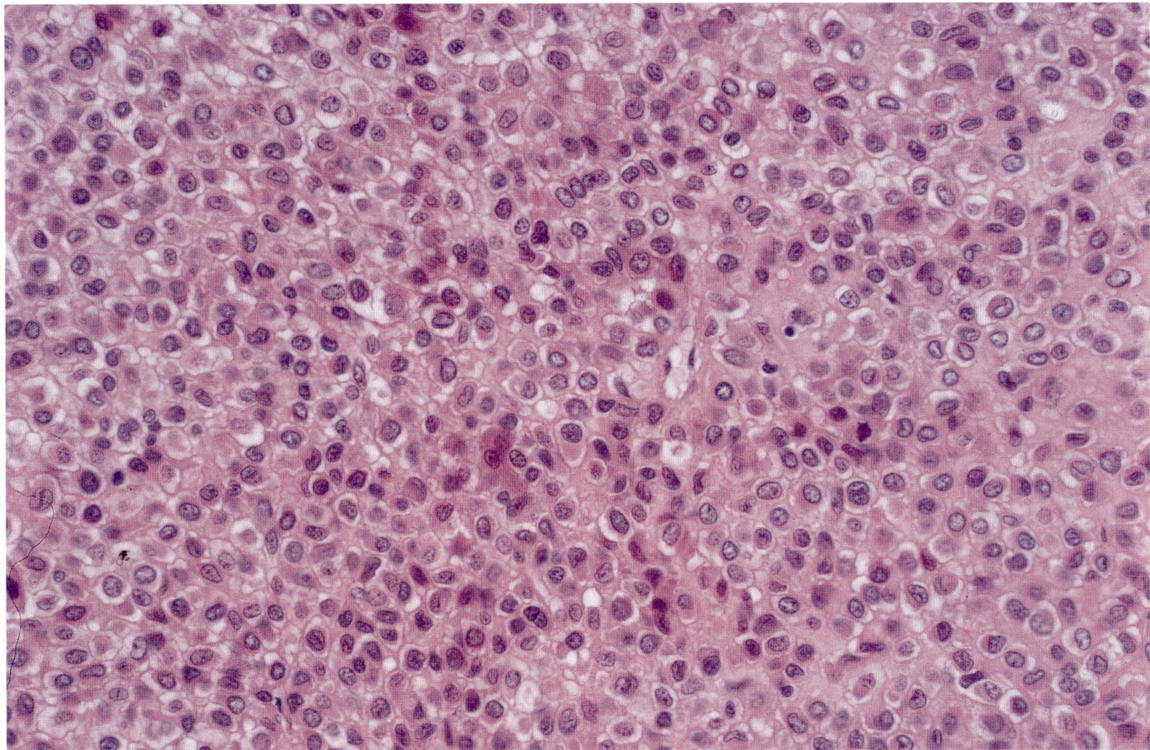

Fig. 12.20

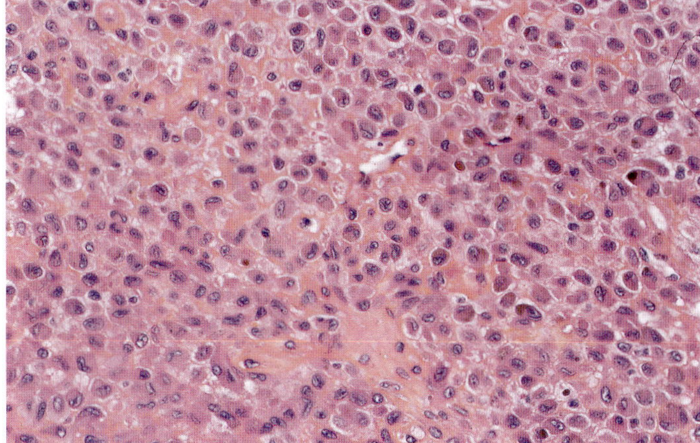

Fig. 12.21

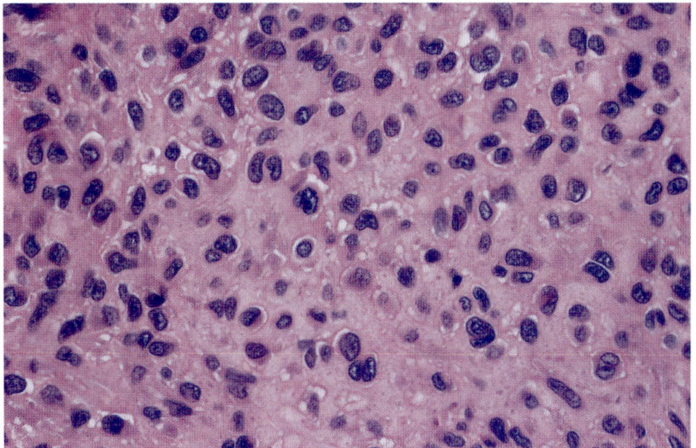

Fig. 12.22

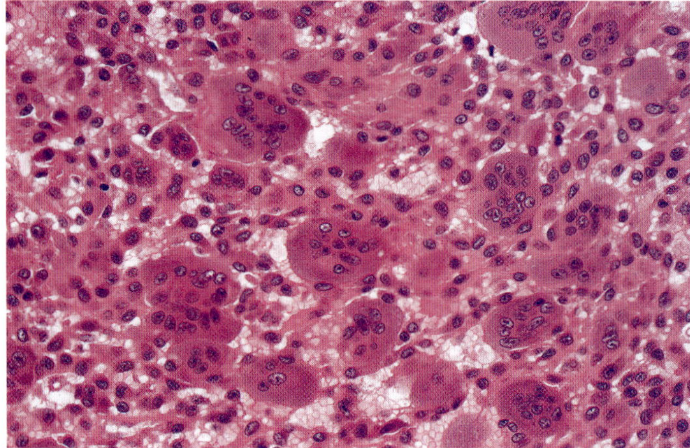

Fig. 12.23

Fig. 12.24

Figs 12.23, 12.24 Chondroblastomas: associated reactive giant cells.

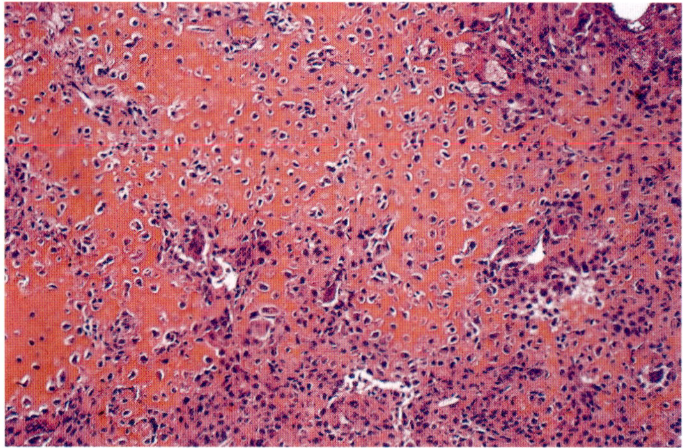

Fig. 12.25

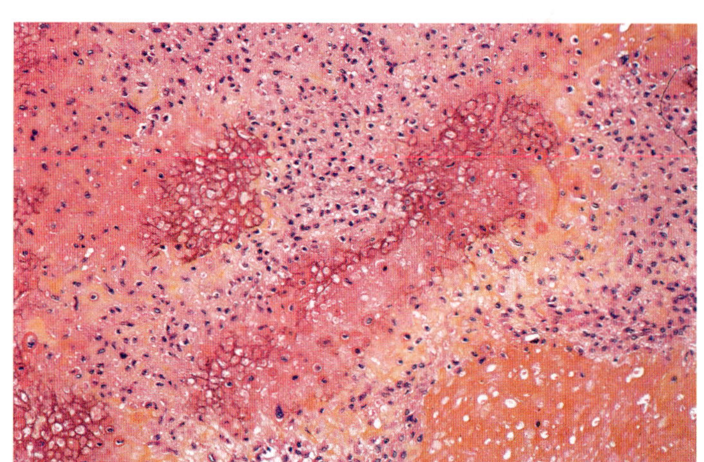

Fig. 12.27

Fig. 12.26

Fig. 12.28

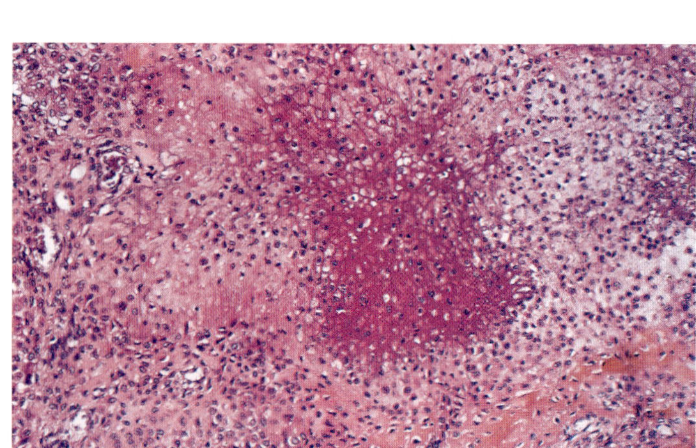

Figs 12.25–12.31 Chondroblastomas: chondroid matrix, necrosis and calcific deposits.

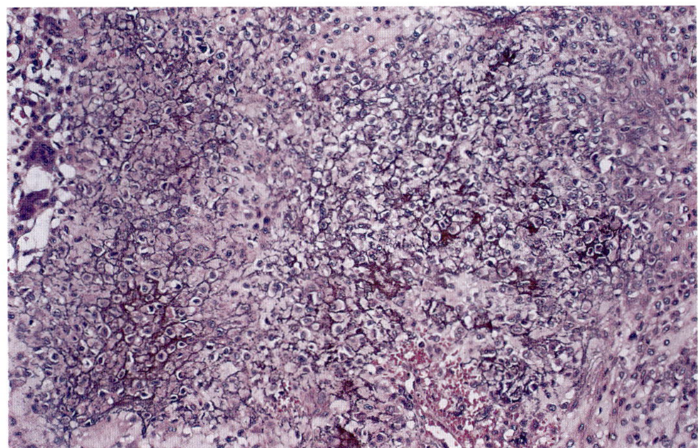

Fig. 12.29

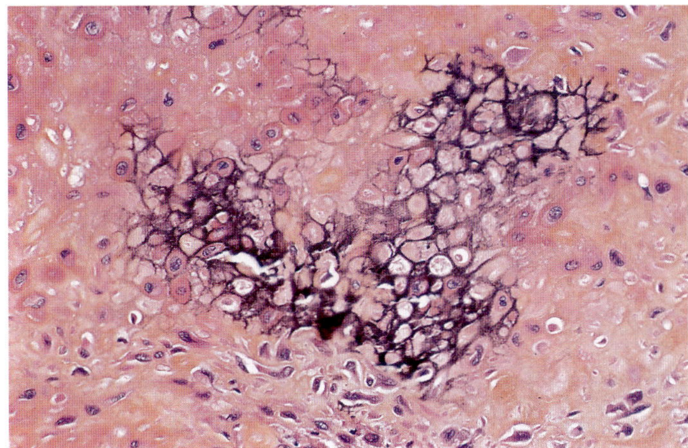

Fig. 12.31

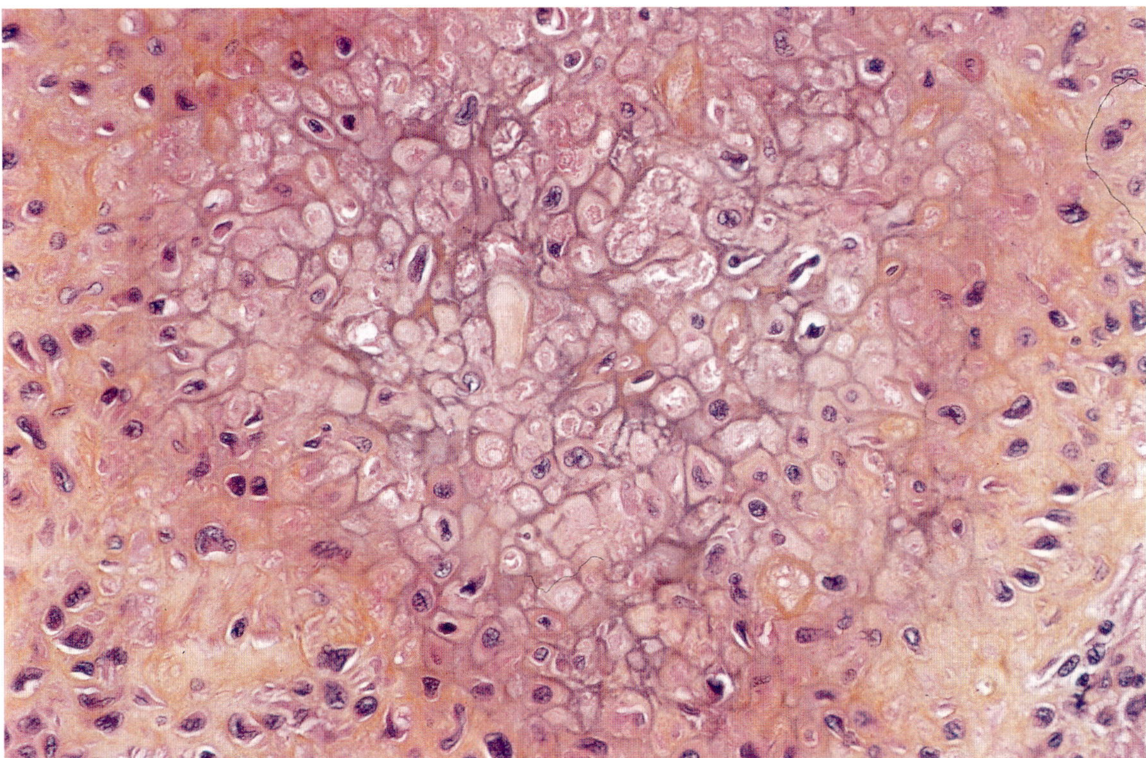

Fig. 12.30

cyst.[8] Small simple cysts are common; more rarely, the tumor appears as a single cavity[5] empty[43] or filled with a serous or hemorrhagic fluid.[24,53,69,70]

HISTOPATHOLOGY

Sheets of relatively uniform-sized cells are characteristic of a chondroblastoma, which is a highly cellular lesion with a scant intercellular matrix (Figs 12.19–12.22). The rounded or polyhedral cells have well-defined cytoplasmic borders, with a small amount of pink cytoplasm. The nuclei are round, oval or reniform or sometimes indented or marked with longitudinal grooves. One or two small nucleoli may be found. The chromatin is evenly distributed. Rare cells may have two or three nuclei. Glycogen granules or hemosiderin pigment may be found in the cytoplasm. Rarely, chondroblast cells may look like epithelioid cells, especially in temporal locations;[71] some cells may appear spindly or present a hyperchromatic and enlarged nucleus.[8,33] Spindle or stellate cells, in rare cases, can mimic a chondromyxoid fibroma.[4,18,64] In 80% of cases, normal mitotic activity is found.[4]

Reactive giant cells are randomly distributed or appear close to areas of necrosis or hemorrhage (Figs 12.23,

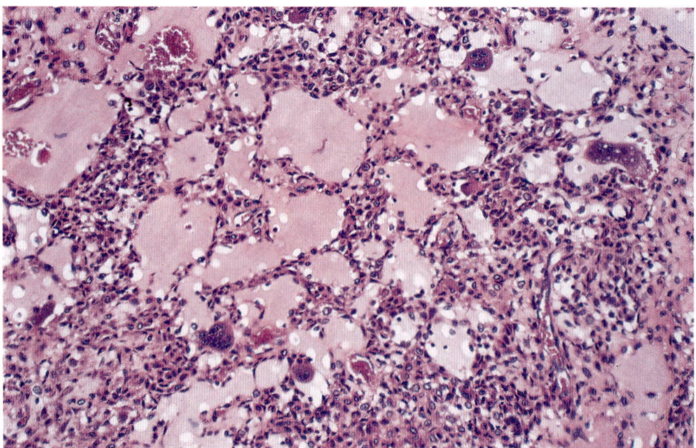

Fig. 12.32

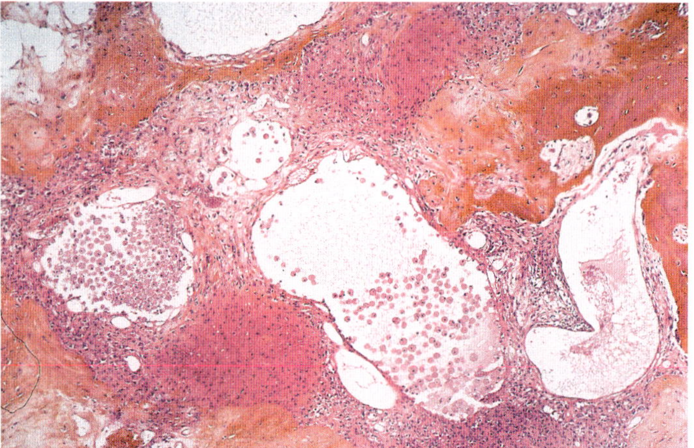

Fig. 12.33

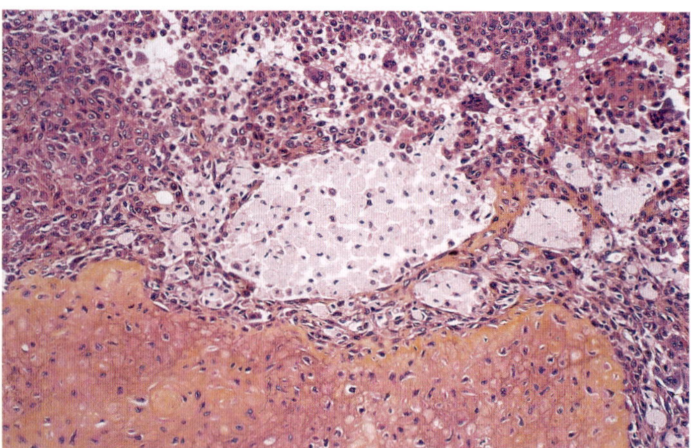

Fig. 12.34

Figs 12.32–12.34 Secondary changes in chondroblastomas with cystic spaces and lipophagic cell collections.

12.24). Foci of cellular necrosis are associated with a deposition of calcium; the calcific deposits around empty lacunae have a lace-like or chicken-wire appearance,[64] highly typical of chondroblastomas[8] (Figs 12.25–12.31). The fibrochondroid or amorphous pinkish chondroid matrix may be sparse or extensive, with calcification or osseous metaplasia.[4,72]

Lichtenstein and Huvos have suggested a staged progression of the lesion, from a highly cellular tumor to a reparative fibrosis, with chondroid and osseous metaplasia.

Cystic changes are not unusual (Figs 12.32–12.34) and large cystic blood spaces suggest a secondary aneurysmal bone cyst-like pattern in many locations, but especially in the small bones of hands and feet.[66,68]

An associated synovitis may resemble that of rheumatoid arthritis, with lymphocytes and plasma cells.

CYTOPATHOLOGY

Smears or imprints are useful in depicting the mononuclear or, less often, binucleate chondroblastic cells, with nuclear longitudinal grooves or deep convolutions[73–75] (Figs 12.35–12.38). Intranuclear pseudoinclusions[76–78] are not specific to chondroblastomas.[79] Reactive giant cells may be numerous.

The chondroid matrix is green to violet with Papanicolaou stain,[74] eosinophilic on Giemsa stain.[75]

IMMUNOHISTOCHEMISTRY AND HISTOCHEMISTRY

The cells of chondroblastoma are strongly positive for S-100 protein[80–87] and there is coexpression of vimentin, fibronectin and NSE[86,87] (Fig. 12.39).

A strong cytokeratin and epithelial membrane antigen expression has been reported in half of the cases,[4,87,88] considered to be an aberrant expression or a biphasic differentiation (Fig. 12.40). Another unusual staining characteristic in some tumors is for smooth muscle or muscle-specific actin.[87]

An immunoreactivity to the proliferating cell nuclear antigen has been found in 100% of cases in one series.[87] There is a lack of histiocytic markers.[82,85] Collagen type II is distributed in the chondroid matrix and type VI in the chondroid matrix and also around the cells.[4]

Abundant PAS-positive diastase-labile glycogen granules, shown also in tissue culture studies, are found in the cytoplasm and the matrix contains Alcian blue-stained acid-sulfated glycosaminoglycans.[86]

ELECTRON MICROSCOPY

Numerous ultrastructural studies have been performed.[28,29,52,76,77,81,89–100] The cells, which have an irregular outline, have numerous microvilli, Golgi complexes, mitochondria and glycogen particles. The multilobulated nuclei show a fibrous lamina closely applied to the inner nuclear membrane.

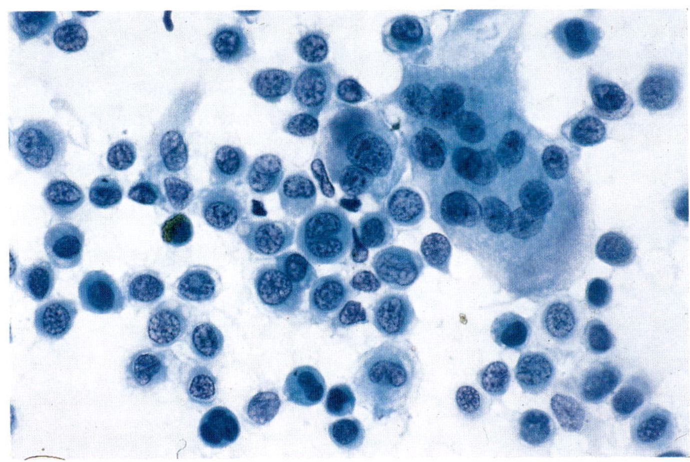

Fig. 12.35

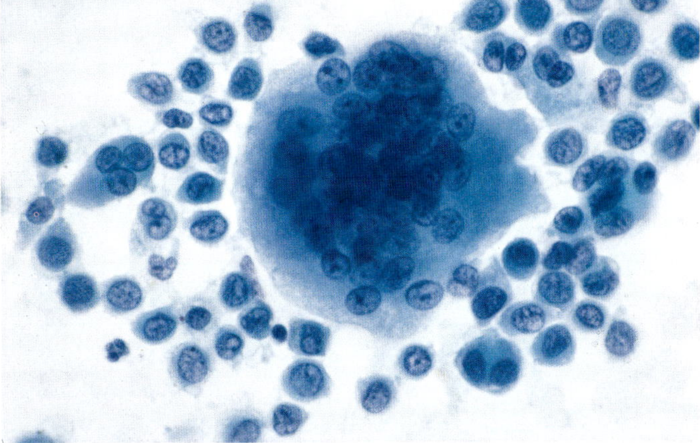

Fig. 12.36

Figs 12.35, 12.36 Imprint cytology of chondroblastoma (Papanicolaou stain).

Ultrastructural cytochemical studies demonstrate proteoglycans and calcium in the matrix.[76,98]

The cells may arise from chondrocytes, most probably related to the epiphyseal cartilage, with various degrees of differentiation. Despite some histological, immunohistochemical and ultrastructural reports[99,100] suggesting a histiocytic lineage, the chondrogenic origin of the tumor is now well established.

FLOW CYTOMETRY

Nuclei of chondroblastoma cells are diploid;[101–104] aneuploidy has been detected in some cases,[105,106] but one case has a possible diagnosis of clear cell chondrosarcoma.[105]

CYTOGENETICS

Some tumors may be cytogenetically normal or show structural anomalies involving 11p15, like those found in giant cell tumors.[107] A further cytogenetic study has shown abnormalities of chromosome 1 and involvement of chromosome 22 in a complex translocation.[108] In an aggressive chondroblastoma, unbalanced translocations have involved chromosomes 2, 5, 8 and 21.[107]

COURSE, TREATMENT AND PROGNOSIS

The treatment is thorough curettage and bone grafting.[3] Chondroblastoma is radiosensitive, but there is a risk of induced sarcomas.[65]

The rate of recurrence (usually within 3 years[5]) ranges from 5% to 22%.[3–5, 33,50,99] A higher rate is not associated with chondroblastomas showing an aneurysmal bone cyst component,[3,5,8,33] contrary to the results of Huvos.[65]

Very rarely bone metastases have been reported,[109] in one case occurring over a 30-year period after local recurrences.[110]

Chondroblastomas may be locally very aggressive[22,49–52,111,112] or, rarely, show malignant transformation.[113] Some malignant chondroblastomas are more probably postradiation sarcomas.[3,5,51] Apart from truly malignant lesions,[114] usually pulmonary metastases exhibit the same histology as the primary tumor, having a limited growth potential[8,50,52,111,115–120] and possibly representing self-limiting lung implants. Some tumors are associated with clusters of tumor cells in small veins and lymphatics at the edge of the primary tumor,[120] but these unusual findings appear to be unrelated to the occurrence of metastases.[3]

There is no histological criterion that reliably predicts the rare worse outcome.[120]

DIFFERENTIAL DIAGNOSIS

Chondroblastomas have to be differentiated from giant cell tumors, clear cell chondrosarcomas and aneurysmal bone cysts; epiphyseal clear cell osteosarcoma is a rarity.

Giant cell tumors exhibit more giant cells and more spindly stromal cells which lack the peculiar nuclei of chondroblastomas. They are also devoid of chondroid matrix, S100 positivity and matrix glycosaminoglycans.

Clear cell chondrosarcomas may have limited areas which are cytologically similar to chondroblastomas and one has to find a cytological component with a prominent water-clear cytoplasm and round vesicular nuclei and associated reactive bone formation.

An aneurysmal bone cyst can almost completely destroy the chondroblastic areas; the diagnosis can be made only on the material obtained via thorough curettage, with a wide histological sampling of the tissue.

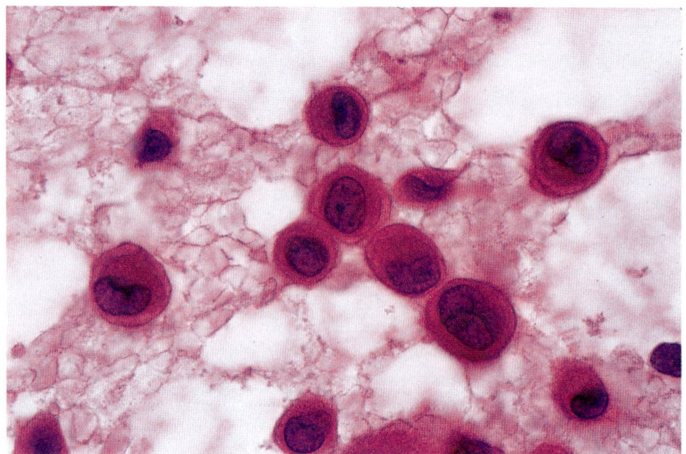

Fig. 12.37

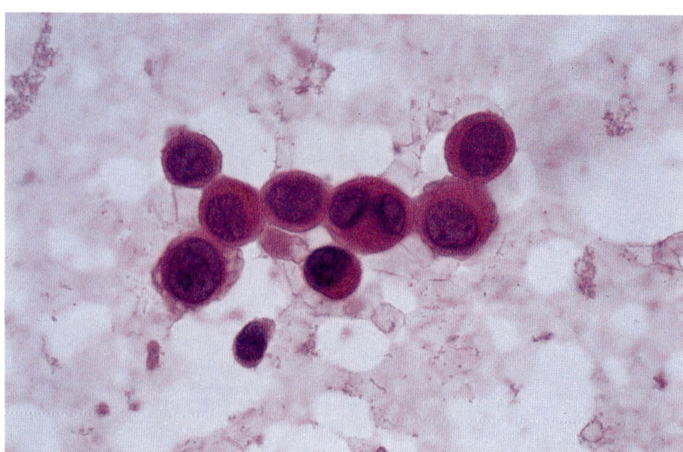

Fig. 12.38

Figs 12.37, 12.38 Imprint cytology of chondroblastoma (H&E stain).

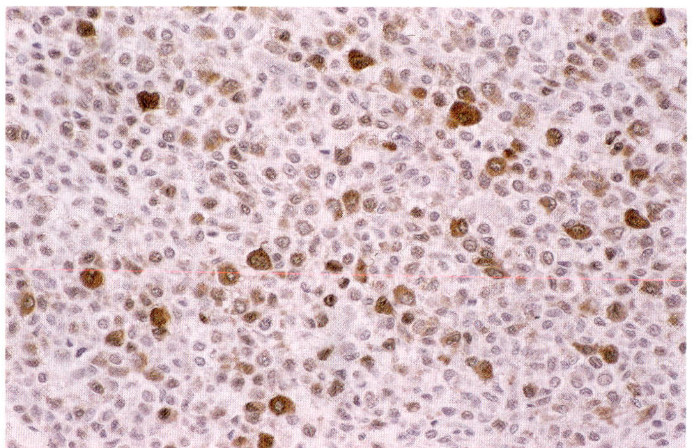

Fig. 12.39 Chondroblastoma: focal immunoreactivity with S-100 protein.

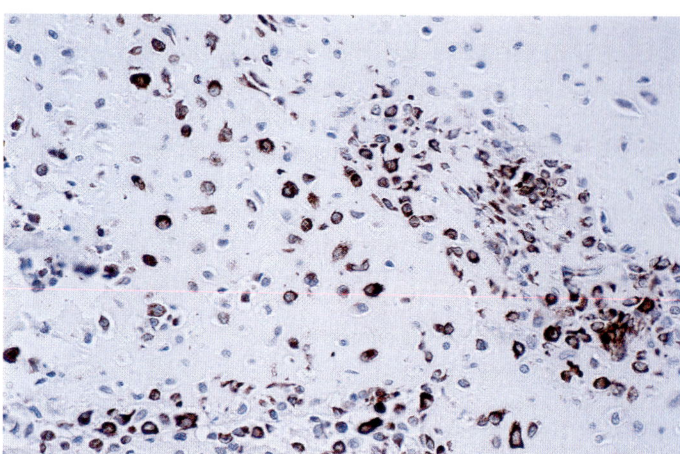

Fig. 12.40 Chondroblastoma: immunoreactivity with cytokeratins.

COMMENTS FOR THE SURGICAL PATHOLOGIST

With respect, one may debate a Mayo Clinic statement that the finding of chondroid islands or chicken-wire calcifications is necessary for a diagnosis of chondroblastoma. In a young patient with an epiphyseal lesion very suggestive of the diagnosis on X-ray, it seems that a diagnosis may be established solely on the cytology of chondroblasts and a positive S-100 protein staining.[38,74,82]

REFERENCES

1. Jaffe H L, Lichtenstein L. Benign chondroblastoma of bone. A reinterpretation of so-called calcifying or chondromatous giant cell tumor. Am J Pathol 1942: 18: 969–991
2. Codman E A. Epiphyseal chondromatous giant cell tumors of the upper end of the humerus. Surg Gynecol Obstet 1931: 52: 543–546 and Clin Orthop 1980: 153: 7–13
3. Turcotte R E, Kurt A M, Sim F H, Unni K K, McLeod R A. Chondroblastoma. Hum Pathol 1993: 24: 944–949
4. Edel G, Ueda Y, Nakanishi J et al. Chondroblastoma of bone. A clinical, radiological, light and immunohistochemical study. Virchows Arch A Pathol Anat Histopathol 1992: 421: 355–366
5. Bloem J L, Mulder J D. Chondroblastoma: a clinical and radiological study of 104 cases. Skeletal Radiol 1985: 14: 1–9
6. Resendes M, Parker B R, Kempson R L, Jones H H, Nagel D A. Case report 663. Unusual chondroblastoma of the scapula. Skeletal Radiol 1991: 20: 222–225
7. Brower A C, Moser R P, Gilkey F W, Kransdorf M J. Chondroblastoma. In: Moser R P, Ed. Carilaginous tumors of the skeleton. AFIP Atlas of radiologic-pathologic correlations II. Philadelphia: Hanley & Belfus, 1990, pp 74–113
8. Kurt A M, Unni K K, Sim F H, McLeod R A. Chondroblastoma of bone. Hum Pathol 1989: 20: 965–976
9. Holt E M, Murphy G J, al-Jafari M. Chondroblastoma of the acromion. Skeletal Radiol 1995: 24: 223–224
10. Kricun M E, Kricun R, Haskin M E. Chondroblastoma of the calcaneus: radiographic features with emphasis on location. AJR 1977: 128: 613–616

11. Moore T M, Roe J B, Harvey J P Jr. Chondroblastoma of the talus: a case report. J Bone Joint Surg (Am) 1977: 59: 830–831
12. Ochsner P E, Von Hochstetter A R, Hilfiker B. Chondroblastoma of the talus: natural development over 9.5 years. Case report. Arch Orthop Trauma Surg 1988: 107: 122–125
13. Neviaser R J, Wilson J N. Benign chondroblastoma in the finger. J Bone Joint Surg (Am) 1972: 54: 389–392
14. Bliss D G, Mann R J. Chondroblastoma of a metacarpal. Report of a case and review of the literature. Clin Orthop 1985: 194: 211–213
15. Assor D. Chondroblastoma of the rib. Report of a case. J Bone Joint Surg (Am) 1973: 55: 208–210
16. Sundaram M, McGuire M H, Naunheim K, Schajowicz F. Case report 467. Cystic chondroblastoma left 4th rib. Skeletal Radiol 1988: 17: 136–140
17. Mayo-Smith W, Rosenberg A E, Khurana J S, Kattapuram S V, Romero L M. Chondroblastoma of the rib. A case report and review of the literature. Clin Orthop 1990: 251: 230–234
18. Kunkel M G, Dahlin D C, Young H H. Benign chondroblastoma. J Bone Joint Surg (Am) 1956: 38: 817–826
19. Hoeffel J C, Brasse F, Schmitt M et al. About one case of vertebral chondroblastoma. Pediatr Radiol 1987: 17: 392–396
20. Howe J W, Baumgard S, Yochum T R, Sladich M A. Case report 449. Chondroblastoma involving C5 and C6. Skeletal Radiol 1988: 17: 52–55
21. Akai M, Tateishi A, Machinami R, Iwano K, Asao T. Chondroblastoma of the sacrum. A case report. Acta Orthop Scand 1986: 57: 378–381
22. Matsuno T, Hasegawa I, Masuda T. Chondroblastoma arising in the triradiate cartilage. Report of two cases with review of literature. Skeletal Radiol 1987: 16: 216–222
23. Abdelwahab I F, Hermann G, Klein M J, Silver A, Kenan S, Lewis M M. Case report 696. Chondroblastoma of the right acetabulum and superior pubic ramus. Skeletal Radiol 1991: 20: 547–549
24. Lewis M M, Bullough P G. An unusual case of cystic chondroblastoma of the patella. Clin Orthop 1976: 121: 188–190
25. Remagen W, Schafer R, Roggatz J. Chondroblastoma of the patella. Arch Orthop Trauma Surg 1980: 96: 157–158
26. Moser R P Jr, Brockmole D M, Vinh T N, Kransdorf M J, Aoki J. Chondroblastoma of the patella. Skeletal Radiol 1988: 17: 413–419
27. Roberts P F, Taylor J G. Multifocal benign chondroblastomas: report of a case. Hum Pathol 1980: 11: 296–298
28. Ohno T, Kadoya H, Park P et al. Case report 382. Benign chondroblastoma of the talus invading calcaneus. Skeletal Radiol 1986: 15: 478–483
29. Rosa M A, Laudati A, Pannone A. Localizzazione epifisaria ed apofisaria del condroblastoma (studio di una casistica di 19 osservazioni). Arch Putti Chir Organi Mov 1990: 38: 363–370
30. Kingsley T C, Markel S F. Extraskeletal chondroblastoma. Cancer 1971: 27: 203–206
31. Abdul-Karim F W, Ayala A G, Spjut H J. Case report 321. Extraosseous chondroblastoma in the subcutaneous tissues of the right shoulder. Skeletal Radiol 1985: 14: 73–75
32. Weinrauch L, Katz M, Pizov G. Primary benign chondroblastoma cutis: extraskeletal manifestation without bone involvement. Arch Dermatol 1987: 123: 24–26
33. Springfield D S, Capanna R, Gherlinzoni F, Picci P, Campanacci M. Chondroblastoma. A review of seventy cases. J Bone Joint Surg (Am) 1985: 67: 748–755
34. Salzer M, Salzer-Kuntschik M, Kretschmer G. Das benigne Chondroblastoma I. Arch Orthop Unfallchirurg 1968: 64: 229–244
35. Schajowicz F, Gallardo H. Epiphyseal chondroblastoma of bone. A clinicopathological study of sixty-nine cases. J Bone Joint Surg (Br) 1970: 52: 205–226
36. McLeod R A, Beabout J W. The roentgenographic features of chondroblastoma. Am J Roentgenol Radium Ther Nucl Med 1973: 118: 464–471
37. Fechner R E, Wilde H D. Chondroblastoma in the metaphysis of the femoral neck. A case report and review of the literature. J Bone Joint Surg (Am) 1974: 56: 413–415
38. Schwinn C P. Differential diagnosis of giant cell lesions of bone. In: Ackerman L V, Spjut H J, Abell M R, Eds. Bone and joints. Baltimore: Williams & Wilkins, 1976, pp 251–255
39. Aronsohn R S, Hart W R, Martel W. Metaphyseal chondroblastoma of bone. AJR 1976: 127: 686–688
40. Nimbkar S A, Sane S Y, Pradhan C G. Benign chondroblastoma (in the metaphysis of the femoral neck) – a case report. J Postgrad Med 1980: 26: 259–260
41. Sotelo-Avila C, Sundaram M, Kyriakos M, Graviss E R, Tayob A A. Case report 373. Diametaphyseal chondroblastoma of the upper portion of the left femur. Skeletal Radiol 1986: 15: 387–390
42. Ippolito E, Tudisco C, Mariani P P. Rare forms of chondroblastoma. Cystic and diaphyseal types. Ital J Orthop Traumatol 1986: 12: 455–460
43. Pignatti G, Nigrisoli M. Case report 537. Chondroblastoma. Skeletal Radiol 1989: 18: 225–227
44. Dwaik M, Devlin P B. Case report: metadiaphyseal chondroblastoma. Clin Radiol 1992: 45: 131–133
45. Vestring T, Edel G, Muller-Miny H et al. Lokalisationsabhangige befundmuster beim chondroblastom. Rofo 1993: 159: 331–336
46. Coleman S S. Benign chondroblastoma with recurrent soft tissue and intra articular lesions. J Bone Joint Surg (Am) 1966: 48: 1554–1560
47. Sundaram T K. Benign chondroblastoma. J Bone Joint Surg (Br) 1966: 48: 92–104
48. Shoji H, Miller T R. Benign chondroblastoma of bone with soft tissue recurrence. N Y State J Med 1971: 71: 2786–2789
49. McLaughin R E, Sweet D E, Webster T, Merritt W M. Chondroblastoma of the pelvis suggestive of malignancy. J Bone Joint Surg (Am) 1975: 57: 549–551
50. Huvos A G, Higinbotham N L, Marcove R C, O'Leary P. Aggressive chondroblastoma. Review of the literature on aggressive behavior and metastases with a report of one new case. Clin Orthop 1977: 126: 266–272
51. Hull M T, Gonzalez-Crussi F, DeRosa G P, Graul R S. Aggressive chondroblastoma. Report of a case with multiple bone and soft tissue involvement. Clin Orthop 1977: 126: 261–265
52. Mirra J M, Ulich T R, Eckardt J J, Bhuta S. 'Aggressive chondroblastoma'. Light and ultramicroscopic findings after en bloc resection. Clin Orthop 1983: 178: 276–284
53. Alexander C. Case report 5. Chondroblastoma of tibia. Skeletal Radiol 1976: 1: 63–64
54. Braunstein E, Martel W, Weatherbee L. Periosteal bone apposition in chondroblastoma. Skeletal Radiol 1979: 4: 34–36
55. Brower A C, Moser R P, Kransdorf M J. The frequency and diagnostic significance of periostitis in chondroblastoma. AJR 1990: 154: 309–314
56. Humphry A, Gilday D L, Brown R G. Bone scintigraphy in chondroblastoma. Radiology 1980: 137: 497–499
57. Hudson T M, Hawkins I F Jr. Radiological evaluation of chondroblastoma. Radiology 1981: 139: 1–10
58. Quint L E, Gross B H, Glazer G M, Braunstein E M, White S J. CT evaluation of chondroblastoma. J Comput Assist Tomogr 1984: 8: 907–910
59. Cohen E K, Kressel H Y, Frank T S, Fallon M, Burk D L Jr, Dalinka M K, Schiebler M L. Hyaline cartilage-origin bone and soft-tissue neoplasms: MR appearance and histologic correlation. Radiology 1988: 167: 477–481
60. Fobben E S, Dalinka M K, Schiebler M L, Burk D L, Fallon M D, Schmidt R G, Kressel H Y. The magnetic resonance imaging appearance at 1.5 tesla of cartilaginous tumors involving the epiphysis. Skeletal Radiol 1987: 16: 647–651
61. Wheatherall P T, Maale G E, Mendelsohn D B, Sherry C S, Erdman W E, Pascoe H R. Chondroblastoma: classic and confusing appearance at MR imaging. Radiology 1994: 190: 467–474
62. Oxtoby J W, Davies A M. MRI characteristics of chondroblastoma. Clin Radiol 1996: 51: 22–26
63. Yamamura S, Sato K, Sugiura H, Iwata H. Inflammatory reaction in chondroblastoma. Skeletal Radiol 1996: 25: 371–376
64. Dahlin D C, Ivins J C. Benign chondroblastoma. Cancer 1972: 30: 401–413

65. Huvos A G, Marcove R C, Erlandson R A, Miké V. Chondroblastoma of bone. A clinicopathologic and electron microscopic study. Cancer 1972: 29: 760–771

66. Abdelwahab I F, Hermann G, Klein M J, Kenan S, Lewis M M. Case report 635. Chondroblastoma of the fourth metatarsal bone with secondary aneurysmal bone cyst. Skeletal Radiol 1990: 19: 539–541

67. Crim J R, Gold R H, Mirra J M, Eckardt J. Case report 748. Chondroblastoma of the femur with an aneurysmal bone cyst. Skeletal Radiol 1992: 21: 403–405

68. Brien E W, Mirra J M, Ippolito V. Chondroblastoma arising from a nonepiphyseal site. Skeletal Radiol 1995: 24: 220–222

69. Barbera C, Pinotti N, Klein M J, Lewis M M. An unusual case of cystic chondroblastoma of the calcaneus: a case report. Bull Hosp Jt Dis Orthop Inst 1988: 48: 88–92

70. Kahmann R, Gold R H, Eckardt J J, Mirra J M. Case report 337. Cystic chondroblastoma of calcaneus. Skeletal Radiol 1985: 14: 301–304

71. Bertoni F, Unni K K, Beabout J W, Harner S G, Dahlin D C. Chondroblastoma of the skull and facial bones. Am J Clin Pathol 1987: 88: 1–9

72. Gravanis M B, Giansanti J S. Benign chondroblastoma: report of four cases with a discussion of the presence of ossification. Am J Clin Pathol 1971: 55: 624–631

73. Troncone G, Vetrani A, Marino G, Palombani L. Il condroblastoma in citologia aspirativa con ago sottile. Isto-citopatologia 1989: 9: 85–90

74. Fanning C V, Sneige N S, Carrasco C H, Ayala A G, Murray J A, Raymond A K. Fine needle aspiration cytology of chondroblastoma of bone. Cancer 1990: 65: 1847–1863

75. Pohar-Marinsek Z, Us-Krasovec M, Lamovec J. Chondroblastoma in fine needle aspirates. Acta Cytol 1992: 36: 367–370

76. Walaas L, Kindblom L G, Gunterberg B, Bergh P. Light and electron microscopic examination of fine-needle aspirates in the preoperative diagnosis of cartilaginous tumors. Diagn Cytopathol 1990: 6: 396–408

77. Ascoli V, Facciolo F, Muda A O, Martelli M, Nardi F. Chondroblastoma of the rib presenting as an intrathoracic mass. Report of a case with fine needle aspiration biopsy, immunohistochemistry and electron microscopy. Acta Cytol 1992: 36: 423–429

78. Hazarika D, Kumar R V, Rao C R, Mukherjee G, Pattabhiraman V, Shekar M C. Fine needle aspiration cytology of chondroblastoma and chondromyxoid fibroma. A report of two cases. Acta Cytol 1994: 38: 592–596

79. Insabato L. Chondrogenic tumors with intranuclear vacuoles. Acta Cytol 1994: 38: 489

80. Nakamura Y, Becker L E, Marks A. S-100 protein in tumors of cartilage and bone. An immunohistochemical study. Cancer 1983: 52: 1820–1824

81. Ushigome S, Takakuwa T, Shinagawa T, Takagi M, Khishimoto H, Mori N. Ultrastructure of cartilaginous tumors and S-100 protein in the tumors, with reference to the histogenesis of chondroblastoma, chondromyxoid fibroma and mesenchymal chondrosarcoma. Acta Pathol Jpn 1984: 34: 1285–1300

82. Monda L, Wick M. S-100 protein immunostaining in the differential diagnosis of chondroblastoma. Hum Pathol 1985: 16: 287–293

83. Weiss A P, Dorfman H D. S-100 protein in human cartilage lesions. J Bone Joint Surg (Am) 1986: 68: 521–526

84. Okajima K, Honda I, Kitagawa T. Immunohistochemical distribution of S-100 protein in tumors and tumor-like lesions of bone and cartilage. Cancer 1988: 61: 792–799

85. Brecher M E, Simon M A. Chondroblastoma: an immunohistochemical study. Hum Pathol 1988: 19: 1043–1047

86. Karabela-Bouropoulou V, Markaki S, Prevedorou D, Vidali N. A combined immunohistochemical and histochemical approach on the differential diagnosis of giant cell epiphyseal neoplasms. Pathol Res Pract 1989: 184: 184–187

87. Hasegawa T, Seki K, Yang P et al. Differentiation and proliferative activity in benign and malignant cartilage tumors of bone. Hum Pathol 1995: 26: 838–845

88. Semmelink H J, Pruszczynski M, Wiersma Van Tilburg A, Smedts F, Ramaekers F C. Cytokeratin expression in chondroblastomas. Histopathology 1990: 16: 257–263

89. Welsh R A, Meyer A T. A histogenetic study of benign chondroblastoma. Cancer 1964: 17: 578–589

90. Wellmann K F. Chondroblastoma of the scapula. A case report with ultrastructural observations. Cancer 1969: 24: 408–416

91. Levine G D, Bensch K G. Chondroblastoma – the nature of the basic cell. A study by means of histochemistry, tissue culture, electron microscopy and autoradiography. Cancer 1972: 29: 1546–1562

92. Meary R, Abelanet R, Forest M et al. Les chondroblastomes bénins des os. Etude anatomo-clinique et ultrastructurale à propos de 11 observations. Rev Chir Orthop Reparatrice Appar Mot 1975: 61: 717–734

93. Steiner G C. Ultrastructure of benign cartilaginous tumors of intraosseous origin. Hum Pathol 1979: 10: 71–86

94. Povysil C, Matejovsky Z. Ultrastructure of benign chondroblastoma. Pathol Res Pract 1979: 166: 80–89

95. De Santis E, Turbacci F, Strazzulo E, Piantelli M. Aspetti ultrastrutturali del condroblastoma dello scheletro. Arch Putti Chir Organi Mov 1980: 30: 79–88

96. Martinez-Tello F J, Martinez-Gonzalez M A. The ultrastructure of the cartilaginous tumors. In: Bonucci E, Motta P M, Eds. Ultrastructure of skeletal tissues. Boston: Kluwer, 1990, pp 191–192

97. Fadda M, Manunta A, Rinonapoli G, Zirattu G, De Santis E. Ultrastructural appearance of chondroblastoma. Int Orthop 1994: 18: 389–392

98. Mii Y, Miyauchi Y, Morishita T et al. Ultrastructural cytochemical demonstration of proteoglycans and calcium in the extracellular matrix of chondroblastomas. Hum Pathol 1994: 25: 1290–1294

99. Higaki S, Takeyama S, Tateishi A, Machinami R, Abe M. Clinicopathological study of twenty-two cases of benign chondroblastoma (in Japanese). Nippon Seikeigeka Gakkai Zasshi 1981: 55: 647–664

100. Morimoto K, Okada S. Electron microscopic and immunohistochemical studies on chondroblastoma (in Japanese). Nippon Seikeigeka Gakkai Zasshi 1992: 66: 668–674

101. Cuvelier C A, Roels H J. Cytophotometric studies of the nuclear DNA content in cartilaginous tumors. Cancer 1979: 44: 1363–1374

102. Schajowicz F, Cabrini R L, Gimenez I. Microspectrophotometric quantitation of DNA in bone tumors with giant cells (osteoclastoma, osteosarcoma and chondroblastoma). Clin Orthop 1981: 156: 91–97

103. Mankin H J, Connor J F, Schiller A L, Permutter N, Alho A, McGuire M. Grading of bone tumors by analysis of nuclear DNA content using flow cytometry. J Bone Joint Surg (Am) 1985: 67: 404–413

104. Scotlandi K, Serra M, Manara M C et al. Clinical relevance of Ki-67 expression in bone tumors. Cancer 1995: 75: 806–814

105. Kreicbergs A, Silversward C, Tribukait B. Flow DNA analysis of primary bone tumors. Relationship between cellular DNA content and histopathologic classification. Cancer 1984: 53: 129–136

106. Xiang J H, Spanier S S, Benson N A, Braylan R C. Flow cytometric analysis of DNA, in bone and soft-tissue tumors using nuclear suspensions. Cancer 1987: 59: 1951–1958

107. Bridge J A, Bhatia P S, Anderson J R, Neff J R. Biological and clinical significance of cytogenetic and molecular cytogenetic abnormalities in benign and malignant cartilaginous lesions. Cancer Genet Cytogenet 1993: 69: 79–90

108. Mark J, Wedell B, Dahlenfors R, Grepp C, Burian P. Human benign chondroblastoma with a pseudodiploid stemline characterized by a complex and balanced translocation. Cancer Genet Cytogenet 1992: 58: 14–17

109. Konstantinov D. Knochen metastasen bei epiphysärem Chondroblastom. Radiol Diagn (Berl) 1984: 25: 81–84

110. Birch P J, Buchanan R, Golding P, Pringle J A. Chondroblastoma of the rib with widespread bone metastases. Histopathology 1994: 25: 583–585

111. Wirman J A, Crissman J D, Aron B F. Metastatic chondroblastoma: report of unusual case treated with radiotherapy. Cancer 1979: 44: 87–93

112. Povysil C, Matejovsky Z, Zidkova H, Trnka V. Agresivni chondroblastom (Czech). Acta Chir Orthop Traumatol Czech 1993: 60: 232–236

113. Reyes C V, Kathuria S. Recurrent and aggressive chondroblastoma of the pelvis with late malignant neoplastic changes. Am J Surg Pathol 1979: 3: 449–455

114. Sirsat M V, Doctor V M. Benign chondroblastoma of bone. Report of a case of malignant transformation. J Bone Joint Surg (Br) 1970: 52: 741–745

115. Van Horn J R, Vincent J G, Wiersma Van Tilburg A M, Pruszczynski M, Slooff T J, Molkenboer J F. Late pulmonary metastases from chondroblastoma of the distal femur. A case report. Acta Orthop Scand 1990: 61: 466–468

116. Kahn L B, Wood F M, Ackerman L V. Malignant chondroblastoma. Report of two cases and review of the literature. Arch Pathol Lab Med 1969: 88: 371–376

117. Riddell R J, Louis C J, Bromberger N A. Pulmonary metastasis from chondroblastoma of the tibia: report of a case. J Bone Joint Surg (Br) 1973: 55: 848–853

118. Green P, Whittaker R P. Benign chondroblastoma. Case report with pulmonary metastasis. J Bone Joint Surg (Am) 1975: 57: 418–420

119. Kyriakos M, Land V J, Penning L, Parker S G. Metastatic chondroblastoma. Report of a fatal case with a review of the literature on atypical, aggressive and malignant chondroblastomas. Cancer 1985: 55: 1770–1789

120. Kunze E, Graewe T, Peitsch E. Histology and biology of metastatic chondroblastoma. Pathol Res Pract 1987: 182: 113–123

13

Chondromyxoid fibroma

M. Forest

INTRODUCTION AND CLINICAL DATA

A chondromyxoid fibroma is a benign cartilaginous tumor characterized by a lobular pattern and spindle or stellate cells in a myxoid or, less often, chondroid stroma. First described in 1948 by Jaffe & Lichtenstein,[1] it accounts for 0.5–1% of all bone tumors and is found in all age groups, but mostly in the second and third decades.[2]

Clinical symptoms are pain and swelling; pathological fractures are uncommon (5%[3]). Occasionally, the tumor may be asymptomatic, especially in rib and ilium sites.[4] It is detected earlier in children.[5] Most of the lesions have a protracted course.[5–8]

SKELETAL DISTRIBUTION

All bones may be involved, the lower extremity accounts for 75–90% of cases:[2] proximal part of the tibia (and even the tibial tuberosity[9]), distal part of the tibia (Figs 13.1–13.3), distal fibula and femur (Figs 13.4–13.5). Overall, long tubular bones are involved in 60% of cases and short tubular bones, such as the metatarsals[11–14] (Fig. 13.6), in 20%.[10]

Tumors are also found in the flat bones, chiefly the ilium[15,16] (Figs 13.7–13.10), ribs[17] and sternum.[18,19,20] The calcaneus may also be involved[21,22] and, less often, the vertebral column and the sacrum.[23–27] Small and flat bone locations are more common in older patients.[4,28] A multicentric tumor has been reported.[29]

IMAGING

In long bones, the location is metaphyseal for most tumors, with eventual extension into the diaphysis or epiphysis. A metaphyseal lesion can extend through an open growth plate.[4] Primary epiphyseal or diaphyseal locations are uncommon.[4,6,10,30]

Cortical or periosteal sites are rare.[1,21,31–36] A surface

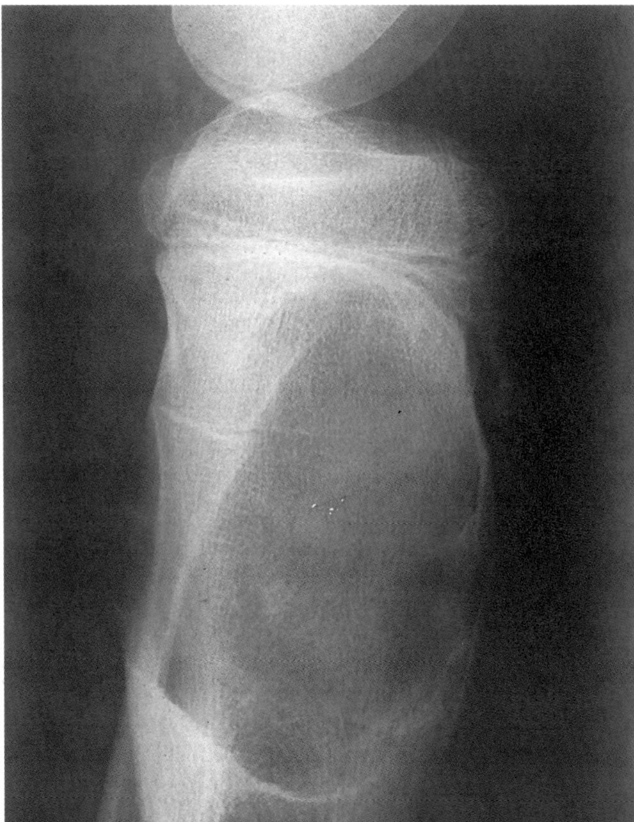

Fig. 13.1

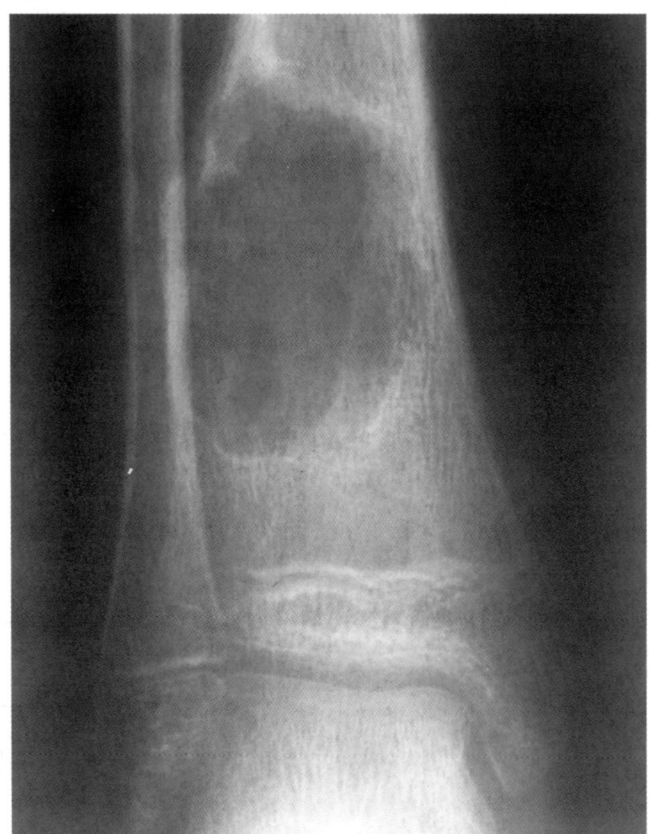

Fig. 13.3

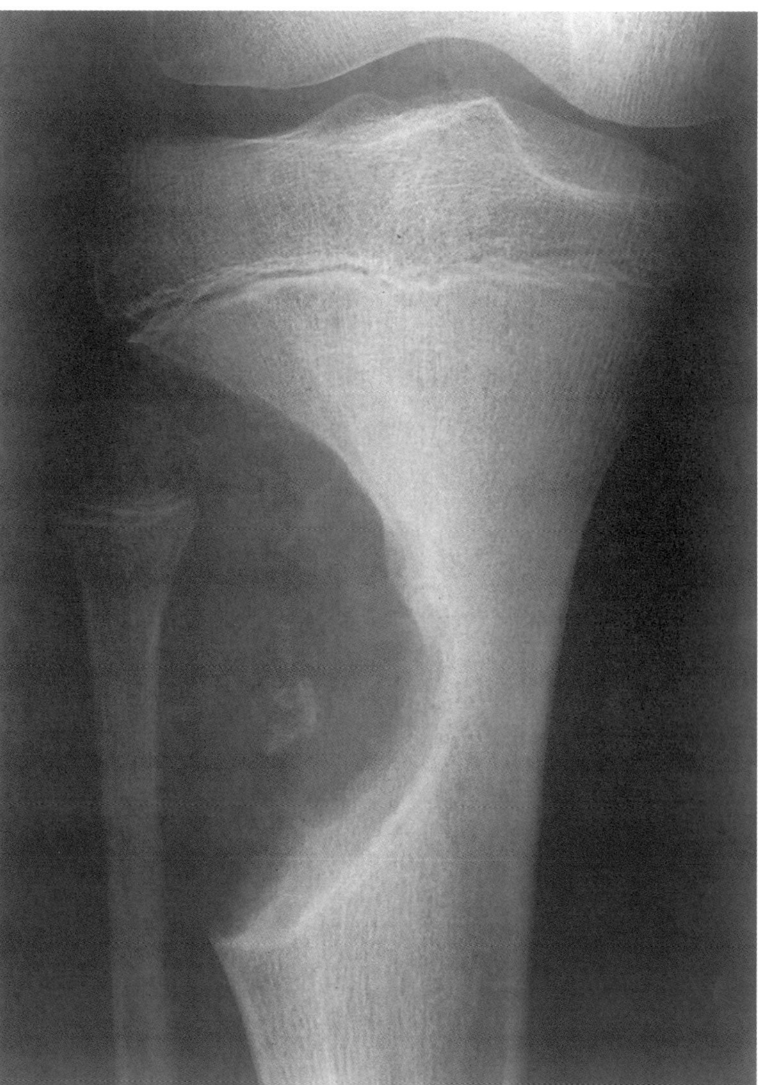

Fig. 13.2

Figs 13.1–13.3 Chondromyxoid fibromas in tibial location.

lesion, with saucerization of the cortex, may mimic a periosteal chondroma (Wilner 1982) in small tubular bones.

The tumor appears as a well-circumscribed radiolucent lesion, located eccentrically in long bones and oriented along the long axis;[8,34,37–39] it looks like a hemispherical 'bite out of the bone'.[4,30] Ridges and grooves of the cortex can look like pseudotrabeculations.[20] Intralesional calcifications are unusual.[4,6,40,41]

The geographic pattern of bone destruction is associated with scalloped internal borders and a thin, well-defined rim of bone sclerosis; the outer surface may have only a shell of periosteal bone, the cortex being expanded, eroded or even absent.[2] A cortical expansion is sometimes related to a secondary aneurysmal bone cyst component.[42]

Periosteal reactions are usually found only if there is a pathologic fracture and are otherwise unusual (2.6%.[10,39])

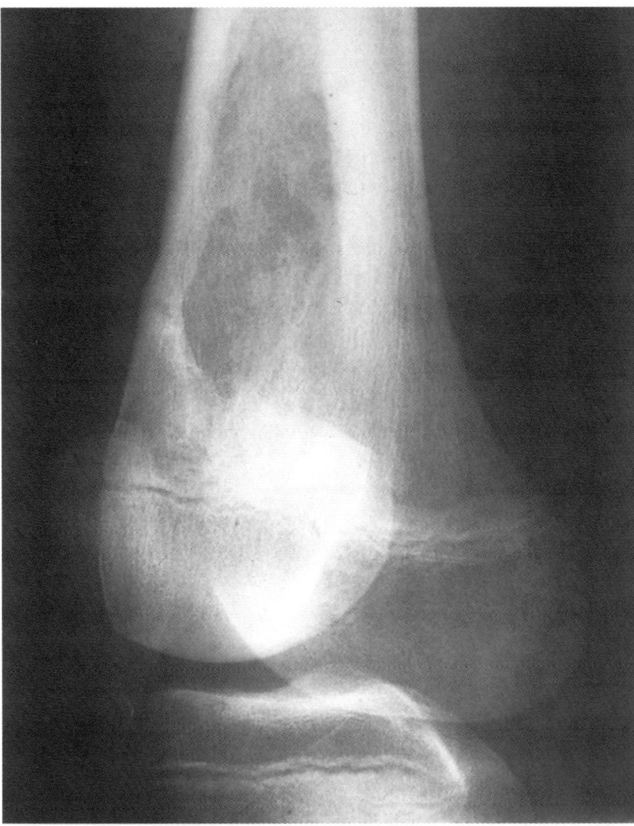

Fig. 13.4

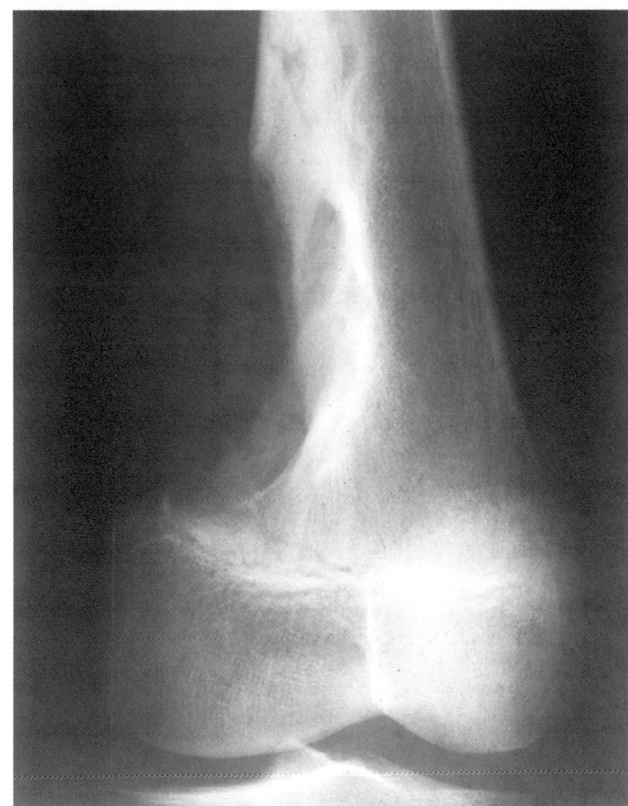

Fig. 13.5

Figs 13.4, 13.5 Chondromyxoid fibromas in femoral location.

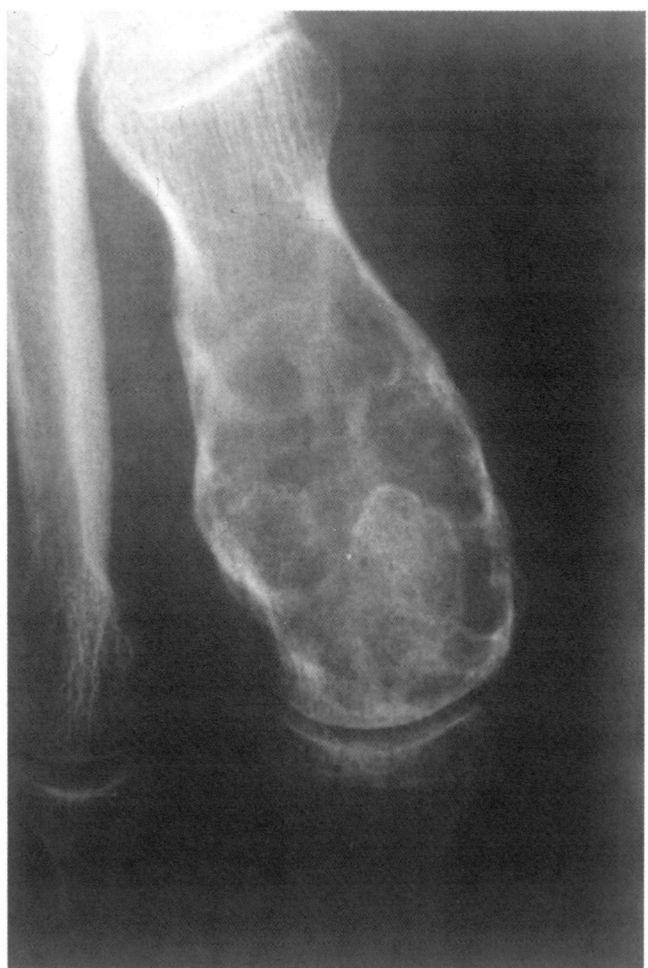

Figs 13.6 Chondromyxoid fibroma of a metatarsal.

In flat bones, the tumor is often loculated, with cortical expansion;[4,8] in small bones, it is centrally located and may fill the entire medullary canal.[8,10] In vertebrae, it has a more aggressive appearance[24–27] and may extend into the spinal canal.

On bone scans, chondromyxoid fibromas are active lesions.[34] Typical MRI signals are hypointensity on T1-weighted images and hyperintensity on T2-weighted images.[13,34,36]

GROSS PATHOLOGY

Tumor size ranges from 1 to 13 cm in the reported cases. The tissue is firm, rubbery, whitish, grayish or bluish-gray, slightly translucent and somewhat lobulated (Fig. 13.11). Small cavities or secondary aneurysmal bone cysts have been reported.[4,6,33,42]

HISTOPATHOLOGY

Chondromyxoid fibroma is a pseudolobulated tumor, the

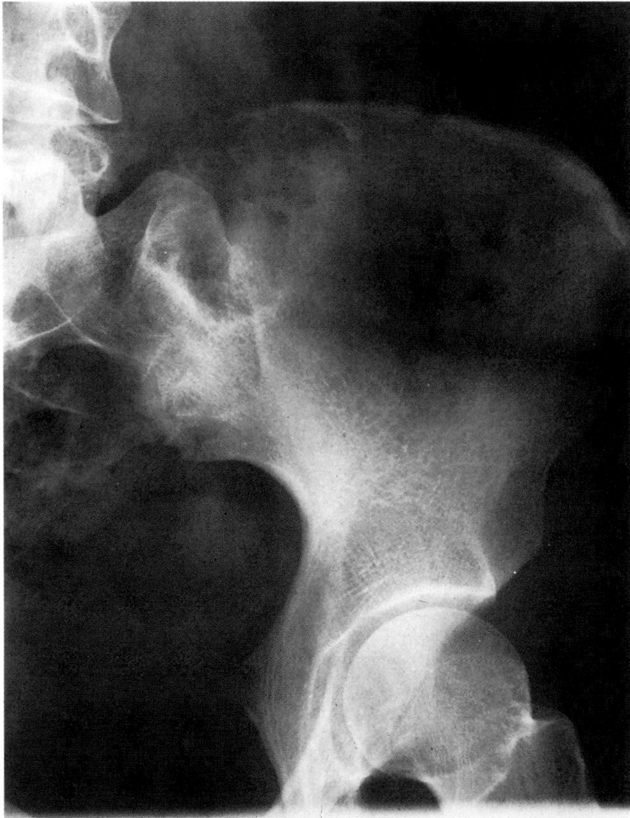

Fig. 13.7

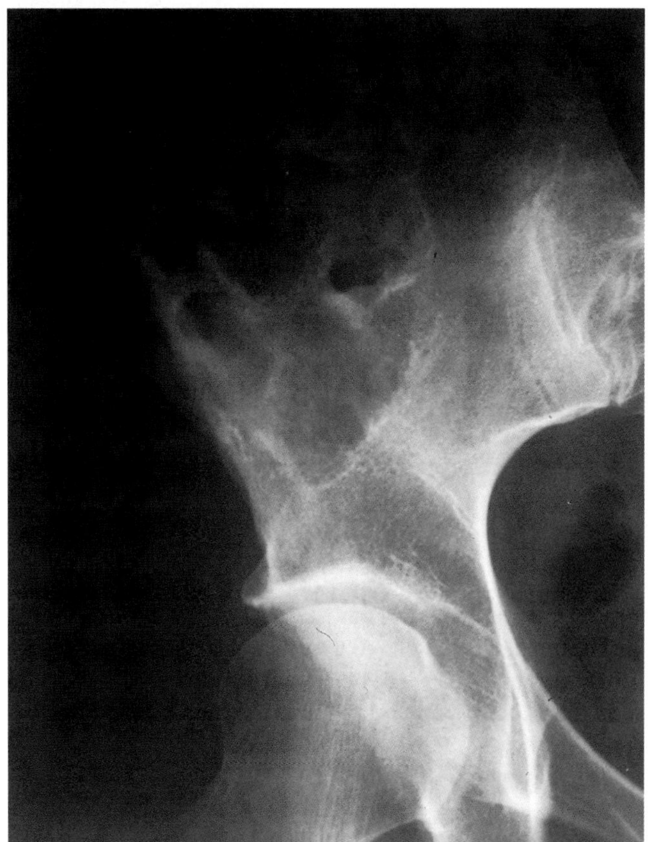

Fig. 13.8

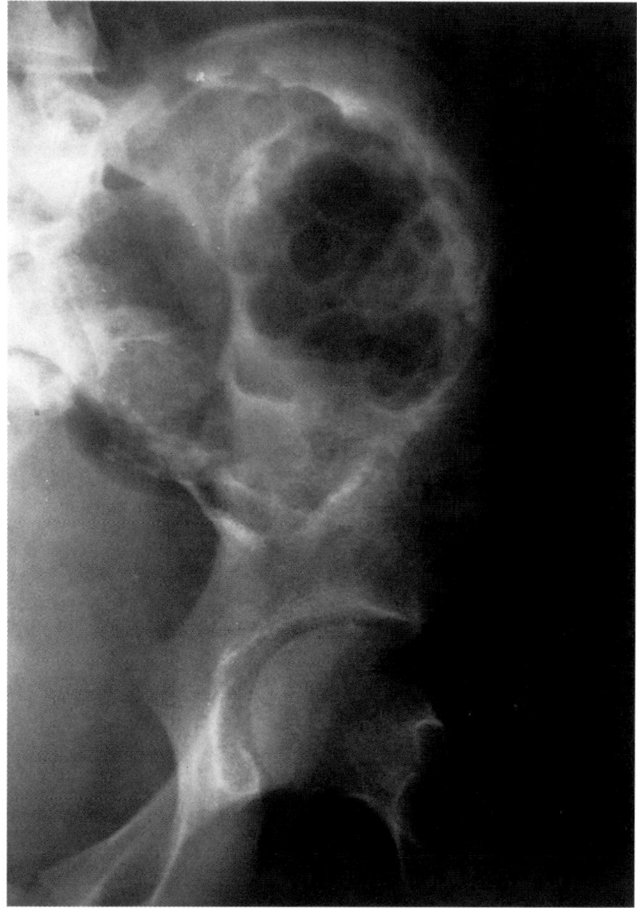

Fig. 13.9

Figs 13.7–13.9 Chondromyxoid fibromas of the iliac wing.

lobules being separated by fibrous tissue (Figs 13.12, 13.13). In the center of the lobules, the cells are spindly or stellate, with long cytoplasmic processes and an eosinophilic cytoplasm showing fairly distinct borders.[6] There is usually a higher density of cells towards the periphery of the lobules (the so-called 'cambium layer'[3]) (Figs 13.14–13.16). Some tumoral cells may be large, with two or three nuclei,[6] and appear as 'bizarre cells' with plump and hyperchromatic nuclei; these findings are not correlated with the recurrence rate. Mitotic activity is very unusual.[4,5]

In the peripheral areas, a cellular component with rounded cells and indented nuclei may resemble a chondroblastoma.[6]

The myxoid matrix of the lobules is predominant,[3] but the lobules may be more fibrous and hypocellular and contain microcysts (Mirra 1989)[7] in long-standing tumors (Fig. 13.17). Well formed hyaline cartilage matrix is sparse or usually absent.[3] Glycogen can be found in the stellate cells and the myxoid areas, which show Alcian blue staining.[43]

Some tumors may present punctate calcifications or

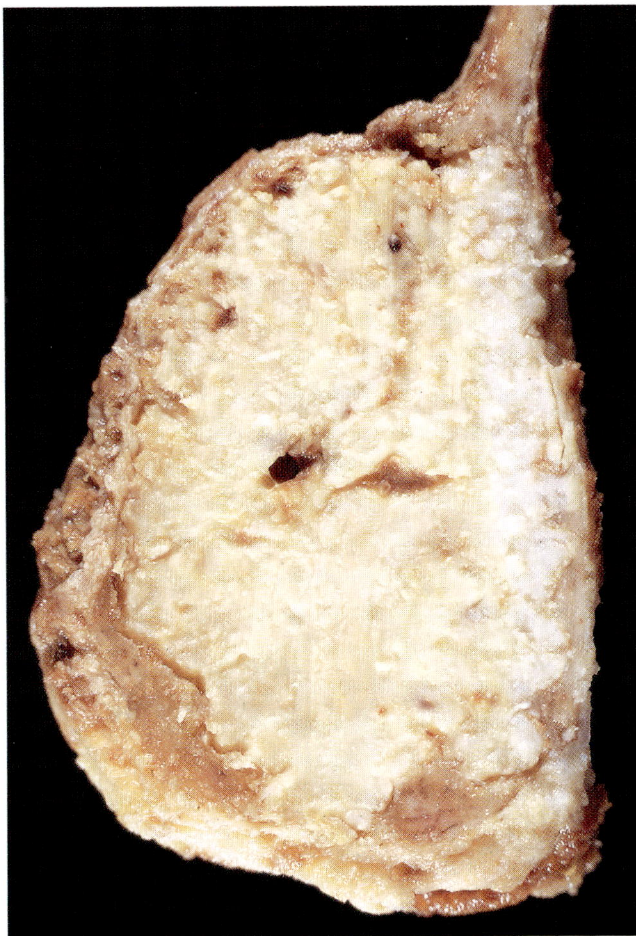

Figs 13.10 Chondromyxoid fibroma of the ilium appearing as a whitish fibrous mass.

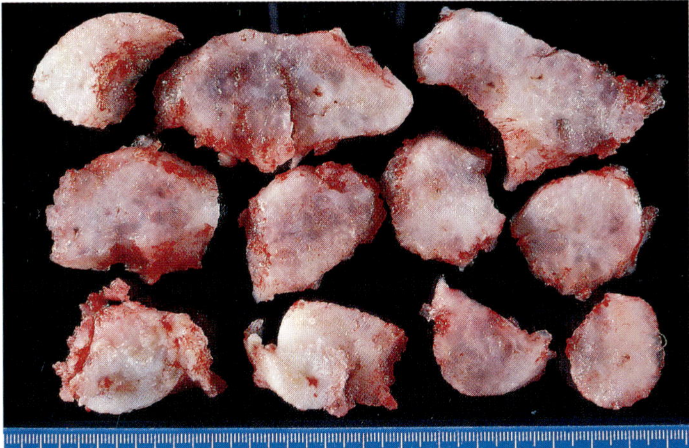

Figs 13.11 Chondromyxoid fibroma of the ilium: glistening chondroid appearance of the tumor fragments.

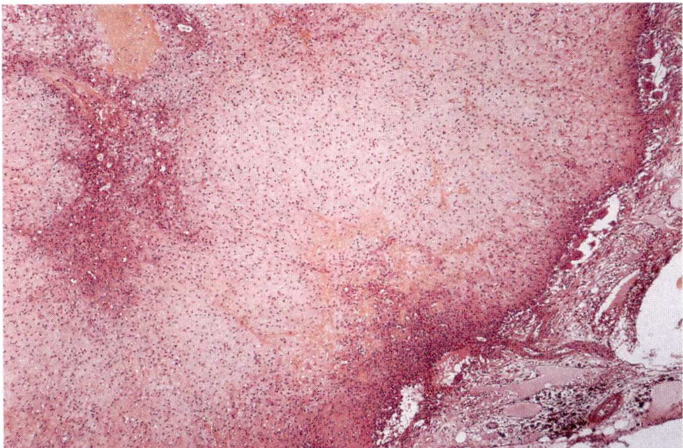

Fig. 13.12

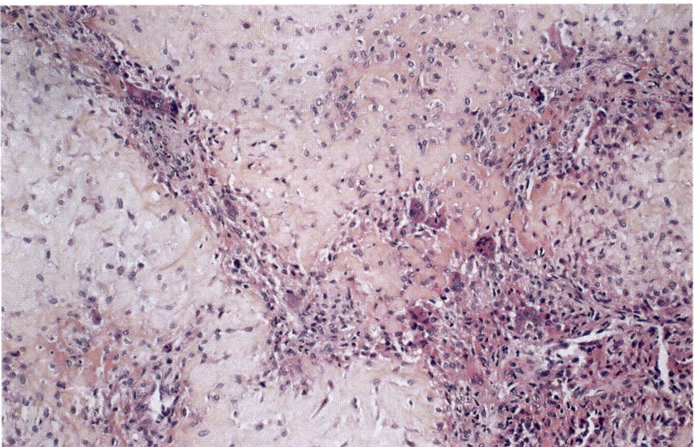

Fig. 13.13

Figs 13.12, 13.13 Pseudolobular architecture of chondromyxoid fibromas.

necrotic areas (Figs 13.18, 13.19). The narrow fibrous septa between the lobules are highly vascularized, with reactive giant cells (Fig. 13.20), macrophages and even osteoid and bone formation. The tumor's lobular growth and the peripheral increased cellularity are the most significant histological patterns[6,16] (Schajowicz 1994).

CYTOPATHOLOGY

On smears or imprints, stellate, spindle and occasional rounded cells are found along with osteoclast-like giant cells, in a myxoid, chondroid or fibrillar background.[44–46] Some tumoral cells may be binucleated or multinucleated or even enlarged with an irregular nucleus and a smudged chromatin (Figs 13.21, 13.22). There is no mitotic activity but in some cases there is considerable nuclear pleomorphism.[45]

IMMUNOHISTOCHEMISTRY

S-100 protein positivity has been found in 25–50% of cells, chiefly in the myxoid areas,[4,47,48] in cells with chondroblastic differentiation as well as in the spindle cells.[49] A negative reaction has been reported in one study, but with

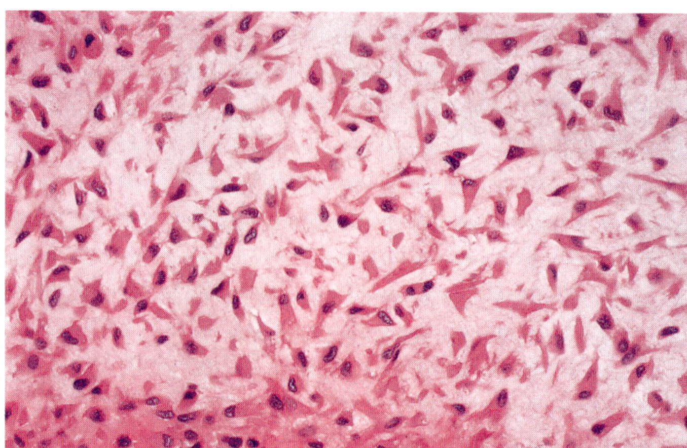

Figs 13.14, 13.15 Chondromyxoid fibroma: spindle or stellate cells in the center of the lobules.

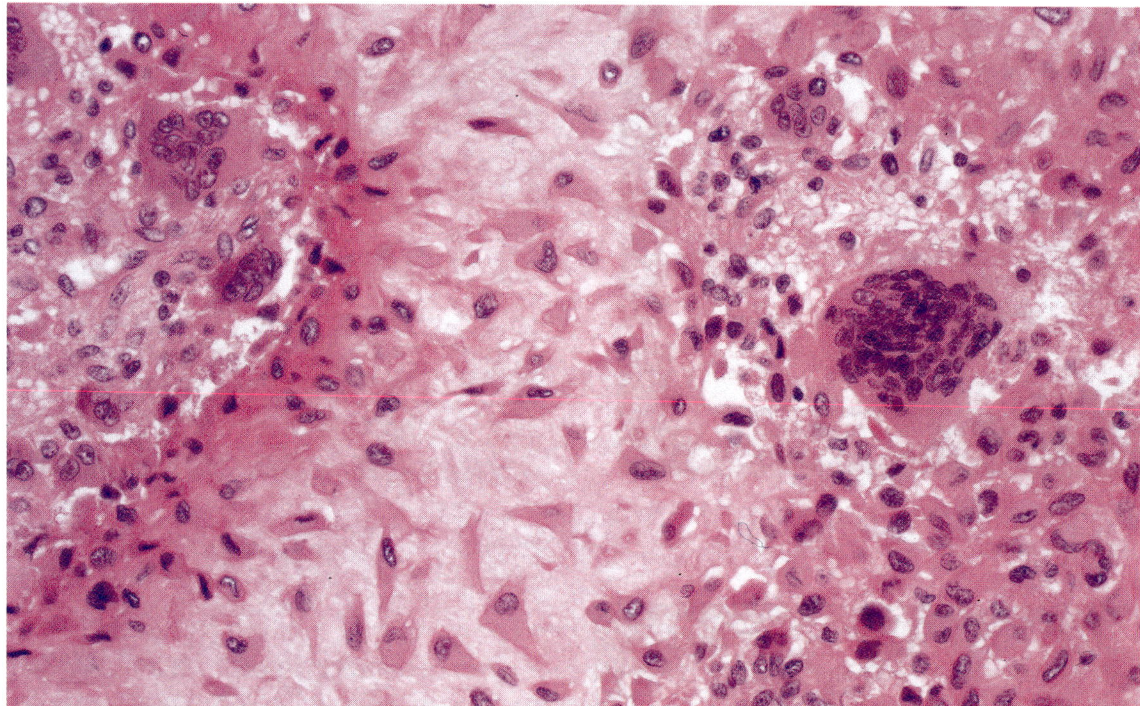

Fig. 13.15

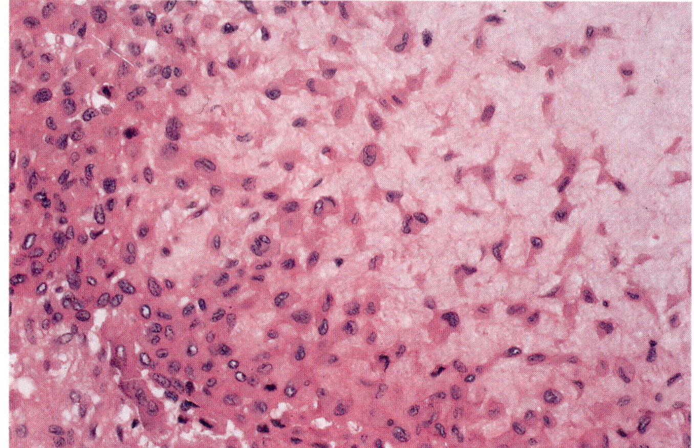

Fig. 13.16 Chondromyxoid fibroma: some cells resemble those of a chondroblastoma, with reniform nuclei.

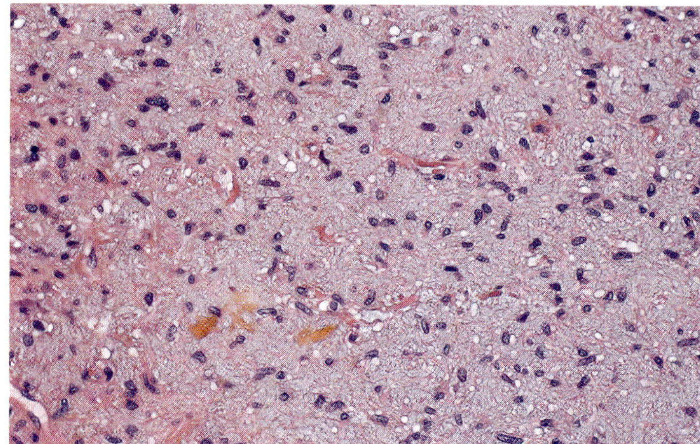

Fig. 13.17 Chondromyxoid fibroma: long-standing case with a lower cellularity.

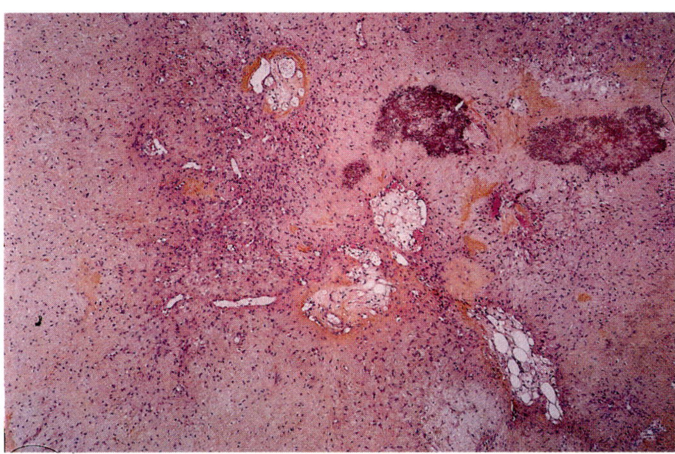

Fig. 13.18

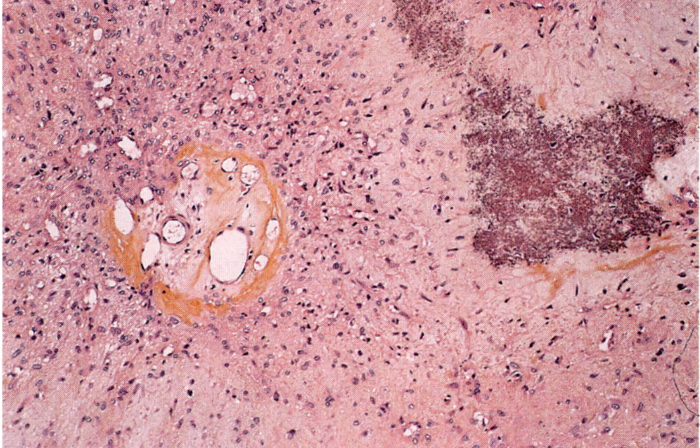

Fig. 13.19

Figs 13.18, 13.19 Chondromyxoid fibroma: secondary changes with microcysts and calcifications.

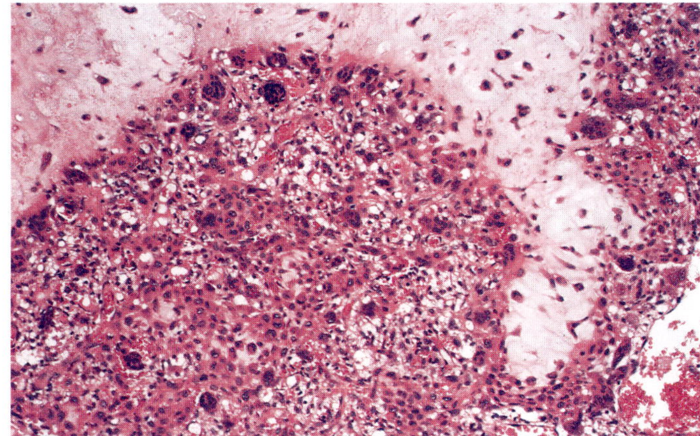

Fig. 13.20 Chondromyxoid fibroma: highly cellular interlobular septa with reactive giant cells.

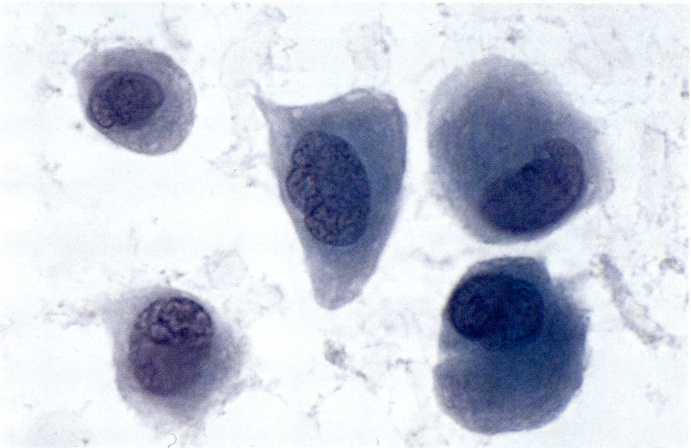

Fig. 13.21

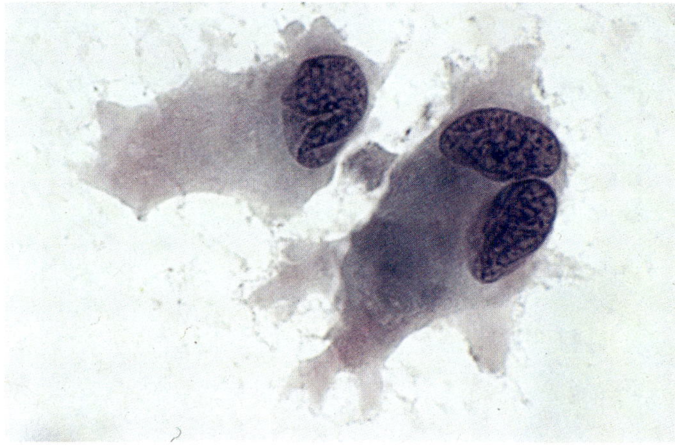

Fig. 13.22

Figs 13.21, 13.22 'Bizarre cells' demonstrated by imprint cytology of a chondromyxoid fibroma.

NSE-positive reaction, probably representing the increased rate of glycolysis.[50] In another report, tumor cells were extensively labeled with all monoclonal antibodies against monocyte–macrophage antigens, suggesting a fibrohistiocytic origin,[51] but the chondroblastic differentiation is well supported by histochemical studies.[43,52]

FLOW CYTOMETRY

The average DNA content is diploid with several tetraploid nuclei.[53]

CYTOGENETICS

Cytogenetical studies have shown clonal chromosomal rearrangements involving chromosomes 2 and 5.[54–56]

ELECTRON MICROSCOPY

At the ultrastructural level, various cells are found including fibroblast-like or chondroblast-like cells.[57] The cells

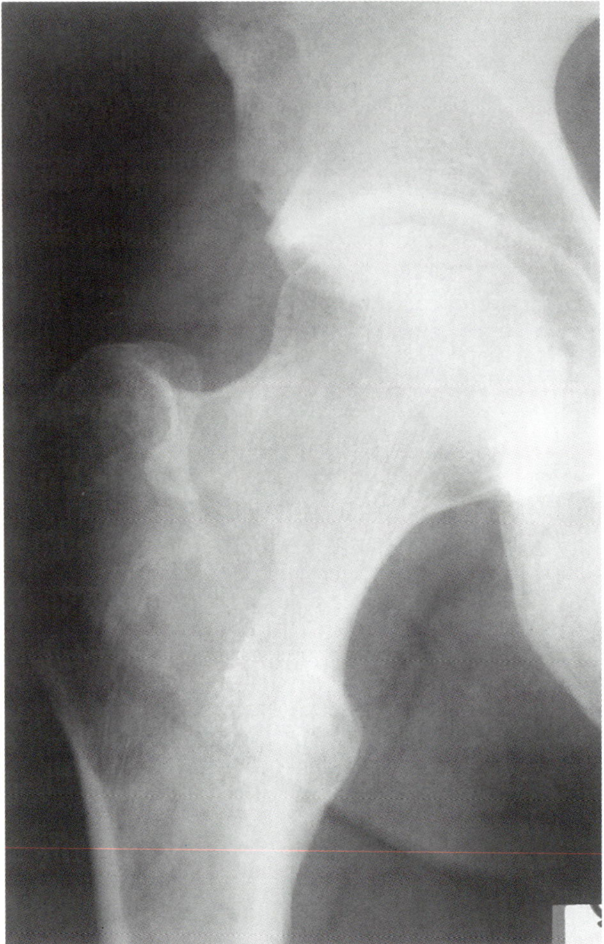

Fig. 13.23

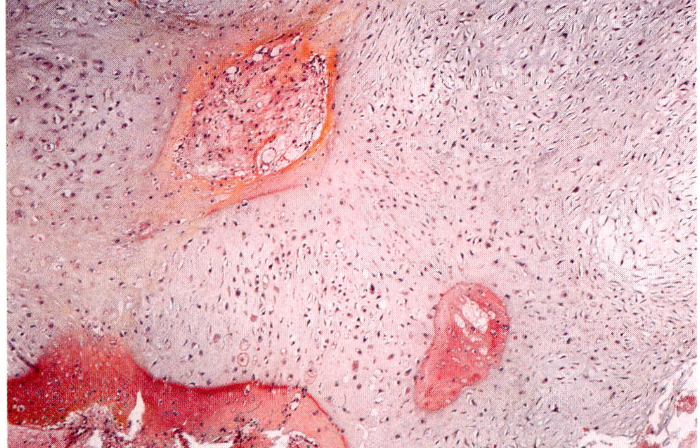

Fig. 13.24

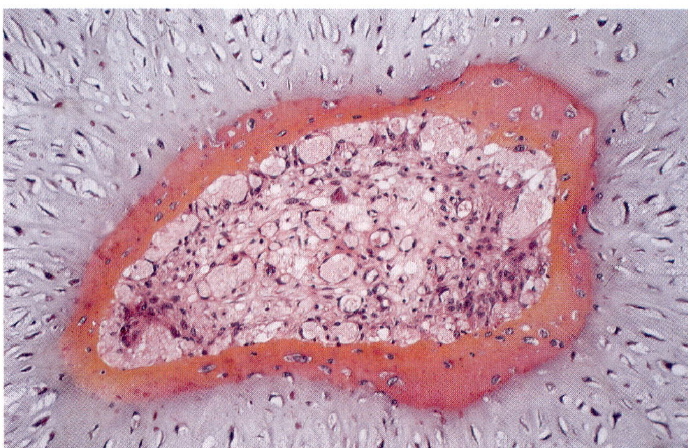

Fig. 13.25

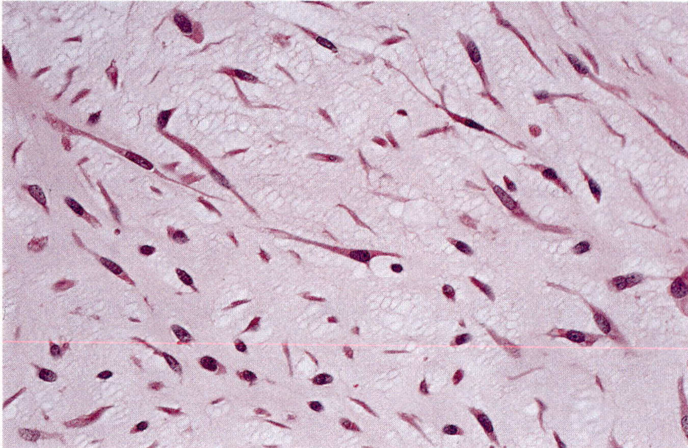

Fig. 13.26

Figs 13.23–13.26 Myxoid chondrosarcoma of the femur initially misdiagnosed as a chondromyxoid fibroma.

in the myxoid areas have an irregular shape, with long cytoplasmic processes; the nuclei are indented with a thick fibrous lamina along the inner nuclear membrane.[16,47,57–60] Intracytoplasmic glycogen is usually found.[4,57]

The matrix has abundant thin fibrils and granules of proteoglycans;[16,58] Long spacing collagen has been reported.[57]

Most investigators report that the tumor originates from cartilage cells derived from the epiphyseal growth plate, despite some reports suggesting a histiocytic origin[61] or even a fibroblastic proliferation with cartilaginous differentiation.[62]

COURSE, TREATMENT AND PROGNOSIS

Rare tumors have an aggressive clinical course,[15,27,63] but most have a slow growth rate or even, in sporadic cases, a spontaneous cessation of growth.[2] Histological findings have no prognostic significance.[4,5] Two cases of malignant transformation have been reported[6,64] but one should remember the very sound statement of Fechner: 'Malignant chondromyxoid fibromas are myxoid chondrosarcomas'.

The misdiagnosis rate is unusually high, ranging from 22%[4] to 28%.[62]

The treatment is curettage with bone grafting or en bloc resection. Radiation therapy is not indicated; a case of radiation-induced sarcoma has been reported.[4] Recurrences are the sole complications,[11,65] appearing in less than 2 years or as long as 19 years later.[66] Implantation in the soft tissues[12,23,66–68] may be iatrogenic, occurring at the time of surgery.

DIFFERENTIAL DIAGNOSIS

Some myxomas or fibromyxomas of bone may well represent chondromyxoid fibromas.[6] Myxoid chondrosarcomas are the most difficult differential diagnosis;[3,69] however, they have a more defined hyaline cartilage matrix,[6] a greater cellular pleomorphism, more calcifications and, most of all, a permeative pattern of growth (Figs 13.23–13.26).

COMMENTS FOR THE SURGICAL PATHOLOGIST

Whatever the name, chondromyxoid fibroma of bone or fibromyxoid chondroma,[70] this bone tumor is one of the most difficult lesions to diagnose.

One should bear in mind the frequency of recurrences, despite the benign course, the possibility of a misdiagnosis (myxoid chondrosarcoma) and the usefulness of studying the whole pattern of the tumor, rather than just the cytology. Despite some reports, this may well exclude needle aspiration or small core biopsies in the search for a well-established diagnosis.

REFERENCES

1. Jaffe H L, Lichtenstein L. Chondromyxoid fibroma of bone, a distinctive benign tumor likely to be mistaken especially for chondrosarcomas. Arch Pathol 1948: 45: 541–551
2. Kreicbergs A, Lonnquist P A, Willems J. Chondromyxoid fibroma. A review of literature and a report on our own experience. Acta Pathol Microbiol Immunol Scand A 1985: 93: 189–197
3. Moser R P, Kransdorf M J, Gilkey F W, Aoki J. Chondromyxoid fibroma. In: Moser R P, Ed. Cartilaginous tumors of the skeleton. AFIP Atlas of radiologic-pathologic correlations II. Philadelphia: Hanley & Belfus, 1990, pp 114–154
4. Zillmer D A, Dorfman H D. Chondromyxoid fibroma of bone: thirty-six cases with clinicopathologic correlation. Hum Pathol 1989: 20: 952–964
5. Gherlinzoni F, Rock M, Picci P. Chondromyxoid fibroma. The experience at the Istituto Ortopedico Rizzoli. J Bone Joint Surg (Am) 1983: 65: 198–204
6. Rahimi A, Beabout J W, Ivins J C, Dahlin D C. Chondromyxoid fibroma: a clinicopathologic study of 76 cases. Cancer 1972: 30: 726–736
7. Salzer M, Salzer-Kuntschik M. Das chondromyxoid fibrom. Langenbecks Arch Klin Chir 1965: 312: 216–231
8. Turcotte B, Pugh D G, Dahlin D C. The roentgenologic aspects of chondromyxoid fibroma of bone. AJR 1962: 87: 1085–1095
9. Kenan S, Abdelwahab I F, Klein M J, Lewis M M. Case report 837. Juxtacortical (periosteal) chondromyxoid fibroma of the proximal tibia. Skeletal Radiol 1994: 23: 237–239
10. Wilson A J, Kyriakos M, Ackerman L V. Chondromyxoid fibroma: radiographic appearance in 38 cases and in a review of the literature. Radiology 1991: 179: 513–518
11. Norman A, Steiner G C. Case report 66. Recurrent chondromyxoid fibroma of 4th metatarsal. Skeletal Radiol 1978: 3: 115–117
12. Van Horn J R, Lemmens J A. Chondromyxoid fibroma of the foot. Report of a missed diagnosis. Acta Orthop Scand 1986: 57: 375–377
13. Mitchell M, Sartoris D J, Resnick D. Case report 713. Chondromyxoid fibroma of the third metatarsal. Skeletal Radiol 1992: 21: 252–255
14. O'Connor P J, Gibbon W W, Hardy G, Butt W P. Chondromyxoid fibroma of the foot. Skeletal Radiol 1996: 25: 143–148
15. Schutt P G, Frost H M. Chondromyxoid fibroma. Clin Orthop 1971: 78: 323–329
16. Montaguti A, Esposito C, Segato P, Melanotte P L, Pennelli N. Chondromyxoid fibroma of the iliac bone. A case report with ultrastructural observations. Tumori 1984: 70: 89–97
17. Lawson J P, Barwick K W. Case report 209. Chondromyxoid fibroma of left first rib. Skeletal Radiol 1982: 9: 53–55
18. Teitelbaum S L, Bessone L. Resection of a large chondromyxoid fibroma of the sternum: report of the first case and review of the literature. J Thorac Cardiovasc Surg 1969: 57: 333–340
19. Wuisman P, Scheld H, Tjan T et al. Chondromyxoid fibroma of the sternum. Case report. Arch Orthop Trauma Surg 1993: 112: 255–256
20. Lyzak J C, Gurley J, Boyle C, Dixon L, Olak J. Chondromyxoid fibroma of the sternum. Skeletal Radiol 1996: 25: 489–492
21. Feldman F, Hecht H L, Johnston A D. Chondromyxoid fibroma of bone. Radiology 1970: 94: 249–260
22. Tang J, Gold R H, Mirra J M. Case report 454. Chondromyxoid fibroma of the calcaneus. Skeletal Radiol 1987: 16: 675–678
23. Benson W R, Bass S. Chondromyxoid fibroma: first report of occurrence of this tumor in vertebral column. Am J Clin Pathol 1955: 25: 1290–1292
24. Nunez C, Bennett T, Bohlman H H. Chondromyxoid fibroma of the thoracic spine: case report and review of the literature. Spine 1982: 7: 436–439
25. Shulman L, Bale P, De Silva M. Sacral chondromyxoid fibroma. Pediatr Radiol 1985: 15: 138–140
26. Rivierez M, Richard S, Pradat P, Devred C. Fibrome chondromyxoïde du rachis cervical. A propos d'un cas traité par vertebrectomie partielle. Neurochirurgie 1991: 37: 264–268
27. Tsuchiya H, Tomita K, Tsuchida T, Ueda Y, Roessner A, Suzuki M. Case report 741. Chondromyxoid fibroma of T2. Skeletal Radiol 1992: 21: 339–342
28. Ribalta T, Ro J Y, Carrasco C H, Heffelman C, Ayala A G. Case report 638. Chondromyxoid fibroma of a sesamoid bone. Skeletal Radiol 1990: 19: 549–551
29. Munzenberg K J, Cremer H. Multizentrisches chondromyxoid-fibrom des knochens mit extraskeletaler beteiligung. Z Orthop 1977: 115: 355–362
30. Beggs I G, Stoker D J. Chondromyxoid fibroma of bone. Clin Radiol 1982: 33: 671–679
31. Schajowicz F. Chondromyxoid fibroma: report of three cases with predominant cortical involvement. Radiology 1987: 164: 783–786
32. Andrew T, Kenwright J, Woods C. Periosteal chondromyxoid fibroma of the tibia: a case report. Acta Orthop Scand 1982: 53: 467–470
33. Bialik V, Kedar A, Ben-Arie Y, Kleinhaus U, Fishman J. Case report 315. Parosteal (periosteal, juxta-cortical) chondromyxoid fibroma of the upper end of the femur. Skeletal Radiol 1985: 13: 323–326
34. Adams M J, Spencer G M, Totterman S, Hicks D G. Case report 776. Chondromyxoid fibroma of femur. Skeletal Radiol 1993: 22: 358–361
35. Kenan S, Abdelwahab I F, Klein M J, Lewis M M. Case report 837. Juxtacortical (periosteal) chondromyxoid fibroma of the proximal tibia. Skeletal Radiol 1994: 23: 237–239

36. Park H R, Lee I S, Lee C J, Park Y K. Chondromyxoid fibroma of the femur: a case report with intra-cortical location. J Korean Med Sci 1995: 10: 51–56

37. Murphy N B, Price C H G. The radiological aspects of chondromyxoid fibroma of bone. Clin Radiol 1971: 22: 261–269

38. Mueller-Miny H, Erlemann R, Roessner A, Wuismann P, Reisner M. Roentgenmorphologie des chondromyxoidfibroms. RÖFO 1989: 150: 390–394

39. Davey H A, Rad F R, Cremin B J, Sinclair Smith C. Case report 625. Chondromyxoid fibroma. Skeletal Radiol 1990: 19: 395–397

40. Dahlin D C. Chondromyxoid fibroma of bone, with emphasis on its morphological relationship to benign chondroblastoma. Cancer 1956: 9: 195–203

41. White P G, Saunders L, Orr W, Friedman L. Chondromyxoid fibroma. Skeletal Radiol 1996: 25: 79–81

42. Adler C P. Case report 338. Chondromyxoid fibroma (CMF) of the radius associated with an aneurysmal bone cyst (ABC). Skeletal Radiol 1985: 14: 305–308

43. Benedetti G B, Canepa G, Garcia M. Il fibroma condromixoide dell'osso. Arch Putti Chir Organi Mov 1962: 17: 44–72

44. Layfield L J, Ferreiro J A. Fine-needle aspiration cytology of chondromyxoid fibroma: a case report. Diagn Cytopathol 1988: 4: 148–151

45. Gupta S, Dev G, Marya S. Chondromyxoid fibroma: a fine-needle aspiration diagnosis. Diagn Cytopathol 1993: 9: 63–65

46. Hazarika D, Kumar R V, Rao C R, Mukherjee G, Pattabhiraman V, Shekar M C. Fine needle aspiration cytology of chondroblastoma and chondromyxoid fibroma. A report of two cases. Acta Cytol 1994: 38: 592–596

47. Ushigome S, Takakuwa T, Shinagawa T, Takagi M, Kishimoto H, Mori N. Ultrastructure of cartilaginous tumors and S-100 protein in the tumors, with reference to the histogenesis of chondroblastoma, chondromyxoid fibroma and mesenchymal chondrosarcoma. Acta Pathol Jpn 1984: 34: 1285–1300

48. Bleiweiss I J, Klein M J. Chondromyxoid fibroma. Report of six cases with immunohistochemical studies. Mod Pathol 1990: 3: 664–666

49. Weiss A P, Dorfman H D. S-100 protein in human cartilage lesions. J Bone Joint Surg (Am) 1986: 68: 521–526

50. Karabela-Bouropoulou V, Markaki S, Milas C. S-100 protein and neuron specific enolase immunoreactivity of normal, hyperplastic and neoplastic chondrocytes in relation to the composition of the extracellular matrix. Pathol Res Pract 1988: 183: 761–766

51. Meyer A, Steinmeier T, Löning T, Radzun H J, Delling G. Histiocytic differentiation in benign and malignant bone tumors. J Cancer Res Clin Oncol 1988: 114: 565–574

52. Baruffaldi O, Benedetti G B. Fibroma condromixoide dell'osso (ricerche istochimiche) Arch Ortop 1966: 79: 101–111

53. Cuvelier C A, Roels H J. Cytophotometric studies of the nuclear DNA content in cartilaginous tumors. Cancer 1979: 44: 1363–1374

54. Bridge J A, Sanger W G, Neff J R. Translocations involving chromosomes 2 and 13 in benign and malignant cartilaginous neoplasms. Cancer Genet Cytogenet 1989: 38: 83–88

55. Bridge J A, Bhatia P S, Anderson J R, Neff J R. Biologic and clinical significance of cytogenetic and molecular cytogenetic abnormalities in benign and malignant cartilaginous lesions. Cancer Genet Cytogenet 1993: 69: 79–90

56. Tarkkanen M, Bohling T, Helio H et al. A recurrent chondromyxoid fibroma with chromosome aberrations in (5;2)(q13;p21p25) and 2p deletion: a case report. Cancer Genet Cytogenet 1993: 65: 141–146

57. Tornberg D N, Rice R W, Johnston A D. The ultrastructure of chondromyxoid fibroma. Its biologic and diagnostic implications. Clin Orthop 1973: 95: 295–299

58. Steiner G C. Ultrastructure of benign cartilaginous tumors of intraosseous origin. Hum Pathol 1979: 10: 71–86

59. Ushigome S, Takakuwa T, Shinigawa T, Kishida H, Yamazaki M. Chondromyxoid fibroma of bone. An electron microscopic observation. Acta Pathol Jpn 1982: 32: 113–122

60. Martinez-Tello F J, Martinez Gonzalez M A. The ultrastructure of the cartilaginous tumors. In: Bonucci E, Motta P M, Eds. Ultrastructure of skeletal tissues. Boston: Kluwer, 1990, pp 193–195

61. Morimoto K, Okada S. Ultrastructural and pathological studies of chondromyxoid fibroma of bone (in Japanase). Nippon Seikeigeka Gakkai Zasshi 1984: 58: 887–894

62. Itoh J, Mizushima M, Miyamoto M, Onada T. Chondromyxoid fibroma, report of a case and review of the Japanese literature (in Japanese). Seikeigeka 1977: 28: 193–202

63. Norman A, Steiner G C. Case report 38. Recurrent chondromyxoid fibroma. Skeletal Radiol 1977: 2: 105–107

64. Sehayik S, Rosman M A. Malignant degeneration of a chondromyxoid fibroma in a child. Can J Surg 1975: 18: 354–357

65. Mikulowski P, Ostberg G. Recurrent chondromyxoid fibroma. Acta Orthop Scand 1971: 42: 385–390

66. Troncoso A, Ro J Y, Edeiken J, Carrasco C H, Murray J A, Ayala A G. Case report 798. Recurrent chondromyxoid fibroma in connective tissue of leg. Skeletal Radiol 1993: 22: 445–448

67. Kyriakos M. Soft tissue implantation of chondromyxoid fibroma. Am J Surg Pathol 1979: 3: 363–372

68. Heydemann J, Gillespie R, Mancer K. Soft tissue recurrence of chondromyxoid fibroma. J Pediatr Orthop 1985: 5: 725–727

69. Bernd L, Ewerbeck V, Mau H, Cotta H. Zur Dignität des Chondromyxoidfibroms: sind maligne Verlaufsformen möglich? Präsentation eigener Fälle und Literarübersicht. Unfallchirurg 1994: 97: 332–335

70. Schajowicz F, Gallardo H. Chondromyxoid fibroma of bone (fibromyxoid chondroma). A clinico-pathological study of thirty-two cases. J Bone Joint Surg (Br) 1971: 53: 198–216

Chondrosarcoma

M. Forest

INTRODUCTION AND CLINICAL DATA

Chondrosarcomas were defined in 1943 by Lichtenstein & Jaffe[1] as sarcomas whose tumor cells are associated with a cartilage matrix, bone formation being only reactive or by enchondral ossification. Location in bone is central (medullary) or peripheral.

Chondrosarcoma is the second most common primary sarcoma of bone after osteosarcoma (11–22%), with a male predominance of 1.5–2:1 (Unni 1996).

Patients are usually between 30 and 70 years old, with a peak incidence in the fifth to seventh decades of life. More than 40% are over 40 years of age (Wilner 1982).

Chondrosarcoma rarely occurs in children;[3–7] only 2.2% of patients are less than 17 years of age in the Mayo Clinic series. In children and adolescents, preferential locations are the upper ends of long bones, particularly the humerus and femur,[7] and the trunk. One-third of cases are secondary chondrosarcomas.[2,7] A rapid onset and a worse outcome may be related to peculiar forms in the young (mesenchymal chondrosarcoma[2,5,8]) or to a misdiagnosed chondroblastic osteosarcoma.[7] Many are low grade with no malignant behavior.[7]

Clinical symptoms of chondrosarcoma are pain and tenderness with or without a mass. Some patients are asymptomatic. Pathologic fractures are rare (3%[9]). The average duration of symptoms is 1–2 years[10] but the growth may be very slow, especially for pelvic tumors.

Eighty percent of affected adults have been shown to have an altered carbohydrate metabolism, with a diabetic glucose tolerance curve;[11] Hypertrophy of the islets of Langerhans has been found in an autopsy study.[12] Chondrosarcoma may also secrete chorionic gonadotrophin[13] and accretion of calcium in the large tumor mass may even induce hypocalcemia.[14]

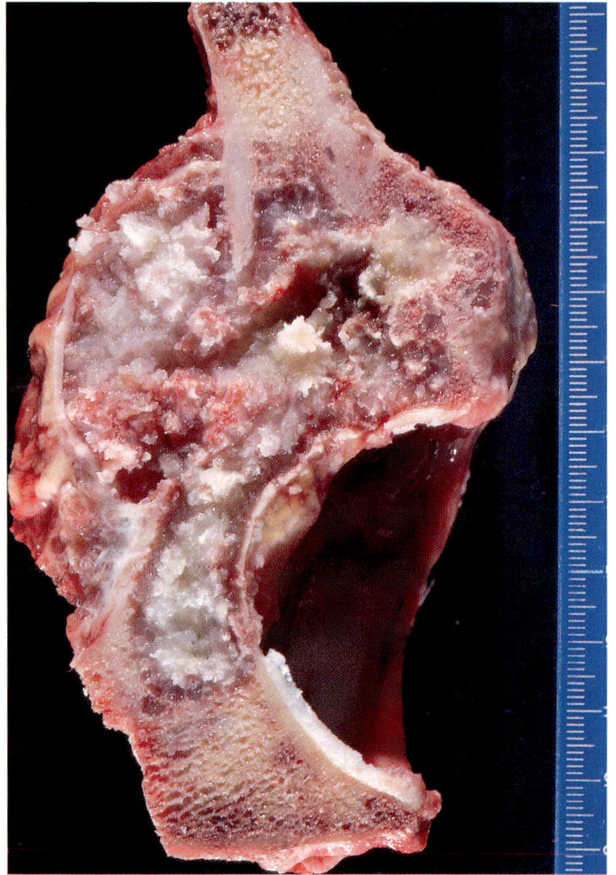

Fig. 14.1

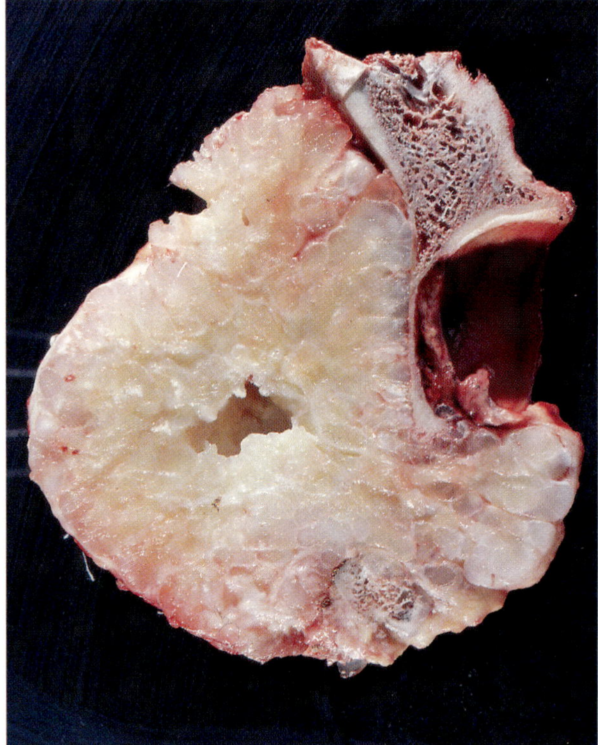

Fig. 14.2

Figs 14.1, 14.2 Chondrosarcomas of the pelvis.

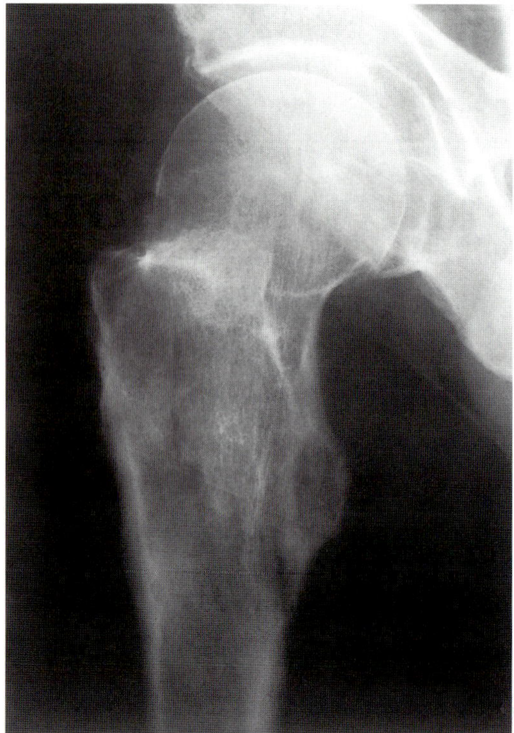

Fig. 14.3

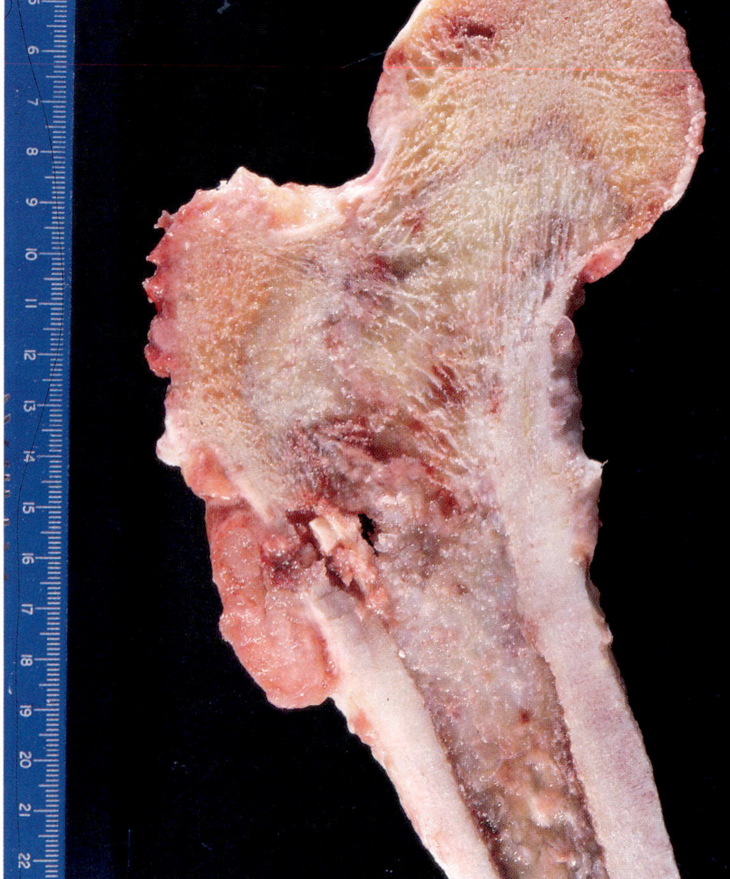

Fig. 14.4

Figs 14.3, 14.4 Chondrosarcoma of the femur.

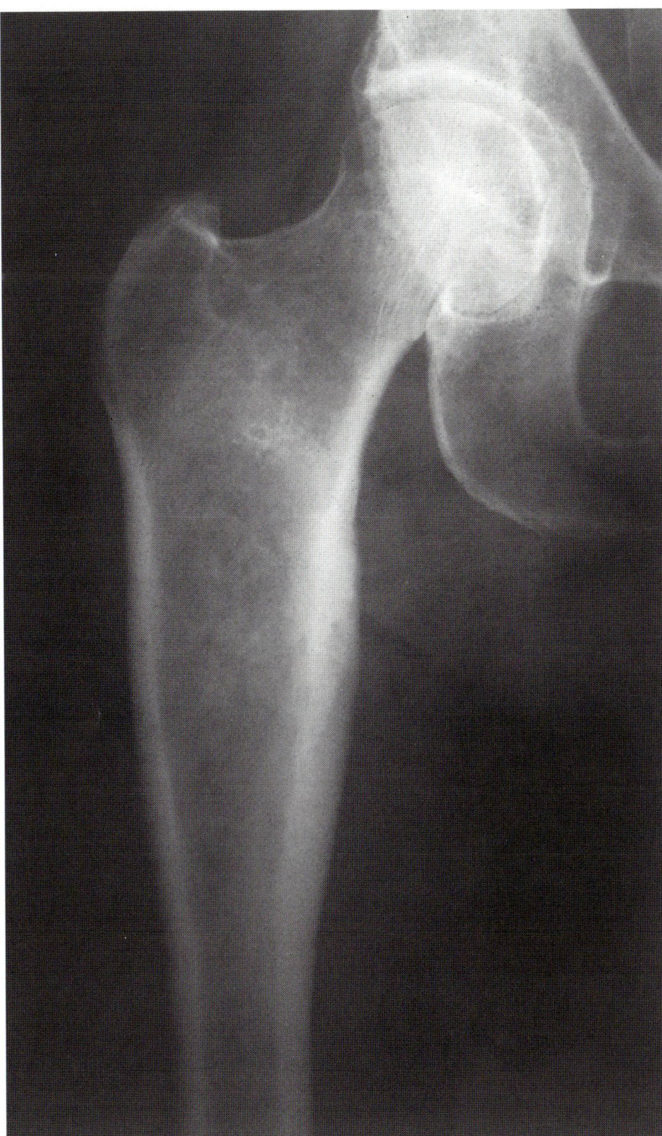

Fig. 14.5

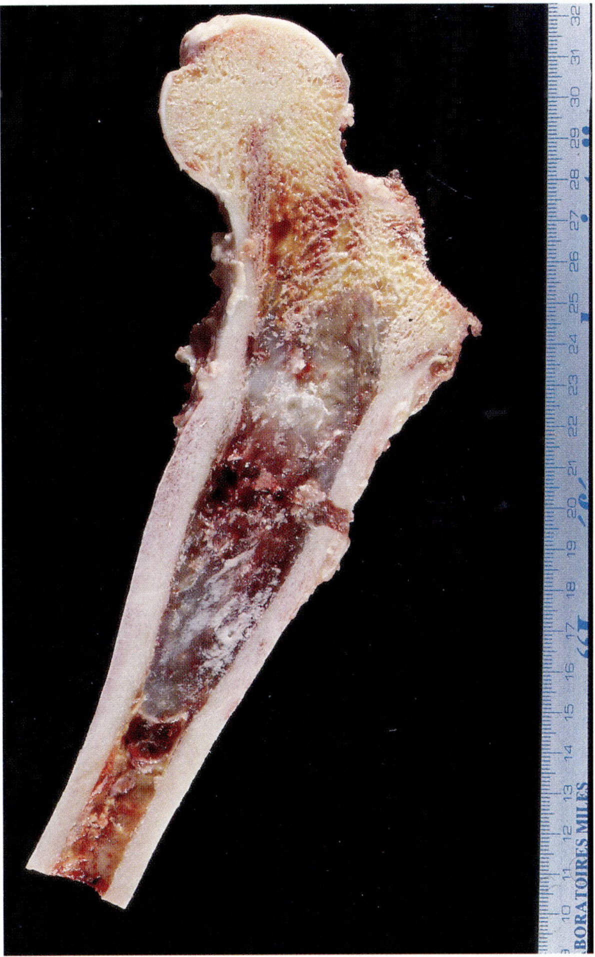

Fig. 14.6

Figs 14.5, 14.6 Chondrosarcoma of the femur.

SKELETAL DISTRIBUTION

The most common sites are the pelvic bones (Figs 14.1, 14.2), the proximal femur and humerus, the distal femur and ribs (Figs 14.3–14.11); 50% of cases are located in the pelvis and upper femur (Wilner 1982). Other sites are the scapula, the sternum, the skull and facial bones.

Involvement of the small bones of the hands (proximal phalanges and metacarpal bones) and feet is rare (incidence of 3% at the Mayo Clinic[15]) (Figs 14.12–14.17). Some are chondrosarcomas from the onset but more often they arise from solitary or multiple enchondromas.[16–19] A fulminant course is a rare event;[20] most are less malignant in these locations.

In the ribs and sternum, the tumor occurs near the costochondral junction.

Four to 7% of cases are located in the spine or sacrum, with a higher incidence in the thoracic spine (Wilner 1982). They may arise in the posterior elements or in the vertebral body.[21]

Central chondrosarcomas predominate in the femur and humerus, peripheral tumors in the pelvis (Figs 14.18–14.20), the extremities, ribs and vertebrae.

IMAGING

The diagnosis can usually be made on plain films[22] but not in all cases.[23]

The growth of chondrosarcomas in long bones begins in the metaphysis and extends to the diaphysis, often with quite extensive intramedullary spread (Figs 14.21–14.23). Extension into the epiphysis is less frequent,[3] as are pri-

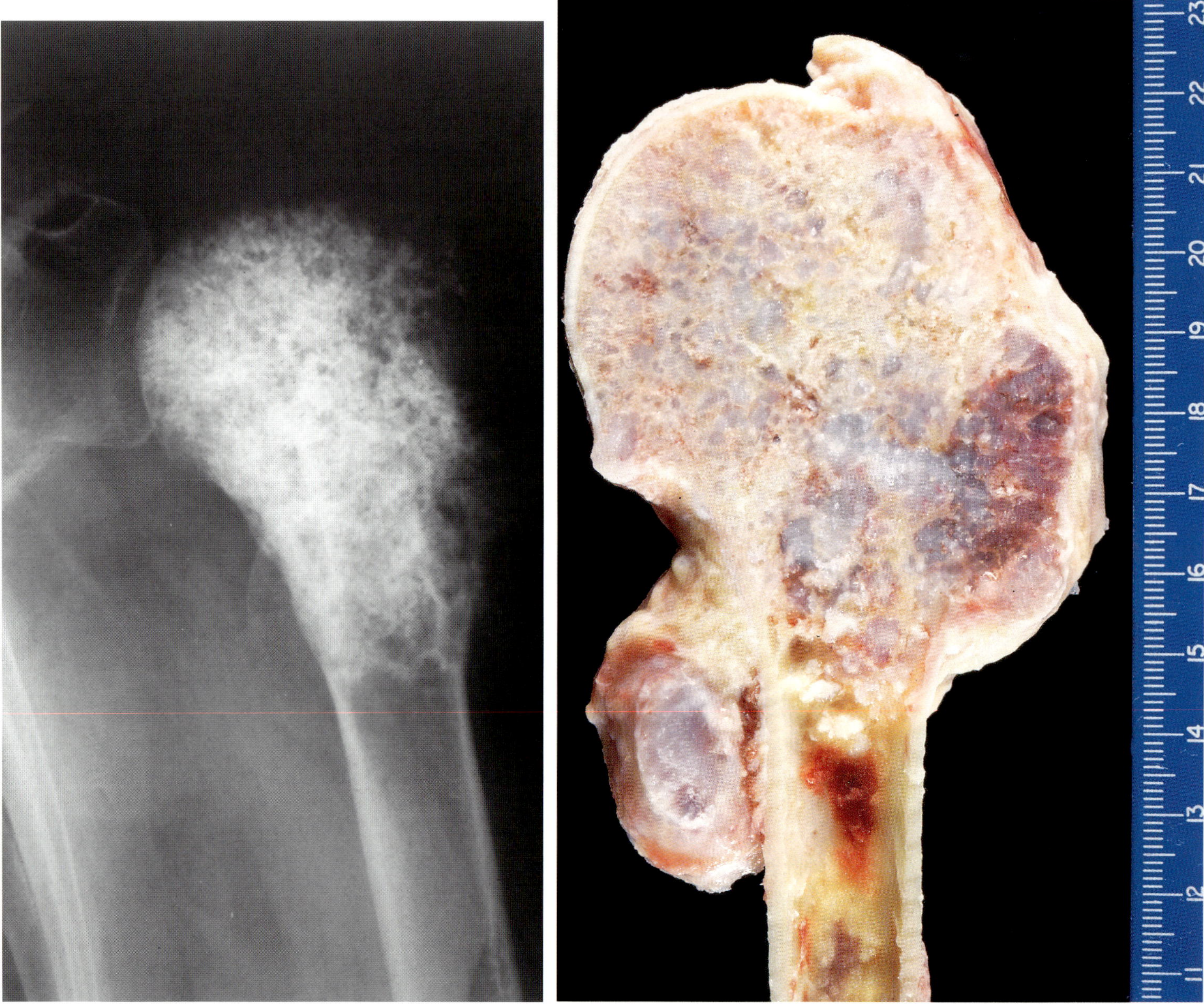

Fig. 14.7

Fig. 14.8

Figs 14.7, 14.8 Chondrosarcoma of the humerus with soft tissue extension.

mary epiphyseal, apophyseal or diaphyseal locations, with eventual transarticular extension[24] (Figs 14.24–14.33).

They appear as osteolytic lesions, usually elongated and well marginated;[25] some may be expansile (Fig. 14.34). The geographic margins are associated with endosteal scalloping (Figs 14.35–14.37), cortical thinning, or thickening by reactive periosteal and endosteal bone formation, which may be diffuse or focal. High-grade tumors show more irregular, ill-defined margins (Figs 14.38–14.40).

In two-thirds of cases, calcifications are found with a variable appearance: amorphous, punctate, small, dense and flocculent. A distinctive ring-like pattern is due to enchondral ossification of the tumor cartilage; it is mostly

found in low-grade tumors[26] which also have widespread dense calcifications uniformly distributed. High-grade tumors have faint amorphous calcifications with large, purely lytic areas.[27,28]

CT is useful to study the endosteal scalloped resorption, the density of mineralization[27] and, chiefly, the intra- and extraosseous extent.[29]

The anatomic staging may also be studied on MRI; soft tissue extension may be well delineated.[30] MRI shows an intermediate signal intensity on T1- weighted images and a high signal intensity on T2-weighted images.[30,31] On T2, a ring and arc pattern of mineralization is enhanced with gadolinium,[32] as are areas of necrosis.[33] MRI can show the

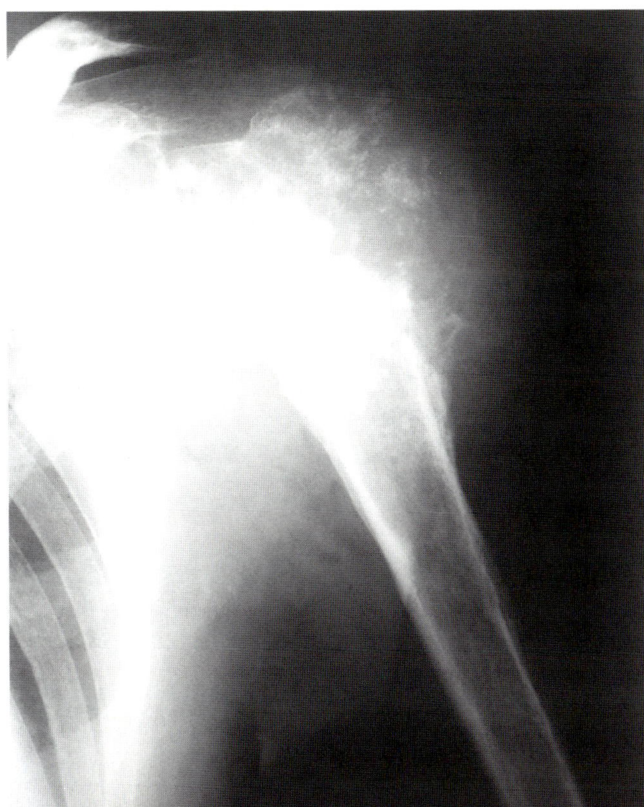

Fig. 14.9

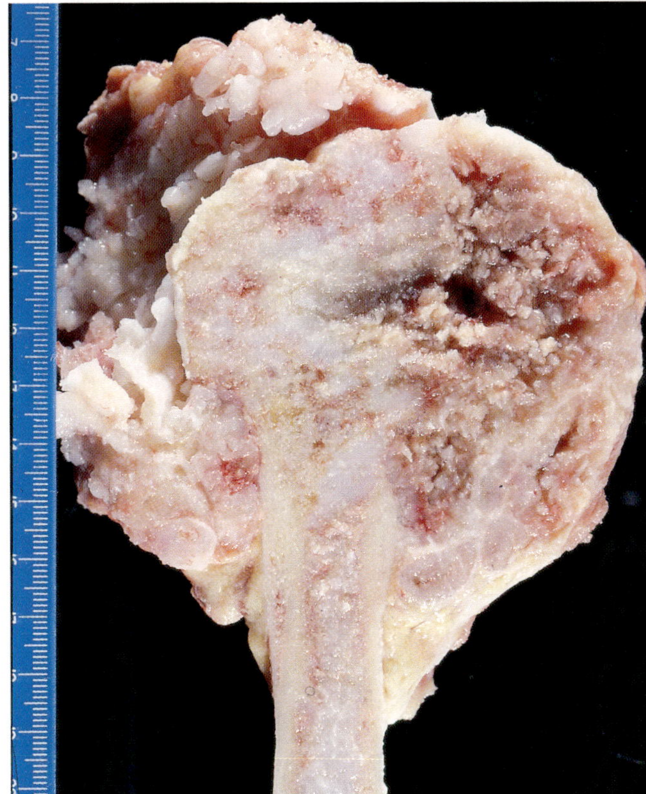

Fig. 14.10

Figs 14.9, 14.10 Chondrosarcoma of the humerus with massive soft tissue extension and involvement of the joint.

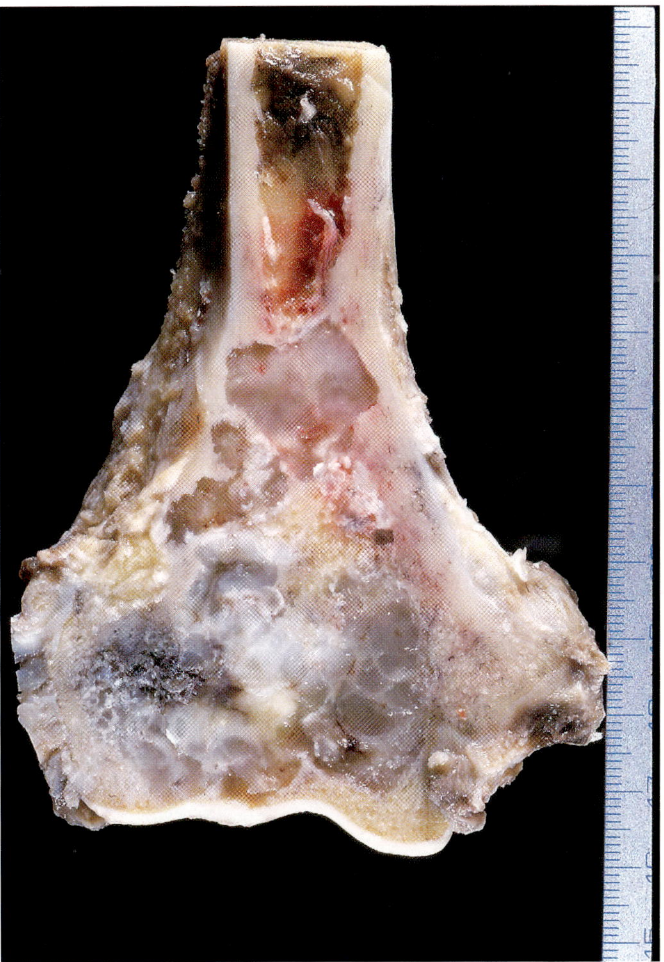

Fig. 14.11 Chondrosarcoma: less frequent localization in the lower end of the humerus.

lobulation of well-differentiated tumors[34] and sometimes the fibrous septa between the lobules.[35,36] Benign and malignant cartilage tumors cannot be distinguished by MR appearance of the matrix alone.[34]

Chondrosarcomas show an intense uptake on bone scans, due to the reactive bone formation and to hyperemia.[37] They are moderately vascular lesions on angiography.[29,38]

GROSS PATHOLOGY

Chondrosarcomas are huge tumors, with a median size of 10–15 cm. The most extensive tumors are found in the flat and irregular bones (Wilner 1982).

The tissue may be firm, translucent, blue-gray or white, with a lobular pattern, especially at the periphery, in well-differentiated tumors. Yellowish and gritty calcifications or foci of enchondral ossification are easily found. High-grade tumors may show extensive myxoid areas with hemorrhages and necrosis.

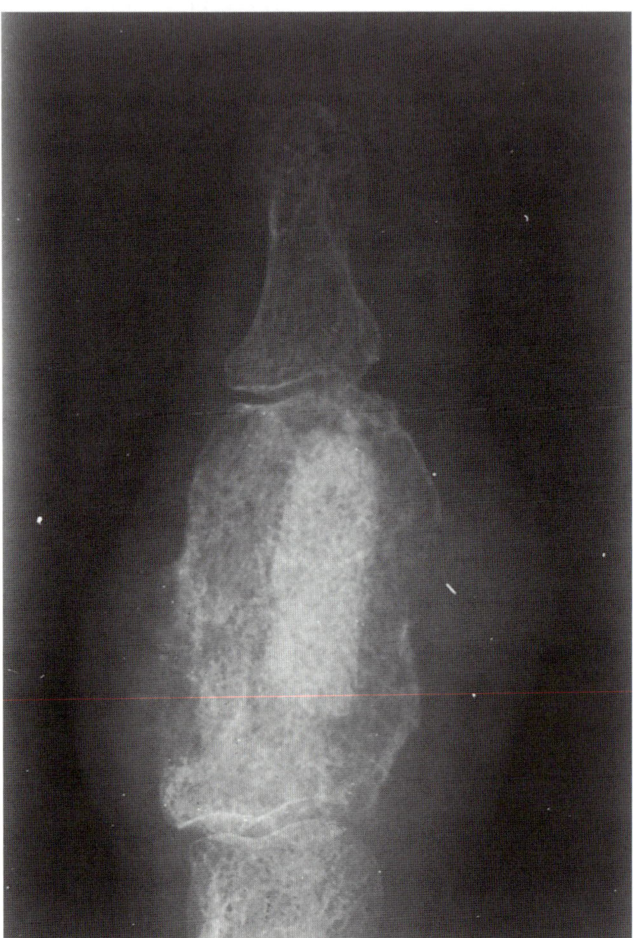

Fig. 14.12

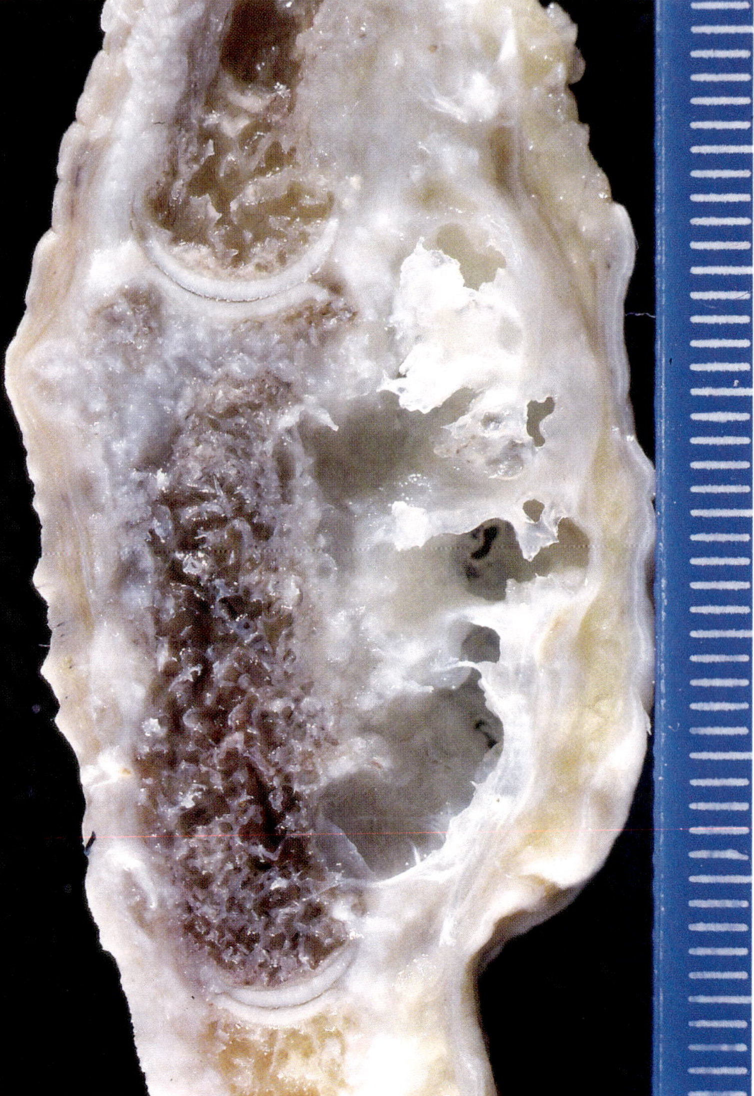

Fig. 14.13

Figs 14.12, 14.13 Chondrosarcoma of a phalanx initially diagnosed as an enchondroma; resorption of the bone graft.

On plain films, the gross extent in the marrow cavity is much greater than expected (Mulder et al 1993).

In central chondrosarcomas, the most significant features are the endosteal scalloping or focal cortical destruction and the cortical thickening (Schajowicz 1994). The soft tissue extension is limited by a pseudocapsule or a shell of periosteal new bone.

Peripheral chondrosarcomas may show a prominent lobulation, with cystic change in the center of the lobules; some such regions are mucoid and gelatinous, others are due to necrosis or tumor liquefaction. One has to search for satellite cartilage nodules in the soft tissues.

HISTOPATHOLOGY

The cytological component has to be studied in viable, non-calcified areas (Lichtenstein 1977). Tumoral chondrocytes have plump and enlarged nuclei,[1] sometimes with nucleoli. They are mononucleated, binucleated or even multinucleated cells. Nuclear pleomorphism and hyperchromasia are obvious in the usual form of chondrosarcoma (Figs 14.41–14.44).

Rare tumors may exhibit intracytoplasmic single large vacuoles, giving a signet-ring appearance to the chondrocytes[39,40] (Fig. 14.45), or PAS-positive eosinophilic droplets demonstrating an autofluorescence (presumably secretory products[41]).

Chondrocytes are distributed in clusters or groups in lobules of variable size and irregular shape, separated by fibrous tissue (Fig. 14.46).

The matrix is chondroid or myxoid. In the myxoid areas, the cells are spindle shaped or stellate (Figs 14.48–14.50).

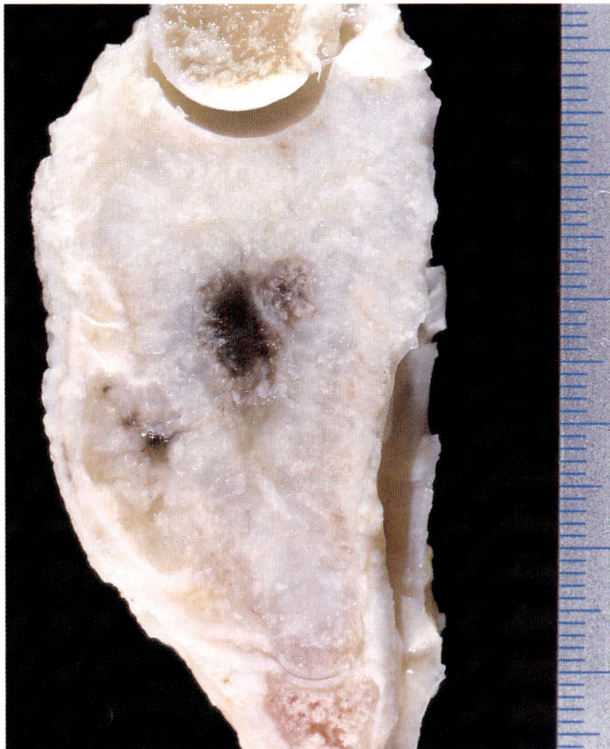

Fig. 14.14

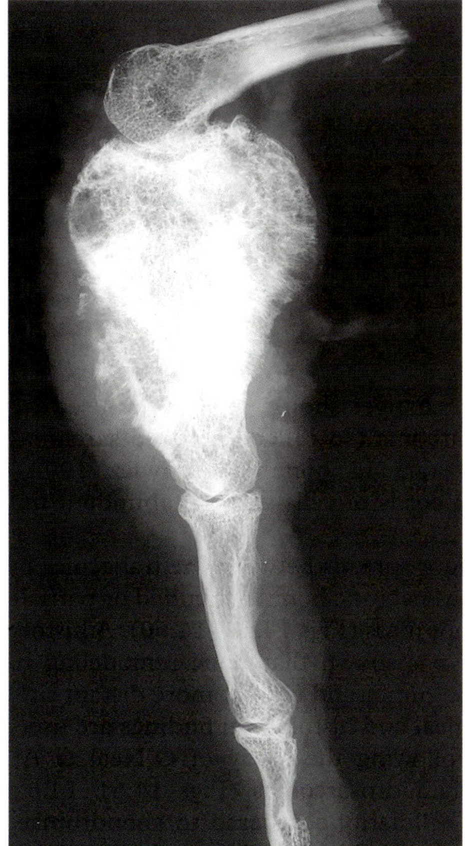

Fig. 14.15

Figs 14.14, 14.15 Chondrosarcoma of a phalanx with a 10-year clinical course.

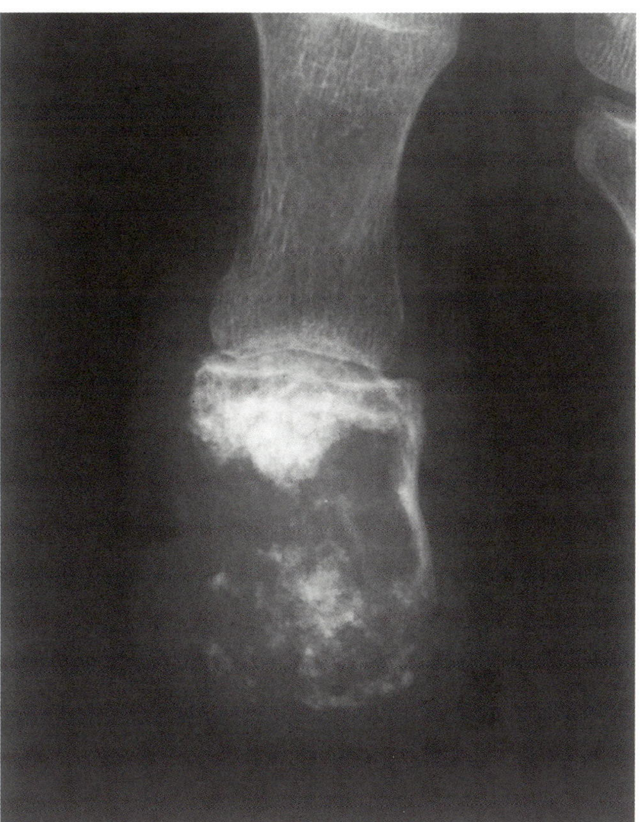

Fig. 14.16

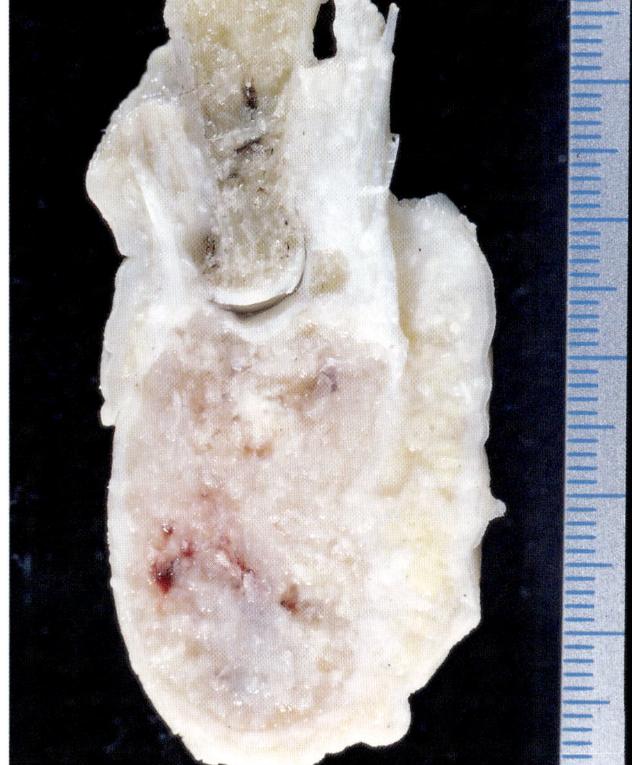

Fig. 14.17

Figs 14.16, 14.17 High-grade chondrosarcoma of the thumb with early pulmonary metastases.

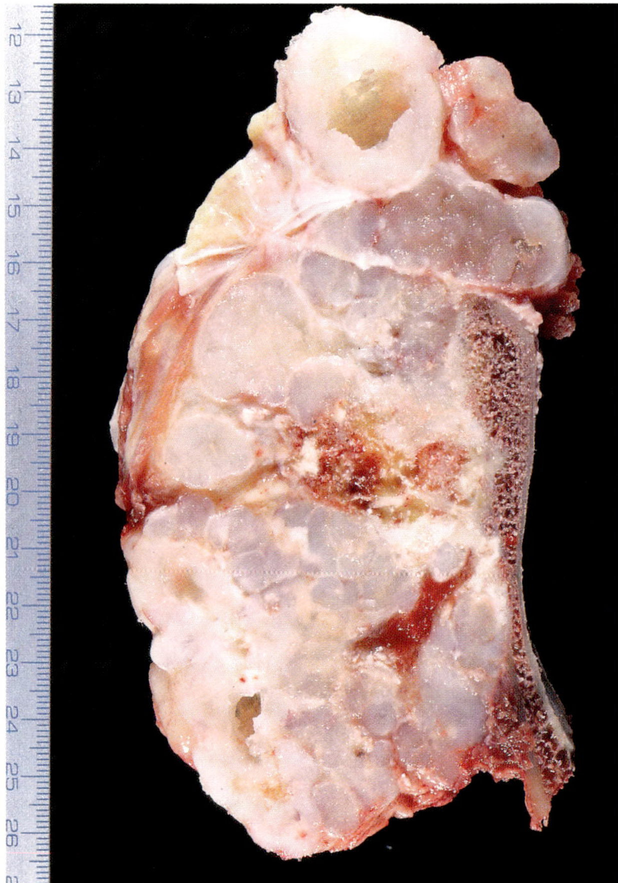

Fig. 14.18

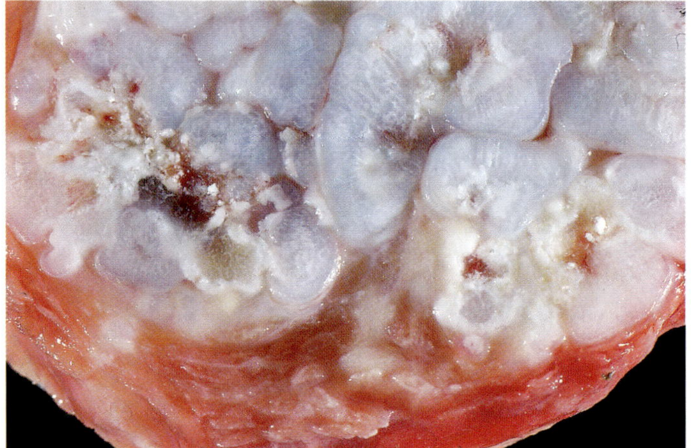

Fig. 14.19

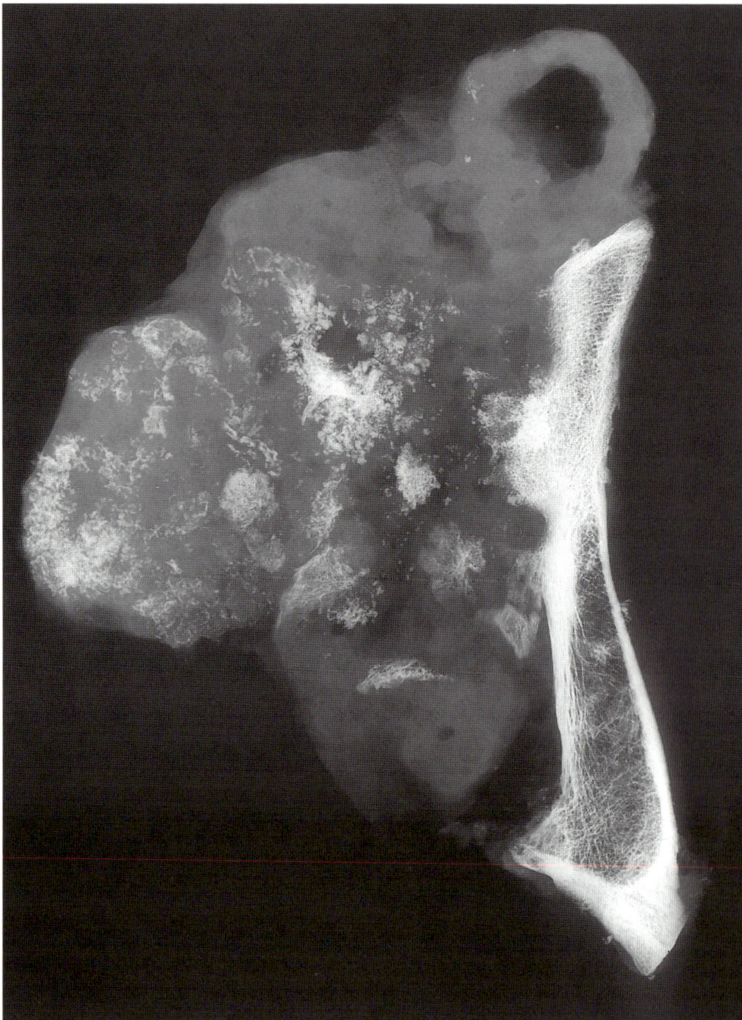

Fig. 14.20

Figs 14.18–14.20 Peripheral chondrosarcomas of the iliac wing.

In the lobules, the cellularity is greater at the periphery, where mitoses may eventually be found (in high-grade tumors). Spindly tumor cells may be located close to the fibrous septa.

Around the lobules, calcifications or woven bone formation may be found as well as reactive bone with osteoblastic rimming (Figs 14.51, 14.52). Enchondral ossification is linked to the vascularity of the fibrous septa with osteoclastic resorption of the calcified cartilage.

Myxoid changes should not be confused with myxoid chondrosarcoma (so-called chordoid sarcoma), which is extremely rare in bone (Schajowicz 1994), showing strands or cords of cells with an abundant mucoid stroma.

The tumor spreads between the trabecular bone and in some places necrotic bone is engulfed or partially resorbed in the tumor mass (Figs 14.53–14.60). A histomorphometric study has shown that bone remodeling is increased close to the tumor and even at more distant sites.[42]

Cytological and histological findings are used for tumor grading, following the study of O'Neal & Ackerman.[43] Grade 1 chondrosarcomas (Figs 14.61–14.64) have an increased cellularity compared to chondromas; chondrocytes are small with a slightly enlarged dense nucleus. The lobules are mostly chondroid, with very little myxoid changes and sometimes extensive calcifications. There is no mitotic activity. Grade 2 chondrosarcomas

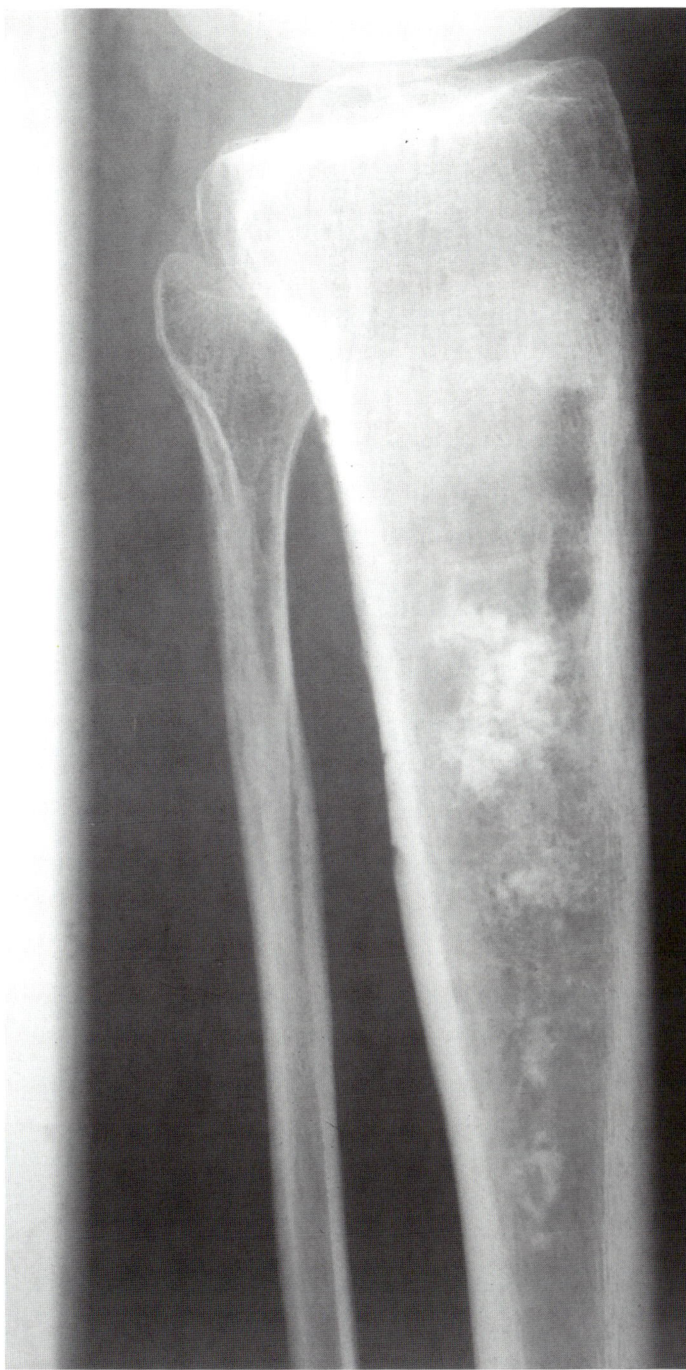

Fig. 14.21

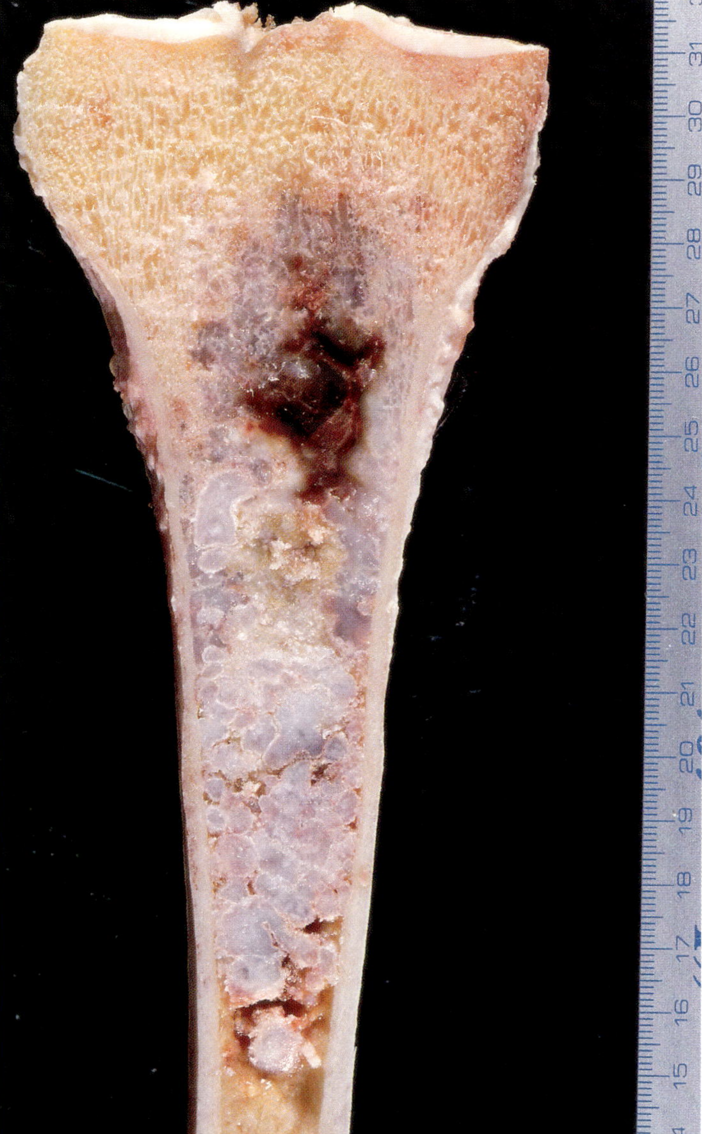

Fig. 14.22

Figs 14.21–14.23 Intramedullary spread of a chondrosarcoma of the tibia.

(Figs 14.65–14.67) are more cellular, especially at the periphery of the lobules where a few mitoses can be found. Nuclei are enlarged and hyperchromatic; cells may be binucleated. Calcification is reduced and a myxoid stroma appears along with necrotic areas. Grade 3 chondrosarcomas (Fig. 14.68) are the most cellular. Pleomorphic nuclei are vesicular; some cells are spindle shaped many are binucleated. Giant multinucleated cells may be found and mitotic activity is present. A myxoid stroma predominates over the chondroid matrix; necrotic changes are frequent and calcification is rare or absent.

Grade 2 tumors are the most frequent (30–60%), followed by grade 1 (26–50%); grade 3 are rarer (8–25%).[9,10,44,45]

A modified schedule of grading has been proposed:[10] besides evaluation of the intercellular matrix and the frequency of binucleate cells, the criteria used were the cellularity, the nuclear size and the mitotic rate. Cellularity and mitotic activity appeared more related to the prognosis than nuclear pleomorphism and hyperchromasia.

These findings are now somewhat disputed; for some authors, cellularity is the main difference between low-

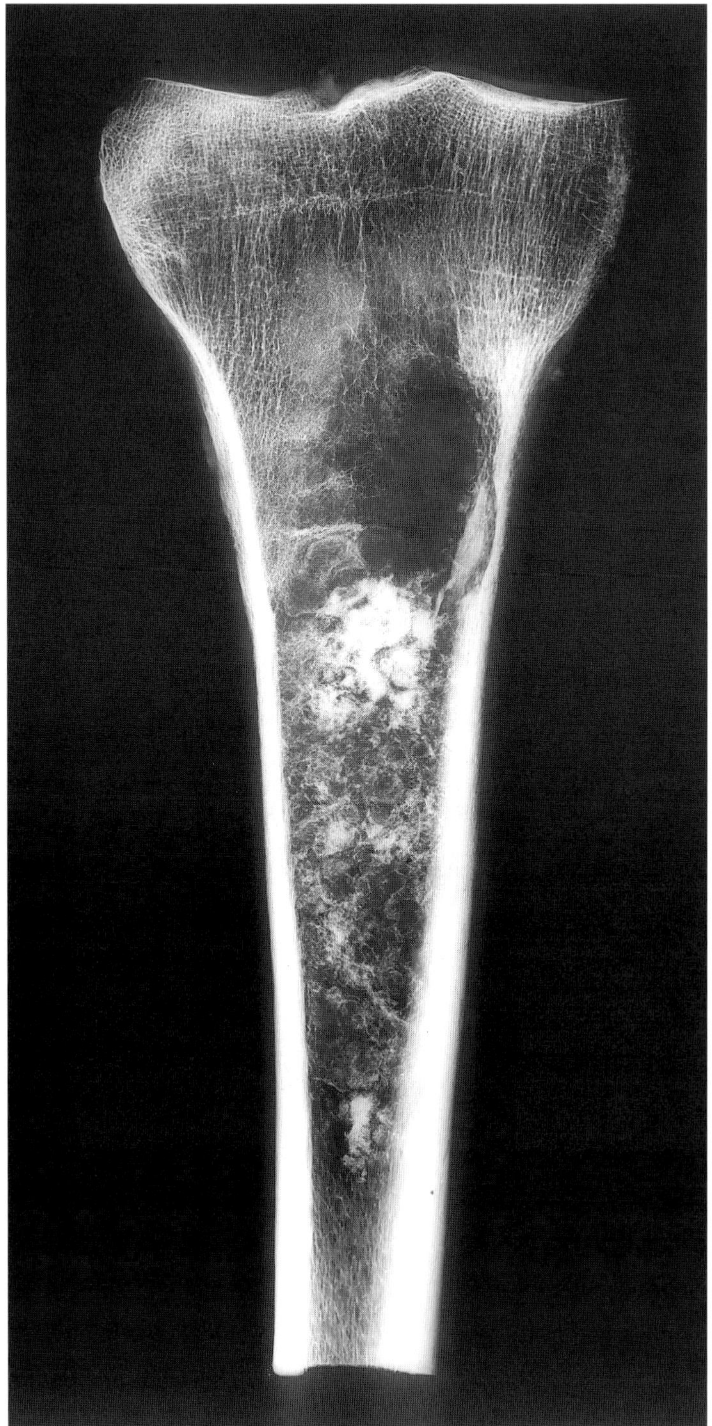

Fig. 14.23

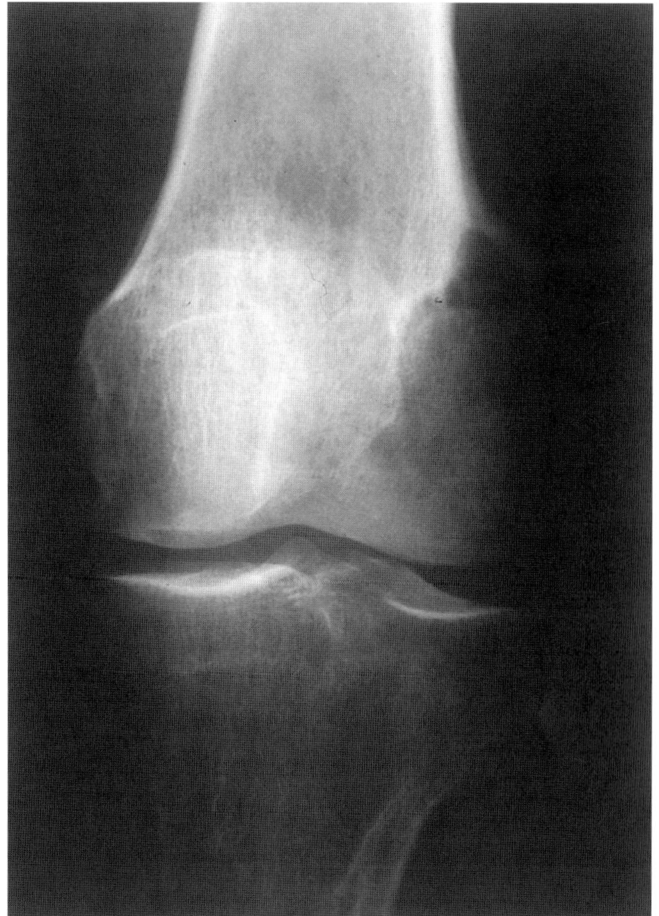

Fig. 14.24

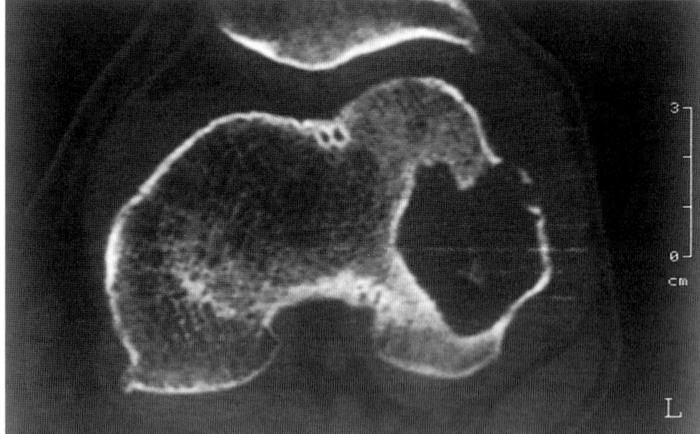

Fig. 14.25

Figs 14.24, 14.25 Epiphyseal chondrosarcoma of the femur mimicking a giant cell tumor on imaging.

grade and high-grade chondrosarcomas and mitotic figures are not easily found in high-grade tumors,[46,47] reflecting our own experience. Cytophotometric studies[48,49] have shown that cellularity is the strongest determinant for grading and the nuclear size seems to be the best prognostic factor. There is no correlation between the mitotic rate and the clinical course.

Other findings may be useful. For Schajowicz, there is an inverse relationship between the glycogen content of chondrocytes and the grade of malignancy; widespread myxoid stroma may be related to a more severe clinical course.[46]

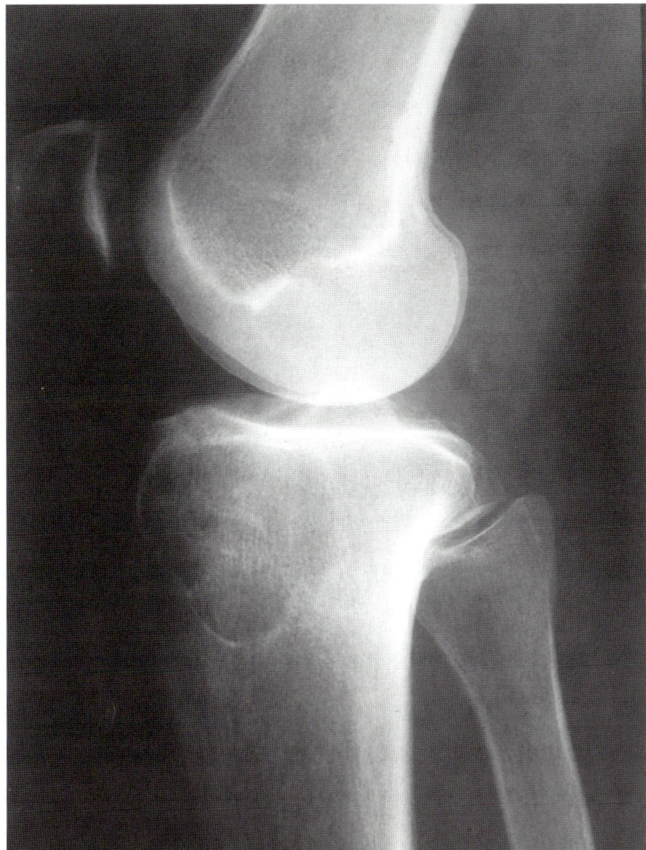

Fig. 14.26

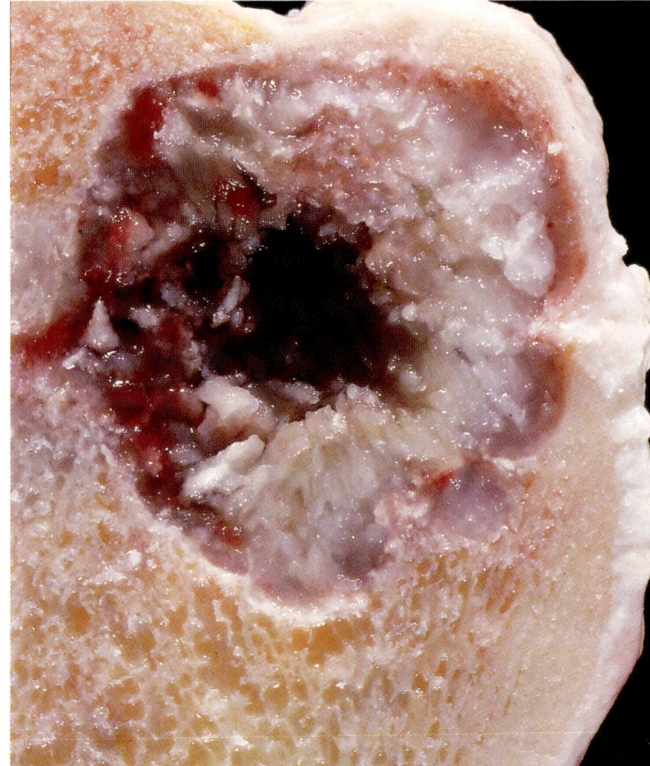

Fig. 14.27

Figs 14.26, 14.27 Epiphyseal chondrosarcoma of the tibia.

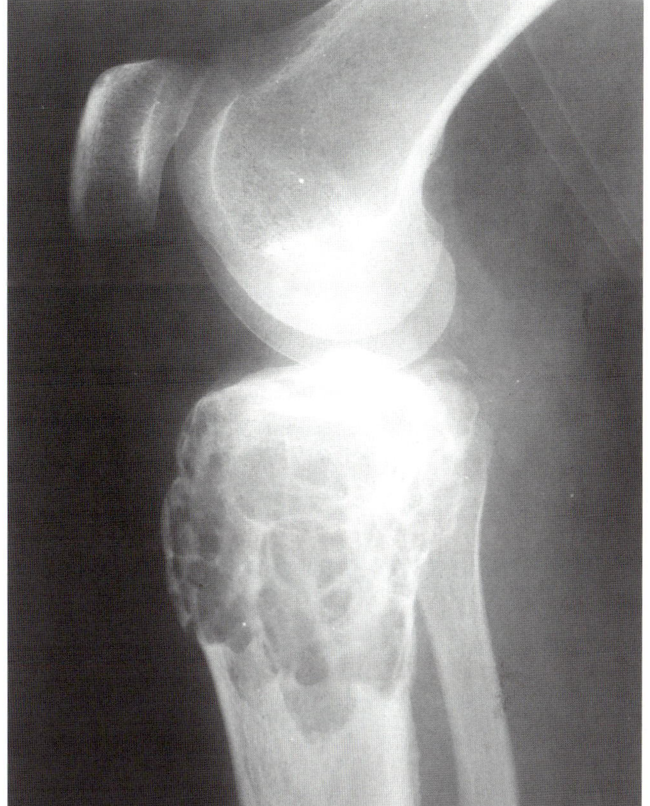

Fig. 14.28

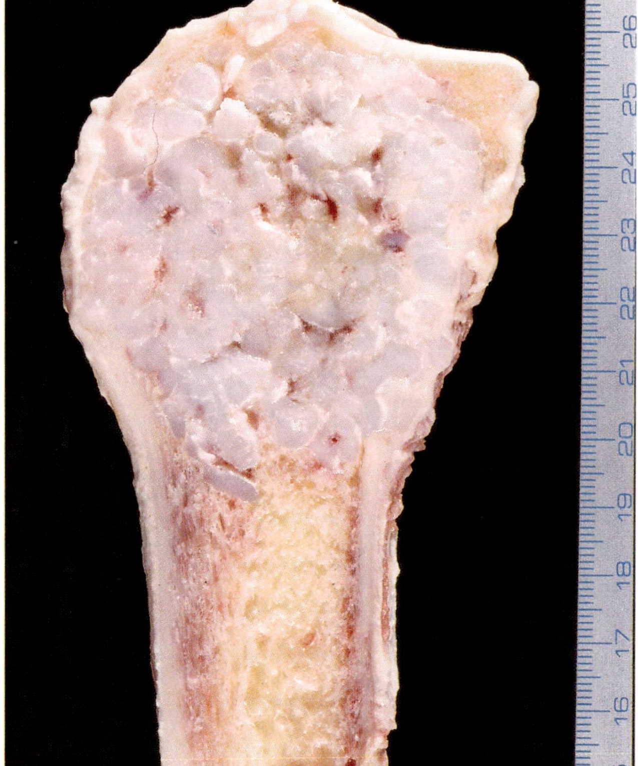

Fig. 14.29

Figs 14.28, 14.29 'Bubbly', epiphyseal well-differentiated chondrosarcoma of the tibia.

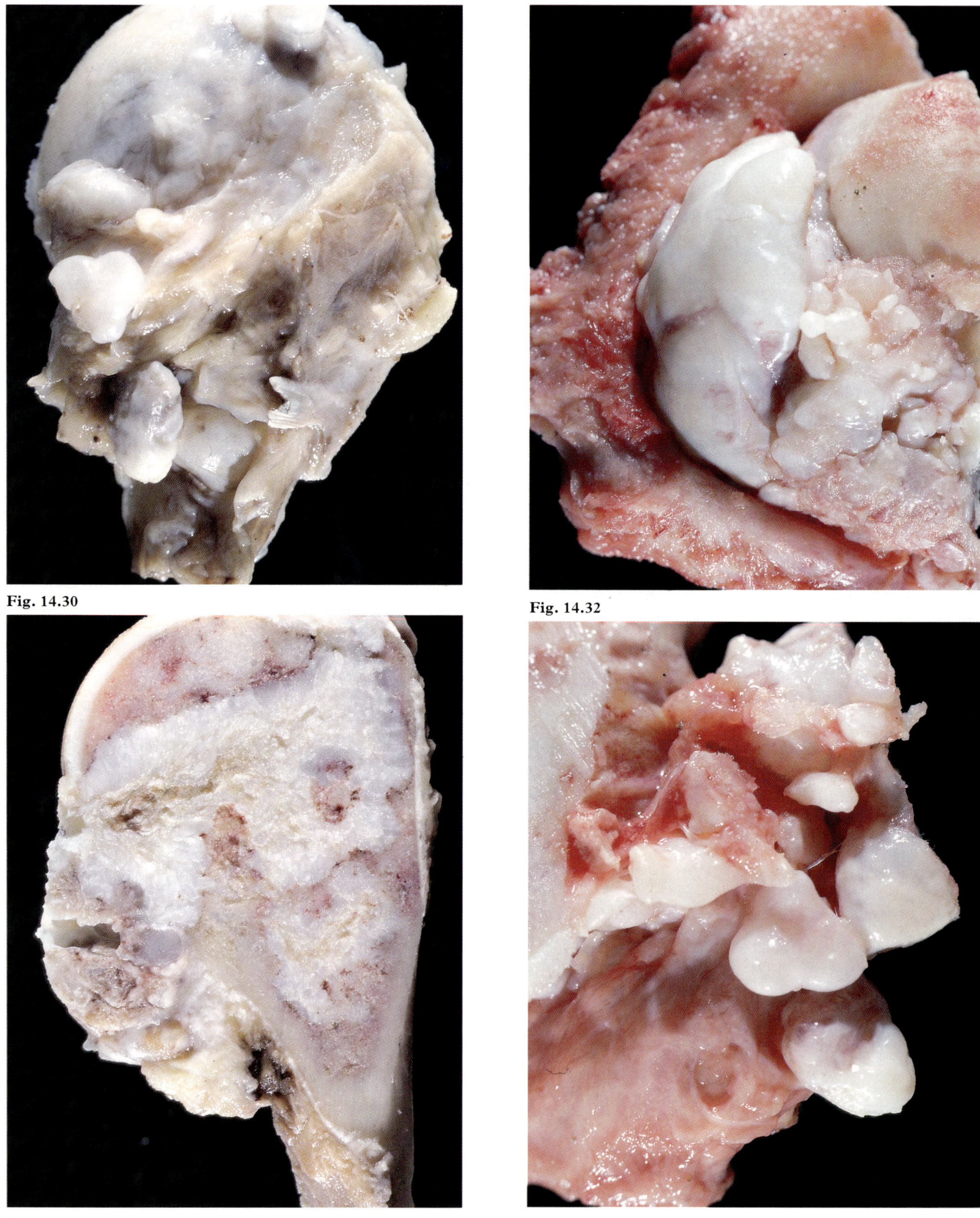

Fig. 14.30

Fig. 14.32

Fig. 14.31

Fig. 14.33

Figs 14.30–14.33 Chondrosarcoma of the humerus with tumoral spread into the joint cavity resembling synovial chondromatosis.

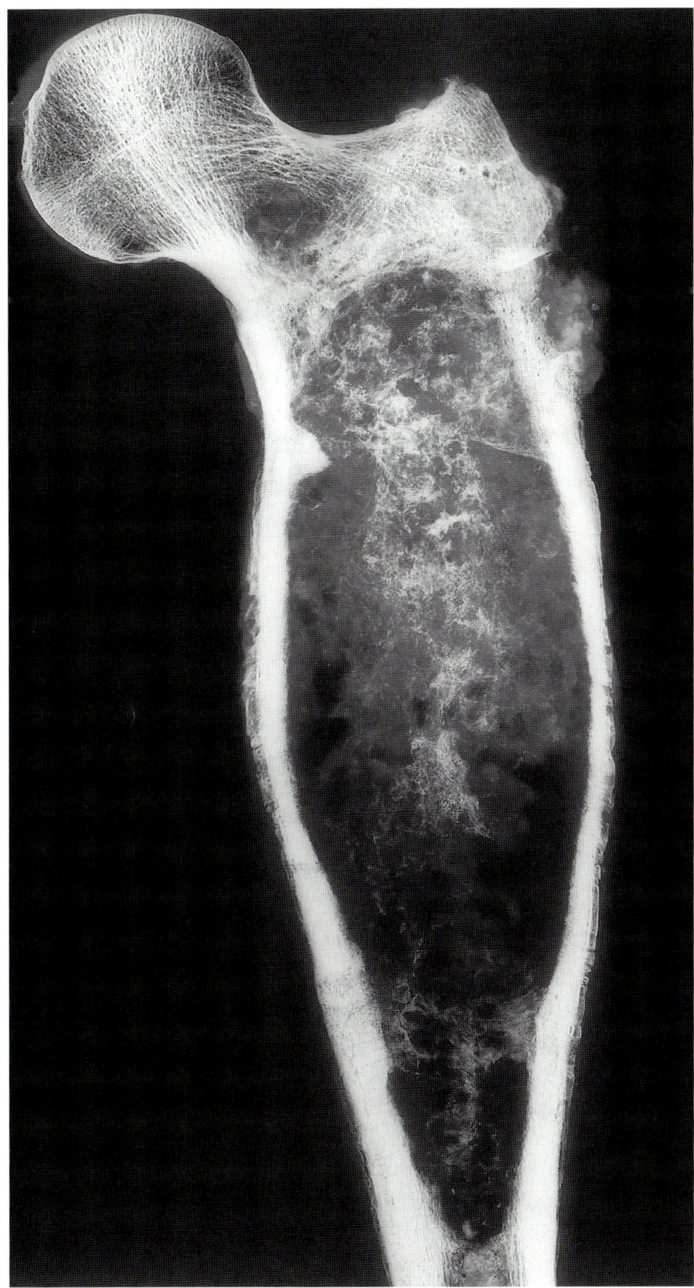

Fig. 14.34 Expansion of the shaft in a chondrosarcoma of the femur.

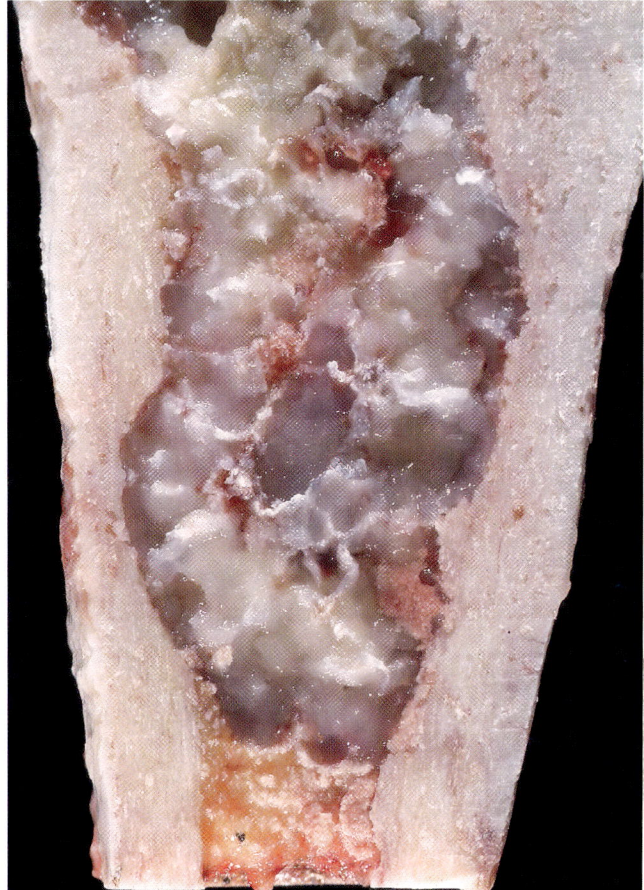

Fig. 14.35 Endosteal erosion in the lower part of a femoral chondrosarcoma.

CYTOPATHOLOGY

Some authors have stressed the usefulness of cytology for diagnosis and also for grading[50-54] (Figs 14.69–14.74). Fine-needle aspiration biopsies may have some utility as the sole technique in the diagnosis of recurrences or metastases of a known tumor.[52] Low-grade chondrosarcomas are very difficult to diagnose,[53] while high-grade tumors usually have a myxoid matrix on smears.[53]

We find tumor imprints very useful as an adjunct to histological sections. Chondrocytes may be dissociated from their matrix with trypsin and clostridium collagenase, retaining their cytologic identity.[55]

Chondrocytes appear in clusters, sheets or loose aggregates.[40] Most often, they are oval or polyhedral; spindle cells are found in high-grade tumors. The cytoplasm, with distinct outlines, is foamy, vacuolated or granular[52] and in rare cases shows a large cytoplasmic vacuole.[40] The nucleus has a finely or coarsely granular, evenly distributed chromatin with a central or eccentric location. Distinct nucleoli are found. There is a variable number of binucleated cells.

The amorphous matrix is intensely metachromatic with on toluidine blue, or Alcian blue staining.[53] S-100 positivity of cells can be very well demonstrated on smears.

BIOCHEMICAL AND HISTOCHEMICAL STUDIES

In organ cultures, as malignancy increases, there is a decrease in collagen synthesis and in the specific activity of hydroxyproline.[56] Size of proteoglycan subunits and tissue concentration of total glycosaminoglycans decrease and keratan sulfate increases with the changes from low-grade to high-grade tumors.[57] Molecular weight of both keratan

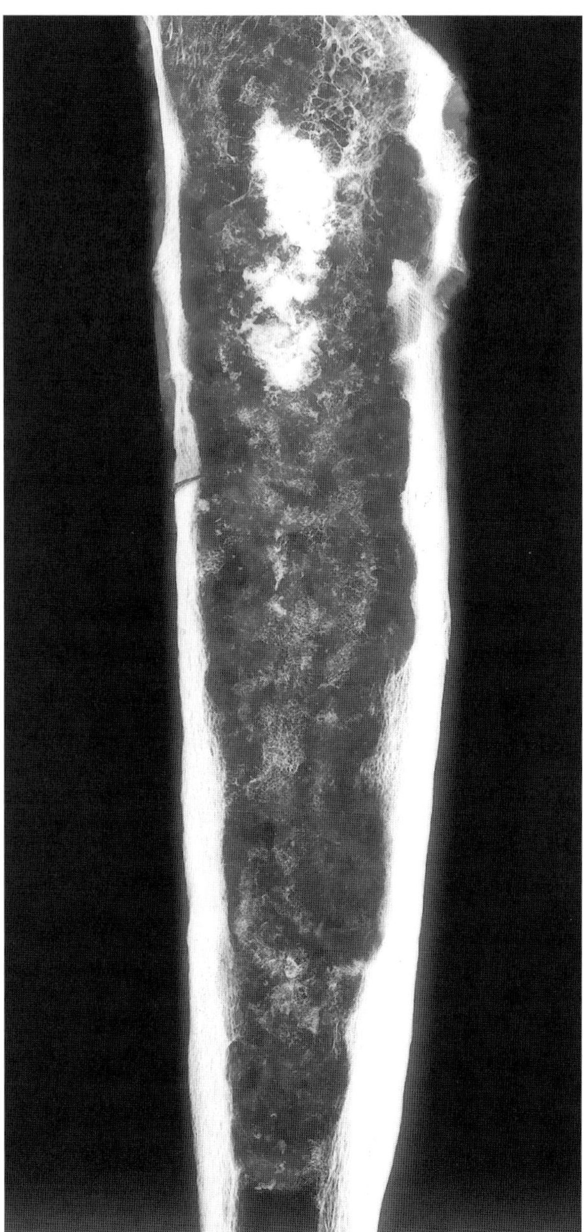

Fig. 14.36 Thinning of the cortex and endosteal scalloping in a chondrosarcoma of the femoral shaft.

sulfate chains[58] and chondroitin sulfate chains decreases with increasing malignancy.

Differences in the chemical composition, compared to mature normal cartilage, have been reported:[58-60] lower collagen content, higher water content,[58] increased amounts of non-collagenous matrix proteins and glycoproteins. Changes in the chemical composition of the proteoglycan monomers appear to be related to the degree of malignancy, particularly the glucosamine–sialate molar ratio.

However, in a very extensive study, Mankin et al conclude that there is marked variability in the biochemical composition of chondrosarcomas, with no clear relationship to the degree of malignancy.[61,62]

Histochemically, low-grade chondrosarcomas show a similar staining to adult cartilage with Alcian blue and toluidine blue at different pHs. Higher grade tumors have the same staining properties as fetal cartilage, containing chondroitin 4- and 6-sulfate but not keratan sulfate.[63]

IMMUNOHISTOCHEMISTRY

S-100 protein immunoreactivity is intense in the cytoplasm of well-differentiated chondrosarcomas but weak or negative in poorly differentiated tumors.[64-68] Vimentin positivity is found in chondrosarcomas; more unusual is staining for desmin, smooth muscle or muscle-specific actins.[69] Tenascin is an extracellular matrix glycoprotein expressed transiently during embryonic development;[70] it has been detected in the periphery of tumor lobules or in the matrix in high-grade chondrosarcomas, corresponding with the distribution of proliferating cell nuclear antigen reactivity.[69] Tenascin can also be found in osteosarcomas.[70]

The maturity of the tumor cells may be demonstrated by the immunohistochemical distribution of different collagen types. Type II collagen is localized predominantly in the cytoplasm; there is a loss of the pericellular distribution of type VI collagen, with additional types of collagen (I, III and V), as opposed to the normal hyaline cartilage.[71] Moreover, there is a correlation of the distribution of collagen types with aggressive behavior: in low-grade chondrosarcomas, the main collagen types are II and VI, as in enchondromas; type III collagen is found predominantly in high-grade tumors, without any rimming of lobules by collagen types I and V, as in enchondromas.[71]

Another study has shown a decrease of collagen types II and IX, compared to enchondromas, with an uneven distribution of collagen type IX; collagen types I, III and V increased with the grade of malignancy.[72]

Besides the proliferating cell nuclear antigen reactivity,[69] the proliferating cells may be labeled with the monoclonal antibody Ki-67 directed against a nuclear antigen present in all the active phases of the cell cycle;[73,74] there is a significant difference in the count of Ki-67-positive nuclei between chondromas and chondrosarcomas, as well as between chondrosarcomas of different grades.

A close relationship of the Ki-67 labeling index has been reported with the demonstration of the nucleolar organizer region-associated proteins,[75] identified as black dots in the nuclei by a silver staining method. Their number and distribution seem to reflect the growth rate of chondrosarcomas.[75]

Immunohistochemical detection of the c-erbB-2 protooncogene is found in chondrosarcomas and not in benign cartilaginous tumors[76] but the prognostic significance is not as well established as the occasionally detected amplification of the c-myc protooncogene.[77]

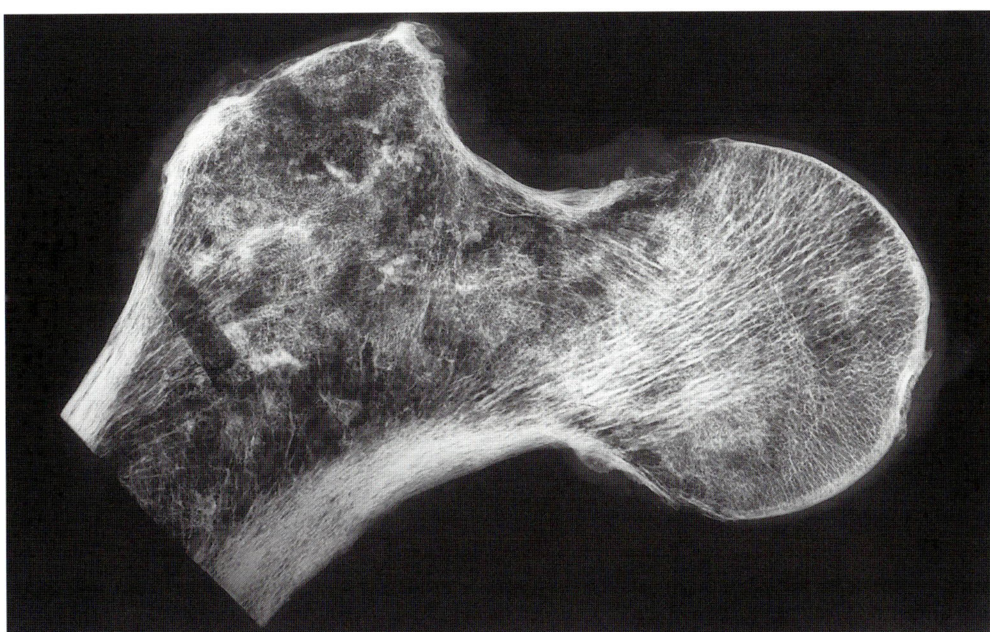

Fig. 14.37 Chondrosarcoma of the femur: thinning, thickening and breakthrough of the cortex.

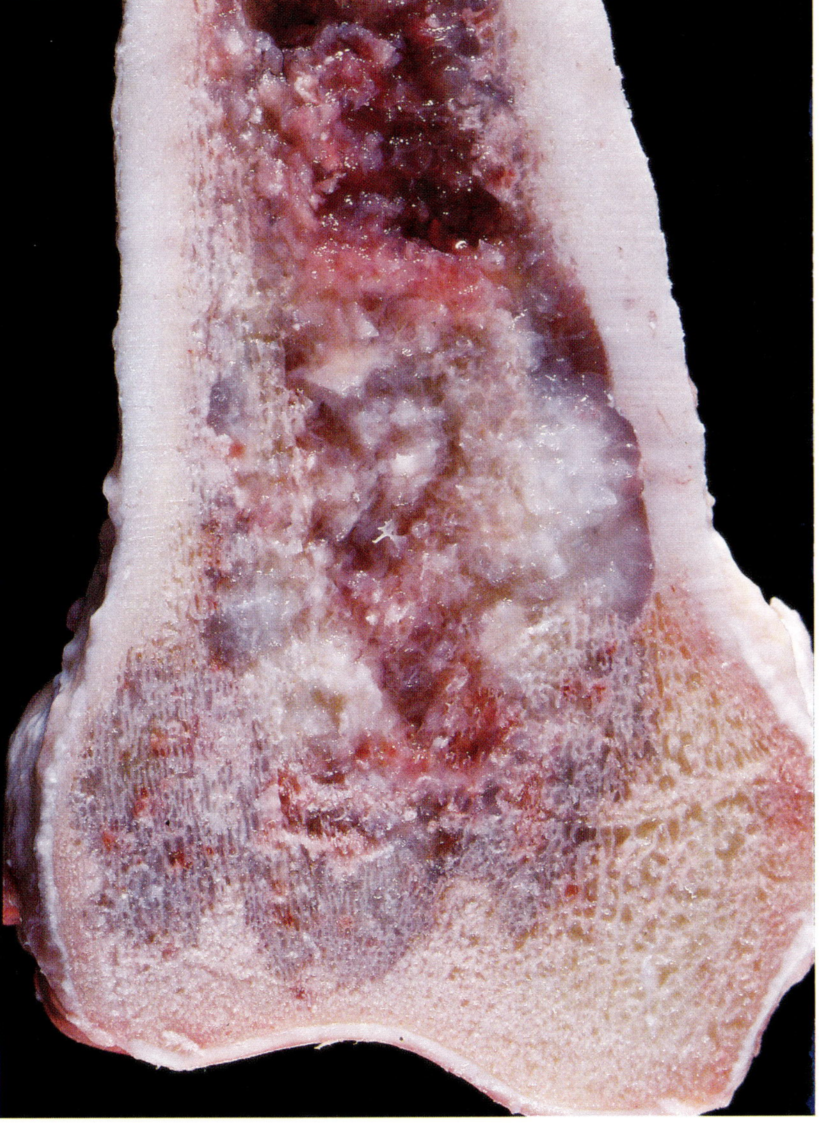

Fig. 14.38 Infiltrative pattern of growth in a high-grade chondrosarcoma of the femur.

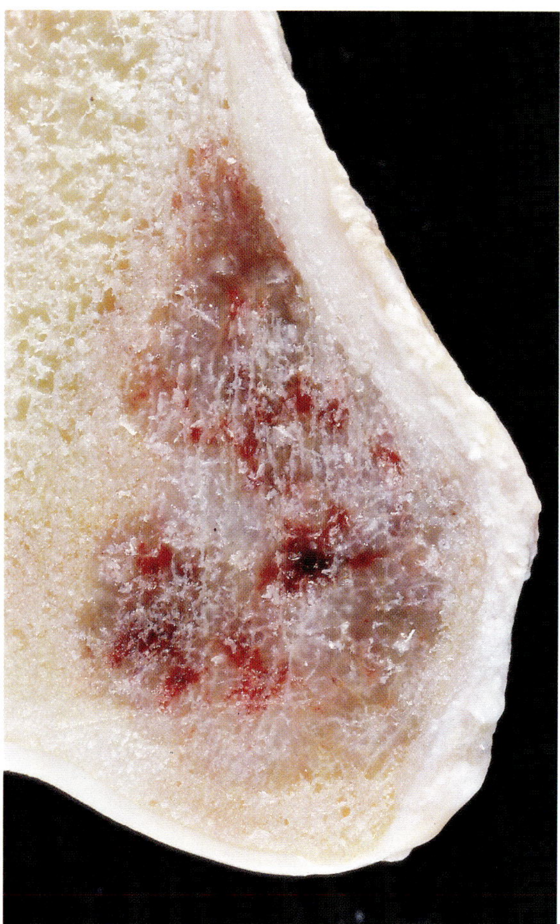

Fig. 14.39

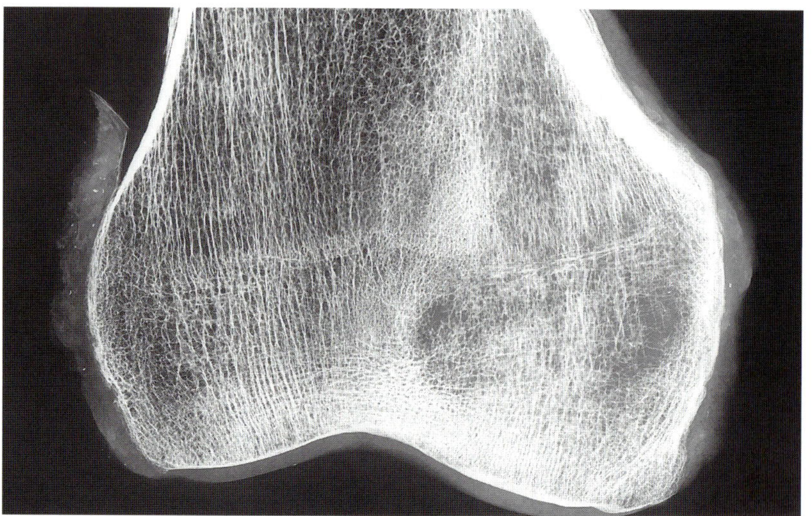

Fig. 14.40

Figs 14.39, 14.40 Infiltrative pattern of growth of a myxoid chondrosarcoma of the femur.

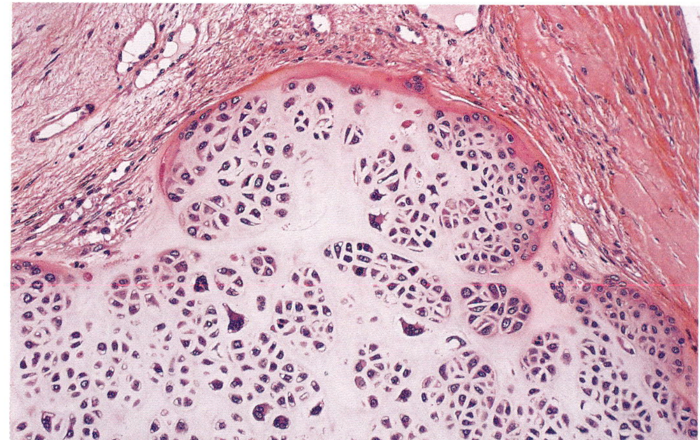

Fig. 14.41

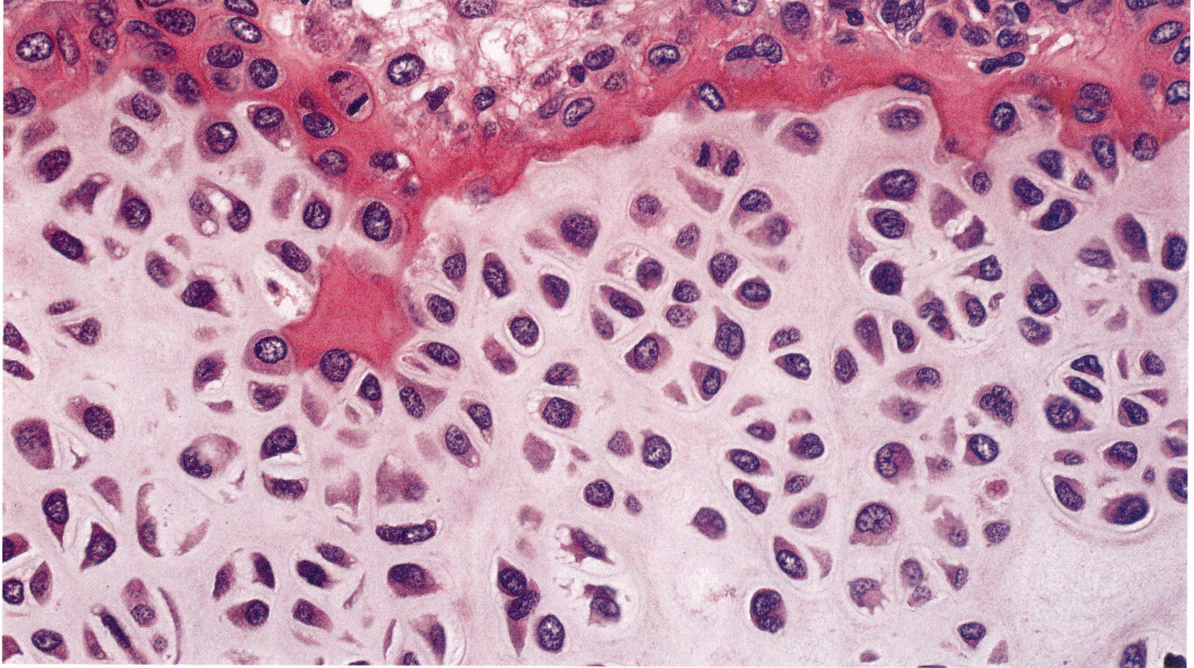

Fig. 14.42

Figs 14.41, 14.42 Soft tissue extension of a chondrosarcoma of the pelvis with high cellularity and a faint peripheral rim of calcification.

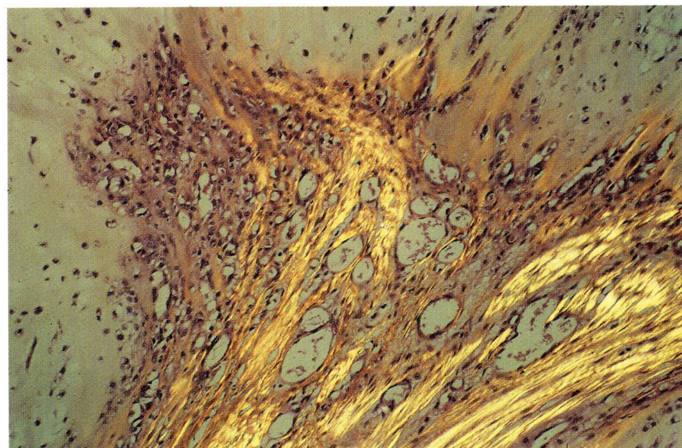

Fig. 14.46 Chondrosarcoma: fibrous tissue separating the lobules of cartilage (polarized light).

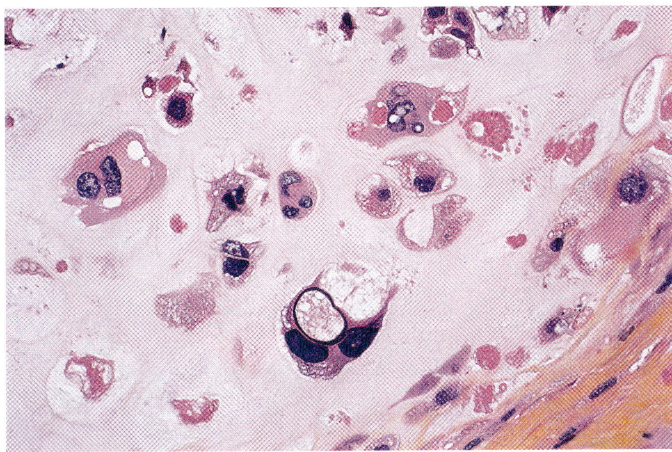

Fig. 14.43 Binucleated chondrocytes and a mitotic figure in a chondrosarcoma of the femur.

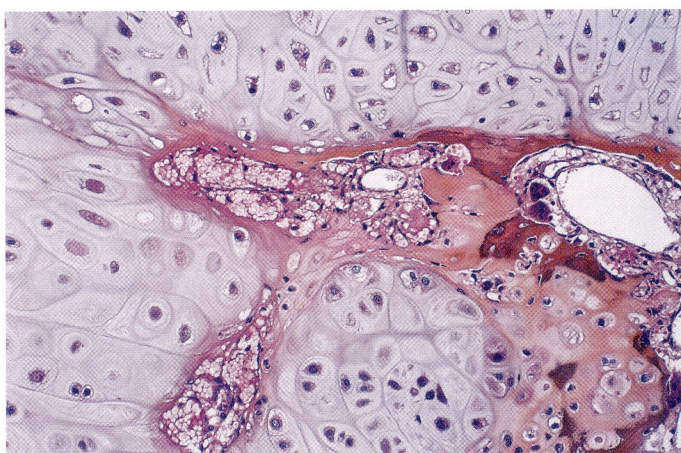

Fig. 14.47 Chondrosarcoma: fibrous septa with calcifications and osteoclastic activity.

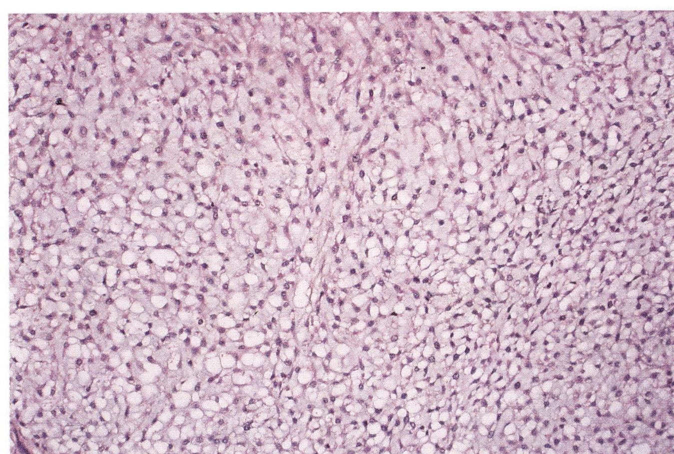

Fig. 14.44 Nuclear abnormalities in a chondrosarcoma, presumably corresponding in part to degenerative changes.

Fig. 14.45 Unusual signet-ring cell appearance of a chondrosarcoma of the humerus.

Overexpression and point mutation of the p53 protein gene have been investigated in a series of chondrosarcomas, immunohistochemically and by direct sequencing of the genomic DNA.[78] Only two cases of 16 showed genotypic and phenotypic alterations, including paradoxically one clear cell chondrosarcoma of low-grade malignancy. In another report, expression of the tumor suppressor gene p53 was studied immunohistochemically along with the histological grade and DNA ploidy. High-grade aneuploid tumors demonstrate higher levels of p53 than low-grade malignant chondrosarcomas or benign cartilage lesions.[79]

FLOW CYTOMETRY

Chondromas are diploid and chondrosarcomas are diploid or hyperploid,[80] so by flow cytometry or cytophotometry,

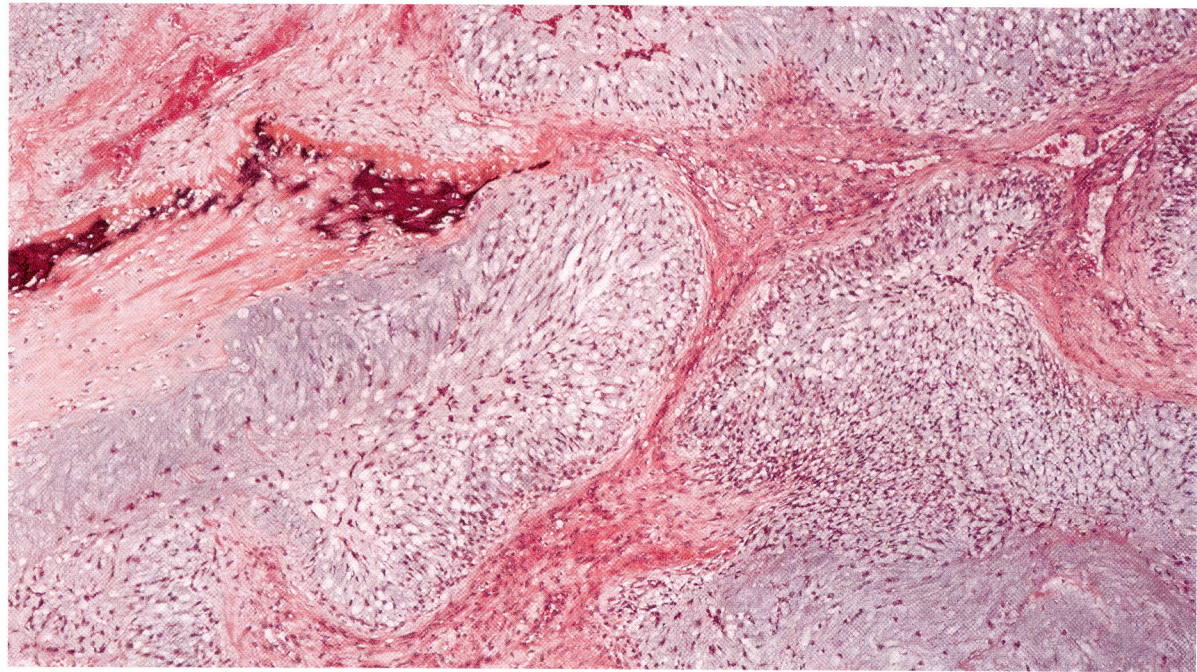

Fig. 14.48

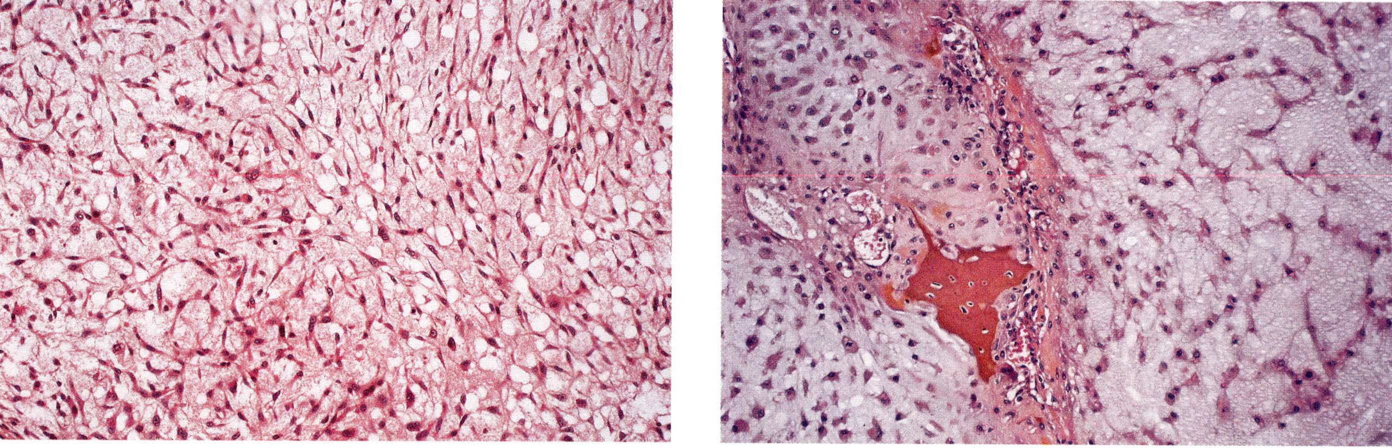

Fig. 14.49

Fig. 14.50

Figs 14.48–14.50 Myxoid chondrosarcoma of the humerus, pelvis and tibia.

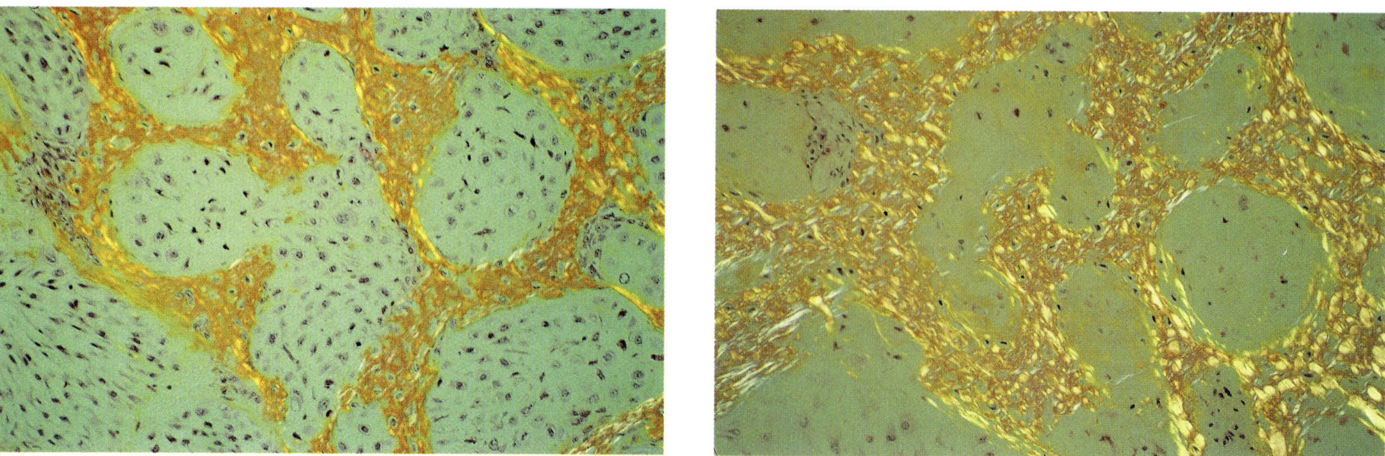

Fig. 14.51

Fig. 14.52

Figs 14.51, 14.52 Chondrosarcoma of the pelvis: immature bone formation around cartilage lobules (polarized light).

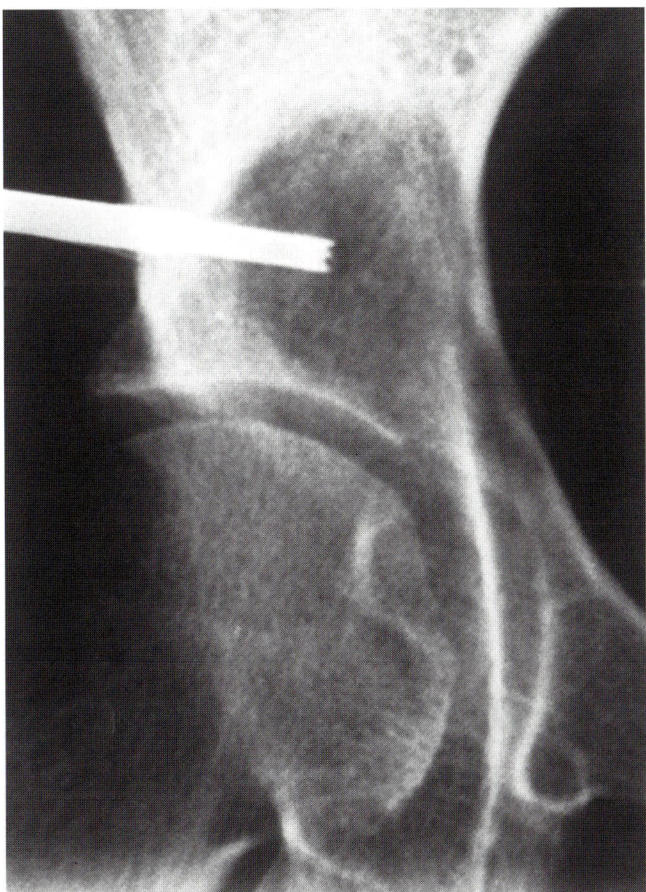

Fig. 14.53

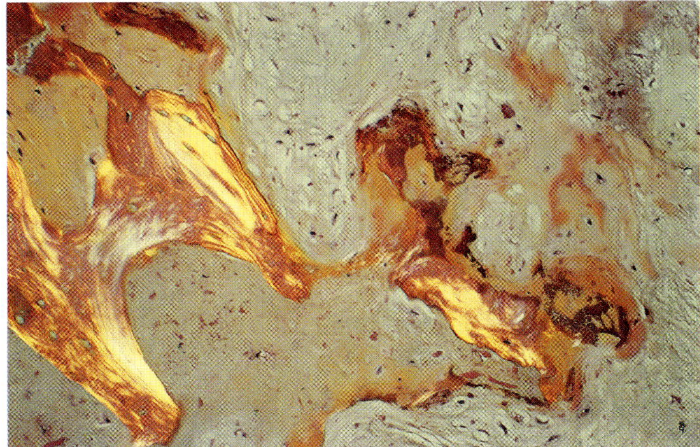

Fig. 14.54

Figs 14.53, 14.54 Chondrosarcoma of the acetabulum: on limited material, resorption and entrapment of residual bone by the tumor is an important finding for the diagnosis (polarized light).

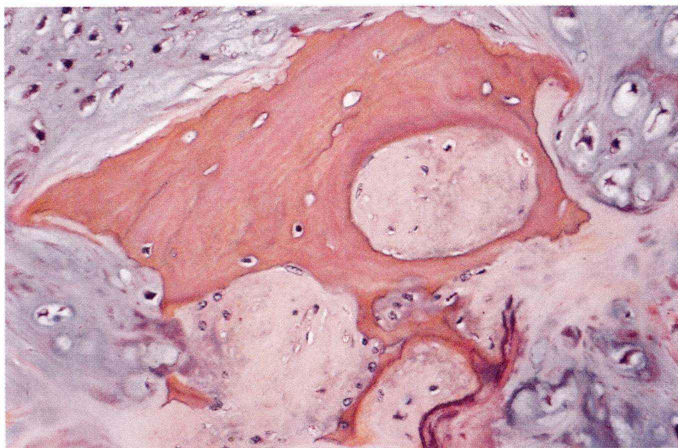

Fig. 14.55

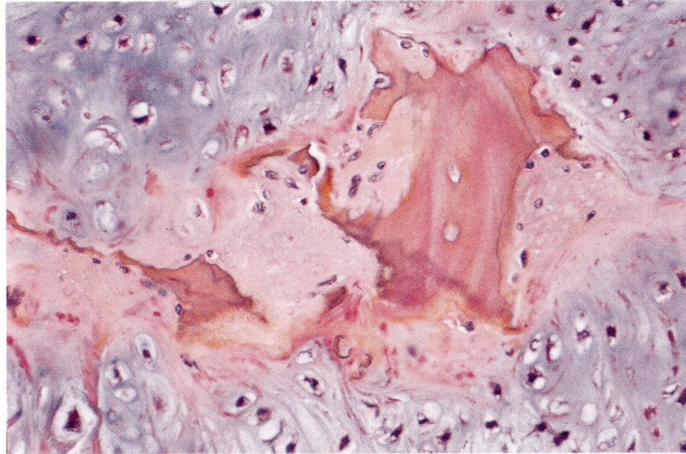

Fig. 14.56

Figs 14.55, 14.56 Entrapment of residual bone in a chondrosarcoma.

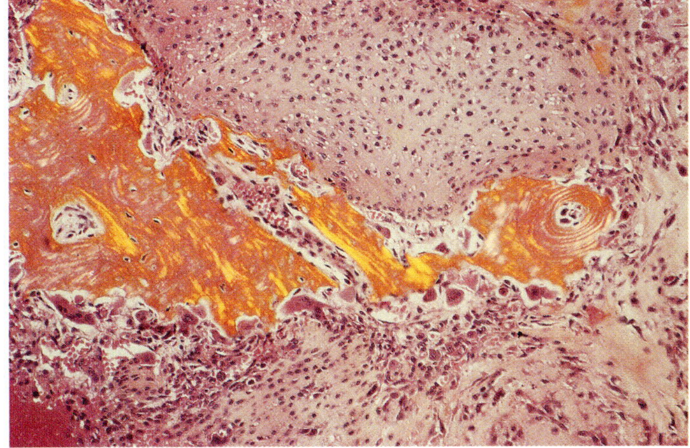

Fig. 14.57 Osteoclastic resorption of bone in front of the chondrosarcomatous lobules.

chondromas cannot be separated from low-grade chondrosarcomas[81,82] but ploidy can detect the tumors with increased metastatic potential.[80,83–85] Higher polyploidy coincides with increased malignancy[81,86–88] whereas diploid chondrosarcomas are associated with a significantly higher 10-year survival rate.

CYTOGENETICS

The pathologist may currently be somewhat lost, with the cytogenetic studies showing variable results. These

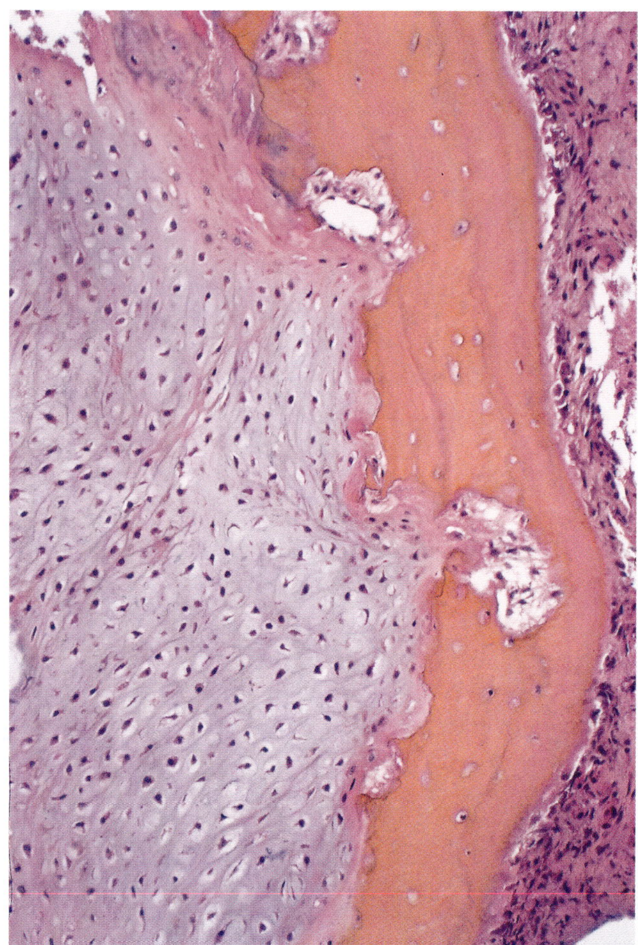

Fig. 14.58 Chondrosarcoma of a phalanx: focal resorption of the cortex.

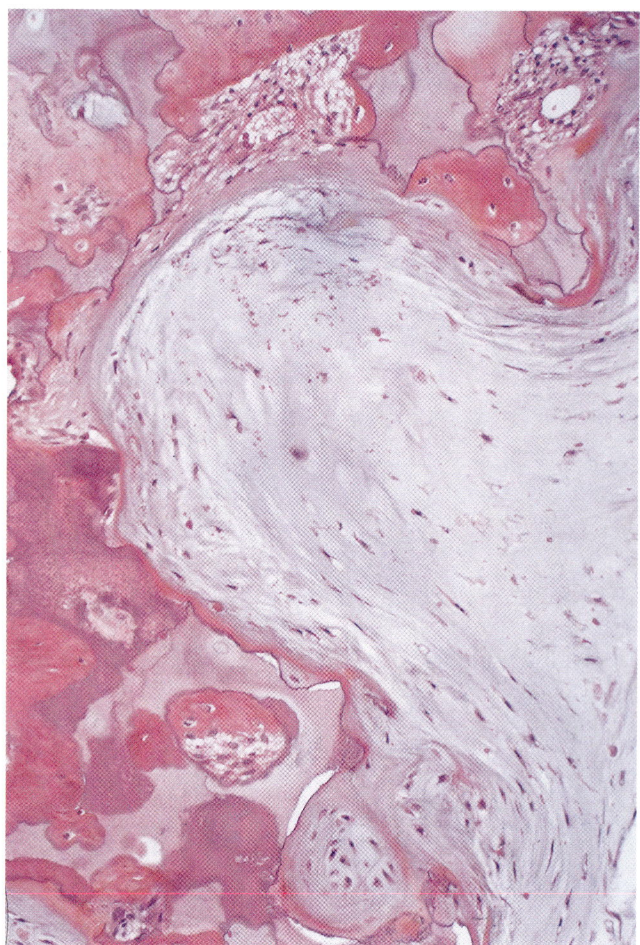

Fig. 14.59 Expanding lobules in a chondrosarcoma of the tibia.

findings reflect the considerable cytogenetic heterogeneity of chondrosarcomas, even in a single tumor.[89]

A common structural change may involve the chromosome 12q13[90] or chromosomes 1, 12 and 15, along with numerical aberrations of chromosomes 5, 7, 8 and 18[91] or monosomy for chromosomes 11, 13 and 22.[89]

The most frequent numerical abnormalities are a loss of chromosome Y, 6, 10 and 13 and a gain of chromosomes 7 and 20[92] or structural abnormalities and even a loss of a whole copy of chromosome 6.[93] Abnormalities of chromosome 9 may be found only in low-grade tumors;[93] a strong correlation between chromosomes, aberrations and grade has even been postulated[91] but numerous structural chromosome aberrations have also been reported in low-grade tumors.[94]

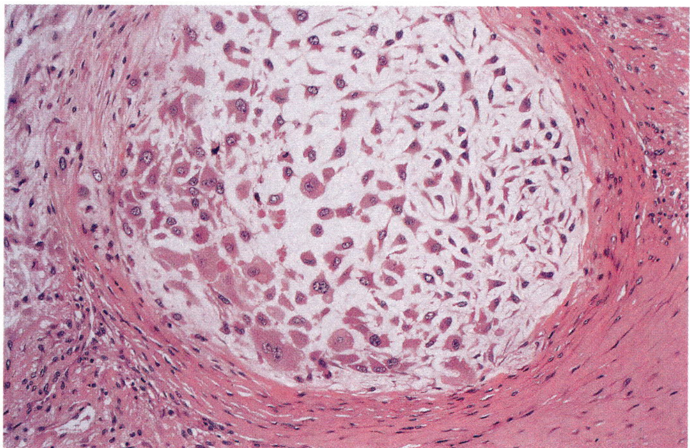

Fig. 14.60 Soft tissue extension in a femoral chondrosarcoma.

ELECTRON MICROSCOPY

Low-grade chondrosarcomas have round or oval nuclei with little atypia.[53,95] The abundant rough endoplasmic reticulum is dilated and Golgi zones are distinct. Glycogen and lipid droplets are found in the cytoplasm which shows microvillous projections.

High-grade chondrosarcomas have fewer cytoplasmic organelles, few glycogen particles and the dilatations of the rough endoplasmic reticulum are less conspicuous.[95–99]

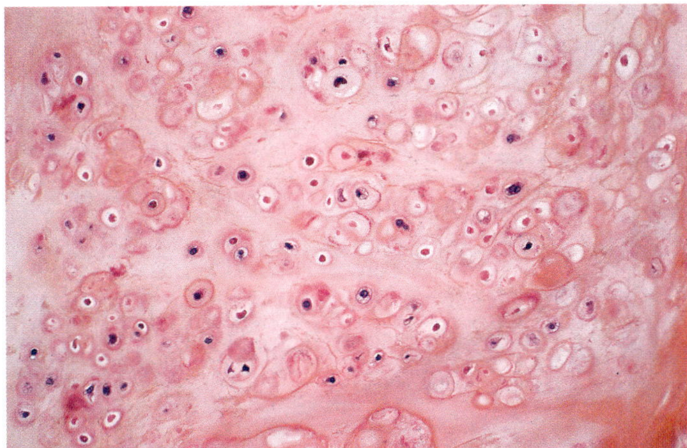

Fig. 14.61

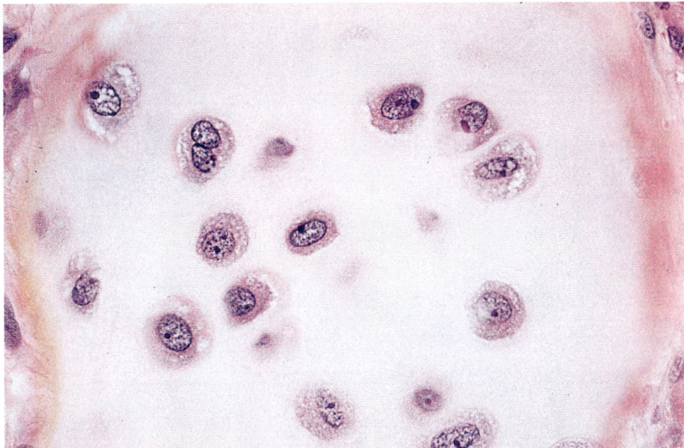

Fig. 14.63

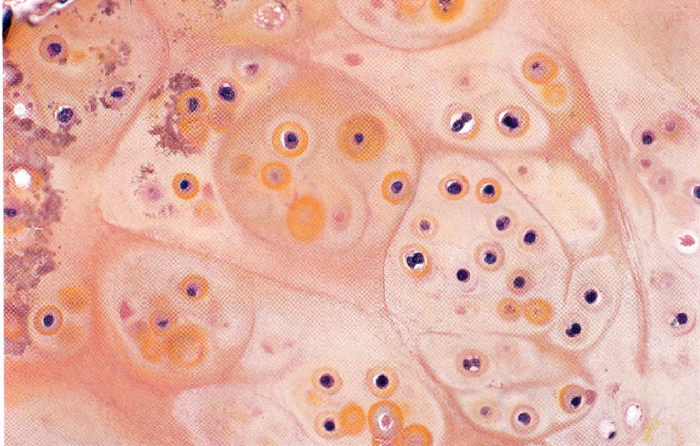

Fig. 14.62

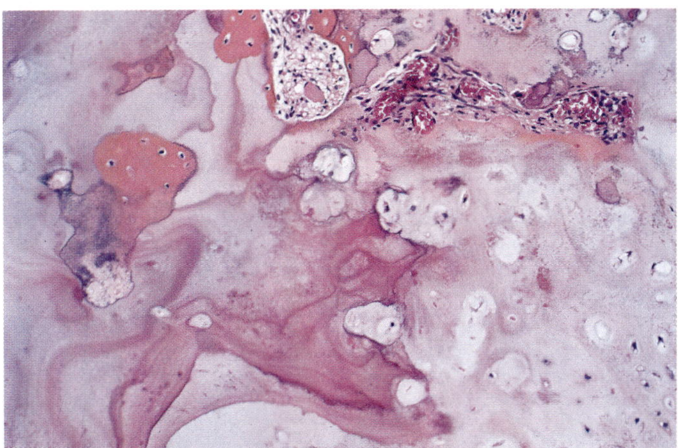

Fig. 14.64

Figs 14.61–14.64 Grade I chondrosarcomas with low cellularity and huge calcifications.

Lipid droplets and cytoplasmic filaments are increased. Nuclei are irregularly shaped with a coarse chromatin pattern and prominent nucleoli.[53,95,97]

Intracytoplasmic droplets may be localized within the rough endoplasmic reticulum, chiefly in low-grade tumors; they are of presumably glycoprotein in nature admixed with lipids, calcium and sulfur.[41]

The intercellular stroma is abundant, with microfibrils, collagen fibrils and granules of proteoglycans.[53,96] Proteoglycan subunits have the same basic structure as proteoglycans synthesized by normal chondrocytes, but with a greater average length of the chondroitin sulfate chains and a shorter mean length of the subunit core filaments; proteoglycan aggregates are smaller than those of normal cartilage.[60]

Amianthoid fibers in the matrix, as well as intramitochondrial paracrystalline inclusions, may correspond to degenerative changes.[98,99]

COURSE, TREATMENT AND PROGNOSIS

Chondrosarcomas of long bones spread in the medullary cavity and may involve soft tissues, into large veins or transarticularly. There is only one report of a skip lesion involving a low-grade tumor.[100]

Metastases (6–12% of cases) occur late in the disease course.[9] They are most commonly found in the lungs. Lymph node metastases are rare,[10] as are those in brain, liver, kidney, heart, skin or bone. Skeletal metastases in the absence of pulmonary dissemination are unusual.[101]

The treatment is en bloc surgical excision with, when feasible, limb salvage procedures in long bones.

Chondrosarcomas are considered to be radioresistant tumors (Huvos 1991, Schajowicz 1994), but a slow clinical regression has been reported in 50% of cases in one series.[102]

Local recurrences are related to surgical control of the primary lesion and not to the tumor grade,[10,44,45] with a rate of 21% in our own series of 180 cases. They usually occur within the first 5 years, but some appear many years after surgery.[103] Despite some findings,[104] most are not of higher grade[10,105] and they do not always result in metastases and death.[106]

An important recent report has shown that low-grade

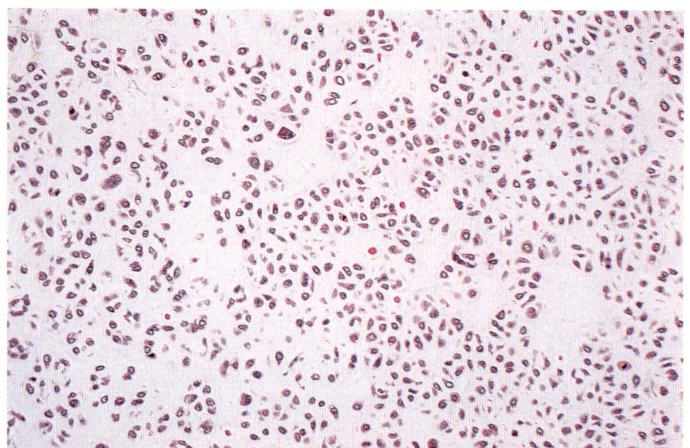

Fig. 14.65

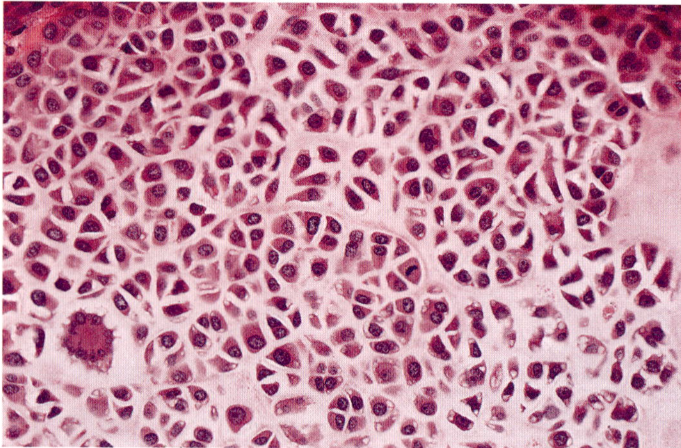

Fig. 14.66

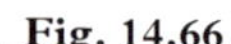

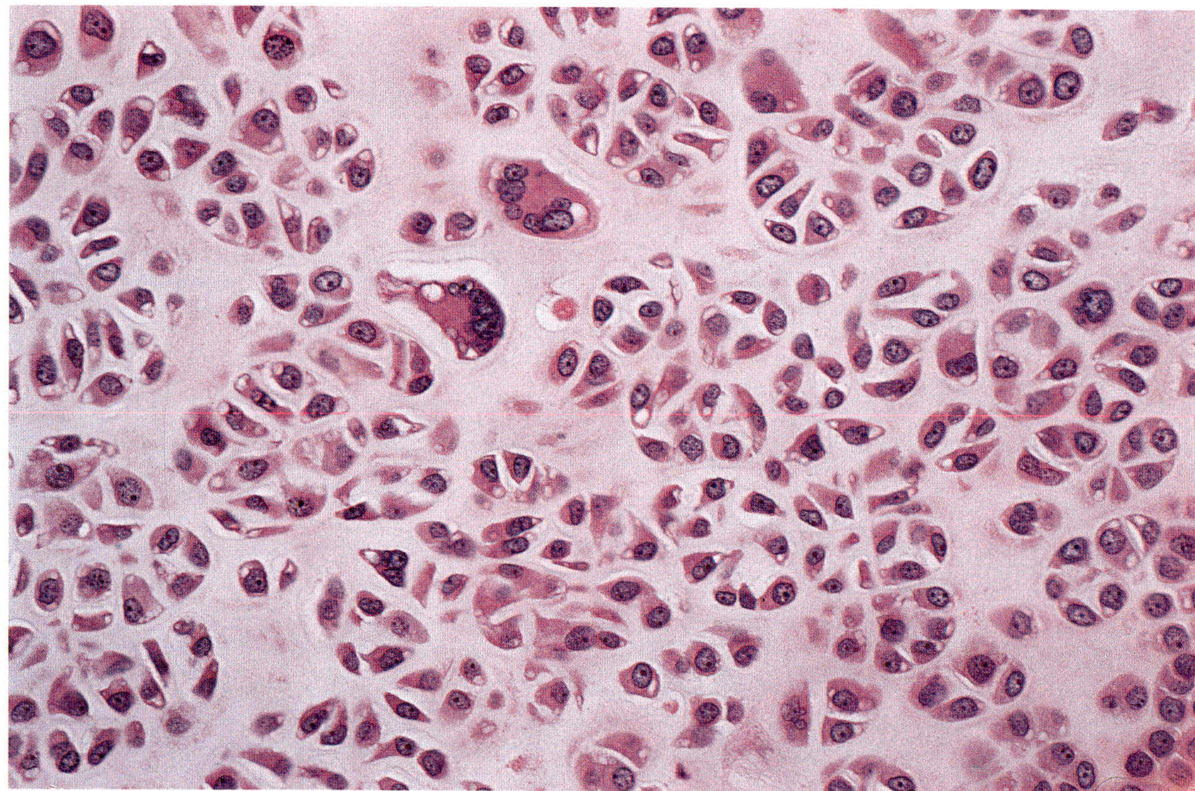

Fig. 14.67

Figs 14.65–14.67 Grade II chondrosarcomas; high cellularity, few mitotic figures and multinucleated cells.

chondrosarcomas in the extremities have a low rate of local recurrences and no metastases, even after non-radical surgery, suggesting a surgical approach limited to curettage and filling of the cavity with autogenous bone or cement.[107]

The prognosis of grade I and II chondrosarcomas is related to the surgical resectability; they may recur locally, but metastases occur late in the clinical course (Huvos 1991). Metastases are related to the histological grade and the metastatic risk for grade III chondrosarcomas ranges from 75% to 85% at 5 years. Survival at 5 years is 83% (grade I), 75% (grade II) and 15% grade III) in our series.[45] In other reports, the survival at 10 years is 71–85% (grade I), 40–59% (grade II) and 28–36% (grade III).[9,10,44,108]

The overall survival is 67–79% of cases at 5 years, 59% after 15 years.

DIFFERENTIAL DIAGNOSIS

Myxoid chondrosarcomas have to be differentiated from chondromyxoid fibromas, the latter showing a less cellular pleomorphism, a more peripheral cellularity in the lobules and fibrous septa with many reactive cells.

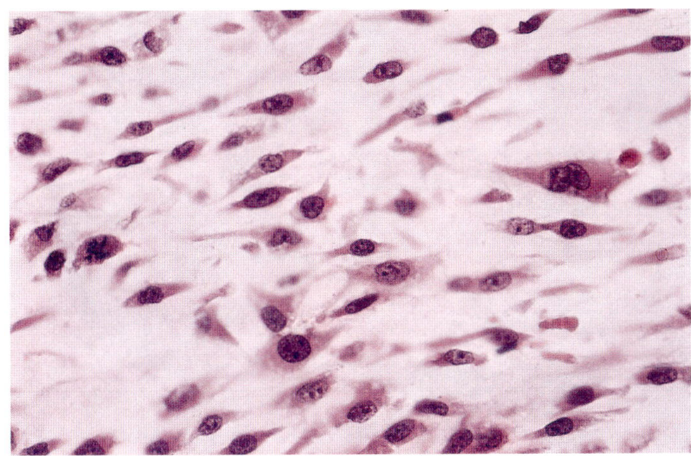

Fig. 14.68 Grade III chondrosarcoma of the femur.

High-grade chondrosarcomas have to be separated from dedifferentiated forms which usually show an abrupt transition between the cartilage areas and the other sarcoma components.

All chondrosarcomas have to be differentiated from chondroblastic osteosarcomas which show, even in limited areas, tumoral bone formation.

An unusual differential diagnosis is tophaceous pseudo-gout (tumoral calcium pyrophosphate dihydrate crystal deposition disease), appearing as a granular calcified mass; the chondroid metaplasia commonly found may show some cellular atypia.[109]

The main differential diagnosis is chondromas and for Mirra,[110] more than 25% of well-differentiated chondrosarcomas have the cytology of these tumors. Double nucleated chondrocytes are of doubtful value, as they only suggest an active growth of cartilage.[110–112]

Morphometric studies show that the relative volume density of tumor cell nuclei and nuclear areas, as well as the cellularity, are useful parameters to discriminate chondromas from chondrosarcomas, except in young patients or in tumors located in the hands.[47,112]

The most useful histological findings are the invasive behavior and the relationship to the host bone found in chondrosarcomas.[46,50,110,111,114]

Chondromas exhibit cartilage lobules separated by bone marrow; the lobules are partially or completely encased by

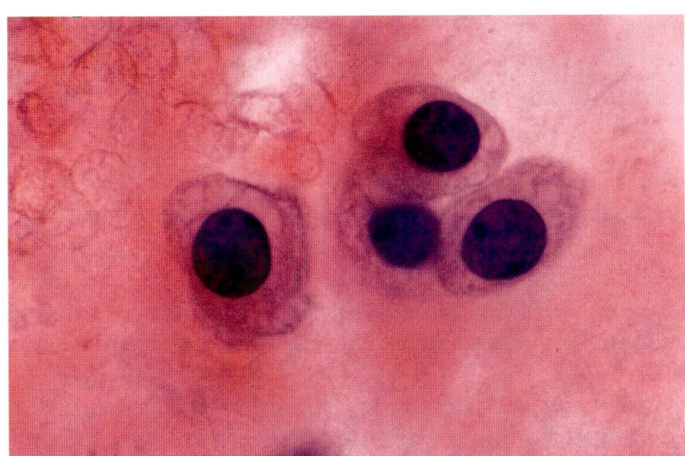

Fig. 14.69

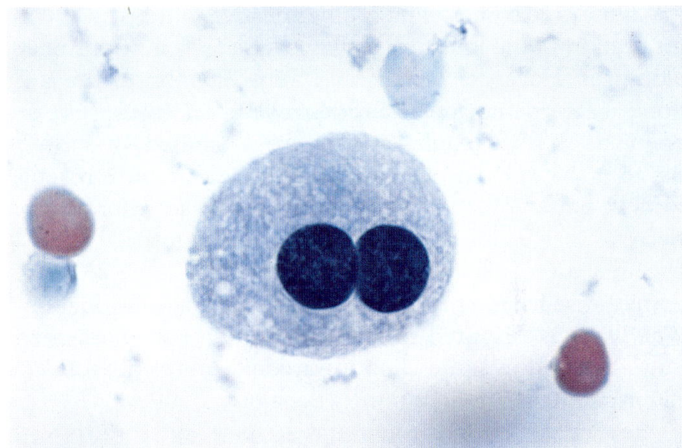

Fig. 14.71

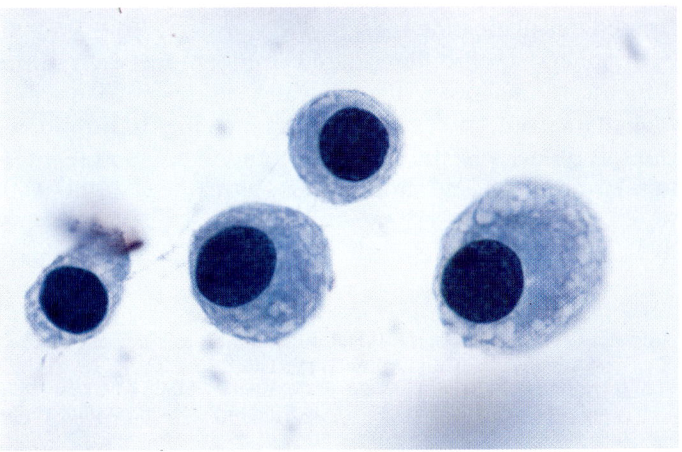

Fig. 14.70

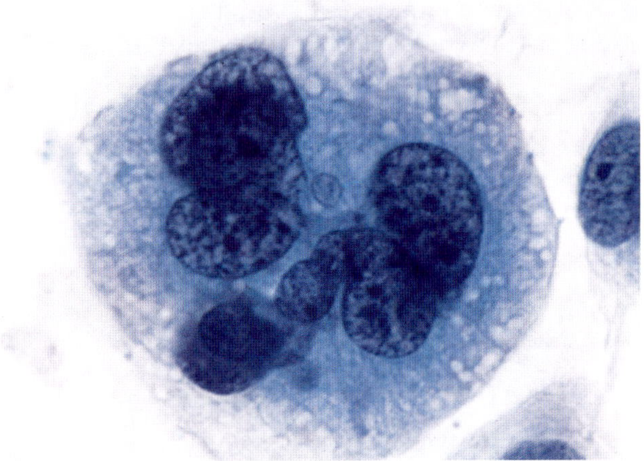

Fig. 14.72

Figs 14.69–14.72 Imprint cytology of chondrosarcomas: high nuclear – cytoplasmic ratio, dense nuclei, binucleated and multinucleated cells.

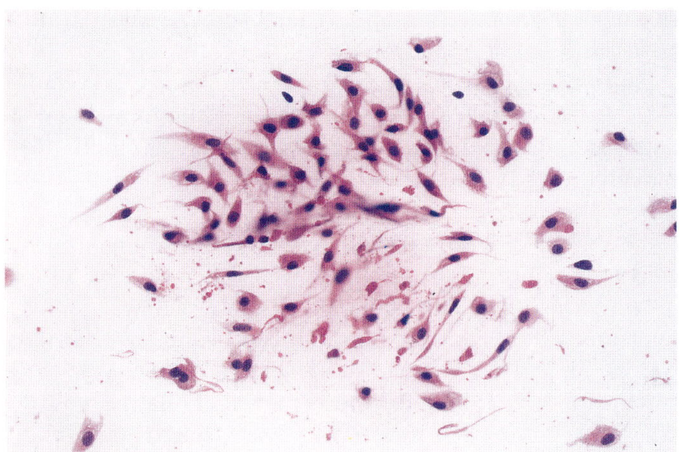

Fig. 14.73

Fig. 14.74

Figs 14.73, 14.74 Imprint cytology of a myxoid chondrosarcoma of the pelvis.

shells of woven or lamellar bone. The hyaline cartilage may show calcifications, but no entrapment of residual bone. In the absence of calcification, necrosis is not found and myxoid areas are rare except in enchondromatosis.[111] Tumor tissue does not abut directly onto pre-existing bone.[50]

Chondrosarcomas exhibit a permeative pattern[50,110] with infiltration of the intertrabecular spaces; they may permeate along the Haversian canals and abut directly on the host bone.[50] Remnants of partially destroyed or necrotic bone are engulfed in the lobules which are separated by fibrous tissue[46,110,113,114] and eventually encircled by pure reactive woven bone.[110,111,114] Focal or widespread chondrocyte necrosis may be found as well as a myxoid stroma.[110,111]

Some authors state that more than half of all chondrosarcomas arise from a preexisting benign cartilage lesion.[110,111] This view is disputed and the enchondroma encasement pattern found in some chondrosarcomas may only reflect a different rate of proliferation[46] (Schajowicz 1994).

'Borderline' chondrosarcomas are cartilage tumors with a cytology resembling enchondromas, but with intermittent pain, endosteal erosions without cortical destruction on X-ray and a clinical outcome that is, local recurrences similar to low-grade chondrosarcomas (Unni 1996). They may well be the initial process of malignant transformation.[115] Their expression of collagen types I, II, III, V and VI has been studied immunohistochemically.[115] Matrix immunoreactivity for collagen types II and VI is predomi-

nant, with immunoreactivity for collagen type II in the cytoplasm of tumor cells. Collagen types I, III and V exhibit a heterogeneous expression. The collagen pattern, reflecting immaturity of cartilage, is similar to that of low-grade chondrosarcoma, perhaps suggesting a similar treatment, that is, wide en bloc resection.[115]

COMMENTS FOR THE SURGICAL PATHOLOGIST

The major practical problem is the diagnosis of borderline cartilaginous tumors. The search for 'histological patterns'[110] excludes a diagnosis made on cytology alone or on limited material. The surgeon has to biopsy the interface between the tumor and the host bone, excluding calcified or necrotic areas, without spilling the tumoral tissue.[110]

In spite of detailed studies, sophisticated immunohistochemical techniques (e.g. on collagens) are not yet common in routine practice and the pathologist has to rely on crude detail: especially adequate fixation and well-performed decalcification.

Peripheral well-differentiated tumors are even more difficult to diagnose histologically, in spite of obvious malignancy on clinical findings and imaging. Infiltration of the soft tissues and the spread of tumoral cells in the interlobular fibrous tissue should be sought.

REFERENCES

1. Lichtenstein L, Jaffe H L. Chondrosarcoma of bone. Am J Path 1943: 19: 553–589
2. Huvos A G, Marcove R C. Chondrosarcoma in the young. A clinicopathologic analysis of 79 patients younger than 21 years of age. Am J Surg Pathol 1987: 11: 930–942
3. Young C L, Sim F H, Unni K K, McLeod R A. Case report 559. Chondrosarcoma of proximal humeral epiphysis. Skeletal Radiol 1989: 18: 403–405
4. Wilkinson R H, Kirkpatrick J A. Case report 14. Low-grade chondrosarcoma of femur. Skeletal Radiol 1976: 1: 127–128
5. Aprin H, Riseborough E J, Hall J E. Chondrosarcoma in children and adolescents. Clin Orthop 1982: 166: 226–232
6. Haygood T M, Teot L, Ward W G, Allen A, Monu J U. Low-grade chondrosarcoma in a 12-year-old boy. Skeletal Radiol 1995: 24: 466–468
7. Young C L, Sim F H, Unni K K, McLeod R A. Chondrosarcoma of bone in children. Cancer 1990: 66: 1641–1648
8. Hermann G, Wagner L D, Klein M J, Faye-Peterson O M,

Lewis M M. Case report 541. Low grade chondrosarcoma. Skeletal Radiol 1989: 18: 241–244

9. Pritchard D J, Lunke R J, Taylor W F, Dahlin D C, Medley B E. Chondrosarcoma: a clinicopathologic and statistical analysis. Cancer 1980: 45: 149–157

10. Evans H L, Ayala A G, Romsdahl M M. Prognostic factors in chondrosarcoma of bone. A clinicopathologic analysis with emphasis on histologic grading. Cancer 1977: 40: 818–831

11. Marcove R C, Francis K C. Chondrosarcoma and altered carbohydrate metabolism. N Engl J Med 1963: 268: 1399–1400

12. Ghosh L, Huvos A G, Miké V. The pancreatic islets in chondrosarcoma. A qualitative and quantitative study in humans. Am J Pathol 1973: 71: 23–32

13. Mack G R, Robey D B, Kurman R J. Chondrosarcoma secreting chorionic gonadotrophin: report of a case. J Bone Joint Surg (Am) 1977: 59: 1107–1111

14. Relkin R. Hypocalcemia resulting from calcium accretion by a chondrosarcoma. Cancer 1974: 34: 1834–1837

15. Dahlin D C, Salvador A H. Chondrosarcomas of bones of the hands and feet. A study of 30 cases. Cancer 1974: 34: 755–760

16. Block R S, Burton R I. Multiple chondrosarcomas in a hand: a case report. J Hand Surg (Am) 1977: 2: 310–313

17. Wu K K, Frost H M, Guise E E. A chondrosarcoma of the hand arising from an asymptomatic benign solitary enchondroma of 40 years' duration. J Hand Surg (Am) 1983: 8: 317–319

18. Nelson D L, Abdul-Karim F W, Makley J T. Chondrosarcoma of small bones of the hand arising from enchondroma. J Hand Surg (Am) 1990: 15: 655–659

19. Landry M M, Sarma D P. In-situ chondrosarcoma of the foot arising in a solitary enchondroma. J Foot Surg 1990: 29: 324–326

20. Karabela-Bouropoulou V, Patra-Malli F, Agnantis N. Chondrosarcoma of the thumb: an unusual case with lung and cutaneous metastases and death of the patient 6 years after treatment. J Cancer Res Clin Oncol 1986: 112: 71–74

21. Hermann G, Sacher M, Lanzieri C F, Anderson P J, Rabinowitz J G. Chondrosarcoma of the spine: an unusual radiographic presentation. Skeletal Radiol 1985: 14: 178–183

22. Jurik A G, Jensen O, Keller J et al. Imaging of chondrosarcoma with histopathological and prognostic correlation. RÖFO 1995: 163: 372–377

23. West O C, Reinus W R, Wilson A J. Quantitative analysis of the plain radiographic appearance of central chondrosarcoma of bone. Invest Radiol 1995: 30: 440–447

24. Pinstein M L, Sebes J I, Scott R L. Transarticular extension of chondrosarcoma. AJR 1984: 142: 779–780

25. Reiter F B, Staple T W, Ackerman L V. Central chondrosarcoma of the appendicular skeleton. Radiology 1972: 105: 525–530

26. Lodwick G S. The radiologist's role in the management of chondrosarcoma. Radiology 1984: 150: 275

27. Rosenthal D I, Schiller A L, Mankin H J. Chondrosarcoma: correlation of radiological and histological grade. Radiology 1984: 150: 21–26

28. Feldman F. Cartilaginous tumors and cartilage-forming tumor-like conditions of the bones and soft tissues. In: Ranniger K, Ed. Encyclopedia of medical radiology, vol 5, pt 6. Berlin: Springer, 1977, pp 83–242

29. Hudson T M, Manaster B J, Springfield D S, Spanier S S, Enneking W F, Hawkins I F Jr. Radiology of medullary chondrosarcoma: preoperative treatment planning. Skeletal Radiol 1983: 10: 69–78

30. Varma D G, Ayala A G, Carrasco C H, Guo S Q, Kumar R, Edeiken J. Chondrosarcoma: M R imaging with pathologic correlation. Radiographics 1992: 12: 687–704

31. Cohen E K, Kressel H Y, Frank T S et al. Hyaline cartilage-origin bone and soft-tissue neoplasms: MR appearance and histologic correlation. Radiology 1988: 167: 477–481

32. Aoki J, Sone S, Fujioka F et al. MR of enchondroma and chondrosarcoma: rings and arcs of Gd-DTPA enhancement. J Comput Assist Tomogr 1991: 15: 1011–1016

33. Hanna S L, Magill H L, Paraham D M, Bowman L C, Fletcher B D. Childhood chondrosarcoma: MR imaging with gadolinium-DTPA. Magn Reson Imaging 1990: 8: 669–672

34. Ragsdale B D, Sweet D E, Vinh T N. Radiology as gross pathology in evaluating chondroid lesions. Hum Pathol 1989: 20: 930–951

35. Geirnaerdt M J, Bloem J L, Eulderink F, Hogendoorn P C, Taminiau A H. Cartilaginous tumors: correlation of gadolinium-enhanced MR imaging and histopathologic findings. Radiology 1993: 186: 813–817

36. De Beuckeleer L H, De Schepper A M A, Ramon F. Magnetic resonance imaging of cartilaginous tumors: is it useful or necessary? Skeletal Radiol 1996: 25: 137–141

37. Hudson T M, Chew F S, Manaster B J. Radionuclide bone scanning of medullary chondrosarcoma. AJR 1982: 139: 1071–1076

38. Yaghmai I. Angiographic features of chondromas and chondrosarcomas. Skeletal Radiol 1978: 3: 91–98

39. Demetrick D J, Kneafsey P D, Hwang W S. Signet-ring chondrosarcoma: a new morphologic entity. Hum Pathol 1991: 22: 1175–1179

40. Olszewski W, Woyke S, Musiatowicz B. Fine needle aspiration biopsy cytology of chondrosarcoma. Acta Cytol 1983: 27: 345–349

41. Del Rosario A D, Bui H X, Singh J, Ginsburg R, Ross J S. Intracytoplasmic eosinophilic hyaline globules in cartilaginous neoplasms: a surgical, pathological, ultrastructural, and electron probe X-ray microanalytic study. Hum Pathol 1994: 25: 1283–1289

42. Gruber H E, Marshall G J, Kirchen M E, Menendez L R, Schwinn C P. Bone remodelling in the presence of chondrosarcoma: histomorphometry. Acta Anat 1993: 148: 1–7

43. O'Neal L W, Ackerman L V. Chondrosarcoma of bone. Cancer 1952: 5: 551–577

44. Gitelis S, Bertoni F, Picci P, Campanacci M. Chondrosarcoma of bone. The experience at the Istituto Ortopedico Rizzoli. J Bone Joint Surg (Am) 1981: 63: 1248–1257

45. Ucla E, Tomeno B, Forest M. Facteurs du pronostic tumoral dans les chondrosarcomes de l'appareil locomoteur. A propos de 180 cas. Rev Chir Orthop 1991: 77: 301–311

46. Feaux de Lacroix W, Dietlein M, Schmidt J, Stützer H. Histological investigation for comparison of cartilaginous tumors of unknown biological course with unequivocal chondrosarcomas. Zentralbl Pathol 1992: 138: 339–343

47. Ishida T, Kikuchi F, Machinami R. Histological grading and morphometric analysis of cartilaginous tumours. Virchows Arch A Pathol Anat Histopathol 1991: 418: 149–155

48. Kreicbergs A, Slezak E, Söderberg G. The prognostic significance of different histomorphologic features in chondrosarcoma. Virchows Arch Pathol Anat Histol 1981: 390: 1–10

49. Zeppa P, Zabatta A, Marino G et al. A morphometric approach to the grading of chondroid tumours on fine-needle smears. Pathol Res Pract 1989: 185: 760–763

50. Sanerkin N G. The diagnosis and grading of chondrosarcoma of bone. A combined cytologic and histologic approach. Cancer 1980: 45: 582–594

51. Salzer-Kuntschik M. Cytologic and cytochemical behaviour of primary malignant bone tumors. In: Grundmann E, Ed. Malignant bone tumors. Berlin: Springer, 1976, pp 152–155

52. Abdul-Karim F W, Wasman J K, Pitlik D. Needle aspiration cytology of chondrosarcomas. Acta Cytol 1993: 37: 655–660

53. Walaas L, Kindblom L G, Gunterberg B, Bergh P. Light and electron microscopic examination of fine needle aspirates in the preoperative diagnosis of cartilaginous tumors. Diagn Cytopathol 1990: 6: 396–408

54. Tunç M, Ekinci C. Chondrosarcoma diagnosed by fine needle aspiration cytology. Acta Cytol 1996: 40: 283–288

55. Mitchell M L, Sokoloff L. A method for cytologic examination of cartilaginous lesions. Arch Pathol Lab Med 1987: 111: 342–345

56. Miller D R, Mankin H J. A comparison of collagen synthesis by different categories of human chondrosarcoma in organ culture. Clin Orthop 1982: 168: 252–257

57. Herwig J, Roessner A, Buddecke E. Isolation and characterization of proteoglycans and glycosaminoglycans from human chondrosarcoma. Exp Mol Pathol 1986: 45: 118–127

58. Pal S, Strider W, Margolis G, Gallo G, Lee-Huang S. Isolation

and characterization of proteoglycans from human chondrosarcomas. J Biol Chem 1978: 253: 1279–1289

59. Rosenberg L C, Pal S, Buckwalter J A. Structural changes related to malignancy in proteoglycans from cartilage neoplasms. Ala J Med Sci 1980: 17: 283–292

60. Buckwalter J A. The structure of human chondrosarcoma proteoglycans. J Bone Joint Surg (Am) 1983: 65: 958–974

61. Mankin H J, Cantley K P, Lippiello L, Schiller A L, Campbell C J. The biology of human chondrosarcoma. I. Description of the cases, grading and biochemical analyses. J Bone Joint Surg (Am) 1980: 62: 160–175

62. Mankin H J, Cantley K P, Schiller A L, Lippiello L. The biology of human chondrosarcoma. II. Variation in chemical composition among types and subtypes of benign and malignant cartilage tumors. J Bone Joint Surg (Am) 1980: 62: 176–188

63. Kindblom L G, Angervall L. Histochemical characterization of mucosubstances in bone and soft tissue tumors. Cancer 1975: 36: 985–994

64. Nakamura Y, Becker L E, Marks A. S-100 protein in tumors of cartilage and bone. An immunohistochemical study. Cancer 1983: 52: 1820–1824

65. Kahn H J, Marks A, Thom H, Baumal R. Role of antibody to S100 protein in diagnostic pathology. Am J Clin Pathol 1983: 79: 341–347

66. Weiss A P, Dorfman H D. S-100 protein in human cartilage lesions. J Bone Joint Surg (Am) 1986: 68: 521–526

67. Okajima K, Honda I, Kitagawa T. Immunohistochemical distribution of S-100 protein in tumors and tumor-like lesions of bone and cartilage. Cancer 1988: 61: 792–799

68. Karabela-Bouropoulou V, Markaki S, Milas C. S-100 protein and neuron specific enolase immunoreactivity of normal, hyperplastic and neoplastic chondrocytes in relation to the composition of the extracellular matrix. Pathol Res Pract 1988: 183: 761–766

69. Hasegawa T, Seki K, Yang P et al. Differentiation and proliferative activity in benign and malignant cartilage tumors of bone. Hum Pathol 1995: 26: 838–845

70. Koukoulis G K, Gould V E, Bhattacharyya A, Gould J E, Howeedy A A, Virtanen I. Tenascin in normal, reactive, hyperplastic, and neoplastic tissues: biologic and pathologic implications. Hum Pathol 1991: 22: 636–643

71. Ueda Y, Oda Y, Tsuchiya H, Tomita K, Nakanishi I. Immunohistological study on collagenous proteins of benign and malignant human cartilaginous tumours of bone. Virchows Arch A Pathol Anat Histopathol 1990: 417: 291–297

72. Kawashima A, Ueda Y, Tsuchiya H, Tomita K, Nagai Y, Nakanishi I. Immunohistochemical localization of collagenous proteins in cartilaginous tumors: characteristic distribution of type IX collagen. J Cancer Res Clin Oncol 1993: 120: 35–40

73. Vollmer E, Roessner A, Wuisman P, Härle A, Grundmann E. The proliferation behavior of bone tumors investigated with the monoclonal antibody Ki-67. In: Roessner A, Ed. Biological characterization of bone tumors. Berlin: Springer, 1989, pp 91–114

74. Scotlandi K, Serra M, Manara M C et al. Clinical relevance of Ki-67 expression in bone tumors. Cancer 1995: 75: 806–814

75. Ohno T, Tanaka T, Takeuchi S, Matsunaga T, Mori H. Silver-stained nucleolar organizer proteins in chondrosarcoma. Virchows Arch B Cell Pathol 1991: 60: 207–211

76. Wrba F, Gullick W J, Fertl H, Amann G, Salzer-Kuntschik M. Immunohistochemical detection of the c-erbB-2 proto-oncogene product in normal, benign and malignant cartilage tissues. Histopathology 1989: 15: 71–76

77. Castresana J S, Barrios C, Gomez L, Kreicbergs A. Amplification of the c-myc proto-oncogene in human chondrosarcoma. Diagn Mol Pathol 1992: 1: 235–238

78. Dobashi Y, Sugimura H, Sato A et al. Possible association of p53 overexpression and mutation with high-grade chondrosarcoma. Diagn Mol Pathol 1993: 2: 257–263

79. Coughlan B, Feliz A, Ishida T, Czerniak B, Dorfman H D. p53 expression and DNA ploidy of cartilage lesions. Hum Pathol 1995: 26: 620–624

80. Kreicbergs A, Zetterberg A, Soderberg G. The prognostic significance of nuclear DNA content in chondrosarcoma. Anal Quant Cytol 1980: 2: 272–278

81. Alho A, Connor J F, Mankin H J, Schiller A L, Campbell C J. Assessment of malignancy of cartilage tumors using flow cytometry. A preliminary report. J Bone Joint Surg (Am) 1983: 65: 779–785

82. Mankin H J, Connor J F, Schiller A L, Perlmutter N, Alho A, McGuire M. Grading of bone tumors by analysis of nuclear DNA content using flow cytometry. J Bone Joint Surg (Am) 1985: 67: 404–413

83. Kreicbergs A, Boquist L, Borssen B, Larsson S E. Prognostic factors in chondrosarcoma. A comparative study of cellular DNA content and clinicopathologic features. Cancer 1982: 50: 577–583

84. Heliö H, Karaharju E, Bôhling T, Kivioja A, Nordling S. Chondrosarcoma of bone. A clinical and DNA flow cytometric study. Eur J Surg Oncol 1995: 21: 408–413

85. Adler C P, Herget G W, Neuburger M. Cartilaginous tumors. Prognostic applications of cytophotometric DNA analysis. Cancer 1995: 76: 1176–1180

86. Cuvelier C A, Roels H J. Cytophotometric studies of the nuclear DNA content in cartilaginous tumors. Cancer 1979: 44: 1363–1374

87. Kreicbergs A, Silfersward C, Tribukait B. Flow DNA analysis of primary bone tumors. Relationship between cellular DNA content and histopathologic classification. Cancer 1984: 53: 129–136

88. Xiang J H, Spanier S S, Benson N A, Braylan R C. Flow cytometric analysis of DNA in bone and soft-tissue tumors using nuclear suspensions. Cancer 1987: 59: 1951–1958

89. Mandahl N, Heim S, Arheden K, Rydholm A, Willen H, Mitelman F. Chromosomal rearrangements in chondromatous tumors. Cancer 1990: 65: 242–248

90. Hirabayashi Y, Yoshida M A, Ikeuchi T et al. Chromosome rearrangements at 12q13 in two cases of chondrosarcomas. Cancer Genet Cytogenet 1992: 60: 35–40

91. Bridge J A, Bhatia P S, Anderson J R, Neff J R. Biologic and clinical significance of cytogenetic and molecular cytogenetic abnormalities in benign and malignant cartilaginous lesions. Cancer Genet Cytogenet 1993: 69: 79–90

92. Örndal C, Mandahl N, Rydholm A, Willen H, Brosjo O, Mitelman F. Chromosome aberrations and cytogenetic intratumor heterogeneity in chondrosarcomas. J Cancer Res Clin Oncol 1993: 120: 51–56

93. Dijkhuizen T, Van Den Berg E, Molenaar W M et al. Cytogenetics as a tool in the histologic subclassification of chondrosarcomas. Cancer Genet Cytogenet 1994: 76: 100–105

94. Fletcher J A, Lipinski K K, Weidner N, Morton C C. Complex cytogenetic aberrations in a well-differentiated chondrosarcoma. Cancer Genet Cytogenet 1989: 41: 115–121

95. Erlandson R A, Huvos A G. Chondrosarcoma: a light and electron microscopic study. Cancer 1974: 34: 1642–1652

96. Povysil C, Matejovsky Z. A comparative ultrastructural study of chondrosarcoma, chordoid sarcoma, chordoma and chordoma periphericum. Pathol Res Pract 1985: 179: 546–559

97. Martinez-Tello F J, Martinez-Gonzalez M A. The ultrastructure of the cartilaginous tumors. In: Bonucci E, Motta P M, Eds. Ultrastructure of skeletal tissues. Boston: Kluwer, 1990, pp 189–205

98. Ghadially F N, Lalonde J M, Yong N K. Amianthoid fibres in a chondrosarcoma. J Pathol 1980: 130: 147–151

99. Jaworski R C. Intramitochondrial paracrystalline inclusions in chondrosarcoma. Pathology 1984: 16: 172–173

100. Pope T L Jr, McLaughin R, Wanebo H J, Williamson B R J, Fechner R E. Case report 281. Low-grade cartilaginous tumor with 'skip lesion'. Skeletal Radiol 1984: 12: 134–138

101. Disler D G, Rosenberg A E, Springfield D, O'Connell J X, Rosenthal D I, Kattapuram S V. Extensive skeletal metastases from chondrosarcoma without pulmonary involvement. Skeletal Radiol 1993: 22: 595–599

102. Harwood A R, Krajbich J I, Fornasier V L. Radiotherapy of chondrosarcoma of bone. Cancer 1980: 45: 2769–2777

103. Marcove R C, Mike V, Hutter R V et al. Chondrosarcoma of the pelvis and upper end of the femur: an analysis of factors influencing survival time in one hundred and thirteen cases. J Bone Joint Surg (Am) 1972: 54: 561–572

104. Kristensen I B, Munk Sunde L M, Jensen O M. Chondrosarcoma. Increasing grade of malignancy in local recurrence. Acta Pathol Microbiol Immunol Scand A 1986: 94: 73–77
105. Lindbom A, Soderberg G, Spjut H J. Primary chondrosarcoma of bone. Acta Radiol 1961: 55: 81–96
106. Ozaki T, Lindner N, Hillmann A, Rôdl R, Blasius S, Winkelmann W. Influence of intralesional surgery on treatment outcome of chondrosarcoma. Cancer 1996: 77: 1292–1297
107. Bauer H C, Brosjö O, Kreicbergs A, Lindholm J. Low risk of recurrence of enchondroma and low-grade chondrosarcoma in extremities. 80 patients followed for 2–25 years. Acta Orthop Scand 1995: 66: 283–288
108. Sanerkin N G, Gallagher P. A review of the behaviour of chondrosarcoma of bone. J Bone Joint Surg (Br) 1979: 61: 395–400
109. Ishida T, Dorfman H D, Bullough P G. Tophaceous pseudogout (tumoral calcium pyrophosphate dihydrate crystal deposition disease). Hum Pathol 1995: 26: 587–593
110. Mirra J M, Gold R, Downs J, Eckardt J J. A new histologic approach to the differentiation of enchondroma and chondrosarcoma of the bones. A clinicopathologic analysis of 51 cases. Clin Orthop 1985: 201: 214–237
111. Schiller A L. Diagnosis of borderline cartilage lesions of bone. Semin Diagn Pathol 1985: 2: 42–62
112. Böhm G, Salzer-Kuntschik M, Lintner F. Morphometric analysis of cartilaginous tumors. Pathol Res Pract 1992: 188: 570–575
113. Barnes R, Catto M. Chondrosarcoma of bone. J Bone Joint Surg (Br) 1966: 48: 729–764
114. Jelthi A, Forest M, Tomeno B, Abelanet R. Resorption et remodelage osseux dans les chondrosarcomes des membres et des ceintures. Valeur diagnostique à propos de 84 cas. Ann Pathol 1987: 7: 198–208
115. Tsuchiya H, Ueda Y, Morishita H et al. Borderline chondrosarcoma of long and flat bones. J Cancer Res Clin Oncol 1993: 119: 363–368

15

Chondrosarcoma: variants

M. Forest

PERIOSTEAL CHONDROSARCOMA

This form of tumor, originally reported by Lichtenstein in 1955,[1] accounts for only 1–2% of all chondrosarcomas. The term 'juxtacortical chondrosarcoma' has been advocated by Jaffe and Schajowicz.

Periosteal chondrosarcomas occur chiefly in the fourth decade[2] and there is a slight male predominance.[3] Clinical symptoms are swelling and pain; some patients may not experience pain.[3]

The reported locations are the femur, humerus, innominate bone, metatarsals[2] and even the hands.[4,5] Like parosteal osteosarcomas, periosteal chondrosarcomas may be found on the posterior aspect of the distal femur.[3]

In long bones (Figs 15.1–15.11), the lesions tend to affect the metaphysis or are metadiaphyseal; the cortex may be eroded, saucerized or thickened, with or without periosteal buttresses. Matrix calcifications are inconstant, appearing as spotty, popcorn or eggshell areas.[2,3]

Grossly, periosteal chondrosarcomas are large masses (average size is more than 11 cm), made of a slightly lobular, grayish-white tissue, with or without yellowish calcifications or ossifications, the irregular surface being covered by a thick fibrous layer. Soft tissues may be invaded, the cortex more rarely.

Histologically, most tumors are well differentiated (grade I or II), eventually showing calcifications or areas of enchondral ossification (Figs 15.12–15.16).

The treatment is wide resection; metastases are uncommon and appear very late in the clinical course.[3] Regional lymph node metastases have been reported in a long-standing case.[6] Only one case of dedifferentiation has been documented, in the form of a malignant fibrous histiocytoma.[7]

Periosteal chondrosarcomas must be differentiated from periosteal chondromas and periosteal osteosarcomas, periosteal chondrosarcomas usually being secondary tumors with, in some cases, the remnants of an osteochondroma.

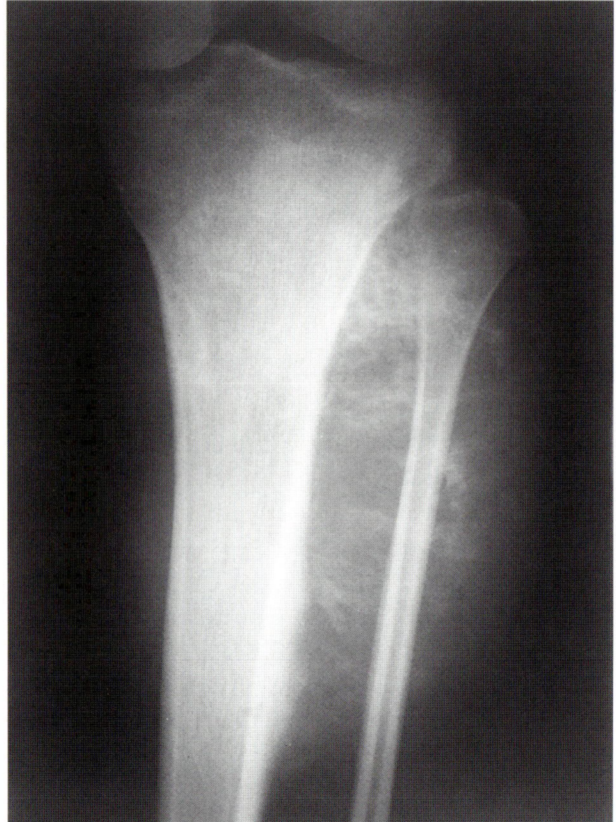

Fig. 15.1

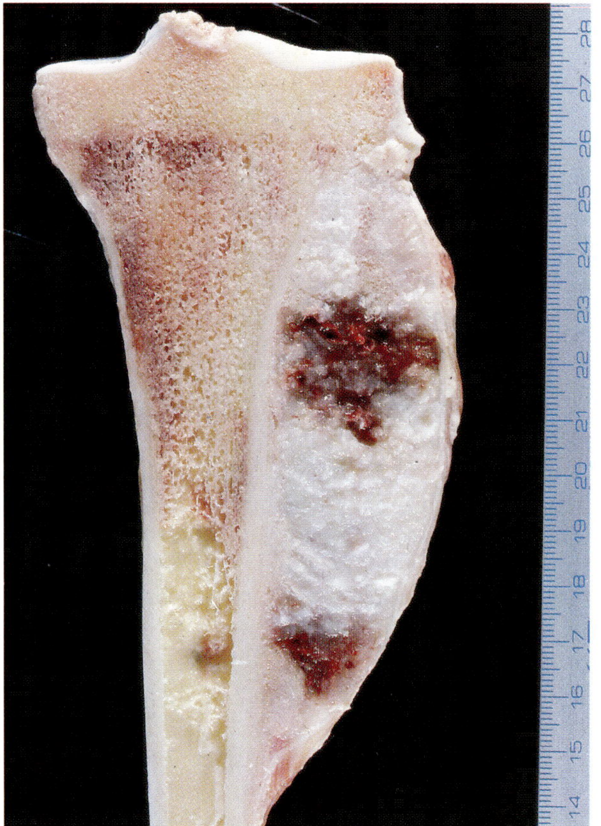

Fig. 15.2

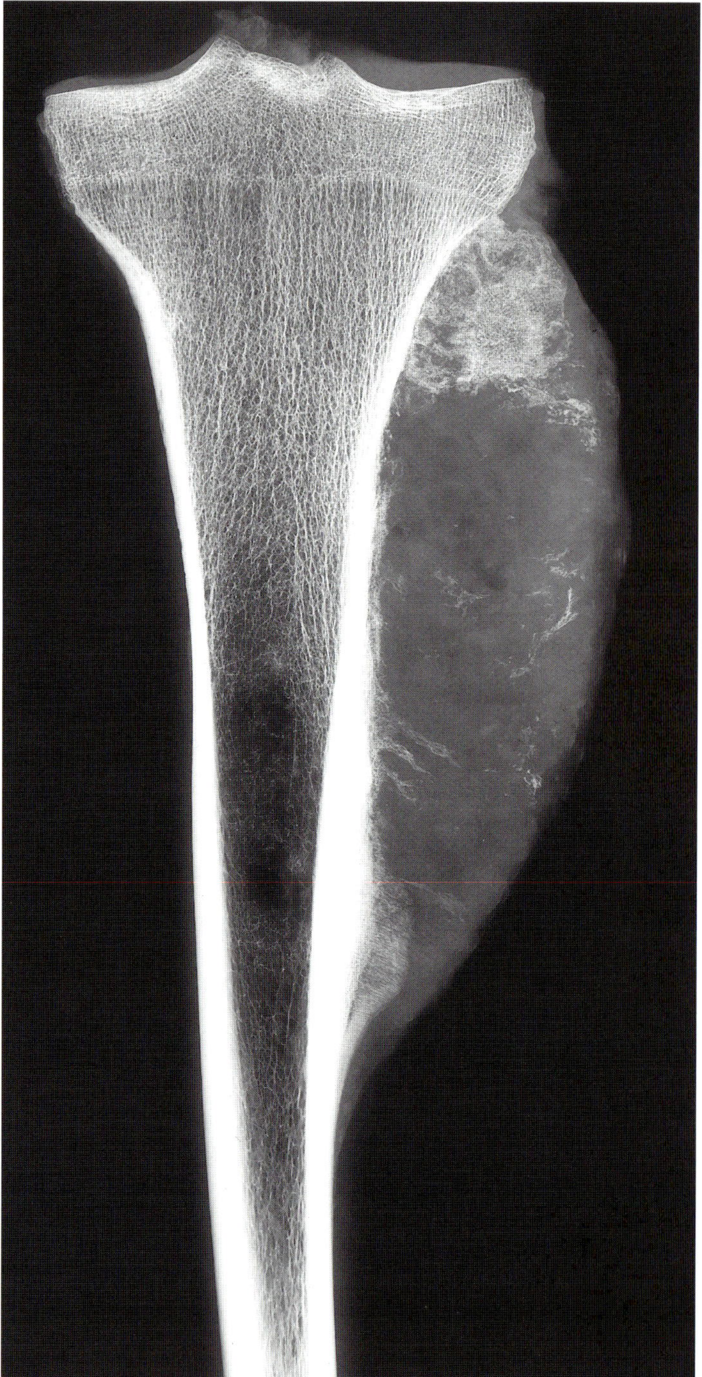

Fig. 15.3

Figs 15.1–15.3 Periosteal chondrosarcoma of the tibia.

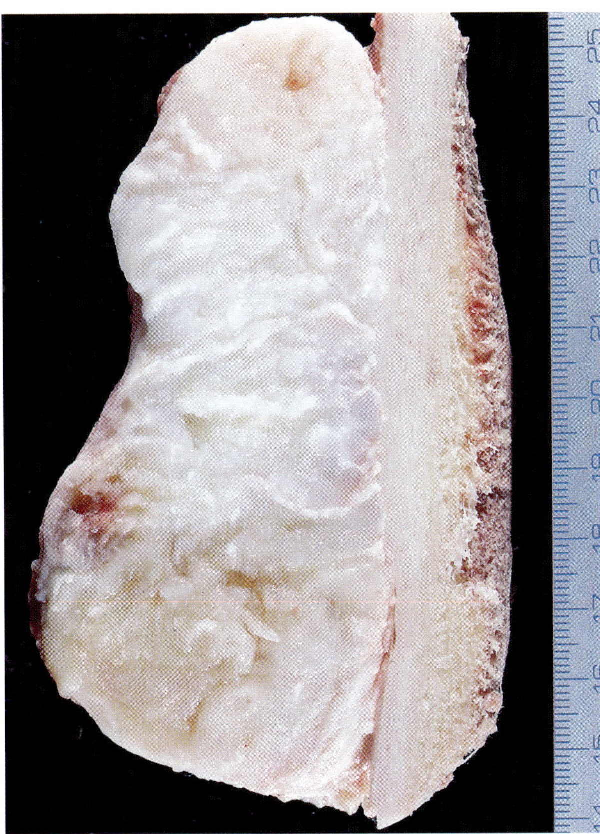

Fig. 15.4 Periosteal chondrosarcoma: posterior aspect of the femur.

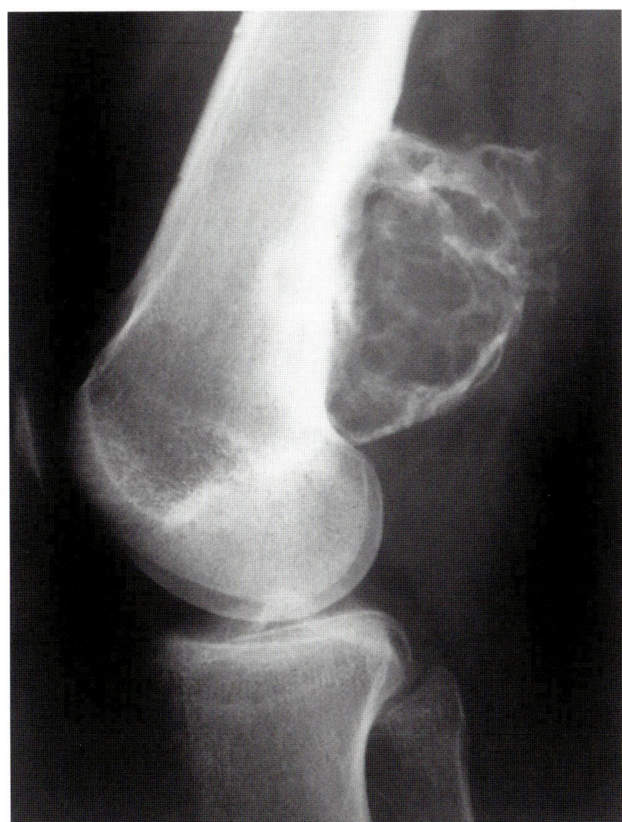

Fig. 15.5

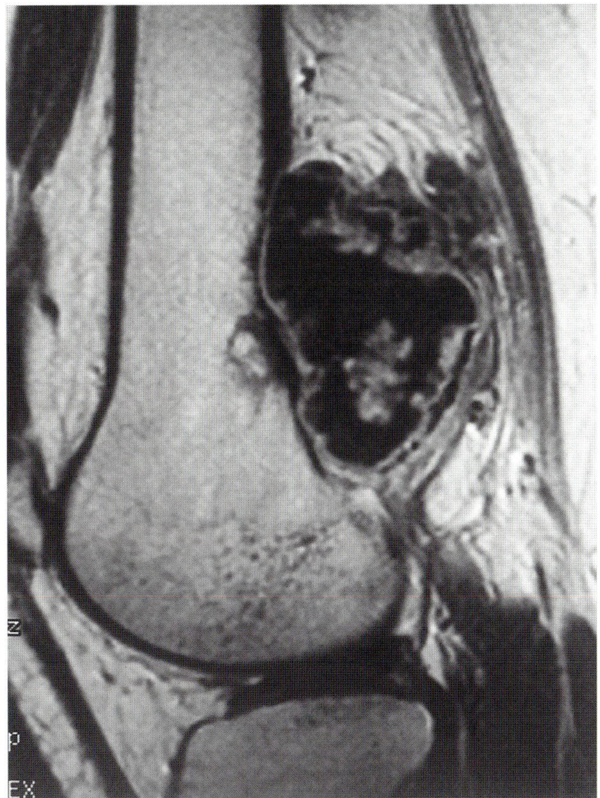

Fig. 15.6

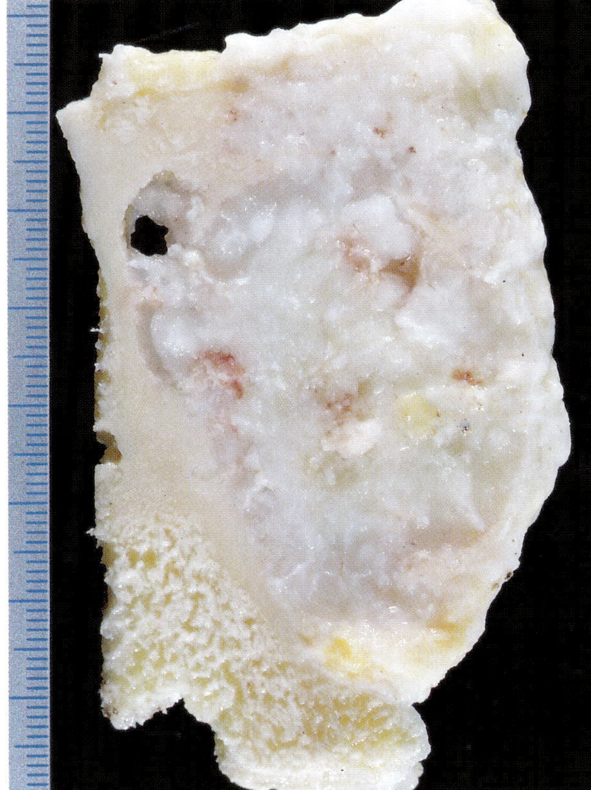

Fig. 15.7

Figs 15.5–15.7 Periosteal chondrosarcoma: posterior aspect of the femur.

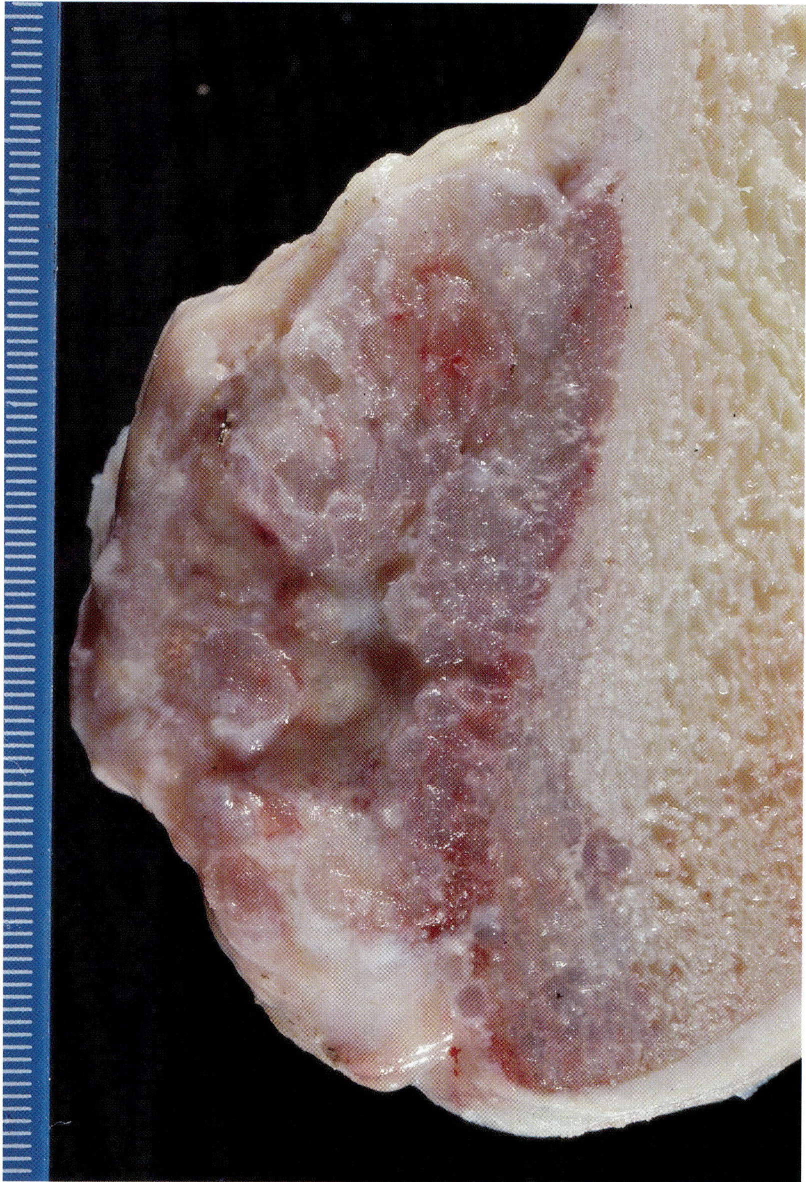

Fig. 15.8 Unusual periosteal chondrosarcoma of the femur centered in the epiphysis.

Periosteal chondromas, occurring in younger patients, are smaller (rarely more than 6 cm). They may be quite cellular, with plump nuclei and binucleate chondrocytes. Malignancy is chiefly assessed by the pattern of infiltration of the surrounding tissues.[2]

The differential diagnosis with periosteal osteosarcomas has caused much debate between Schajowicz,[8] the Mayo Clinic and the Rizzoli Institute.[2,3] For Schajowicz, the diagnosis could only be made after a complete study of the resection specimen[9,10], insuring that the lace-like tumoral osteoid is not confused with strands of calcified cartilage or areas of enchondral ossification.[11] The patients are younger and exhibit more pain than periosteal chondrosarcomas. Periosteal osteosarcomas are more fusiform lesions, occurring in the midshaft of long bones. On X-ray, spicules of reactive bone are perpendicular to the cortex and may be associated with Codman's triangles.

Histologically, the tumors are more cellular, with a cartilage component of grade II–III,[3] showing a spindling of cells at the periphery of the lobules.[2] The diagnosis is made on the finding of tumoral lace-like osteoid. A double immunohistochemical staining using proliferative cell nuclear antigen and S-100 protein has shown that in periosteal chondrosarcomas, the cartilage cells are the proliferative component.[12]

MESENCHYMAL CHONDROSARCOMA

This tumor, first described by Lichtenstein & Bernstein in 1959,[13] combines an undifferentiated cell component with

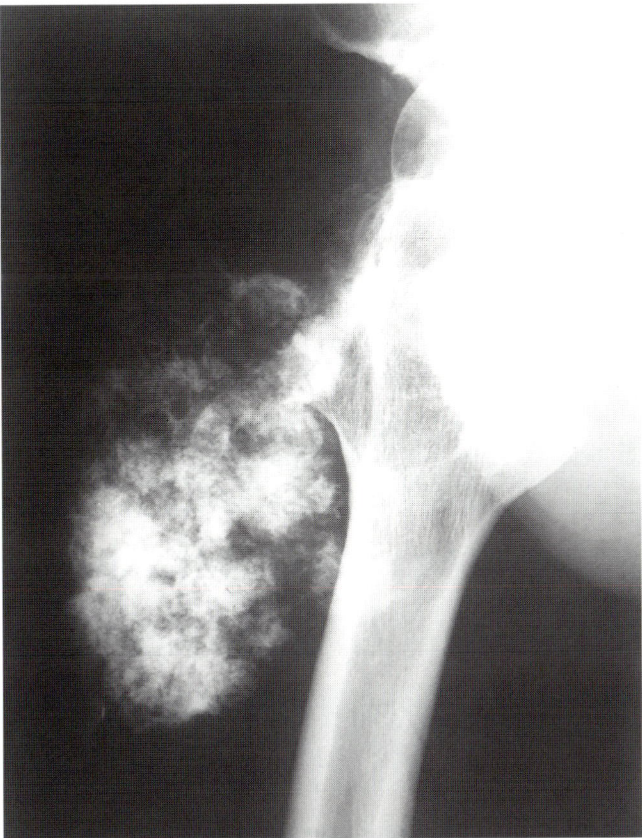

Fig. 15.9

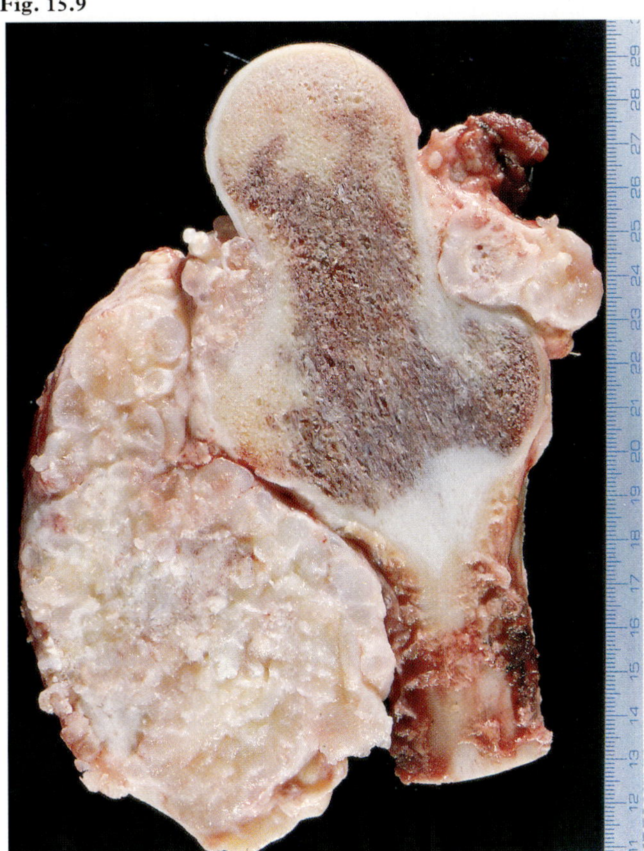

Fig. 15.10

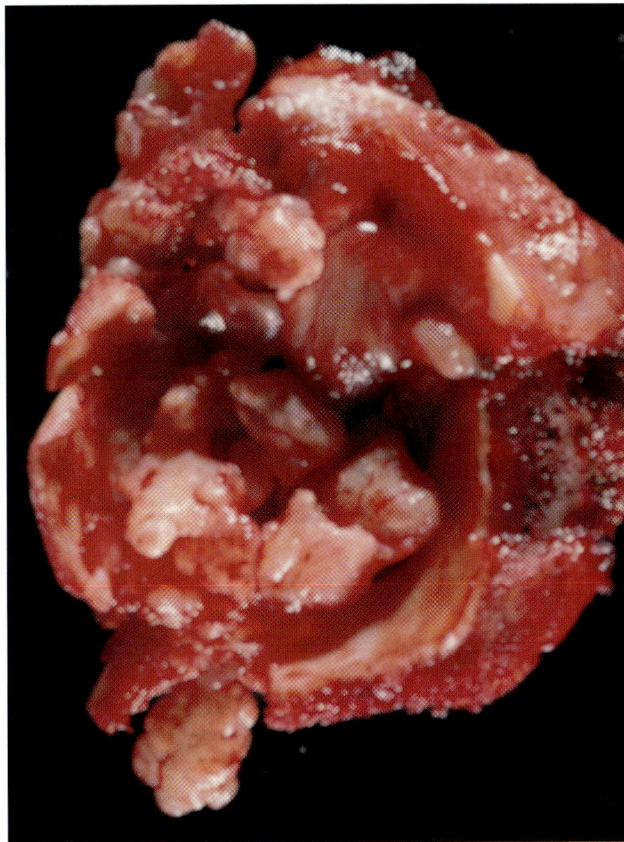

Fig. 15.11

Figs 15.9–15.11 Periosteal chondrosarcoma of the femur with involvement of the hip joint and synovial implantation.

well-differentiated cartilaginous areas of variable quantity. It accounts for about 2% of all chondrosarcomas.[14] Sixty percent of patients are in the second and third decades of life,[15] with an average age of 26 years;[16] the tumors being rare in the first decade.[17–19] Clinical symptoms are pain and swelling, with a duration from a few days to years.[20]

Common skeletal sites are the femur, the craniofacial bones, pelvic bones, ribs and vertebrae[16] (Figs 15.17–15.20). About one-third of cases involve extraosseous sites: brain, meninges or soft tissues of the lower extremities.[16] Multifocal synchronous or metasynchronous involvement of bone or bone and soft tissues has been reported,[15,16,18] as well as a radiation-induced sarcoma[21] and occurrence in fibrous dysplasia.[22]

At initial presentation, most tumors are large and destructive lesions, predominantly lytic, with ill-defined borders, destruction of the cortex and extension into the soft tissues;[15] some may show a purely lytic pattern, but stippled calcifications or irregularly calcified masses can be found in the tumor itself or in the soft tissue extension. There is usually little periosteal reaction.[14]

The location in long bones may be epiphyseal, diaphyseal[16,17] or even periosteal;[14,17] in some cases, the expansion of bone is associated with cortical thickening[14] or

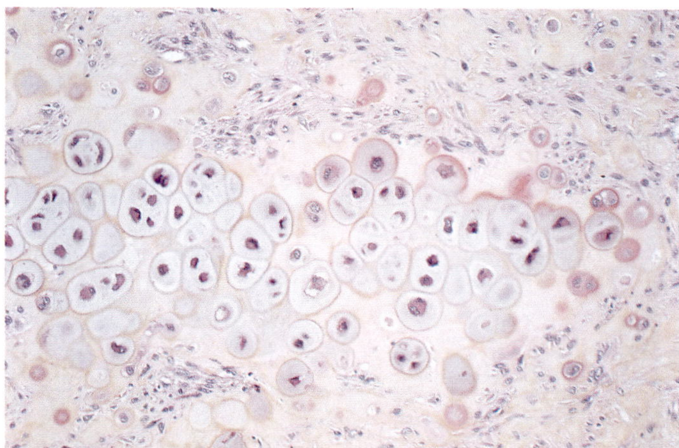

Fig. 15.12

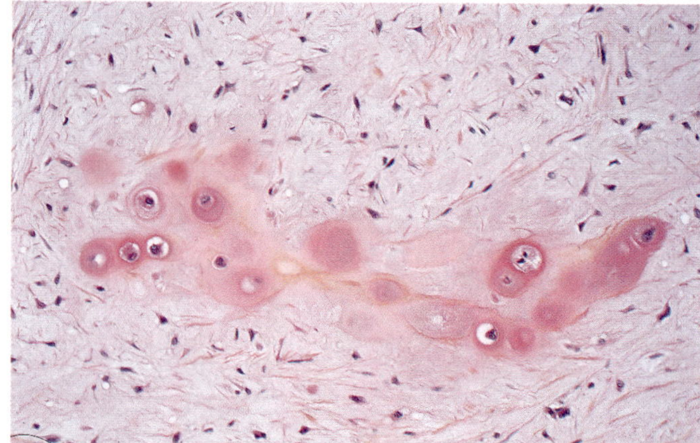

Fig. 15.13

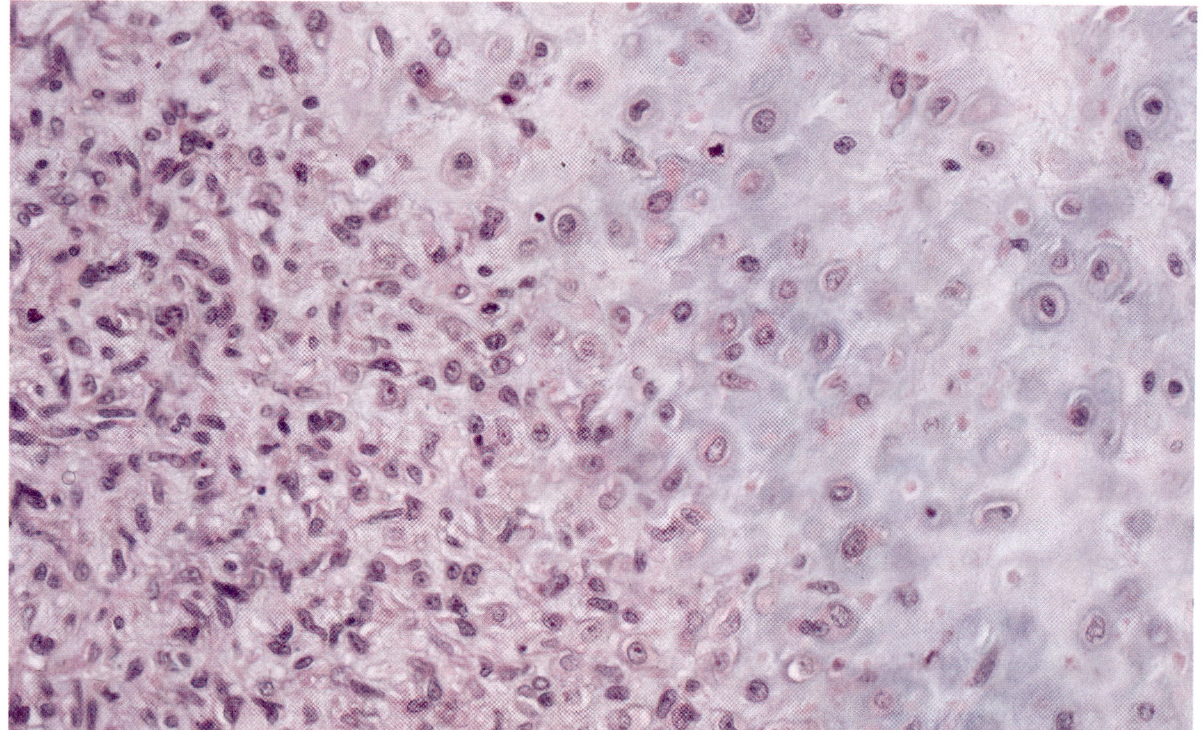

Fig. 15.15

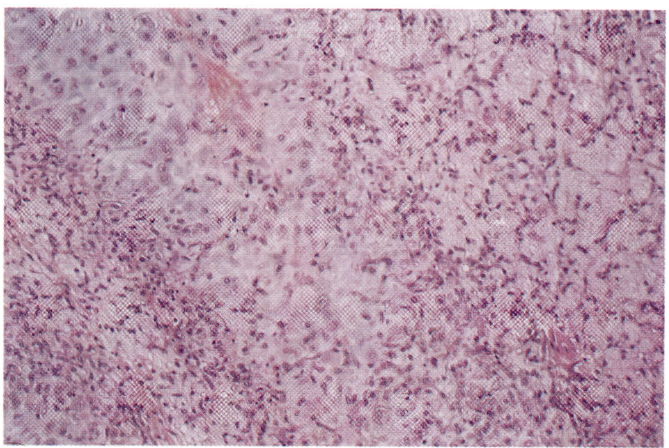

Fig. 15.14

Figs 15.12–15.15 Histology of periosteal chondrosarcoma with peripheral oval or spindle cell tumoral component.

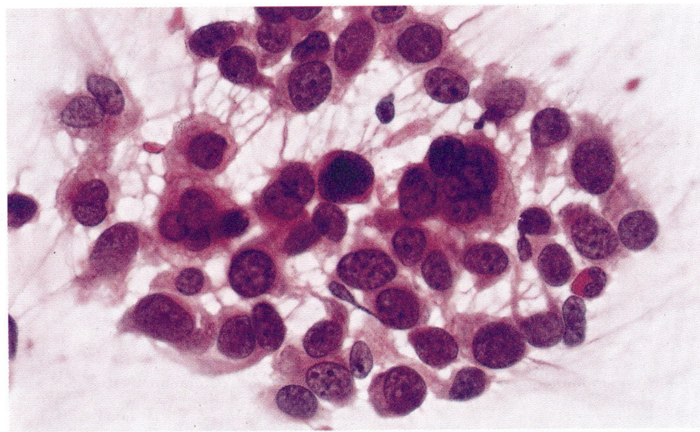

Fig. 15.16 Periosteal chondrosarcoma of the tibia: imprint cytology.

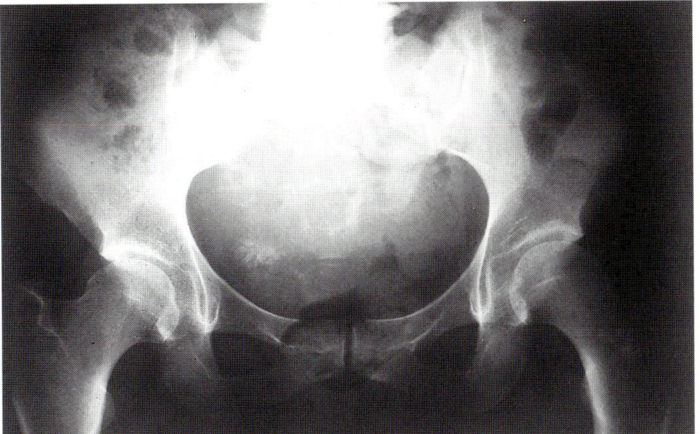

Fig. 15.17 Mesenchymal chondrosarcoma of the sacrum appearing as a purely lytic lesion.

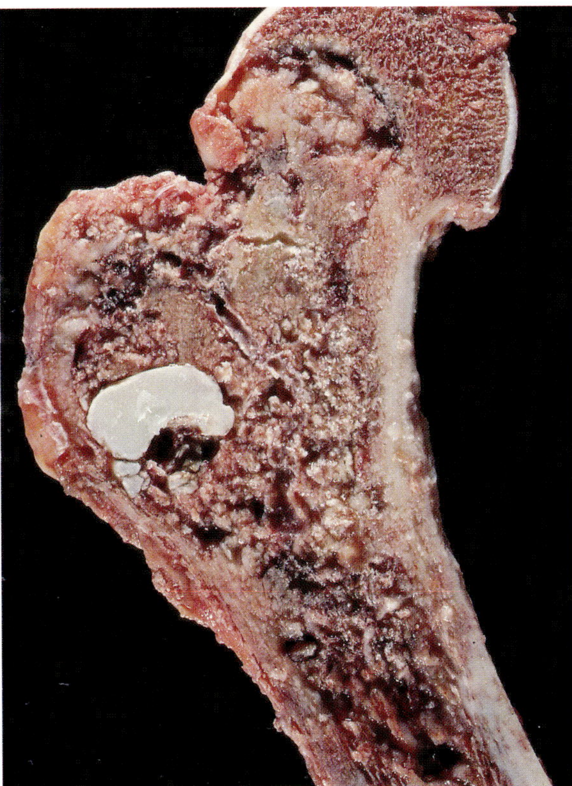

Fig. 15.19

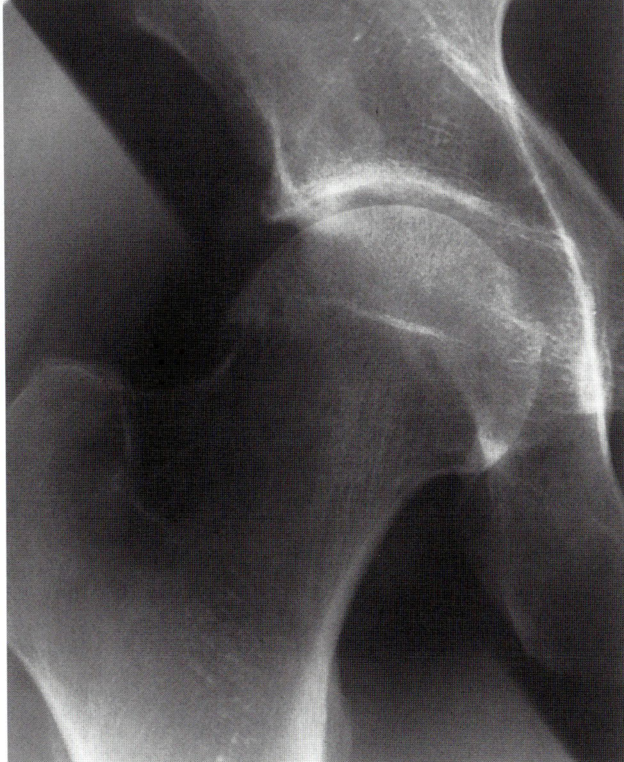

Fig. 15.18

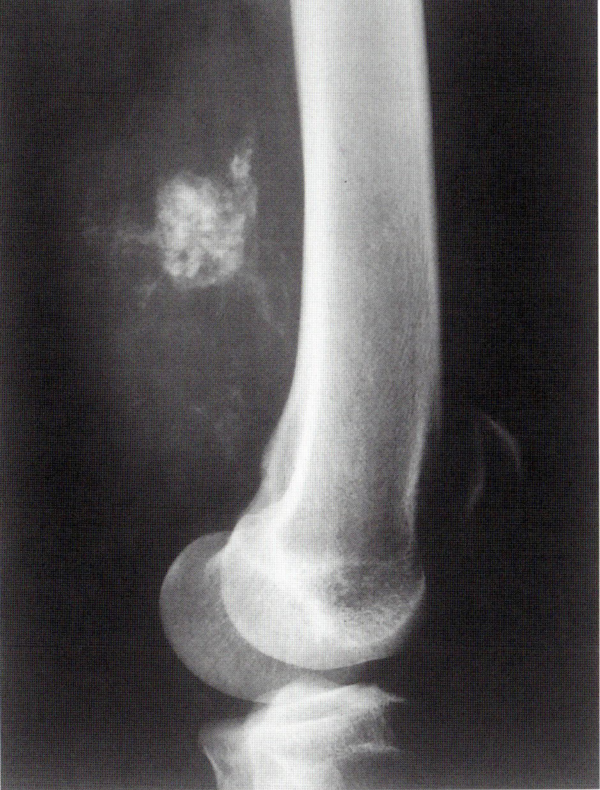

Fig. 15.20

Figs 15.18–15.20 Mesenchymal chondrosarcoma of the femur associated at initial presentation with a soft-tissue involvement in the thigh.

the tumor may appear as a saucer-like destruction in the midshaft.[18]

Grossly, the tumoral tissue is soft or firm, gray or reddish, with an average size of 12 cm,[16] eventually showing cartilage areas, calcifications, necrosis, hemorrhage or cyst formation.

Histologically (Figs 15.21–15.27), mesenchymal chondrosarcomas are highly cellular tumors, sometimes lobulated.[17] Most of the undifferentiated cells are small and lymphocyte-like, with scant cytoplasm and hyperchromatic nuclei of fairly uniform size; nucleoli are small and the mitotic activity is variable.[15] The cells may be larger, with a small rim of cytoplasm, or elongated.[15,16] Glycogen granules may be found in the cytoplasm.

The small or large chondroid areas are composed of low-grade tumor cartilage, the transition with the undifferentiated parts being sharp or less commanly gradual.[14,15] Some tumors may show extensive calcifications and enchondral ossification,[23] mineralization occurring in about 75% of cases. Necrosis may be prominent in a few cases.[17]

The vascularization comprises a capillary network and cleft-like spaces resembling those of hemangiopericytomas.[16,23]

Some authors suggest that the histological tissue pattern closely mimics early chondrogenesis.[24]

On smears, the small cells have a sparse cytoplasm; the nucleus is round, oval or elongated, with a coarse chromatin and one or more small nucleoli. Large chondroid tumor cells may be found, with a finely vacuolar cytoplasm and one or two rounded hyperchromatic nuclei.[25] The diagnosis, as well as the differential diagnosis with small cell osteosarcoma, is quite difficult on cytological findings alone.[25]

Immunohistochemically, the cartilage islands show S-100 protein positivity, but the small undifferentiated cells do not express the staining.[25–26] Isolated S-100-positive round cells can be found in the poorly differentiated areas; they are definitely cartilaginous.[27] Immunoreactivity for Leu-7 antigen, vimentin and in some cases for neuron-specific enolase is demonstrated,[28,29] the immunophenotype resembling that of embryonic cartilage. An unusually strong immunoreactivity for desmin and a scattered immunoreactivity for muscle-specific actin and smooth-muscle actin have been reported.[29] In rare cases of mesenchymal chondrosarcoma, immunodetection of the glycoprotein p30/32 MIC2 antigen, known to be specific for Ewing's sarcoma and primitive neuroectodermal tumors, gives positive results.[30]

On a cytophotometric study of DNA, tumors are aneuploid.[31]

A cytogenetic study has shown a highly abnormal hyper-tetraploid chromosomal pattern with numerous clonal abnormalities.[29,32] In culture, a reciprocal translocation t(11;22)(q24;12), characterizing Ewing's sarcoma and primitive neuroectodermal tumors, has been reported, suggesting that mesenchymal chondrosarcoma could be related to Ewing's sarcoma.[33]

Ultrastructurally, undifferentiated cells are similar in size and shape,[29,34,35] with a moderate number of organelles in a scant cytoplasm containing small amounts of glycogen[34,36] and lipid vacuoles. The nuclei are round or oval,[36] with a dispersed chromatin and small or large nucleoli. The intercellular matrix is very sparse.[14,34]

A transition of undifferentiated cells to chondrocytes has been reported,[38] as well as round cells resembling neoplastic cartilage cells in the undifferentiated areas.[27] Ultrastructural findings support the view of Lichtenstein: undifferentiated cells are derived from the primitive mesenchyme involved in chondroblastic differentiation.[27,36]

Metastases are chiefly located in the lung;[15] they may involve bone, soft tissues and regional or distant lymph nodes, in some cases appearing years after treatment.[15,39]

The treatment is radical surgery; in cases of inadequate tumor removal, surgery is combined with chemotherapy and radiotherapy,[16,39] but the course is particularly aggressive and the 10-year survival is only 28%.[15,16] It has been stated that the hemangiopericytoma-like variant seems to respond to a multidrug chemotherapy used for osteosarcomas, in addition to surgical treatment, and the small cell variant to a combination of chemotherapy and irradiation as in Ewing's sarcoma.[16] This view is disputed.[15]

A secure diagnosis is only made on the biphasic pattern: anaplastic cells and well-differentiated tumoral cartilage. There is now some doubt about the specificity of immunohistochemistry in differentiating mesenchymal chondrosarcoma from Ewing's sarcoma[30] and one has to rely on the presence or absence of the chondroid component.

In the same way, small cell osteosarcomas are diagnosed on the tumoral bone production. In dedifferentiated chondrosarcoma, the sarcoma component associated with the well-differentiated cartilage exhibits a broad histological pattern ranging from fibrosarcoma, malignant fibrous histiocytoma, osteosarcoma to even muscular tumors.

CLEAR CELL CHONDROSARCOMA

These cartilage tumors, accounting for less than 2% of all chondrosarcomas,[40,41] are distinguished by their cytology, epiphyseal location in long bones and protracted course.[40]

Most patients are in their third and fourth decades and there is a male predominance (2.6:1[42]). Clinical symptoms are local pain and swelling or may be related to the adjacent joint; the clinical course is usually of long duration, ranging from 1 to 23 years.[43,44] Some tumors may be an incidental finding.[45] Pathological fractures have been reported in about a quarter of cases.[46–49]

The most common sites in long bones (85% of cases) are the proximal femur (head and neck region[42,48]) (Figs 15.28–15.40), followed by the proximal humerus

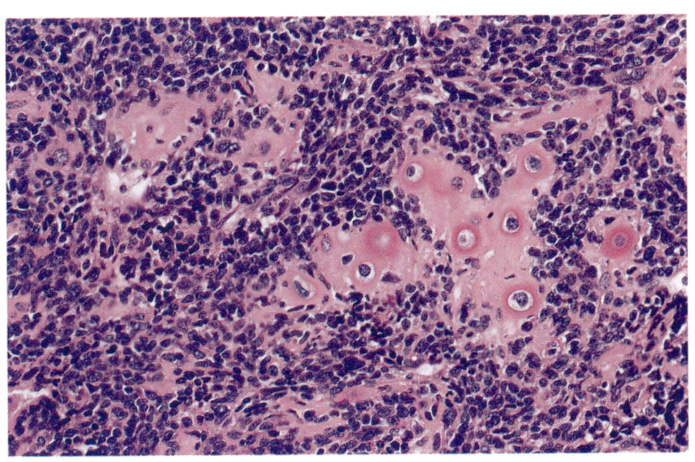

Fig. 15.21

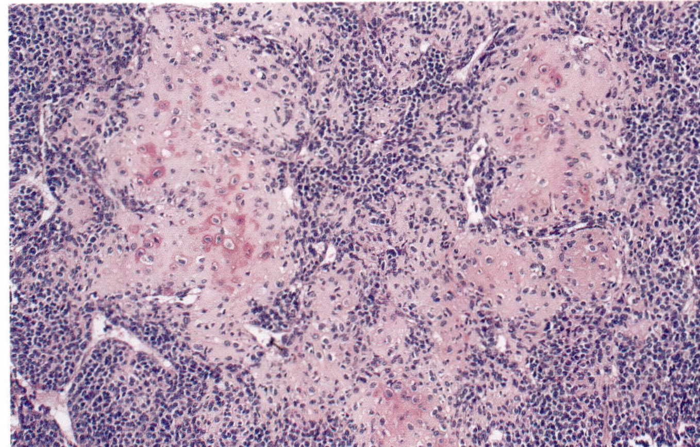

Fig. 15.23

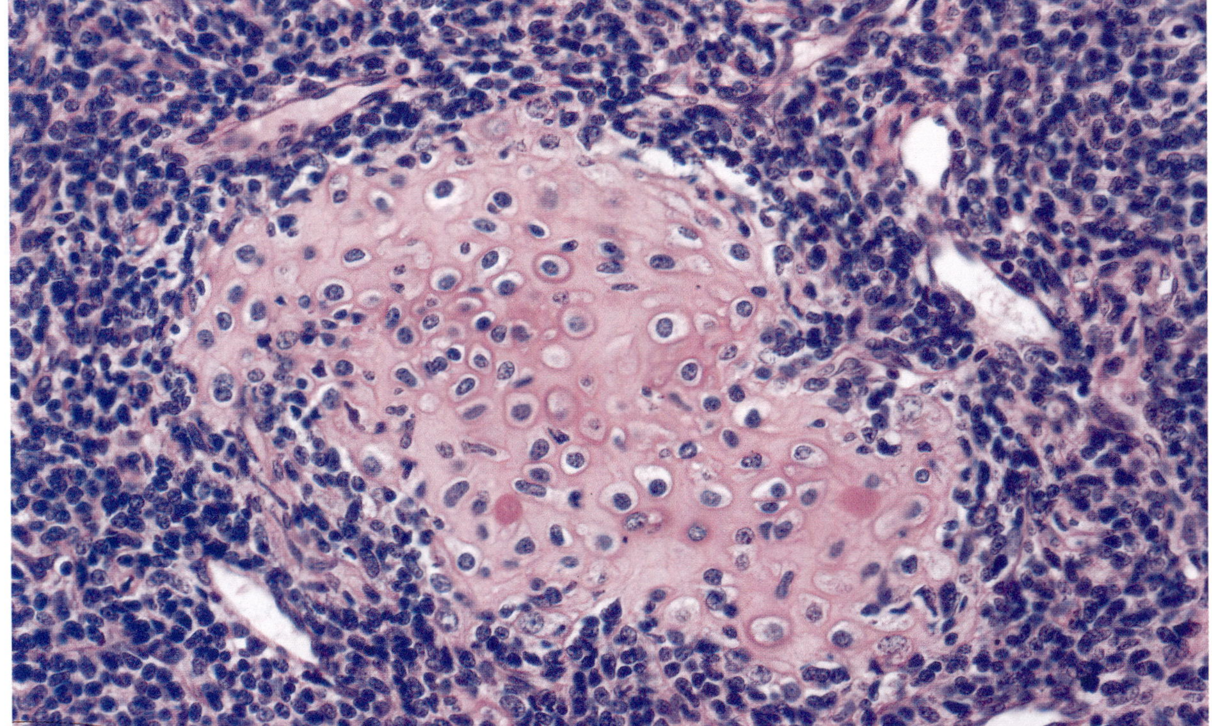

Fig. 15.22

Figs 15.21–15.24 Mesenchymal chondrosarcoma: undifferentiated small cell component with areas of well-differentiated cartilage.

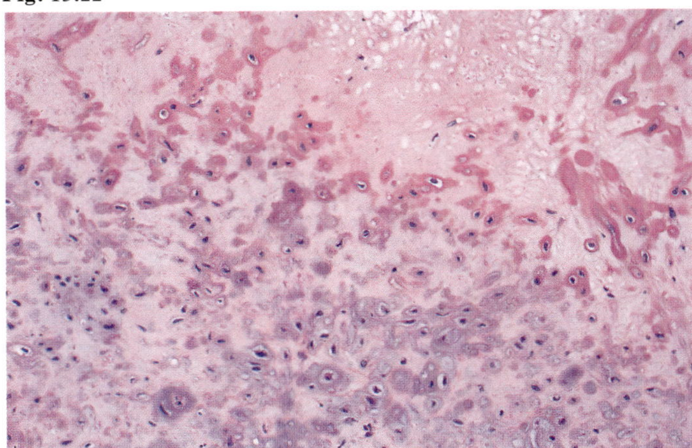

Fig. 15.24

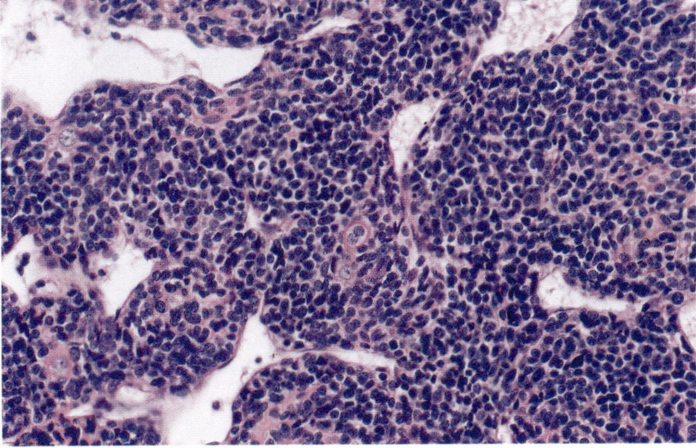

Fig. 15.25 Mesenchymal chondrosarcoma: vascularization resembling that of a hemangiopericytoma.

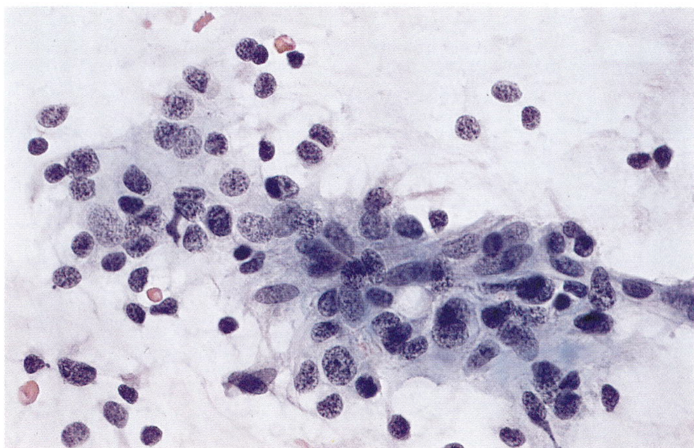

Fig. 15.26 Mesenchymal chondrosarcoma: imprint cytology demonstrating the undifferentiated cell component.

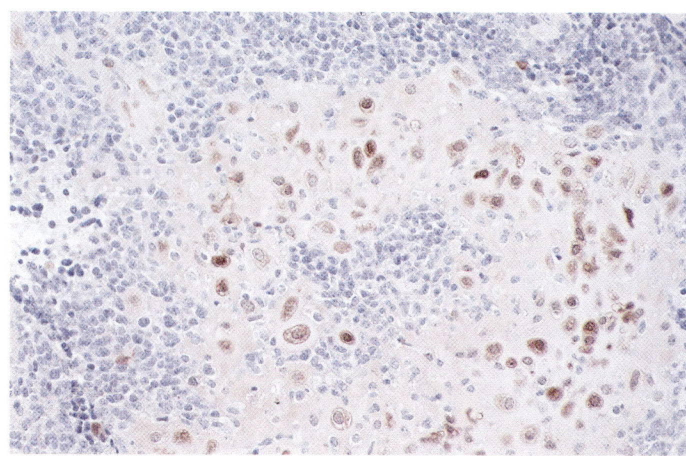

Fig. 15.27 Mesenchymal chondrosarcoma: undifferentiated cells do not express S-100 protein.

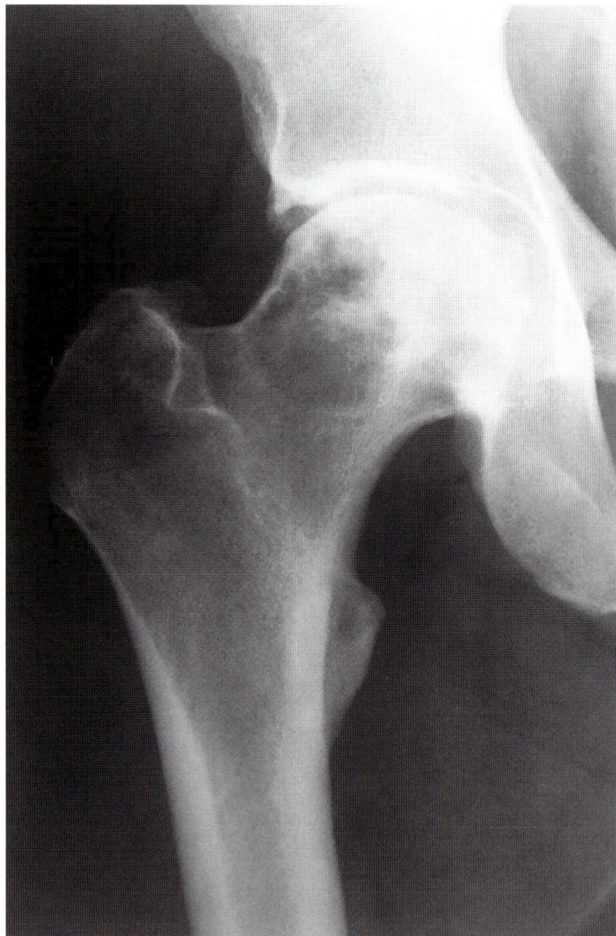

Fig. 15.28

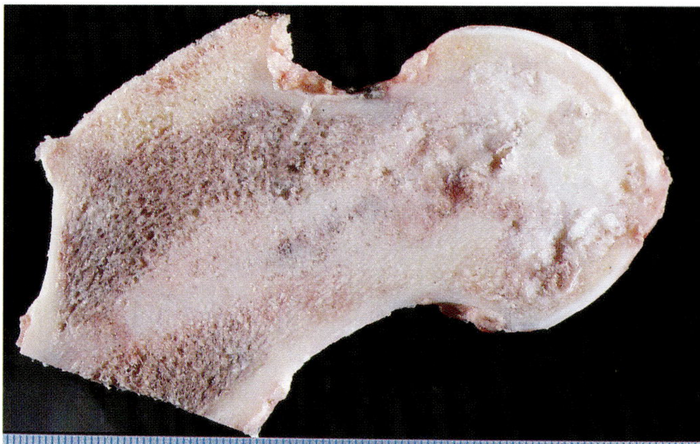

Fig. 15.29

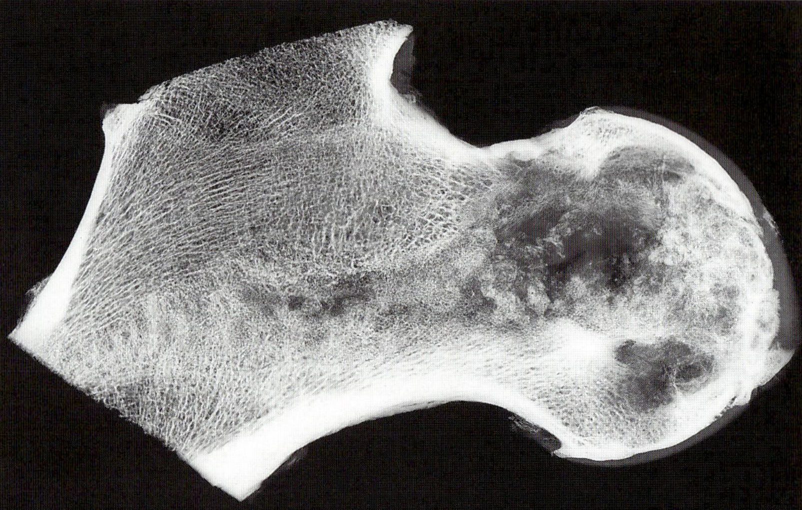

Figs 15.28–15.30 Small clear cell chondrosarcoma of the femur.　**Fig. 15.30**

(Figs 15.41–15.44) and the tibia[50] (Figs 15.45–15.49). Rarer sites are the vertebrae, ribs, scapula, skull, maxilla, pubic bone and small bones of hands and feet.[41,50,51] Multiple simultaneous or metachronous sites of involvement have been described.[40]

In long bones, clear cell chondrosarcomas are located in the epiphysis, with extension to the metaphysis in large lesions. Primary involvement of the metaphysis or diaphysis is unusual,[42,52] as are subperiosteal locations (Mulder et al 1993). In most cases, they appear as sharply delineated osteolytic lesions but indistinct or, more rarely, sclerotic borders have been described. The cortex may be

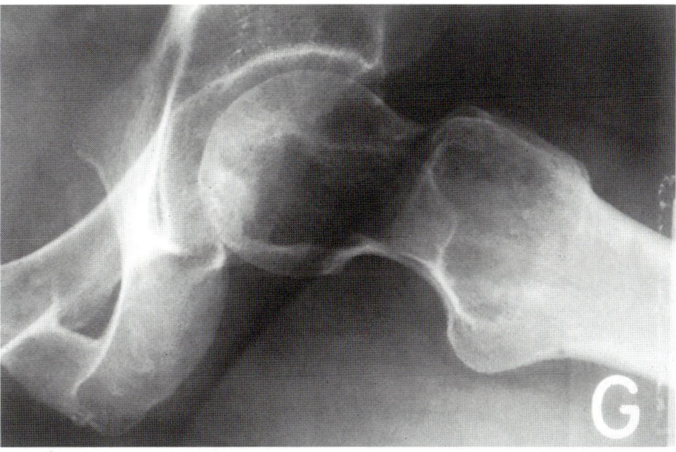

Fig. 15.31

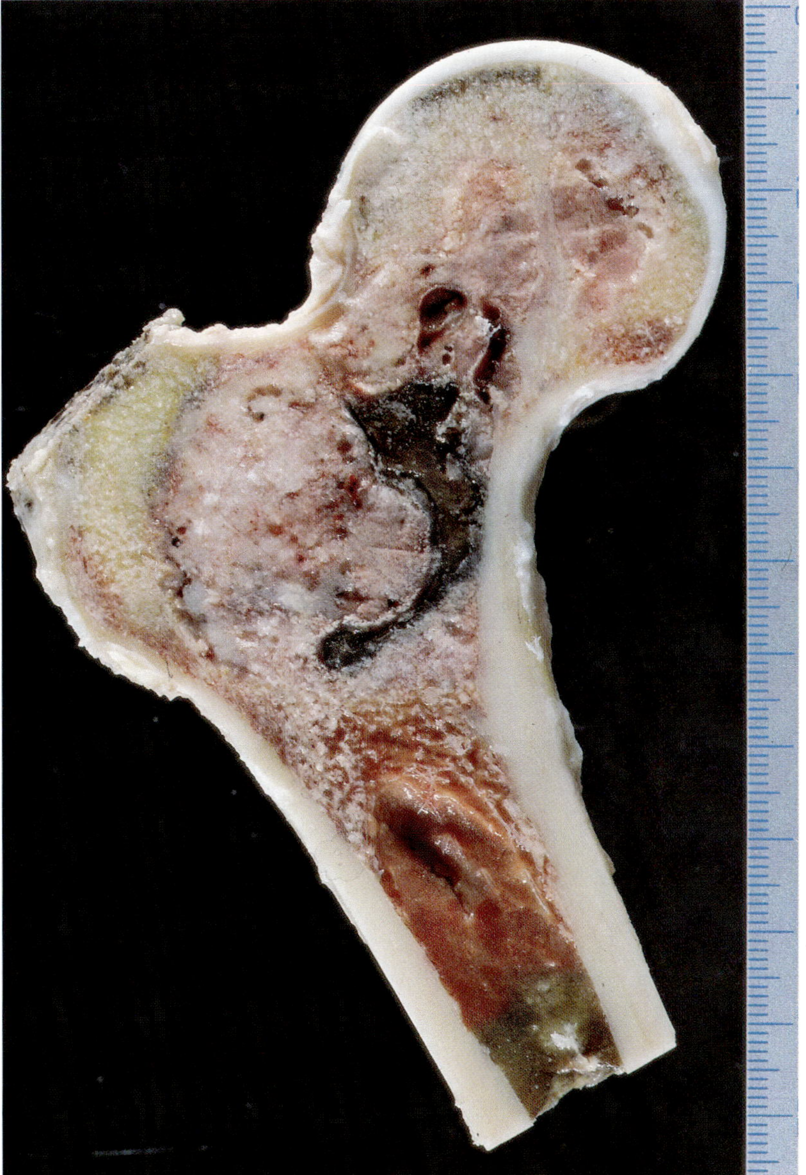

Fig. 15.32

Figs 15.31–15.33 Epiphyseal clear cell chondrosarcoma of the femur extending to the metaphysis.

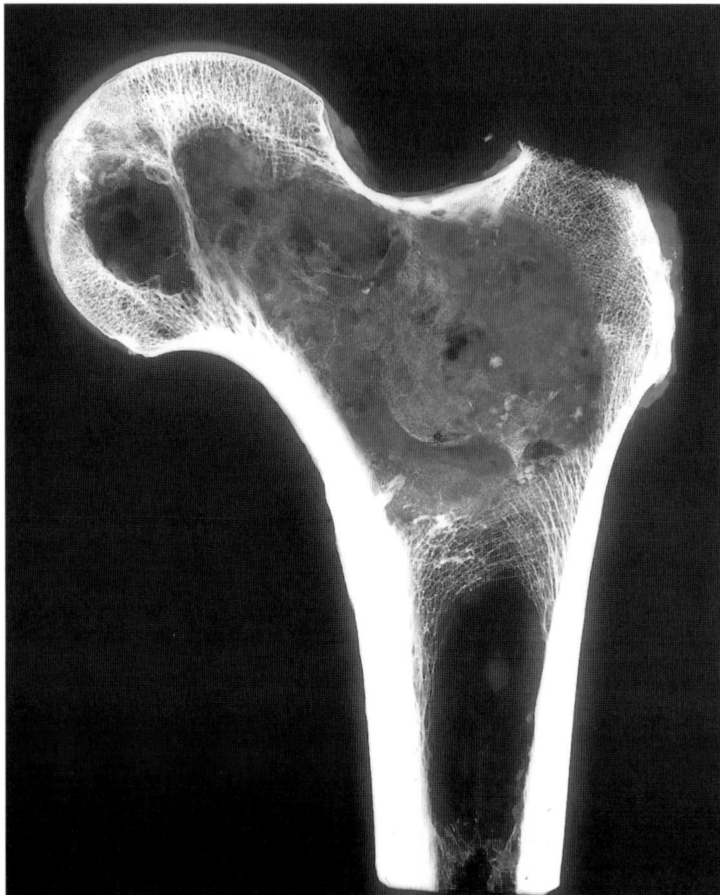

Fig. 15.33

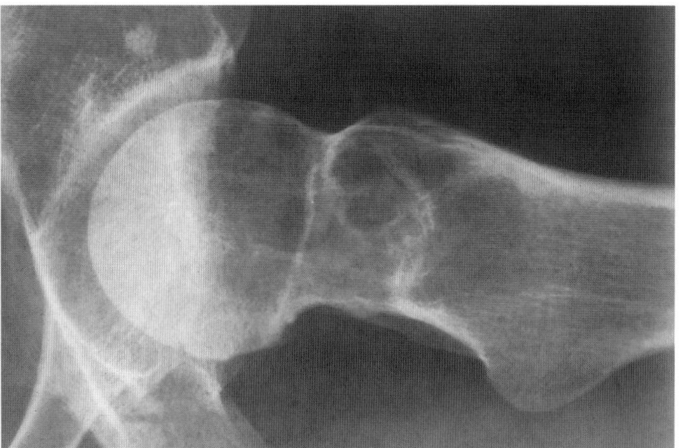

Fig. 15.34

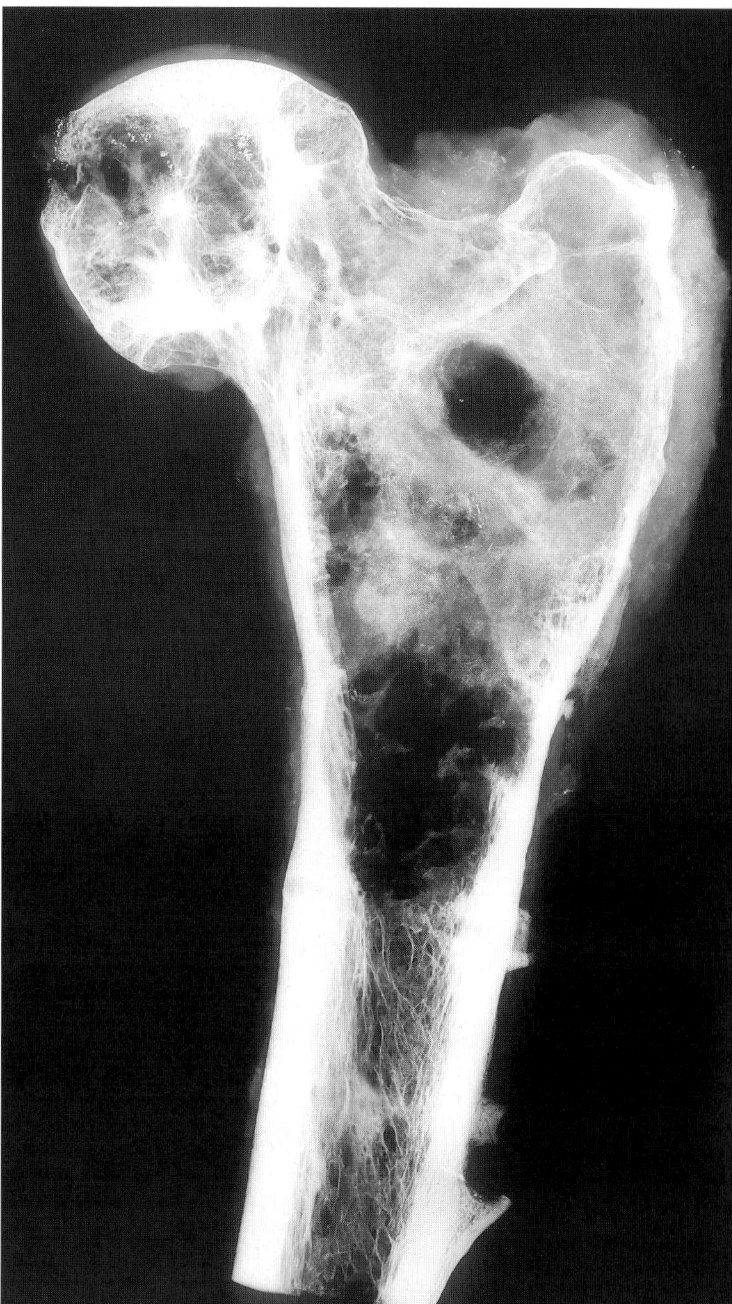

Fig. 15.35

Figs 15.34, 15.35 Protracted course of a clear cell chondrosarcoma of the femur, with involvement of the metaphysis, after initial curettage.

thinned or may show endosteal erosions; infiltration is rare, as is extension into the soft tissues. Periosteal reactions are very unusual. Some tumors may be expansile or present a multicystic appearance.[41] Punctate or prominent calcifications are found in 30–35% of cases.[45,48]

CT may be useful to depict the lobulated margins and calcified matrix.[53,54]

On MRI, there is an increased signal intensity on moderately T2-weighted images[55] and a heterogeneous intermediate signal intensity on T2-weighted images, differing from chondromas and chondrosarcomas.[56]

On gross examination, most tumors lack the bluish chondroid appearance of typical chondrosarcomas. The tissue is soft or firm, granular, appearing as a gray or red-brown material with highly vascularized or hemorrhagic areas and eventually small or large cysts. A cartilage component is found in rare cases.[40,52]

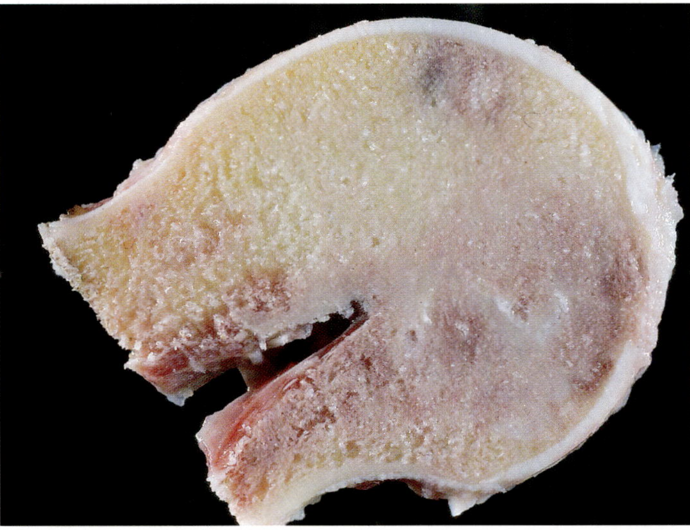

Fig. 15.36 Clear cell chondrosarcoma of the femur appearing at initial presentation as two separate foci.

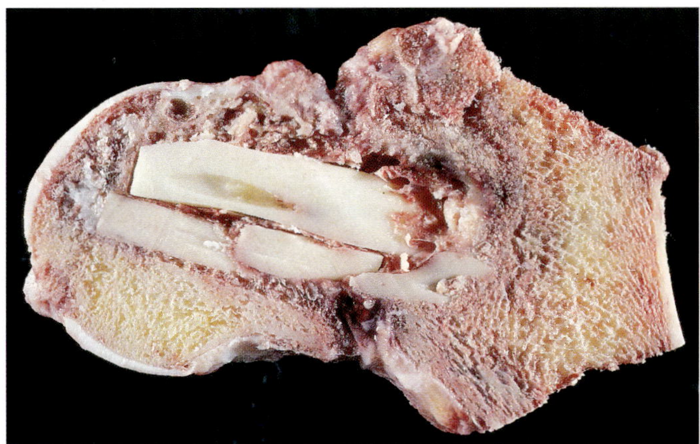

Fig. 15.37 Pathological fracture of the femur. The clear cell chondrosarcoma had been misdiagnosed.

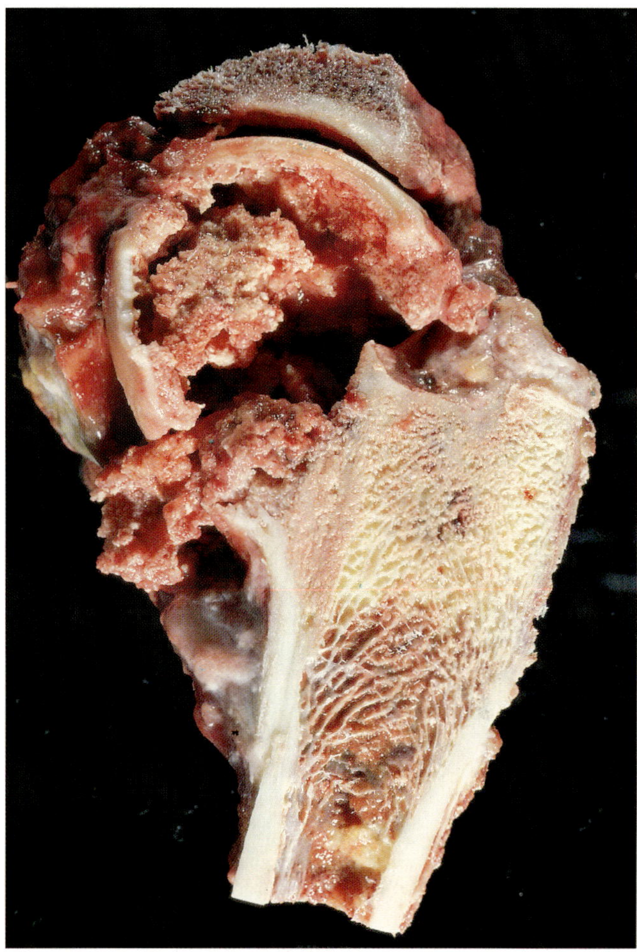

Fig. 15.38 Clear cell chondrosarcoma of the femur misdiagnosed as a femoral head necrosis. Treatment by cup arthroplasty. Pathologic fracture.

Histologically (Figs 15.50–15.62), most of the tumor cells have an abundant and clear cytoplasm. The cytoplasm may appear condensed near the cell membrane or the nucleus or may be eosinophilic in smaller cells. The nucleus is centrally located and hyperchromatic, with an even chromatin distribution[42] or it may look vesicular, with prominent nucleoli.[48] Some clear cells are binucleated. Mitotic activity is extremely rare.

The cells are distributed in sheets or in a lobular or microlobular pattern with thin fibrovascular septa.[50] Scattered osteoclast-like giant cells may be numerous.

In most cases, a reactive woven bone formation is found, in some fields, with the trabeculae showing rimming by osteoblasts and some osteoclastic resorption. There is a wide range of bone formation, even in the same tumor, from minute foci of osteoid to huge areas of reactive lamellar bone.

In the clear cell areas, the matrix is sparse; the chondroid material may be partially calcified or fine lines of amorphous calcifications are found between the cells. Associated areas of typical chondrosarcoma are randomly distributed in about half the cases[40,50] (Figs 15.63–15.66); a peripheral distribution of the clear cell component has been described.[57] The chondrosarcoma component is grade II;[41] higher grades or myxoid-like areas are very unusual.[57]

Secondary changes in these quite vascularized tumors are focal areas of necrosis, simple cystic change or an aneurysmal bone cyst-like formation,[40,48] (Fig. 15.67). Small foci of clear cells may be found in the bone marrow, close to the main tumor, without bone-resorbing activity; a microinfiltrative pattern of growth has been described.[58]

Immunohistochemically, clear cell chondrosarcoma shows a strong positivity for S-100 protein,[41,47,59–62] especially near the areas of matrix mineralization.[60]

Ultrastructurally, the chondroid cells appear closely packed,[61–66] exhibiting different stages of differentia-

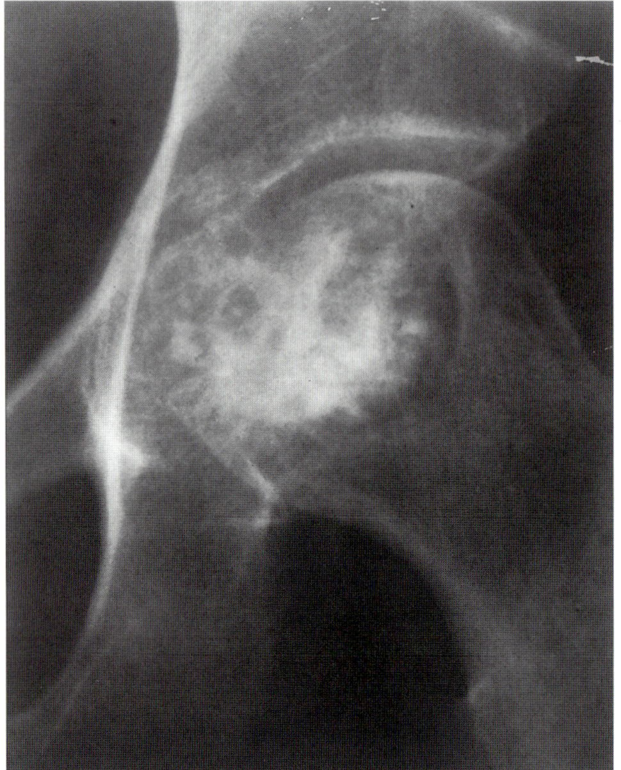

Fig. 15.39

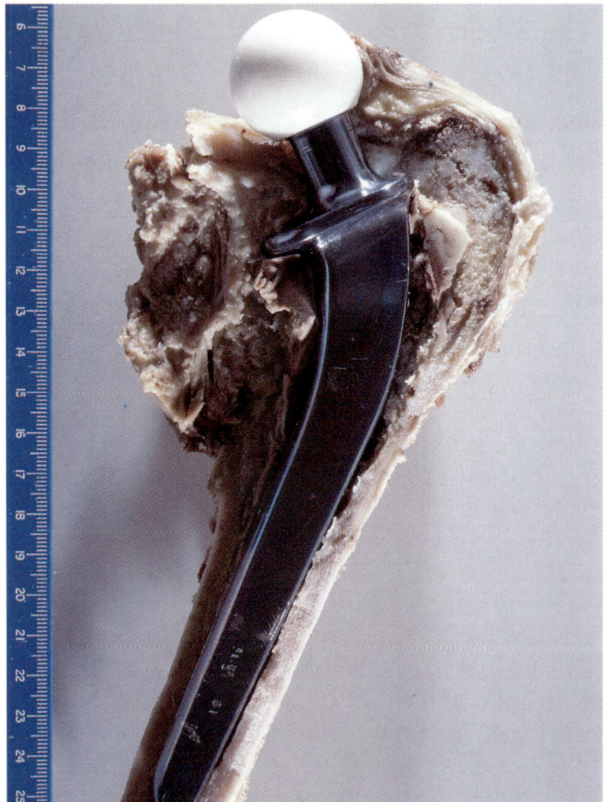

Fig. 15.40

Figs 15.39, 15.40 Clear cell chondrosarcoma misdiagnosed as femoral head necrosis. Treatment by a total hip replacement. Huge tumoral recurrence.

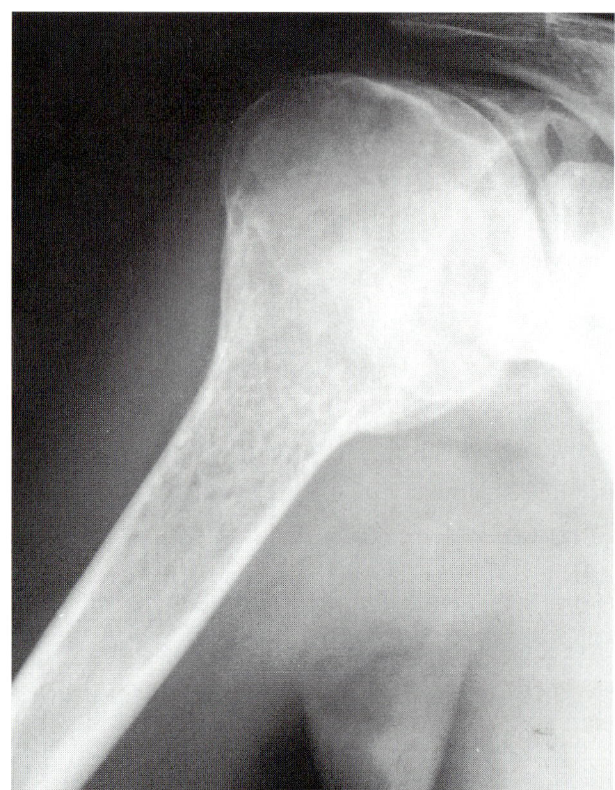

Fig. 15.41

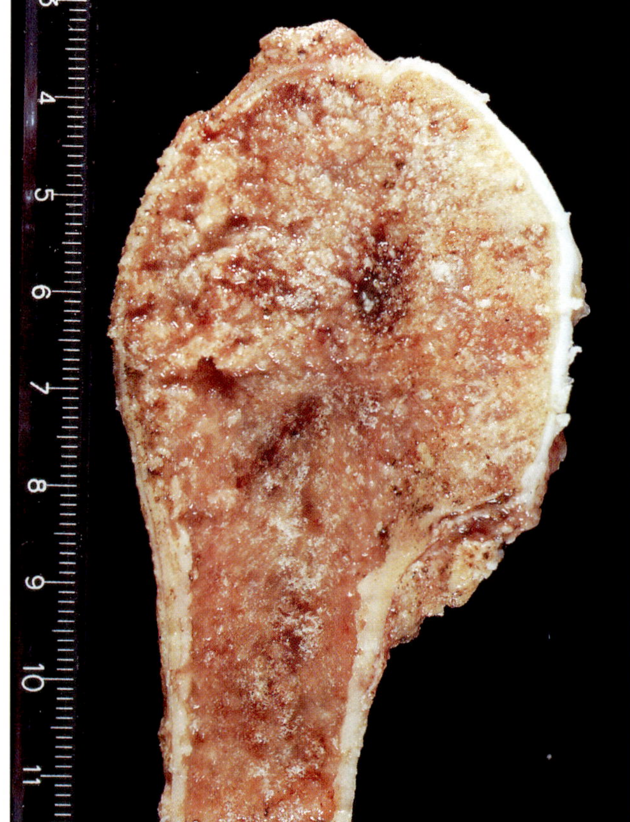

Fig. 15.42

Figs 15.41, 15.42 Clear cell chondrosarcoma of the humerus.

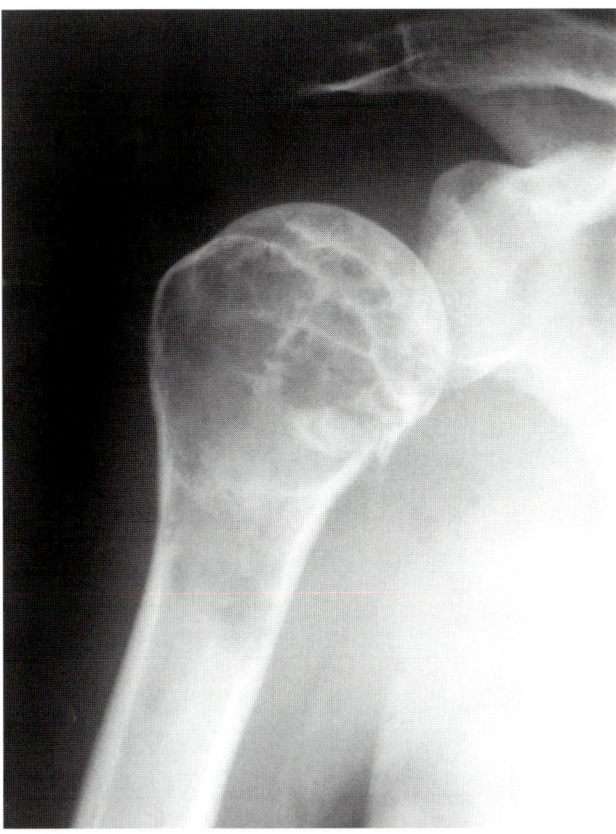

Fig. 15.43

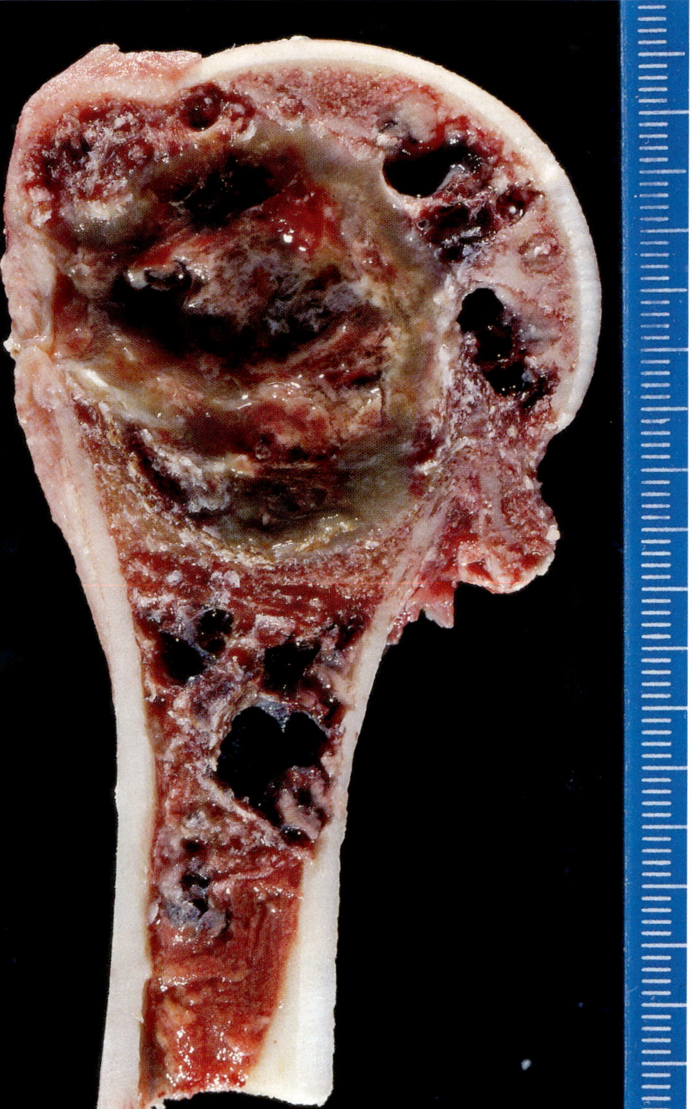

Fig. 15.44

Figs 15.43, 15.44 Clear cell chondrosarcoma of the humerus with cyst formation.

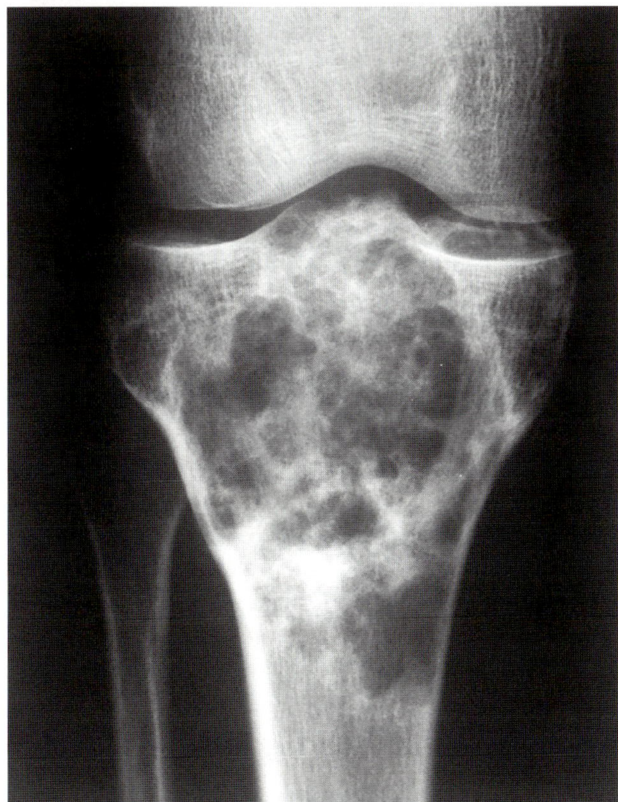

Fig. 15.45

Fig. 15.45 Clear cell chondrosarcoma of the tibia.

tion.[61,63] The features of chondroblasts are found with numerous cytoplasmic microvilli, widely dilated rough endoplasmic reticulum[61,63–66] and bundles of actin-like filaments.[63]

The clear cells have sparse organelles mostly distributed in the perinuclear region,[63] the cytoplasm being almost completely occupied by glycogen[63–69] or a low-density granular material.[70] The nucleus is lobulated; some cells are binucleated, others have a more irregular nucleus with prominent nucleoli. Multinucleated reactive giant cells resemble osteoclasts.[63]

Complex structures of regularly alternating mitochondria and rough endoplasmic reticulum, similar to those found in chordomas, have been described.[67] The intercel-

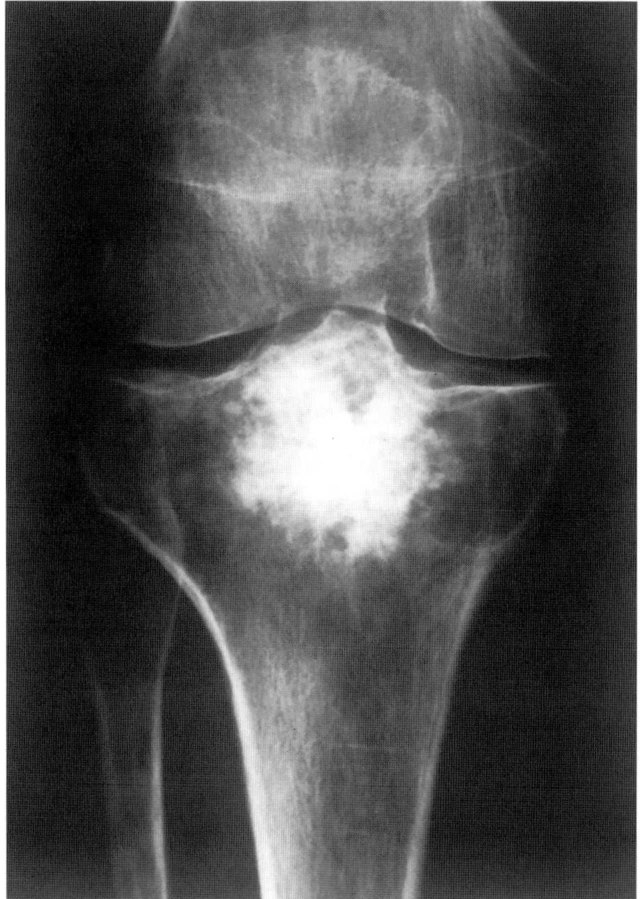

Fig. 15.46

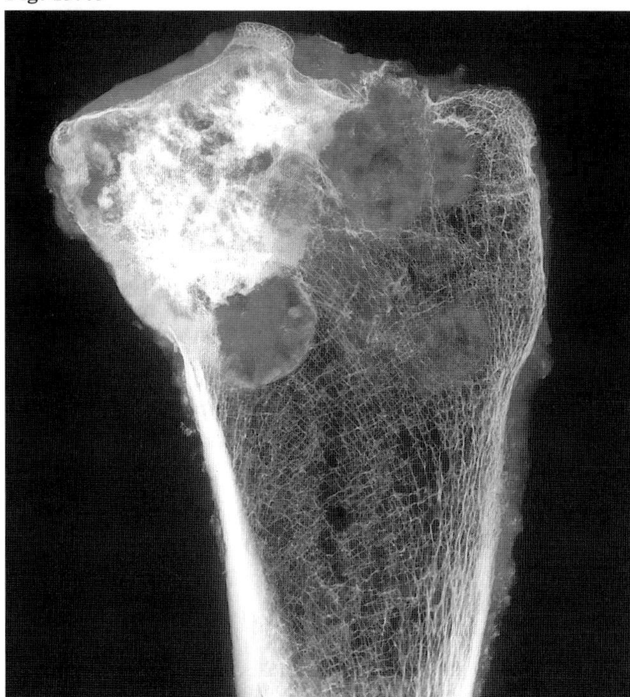

Fig. 15.47

Figs 15.46, 15.47 Clear cell chondrosarcoma of the tibia: extensive calcifications.

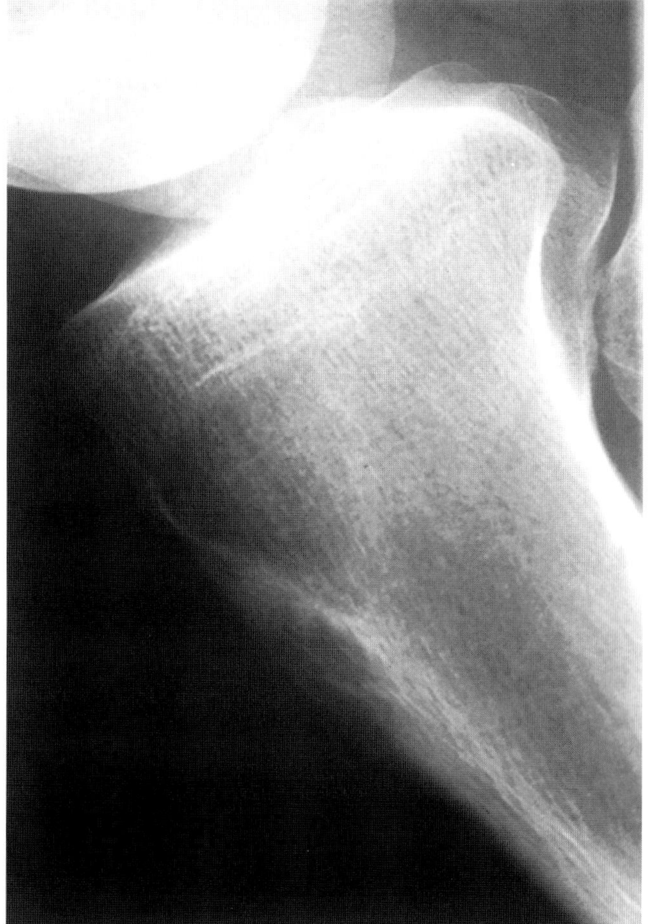

Fig. 15.48

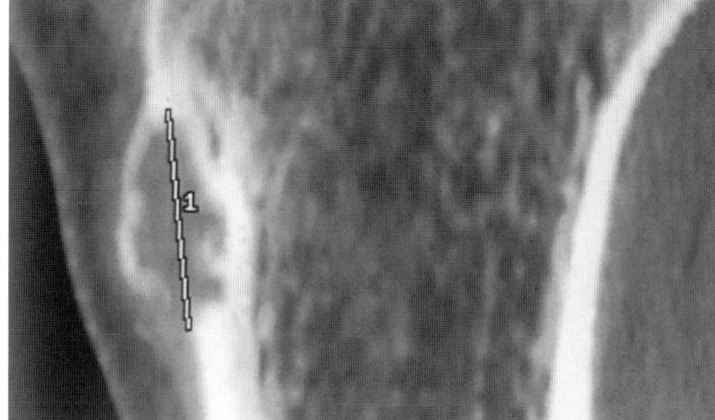

Fig. 15.49

Figs 15.48, 15.49 Periosteal clear cell chondrosarcoma of the tibia.

lular matrix is sparse, with a variable amount of collagen.[63,64,67]

Some authors have suggested that the clear cell appearance could be related to the lack of development of Golgi complexes: the intercellular matrix bony is synthesized by

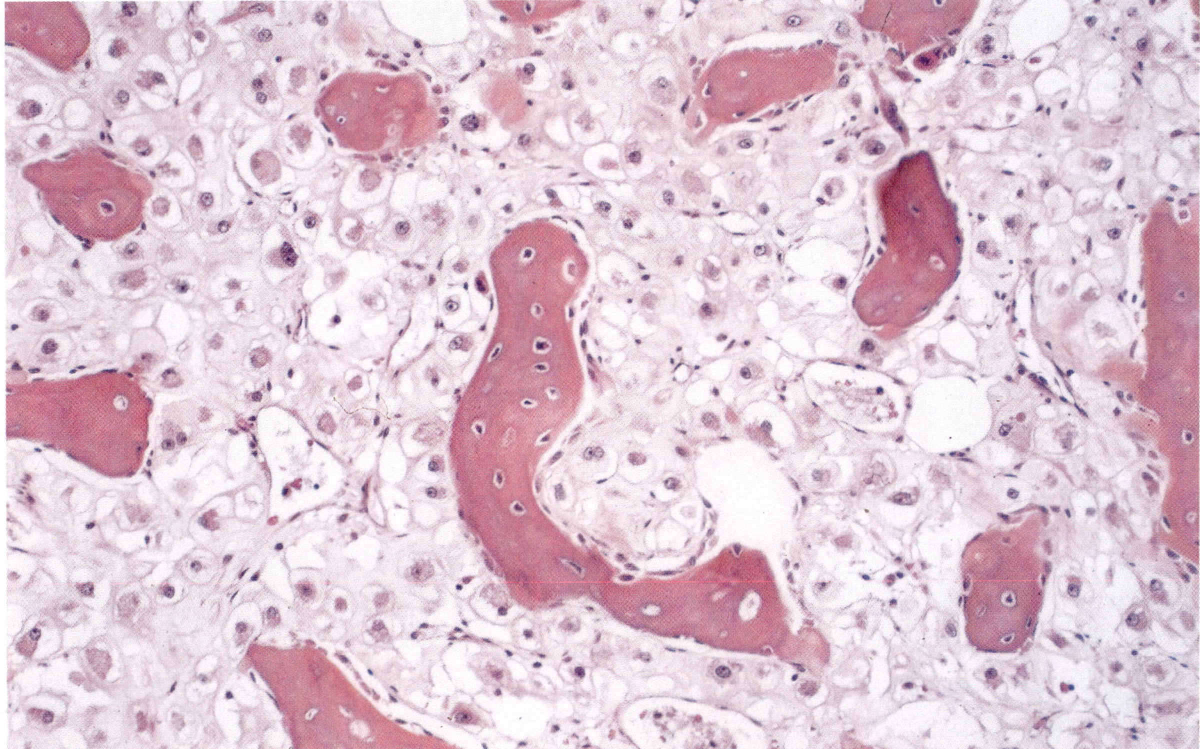

Fig. 15.50

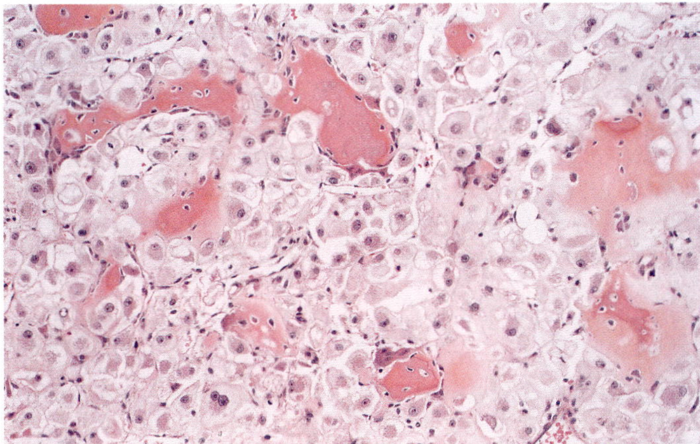

Fig. 15.51

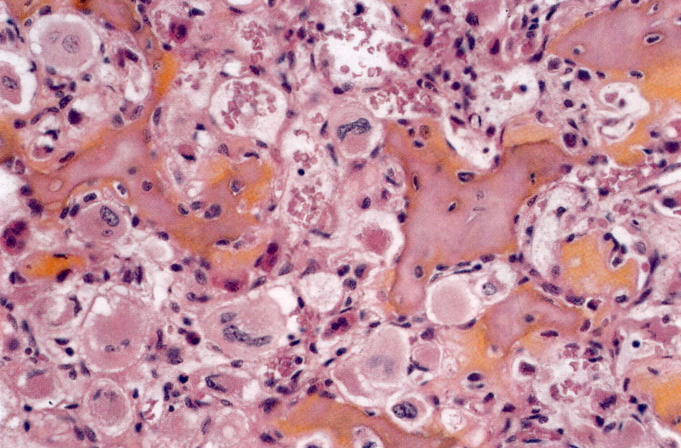

Fig. 15.52

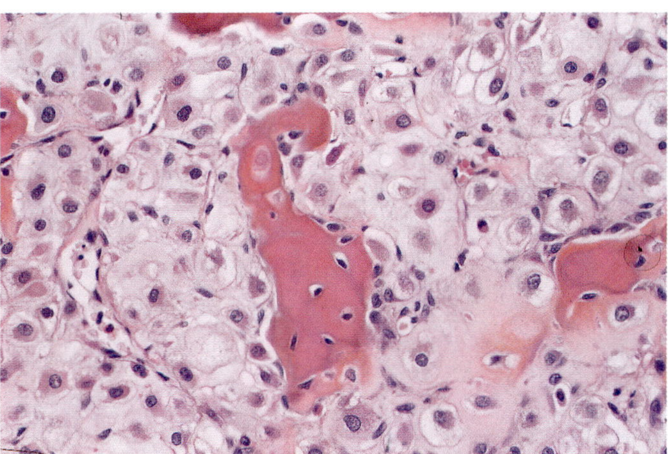

Fig. 15.53

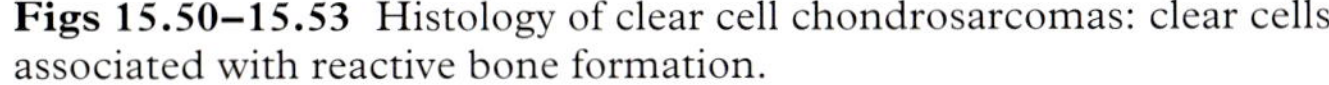

Figs 15.50–15.53 Histology of clear cell chondrosarcomas: clear cells associated with reactive bone formation.

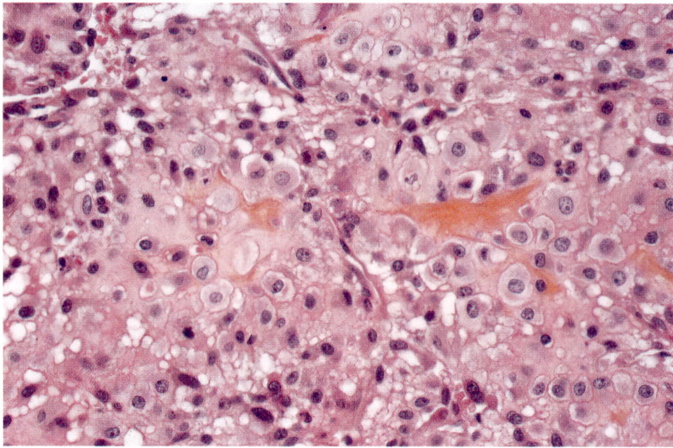

Fig. 15.54

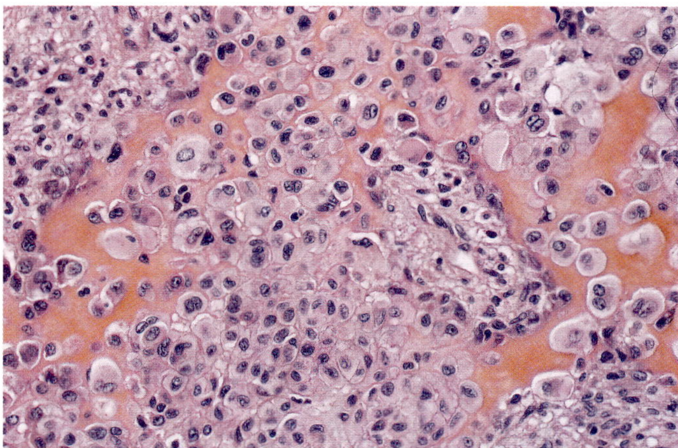

Fig. 15.55

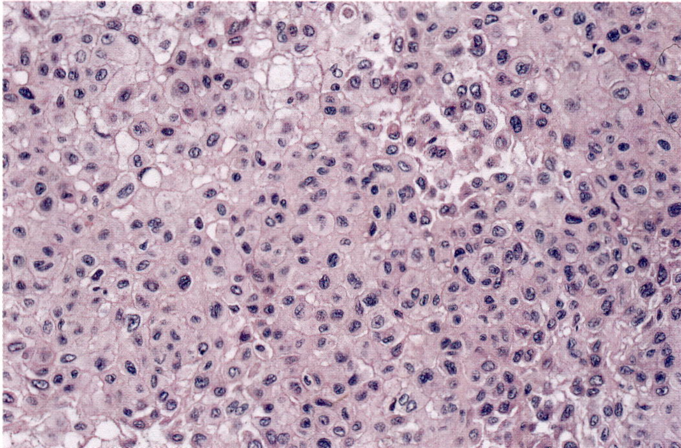

Fig. 15.56

Figs 15.54–15.56 Clear cell chondrosarcomas: cartilage cells with an acidophilic or smaller cytoplasm which may be confused with the cytology of chondroblastomas.

the rough endoplasmic reticulum, but unable to be transported into the extracellular spaces.[61,64,68]

Clear cell chondrosarcomas may exhibit some very unexpected findings. A case developing at the site of a repetitive low-impact trauma over a period of 24 years has been reported.[71] Biochemically, clear cell chondrosarcomas, unlike typical tumors, have a very low water content, a low concentration of collagen and a high ash content.[72] A strong immunoexpression of osteonectin has been reported in clear cells as well as in the chondroid and osseous areas, seeming to indicate an osteogenic rather than chondrogenic origin.[73] Overexpression and point mutation of the p53 protein/gene have been found in a clear cell chondrosarcoma of the pelvis, as in high-grade tumors.[74]

An unusual karyotypic finding is a near haploid chromosome count, characterized by numerical changes and not by structural abnormalities.[75]

Clear cell chondrosarcomas are slow-growing tumors and extension into the soft tissues or adjacent joint is quite unusual.[69]

The treatment is surgical resection. A 5-year survival rate of 92% has been reported;[47] in the Mayo Clinic series, metastases occur in 15% of cases, usually during the first decade after treatment[42] but the delay may be as long as 23 years.[43] Metastases are found in the lungs, brain and bones.[42] Rarely, clear cell chondrosarcoma can dedifferentiate.[66]

As for the differential diagnosis, conventional chondrosarcomas may be confused with the clear cell variant if the characteristic cell component is not found in a limited biopsy or, more rarely, if the tumor has a signet-ring cell cytology, the moderately sized round cell showing a large, clear, central fat vacuole.[76]

Rare osteosarcomas can be located in the epiphysis, the cytoplasm of the tumor cells being clear or finely granular and eosinophilic,[77,78] caused by vacuolar degeneration or exaggerated glycogen deposits.[79] The S-100 protein staining is negative.

Metastatic clear cell carcinomas have to be differentiated on histological findings alone; Fechner & Mills (1993) have stressed the limited value of the immunohistochemical reactions: chondrosarcomas may show cytokeratin and epithelial membrane antigen immunopositivity, while metastatic renal carcinomas may exhibit vimentin and S-100 protein positivities.

The differential diagnosis with chondroblastoma is more difficult and for some authors, clear cell chondrosarcoma may well be the malignant counterpart of the benign tumor (Schajowicz 1994).[80] Chondroblastomas are found in younger patients, with a more restricted epiphyseal location in long bones. The cells are much smaller, oval or spindly, with a grooved nucleus and a sparse eosinophilic cytoplasm. Neither significant reactive bone formation nor conventional chondrosarcoma areas are found.

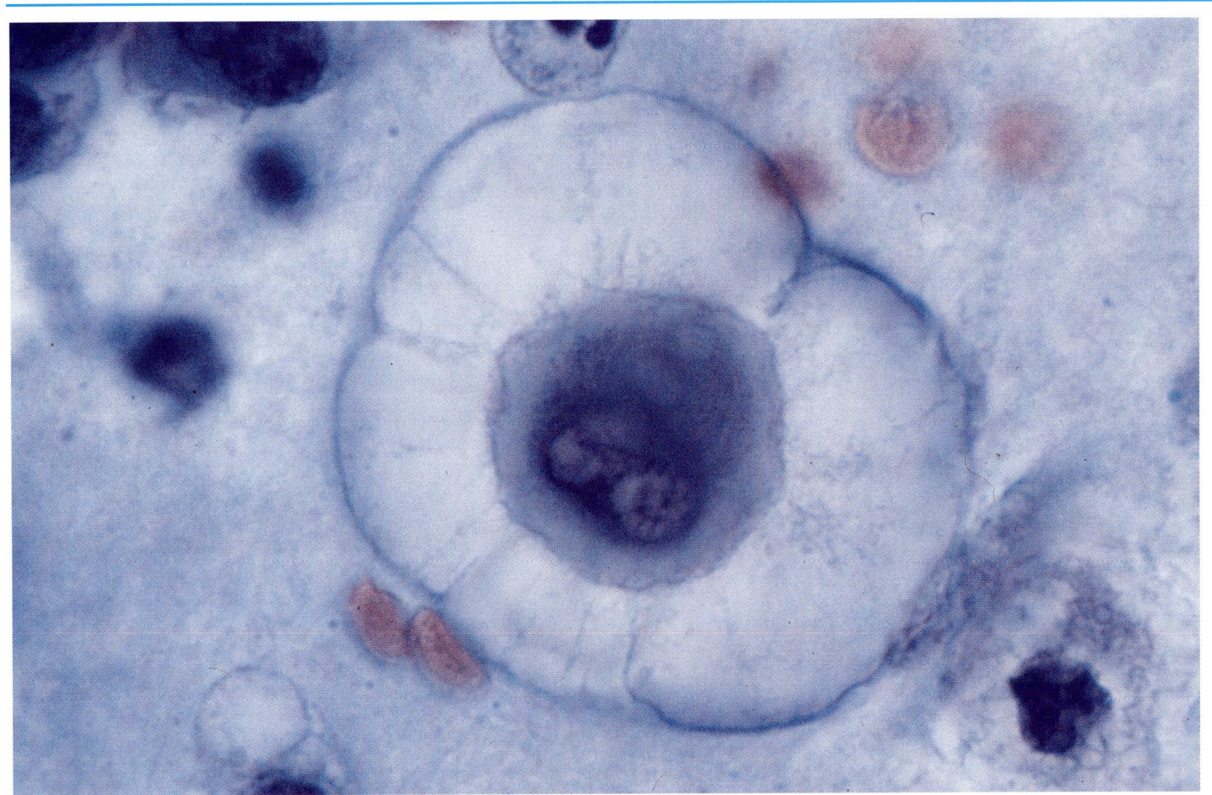

Figs 15.57–15.62 Clear cell chondrosarcomas: imprint cytology demonstrating the watery cytoplasm, binucleated chondrocytes, acidophilic cells, reactive giant cells and tumoral multinucleated cells.

Fig. 15.57

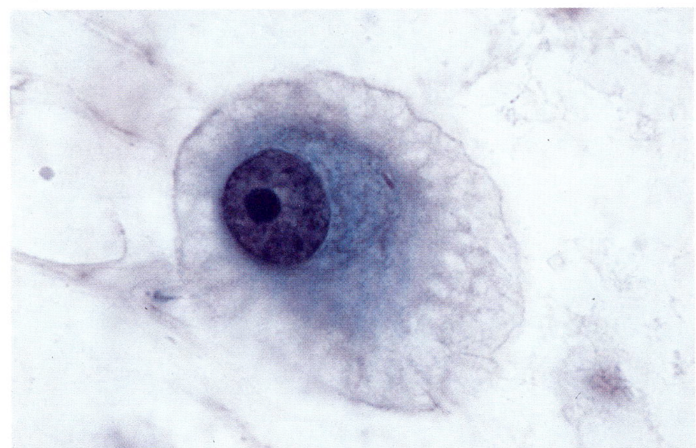

Fig. 15.58

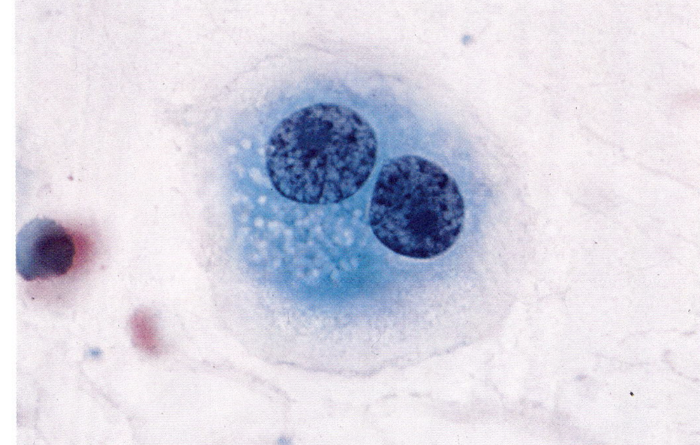

Fig. 15.59

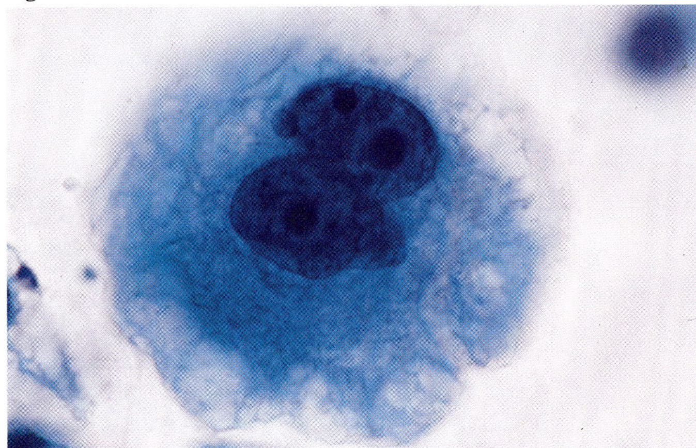

Fig. 15.60

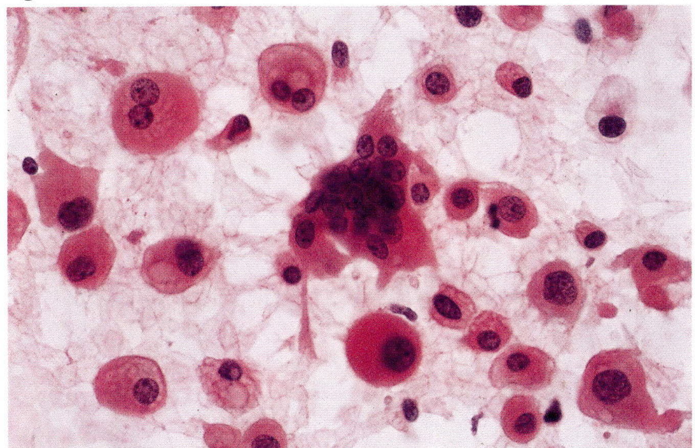

Fig. 15.61

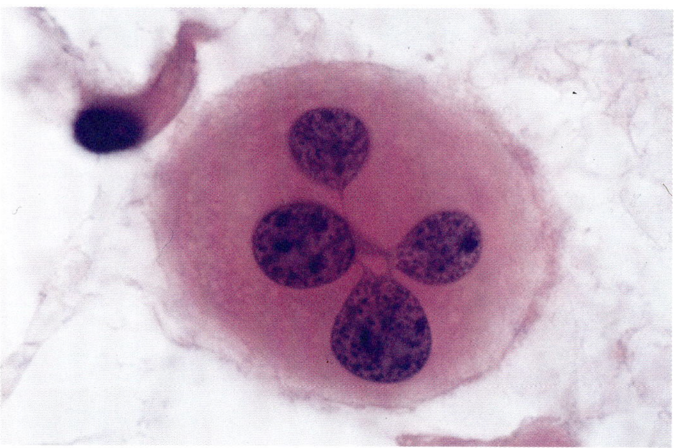

Fig. 15.62

SKELETAL MYXOID CHONDROSARCOMA

This is a very rare variant in bone,[81–86] known as chordoid sarcoma when it appears in the soft tissues.

Stellate or round cells with a moderate amount of cytoplasm are distributed in cords, strands, nests or even tubular structures within a myxoid stroma. The nuclei may be hyperchromatic, with occasional nucleoli. Abundant granules of glycogen are found in the cytoplasm. There is no mitotic activity.[85]

Ultrastructurally, the cells have scalloped cytoplasmic membranes, a variable amount of glycogen, round or oval nuclei. Crystalline arrays of microtubules within the dilated rough endoplasmic reticulum have been reported,[85] found also in extraskeletal locations, in chondroid chordomas and osteosarcomas.

DEDIFFERENTIATED CHONDROSARCOMA

This was defined as a distinct clinicopathologic entity by Dahlin & Beabout in 1971:[87] a usually low-grade chondrosarcoma is associated with non-chondroid high-grade sarcoma. More recently, the term 'chondrosarcoma with additional mesenchymal component' has been suggested.[88]

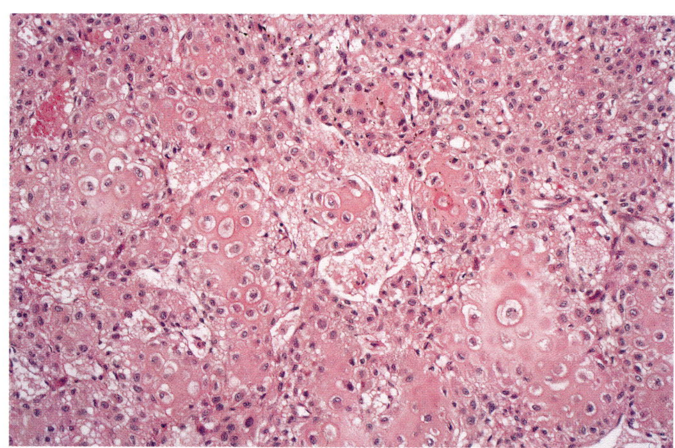

Fig. 15.63

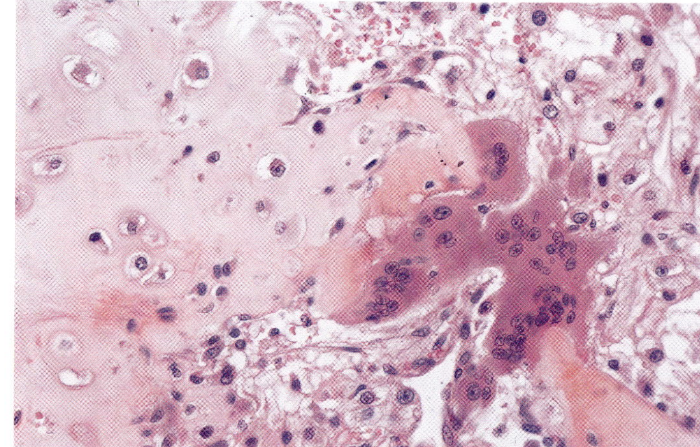

Fig. 15.65

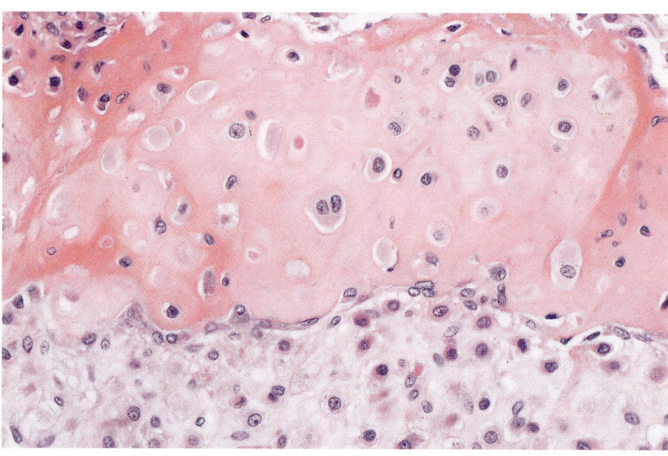

Fig. 15.64

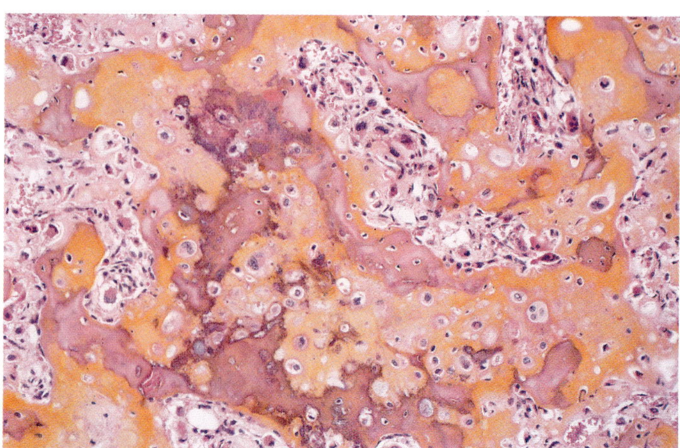

Fig. 15.66

Figs 15.63–15.66 Clear cell chondrosarcomas: associated typical chondrosarcoma component.

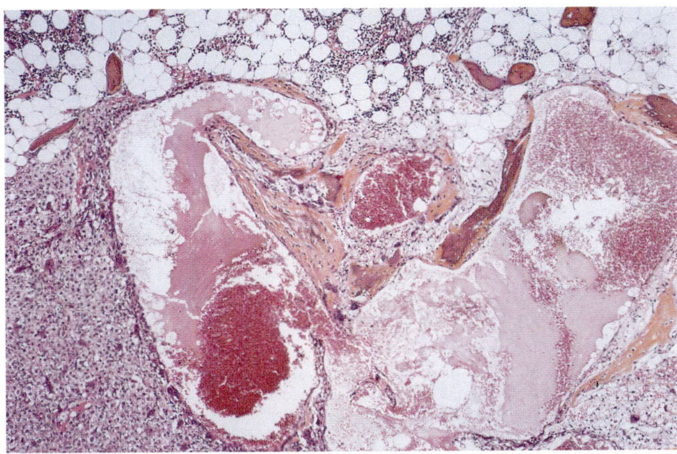

Fig. 15.67 Clear cell chondrosarcoma of the humerus: cystic changes.

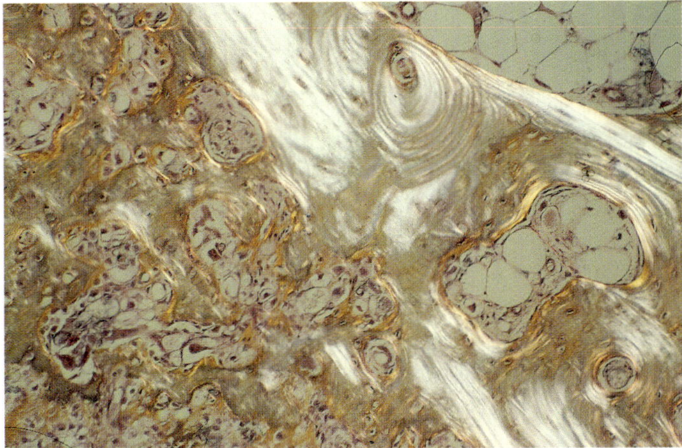

Fig. 15.68 Clear cell chondrosarcoma of the femur abutting cancellous bone, without active resorption (polarized light).

This lesion accounts for 6%[88] to 11% of all chondrosarcomas.[89,90] The peak incidence is in the fifth to seventh decades,[91] with no significant sex predilection[92] or a male-to-female ratio of 1.5:1[88] to 2:1.[93]

The biphasic tumor is diagnosed at initial presentation (86% of cases) or on recurrence after resection of the chondrosarcoma (14% of cases[92]).

Clinical symptoms are pain, swelling and pathologic fracture,[94] with an incidence ranging from 13%[92] to 38% of cases.[90] There is wide variation in duration of the symptoms: a few months if the high-grade component is present at initial presentation or years for a low-grade cartilaginous tumor.[93]

Reports describing osteosarcomas, fibrosarcomas or malignant fibrous histiocytomas arising in enchondromas, enchondromatosis and osteochondromas presumably represent dedifferentiated chondrosarcomas.[95–103]

The significance of the dual components has provoked controversy with conflicting results in immunohistochemi-

cal and ultrastructural studies. Some views are not well supported, such as the direct transformation of the well-differentiated chondrosarcoma[87,94] or the originate of the high-grade sarcoma from a reparative process around necrotic and calcific enchondromas.[96]

There is no loss of differentiation of mature cartilaginous cells. Some authors suggest that separate clones of cells differentiate in low-grade and high-grade sarcomas,[88,91,104–107] reflecting the genetic instability of the tumor.[106] However, immunohistochemical and ultrastructural studies show that the high-grade sarcoma may retain some chondroid features, supporting the view of a progression of the cartilaginous tumor, as has been suggested by some authors (Mirra 1989),[108] with all the steps from an enchondroma to a highly anaplastic sarcoma.[109–111]

The most common locations are the femur (proximal and distal), the acetabular regions and the proximal humerus[88–90,92] (Figs 15.69–15.76). The scapula, ilium and ribs are less often involved and vertebral locations are unusual.[112] In 10% of cases, dedifferentiated chondrosarcomas are found on peripheral cartilaginous lesions, chondrosarcomas[7,112] or, most often, osteochondromas or osteochondromatosis.[87,89,110,113–115]

On imaging, these lesions are rapidly destructive with a metaphyseal or diaphyseal location in long bones.[112] The osteolytic lesion may predominate with no cartilaginous component on X-ray,[89] but usually a cartilaginous tumor is diagnosed, chondroid calcifications being located in the medullary cavity.

The purely lytic areas are clearly demarcated from the cartilaginous tumor, associated with a cortical permeation or destruction and an extraosseous extension appearing in most cases as a large mass.[110]

CT is useful to delineate the non-chondroid component,[110] as well as the areas of cartilage and osseous destruction in peripheral tumors.[114]

Grossly, the anaplastic component may be extensive or only found in small areas; it can also appear as a large mass in the soft tissues.[89] The tissue is fleshy, gray or brown, with hemorrhage and necrosis. The transition with the typical cartilaginous tumor is abrupt.

Histologically (Figs 15.77–15.82), the cartilaginous tumor is often of low grade or may even be a borderline chondrosarcoma;[87–89] some series include higher grades, II or III.[89,90] In most cases, there is a fairly sharp transition with the high-grade sarcoma, but spindling of the cartilaginous cells and a gradual transition have also been described.[111] A malignant fibrous histiocytoma is the most common type of sarcoma,[88,94,106] supporting the view that this tumor may be the final common pathway in tumor progression.[116] In the Mayo Clinic studies, osteosarcomas and fibrosarcomas predominate.[89]

Rare cases show the association of malignant fibrous histiocytoma and osteosarcoma.[110]

Muscular tumors have also been reported,[88,91,117–123]

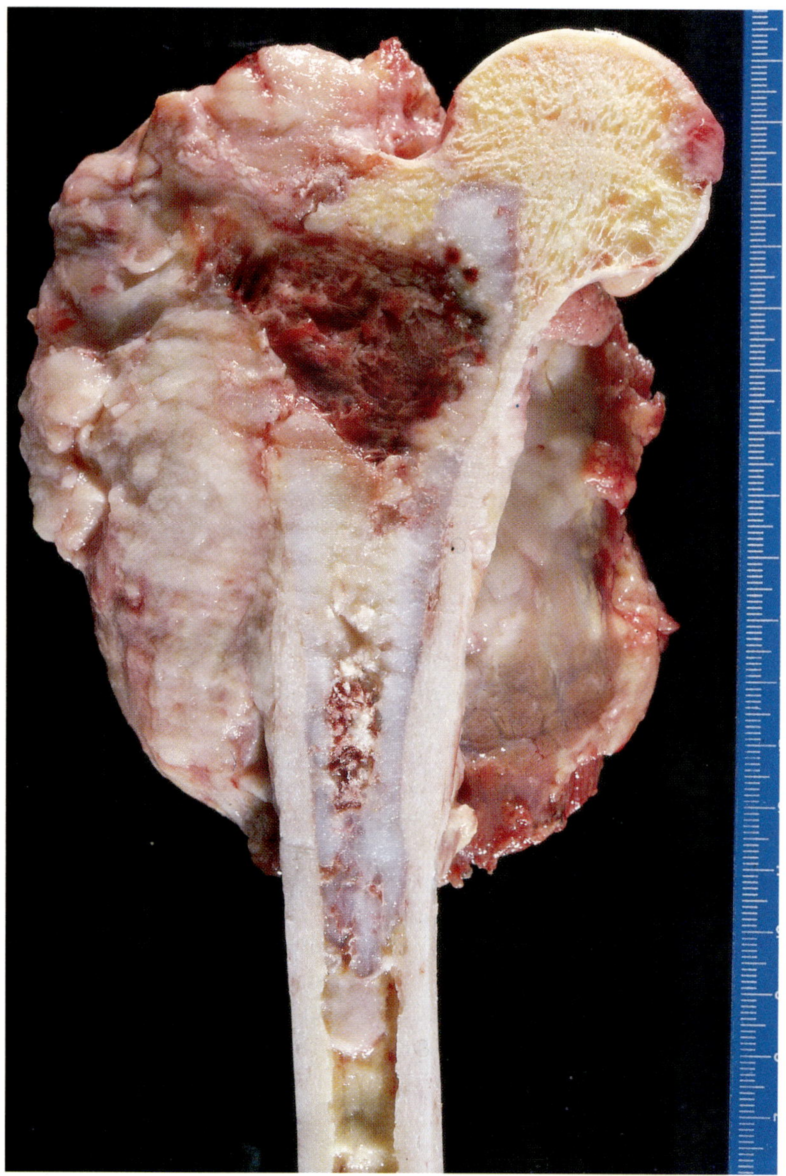

Fig. 15.69

Fig. 15.70

Figs 15.69, 15.70 Dedifferentiated chondrosarcoma of the femur.

with an estimated incidence of 10–20% of cases,[123] as well as rare angiosarcomas.[90] Some are undifferentiated sarcomas but all, with very few exceptions,[88] are high-grade tumors.

Rare tumors may have a predominant reactive giant cell component simulating the histologic appearance of a giant cell tumor,[88,124,125] but the malignant stroma background is that of a giant cell-rich malignant fibrous histiocytoma.[126] They have to be differentiated from the very unusual finding of chondromas close to giant cell tumors, both being independent lesions.[127]

On smears (Figs 15.83, 15.84), the cytologic and immunocytochemical features may be those of a malignant fibrous histiocytoma: pleomorphic spindle-shaped cells with multinucleated forms. Some cells can exhibit an S-100 immunoreactivity.[128]

Immunohistochemically, the non-chondroid component in most cases is S-100 protein negative[91] but occasional cells may be positive,[105,106] presumably by persistence of some chondroid characteristics.

A fibrohistiocytic differentiation can be established,[91,105,106,121] as well as a muscle differentiation.[117–120,123] A cytokeratin positivity has been reported in rare cases.[120,121]

The expression of p53, along with that of ki-67 and PCNA, has been studied.[129] The percentage of p53 positive staining is roughly parallel to the proliferating fraction of cells in the various components: the high-grade, non-

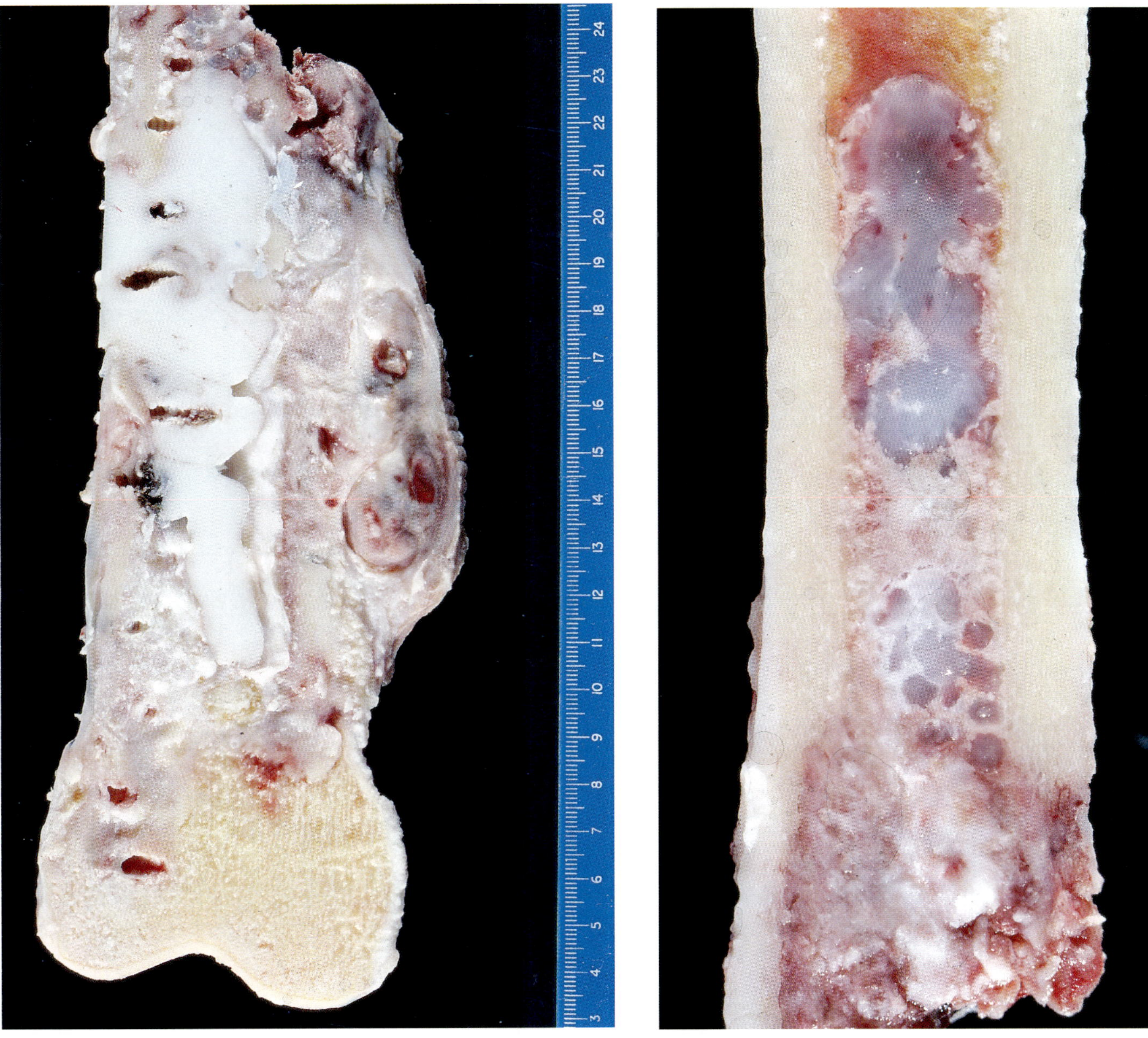

Fig. 15.71

Fig. 15.72

Figs 15.71, 15.72 Dedifferentiated chondrosarcoma of the femur. Initially diagnosed as an enchondroma and curetted. The cavity has been packed with cement.

cartilaginous component shows a strong nuclear staining for p53, as well as some high-grade cartilaginous areas, while the low-grade tumoral cartilage is almost negative.[129]

Ultrastructurally, the cells of the non-chondroid component resemble immature mesenchymal cells.[91,130] They may have the features of malignant fibrous histiocytomas or show muscular[91,117,123] or myofibroblastic differentiation.[105] In only one report, the cells of the spindle cell component had features similar to those seen within the cartilaginous tumor.[131]

Variegated cytogenetic abnormalities have been described: translocation t(9;22)(q34;q11–13), as in myx-

oid chondrosarcomas;[132] breaks in the short arms of both chromosomes 1, resulting in deletion in one homolog and recombination in the other;[133] structurally aberrant chromosome 17 and extra copies of chromosomes 5, 7, 12 and 20.[122] An important finding is that combined cytogenetic and immunohistochemical studies of the abnormal cells in the chondroid and non-chondroid components have shown a common abnormal clone.[122]

The treatment is surgical resection with wide or radical margins and adjuvant chemotherapy or radiotherapy, but the tumor appears to be resistant to chemotherapy.[88,110] The prognosis is very poor, with an overall survival rate at

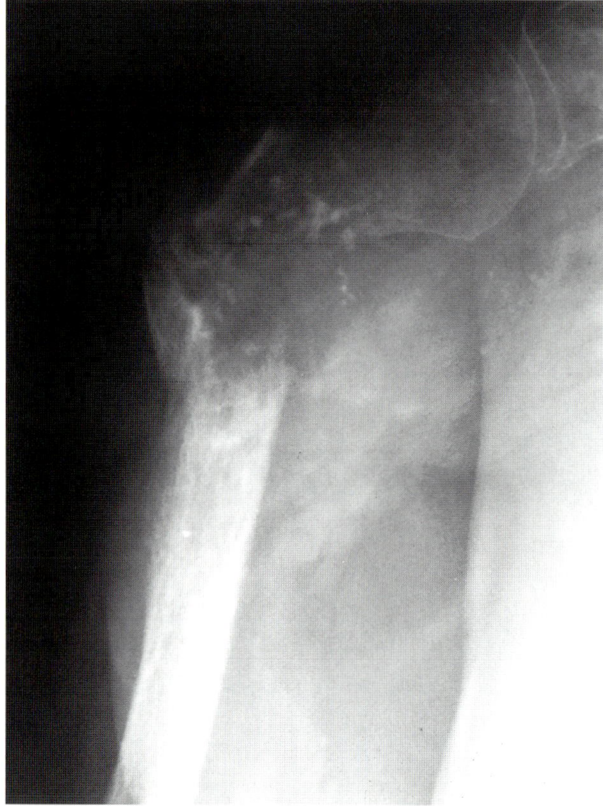

Fig. 15.73

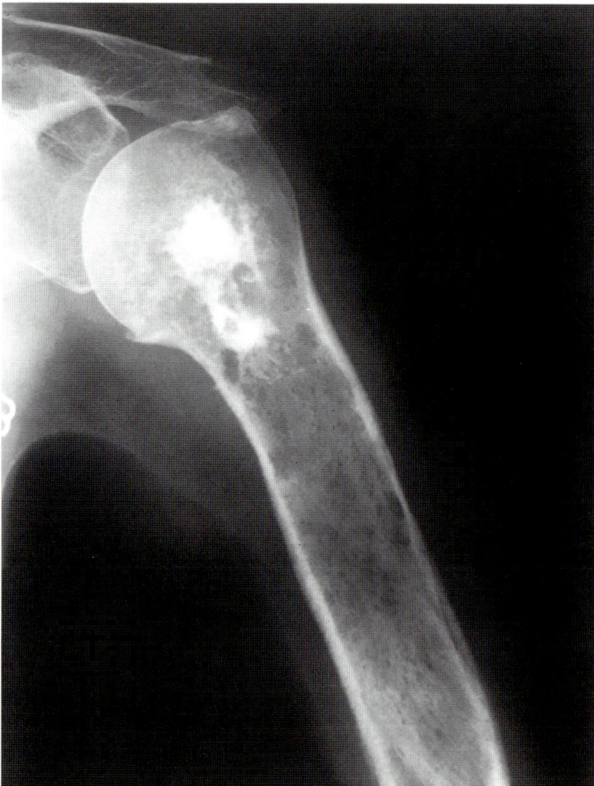

Fig. 15.74

Figs 15.73, 15.74 Dedifferentiated chondrosarcomas in humeral location.

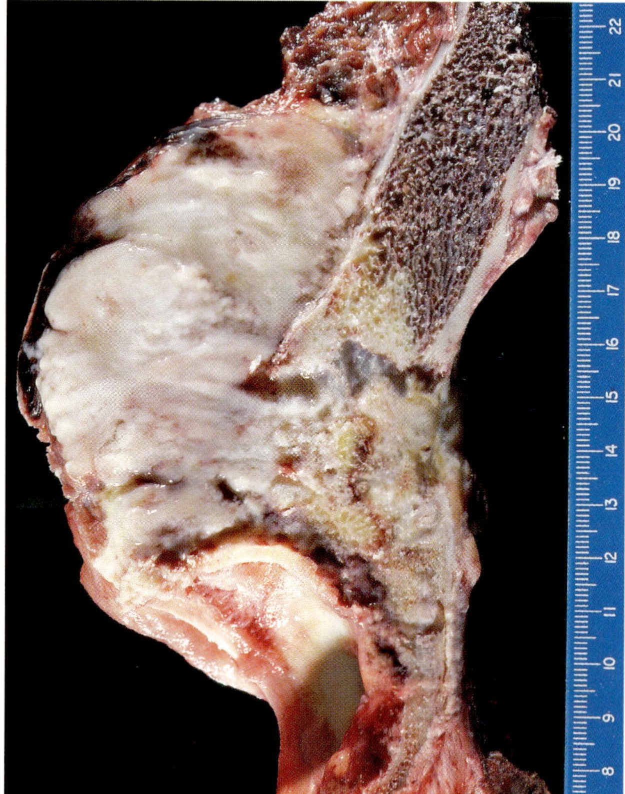

Fig. 15.75

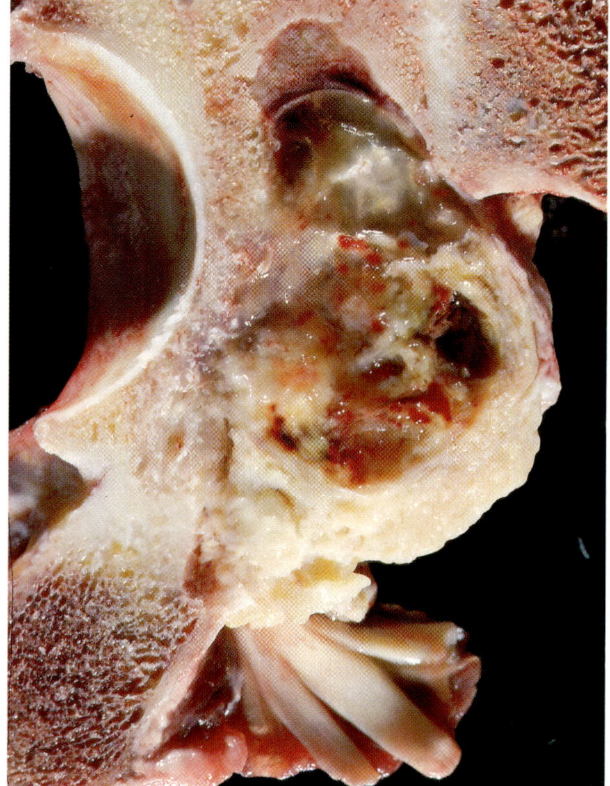

Fig. 15.76

Figs 15.75, 15.76 Dedifferentiated chondrosarcomas in acetabular locations.

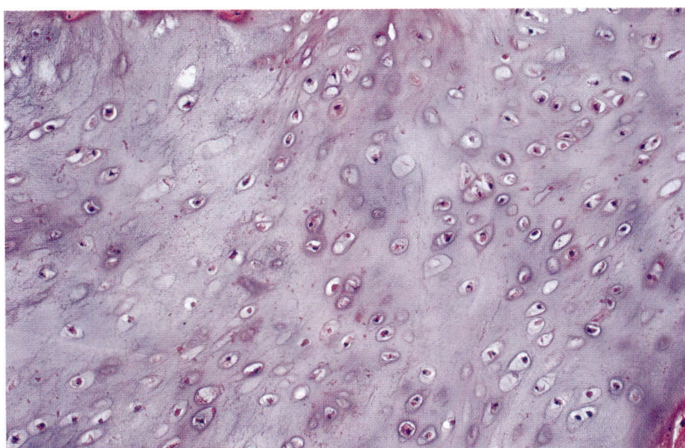

Fig. 15.77

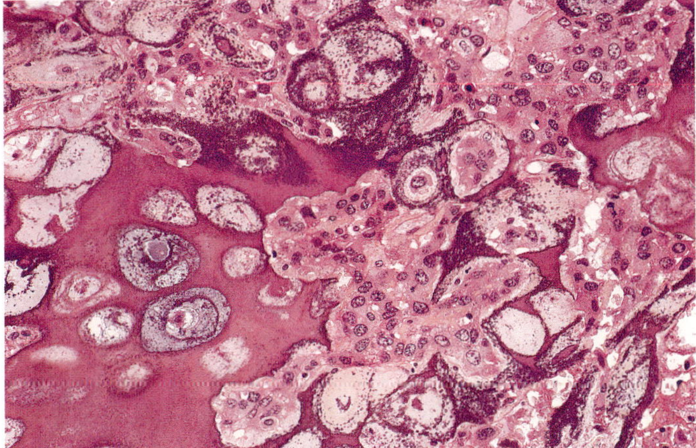

Fig. 15.78

Figs 15.77, 15.78 Well-differentiated chondrosarcoma components partly invaded by the sarcoma (Fig. 15.78).

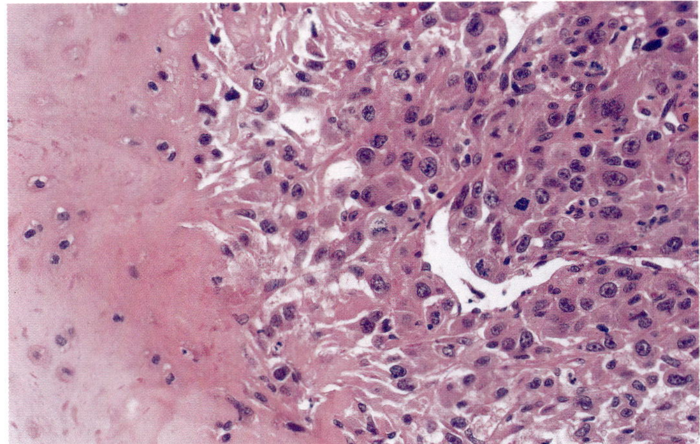

Fig. 15.79 Dedifferentiated chondrosarcoma of the sacrum: interface between the tumoral cartilage and the osteosarcoma component.

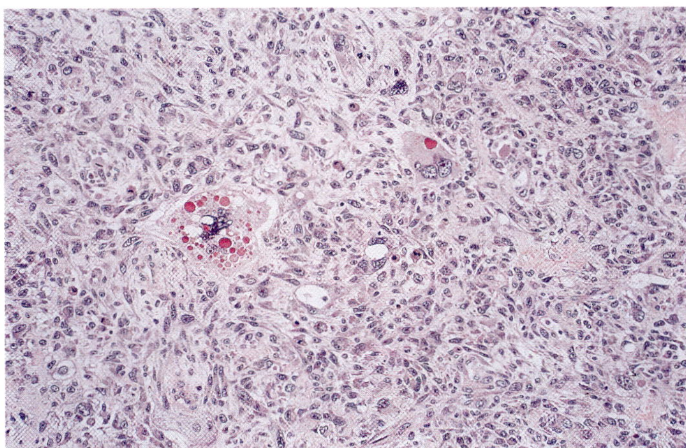

Fig. 15.80 Dedifferentiated chondrosarcoma of the tibia: malignant fibrous histiocytoma component.

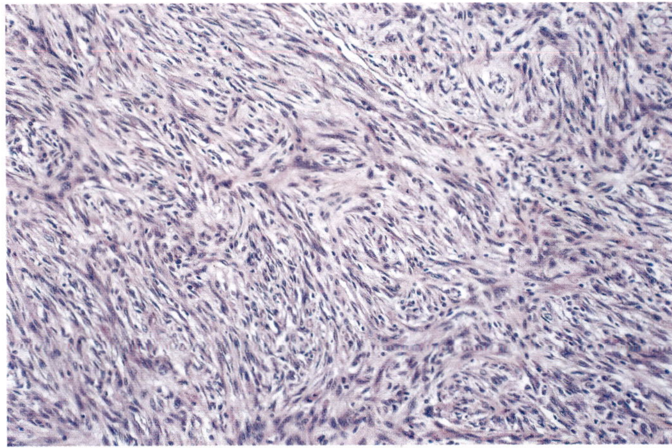

Fig. 15.81 Dedifferentiated chondrosarcoma of the femur: malignant fibrous histiocytoma component.

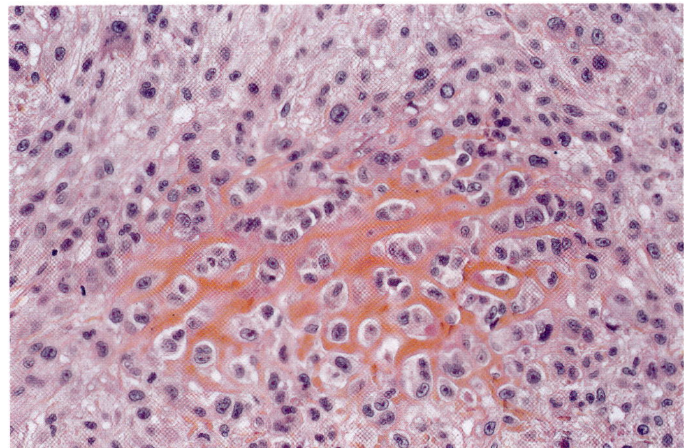

Fig. 15.82 Dedifferentiated chondrosarcoma of the humerus: osteosarcoma component.

5 years of only 8.5–13%.[89,110] Rare cases with a low-grade fibrosarcoma as a non-chondroid component have a better outcome.[88] There are no survivors in cases of associated osteosarcoma.[89]

The metastases, comprising exclusively the high-grade non-cartilaginous component, are found in the lungs, bones[94] and visceral organs.[89]

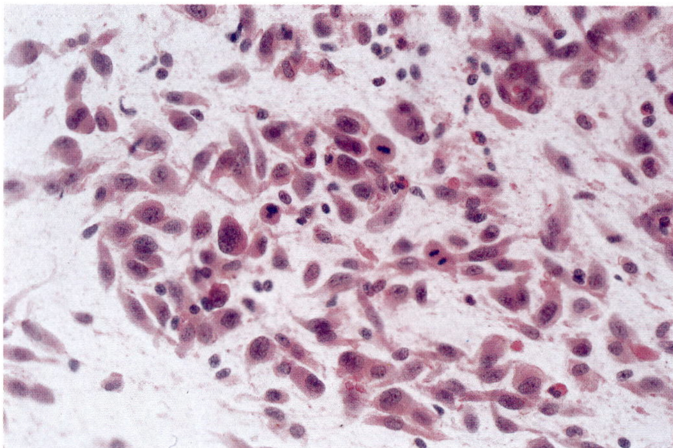

Fig. 15.83

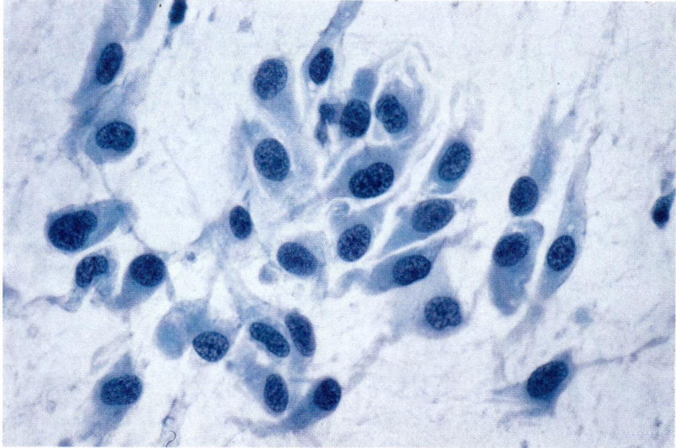

Fig. 15.84

Figs 15.83, 15.84 Dedifferentiated chondrosarcoma: imprint cytology of the malignant fibrous histiocytoma component.

Dedifferentiated chondrosarcomas may be confused with high-grade chondrosarcomas and according to Schajowicz, the distinction is not even justified. In grade III chondrosarcomas, one can find zones of transition made of spindle cells in the anaplastic areas, with no other osseous, fibrous or fibrohistiocytic pattern of differentiation.

In the same way, chondroblastic osteosarcomas[134] do not present an abrupt transition between the two tumor components.

Mesenchymal chondrosarcomas exhibit only a lymphocyte-like anaplastic component and obviously, malignant fibrous histiocytomas or fibrosarcomas are devoid of tumoral cartilage.

On imaging, a most unusual differential diagnosis is a metastases localized to a chondrosarcoma.[135]

SECONDARY CHONDROSARCOMA

Most secondary chondrosarcomas are engrafted on preexisting benign cartilaginous tumors (Figs 15.85–15.91).

In enchondromas, clinical symptoms are pain unrelated

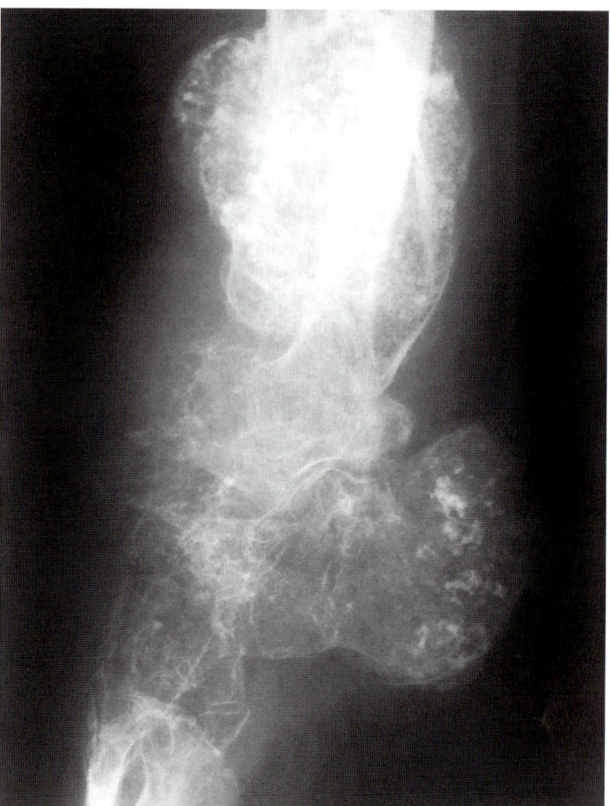

Fig. 15.85 Chondrosarcoma of the foot in Ollier's disease.

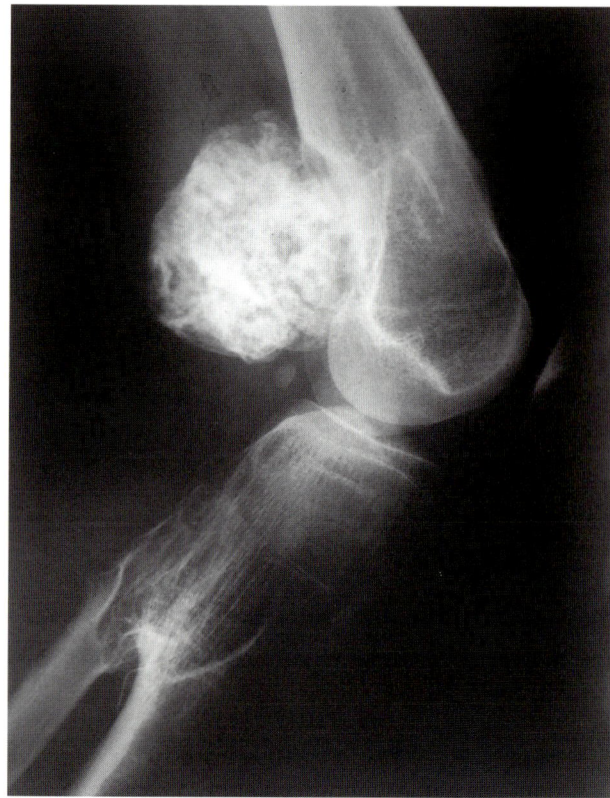

Fig. 15.86 Secondary chondrosarcoma of the femur (osteochondromatosis).

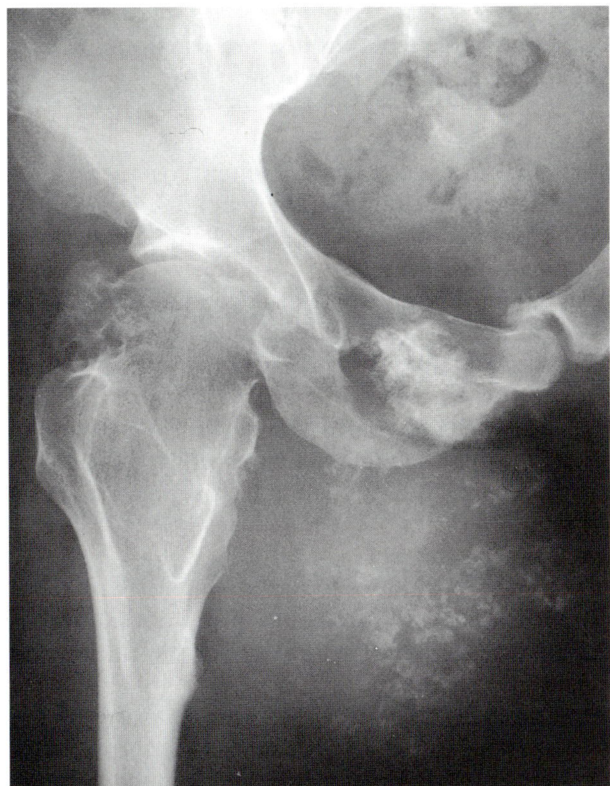

Fig. 15.87

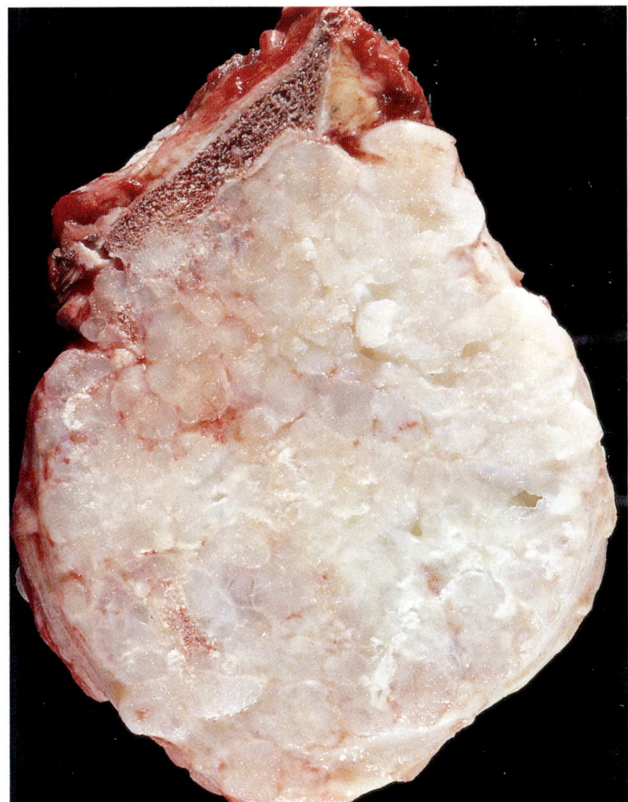

Fig. 15.88

Figs 15.87, 15.88 Secondary chondrosarcoma of the pubis (osteochondromatosis).

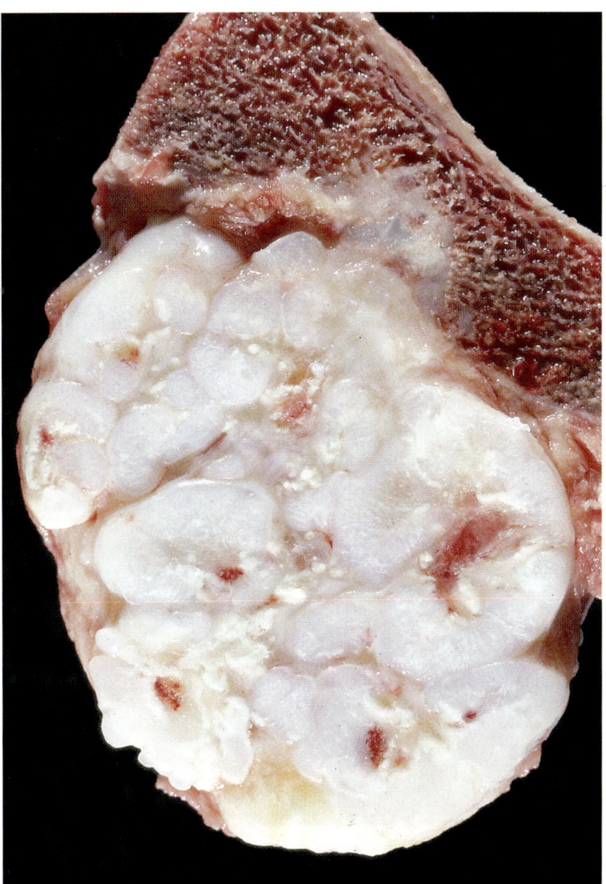

Fig. 15.89

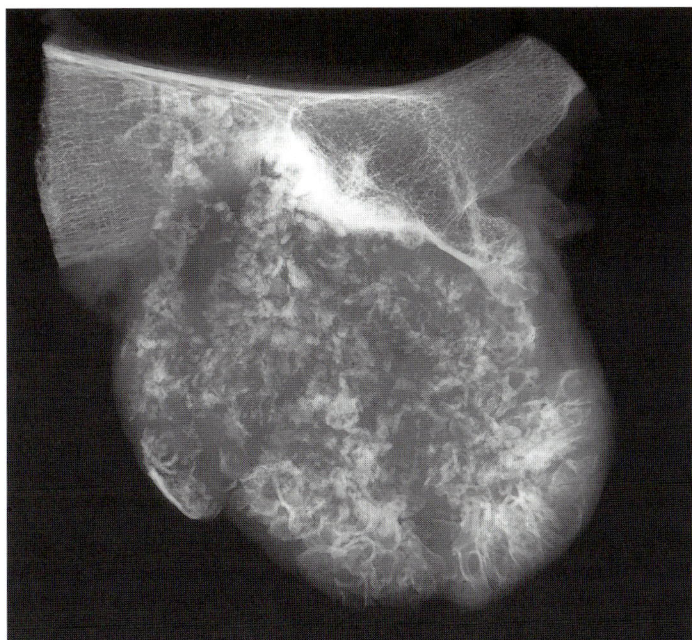

Fig. 15.90

Figs 15.89, 15.90 Secondary pelvic chondrosarcoma (osteochondromatosis).

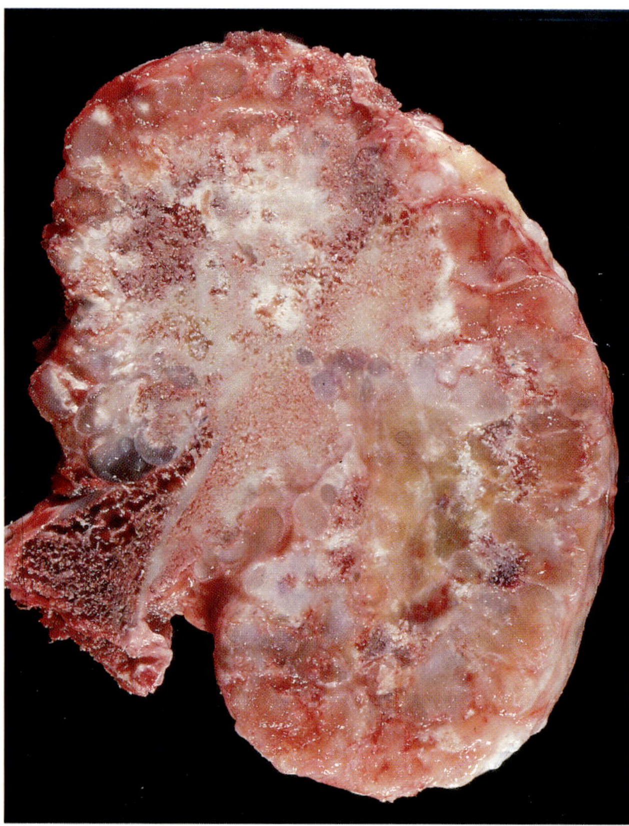

Fig. 15.91 Secondary chondrosarcoma of the iliac wing (osteochondromatosis).

to fracture and a rapidly growing mass. On X-ray, a zone of radiolucency is found in the mineralized lesion, with scalloping or destruction of the cortex and extension into the soft tissue.[136]

However, one has to remember that in Ollier's and Maffucci's diseases, masses of benign cartilage may be located in cortical or periosteal locations, showing hypercellularity and even myxoid areas. Similarly, in a short tubular bone, an enchondroma may induce a progressive

thinning and even disappearance of part of the cortex. More cellular benign enchondromas are also found in children, in the hand and in periosteal chondromas.

Rare multiple secondary chondrosarcomas have been described in the hands.[137]

Chondrosarcomas secondary to solitary osteochondromas[138,139] involve the long and flat bones, while those engrafted on osteochondromatosis involve chiefly the flat bones (ilium, pubis, scapula).[140] Malignant transformation appears to be very unusual in the hand.[141]

Early radiographic changes are a poorly mineralized or less mineralized area in the cartilage cap with indistinct margins or scattered calcifications in the cap, separated from the heavily calcified part.[142] However, at the time of diagnosis, most tumors are huge lesions which may entirely destroy the preexisting osteochondroma, appearing as a partially mineralized soft tissue mass.

Many tumors are low grade on histology.[140]

Formation of bursa around the chondrosarcoma has been described, the bursal sac being filled with numerous malignant nodules shed from the cap of the tumor and appearing as a soft tissue mass.[143]

Ultrastructural findings in these secondary tumors are unremarkable: irregular cell borders with numerous cytoplasmic processes, Golgi complexes and abundant rough endoplasmic reticulum, collagen fibrils, lipid droplets and glycogen granules.[144]

Chondrosarcomas may develop on unrelated conditions, such as unicameral bone cyst[145] or osteopoikilosis.[146] Others are induced by Thorotrast[147] or radiation.[148–151] They are rarely found in the course of Paget's disease.

Chondrosarcomas may be identified in fibrous dysplasia,[152–156] some being radiation-induced sarcomas; they have to be differentiated from the large amounts of hyaline and atypical cartilage found in some cases of fibrous dysplasia and known as fibrochondrodysplasia.[157,158]

Chondrosarcomas have been reported as unrelated malignancies in children treated successfully for malignant tumors of soft tissues.[159]

REFERENCES

1. Lichtenstein L. Tumors of periosteal origin. Cancer 1955: 8: 1060–1069
2. Nojima T, Unni K K, McLeod R A, Pritchard D J. Periosteal chondroma and periosteal chondrosarcoma. Am J Surg Pathol 1985: 9: 666–677
3. Bertoni F, Boriani S, Laus M, Campanacci M. Periosteal chondrosarcoma and periosteal osteosarcoma. Two distinct entities. J Bone Joint Surg (Br) 1982: 64: 370–376
4. Jockl P, Albright J A, Goodman A H. Juxtacortical chondrosarcoma of the hand. J Bone Joint Surg (Am) 1971: 53: 1370–1376
5. Wu K K, Kelly A P. Periosteal (juxtacortical) chondrosarcoma: report of a case occurring in the hand. J Hand Surg (Am) 1977: 2: 314–315
6. Matsumoto K, Hukuda S, Ishizawa M, Saruhashi Y, Okabe H, Asano Y. Parosteal (juxtacortical) chondrosarcoma of the humerus associated with regional lymph node metastasis. A case report. Clin Orthop 1993: 290: 168–173
7. Mitchell A, Rudan J R, Fenton P V. Juxtacortical dedifferentiated chondrosarcoma from a primary periosteal chondrosarcoma. Mod Pathol 1996: 9: 279–283
8. Schajowicz F. Juxtacortical chondrosarcoma. J Bone Joint Surg (Br) 1977: 59: 473–480
9. Schajowicz F. Current trends in the diagnosis and treatment of malignant bone tumors. Clin Orthop 1983: 180: 220–252
10. Schajowicz F, McGuire M H. Diagnostic difficulties in skeletal pathology. Clin Orthop 1989: 240: 281–310
11. Schajowicz F, McGuire M H, Santini Araujo E, Muscolo DL, Gitelis S. Osteosarcomas arising on the surfaces of long bones. J Bone Joint Surg (Am) 1988: 70: 555–564
12. Chano T, Matsumoto K, Ishizawa M, Morimoto S, Hukuda S, Okabe H. Periosteal osteosarcoma and parosteal chondrosarcoma evaluated by double immunohistochemical staining. Report of 2 cases. Acta Orthop Scand 1994: 65: 355–358
13. Lichtenstein L, Bernstein D. Unusual benign and malignant

chondroid tumors of bone: a survey of some mesenchymal cartilage tumors and malignant chondroblastic tumors, including a few multicentric ones as well as many atypical benign chondroblastomas and chondromyxoid fibromas. Cancer 1959: 12: 1142–1157

14. Bertoni F, Picci P, Bacchini P et al. Mesenchymal chondrosarcoma of bone and soft tissues. Cancer 1983: 52: 533–541

15. Nakashima Y, Unni K K, Shives T C, Swee R G, Dahlin D C. Mesenchymal chondrosarcoma of bone and soft tissue: a review of 111 cases. Cancer 1986: 57: 2444–2453

16. Huvos A G, Rosen G, Dabska M, Marcove R C. Mesenchymal chondrosarcoma. A clinicopathologic analysis of 35 patients with emphasis on treatment. Cancer 1983: 51: 1230–1237

17. Salvador A H, Beabout J W, Dahlin D C. Mesenchymal chondrosarcoma – observations on 30 new cases. Cancer 1971: 28: 605–615

18. Dabska M, Huvos A G. Mesenchymal chondrosarcoma in the young. Virchows Arch A Pathol Anat Histopathol 1983: 399: 89–104

19. Castello M A, Clerico A, Dominici C, Capocaccia P, Helson L. Mesenchymal chondrosarcoma. A case report in a four year old girl. Eur Paediatr Haematol Oncol 1985: 2: 209–215

20. Bertoni F, Bacchini P, Picci P, Gherlinzoni F. Case report 517. Mesenchymal chondrosarcoma of the femur. Skeletal Radiol 1989: 18: 221–224

21. Sears W P, Tefft M, Cohen J. Post-irradiation mesenchymal chondrosarcoma. A case report. Pediatrics 1967: 40: 254–258

22. Blackwell J B. Mesenchymal chondrosarcoma arising in fibrous dysplasia of the femur. J Clin Pathol 1993: 46: 961–962

23. Dahlin D C, Henderson E D. Mesenchymal chondrosarcoma: further observations on a new entity. Cancer 1962: 15: 410–417

24. Vilanova J R, Simon-Marin R, Burgos-Bretones J, Ramirez M M, Rivera-Pomar JM. Non-conventional chondrosarcomas and chondrogenesis. Histopathology 1985: 7: 719–728

25. Walaas L, Kindblom L G, Gunterberg B, Bergh P. Light and electron microscopic examination of fine needle aspirates in the preoperative diagnosis of cartilaginous tumors. Diagn Cytopathol 1990: 6: 396–408

26. Nakamura Y, Becker L E, Marks A. S100 protein in tumors of cartilage and bone. An immunohistochemical study. Cancer 1983: 52: 1820–1824

27. Ushigome S, Takakuwa T, Shinagawa T, Tagaki M, Kishimoto M, Mori N. Ultrastructure of cartilaginous tumors and S-100 protein in the tumors. With reference to the histogenesis of chondroblastoma, chondromyxoid fibroma and mesenchymal chondrosarcoma. Acta Pathol Jpn 1984: 34: 1285–1300

28. Swanson P E, Lillemoe T J, Manivel J C, Wick M R. Mesenchymal chondrosarcoma. An immunohistochemical study. Arch Pathol Lab Med 1990: 114: 943–948

29. Dobin S M, Donner L R, Speights V O Jr. Mesenchymal chondrosarcoma. A cytogenetic, immunohistochemical and ultrastructural study. Cancer Genet Cytogenet 1995: 83: 56–60

30. Devaney K, Abbondanzo S L, Shekitka K M, Wolov R B, Sweet D E. MIC2 detection in tumors of bone and adjacent soft tissues. Clin Orthop 1995: 310: 176–187

31. Welkerling H, Wolf E, Delling G. Morphologische Besonderheiten und Differentialdiagnose des zentralen mesenchymalen Chondrosarkoms-eine Analyse an 15 Fällen. Pathologe 1993: 14: 78–83

32. Mandahl N, Heim S, Arheden K, Rydholm A, Willen H, Mitelman F. Chromosomal rearrangements in chondromatous tumors. Cancer 1990: 65: 242–248

33. Sainati L, Scapinello A, Montaldi A et al. A mesenchymal chondrosarcoma of a child with the reciprocal translocation (11;22)(q24;q12). Cancer Genet Cytogenet 1993: 71: 144–147

34. Martinez-Tello F J, Navas-Palacios J J. Ultrastructural study of conventional chondrosarcoma and myxoid and mesenchymal chondrosarcomas. Virchows Arch A Pathol Anat Histol 1982: 396: 197–211

35. Mawad J K, MacKay B, Raymond A K, Ayala A G. Electron microscopy in the diagnosis of small round cell tumors of bone. Ultrastruct Pathol 1994: 18: 263–268

36. Steiner G C, Mirra J M, Bullough P G. Mesenchymal chondrosarcoma. A study of the ultrastructure. Cancer 1973: 32: 926–939

37. Mandalenakis N. Chondrosarcome mesenchymateux. Etude histologique et ultrastructurale. Ann Anat Pathol (Paris) 1974: 19: 175–188

38. Mikata A, Iri H, Inuyama Y. Mesenchymal chondrosarcoma – a case report with an ultrastructural study and review of Japanese literature. Acta Pathol Jpn 1977: 27: 93–109

39. Harwood A R, Krajbich J I, Fornasier V L. Mesenchymal chondrosarcoma: a report of 17 cases. Clin Orthop 1981: 158: 144–148

40. Unni K K, Dahlin D C, Beabout J W, Sim F H. Chondrosarcoma: clear-cell variant. A report of sixteen cases. J Bone Joint Surg (Am) 1976: 58: 676–683

41. Present D, Bacchini P, Pignatti G, Picci P, Bertoni F, Campanacci M. Clear cell chondrosarcoma of bone. A report of 8 cases. Skeletal Radiol 1991: 20: 187–191

42. Bjornsson J, Unni K K, Dahlin D C, Beabout J W, Sim F H. Clear cell chondrosarcoma of bone. Observations in 47 cases. Am J Surg Pathol 1984: 8: 223–230

43. Bagley L, Kneeland J B, Dalinka M K, Bullough P, Brooks J. Unusual behavior of clear cell chondrosarcoma. Skeletal Radiol 1993: 22: 279–282

44. Bejui J, Carret J P, Caille J P et al. Le chondrosarcome à cellules claires. A propos de quatre observations. Ann Chir 1982: 36: 303–306

45. Taconis W K. Clear cell chondrosarcoma: report of three cases and review of the literature. Diagn Imag Clin Med 1986: 55: 219–227

46. Salzer-Kuntschik M. Clear cell chondrosarcoma. J Cancer Res Clin Oncol 1981: 101: 171–176

47. Yamaguchi H, Isu K, Ubayama Y et al. Clear cell chondrosarcoma. Acta Pathol Jpn 1986: 36: 1577–1585

48. Weiss A P, Dorfman H D. Clear cell chondrosarcoma: a report of ten cases and review of the literature. Surg Pathol 1988: 1: 123–129

49. Gilbert T J, Goswitz J J, Griffiths H. Radiologic case study. Clear-cell chondrosarcoma. Orthopedics 1995: 18: 407, 410–412

50. Dahlin D C. Case report 54. Clear cell chondrosarcoma of humerus. Skeletal Radiol 1978: 2: 247–249

51. Ogose A, Motoyama T, Hotta T et al. Clear cell chondrosarcomas arising from rare sites. Pathol Int 1995: 45: 684–690

52. Campanacci M, Bertoni F, Laus M. Clear-cell chondrosarcoma. Ital J Orthop Traumatol 1980: 6: 365–372

53. Leggon R E Jr, Unni K K, Beabout J W, Sim F H. Clear cell chondrosarcoma. Orthopedics 1990: 13: 593–596

54. Kumar R, David R, Cierney G 3rd. Clear cell chondrosarcoma. Radiology 1985: 154: 45–48

55. Fobben E S, Dalinka M K, Schiebler M L et al. The magnetic resonance imaging appearance at 1.5 tesla of cartilaginous tumors involving the epiphysis. Skeletal Radiol 1987: 16: 647–651

56. Cohen E K, Kresell H Y, Frank T S et al. Hyaline-cartilage origin bone and soft tissue neoplasms: MR appearance and histologic correlation. Radiology 1988: 167: 477–481

57. Ding J, Hashimoto H, Tsuneyoshi M, Enjoji M, Masuda S, Ushijima M. Clear cell chondrosarcoma. A case report with topographic analysis. Acta Pathol Jpn 1989: 39: 533–538

58. Present D A, Bonar S F, Greenspan A, Paonessa K. Clear cell chondrosarcoma. An unusual case complicated by a microinfiltrative pattern of bone marrow involvement and postsurgical myositis ossificans. Clin Orthop 1988: 237: 164–169

59. Monda L, Wick M R. S-100 protein immunostaining in the differential diagnosis of chondroblastoma. Hum Pathol 1985: 16: 287–293

60. Weiss A P, Dorfman H D. S-100 protein in human cartilage lesions. J Bone Joint Surg (Am) 1986: 68: 521–526

61. Chan Y F, Yeung S H, Chow T C, Ma L. Clear cell chondrosarcoma: case report and ultrastructural study. Pathology 1989: 21: 134–137

62. Wang L T, Liu T C. Clear cell chondrosarcoma of bone. A report of three cases with immunohistochemical and affinity histochemical observations. Pathol Res Pract 1993: 189: 411–415

63. Faraggiana T, Sender B, Glicksman F. Light and electron microscopic study of clear cell chondrosarcoma. Am J Clin Pathol 1981: 75: 117–121

64. Ohno T, Park P, Oguro K et al. Ultrastructural study of a clear cell chondrosarcoma. Ultrastruct Pathol 1986: 10: 321–330

65. Forest M, Le Charpentier Y, Postel M et al. Une nouvelle variété de chondrosarcome: les chondrosarcomes dits 'chondroblastiques' ou chondrosarcomes à 'cellules claires'. Etude anatomo-clinique et ultrastructurale de 5 observations. Arch Anat Cytol Pathol 1978: 26: 5–11

66. Le Charpentier Y, Forest M, Postel M, Tomeno B, Abelanet R. Clear cell chondrosarcoma: a report of five cases including ultrastructural study. Cancer 1979: 44: 622–629

67. Povysil C, Matejovsky Z. A comparative ultrastructural study of chondrosarcoma, chordoid sarcoma, chordoma and chordoma periphericum. Pathol Res Pract 1985: 179: 546–559

68. Volpe R, Mazabraud A, Thiery J P. Clear cell chondrosarcoma. Report of a new case and review of the literature. Pathologica 1983: 75: 775–787

69. Duparc J, Badelon O, Bocquet L, Grossin M, Feldmann G. Un cas inhabituel de chondrosarcome à cellules claires avec des localisations tumorales intra-synoviales. Rev Chir Orthop Reparatrice Appar Mot 1985: 71: 127–131

70. Angervall L, Kindblom L G. Clear cell chondrosarcoma. A light and electron microscopic and histochemical study of two cases. Virchows Arch A Path Anat and Histol 1980: 389: 27–41

71. Ron I G, Amir G, Inbar M J, Chaitchik S. Clear cell chondrosarcoma of rib following repetitive low-impact trauma. Am J Clin Oncol 1995: 18: 87–89

72. Mankin H J, Cantley K P, Schiller A L, Lippiello L. The biology of human chondrosarcoma. II Variation in chemical composition among types and subtypes of benign and malignant cartilage tumors. J Bone Joint Surg (Am) 1980: 62: 176–188

73. Bosse A, Ueda Y, Wuisman P, Jones D B, Vollmer E, Roessner A. Histogenesis of clear cell chondrosarcoma. An immunohistochemical study with osteonectin, a non-collagenous structure protein. J Cancer Res Clin Oncol 1991: 117: 43–49

74. Dobashi Y, Sugimura H, Sato A et al. Possible association of p53 overexpression and mutation with high-grade chondrosarcoma. Diagn Mol Pathol 1993: 2: 257–263

75. Sreekantaiah C, Leong S P, Davis J R, Sandberg A A. Cytogenetic and flow cytometric analysis of a clear cell chondrosarcoma. Cancer Genet Cytogenet 1991: 52: 193–199

76. Demetrick D J, Kneafsey P D, Hwang W S. Signet-ring chondrosarcoma: a new morphologic entity. Hum Pathol 1991: 22: 1175–1179

77. Tsuneyoshi M, Dorfman H D. Epiphyseal osteosarcoma: distinguishing features from clear cell chondrosarcoma, chondroblastoma and epiphyseal enchondroma. Hum Pathol 1987: 18: 644–651

78. Raymond A K, Murphy G F, Rosenthal D I. Case report 425. Chondroblastic osteosarcoma: clear cell variant of femur. Skeletal Radiol 1987: 16: 336–341

79. Povysil C, Matejovsky Z, Zidkova H. Osteosarcoma with a clear-cell component. Virchows Arch A Pathol Anat Histopathol 1988: 412: 273–279

80. Komiya S, Inoue A, Nakashima M et al. Clear cell chondrosarcoma. A case report suggesting a malignant variation of chondroblastoma. Kurume Med J 1986: 33: 131–137

81. Fu Y S, Kay S. A comparative ultrastructural study of mesenchymal chondrosarcoma and myxoid chondrosarcoma. Cancer 1974: 33: 1531–1542

82. Bender B L, Barnes L, Yunis E J. Intra osseous 'chordoid' sarcoma, chondroblastic or lipoblastic origin? Virchows Arch A Pathol Anat Histol 1980: 387: 241–249

83. Pardo-Mindan F J, Guillen F J, Villas C, Vazquez J J. A comparative ultrastructural study of chondrosarcoma, chordoid sarcoma, and chordoma. Cancer 1981: 47: 2611–2619

84. Steiner G C, Greenspan A, Jahss M, Norman A. Myxoid chondrosarcoma of the os calcis: a case report. Foot Ankle 1984: 5: 84–91

85. Wolford J F, Bedetti C D. Skeletal myxoid chondrosarcoma with microtubular aggregates within rough endoplasmic reticulum. Arch Pathol Lab Med 1988: 112: 77–81

86. Abramovici L C, Steiner G C, Bonar F. Myxoid chondrosarcoma of soft tissue and bone: a retrospective study of 11 cases. Hum Pathol 1995: 26: 1215–1220

87. Dahlin D C, Beabout J W. Dedifferentiation of low-grade chondrosarcomas. Cancer 1971: 28: 461–466

88. Johnson S, Tetu B, Ayala A G, Chawla S P. Chondrosarcoma with additional mesenchymal component (dedifferentiated chondrosarcoma). I. A clinicopathologic study of 26 cases. Cancer 1986: 58: 278–286

89. Frassica F J, Unni K K, Beabout J W, Sim F H. Dedifferentiated chondrosarcoma. A report of clinicopathological features and treatment of seventy-eight cases. J Bone Joint Surg (Am) 1986: 68: 1197–1205

90. Capanna R, Bertoni F, Bettelli G et al. Dedifferentiated chondrosarcoma. J Bone Joint Surg (Am) 1988: 70: 60–69

91. Tetu B, Ordonez N G, Ayala A G, Mackay B. Chondrosarcoma with additional mesenchymal component (dedifferentiated chondrosarcoma). II. An immunohistochemical and electron microscopic study. Cancer 1986: 58: 287–298

92. Daly P J, Sim F H, Wold L E. Dedifferentiated chondrosarcoma of bone. Orthopedics 1989: 12: 763–767

93. Campanacci M, Bertoni F, Capanna R. Dedifferentiated chondrosarcomas. Ital J Orthop Traumatol 1979: 5: 331–341

94. McCarthy E F, Dorfman H D. Chondrosarcoma of bone with dedifferentiation: a study of eighteen cases. Hum Pathol 1982: 13: 36–40

95. Rockwell M A, Enneking W F. Osteosarcoma developing in solitary enchondroma of the tibia. J Bone Joint Surg (Am) 1971: 53: 341–344

96. Sanerkin N G, Woods C G. Fibrosarcomata and malignant fibrous histiocytomata arising in relation to enchondromata. J Bone Joint Surg (Br) 1979: 61: 366–372

97. Smith G D, Chalmers J, McQueen M M. Osteosarcoma arising in relation to an enchondroma. A report of three cases. J Bone Joint Surg (Br) 1986: 68: 315–319

98. Braddock G T, Hadlow V D. Osteosarcoma in enchondromatosis (Ollier's disease). Report of a case. J Bone Joint Surg (Br) 1966: 48: 145–149

99. Schweitzer G, Pirie D. Osteosarcoma arising in a solitary osteochondroma. S Afr Med J 1971: 45: 810–811

100. Slullitel J A, Schajowicz F, Slullitel J. Osteochondrome solitaire avec degenerescence maligne vers un sarcome osteogénique. Rev Chir Orthop Reparatrice Appar Mot 1971: 57: 471–478

101. Van Lerberghe E, Van Damme B, Van Hosbeeck M, Burssens A, Hoogmartens M. Case report 626. Osteosarcoma arising in a solitary osteochondroma of the femur. Skeletal Radiol 1990: 19: 594–597

102. Nojima T, Yamashiro K, Fujita M, Isu K, Ubayama Y, Yamawaki S. A case of osteosarcoma arising in a solitary osteochondroma. Acta Orthop Scand 1991: 62: 290–292

103. Tsuchiya H, Morikawa S, Tomita K. Osteosarcoma arising from multiple exostoses lesions: case report. Jpn J Clin Oncol 1990: 20: 296–298

104. Fechner R E, Huvos A G, Mirra J M, Spjut H J, Unni K K. A symposium on the pathology of bone tumors. Pathol Annu 1984: 19: 125–194

105. Abenoza P, Neumann P, Manivel J C, Wick M R. Dedifferentiated chondrosarcoma: an ultrastructural study of two cases, with immunocytochemical correlations. Ultrastruct Pathol 1986: 10: 529–538

106. Wick M R, Siegal G P, Mills S E, Thompson R C, Sawhney D, Fechner R E. Dedifferentiated chondrosarcoma of bone. An immunohistochemical and lectin-histochemical study. Virchows Arch A Pathol Anat Histopathol 1987: 411: 23–32

107. Rywlin A M. Chondrosarcoma of bone with 'dedifferentiation'. Hum Pathol 1982: 13: 963–964

108. Meis J M. 'Dedifferentiation' in bone and soft-tissue tumors. A histological indicator of tumor progression. Pathol Annu 1991: 26: 37–62

109. McFarland G B Jr, McKinley L M, Reed R J. Dedifferentiation of low grade chondrosarcomas. Clin Orthop 1977: 122: 157–164

110. Mercuri M, Picci P, Campanacci L, Rulli E. Dedifferentiated chondrosarcoma. Skeletal Radiol 1995: 24: 409–416
111. Mirra J M, Marcove R C. Fibrosarcomatous dedifferentiation of primary and secondary chondrosarcoma. J Bone Joint Surg (Am) 1974: 56: 285–296
112. DeLange E E, Pope T L Jr, Fechner R E. Dedifferentiated chondrosarcoma: radiographic features. Radiology 1986: 161: 489–492
113. Sissons H A. Case report 83. Dedifferentiated chondrosarcoma of the tibia. Skeletal Radiol 1979: 3: 257–260
114. Bertoni F, Present D, Bacchini P et al. Dedifferentiated peripheral chondrosarcomas. A report of seven cases. Cancer 1989: 63: 2054–2059
115. Park Y K, Yang M H, Fyu K N, Chung D W. Dedifferentiated chondrosarcoma arising in an osteochondroma. Skeletal Radiol 1995: 24: 617–619
116. Brooks J J. The significance of double phenotypic patterns and markers in human sarcomas. A new model of mesenchymal differentiation. Am J Pathol 1986: 125: 113–123
117. Astorino R N, Tesluk H. Dedifferentiated chondrosarcoma with a rhabdomyosarcomatous component. Hum Pathol 1985: 16: 318–320
118. Niezabitowski A, Edel G, Roessner A, Grundmann E, Timm C, Wuisman P. Rhabdomyosarcomatous component in dedifferentiated chondrosarcoma. Pathol Res Pract 1987: 182: 275–282
119. Munk P L, Connell D G, Quenville N F. Dedifferentiated chondrosarcoma of bone with leiomyosarcomatous mesenchymal component: a case report. Can Assoc Radiol J 1988: 39: 218–220
120. Dervan P A, O'Loughlin J, Hurson B J. Dedifferentiated chondrosarcoma with muscle and cytokeratin differentiation in the anaplastic component. Histopathology 1988: 12: 517–526
121. Karabela-Bouropoulou V, Markaki S, Kypparidou L, Stefis A, Prevedorou D. Dedifferentiated chondrosarcoma: a clinicopathological and immunohistochemical study of six cases. Arch Anat Cytol Pathol 1988: 36: 218–225
122. Bridge J A, DeBoer J, Travis J et al. Simultaneous interphase cytogenetic analysis and fluorescence immunophenotyping of dedifferentiated chondrosarcoma. Implications for histopathogenesis. Am J Pathol 1994: 144: 215–220
123. Reith J D, Bauer T W, Fischler D F, Joyce M J, Marks K E. Dedifferentiated chondrosarcoma with a rhabdomyosarcomatous differentiation. Am J Surg Pathol 1996: 20: 293–298
124. Sissons H A, Matlen J A, Lewis M M. Dedifferentiated chondrosarcoma. Report of an unusual case. J Bone Joint Surg (Am) 1991: 73: 294–300
125. Ishida T, Dorfman H D, Habermann E T. Dedifferentiated chondrosarcoma of humerus with giant cell tumor-like features. Skeletal Radiol 1995: 24: 76–80
126. Bonfiglio M, Platz C E. Case report 141. Malignant fibrous histiocytoma associated with enchondroma of bone. Skeletal Radiol 1981: 6: 127–130
127. Ruckstuhl H J, Morscher E, Remagen W, Ganz R, Beffa X. Giant cell tumors in combination with other primary bone tumors. Arch Orthop Trauma Surg 1981: 98: 1–6
128. Dee S, Meneses M, Ostrowski M L, Murakami M, Horowitz M, Graf W. Pleomorphic ('dedifferentiated') chondrosarcoma. Report of a case initially examined by fine needle aspiration biopsy. Acta Cytol 1991: 35: 467–471
129. Simms W W, Ordonez N G, Johnston D, Ayala A G, Czerniak B. p53 expression in dedifferentiated chondrosarcoma. Cancer 1995: 76: 223–227
130. Kahn L B. Chondrosarcoma with dedifferentiated foci. A comparative and ultrastructural study. Cancer 1976: 37: 1365–1375
131. Jaworski R C. Dedifferentiated chondrosarcoma. An ultrastructural study. Cancer 1984: 53: 2674–2678
132. Tarkkanen M, Wiklund T, Virolainen M, Elomaa I, Knuutila S. Dedifferentiated chondrosarcoma with t(9;22)(q34;q11–12). Genes Chromosomes Cancer 1994: 9: 136–140
133. Zalupski M M, Ensley J F, Ryan J, Selvaggi S, Baker L H, Wolman S R. A common cytogenetic abnormality and DNA content alterations in dedifferentiated chondrosarcoma. Cancer 1990: 66: 1176–1182
134. Remagen W, Jani L, Lüthi A, Schuman L. Atypical (dedifferentiated) chondrosarcoma or osteosarcoma with preponderant chondroblastic differentiation? J Cancer Res Clin Oncol 1981: 101: 177–182
135. Hollander J L, Dahlin D C, Sim F H. Adenocarcinoma metastatic to chondrosarcoma: a case report. J Bone Joint Surg (Am) 1978: 60: 543–545
136. Howie F M, Davidson J K. Case report 492. Chondrosarcoma of right ischium developing in a patient with Maffucci syndrome. Skeletal Radiol 1988: 17: 368–374
137. Block R S, Burton R I. Multiple chondrosarcomas in a hand. A case report. J Hand Surg (Am) 1977: 2: 310–313
138. Lewis M M, Marcove R C, Bullough P G. Chondrosarcoma of the foot. A case report and review of the literature. Cancer 1975: 36: 586–589
139. Stoker D J, Pringle J. Case report 168. Chondrosarcomatous transformation in a cartilage-capped exostosis. Skeletal Radiol 1981: 7: 135–138
140. Garrison R C, Unni K K, McLeod R A, Pritchard D J, Dahlin D C. Chondrosarcoma arising in osteochondroma. Cancer 1982: 49: 1890–1897
141. Ostlere S J, Gold R H, Mirra J M, Perlman R D. Case report 658. Chondrosarcoma of the proximal phalanx of right fourth finger secondary to multiple hereditary exostoses (MHE). Skeletal Radiol 1991: 20: 145–148
142. Norman A, Sissons H A. Radiographic hallmarks of peripheral chondrosarcoma. Radiology 1984: 151: 589–596
143. Josefczyk M A, Huvos A G, Smith J, Urmacher C. Bursa formation in secondary chondrosarcoma with intrabursal chondrosarcomatosis. Am J Surg Pathol 1985: 9: 309–314
144. Fadda M, Zirattu G, Espa E. Peripheral chondrosarcoma: ultrastructural investigation by transmission and scanning electron microscopy. Ital J Orthop Traumatol 1991: 17: 381–385
145. Grabias S, Mankin H J. Chondrosarcoma arising in histologically proved inicameral bone cyst: a case report. J Bone Joint Surg (Am) 1974: 56: 1501–1509
146. Grimer R J, Davies A M, Starkie C M, Sneath R S. Chondrosarcome chez un patient porteur d'osteopoikilie. A propos d'un cas. Rev Chir Orthop 1989: 75: 188–190
147. Schajowicz F, Defilippi-Novoa C A, Firpo C A. Thorotrast induced chondrosarcoma of the axilla. Am J Roentgenol Radium Ther Nucl Med 1967: 100: 931–937
148. Hatfield P M, Schulz M D. Post-irradiation sarcoma. Including 5 cases after X-ray therapy of breast carcinoma. Radiology 1970: 96: 593–602
149. Fitzwater J E, Cabaud H E, Farr G H. Irradiation-induced chondrosarcoma. A case report. J Bone Joint Surg (Am) 1976: 58: 1037–1039
150. Peimer C A, Yuan H A, Sagerman R H. Postradiation chondrosarcoma. A case report. J Bone Joint Surg (Am) 1976: 58: 1033–1036
151. Aprin H, Calandra J, Mir R, Lee J Y. Radiation-induced chondrosarcoma of the clavicle complicating Hodgkin's disease. Clin Orthop 1986: 209: 189–193
152. Huvos A G, Higinbotham N L, Miller T R. Bone sarcomas arising in fibrous dysplasia. J Bone Joint Surg (Am) 1972: 54: 1047–1056
153. Feintuch T A. Chondrosarcoma arising in a cartilaginous area of previously irradiated fibrous dysplasia. Cancer 1973: 31: 877–881
154. De Smet A A, Travers H, Neff J R. Chondrosarcoma occurring in a patient with polyostotic fibrous dysplasia. Skeletal Radiol 1981: 7: 197–201
155. Halawa M, Aziz A A. Chondrosarcoma in fibrous dysplasia of the pelvis. Case report and review of the literature. J Bone Joint Surg (Br) 1984: 66: 760–764
156. Ruggieri P, Sim F H, Bond J R, Unni K K. Malignancies in fibrous dysplasia. Cancer 1994: 73: 1411–1424
157. Pelzmann K S, Nagel D Z, Salyer W R. Case report 114. Polyostotic fibrous dysplasia and fibrochondrodysplasia. Skeletal Radiol 1980: 5: 116–118
158. Unni K K, Dahlin D C. Premalignant tumors and conditions of bone. Am J Surg Pathol 1979: 3: 47–60
159. Vanel D, Coffre C, Zemoura L, Oberlin O. Chondrosarcoma in children subsequent to other malignant tumours in different locations. Skeletal Radiol 1984: 11: 96–101

16

Fibrous cortical defect and non-ossifying fibroma

M. Forest

INTRODUCTION AND CLINICAL DATA

Although usually classed as bone tumors, fibrous cortical defects are presumably development abnormalities composed of a fibrohistiocytic cellular component, located in the metaphyseal region of long bones and discovered in children and adolescents.

The term 'fibrous metaphyseal defect' has been proposed by Schajowicz to describe fibrous cortical defects as well as the non-ossifying fibromas of long bones discussed in the original study of Jaffe & Lichtenstein.[1] The same lesions are reported under the term 'fibroxanthoma'.

Although there are some differences in size and location during the course of the lesion,[2] fibrous cortical defects and non-ossifying fibromas have the same histologic structure. Their frequent association or a gradual transition from one lesion to another on imaging studies are other reasons to suggest that they are either the same or closely related entities.[3]

Fibrous metaphyseal defects are found in patients between the ages of 2 and 22, with a mean age of 14 years.[4] There is a male predominance with a ratio of 4:3 to 2:1.

The incidence is somewhat difficult to assess. Many are clinically asymptomatic but in radiological screening studies, lesions are found in 35% of children between 2 and 12.[5] A higher incidence has been reported: a quarter of young females and more than half of young males between 2 and 18.[6] Despite the lower incidence found in German studies,[4,7] this is a very common lesion and one of the most characteristic on radiological grounds.

SKELETAL DISTRIBUTION

The most common sites are in the lower extremity: distal femur (40%), distal and proximal tibia (40%), fibula (10%) (Figs 16.1–16.4); rarer sites are in the upper

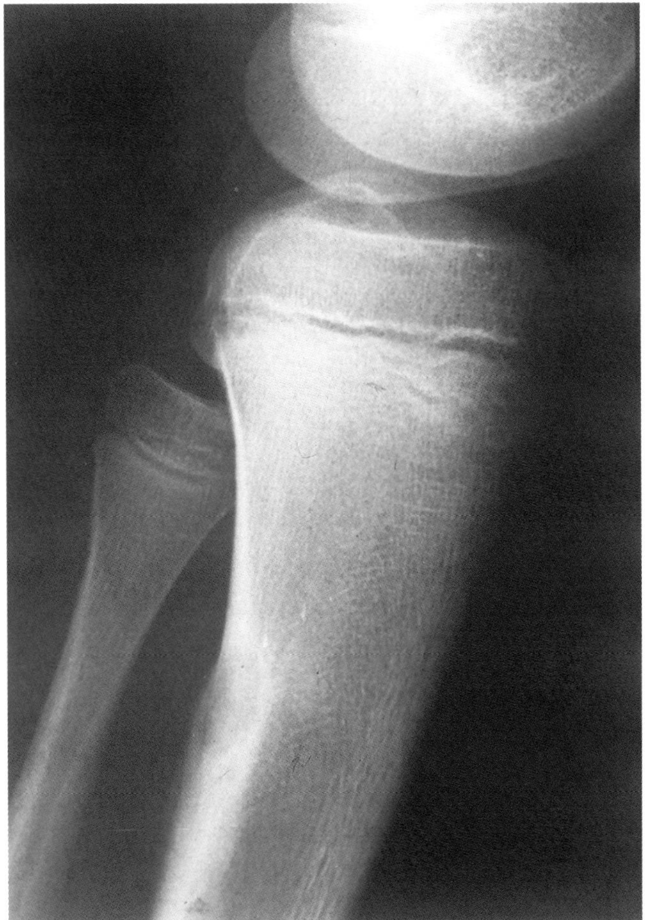

Fig. 16.1

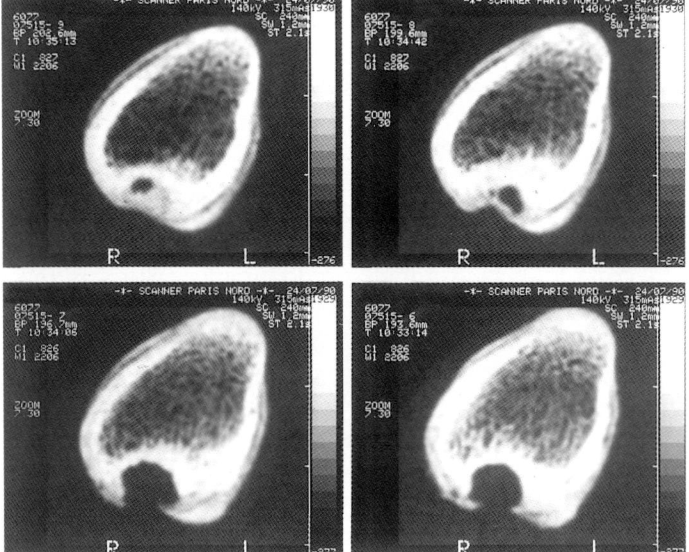

Fig. 16.2

Figs 16.1, 16.2 Fibrous metaphyseal defect of the tibia: cortical location well demonstrated on CT scans.

extremity (humerus). A few cases involve unusual locations such as the clavicle,[8] the ilium,[9] ribs, vertebrae, scapula, skull, mandible or even the small bones of the

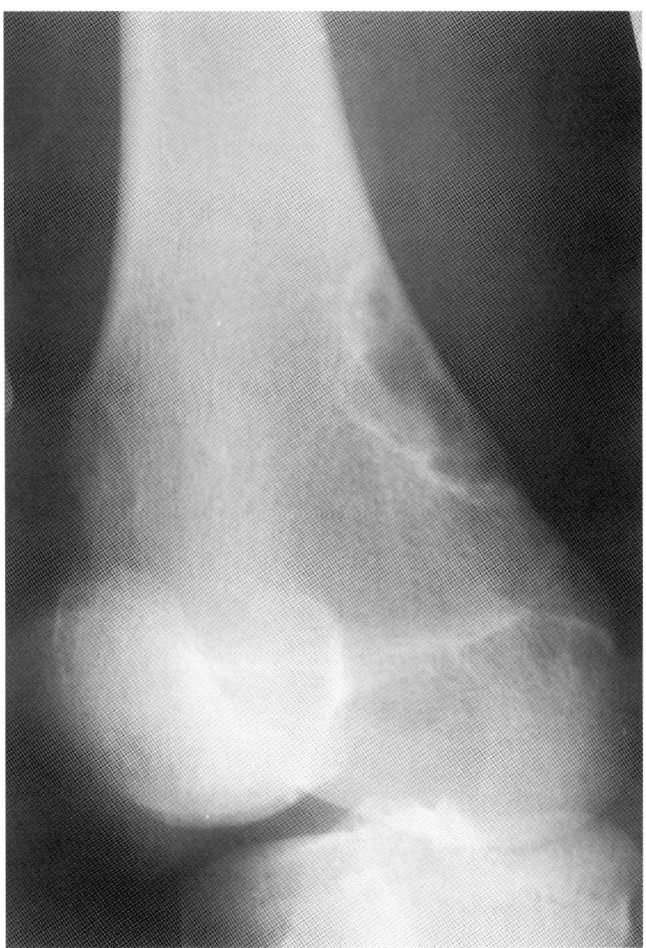

Fig. 16.3 Fibrous metaphyseal defect of the femur.

hand and feet. These lesions are now viewed as benign fibrous histiocytomas.

IMAGING

On plain films, fibrous cortical defects of tubular bones are metaphyseally located, close to the epiphyseal plate. They appear as an eccentrically located radiolucent area of circular or oval shape, the long axis being parallel to the axis of bone, with a size ranging from a few millimeters to 2 cm.[10] The margins are smooth or lobulated, in most cases well delineated with a thin rim of sclerosis.

Recent radiological studies have shown that most lesions occur very close to the tendon attachment sites for either the perichondrium of the epiphysis,[11] or, for the posteromedial site of the distal femur, the extensor tendon of the adductor magnus muscle or the medial head of the gastrocnemius.[10,11] This finding could suggest some etiological role of stress or trauma for these lesions. Similarly, metaphyseal cortical defects may constitute a weak site of muscle attachment and they have been reported with a periosteal reaction after an avulsion injury.[12]

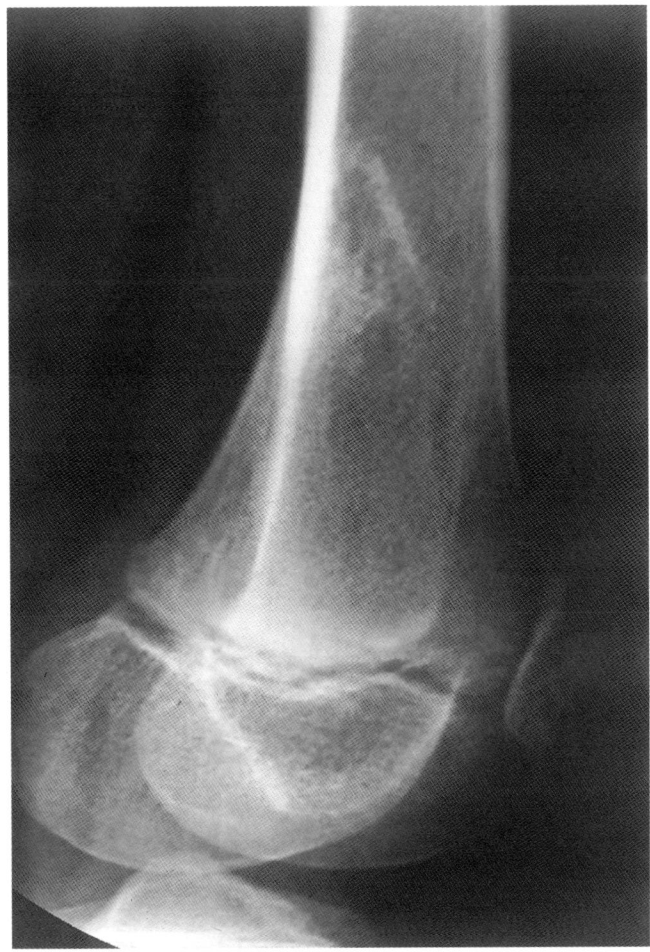

Fig. 16.4 Involuted fibrous cortical defect of the femur.

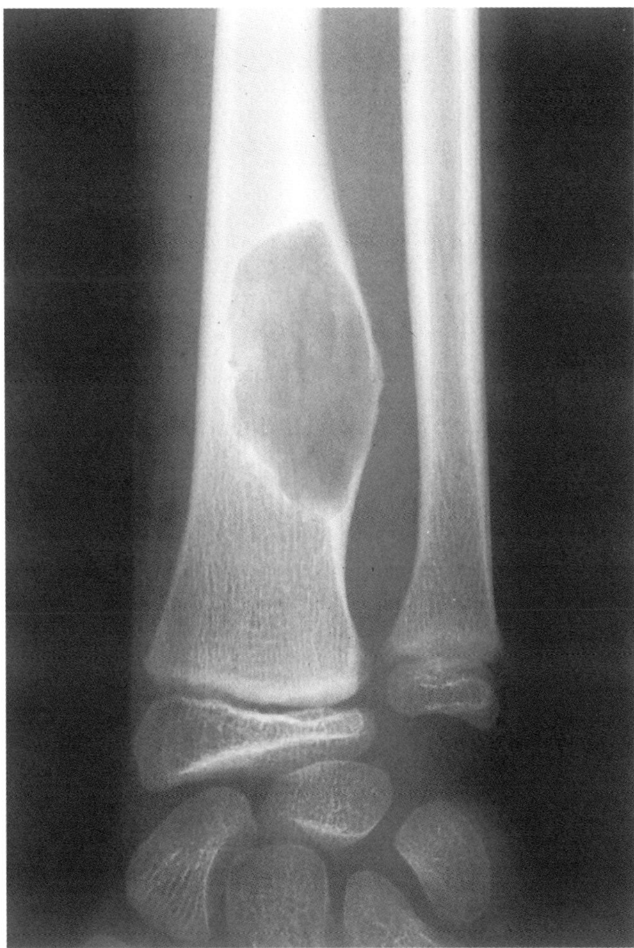

Fig. 16.5 Non-ossifying fibroma of the radius.

Radiological findings are closely related to the natural history of the lesions. Arising during the growth period, most of them persist with an average duration of 29 months.[11] Regression appears as a progressive peripheral ossification starting from the diaphyseal side and resulting in a homogeneous sclerosis,[11] which may be denser than the surrounding bone. Involution and total disappearance may be due to the physiological remodeling process of bone.

With bone growth, other lesions may move into the diaphysis; the cortex is expanded but the medullary cavity is not invaded. They appear as a fusiform expanding lytic defect located further away from the epiphyseal plate, with sclerotic borders and a thinning of the cortex. This intermediate stage of development has been aptly named a fibrous endosteal defect by Wilner.

Some lesions may grow into the medullary cavity, achieving a size of several centimeters, and are then known as non-ossifying fibromas[13] (Figs 16.5–16.8). Most of them occur between the ages of 10 and 20. The osteolytic areas with geographic borders are also eccentrically located and oval in shape. Some may have a multilocular appearance or ridges in the bony wall, corresponding to septa or trabeculations (Wilner 1982) (Figs 16.9, 16.10). Sclerotic scalloped borders are a frequent finding; the cortex may be thinned, eroded or slightly expanded. In small tubular bones, the lesion is usually central, with a moderate expansion of the cortex.

Non-ossifying fibromas may also involute, being filled by new bone in a few years (Wilner 1982), resulting in a ground glass or sclerotic appearance (Mulder et al 1993).

X-ray findings are so typical that other imaging techniques are seldom needed. CT may be useful for delineating the cortical involvement in rare doubtful cases, the lesion showing a non-specific attenuation value (Hudson 1987).

On MRI, both T1- and T2-weighted images show either a low signal intensity[14] or a high signal intensity on T2 surrounded by a low signal intensity rim representing marginal sclerosis.[10,15]

On radionuclide bone imaging, there is low or mild activity,[16] chiefly related to the new bone formation around the lesion (Hudson 1987).

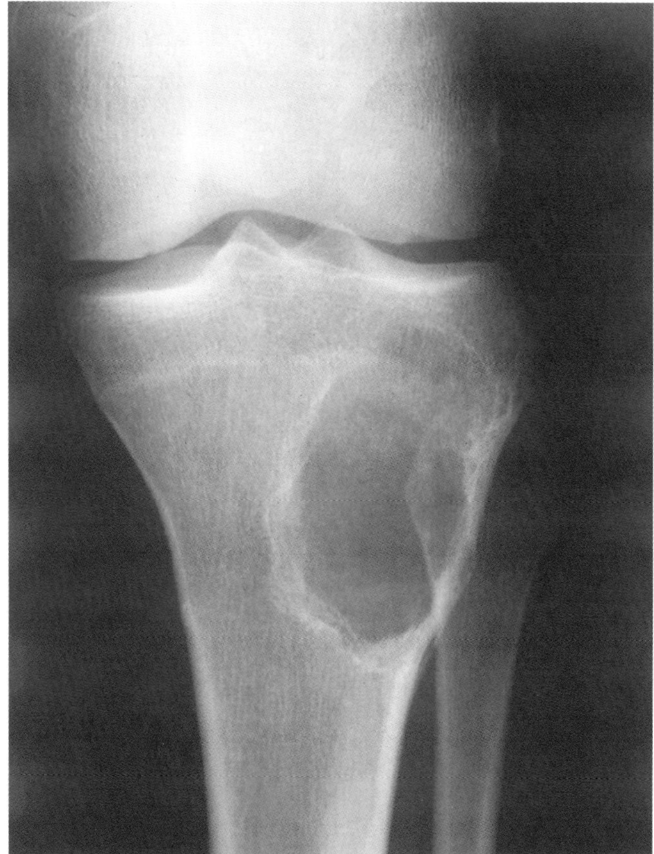

Fig. 16.6

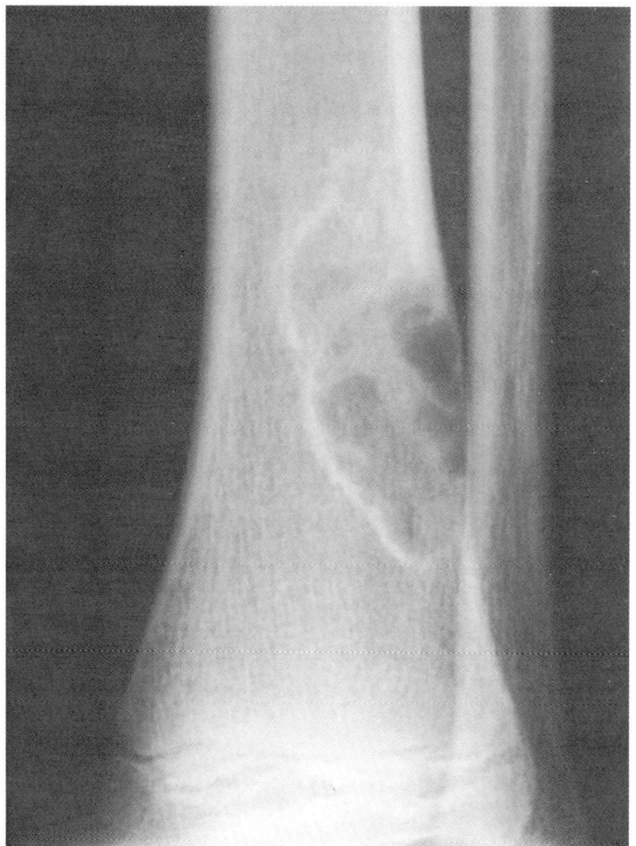

Fig. 16.7

Figs 16.6, 16.7 Non-ossifying fibromas of the tibia.

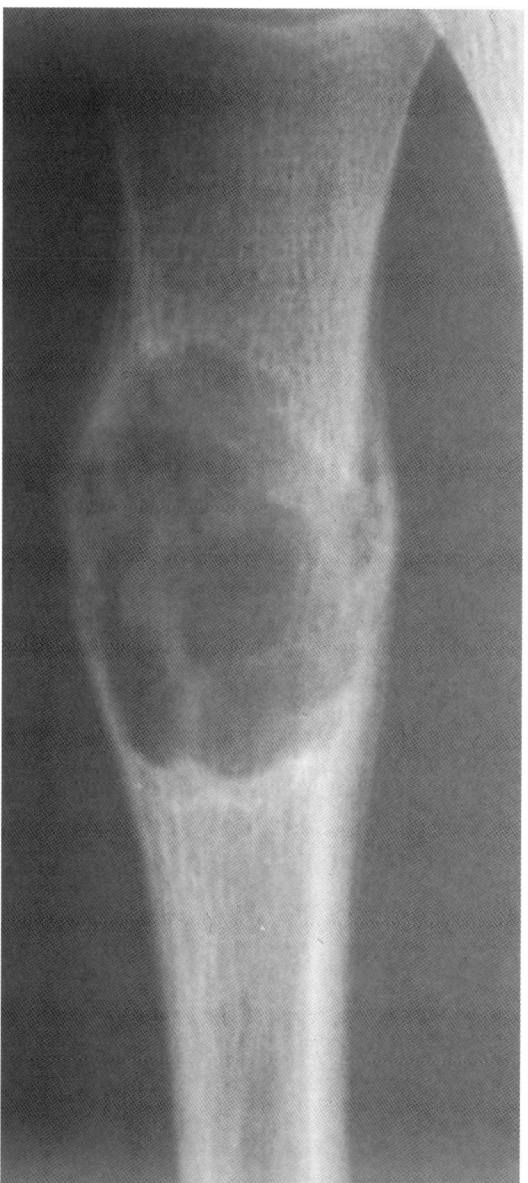

Fig. 16.8 Non-ossifying fibroma of the fibula.

MULTIPLE FIBROUS METAPHYSEAL DEFECTS

In about 8% of patients one can identify more than one lesion, with an average of three, most commonly presenting in the lower extremities (femur, tibia, fibula)[17] (Figs 16.11, 16.12). Some studies show an incidence as high as 50%.[18] Fibrous cortical defects are more often multiple than non-ossifying fibromas. With a size ranging from 0.5 to 10 cm, they are often bilateral and symmetrically distributed.[19] They may be clustered or coalescent; some may appear during the clinical course in a previously unaffected bone.[17]

In 5% of patients presenting with multiple lesions, neurofibromatosis lesions are identified.[20,21] Jaffe has described a new syndrome which comprises café au lait spots without evidence of neurofibromatosis; this entity was further studied by Campanacci et al[22] who described

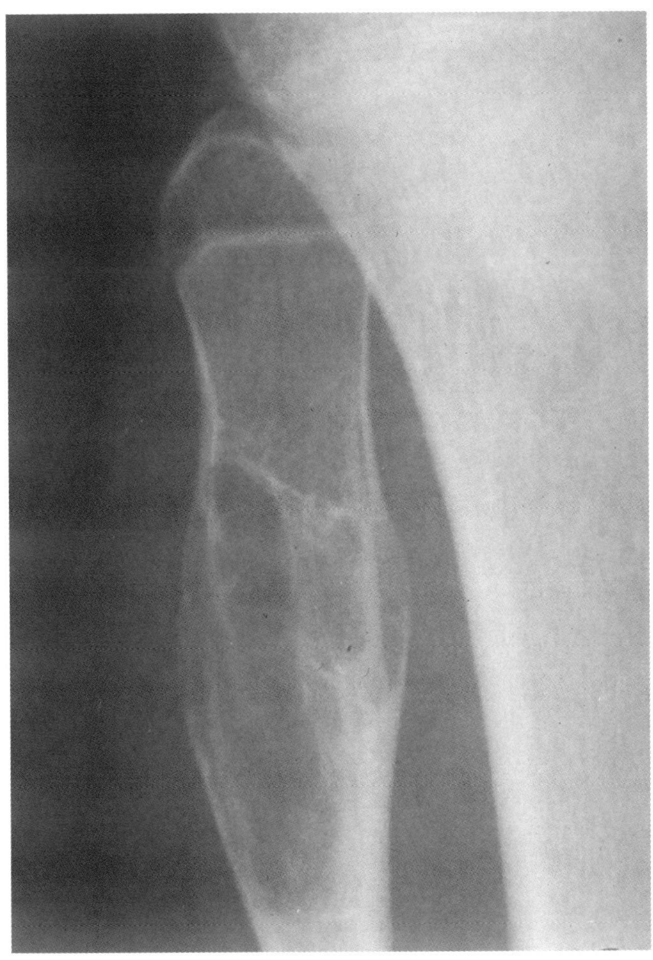

Fig. 16.9

Figs 16.9, 16.10 Non-ossifying fibroma of the fibula: trabeculations responding to ridges in the bony wall.

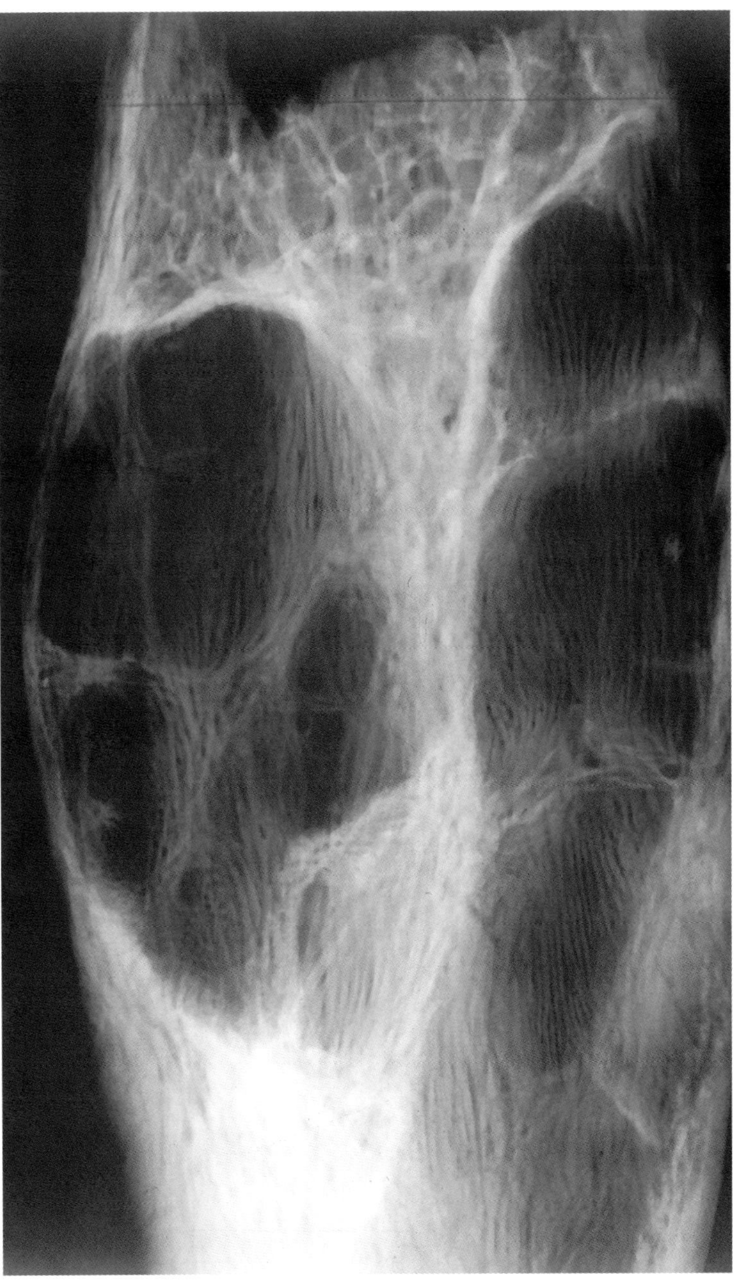

Fig. 16.10

associated jaw lesions, mental retardation, congenital blindness, kyphoscoliosis and precocious puberty. For this clinicopathological syndrome, Mirra has advocated the term 'Jaffe–Campanacci syndrome' and has stressed the histological similaraties between the giant cell reparative granulomas of the jaws and non-ossifying fibromas.[23]

Some cases with multifocal non-ossifying fibromas have been reported with a familial incidence.[24]

GROSS PATHOLOGY

The pathologist is usually dealing with the material of a curettage. Whole lesions may be found in amputation or resection specimens for malignant tumors, as an incidental finding.[25] The tissue appears red, gray or yellow, soft or rubbery. The cortical wall may show some scalloped borders.

HISTOPATHOLOGY

In most cases, metaphyseal fibrous defects appear as a fibroblastic proliferation with a high cellularity. Spindle-shaped fibroblasts do not present any nuclear pleomorphism, but some mitotic activity may be found, without atypical forms. The cellular component is distributed in a whorled or storiform pattern (Figs 16.13, 16.14). The associated collagen production, appearing as bundles of thin collagen fibers, is variable from field to field but more abundant in long-standing cases.

Foam cells or xanthoma cells are distributed in small

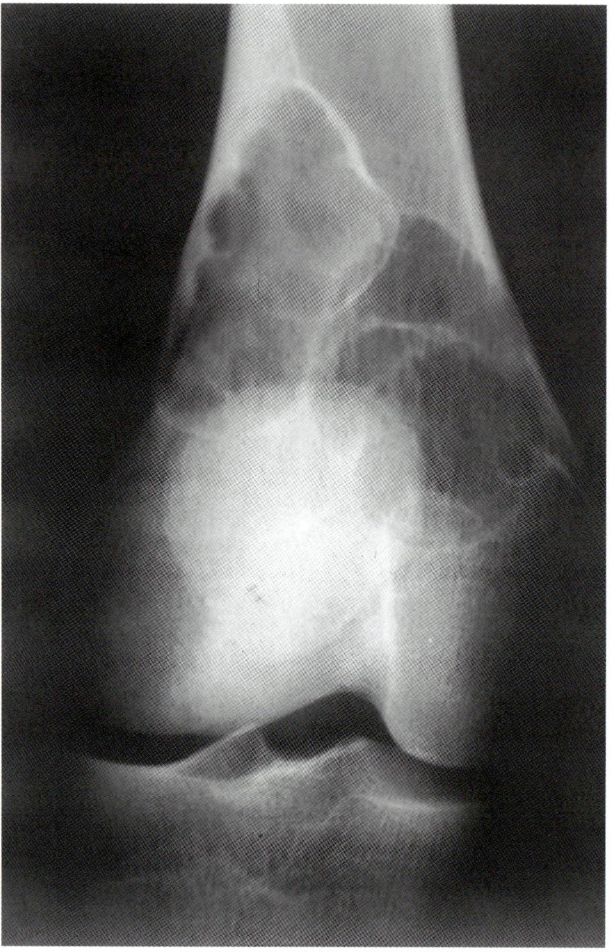

Fig. 16.11

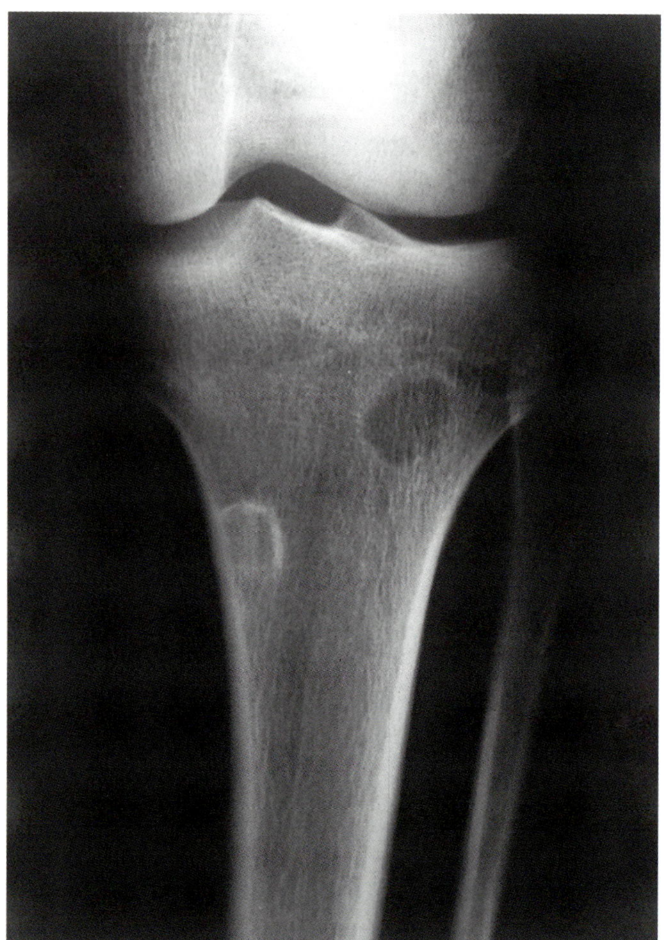

Fig. 16.12

Figs 16.11, 16.12 Case of multiple non-ossifying fibromas.

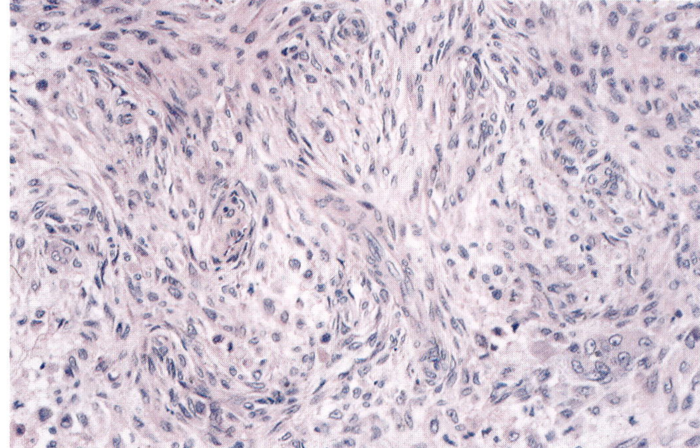

Fig. 16.13

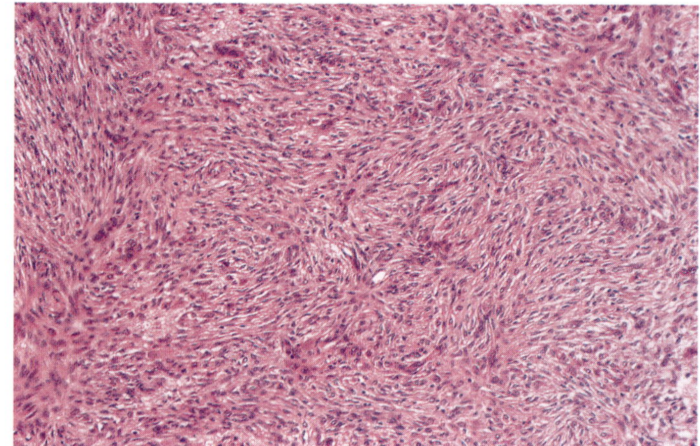

Fig. 16.14

Figs 16.13, 16.14 Non-ossifying fibroma: fibroblastic proliferation with a storiform pattern.

nests, related to hemosiderin pigment or lipid and cholesterol crystals (Figs 16.15–16.17). Haphazardly placed giant cells are common, sometimes clustered around stromal hemorrhages (Figs 16.18, 16.19).

Scattered lymphocytes are frequently found in the peripheral as well as the central parts of the lesion (Figs 16.16, 16.17).

Reactive bone formation is another common finding in peripheral areas (Figs 16.20), prompted by a pathologic facture. One study stressing bone production in a non-ossifying fibroma[26] may well represent a case of osteofibrous dysplasia (Wilner 1982). Obviously, healing lesions with extensive bone formation are never submitted to histological examination.

Unusual findings have been reported. Some lesions may be partially cystic and filled with a yellow liquid.[11,27] Other lesions have shown unexpected epithelioid cell granulomas whose significance is unclear: they could represent a

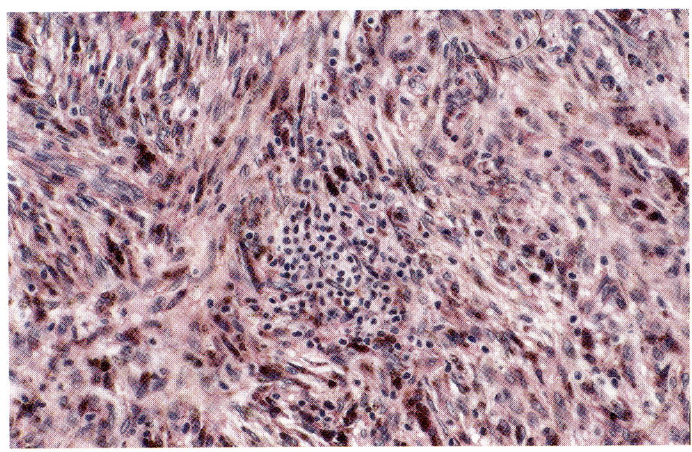

Fig. 16.17 Non-ossifying fibroma: hemosiderin pigment and lymphocytic infiltrate.

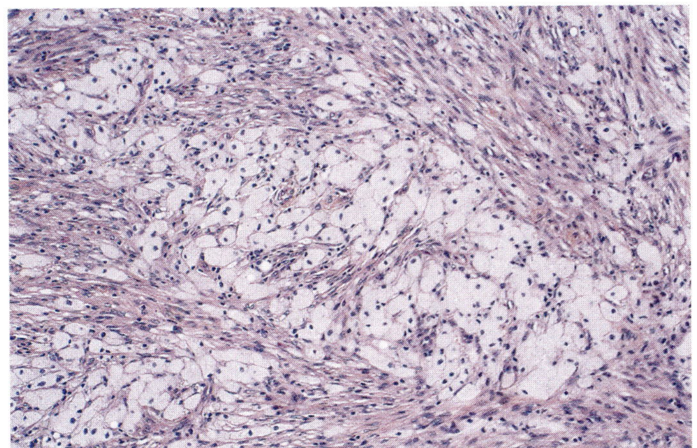

Fig. 16.15

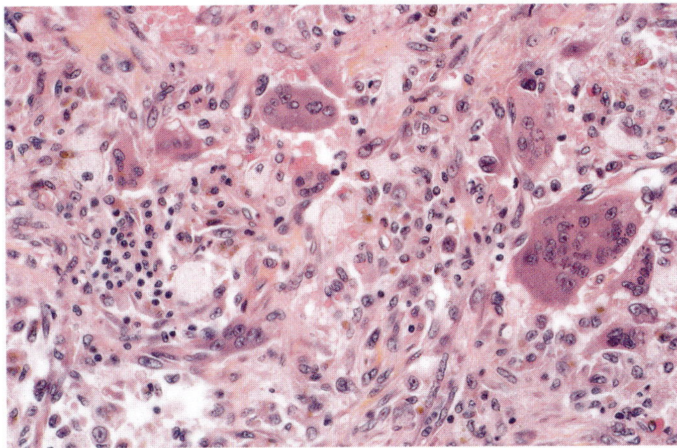

Fig. 16.18

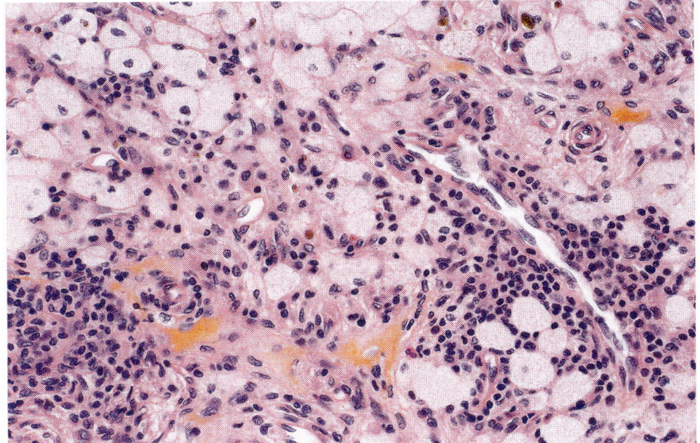

Fig. 16.16

Figs 16.15, 16.16 Non-ossifying fibroma: foam cells and lymphocytic infiltrates.

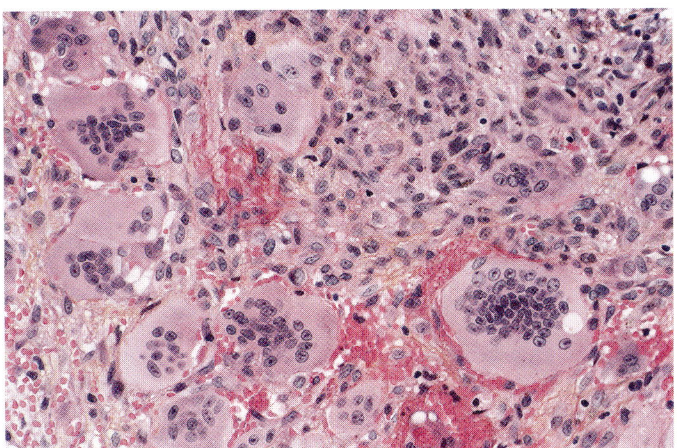

Fig. 16.19

Figs 16.18, 16.19 Non-ossifying fibroma: associated reactive giant cells.

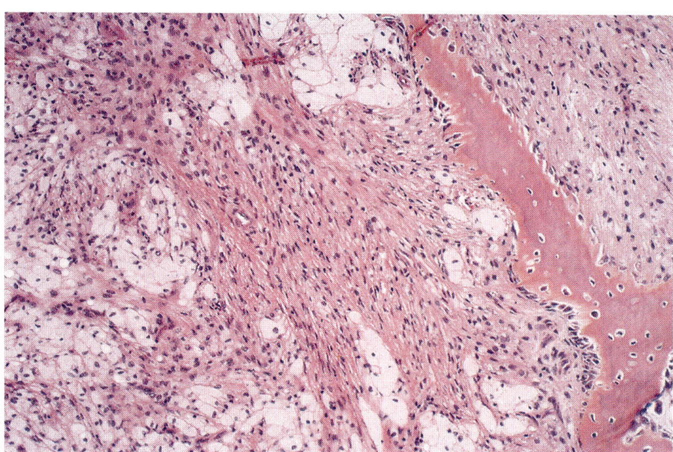

Fig. 16.20 Non-ossifying fibroma: peripheral reactive bone formation.

reaction to hemorrhage or a hypersensitivity response to drugs.[28]

CYTOPATHOLOGY

Clusters of fibroblast-like cells are associated with foam cells and some osteoclast-like giant cells.[29]

ELECTRON MICROSCOPY AND IMMUNOHISTOCHEMISTRY

The basic cells are fibroblast-like and many have myo-fibroblastic features with actin-like microfilaments;[30–33] progressively loaded with lipids, they transform into foam cells or present intracytoplasmic hemosiderin deposits located in lysosomes.[30,31] They resemble normal fibroblasts in different stages of proliferation and elaboration of extra-cellular material.[30]

Giant cells are similar to those of giant cell tumors and to osteoclasts, but there is no ruffled border.[30]

One study supports a histiocytic proliferation, based on the extensive pinocytotic activity and the large number of lysosomal bodies and lipid droplets, stressing the ability of histiocytes to behave as facultative fibroblasts.[34] A more unusual interpretation of fibroblast-like cells gradually accumulating lipids and forming xanthoma or foam cells is the similarity to primitive mesenchymal cells showing a partial maturation to lipoblasts, leading to the very unexpected name of 'benign lipoblastoma of bone'.[32]

A more recent immunohistochemical investigation corroborates the findings of Roessner et al.[35] Foam cells in non-ossifying fibromas stain strongly for LCA, CD68 and HLA-DR, indicating that they are not fibroblasts but macrophages, most probably part of the reactive mononu-clear histiocytic component of the lesion.[36]

COURSE, TREATMENT AND PROGNOSIS

Most of the fibrous cortical defects and many non-ossifying fibromas regress spontaneously through periph-eral ossification. In huge lesions, pathologic fractures occur in about 20% of cases;[18,37,38] they may heal spon-taneously.

Curettage and bone grafting are performed to prevent the fracture if the transverse diameter of the lesion is greater than 50% of the width of bone.[38]

A few cases have been reported in association with malignant tumors, chiefly with osteosarcomas;[39–43] they have been thoroughly discussed by Kyriakos & Murphy[43] and must be considered as a coexistence of two distinct lesions, as in the isolated report of an associated osteoid osteoma.[44] Some may be radiation-induced sarcomas.

DIFFERENTIAL DIAGNOSIS

Usually, the histological diagnosis is straightforward, espe-cially when the pathologist knows the radiological findings.

The most frequent pitfall is diagnosis of a giant cell tumor, due to the finding of many giant cells and fibro-blastic areas with a storiform pattern, also common in giant cell tumors. In fibrous metaphyseal defects, giant cells are less numerous, haphazardly distributed and not associated with a mononuclear cell component; the lesions occur at a younger age with a metaphyseal, not epiphyseal, location.

The differential diagnosis with benign fibrous histiocy-toma relies on clinical findings (pain) and chiefly on unusual locations, sometimes with an associated aggres-sive growth.

A prominent fibrous component may also mimic fibrous dysplasia, but the bone formation in fibrous cortical defects is only reactive, with frequent osteoblastic rim-ming.

In involuted lesions, the huge infiltration by foamy cells may resemble a xanthogranuloma or the end stage of an eosinophilic granuloma.

Parosteal or juxtacortical 'desmoids' may be considered as a hypocellular variant of a fibrous metaphyseal defect (Unni 1996, Wilner 1982), although Schajowicz relates the lesion to desmoplastic fibromas. Parosteal desmoid appears as a benign fibrous lesion beneath the periosteum, most often found at the site of insertion of the adductor magnus muscle.[45–49] It almost always involves the distal end of the femur (posterior medial surface of the medial femoral condyle) and is usually found in boys between 10 and 20 years. It may be bilateral and of small size, although some may be quite large.[50] Clinical symptoms, if present, are a localized soft tissue swelling or pain.

Juxtacortical desmoids are closely related to avulsive cortical irregularities believed to result from chronic stress with reactive bone formation.[48,51,52] On imaging, the radi-olucent cortical erosion or excavation may be associated with a compact periosteal reaction. Computed tomography is useful in doubtful cases.[53] Occasional reactive small bone spiculations may mimic malignancy[48,49,54] but on bone scintigraphy the uptake is negative[54] or slightly increased.[55] A stress fracture may also simulate a periosteal desmoid;[55] MRI shows the fracture line as well as the bone marrow edema.[56]

Histologically, dense fibrous tissue, continuous with the periosteum, may engulf some scattered fragments of bone, with osteoclastic resorption of the cortex.[57]

REFERENCES

1. Jaffe H L, Lichtenstein L. Non osteogenic fibroma of bone. Am J Pathol 1942: 18: 205–221
2. Skrede O. Non osteogenic fibroma of bone. Acta Orthop Scand 1970: 41: 362–380
3. Maudsley R H, Stanfeld A G. Non osteogenic fibroma of bone (fibrous metaphyseal defect). J Bone Joint Surg (Br) 1956: 38: 714–733
4. Freyschmidt J, Saure D, Dammenhain S. Der fibrose metaphysare Defekt (fibroser Kortikalisdefekt nicht-ossifizierendes Knochenfibrom). RÖFO 1981: 134: 169–177, 392–400
5. Caffey J. On fibrous defects in cortical walls of growing tubular bones. Their radiologic appearance, structure, prevalence, natural course, and diagnostic significance. Adv Pediatr 1955: 7: 13–51
6. Sontag L W, Pyle S I. The appearance and nature of cyst-like areas in the distal femoral metaphyses of children. Am J Roentgenol Radium Ther 1941: 46: 185–188
7. Schmidt M, Thiel H J, Spitz J. Der fibrose Kortikalisdefekt. RÖFO 1978: 128: 521–524
8. Gardiner G A, Linda L. Clavicular non osteogenic fibroma. An old tumor in a new location. Am J Dis Child 1974: 127: 734–735
9. Magliato H J, Nastasi A. Non osteogenic fibroma occurring in the ilium. Report of a case. J Bone Joint Surg 1967: 49: 384–386
10. Araki Y, Tanaka H, Yamamoto H et al. MRI of fibrous cortical defect of the femur. Radiat Med 1994: 12: 93–98
11. Ritschl P, Karnel P, Hajek P. Fibrous metaphyseal defects – determination of their origin and natural history using a radiomorphological study. Skeletal Radiol 1988: 17: 8–15
12. Kumar R, Swischuk L E, Madewell J E. Benign cortical defect: site for an avulsive fracture. Skeletal Radiol 1986: 15: 553–555
13. Young J W, Levine A M, Dorfman H D. Case report 293. Nonossifying fibroma (NOF) of the upper diametaphysis with considerable increase in size over a three-year period. Skeletal Radiol 1984: 12: 294–297
14. Kransdorf M J, Utz J A, Gilkey F W, Berrey B H. MR appearance of fibroxanthoma. J Comput Assist Tomogr 1988: 12: 612–615
15. Ritschl P, Hajek P C, Pechmann U. Fibrous metaphyseal defects. Magnetic resonance imaging appearances. Skeletal Radiol 1989: 18: 253–259
16. Brenner R J, Hattner R S, Lillien D L. Scintigraphic features of non osteogenic fibroma. Radiology 1979: 131: 727–730
17. Moser R P Jr, Sweet D E, Haseman D B, Madewell J E. Multiple skeletal fibroxanthomas. Radiologic-pathologic correlations of 72 cases. Skeletal Radiol 1987: 16: 353–359
18. Blau R A, Zwick D L, Westphal R A. Multiple non-ossifying fibromas. A case report. J Bone Joint Surg (Am) 1988: 70: 299–304
19. Kozlowski K, Harrington C, Lees R. Multiple symmetrical non-ossifying fibromata without extraskeletal anomalies: report of two related cases. Pediatr Radiol 1993: 23: 311–313
20. Gross M L, Soberman N, Dorfman H D, Seimon L P. Case report 556. Multiple non-ossifying fibromas of long bones in a patient with neurofibromatosis. Skeletal Radiol 1989: 18: 389–391
21. Mandell G A, Dalinka M K, Coleman B G. Fibrous lesions in the lower extremities in neurofibromatosis. AJR 1979: 133: 1135–1138
22. Campanacci M, Laus M, Boriani S. Multiple non ossifying fibromata with extraskeletal anormalities: a new syndrome? J Bone Joint Surg (Br) 1983: 65: 627–632
23. Mirra J M, Gold R H, Rand F. Disseminated non ossifying fibromas in association with café au lait spots (Jaffe–Campanacci syndrome). Clin Orthop 1982: 168: 192–205
24. Evans G A, Park W M. Familial multiple non osteogenic fibromata. J Bone Joint Surg (Br) 1978: 60: 416–419
25. Mubarak S, Saltzstein S L, Daniel D M. Non ossifying fibroma. Report of an intact lesion. Am J Clin Pathol 1974: 61: 697–701
26. Morton K S. Bone production in non osteogenic fibroma. J Bone Joint Surg (Br) 1964: 46: 233–243
27. Hoeffel J C, Metaizeau J P, Lascombes P, Aymard B, Galloy M A. Cystic degeneration in non-ossifying fibroma. Eur J Pediatr Surg 1992: 2: 374–377
28. Cozzutto C, Comelli A. Epithelioid granulomata in a nonossifying fibroma. The possible drug induced mechanism. Virchows Arch Pathol Anat Histol 1982: 397: 61–66
29. Troncone G, Vetrani A, Boschi R, Marino G. Il difetto fibroso metafisario in biopsia aspirativa per ago sottile. Isto-cytopatologia 1988: 10: 113–119
30. Steiner G C. Fibrous cortical defect and nonossifying fibroma of bone. A study of the ultrastructure. Arch Pathol 1974: 97: 205–210
31. Llombart-Bosch A, Peydro Olaya A, Lopez Fernandez A. Non ossifying fibroma of bone. A histochemical and ultrastructural characterization. Virchows Arch Path Anat Histol 1974: 362: 13–21
32. Lazarus S S, Trombetta L D. Non-ossifying fibroma or benign lipoblastoma of bone. An electron-microscopic and histochemical study. Histopathology 1982: 6: 793–805
33. Peuchmaur M, Forest M, Tomeno B, Abelanet R. Multifocal nonosteogenic fibroma: report of a case with ultrastructural findings. Hum Pathol 1985: 16: 751–753
34. Herrera G A, Reimann B E, Scully T J, Difiore R J. Nonossifying fibroma. Electron microscopic examination of two cases supporting a histiocytic rather than a fibroblastic origin. Clin Orthop 1982: 167: 269–276
35. Roessner A, Zwadlo G, Vollmer E, Sorg C, Grundmann E. Biologic characterization of human bone tumors. IX Occurrence of macrophages. Pathol Res Pract 1987: 182: 336–343
36. Doussis I A, Puddle B, Athanasou N A. Immunophenotype of multinucleated and mononuclear cells in giant cell lesions of bone and soft tissue. J Clin Pathol 1992: 45: 398–404
37. Drennan D B, Maylahn D J, Fahey J J. Fractures through large non ossifying fibromas. Clin Orthop 1974: 103: 82–88
38. Arata M A, Peterson H A, Dahlin D C. Pathological fractures through non-ossifying fibromas. Review of the Mayo Clinic experience. J Bone Joint Surg (Am) 1981: 63: 980–988
39. Katz J F, Marek F M. Case of coexistent benign and malignant bone tumors. J Mt Sinai Hosp NY 1950: 17: 187–191
40. Hastrup J, Jensen T S. Osteogenic sarcoma arising in a non-osteogenic fibroma of bone. Acta Pathol Microbiol Scand 1965: 63: 493–499
41. Bhagwajwandeen S B. Malignant transformation of a non osteogenic fibroma of bone. J Pathol Bacteriol 1966: 92: 562–564
42. Koppers B, Rakow D, Schmid L. Monostotische Kombination eines osteogenen Sarkoms mit einem nicht-ossifzierenden Knochenfibrom. Rontgenblatter 1977: 30: 261–266
43. Kyriakos M, Murphy W A. Concurrence of metaphyseal fibrous defect and osteosarcoma. Report of a case and review of the literature. Skeletal Radiol 1981: 6: 179–186
44. Fenton R L, Hoffman B P. Osteoid osteoma and nonossifying fibromas co-existing in one femur: case report. Bull Hosp Jt Dis 1953: 14: 217–220
45. Kimmelstiel P, Rapp I H. Cortical defect due to periosteal desmoid. Bull Hosp Jt Dis 1951: 12: 286–297
46. Marek F. Fibrous cortical defect (periosteal desmoid). Bull Hosp Jt Dis 1955: 16: 77–87
47. Melanotte P L. Il desmoide parostale. Clin Ortop 1960: 12: 436–444
48. Barnes G R Jr, Gwinn J L. Distal irregularities of the femur

simulating malignancy. Am J Roentgenol Radium Ther Nucl Med 1974: 122: 180–185

49. Craigen M A, Bennet G C, Mackenzie J R, Reid R. Symptomatic cortical irregularities of the distal femur simulating malignancy. J Bone Joint Surg (Br) 1994: 76: 814–817

50. Kirkpatrick J A, Wilkinson R H. Case report 52. Post-traumatic fibrous lesion distal end of the femur – parosteal (juxtacortical) desmoid. Skeletal Radiol 1978: 2: 189–190

51. Resnick D, Greenway G. Distal femoral cortical defects, irregularities, and excavations. Radiology 1982: 143: 345–354

52. Sklar D H, Phillips J J, Lachman R S. Case report 683. Distal metaphyseal femoral defect (cortical desmoid; distal femoral cortical irregularity). Skeletal Radiol 1991: 20: 394–396

53. Pennes D R, Braunstein E M, Glazer G M. Computed tomography of cortical desmoid. Skeletal Radiol 1984: 12: 40–42

54. Feine U, Ahlemann L M. Das periostale Desmoid im metaphysenbereich und seine differentialdiagnostische Abgrenzung von bösartigen Knochentumoren durch das Knochenszintigramm. RÖFO 1981: 135: 193–196

55. Dunham W K, Marcus N W, Enneking W F, Haun C. Developmental defects of the distal femoral metaphysis. J Bone Joint Surg (Am) 1980: 62: 801–806

56. Pistolesi G F, Caudana R, D'Attoma N, Residori E, Pregarz M. Case report 686. Stress fracture at distal end of femur simulating 'periosteal desmoid'. Skeletal Radiol 1991: 20: 454–457

57. Brower A C, Culver J E Jr, Keats T E. Histological nature of the cortical irregularity of the medial posterior distal femoral metaphysis in children. Radiology 1971: 99: 389–392

Desmoplastic fibroma of bone

M. Forest

INTRODUCTION AND CLINICAL DATA

Desmoplastic fibroma of bone, first described by Jaffe in 1958, is the osseous counterpart of desmoid tumors of the soft tissues.

It accounts for 0.3% of all benign bone tumors in the Mayo Clinic files. There is a male predominance in some series,[1] but no sex predilection in others.[2,3] It can occur at any age, but is most common in the first three decades of life,[4,5] with a mean age of 24 years.[1]

Some tumors are incidental findings,[4,6] the tumor being asymptomatic.[7] The growth may be insidious[8] with long-standing symptoms of swelling, tenderness or aching pain. Pathologic fractures are reported with an incidence of 10–15%; they can heal spontaneously.[9]

Desmoplastic fibromas have been reported in association with fibrous dysplasia[10,11] and Paget's disease.[12]

SKELETAL DISTRIBUTION

The common sites are the mandible,[1,2] the pelvis, chiefly the ilium[2] (Figs 17.1–17.3), and the femur,[13] followed by the humerus, tibia, radius, os calcis,[14] maxilla and skull. Almost any bone may be involved;[2] less frequent locations are the ribs,[15] the scapula, clavicle, sternum,[16] vertebrae[17–19] and small bones of hands and feet.[20–23] Two-thirds of the tumors involve the long bones. An unusual multicentric lesion has been reported.[4]

IMAGING

In long bones, most tumors are located in the metaphysis. They may reach a considerable size, up to 20 cm, with an epiphyseal extension;[1,24] a midshaft involvement is unusual.[8]

They appear as centrally located, purely lytic lesions, well defined by reactive sclerotic borders. A delicate trabeculated, soap bubble or honeycomb pattern is frequent,

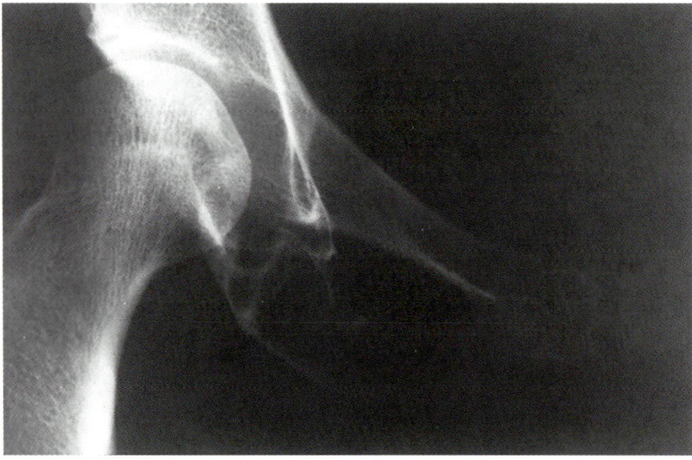

Fig. 17.1

Fig. 17.3

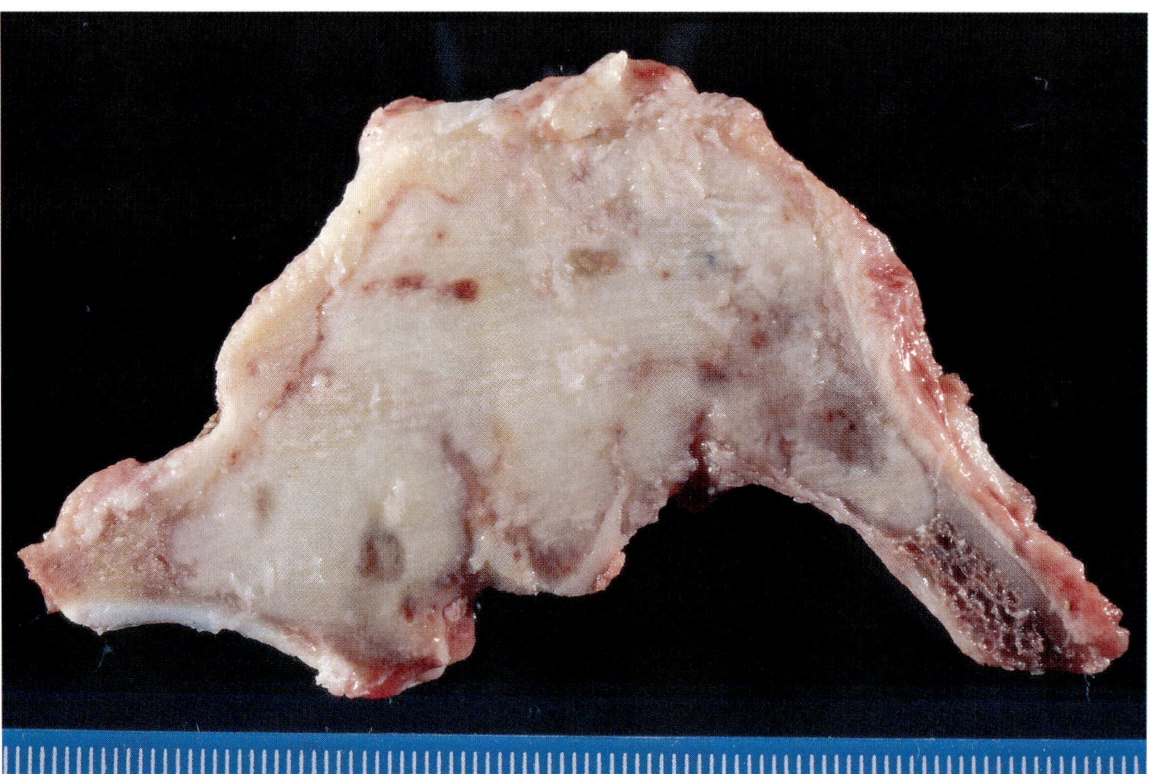

Fig. 17.2

Figs 17.1–17.3
Desmoplastic fibroma of the ischium. Honeycomb appearance due to bony ridges of the cortex.

pseudolobulations corresponding to bony ridges of the cortical wall (Wilner 1982). A polycystic aspect is mostly seen in pelvic bones or in the scapula.[3]

There may be thinning or expansion of the cortex, but periosteal reactions are very unusual.[2]

Occasionally, the tumor presents a permeative or moth-eaten patterns of bone destruction with cortical erosion or destruction and a soft tissue mass.[25]

CT imaging appears to be the best technique, especially in flat bones, to show the expansile lesion with well-defined margins or cortical breakthrough and soft tissue extension.[8,26–29]

MRI seems to add little to the diagnosis, but imaging of the intramedullary extent of the tumor,[28] as well as the extraosseous tumor component, may be useful for surgical planning.[29] There is an intermediate or low signal on T1- and T2-weighted images[6] or an inhomogeneous increased signal intensity on T2, representing areas of cystic necrosis.[7]

The tumor is hypovascular on angiography[2,29] and shows an increased uptake on radionuclide bone scans.

GROSS PATHOLOGY

The tumor appears as a firm, rubbery, dense mass, gray-white, sometimes with a whorled appearance and some authors describe it as peeling away easily from bone.[4,25] Occasionally, cysts may be found.[30] The adjacent cortex shows erosions or excavations.

HISTOPATHOLOGY

Uniform, small, spindle fibroblasts are distributed in sheets or haphazardly. Nuclei are ovoid or elongated, with a vesicular chromatin pattern.[1] Some nuclei may be prominent or hyperchromatic, but nucleoli and mitotic figures are absent.

Collagen fibers are usually abundant, appearing as thick bundles (Figs 17.4, 17.5). Rarely, some bone remnants may be trapped in the tumor. Foci of lymphocytes or mast cells have been found in some cases.[4] Reactive and usually peripheral bone appears in cases of pathologic fractures.

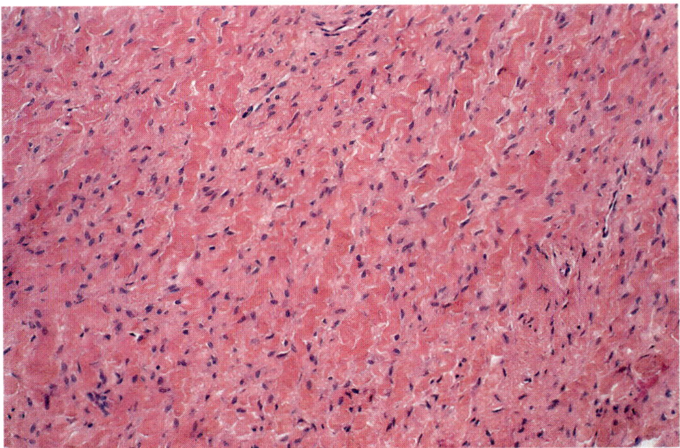

Fig. 17.4

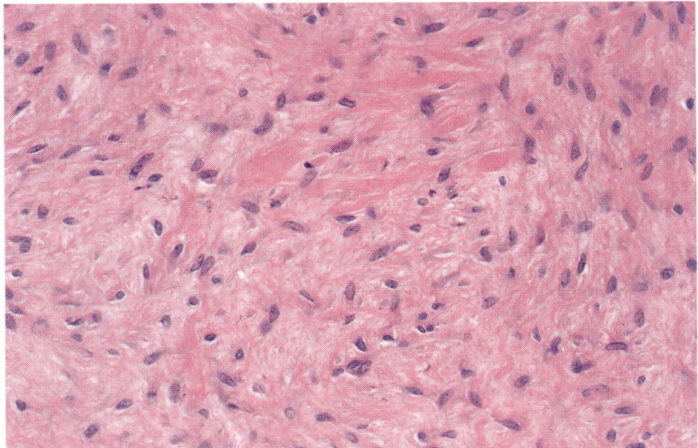

Fig. 17.5

Figs 17.4, 17.5 Desmoplastic fibroma of bone: small spindle fibroblasts and abundant collagen fibers.

Tongues of tumor may be found infiltrating bone. Some areas may be more cellular and less collagenous, but this has no prognostic significance.

IMMUNOHISTOCHEMISTRY

Most tumor cells exhibit a vimentin positivity while a few are weakly positive with antiactin.[29]

Five percent and 20% of the cells were labeled as proliferating cells in two cases with MIB-1 immunostaining.[29]

FLOW CYTOMETRY

In two cases, the tumors were diploid, but with indices of proliferation higher than that of extraosseous desmoid tumors, corresponding presumably to more aggressive growths.[29]

CYTOGENETICS

In a case of desmoplastic fibroma associated with fibrous dysplasia, a primary abnormal clone trisomic for both chromosomes 3 and 5 and two subclones, one trisomic for chromosome 3, one for chromosome 5, have been described.[11] Chondromyxoid fibroma shows an identical numerical abnormality (trisomy 5).[11]

ELECTRON MICROSCOPY

Some tumors exhibit the usual cellular features of fibroblasts[5,8] but myofibroblasts appear to be the predominent cell component,[31–33] associated with undifferentiated mesenchymal cells. It has been suggested that myofibroblasts could be linked to a better prognosis.[32]

COURSE, TREATMENT AND PROGNOSIS

The prognosis is dominated by recurrences following surgical treatment. There are no metastases. A recurrence rate as high as 42% has been reported following curettage;[4] there is no recurrence with a wide or marginal resection.[8,25]

Recurrences, appearing with an average interval of 2.7 years, have the same histological appearance.[4,5,8] The cellularity of the lesion has no correlation with the incidence of recurrence.[1]

Other modalities of treatment have been suggested: thorough curettage followed by cryosurgery (Huvos 1991) or, if feasible, en bloc resection.[6]

DIFFERENTIAL DIAGNOSIS

Rare cases of parosteal, juxtacortical or interosseous tumors have been reported[2,6,34] (Schajowicz 1994), demonstrating

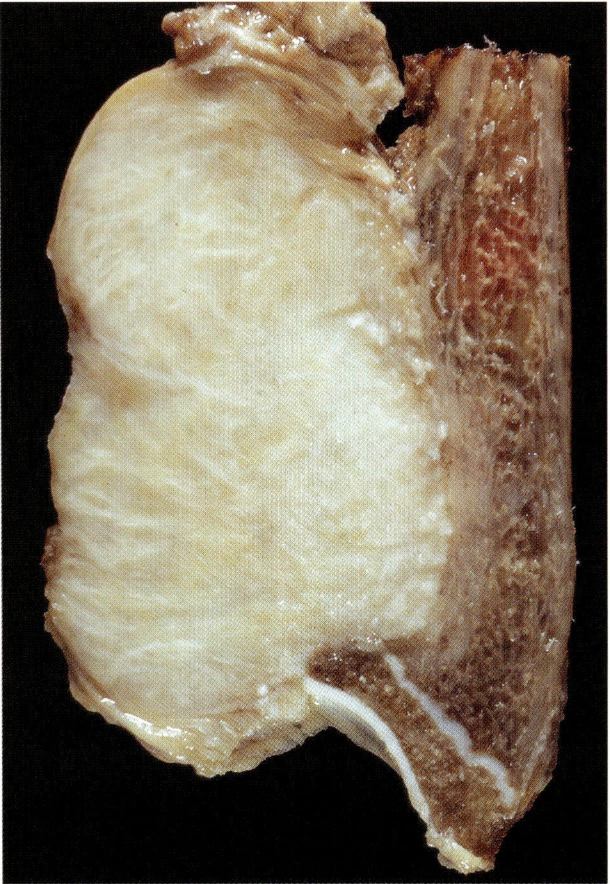

Fig. 17.6

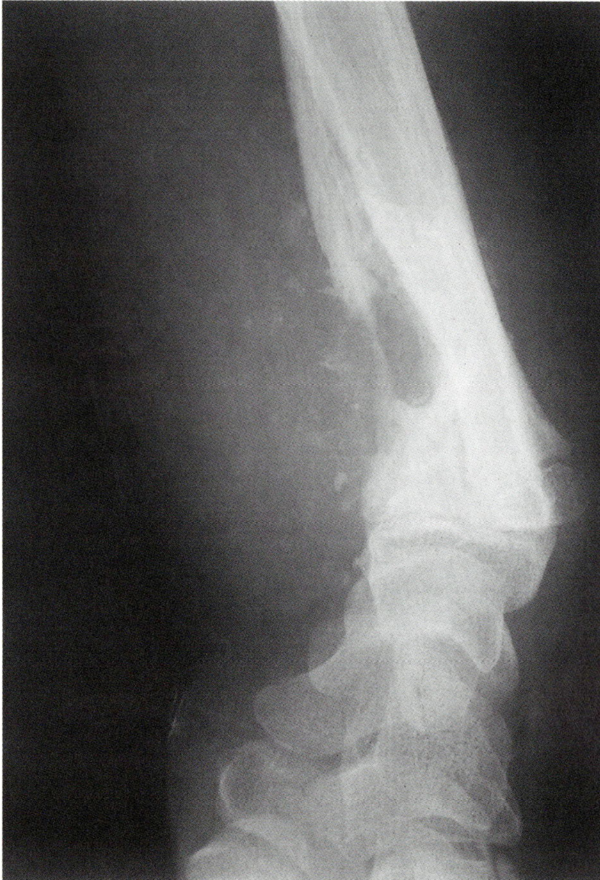

Fig. 17.7

Figs 17.6, 17.7   Recurrence of a soft tissue desmoplastic fibroma invading the radius.

a concave saucerization of the cortex with sclerotic borders (Figs 17.6, 17.7). They have to be differentiated from the small periosteal desmoids linked to the cortical irregularity syndrome (Figs 17.8–17.11).

Soft tissue fibromatosis arising periostally shows no overhanging edges of cortical bone on imaging studies.[27]

Congenital fibromatosis may be generalized or isolated in the skeleton,[35-42] with either a high incidence of recurrence or spontaneous regression.[35] Many of these lesions may well represent a myofibromatosis.[42]

Infantile myofibromatosis appears as multiple, well-marginated lytic bone areas.[43] Spindle cells are arranged in a whorled pattern with a collagenized background; some appear more typical of smooth muscular cells.

Solitary myofibromatosis[44-47] appears as a purely osteolytic lesion with a sclerotic rim; plump spindle-shaped cells alternate with fibroblastic and smooth-muscle cells, arranged in hyalinized or cellular nodules in short bundles or a whorled pattern and sometimes a chondroid-like matrix.[45] There is immunoreactivity for vimentin and α smooth-muscle actin and on ultrastructural exam-

ination, microfilaments with dense bodies in the fibroblast-like tumor cells are identified.[46] The lesions are cured by local excision or curettage; some may regress spontaneously.[44]

Solitary fibrous tumor of the periosteum[48] is a very rare lesion, appearing as a soft tissue mass attached to the periosteum (Figs 17.12–17.14). Hyalinized collagen fibers are associated with aggregates of fragmented elastic fibers. On ultrastructural study, fibroblasts are the sole cytological component.

Fibrous dysplasia, as well as intramedullary well-differentiated osteosarcoma, shows peculiar 'alphabetic' or metaplastic bone production or long strands of bone formation leading to the diagnosis.

Low-grade fibrosarcoma is a well-known and most difficult differential diagnosis, but the clinical course is similar (mostly recurrences). A well-differentiated fibrosarcoma may present a 'herringbone' pattern, slight pleomorphism and hyperchromasia of the cellular component and clumping of the chromatin in enlarged nuclei with nucleoli and few mitoses.

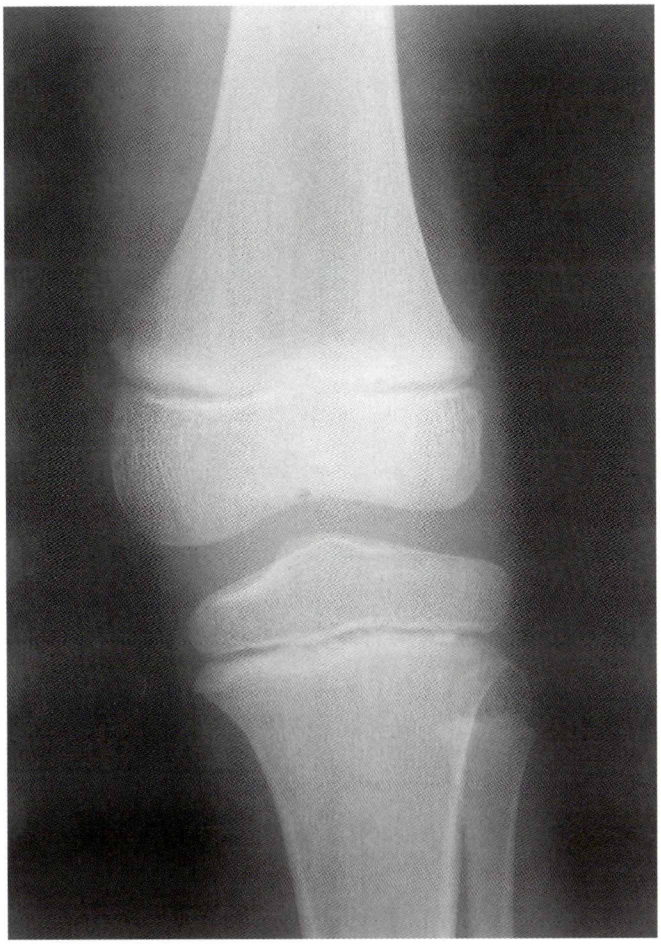

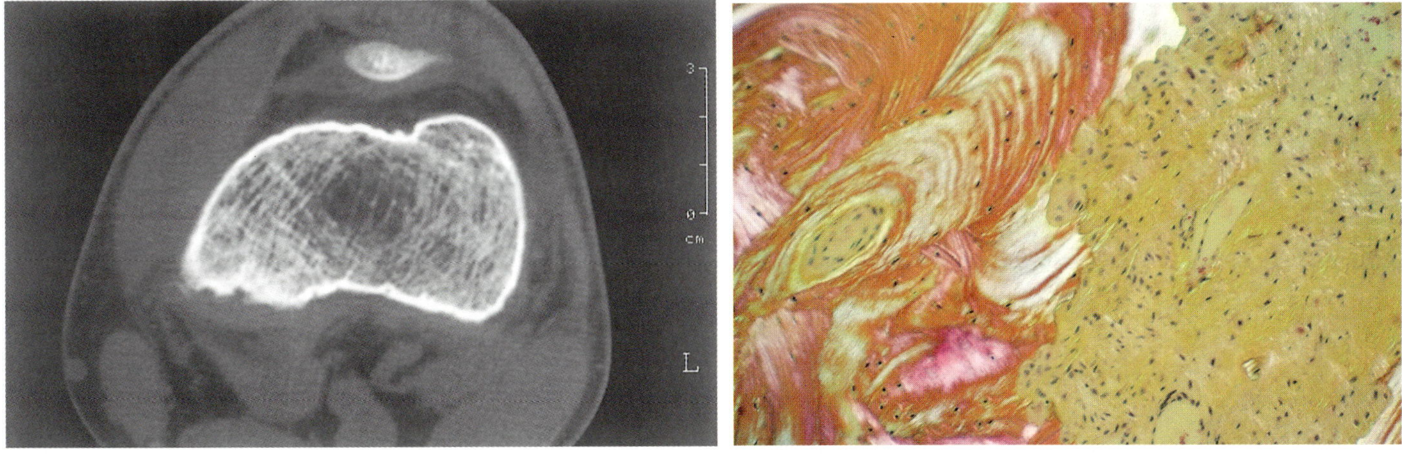

Fig. 17.8

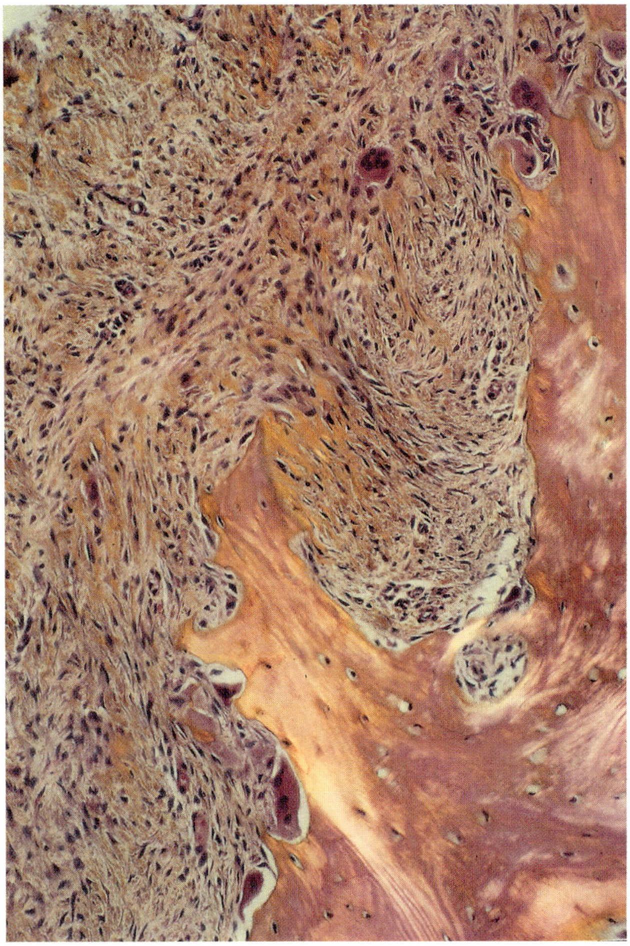

Fig. 17.9

Figs 17.8, 17.9 Periosteal 'desmoid' of the femur exhibiting fibrous tissue with osteoclastic resorption of the outer cortex (polarized light).

Fig. 17.10

Fig. 17.11

Figs 17.10, 17.11 Cortical irregularity syndrome of the femur demonstrating the same histologic features of periosteal 'desmoids' (polarized light).

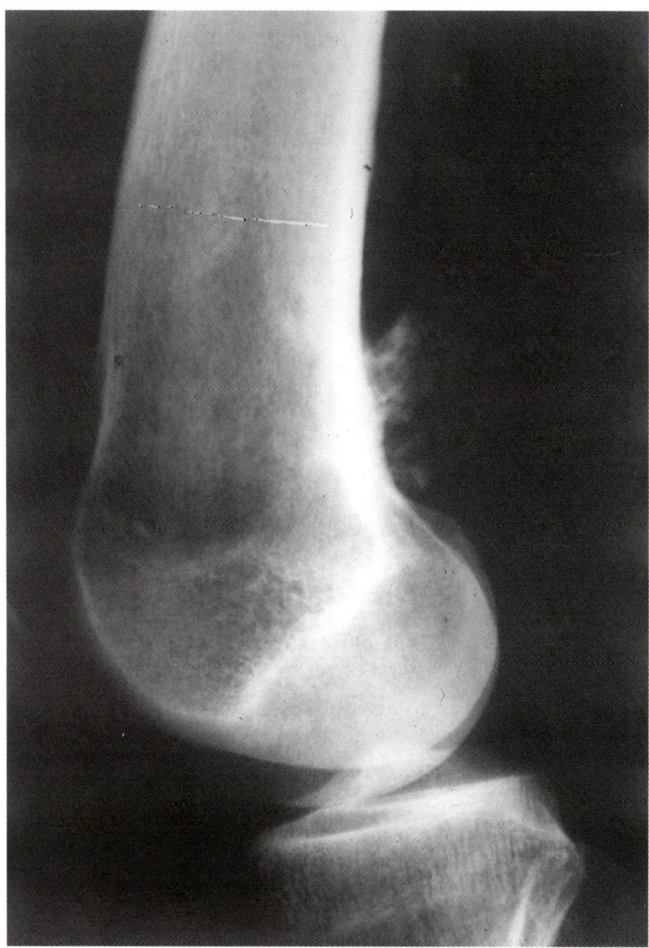

Fig. 17.12

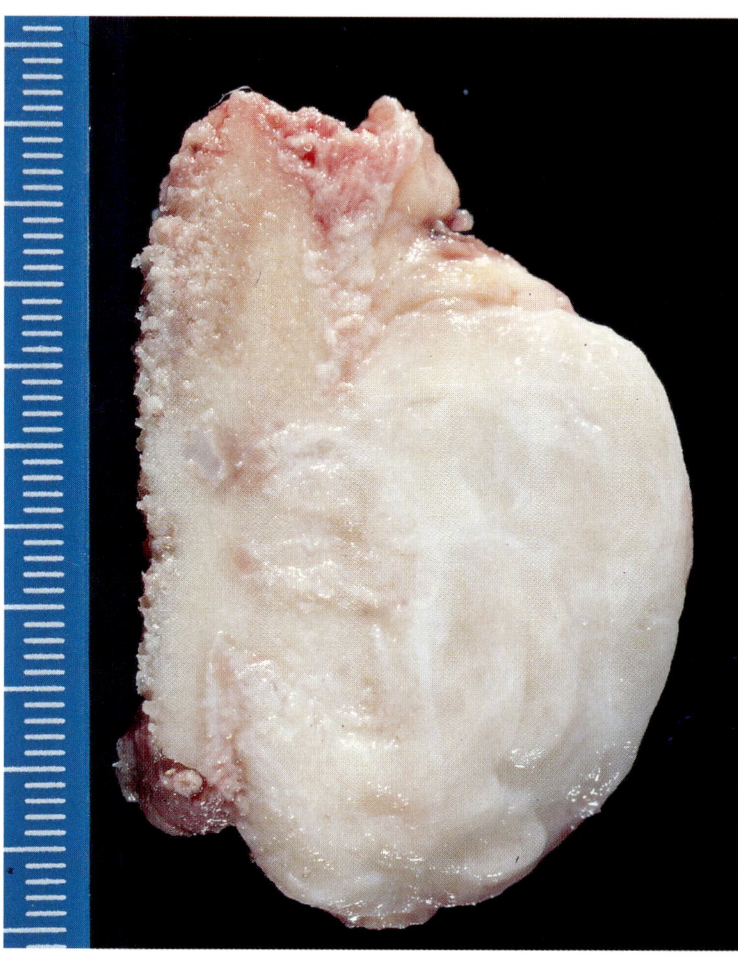

Fig. 17.13

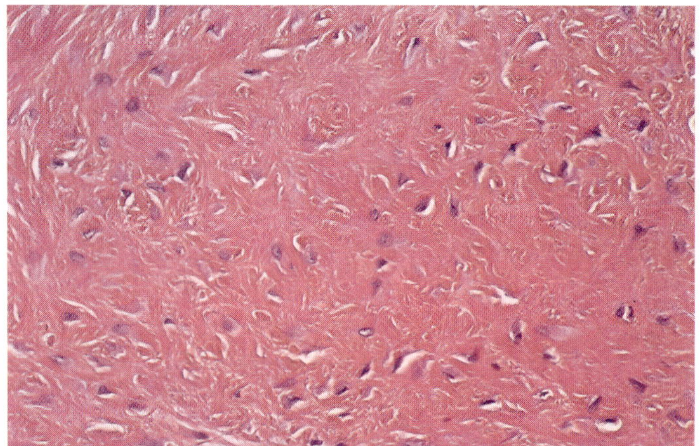

Fig. 17.14

Figs 17.12–17.14 Unusual surface lesion of the femur mimicking a parosteal osteosarcoma but histologically, only bland and scarce fibroblasts are associated with hyalinized collagen fibers (fibrous tumor of the periosteum?).

REFERENCES

1. Inwards C Y, Unni K K, Beabout J W, Sim F H. Desmoplastic fibroma of bone. Cancer 1991: 68: 1978–1983
2. Crim J R, Gold R H, Mirra J M, Eckardt J J, Bassett L W. Desmoplastic fibroma of bone: radiographic analysis. Radiology 1989: 172: 827–832
3. Nilsonne U, Göthlin G. Desmoplastic fibroma of bone. Acta Orthop Scand 1969: 40: 205–215
4. Gebhardt M C, Campbell C J, Schiller A L, Mankin H J. Desmoplastic fibroma of bone. A report of eight cases and review of the literature. J Bone Joint Surg (Am) 1985: 67: 732–747
5. Sugiura I. Desmoplastic fibroma. Case report and review of the literature. J Bone Joint Surg (Am) 1976: 58: 126–130
6. Taconis W K, Schütte H E, Van Der Heul R O. Desmoplastic fibroma of bone: a report of 18 cases. Skeletal Radiol 1994: 23: 283–288

7. Greenspan A, Unni K K. Case report 787. Desmoplastic fibroma. Skeletal Radiol 1993: 22: 296–299

8. Bertoni F, Calderoni P, Bacchini P, Campanacci M. Desmoplastic fibroma of bone. A report of six cases. J Bone Joint Surg (Am) 1984: 66: 265–268

9. Specchiulli F, Florio U. Desmoplastic fibroma of bone. A study of three cases. Ital J Orthop Traumatol 1976: 2: 141–150

10. West R, Huvos A G, Lane J M. Desmoplastic fibroma of bone arising in fibrous dysplasia. Am J Clin Pathol 1983: 79: 630–633

11. Bridge J A, Rosenthal H, Sanger W G, Neff J R. Desmoplastic fibroma arising in fibrous dysplasia. Chromosomal analysis and review of the literature. Clin Orthop 1989: 247: 272–278

12. Hillmann J S, Mesgarzadeh M, Tang C K, Bonakdarpour A, Reyes T G. Case report 481. Benign intraosseous fibroma (desmoplastic fibroma), associated with Paget disease of the iliac bone. Skeletal Radiol 1988: 17: 356–359

13. Graudal N. Desmoplastic fibroma of bone. Case report and literature review. Acta Orthop Scand 1984: 55: 215–219

14. Yu J S, Lawrence S, Pathria M, Resnick D, Haghighi P. Desmoplastic fibroma of the calcaneus. Skeletal Radiol 1995: 24: 451–454

15. Butters M, Hamann H, Mohr W. Desmoplastic fibroma of the rib. Thorac Cardiovasc Surg 1985: 33: 317–318

16. Obaro R O. Case report: desmoplastic fibroma of the sternum. Clin Radiol 1992: 46: 359–360

17. Fuji T, Hamada H, Masuda T et al. Desmoplastic fibroma of the axis. A case report. Clin Orthop 1988: 234: 16–20

18. Krakovits G E, Julow J, Illyes G. Desmoplastic fibroma in the spine. A case report. Spine 1991: 16: 481–482

19. Shinomiya K, Furuya K, Mutoh N. Desmoplastic fibroma in the thoracic spine. J Spinal Disord 1991: 4: 229–233

20. Di Stefano A, Pinelli G, Asquasciati G, Guarino M. Il fibroma demoplastico. Descrizione del primo caso della letteratura localizzato al metatarso. Desmoplastic fibroma. Minerva Pediatr 1981: 33: 577–582

21. Beskin J L, Haddad R J Jr. Desmoplastic fibroma of the first metatarsal. A case report. Clin Orthop 1985: 195: 299–303

22. El-Tabbakh A O, Al-Arabi K M. Desmoplastic fibroma – a rare tumor in a rare site. Int Orthop 1986: 10: 261–263

23. Hadjipavlou A, Lander P H, Begin L R, Eibel P. Desmoplastic fibroma of a metatarsal. Case report. J Bone Joint Surg (Am) 1986: 68: 459–461

24. Whitesides T E, Ackerman L V. Desmoplastic fibroma. J Bone Joint Surg (Am) 1960: 42: 1143–1155

25. Rabhan W N, Rosai J. Desmoplastic fibroma. Report of ten cases and review of the literature. J Bone Joint Surg (Am) 1968: 50: 487–502

26. Goldman A B, Bohne W H, Bullough P G. Case report 91. Desmoplastic fibroma of the ilium. Skeletal Radiol 1979: 4: 102–105

27. Young J W, Aisner S C, Levine A M, Resnik C S, Dorfman H D. Computed tomography of desmoid tumors of bone: desmoplastic fibroma. Skeletal Radiol 1988: 17: 333–337

28. Haney J, Olson P N, Griffiths H J. Radiologic case study. The clinical and radiologic features of desmoplastic fibroma of bone. Orthopedics 1994: 17: 80–85, 88

29. Böhm P, Kröber S, Greschniok A, Laniado M, Kaiserling E. Desmoplastic fibroma of the bone. Cancer 1996: 78: 1011–1023

30. Lichtman E A, Klein M J. Case report 302. Desmoplastic fibroma of the proximal end of the left femur. Skeletal Radiol 1985: 13: 160–163

31. Meerbach W. Das desmoplastische Fibrom als seltener Knochentumor. Zentralbl Allg Pathol 1987: 133: 243–248

32. Lagacé R, Delage C, Bouchard H L, Seemayer T A. Desmoplastic fibroma of bone. An ultrastructural study. Am J Surg Pathol 1979: 3: 423–430

33. Thirupathi R G, Vuletin J C, Wadwa R, Ballah S. Desmoplastic fibroma of the ulna. A case report. Clin Orthop 1983: 179: 231–238

34. Dong P R, Seeger L L, Eckardt J J, Mirra J M. Case report 847. Juxtacortical aggressive fibromatosis (desmoplastic fibroma) of the forearm. Skeletal Radiol 1994: 23: 560–563

35. Heiple K G, Perrin E, Aikawa M. Congenital generalized fibromatosis. A case limited to osseous lesions. J Bone Joint Surg (Am) 1972: 54: 663–669

36. Kindblom L G, Angervall L. Congenital solitary fibromatosis of the skeleton. Case report of a variant of congenital generalized fibromatosis. Cancer 1978: 41: 636–640

37. Faure C, Gruner M, Boccon-Gibod L. Case report 149. Infantile congenital fibrosarcoma of humerus. Skeletal Radiol 1981: 6: 208–211

38. Dahlin D C. Case report 189. Infantile fibrosarcoma (congenital fibrosarcoma-like fibromatosis). Skeletal Radiol 1982: 8: 77–78

39. Capusten B M, Azouz E M, Rosman M A. Fibromatosis of bone in children. Radiology 1984: 152: 693–694

40. Gold R H, Mirra J M. Case report 339. Congenital multiple fibromatosis. Skeletal Radiol 1985: 14: 309–311

41. Bolano L E, Yngve D A, Altshuler G. Solitary fibromatosis of bone. A rare variant of congenital generalized fibromatosis. Clin Orthop 1991: 263: 238–241

42. Wuisman P, Roessner A, Blasius S, Edel G, Vestring T, Winkelmann W. Case report 832. Solitary congenital or infantile (desmoid-type) fibromatosis of the proximal end of the tibia. Skeletal Radiol 1994: 23: 380–384

43. Present D A, Abdelwahab I F, Zwass A, Klein M J. Case report 575. Infantile myofibromatosis. Skeletal Radiol 1989: 18: 557–560

44. Beyer W F, Kraus J, Glückert K, Goldmann A R. Solitare infantile Myofibromatose des Os sacrum. Z Orthop 1990: 128: 473–476

45. Inwards C Y, Unni K K, Beabout J W, Shives T C. Solitary congenital fibromatosis (infantile myofibromatosis) of bone. Am J Surg Pathol 1991: 15: 935–941

46. Hasegawa T, Hirose T, Seki K, Hizawa K, Okada J, Nakanishi H. Solitary infantile myofibromatosis of bone. An immunohistochemical and ultrastructural study. Am J Surg Pathol 1993: 17: 308–313

47. Asirvatham R, Moreau P G, Antonius J I. Solitary infantile myofibromatosis of the axis. A case report. Spine 1994: 19: 80–82

48. O'Connell J X, Logan P M, Beauchamp C P. Solitary fibrous tumor of the periosteum. Hum Pathol 1995: 26: 460–462

18

Fibrosarcoma

M. Forest

INTRODUCTION AND CLINICAL DATA

Fibrosarcoma of bone displays proliferation of malignant, spindle-shaped, fibroblast-like cells and a matrix production of collagen fibers, with no cartilage or bone formation or acid phosphatase activity on histochemical or cytochemical study.[1] It accounts for 4–5% of all malignant bone tumors.[2,3]

Secondary fibrosarcomas have been reported in various conditions such as Paget's disease, giant cell tumors, fibrous dysplasia, irradiation,[5] bone infarcts,[6,7] and osteomyelitis, with an overall incidence of 20–23.9%.[4,8] More unusual presentations are in association with enchondromas[9] or in the area of a joint replacement.[10]

Fibrosarcomas of bone may rarely be multifocal,[11–14] representing for some authors malignant fibrous histiocytomas, despite ultrastructural findings of fibroblastic cells and collagen fibers.[13] Some tumors are congenital,[15] with a better prognosis in the few cases published; a familial case has also been quoted (Mulder et al. 1993).

In some series, a slight female preponderance[16] or male preponderance[17] is found, but usually there is no sex predilection.[2,18,19] Tumors occur in the second to seventh decades, with a median age of 41 years.[19]

The tumor may be slow growing[20] and clinical symptoms are non-specific: pain, swelling, a palpable mass or a pathologic fracture in 19–27% of cases[17] (Mulder et al 1993).

SKELETAL DISTRIBUTION

The most common sites are the long tubular bones:[20–23] lower end of the femur, upper end of the tibia or proximal humerus in 50% of cases (Figs 18.1–18.7). The incidence of pelvic locations (iliac bone) is about 10%. Any bone may be affected, but fibrosarcomas are rarely found in the spine.

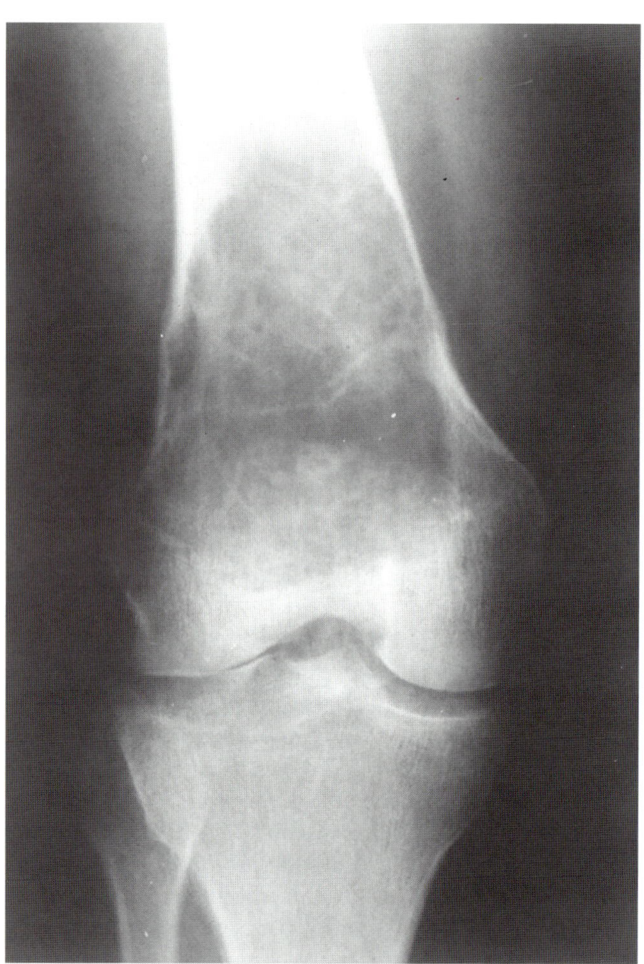

Fig. 18.1

Fig. 18.2

Figs 18.1, 18.2 Fibrosarcoma of the lower end of the femur.

IMAGING

Fibrosarcoma appears in most cases as a purely lytic lesion, with a permeative or moth-eaten pattern and ill-defined borders. In long bones, the tumor is located in the metaphysis, eventually with an epiphyseal or diaphyseal extension. Purely diaphyseal lesions account for about 7% of cases.[19] The cortex is thinned or disrupted and soft tissue invasion is detected in up to 86% of cases.[17] There is little or no periosteal reaction.

A few low-grade tumors present with a 'soap bubble' or trabeculated appearance, associated with slightly sclerotic and well-defined margins.[17]

CT is useful to delineate the cortical erosion or penetration, as well as the soft tissue mass (Hudson 1987), the lesion itself presenting a non-specific tumor attenuation.

GROSS PATHOLOGY

Tumors show a non-specific aspect similar to soft tissue sarcomas. The tissue is grayish-white, firm and rubbery or soft and friable in high-grade tumors which may exhibit hemorrhages, necrosis, cystic degeneration or myxoid areas.[18]

HISTOPATHOLOGY

Usually, the diagnosis is straightforward (Figs 18.8–18.10). The spindle cells, with a fine or granular chromatin and often with nucleoli, are distributed in interlacing fascicles or in the well-known 'herringbone' pattern. Collagen production is related to the tumor grade and may be massive or even hyalinized in well-differentiated sarcomas. Accessory findings are a few scattered giant cells or residual bone trabeculae entrapped by the tumor in low-grade fibrosarcomas.[17]

The grading of the tumor is important for prognosis. The well-known Broder's method with four grades is advocated by the pathologists of the Mayo Clinic;[23–25]

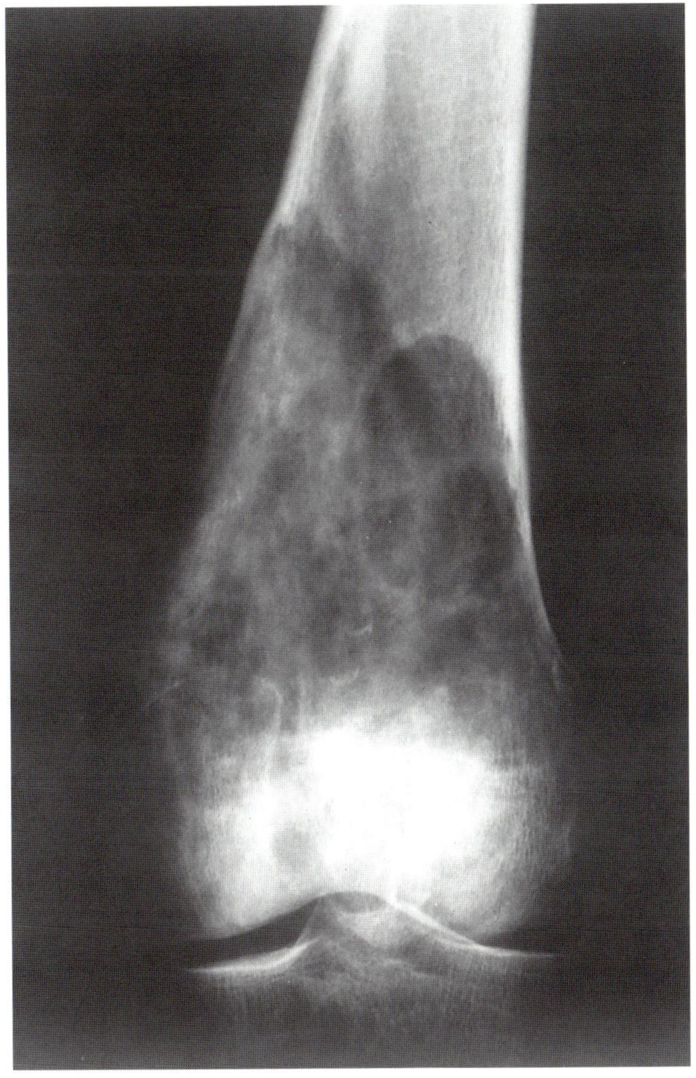

Fig. 18.3

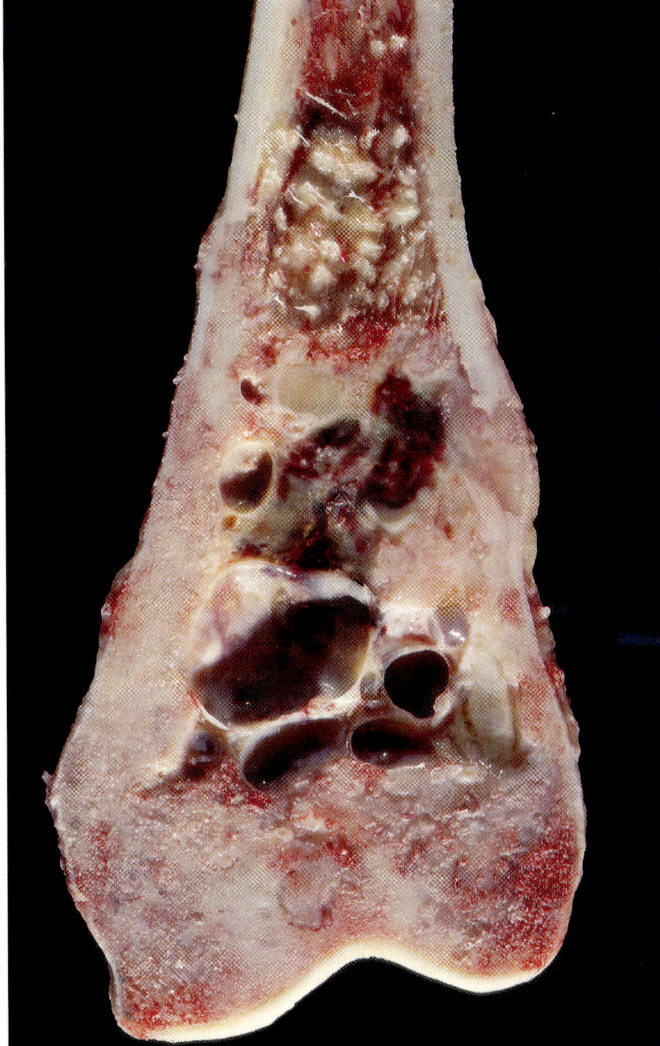

Fig. 18.4

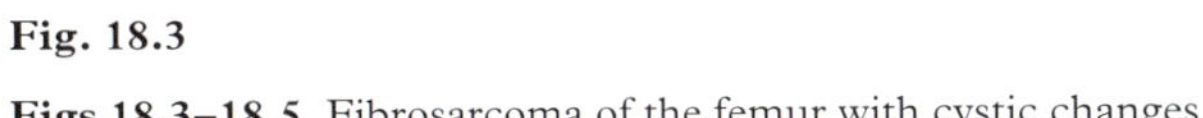

Figs 18.3–18.5 Fibrosarcoma of the femur with cystic changes.

some authors[17,19] (Schajowicz 1994) have suggested a simpler method with two or three grades.

Well-differentiated or low-grade tumors (Broder's 1–2) exhibit fibroblastic spindle cells with ovoid or elongated nuclei, some of them being plump and hyperchromatic; collagen fibers are relatively abundant, even hyalinized in some areas. Very few mitoses are found. Poorly differentiated fibrosarcomas (Broder's 3–4) are very cellular tumors with an overt mitotic activity. The nuclei are hyperchromatic and pleomorphic; some cells are multinucleated. The collagen production is scarce; areas of necrosis and hemorrhage or a myxoid stroma are usual.

Most fibrosarcomas are moderately differentiated (65% [14,19]); well-differentiated tumors account for about 5%, high-grade poorly differentiated for 30–36%.[14,19]

CYTOPATHOLOGY

On smears, tumor cells are fusiform, with elongated nuclei. Poorly differentiated fibrosarcomas have cells of irregular shape, rounded, polyhedral or with huge and multiple nuclei (Sanerkin & Jeffree 1980). Although malignancy is obvious in high-grade tumors, well-differentiated fibrosarcomas are characterized by scarce cytological material and the diagnosis relies on histopathological findings.

FLOW CYTOMETRY

Aneuploid stemlines have been found on most of the studied tumors. High rates of aneuploidy and proliferation are about the same as in osteosarcomas. There is no significant difference between primary and secondary fibrosarcomas.[26]

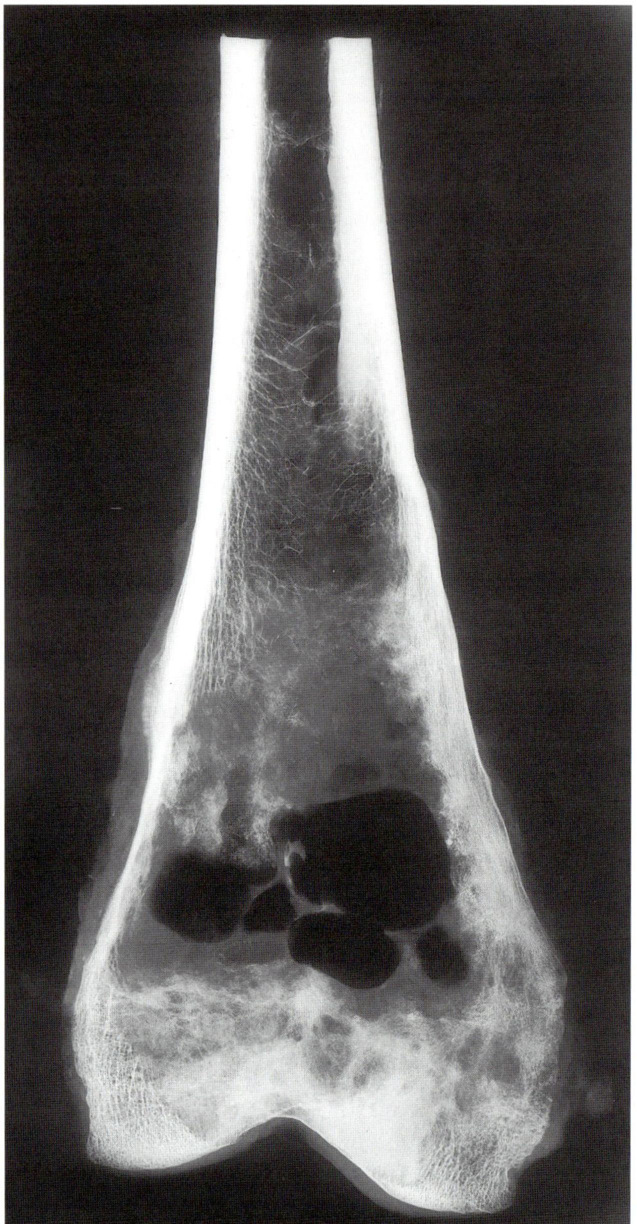

Fig. 18.5

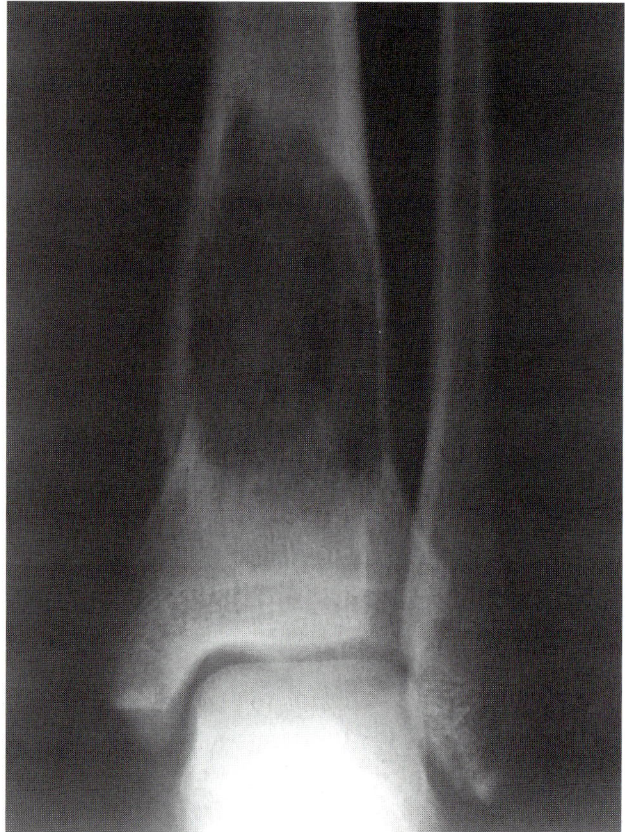

Fig. 18.6

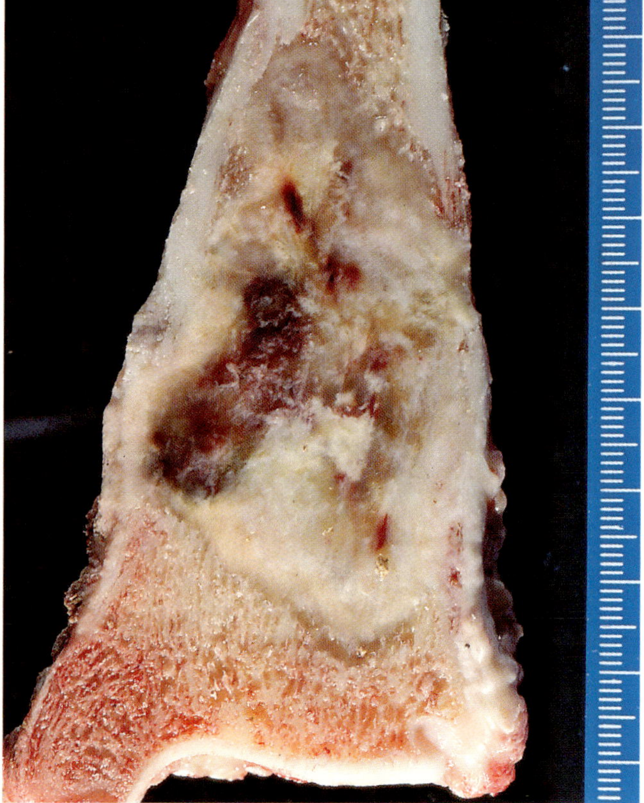

Fig. 18.7

COURSE, TREATMENT AND PROGNOSIS

Metastases are found in the lungs, but they appear later and are fewer than metastases of osteosarcomas.[16] There are more extrapulmonary metastases: bone, muscle, subcutaneous tissues.[16]

The survival rate can be linked to the imaging findings and histology. Favorable radiographic signs are a geographic pattern of destruction or an eccentric location involving no more than two quadrants of the bone circumference.[19] Local recurrences, after amputation, imply a bad pro-

Figs 18.6, 18.7 Fibrosarcoma of the lower end of the tibia with necrotic and hemorrhagic changes.

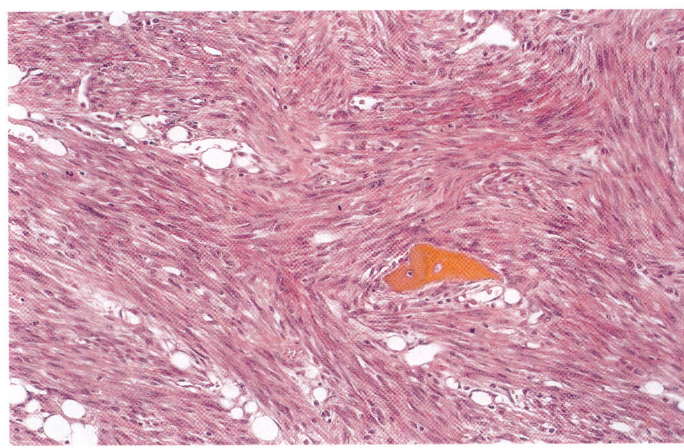

Fig. 18.8

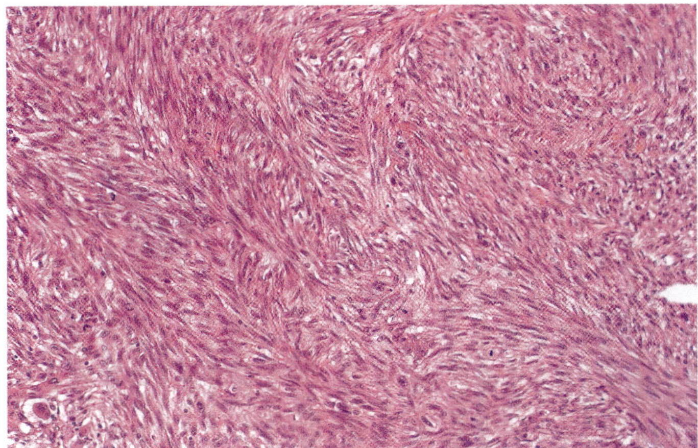

Fig. 18.9

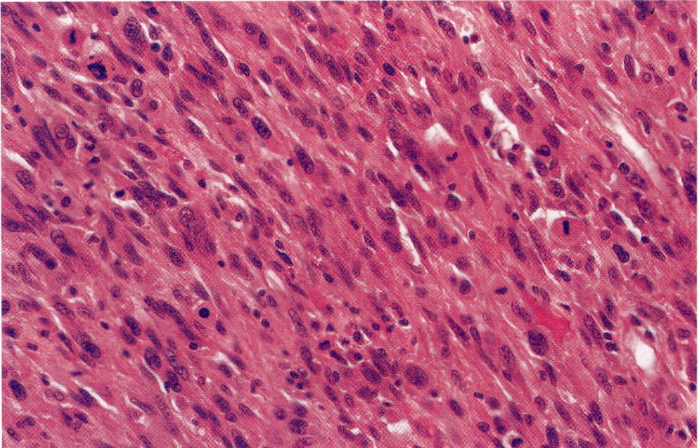

Fig. 18.10

Figs 18.8–18.10 Fibrosarcomas of bone: varied degrees of cellular abnormalities and collagen production.

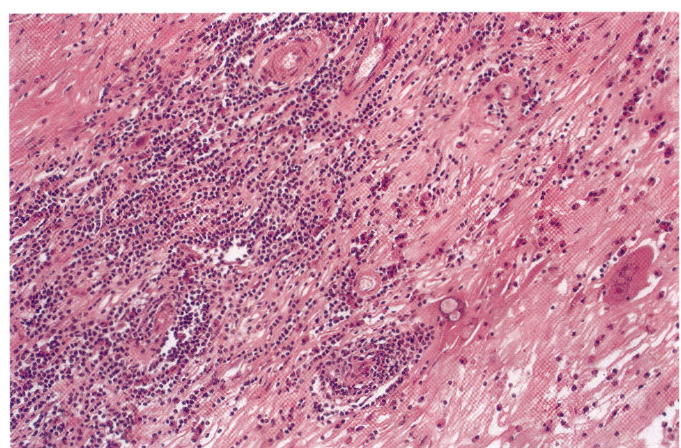

Fig. 18.11 Response of a high-grade fibrosarcoma of the femur to intraarterial chemotherapy: drop-out of cells, degenerative changes and lymphocytic infiltrates.

gnosis.[17] The histological grade is also a significant prognostic factor.[17,23] The overall survival rate at 10 years is 21.8–34%;[19,23] in grade I tumors, it can be 64%[19] to 83%.[17]

The treatment is segmental resection in well-differentiated tumors or pre- and adjuvant chemotherapy in poorly differentiated ones (Fig. 18.11). Radiation therapy appears to be ineffective.[17]

DIFFERENTIAL DIAGNOSIS

The main problem for the surgical pathologist is confusing a well-differentiated fibrosarcoma with a desmoplastic fibroma. One has to rely on the nuclear pleomorphism, the slight mitotic activity and a 'herringbone' pattern in the case of fibrosarcoma. However, the treatment and prognosis are the same.

A fibrosarcoma may be confused with a malignant fibrous histiocytoma of bone. In one series, nearly half of the tumors showed extensive areas of tumor resembling a malignant fibrous histiocytoma.[27] However, there is no significant difference in the behavior and incidence of lung metastases.[27]

One should remember the differential diagnosis of fibroblastic osteosarcoma (tumoral bone production). Spindle cell carcinoma (Fechner & Mills 1993) or spindle cell melanoma are easily distinguished by immunohistochemical techniques.

More unusual periosteal fibrosarcomas have to be differentiated from extraosseous soft tissue sarcomas eroding the cortex. In that location, fibrosarcomas appear to have a better prognosis.[3,19]

REFERENCES

1. Sanerkin N G. Definitions of osteosarcoma, chondrosarcoma and fibrosarcoma of bone. Cancer 1980: 46: 178–185
2. Dahlin D C, Ivins J C. Fibrosarcoma of bone. A study of 114 cases. Cancer 1969: 23: 35–41
3. Huvos A G, Higinbotham N L. Primary fibrosarcoma of bone. A clinicopathologic study of 130 patients. Cancer 1975: 35: 837–847
4. André S, Tomeno B, Forest M, Carlioz A. Fibrosarcomes des os. Rev Chir Orthop Reparatrice Appar Mot 1983: 69: 107–116
5. Morrison M J, Ivins J C. Case report 57. Radiation-induced fibrosarcoma of the distal end of femur. Skeletal Radiol 1978: 2: 258–260
6. Furey J G, Ferer-Torells M, Reagan JW. Fibrosarcoma arising at the site of bone infarcts. J Bone Joint Surg (Am) 1960: 42: 802–810
7. Dorfman H D, Norman A, Wolff H. Fibrosarcoma complicating bone infarction in a caisson worker. A case report. J Bone Joint Surg (Am) 1966: 48: 528–532
8. Akbarnia B A, Wirth C R, Colman N. Fibrosarcoma arising from chronic osteomyelitis. Case report and review of the literature. J Bone Joint Surg (Am) 1976: 58: 123–125
9. Sanerkin N G, Woods C G. Fibrosarcomata and malignant fibrous histiocytomata arising in relation to enchondromata. J Bone Joint Surg (Br) 1979: 61: 366–372
10. Eckstein F S, Vogel U, Mohr W. Fibrosarcoma in association with a total knee joint prosthesis. Virchows Arch A Pathol Anat Histopathol 1992: 421: 175–178
11. Steiner E. Multiple diffuse fibrosarcoma of bone. Am J Pathol 1944: 20: 877–893
12. Nielsen A R, Poulsen H. Multiple diffuse fibrosarcomatosis of the bones. Acta Pathol Microbiol Scand 1962: 55: 265–272
13. Hernandez F J, Fernandez B B. Multiple diffuse fibrosarcoma of bone. Cancer 1976: 37: 939–945
14. Campanacci M, Olmi R. Fibrosarcoma of bone. A study of 114 cases. Ital J Orthop Traumatol 1977: 3: 199–206
15. Bernado L, Admella C, Lucaya J, Sanchez De Toledo J, Bosch J. Infantile fibrosarcoma of femur. Pediatr Pathol 1987: 7: 201–207
16. Jeffree G M, Price C H. Metastatic spread of fibrosarcoma of bone. A report of forty-nine cases, and a comparison with osteosarcoma. J Bone Joint Surg (Br) 1976: 58: 418–425
17. Bertoni F, Capanna R, Calderoni P, Bacchini P, Campanacci M. Primary central (medullary) fibrosarcoma of bone. Semin Diagn Pathol 1984: 1: 185–198
18. Frassica F J, Sim F H, Wold L E. Case report 462. Grade 2 myxoid fibrosarcoma of femur. Skeletal Radiol 1988: 17: 77–80
19. Taconis W K, Mulder J D. Fibrosarcoma and malignant fibrous histiocytoma of long bones: radiographic features and grading. Skeletal Radiol 1984: 11: 237–245
20. Eyre-Brook A L, Price C H G. Fibrosarcoma of bone. Review of fifty consecutive cases from the Bristol Bone Tumour Registry. J Bone Joint Surg (Br) 1969: 51: 20–37
21. De Santis E. Fibrosarcoma primitivo dell'osso. Arch Putti Chir Organi Mov 1986: 36: 183–193
22. Larsson S E, Lorentzon R, Boquist L. Fibrosarcoma of bone. A demographic, clinical and histopathological study of all cases recorded in the Swedish cancer registry from 1958 to 1968. J Bone Joint Surg (Br) 1976: 56: 412–417
23. Pritchard D J, Sim F H, Ivins J C, Soule E H, Dahlin D C. Fibrosarcoma of bone and soft tissues of the trunk and extremities. Orthop Clin North Am 1977: 8: 869–881
24. Unni K K, Dahlin D C. Grading of bone tumors. Semin Diagn Pathol 1984: 1: 165–172
25. Inwards C Y, Unni K K. Classification and grading of bone sarcomas. Hematol Oncol Clin North Am 1995: 9: 545–569
26. Mellin W, Dierschauer W, Hiddemann W et al. Flow cytometric DNA analysis of bone tumors. Curr Top Pathol 1989: 80: 115–152
27. Taconis W K, Van Rijssel T G. Fibrosarcoma of long bones. A study of the significance of areas of malignant fibrous histiocytoma. J Bone Joint Surg (Br) 1985: 67: 111–116

Benign fibrous histiocytoma

M. Forest

INTRODUCTION AND CLINICAL DATA

Benign fibrous histiocytoma is histologically similar to non-ossifying fibromas: fibroblasts are associated with mononuclear or multinucleated cells resembling histiocytes, but it differs in the clinical features (age and pain), as well as in the radiological findings (unusual location for a non-ossifying fibroma).[1,2]

This tumor is unusual. More than 50 cases have been reported, with no sex predominance. Patient age ranges from 5 to 75 years; some cases involve children[3,4] but benign fibrous histiocytoma appears mostly as a tumor of adulthood, with a mean age of 37 years.[5,6] The main clinical feature is local pain with or without swelling, in the absence of fracture.[7] The tumor is slow growing, but a pathologic fracture may occur.[5,8]

SKELETAL DISTRIBUTION

More than 30% of cases involve the wing of the ilium, the pubis, sacrum and femur.[7,9] Various other sites have been reported including the tibia,[5] ulna,[1] humerus,[10] vertebrae,[11–14] clavicle,[15] scapula, ribs,[1,16,17] mandible and even the patella.[1]

IMAGING

In long bones, the tumor is centered on the epiphysis and not the metaphysis[6] (Fig. 19.1); if the location is metaphyseal, the tumor tends to involve the epiphysis.[1,5] In epiphyseal locations, it resembles a giant cell tumor.[6,8,18–21] Diaphyseal tumors[10] (Unni 1996) have been described in the femur and humerus, maybe representing unresolved non-ossifying fibromas of childhood.[6]

The initial lesion is generally centrally located, unlike non-ossifying fibromas. However, some tumors are eccentrically located.[22]

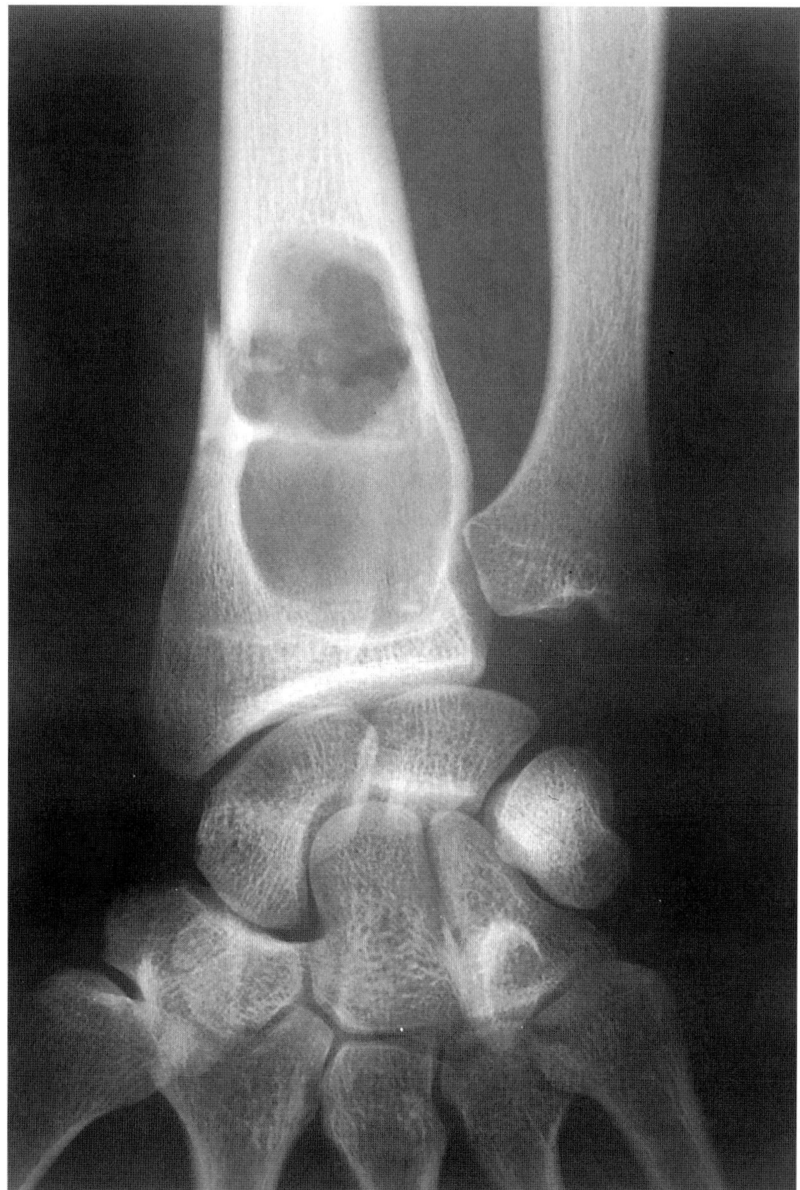

Fig. 19.1 Benign fibrous histiocytoma of the radius with pathologic fracture.

All tumors are lytic lesions, with no demonstrable matrix[5] (Fig. 19.2). Eventually a sclerotic rim,[5,22] well demonstrated on CT,[7] or a soap-bubble appearance may occur.[22] The bone may be expanded, with thinning or breach of the cortex. There is no periosteal reaction.

The lesion exhibits a pronounced scintigraphic and MR signal intensity, particularly in the late phase.[23]

GROSS PATHOLOGY

The tumoral tissue may be red, brown and yellow, resembling a giant cell tumor[5,22] (Fig. 19.3), or gray-white and firm. Cyst formation with a yellowish or hemorrhagic fluid has been described.[5]

HISTOPATHOLOGY

Like a non-ossifying fibroma, a benign fibrous histiocytoma is usually highly cellular (Figs 19.4–19.8). Spindle-shaped cells are distributed in whorls, forming a characteristic storiform pattern, at least in some fields. Fibroblastic cells are associated with histiocytic or even multinucleated cells; lipid-filled cells appearing as xanthoma cells may be numerous. A few scattered reactive giant cells are found. Whatever the predominant cell component, there is no nuclear atypia and normal-appearing mitoses are very few. Secondary changes are cholesterol clefts, hemosiderin deposits or reactive bone formation, usually peripherally located.[5] The tumor may infiltrate the medullary spaces.

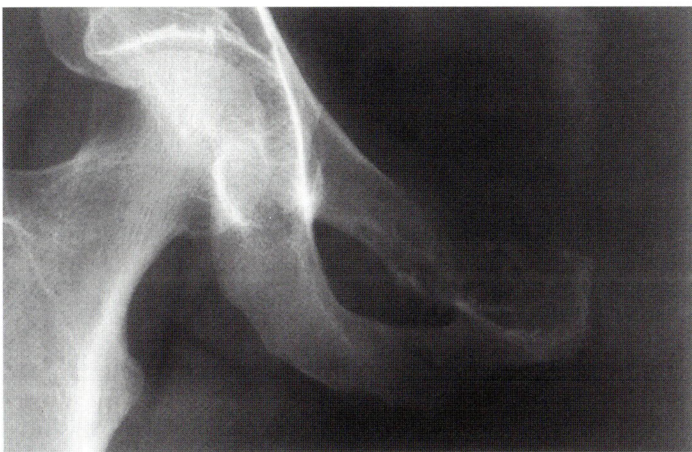

Fig. 19.2

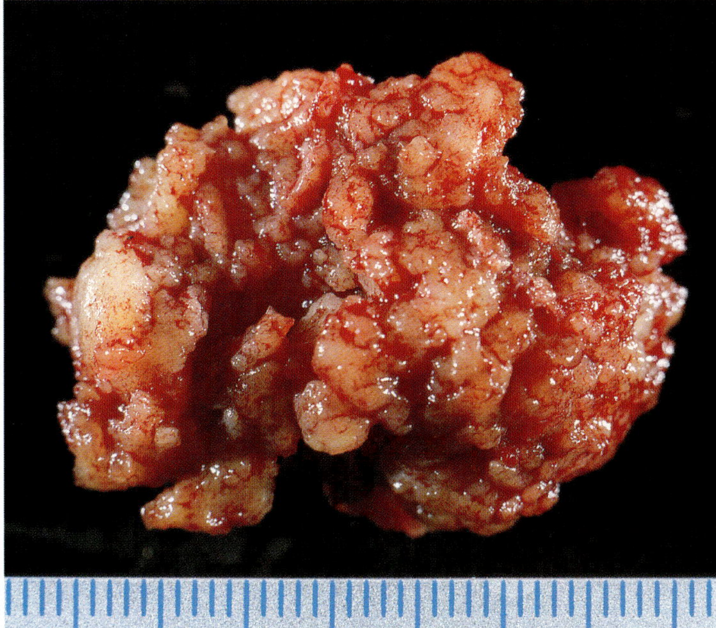

Fig. 19.3

Figs 19.2, 19.3 Benign fibrous histiocytoma of the iliopubic ramus.

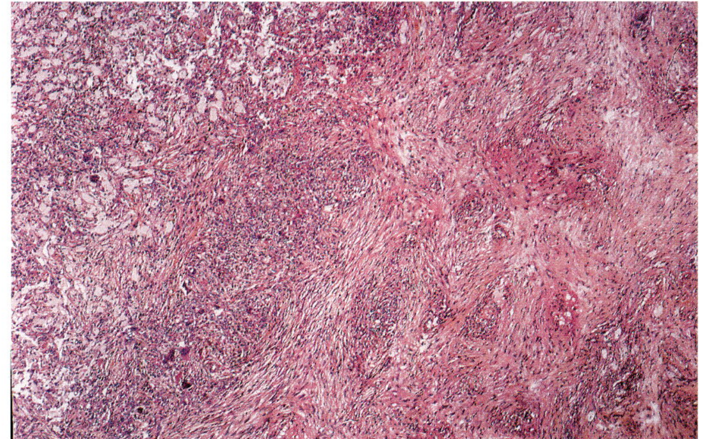

Fig. 19.4 Benign fibrous histiocytoma: spindle-shaped and xanthoma cells.

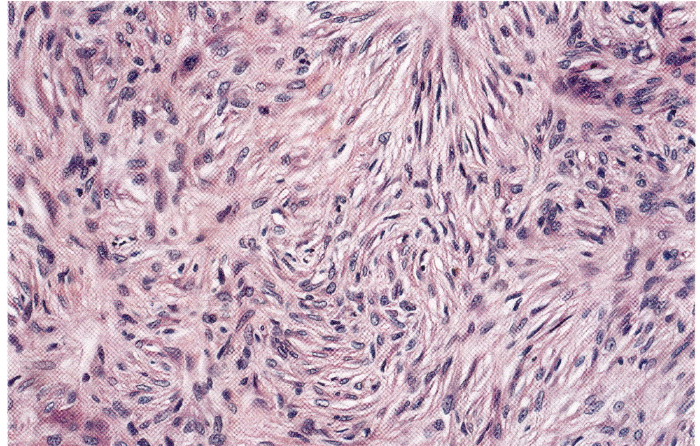

Fig. 19.5

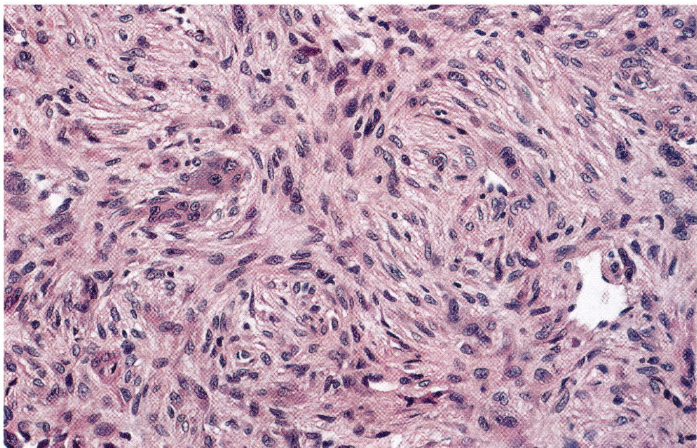

Fig. 19.6

Figs 19.5, 19.6 Benign fibrous histiocytoma: fibroblastic cells with a storiform pattern.

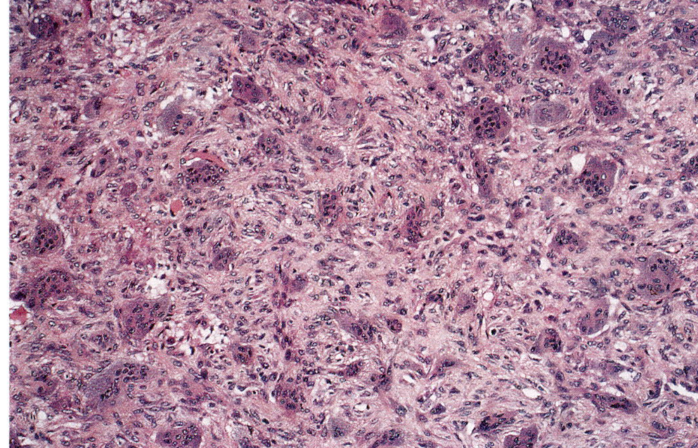

Fig. 19.7 Benign fibrous histiocytoma: reactive giant cells.

IMMUNOHISTOCHEMISTRY

Reactions with antibodies to α 1-antitrypsin, α 1-antichymotrypsin and lysozyme have been performed, to define the histiocytic cellular component[24] (Huvos 1991), but the use-

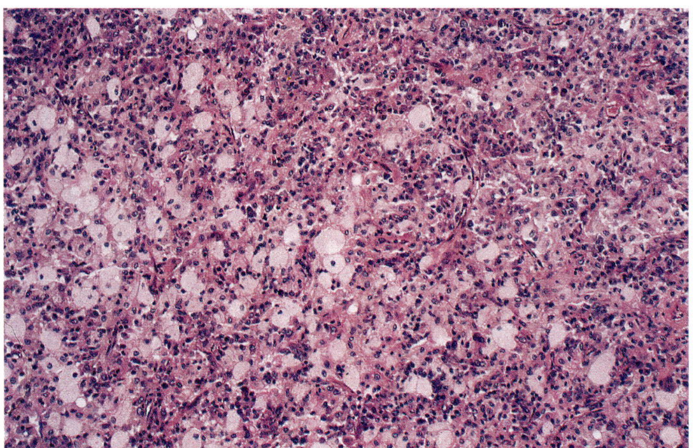

Fig. 19.8 Benign fibrous histiocytoma: lipid-filled cells with some scattered lymphocytes.

fulness of immunohistochemical findings is discussed by Schajowicz (1994).

ELECTRON MICROSCOPY

The ultrastructural features are very similar to those of non-ossifying fibroma: elongated fibroblast-like cells with a prominent rough endoplasmic reticulum, histiocytic cells with a more irregular outline, prominent Golgi apparatus and lipid droplets[5,12,24] and undifferentiated mesenchymal cells. The xanthomatous and giant cells derive from the histiocytic component.[12]

As with all fibrohistiocytic lesions, there is some debate about the cell of origin: histiocytic cells acting as facultative fibroblasts (Huvos 1991) or fibroblastic cells looking and acting like facultative histiocytes.[1,6]

COURSE, TREATMENT AND PROGNOSIS

A benign fibrous histiocytoma exhibits more aggressive bone destruction than non-ossifying fibromas.[21] Locally destructive and invasive growth has been described, especially in the spine,[12] but there is no metastasis or progression to malignant fibrous histiocytoma.

The treatment is usually conservative: curettage and bone grafting or marginal excision with a rim of peripheral bone. However, in short series, an unusually high rate of recurrence has been established,[5,6] leading to a more aggressive surgical approach, i.e. wide local resection. There is no histological feature that predicts the incidence of recurrence.[5]

DIFFERENTIAL DIAGNOSIS

Non-ossifying fibromas affect younger patients and are painless lesions, metaphyseally located, with less bone destruction.

So-called 'atypical' benign fibrous histiocytomas[25] (Unni 1996) are rare lesions with cytological atypia and more numerous mitoses; spindle cells are also present in a storiform pattern. Ultrastructural findings are the same as those of the usual form.[25] Schajowicz considers these tumors to be low-grade malignant fibrous histiocytomas.

A malignant fibrous histiocytoma is a much more pleomorphic tumor, with atypical mitoses and an obvious permeative pattern of bone destruction. Highly collagenized tumors show paradoxically less cellularity than benign fibrous histiocytomas.[6]

Desmoplastic fibroma has a lower cellularity with no giant cells, histiocytic cells or storiform pattern.

Fibrous dysplasia can easily be ruled out by the absence of the characteristic metaplastic bone formation.

Low-grade fibrosarcomas show mild mitotic activity and are devoid of any histiocytic component or storiform pattern.

Late stages of eosinophilic granulomas present as scar-like fibrous tissue. Some histiocytes and eosinophilic cells may be found but there is no storiform pattern.

Brown tumors of hyperparathyroidism should be ruled out by the biochemical findings, inconspicuous giant cells and hemorrhages.

The most difficult differential diagnosis is a giant cell tumor. A benign fibrous histiocytoma may closely mimic the so-called secondary regressive changes found extensively or focally in giant cell tumors, i.e. fibrotic areas with a storiform pattern. Radiological findings may be similar.

A thorough sampling of the tumor is necessary to find diffuse and larger giant cells, packed round or oval stromal cells and eventually areas of necrosis.[5,6,21,22] Mirra considers that benign fibrous histiocytomas are giant cell tumors with a massive fibrohistiocytic repair and in a series of 350 giant cell tumors, Bertoni found 10 cases histologically similar to a benign fibrous histiocytoma.[22]

REFERENCES

1. Spjut H J, Fechner R E, Ackerman L V. Tumors of bone and cartilage. Atlas of tumor pathology, fasc 5, second series (suppl). Washington: AFIP, 1981, pp 16–18
2. De Santis E, Serra F. Il fibroma non osteogenico delle ossa lunghe. Considerazioni clinicopatologiche e terapeutiche della rassegna di 18 casi. Ipotesi di possible identificazione nell'istiocitoma fibroso benigno. Arch Putti Chir Organi Mov 1980: 30: 99–116
3. Magliato H J, Nastasi A. Non osteogenic fibroma occurring in the ilium. Report of a case. J Bone Joint Surg 1967: 49: 384–386
4. Azouz E M. Benign fibrous histiocytoma of the proximal tibial epiphysis in a 12-year-old girl. Skeletal Radiol 1995: 24: 375–378
5. Clarke B E, Xipell J M, Thomas D P. Benign fibrous histiocytoma of bone. Am J Surg Pathol 1985: 9: 806–815
6. Fechner R E, Spjut H J, Haggitt R C. Giant cell tumor with areas

resembling benign fibrous histiocytoma. In: Diseases of bones and joints. Chicago: ASCP Press, 1985, pp 12–17

7. Hamada T, Ito H, Araki Y, Fujii K, Inoue M, Ishida O. Benign fibrous histiocytoma of the femur: review of three cases. Skeletal Radiol 1996: 25: 25–29

8. Hermann G, Steiner G C, Sherry H H. Case report 465. Benign fibrous histiocytoma (BHF). Skeletal Radiol 1988: 17: 195–198

9. Ramos J V, Daumen-Legre V, Garbe L, Kelberine F, Schiano A, Serratrice G. Histiocytofibrome bénin osseux. Rhumatologie 1993: 45: 85–88

10. Nunnery E W, Kahn L B, Guilford W B. Locally aggressive fibrous histiocytoma of bone. A case report. S Afr Med J 1979: 55: 763–767

11. Destouet J M, Kyriakos M, Gilula L A. Fibrous histiocytoma (fibroxanthoma) of a cervical vertebra. A report with a review of the literature. Skeletal Radiol 1980: 5: 241–246

12. Roessner A, Immenkamp M, Weidner A, Hobik H P, Grundmann E. Benign fibrous histiocytoma of bone. Light and electron-microscopic observations. J Cancer Res Clin Oncol 1981: 101: 191–202

13. Fabris D, Candiotto S, Mammano S, Ferraro C, Agostini S. Antalgic scoliosis due to nonosteogenic fibroma of the L1 neural arch: report of a case. J Pediatr Orthop 1986: 6: 103–106

14. Hoeffel J C, Boman-Ferrand F, Tachet F, Lascombes P, Czorny A, Bernard C. So-called benign fibrous histiocytoma: report of a case. J Pediatr Surg 1992: 27: 672–674

15. Gardiner G A, Linda L. Clavicular non osteogenic fibroma. An old tumor in a new location. Am J Dis Child 1974: 127: 734–735

16. Clark T D, Stelling C B, Fechner R E. Case report 328. Benign fibrous histiocytoma of the left 8th rib. Skeletal Radiol 1985: 14: 149–151

17. Friedman L, Patel M, Lew E, Silberberg P. Benign histiocytic fibroma of rib with CT correlation. Can Assoc Radiol J 1989: 40: 114–116

18. Dominok G W, Eisengarten W. Benignes fibroses Histiozytom des Knochens. Zentralbl Allg Pathol 1980: 124: 77–83

19. Bertoni F, Capanna H, Calderoni P, Bacchini P, Case report 223. Benign fibrous histiocytoma. Skeletal Radiol 1983: 9: 215–217

20. Schwesinger G, Seide H W, Seidlein H. Das benigne fibröse histiozytom des knochens. Beitr Orthop Traumatol 1990: 37: 65–70

21. Matsuno T. Benign fibrous histiocytoma involving the ends of long bone. Skeletal Radiol 1990: 19: 561–566

22. Bertoni F, Calderoni P, Bacchini P et al. Benign fibrous histiocytoma of bone. J Bone Joint Surg (Am) 1986: 68: 1225–1230

23. Exner G U, Von Hochstetter A R, Uehlinger K. 'Benignes fibröses histiozytom' der distalen femurmetaphyse. Differentialdiagnose zwischen Neoplasie und Wachstermsstorung bei identischen Morphologie. Z Orthop 1990: 128: 308–312

24. Statz E M, Pochebit S M, Cooper A, Philipps E, Leslie B M. Case report 525. Benign fibrous histiocytoma (BFH) of thumb. Skeletal Radiol 1989: 18: 299–302

25. Saito R, Caines M J. Atypical fibrous histiocytoma of the humerus. A light and electron microscopic study. Am J Clin Pathol 1977: 68: 409–415

20

Malignant fibrous histiocytoma

M. Forest

INTRODUCTION AND CLINICAL DATA

'Be that as it may, I have at least four primary tumors of bone in my consultation files that appear to satisfy the pathologic citeria for the diagnosis of malignant fibrous histiocytoma' (Lichtenstein 1977). These words should remind the surgical pathologist that not all undifferentiated bone sarcomas are synonymous with malignant fibrous histiocytomas,[1] the same problem being stressed in a recent work by Fletcher[2] about soft tissue locations.

The most pertinent definition appears to be that of Fechner & Mills: a sarcoma whose cells are fibroblasts, myofibroblasts and cells resembling histiocytes, reflecting a growing trend towards a fibroblastic phenotype,[3] or even a primitive 'embryonal' form of fibrosarcoma.[4]

Malignant fibrous histiocytoma has been reported in bone; Feldman & Norman first mentioned nine cases in 1972.[5,6] It accounts for less than 1% of primary bone tumors in the Mayo Clinic files and for 5% in the Netherlands Registry of Bone Tumors (Mulder et al 1993). It appears to be ten less frequent than osteosarcoma.[7]

There is a relative predilection for male patients, with a ratio of about 1.6:1,[8–11] although Schajowicz reports a slight female predominance. It occurs at all ages, but is more common in the six and seventh decades, with a median age ranging from 40 to 52 years.[7,12]

Clinical symptoms are non-specific, with a duration from a few weeks to some months: pain, swelling or pathologic fracture occurs in 20–25% of cases.[7,10]

Multiple malignant fibrous histiocytomas have been reported,[1,7,13–15,16] even in one family,[17] and some authors believe that cases of multiple diffuse bone fibrosarcomas[18] could be malignant fibrous histiocytomas. They may be synchronous or metachronous tumors or metastases;[15] in one case, the tumors were histologically dissimilar[19] without lung lesions.

SECONDARY MALIGNANT FIBROUS HISTIOCYTOMAS OF BONE

These lesions should be kept in mind by the pathologist because the frequency is high, ranging from 20%[20,21] to 28% in Huvos' study.[7] Preexisting bone conditions are varied, but the tumors seem to be linked to some background of a reparative or remodeling process or to reflect dedifferentiation or progression of a preexisting sarcoma.

More than 15% are radiation-induced sarcomas.[22-27] The most common sites are pelvic bones following irradiation of a cervical uterine cancer or head of the humerus in the case of an irradiated breast cancer.[27] Average age peaks are in the fifth decade of life, with a mean latent period of 16.5 years and a mean radiation dose of 6040 rads. Survival at 3 years is no more than 58% and the prognosis is worse following incidental irradiation directed against a non-osseous condition.[27] The development of sarcomas may be caused both by the infarcts produced by irradiation and the carcinogenicity of radiation per se.[23]

Malignant fibrous histiocytomas may develop in bone infarcts;[28-36] most patients have large, multiple and usually symmetric medullary infarcts[30] in the diaphyseal-metaphyseal regions of long bones, particularly the femur and the tibia. It has been suggested that the chronic reparative process could produce some pluripotential primitive cells, leading to sarcoma.[28,29,33] The prognosis is poor, with a mean survival time of 18 months and a hematogenous spread of metastases to lung, bone or even lymph nodes.[33]

A chronic reparative process may well be involved in sarcomas complicating osteomyelitis[37,38] as well as rare cases following metal implants[39,40] or total joint replacement.[41-44]

Tumors may be linked to a remodeling process (Paget's disease or fibrous dysplasia[45,46]) or reflect a progression in cases of chondromas, chondrosarcomas or chordomas[47-51] with, in some cases, a role for irradiation.[50] They may appear as a secondary malignancy.[52]

Malignant fibrous histiocytomas may have no relationship with the underlying condition, as in melorrheostosis.[53]

On the whole, secondary tumors involve older patients[10,27] and the prognosis is worse.[10]

SKELETAL DISTRIBUTION

The appendicular skeleton is most frequently involved; 75% of cases are located in long tubular bones,[21] chiefly the distal femur, proximal tibia and humerus (Figs 20.1–20.6). Malignant fibrous histiocytoma is not uncommon in the flat bones of the pelvis but rare in the ribs,[54] hand[55-57] and spine.[58-60] It has even been reported in the patella.[61,62]

IMAGING

Tumor involving the long bones is located mostly in the metadiaphyseal region, followed by a metaepiphyseal location. Diaphyseal tumors have an incidence of 10–27% of cases. The lesion is most often centrally located; subperiosteal location is unusual, with erosion and scalloping of the cortex.[1,63]

The lesion is mostly lytic or may have a few internal calcifications, with a moth-eaten or permeative pattern of bone destruction. The cortex is destroyed in up to 85% of cases and there is soft tissue extension in 88%.[10] The osteolytic lesion is highly destructive.[64,65] A few tumors may have a geographic pattern of bone destruction (Mulder et al 1993) or even appear well circumscribed.[1,14]

Mineralization in the soft tissue mass suggests calcific deposits on collagen fibers or reactive periosteal bone.

On bone scans, the tumor exhibits a non-specific increased uptake, centrally or eccentrically located. On angiography, the tumor is hypervascular, with diffuse tumor blushes and malignant tumor vessels.[66]

CT is useful for evaluating the cortical erosion or destruction and the soft tissue mass, MRI for showing the marrow and soft tissue extension or the joint invasion.[21]

There is no periosteal reaction in the majority of cases,[10] but bone extension of tumors of soft tissue origin may induce a periosteal reaction.[5,6]

GROSS PATHOLOGY

Malignant fibrous histiocytomas are usually huge tumors with a mean diameter of 10 cm and the cortical destruction and medullary extension are more important than that reflected on imaging studies.[11] The soft tissue involvement may contain associated nodules.[6] Skip lesions may be found in bone and joint involvement has been reported.[64,6]

The tumoral tissue is gray or grayish-white, with yellow streaks corresponding to necrosis.[7] It may be quite extensive, firm or soft, with hemorrhages. Some necrotic bone may be engulfed by the tumor.

HISTOPATHOLOGY

The spindly fibroblast-like cells and the histiocyte-like cells appear in most tumors with a biphasic pattern of growth, but one component or the other may predominate, even in different fields of the same tumor (Figs 20.7–20.14). Plump fibroblastic cells have an oval or elongated vesicular or dense nucleus. They are arranged in fascicles or a cartwheel or storiform pattern. Varying degrees of collagen production may be present, which is sometimes hyalinized; the collagen may be very coarse or have a lace-like pattern, mimicking osteoid.[14]

Histiocyte-like cells are mononuclear, multinucleated or

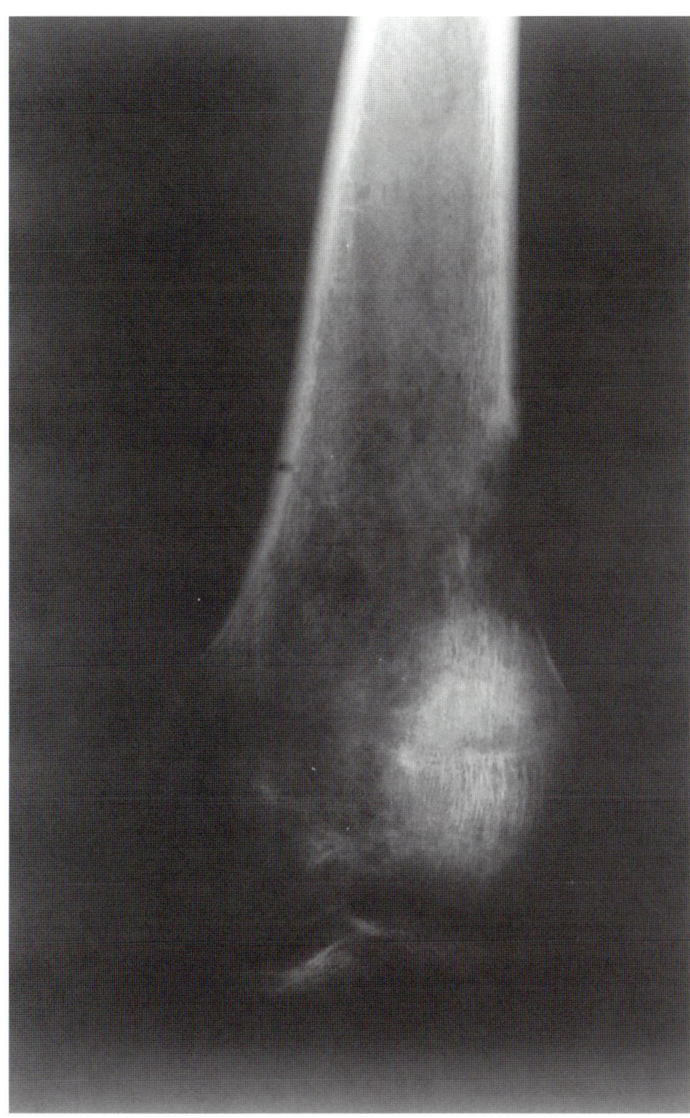

Fig. 20.1

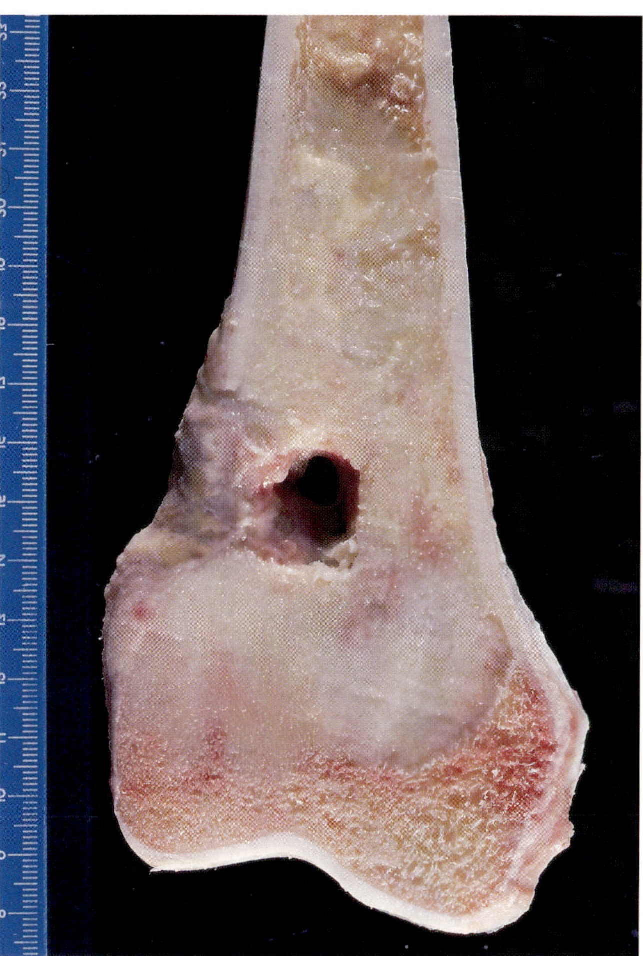

Fig. 20.2

Figs 20.1, 20.2 Malignant fibrous histiocytoma of the femur.

polygonal with abundant eosinophilic cytoplasm and well-defined borders. The nuclei are grooved, indented or multilobulated, with one or more prominent nucleoli.[14] Prominent mitotic activity is usually found in the histiocytic component.[67] Phagocytic activity is obvious in some tumors: red blood cells, hemosiderin and mostly lipids leading to foam or xanthoma cells or even bizarre pleomorphic cells.

Multinucleated giant cells of the osteoclast type are haphazardly distributed.

A conspicuous infiltration of inflammatory cells is frequent: lymphocytes predominate, mixed with eosinophils, neutrophils or plasma cells.[64,65]

Secondary changes are cholesterol clefts, hemorrhages or extensive necrosis.

Some tumors may present a hemangiopericytomatous pattern, at least focally,[14,68,69] with cells in clusters or bundles around vascular spaces.[14]

The majority of tumors are of the storiform-pleomorphic subtype with a storiform appearance; the histiocytic or xanthomatous type is less frequent. A giant cell pattern is rare[10,70] with osteoclast-like giant cells or malignant giant cells.[7] The angiomatoid form with hemorrhagic or cyst-like spaces is also unusual.[10,70]

The various histological subtypes have no correlation with clinical behavior.[7] Most tumors are high grade, Broder's 3–4.[7,10]

Quantitative morphometry of bone changes during tumoral invasion has shown activity affecting bone formation but not resorption.[71]

CYTOPATHOLOGY

Smears display plump, spindle-shaped cells, irregular cells with enlarged nuclei, foamy pleomorphic histiocytic cells or multinucleated tumoral giant cells[72]

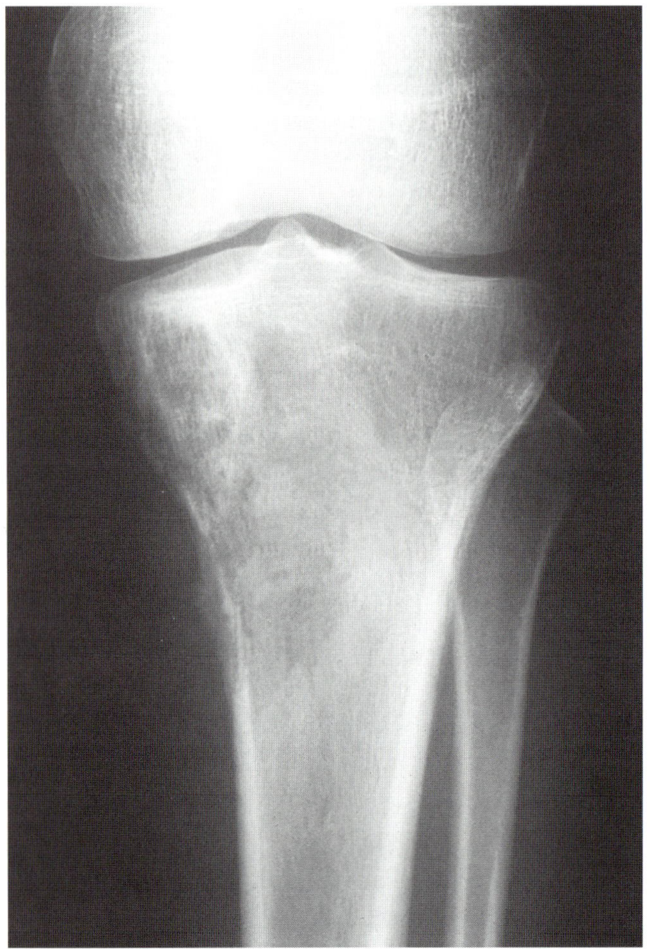

Fig. 20.3

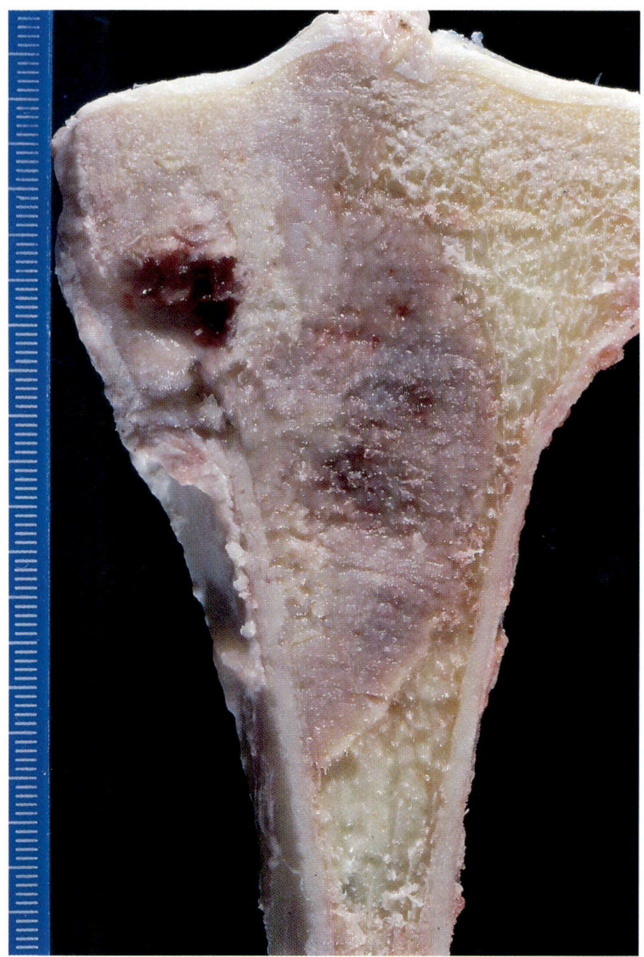

Fig. 20.4

Figs 20.3, 20.4 Malignant fibrous histiocytoma of the tibia.

(Figs 20.15, 20.16), but the diagnosis relies on histological findings.

IMMUNOHISTOCHEMISTRY

The usual and not very specific histiocytic markers are positive in the histiocytic areas, negative in the fibroblastic or myxoid areas.[7,73,74] Enzinger & Weiss suggest that soft tissue tumors do not express CD68, a panhistiocytic marker, or CD45. On cell lines grown from soft tissue and bone sarcomas, the cells display histiocytic functional markers, but CD14 and CD15, recognizing the cells of the monocyte-macrophage lineage, are negative.[73]

A homogeneous vimentin reactivity[74] is associated with a mesenchymal antigen (Fu-3), distributed among perivascular cells and fibroblasts.[75]

Malignant fibrous histiocytomas of bone may show a coexpression of cytokeratin and vimentin[76] and some focal positivity for desmin, myoglobin and anti-muscle antigen (HHF35), presumably related to a myofibroblastic differentiation,[74] as in the soft tissue tumors.[77]

A double-labeling immunohistochemical technique associating different monoclonal antibodies with the mononuclear phagocyte system, HLA-DR antigens and a proliferation-associated nuclear antigen (Ki-67) clearly demonstrated that the fibroblast-like mesenchymal cells are the proliferating tumor cells originating from local mesenchymal cells and not from the mononuclear phagocyte system.[78,79]

In vitro also, the tumors show a mesenchymal differentiation and neoplastic fibroblasts may be 'facultative histiocytes' associated with reactive histiocytes deriving from the monocyte-macrophage lineage and showing active phagocytosis with siderophages and foam cells.[73]

In one series, an overexpression of p53 protein has been found in 50% of cases.[12]

FLOW CYTOMETRY

Tumors of soft tissue have all been shown to have an abnormal DNA content (mostly hyperploid and hypotetraploid); a few cases of malignant fibrous histiocytoma of

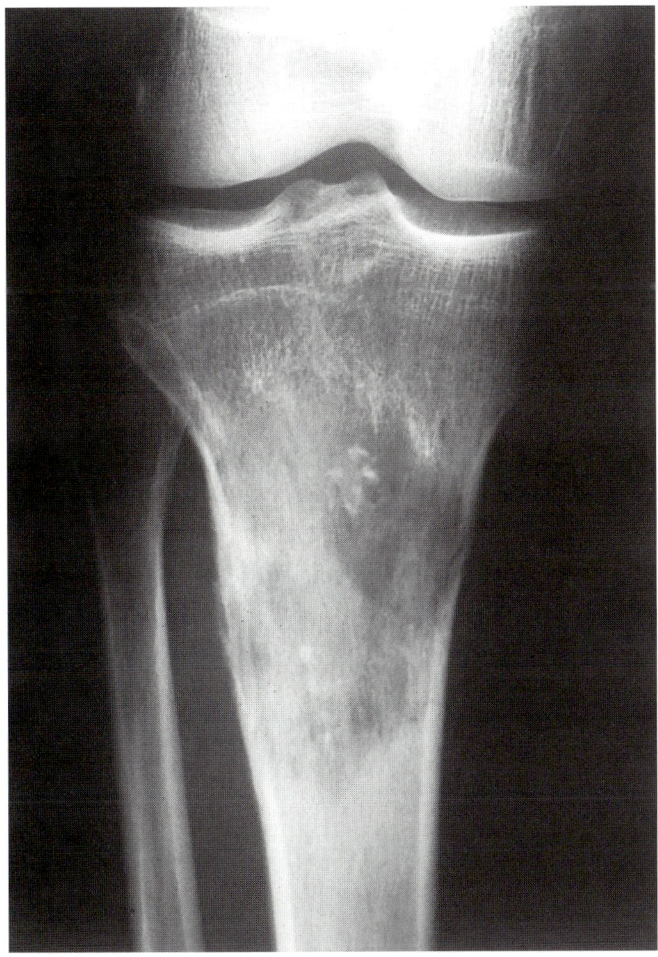

Fig. 20.5

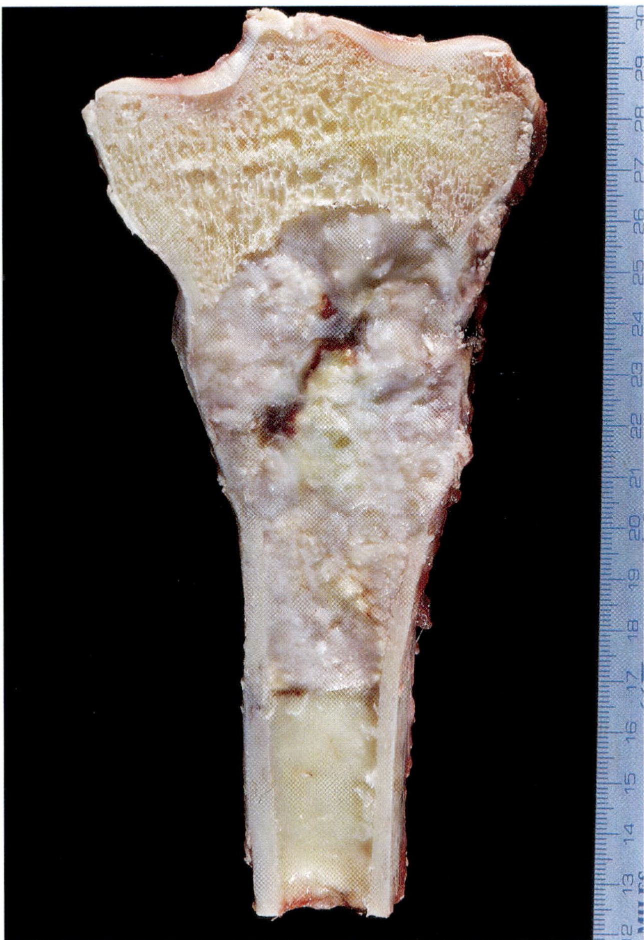

Fig. 20.6

Figs 20.5, 20.6 Malignant fibrous histiocytoma of the tibia with breaching of the cortices.

bone have been investigated on flow cytometric DNA analysis, the kinetic parameters suggesting a better prognosis compared to osteosarcoma.[80]

CYTOGENETICS

Some clonal and non-clonal chromosomal aberrations similar to those described in giant cell tumors have been reported (aberrations involving 8p11, 19q13 and 20q13).[81] Structural abnormalities involve chromosomes 1, 3, 5, 10, 11, 13, 15, 16 and 17; numeric chromosome abnormalities are found for all chromosomes, except chromosomes 2, 4 and 16.[82]

ELECTRON MICROSCOPY

Numerous studies identify very similar cellular components, but with divergent histogenetic interpretations.[14,57,67,69,70,83–92] Undifferentiated cells are found as well as cells of intermediate differentiation, showing both histiocytic and fibrocytic features.[14,86,88,90]

Histiocyte-like cells have a ruffled or villous plasma membrane; organelles are sparse and lysosomes are found as well as a Golgi apparatus. Rough endoplasmic reticulum is scant and many cells are lipid filled.[90] Multinucleated giant cells of the Touton type and xanthomatous cells are identified.[84]

Fibroblast-like cells have a rich endoplasmic reticulum and a well-developed Golgi apparatus.[90]

Spindle-shaped cells with an abundance of myofilaments and dense body-like structures are myofibroblastic cells[23,69,70,74,88,89] although sometimes simulating pleomorphic malignant histiocytic cells.[74]

Histiocytic-like cells predominate in one study[70] and fibroblast-like cells and myofibroblastic-like cells in another,[74] leading to the concept that the tumor is composed of fibroblasts and myofibroblasts with a considerable reactive infiltration of mature tissue macrophages and osteoclast-like giant cells.[87]

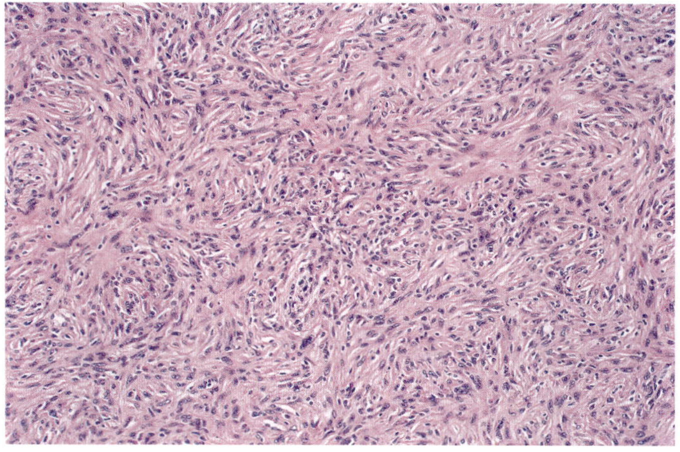

Fig. 20.7

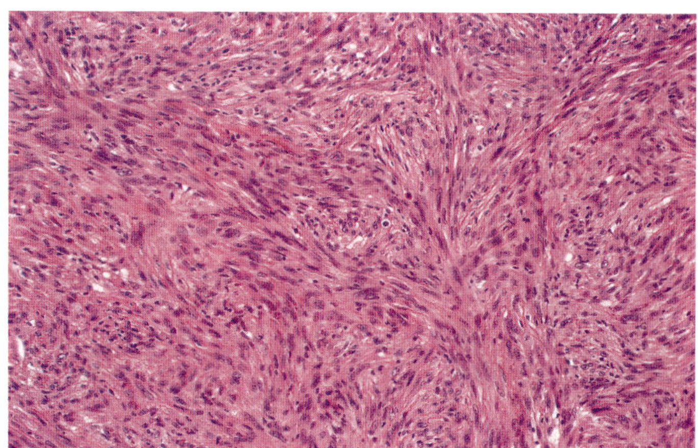

Fig. 20.8

Figs 20.7, 20.8 Malignant fibrous histiocytoma of bone: fibroblast cells.

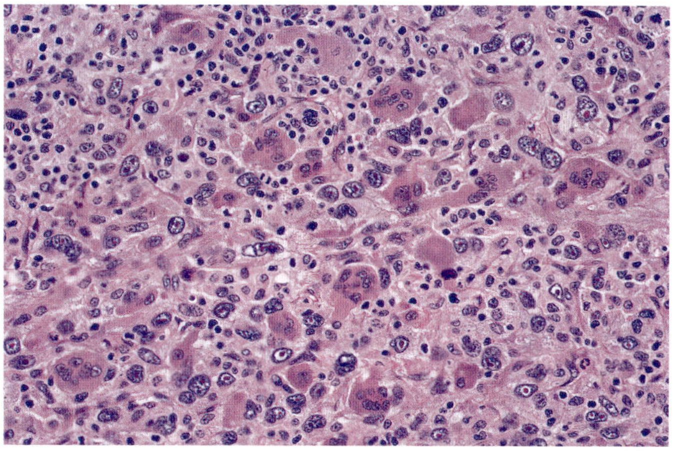

Fig. 20.9

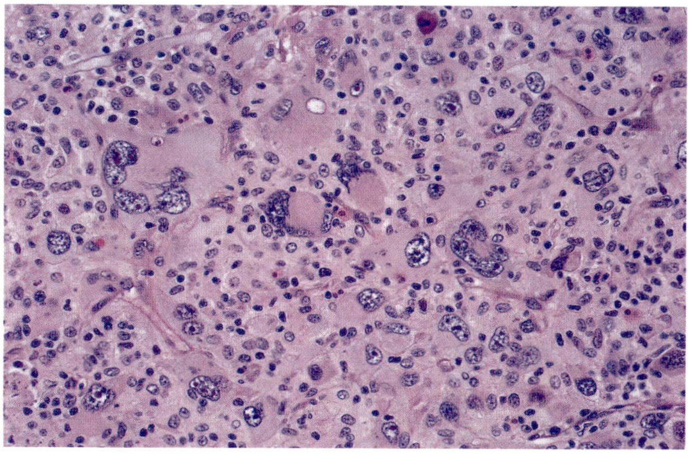

Fig. 20.10

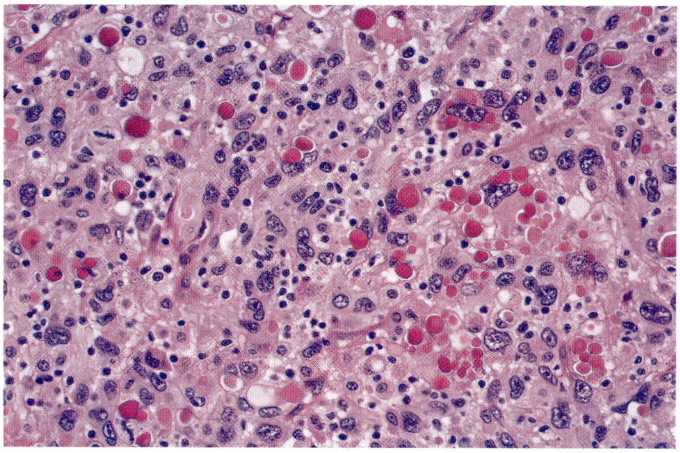

Fig. 20.11

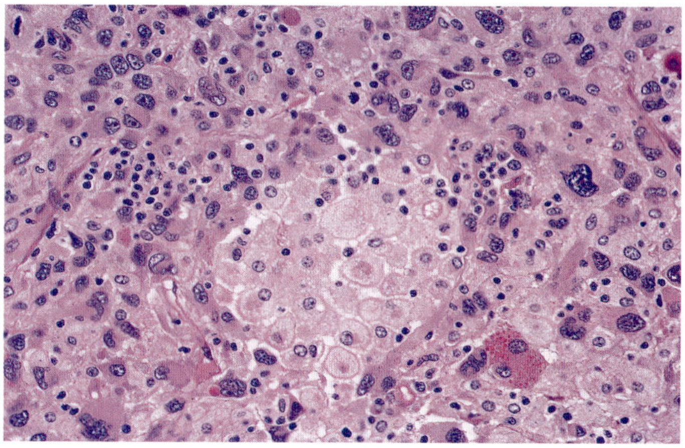

Fig. 20.12

Figs 20.9–20.12 Malignant fibrous histiocytoma of bone: histiocyte-like cells.

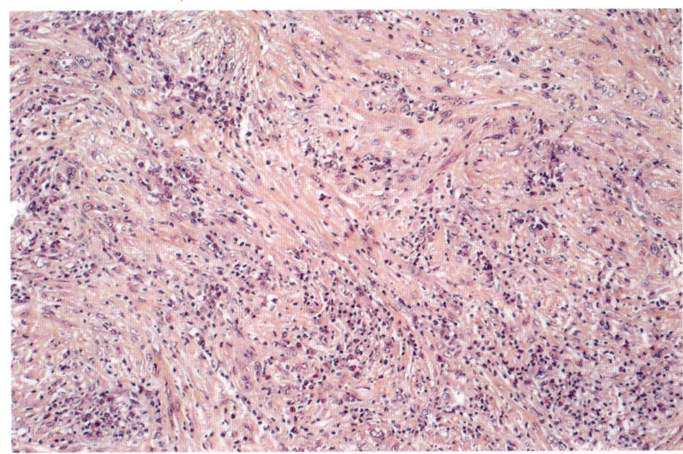

Fig. 20.13 Malignant fibrous histiocytoma of bone: infiltration by inflammatory cells.

A very unusual view on histochemical and ultrastructural findings is that fibroblast-like cells may also differentiate into osteoblasts.[92] Other unusual features are Gaucher's body-like large lysosomes,[70] asteroid bodies,[84] Langerhans organelles[83] or a fibrous long-spacing collagen.[23,89]

COURSE, TREATMENT AND PROGNOSIS

Metastases develop within the first 2 years and hematoge-nous dissemination leads to lung and bone metastases. Regional lymph node spread is well recognized but less frequent, about 5% of cases.[7,10,64,65,70,93]

For most authors, the survival is not related to histology, if one excepts rare cases of low-grade sarcoma. It has been suggested that desmoplasia could be linked with a worse prognosis and chronic inflammatory infiltration with pro-longed survival,[94] but other studies do not corroborate these findings.[12]

In earlier reports, the prognosis was very poor,[64,65] with an average survival of 1 year. Now, adjuvant and neoadju-vant chemotherapy combined with adequate (radical) surgery has improved the survival rate to 63% at 5 years.[94] The usefulness of chemotherapy is stressed in many reports.[94–98] Radiation therapy is used in inoperable tumors only, with some good results, but there is a risk of radiation-induced sarcoma.[1,4,10,30] Local recurrence (31% of cases) is a bad prognostic factor,[10] as are most sec-ondary forms.[7,10]

DIFFERENTIAL DIAGNOSIS

The malignant fibrous histiocytoma subtype of osteosar-coma, or MFH-like osteosarcoma[99] (Mirra 1989, Unni 1996), is defined by the finding of a network of osteoid with marginated or encased tumoral osteoblasts or even minute foci of primitive bone (Huvos 1991), but Fechner

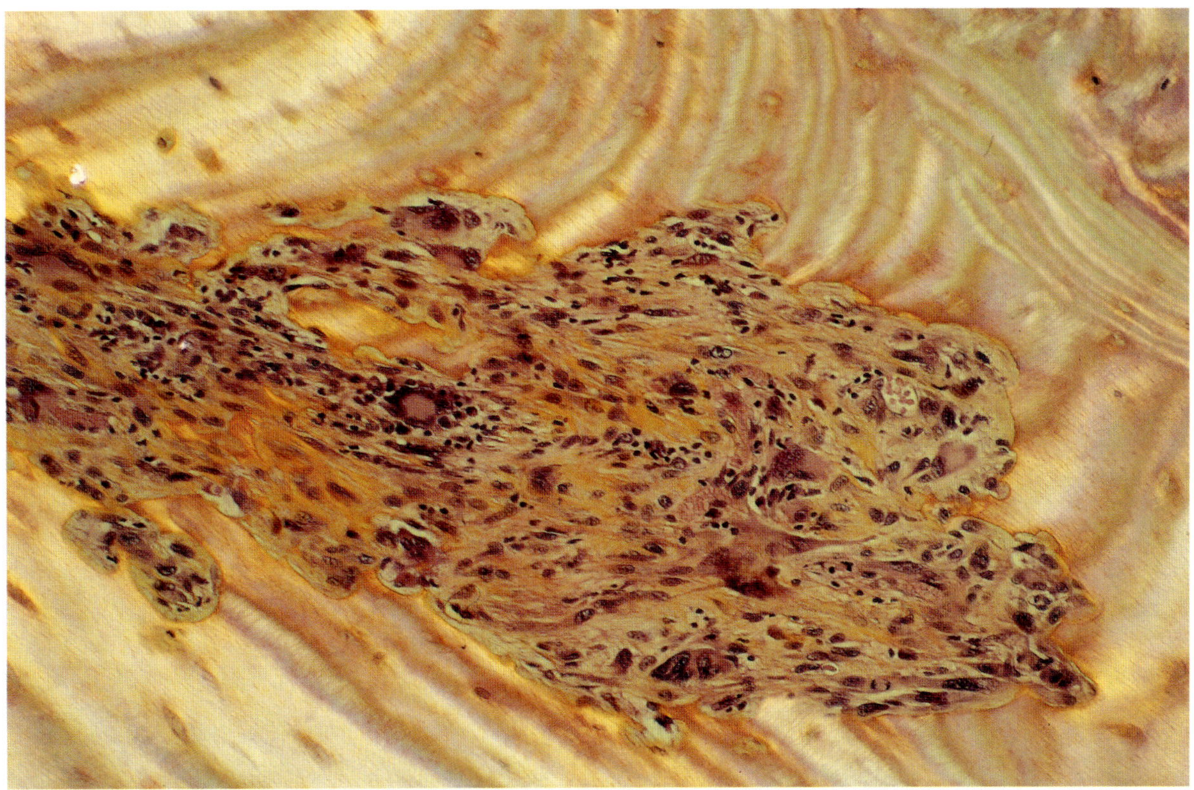

Fig. 20.14 High-grade malignant fibrous histiocytoma of bone invading the cortex (polarized light).

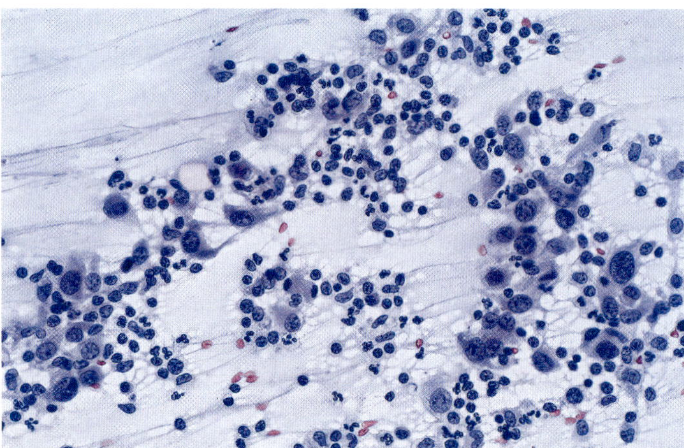

Fig. 20.15

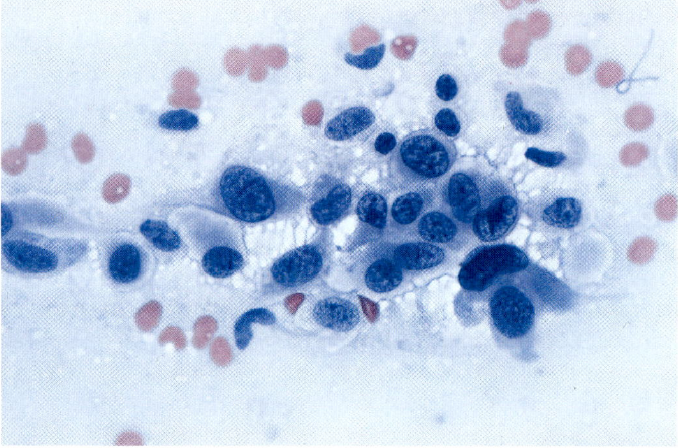

Fig. 20.16

Figs 20.15, 20.16 Malignant fibrous histiocytoma of bone: imprint cytology.

suggests that this last component should not prevent a straightforward diagnosis of malignant fibrous histiocytoma. For some authors, the tumoral bone formation may even be a normal component[92] and ultrastructurally, calcific deposits may be found in the ground substance.[87] ALPase activity[26,90] is detected in some malignant fibrous histiocytomas;[100,101] conversely, so-called histiocytic markers may be demonstrated in osteoblastic osteosarcomas.[101]

A bone sarcoma may exhibit malignant fibrous histiocytoma features in the soft tissue mass and osteosarcoma features in the osseous component.[100,101] MFH-like areas in osteosarcoma may vary from 7% to 55% of the sarcoma bulk and are found in 5–30% of all osteosarcomas.[102]

MFH-like osteosarcomas express vimentin, antibodies against collagen type I and factor XIIIa, aminopeptidase (APm) and dipeptidylpeptidase IV (DDP IV) for fibroblasts and osteoblasts.[102] Osteocalcin may be demonstrated even in tumors devoid of tumoral osteoid and appears as an important guide for further additional sampling of the tumor;[101] it is not demonstrated in malignant fibrous histiocytomas and fibrosarcomas.

Ultrastructurally, MFH-like osteosarcomas display cells with pronounced phagocytic structures and well-developed lysosomes and round or spindle cells resembling osteoblasts.[87,100,102]

High-grade fibrosarcomas can be confused with malignant fibrous histiocytomas: the prognosis and survival for both tumors appear very similar.[11,103] Fibrosarcomas exhibit a 'herring bone' pattern, a less cellular pleomorphism, rare multinucleated giant cells and no histiocytic component. The degree of collagen production is linked to the differentiation of the tumor; one has to remember that most heavily collagenized or even hyalinized spindle cell bone sarcomas represent malignant fibrous histiocytomas (Huvos 1991).

Some malignant fibrous histiocytomas may contain a prominent component of osteoclast-type, benign looking giant cells[67] and the differential diagnosis with a malignant giant cell tumor appears quite difficult theoretically; in practice, one could consider that the two entities are closely-related, if not identical tumors (Huvos 1991).

Leiomyosarcomas have elongated cells with blunt-ended nuclei, arranged in fascicles. Striations on trichrome stains and myofilaments on ultrastructural examination are demonstrated, as well as immunoreactivity for desmin, actin, Leu 7 and even S-100 protein and myelin basic protein (Huvos 1991). However, desmin and muscle common actin may be found in malignant fibrous histiocytomas.

Rare angiomatoid malignant fibrous histiocytomas may be confused with hemangiopericytomas.

Clusters of histiocyte-like cells can mimic a metastatic carcinoma.[14] The differential diagnosis is broad, including giant cell carcinoma of the thyroid or hepatocarcinomas, but mostly renal or lung carcinomas with sarcomatous features,[100] which Huvos found with an unusual incidence in the proximal end of the humerus.[7]

Lymphomas or Hodgkin's disease in bone are easily ruled out by immunohistochemistry.

Dedifferentiated chondrosarcomas or chordomas should be excluded by the radiological findings and a thorough sampling of the tumor.

Bone involvement by a malignant fibrous histiocytoma of the soft tissues is established by the radiological and gross findings.

REFERENCES

1. Dahlin D C, Unni K K, Matsuno T. Malignant (fibrous) histiocytoma of bone. Fact or fancy? Cancer 1977: 39: 1508–1516

2. Fletcher C D M. Pleomorphic malignant fibrous histiocytoma: fact or fiction? A critical reappraisal based on 159 tumors diagnosed as pleomorphic sarcoma. Am J Surg Pathol 1992: 16: 213–228

3. Wood G S, Beckstead J H, Turner R R, Hendrickson M, Kempson R, Warnke R A. Malignant fibrous histiocytoma tumor cells resemble fibroblasts. Am J Surg Pathol 1986: 10: 323–335

4. Meister P. Malignant fibrous histiocytoma: a 'fibrohistiocytic' or primitive, fibroblastic sarcoma. Curr Top Pathol 1995: 89: 193–214

5. Feldman F, Norman D. Intra and extraosseous malignant histiocytoma (malignant fibrous xanthoma). Radiology 1972: 104: 497–508

6. Feldman F, Lattes R. Primary malignant fibrous histiocytoma (fibrous xanthoma) of bone. Skeletal Radiol 1977: 1: 145–160

7. Huvos A G, Heilweil M, Bretsky S S. The pathology of malignant fibrous histiocytoma of bone. A study of 130 patients. Am J Surg Pathol 1985: 9: 853–871

8. Dunham W K, Wilborn W H. Malignant fibrous histiocytoma of bone. Report of two cases and review of the literature. J Bone Joint Surg (Am) 1979: 61: 939–942

9. Freyschmidt J, Ostertag H, Majewski A, Korvalian Z. Das maligne fibröse Histiozytom des Knochens (MFH): eine neue Tumorentität? RÖFO 1981: 135: 1–12

10. Capanna R, Bertoni F, Bacchini P, Bacci G, Guerra A, Campanacci M. Malignant fibrous histiocytoma of bone. The experience at the Rizzoli Institute: report of 90 cases. Cancer 1984: 54: 177–187

11. Taconis W K, Mulder J D. Fibrosarcoma and malignant fibrous histiocytoma of long bones. Radiographic features and grading. Skeletal Radiol 1984: 11: 237–245

12. Naka T, Fukuda T, Shinohara N, Iwamoto Y, Sugioka Y, Tsuneyoshi M. Osteosarcoma versus malignant fibrous histiocytoma of bone in patients older than 40 years. A clinicopathologic and immunohistochemical analysis with special reference to malignant fibrous histiocytoma-like osteosarcoma. Cancer 1995: 76: 972–984

13. Chen K T. Multiple fibroxanthosarcoma of bone. Cancer 1978: 42: 770–773

14. McCarthy E F, Matsuno T, Dorfman H D. Malignant fibrous histiocytoma of bone: a study of 35 cases. Hum Pathol 1979: 10: 57–70

15. Castillo M, Tehranzadeh J, Becerra J, Mnaymneh W. Case report 408. Malignant fibrous histiocytoma of innominate bones and femur (multicentric). Skeletal Radiol 1987: 16: 74–77

16. Walter H, Schneider-Stock R, Mellin W, Günther T, Nebelung W, Roessner A. Synchronous multifocal bone sarcomas – a case report and molecular pathologic investigation. Gen Diagn Pathol 1995: 141: 67–74

17. Finci R, Gunham O, Uçmakli E, Sarlak O. Multiple and familial malignant fibrous histiocytoma of bone. A report of two cases. J Bone Joint Surg (Am) 1990: 72: 295–298

18. Steiner P E. Multiple diffuse fibrosarcoma of bone. Am J Pathol 1944: 20: 877–893

19. Ozaki T, Taguchi K, Sugihara S, Inoue H. Multiple malignant fibrous histiocytoma of bone. A case report. Acta Orthop Scand 1994: 65: 209–211

20. Smith J. Radiation-induced sarcoma of bone; clinical and radiographic findings in 43 patients irradiated for soft tissue neoplasms. Clin Radiol 1982: 33: 205–221

21. Murphey M D, Gross T M, Rosenthal H G. From the archives of the AFIP. Musculoskeletal malignant fibrous histiocytoma: radiologic-pathologic correlation. Radiographics 1994: 14: 807–828

22. Meister P, Konard E. Malignes fibroses Histiozytom des Knochens (8 Jahre nach Strahlenexposition). Arch Orthop Unfallchir 1977: 90: 95–101

23. Angervall L, Johansson B, Kindblom L G, Säve-Soderberg J. Primary malignant fibrous histiocytoma of bone after irradiation. Acta Pathol Microbiol Scand A 1979: 87: 437–446

24. Pinkston J A, Sekine I. Postirradiation sarcoma (malignant fibrous histiocytoma) following cervix cancer. Cancer 1982: 49: 434–438

25. Vanel D, Hagay C, Rebibo G, Oberlin O, Masselot J. Study of three radio-induced malignant fibrohistiocytomas of bone. Skeletal Radiol 1983: 9: 174–178

26. Bayer Kristensen I, Myrhe Jensen O. Malignant fibrous histiocytoma of bone. A clinicopathologic study of 9 cases. Acta Pathol Microbiol Immunol Scand A 1984: 92: 205–210

27. Huvos A G, Woodard H Q, Heilweil M. Post radiation malignant fibrous histiocytoma of bone. A clinicopathologic study of 20 patients. Am J Surg Pathol 1986: 10: 9–18

28. Mirra J M, Bullough P G, Marcove R C, Jacobs B, Huvos A G. Malignant fibrous histiocytoma and osteosarcoma in association with bone infarcts. Report of four cases, two in caisson workers. J Bone Joint Surg (Am) 1974: 56: 932–940

29. Mirra J M, Gold R H, Marafiote R. Malignant (fibrous) histiocytoma arising in association with a bone infarct in sickle-cell disease: coincidence or cause and effect? Cancer 1977: 39: 186–194

30. Galli S J, Weintraub H P, Proppe K H. Malignant fibrous histiocytoma with pleiomorphic sarcoma in association with medullary bone infarcts. Cancer 1978: 41: 607–619

31. Heselson N G, Price S K, Mills E E, Conway S S, Marks R K. Two malignant fibrous histiocytoma in bone infarcts. Case report. J Bone Joint Surg (Am) 1983: 65: 1166–1171

32. Abrahams T G, Hull M. Case report 394. Malignant fibrous histiocytoma (MFH) arising in an infarct of bone. Skeletal Radiol 1986: 15: 578–583

33. Breen T F, Healy W L. Malignant fibrous histiocytoma arising in medullary long bone infarcts. A case report. Orthopedics 1987: 10: 1169–1173

34. Frierson H F Jr, Fechner R E, Stallings R G, Wang G J. Malignant fibrous histiocytoma in bone infarct. Association with sickle cell trait and alcohol abuse. Cancer 1987: 59: 496–500

35. Gaucher A A, Regent D M, Gillet P M, Pere P G, Aymard B M, Clement V. Case report 656. Malignant fibrous histiocytoma in a previous bone infarct. Skeletal Radiol 1991: 20: 137–140

36. Desai P, Perino G, Present D, Steiner G C. Sarcoma in association with bone infarcts. Report of five cases. Arch Pathol Lab Med 1996: 120: 482–489

37. Kennedy C, Stocker D J. Malignant fibrous histiocytoma complicating chronic osteomyelitis. Clin Radiol 1990: 41: 435–436

38. Helio H, Kivioja A, Karaharju E O, Elomaa I, Knuutila S. Malignant fibrous histiocytoma arising in a previous site of fracture and osteomyelitis. Eur J Surg Oncol 1993: 19: 479–484

39. Lee Y S, Pho R W H, Nather A. Malignant fibrous histiocytoma at site of metal implant. Cancer 1984: 54: 2286–2289

40. Lindeman G, McKay M J, Taubman K L, Bilous A M. Malignant fibrous histiocytoma developing in bone 44 years after shrapnel trauma. Cancer 1990: 66: 2229–2232

41. Bago-Granell J, Aguirre-Canyadell M, Nardi J, Tallada N. Malignant fibrous histiocytoma of bone at the site of a total hip arthroplasty. J Bone Joint Surg (Br) 1984: 66: 38–40

42. Vives P, Sevestre H, Grodet H, Marie F. Histiocytome fibreux malin du fémur après prothèse totale de hanche. A propos d'un cas. Rev Chir Orthop 1987: 73: 407–409

43. Haag M, Adler C P. Malignant fibrous histiocytoma in association with a hip replacement. J Bone Joint Surg (Br) 1989: 71B: 701

44. Troop J K, Mallory T H, Fisher D A, Vaughn B K. Malignant fibrous histiocytoma after total hip arthroplasty. A case report. Clin Orthop 1990: 253: 297–300

45. Ruggieri P, Biagini R. Istiocitoma fibroso maligno in m. di Paget. Chir Organi Mov 1984: 69: 97–100

46. Ishida T, Machinami R, Kojima T, Kikuchi F. Malignant fibrous histiocytoma and osteosarcoma in association with fibrous dysplasia of bone. Report of three cases. Pathol Res Pract 1992: 188: 757–763

47. Sanerkin N G, Woods C G. Fibrosarcomata and malignant fibrous histiocytomata arising in relation to enchondromata. J Bone Joint Surg (Br) 1979: 61: 366–372

48. Makek M, Leu H J. Malignant fibrous histiocytoma arising in a recurrent chordoma. Case report and electron microscopic findings. Virchows Arch A Pathol Anat Histol 1982: 397: 241–250

49. Miettinen M, Lehto V P, Virtanen I. Malignant fibrous histiocytoma within a recurrent chordoma. A light microscopic, electron microscopic and immunohistochemical study. Am J Clin Pathol 1984: 82: 738–743

50. Halpern J, Kopolovic J, Catane R. Malignant fibrous histiocytoma

developing in irradiated sacral chordoma. Cancer 1984: 53: 2661–2662

51. Belza M G, Urich H. Chordoma and malignant fibrous histiocytoma. Evidence for transformation. Cancer 1986: 58: 1082–1087

52. Siegel S E, Stanley P, Shimada H, Bernstein S, Soni D, Hays D M. Malignant fibrous histiocytoma of bone following primitive neuroectodermal tumor of bone. Med Pediatr Oncol 1994: 22: 341–347

53. Baer S C, Ayala A G, Ro J Y, Yasco A W, Raymond A K, Edeiken J. Case report 843. Malignant fibrous histiocytoma of the femur arising in melorheostosis. Skeletal Radiol 1994: 23: 310–314

54. Laverdiere J T, Abrahams T G, Jones M A. Primary osseous malignant fibrous histiocytoma involving a rib. Skeletal Radiol 1995: 24: 152–154

55. Mutale C B, Patil P S, Patel J B. Malignant fibrous histiocytoma of the second metacarpal. J Hand Surg (Br) 1986: 11: 149–150

56. Hankin F M, Hankin R C, Louis D S. Malignant fibrous histiocytoma involving a digit. J Hand Surg (Am) 1987: 12: 83–86

57. Dock W, Hajek P, Wittich G, Kumpan W, Grabenwoger F. Primary malignant fibrous histiocytoma of a metacarpal bone: a new localization. Br J Radiol 1989: 62: 940–942

58. Rechtine G R, Hassan M O, Bohlman H H. Malignant fibrous histiocytoma of the cervical spine. Report of an unusual case and description of light and electron microscopy. Spine 1984: 9: 824–830

59. Bidwell J K, Young J W, Saylor L. Malignant fibrous histiocytoma of the spine: computed tomography appearance and review of the literature. J Comput Tomogr 1987: 11: 355–358

60. Sturm P F, Abramowitz J, Wagner C, Ferguson R, Walker S. Malignant fibrous histiocytoma of the spine. A case report and review of the literature. Spine 1992: 17: 975–977

61. Lopez-Barea F, Rodriguez-Peralto J L, Burgos-Lizalde E, Gonzalez-Lopez J, Sanchez-Herrera S. Case report 639. Malignant fibrous histiocytoma (MFH) of the patella. Skeletal Radiol 1991: 20: 125–128

62. Roger D J, Uhl R L, Carl A. Malignant fibrous histiocytoma of the patella. Orthopedics 1994: 17: 189–192

63. Kemp H B, Byers P D. Case report 444. Subperiosteal malignant fibrous histiocytoma (MFH) of thigh, with involvement of femur. Skeletal Radiol 1987: 16: 584–588

64. Spanier S S, Enneking W F, Enriquez P. Primary malignant fibrous histiocytoma of bone. Cancer 1975: 36: 2084–2098

65. Spanier S S. Malignant fibrous histiocytoma of bone. Orthop Clin North Am 1977: 8: 947–961

66. Hudson T M, Hawkins I F Jr, Spanier S S, Enneking W F. Angiography of malignant fibrous histiocytoma of bone. Radiology 1979: 131: 9–15

67. Kahn L B, Webber B, Mills E, Anstey L, Heselson N G. Malignant fibrous histiocytoma (malignant fibrous xanthoma; xanthosarcoma) of bone. Cancer 1978: 42: 640–651

68. Terashima K, Suda A, Imai Y et al. Malignant fibrous histiocytoma of bone associated with focal hemangiopericytomatous pattern. Acta Pathol Jpn 1981: 31: 1063–1078

69. Martinez-Tello F J, Navas Palacios J, Calvo-Asensio M, Loizaga-Iriondo J M. Malignant fibrous histiocytoma of bone. A clinicopathological and electron microscopical study. Pathol Res Pract 1981: 173: 141–158

70. Nakashima Y, Morishita S, Kotoura Y et al. Malignant fibrous histiocytoma of bone. A review of 13 cases and an ultrastructural study. Cancer 1985: 55: 2804–2811

71. Gruber H E, Marshall G J, Moore T M, Schwinn C P, Kirchen M E, Massry G S. Alteration in osteoblast cell number and cell activity in the presence of invading malignant fibrous histiocytoma. Cancer 1987: 59: 755–760

72. Kannan V, Von Ruden D. Malignant fibrous histiocytoma of bone: initial diagnosis by aspiration biopsy cytology. Diagn Cytopathol 1988: 4: 262–264

73. Iwasaki H, Isayama T, Ohjimi Y et al. Malignant fibrous histiocytoma. A tumor of facultative histiocytes showing mesenchymal differentiation in cultured cell lines. Cancer 1992: 69: 437–447

74. Martorell M, Galabuig C, Peydro Olaya A, Llombart-Bosch A, Terrier-Lacombe M J, Contesso G. Fibroblast and myofibroblast participation in malignant fibrous histiocytoma (MFH) of bone. Ultrastructural study of eight cases with immunohistochemical support. Pathol Res Pract 1989: 184: 582–590

75. Perez-Bacete M J, Llombart-Bosch A. FU-3 monoclonal antibody: a specific marker for malignant fibrous histiocytoma? An analysis of 32 malignant soft tissue and bone sarcomas. Virchows Arch 1994: 424: 243–247

76. Weiss S W, Bratthauer G L, Morris P A. Postirradiation malignant fibrous histiocytoma expressing cytokeratin. Implications for the immunodiagnosis of sarcomas. Am J Surg Pathol 1988: 12: 554–558

77. Rosenberg A E, O'Connell J X, Dickersin G R, Bhan A K. Expression of epithelial markers in malignant fibrous histiocytoma of the musculoskeletal system. An immunohistochemical and electron microscopic study. Hum Pathol 1993: 24: 284–293

78. Roessner A, Zwadlo G, Vollmer E, Sorg C, Grundmann E. Biologic characterization of human bone tumors. IX. Occurrence of macrophages. Pathol Res Pract 1987: 182: 336–343

79. Roessner A, Vassallo J, Vollmer E, Zwadlo G, Sorg C, Grundmann E. Biological characterization of human bone tumors. X. The proliferation behavior of macrophages as compared to fibroblastic cells in malignant fibrous histiocytoma and giant cell tumor of bone. J Cancer Res Clin Oncol 1987: 113: 559–562

80. Mellin W, Dierschauer W, Hiddemann W et al. Flow cytometric DNA analysis of bone tumors. Curr Top Pathol 1989: 80: 115–152

81. Molenaar W M, Van Den Berg E, Veth R P, Dijhuizen T, De Vries E G E. Tumor progression in a giant cell type malignant fibrous histiocytoma of bone: clinical, radiologic, histologic, and cytogenetic evidence. Genes Chromosomes Cancer 1994: 10: 66–70

82. Bridge J A, Sanger W G, Neff J R, Hess M M. Cytogenetic findings in a primary malignant fibrous histiocytoma of bone and the lung metastasis. Pathology 1990: 22: 16–19

83. Newland R C, Harrison M A, Wright R G. Fibroxanthosarcoma of bone. Pathology 1975: 7: 203–208

84. Inada O, Yumoto T, Furuse K, Tanaka T. Ultrastructural features of malignant fibrous histiocytoma of bone. Acta Pathol Jpn 1976: 26: 491–501

85. Saito R, Caines M J. Atypical fibrous histiocytoma of the humerus. A light and electron microscopic study. Am J Clin Pathol 1977: 68: 409–415

86. Johnson W W, Coburn T P, Pratt C B, Smith J W, Kumar A P, Dahlin D C. Ultrastructure of malignant histiocytoma arising in the acromion. Hum Pathol 1978: 9: 199–209

87. Roessner A, Hobik H P, Grundmann E. Malignant fibrous histiocytoma of bone and osteosarcoma. A comparative light and electron microscopic study. Pathol Res Pract 1979: 164: 385–401

88. Shapiro F. Malignant fibrous histiocytoma of bone. An ultrastructural study. Ultrastruct Pathol 1981: 2: 33–42

89. Katenkamp D, Stiller D. Malignant fibrous histiocytoma of bone. Light microscopic and electron microscopic examination of four cases. Virchows Arch A Pathol Anat Histol 1981: 391: 323–335

90. Ghandur-Mnaymneh L, Zych G, Mnaymneh W. Primary malignant fibrous histiocytoma of bone; report of six cases with ultrastructural study and analysis of the literature. Cancer 1982: 49: 698–707

91. Stiller D, Katenkamp D. Das maligne fibröse Histiozytom des Knochens. Klinische Pathologie und histologisch Diagnose. Zentralbl Allg Pathol 1983: 128: 5–20

92. Komiya S, Inoue A, Ikuta H, Nagata K. A study on the osseous elements in malignant fibrous histiocytoma of bone. Nippon Seikeigeka Gakkai Zasshi 1985: 59: 67–73

93. Yuen W W, Saw D. Malignant fibrous histiocytoma of bone. J Bone Joint Surg (Am) 1985: 67: 482–486

94. Yokoyama R, Tsuneyoshi M, Enjoji M, Shinohara N, Masuda S. Prognostic factors of malignant fibrous histiocytoma of bone. A clinical and histopathologic analysis of 34 cases. Cancer 1993: 72: 1902–1908

95. Weiner M, Sedlis M, Johnston A D, Dick H M, Wolff J A.

Adjuvant chemotherapy of malignant fibrous histiocytoma of bone. Cancer 1983: 51: 25–29

96. Urban C, Rosen G, Huvos A G, Caparros B, Cacavio A, Nirenberg A. Chemotherapy of malignant fibrous histiocytoma of bone. A report of five cases. Cancer 1983: 51: 795–802

97. Den Heeten G J, Schraffordt Koops H, Kamps W A, Oosterhuis J W, Sleijfer D T, Oldhoff J. Treatment of malignant fibrous histiocytoma of bone. A plea for primary chemotherapy. Cancer 1985: 56: 37–40

98. Bacci G, Springfield D, Capanna R, Picci P, Bertoni F, Campanacci M. Adjuvant chemotherapy for malignant fibrous histiocytoma in the femur and tibia. J Bone Joint Surg (Am) 1985: 67: 620–825

99. Ballance W A Jr, Mendelsohn G, Carter J R, Abdul-Karim F W, Jacobs G, Makley J T. Osteogenic sarcoma. Malignant fibrous histiocytoma subtype. Cancer 1988: 62: 763–771

100. Ushigome S, Hirota T. Malignant fibrous histiocytoma with special reference to its differential diagnosis. Acta Pathol Jpn 1980: 30: 799–813

101. Ushigome S, Takakuwa T, Shimoda T, Nakajima M, Fukunaga M. Immunocytochemical aspects of the differential diagnosis of osteosarcoma and malignant fibrous histiocytoma. Surg Pathol 1988: 1: 347–357

102. Yoshida H, Yumoto T, Minamizaki T. Osteosarcoma with features mimicking malignant fibrous histiocytoma. Virchows Arch A Pathol Anat Histopathol 1992: 421: 229–238

103. Taconis W K, Van Rijssel T G. Fibrosarcoma of long bones. A study of the significance of areas of malignant fibrous histiocytoma. J Bone Joint Surg (Br) 1985: 67: 111–116

Lipoma and liposarcoma

M. Forest

INTRAMEDULLARY LIPOMAS

Introduction and clinical data

Lipomas are hamartomatous lesions, the incidence of which appears very low in bone,[1] ranging from 0.1% (Wilner 1982, Unni 1996) to 2.5% of all bone tumors.[2] However, the majority of them are asymptomatic.

They have been found in patients from 5 to 70 years old, with a median age of 37 years.[3,4] Males and females are equally affected,[5] although there is a slight male predominance in the huge series of Milgram.[3,4]

Nearly half of the lesions are incidental findings.[6–12] Clinical symptoms are a mild pain or a non-tender small mass, rarely a pathologic fracture.[13,14]

Skeletal distribution

Any bone may be involved, but the most frequent locations are the long bones (Figs 21.1–21.7): the femur in a quarter of cases,[3,4] tibia,[6] fibula,[15,16] radius, humerus, calcaneus[17–22] (Figs 21.8, 21.9) and the pelvis[23–25] (Fig. 21.10). The sacrum and coccyx may be involved[26–28] but vertebral sites are unusual,[29] as are locations in the ribs[30] or the bones of the hands and feet.[31]

Imaging

In long bones, the lesion is usually metaphyseal but occurs in epiphyseal or diaphyseal regions in 25% of cases.[11] Proximal femoral intertrochanteric or subtrochanteric involvement is more usual than a femoral head location.[32,33]

An aggressive appearance is rare.[34] Lipomas appear as a well-circumscribed radiolucent lesion, with a geographic pattern of destruction, a narrow zone of transition and sometimes lobulated edges or sclerotic borders.[17,23] Some may exhibit bony ridges[11] or central, round or oval opacities simulating a sequestrum.[16,18,35] The lesion is frequent-

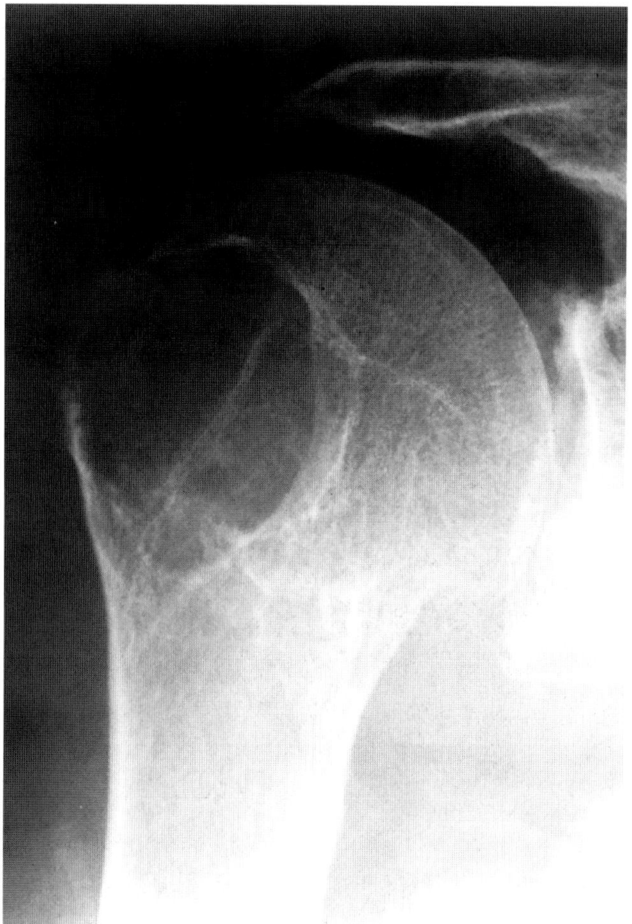

Fig. 21.1 Lipoma of the humeral head.

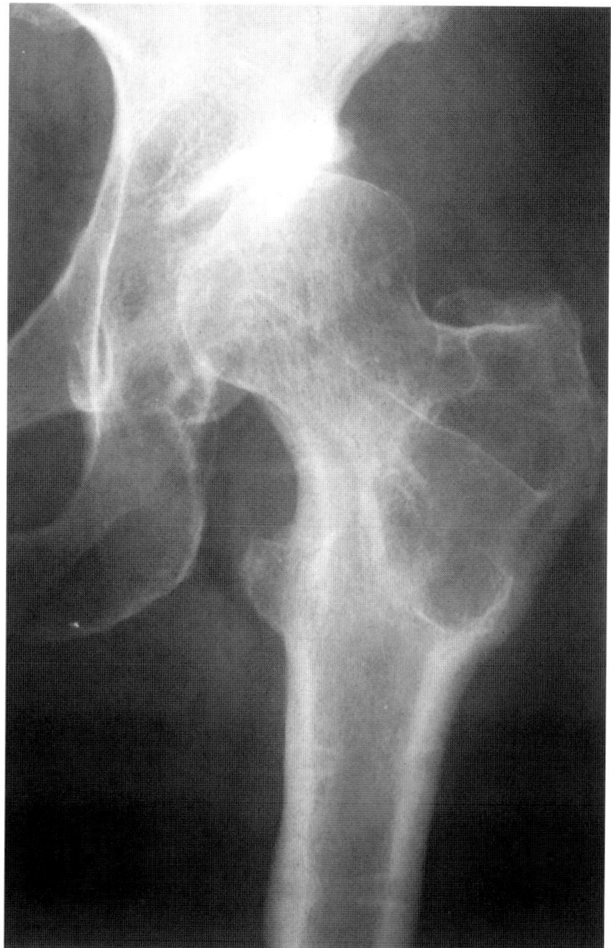

Fig. 21.2 Lipoma of the upper metaphysis of the femur.

ly eccentric in long bones, with an ovoid, elongated appearance.[6]

The cortex is thinned, but remains intact.[36] Nearly half of the cases are expansile lesions with or without a bubbly appearance,[5,36] usually asymmetrical.[6] A large expanding radiolucent mass involving almost all the sacrum has been reported.[28]

On radionuclide bone scans, there is no abnormal uptake.[12,29]

On CT examination, the low density is characteristic of fat[9,10,12,24,25,27,36] and the distinct margins and the intact or thinned cortices are well delineated. Cortical disruption is found in a very small number of cases.

On MRI, increased intensities on T1- and T2-weighted images are a signal of fat, allowing a preoperative diagnosis[12,37] and the delineation of medullary extension. Reactive bone, cyst formation or myxoid degeneration may cause some diagnostic problems.[38]

Gross pathology

The glistening bright, yellow, mass of fat is well circum-scribed, even lobulated[39] and calcium deposits or cysts may be found. A few trabeculae of bone may be engulfed in the fatty tissue.

Histopathology

The pathologist is usually familiar with lesional adipose tissue devoid of hematopoietic elements. The well-differentiated lobulated fat may, however, present secondary changes important in the differential diagnosis (Figs 21.11–21.14).

A thorough radiologic-pathologic correlation, established by Milgram and followed by others,[2] delineates three evolutionary stages.

In stage 1, the preexisting bone is resorbed, the mature and enlarged fat cells are viable, with fine fibrovascular septa. In about half of the cases, atrophic, viable or necrotic bone trabeculae may be found. On plain films, the lesion is radiolucent.

In stage 2, focal fat necrosis is partially calcified or associated with ischemic bone formation appearing as dark-stained woven bone with hematoxylin. An

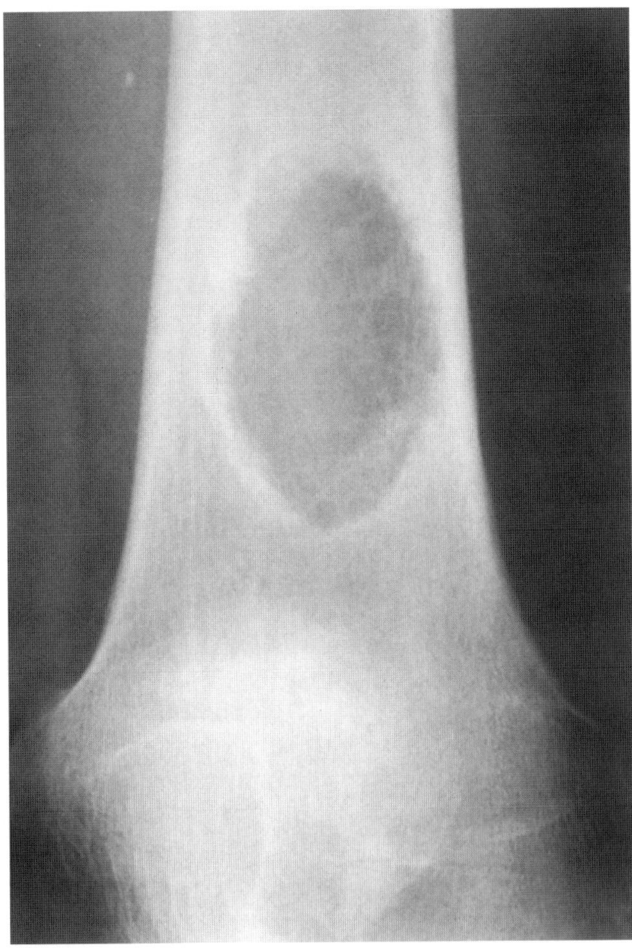

Fig. 21.3 Lipoma of the lower metaphysis of the femur.

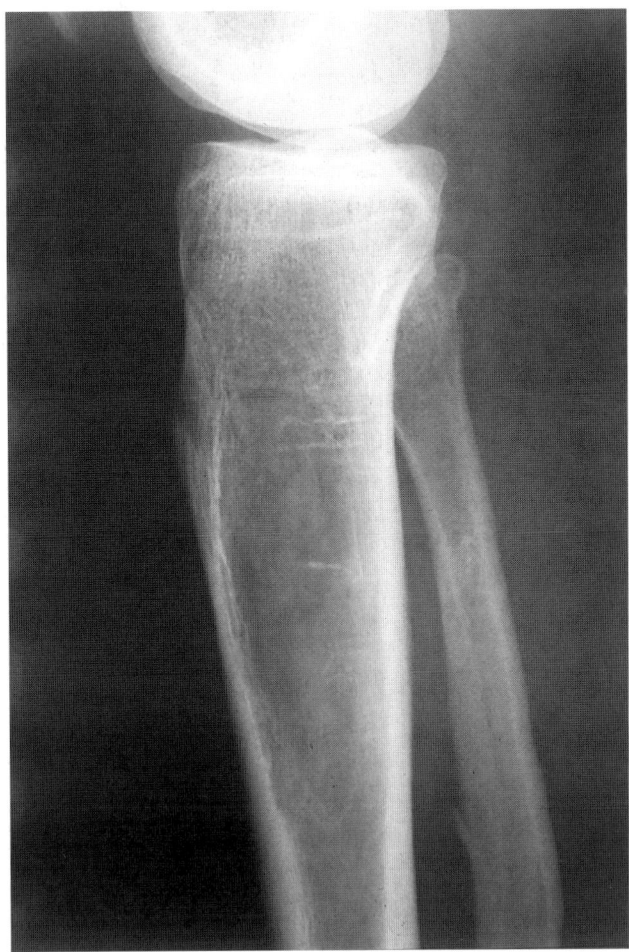

Fig. 21.4 Lipoma of the tibia shaft.

eosinophilic, globular, osteoid-like substance with varying degrees of calcification[2] mimics the 'fibrin-like coagulum' usually found in solitary bone cysts.[40] Other calcifications have a Liesegang ring-like pattern (Mirra 1989). On plain films, the sclerotic regions are distributed centrally or marginally.

Stage 3 is marked by extensive areas of eosinophilic necrotic fat and massive ischemic bone formation and calcification.[2,3,4] The extensive production of immature woven bone is associated with inconspicuous or absent osteoblastic activity. Secondary changes include aggregates of foamy histiocytes, myxoid degeneration and thin-walled cystic cavities. On plain films, an unusual calcified mass may be associated with very dense borders.

Course, treatment and prognosis

The treatment is conservative, usually curettage and packing with bone chips. A rare malignant transformation has been reported as high-grade liposarcoma and malignant fibrous histiocytoma.[41]

Differential diagnosis

Localized osteoporosis and circumscribed areas of fatty marrow (Fig. 21.15), especially in the vertebral bodies, should be ruled out[42] (Schajowicz 1994).

The ischemic bone found in lipomas is quite similar to that found in bone infarcts, but in infarcts, calcification is peripheral, the bone is not resorbed and there is no expansion of the lesion.[3,4,6,14]

The differential diagnosis with solitary bone cysts, especially in the calcaneus where imaging and location are the same, is particularly difficult, relying mostly on operative findings.

Bone infarcts may be cystic also, but usually there are no calcium deposits in the wall of a bone cyst.[19]

PAROSTEAL LIPOMAS

A very rare intracortical lipoma in the femur has been described.[43] The incidence of parosteal or periosteal lipomas,[44] is difficult to establish but about 150 cases have

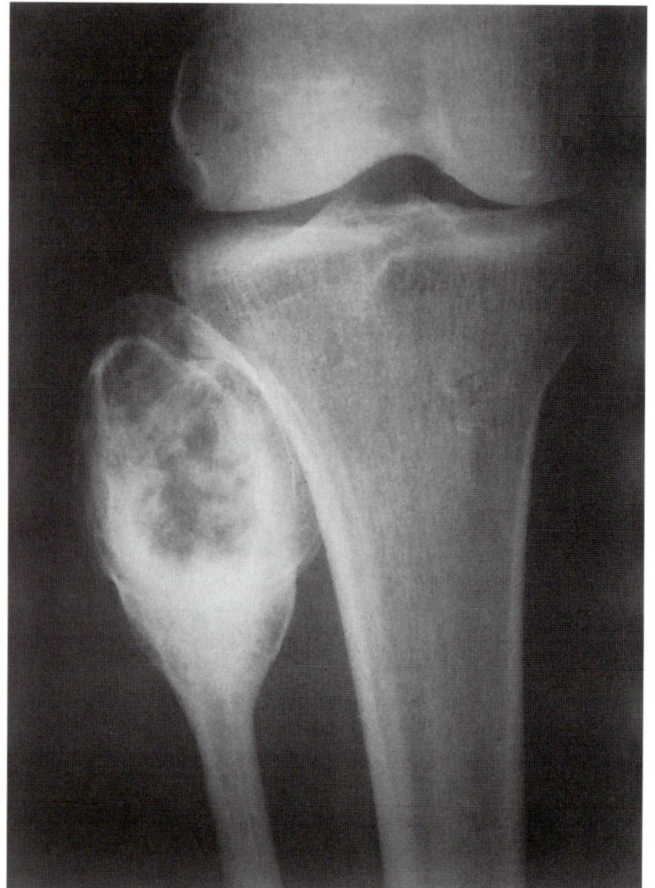

Fig. 21.5

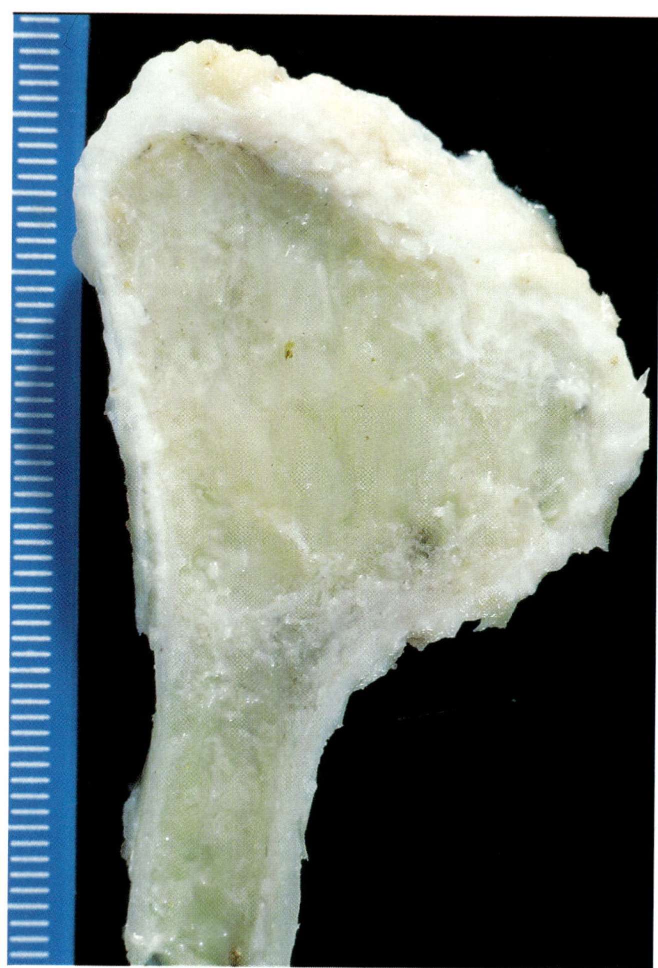

Fig. 21.6

Figs 21.5–21.7 Lipoma of the fibula.

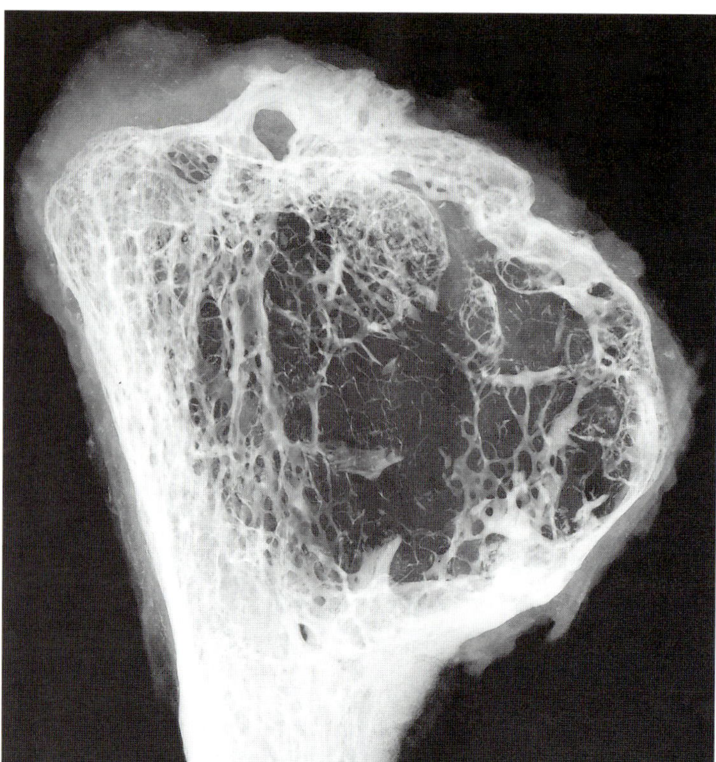

Fig. 21.7

been reported.[45] They can be found at any age, but most involve patients over 40,[46] with no sex predominance.

Some are asymptomatic[47] despite a rather large size. Others may present with a palpable mass which is firm and fixed to the underlying bone,[48] with occasional local pain, tenderness or even limitation of joint movement.

A parosteal lipoma (Fig. 21.16) is always solitary and may involve any part of the skeleton, but mostly the extremities: thigh, calf, arm and forearm, but also the scapula, clavicle, ribs, pelvis and even metacarpals and metatarsals.[44,48] The proximal radius is a particularly frequent site.[46,49–51] Some tumors may be associated with an intramuscular lipoma.[52]

On imaging, in long bones, lesions are most frequently located on the diaphysis[47] or have a broad diametaphysial base of attachment.[52] The outer cortex may be eroded or saucerized; soft tissue lipomas may also cause pressure erosion of bone. In nearly half of the cases, bone changes include cortical erosion, bowing (tibia) and bone production;[44,53] the lobulated radiolucent area presents characteristic bony excrescences.[48,54]

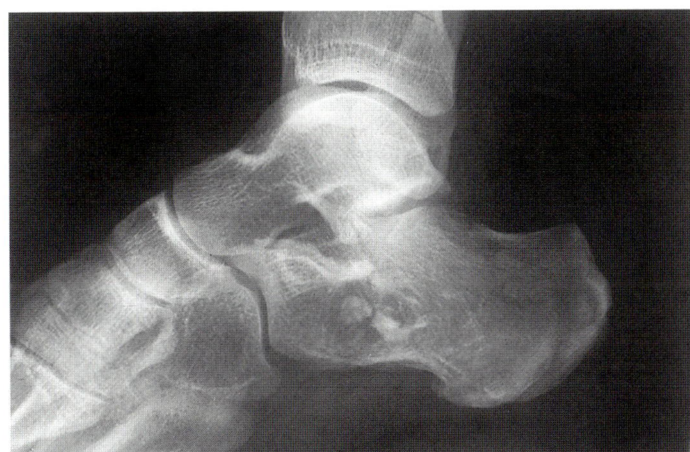

Fig. 21.8

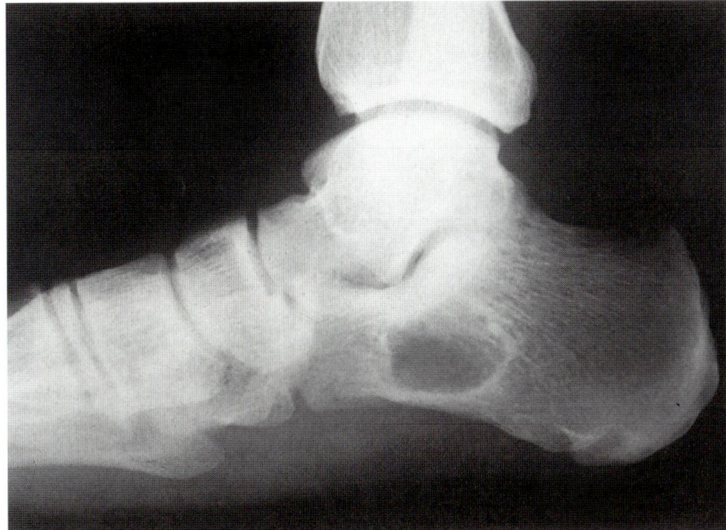

Fig. 21.9

Figs 21.8, 21.9 Lipomas of the calcaneus.

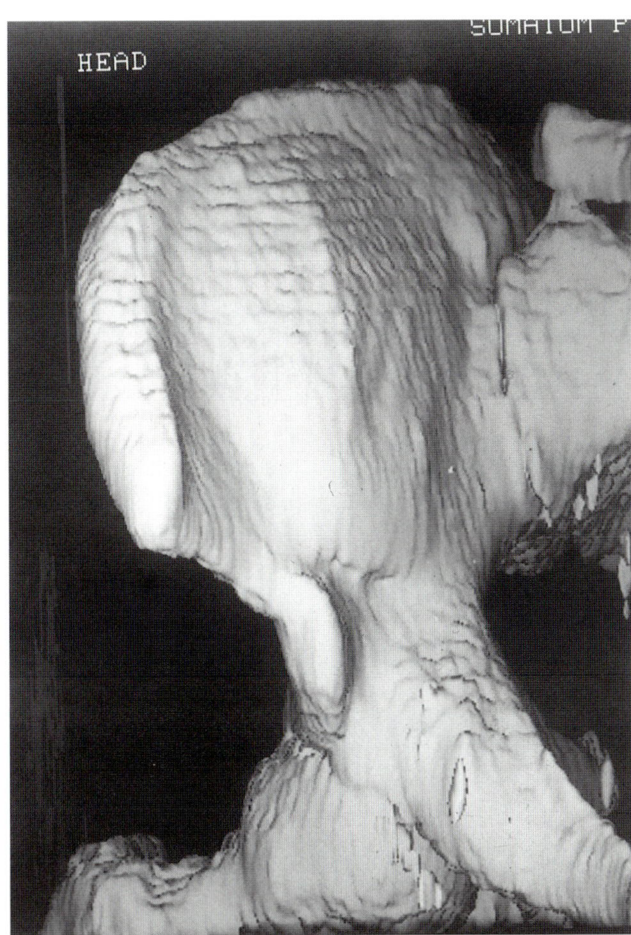

Fig. 21.10 Lipoma of the iliac wing: 3-D CT scan.

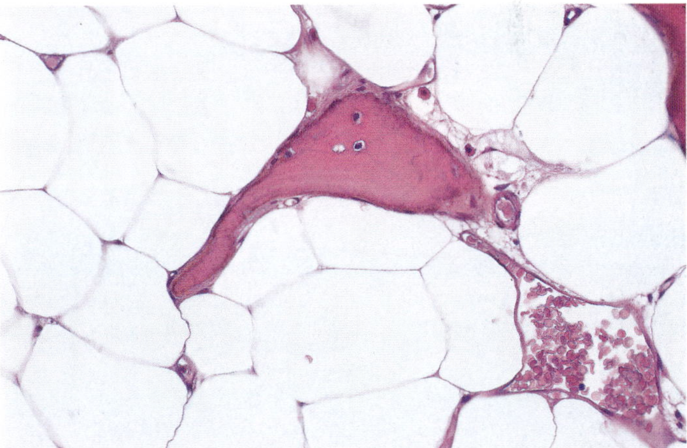

Fig. 21.11 Lipoma of the tibia: well-differentiated fat with peripheral atrophic cancellous bone.

On CT, the low density of the lesion is equivalent to that of fat; a cartilaginous lining may be found between fat and the ossification.[55,56]

On MRI, the imaging signal intensity approximates that of both subcutaneous and bone marrow fat.[56,57] Linear densities may correspond to fibrous septa, calcifications or ossifications.[48,58]

Histologically, the lesion may consist entirely of mature fat separated by strands of connective tissue.[59] More often there is formation of metaplastic bone or cartilage, sometimes radiating from the adjacent periosteum.[44,47,54,55,58,60,61] The metaplastic cartilage attachment may mimic an osteochondroma, undergoing enchondral ossification.[46,56] It may even appear as a sessile formation[47] or a bony, pedunculated mass with a lipomatous cap.

Cytogenetic findings in one case revealed a t(3;12) (q28;q14) translocation characteristic of soft tissue lipomas.[62]

LIPOMATOSIS

Rare cases have been reported with multiple lesions of the lumbar spinous processes,[2] of the femur, tibia, tarsal, metatarsal or talar bones[63,64] and in two cases associated with type IV hyperlipoproteinemia[65] and Paget's disease.[66]

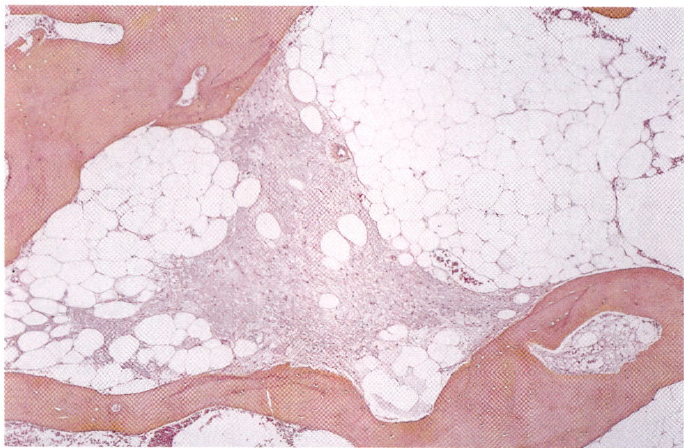

Fig. 21.12 Lipoma of the iliac wing: remodeling of bone around the lobulated fat.

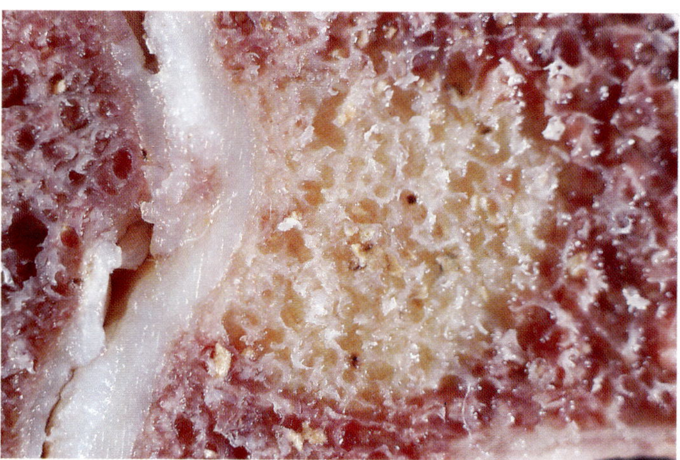

Fig. 21.15 Incidental findings of an adipose area close to the sacroiliac joint (resection of a chondrosarcoma).

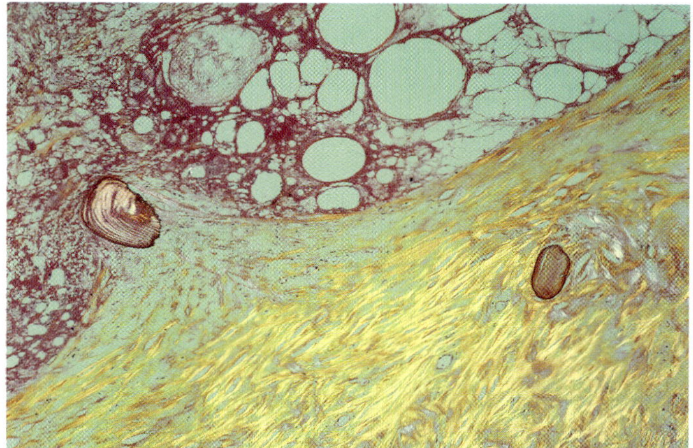

Fig. 21.13

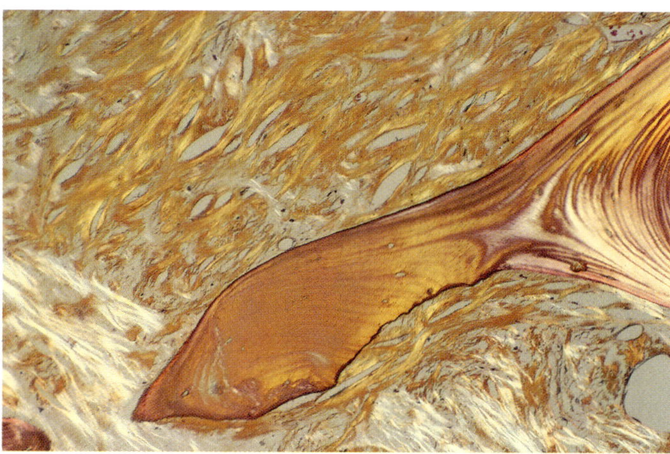

Fig. 21.14

Figs 21.13, 21.14 Necrotic changes in a lipoma of the femur (polarized light).

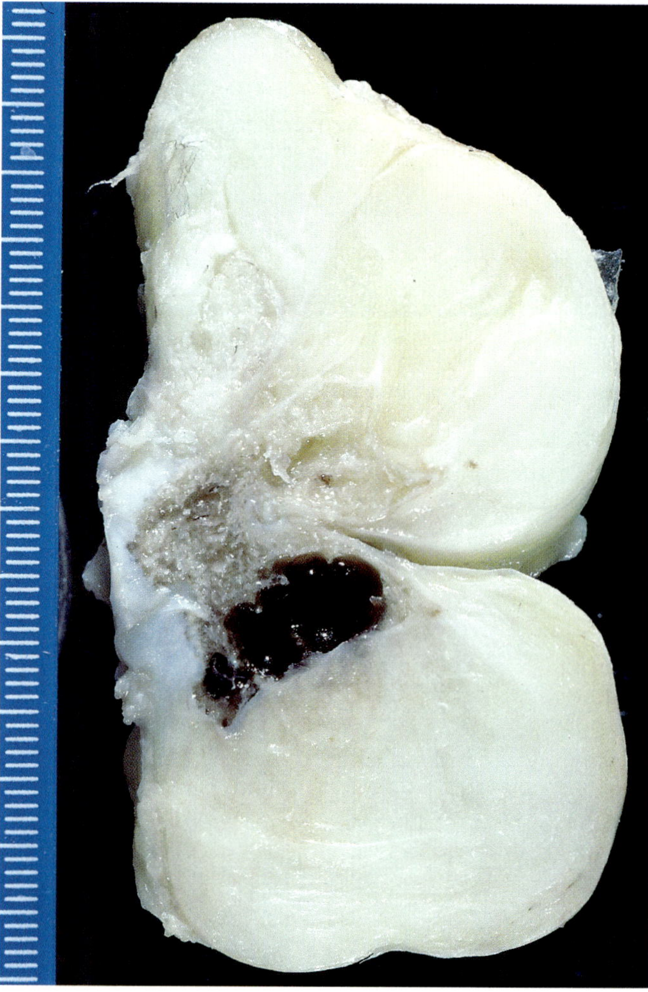

Fig. 21.16 Parosteal lipoma of the lower metaphysis of the femur.

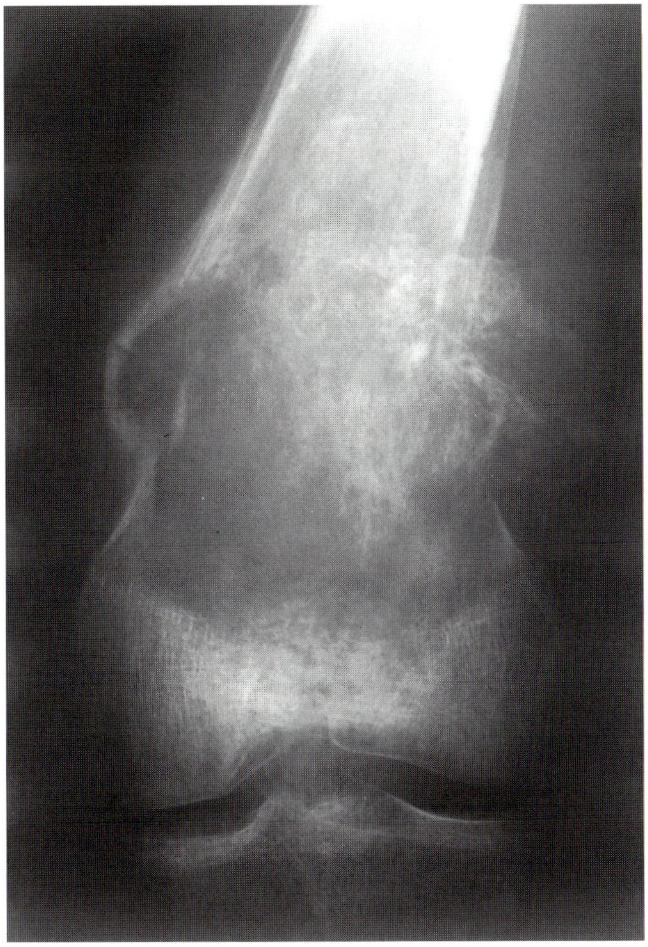

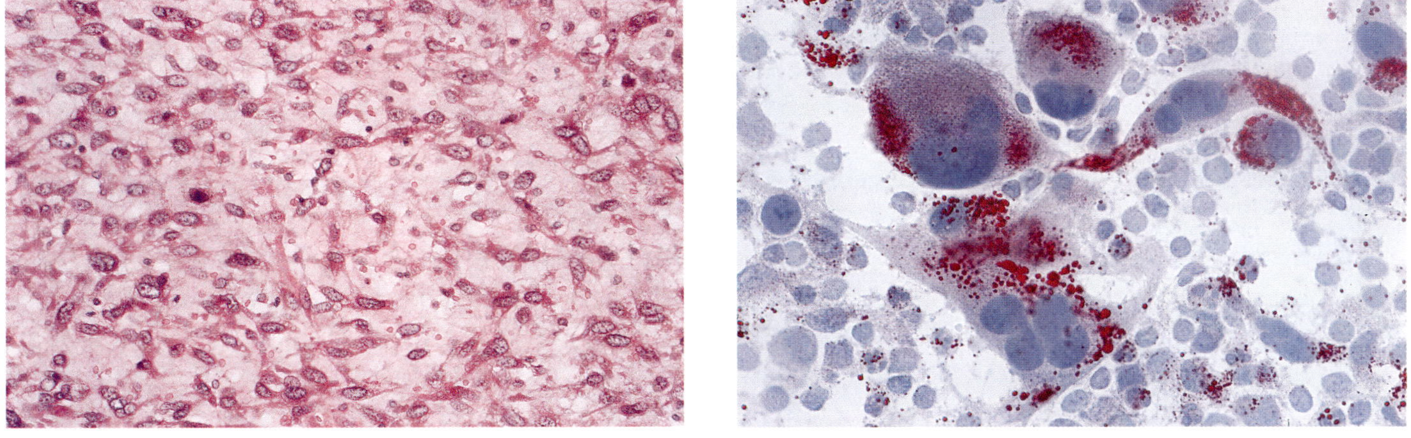

Fig. 21.17

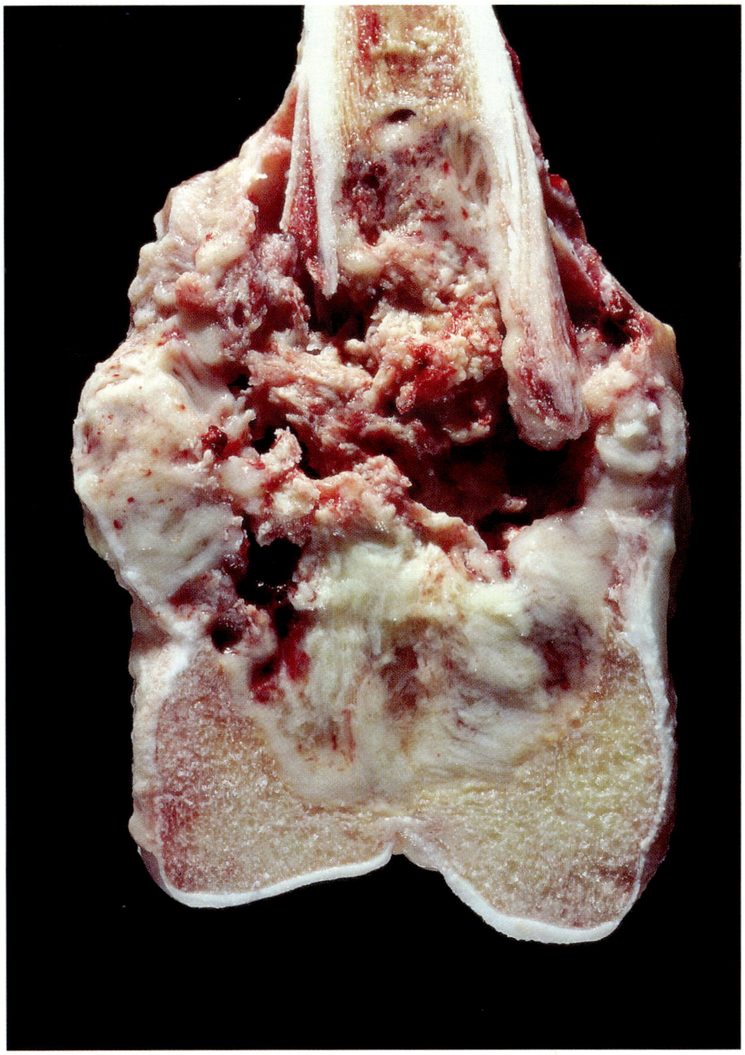

Fig. 21.18

Fig. 21.19

Fig. 21.20

Figs 21.17–21.20 Liposarcoma of the femur with pathologic fracture, high-grade pleomorphic type with intracytoplasmic fat droplets on imprint cytology (oil red O staining).

Some cases exhibiting a membranous material, as well as some reports in the Japanese literature, may well represent membranous lipodystrophy of bone.[67]

LIPOSARCOMA

About 40 cases of liposarcomas with the greater part of the tumor located in bone have been reported.[68–70] Most patients are in their third to fourth decades (Wilner 1982) with no sex predilection. Clinical symptoms are a dull pain, a soft tissue swelling or a pathologic fracture.

The most frequent sites are the medullary canals of the tibia,[69,71] the femur[72–74] (Schajowicz 1994) (Figs 21.17–21.20) and the humerus;[75,76] 60% of cases are located in the lower extremity.

On plain films, a liposarcoma of bone appears as a radiolucent destructive and ill-defined tumor with a moth-eaten type of bone destruction (Wilner 1982). The cortex is expanded, thinned or destroyed with a soft tissue extension.

Juxtacortical liposarcomas[77] are large soft tissue masses with superficial cortical erosion or scalloping and no medullary involvement. They have to be differentiated from soft tissue sarcomas adjacent to the cortex, which seldom infiltrate bone.[71,78]

Grossly, a liposarcoma of bone is a soft or rubbery, yellow, white or gray mass, sometimes with a lobular appearance.[75,78]

Histologically, rare cases are of the low-grade myxoid type,[79] but most are of a high-grade pleomorphic type, appearing as very cellular tumors with small spindle cells, large polyhedral acidophilic or multi- and univacuolated cells. The cytoplasmic fat is demonstrated by the usual stains or ultrastructural examination,[75,80] demonstrating multiple lipid droplets and a lipoblastic differentiation.

The average survival time is 1 or 2 years, with metastases to the lung. Liposarcomas are radiosensitive, but the therapeutic schedules are not well established. Some recent cases were treated by en bloc surgical resection with pre- and postoperative chemotherapy.

Liposarcoma involving bone has to be differentiated from bone metastases of liposarcomas and from malignant mesenchymomas (osteoliposarcomas). A case has been reported showing an osteosarcomatous pattern in the lung metastases.[81]

REFERENCES

1. Döhler R, Harms D. Intraossäre lipome. Z Orthop Ihre Grenzgeb 1981: 119: 138–141
2. Chow L T, Lee K C. Intraosseous lipoma. Am J Surg Pathol 1992: 16: 401–410
3. Milgram J W. Intraosseous lipomas: radiologic and pathologic manifestations. Radiology 1988: 167: 155–160
4. Milgram J W. Intraosseous lipomas. Clin Orthop 1988: 231: 277–302
5. Hart J A. Intraosseous lipoma. J Bone Joint Surg (Am) 1973: 55: 624–632
6. Goldman A B, Marcove R C, Huvos A G, Smith J. Case report 280. Intraosseous lipoma of the tibia. Skeletal Radiol 1984: 12: 209–212
7. Manitz U, Lossnitzer A. Ein weiterer Fall eines intraossären Lipoms der proximalen Tibia. Beitr Orthop Traumatol 1985: 32: 204–206
8. Lemerle R, Gaulier A, Zucman J. Un cas de lipome intra-osseux de l'extremité supérieure du fémur. Rev Chir Orthop Reparatrice Appar Mot 1985: 71: 275–277
9. Ramos A, Castello J, Sartoris D J, Greenway G D, Resnick D, Haghighi P. Osseous lipoma: CT appearance. Radiology 1985: 157: 615–619
10. Reig-Boix V, Guinot-Tormo J, Risent-Martinez F, Aparisi Rodriguez F, Ferrer-Jimenez R. Computed tomography of intraosseous lipoma of os calcis. Clin Orthop 1987: 221: 286–291
11. Noble J S, Leeson M C. Intra-osseous lipoma of the humerus. Orthopedics 1992: 15: 51–54
12. Barcelo M, Pathria M N, Abdul-Karim F W. Intraosseous lipoma. Arch Pathol Lab Med 1992: 116: 947–950
13. Mueller M C, Robbins J L. Intramedullary lipoma of bone. J Bone Joint Surg (Am) 1960: 42: 517–520
14. Hanelin L G, Sclamberg E L, Bardsley J L. Intraosseous lipoma of the coccyx. Radiology 1975: 114: 343–344
15. Lagier R. Fibular lipoma with areas of bone infarct calcifications. Eur J Radiol 1985: 5: 226–227
16. Gero M J, Kahn L B. Case report 498. Intraosseous lipoma of the distal end of the fibula with focal infarction. Skeletal Radiol 1988: 17: 443–446
17. Appenzeller J, Weitzner S. Intraosseous lipoma of os calcis. Case report and review of literature of intraosseous lipomas of extremities. Clin Orthop 1974: 101: 171–175
18. Poussa M, Holmström T. Intraosseous lipoma of the calcaneus. Acta Orthop Scand 1976: 47: 570–574
19. Lagier R. Case report 128. Lipoma of the calcaneus with bone infarct. Skeletal Radiol 1980: 5: 267–269
20. Lagier R. Calcaneous lipoma with bone infarct. An anatomoradiological study. RÖFO 1985: 142: 472–474
21. Rosenblatt E M, Mollin J, Abdelwahab I F. Bilateral calcaneal intraosseous lipomas. Mt Sinai J Med 1990: 57: 174–176
22. Regi L, Panzarola P, Pazzaglia G, Barzi F. Il lipoma intraosseo del calcagno. Radiol Med (Torino) 1994: 87: 701–704
23. Buckley S L, Burkus J K. Intraosseous lipoma of the ilium. Clin Orthop 1988: 228: 297–301
24. Bertin P, Boncoeur-Martel M P, Traoré A et al. Scanner et imagerie par résonance magnétique nucléaire d'un lipoma intra osseux iliaque. Sem Hôp Paris 1993: 69: 125–128
25. Coquerelle P, Cotten A, Flipo R M, Chastanet P, Duquesnoy B, Delcambre B. Intraosseous lipoma: role and limitations of modern imaging techniques. Rev Rhum Engl Ed 1995: 62: 147–150
26. Zorn D T, Cordray D R, Randels P H. Intraosseous lipoma of bone involving the sacrum. J Bone Joint Surg (Am) 1971: 53: 1201–1204
27. Ehara S, Kattapuram S V, Rosenberg A E. Case report 619. Intraosseous lipoma of the sacrum. Skeletal Radiol 1990: 19: 375–376
28. Milgram J W. Involuted intraosseous lipoma of the sacrum. Spine 1991: 16: 243–245
29. Matsubayashi I, Nakajima M, Tsukada M. Case report 118. Intraosseous lipoma involving the spinous process of 4th lumbar vertebra. Skeletal Radiol 1980: 5: 131–133
30. Hall F M, Cohen R B, Grumbach K. Case report 377. Intraosseous lipoma (angiolipoma) of right third rib. Skeletal Radiol 1986: 15: 401–403
31. Fox I M. Intraosseous lipoma of the fifth metatarsal. J Foot Ankle Surg 1994: 33: 138–140
32. Milgram J W. Intraosseous lipomas with reactive ossification on the proximal femur. Skeletal Radiol 1981: 7: 1–13

33. Latham P D, Athanasou N A. Intraosseous lipoma within the femoral head. Clin Orthop 1991: 265: 228–232
34. Caruolo J E, Dahlin D C. Lipoma involving bone and simulating malignant bone tumor. Proc Staff Mayo Clin 1953: 28: 361–363
35. Gunterberg B, Kindblom L G. Intraosseous lipoma. Acta Orthop Scand 1978: 49: 95–97
36. Leeson M C, Kay D, Smith B S. Intra-osseous lipoma. Clin Orthop 1983: 181: 186–190
37. Levin M F, Vellet A D, Munk P L, McLean C A. Intraosseous lipoma of the distal femur: MRI appearance. Skeletal Radiol 1996: 25: 82–84
38. Blacksin M F, Ende N, Benevenia J. Magnetic resonance imaging of intraosseous lipomas: a radiologic-pathologic correlation. Skeletal Radiol 1995: 24: 37–41
39. Dickson A B, Ayers W W, Hason M V, Miller W R. Lipoma of bone of intra osseous origin. J Bone Joint Surg (Am) 1951: 33: 257–261
40. Ragsdale B D, Sweet D E. Intraosseous lipoma. Am J Surg Pathol 1993: 17: 209–211
41. Milgram J W. Malignant transformation in bone lipomas. Skeletal Radiol 1990: 19: 347–352
42. Salzer M, Salzer-Kuntschik M. Zur Frage der sogenannten zentralen Knochenlipome. Beitr Pathol 1965: 132: 365–375
43. Downey E F Jr, Brower A C, Holt R B. Case report 243. Cortical ossifying lipoma of femur. Skeletal Radiol 1983: 10: 189–191
44. Fleming R J, Alpert M, Garcia A. Parosteal lipoma. Am J Roentgenol Radium Ther Nucl Med 1962: 87: 1075–1084
45. LeMinor J M, Bourjat P, Archer F. Parosteal lipoma of the first metacarpal: CT demonstration. RÖFO 1992: 157: 429–430
46. Krajewska I, Vernon-Roberts B, Sorby-Adams G. Parosteal (periosteal) lipoma. Pathology 1988: 20: 179–183
47. Miller M D, Ragsdale B D, Sweet D E. Parosteal lipomas: a new perspective. Pathology 1992: 24: 132–139
48. Kawashima A, Magid D, Fishman E K, Hruban R H, Ney D R. Parosteal ossifying lipoma: CT and MR findings. J Comput Assist Tomogr 1993: 17: 147–150
49. Moon N, Marmor L. Parosteal lipoma of the proximal part of the radius. J Bone Joint Surg (Am) 1964: 46: 608–614
50. Kurland K Z, Kennard J W. Parosteal lipoma arising from the proximal radius. Clin Orthop 1965: 41: 140–144
51. Lidor C, Lotem M, Hallel T. Parosteal lipoma of the proximal radius. J Hand Surg (Am) 1992: 17: 1095–1097
52. Goldman A B, DiCarlo E F, Marcove R C. Case report 774. Coincidental parosteal lipoma with osseous excresence and intramuscular lipoma. Skeletal Radiol 1993: 22: 138–145
53. Asirvatham R, Linjawi T. Ossifying parosteal lipoma with exuberant cortical reaction. Int Orthop 1994: 18: 55–56
54. Jacobs P. Parosteal lipoma with hyperostosis. Clin Radiol 1972: 23: 196–198
55. Demos T C, Bruno E, Armin A, Dobozi W R. Parosteal lipoma with enlarging osteochondroma. AJR 1984: 143: 365–366
56. Jones J G, Habermann E T, Dorfman H D. Parosteal ossifying lipoma of femur. Case report 553. Skeletal Radiol 1989: 18: 537–540
57. Laorr A, Greenspan A. Parosteal lipoma with hyperostosis. Can Assoc Radiol J 1993: 44: 285–290
58. Murphey M D, Johnson D L, Bhatia P S, Neff J R, Rosenthal H G, Walker C W. Parosteal lipoma: MR imaging characteristics. AJR 1994: 162: 105–110
59. Liapi-Avgeri G, Markakis P, Kokka H, Karajannis S, Christophidou E, Karabela-Bouropoulou V. Intraosseous lipoma. Arch Anat Cytol Pathol 1994: 42: 334–338
60. Kenin A, Levine J, Spinner M. Parosteal lipoma. J Bone Joint Surg (Am) 1959: 41: 1122–1126
61. Rodriguez-Peralto J L, Lopez-Barea F, Gonzalez-Lopez J, Lamas-Lorenzo M. Case report 821. Parosteal ossifying lipoma of femur. Skeletal Radiol 1994: 23: 67–69
62. Bridge J A, DeBoer J, Walker C W, Neff J R. Translocation t(3;12)(q28;q14) in parosteal lipoma. Genes Chromosomes Cancer 1995: 12: 70–72
63. Döhler R, Poser H L, Harms D, Wiedemann H R. Systemic lipomatosis of bone. J Bone Joint Surg (Br) 1982: 64: 84–87
64. Szendroi M, Karlinger K, Gonda A. Intraosseous lipomatosis. J Bone Joint Surg (Br) 1991: 73: 109–112
65. Freiberg R A, Air G W, Glueck C H, Ishikawa T, Abrams N R. Multiple intraosseous lipomas with type IV hyperlipoproteinemia. J Bone Joint Surg (Am) 1974: 56: 1729–1732
66. Robbie M J. Intraosseous lipomata in Paget's disease: an unusual CT appearance. Australas Radiol 1991: 35: 268–270
67. Pazzaglia U E. Fatty lesions in bone. J Bone Joint Surg (Br) 1991: 73: 870
68. Retz L D. Primary liposarcoma of bone. J Bone Joint Surg (Am) 1961: 43: 123–129
69. Catto M, Stevens J. Liposarcoma of bone. J Pathol Bacteriol 1963: 86: 248–253
70. Goldman R L. Primary liposarcoma of bone. Am J Clin Pathol 1964: 42: 503–508
71. Schwartz A, Shuster M, Becker S M. Liposarcoma of bone. J Bone Joint Surg (Am) 1970: 52: 171–177
72. Dawson E K. Liposarcoma of bone. J Pathol Bacteriol 1955: 70: 513–520
73. Honore D, Rogister G, Delvigne-Van Lancker M. A propos d'un cas de liposarcoma intra osseux. Acta Chir Belg 1963: 62: 887–895
74. Larsson S E, Lorentzon R, Boquist L. Primary liposarcoma of bone. Acta Orthop Scand 1975: 46: 869–876
75. Pardo-Mindan F J, Ayala H, Joly M, Gimeno E, Vazquez J J. Primary liposarcoma of bone. Light and electron microscopic study. Cancer 1981: 48: 274–280
76. Addison A K, Payne S R. Primary liposarcoma of bone. J Bone Joint Surg (Am) 1982: 64: 301–304
77. Kenan S, Klein M, Lewis M M. Juxtacortical liposarcoma. Clin Orthop 1989: 243: 225–229
78. Torok G, Meller Y, Maor E. Primary liposarcoma of bone. Bull Hosp Jt Dis Orthop Inst 1983: 43: 28–37
79. Kenan S, Lewis M M, Abdelwahab I F, Hermann G, Klein M J. Case report 652. Primary intraosseous low grade myxoid sarcoma of the scapula (myxoid liposarcoma). Skeletal Radiol 1991: 20: 73–75
80. Schneider H M, Wunderlich T, Puls P. The primary liposarcoma of the bone. Arch Orthop Trauma Surg 1980: 96: 235–239
81. Downey E F Jr, Worsham G F, Brower A C. Liposarcoma of bone with osteosarcomatous foci. Skeletal Radiol 1982: 8: 47–50

Vascular tumors

M. Forest

HEMANGIOMAS

The clinical incidence of capillary or cavernous vascular lesions in bone is low, ranging from 0.8% (Wilner) to 1.2% (Schajowicz) of all bone tumors, contrasting with the high incidence of vertebral hemangiomas on autopsy material, some being considered as focal telangiectasias.[1] Most patients are over the age of 40 and there is a female predominance of about 2 to 1.[1] Many lesions are asymptomatic but progressive pain is the main clinical symptom and, in vertebral locations, neurological symptoms or a collapse of the vertebral body.

In more than 75% of cases hemangiomas are located in the vertebra and the skull, 10% in long bones and 5% in ribs.

Histological findings are straightforward, demonstrating capillary vessels, dilated cavernous spaces, arterioles or veins with thick walls. Bone trabeculae are resorbed, atrophic or enlarged, sometimes with some woven bone, but active bone remodeling is unusual. The lesional vessels can expand through the intertrabecular spaces. Very rare vertebral vascular lesions have been described: hemangioblastoma[2] and epidural angiolipomas involving bone.[3,4]

Vertebral hemangiomas (Figs 22.1, 22.2) are located mostly at the thoracic level (T6 and T8) and two or more vertebrae may be involved (Wilner 1982). In about 1% of cases, the neural compression may be associated with compression fractures, hematoma, epidural extension or 'ballooning' of bone.[5,6]

On plain films, thick vertical trabeculae appear as vertical striations ('corduroy cloth' or honeycomb pattern). Many lesions are confined to the vertebral body, sparing the cortices and the disc spaces, but some may extend to the lamina, spinous and transverse processes or even the ribs.[1]

On CT scans, the cross-sections of the trabeculae give a coarsened appearance. On MRI, the signal intensities are

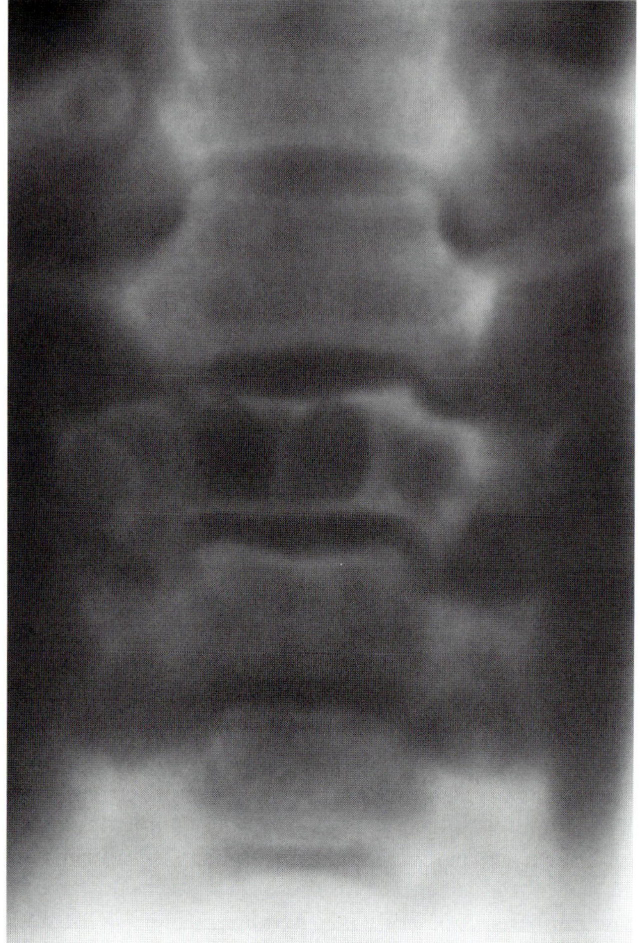

Fig. 22.1

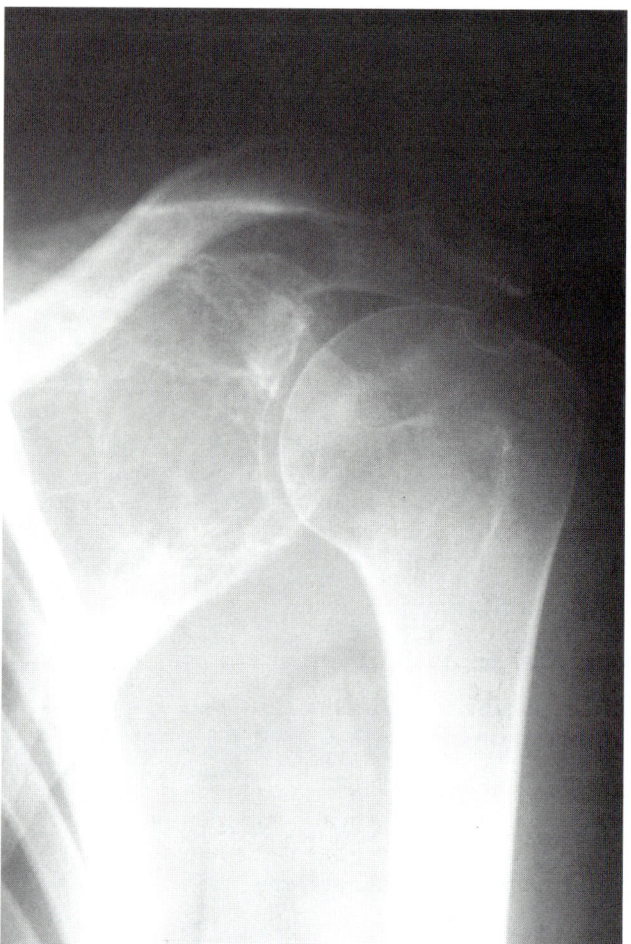

Fig. 22.3

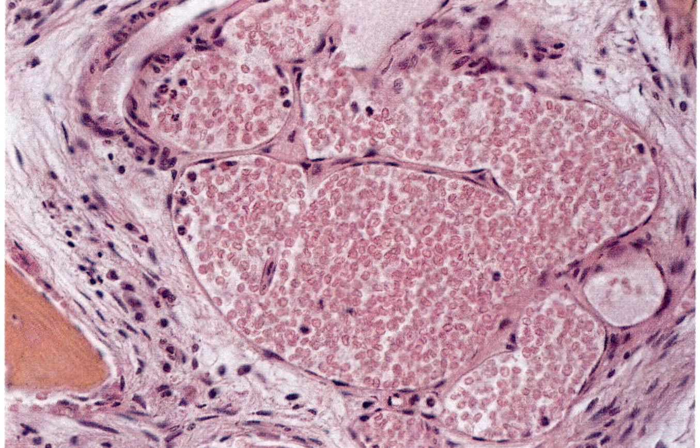

Fig. 22.2

Figs 22.1, 22.2 Spinal hemangioma with collapse of the vertebral body.

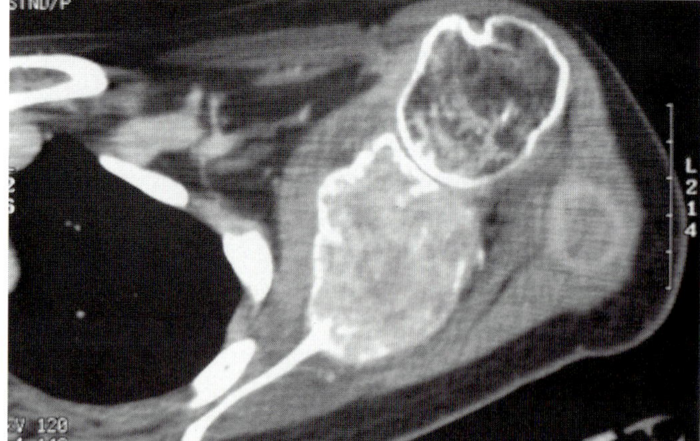

Fig. 22.4

Figs 22.3, 22.4 Hemangioma of the scapula.

increased in T1 and T2-weighted images.[7] On angiography, hemangiomas are fed by the intercostal arteries, showing a prominent tumor blush. Radionuclide bone scans are useful to locate multiple lesions; some may be negative.

The treatment is irradiation with or without laminectomy, embolization and laminectomy or radical tumor resection with spinal reconstruction and stabilization.

Hemangiomas of flat bones (Figs 22.3, 22.4) may demonstrate on imaging a sunburst appearance on the innominate bone,[1] expansion or huge bone formation on the ribs (Wilner 1982)[8] or even cortical destruction and soft tissue mass or a honeycomb pattern on the clavicle (Wilner 1982).

Medullary hemangiomas of long bones (Figs 22.5–22.8) are rarely purely lytic on X-ray,[9] presenting a coarsely loculated appearance or a soap bubble or honeycomb pattern.[10] Most of those of the cavernous type are located in the metaphyseal region.[10] On MRI, the signal intensity is low in T1-weighted images, high in T2-weighted images.[11]

Periosteal hemangiomas of long bones are unusual[12–17] (Figs 22.9, 22.10). All cases involve the midshaft of long tubular bones with a soft tissue mass associated with cortical thickening or a cup-shaped depression of the outer cortex. A prominent sclerosis may mimic an osteoid osteoma.[1] Soft tissue hemangiomas may also induce a periosteal reaction.[18]

Cortical hemangiomas of long bones are extremely rare.[10,19–21] Most of them are located in the tibia shaft[22] and on imaging they mimic an osteoid osteoma or a Brodie's abscess. MRI demonstrates an area of cortical thickening with a 'nidus' of intermediate signal intensity in T1 and T2-weighted images. A radiologic-pathologic study from the AFIP has demonstrated that periosteal hemangiomas have a cortical component in all cases, suggesting the name 'surface-based hemangiomas' for lesions centered on the periosteum, the subperiosteal zone or the cortex[22] (Figs 22.11, 22.12).

CYSTIC ANGIOMATOSIS OF BONE

This rare disease[23,24] may be considered as a vascular hamartoma.[25] Most patients are in the first two decades of life.[26] and men are affected twice as often as women.[27] Bone lesions may be an incidental finding or may induce pain, swelling or a pathologic fracture.[26]

The widespread cystic lesions (Figs 22.13, 22.14) have to be differentiated from multiple hemangiomas restricted to one or two bones, usually in an extremity.[28]

In 60–70% of cases, bone lesions are associated with visceral involvement, particularly the spleen but also the liver, lungs and soft tissues, which is responsible for most clinical symptoms and indicative of the prognosis.[29]

Most common locations are the ribs, pelvis, femur, humerus, vertebrae and skull. Involvement of the bones of hands and feet is unusual.[30,31] The lytic defects may be located anywhere within the bone. Widespread lesions may show a honeycomb pattern, specially in the pelvis,[25] and reactive bone formation may be prominent, mimicking osteoblastic metastases.[29,32] The features on MR imaging indicate vascular, fibrous and fatty structures.[33]

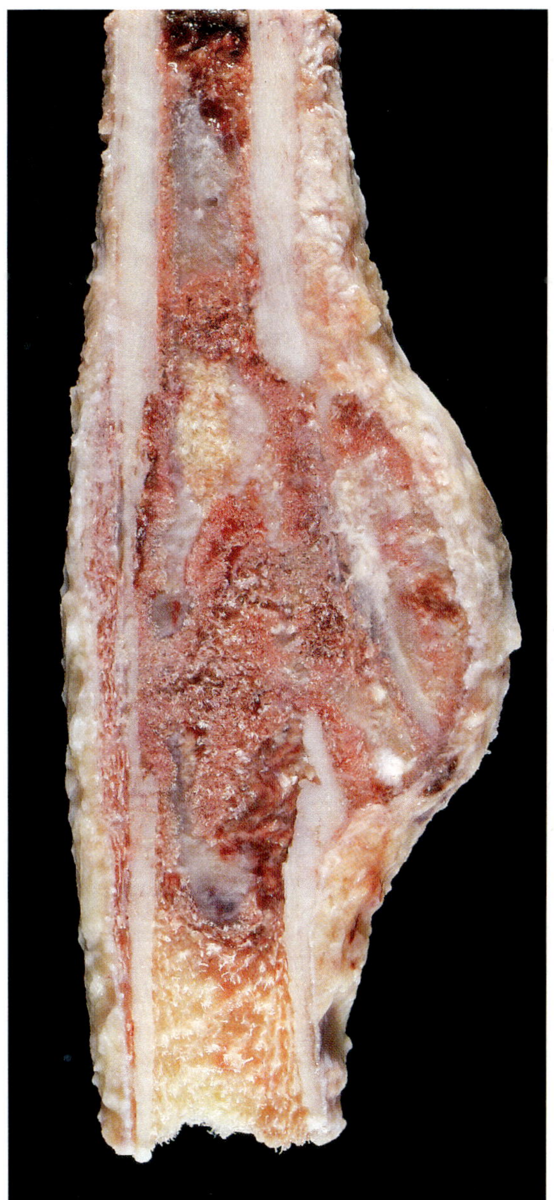

Fig. 22.5

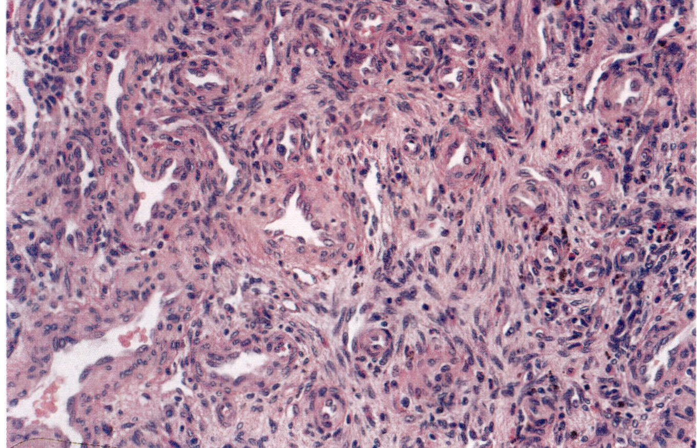

Fig. 22.6

Figs 22.5, 22.6 Hemangioma of the femur (recurrence and resorption of the bone grafts).

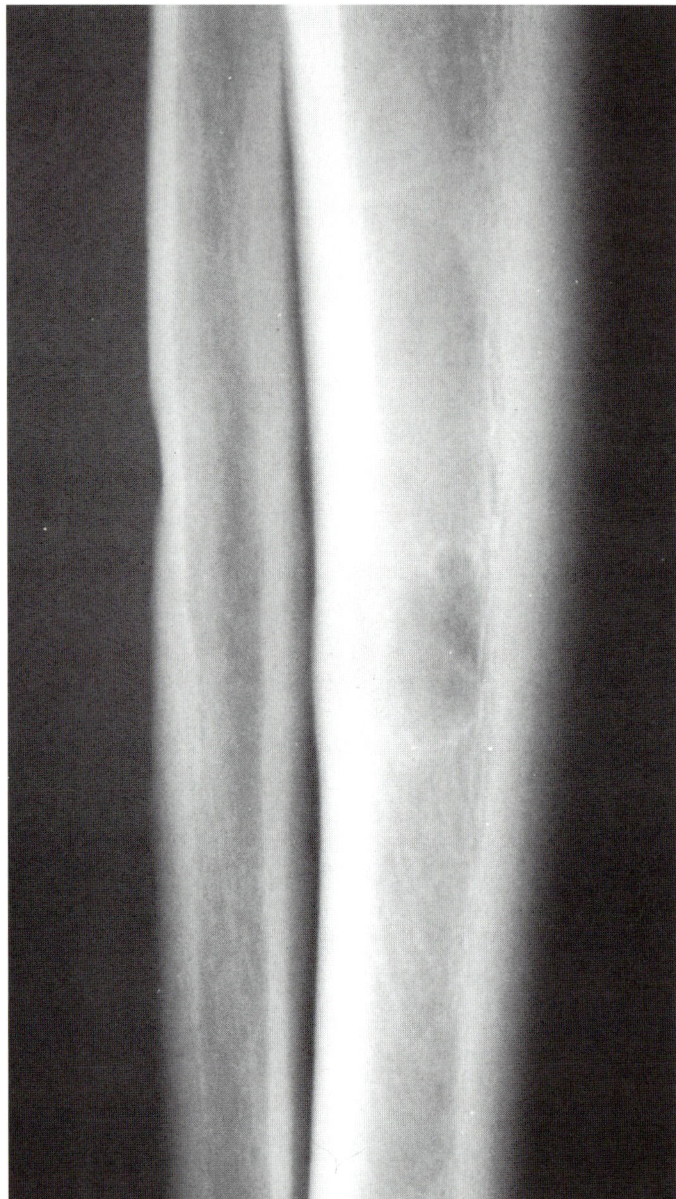

Fig. 22.7

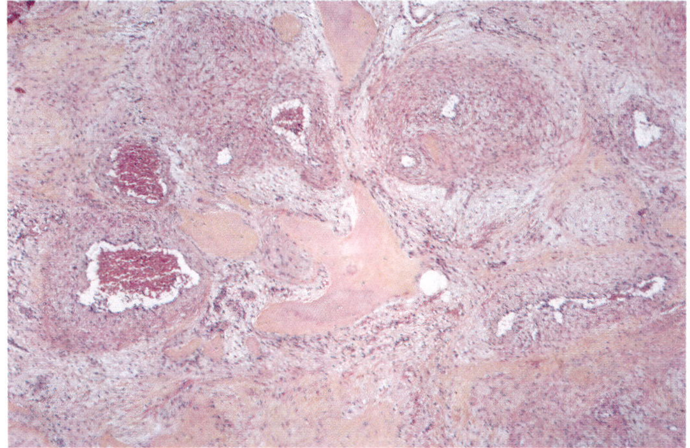

Fig. 22.8

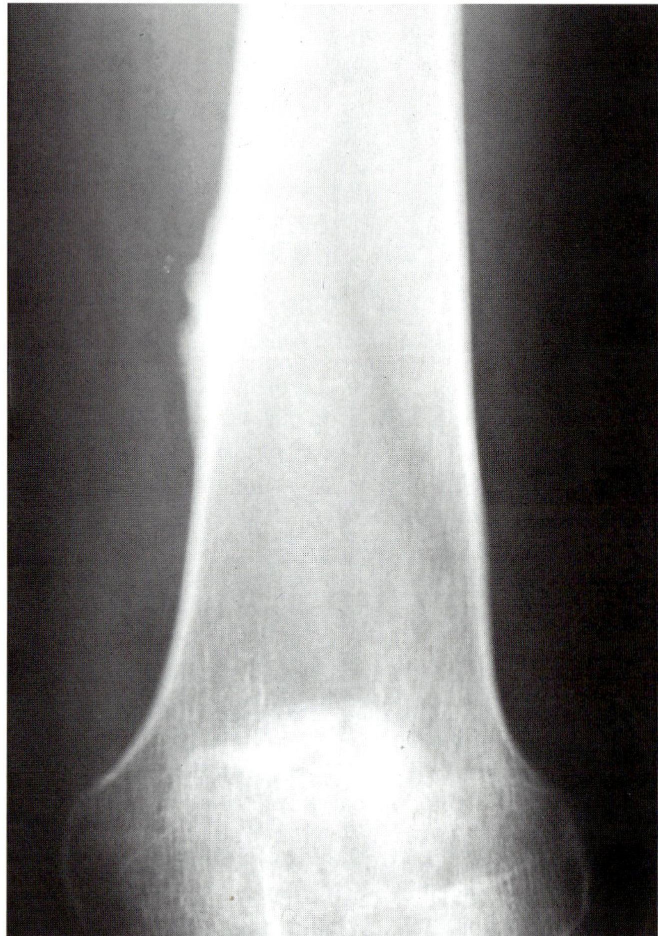

Fig. 22.9

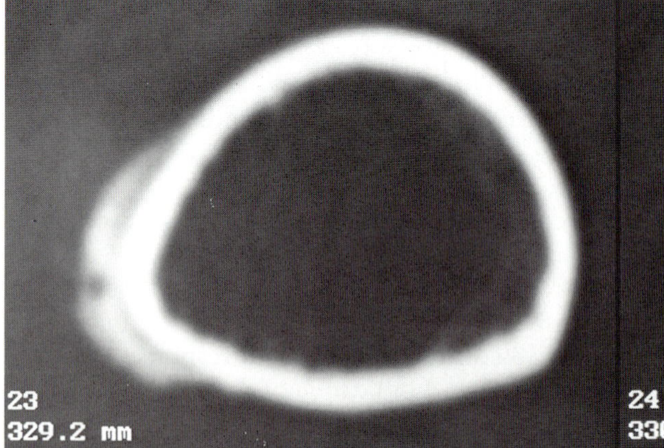

Fig. 22.10

Figs 22.9, 22.10 Periosteal hemangioma of the femur mimicking an osteoid osteoma.

Figs 22.7, 22.8 Hemangioma of the tibial shaft.

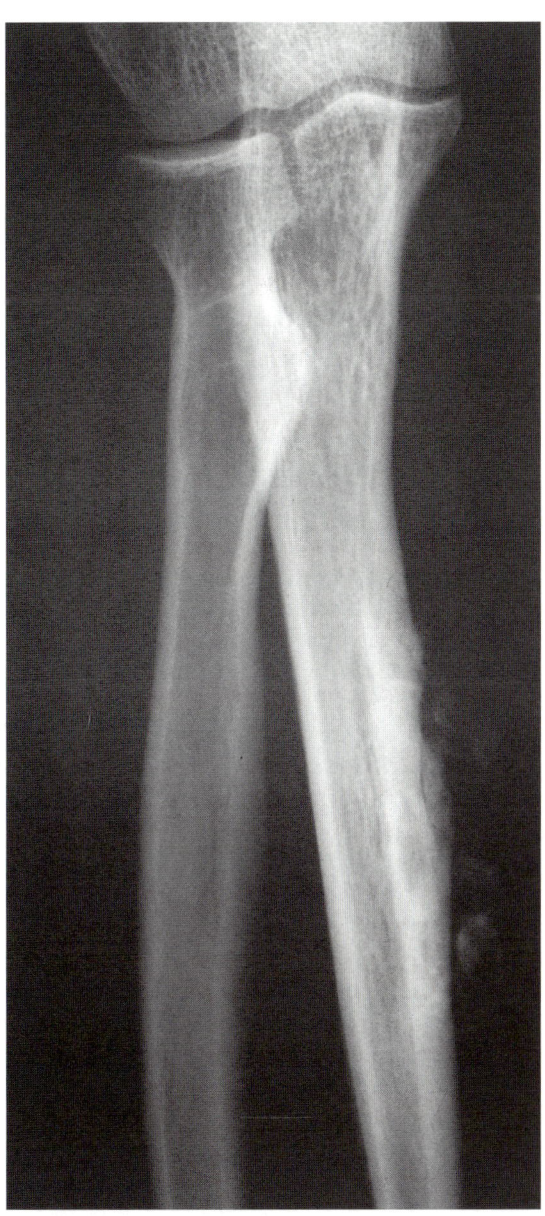

Figs 22.11 'Surface-based' hemangioma of the ulna.

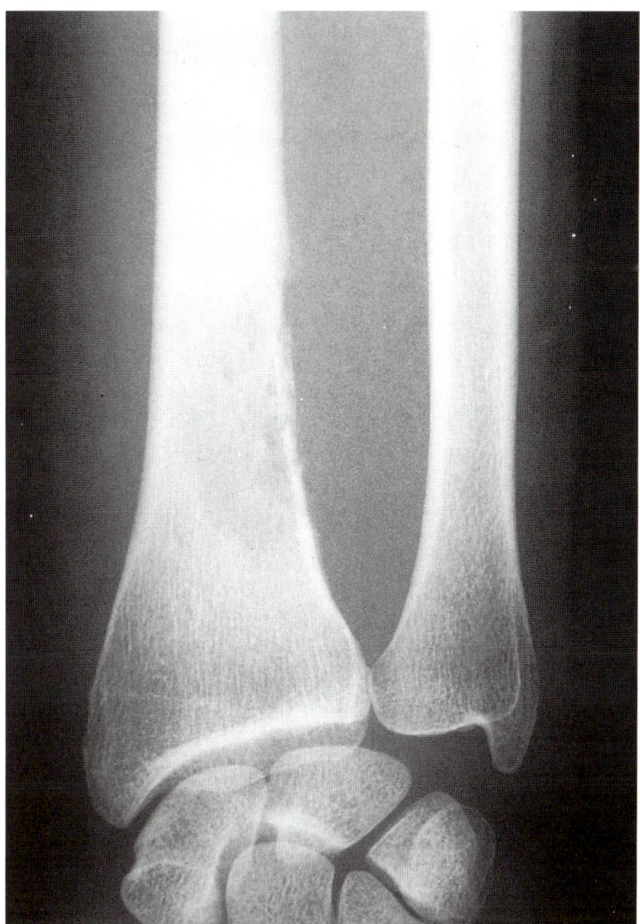

Fig. 22.12 'Surface-based' hemangioma of the radius.

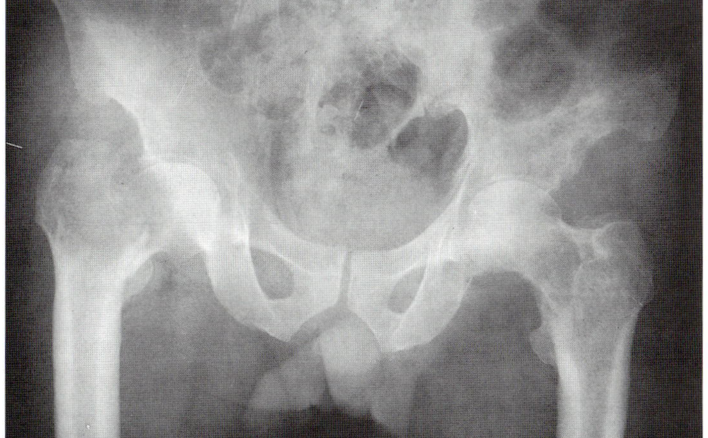

Fig. 22.13

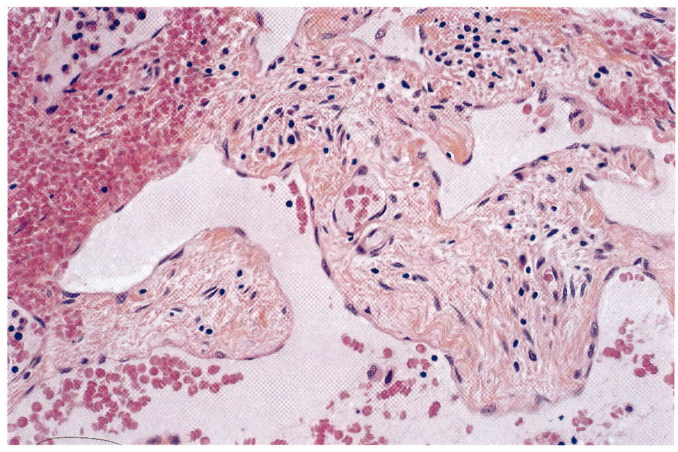

Fig. 22.14

Figs 22.13, 22.14 Widespread angiomatosis of the pelvis and femurs.

Histologically, lesions are similar to capillary or mostly cavernous hemangiomas; in some cases, lymphatic channels may be associated.[25,34–36]

The lesions may appear synchronously or metasynchronously. Some may enlarge or regress with progressive sclerosis and cyst obliteration.[31]

SOLITARY LYMPHANGIOMAS AND LYMPHANGIOMATOSIS OF BONE

These are usually discovered in childhood.[37–44] Solitary cystic lymphangiomas are extremely rare in bone, involving the spine, ilium and long bones as well as the small bones of the hands. Lymphangiomatosis of bone is associated in many cases with widespread visceral and soft tissue involvement. Bone lesions may be revealed by a pathologic fracture.[45] Lymphography demonstrates abnormal and dilated vessels filling the bone lesions.[46,47]

Histologically, cavernous spaces, empty or filled with a proteinaceous material, are lined with a single layer of flattened endothelial cells. Lymphoid aggregates can be found in the interstitium. The differential diagnosis with a hemangioma may be quite difficult,[36] relying chiefly on the finding, at surgery, of a clear, milky or yellow fluid.

The lesions grow slowly and some may regress.[26] Most cases with soft tissue and visceral involvement have a poor prognosis but exclusive involvement of lower limbs or limb girdles seems to herald a better prognosis.[48] The treatment is curettage, grafting and irradiation.

MASSIVE OSTEOLYSIS

Massive osteolysis, also called disappearing bone disease, phantom bone disease and Gorham disease, is a rare condition leading to extensive destruction of bone in adolescents or young adults[49–51] (Figs 22.15–22.18).

The disease most often involves the long bones,[52] the pelvis, the scapula[53] and vertebrae.[54] The lesions may be monocentric or multicentric,[55] originating from bone or from the adjacent soft tissues, with a narrowing of the contour of the bone ('tapering'[56]), resulting in a concentric shrinkage.[52] The osteolytic process may appear as multiple radiolucent areas or as a patchy osteoporosis. Arteriography demonstrates only a faint blush[57] while CT scans are useful to delineate the soft tissue extension.[58,59]

Histologically, numerous thin-walled capillary-like vessels and a few thick-walled vessels have been described in bone as well as in the surrounding connective tissue and even muscle;[49,56,60,61] lymphatic vessels are unusual. Bone is replaced by dense fibrous tissue[49,62,63] with some anastomosing blood-filled spaces. Very few osteoclasts are found,[49,52,61–64] if any.

Histochemical studies have demonstrated strong acid phosphatase and leucine aminopeptidase activities in endothelial cells[62,63] and in perivascular mononuclear cells, presumably pericytes, close to the remaining bone, suggesting that these cells may be involved in the process of bone resorption.

Ultrastructurally, the osteoblasts present a decreased synthetic activity and osteoclasts are rare; numerous mononuclear cells are probably macrophages.[63]

The widespread involvement of ribs or vertebrae may lead to death but usually, despite bone destruction and deformities, the prognosis is good.[49,65] Surgical treatment is often ineffective and in some cases radiation therapy can halt the process of bone lysis.[50,66,67]

INTRAOSSEOUS GLOMUS TUMORS

Glomus tumors or glomangiomas are unusual in intraosseous locations. In most cases, it is a tumor of adulthood with a female predominance[68] (Wilner 1982). Clinical symptoms are characteristic: point tenderness or persistent and excruciating pain.

The erosion of bone by a soft tissue lesion, mostly in the subungual region of the fingers, is common, rarely involving the metacarpal joint.[69]

Unusual true intraosseous tumors predominate in the distal phalanges, with a few cases in the middle phalanges,[70] the metacarpals and even the long tubular bones, ulna[71] and femur (Huvos 1991).

Precoccygeal glomus tumors have been described close to the coccyx, with no bone involvement,[72,73] or located in the coccyx[74] or the sacrum.[75] However, the glomus coccygeum, a normal structure located at the tip of the coccyx, when removed incidentally shows striking similarities with glomus tumors; the latter may simply represent some very large variant of normal glomus bodies.[76–78]

On X-ray, a glomus tumor appears as a well-demarcated, punched out lytic lesion, with thinning or eventually some expansion of the cortex.

Grossly, the tumor has a diameter ranging from a few millimeters to less than 1 cm, appearing as reddish vascular tissue.

Histologically, the tumor cells are fairly uniform, oval or polygonal or even spindle shaped, with well-defined cytoplasmic borders and an epithelioid appearance. They are distributed in sheets, with a rich network of reticulin fibers around capillary spaces.[68] Associated large vessels may predominate. The stroma can be profusely hyalinized or myxoid. Non-myelinated nerve fibers have been described.[79]

Immunohistochemically, there is positive staining with vimentin and muscle-specific actin;[80] desmin staining gives variable results.

On electron microscopy, tumoral cells appear as modified smooth muscle cells with a thick basement membrane distributed around individual cells.[74,80]

Usually excision or curettage, with or without grafting, is performed,[68,80] without recurrence if the surgical treatment is complete.

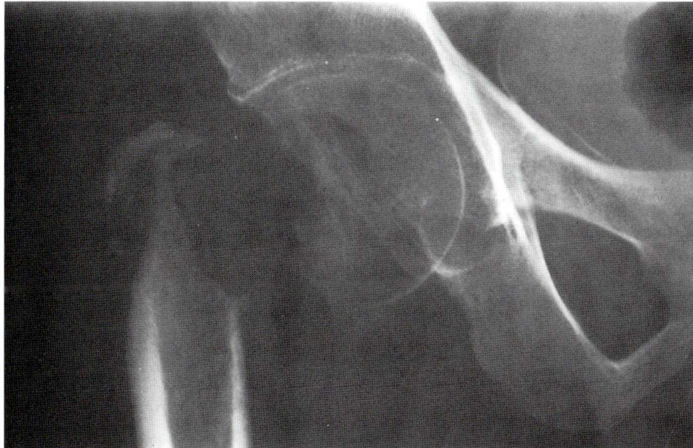

Fig. 22.15

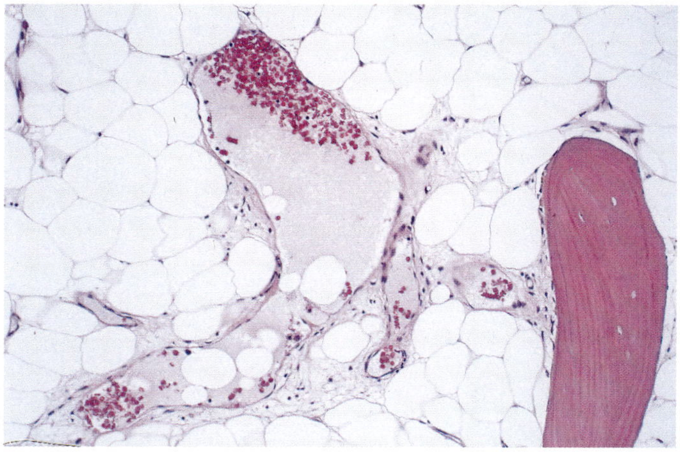

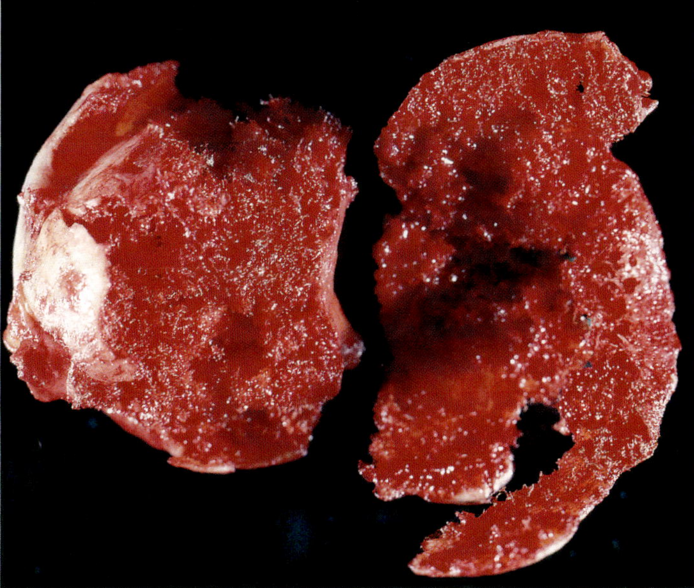

Fig. 22.16

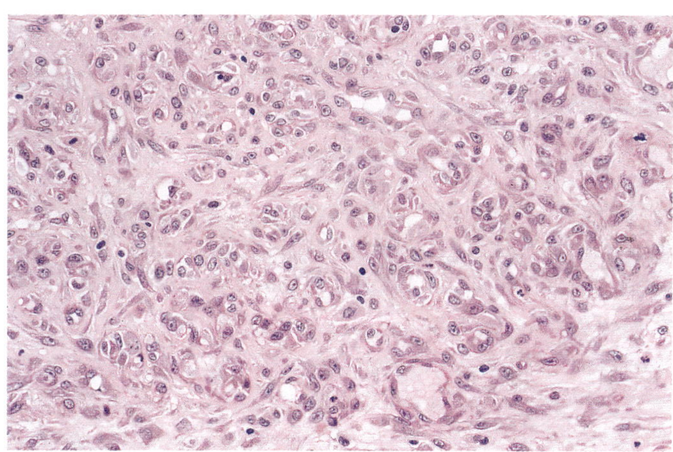

Fig. 22.17

Fig. 22.18

Figs 22.15–22.18 Gorham's disease of the upper end of the femur, with dilated blood vessels in bone and neovascularization of the soft tissues.

HEMANGIOPERICYTOMAS OF BONE

Hemangiopericytomas, with neoplastic cells related to smooth muscle cells and a rich network of capillaries, are uncommon in bone. About 50 cases have been reported, with a wide age range[81] but with a peak incidence in the fourth and fifth decades and a male to female ratio of 1.8:1.[81]

Clinical symptoms are local tenderness or regional pain; the growth of the tumor may be indolent, with a protracted course of years.[81,82] Thirty-five percent of the skeletal tumors associated with oncogenic osteomalacia are hemangiopericytomas.[83–87]

Almost any bone may be involved, even the small bones of the hand [88] or the sternum,[89] but the most common sites are the pelvis,[90,91] the spine and sacrum,[92–94] long bones in proximal locations[95] and the mandible (Figs 22.19–22.22). Rare multicentric cases have been reported[86] (Mulder et al 1993).

On X-ray, hemangiopericytoma is predominantly a lytic lesion (Huvos 1991). Some tumors are fairly well circumscribed, with sclerotic borders (Wilner 1982), trabeculations or even sclerosis. Others may exhibit a mild expansion of bone, with a honeycomb or bubbly appearance.[81] Cortical destruction and a soft tissue mass are usually found in flat bones. A periosteal reaction is found in one-third of cases.[81] Radially arranged branching vessels can be demonstrated by angiography.[96]

Histologically, the proliferating cells are ovoid or spindle shaped; the eosinophilic cytoplasm is scant or profuse and the nucleus is round or oval, vesicular or hyperchromatic. The cells are distributed in cords or sheets, sometimes sur-

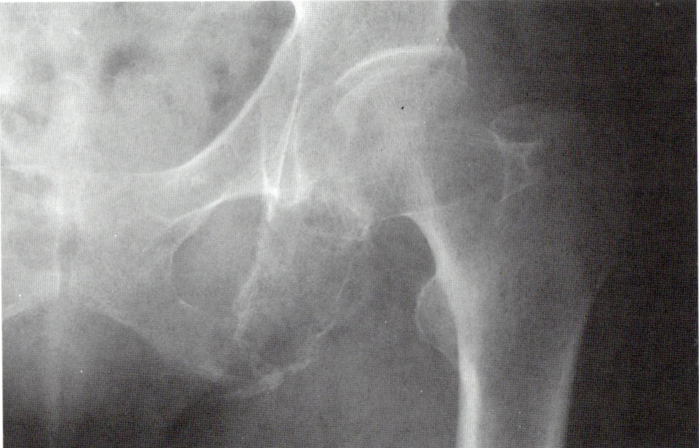

Fig. 22.19

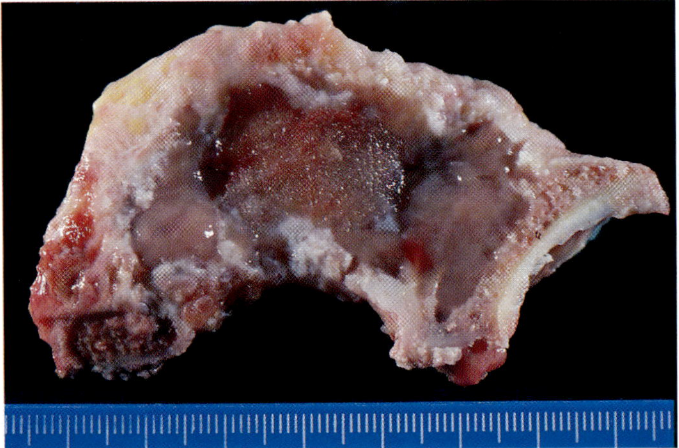

Fig. 22.20

Figs 22.19, 22.20 Hemangiopericytoma of the ischium.

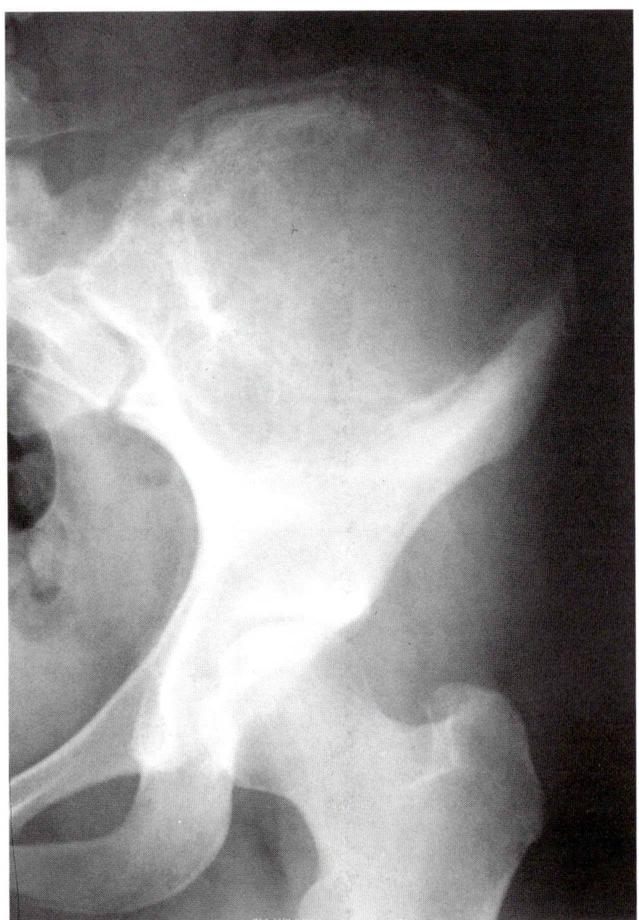

Fig. 22.21 Hemangiopericytoma of the iliac wing.

rounded by a hyaline matrix,[97] but in all tumors reticulin fibers surround individual cells or small groups of cells, external to the vascular channels (Figs 22.23–22.26).

The abundant ramifying thin-walled blood vessels are lined by flat, normal-appearing endothelial cells. The growth of the cells may be circumferential around the vascularization ('onion-skin' pattern) or associated with branching vascular channels ('antler'-like pattern).

Tumors associated with osteomalacia may exhibit lattice-like, fine trabecular or spotty and punctate calcifications[87] or even prominent osteoid and bone formation.[86]

Attempts at histological grading are based on cellularity, the size of the nucleus or atypia, and mitotic activity, the finding of necrosis and hemorrhages in order to distinguish benign, intermediate and malignant tumors.[81,91]

Immunohistochemically, the endothelial cells are weakly positive with Ulex Europaeus staining.[86] Immunoreactivity of tumor cells is variable with vimentin and negative with desmin and FVIIIRag stainings. In soft tissue tumors, positivity has been demonstrated for vimentin, CD34, factor XIIIa, HLA-DR antigen and even S-100 protein, L7 and myelin-associated glycoprotein.

Ultrastructural studies demonstrate that tumor cells surrounded by a basement-like material exhibit the features of pericytes.[86,93,97] No secretory granules have been identified in tumors associated with oncogenic osteomalacia.[85,86]

The prognosis appears unpredictable on morphological analysis. Survival rates are about 75% at 5 years, 44% at 10 years.[81] Recurrences may appear late in the clinical course[91] and the most common site of metastases is the lung. The treatment is adequate surgical removal; if this is not possible, radiation therapy[81] or even amputation[82] may be necessary. Chemotherapy gives poor results.[95]

As for the differential diagnosis, metastases from extraskeletal hemangipericytomas can occur in bone, specially from intracranial lesions.[98,99] Soft tissue tumors may cause pressure erosions or eventually invade bone. Mesenchymal chondrosarcomas, dedifferentiated chondrosarcomas, malignant fibrous histiocytomas, phosphaturic mesenchymal tumors and even small cell osteosarcomas can present focally with a hemangiopericytoma pattern. A thorough sampling is necessary to demonstrate the tumoral

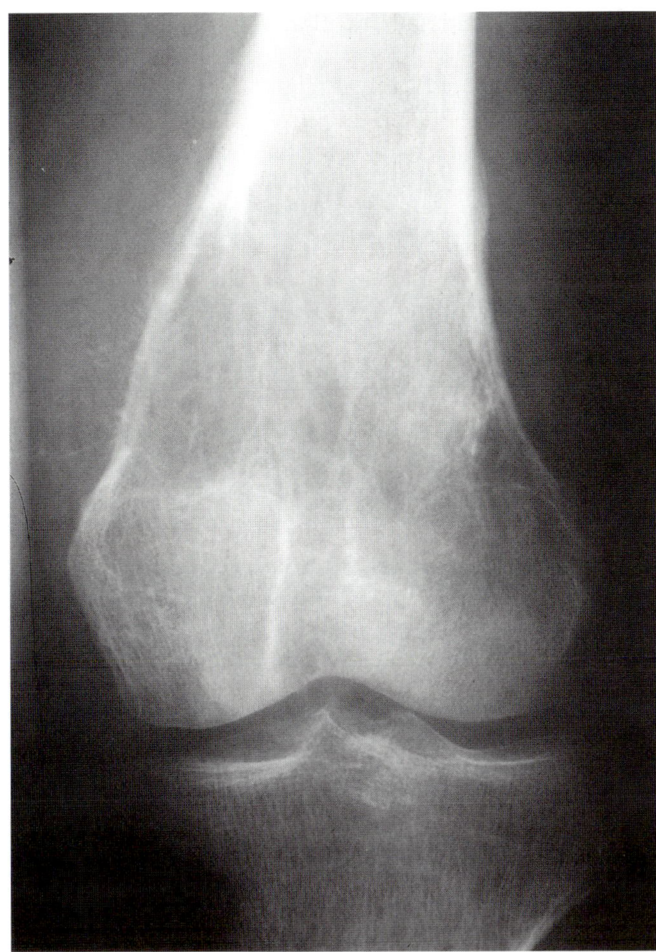

Fig. 22.22 Hemangiopericytoma of the femur with a permeative pattern of bone destruction.

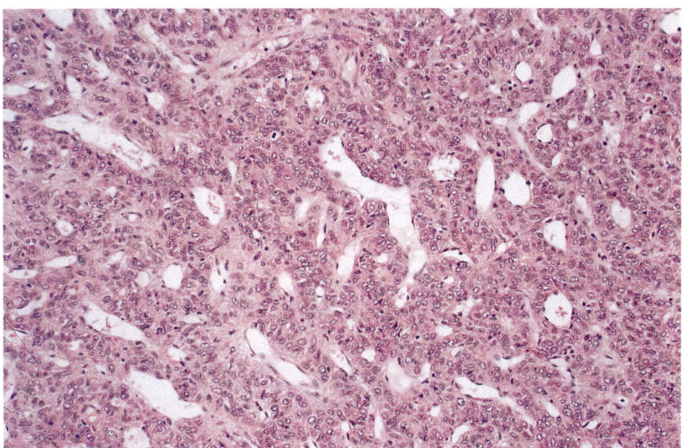

Fig. 22.24

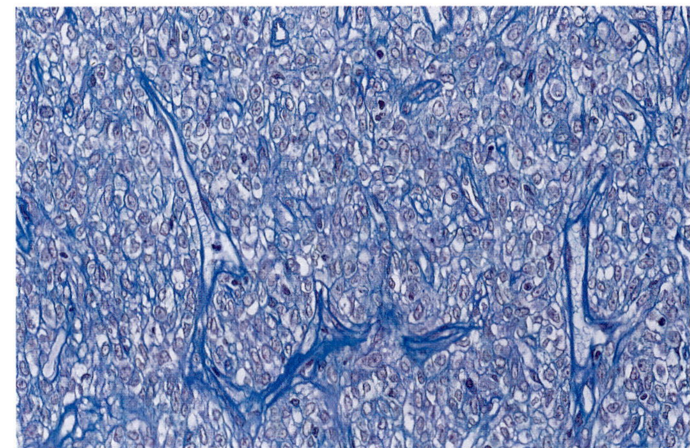

Fig. 22.25

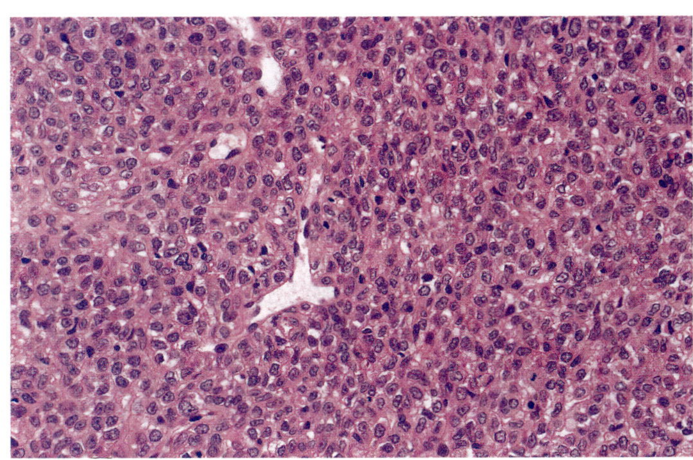

Fig. 22.23

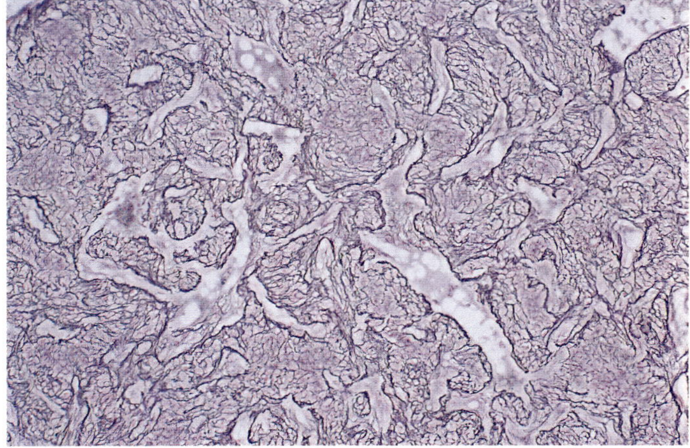

Fig. 22.26

Figs 22.23–22.26 Hemangiopericytomas of bone: ovoid or spindle-shaped cells with ramifying thin-walled vessels and a reticulin network surrounding small groups of cells.

cartilage, tumoral bone or a predominantly storiform pattern.

HEMANGIOENDOTHELIOMA OF BONE

Apart from the common hemangiomas, vascular tumors in bone exhibit a wide range of radiological and histological features as well as great variability in the clinical course and prognosis.

The rarity of such lesions (less than 1% of all malignant bone tumors)[100] and the variegated and confusing terminology necessitate a careful analysis of most reported studies which do not follow the recent scheme of the WHO classification on bone tumors, considering hemangioendotheliomas as tumors of intermediate or borderline malignancy without any metastatic potential.

The disease-free survival appears to be closely related to the histological findings[101–104] and in correlation with the radiological findings, three grades have been delineated[102–104] based on the degree of vasoformative appearance, the pleomorphism of cells, aspects of the nuclei and nucleoli, chromatin pattern and mitotic activity.

Grade I tumors are purely osteolytic lesions, with various degrees of peripheral sclerosis or a honeycomb pattern; periosteal reactions are unusual. Numerous well-differentiated vascular spaces are lined by crowded endothelial cells with mild hyperchromasia and slight variation in size; mitotic figures are rare. The cells are larger and plumper than those of hemangiomas.[104] The tumors exhibit an indolent course,[103] despite frequent multicentric locations,[105] and the overall survival is 95%.[100,103]

In grade II tumors, histologically, solid areas are more prominent;[104] nuclei are larger, plumper and hyperchromatic and mitotic activity is found.

Grade III tumors are high-grade sarcomas with undifferentiated areas or a spindling of cells mimicking a fibrosarcoma.[103,104]

Another approach relies on the prognostic significance of Ag-NOR proteins and of cathepsin proteolytic enzymes in bone hemangioendotheliomas. The mean nucleolar organizer region (NOR) has been found to be significantly higher in high-grade tumors; poorly differentiated tumors exhibit a discontinuous distribution of laminin and type IV collagen, reflecting the disorganized architecture of the basement membrane, along with an increased cell proliferation and a tumoral secretion of cathepsin D and G involved in tumor invasion.[106]

The term 'hemangioendothelioma' is considered to embrace grade I and II vascular tumors of bone and there is a definite trend to assimilate some of them as hemangiomas,[107–109] despite some diagnoses of low-grade malignant hemangioendotheliomas or hemangioendotheliomas.[105,107]

Histiocytoid or epithelioid hemangiomas or hemangioendotheliomas have been delineated in bone by Rosai et al[110] on cytological and architectural findings (Figs 22.27–22.38). They have also been found in skin, subcutaneous tissue, vessels, heart, embracing angiolymphoid hyperplasia with eosinophilia[111] and mainly relating to the epithelioid hemangioendotheliomas of soft tissues described by Weiss and Enzinger.[112,113]

Patients are usually 10–30 years old, but the tumors may be found in later life;[114] a mean age of 46 years has been established.[108] There is a male predominance.[115] The clinical symptom is pain, with or without a pathologic facture. The clinical course is protracted,[116] with no aggressive local growth and no metastases. An unusual presentation is the association with an osteoblastoma on two separate vertebrae.[117]

Various sites have been reported including clavicle, ribs, sternum, sacrum, ilium, pelvis, radius, femur and tibia; the majority of cases are found in the calvaria, axial skeleton and lower extremities. Multifocal lesions account for 50–64% of cases, specially in the lower limb or in the hand;[115,118,119] they may occur in a single bone, in bones of the same extremity or widely separated.

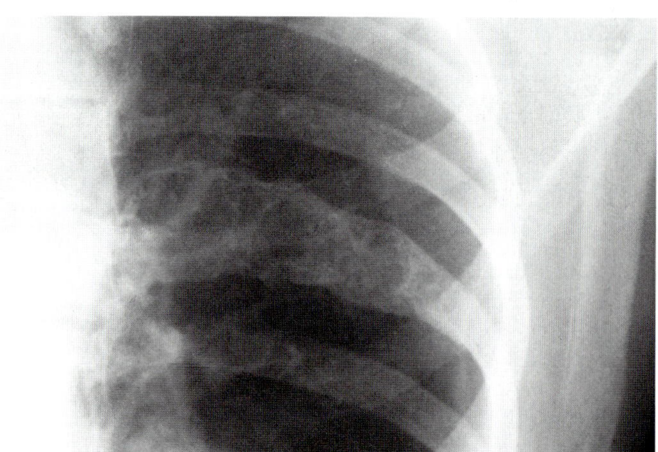

Fig. 22.27

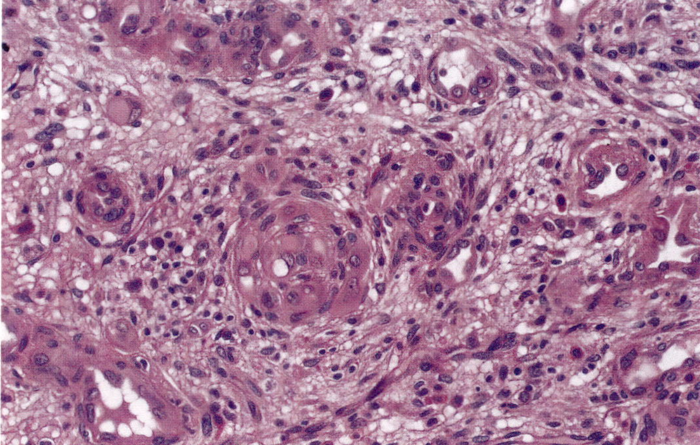

Fig. 22.28

Figs 22.27, 22.28 Epithelioid hemangioma of the fifth rib.

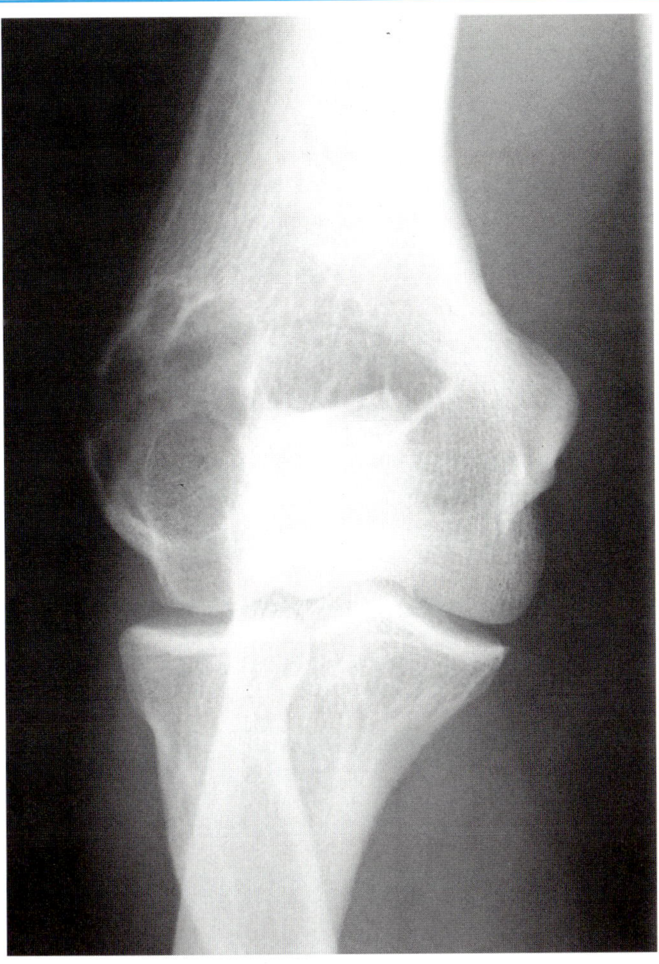

Fig. 22.29

On imaging, in long bones, location is epiphyseal, metaphyseal or diaphyseal.[116] A periosteal tumor has been reported.[120] The lytic lesions are sharply demarcated with peripheral sclerosis.[114,115] The multiple lesions are more or less confluent, without periosteal reaction in the absence of a pathologic fracture. Some tumors may induce a bone expansion or appear as a soap bubble lesion. Radiological findings are well correlated with the degree of histological differentiation.[114]

CT scans are performed to determine the extent of the lesion.[107] On MRI, short T1 and long T2 spin-echo signals are fundamental characteristics.[114]

Grossly, the tumoral tissue appears as a spongy, reddish, lobular mass, well circumscribed, soft and hemorrhagic.

Histologically, the endothelial cells are isolated or arranged in clusters, compact nests or cords. The intracytoplasmic vacuolization with a signet-ring configuration corresponds to a central lumen formation sometimes containing red blood cells.[110,115]

The cells are plump, round, oval or cuboidal with an abundant, well-defined eosinophilic cytoplasm. The nucleus, often peripheral,[121] is large, oval and bilobed, with the nuclear membrane showing grooves, folds or sharp indentations.[110] Distinct nucleoli are found.[121] There is absent or reduced mitotic activity. Lumina are formed by cellular coalescence[122] and well-defined and even dilated vessels may be found with subendothelial thickening,[110,115] but

Figs 22.29, 22.30 Epithelioid hemangioma of the humerus.

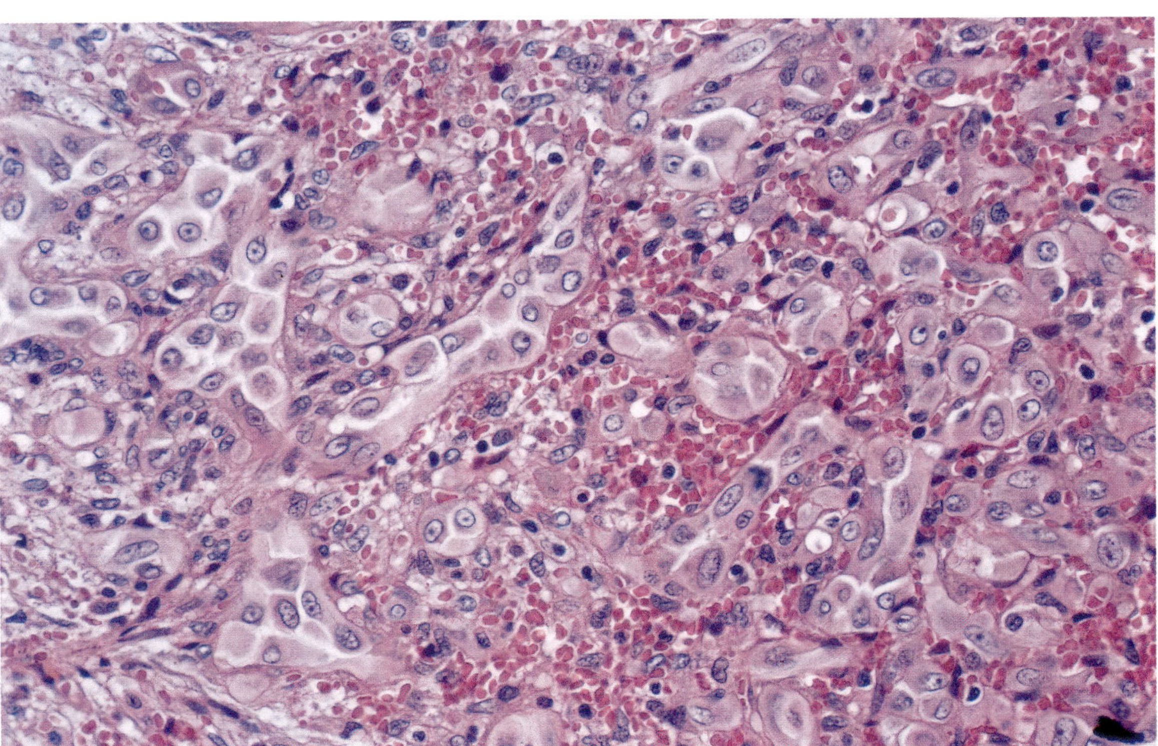

Fig. 22.30

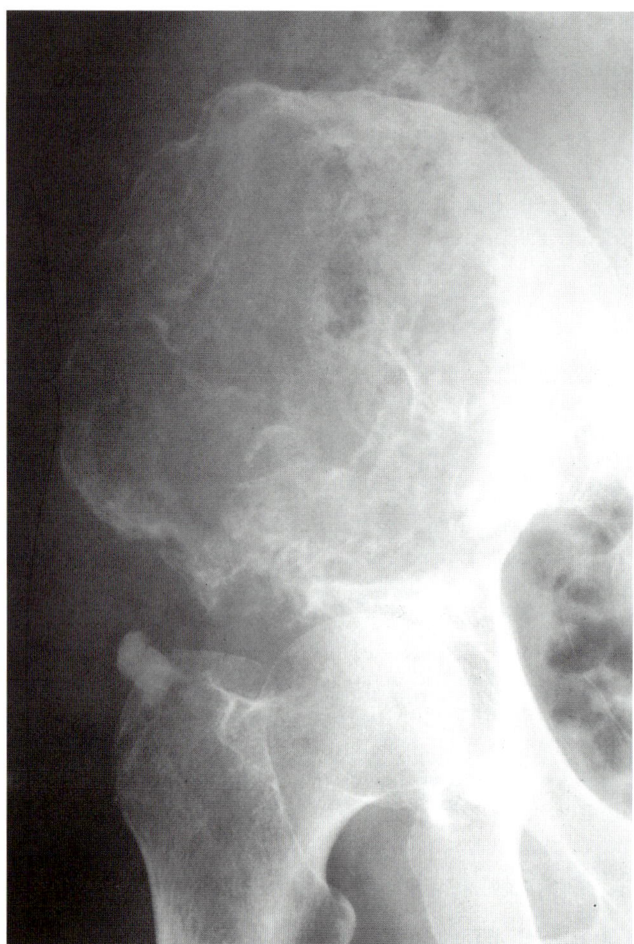

Fig. 22.31

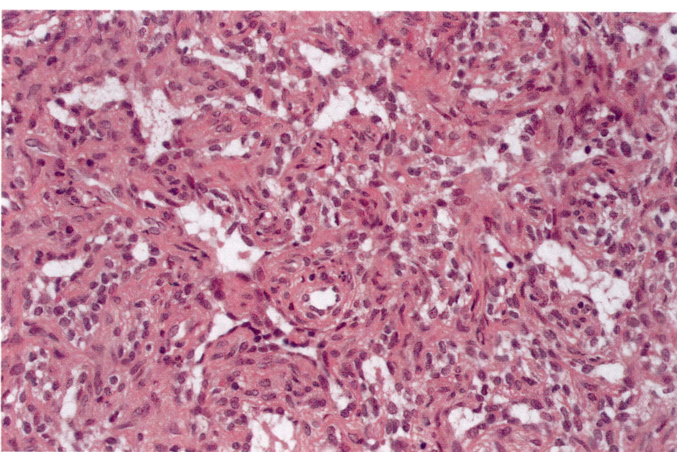

Fig. 22.32

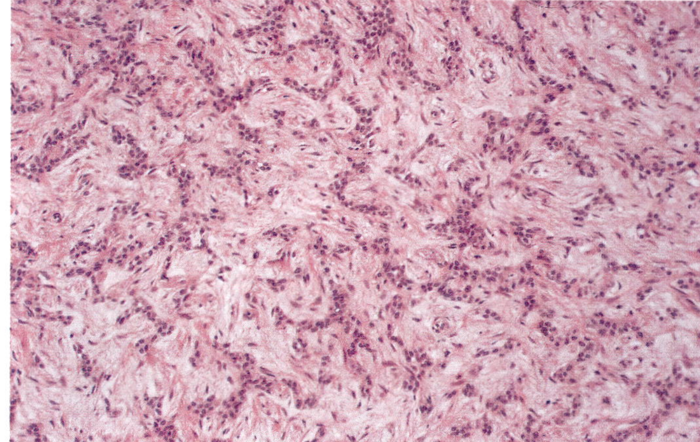

Fig. 22.33

Figs 22.31–22.33 Epithelioid hemangioma of the iliac wing, with well-differentiated vessels and cords of primitive cells in a fibrous stroma.

there is no vasocentric growth involving veins such as is usually found in soft tissue tumors.[121]

The stroma is myxoid or appears as a hyaline cartilage-like matrix.[115,121,123] Inflammatory infiltrates are composed of hemosiderin-laden macrophages, lymphocytes, neutrophils and plasma cells but eosinophils predominate.

Rare cases may be associated with abundant intralesional reactive woven bone.[108] Delicate reticulin fibers surround individual cells or nests of cells.[115,121] Alcian blue staining is negative, but PAS staining may be slightly positive on the vacuolar membranes.[121]

Angioglomoid tumor of bone,[124] *myxoid angioblastoma* and *myxoid angioblastomatosis*[125–127] are similar lesions. Individual cells, nests or branching cords of cells are distributed in a myxoid or fibromyxoid matrix containing mucopolysaccharides; spindle cells exhibit intracytoplasmic vacuoles representing lumina with erythrocytes.

Some epithelioid hemangioendotheliomas may present a more primitive vascular differentiation indicative of a more aggressive course, with atypical cells, hyperchromatic nuclei, prominent nucleoli and solid areas with spindle cells.[108,128]

Immunoreactivity for endothelial markers (FVIIIRag and Ulex Europeaus agglutinin I) is expressed, sometimes with a patchy distribution, along with a strong positivity for vimentin.[115,121,129] Positivity for epithelial membrane antigen and polyclonal or monoclonal cytokeratins is found in 30–50% of cells,[108,121,130] coexpression with FVIIIRag being demonstrated by step sections.[121] In one case, tumor cells expressed HLA-DR antigen.[131]

All ultrastructural studies confirm the endothelial origin of the tumor.[111,115,121,123,126,129,131] The cells are polygonal or spindle shaped with small folds projecting into the vascular lumen. A typical discontinuous basement membrane material surrounds the cells which are connected by junctional complexes. A considerable number of organelles, intermediate filaments and pinocytotic vesicles are found in the cytoplasm.

Leptomeric fibrils and crystal-like filamentous aggregates may indicate a smooth muscle cell differentiation.[120]

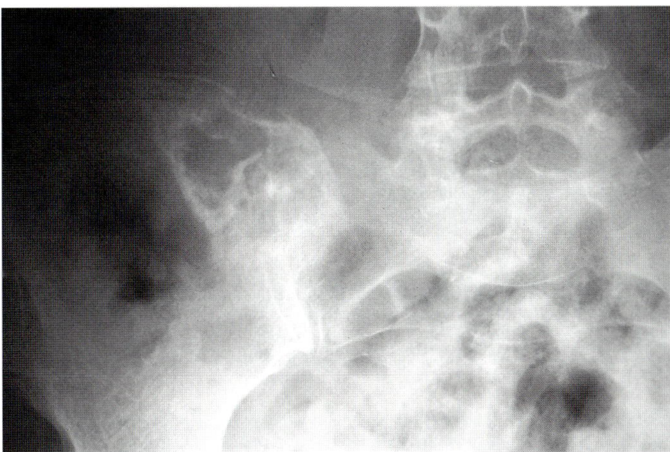

Fig. 22.34

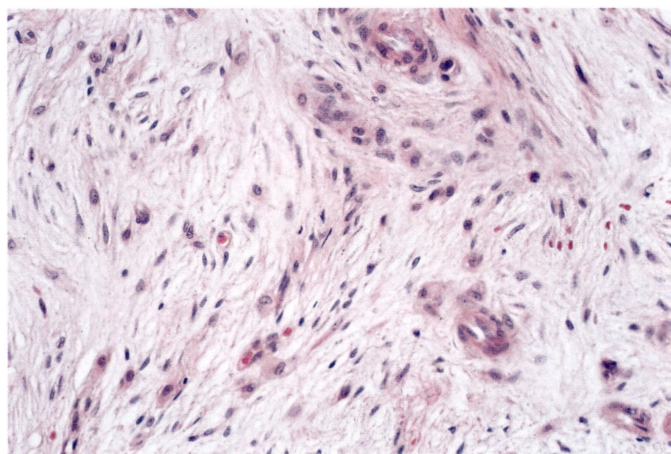

Fig. 22.37

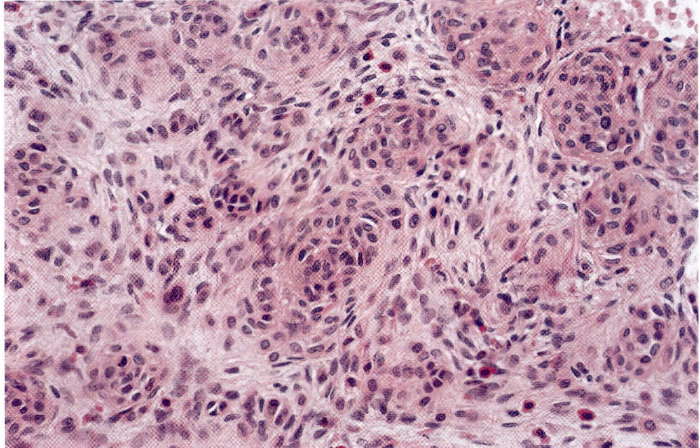

Fig. 22.35

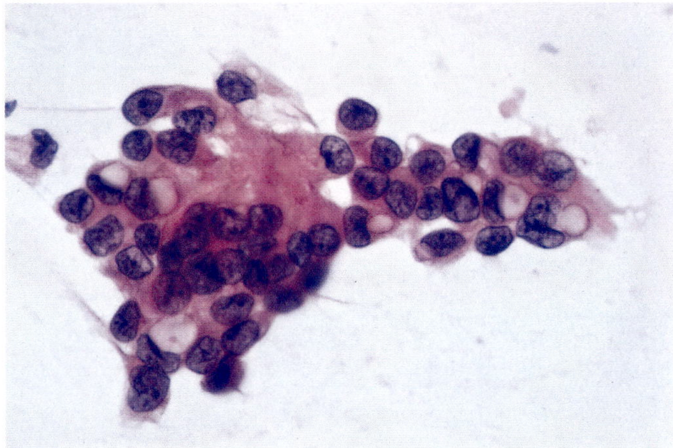

Fig. 22.38

Figs 22.34–22.38 Epithelioid hemangioma of the iliac wing: strands and nests of cells in a myxoid stroma, exhibiting cytoplasmic vacuolization well demonstrated on imprint cytology.

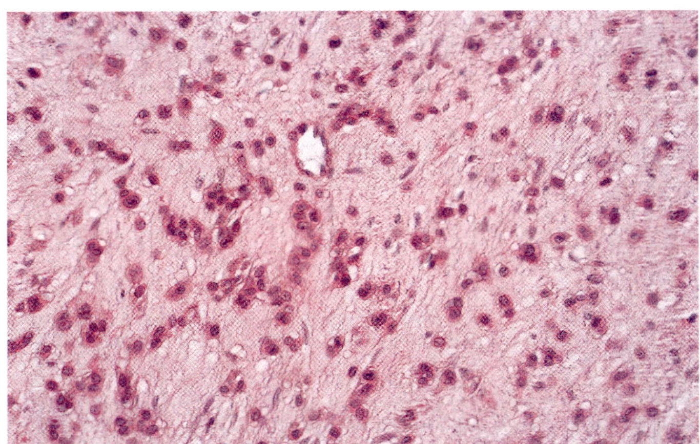

Fig. 22.36

Weibel–Palade bodies appear as rod-shaped structures with an internal parallel array of fine filaments.

The nucleus has irregularities of the nuclear envelope, with a prominent nucleolus. On the whole, vasoformative differentiation is demonstrated with various degrees of maturation,[115] from slit-like spaces to larger vascular channels lined with one or more layers of epithelioid cells.[121]

As for the differential diagnosis, epithelioid angiosarcoma is an overt sarcoma, composed of solid sheets of pleomorphic, large, irregular cells with a high nuclear–cytoplasmic ratio, a coarsely clumped chromatin, numerous atypical mitoses and primitive branching channels.[108] Necrosis is prominent but may also be present in histiocytoid hemangioendotheliomas without suggesting a worse course.[132]

ANGIOSARCOMAS OF BONE

Whatever the name, hemangiosarcoma, hemangioendothelial sarcoma, malignant hemangioendothelioma or even hemangioendothelioma, these tumors, composed of endothelial cells, are not defined by the multicentricity, the intracytoplasmic vacuoles indicating early stages of

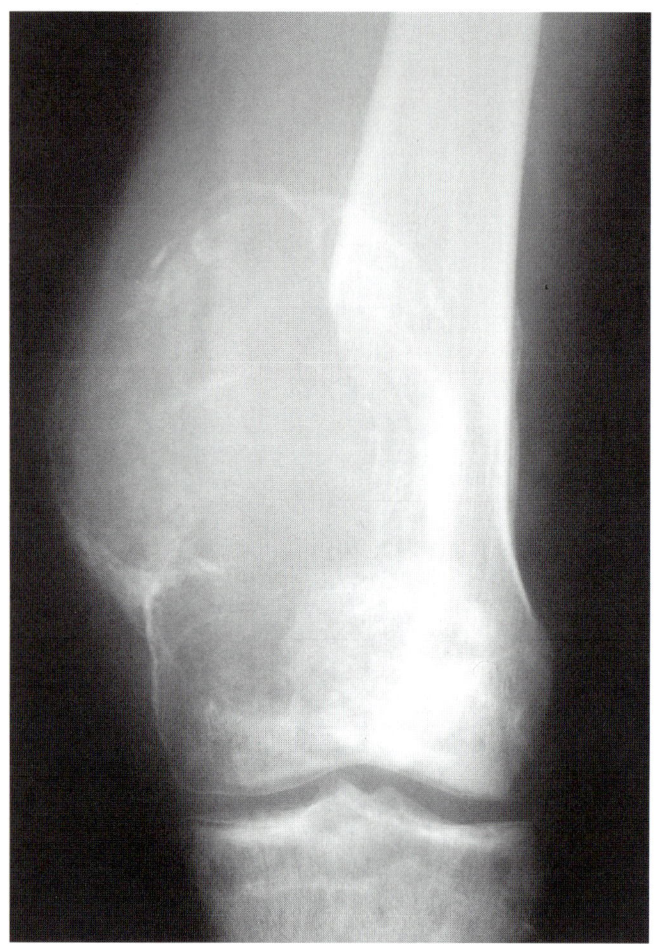

Fig. 22.39

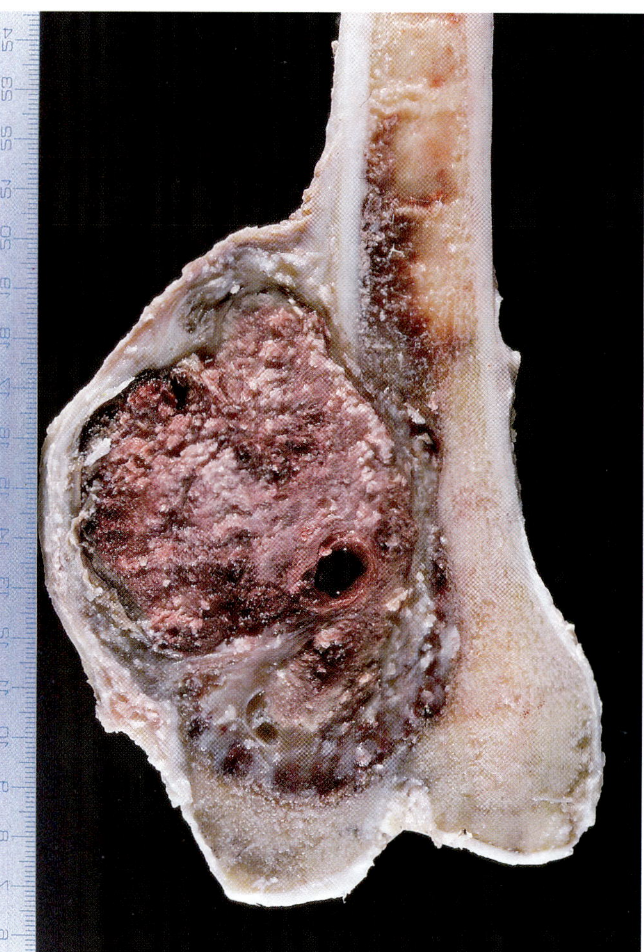

Fig. 22.40

Figs 22.39, 22.40 Angiosarcoma of the femur

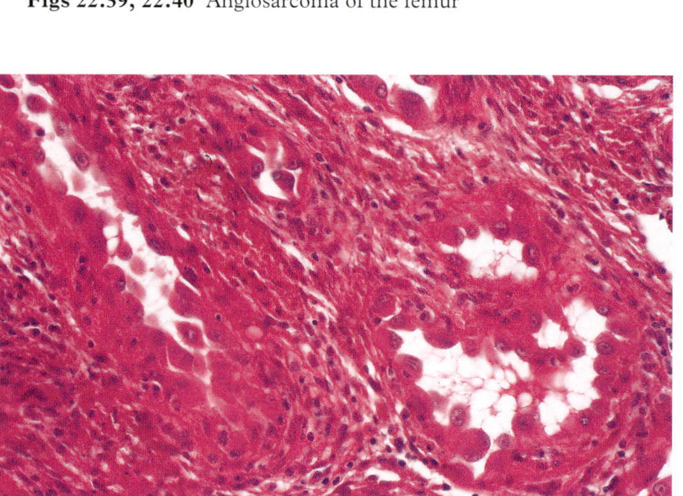

Figs 22.41 Angiosarcoma of the femur with intravascular papillary tufting.

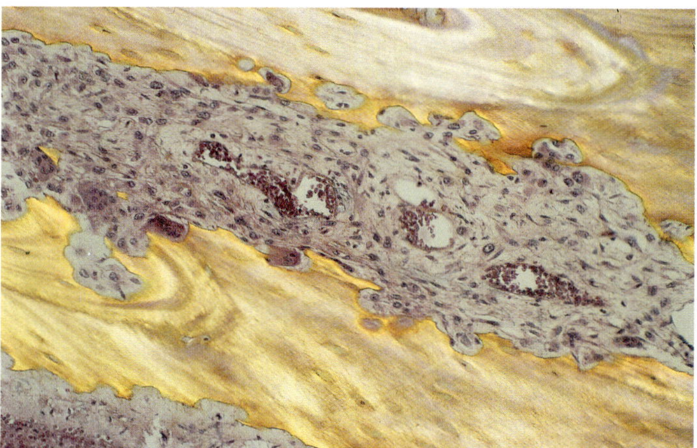

Fig. 22.42 Angiosarcoma of the cuboid bone: widespread resorption of the cortex (polarized light).

angiogenesis or epithelioid-histiocytoid cells, features of both benign and malignant tumors,[133] but by the histologic degree of anaplasia, the radiologic aggressive appearance, the rapid progression of the disease[102,134,135] and a full metastatic potential (Figs 22.39–22.42).

Angiosarcoma is a grade III vascular tumor as defined

by Wold et al[102,103] and Campanacci et al.[104] In some cases, an indolent course may well indicate a hemangioendothelioma.[136]

Some may be associated with Paget's disease,[137] bone infarcts,[138–140] osteomyelitis,[141,142] plates, metallic corrosion products[143] or total hip or knee prosthesis.[144,145] They may also be associated with low-grade dedifferentiated chondrosarcomas.[104]

On gross examination, gray areas are associated with a dark red tissue of spongy consistency (Fechner & Mills 1993).

Histologically, the cellular pleomorphism is obvious with numerous mitotic figures. Solid sheets are composed of fibroblast-like cells,[104] multinucleated or undifferentiated cells. Intravascular papillary tufting is an unusual finding.[103,146] The reticulin stain demonstrates that the proliferative cells are within the basement membrane,[146] delineating anastomotic vascular channels. The eosinophilic infiltration is the same as in benign vascular lesions.[103]

On smears, large pleomorphic or spindle-shaped cells appear isolated or in clusters or rosette-like aggregates, with a hemorrhagic background. More differentiated tumors may exhibit vascular structures or cytoplasmic vacuoles with erythrophagocytosis, but the diagnosis is quite difficult on fine-needle aspiration.[147,148]

Immunoreactivity is positive for factor VIIIRag, but may be weakly or focally positive for Ulex Europaeus.[108,149]

On electron microscopy, the tumor vessels are lined with large endothelial cells, with endothelial gaps and occasional cytoplasmic protrusions.[150] The cells are surrounded by a basement membrane and the cytoplasm comprises Weibel–Palade bodies, myofilaments and pinocytotic vesicles.[148,150,151]

Metastases can occur in the skeleton, lung and pleura[146] and some tumors may spread through the lymphatics.[103,152] The overall survival rate is about 20%.[102] The tumors are moderately radiosensitive and there is a risk of postradiation sarcoma. The main treatment is surgical resection,[102] with adjuvant chemotherapy.[104]

REFERENCES

1. Dorfman H D, Steiner G C, Jaffe H L. Vascular tumors of bone. Hum Pathol 1971: 2: 349–376
2. Stevens J, Love S, Davis C, Kendall B E. Capillary haemangioblastoma of bone resembling vertebral haemangioma. Br J Radiol 1983: 56: 571–575
3. Gonzalez-Crussi F, Enneking W F, Arean V M. Infiltrating angiolipoma. J Bone Joint Surg (Am) 1966: 48: 1111–1124
4. Von Hanwehr R, Apuzzo M L, Ahmadi J, Chandrasoma P. Thoracic spinal angiolipoma. Neurosurgery 1985: 16: 406–411
5. Healy M, Herz D A, Pearl L. Spinal hemangiomas. Neurosurgery 1983: 13: 689–691
6. Baker N D, Klein M J, Greenspan A, Neuwirth M. Symptomatic vertebral hemangiomas: a report of four cases. Skeletal Radiol 1986: 15: 458–463
7. Ross J S, Masaryk T J, Modic M T, Carter J R, Mapstone T, Dengel F H. Vertebral hemangiomas: MR imaging. Radiology 1987: 165: 165–169
8. Feldman F. Case report 104. Sclerosing hemangioma of right seventh rib. Skeletal Radiol 1979: 4: 245–248
9. Sherman R S, Wilner D. The roentgen diagnosis of hemangioma of bone. Am J Roentgenol Radium Ther Nucl Med 1961: 86: 1146–1159
10. Kenan S, Abdelwahab I F, Klein M J, Lewis M M. Hemangiomas of the long tubular bone. Clin Orthop 1992: 280: 256–260
11. Weiss K S, Sabogal J, Carter J R. Intramedullary hemangioma of the tibia and the value of MRI in its detection. Orthopedics 1990: 13: 89–90
12. Loxley S S, Thiemeyer J S Jr, Ellsasser J C. Periosteal hemangioma. Clin Orthop 1972: 85: 151–154
13. Sugiura I. Tibial periosteal hemangioma. Clin Orthop 1975: 106: 242–244
14. Hall F M, Goldberg R P, Kasdon E J, White A A 3rd. Case report 131. Periosteal hemangioma of the fibula. Skeletal Radiol 1980: 5: 275–278
15. Pena J M, Calone J A, Ortega F, Marco A, Martinez A, Saez F. Case report 324. Periosteal hemangioma of left fibula. Skeletal Radiol 1985: 14: 133–135
16. Kenan S, Bonar S, Jones C, Lewis M M. Subperiosteal hemangioma. Clin Orthop 1988: 232: 279–283
17. Yao L, Lee J K. Case report 494. Hemangioma of surface of ulna with prominent sclerosis. Skeletal Radiol 1988: 17: 378–381
18. De Filippo J K, Yu J S, Weis L, Lucas J. Soft tissue hemangioma with adjacent periosteal reaction simulating a primary bone tumor. Skeletal Radiol 1996: 25: 174–177
19. Schajowicz F, Rebecchini A C, Bosch-Mayol G. Intracortical haemangioma simulating osteoid osteoma. J Bone Joint Surg (Br) 1979: 61: 94–95
20. Willinsky R A, Rubenstein J D, Cruickshank B. Case report 216. Intracortical hemangioma of tibia. Skeletal Radiol 1982: 9: 137–139
21. Seeff J, Blacksin M F, Lyons M, Benevenia J. A case report of intracortical hemangioma. A forgotten intracortical lesion. Clin Orthop 1994: 302: 235–238
22. Devaney K, Vinh T N, Sweet D E. Surface-based hemangiomas of bone. Clin Orthop 1994: 300: 233–240
23. Levey D S, MacCormack L M, Sartoris D J, Haghighi P, Resnick D, Thorne R. Cystic angiomatosis: case report and review of the literature. Skeletal Radiol 1996: 25: 287–293
24. Lateur L, Simoens C J, Gryspeerdt S, Samson I, Mertens V, Van Damme B. Skeletal cystic angiomatosis. Skeletal Radiol 1996: 25: 92–95
25. Schajowicz F, Aiello C L, Francone M V, Giannini R E. Cystic angiomatosis (hamartous haemolymphangiomatosis) of bone. J Bone Joint Surg (Br) 1978: 60: 100–106
26. Gutierrez R M, Spjut H J. Skeletal angiomatosis. Clin Orthop 1972: 85: 82–97
27. Boyle W J. Cystic angiomatosis of bone. J Bone Joint Surg (Br) 1972: 54: 626–636
28. Karlin C A, Brower A C. Multiple primary hemangiomas of bone. AJR 1977: 129: 162–164
29. Brower A C, Culver J E Jr, Keats T E. Diffuse cystic angiomatosis of bone. Am J Roentgenol Radium Ther Nucl Med 1973: 118: 456–463
30. Graham D Y, Gonzales J, Kothari S. Diffuse skeletal angiomatosis. Skeletal Radiol 1978: 2: 131–135
31. Reid A B, Reid I L, Johnson G, Hamonic M, Major P. Familial diffuse cystic angiomatosis of bone. Clin Orthop 1989: 238: 211–218
32. Ishida T, Dorfman H D, Steiner G C, Norman A. Cystic angiomatosis of bone with sclerotic changes mimicking osteoblastic metastases. Skeletal Radiol 1994: 23: 247–252
33. Bergman A G, Rogero G W, Hellman B H, Lones M A. Case report 841. Skeletal cystic angiomatosis. Skeletal Radiol 1994: 23: 303–305

34. Jacobs J E, Kimmelstein P. Cystic angiomatosis of the skeletal system. J Bone Joint Surg (Am) 1953: 35: 409–420
35. Gramiak R, Ruiz G, Campeti F L. Cystic angiomatosis of bone. Radiology 1967: 69: 343–353
36. Devaney K, Vinh T N, Sweet D E. Skeletal-extraskeletal angiomatosis. J Bone Joint Surg (Am) 1994: 76: 878–891
37. Bickel W H, Broders A C. Primary lymphangioma of the ilium. J Bone Joint Surg 1947: 29: 517–522
38. Falkmer S, Tilling G. Primary lymphangioma of bone. Acta Orthop Scand 1956: 26: 99–110
39. Schopfner C E, Allen R P. Lymphangioma of bone. Radiology 1961: 76: 449–453
40. Rosenquist C, Wolfe D C. Lymphangioma of bone. J Bone Joint Surg (Am) 1968: 50: 158–162
41. Steiner G M, Farman J, Lawson J P. Lymphangiomatosis of bone. Radiology 1969: 93: 1093–1098
42. Bullough P G, Goodfellow J W. Solitary lymphangioma of bone. J Bone Joint Surg (Am) 1976: 58: 418–419
43. Martinat P, Cotten A, Singer B, Petyt L, Chastanet P. Solitary cystic lymphangioma. Skeletal Radiol 1995: 24: 556–558
44. Sökmensüer C, Sungur A, Tokgözoglu M, Ruacan S. Lymphangiomatosis of bone. Int Orthop 1995: 19: 63–64
45. Jumbelic M, Feuerstein I M, Dorfman H D. Solitary intraosseous lymphangioma. J Bone Joint Surg (Am) 1984: 66: 1479–1481
46. Nixon G W. Lymphangiomatosis of bone demonstrated by lymphangiography. Am J Roentgenol Radium Ther Nucl Med 1970: 110: 582–586
47. Winterberger A R. Radiographic diagnosis of lymphangiomatosis of bone. Radiology 1972: 102: 321–324
48. Gomez C S, Calonje E, Ferrar D W, Browse N L, Fletcher C D. Lymphangiomatosis of the limbs. Am J Surg Pathol 1995: 19: 125–133
49. Heyden G, Kindblom L G, Nielsen J M. Disappearing bone disease. J Bone Joint Surg (Am) 1977: 59: 57–61
50. Shives T C, Beabout J W, Unni K K. Massive osteolysis. Clin Orthop 1993: 294: 267–276
51. Bullough P G. Massive osteolysis. N Y State J Med 1971: 71: 2267–2278
52. Friedman L, Horwitz T, Beck M, Sinn R. Case report 672. Gorham's disease. Skeletal Radiol 1991: 20: 307–309
53. Damron T A, Brodke D S, Heiner J P, Swan J S, DeSouky S. Case report 803. Gorham's disease (Gorham–Stout syndrome) of scapula. Skeletal Radiol 1993: 22: 464–467
54. Edwards W H Jr, Thompson R C Jr, Varsa E W. Lymphangiomatosis and massive osteolysis of the cervical spine. Clin Orthop 1983: 177: 222–229
55. Tauro B. Multicentric Gorham's disease. J Bone Joint Surg (Br) 1992: 74: 928–929
56. Halliday D R, Dahlin D C, Pugh D G, Young H H. Massive osteolysis and angiomatosis. Radiology 1964: 82: 637–644
57. Cannon S R. Massive osteolysis. J Bone Joint Surg (Br) 1986: 68: 24–28
58. Vinee P, Tanyü M O, Hauenstein K H, Sigmund G, Stöver B, Adler C P. C T and MRI of Gorham syndrome. J Comput Assist Tomogr 1994: 18: 985–989
59. Assoun J, Richardi G, Railhac J J et al. C T and MRI of massive osteolysis of Gorham. J Comput Assist Tomogr 1994: 18: 981–984
60. Fornasier V L. Hemangiomatosis with massive osteolysis. J Bone Joint Surg (Br) 1970: 52: 444–451
61. Gorham L W, Stout A P. Massive osteolysis (acute spontaneous absorption of bone, phantom bone, disappearing bone); its relation to hemangiomatosis. J Bone Joint Surg (Am) 1955: 37: 985–1004
62. Dickson G R, Mollan R A, Carr K E. Cytochemical localization of alkaline and acid phosphatase in human vanishing bone disease. Histochemistry 1987: 87: 569–572
63. Dickson G R, Hamilton A, Hayes D, Carr K E, Davis R, Mollan R A. An investigation of vanishing bone disease. Bone 1990: 11: 205–210
64. Johnson P M, McClure J G. Observations on massive osteolysis. Radiology 1958: 71: 28–42
65. Campbell J, Almond H G, Johnson R. Massive osteolysis of the humerus with spontaneous recovery. J Bone Joint Surg (Br) 1975: 57: 238–240
66. Choma N D, Biscotti C V, Bauer T W, Mehta A C, Licata A A. Gorham's syndrome. Am J Med 1987: 83: 1151–1156
67. Dunbar S F, Rosenberg A, Mankin H, Rosenthal D, Suit H D. Gorham's massive osteolysis: the role of radiation therapy and a review of the literature. Int J Radiat Oncol Biol Phys 1993: 26: 491–497
68. Sunderraj S, al-Khalifa A A, Pal A K, Pim H P, Sabri S H. Primary intraosseous glomus tumor. Histopathology 1988: 14: 532–536
69. Serra J M, Muiragui A, Tadjalli H. Glomus tumor of the metacarpophalangeal joint. J Hand Surg (Am) 1985: 10: 142–143
70. Björkengren A G, Resnick D, Haghighi P, Sartoris D J. Intraosseous glomus tumor. AJR 1986: 147: 739–741
71. Rozmaryn L M, Sadler A H, Dorfman H D. Intraosseous glomus tumor of the ulna. Clin Orthop 1987: 220: 126–129
72. Ho K L, Pak M S. Glomus tumor of the coccygeal region. J Bone Joint Surg (Am) 1980: 62: 141–142
73. Pambakian H, Smith M A. Glomus tumours of the coccygeal body associated with coccydynia. J Bone Joint Surg (Br) 1981: 63: 424–426
74. Duncan L, Halverson J, DeSchryver-Kecskemeti K. Glomus tumor of the coccyx. A curable cause of coccygodynia. Arch Pathol Lab Med 1991: 115: 78–80
75. Kobayashi Y, Kawaguchi T, Imoto K, Yamamoto T. Intraosseous glomus tumor in the sacrum. Acta Pathol Jpn 1990: 40: 856–859
76. Bell R S, Goodman S B, Fornasier V L. Coccygeal glomus tumors: a case of mistaken identity? J Bone Joint Surg (Am) 1982: 64: 595–597
77. Albrecht S, Zbieranowski I. Incidental glomus coccygeum. When a normal structure looks like a tumor. Am J Surg Pathol 1990: 14: 922–924
78. Albrecht S, Hicks M J, Antalffy B. Intracoccygeal and pericoccygeal glomus bodies and their relationship to coccygodynia. Surgery 1994: 115: 1–6
79. Sugiura I. Intraosseous glomus tumour. J Bone Joint Surg (Br) 1976: 58: 245–247
80. Simmons T J, Bassler T J, Schwinn C P, Forrester D M. Case report 749. Primary glomus tumor of bone. Skeletal Radiol 1992: 21: 407–409
81. Tang J S, Gold R H, Mirra J M, Eckardt J. Hemangiopericytoma of bone. Cancer 1988: 62: 848–859
82. Vang P S, Falk E. Hemangiopericytoma of bone. Acta Orthop Scand 1980: 51: 903–907
83. Linovitz R J, Resnick D, Keissling P et al. Tumor-induced osteomalacia and rickets: a surgically curable syndrome. J Bone Joint Surg (Am) 1976: 58: 419–423
84. Robertson A. Hypophosphatemic osteomalacia secondary to hemangiopericytoma of right femur. Semin Roentgenol 1983: 18: 5–6
85. McClure J, Smith P S. Oncogenic osteomalacia. J Clin Pathol 1987: 40: 446–453
86. Nuovo M A, Dorfman H D, Sun C C, Chalew S A. Tumor-induced osteomalacia and rickets. Am J Surg Pathol 1989: 13: 588–599
87. Park Y R, Unni K K, Beabout J W, Hodgson S F. Oncogenic osteomalacia: a clinicopathologic study of 17 bone lesions. J Korean Med Sci 1994: 9: 289–298
88. Vathana P. Primary hemangiopericytoma of bone in the hands. J Hand Surg (Am) 1984: 9: 761–764
89. Sellke F W, Laszewski M J, Robinson R A, Davis R, Rossi N P. Hemangiopericytoma of the sternum. Arch Pathol Lab Med 1991: 115: 242–244
90. Spagnolo R, Torelli L, Brusamolino R, Bono A, Rossi N, Zurrida S. Primary haemangiopericytoma of bone. Int J Oncol 1993: 2: 601–606
91. Wold L E, Unni K K, Cooper K L, Sim F H, Dahlin D C. Hemangiopericytoma of bone. Am J Surg Pathol 1982: 6: 53–58
92. Fathie K. Hemangiopericytoma of the thoracic spine. J Neurosurg 1970: 32: 371–374
93. Stern M B, Grode M L, Goodman M D. Hemangiopericytoma of the cervical spine. Clin Orthop 1980: 151: 201–204

94. Muraszko K M, Antunes J L, Hilal S K, Michelsen W J. Hemangiopericytoma of the spine. Neurosurgery 1982: 10: 473–479

95. Giunti A, Calderoni P, Martucci E. Haemangiopericytoma of bone. Ital J Orthop Traumatol 1982: 8: 345–349

96. Yaghmai I. Angiographic manifestations of soft tissue and osseous hemangiopericytomas. Radiology 1978: 126: 653–659

97. Kahn L B, Nunnery E W, Lipper S, Reddick R L. Case report 144. Primary hemangiopericytoma of the right radius. Skeletal Radiol 1981: 6: 139–143

98. Anderson C, Rorabeck C H. Skeletal metastases of an intracranial malignant hemangiopericytoma. J Bone Joint Surg (Am) 1980: 62: 145–148

99. Dahlin D C. Case report 160. Malignant hemangiopericytoma of femur, metastatic from intracranial lesion. Skeletal Radiol 1981: 6: 303–305

100. Beauchamp C P, Wold L E, Sim F H. Hemangioendothelial sarcoma. Orthopedics 1986: 9: 1575–1577

101. Unni K K, Ivins J C, Beabout J W, Dahlin D C. Hemangioma, hemangiopericytoma, and hemangioendothelioma (angiosarcoma) of bone. Cancer 1971: 27 : 1403–1414

102. Wold L E, Unni K K, Beabout I W, Ivins J C, Bruckman J E, Dahlin D C. Hemangioendothelial sarcoma of bone. Am J Surg Pathol 1982: 6: 59–70

103. Wold L E, Swee R G, Sim F H. Vascular lesions of bone. Pathol Annu 1985: 20 Pt 2: 101–137

104. Campanacci M, Boriani S, Giunti A. Hemangioendothelioma of bone: a study of 29 cases. Cancer 1980: 46: 804–814

105. Hartmann W H, Stewart F W. Hemangioendothelioma of bone. Unusual tumor characterized by indolent course. Cancer 1962: 15: 846–854

106. Benassi M S, Gamberi G, Ragazzini P et al. Bone hemangioendothelioma: an immunohistochemical study related to histological malignancy and proliferative activity (NORs). Tumori 1995: 81: 179–184

107. Jaffe J W, Mesgarzadeh H, Bonakdarpour A, Edmonds P R. Case report 519. Histiocytoid hemangioendothelioma of right 10th rib. Skeletal Radiol 1989: 18: 50–54

108. O'Connell J X, Kattapuram S V, Mankin H J, Bhan A K, Rosenberg A E. Epithelioid hemangioma of bone. A tumor often mistaken for low-grade angiosarcoma or malignant hemangioendothelioma. Am J Surg Pathol 1993: 17: 610–617

109. Ben Romdhane K, Khattech R, Ben Othman M. Epithelioid hemangioma of bone. Am J Surg Pathol 1994: 18: 1270–1271

110. Rosai J, Gold J, Landy R. The histiocytoid hemangiomas. A unifying concept embracing several previously described entities of skin, soft tissue, large vessels, bone and heart. Hum Pathol 1979: 10: 707–730

111. Fornasier V L, Finkelstein S, Gardiner G W, Wong D. Angiolymphoid hyperplasia with eosinophilia: a bone lesion pathologically resembling Kimura's disease of skin. Clin Orthop 1982: 166: 243–248

112. Weiss S W, Enzinger F M. Epithelioid hemangioendothelioma: a vascular tumor often mistaken for a carcinoma. Cancer 1982: 50: 970–981

113. Weiss S W, Ishak K G, Dail D H, Sweet D E, Enzinger F M. Epithelioid hemangioendothelioma and related lesions. Semin Diagn Pathol 1986: 3: 259–287

114. Abrahams T G, Bula W, Jones M. Epithelioid hemangioendothelioma of bone. Skeletal Radiol 1992: 21: 509–513

115. Tsuneyoshi M, Dorfman H D, Bauer T W. Epithelioid hemangioendothelioma of bone. A clinicopathologic, ultrastructural and immunohistochemical study. Am J Surg Pathol 1986: 10: 754–764

116. Cone R O, Hudkins P, Nguyen V, Merriwether W A. Histiocytoid hemangioma of bone: a benign lesion which may mimic angiosarcoma. Skeletal Radiol 1983: 10: 165–169

117. Lange T A, Zoltan D, Hafez G R. Simultaneous occurrence in the spine of osteoblastoma and hemangioendothelioma. Spine 1986: 11: 92–95

118. Boutin R D, Spaeth H J, Mangalik A, Sell J J. Epithelioid hemangioendothelioma of bone. Skeletal Radiol 1996: 25: 391–395

119. Finsterbush A, Husseini N, Rousso M. Multifocal hemangioendothelioma of bones in the hand. J Hand Surg (Am) 1981: 6: 353–356

120. Hirose T, Sano T, Shinomiya S, Hizawa K, Endo H, Henmi T. Periosteal epithelioid hemangioendothelioma with leptomeric fibrils. Ultrastruct Pathol 1987: 11: 405–410

121. Van Haelst U J, Pruszczynski M, Ten Cate L N, Mravunac M. Ultrastructural and immunohistochemical study of epithelioid hemangioendothelioma of bone: coexpression of epithelial and endothelial markers. Ultrastruct Pathol 1990: 14: 141–149

122. De Smet A A, Inscore D, Neff J R. Case report 521. Histiocytoid hemangioma of the distal end of the right humerus. Skeletal Radiol 1989: 18: 60–65

123. Martinez-Tello F J, Marcos-Robles J, Blanco-Lorenzo F. Case report 520. Primary epithelioid hemangioendothelioma of bone (polyostotic). Skeletal Radiol 1989: 18: 55–59

124. Tang T T, Zuege R C, Babbitt D P, Blount W P, McCreadie S R. Angioglomoid tumor of bone. J Bone Joint Surg (Am) 1976: 58: 873–876

125. Reed R J. Malignant myxoid angioblastoma of bone. Am J Surg Pathol 1982: 6: 159–163

126. Mirra J M, Kameda N. Myxoid angioblastomatosis of bone. Am J Surg Pathol 1985: 9: 450–458

127. Mirra J M, Kameda N. Case report 366. Myxoid angioblastomatosis of bone (disseminated). Skeletal Radiol 1986: 15: 323–326

128. Bohn L E, Dehner L P, Walker H C Jr. Case report 204. Multicentric angiosarcoma of bone involving the right lower extremity. Skeletal Radiol 1982: 8: 303–305

129. Ose D, Vollmer R, Shelburne J, McComb R, Harrelson J. Histiocytoid hemangioma of the skin and scapula. A case report with electron microscopy and immunohistochemistry. Cancer 1983: 51: 1656–1662

130. Gray M H, Rosenberg A E, Dickersin G R, Bhan A K. Cytokeratin expression in epithelioid vascular neoplasms. Hum Pathol 1990: 21: 212–217

131. Maruyama N, Kumagai Y, Ishida Y et al. Epithelioid haemangioendothelioma of the bone tissue. Virchows Arch A Pathol Anat Histopathol 1985: 407: 159–165

132. Vinuela A, Fernandez-Rojo F, Gonzalez-Nunez A. Hemangioendothelioma of bone. A case report with massive tissular necrosis. Pathol Res Pract 1984: 178: 297–300

133. Markaki S, Kokka H, Kyparidou E, Bouropoulou V. Primary vascular bone sarcomas. Arch Anat Cytol Pathol 1990: 38: 163–167

134. Carmody E, Loftus B, Corrigan J, O'Sullivan T, Leader M, Keeling F. Case report 759. Malignant epithelioid haemangioendothelioma of bone. Skeletal Radiol 1992: 21: 538–541

135. Wu K K, Guise E R. Malignant hemangioendothelioma of bone. Orthopedics 1981: 4: 58–64

136. Craver W L, Brown B S. Hemangioendothelioma of bone with pulmonary metastases: a 25-year course. Cancer 1979: 43: 1917–1923

137. Chen K T. Hemangiosarcoma complicating Paget's disease of the bone. J Surg Oncol 1985: 28: 187–189

138. Abdelwahab I F, Kenan S, Klein M J, Lewis M M. Case report: angiosarcoma occurring in a bone infarct. Clin Radiol 1992: 45: 412–414

139. Pins M R, Mankin H J, Xavier R J, Rosenthal D I, Dickersin G R, Rosenberg A E. Malignant epithelioid hemangioendothelioma of the tibia associated with a bone infarct in a patient who had Gaucher disease. J Bone Joint Surg (Am) 1995: 77: 777–781

140. Matsuno T, Kaneda K, Takeda N. Development of angiosarcoma at the site of a bone infarct. Clin Orthop 1996: 327: 259–263

141. Olmi R, Rubbini L. Angiosarcoma in osteomielite cronica. Chir Organi Mov 1975: 61: 765–768

142. Bacchini P, Calderoni P, Gherlinzoni F, Gualtieri G. Angiosarcoma in chronic osteomyelitis. Ital J Orthop Traumatol 1984: 10: 393–398

143. Dube V E, Fisher D E. Hemangioendothelioma of the leg following metallic fixation of the tibia. Cancer 1972: 30: 1260–1266

144. Van der List J J, Van Horn J R, Slooff T J, Ten Cate N L. Malignant epithelioid hemangioendothelioma at the site of a hip prosthesis. Acta Orthop Scand 1988: 59: 328–330

145. Himmer O, Lootvoet L, Deprez P, Monfort L, Ghosez J P. Angiosarcome après prothèse totale du genou. Rev Chir Orthop Reparatrice Appar Mot 1991: 77: 125–129

146. Volpe R, Mazabraud A. Hemangioendothelioma (angiosarcoma) of bone. A distinct pathologic entity with unpredictable course? Cancer 1982: 49: 727–736

147. Jayaram G, Kapoor R, Saha M M. Hemangioendothelioma. Cytologic appearances in two cases presenting with multiple soft tissue and bone lesions. Acta Cytol 1987: 31: 497–501

148. Khiyami A, Green L K, Gyorkey F, Landon G. Primary angiosarcoma of the cuboidal bone. Diagn Cytopathol 1991: 7: 520–523

149. Hultberg B M, Daugaard S, Johansen H F, Mouridsen H T, Hou-Jensen K. Malignant haemangiopericytomas and haemangioendotheliosarcomas: an immunohistochemical study. Histopathology 1988: 12: 405–414

150. Steiner G C, Dorfman H D. Ultrastructure of hemangioendothelial sarcoma of bone. Cancer 1972: 29: 122–135

151. Adler C P, Reichelt A. Haemangiosarcoma of bone. Int Orthop 1985: 8: 273–279

152. Volpe R, Carbone A, Manconi R, Santi L. Hemangioendothelioma of bone. A report of an unusual case with lymph node metastasis. Pathol Res Pract 1985: 180: 521–525

23

Muscular tumors

M. Forest

LEIOMYOMAS OF BONE

A few cases have been described in the mandible or the maxilla[1-3] but leiomyoma of bone is exceedingly rare in extragnathic locations. Cases have been reported in the periosteum (Mirra 1989), the tibia[4] and the femoral neck, the latter being a possible manifestation of a peritoneal leiomyomatosis.[5,6] An osteolytic lesion in the pubic bone, initially diagnosed as a leiomyosarcoma, may also be a leiomyoma.[7]

Rare cases of angioleiomyomas have been reported in the mandibular region.[8] A single case in an extragnathic site involved the proximal tibia;[9] tortuous vascular channels with thick muscular walls were associated with interlacing smooth muscle fibers, bundles of nerve fibers, foci of calcification and myxoid changes.

LEIOMYOSARCOMAS OF BONE

Introduction and clinical data

In bone, a spindle cell sarcoma exhibiting smooth muscle differentiation in a proximal tibial lesion was first described by Evans & Sanerkin in 1965.[10] It was presumed to arise from the smooth muscle cells of the intraosseous blood vessels,[11,12] from fibroblasts or myofibroblasts[13,14] or from perivascular primitive mesenchymal cells.[12,15]

Fewer than 70 cases have been reported, accounting for 0.64% of all primary bone tumors.[11] There is a wide age range[16] but most patients are in their fifth or sixth decades[17] with a median age of 50 years.[18] Men are affected about twice as often as women.[18,19]

Clinical presentations are pain, a palpable mass or a pathologic fracture. Two cases have been reported as radiation-induced sarcomas[18,20] and one as a second malignancy long after the excision of a retinoblastoma.[21]

Skeletal location

The most common extragnathic sites are the distal femur, followed by the proximal tibia (slightly more than 50% of cases) and the proximal humerus. Tumors have been described in numerous locations including the pelvis, clavicle, ribs and even the os calcis[22] and the spine.[23]

Imaging

In long bones, most cases are in the metaphysis[24] but metaepiphyseal, or diaphyseal tumors are not unusual[18] (Figs 23.1–23.4). The poorly defined osteolytic lesion with a moth-eaten appearance is non-specific and may be indistinguishable from a fibrosarcoma or a malignant fibrous histiocytoma.[17] Some tumors exhibit a geographic osteolysis without sclerosis.[11] The cortex is frequently destroyed with soft tissue extension[17] and periosteal new bone formation.

Gross pathology

The cut surface of the tumoral tissue appears gray, tan or white, with focal areas of necrosis. The size ranges from 2 to 12 cm. Most tumors have extension into the soft tissues.

Histopathology

Most leiomyosarcomas in bone are high-grade tumors. Broad interlacing bundles of plump spindle cells are associated with a collagenized or myxoid stroma (Figs 23.5–23.7). The cytoplasm is prominent, eosinophilic and fibrillar; the blunt-ended nuclei are elongated. A non-specific storiform pattern may be found (Fechner & Mills 1993). Occasionally, tumor cells may be rounded, with a clear cytoplasm,[17] or multinucleated, with bizarre nuclei and prominent nucleoli.[19] Some fields even have an epithelioid appearance.

The tumors can be associated with a prominent reactive osteoclast-like giant cell component.[11,17,25] Mitotic figures are easily found, as well as areas of necrosis.

Reticulin fibers encircle individual cells.[11] The cytoplasm is intensely red on trichrome stain and myofibrils

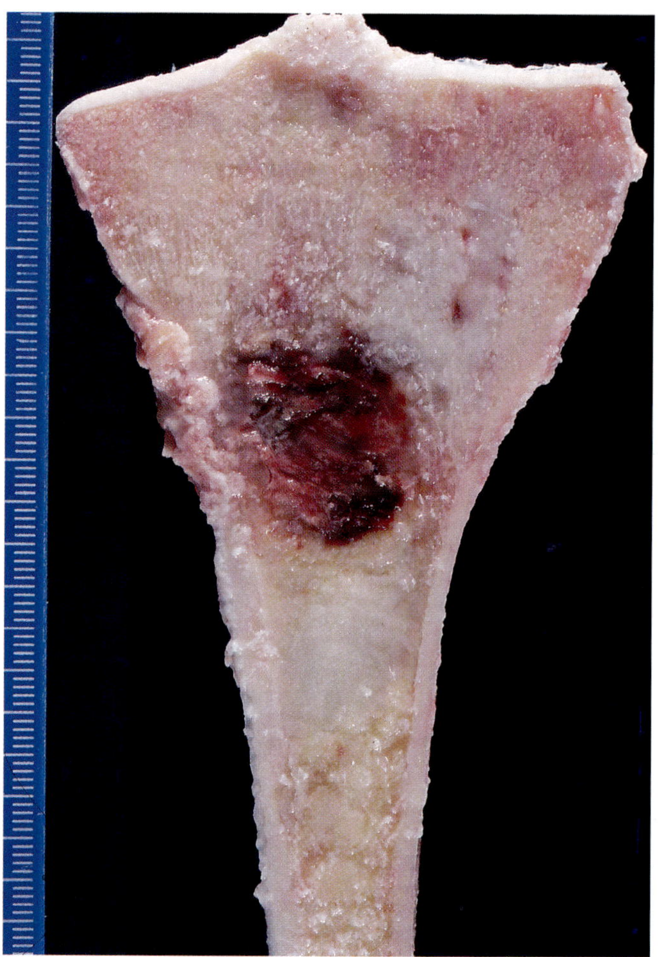

Fig. 23.1

Fig. 23.2

Figs 23.1, 23.2 Leiomyosarcoma of the tibia.

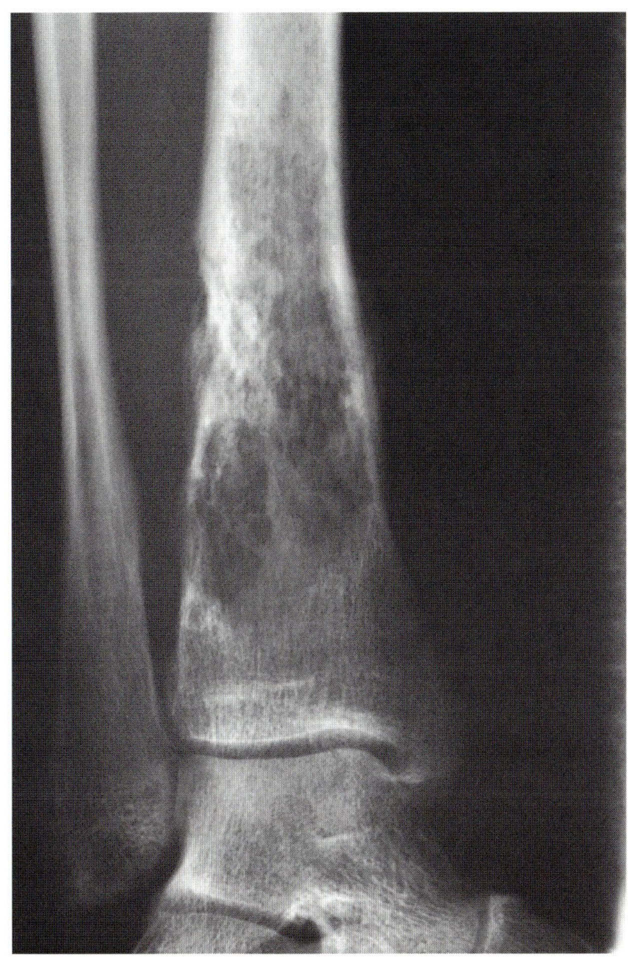

Fig. 23.3

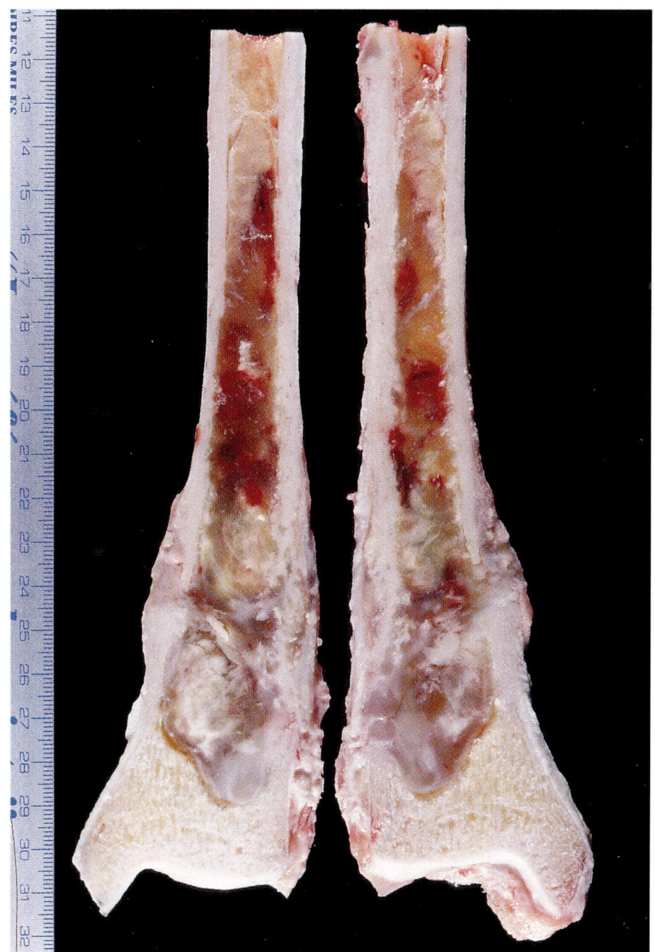

Fig. 23.4

Figs 23.3, 23.4 Leiomyosarcoma of the tibia.

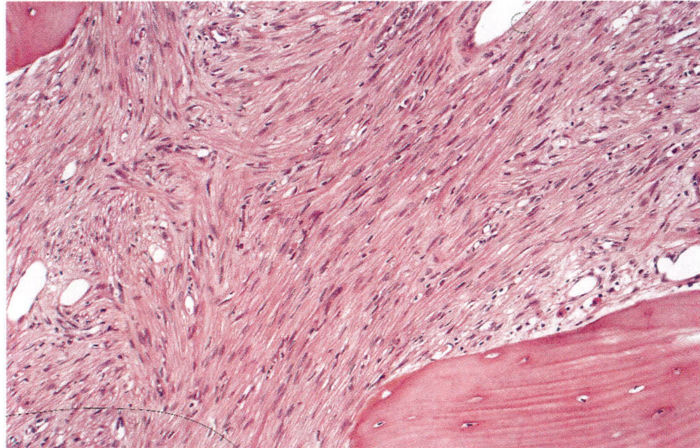

Fig. 23.5

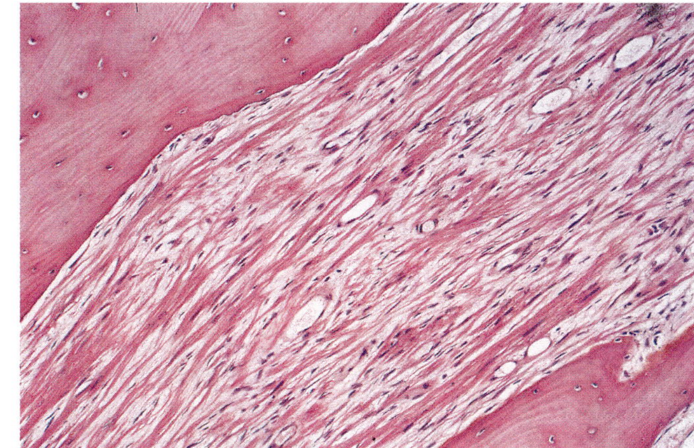

Fig. 23.6

Figs 23.5, 23.6 Leiomyosarcomas of bone: bundles of plump spindled cells with blunt-ended nuclei and eosinophilic cytoplasm.

may be demonstrated by Mallory's phosphotungstic acid-hematoxylin stain, but some authors feel that conventional special stains are not very useful.[19]

Cytopathology

The eosinophilic cytoplasm is unusually elongated; the

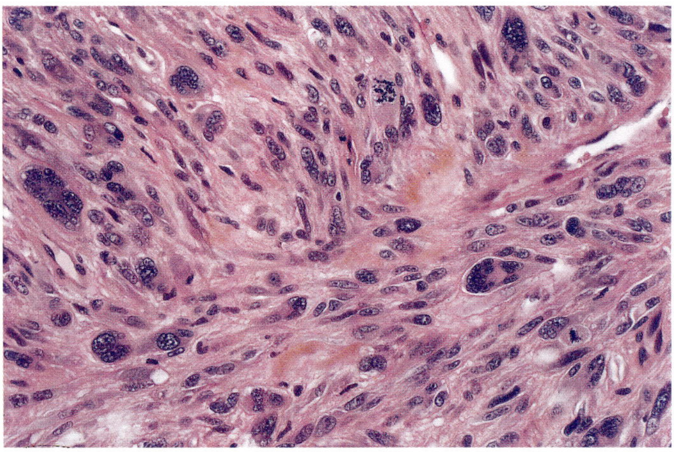

Fig. 23.7 Leiomyosarcoma of bone: pleomorphic cells with multinucleated forms.

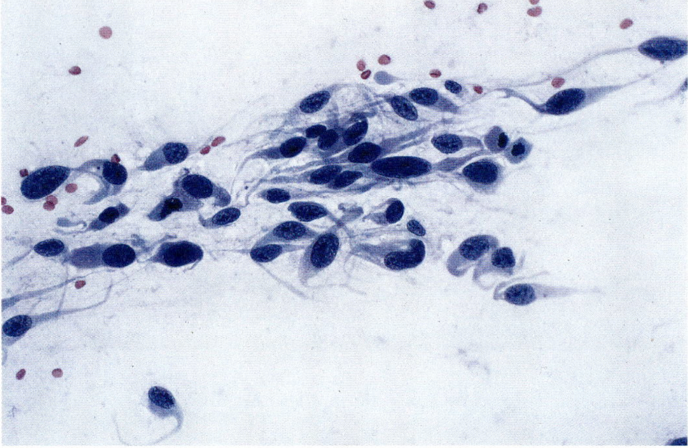

Fig. 23.8 Poorly differentiated leiomyosarcoma of bone on imprint cytology.

nucleus is ovoid or cigar shaped, elongated with blunt or rounded ends.[13] In less well-differentiated sarcomas, the cytology is that of a pleomorphic tumor (Fig. 23.8).

Immunohistochemistry

The reaction patterns are those of a vascular musculature.[11] Positivity is found with antibodies directed against muscle-specific actin,[11,17,19,26] antimyosin,[19,27] desmin with intense or variable results,[11,17–19] type IV collagen (basement membrane component),[11] laminin and vimentin in most cases.[17] In 50% of cases positivity may be demonstrated for cytokeratin[11,17] and even S-100 protein in few cases.[11]

Electron microscopy

Ultrastructural examination is now somewhat over-taken by immunohistochemistry, but all reports show most features of a smooth muscle cell differentiation.[12–15, 17,18,19,25–32]

The cells, with typical features of smooth muscle cells, are spindle shaped, with thin myofilaments parallel to the long axis of the cell, or they may appear more rounded with thicker filaments,[12,14,19] with pinocytotic vesicles, attachment plaques and an incomplete basal lamina enveloping some cells.[17,19] Varying amounts of glycogen and lipids[28] are located in the cytoplasm.

Course, treatment and prognosis

Some authors suggest that the histological grading of tumor differentiation, the mitotic activity and the extent of necrosis are important prognostic factors[18] but in some series, there is no correlation with survival.[11]

Most tumors have an aggressive course with rapid local extension. The mortality rate is 48% and the mean survival 3.4 years,[17,18] with mostly pulmonary or even cutaneous metastases.[18]

The treatment is early wide surgical resection, with chemotherapy and/or radiotherapy.[11]

Differential diagnosis

Primary soft tissue leiomyosarcomas may involve bone. Metastatic leiomyosarcomas, mostly from the uterus (Fig. 23.9) but occasionally from the gastrointestinal tract, have to be excluded.[17, 33] They are sometimes located in unusual sites for a primary tumor, such as the skull, the spine or the scapula. Fibrosarcomas usually display a herring-bone or fascicular pattern.

Some cases of leiomyosarcoma have initially been diagnosed as malignant fibrous histiocytoma on the grounds of a storiform pattern and bizarre multinucleated giant cells,[17,28,30] but the immunostaining for desmin and muscle-specific actin is positive.

Spindle cell carcinomas cannot be ruled out with certitude, as some leiomyosarcomas may show a cytokeratin positivity.

RHABDOMYOSARCOMAS OF BONE

Except for some cases localized in craniofacial bones, rhabdomyosarcoma in bone is extremely rare. Five cases have been reported in the tibia,[34–36] five in the femur,[36–40] one in the iliac bone[41] and one in the spine,[42] with histological variants including spindle cell rhabdomyosarcomas, embryonal rhabdomyosarcomas or mixed pleomorphic-embryonal rhabdomyosarcomas.[40]

There is clearly a differential diagnosis. Primary soft tissue tumors may involve bones[43] (Fig. 23.10). Rhabdomyosarcoma may represent the high-grade malignant

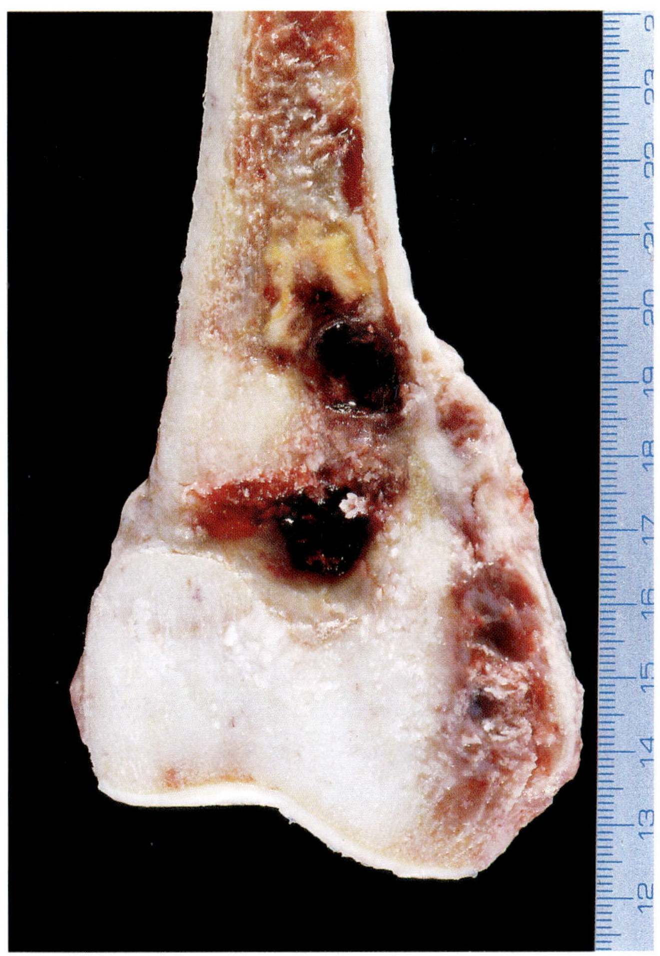

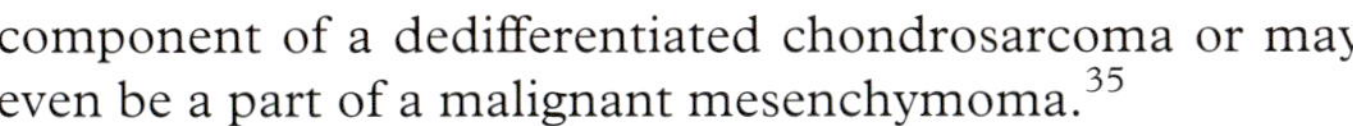

Fig. 23.9 Metastatic leiomyosarcoma of the uterus involving the femur.

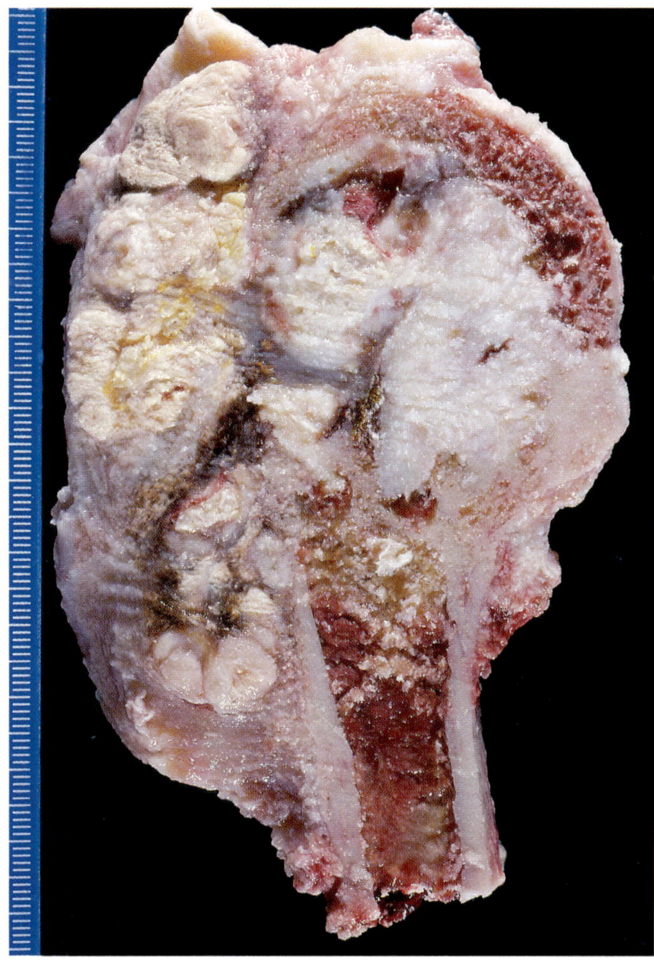

Fig. 23.10 Involvement of the humerus by a rhabdomyosarcoma of the soft tissues.

component of a dedifferentiated chondrosarcoma or may even be a part of a malignant mesenchymoma.[35]

Exceptionally, alveolar rhabdomyosarcomas may pre-

sent with diffuse bone marrow involvement;[44–46] skeletal metastases of disseminated rhabdomyosarcomas may even be encountered in the absence of obvious primary sites.[47]

REFERENCES

1. Rhatigan R M, Kim Z E. Leiomyoma arising adjacent to a maxillary tooth socket: an intraosseous leiomyoma presenting as an odontogenic lesion. South Med J 1976: 69: 493–494
2. Goldblatt L I, Edesess R B. Central leiomyoma of the mandible. Oral Surg Oral Med Oral Pathol 1977: 43: 591–597
3. McMillan M D, Ferguson J W, Kardos T B. Mandibular vascular leiomyoma. Oral Surg Oral Med Oral Pathol 1986: 62: 427–433
4. Taxy J B, Conklin J, Mann J J, Brooker A. Case report 147. Leiomyoma of the periosteum of the tibia. Skeletal Radiol 1981: 6: 153–154
5. Wagner T, Braun W, Kotter A. Das Ossäare Leiomyom-Eine Erstbeschreibung. Chirurg 1992: 63: 432–434
6. Braun W, Kotter A, Kundel K, Wiedemann M, Wagner T. Intraosseous leiomyoma of the neck of the femur. Int Orthop 1994: 18: 47–49
7. Takami K M, Ishida T, Iguchi M, Kuniyoshi Y, Wakasa K, Sakurai M. Primary leiomyosarcoma or leiomyoma of the public bone? Int Orthop 1994: 18: 248–251
8. White D K, Selinger L R, Miller A S, Behr M M, Damm D D.

Primary angioleiomyoma of the mandible. J Oral Maxillofac Surg 1985: 43: 640–644
9. Tomoda K, Iyama K. A case of intraosseous angioleiomyoma. Acta Orthop Scand 1992: 63: 568–570
10. Evans D M, Sanerkin N G. Primary leiomyosarcoma of bone. J Pathol Bacteriol 1965: 90: 348–350
11. Jundt G, Moll C, Nidecker A, Schilt R, Remagen W. Primary leiomyosarcoma of bone: report of eight cases. Hum Pathol 1994: 25: 1205–1212
12. Wang T Y, Erlandson R A, Marcove R C, Huvos A G. Primary leiomyosarcoma of bone. Arch Pathol Lab Med 1980: 104: 100–104
13. Sanerkin N G. Primary leiomyosarcoma of the bone and its comparison with fibrosarcoma. Cancer 1979: 44: 1375–1387
14. Overgaard J, Fredericksen P, Helmig O, Jensen O M. Primary leiomyosarcoma of bone. Cancer 1977: 39: 1664–1671
15. Von Hochstetter A R, Eberle H, Ruttner J R. Primary leiomyosarcoma of extragnathic bones. Cancer 1984: 53: 2194–2200
16. Abdelwahab I F, Hermann G, Kenan S, Klein M J, Lewis M M.

Case report 794. Primary leiomyosarcoma of the right femur. Skeletal Radiol 1993: 22: 379–381

17. Myers J L, Arocho J, Bernreuter W, Dunham W, Mazur M T. Leiomyosarcoma of bone. Cancer 1991: 67: 1051–1056

18. Berlin Ö, Angervall L, Kindblom L G, Berlin I C, Stener B. Primary leiomyosarcoma of bone. Skeletal Radiol 1987: 16: 364–376

19. Kawai T, Suzuki M, Mukai M, Hiroshima K, Shinmei M. Primary leiomyosarcoma of bone. An immunohistochemical and ultrastructural study. Arch Pathol Lab Med 1983: 107: 433–437

20. Abdelwahab I F, Kenan S, Hermann G, Klein M J, Lewis M M. Radiation-induced leiomyosarcoma. Skeletal Radiol 1995: 24: 81–83

21. Guse T R, Weis L D. Leiomyosarcoma of the femur in a patient with a history of retinoblastoma. J Bone Joint Surg (Am) 1994: 76: 904–906

22. Marymont J V, Clanton T O. Leiomyosarcoma of the os calcis. Foot Ankle 1990: 10: 239–242

23. Lo T H, Van Rooij W J, Teepen J L, Verhagen I T. Primary leiomyosarcoma of the spine. Neuroradiology 1995: 37: 465–467

24. Young C L, Wold L E, McLeod R A, Sim F H. Primary leiomyosarcoma of bone. Orthopedics 1988: 11: 615–618

25. Angervall L, Berlin O, Kindblom L G, Stener B. Primary leiomyosarcoma of bone: a study of five cases. Cancer 1980: 46: 1270–1279

26. Kameda N, Kagesawa M, Hiruta N, Akima M, Ohki M, Matsumoto T. Primary leiomyosarcoma of bone. Acta Pathol Jpn 1987: 37: 291–303

27. Meister P, Konrad E, Gokel J M, Remberger K. Case report 59. Leiomyosarcoma of the humerus. Skeletal Radiol 1978: 2: 265–267

28. Shamsuddin A K, Reyes F, Harvey J W, Toker C. Primary leiomyosarcoma of bone. Hum Pathol 1980: 11(suppl): 581–583

29. Trojani M, Coquet M, Peres P, Coindre J M, Ragni R, Meuge-Moraw C. Leiomyosarcome primitif de l'os. Arch Anat Cytol Pathol 1982: 30: 197–201

30. Gould V E, Patel N S, Dardi L E, Memoli V A. Painful lytic lesion of the left femur in an adult male. Ultrastruct Pathol 1982: 3: 301–307

31. Eady J L, McKinney J D, McDonald E C. Primary leiomyosarcoma of bone. J Bone Joint Surg (Am) 1987: 69: 287–289

32. Young M P, Freemont A J. Primary leiomyosarcoma of bone. Histopathology 1991: 19: 257–262

33. Fornasier V L, Paley D. Leiomyosarcoma in bone: primary or secondary? Skeletal Radiol 1983: 10: 147–153

34. Deb H K, Kundu A. Rhabdomyosarcoma of tibia. J Indian Med Assoc 1982: 78: 117–118

35. Lamovec J, Zidar A, Bracko M, Golouh R. Primary bone sarcoma with rhabdomyosarcomatous component. Pathol Res Pract 1994: 190: 51–60

36. Hai-Shan Y, Gee W Q, Gee C W et al. X-ray diagnosis of primary rhabdomyosarcoma of long bone. Chin J Radiol 1989: 23: 165–167

37. Pasquel P M, Levet S N, De Leon B. Primary rhabdomyosarcoma of bone. J Bone Joint Surg (Am) 1976: 58: 1176–1178

38. Hsueh S, Hsih S N, Kuo T T. Primary rhabdomyosarcoma of long bone. Orthopedics 1986: 9: 705–707

39. Rashid A, Dickersin G R, Rosenthal D I, Mankin H, Rosenberg AE. Rhabdomyosarcoma of the long bone in an adult. Int J Surg Pathol 1994: 1: 253–260

40. Lucas D R, Ryan J R, Zalupski M M, Gross M L, Ravindranath Y, Ortman B. Primary embryonal rhabdomyosarcoma of long bone. Am J Surg Pathol 1996: 20: 239–244

41. Oda Y, Tsuneyoshi M, Hashimoto H et al. Primary rhabdomyosarcoma of the iliac bone in an adult: a case mimicking fibrosarcoma. Virchows Arch A Pathol Anat Histopathol 1993: 423: 65–69

42. Ghosez J P, Himmer O, Lootvoet L, Beugnies A, Devyver B. Rhabdomyosarcome osseux primitif. A propos d'une localisation vertebrale. Rev Chir Orthop Reparatrice Appar Mot 1993: 79: 70–73

43. Ruymann F B, Newton W A, Jr, Ragab A H, Donaldson M H, Foulkes M. Bone marrow metastases at diagnosis in children and adolescents with rhabdomyosarcoma. Cancer 1984: 53: 368–373

44. Nunez C, Abboud S L, Lemon N C, Kemp J A. Ovarian rhabdomyosarcoma presenting as leukemia. Cancer 1983: 52: 297–300

45. Almanaseer I Y, Trujillo Y P, Taxy J B, Okuno T. Systemic rhabdomyosarcoma with diffuse bone marrow involvement. Am J Clin Pathol 1984: 82: 349–353

46. Cho K R, Olson J L, Epstein J I. Primitive rhabdomyosarcoma presenting with diffuse bone marrow involvement. An immunohistochemical and ultrastructural study. Mod Pathol 1988: 1: 23–28

47. Henderson D W, Raven J L, Pollard J A, Walters M N. Bone marrow metastases in disseminated alveolar rhabdomyosarcoma: case report with ultrastructural study and review. Pathology 1976: 8: 329–341

24

Schwannoma

M. Forest

INTRODUCTION AND CLINICAL DATA

Schwannoma, also called neurilemmoma or neurinoma, is a benign tumor of nerve sheath origin with a very low incidence in bone,[1,2] accounting for less than 0.2% of all bone tumors.

Patient age ranges from the second to the sixth decades of life, with no sex predilection[3] or a slight predominance of females in some series.

Clinical symptoms are localized pain or tenderness,[4] localized swelling or even a pathologic fracture. In vertebral locations, early compression of the spinal cord may occur. In the sacrum, despite the large size and the bone destruction, neurologic deficits are not significant.[5]

Neurofibromatosis can induce secondary erosion of bone by the hyperplasia of peripheral nerves[6] but schwannomas of bone associated with neurofibromatosis are uncommon.[7,8]

A schwannoma, usually solitary, may appear as an extraosseous tumor eroding bone or it may be located close to the nutrient canal with a dumbbell-shaped appearance, but most tumors are centrally located in bone.[3,8,9]

SKELETAL LOCATION

Any bone may be involved, but the mandible is the most commonly affected site, followed by the sacrum (Figs 24.1–24.6) and humerus.[5,10–15] Other reported locations are the vertebral bodies,[16–18] femur, tibia, ulna, radius (Figs 24.7, 24.8), fibula, patella, scapula, pubis and even the small bones of the hands[20,21] (Schajowicz 1994).

IMAGING

The tumors are virtually always lytic, with a narrow zone of transition.[22] Some may exhibit a sclerotic border while others may expand the bone with cortical thinning[3] or cortical erosion, but without periosteal new bone formation. Huge lesions are found in the sacrum.

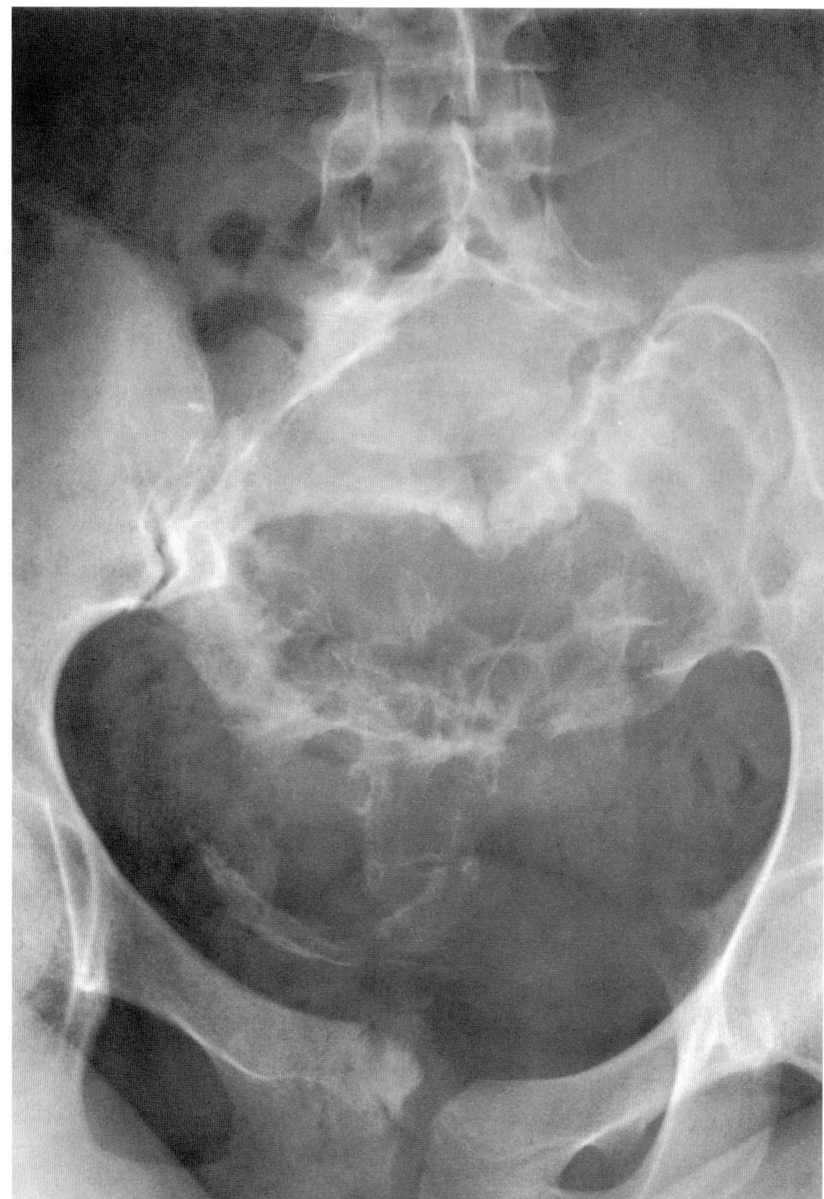

Fig. 24.1 Schwannoma of the sacrum with a faint peripheral shell of reactive bone.

The well-delineated radiolucent areas on MRI present as a mass isointense with the nerve on T1 and T2-weighted images or a hyperintense signal on T2-weighted images.[14]

GROSS PATHOLOGY

The tumor is well circumscribed and pseudoencapsulated, appearing as a firm gray or yellowish tissue, with hemorrhages or cyst formation,[3] especially in old schwannomas also exhibiting calcified areas.[5]

In the sacrum, the huge expanding mass may induce erosion of the anterior cortex and involvement of the retrorectal space, without periosteal reaction.[10,11]

It has been suggested that schwannomas are more prone to develop in nerves running for a long distance in bone (mandible, sacrum),[9] but in some cases, there is no direct continuity between the tumors and the nerve trunks.[3]

HISTOPATHOLOGY

Schwannomas in bone have the usual Antoni A or B pattern (Figs 24.9–24.16). Bland compact spindle cells with twisted nuclei and indistinct cytoplasmic borders are arranged in prominent nuclear palissading, with Verocay bodies and thick-walled blood vessels. Mitotic activity is absent or very sparse. In the type B pattern, the tumor is hypocellular with an edematous fibrocollagenous tissue.

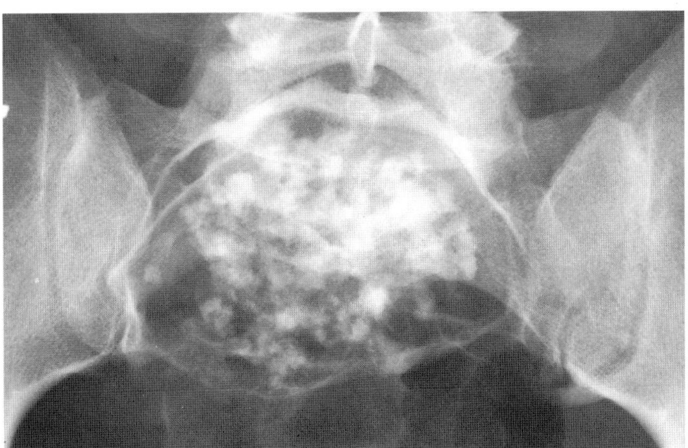

Fig. 24.2

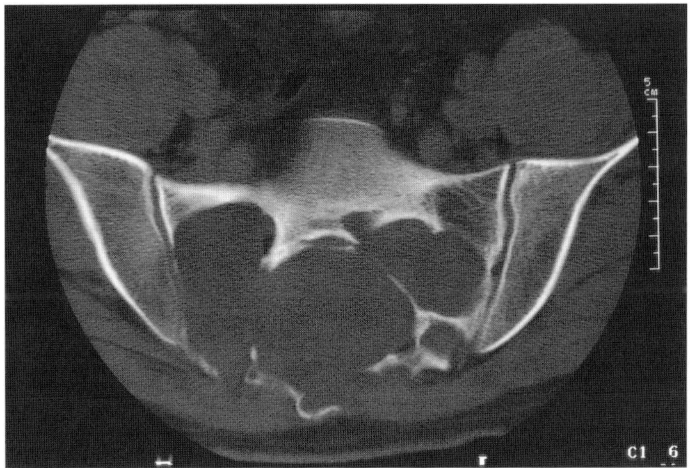

Fig. 24.4

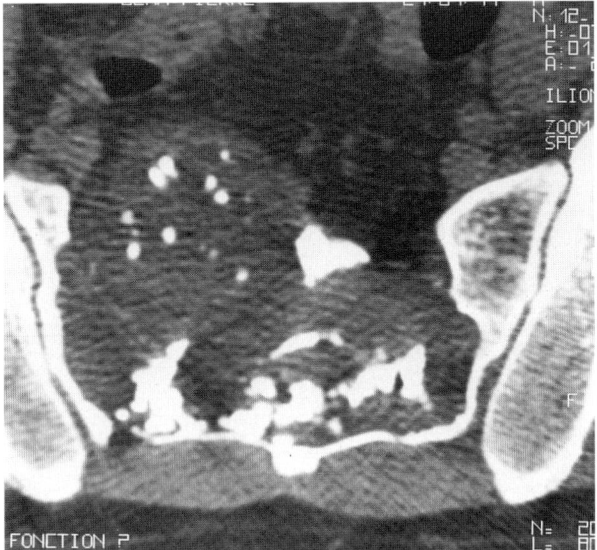

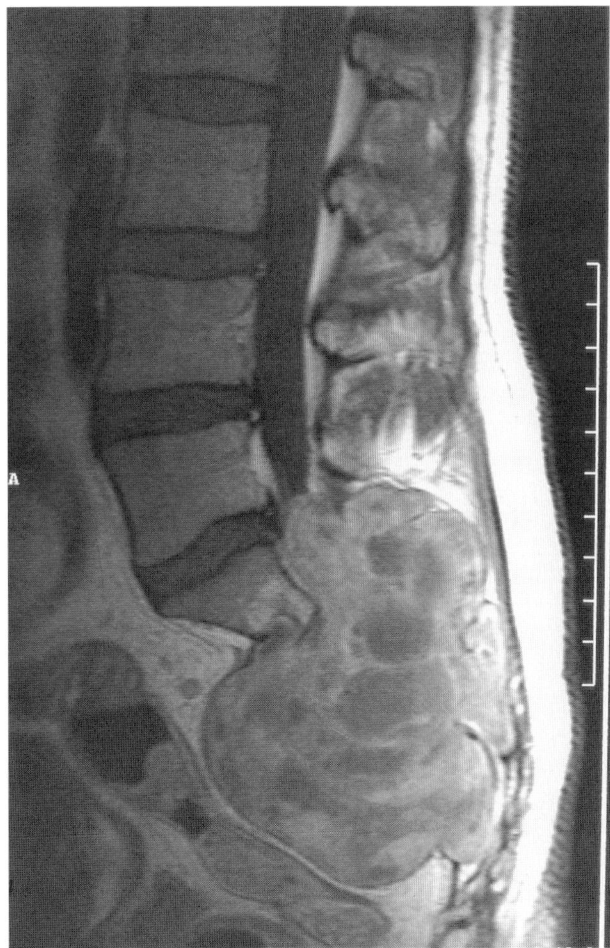

Fig. 24.5

Figs 24.4–24.6 Schwannoma of the sacrum appearing as a lytic lesion on CT scan and demonstrating fluid–fluid levels on MRI.

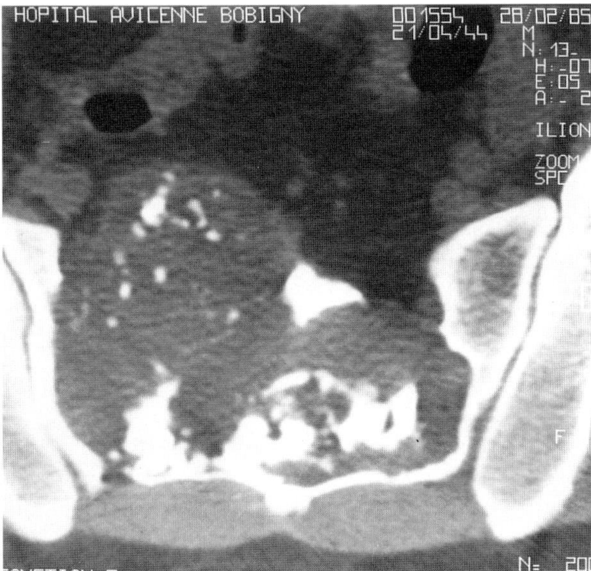

Fig. 24.3

Figs 24.2, 24.3 Unusual calcifications of fat and necrotic areas in a schwannoma of the sacrum.

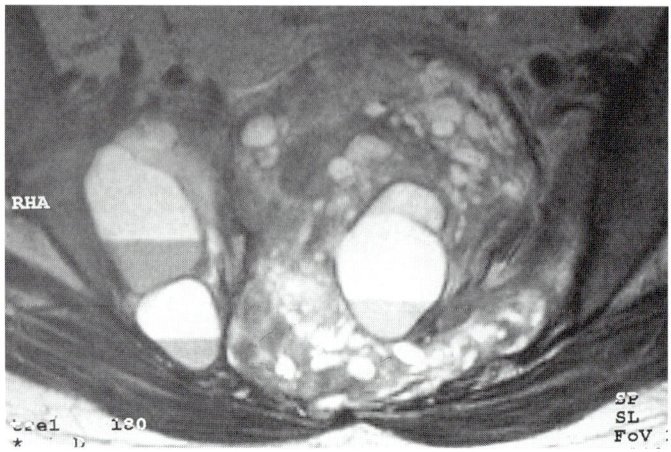

Fig. 24.6

Variable numbers of histiocytes, hemosiderin-laden or foamy macrophages, lymphocytes and mast cells may be found.[3] Microcyst formation is prominent in large lesions, especially in the sacrum.[11,14]

Some tumors may exhibit a high degree of cellularity or cellular pleomorphism, with hyperchromatic nuclei, in response to degenerative changes.[8,9]

IMMUNOHISTOCHEMISTRY

All tumors are immunoreactive for S-100 protein and vimentin. Most are positive with Leu-7 (CD57) and a few for the glial fibrillary acidic protein.

ELECTRON MICROSCOPY

Schwannomas in bone exhibit the same ultrastructural features as their soft tissue counterparts.[3,5] Spindle cells have an irregularly shaped nucleus, with prominent nuclear invaginations and a single nucleolus. Abundant thin cytoplasmic processes are distributed in a parallel arrangement. The cytoplasmic membrane is coated by amorphous bands of basal lamina. A long spacing collagen is found in the extracellular spaces.

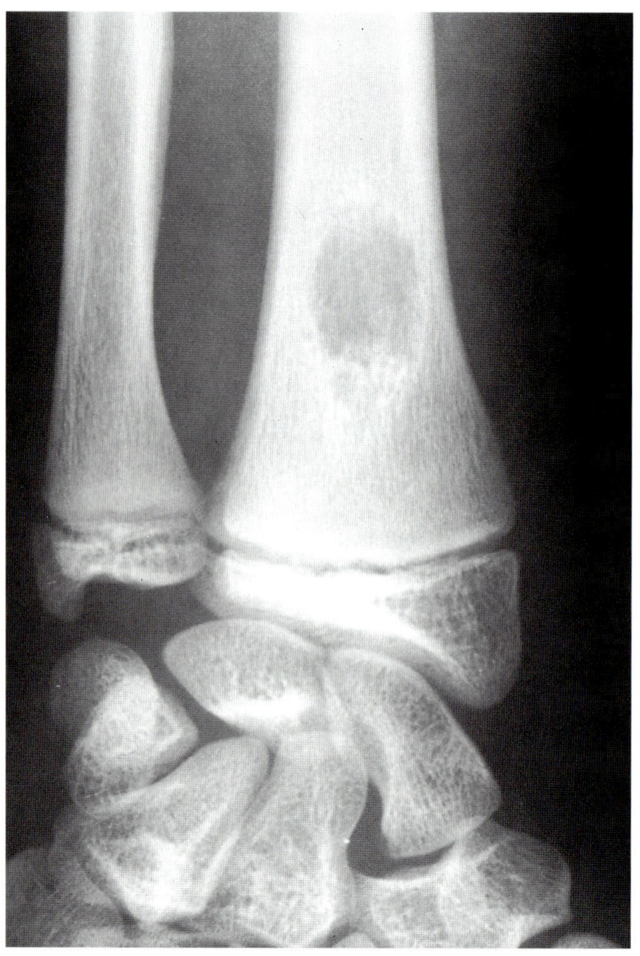

Fig. 24.7

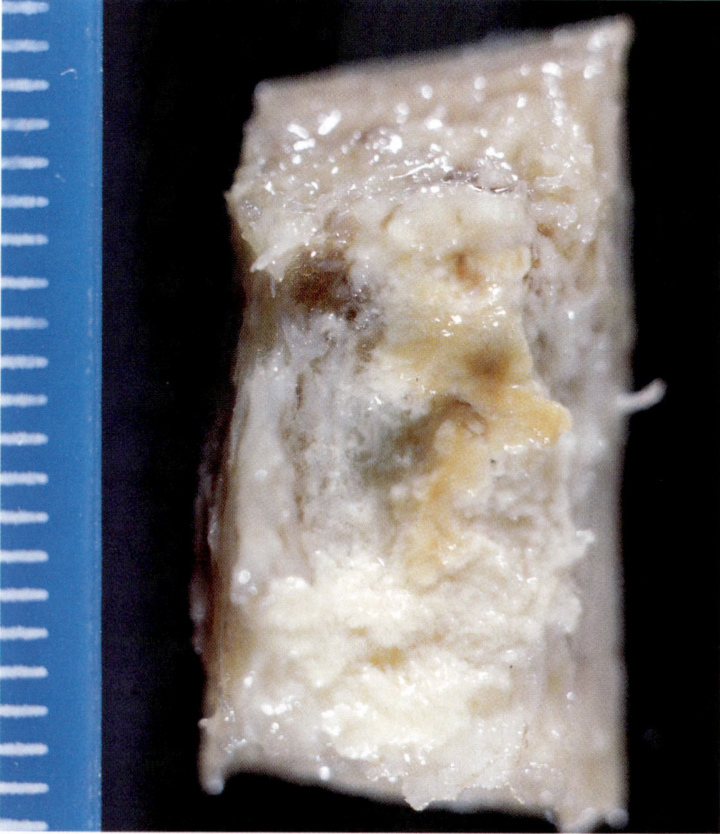

Fig. 24.8

Figs 24.7, 24.8 Schwannoma of the radius.

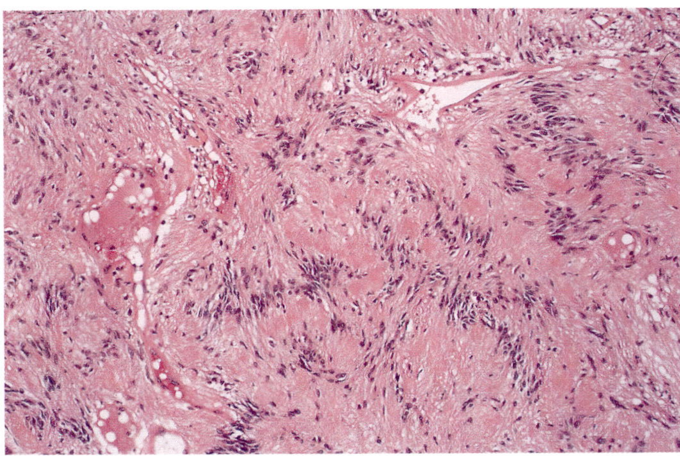

Fig. 24.9 Schwannoma of the sacrum: spindle cells with nuclear palissading.

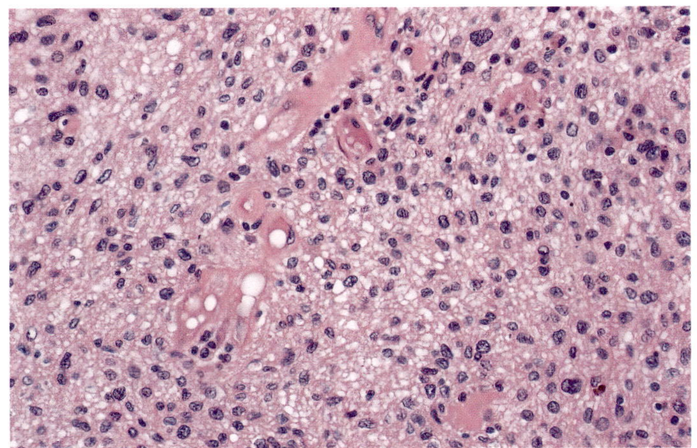

Fig. 24.10 Schwannoma of the sacrum: oval or rounded nuclei and lipid droplets.

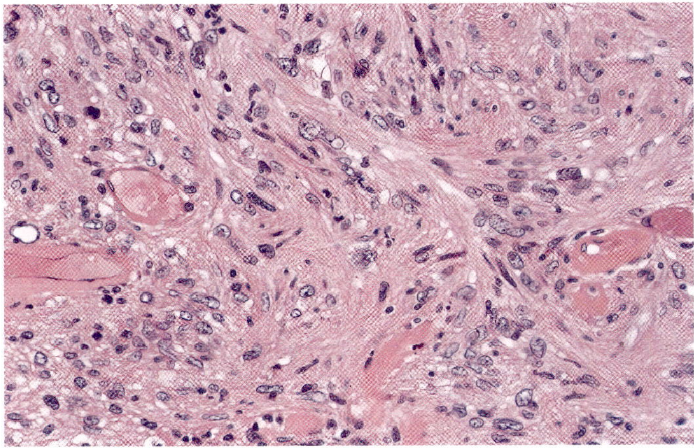

Fig. 24.11 Schwannoma of the sacrum: slight nuclear irregularities.

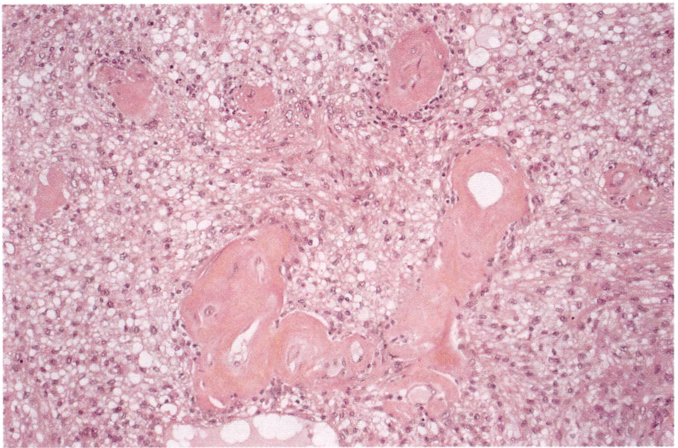

Fig. 24.12

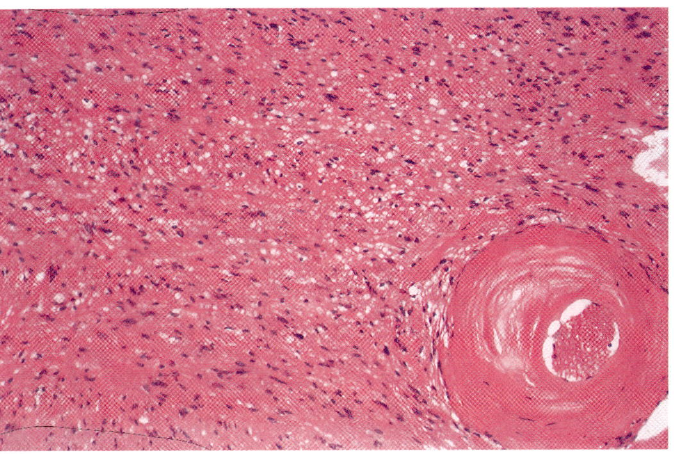

Fig. 24.13

Figs 24.12, 24.13 Schwannoma of the sacrum: hyalinized vessels.

COURSE, PROGNOSIS AND TREATMENT

Excision or thorough curettage appears to be the appropriate therapy, with very rare recurrences. However, in the sacrum, a complete surgical resection has been advocated to prevent local recurrences which may be as high as 54% of cases.[5,10,14]

DIFFERENTIAL DIAGNOSIS

An uncommon variant is the melanotic or melanocytic schwannoma, described in the ilium.[23] The highly pigmented brown tumor is composed of plump spindle cells with a granular eosinophilic cytoplasm and a centrally located nucleus; cells are arranged in compact interlacing fascicles, with a vague nuclear palisading. The abundant finely granular brown intracytoplasmic pigment is made of melanin and hemosiderin. Laminated calcified concretions resembling psammoma bodies are found.

The tumor cells are S-100 protein, vimentin and HMB45 positive. Ultrastructurally, the bipolar spindle

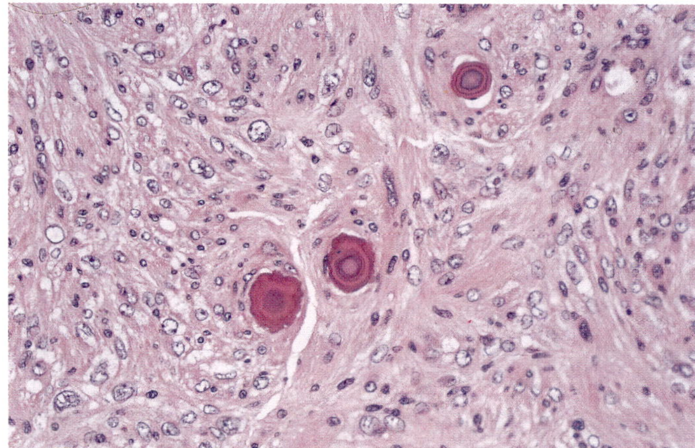

Fig. 24.14

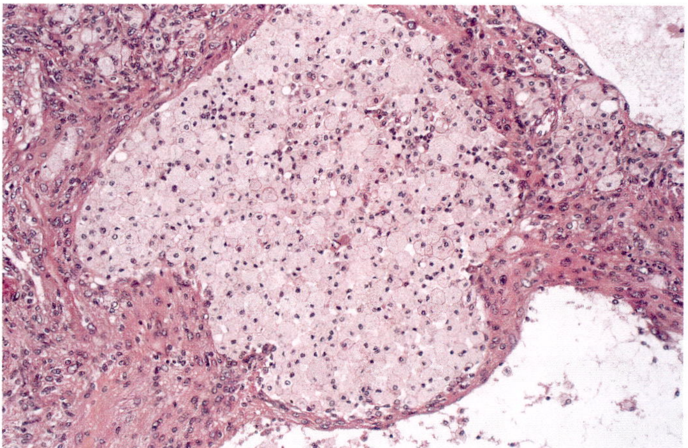

Fig. 24.15

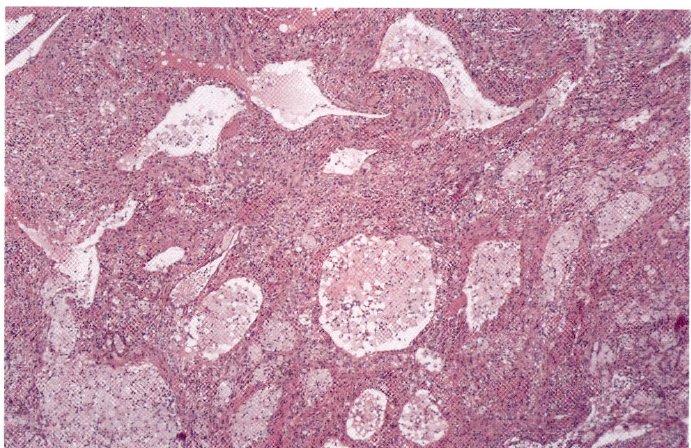

Fig. 24.16

Figs 24.14–24.16 Schwannomas of the sacrum. Secondary changes: microcalcifications, lipid-laden macrophages and microcystic formation.

cells have slender interdigitating cytoplasmic processes and a basal lamina. Nuclei are irregularly shaped; numerous cells exhibit melanosomes or degenerative changes of the mitochondria.[23] Melanotic schwannoma may be part of a complex familial syndrome (Carney syndrome).

Most of the neurofibromas in bone are associated with the lesions of neurofibromatosis; spindle-shaped or stellate cells with elongated nuclei are associated with an edema-tous stroma staining positively for mucopolysaccharides and containing bundles of collagen fibers.

Intraosseous malignant peripheral nerve sheath tumors have been reported in the femur, ulna and humerus.[24] Spindle or polygonal cells with an eosinophilic cytoplasm are distributed in myxoid areas, demonstrating a nuclear pleomorphism and a mitotic activity. Tumor cells are immunoreactive for S-100 protein and neuron-specific enolase. On ultrastructural examination, mesenchymal cells exhibit a perineural differentiation.

Only one case of juxtacortical malignant schwannoma has been described in a femoral location,[25] with no clinical symptoms of neurofibromatosis but presenting osteoid, chondroid and rhabdoid tumoral areas.

Ganglioneuromas are slow-growing tumors which may invade bone in the lumbosacral region or sacrum.[26–28] Mature ganglion cells have a pink cytoplasm and one or more nuclei with prominent nucleoli. Nissl granules are found in large cells. Ganglion cells are associated with coarse interlacing fascicles of Schwann cells. Ultrastructural findings are characteristic, combining neurofilaments and microtubules with dense-core vesicles.

REFERENCES

1. Samter T G, Vellios F, Shafer W G. Neurilemmoma of bone. Radiology 1960: 75: 215–222
2. Wirth W A, Bray C B Jr. Intraosseous neurilemmoma. J Bone Joint Surg (Am) 1977: 59: 252–255
3. De La Monte S M, Dorfman H D, Chandra R, Malawer M. Intraosseous schwannoma: histologic features, ultrastructure and review of the literature. Hum Pathol 1984: 15: 551–558
4. Dalinka M K, Cannino C, Patchewsky A S, Romisher G P. Case report 12. Intraosseous neurilemmoma of the tibia. Skeletal Radiol 1976: 1: 123–124
5. Turk P S, Peters N, Libbey P, Wanebo H J. Diagnosis and management of giant intrasacral schwannoma. Cancer 1992: 70: 2650–2657
6. Hunt J C, Pugh D G. Skeletal lesions in neurofibromatosis. Radiology 1961: 76: 1–20
7. Morrison M J, Ivins J C. Case report 47. Benign intraosseous neurilemmoma of the femur. Skeletal Radiol 1978: 2: 177–178
8. Fawcett K J, Dahlin D C. Neurilemmoma of bone. Am J Clin Pathol 1967: 47: 759–766
9. Gordon E J. Solitary intraosseous neurilemmoma of the tibia. Clin Orthop 1976: 117: 271–282
10. Abernathey C D, Onofrio B M, Scheithauer B, Pairolero P C, Shives T C. Surgical management of giant sacral schwannomas. J Neurosurg 1986: 65: 286–295
11. Abdelwahab I F, Hermann G, Stollman A, Wolfe D, Lewis M, Zawin J. Case report 564. Giant intraosseous schwannoma. Skeletal Radiol 1989: 18: 466–469

12. Santi M D, Mitsunaga M M, Lockett J L. Total sacrectomy of a giant sacral schwannoma. Clin Orthop 1993: 294: 285–289

13. Salvant J B Jr, Young H F. Giant intrasacral schwannoma: an unusual cause of lumbosacral radiculopathy. Surg Neurol 1994: 41: 411–413

14. Aaron A D, Nelson M C, Layug J M, Lage J M. Intraforaminal schwannoma of the sacrum. Skeletal Radiol 1995: 24: 458–461

15. Ortolan G, Sola C A, Gruenberg M F, Vazquez F C. Giant sacral schwannoma. Spine 1996: 21: 522–526

16. Dickson J H, Waltz T A, Fechner R E. Intraosseous neurilemmoma of the third lumbar vertebra. J Bone Joint Surg (Am) 1971: 53: 349–355

17. Hibri N S, El-Khouri G Y. Case report 113. Intraosseous neurilemmoma of vertebral body of T6. Skeletal Radiol 1980: 5: 112–115

18. Wells F, Thomas T L, Matthewson M H, Holmes A E. Neurilemmoma of the thoracic spine. Spine 1982: 7: 66–70

19. Divertie M B, Dahlin D C. Neurilemmoma of rib. Dis Chest 1963: 44: 635–637

20. Seth H N, Rao B D, Kathpalia P M. Neurilemmoma of bone. J Bone Joint Surg (Br) 1963: 45: 382–383

21. Lewis H H, Kobrin H I. Neurilemmoma of the first metacarpal. Clin Orthop 1972: 82: 67–69

22. Agha F P, Lilienfeld R M. Roentgen features of osseous neurilemmoma. Radiology 1972: 102: 325–326

23. Myers J L, Bernreuter W, Dunham W. Melanotic schwannoma of bone: clinicopathologic, immunohistochemical and ultrastructural features of a rare primary bone tumor. Am J Clin Pathol 1990: 93: 424–429

24. Bullock M J, Bedard Y C, Bell R S, Kandel R. Intraosseous malignant peripheral nerve sheath tumor. Arch Pathol Lab Med 1995: 119: 367–370

25. Andrew S M, Freemont A J. Juxtacortical malignant schwannoma with heterologous elements. Histopathology 1993: 23: 280–282

26. Wilber M C, Woodcock J A. Ganglioneuromata in bone. J Bone Joint Surg (Am) 1957: 39: 1385–1388

27. Leeson M C, Hite M. Ganglioneuroma of the sacrum. Clin Orthop 1989: 246: 102–105

28. Richardson R R, Reyes R, Sanchez R A, Torres H, Vela S. Ganglioneuroma of the sacrum. Spine 1986: 11: 87–89

25

Myxoma and xanthoma

M. Forest

FIBROMYXOMAS OR MYXOMAS OF BONE

These rare tumors are composed of mesenchymal stellate or spindle-shaped cells, with an abundant myxoid ground substance.[1-3]

The age range of the patients is wide, but the average age is 50 years, with no sex predominance. Pain is the main clinical symptom.

One-third of cases are located in the femur, followed by the pelvic bones, the tibia, ulna and various other locations such as metatarsals or phalanges. A periosteal tumor on the shaft of the femur has been reported.[4]

On imaging, the tumor is metaphyseally located in long bones but may extend to the epiphysis or diaphysis. The lesion is lytic and well circumscribed; some tumors may expand the cortex which can eventually be destroyed.

Grossly, the tumor is soft, translucent and mucoid or may have fibrous and rubbery areas or cyst formation.

Histologically, the stromal cells are uniform, without mitotic activity. They are stellate or spindle shaped and the nucleus is small and sometimes hyperchromatic;[5] the cytoplasm may be foamy or vacuolated. The loose myxoid stroma is poorly vascularized and contains mucopolysaccharides; it stains for mucin. Some tumors exhibit areas of collagenization, calcifications[6-9] or some reactive woven bone.[10] A secondary aneurysmal bone cyst formation has been reported.[6]

The treatment is curettage or en bloc excision if there is extension into the soft tissues.[7]

Many reported cases represent chondromyxoid fibromas[11] which are the main diagnostic problem if one rules out some intraosseous ganglions, which are usually limited by a fibrous capsule, and also involuted forms of fibrous dysplasia.[12] Chondromyxoid fibromas involve younger patients, are more eccentrically located in long bones and exhibit sclerotic borders; histologically a lobular pattern is associated with a peripheral condensation of cells and very cellular fibrous septa. A chondroid matrix and 'bizarre cells' are not found in fibromyxomas or myxomas.

XANTHOMAS OF BONE

These tumors, composed of lipid-laden cells, are a somewhat disputed entity and Fechner & Mills suggest that xanthomas or fibroxanthomas are within the range of some benign fibrous histiocytomas with a major component of foam cells.

In the most important series of these unusual tumors, men are mainly involved,[13] clinical symptoms are pain, neurological symptoms or a pathologic fracture.[14] Some tumors are incidental findings. They have been reported in association with hyperlipoproteinemia.[14–18]

Main locations are the ilium and the femur, followed by ribs, skull, vertebral bodies, humerus, tibia and small bones of the hands.

On imaging, the lesions are well-defined, round or oval radiolucent areas; some may be expansile or with distinct sclerotic margins.

Grossly, the lesional tissue is soft, granular and yellow; it may contain cysts with fluid.[13]

Histologically, xanthoma cells may be associated with giant cells, cholesterol clefts and iron pigment in fibrous areas.[13,14]

The treatment is complete or even partial removal of the lesion.[13]

As for the differential diagnosis, many more common lesions have to be excluded, including xanthogranulomatous osteomyelitis, end stages of eosinophilic granulomas and involuted forms of fibrous dysplasia. The diagnosis may be quite difficult.

Rare cases of Erdheim–Chester disease usually exhibit a symmetrical involvement in long bones and histologically, chronic inflammatory cells, fibrosis and new bone formation.

Even rarer cases of Rosai–Dorfman disease in bone appear as ill-defined lesions which contain histiocytes with an abundant pale cytoplasm, phagocytosed lymphocytes or neutrophils, plasma cells and lymphocytes.

REFERENCES

1. Bauer W H, Harell A. Myxoma of bone. J Bone Joint Surg (Am) 1954: 36: 263–266
2. Soren A. Myxoma in bone. Clin Orthop 1964: 37: 145–150
3. McClure D K, Dahlin D C. Myxoma of bone. Mayo Clin Proc 1977: 52: 249–253
4. Chacha P B, Tan K K. Periosteal myxoma of the femur. J Bone Joint Surg (Am) 1972: 54: 1091–1094
5. Perou M L, Kolis J A, Zaeske E V, Borja S R. Myxoma of the toe. Cancer 1967: 20: 1030–1034
6. Marcove R C, Kambolis C, Bullough P G, Jaffe H L. Fibromyxoma of bone. Cancer 1964: 17: 1209–1213
7. Marcove R C, Lindeque B G, Huvos A G. Fibromyxoma of the bone. Surg Gynecol Obstet 1989: 169: 115–118
8. Adler C P. Fibromyxoma of the femoral neck. J Cancer Res Clin Oncol 1981: 101: 183–189
9. Abdelwahab I F, Hermann G, Klein M J, Kenan S, Lewis M M. Fibromyxoma of bone. Skeletal Radiol 1991: 20: 95–98
10. Goldman A B, Vigorita V J. Case report 245. Fibromyxoma of the femur. Skeletal Radiol 1983: 10: 197–200
11. Scaglietti O, Stringa G. Myxoma of bone in childhood. J Bone Joint Surg (Am) 1961: 43: 67–80
12. Caballes R L. Fibromyxoma of bone. Radiology 1979: 130: 97–99
13. Bertoni F, Unni K K, McLeod R A, Sim F H. Xanthoma of bone. Am J Clin Pathol 1988: 90: 377–384
14. Inserra S, Einhorn T A, Vigorita V J, Smith A G. Intraosseous xanthoma associated with hyperlipoproteinemia. Clin Orthop 1984: 187: 218–222
15. Siegelman S S, Schlossberg I, Becker N H, Sachs B A. Hyperlipoproteinemia with skeletal lesions. Clin Orthop 1972: 87: 228–232
16. Hamilton W C, Ramsey P L, Hanson S M, Schiff D C. Osseous xanthoma and multiple hand tumors as a complication of hyperlipidemia. J Bone Joint Surg (Am) 1975: 57: 551–553
17. Yaghmai I. Intra and extraosseous xanthomata associated with hyperlipidemia. Radiology 1978: 128: 49–54
18. Yokoyama K, Shinohara N, Wada K. Osseous xanthomatosis and a pathologic fracture in a patient with hyperlipidemia. Clin Orthop 1988: 236: 307–310

26

Hamartoma and mesenchymoma

M. Forest

MESENCHYMAL HAMARTOMA OF THE CHEST WALL

Vascular and cartilaginous hamartomas are rare benign lesions occurring in the chest wall of young male infants.[1–3] The tumors are present from birth and most are recognized within the first year.[4,5] Some are incidental findings while others present with a symptomless swelling or more rarely with respiratory distress.

The tumor, which may be bilateral or multicentric, is located in the central portion of one or more lateral ribs; bone is eroded, destroyed or enlarged by a well-delineated red-brown mass, up to 8 cm in diameter.[6] On section, the lobulated tumor contains fibrous tissue, small islands of cartilage and dilated spaces filled with blood.

Histologically, in some cases a bland spindle cell proliferation may mimic the features of a nodular fasciitis.[6] In the spindle cell stroma, numerous islands of mature hyalin cartilage exhibit focal chickenwire calcifications, similar to chondroblastoma,[6] or an epiphyseal cartilaginous plate-like pattern with calcification. Reactive new bone may have a prominent osteoblastic rim.[6] Cystic spaces have the structure of aneurysmal bone cysts.[5–7]

The spindle cell positivity for vimentin and α smooth muscle actin may suggest that the basic cell components are fibroblasts and myofibroblasts.[6] FVIIIRag immunostaining is negative in the aneurysmal bone cyst spaces.[8]

After an initial period of rapid growth, some lesions may reduce in size.[4] The treatment is surgical resection, with no recurrences or metastases.

FIBROCARTILAGINOUS MESENCHYMOMA OF BONE

This tumoral entity, which is somewhat debated, was described in 1984 from the study of cases of fibrous dysplasia, showing a peculiar clinical behavior, unusual radi-

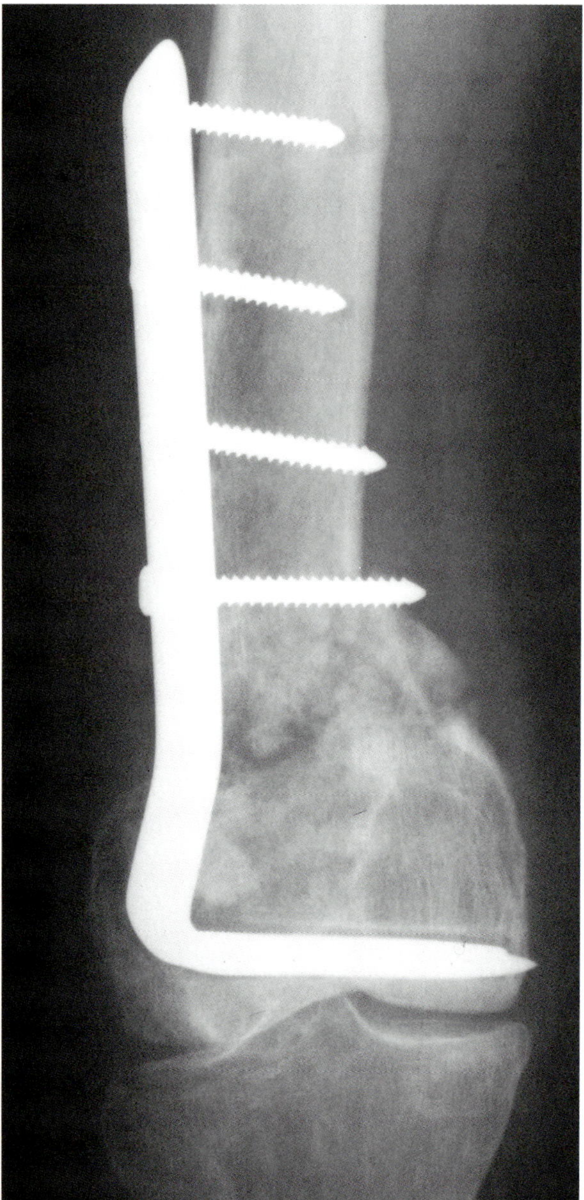

Fig. 26.1

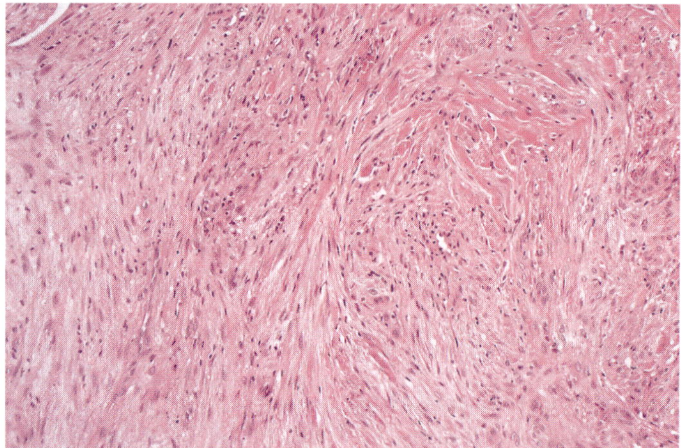

Fig. 26.2

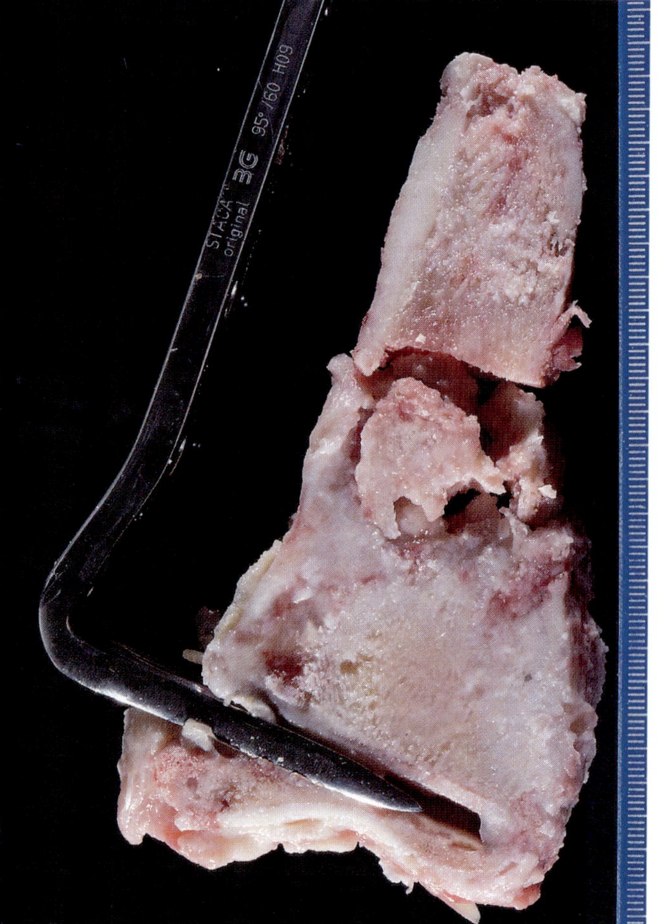

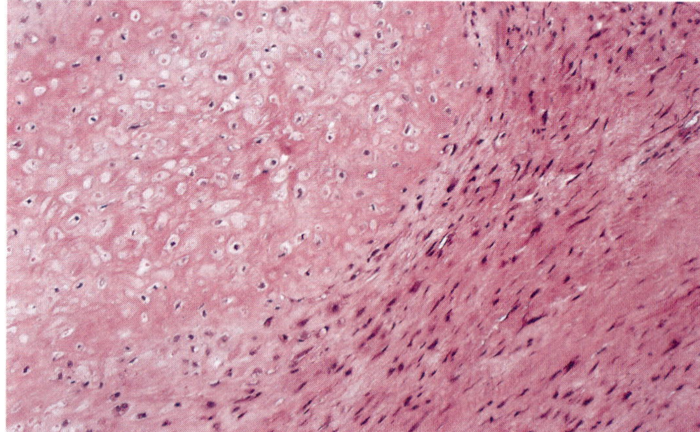

Fig. 26.4

Figs 26.1–26.4 So-called 'fibrocartilaginous mesenchymoma' of bone, with a pathologic fracture. A low-grade fibroblastic tumoral component is associated with islands of well-differentiated cartilage.

Fig. 26.3

ographic features and a low-grade malignant spindle cell component[9] (Figs 26.1–26.14).

Patients are young with a mean age of 13 years,[9] presenting with pain, swelling or both. One-third of cases involve the fibula;[10] other locations include the tibia, humerus, vertebra,[11] iliac bone, pubis, ribs and metatarsals.

In long bones, the lesion is metaphyseal, abutting the growth plate or the articular cartilage, predominantly lucent on X-ray or showing fuzzy or ring-like mineralization. The cortex may be thinned or destroyed and some tumors gain a considerable size.[10,12] There is no periosteal reaction.

Grossly, the tumor exhibits poorly defined fibrous tissue looking like a desmoplastic fibroma or a low-grade fibrosarcoma, but many cartilaginous islands are found, associated with eventual cyst formation.[9]

Histologically, spindle cells are distributed in bundles or fascicles, sometimes with heavy production of collagen. A slight nuclear irregularity or hyperchromatism can be found,[10,11] as well as a few mitoses. Reactive giant cells and aneurysmal bone cyst formation have been reported.[10] Well-circumscribed and usually prominent cartilage lobules display a pattern of long parallel columns with hypertrophic changes and enchondral ossification; some may have an irregular shape, but the appearance is that of an epiphyseal plate.[9]

An ultrastructural study has not been particularly helpful.[12]

In the few cases reported, the tumor appears to be only locally aggressive, with clinical behavior similar to that of a desmoplastic fibroma; that is, recurrence after intralesional excision but no metastatic potential.

We concur with Mirra in his belief that cartilage islands are remnants of the epiphyseal growth plate which have been displaced and grow into various tumors: desmoplastic fibroma, fibrous dysplasia or low-grade fibrosarcomas. All these lesions may well be differential diagnoses, if one accepts the much disputed concept of a fibrocartilaginous mesenchymoma.

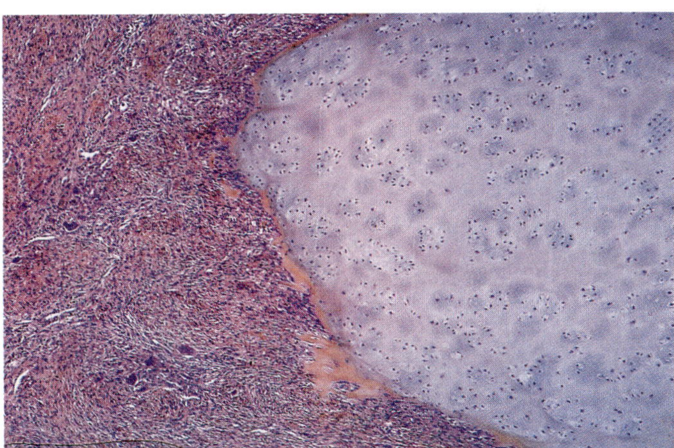

Fig. 26.6

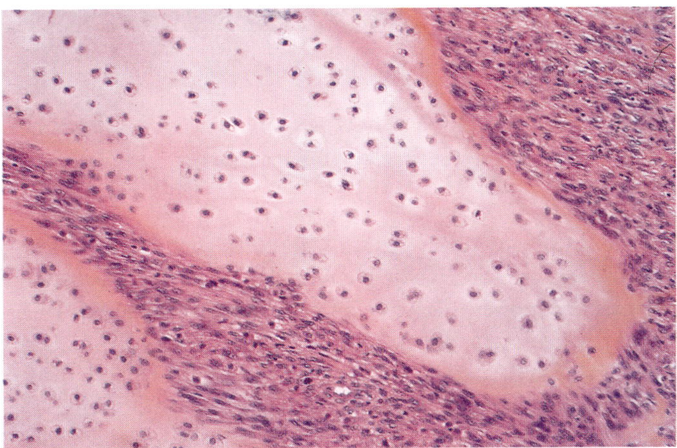

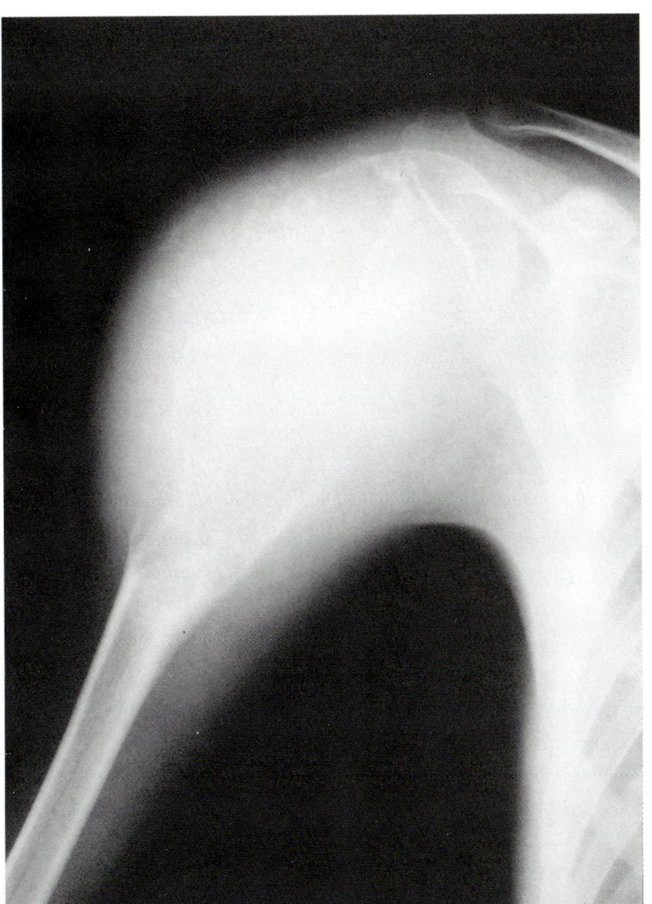

Fig. 26.5

Fig. 26.7

Figs 26.5–26.10 So-called 'fibrocartilaginous mesenchymoma' of bone in a humeral location. Wide areas of cartilage resembling a growth plate are embedded in and partially destroyed by a fibroblastic tumor (presumably a low-grade fibrosarcoma). (Fig. 26.5 courtesy of A. Jelthi, Rabat, Morocco.)

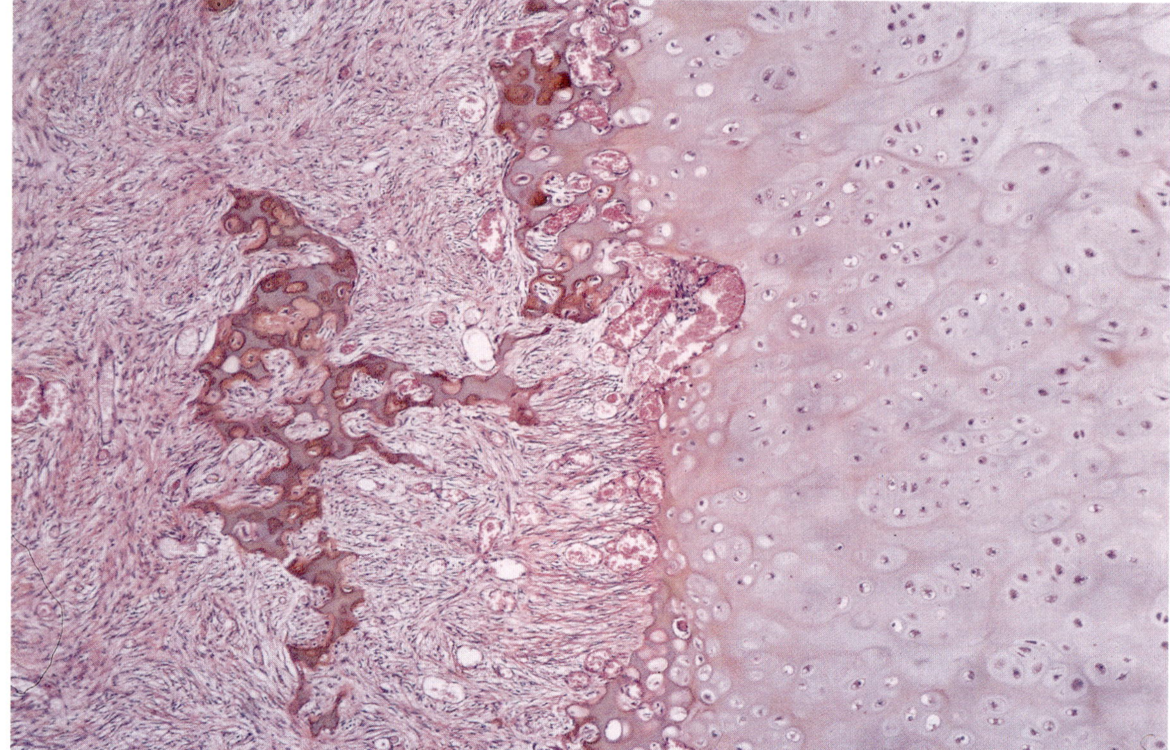

Fig. 26.8

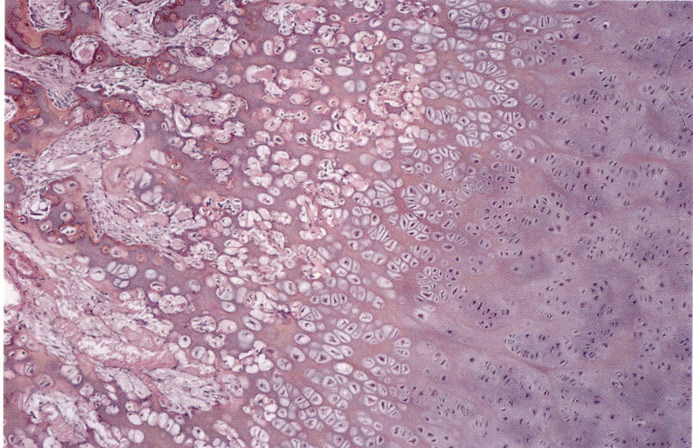

Fig. 26.9

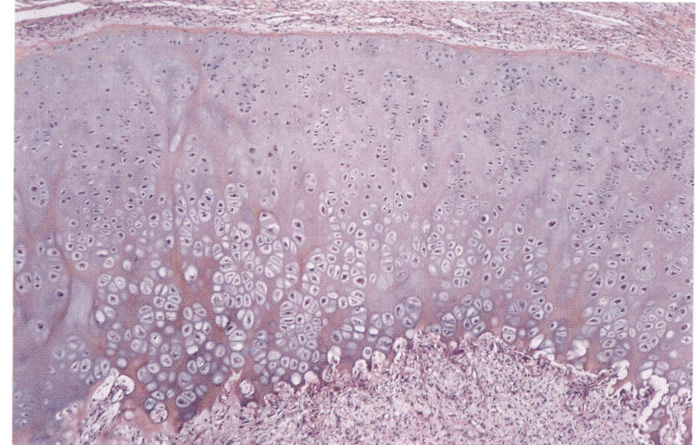

Fig. 26.10

MALIGNANT MESENCHYMOMA OF BONE

Primitive multipotential primary sarcomas of bone, with two or more unrelated tissue elements other than a fibrosarcomatous component, have been reported in two series[13,14] and in a few isolated case reports.

A well-differentiated cartilage component has been described with a less well-differentiated epithelial component.[15]

A tumor probably originating from multipotential cells has shown association of round cell areas resembling a lymphoma and areas of epithelial differentiation as well as osteosarcomatous foci.[16]

A very rare but more obvious malignant mesenchymoma is the osteoliposarcoma, first described by Schajowicz.[17] Only 12 cases have been reported.[18–24] However, some tumors described as liposarcomas may well represent osteoliposarcomas.[23]

These tumors are mostly located in the metaphysis of the long bones of the lower extremity. The lipoblastic component appears as a pleomorphic liposarcoma.

The clinical course is extremely rapid,[22] with early pulmonary metastases and a survival of less than 3 years.

Some exceedingly rare primary rhabdomyosarcomas of bone may also exhibit an osteosarcomatous component[23] and the differential diagnosis also includes dedifferentiated chondrosarcomas.[25,26]

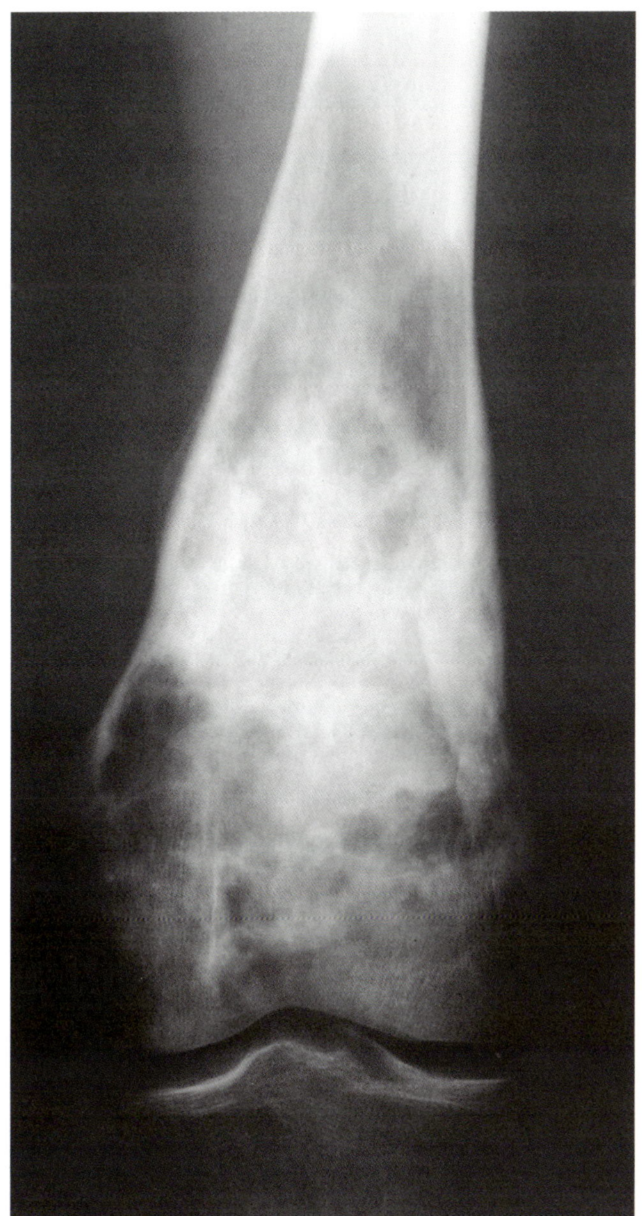

Fig. 26.11

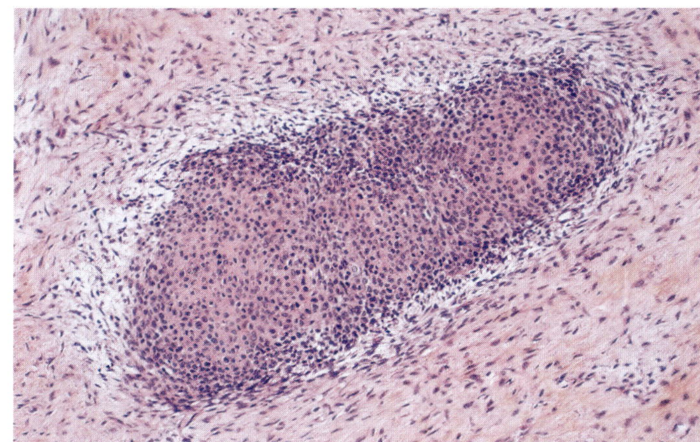

Fig. 26.13

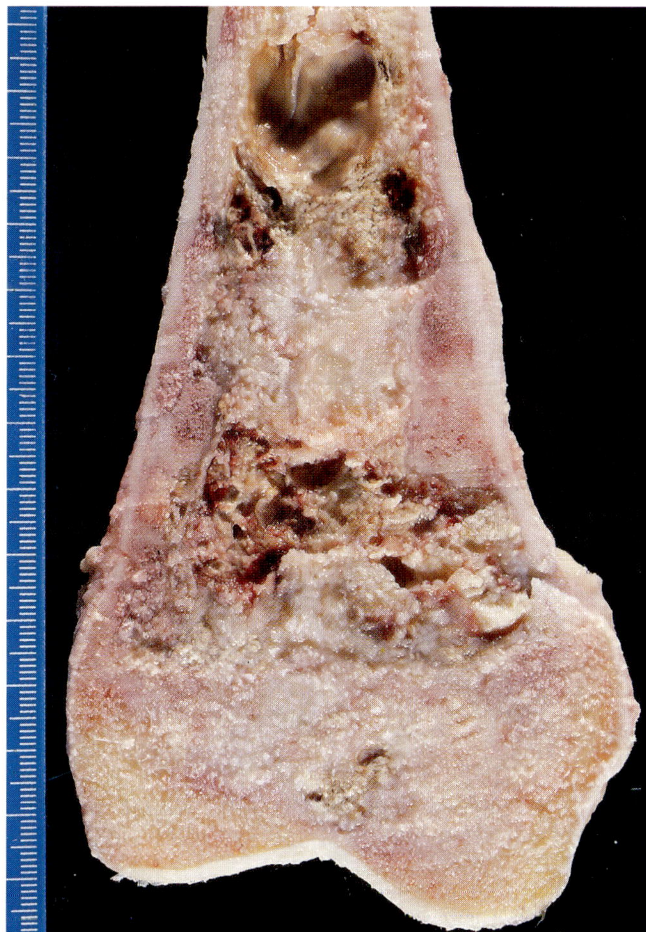

Fig. 26.12

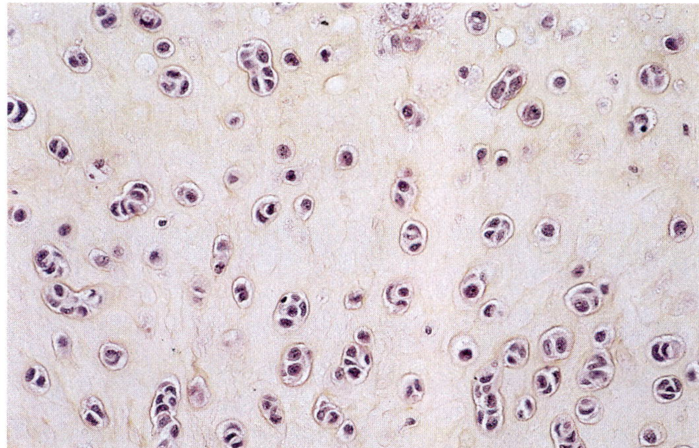

Fig. 26.14

Figs 26.11–26.14 Unusual low-grade fibroblastic sarcoma of the femur presenting numerous islands of immature cartilage.

REFERENCES

1. Campbell A N, Wagget J, Mott M G. Benign mesenchymoma of the chest wall in infancy. J Surg Oncol 1982: 21: 267–270
2. Cohen M C, Drut R, Garcia C, Kaschula R O. Mesenchymal hamartoma of the chest wall. Pediatr Pathol 1992: 12: 525–534
3. Dounies R, Chwals W J, Lally K P et al. Hamartomas of the chest wall in infants. Ann Thorac Surg 1994: 57: 868–875
4. Davies R I, Macloon J, Sloan J M. Vascular and cartilaginous hamartoma. Histopathology 1992: 20: 269–270
5. McCarthy E F, Dorfman H D. Vascular and cartilaginous hamartomas of the ribs in infancy with secondary aneurysmal bone cyst formation. Am J Surg Pathol 1980: 4: 247–253
6. Ayala A G, Ro J Y, Bolio-Solis A, Hernandez-Batres F, Eftekhari F, Edeiken J. Mesenchymal hamartoma of the chest wall in infants and children: a clinicopathological study of five patients. Skeletal Radiol 1993: 22: 569–576
7. McLeod R A, Dahlin D C. Hamartoma (mesenchymoma) of the chest wall in infancy. Radiology 1979: 131: 657–661
8. Odell J M, Benjamin D R. Mesenchymal hamartoma of the chest wall in infancy: natural history of two cases. Pediatr Pathol 1986: 5: 135–146
9. Dahlin D C, Bertoni F, Beabout J W, Campanacci M. Fibrocartilaginous mesenchymoma with low-grade malignancy. Skeletal Radiol 1984: 12: 263–269
10. Bulychova I V, Unni K K, Bertoni F, Beabout J W. Fibrocartilaginous mesenchymoma of bone. Am J Surg Pathol 1993: 17: 830–836
11. Gibson J N, Reid R, McMaster M J. Fibrocartilaginous mesenchymoma of the fifth lumbar vertebra treated by vertebrectomy. Spine 1994: 19: 1992–1997
12. Cozzutto C, Cornaglia-Ferraris P. Fibrocartilaginous mesenchymoma of bone. Pathol Res Pract 1991: 187: 279–283
13. Hutter R V, Foote F W Jr, Francis K C, Sherman R S. Primitive multipotential primary sarcoma of bone. Cancer 1966: 19: 1–25
14. Jacobson S A. Polyhistioma. A malignant tumor of bone and extraskeletal tissues. Cancer 1977: 40: 2116–2130
15. Ling L L, Steiner G C. Primary multipotential malignant neoplasm of bone. Chondrosarcoma associated with squamous cell carcinoma. Hum Pathol 1986: 17: 317–320
16. Frydman C P, Klein M J, Abdelwahab I F, Zwass A. Primitive multipotential primary sarcoma of bone. Mod Pathol 1991: 4: 768–772
17. Schajowicz F, Cuevillas A R, Silberman F S. Primary malignant mesenchymoma of bone. A new tumor entity. Cancer 1966: 19: 1423–1428
18. Ross C F, Hadfield G. Primary osteoliposarcoma of bone (malignant mesenchymoma). J Bone Joint Surg (Br) 1968: 50: 639–643
19. Bertoni F, Laus M. Primary malignant mesenchymoma of bone. Ital J Orthop Traumatol 1978: 4: 105–108
20. Cremer H, Koischwitz D, Tismer R. Primary osteoliposarcoma of bone. J Cancer Res Clin Oncol 1981: 101: 203–211
21. Downey E F Jr, Worsham G F, Brower A C. Liposarcoma of bone with osteosarcomatous foci. Skeletal Radiol 1982: 8: 47–50
22. Bosman C, Boldrini R, Guzzanti V. Primary osteoliposarcoma of bone. First observation in the pediatric age group. Appl Pathol 1988: 8: 56–60
23. Marcial-Seoane R A, Marcial-Seoane M A, Davila-Toro F J, Marcial-Rojas R A. Bone tumors of mixed origin: osteoliposarcoma and osteo-rhabdomyosarcoma. Bol Asoc Med PR 1990: 82: 378–393
24. Reijnierse M, Kroon H M, Van Der Heul R O, Mulder J D. Mesenchymoma of bone. J Bone Joint Surg (Am) 1993: 75: 112–115
25. Scheele P M Jr, Von Kuster L C, Krivchenia G 2nd. Primary malignant mesenchymoma of bone. Arch Pathol Lab Med 1990: 114: 614–617
26. Sathaphatayavongs B, Sirikulchayanonta V, Virat C I. Roentgenographic findings in malignant mesenchymoma of bone. J Med Assoc Thai 1987: 67: 678–684

Adamantinoma

M. Forest

INTRODUCTION AND CLINICAL DATA

Adamantinoma of long bones is a low-grade malignant tumor, presumably of epithelial origin and located predominantly in the tibia. Its name is based on histological features resembling those of an ameloblastoma of the jaws.[1]

About 300 cases have been reported and it accounts for 0.33–1% of all primary malignant bone tumors (Schajowicz 1994, Unni 1996).

There is a wide age range but most patients are in their second to fifth decades. About 3% of cases are found in children;[2] the mean age in one series was 29 years.[3] There is a slight male predominance.[4,5]

Pain and/or swelling may be present for years.[5–7] Pathologic fractures occur in 10–13% of cases,[3,5] more frequently in children.[8] Some cases may be associated with severe paraneoplastic hypercalcemia.[9,10]

A history of trauma is reported in many cases (from 28% to 57%), but usually the short interval between trauma and clinical symptoms excludes a causal relationship.[3] Rare cases have been described in association with Paget's disease or osteomyelitis.[3]

HISTOGENESIS

The most recent ultrastructural and immunohistochemical studies demonstrate the epithelial nature of the osseous tumor. In his original report in 1913, Fischer[1] suggested the role of misplaced nests of basal epithelium during embryonic development. A traumatic basis for such inclusions has also been put forward.[12–13] Some authors stress the link between the tibial location and the close relationship with the epidermis or epidermal anlages.[14–15]

There are many morphologic, ultrastructural, histochemical and immunohistochemical similarities with cutaneous eccrine carcinomas[16,17] and Lichtenstein has firmly stressed the resemblance with basal cell carcinomas, as

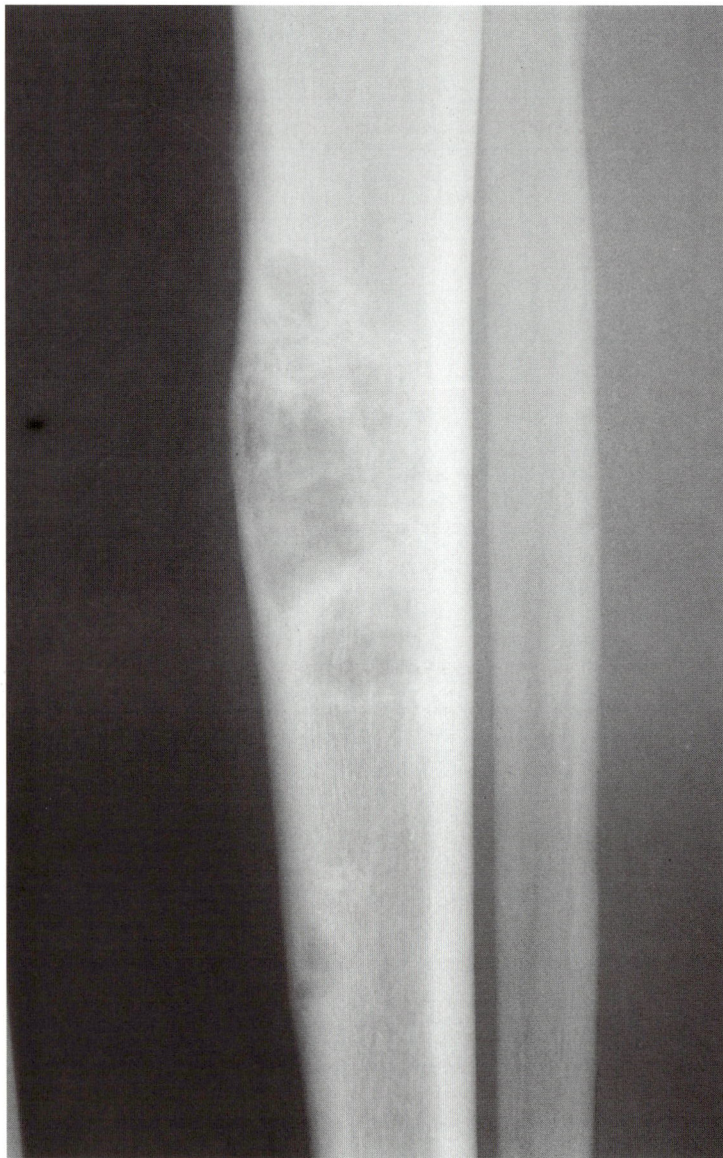

Fig. 27.1

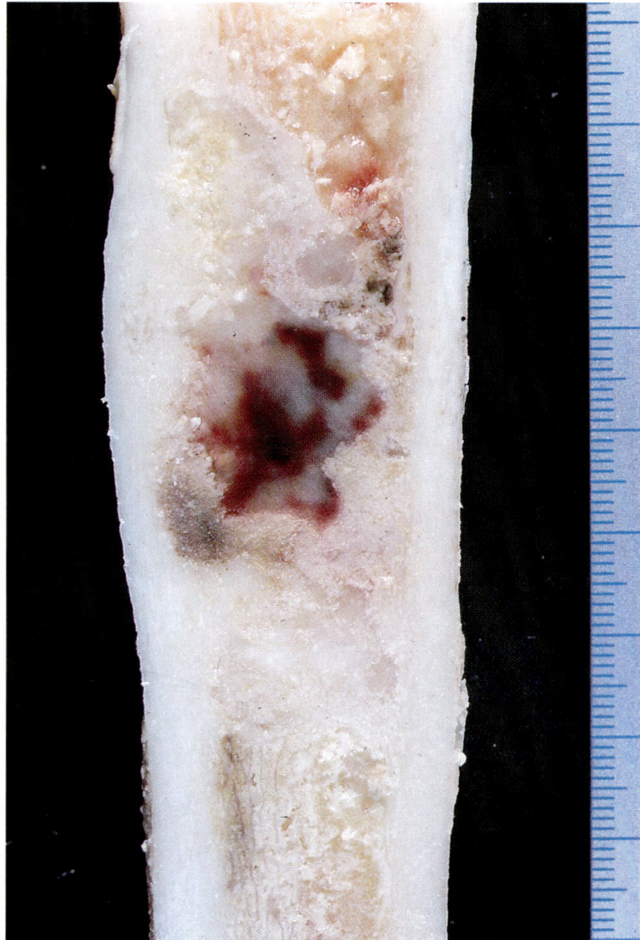

Fig. 27.2

Figs 27.1, 27.2 Adamantinoma of the tibia: polycystlic lesion with thinning of the cortex.

well as with adnexal skin tumors of sweat gland origin, advocating the term 'dermal inclusion tumor'.

A vascular origin has been proposed on morphological, ultrastructural, enzyme histochemical and culture studies[18–23] but this view is now somewhat disputed, as is a synovial origin based on the biphasic morphological pattern.[24,25]

It has also been suggested that adamantinomas could derive from a stem cell, giving rise to a low-grade biphasic epithelial mesenchymal tumor.[26,27]

SKELETAL DISTRIBUTION

Most tumors are located in the tibia (90%), but ada-

mantinomas have been reported in the humerus,[28–31] ulna,[7,32–34] radius,[35] femur[4,5,31,36–38] (Lichtenstein 1977, Mulder et al 1993, Schajowicz 1994), fibula[5,39] (Mulder et al 1993), spine,[40] pelvis,[41] ischium[42] (Lichtenstein 1977), ribs[43,44] (Schajowicz 1994) and even the small bones of the hands and feet.[45]

In most cases, the fibula is involved by contiguous extension from the tibia[4,46,47] (Mulder et al 1993). Multicentric lesions have been reported in 5% of cases[5,6,48] (Mulder et al 1993, Schajowicz 1994).

Pretibial soft tissue adamantinomas have been described without osseous extension,[49–51] but with secondary bone erosion and remodeling.[51] It has been suggested that intraosseous adamantinomas may begin as tumors located peripherally to the periosteum, with subsequent invasion of the medullary cavity.[50]

IMAGING

In the tibia, most cases are located in the diaphyseal portion of bone (anterior mid-diaphysis) (Figs 27.1–27.6). Involvement of the metaphysis is less common and no

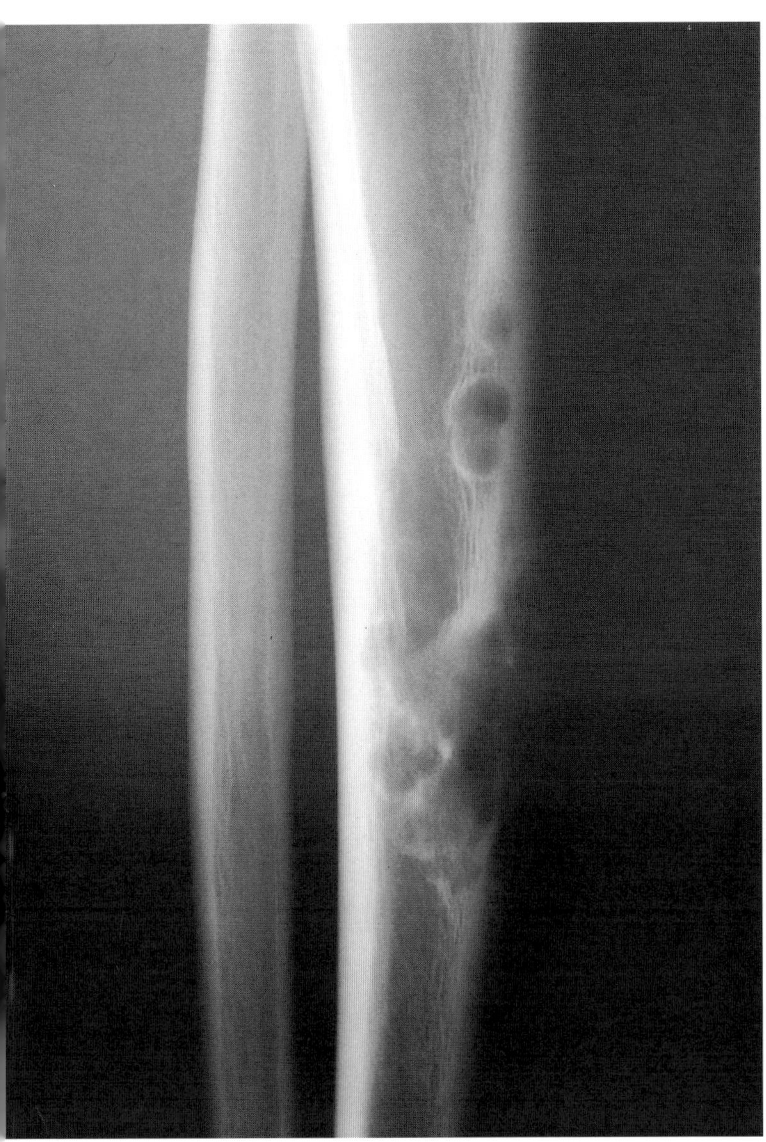

Fig. 27.3

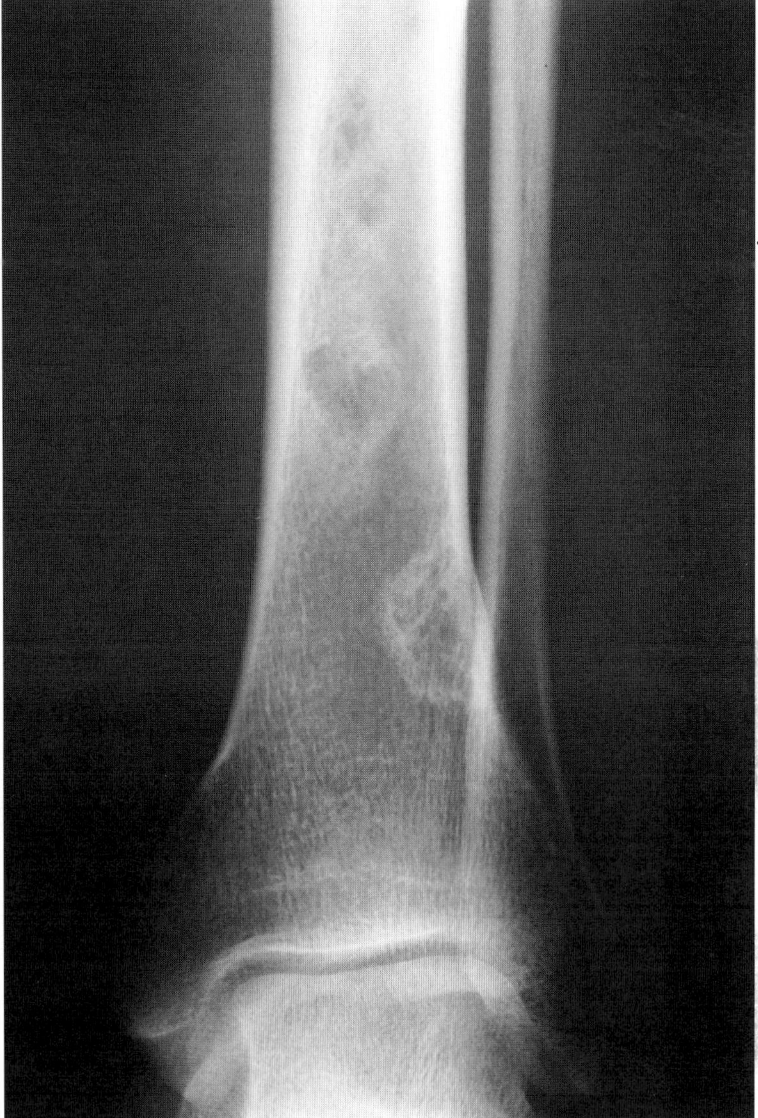

Fig. 27.4

Figs 27.3, 27.4 Adamantinomas of the tibia: multiple lucent areas, some of them intracortical.

purely epiphyseal tumors have been reported (Wilner 1982).

Small adamantinomas are eccentrically located or predominantly intracortical in 10% of cases, responding to an early phase of evolution.[5,7,50,52,53] In 50% of cases, both cortical and medullary portions are involved.

Single or multiple lucent areas are sharply defined, appearing as longitudinal lesions with an average size of 11 cm[55] and a significant thickening of the cortex.[7] One of the lytic areas may appear larger and more destructive with thinning of the cortex.[7] Larger tumors may exhibit a soap bubble or multiloculated appearance.

The cortex is asymmetrically expanded, chiefly on the anterior surface. In 15% of cases, it is destroyed, with a soft tissue tumoral component.[5] Perilesional sclerosis may be prominent and in long-standing cases, most of the shaft can be involved.[5,7,52] Rarely, the tumor appears as multiple lesions separated by uninvolved bone.[5] In juxtacortical locations, the erosion or thickening of the outer cortex is associated with extensive soft tissue involvement.[5,22,3

MRI and CT scans do not add to the differential diagnosis but show more accurately the true extent and invasiveness of the tumor,[39,55,56] intratumoral septa,[57] cystic spaces (Mulder et al 1993) or bony loculations. On MRI, the signal intensity exhibits some increase on T1-weighted images and is markedly increased on T2-weighted images,[57,58] with enhancement following gadolinium administration.[55]

For Wilner, radiologic findings are dependent on the primary location of the tumor, but also on the predomi-

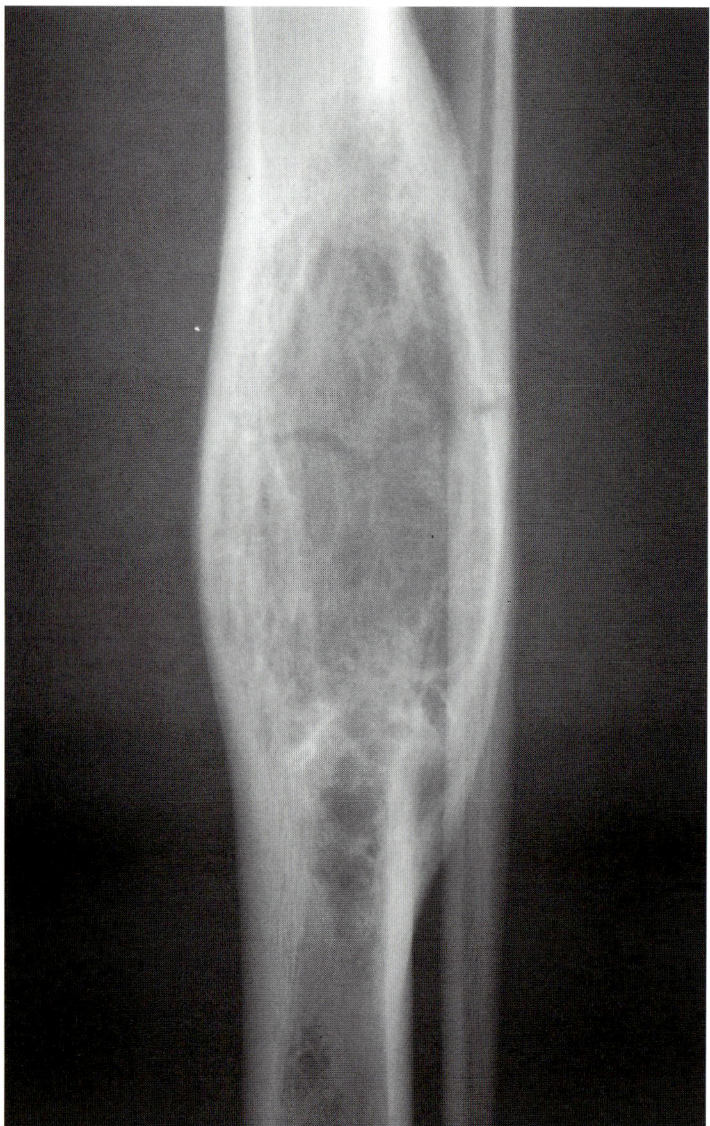

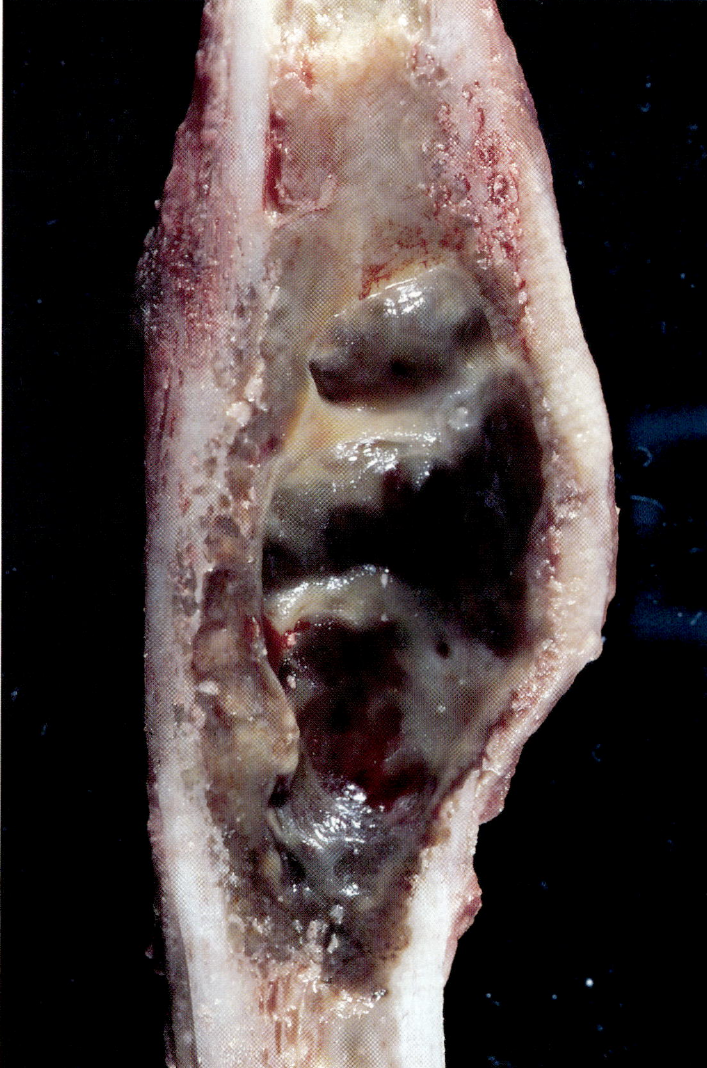

Fig. 27.5

Fig. 27.6

Figs 27.5, 27.6 Adamantinoma of the tibia: cyst formation and pathologic fracture.

nant histological pattern. Epithelial tumors appear as slow-growing and well-demarcated lesions, predominantly tubular tumors display a coarsely septate or honeycomb appearance and tumors with large collagenized areas show frank destruction of bone, cortical penetration and soft tissue extension.

GROSS PATHOLOGY

More than 80% of tumors are at least 5 cm in length.[5] They appear sharply demarcated from bone, sometimes with a lobular configuration. The tumoral tissue is gray, white or pink, fleshy or fibrous and granular (Figs 27.7–27.9), with intralesional hemorrhages and fre-

quent cystic spaces filled with a yellow or blood-like fluid. The tumors may be largely cystic[6] (Schajowicz 1994).

HISTOPATHOLOGY

An adamantinoma is composed of a mesenchymal-like and an epithelial-like component, with great histological diversity from one tumor to another or even within the same tumor (Figs 27.10–27.15). Most descriptions follow basic histologic patterns which have been delineated in recent studies.[4,5,26]

The basaloid pattern is made of lobules or nests of cuboid or columnar cells;[26] central cells exhibit a stellate or reticular arrangement.

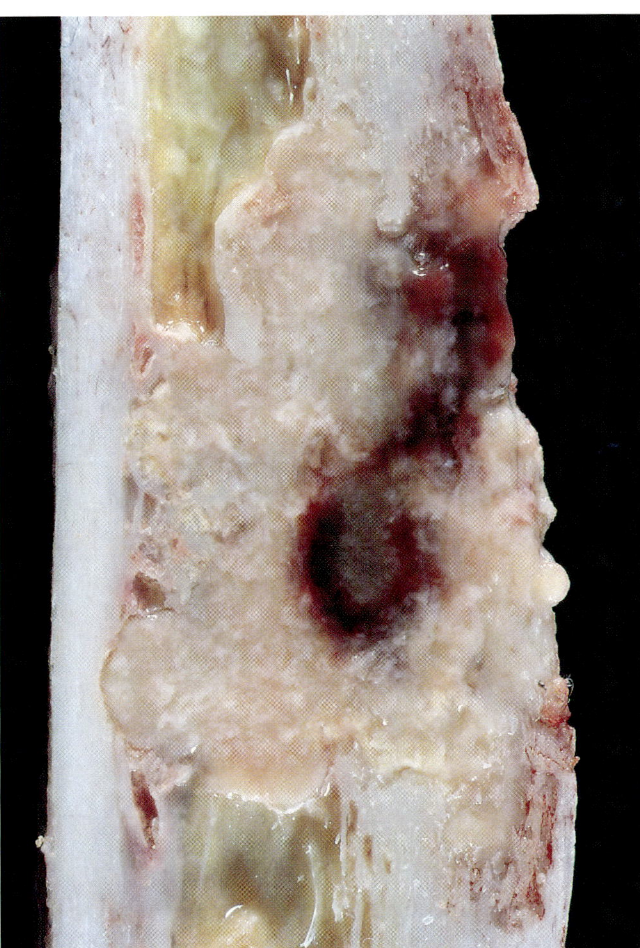

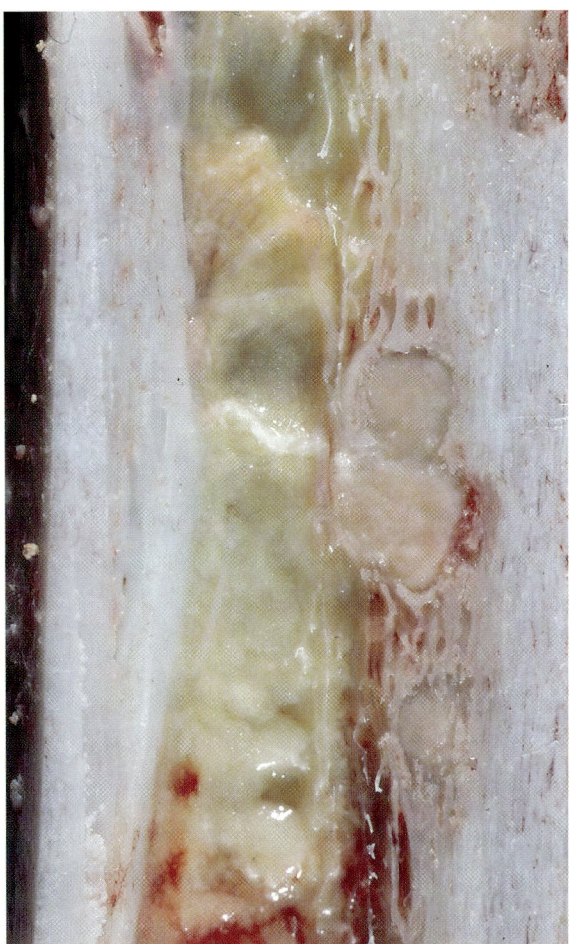

Fig. 27.7

Fig. 27.8

Figs 27.7, 27.8 Adamantinoma of the tibia: involvement of the medullary cavity and cortex.

The squamoid pattern corresponds to areas of squamous differentiation, with keratohyalin granules or overt keratinization.

Small flattened cells may line vascular-like tubular structures which look like capillary or small cavernous spaces.[26]

The spindle cell pattern is represented by cells distributed in a fascicular or herring-bone arrangement in the loose fibrous tissue.

The fibrous dysplasia-like pattern[59] combines collagenized tissue and foci of woven bone which are part of the tumor[6] (Fig. 27.16).

Small nests of cells or small tubular structures may exist in an osteofibrous-like pattern;[61] loose fascicles of elongated cells are associated with trabeculae of bone exhibiting an osteoblastic rim. Both osteofibrous and fibrous dysplasia-like areas must be differentiated from reactive ossification around the tumoral areas, which is usually quite prominent.[61]

Large areas may only contain spindle cells in a storiform or cartwheel pattern;[4,5,7,62] some may be hypocellular and heavily collagenized and over the years, an intercellular osteoid-like material may even develop.[6,63] Reactive giant cells can be found, usually near the hemorrhagic areas[4,6] (Fig. 27.17).

Whatever the histologic pattern, the nuclei are usually bland or display slight atypia and mitotic figures are rare. Currently, there are no histological rules for grading adamantinomas.[5]

Ewing-like adamantinoma appears to be a clearly distinct variant of adamantinoma. A few cases have been reported involving the femur,[64] the humerus,[65] the humerus in a juxtacortical location,[66] the metatarsals[67] and the radial head and neck.[68]

Areas of poorly or well-differentiated adamantinoma are associated with small cells resembling Ewing's sarcoma. The latter component is arranged in compact masses, anastomosing trabeculae or a cord-like pattern with a hyalinized stroma. The cytoplasm is scanty and glycogen granules may be found. Ultrastructural findings show tonofilaments, desmosomes and basement membrane,[65,66,68] as well as large amounts of intracytoplasmic glycogen.[66] Immuno-

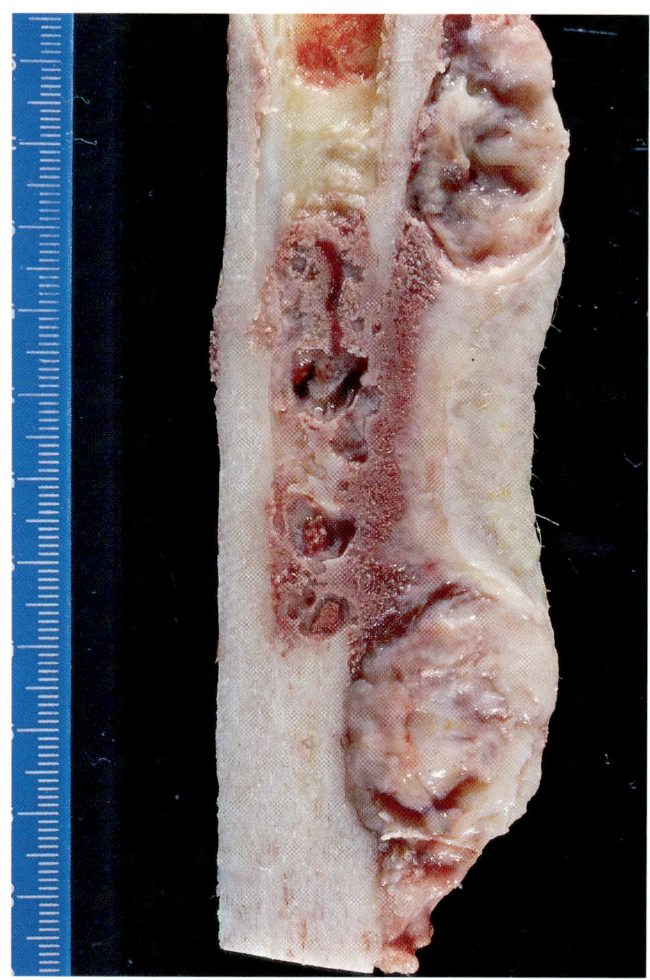

Figs 27.9 Adamantinoma of the tibia: extensive juxtacortical tumoral component.

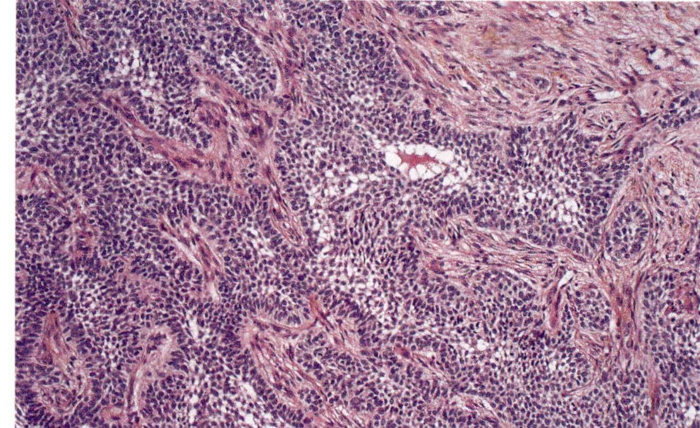

Fig. 27.10

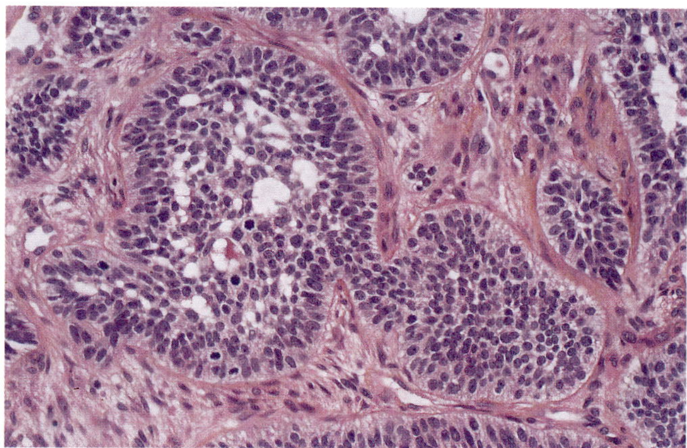

Fig. 27.12

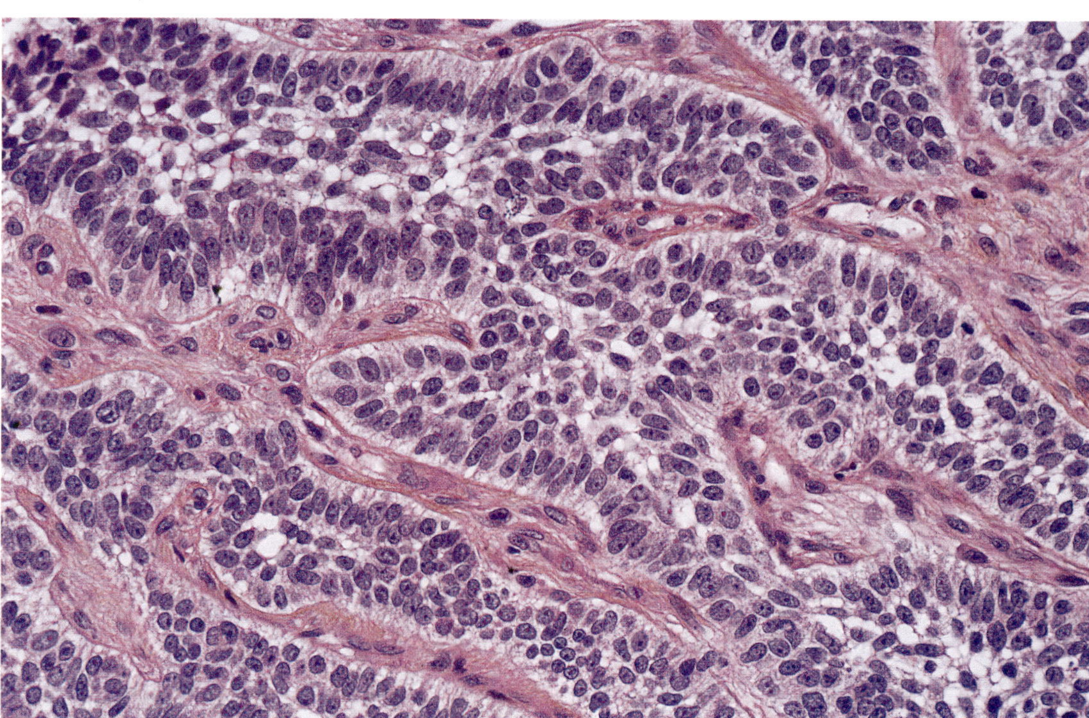

Fig. 27.11

Figs 27.10–27.12
Adamantinoma of the tibia:
basaloid pattern.

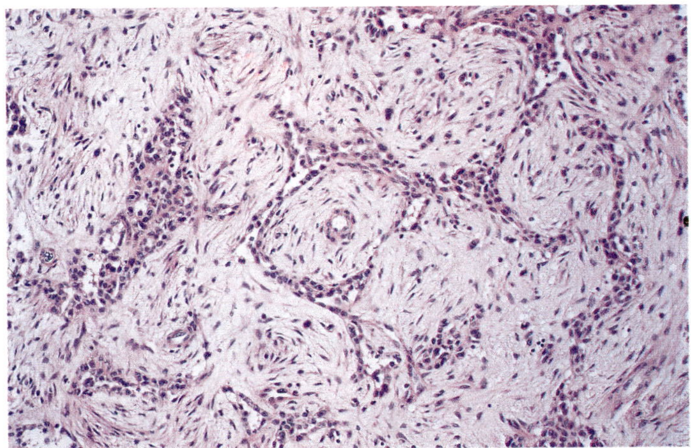

Fig. 27.13

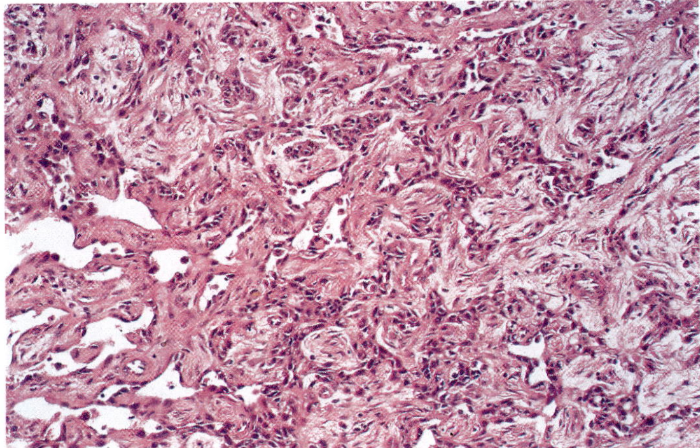

Fig. 27.14

Figs 27.13, 27.14 Adamantinoma of the tibia: vascular-like structures lined by flattened cells.

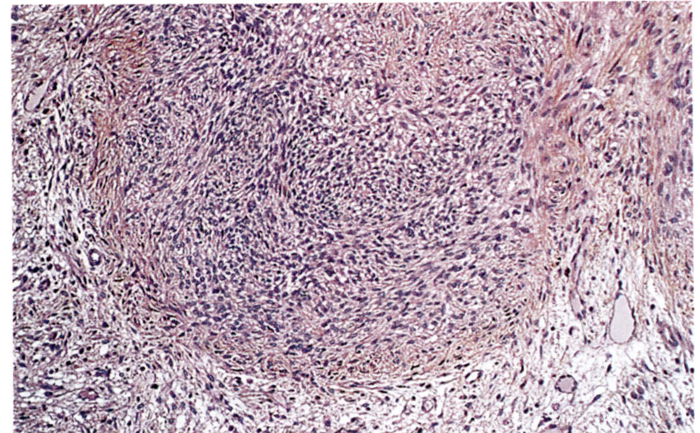

Fig. 27.15 Adamantinoma of the tibia: spindle cell pattern.

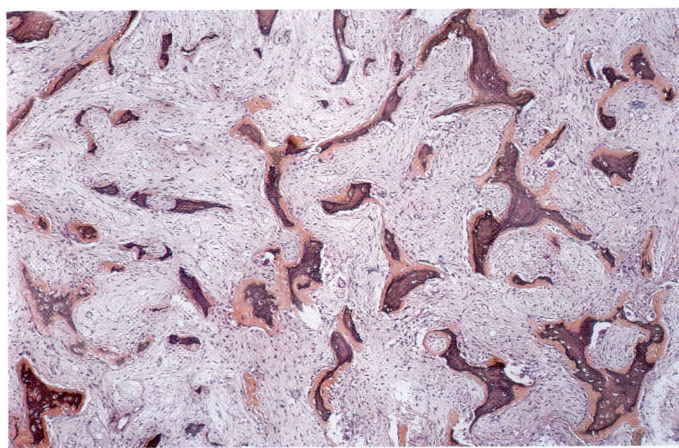

Fig. 27.16 Adamantinoma of the tibia: fibrous dysplasia-like areas.

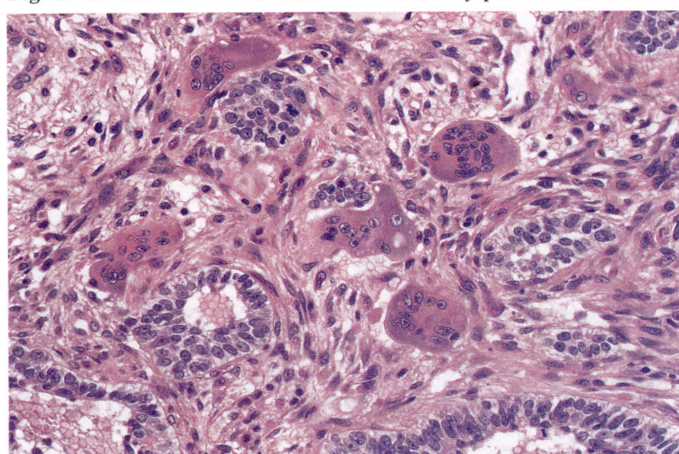

Fig. 27.17 Adamantinoma of the tibia: reactive giant cells.

histochemically, the cells are positive for EMA and vimentin, negative for cytokeratins.

A recently described tumor in the tibia may well represent a *granular cell variant of long bone adamantinoma*:[69] groups, cords or nests of undifferentiated round or granular cells are distributed in a fibrous stroma and there is isolated immunoreactivity for EMA and vimentin. Ultrastructural features are suggestive of an epithelial differentiation.

Differentiated adamantinomas[60] or 'juvenile' adamantinomas (Mirra 1989) are tumors occurring at an earlier age. They are confined to the anterolateral cortex of the tibia. The associated prominent lesions of osteofibrous dysplasia may represent regression or a reparative process of the adamantinoma, but in some cases there is progression to a clearcut adamantinoma,[31] supported by immunohistochemical findings (Chapter 45).

CYTOPATHOLOGY

On smears, the cells are distributed singly or in small clusters;[70–73] they are small, round, oval or fusiform or large and polyhedral (Fig. 27.18). Nuclear pleomorphism is not prominent and mitotic figures are rare. Intercellular strands of hyaline-like PAS-positive material presumably represent tonofilaments.

On smears, the cells exhibit positivity for keratin markers AE1, AE3, like skin and adnexal structures,[73] and are negative for FVIIIRag and Ulex Europaeus.

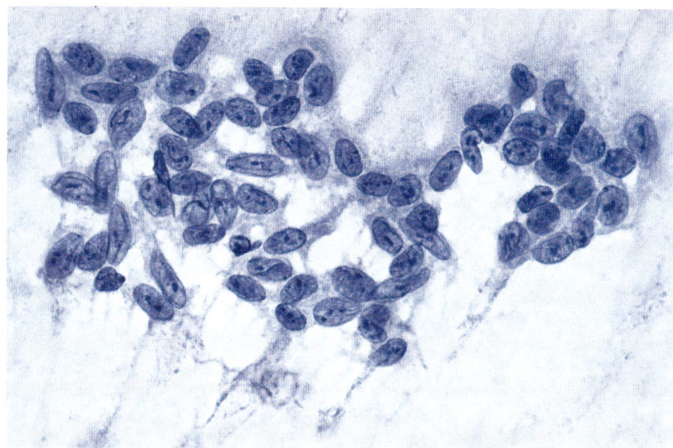

Fig. 27.18 Adamantinoma of the tibia: imprint cytology.

IMMUNOHISTOCHEMISTRY AND ENZYME HISTOCHEMISTRY

Numerous studies demonstrate the intense positivity for cytokeratins and vimentin[60,74–80] in the spindle cell component, as well as the negative staining for FVIIIRag which is confined to the endothelial cells. The cells appear to be positive for CEA[18] and negative for EMA.[31] A focal positivity for actin has been found[60] in some fibroblast-like cells, as well as epithelial ones.[78]

A study of the expression and distribution of the cytokeratin subtypes has shown that the epithelial and mesenchymal components may have the same origin and that adamantinomas and osteofibrous dysplasia may be lesions of a similar histogenesis.[80] Similarly, it has been shown with monoclonal antibodies that the pattern of immunoreactivity suggests a basal epithelial cell-like differentiation of adamantinoma.[79,80]

Enzyme histochemistry has demonstrated the similar reactivity between the tumor and normal eccrine structures: amylophosphorylase, succinic dehydrogenase, β-glucuronidase, leucine aminopeptidase, alkaline and acid phosphatase patterns are in favor of an eccrine differentiation.[17]

Immunohistochemistry for p53 has shown a moderate or strong reactivity restricted to the epithelial cells.[81]

FLOW CYTOMETRY

An aneuploid DNA index has been found in 40% of cases analyzed by flow cytometry.[81] On image cytometry with Feulgen-stained paraffin sections, aneuploid nuclei are found only in cells with an epithelial phenotype.[81]

CYTOGENETICS

A translocation t(7;13)(q32q14) has been described on a lung metastasis, being the first evidence for direct transmission of a translocation involving chromosome 12q14 from a father to a child.[82]

A pseudodiploid tumor karyotype has been established containing two seemingly balanced rearrangements – one three-way translocation involving chromosomes 1, 13 and 22 and another between chromosomes 15 and 17.[83]

ELECTRON MICROSCOPY

An angioblastic origin of adamantinoma has been suggested by the finding of channels appearing as capillaries lined by prominent cells of endothelial appearance and even rod-shaped bodies of the Weibel–Palade type.[23] In another study, tumor cells showing a high phosphatase activity tended to line clefts and resembled endothelial cells with large processes, fenestrations and Weibel–Palade body-like inclusions but they were also interconnected by desmosomes with tonofilaments and exhibited numerous bundles of microfilaments.[27]

Most current studies demonstrate a clearcut epithelial derivation.[3,6,12,13,15,17,26,75,78,84–90] Epithelial features include microvillous processes, tonofilaments, desmosomes and a basement membrane material. Peculiar findings are actin-like filaments in the cells of the epithelial nests,[12,13,89] myofibroblasts in the stroma,[77,89] cells with membrane-limited lipid droplets[23,26] and thin fibrils identical to oxytalan fibrils described in adamantinomas of the jaws.[77]

COURSE, TREATMENT AND PROGNOSIS

The treatment is wide excision with bone grafting;[8] en bloc resection may control local disease in 80% of cases.[8] Curettage leads to local recurrence and implants in the soft tissues in 60% of patients[5] (Fig. 27.19). Chemotherapy gives poor results and the tumors are highly radioresistant, in spite of some partial regression.[21,92]

Long-term follow-up is necessary because recurrences as well as metastases can develop years after the initial surgical treatment,[5,9,34] the local recurrence rate being about 30% of cases.[5]

Metastases are found in the lung,[92, 93] bones, lymph nodes and abdominal viscera, with an incidence ranging from 18%[8] to 29%.[3] Metastases may exhibit the same aspect as the primary tumor: a sarcomatous appearance, increased mitotic activity or a shift towards a spindle cell subtype.[26] The overall mortality rate ranges from 10%[6] to 18%.[2]

There are few if any reliable histologic features relating to the metastatic potential or increased recurrence rate:[5,78] a lack of squamous differentiation has been suggested.[5] The most important risk factor is an intralesional or marginal excision[3,78] and male patients may experience a more aggressive course.[2,3,5,78] Some authors have suggested short duration of symptoms and extreme pain as prognostic factors.[5]

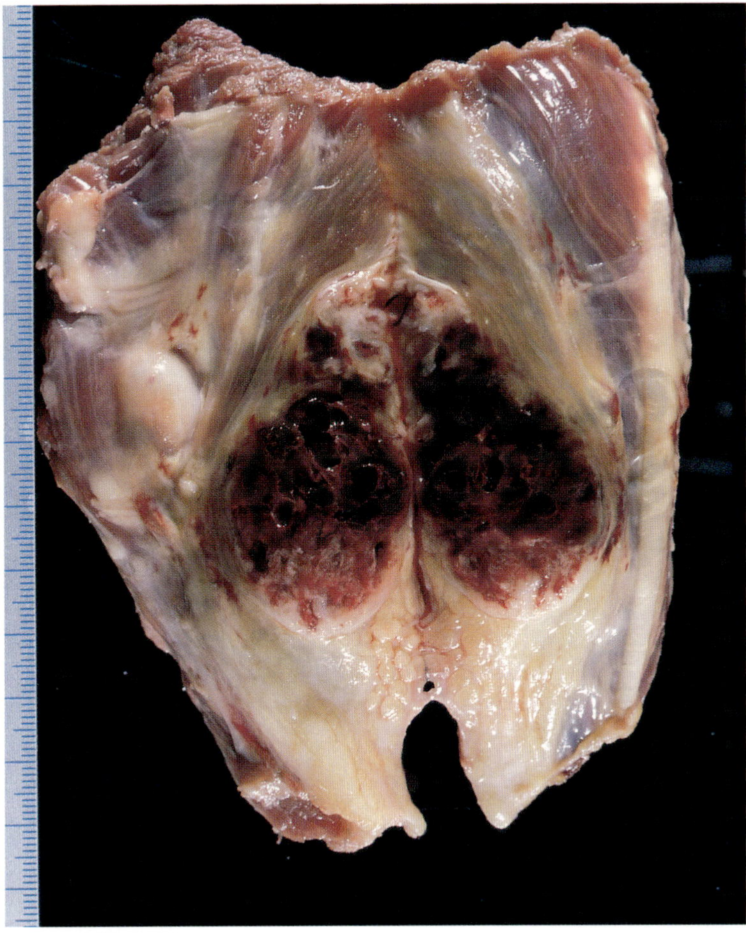

Fig. 27.19 Recurrence in the calf of a tibial adamantinoma treated by resection.

DIFFERENTIAL DIAGNOSIS

Osteofibrous dysplasia is also located in the shaft of the tibia, appearing as an intracortical single or multiple eccentric radiolucent lesion, associated with anterior bowing. Scattered cells or nests of cells may show cytokeratin positivity and spindle cells are vimentin positive. Classic adamantinomas may exhibit an osteofibrous dysplasia-like pattern at the periphery of the lesions[31,94] and a few cases of osteofibrous-like adamantinomas have shown full-blown adamantinomas on recurrence.[3] Moreover, adamantinoma has been confused with osteofibrous dysplasia or fibrous dysplasia.[46,95,96] The differential diagnosis relies on the finding of fully developed epithelial structures for an adamantinoma.

A metastatic carcinoma has to be ruled out by the bland cytologic appearance.

Basal cell carcinomas are not so deeply located and do not exhibit a fibroblastic stroma;[50] in the same way, sweat gland carcinomas are more pleomorphic and are rare in the lower limb.[50] A chondroid syringoma may easily be excluded, although it has been rarely described in bone locations.[97,98]

The lack of endothelial markers rules out vascular tumors and especially epithelioid hemangioendotheliomas.

The biphasic appearance may be reminiscent of a synovial sarcoma, but this tumor shows marked cellularity, pleomorphism and extracellular hyaluronic acid production.

On limited biopsy material, adamantinomas may be confused with a non-ossifying fibroma or even a malignant fibrous histiocytoma[62] if the clearcut epithelial areas are not discovered.

REFERENCES

1. Fischer B. Uber ein primares Adamantinom der Tibia. Frankf Z Pathol 1913: 12: 422–441
2. Moon N F, Mori H. Adamantinoma of the appendicular skeleton – updated. Clin Orthop 1986: 204: 215–237
3. Hazelbag H M, Taminiau A H, Fleuren G J, Hogendoorn P C. Adamantinoma of the long bones. J Bone Joint Surg (Am) 1994: 76: 1482–1499
4. Campanacci M, Giunti A, Bertoni F, Laus M, Gitelis S.

Adamantinoma of the long bones. The experience of the Istituto Ortopedico Rizzoli. Am J Surg Pathol 1981: 5: 533–542

5. Keeney G L, Unni K K, Beabout J W, Pritchard D J. Adamantinoma of long bones. Cancer 1989: 64: 730–737

6. Unni K K, Dahlin D C, Beabout J W, Ivins J C. Adamantinomas of long bones. Cancer 1974: 34: 1796–1805

7. Rock M G, Beabout J W, Unni K K, Sim F H. Adamantinoma. Orthopedics 1983: 6: 472–477

8. Moon N F. Adamantinoma of the appendicular skeleton in children. Int Orthop 1994: 18: 379–388

9. Altmannsberger M, Poppe H, Schauer A. An unusual case of adamantinoma of long bones. J Cancer Res Clin Oncol 1982: 104: 315–320

10. Van Schoor J X, Vallaeys J H, Joos G F, Roels H J, Pauwels R A, Van Der Straeten M E. Adamantinoma of the tibia with pulmonary metastases and hypercalcemia. Chest 1991: 100: 279–281

11. Ryrie B J. Adamantinoma of the tibia: etiology and pathogenesis. Br J Med 1932: 2: 1000–1003

12. Mori H, Shima R, Nakanishi H, Yoshida A, Fukunishi R. Adamantinoma of the tibia. Acta Pathol Jpn 1981: 31: 701–709

13. Mori H, Yamamoto S, Hiramatsu K, Miura T, Moon N F. Adamantinoma of the tibia. Ultrastructural and immunohistochemical study with reference to histogenesis. Clin Orthop 1984: 190: 299–310

14. Baker P L, Dockerty M B, Coventry M B. Adamantinoma (so-called) of long bones. J Bone Joint Surg (Am) 1954: 36: 704–720

15. Rosai J. Adamantinoma of the tibia. Electron microscopic evidence of its epithelial origin. Am J Clin Pathol 1969: 51: 786–792

16. Brandt H, Albores-Saavedra J, Mora-Tiscareno A. Eccrine sweat gland carcinoma. Its microscopic and ultrastructural similarity to adamantinoma of long bones. Patologia 1977: 15: 33–43

17. Eisenstein W, Pitcock J A. Adamantinoma of the tibia. An eccrine carcinoma. Arch Pathol Lab Med 1984: 108: 246–250

18. Changus G W, Speed J S, Stewart F W. Malignant angioblastoma of bone: a reappraisal of adamantinoma of long bone. Cancer 1957: 10: 540–559

19. Eliott G B. Malignant angioblastoma of long bone. So-called 'tibial adamantinoma'. J Bone Joint Surg (Br) 1962: 44: 25–33

20. Rosen R S, Schwinn C P. Adamantinoma of limb bone. Malignant angioblastoma. Am J Roentgenol Radium Ther Nucl Med 1966: 97: 727–732

21. Zand A, Chambers G H, Street D M. So-called 'adamantinoma of long bone'. Clin Orthop 1972: 86: 178–182

22. Huvos A G, Marcove R C. Adamantinoma of long bones. J Bone Joint Surg (Am) 1975: 57: 148–154

23. Llombart-Bosch A, Ortuno-Pacheco G. Ultrastructural findings supporting the angioblastic nature of the so-called adamantinoma of the tibia. Histopathology 1978: 2: 189–200

24. Lederer H, Sinclair A J. Malignant synovioma simulating 'adamantinoma of the tibia'. J Pathol Bacteriol 1954: 67: 163–168

25. Hicks J D. Synovial sarcoma of the tibia. J Pathol Bacteriol 1956: 67: 115–161

26. Weiss S W, Dorfman H D. Adamantinoma of long bone. Hum Pathol 1977: 8: 141–153

27. Povysil C, Matejovsky Z. Ultrastructure of adamantinoma of long bones. Virchows Arch A Pathol Anat Histol 1981: 393: 233–244

28. Besemann E F, Perez M A. Malignant angioblastoma, so-called adamantinoma involving the humerus. Am J Roentgenol Radium Ther Nucl Med 1967: 100: 538–541

29. Shah I C, Castro E B, Miller T R, Gerson G N. Malignant angioblastoma (so-called adamantinoma) of humerus. Int Surg 1972: 57: 753–755

30. Clarke R P, Leonard J R, Von Kuster L, Wesseler T A. Adamantinoma of the humerus with early metastases and death. Orthopedics 1989: 12: 1121–1125

31. Ishida T, Iijima T, Kikuchi F et al. A clinicopathological and immunohistochemical study of osteofibrous dysplasia, differentiated adamantinoma, and adamantinoma of long bones. Skeletal Radiol 1992: 21: 493–502

32. Anderson C E, Saunders J M. Primary adamantinoma of the ulna. Surg Gynecol Obstet 1942: 75: 351–356

33. Trifaud A, Payan H, Bureau H, Legre G. Adamantinome du cubitus. Rev Chir Orthop Reparatrice Appar Mot 1960: 46: 97–103

34. Soucacos P N, Hartofilakidis G K, Touliatos A S, Theodorou V. Adamantinoma of the olecranon. Clin Orthop 1995: 310: 194–199

35. Bourne M H, Wood M B, Shives T C. Adamantinoma of the radius. Orthopedics 1988: 11: 1565–1566

36. Bell A L. A case of adamantinoma of the femur. Br J Surg 1942: 30: 81–82

37. Thurner J, Marcacci M. Ein sog. Adamantinom des rechten Femurs. Zentralbl Allg Pathol 1976: 120: 398–405

38. Carpintero Benitez P, Mesa Ramos M, Carpintero Gomez J, Toro Rojas M, Carpintero Renedo A. Adamantinoma de los huesos largos: communicacion de un caso de localizacion femoral. Rev Esp de Cir Ost 1985: 20: 223–228

39. Sowa D T, Dorfman H D. Unusual localization of adamantinoma of long bones. Report of a case of isolated fibular involvement. J Bone Joint Surg (Am) 1986: 68: 293–296

40. Nerubay J, Chechick A, Horoszowski H, Engelberg S. Adamantinoma of the spine. J Bone Joint Surg (Am) 1988: 70: 467–469

41. Vasin V A, Skotnikov V I, Khazov P D, Shavyrin A V. An adamantinoma located in the pelvic bones (in Russian). Vrach Delo 1990: 6: 96–98

42. Lasda N A, Hughes E C Jr. Adamantinoma of the ischium. J Bone Joint Surg (Am) 1979: 61: 599–600

43. Plump D, Haponik E F, Katz R S, Tipton-Donovan A. Primary adamantinoma of rib: thoracic manifestations of a rare bone tumor. South Med J 1986: 79: 352–355

44. Beppu H, Yamaguchi H, Yoshimura N, Atarashi K, Tsukimoto K, Nagashima Y. Adamantinoma of the rib metastasizing to the liver. Intern Med 1994: 33: 441–445

45. Dieperveen W P, Hjort G H, Pock-Stean O C. Adamantinoma of the capitate bone. Acta Radiol (Stockh) 1960: 53: 377–384

46. Adler C P. Case report 587. Adamantinoma of the tibia mimicking osteofibrous dysplasia. Skeletal Radiol 1990: 19: 55–58

47. Benevenia J, Abdul-Karim F W, Joyce M J, Dicke T. Multifocal adamantinoma of the tibia and fibula. Orthop Rev 1992: 21: 996–1000

48. Bullough P G, Goldberg V M. Multicentric origin of adamantinoma of the tibia. Rev Hosp Spec Surg 1971: 1: 71–74

49. Bambirra E A, Margarida A, Nogueira A M, Miranda D. Adamantinoma of the soft tissue of the leg. Arch Pathol Lab Med 1983: 107: 500–501

50. Mills S E, Rosai J. Adamantinoma of the pretibial soft tissue. Am J Clin Pathol 1985: 83: 108–114

51. Bertoni F, Zucchi V, Mapelli S, Bacchini P. Case report 506. Adamantinoma of the soft tissues of leg. Skeletal Radiol 1988: 17: 522–526

52. Tehranzadeh J, Fanney D, Ghandur-Mnaymneh L, Ganz W, Mnaymneh W. Case report 517. Ulcerating adamantinoma of the tibia. Skeletal Radiol 1989: 17: 614–619

53. Zehr R J, Recht M P, Bauer T W. Adamantinoma. Skeletal Radiol 1995: 24: 553–555

54. Bohndorf K, Nidecker A, Mathias K, Zidkova H, Kaufmann H, Jundt G. Radiologische Befunde beim Adamantinom der langen Röhrenknochen. RÖFO 1992: 157: 239–244

55. Vanhoenacker F, Van Ongeval C, Ceulemans R, Wouters W, Lateur L. Adamantinoma of the tibia. MRI documentation. J Belge Radiol 1993: 76: 154–156

56. Garces P, Romano C C, Vellet A D, Alakija P, Schachar N S. Adamantinoma of the tibia: plain film, computed tomography and magnetic resonance imaging appearance. Can Assoc Radiol J 1994: 45: 314–317

57. Young J W, Aisner S C, Resnik CS , Levine A M, Dorfman H D, Whitley N O. Case report 660. Adamantinoma of the tibia. Skeletal Radiol 1991: 20: 152–156

58. Vandermarcq P, Defaux F, Ferrie J C et al. Adamantinome du tibia. Etude tomodensitométrique et par IRM. J Radiol 1993: 74: 35–38

59. Cohen D M, Dahlin D C, Pugh D G. Fibrous dysplasia associated with adamantinoma of the long bones. Cancer 1962: 15: 515–521

60. Czerniak B, Rojas-Corona R R, Dorfman H D. Morphologic diversity of long bone adamantinoma. The concept of differentiated (regressing) adamantinoma and its relationship to osteofibrous dysplasia. Cancer 1989: 64: 2319–2334

61. Konrad E A, Meister P, Stotz S. 'Adamantinom' der Tibia und

reaktive Knochenveränderungen. Arch Orthop Trauma Surg 1978: 92: 297–301

62. Levack B, Revell P A, Roper B A. Adamantinoma associated with fibrous dysplasia. Int Orthop 1986: 10: 253–259

63. Donner R, Dikland R. Adamantinoma of the tibia. A long standing case with unusual histological features. J Bone Joint Surg (Br) 1966: 48: 138–144

64. Grundmann E. Gemischtzelliges sarkom. Verh Dtsch Ges Pathol 1974: 58: 265–270

65. Meister P, Konrad E, Hübner G. Malignant tumor of humerus with features of 'adamantinoma' and Ewing's sarcoma. Pathol Res Pract 1979: 166: 112–122

66. Ishida T, Kikuchi F, Oka T et al. Case report 727. Juxtacortical adamantinoma of humerus (simulating Ewing tumor). Skeletal Radiol 1992: 21: 205–209

67. Van Haelst U J, De Haas Van Dorsser A H. A perplexing malignant bone tumor. Highly malignant so-called adamantinoma or non-typical Ewing's sarcoma. Virchows Arch A Pathol Anat Histol 1975: 365: 63–74

68. Lipper S, Kahn L B. Case report 235. Ewing-like adamantinoma of the left radial head and neck. Skeletal Radiol 1983: 10: 61–66

69. Schofield D E, Conrad E U, Liddell R M, Yunis E J. An unusual round cell tumor of the tibia with granular cells. Am J Surg Pathol 1995: 19: 596–603

70. Tabei S Z, Abdollahi B, Nili F. Diagnosis of metastatic adamantinoma of the tibia by pulmonary brushing cytology. Acta Cytol 1988: 32: 579–581

71. Hales M S, Ferrell L D. Fine-needle aspiration biopsy of tibial adamantinoma. Diagn Cytopathol 1988: 4: 67–70

72. Galera-Davidson H, Fernandez-Rodriguez A, Torres-Olivera F J, Gomez-Pascual A, Moreno-Fernandez A. Cytologic diagnosis of a case of recurrent adamantinoma. Acta Cytol 1989: 33: 635–638

73. Laucirica R, Mody D, MacLeay L, Kearns R J, Ramzy I. Adamantinoma. A case report with aspiration cytology and differential diagnosis and immunohistochemical considerations. Acta Cytol 1992: 36: 951–956

74. Rosai J, Pinkus G S. Immunohistochemical demonstration of epithelial differentiation in adamantinoma of the tibia. Am J Surg Pathol 1982: 6: 427–434

75. Knapp R H, Wick M R, Scheithauer B W, Unni K K. Adamantinoma of bone. An electron microscopic and immunohistochemical study. Virchows Arch A Pathol Anat Histopathol 1982: 398: 75–86

76. Muretto P, Raspugli P. 'Angioblastic' adamantinoma of the tibia. An immunohistochemical study. Tumori 1985: 71: 387–390

77. Perez-Atayde A R, Kozakewich H P, Vawter G F. Adamantinoma of the tibia. An ultrastructural and immunohistochemical study. Cancer 1985: 55: 1015–1023

78. Jundt G, Remberger K, Roessner A, Schulz A, Bohndorf K. Adamantinoma of long bones. Pathol Res Pract 1995: 191: 112–120

79. Benassi M S, Campanacci L, Gamberi G et al. Cytokeratin expression and distribution in adamantinoma of the long bones and osteofibrous dysplasia of the tibia and fibula. An immunohistochemical study correlated to histogenesis. Histopathology 1994: 25: 71–76

80. Hazelbag H M, Fleuren G J, Van Der Broek L J, Taminiau A H, Hogendoorn P C. Adamantinoma of the long bones: keratin subclass immunoreactivity pattern with reference to its histogenesis. Am J Surg Pathol 1993: 17: 1225–1233

81. Hazelbag H M, Fleuren G J, Cornelisse C J, Van Der Broek L J, Taminiau A H, Hogendoorn P C. DNA aberrations in the epithelial cell component of adamantinoma of long bones. Am J Pathol 1995: 147: 1770–1779

82. Sozzi G, Miozzo M, Di Palma S et al. Involvement of the region 13q14 in a patient with adamantinoma of the long bones. Hum Genet 1990: 85: 513–515

83. Mandahl N, Heim S, Rydholm A, Willen H, Mitelman F. Structural chromosome aberrations in an adamantinoma. Cancer Genet Cytogenet 1989: 42: 187–190

84. Albores-Saavedra J, Dias Gutierrez D, Altamirano Dimas M. Adamantinoma de la tibia: observaciones ultraestructurales. Rev Med Hosp Gen Mex 1968: 31: 241–252

85. Schajowicz F, Cabrini R L, Simes T J. Microscopia electronica del 'adamantinoma' de los huesos largos. Rev Ortop Trauma Lat Amer 1971: 16: 185–194

86. Yoneyama T, Winter W G, Milsow L. Tibial adamantinoma: its histogenesis from ultrastructural studies. Cancer 1977: 40: 1138–1142

87. Ectors P, Muanza E, Heimann R, Ketelbant-Balasse P, Danis A. L'adamantinome du tibia: aspects ultrastructuraux, artériographiques et isotopiques. Acta Orthop Belg 1979: 45: 577–586

88. Aragona F, Emmola P, Casano R, Franco V, De Feo G. Su di un caso di c.d. adamantinoma recidivato della tibia. Arch De Vecchi Anat Patol 1980: 64: 124–156

89. Pieterse A S, Smith P S, McClure J. Adamantinoma of long bones, clinical, pathological and ultrastructural features. J Clin Pathol 1982: 35: 780–786

90. De Santis E, Miceli C, Porfiri B. Studio clinico patologico ed elettronmicroscopico di un caso di adamantinoma della tibia. Riv Anat Pat Oncol 1984: 43: 105–115

91. Gebhardt M C, Lord F C, Rosenberg A E, Mankin H J. The treatment of adamantinoma of the tibia by wide resection and allograft bone transplantation. J Bone Joint Surg (Am) 1987: 69: 1177–1188

92. Lokich J. Metastatic adamantinoma of bone to the lung. Am J Clin Oncol 1994: 17: 157–159

93. Naji A F, Murphy J A, Stasney R J, Neville W E, Chrenka P. So-called adamantinoma of long bones. Report of a case with massive pulmonary metastasis. J Bone Joint Surg (Am) 1964: 46: 151–158

94. Ueda Y, Roessner A, Bosse A, Edel G, Bocker W, Wuisman P. Juvenile intracortical adamantinoma of the tibia with predominant osteofibrous dysplasia-like features. Pathol Res Pract 1991: 187: 1039–1043, 1043–1044

95. Beabout J W. Case report 29. Adamantinoma of the tibia. Skeletal Radiol 1977: 1: 257–258

96. Schajowicz F, Santini-Araujo E. Adamantinoma of the tibia masked by fibrous dysplasia. Clin Orthop 1989: 238: 294–301

97. Wagoner W L, Spencer R B, Ramos R P. Chondroid syringoma. A rare occurrence in the hallux. J Am Podiatr Med Assoc 1993: 83: 424–425

98. Barreto C A, Lipton M N, Smith H B, Potter G K. Intraosseous chondroid syringoma of the hallux. J Am Acad Dermatol 1994: 30: 374–378

Chordoma

M. Forest

INTRODUCTION AND CLINICAL DATA

A chordoma is a slow-growing malignant tumor with a metastatic potential, developing from notochord remnants. The incidence is about 1% of all malignant bone tumors (Huvos 1991, Schajowicz 1994), with a male-to-female ratio of 1:1[1] to 2:1.[2]

Most patients are in their fifth to seventh decades and the median age in one series is 55 years.[3] Patients presenting with skull or vertebral tumors are younger, with a mean age of 47 years.[4] Chordomas are uncommon before the age of 20 years (less than 5% of cases[5]), with a mean age from 6 to 8 years,[6,7] exhibiting a more malignant behavior, a shorter period of survival and a greater tendency to metastasize.[6,7,8]

Chordomas have a protracted course and symptoms are usually present for more than 1 year, if one rules out vertebral chordomas with earlier signs.[9] The symptoms related to the size and location of the tumor are varied: headache, increased intracranial pressure or cranial nerve involvement for sphenooccipital tumors; pain and neurologic symptoms or even herniated lumbar disc-like symptoms for vertebral tumors;[3] pain, mass, neurologic symptoms or rectal and bladder dysfunction for sacral and sacrococcygeal tumors.

Intracranial chordomas have been described, associated with Maffucci's syndrome,[10] hemangiopericytomas, neurofibromatosis or tuberous sclerosis[11] or presenting as a second primary malignant lesion.[12]

HISTOGENESIS

The notochord forms the first axial skeleton during embryogenesis:[13] a rod of ectodermal cells is presumed to act as an embryonic organizer for the chondrification and segmentation of the mesenchymal elements of the vertebral bodies. During the fifth week, this becomes enclosed within the developing vertebral column and is divided in segments[14] (Fig. 28.1).

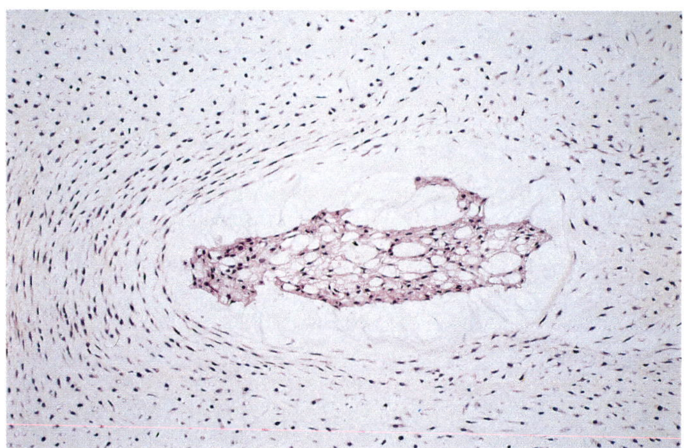

Fig. 28.1 Notochord (8th week).

The notochord regresses during fetal life but there are variations in its persistance or regression, particularly in the sacrococcygeal areas;[15] remnants of notochord tissue can be identified in the fetus as late as the sixth month of gestation.[14] Remnants are left in the nucleus pulposus, particularly in the upper and lower ends of the column,[15] and also in the midline of the sphenooccipital region. It has been suggested that notochordal tissue may produce the mesenchymal tissue corresponding to the structure of the nucleus pulposus,[14] but this view is disputed.[16]

The progressive degeneration of the notochord has been studied ultrastructurally.[17] A three-dimensional reconstruction has also been performed on human embryos, demonstrating the complex anatomy of the caudal and rostral ends of the notochord. The splitting of the ends with separate fragments of chordal tissue is an explanation for the notochord cell nests in the basicranial and sacrococcygeal regions.[18,19]

Heterotopic nests of notochordal cells may be found in adults anywhere along the axial skeleton, outside the sacral and clival areas, including the vertebral bodies and the coccyx.[20]

Notochordal remnants were first described by Luschka

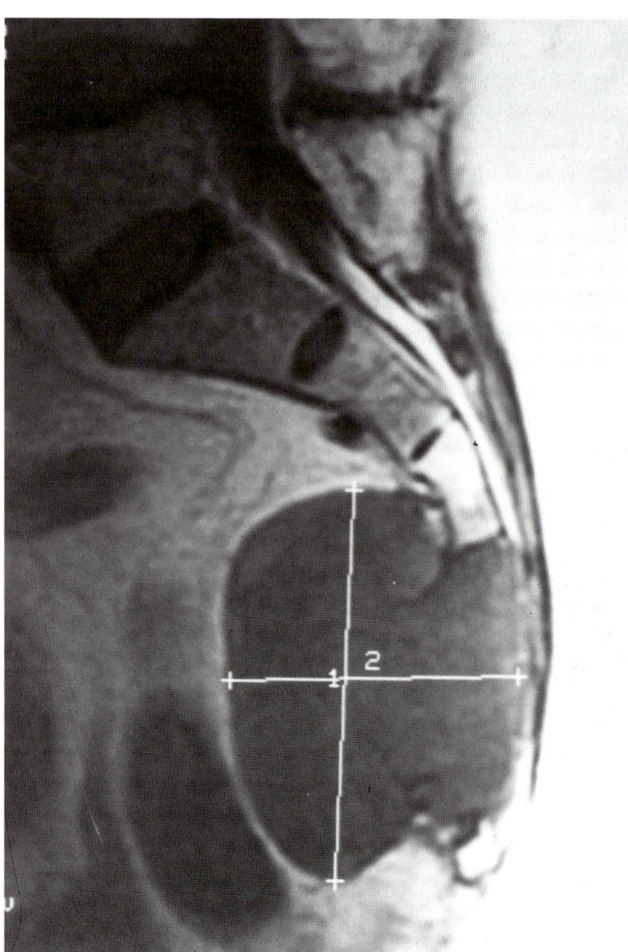

Fig. 28.2

Fig. 28.3

Figs 28.2, 28.3 Sacrococcygeal chordoma appearing as an anterior mass.

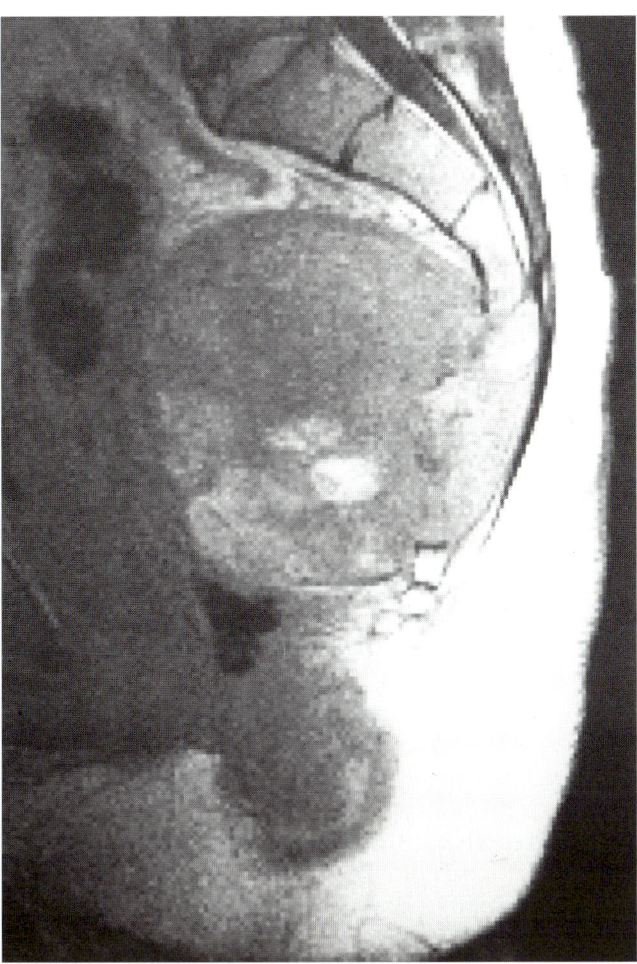

Fig. 28.4

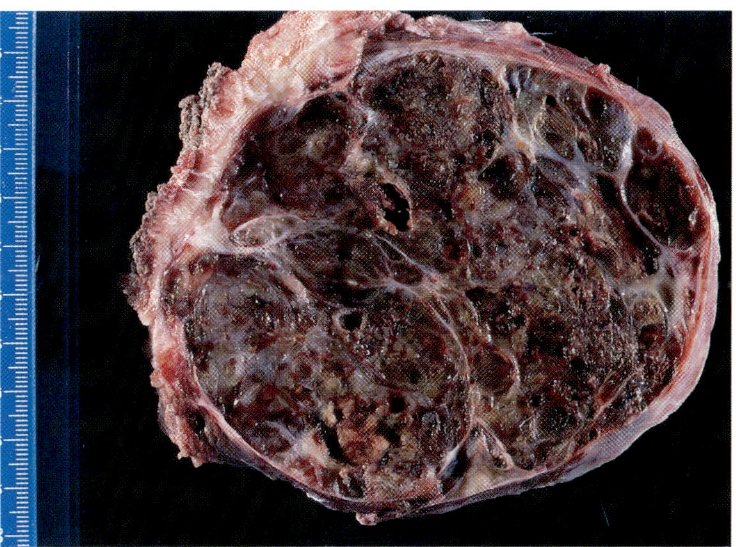

Fig. 28.5

Figs 28.4, 28.5 Sacrococcygeal chordoma with minimal bone involvement.

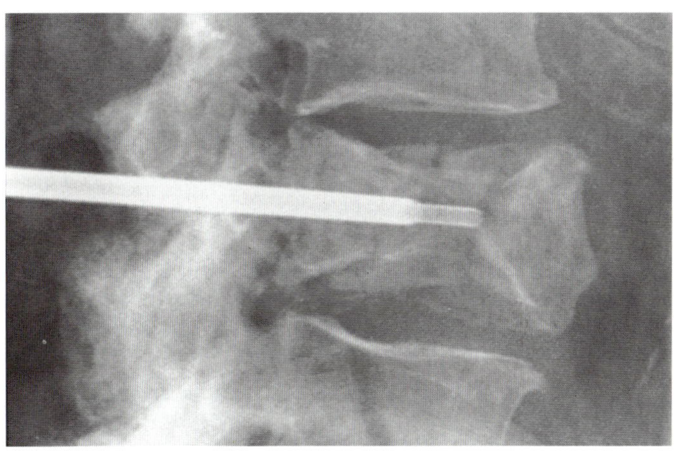

Fig. 28.6 Chordoma at the L3 level: collapse of the vertebral body.

in 1856, on the clivus at the base of the skull. Virchow gave the first histologic description, believing they were derived from the sphenooccipital synchondrosis. Shortly after, Muller found them in a number of sites, including the base of the skull, odontoid process of the axis and coccyx, and gave them the name 'ecchordosis physaliphora', presuming they were derived from the notochord. The current term 'chordoma' was suggested by Ribbert, who produced masses similar to chordomas by puncture of the annulus fibrosus in rabbits.

Ecchordosis physaliphora is a small gelatinous excrescence, presenting as a soft pedunculated mass usually a few millimeters wide at the base of the skull, the sacrococcygeal region, the vertebral body or rarely the nasopharyngeal submucosa. It is usually discovered incidentally at autopsy (1.5–2%[15,20,21]); it may be symptomatic.[21-24] Ultrastructural features of ecchordoses are similar to those of the notochord and chordomas;[25-31] immunohistochemical reactions are also the same,[24] demonstrating the embryologic derivation from fetal notochord.

Chordomas arise from aberrant chordal vestiges rather than from the chordal remnants within the nucleus pulposus of the intervertebral disc.[18,29]

SKELETAL DISTRIBUTION

On the spinal axis, 48–60% are located in the sacrococcygeal region (Figs 28.2–28.5), 13–20% in the mobile spine[32] (Figs 28.6–28.8) and 39% in the sphenooccipital region.[2,33] In vertebrae, almost half of the tumors involve the cervical vertebrae, particularly the second cervical vertebra;[34] the lumbar area is involved in 35% of cases and the thoracic vertebrae in 17%. In children, most tumors are found in the skull or the cervical spine.

Multiple locations are very unusual.[35-37] Rarely, chordomas may arise in ectopic locations, without apparent bone destruction,[38] but most cases of extraaxial chordomas arising in the soft tissues represent extension of bone

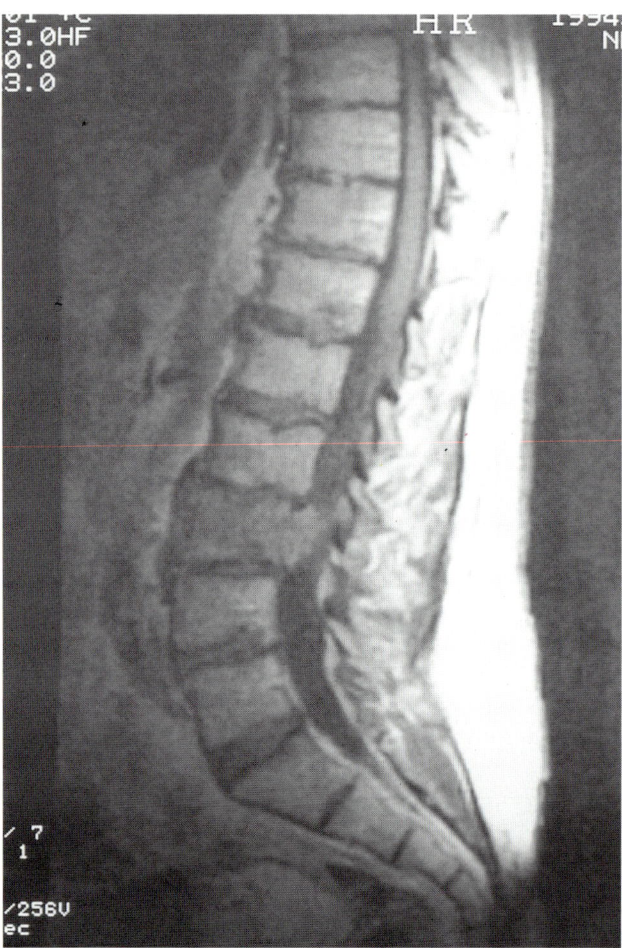

Fig. 28.7

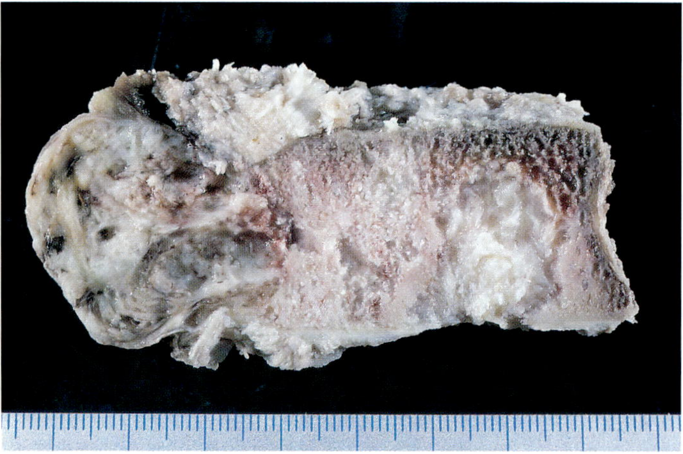

Fig. 28.8

Figs 28.7, 28.8 Chordoma at the L3 level: lateral and posterior tumoral extension.

tumors,[39] especially near the spinal column. In children also, rare extraskeletal locations have been described in the retropharyngeal and gluteal regions and presacral soft tissues.

IMAGING

In rare cases, a sacrococcygeal chordoma may appear as a mass clearly separated from the sacrum, without any bone destruction[40] (Mulder et al 1993), but usually there is destruction of several segments of the sacrum, with a centrally located soft tissue tumor mass.[40] Margins are clearly defined, with pseudolobulation or even a honeycomb pattern. The tumor appears to arise from the more caudal segments of the sacrum, S3–S5, and the coccyx.[40]

Osseous expansion, anterior soft tissue mass and osteosclerosis are associated with calcifications in 50–70% of cases; the calcifications are amorphous and mostly peripheral.

Spinal chordomas generally arise in the vertebral body but may extend into the posterior elements. Rarely, chordomas are confined to a vertebral transverse process.[41,42] In vertebrae, the destruction of bone is associated with osteosclerosis located peripherally or involving the entire vertebral body[34] (Mulder et al 1993). Reactive new bone formation may be related to the slow progressive growth.[43] Initially, the destruction of the vertebral body is not accompanied by loss of the adjacent intervertebral discs,[9] but a narrowing of the disc space may occur[34,43] and contiguous vertebral bodies may be involved, especially in the cervical area.

A paravertebral soft tissue mass eventually exhibits calcifications[1,12] and epidural extension is demonstrated in more than 90% of patients by myelography.[9]

On radionuclide scanning, most of the tumor is cold;[44] the peripheral margins show increased activity.[3] Sacrococcygeal chordomas demonstrate no abnormal vascularity on angiography[1] but on spinal angiography the tumor may be avascular or have considerable neovascularity.[43]

The bone destruction and the soft tissue mass are shown on CT scans in 90% of cases, along with calcified debris.[3] CT is the best method for the evaluation of chordomas,[3,45] demonstrating the peripheral reactive sclerosis,[46,47] the degree of extension and calcification,[48] and necrosis and mucoid collections appearing as hypodense lesions.[49]

MRI is, however, superior for the detection of small polypoid soft tissue mass extension,[44,45] for longitudinal extent and the involvement of sacral nerve roots. Chordomas exhibit a low signal intensity on T1 and a high signal intensity on T2-weighted images.[41,45]

GROSS PATHOLOGY

Vertebral chordomas have a small to moderate size, but sacrococcygeal tumors are usually bulky masses, from 5 to 20 cm in diameter[50] (Figs 28.9–28.12). Most of them exhibit a lobulated configuration and may remain encapsulated or pseudoencapsulated for a long time; the soft tissue component may be covered by a layer of periosteal

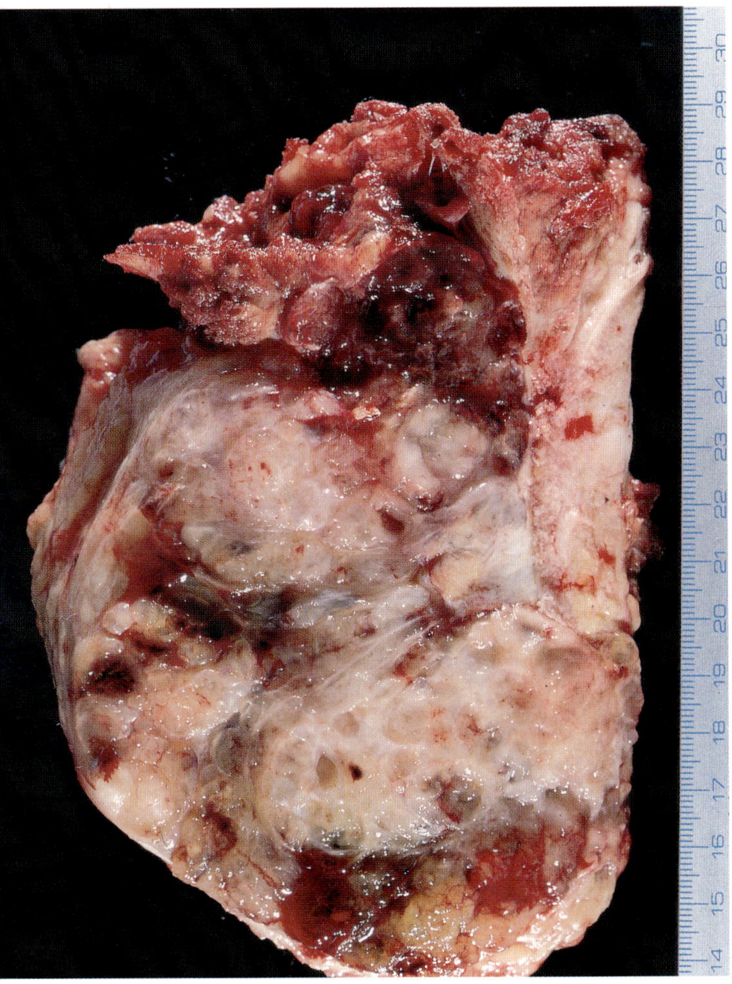

Fig. 28.9

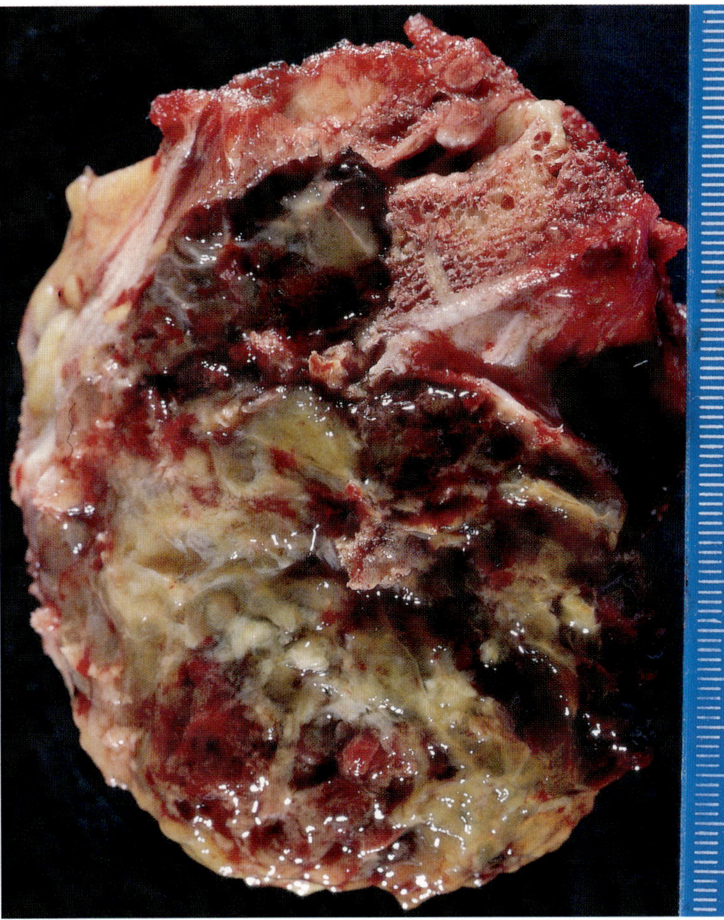

Fig. 28.10

Figs 28.9, 28.10 Sacrococcygeal chordomas: glistening and mucoid, hemorrhagic and necrotic aspects.

bone, but the tumor can extend beyond these boundaries. Intraosseous margins are less distinct.

Tumoral nodules are gelatinous or myxoid, grayish or bluish-white; hemorrhages, cyst formation, areas of necrosis, dystrophic calcifications or remnants of bone engulfed in the tumor are not uncommon.

HISTOPATHOLOGY

Most tumors have a lobular architecture;[33] fibrous septa have thin-walled vessels and sometimes lymphocytic infiltrates. In spite of the usual large lakes of extracellular mucin, there is great variation in the architectural pattern and cells may be arranged in cords, columns, sheets or trabeculae (Figs 28.13–28.25).

Large cells with distinct borders and multiple intracytoplasmic vacuoles are the well-known physaliphorous cells; the nucleus is centrally or eccentrically located. These bubble-like cells may be sparse and difficult to find in some tumors.[2]

Many cells exhibit compact epithelioid growth, with an eosinophilic cytoplasm; they may be arranged in concentric spherical formations.[50] Some are binucleated or even multinucleated.

The cells may be stellate, round or spindle shaped, often in a syncytial cord arrangement, appearing as small immature cells.

Nuclei are variable in shape and size and the nucleoli are often prominent. Mitotic activity is very scarce or absent.[2,50] In about 5% of cases, tumoral cells may exhibit hyperchromatic nuclei or pleomorphism or even appear as large bizarre cells.[2] More usually, the large cells have apparently degenerating nuclei (so-called ghost cells[50]).

Glycogen granules are easily found and are more abundant in eosinophilic cells;[51] reticulin fibers support the tumor cells.[11]

Areas of necrosis, correlated to tumor size, are found in approximately 2% of cases.[2] The peripheral fibrous encapsulation or reactive bone shell may be infiltrated by the tumor. In bone, nodules can be found in the bone marrow.

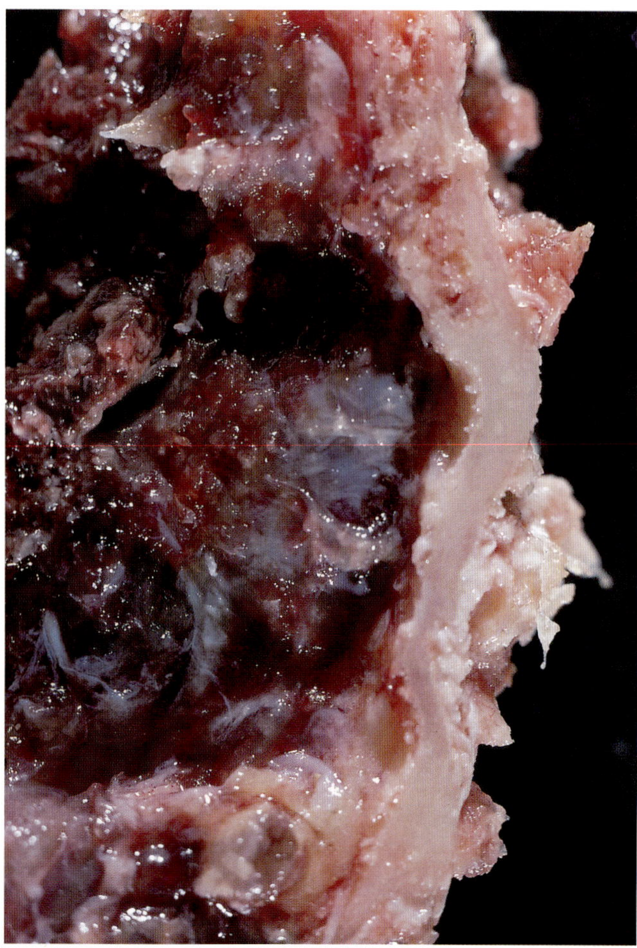

Fig. 28.11 Sacrococcygeal chordoma: reactive peripheral bone shell.

The variations in histologic appearance do not have any prognostic significance.[2,50]

In children, classic chordomas have a greater range of cellularity.[7] Atypical or sarcomatoid variants have been reported, with round, spindle-shaped or epithelioid cells; the diagnosis of chordoma for these primitive tumors has been discussed by Dahlin & Unni.[51]

CHONDROID CHORDOMAS

First described by Falconer et al in 1968,[52] chordomas in the sphenoocciput showing focally cartilaginous features have been associated with a markedly prolonged survival in a study from the Mayo Clinic, the authors suggesting the term 'chondroid chordoma'.[53]

The chondroid variant accounts for 28% of the chordomas of the base of the skull,[54] but they have also been reported in sacrococcygeal or spinal locations.[55–58]

In chondroid areas, which may be small or extensive, cells with mild cellular atypia and hypercellularity are located in lacunae embedded in an amorphous blue ground substance.[57] On smears from aspirate, numerous single or clustered physaliphorous cells are associated with atypical cartilaginous cells, in a myxoid background.[59]

Some immunohistochemical, enzymatic and ultrastructural studies have led to the firm conclusion that chondroid chordomas are a form of low-grade chondrosarcoma,[60–63] the most important finding being the negative immunostaining with epithelial markers. In other reports, the staining was confined to chordomatous areas[31,55] and it has been suggested that the epithelial characteristics are lost as the tumor undergoes a chondroid differentiation[31] or that these findings reflect a mixed epithelial-mesenchymal nature.[64] However, in many studies, cartilaginous regions demonstrate staining for epithelial markers[56–58,65–68] and ultrastructurally, both chordoid and chondroid areas present tonofilaments and desmosomes.[56,67–69] One case, formed only by neoplastic cartilage, has shown cells with epithelial markers.[57]

It has been suggested recently that most cases reported as chondroid chordomas with negative immunohistochemical and ultrastructural epithelial differentiation represent true myxoid chondrosarcomas,[54,58,70] the cord-like arrangement mimicking a chordoma. Furthermore, some authors suggest that focal chondroid differentiation is not unusual in chordomas[58] and the tumors retain their epithelial phenotype.[67] Coexpression of glial fibrillary acidic protein and vimentin has been postulated to be a reflection of the early chondroid differentiation in conventional chordomas.[71]

The term 'hyalinized chordoma' has recently been proposed.[67]

There is no significant survival difference between cartilage-containing tumors that are cytokeratin positive or negative,[70,72] but in children and young adults, a poorer outcome has been reported for those presenting with chondroid chordomas.[5]

DEDIFFERENTIATED CHORDOMAS

These bimorphic tumors, more common in sacrococcygeal locations, combine a classic or even a chondroid chordoma[73] with a spindle cell tumoral component. Accounting for approximately 9% of all chordomas,[74,75] they presumably reflect a tumor progression.

Most of them are discovered on recurrence over long periods[76–78] and a progressive transformation has been well documented over a 7-year period.[79] Many dedifferentiated chordomas arise on irradiated tumors but the time interval after the radiation therapy is relatively short, from 3 to 5 years.[73,77,78,80,82] Some cases exhibit spontaneous progression.[73–75,83]

A biphasic pattern can be diagnosed on aspirates, demonstrating physaliphorous cells and a pleomorphic or anaplastic component.[84–86] Histologically, they have to be differentiated from focal areas in conventional chordomas, showing some spindle-shaped cells with atypical nuclei.

The high-grade sarcoma may be distinctly demarcated

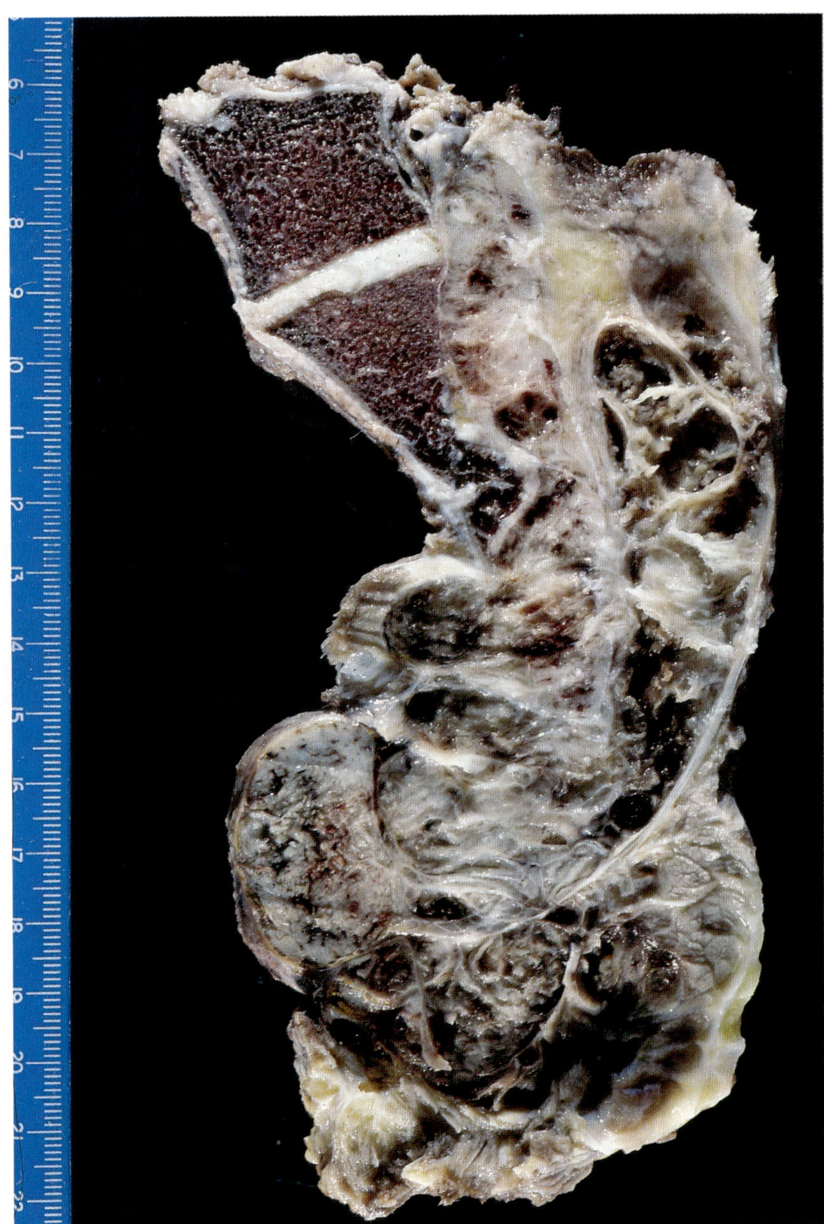

Fig. 28.12 Total involvement of the sacrum by a chordoma.

from the chordoma, with no proof of transition, even on ultrastructural examination.[76,77] Some cases demonstrate a gradual transition, spindle or giant cells being reactive for cytokeratin, EMA and vimentin or keratin-negative cells containing large amounts of glycogen;[73,79,87] ultrastructurally, the spindle cell component may exhibit epithelial features with desmosomes and tonofilaments.[78]

Malignant fibrous histiocytoma is the most common sarcomatous component,[74–82] followed by osteosarcoma,[82,87] fibrosarcoma[40,82] or pleomorphic spindle cell sarcoma.[83,88]

On flow cytometry, dedifferentiated chordomas are all aneuploid or multiploid.[73,89]

The clinical course is rapidly fatal, with recurrences and pulmonary metastases in about 90% of cases,[74,78,81] even if temporary remission has been achieved with aggressive chemotherapy.[89] The purely dedifferentiated component is present in pulmonary metastases or associated with fields of conventional chordomas; some very unusual metastases may exhibit only a classic chordoma.[75]

INTRASKELETAL SO-CALLED 'PARACHORDOMAS'

Rare soft tissue tumors arising in the deep soft tissues of the extremities have been named 'parachordomas'.[90] They have to be separated from the more common chordoid sarcomas which are clearly extraskeletal myxoid chon-

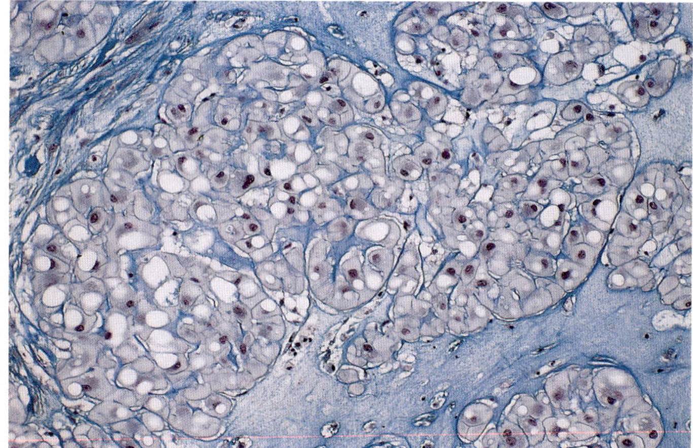

Fig. 28.13

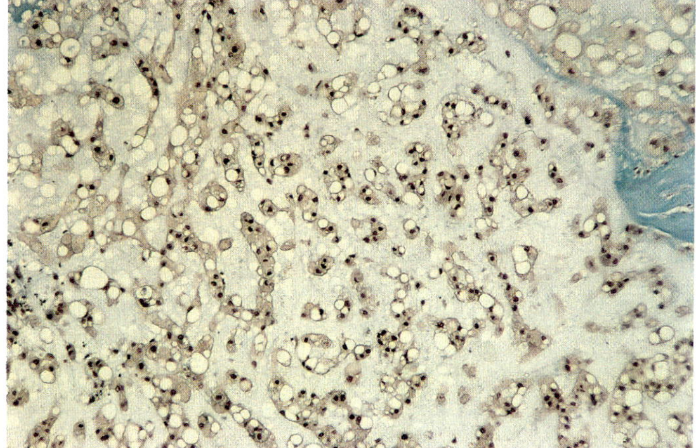

Fig. 28.14

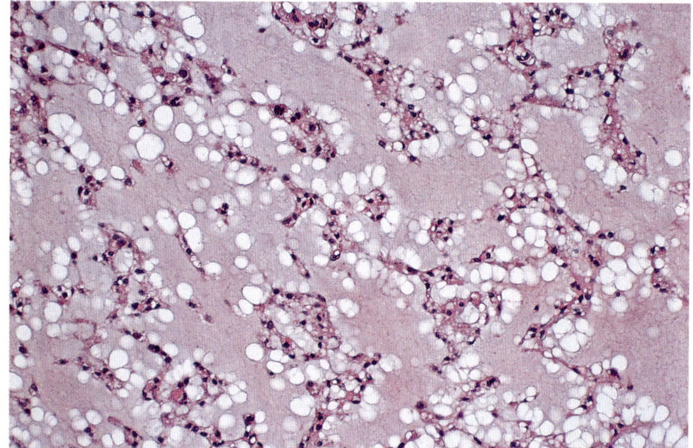

Fig. 28.15

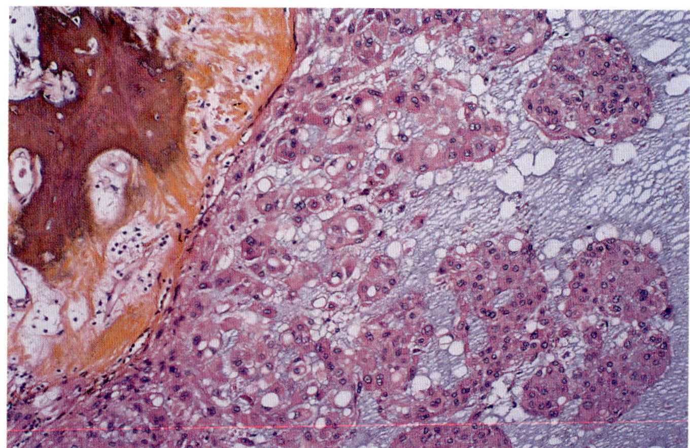

Fig. 28.16

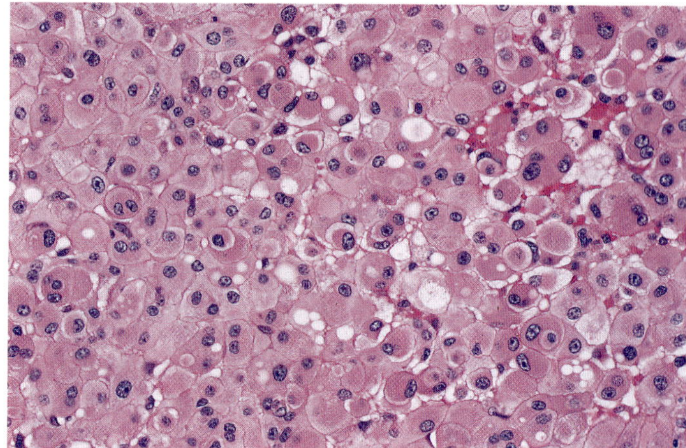

Fig. 28.17

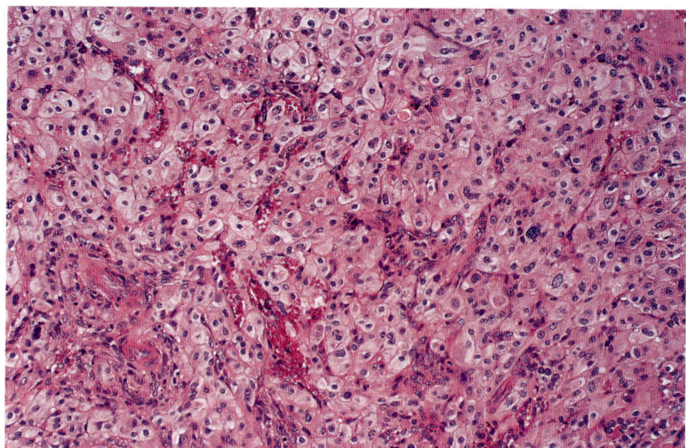

Fig. 28.18

Figs 28.13–28.15 Sacrococcygeal chordomas: variations in the architectural pattern with intra- and extracellular mucin.

Figs 28.16–28.18 Sacrococcygeal chordomas: cells with an epithelioid growth and acidophilic cytoplasms.

drosarcomas,[91] even if some of them exhibit an epithelial antigen.[92]

The real soft tissue parachordomas have histological and ultrastructural features similar to those of chordo-

mas[93] but immunohistochemically, they are similar to chondroid cells.[94] Only two cases of tumors resembling parachordomas have been described in the appendicular skeleton; in one case, the tumor was unexpectedly related

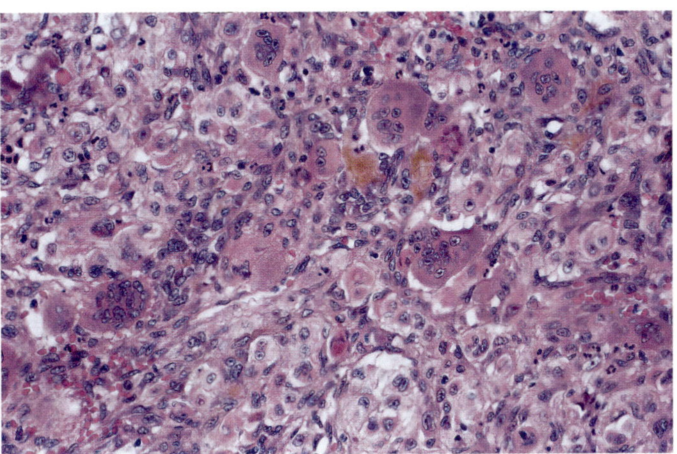

Fig. 28.19 Reactive giant cells in a chordoma of the cervical spine.

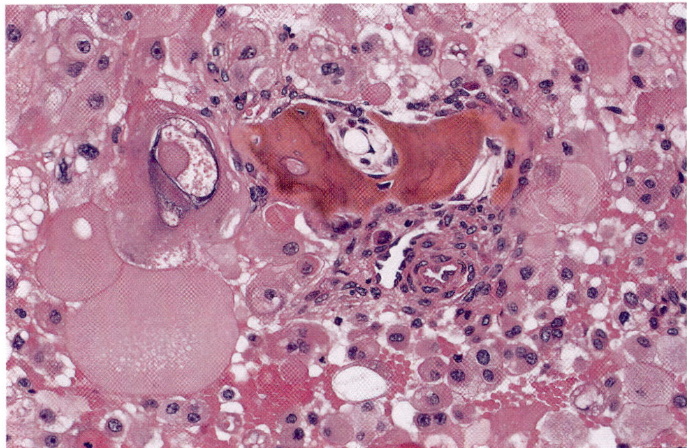

Fig. 28.20 Degenerative cellular changes in a chordoma of a lumbar vertebra.

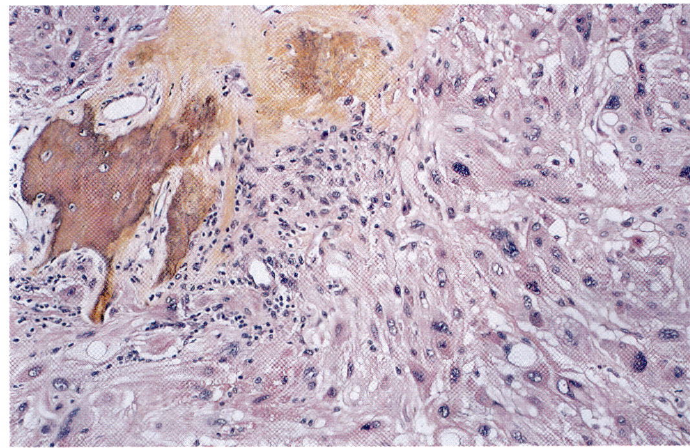

Fig. 28.21 Nuclear abnormalities in a chordoma of a lumbar vertebra.

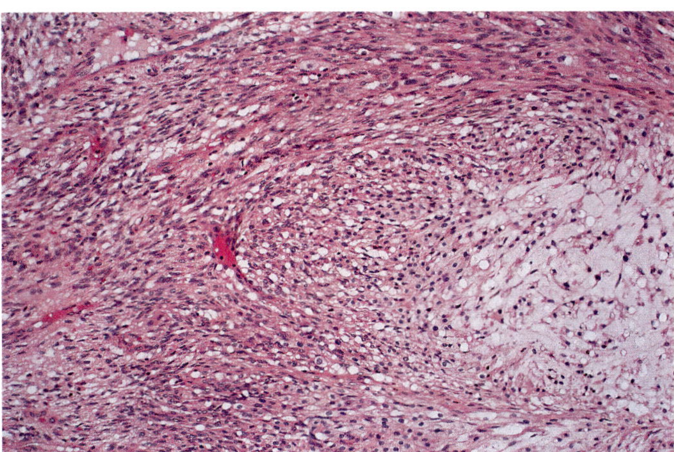

Fig. 28.22 Spindle cells in a chordoma of a lumbar vertebra.

to a brown fat origin,[95] while the other case showed all the ultrastructural features of a true peripheral chordoma.[30]

CYTOPATHOLOGY

Vacuolated cells in a background of myxoid stroma (Figs 28.26–28.32) can be identified on aspirate, squash-smears,[59] touch imprints[96–98] or on cerebrospinal fluid.[99,100] The cells may be isolated or distributed in sheets, aggregates, cords or syncytial clusters.[101]

Physaliphorous cells, mononuclear or binucleated, are not uniformly seen.[98,102,103] The cytoplasm is well demarcated, showing multiple finely septate vacuoles radially arranged around the central nucleus[104,105] with one or two prominent nucleoli[105] and occasional nuclear inclusions or pseudoinclusions.[103,105,106] The cells may present a single vacuole, with a signet-ring form, or may look like multinucleated giant cells.[103]

Some tumors exhibit bland nuclear features[107] with a low nuclear–cytoplasmic ratio and a finely granular chromatic pattern.[103,104]

The vacuolated cells can be associated or replaced by non-vacuolated smaller cells.[102,108,109] Smaller stellate or spindle-shaped cells can be grouped in sheets or in a syncytial arrangement, with a scant eosinophilic cytoplasm.[98,105,106,110,111]

Cell-within-cell arrangements (cannibalism) are a common finding[96,102–104] with a concentric pearl-like formation.[96,106]

May-Grunwald-Giemsa staining appears superior to Papanicolaou staining for demonstrating the purplish-red mucoid matrix and the vacuolated cytoplasm.[105] With Papanicolaou staining, the matrix is gray to green[109] and is intensely metachromatic on Diff-Quick-stained smears.[103]

The matrix stains metachromatically red with toluidine blue[105] and the strong intra- and extracellular staining with alcian blue at p.H 2.5 and 1.0 is almost completely

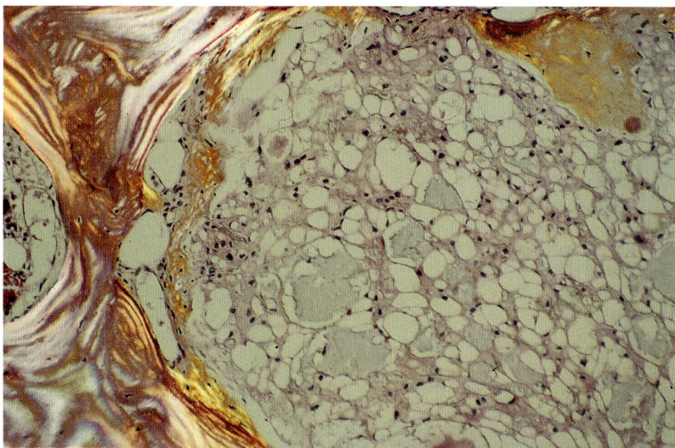

Fig. 28.23

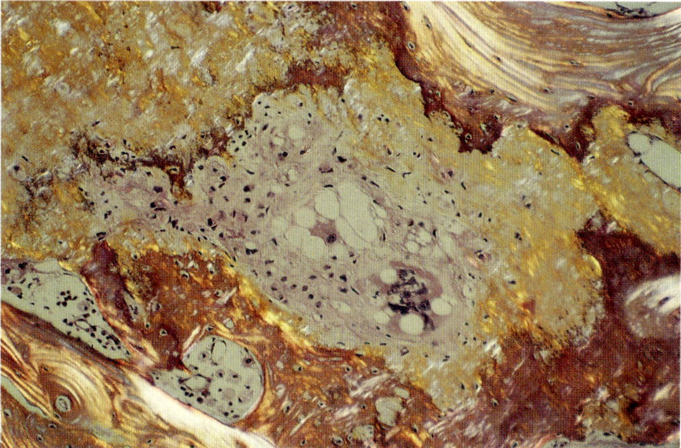

Fig. 28.24

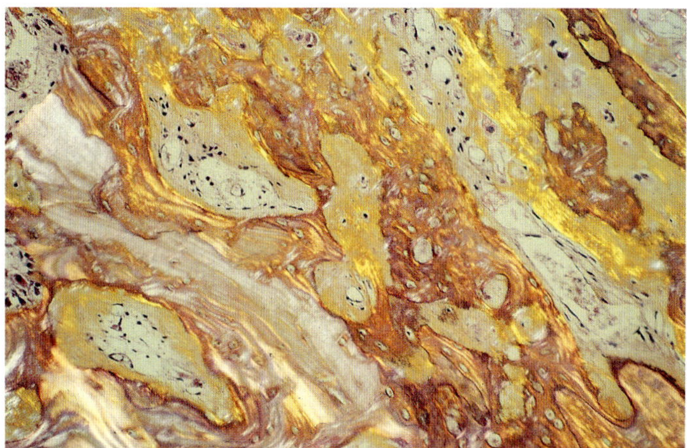

Fig. 28.25

Figs 28.23–28.25 Vertebral chordoma: remodeling of bone with some areas of extensive bone formation (polarized light).

digested by testicular hyaluronidase, responding to 'acidic' mucins. On smears, intracytoplasmic and matrix PAS staining is removed by diastase digestion, responding to glycogen.[103,104,106]

HISTOCHEMISTRY AND ENZYME HISTOCHEMISTRY

On section, chordoma cells and extracellular ground substance are both stained by PAS and alcian blue.[60,104,112] Intracytoplasmic glycogen is present in large amounts.[113,114] Chordomas are not stained with phosphotungsten acid hematoxylin, unlike cartilage lesions.[112]

The extracellular matrix is composed of a collagenous framework and a heterogeneous family of glycosaminoglycans with a prevalence of chondroitin-4 and chondroitin-6-sulfate chains and a lower quantity of keratan sulfate and hyaluronic acid,[114–116] like the early nucleus pulposus extracellular matrix.[114]

Chordomas exhibit a strong 5'nucleotidase positivity localized on the plasma membrane.[60] There is an α-naphtyl acetate esterase (non-specific esterase) activity in chordomas, notochord and chondrosarcomas[13] which is not found in normal cartilage. The tumors are rich in oxydoreductive enzymes, but also in enzymes leading to the synthesis of stromal glycosaminoglycans from glycogen.[116]

On lectin histochemistry, the lectin-binding pattern (sialic acid, sialoglycoproteins) closely reflects that of the human fetal notochord.[117]

IMMUNOHISTOCHEMISTRY

Cytokeratin positivity, first demonstrated with an immunofluorescence technique and polyclonal antibody,[118] is detected in 90–100% of cases with principally low molecular weight keratins; chordomas exhibit immunopositivity with the monoclonal antibody CAM5–2, recognizing three cytokeratin polypeptides.[13] Detailed immunohistochemical characterization of different cytokeratins subclasses demonstrates that the simple epithelial cytokeratins and cytokeratins characteristic of squamous differentiation are generally lacking.[119]

Positivity with the monoclonal antibody HMFG-2 (human milk fat globule protein), recognizing an oligosaccharide sequence present on the cell surface of secretory epithelia, is found in chordomas and notochord but not in normal cartilage.[13,31,56] EMA positivity is found in 80–100% of cases.[56,63,106,120–122]

The coexpression of cytokeratins and vimentin is now well established,[63,65,118–123] in all cell types but not in the intra- or extracellular vacuoles or the mucoid matrix,[122] with an incidence from 30 to 100% of cases. Immunocytochemically, the staining is intense around the cytoplasmic vacuoles.[105] The same coexpression is demonstrated in nucleus pulposus cells,[124] human fetal notochord[13] and ecchordosis physaliphora.[24,125]

S-100 positivity is found in 80–100% of cases.[56,63,120,126,127] The immunoreactivity of chordoma cells seems to correlate with their morphology and meta-

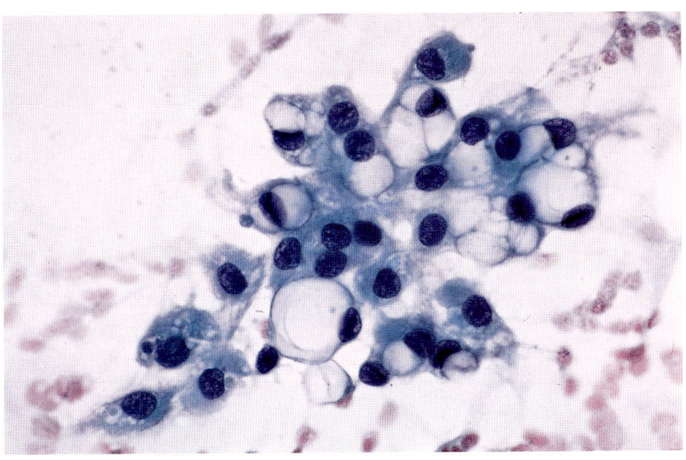

Fig. 28.26

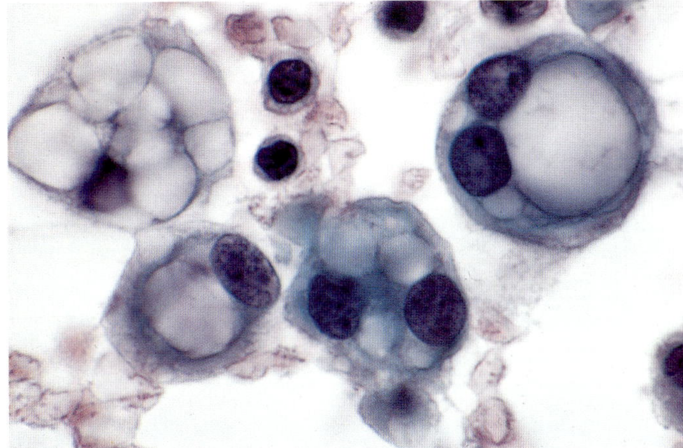

Fig. 28.28

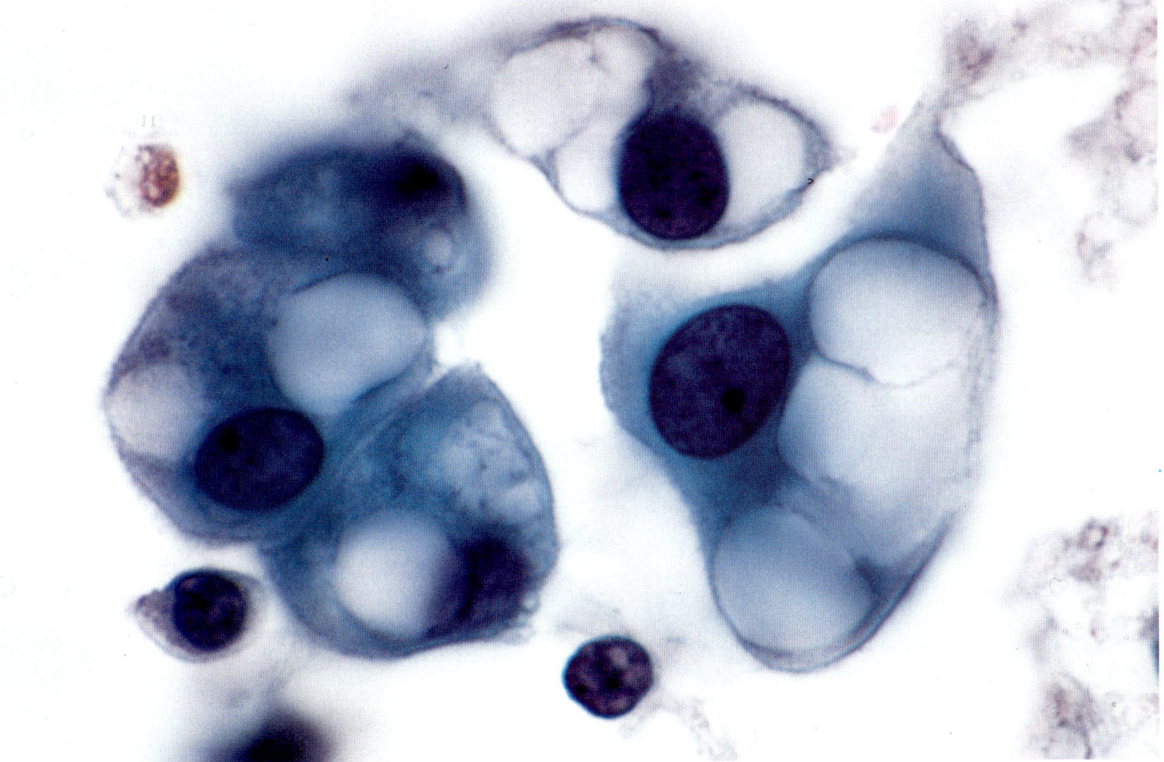

Fig. 28.27

Figs 28.26–28.32 Sacrococcygeal chordomas. Imprint cytology demonstrating vacuolated cells, concentric pearl-like formation and non-vacuolated cells with binucleated forms.

bolic activity as well as the type of extracellular matrix.[128] Stellate cells which are the stem cells as well as the cells of the notochord are S-100 negative and the stroma is devoid of mucosubstances or contains small amounts of hyaluronic acid. Cells with abundant glycogen particles, physaliphorous cells, in areas of stromal GAG and sulfated mucopolysaccharides demonstrate a strong reaction;[128] there is no nuclear staining, unlike chondrosarcomas.[106]

NSE positivity has been found in all cell types, but par-

ticularly in cells with high metabolic activity[106,120,128,129] and in tumor giant cells.[122,130]

CEA immunostaining has been reported as strongly positive as well as alpha foetoprotein,[120] or negative in some series.[7,24,103,131–133]

Neurofilament staining is also variable;[122,123] glial fibrillary acidic expression is sometimes positive[134] but negative in most reports. Expression of melanoma-associated antigens may be entirely negative[67] or exist in more than half

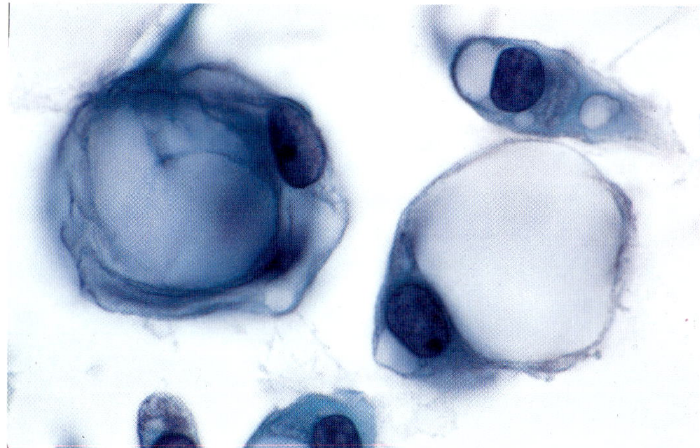

Fig. 28.29

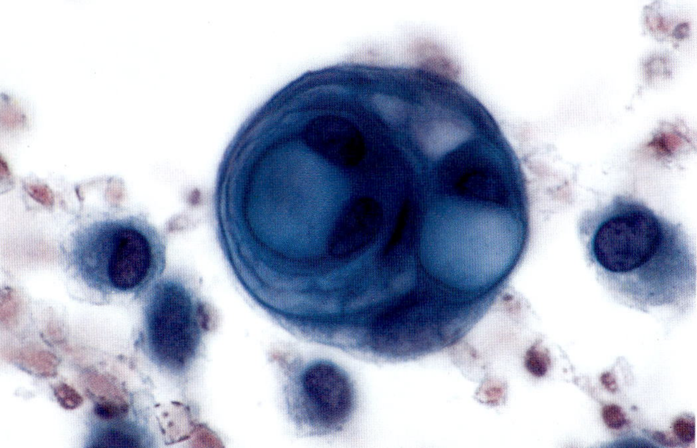

Fig. 28.30

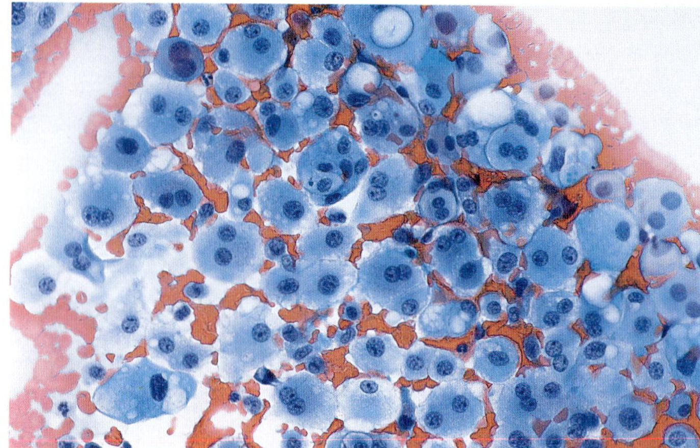

Fig. 28.31

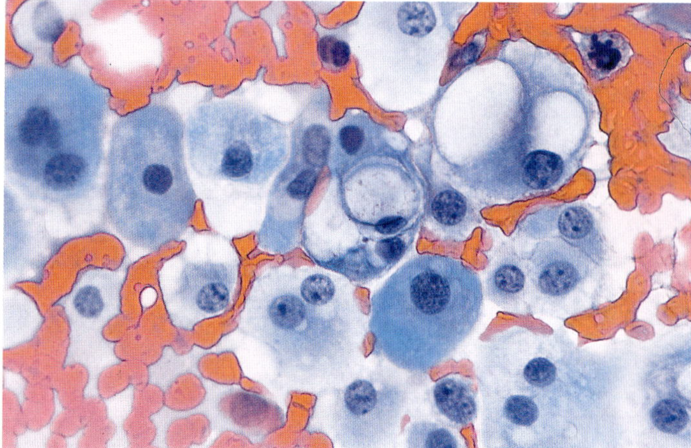

Fig. 28.32

of the cases.[31,63] There is no immunostaining with desmin, but chordomas may express some muscle-like antigens, such as myoglobin.[135]

A strong immunoreactivity for fibronectin has been reported[120] and a tissue polypeptide antigen may be identified,[56,136] corresponding to intermediate filaments containing 'non-epidermal' keratins.

Less specific staining with α-antichymotrypsin is found in 80% of cases;[121] lysozyme is absent or detected in few cases. Epithelial growth factor (EGF) receptor and C-neu oncogene products have been demonstrated.[137]

Collagen is the main structural component of the extracellular matrix of chordomas and notochord. Chordomas contain a predominant collagenous protein type I[138] and basement membrane proteins such as type IV collagen and laminin.[139] In the notochord, type II collagen is widespread, but the biochemical analysis of the collagenous proteins is similar to chordomas, supporting the notochordal origin of the tumors.[138]

The constant coexpression of cytokeratin, vimentin and S-100 protein is a distinctive feature of chordomas[140] and coexpression of cytokeratin, vimentin and neurofilaments is shared only by choroid plexus tumors.[122]

FLOW CYTOMETRY

Ploidy has been studied on flow cytometry or on Feulgen-stained tissue.[72,141–143] Most conventional chordomas are diploid;[141] 20–27% of chordomas exhibit an aneuploid-multiploid DNA content and both typical and chondroid chordomas have the same proportion of diploid and tetraploid tumors.[72]

Whatever the location, DNA aneuploidy appears to be correlated with the clinical outcome, as there is a strong relationship with decreased survival.[141,142] The proliferative activity, as investigated by DNA flow cytometry, MIB-1 labeling index and p53 overexpression, seems related to a diffuse syncytial pattern of chordoma cells, with high-grade nuclear atypias.[143] Conversely, there is no significant correlation between the prognosis and the count of silver-stained nucleolar organizing region-associated proteins (AgNORs).[142]

CYTOGENETICS

Chordomas may be cytogenetically normal or exhibit distinct abnormal clones with an involvement of the Y chromosome in a structural rearrangement.[144] Most cases are hypoploid, with predominant loss of chromosomes 3 and 4 and several complex structural anomalies involving particularly chromosome 1.[144–148] However, it appears that there is a lack of general chromosomal abnormality in chordomas.[149]

ELECTRON MICROSCOPY

The stem cells have a stellate appearance, with a high nuclear–cytoplasmic ratio.[150,151] Physaliphorous cells up to 50 µu in diameter develop from the stellate cells[150,152] and transitional cells are found in most studies.[26,29,150,152]

Microvillous projections of the cytoplasmic membrane have been described.[30,105,119] The nucleus is irregular in size and contour and may present cytoplasmic inclusions,[25,30,150] usually with a single prominent nucleolus. Some cells are binucleated.[30,150,153] Desmosomes may be occasionally present or well developed.[154,155] Abundant bundles of prominent tonofilaments are located in the cytoplasm. Pinocytotic vesicles[56,151,155] or a few scattered lipid droplets have been described; glycogen is often found in great quantity.[113]

A constant association of mitochondria and endoplasmic reticulum in a structurally ordered complex was first described by Erlandson[152] and confirmed by others[30,105,129] but this 'complex' may be found in well-differentiated chondrosarcomas or clear cell chondrosarcomas.[30]

Microtubular aggregates within the rough endoplasmic reticulum have been described in chondroid chordomas,[69] as well as in classic clival or sacrococcygeal tumors[155–157] or even myxoid chondrosarcomas or osteosarcomas, presumably representing some crystallized mucoprotein precursors.[156]

Two types of vacuoles have been described in chordoma cells. Some are smooth walled[150] and full of glycogen[30,113,152] and these are considered as cytolysosomes.[30] Small vacuoles have been described as originating from the rough endoplasmic reticulum,[26,150,158] from the smooth endoplasmic reticulum[25,28,113] or from both.[29,152]

Large vacuoles displace the nucleus and organelles to the cell periphery.[152] Lined by numerous structureless microvilli,[56,105,129,153] they may represent a herniation or a sequestration of the interstitial matrix.[26,29,113,154] Large vacuoles do not participate in the synthesis and storage of sulfated glycosaminoglycans or proteoglycans[116] which are located in the Golgi saccules or Golgi-derived mature secretory vesicles, contrary to some findings.[150,158–160] The large vacuoles may also be viewed as the result of the utilization and breakdown of membrane-bound glycogen by the glycogenolytic enzymes;[116] that is, as a degenerate terminal stage,[120] with membrane destruction of cell organelles.[114,150,154]

The extracellular matrix is fibrogranular, with abundant proteoglycan particles and scarce collagen fibers or lipid droplets.

COURSE, TREATMENT AND PROGNOSIS

The natural history of chordoma is a slow local growth and local invasion; death is most often caused by the consequences of tumoral growth due to incomplete excision.

The best treatment is wide surgical excision, usually followed by high-dose radiation[161] or even cryosurgery in unresectable tumors,[162] but the tumor is relatively radioresistant[11,33,163] and irradiation does not prevent recurrences.[12] Chemotherapy appears ineffective.[12,164,165]

The recurrence rate ranges from 28%[33] to 80% of cases,[3] depending on whether the tumor has been entered at surgery.[33]

The average time of occurrence of metastases is 3 years; they may be present at initial presentation or occur many years later.[11] The mean rate is about 30%.[1,3,11,33] The predominant sites are the lungs, lymph nodes and liver; rarer sites are the bones and the skin, but in some cases they may be widespread.[165–167] Nine to eleven percent of chordomas exhibit skin involvement;[168,169] occasionally, the cutaneous finding is the initial sign of chordoma and the term 'chordoma cutis' has been proposed.[169,170] Metastases to the skeleton without evidence of any other metastases are rare;[34,170,171] the most common skeletal site is the spine.

Sacrococcygeal chordomas metastasize with the greatest frequency. The rate of metastases from vertebral tumors ranges from 5% to 37%.[2,4,9] The actuarial survival rate at 5 years for patients treated by surgery alone is 76%[11] and at 10 years, 28%.[3]

DIFFERENTIAL DIAGNOSIS

Metastatic signet-ring cell or mucinous adenocarcinomas, coming mostly from the rectum, may cause some difficulties[105,129] but there is more cellular pleomorphism[105,110,111] and a higher mitotic rate. One has to rely on the finding of an acinar or glandular configuration, on the presence of neutral rather than acidic mucins and on the absence of physaliphorous cells, rather than on the overlapping findings of immunohistochemistry. Cells with large vacuoles in chordomas are not true signet-ring cells as there is a flap of cytoplasm between the nucleus and cell border opposite the vacuole.[107]

Renal cell carcinomas have some immunohistochemical features in common with chordomas, such as the cytokeratin and in some cases vimentin and S-100 positivity.[172] The fine cytoplasmic vacuoles of renal carcinomas are mucin negative,[126] exhibit a diastase-labile PAS reaction and are stained with oil red O.[104,107]

Myxoid chondrosarcomas are cytokeratin and EMA negative[13] and vimentin, S-100 and lysozyme positive; some chordoid sarcomas may express EMA but not cytokeratin[92] and poorly differentiated chondrosarcomas can ultrastructurally exhibit prominent intermediate filaments or cell-to-cell junctions resembling desmosomes.[118] In some chondrosarcoma cells, large vacuoles may displace the nucleus, but physaliphorous cells are lacking;[173] the cells are more frequently binucleated with plump and hyperchromatic nuclei.[103,111]

Very unusual chondromas in vertebral locations may have a few nests of cells resembling chordomas.[174]

Myxoid liposarcomas lack bubbly cytoplasm[103] and the nuclei are larger with indentations of the vacuoles.[105] PAS and alcian blue stains are abolished by enzymatic digestion with diastase and hyaluronidase.[104] Liposarcomas may be S-100 positive, but lack epithelial markers. Fat stains are not found in chordomas.

Myxopapillary sacrococcygeal ependymomas have spindle or stellate cells with long tapering cytoplasmic processes, arranged in clusters or in papillary or rosette formation, in an abundant mucinous stroma. The electron microscopic features are the presence of cilia and basal bodies, as well as the orientation of the cells to a basal lamina.[105] They are reactive for vimentin and, in half of the cases, for S-100 protein.[126] Strong reactivity for glial fibrillary acidic protein may be found in some chordomas, so the coexpression with cytokeratin is useful for diagnosing the latter.[118]

REFERENCES

1. Ericksson B, Gunterberg B, Kindblom L G. Chordoma: a clinicopathologic and prognostic study of a Swedish national series. Acta Orthop Scand 1981: 52: 49–58
2. Bjornsson J, Wold L E, Ebersold M J, Laws E R. Chordoma of the mobile spine. Cancer 1993: 71: 735–740
3. Smith J, Ludwig R L, Marcove R C. Sacrococcygeal chordoma. Skeletal Radiol 1987: 16: 37–44
4. Sundaresan N. Chordomas. Clin Orthop 1986: 204: 135–142
5. Wold L E, Laws E R Jr. Cranial chordomas in children and young adults. J Neurosurg 1983: 59: 1043–1047
6. Sibley R K, Day D L, Dehner L P, Trueworthy R C. Metastasising chordoma in early childhood; a pathological and immunohistochemical study with review of the literature. Pediatr Pathol 1987: 7: 287–301
7. Coffin C M, Swanson P E, Wick M R, Dehner L P. Chordoma in childhood and adolescence. Arch Pathol Lab Med 1993: 117: 927–933
8. Kaneko Y, Sato Y, Iwaki T, Shin R W, Tateishi J, Fukui M. Chordoma in early childhood: a clinicopathological study. Neurosurgery 1991: 29: 442–446
9. Sundaresan N, Galicich J H, Chu F C, Huvos A G. Spinal chordomas. J Neurosurg 1979: 50: 312–319
10. Nakayama Y, Takeno Y, Tsugu H, Tomonaga M. Maffucci's syndrome associated with intracranial chordoma. Neurosurgery 1994: 34: 907–909
11. Rich T A, Schiller A, Suit H D, Mankin H J. Clinical and pathological review of 48 cases of chordoma. Cancer 1985: 56: 182–187
12. Walsh T M, Mayer P J. Chordoma of the thoracic spine presenting as a second primary malignant lesion. Spine 1992: 17: 1524–1528
13. Salisbury J R, Isaacson P G. Demonstration of cytokeratins and an epithelial membrane antigen in chordomas and human fetal notochord. Am J Surg Pathol 1985: 9: 791–797
14. Heaton J M, Turner D R. Reflections on notochordal differentiation arising from a study of chordomas. Histopathology 1985: 9: 543–550
15. Horwitz T. Chordal ectopia and its possible relation to chordoma. Arch Pathol 1941: 31: 354–362
16. Pazzaglia U E, Salisbury J R, Byers P D. Development and involution of the notochord in the human spine. J R Soc Med 1989: 82: 413–415
17. Panattoni G L, Corvetti G, Sisto-Daneo L. Relations between subcellular events in the degenerating notochord and histopathological features of the spinal chordomas. Panminerva Med 1992: 34: 155–159
18. Salisbury J R. The pathology of the human notochord. J Pathol 1993: 171: 253–255
19. Salisbury J R, Deverell M H, Cookson M J, Whimster W F. Three-dimensional reconstruction of human embryonic notochords: clue to the pathogenesis of chordoma. J Pathol 1993: 171: 59–62
20. Ulich T R, Mirra J M. Ecchordosis physaliphora vertebralis. Clin Orthop 1982: 163: 282–289
21. Kurakowa H, Miura S, Goto T. Ecchordosis physaliphora arising from the cervical vertebra. The CT and MRI appearance. Neuroradiology 1988: 30: 81–83
22. Mapstone T B, Kaufman B, Ratcheson R A. Intradural chordoma without bone involvement: nuclear magnetic resonance (NMR) appearance. J Neurosurg 1983: 59: 535–537
23. Wolfe J T 3rd, Scheithauer B W. 'Intradural chordoma' or 'giant ecchordosis physaliphora'. Clin Neuropathol 1987: 6: 98–103
24. MacDonald R L, Deck J H. Immunohistochemistry of ecchordosis physaliphora and chordoma. Can J Neurol Sci 1990: 17: 420–423
25. Spjut H J, Luse S A. Chordoma: an electron microscopic study. Cancer 1964: 17: 643–656
26. Pena C E, Horvat B L, Fisher E R. The ultrastructure of chordoma. Am J Clin Pathol 1970: 53: 544–551
27. Wyatt R B, Schochet S S Jr, McCormick W F. Ecchordosis physaliphora. An electron microscopic study. J Neurosurg 1971: 34: 672–677
28. Horten B C, Montague S R. Human ecchordosis physaliphora and chick embryonic notochord: a comparative electron microscopic study. Virchows Arch A Pathol Anat Histol 1976: 371: 295–303
29. Ho K L. Ecchordosis physaliphora and chordoma: a comparative ultrastructural study. Clin Neuropathol 1985: 4: 77–86
30. Povysil C, Matejovsky Z. A comparative ultrastructural study of chondrosarcoma, chordoid sarcoma, chordoma and chordoma periphericum. Pathol Res Pract 1985: 179: 546–559
31. Rutherfoord G S, Davies A G. Chordomas. Ultrastructure and immunohistochemistry. Histopathology 1987: 11: 775–787
32. Pinto R S, Lin J P, Firooznia H, Lefleur R S. The osseous and angiographic features of vertebral chordomas. Neuroradiology 1975: 9: 231–241
33. Kaiser T E, Pritchard D J, Unni K K. Clinicopathologic study of sacrococcygeal chordoma. Cancer 1984: 53: 2574–2578
34. Abdelwahab I F, O'Leary P F, Steiner G C, Zwass A. Case report 357. Chordoma of the fourth lumbar vertebra metastasizing to the thoracic spine and ribs. Skeletal Radiol 1986: 15: 242–246
35. Anderson W B, Meyers H I. Multicentric chordoma. Cancer 1968: 21: 126–128
36. Bellet M, Grelet P, Azaloux H, Tavernier J, Reboul J. Chordome vertebral à double localisation. Ann Radiol (Paris) 1971: 14: 121–130
37. Risio M, Bagliani C, Leli R, Digirolamo P, Del Pero M, Coverliza S. Sacrococcygeal and vertebral chordomas. J Neurosurg Sci 1985: 29: 211–227
38. Suster S, Moran C A. Chordomas of the mediastinum: clinicopathologic, immunohistochemical, and ultrastructural study of six cases presenting as posterior mediastinal masses. Hum Pathol 1995: 26: 1354–1362
39. Cesirano A M, Maiorana A, Collina G, Fano R A. Extra-axial chordoma. Pathologica 1993: 85: 755–760
40. Smith J, Reuter V, Demas B. Case report 576. Anaplastic sacrococcygeal chordoma (dedifferentiated chordoma). Skeletal Radiol 1989: 18: 561–564
41. Yuh W T, Flickinger F W, Barloon T J, Montgomery W J. MR

imaging of unusual chordomas. J Comput Assist Tomogr 1988: 12: 30–35

42. Kamal M F, Farah G R, Malkawi H M, Khammash H M. Chordoma in a lumbar vertebral transverse process. Clin Oncol 1984: 10: 167–172

43. Heaston D K, Gelman M I. Case report 74. Chordoma of the 4th lumbar vertebral body with extension into L3–4 intervertebral disk space. Skeletal Radiol 1978: 3: 186–190

44. Hudson T M, Galceran M. Radiology of sacrococcygeal chordoma: difficulties in detecting soft tissue extension. Clin Orthop 1983: 175: 237–242

45. Rosenthal D I, Scott J A, Mankin H J, Wismer G L, Brady T J. Sacro-coccygeal chordoma: magnetic resonance imaging and computed tomography. AJR 1985: 145: 143–147

46. Firooznia H, Golimbu C, Rafii M, Reede D L, Kricheff H, Bjorkengren A. Computed tomography of spinal chordomas. J Comput Tomogr 1986: 10: 45–50

47. Roddie M, Adam A, Lambert H, Pickering D, Barker F. Case report 516. Lumbar vertebral chordoma causing sclerosis of affected vertebra (3rd lumbar vertebra). Skeletal Radiol 1989: 17: 611–613

48. Krol G, Sundaresan N, Deck M. Computed tomography of axial chordomas. J Comput Assist Tomogr 1983: 7: 286–289

49. Meyer J E, Lepke R A, Lindfors K K et al. Chordomas: their C T appearance in the cervical, thoracic and lumbar spine. Radiology 1984: 153: 693–696

50. Volpe R, Mazabraud A. A clinicopathologic review of 25 cases of chordoma (a pleomorphic and metastasizing neoplasm). Am J Surg Pathol 1983: 7: 161–170

51. Dahlin D C, Unni K K. Chordoma. Arch Pathol Lab Med 1994: 118: 596–597

52. Falconer M A, Bailey I C, Duchen L W. Surgical treatment of chordoma and chondroma of the skull base. J Neurosurg 1968: 29: 261–275

53. Heffelfinger M J, Dahlin D C, MacCarthy C S, Beabout J W. Chordomas and cartilaginous tumors of the skull base. Cancer 1973: 32: 410–420

54. Rosenberg A E, Brown G A, Bhan A K, Lee J M. Chondroid chordoma – a variant of chordoma. Am J Clin Pathol 1994: 101: 36–41

55. Chu T A. Chondroid chordoma of the sacrococcygeal region. Arch Pathol Lab Med 1987: 111: 861–864

56. Persson S, Kindblom L G, Angervall L. Classical and chondroid chordoma. Pathol Res Pract 1991: 187: 828–838

57. Wojno K J, Hruban R H, Garin-Chesa P, Huvos A G. Chondroid chordomas and low grade chondrosarcomas of the craniospinal axis. Am J Surg Pathol 1992: 16: 1144–1152

58. Ishida T, Dorfman H D. Chondroid chordoma versus low-grade chondrosarcoma of the base of the skull: can immunohistochemistry resolve the controversy? J Neurooncol 1994: 18: 199–206

59. Nguyen G K, Johnson E S, Mielke B W. Chondroid chordoma of the skull base diagnosed by squash-smear technique. Diagn Cytopathol 1985: 1: 161–163

60. Bottles K, Beckstead J H. Enzyme histochemical characterization of chordomas. Am J Surg Pathol 1984: 8: 443–447

61. Brooks J J, LiVolsi V A, Trojanowski J Q. Does chondroid chordoma exist? Acta Neuropathol (Berl) 1987: 72: 229–235

62. Brooks J J, Trojanowski J Q, LiVolsi V A. Chondroid chordoma: a low-grade chondrosarcoma and its differential diagnosis. Curr Top Pathol 1989: 80: 165–181

63. Walker W P, Landas S K, Bromley C M, Sturm M T. Immunohistochemical distinction of classic and chondroid chordomas. Mod Pathol 1991: 4: 661–666

64. Niwa J, Hashi K, Minase T. Immunohistochemical and electron microscopic studies on intracranial chordomas: difference between typical chordomas and chondroid chordomas. Noshuyo Byori 1994: 11: 15–21

65. Abenoza P, Sibley R K. Chordoma: an immunohistochemical study. Hum Pathol 1986: 17: 744–747

66. Salisbury J R. Demonstration of cytokeratin and an epithelial membrane antigen in chondroid chordoma. J Pathol 1987: 153: 37–40

67. Jeffrey P B, Biava C G, Davis R L. Chondroid chordoma. A hyalinized chordoma without cartilaginous differentiation. Am J Clin Pathol 1995: 103: 271–279

68. Mierau G W, Weeks D A. Chondroid chordoma. Ultrastruct Pathol 1987: 11: 731–737

69. Valderrama E, Kahn L B, Lipper S, Marc J. Chondroid chordoma. Am J Surg Pathol 1983: 7: 625–632

70. O'Connell J X, Renard L G, Liebsch N J, Efird J T, Munzenrider J E, Rosenberg A E. Base of skull chordoma. Cancer 1994: 74: 2261–2267

71. Wittchow R, Landas S K. Glial fibrillary acidic protein expression in pleomorphic adenoma, chordoma and astrocytoma. Arch Pathol Lab Med 1991: 115: 1030–1033

72. Mitchell A, Scheithauer B W, Unni K K, Forsyth P J, Wold L E, McGivney D J. Chordoma and chondroid neoplasms of the spheno-occiput. Cancer 1993: 72: 2943–2949

73. Hruban R H, May M, Marcove R C, Huvos A G. Lumbo-sacral chordoma with high-grade malignant cartilaginous and spindle cell components. Am J Surg Pathol 1990: 14: 384–389

74. Meis J M, Raymond A K, Evans H L, Charles R E, Giraldo A A. 'Dedifferentiated' chordoma. Am J Surg Pathol 1987: 11: 516–525

75. Meis J M. 'Dedifferentiation' in bone and soft-tissue tumors. A histological indicator of tumor progression. Pathol Annu 1991: 26 Pt 1: 37–62

76. Makek M, Leu H J. Malignant fibrous histiocytoma arising in a recurrent chordoma. Virchows Arch A Pathol Anat Histol 1982: 397: 241–250

77. Miettinen M, Lehto V P, Virtanen I. Malignant fibrous histiocytoma within a recurrent chordoma. Am J Clin Pathol 1984: 82: 738–743

78. Miettinen M, Karaharju E, Jarvinen H. Chordoma with massive spindle-cell sarcomatous transformation. Am J Surg Pathol 1987: 11: 563–570

79. Belza M G, Urich H. Chordoma and malignant fibrous histiocytoma. Evidence for transformation. Cancer 1986: 58: 1082–1087

80. Halpern J, Kopolovic J, Catane R. Malignant fibrous histiocytoma developing in irradiated sacral chordoma. Cancer 1984: 53: 2661–2662

81. Nanda A, Hirsch L F, Antoiniades K. Malignant fibrous histiocytoma in a recurrent thoracic chordoma. Neurosurgery 1991: 28: 588–592

82. Fukuda T, Aihara T, Ban S, Nakajima T, Machinami R. Sacrococcygeal chordoma with a malignant spindle cell component. Acta Pathol Jpn 1992: 42: 448–453

83. Knechtges T C. Sacrococcygeal chordoma with sarcomatous features (spindle cell metaplasia). Am J Clin Pathol 1970: 53: 612–616

84. Rone R, Ramzy I, Duncan D. Anaplastic sacrococcygeal chordoma: fine needle aspiration cytologic findings and embryologic considerations. Acta Cytol 1986: 30: 183–188

85. Apaja-Sarkkinen M, Vaananen K, Curran S, Siponen P, Autio-Harmainen H. Carcinomatous features of cervical chordoma in a fine needle aspirate. Acta Cytol 1987: 31: 769–773

86. Nijhawan V S, Rajwanshi A, Das A, Jayaram N, Gupta S K. Fine-needle aspiration cytology of sacrococcygeal chordoma. Diagn Cytopathol 1989: 5: 404–407

87. Choi Y J, Kim T S. Malignant fibrous histiocytoma in chordoma. Immunohistochemical evidence of transformation from chordoma to malignant fibrous histiocytoma. Yonsei Med J 1994: 35: 239–243

88. Gmur W, Von Hochstetter A R. Chordome und Chordom-ähnliche Neoplasien. Pathologe 1988: 9: 268–275

89. Fleming G F, Heimann P S, Stephens J K et al. Dedifferentiated chordoma. Response to aggressive chemotherapy in two cases. Cancer 1993: 72: 714–718

90. Dabska M. Parachordoma. A new clinicopathologic entity. Cancer 1977: 40: 1586–1592

91. Weiss S W. Ultrastructure of the so-called 'chordoid sarcoma'. Evidence supporting cartilaginous differentiation. Cancer 1976: 37: 300–306

92. Wick M R, Burgess J H, Manivel J C. A reassessment of 'chordoid

sarcoma'. Ultrastructural and immunohistochemical comparison with chordoma and skeletal myxoid chondrosarcoma. Mod Pathol 1988: 1: 433–443

93. Shin H J, MacKay B, Ichinose H, Ayala A, Romsdahl M M. Parachordoma. Ultrastruct Pathol 1994: 18: 249–256

94. Ishida T, Oda H, Oka T, Imamura T, Machinami R. Parachordoma: an ultrastructural and immunohistochemical study. Virchows Arch A Pathol Anat Histopathol 1993: 422: 239–245

95. Bender B L, Barnes L, Yunis E J. Intraosseous 'chordoid' sarcoma, chondroblastic or lipoblastic origin? Virchows Arch A Path Anat Histol 1980: 387: 241–249

96. Lefer L G, Rosier R P. The cytology of chordoma. Acta Cytol 1978: 22: 51–53

97. Gandolfi A. Vertebral chordoma: intraoperative cytological diagnosis. Acta Neurol (Napoli) 1979: 1: 156–160

98. Elliott E C, McKinney S, Banks H, Fulks R M. Aspiration cytology of metastatic chordoma. Acta Cytol 1983: 27: 658–662

99. Marigil M A, Pardo-Mindan F J, Joly M. Diagnosis of chordoma by cytologic examination of cerebrospinal fluid. Am J Clin Pathol 1983: 80: 402–404

100. Ali S Z, Semmelmeier S B, Urmacher C. Cytology of cervical chordoma in cerebrospinal fluid from a child. Acta Cytol 1995: 39: 766–769

101. Angelopulos N, Ceppi M, Serio G. Sacrococcygeal chordoma. Pathologica 1990: 82: 167–171

102. Caballero C, Fontaniere B. Sacrococcygeal chordoma: fine needle aspiration cytological findings and differential diagnosis. Cytopathology 1993: 4: 311–313

103. Finley J L, Silverman J F, Dabbs D J et al. Chordoma: diagnosis by fine-needle aspiration biopsy with histologic, immunocytochemical and ultrastructural confirmation. Diagn Cytopathol 1986: 2: 330–337

104. O'Dowd G J, Schumann G B. Aspiration cytology and cytochemistry of coccygeal chordoma. Acta Cytol 1983: 27: 178–183

105. Walaas L, Kindblom L G. Fine-needle aspiration biopsy in the preoperative diagnosis of chordoma: a study of 17 cases with application of electron microscopic, histochemical, and immunocytochemical examination. Hum Pathol 1991: 22: 22–28

106. Kontozoglou T, Qizilbash A H, Sianos J, Stead R. Chordoma: cytologic and immunocytologic study of four cases. Diagn Cytopathol 1986: 2: 55–61

107. Clark S A, Bloch T, Edwards M K, Hall P V. Diagnosis of cervical chordoma by fine needle aspiration biopsy. Acta Cytol 1987: 31: 765–768

108. Carvalho G, Coelho L H. Chordoma of rhinopharynx. Acta Cytol 1974: 18: 425–428

109. Hughes D E, Lamb J, Salter D M, al-Nafussi A. Fine-needle aspiration cytology in a case of chordoma. Cytopathology 1992: 3: 129–133

110. Thompson S K, Callery R T. Cytologic diagnosis of a chordoma without physaliforous cells. Diagn Cytopathol 1988: 4: 144–147

111. Perasole A, Infantolino D, Spigariol F. Aspiration cytology and immunocytochemistry of sacral chordoma with liver metastases. Diagn Cytopathol 1991: 7: 277–281

112. Crawford T. The staining reactions of chordoma. J Clin Pathol 1958: 11: 110–113

113. Murad T M, Murphy M S. Ultrastructure of a chordoma. Cancer 1970: 25: 1204–1215

114. Marotta M, Nappi O, Carillo G, Belli F, Rosati P. Sacrococcygeal chordoma: histochemical findings. Appl Pathol 1985: 3: 186–192

115. Sweet M B, Thonar E J, Berson S D, Skikne M I, Immelman A R, Kerr W A. Biochemical studies of the matrix of craniovertebral chordoma and a metastasis. Cancer 1979: 44: 652–660

116. Lam R. The nature of cytoplasmic vacuoles in chordoma cells. A correlative enzyme and electron microscopic histochemical study. Pathol Res Pract 1990: 186: 642–650

117. Kaneko Y, Iwaki T, Fukui M. Lectin histochemistry of human fetal notochord, ecchordosis physaliphora and chordomas. Arch Pathol Lab Med 1992: 116: 60–64

118. Miettinen N, Lehto V P, Dahl D, Virtanen I. Differential diagnosis of chordoma, chondroid, and ependymal tumors as aided by anti-intermediate filament antibodies. Am J Pathol 1983: 112: 160–169

119. Heikinheimo K, Persson S, Kindblom L G, Morgan P R, Virtanen I. Expression of different cytokeratin subclasses in human chordoma. J Pathol 1991: 164: 145–150

120. Bouropoulou V, Bosse A, Roessner A et al. Immunohistochemical investigation of chordomas: histogenetic and differential diagnostic aspects. Curr Top Pathol 1989: 80: 183–203

121. Meis J M, Giraldo A A. Chordoma. An immunohistochemical study of 20 cases. Arch Pathol Lab Med 1988: 112: 553–556

122. Maiorano E, Renzulli G, Favia G, Ricco R. Expression of intermediate filaments in chordomas. Pathol Res Pract 1992: 188: 901–907

123. Coindre J M, Rivel J, Trojani M, De Mascarel I, De Mascarel A. Immunohistological study in chordomas. J Pathol 1986: 150: 61–63

124. Stosiek P, Kasper M, Karsten U. Expression of cytokeratin and vimentin in nucleus pulposus cells. Differentiation 1988: 39: 78–81

125. Sarasa J L, Fortes J. Ecchordosis physaliphora: an immunohistochemical study of two cases. Histopathology 1991: 18: 273–275

126. Coffin C M, Swanson P E, Wick M R, Dehner L P. An immunohistochemical comparison of chordoma with renal carcinoma, colorectal adenocarcinoma, and myxopapillary ependymoma; a potential diagnostic dilemma in the diminutive biopsy. Mod Pathol 1993: 6: 531–538

127. Nakamura Y, Becker L E, Marks A. S-100 protein in human chordoma and human and rabbit notochord. Arch Pathol Lab Med 1983: 107: 118–120

128. Karabela-Bouropoulou V, Kontogeorgos G, Papamichales G et al. S-100 protein and neuron specific enolase (NSE) expression by chordomas in relation to the composition of their stromal mucosubstances. Pathol Res Pract 1988: 183: 256–261

129. Plaza J A, Ballestin C, Perez-Barrios A, Martinez M A, De Agustin P. Cytologic, cytochemical, immunocytochemical and ultrastructural diagnosis of a sacrococcygeal chordoma in a fine needle aspiration biopsy specimen. Acta Cytol 1989: 33: 89–92

130. Vinores S A, Bonnin J M, Rubinstein L J, Marangos P J. Immunohistochemical demonstration of neuron specific enolase in neoplasms of the CNS and other tissues. Arch Pathol Lab Med 1984: 108: 536–540

131. Harrowe D J, Taylor C R. Immunoperoxidase staining for carcinoembryonic antigen in colonic carcinoma, osteosarcoma, and chordoma. J Surg Oncol 1981: 16: 1–6

132. Miettinen M. Chordoma. Antibodies to epithelial membrane antigen and carcinoembryonic antigen in differential diagnosis. Arch Pathol Lab Med 1984: 108: 891–892

133. Tamayama C, Miyauchi M, Maruyama K. Expression of embryonal and differentiational proteins in chordomas and in the notochord (in Japanese). Gan No Rinsho 1990: 36: 7–12

134. Kasantikul V, Shuangshoti S. Positivity to glial fibrillary acidic protein in bone, cartilage and chordoma. J Surg Oncol 1989: 41: 22–26

135. Carson H J, Streib E W. Myasthenia gravis in a man with a history of chordoma: observations of muscle-like antigens in chordomas. Hum Pathol 1993: 24: 339–342

136. Burger P C, Makek M, Kleihues P. Tissue polypeptide antigen staining of the chordoma and notochord remnants. Acta Neuropathol (Berl) 1986: 70: 269–272

137. Tamayama C, Maruyama K. Expression of EGF receptor and c-neu oncogene product in chordomas (in Japanese). Gan No Rinsho 1990: 36: 773–776

138. Taniguchi K, Tateishi A, Higaki S et al. Type of collagen in chordoma. Nippon Seikeigeka Gakkai Zasshi 1984: 58: 829–834

139. Ueda Y, Oda Y, Kawashima Y, Tsuchiya H, Tomita K, Nakanishi I. Collagenous and basement membrane proteins of chordomas: immunohistochemical analysis. Histopathology 1992: 21: 345–352

140. Plate K H, Bittinger A. Value of immunocytochemistry in aspiration cytology of sacrococcygeal chordoma. Acta Cytol 1992: 36: 87–90

141. Hruban R H, Traganos F, Reuter V E, Huvos A G. Chordomas

with malignant spindle cell components. A DNA flow cytometric and immunohistochemical study with histogenetic implications. Am J Pathol 1990: 137: 435–447

142. Schoedel K E, Martinez A J, Mahoney T M, Contis L, Becich M J. Chordomas: pathologic features, ploidy and silver nucleolar organizing region analysis. Acta Neuropathol (Berl) 1995: 89: 139–143

143. Naka T, Fukuda T, Chuman H, Iwamoto Y, Sugioka Y, Fukui M, Tsuneyoshi M. Proliferative activities in conventional chordoma: a clinicopathologic, DNA flow cytometric and immunohistochemical analysis of 17 specimens with special reference to anaplastic chordoma showing a diffuse proliferation and nuclear atypia. Hum Pathol 1996: 27: 381–388

144. Persons D L, Bridge J A, Neff J R. Cytogenetic analysis of two sacral chordomas. Cancer Genet Cytogenet 1991: 56: 197–201

145. Mertens F, Kreicbergs A, Rydholm A et al. Clonal chromosome aberrations in three sacral chordomas. Cancer Genet Cytogenet 1994: 73: 147–151

146. Gibas Z, Miettinen M, Sandberg A A. Chromosomal abnormalities in two chordomas. Cancer Genet Cytogenet 1992: 58: 169–173

147. DeBoer J M, Neff J R, Bridge J A. Cytogenetics of sacral chordoma. Cancer Genet Cytogenet 1992: 64: 95–96

148. Bridge J A, Pickering D, Neff J R. Cytogenetic and molecular cytogenetic analysis of sacral chordoma. Cancer Genet Cytogenet 1994: 75: 23–25

149. Butler M G, Dahir G A, Hedges L K, Juliao S F, Sciadini M F, Schwartz H S. Cytogenetic, telomere, and telomerase studies in five surgically managed lumbosacral chordomas. Cancer Genet Cytogenet 1995: 85: 51–57

150. Friedman I, Harrison D F, Bird E S. The fine structure of chordoma with particular reference to the physaliphorous cells. J Clin Pathol 1962: 15: 116–125

151. Pardo-Mindan F J, Guillen F J, Villas C, Vazquez J J. A comparative ultrastructural study of chondrosarcoma, chordoid sarcoma and chordoma. Cancer 1981: 47: 2611–2619

152. Erlandson R A, Tandler B, Lieberman P H, Higinbotham N L. Ultrastructure of human chordoma. Cancer Res 1968: 28: 2115–2125

153. Cancilla P, Morecki R, Hurwitt E S. Fine structure of a recurrent chordoma. Arch Neurol 1964: 11: 289–295

154. Kay S, Schatzki P F. Ultrastructural observations of a chordoma arising in the clivus. Hum Pathol 1972: 3: 403–413

155. Ueda Y, Nakanishi I, Tsuchiya H, Tomita K. Microtubular aggregates in the rough endoplasmic reticulum of sacrococcygeal chordoma. Ultrastruct Pathol 1991: 15: 77–82

156. Jeffrey P B, Davis R L, Biava C, Rosenblum M. Microtubule aggregates in a clival chordoma. Arch Pathol Lab Med 1993: 117: 1055–1057

157. Bégin L R. Intracisternal microtubular aggregates in classic (non chondroid) chordoma. J Submicrosc Cytol Pathol 1995: 27: 295–301

158. Gessaga E C, Mair W G P, Grant D N. Ultrastructure of a sacrococcygeal chordoma. Acta Neuropathol (Berl) 1973: 25: 27–35

159. Fu Y S, Pritchett P S, Young H F. Tissue culture study of a sacrococcygeal chordoma. Acta Neuropathol (Berl) 1975: 32: 225–233

160. Mikuz G, Mydla F, Gutter W. Ultrastrukturelle biochemische und cytomorphometrische Befunde beim Chordom. Beitr Pathol 1977: 161: 150–165

161. Higinbotham N L, Phillips R F, Farr H W, Hustu H O. Chordoma thirty-five-year study at Memorial Hospital. Cancer 1967: 20: 1841–1850

162. DeVries J, Oldhoff J, Hadders H N. Cryosurgical treatment of sacrococcygeal chordoma. Cancer 1986: 58: 2348–2354

163. Magrini S M, Papi M G, Marletta F et al. Chordoma – natural history, treatment and prognosis. Acta Oncol 1992: 31: 847–851

164. Cummings B J, Esses S, Harwood A R. The treatment of chordomas. Cancer Treat Rev 1982: 9: 299–311

165. Ashwood N, Hoskin P J, Saunders M I. Metastatic chordoma: pattern of spread and response to chemotherapy. Clin Oncol R Coll Radiol 1994: 6: 341–342

166. Wang C C, James A E Jr. Chordoma: brief review of the literature and report of a case with widespread metastases. Cancer 1968: 22: 162–167

167. Yarom R, Horn Y. Sacrococcygeal chordoma with unusual metastases. Cancer 1970: 25: 659–662

168. Gagne E J, Su W P. Chordoma involving the skin: an immunohistochemical study of 11 cases. J Cutan Pathol 1992: 19: 469–475

169. Su W P, Louback J B, Gagne E J, Scheithauer B W. Chordoma cutis: a report of nineteen patients with cutaneous involvement of chordoma. J Am Acad Dermatol 1993: 29: 63–66

170. Chambers P W, Schwinn C P. Chordoma. A clinicopathologic study of metastasis. Am J Clin Pathol 1979: 72: 765–776

171. Resnik C S, Young J W, Levine A M, Aisner S C. Case report 544. Metastatic chordoma to humeri (originating in sacrum). Skeletal Radiol 1989: 18: 303–305

172. Takashi M, Haimoto H, Murase T, Mitsuya H, Kato K. An immunochemical and immunohistochemical study of S100 protein in renal carcinoma. Cancer 1988: 61: 889–895

173. Byers P D. A study of histological features distinguishing chordoma from chondrosarcoma. Br J Cancer 1981: 43: 229–232

174. Herndon J H, Cohen J. Chondroma of a lumbar vertebral body in a child. An unusual tumor resembling a chordoma. J Bone Joint Surg (Am) 1970: 52: 1241–1247

Giant cell tumor

M. Forest

INTRODUCTION AND CLINICAL DATA

Giant cell tumors are composed of connective tissue stromal cells having the capacity to recruit and interact with multinucleated giant cells that exhibit the phenotypic features of osteoclasts.[1-3] They are benign tumors but are locally aggressive, with a tendency for local recurrence.

The incidence is about 4–5% of all primary bone tumors[4,5] and 21% of all benign bone tumors (Unni 1996). Giant cell tumors account for 20% of all primary bone tumors in China.[6]

There is a distinct female predominance, with a ratio of 1.3 or 1.5:1.[5,7]

More than 80% of patients are older than 18 years[7] and there is a peak incidence in the third decade,[5] but the age range is wide. Incidence of giant cell tumors in skeletally immature patients ranges from 1.7%[8] to 5.7%[9] and even 10.6% for the Netherlands Committee on Bone Tumors.[10] In children and adolescents, there is also a predominance of female patients.

The symptoms are non-specific and the duration of symptoms may be prolonged.[7] Pain is the major complaint[11] and also tenderness, which may or may not be associated with a mass or a limitation of joint motion. Rarely, patients are asymptomatic.[11] The incidence of pathologic fractures ranges from 11% to 37% of cases,[11-14] appearing as a subtle cortical breakthrough or infraction rather than as a complete fracture. They are unusual in the upper extremity[4] and may be associated with intraarticular effusions in the knee.

Giant cell tumors have been described in association with polyostotic or monostotic Paget's disease,[15-19] patients being older and with a male predominance; the skull, facial bones and axial skeleton are more usually involved than the extremities. Lesions of Paget's disease may be evident or, more rarely, found only on histology.[20,21] A familial and geographic clustering in southern Italy has been reported.[22]

Giant cell tumors may rarely be associated with other benign bone tumors.[23]

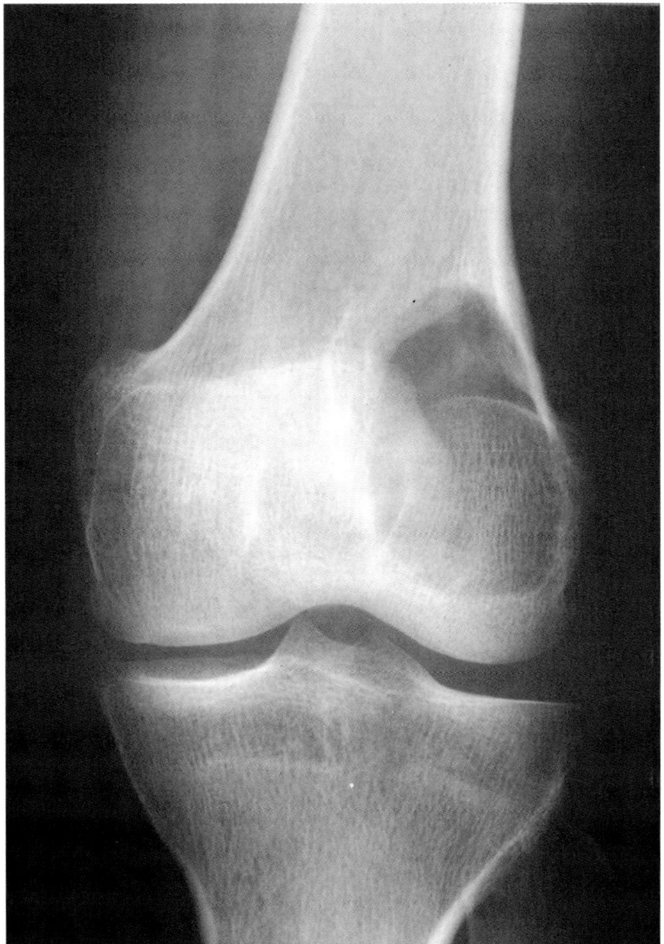

Fig. 29.1

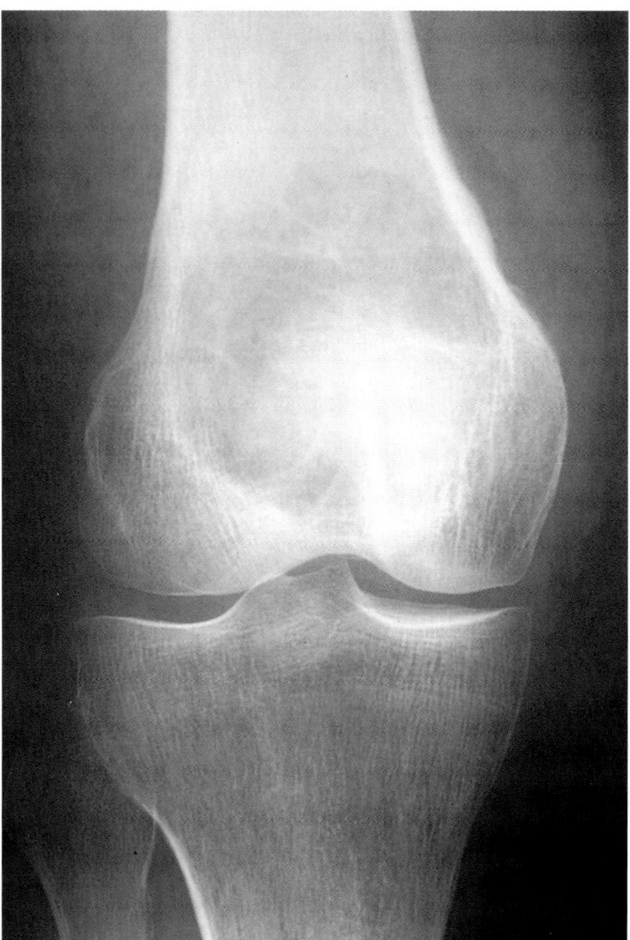

Fig. 29.2

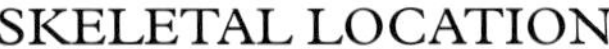

Figs 29.1, 29.2 Giant cell tumors of the distal femur.

SKELETAL LOCATION

Giant cell tumors are located in long bones in more than 80% of cases and 66% of cases involve the distal femur, proximal tibia, distal radius and proximal humerus[5] (Figs 29.1–29.8). The third and fourth most common locations are the distal radius[7,24,25] and the sacrum.[26]

Sacral tumors predominate over vertebral lesions[27] (Figs 29.9, 29.10). Incidence in the spine ranges from 2.7% to 9.3%.[24,28,29] Lumbar, thoracic and cervical regions are involved with decreasing frequency.

In the pelvis (Figs 29.11–29.13), the ilium is the most frequent site. Involvement of ribs, scapula,[30] clavicle or manubrium is unusual (about 1% of cases).

Two percent of giant cell tumors occur in the hands[31] and they account for 20% of all benign bone tumors of the foot. Metacarpal involvement (Figs 29.14, 29.15) is less frequent than phalangeal location; in the foot, metatarsal tumors are more common than phalangeal ones and the calcaneus and talus may be involved.[5] In the hand, they occur in younger patients, with a greater propensity for local recurrence.[31,32]

In children and adolescents, long and short tubular bones are involved,[33,34] more rarely the pelvis, the spine and ribs. The tibia is the most common bone affected,[9,10] followed by the femur and fibula.

Multicentric giant cell tumors occur with a frequency of 0.4% to 1%,[35–40] appearing synchronously or meta-synchronously with an interval of 4 months to 20 years.[41] Giant cell tumors located in the hand are frequently multifocal or associated with tumors in other skeletal sites.[5,31,32,42]

Obviously, one has to exclude the bone lesions of hyper-parathyroidism and search for a polyostotic Paget's disease.[19] Nine to ten tumors have even been reported in one person.[37,43,44] Patients are younger and tumors are more often associated with a pathologic fracture.[45] Some tumors may appear as symmetrical double lesions with a slow clinical course or exhibit varied histologic patterns.[46]

IMAGING

Giant cell tumors are purely lytic lesions, with absent

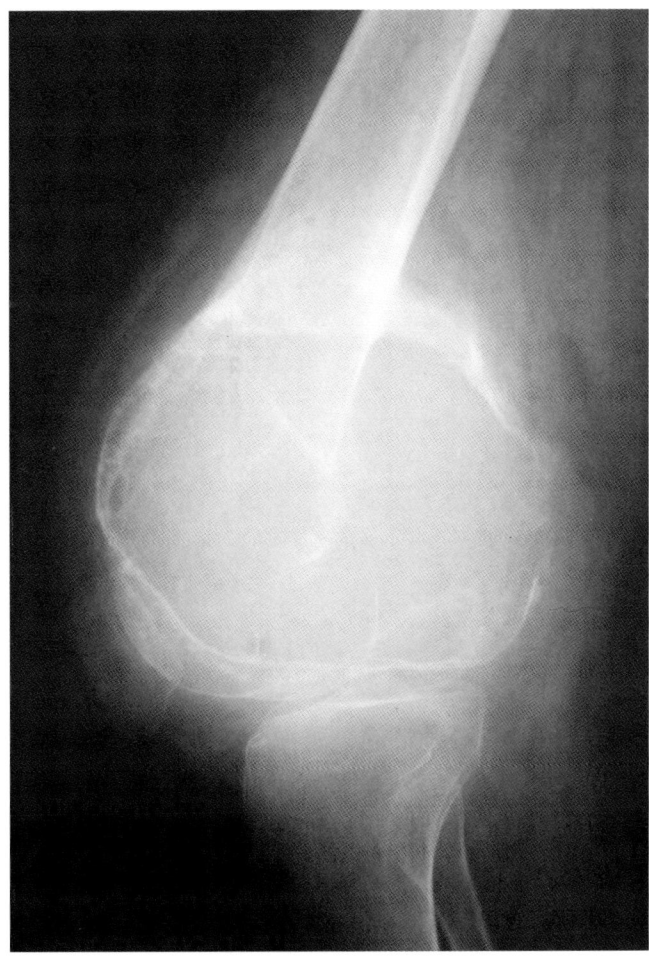

Fig. 29.3

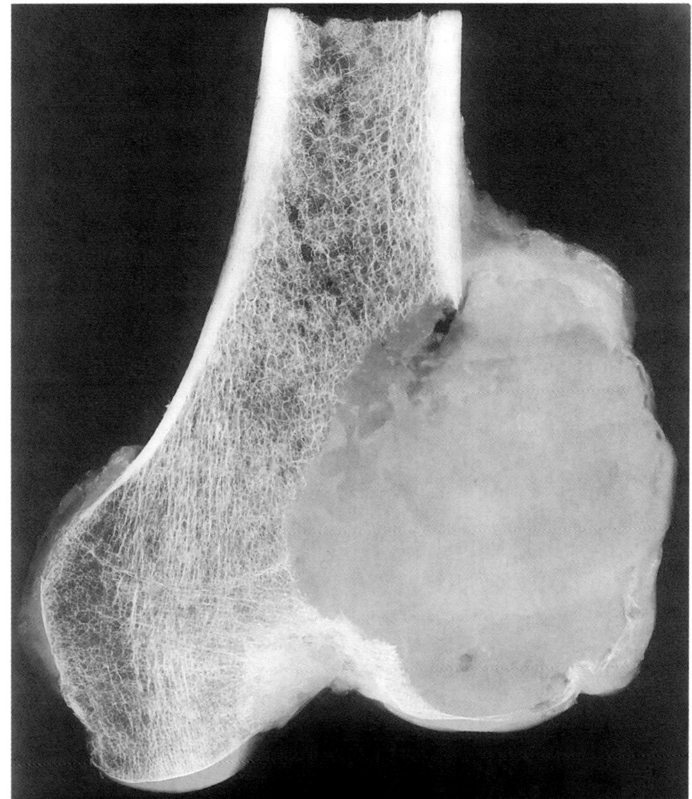

Fig. 29.4

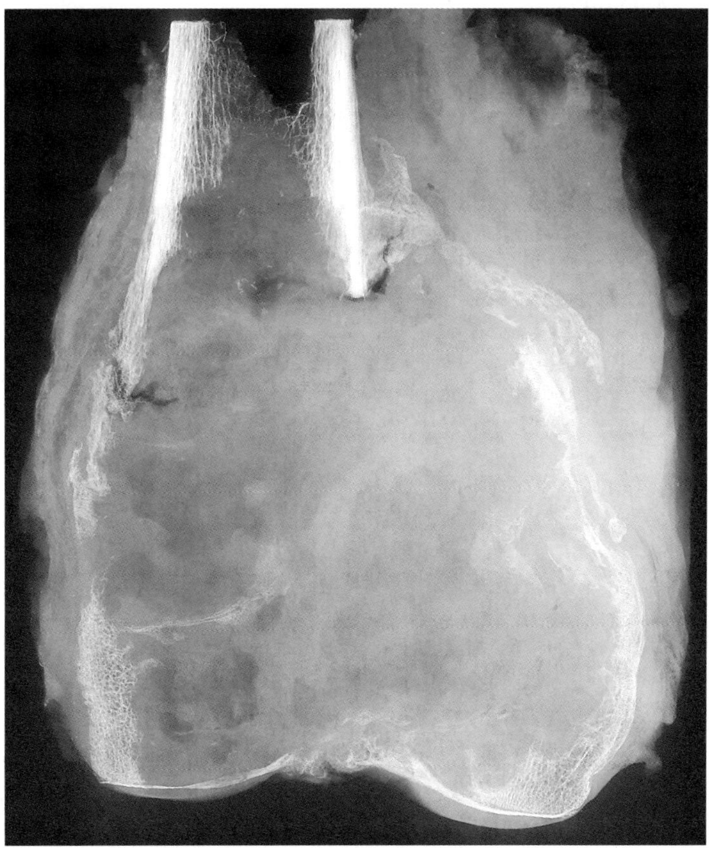

Fig. 29.5

Figs 29.3–29.5 Expanding giant cell tumors of the distal femur.

or, rarely, incomplete surrounding sclerosis[4,12] and no periosteal reaction in the absence of fracture, even in large tumors.[4] A lytic geographic pattern of bone destruction is the most frequent, with a narrow transition zone.[26] In some tumors, aggressive behavior is reflected by poor margination, cortical breakthrough and soft tissue extension.

Expansion of bone is fairly common[7] and a multiloculated appearance indicates the non-uniform resorption of the cortical wall[4,11] (Fig. 29.16).

In a long bone, the tumor essentially involves the epiphysis, extending to the subarticular cortex, often with an eccentric epicenter[26] and thinning of the cortex.

In 1.2% of cases, giant cell tumors involve the metaphysis or the diaphysis, without epiphyseal involvement[47–55] (Figs 29.17, 29.18), and many such cases are seen in skeletally immature bones. In children, tumors almost always involve the metaphysis[8,9] and epiphyseal involvement increases with age.[10]

In adults, early giant cell tumors may be entirely metaphyseal[26] and some authors suggest that they originate in

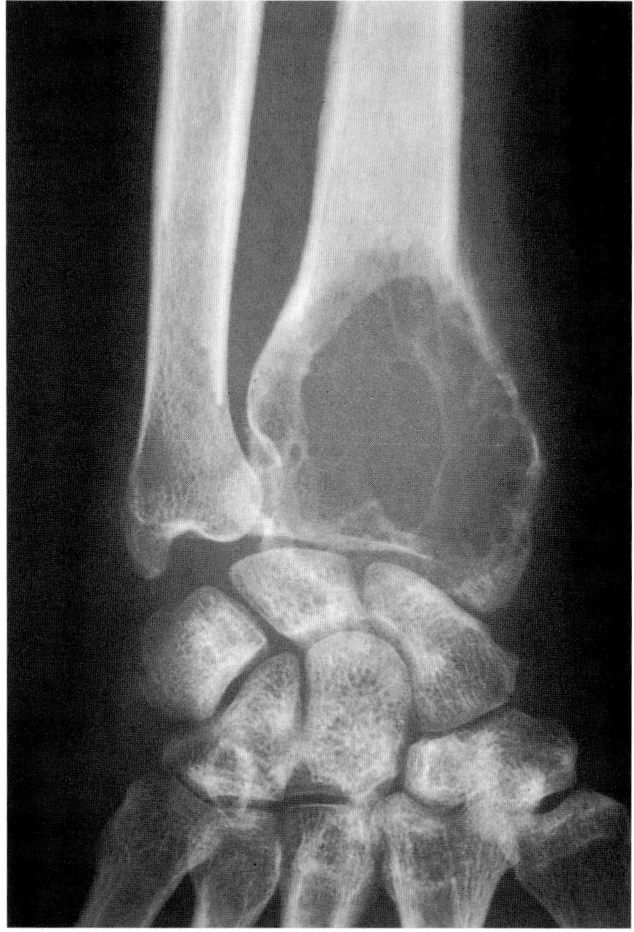

Fig. 29.6 Giant cell tumor of the distal radius.

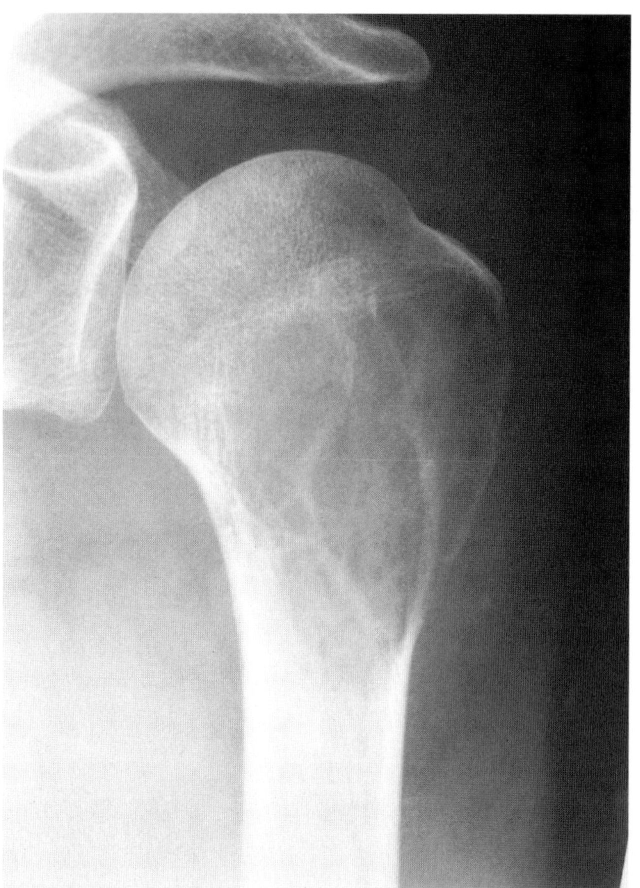

Fig. 29.7 Giant cell tumor of the proximal humerus.

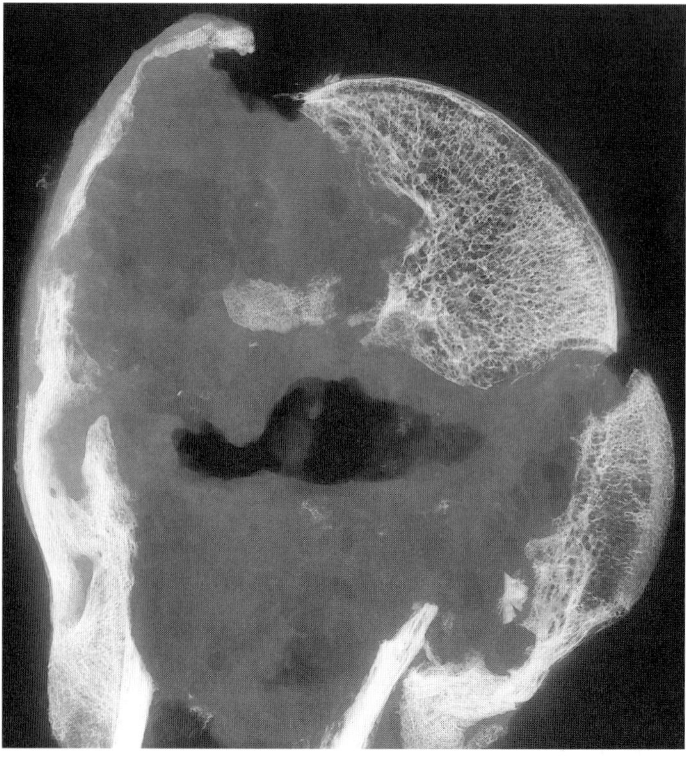

Fig. 29.8 Expanding giant cell tumor of the proximal humerus.

the metaphysis of tubular bones and extend to the epiphysis, after or sometimes before the closure of the growth plate.[9,50,55] Rare diaphyseal lesions are located in most cases in the femur and humerus.[5]

In the hands, giant cell tumors extend to the subarticular bone with expansion or mild trabeculation.[32]

In the spine, the tumor originates usually in the vertebral body, with subsequent involvement of the vertebral arch or even adjacent vertebrae.[29]

In flat bones, there is a frequent cystic component and a sizable soft tissue mass delimited by a continuous or interrupted periosteal bone shell.[30]

In skeletally immature patients, solid periosteal reactions due to microfractures, expansion of bone or secondary aneurysmal bone cyst formation are frequent.[9]

Most radiological features are shown on plain films,[26] but CT scans are useful to evaluate cortical integrity or penetration of the cortex, the soft tissue extension and the extent of spinal, sacral or pelvic tumors.[4,12,26,56,57] Some peripheral sclerosis may be seen in up to 20% of patients, most commonly in the distal femur and proximal tibia.[26,56,57]

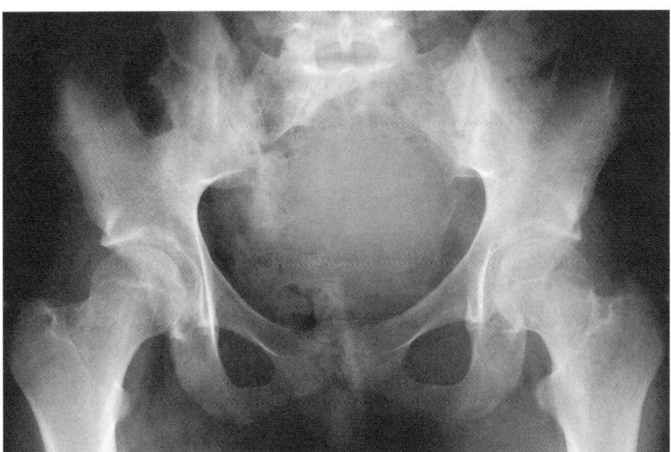

Fig. 29.9

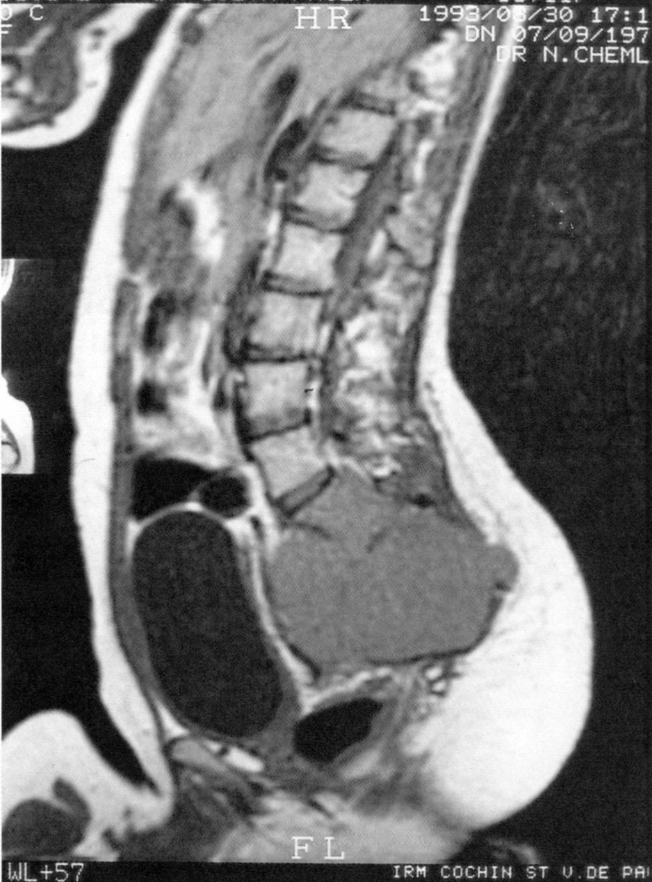

Fig. 29.10

Figs 29.9, 29.10 Huge giant cell tumor of the sacrum.

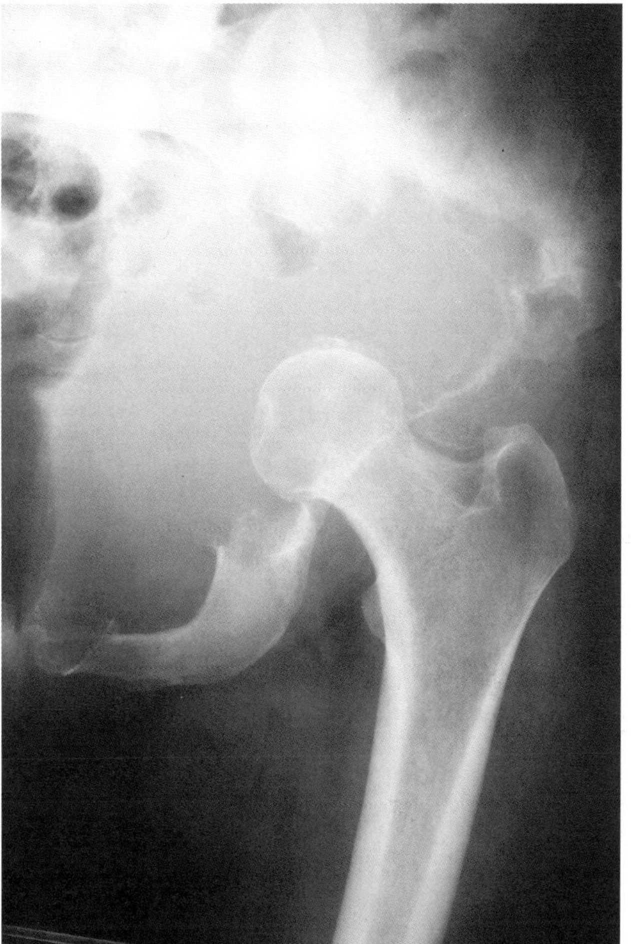

Fig. 29.11 Massive osteolysis of the pelvis induced by a giant cell tumor.

MRI is not useful for diagnosis[4,26,58] but may help to demonstrate areas of soft tissue inhomogeneity within the tumor and soft tissue or intraarticular tumor spread, with a homogeneous diminished signal on T1 and a iso- or hyperintense signal on T2-weighted images. Hemosiderin accumulation may produce markedly reduced signals.[59,60]

Fluid–fluid levels demonstrated on CT scans[61,62] or on MRI[63,64] may correspond to secondary aneurysmal bone cyst-like formation.

Angiography[65] has now been replaced by CT scans, although it may be useful for differentiating the tumors from aneurysmal bone cysts which are predominantly hypovascular;[65,66] the hyperemia often extends to the synovium, simulating an intraarticular extension. Similar errors may occur with gadolinium-enhanced MR imaging.[26]

On radionuclide bone imaging,[67] in some cases the increased peripheral tracer uptake may be beyond the true limits, giving misleading indications of the tumor extent.[68]

A surgical staging system relying on imaging and morphological patterns of extension or on imaging only[14] appears more reliable than histologic findings alone for predicting tumor behavior and especially recurrence.

Latent or 'calm' giant cell tumors have a slow growth; there is no expansion of bone or hypervascularity and the lesion is limited by a reactive rim of mature bone (stage I).

Symptomatic or 'active' tumors are hypervascularized

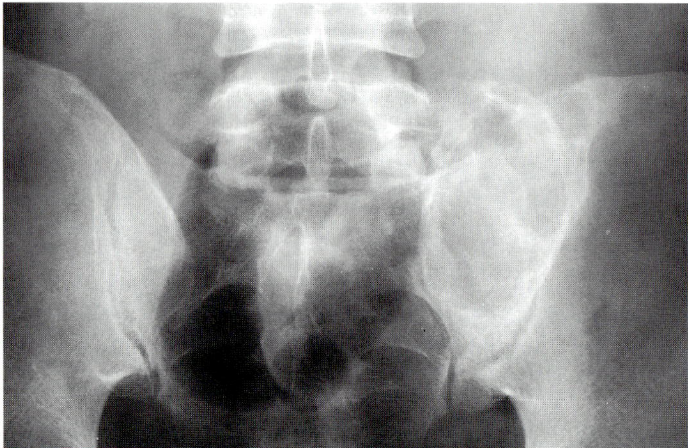

Fig. 29.12

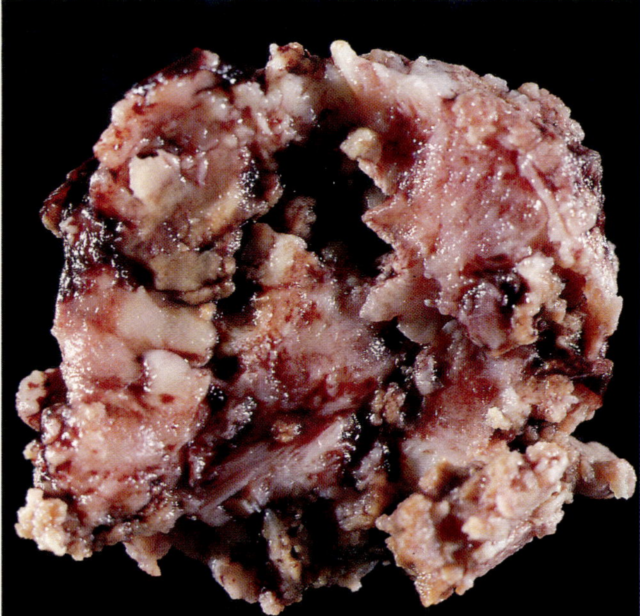

Fig. 29.13

Figs 29.12, 29.13 Giant cell tumor of the ilium with peripheral reactive bone formation.

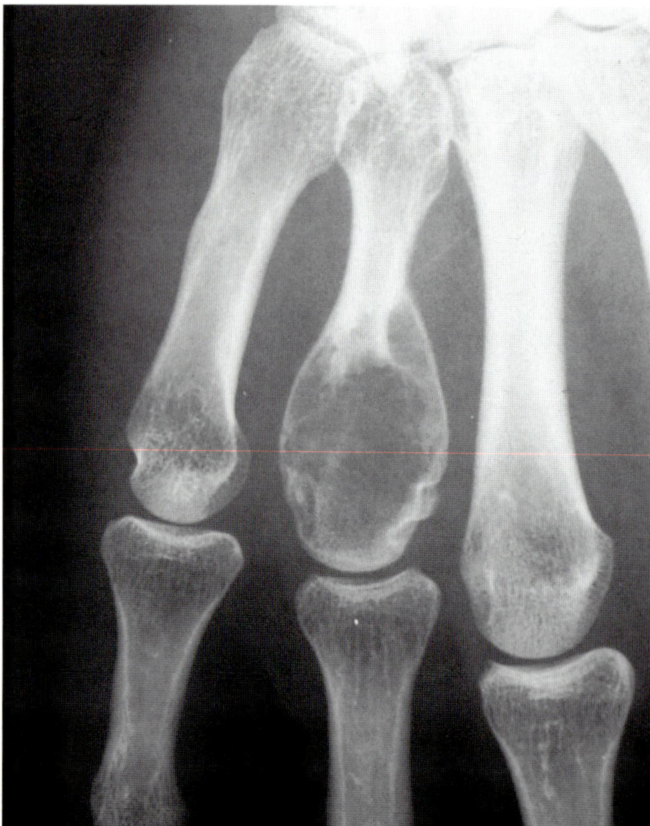

Fig. 29.14

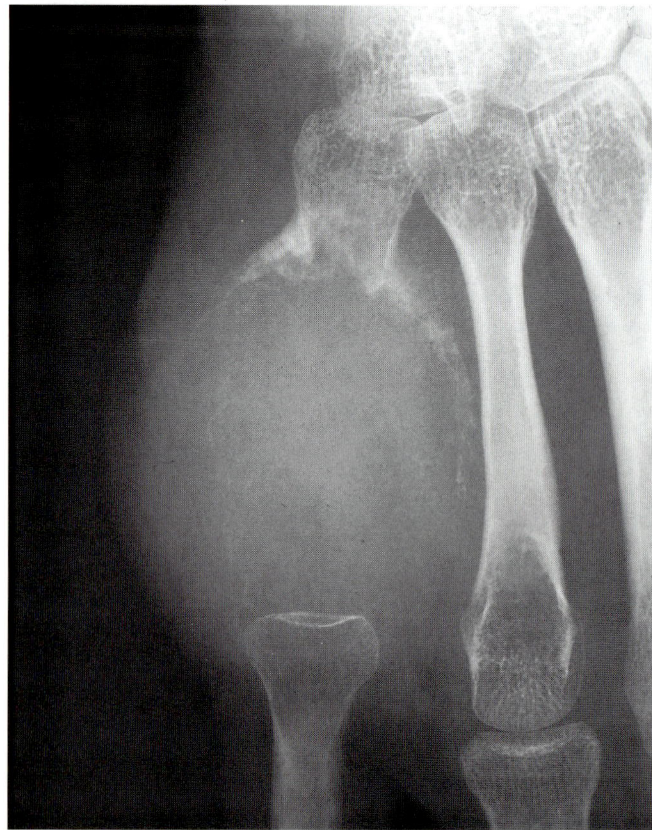

Fig. 29.15

with an increased uptake on bone scintigrams; the periosteal reactive bone or the peripheral capsule is not invaded (stage II).

Aggressive tumors are poorly marginated destructive lesions with a high incidence of pathologic fractures, cortical breakthrough and soft tissue extension. The tumors are hypervascularized with an intense activity on bone scintigrams (stage III).

In the Mayo Clinic studies, the incidence of recurrence is respectively 7%, 26% and 41%;[7] all benign metastasizing giant cell tumors are stage III.[69] The great majority of tumors are stage II.[14] However, some authors believe that

Figs 29.14, 29.15 Giant cell tumors in metacarpal locations.

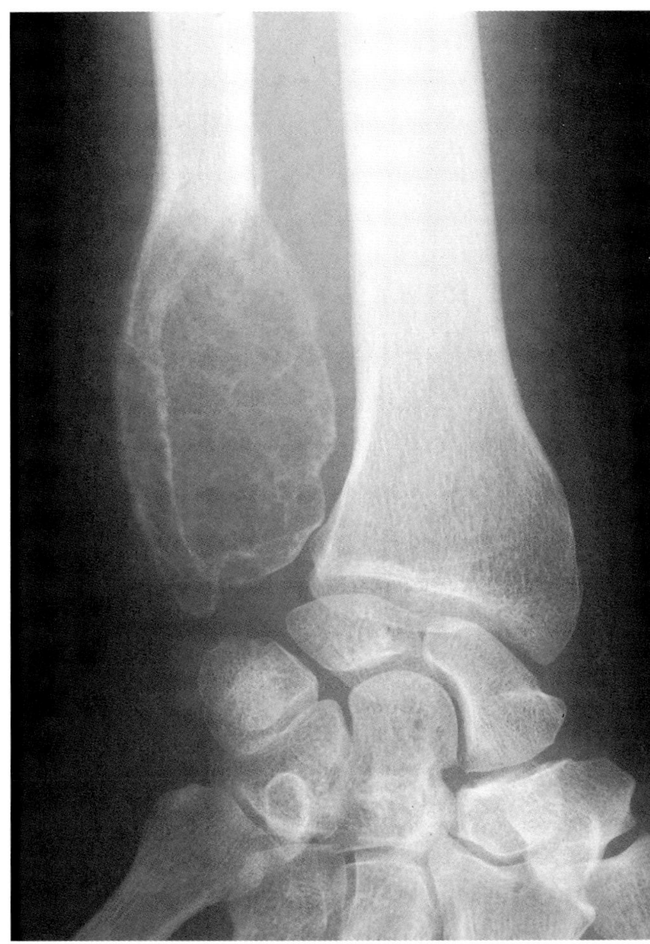

Figs 29.16 Giant cell tumor of the distal ulna: faint trabeculations corresponding to internal cortical ridges.

X-ray findings are of limited value for the evaluation of the prognosis.[11]

GROSS PATHOLOGY

In nearly half of cases, the tumor is large at initial presentation, exceeding 6 cm in length[11] (Figs 29.19–29.24). The tumor is usually eccentric in the long axis of bone, but may be centrally located, involving the epiphysiometaphyseal region with extension to the adjacent cartilage which remains intact.

The invasion of the joint space is by way of the synovial and capsule tissues. The overlying cortex is usually eroded with expansion of bone. The tumor is covered by a thin shell of periosteal new bone. In the upper metaphyseal bone area, the margins are sharp and 'skip' lesions are never found.

The tumoral tissue is soft, fleshy, tan or red-brown, with eventual gray areas of fibrosis, yellow xanthema-like

Figs 29.17, 29.18 Giant cell tumors of the femur in metaphyseal locations.

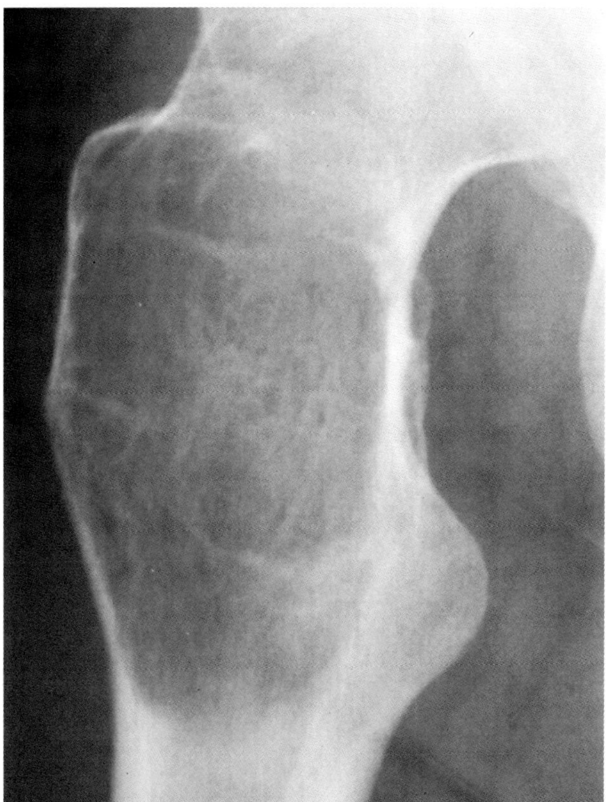

Fig. 29.17

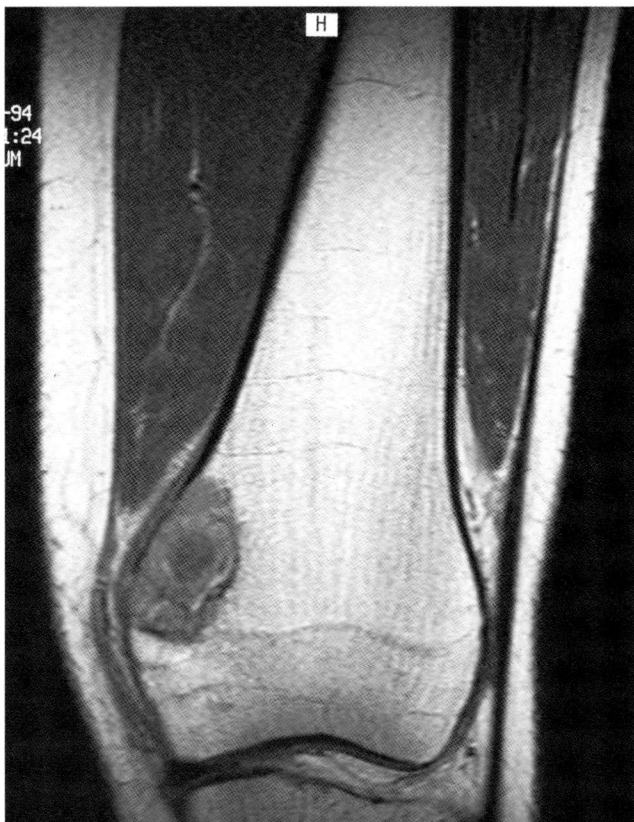

Fig. 29.18

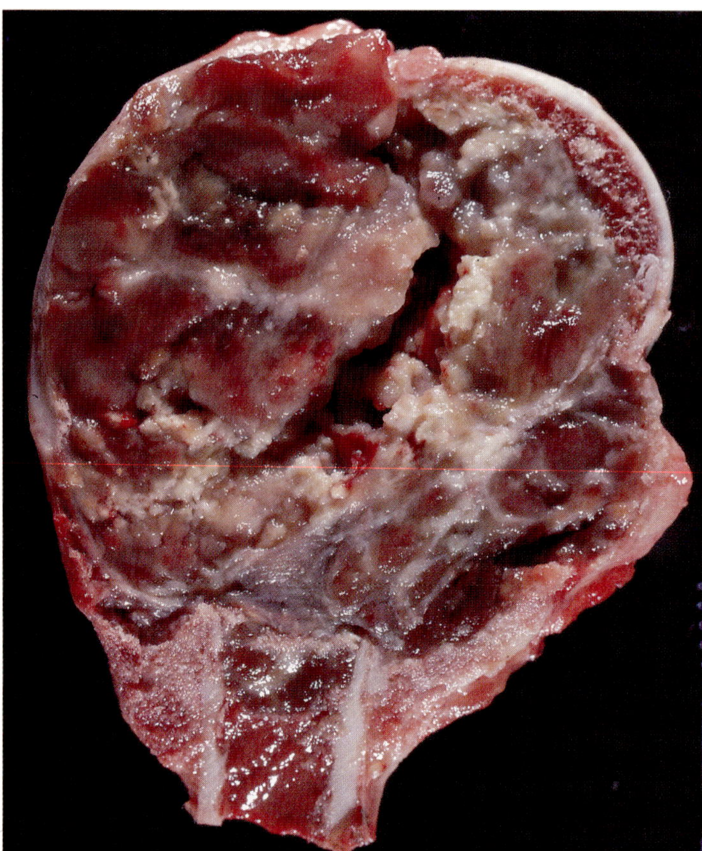

Fig. 29.19

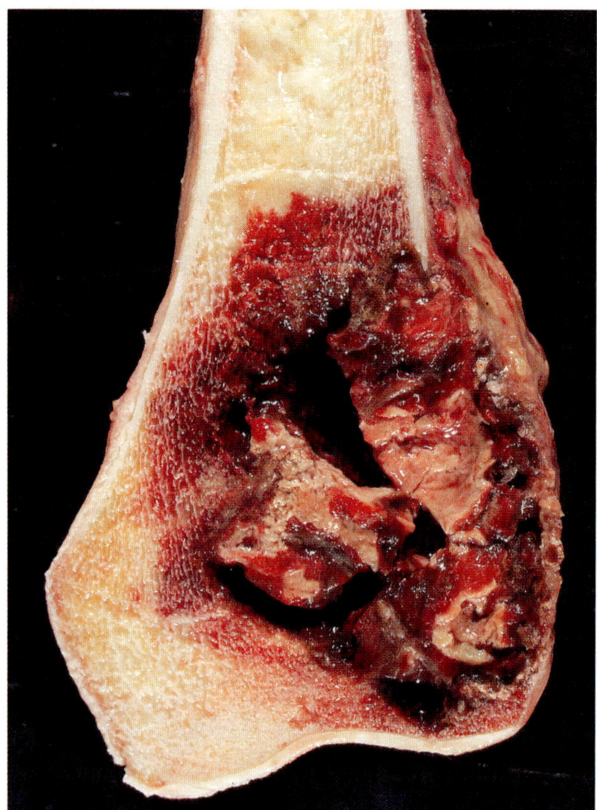

Fig. 29.20

Figs 29.19, 29.20 Giant cell tumors of the humerus and femur exhibiting a fleshy red-brown tissue with some yellow xanthema-like areas.

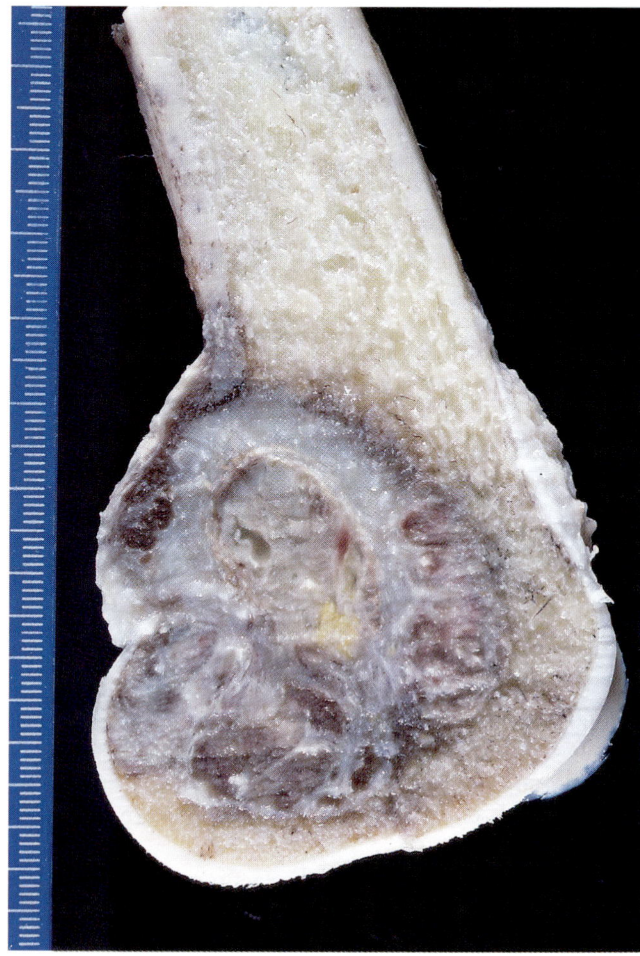

Figs 29.21 Grayish areas in a giant cell tumor of the femur corresponding to fibrous tissue.

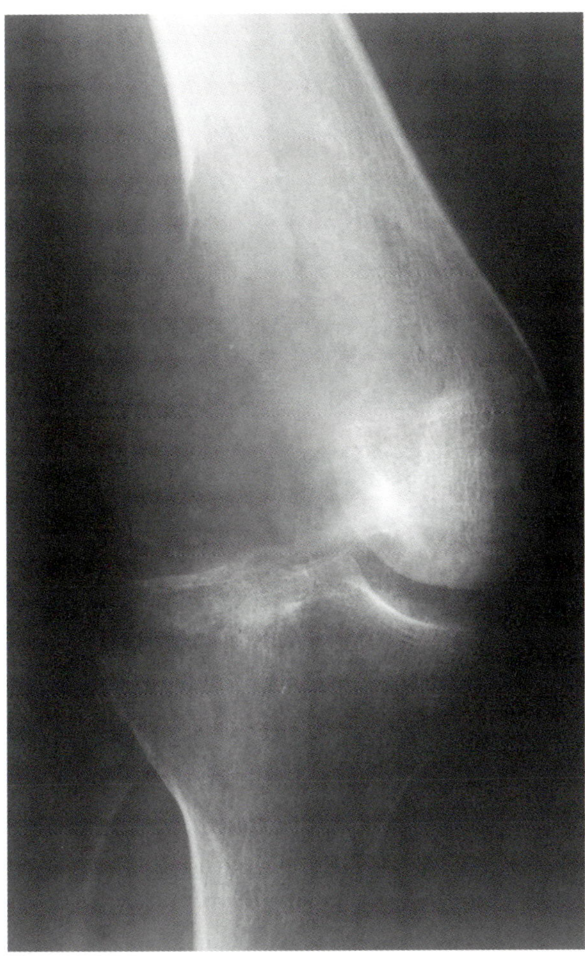

Fig. 29.22

Figs 29.22, 29.23 Giant cell tumor of the femur with sclerotic and necrotic changes.

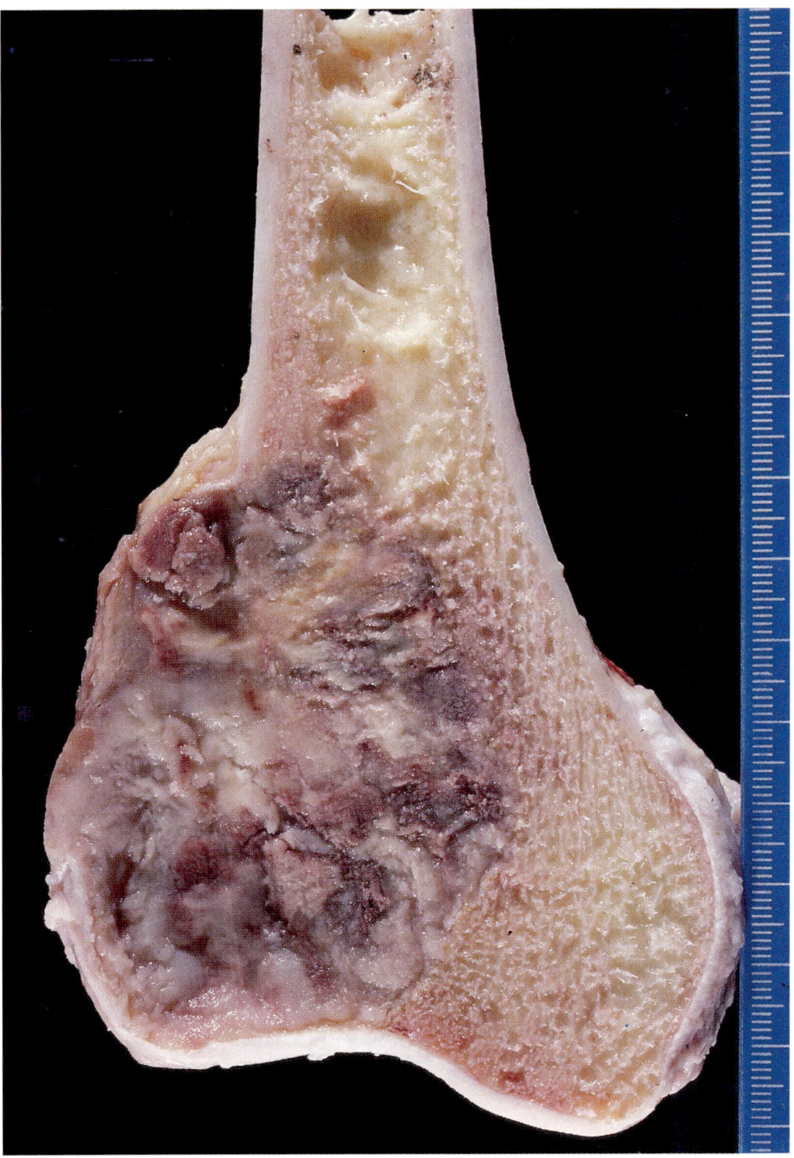

Fig. 29.23

areas or necrosis or cyst formation, resembling in some cases aneurysmal bone cyst,[64] with a serosanguinous fluid.

HISTOPATHOLOGY

In almost all cases, a giant cell tumor appears as very cellular tissue, exhibiting the association of stromal mononuclear cells and multinucleated giant cells (Figs 29.25–29.31).

Mononuclear cells are round, oval or spindle shaped, usually with a sparse acidophilic cytoplasm which may be well delineated or have indistinct margins. Some cells may be binucleate. Mitotic activity may be prominent, without atypical forms.

Giant cells are diffusely distributed, with numerous nuclei usually centrally located. Nuclei are similar to those

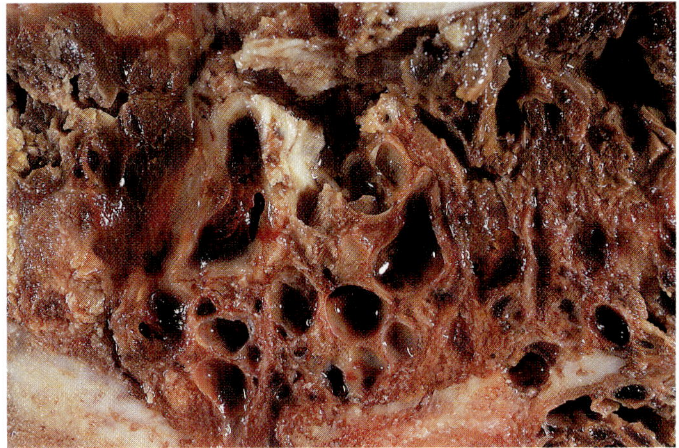

Fig. 29.24 Aneurysmal bone cyst-like changes in a giant cell tumor of the distal femur.

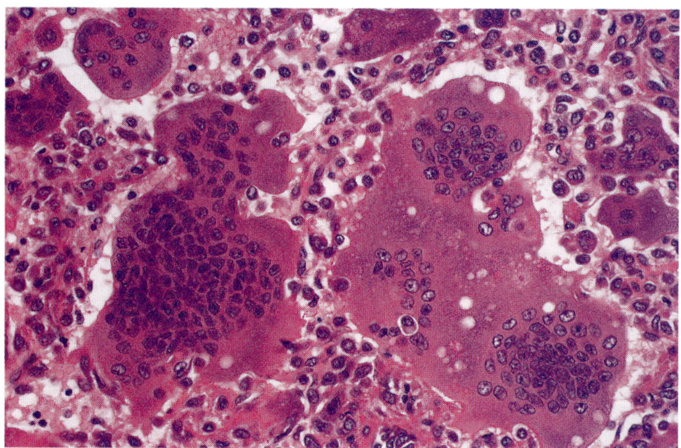

Fig. 29.25

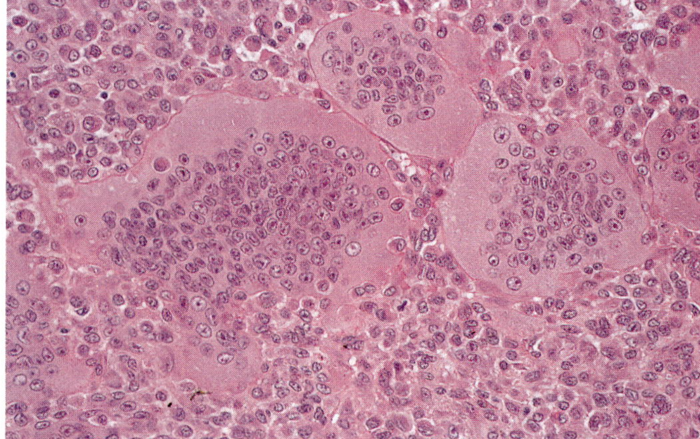

Fig. 29.26

Figs 29.25, 29.26 Giant cell tumors: giant cells with numerous nuclei, engulfing some mononuclear cells.

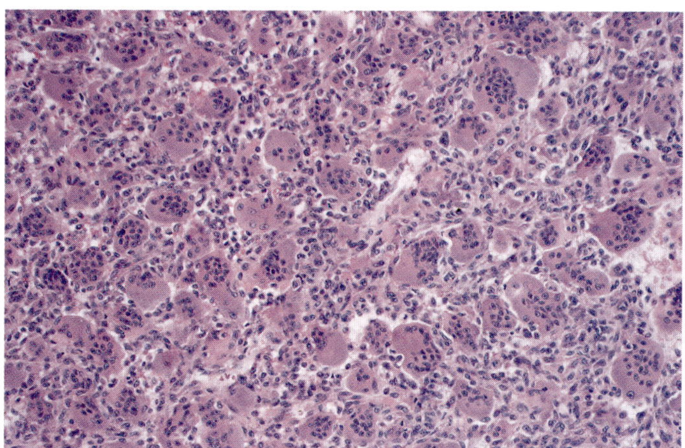

Figs 29.27 Giant cell tumor: diffuse distribution of the giant cells.

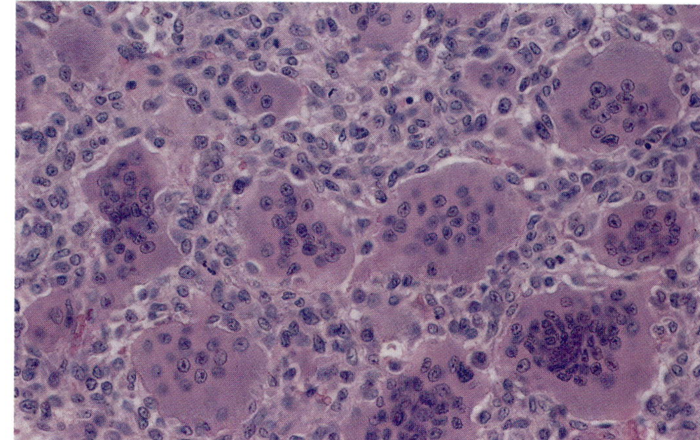

Fig. 29.29

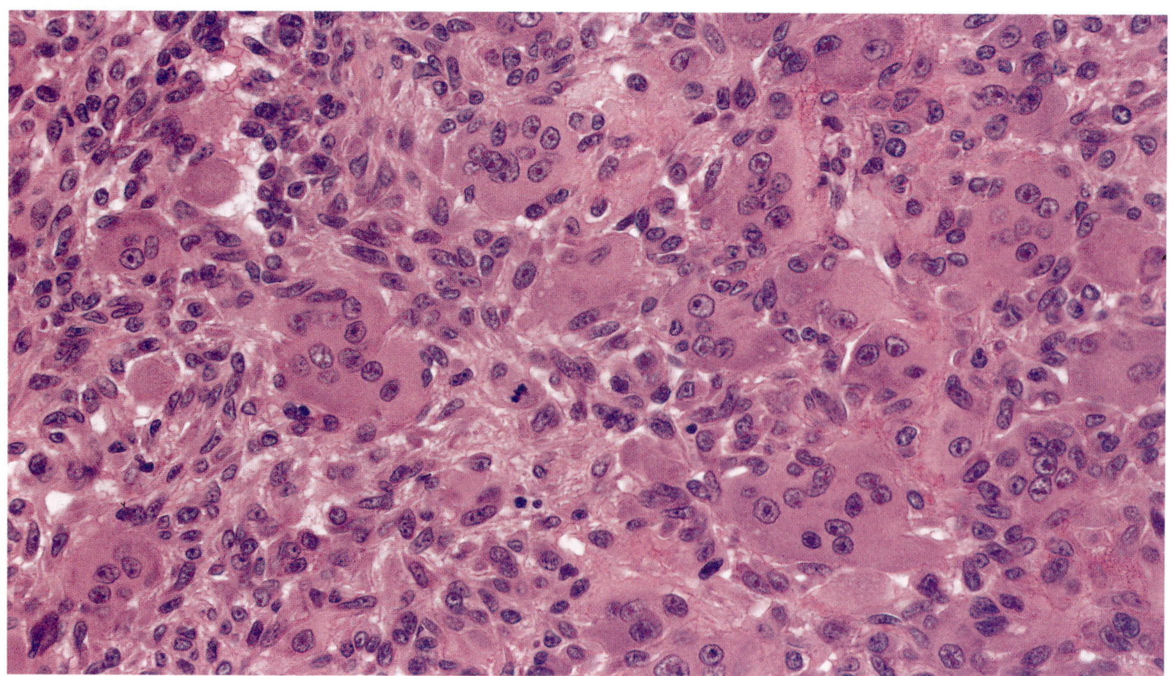

Fig. 29.28

Figs 29.28, 29.29 Giant cell tumors: mononuclear round, oval or spindle cells with some normal mitotic figures.

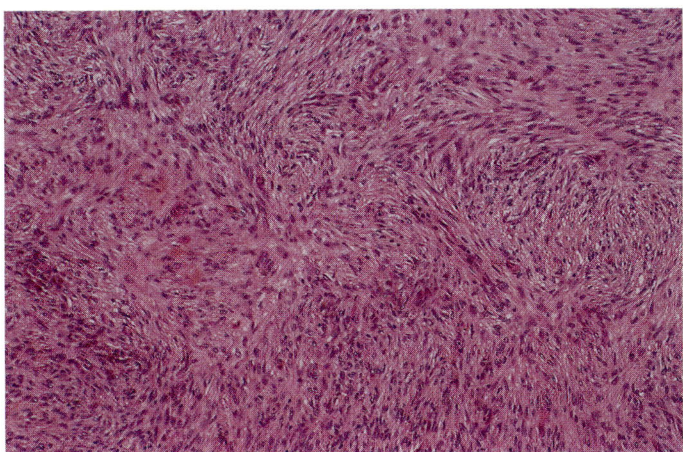

Fig. 29.30 Giant cell tumor: tumoral field with spindle cells and a storiform pattern.

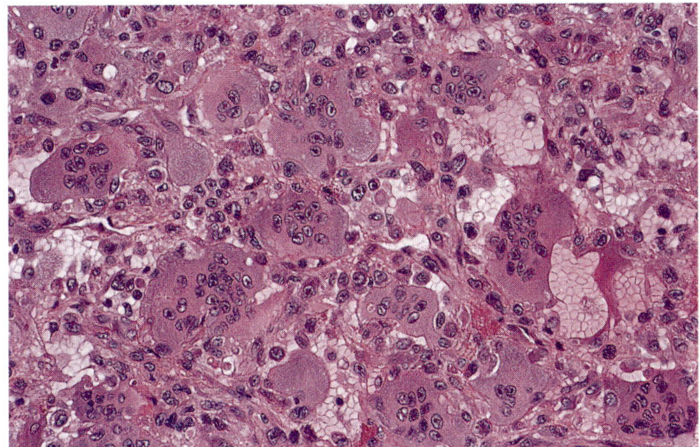

Fig. 29.31 Giant cell tumor: vascular spaces lined by giant cells.

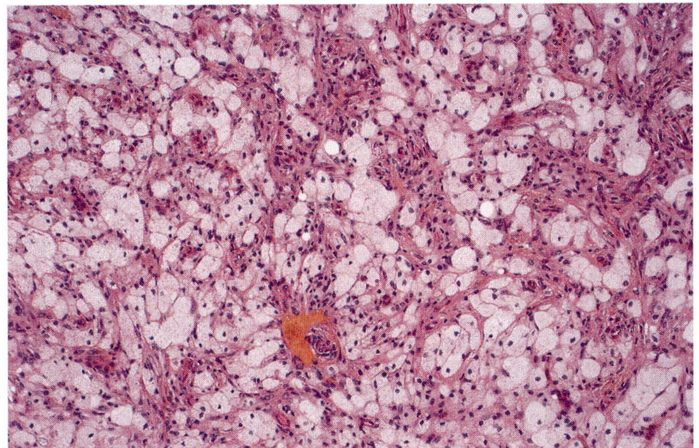

Fig. 29.32 Infiltration of a giant cell tumor by foamy macrophages.

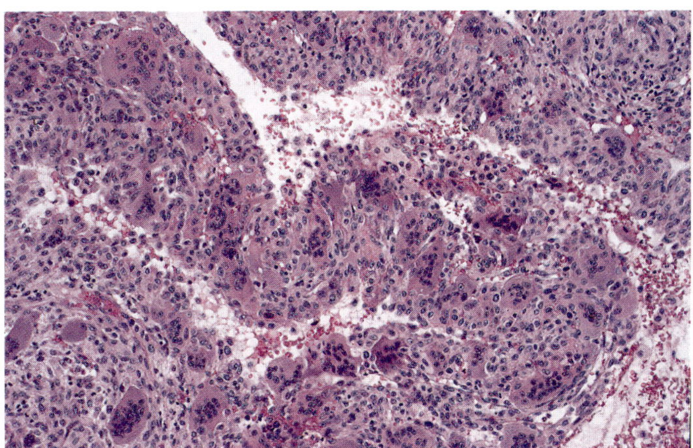

Fig. 29.33 Aneurysmal bone cyst formation in a giant cell tumor of a metacarpal.

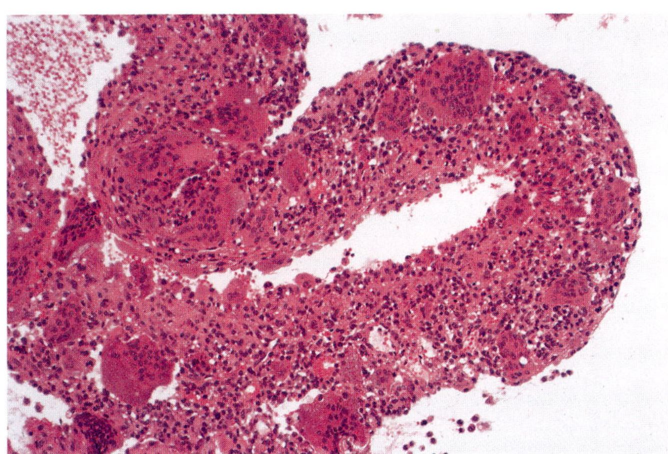

Fig. 29.34 Aneurysmal bone cyst formation in the soft tissue recurrence of a giant cell tumor of the radius.

of mononucleated cells, round or oval, with a prominent or small nucleolus. The cytoplasm can be vacuolated. Mononuclear cells encroach on the cytoplasm of giant cells or may be engulfed. Giant cells may present degenerative changes, pyknotic nuclei being associated with shrinkage of the acidophilic cytoplasm. They are devoid of mitotic activity.

Large tumoral fields may be composed of only mononuclear cells. Other fields may have many spindle cells with few giant cells and broad bands of fibrous tissue; the storiform pattern usually found may mimic a benign fibrous histiocytoma. Such fields have been viewed by Mirra as a regressive, involuted pattern but, while some of them contain large collagenized foci, others may be quite cellular with mitotic activity.

Giant cell tumors have an important network of thin-walled capillaries or small spaces lined directly by the mononuclear cells or mostly by the giant cells.

Secondary changes are usual and more prominent in recurrences. Infiltration by foamy or hemosiderin-laden macrophages,[70] stromal hemorrhages or secondary aneurysmal bone cyst formation is seen in about 15% of cases (Figs 29.32–29.34).

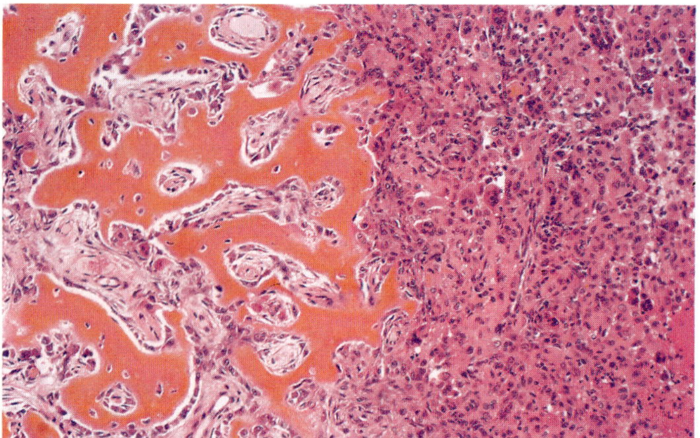

Fig. 29.35

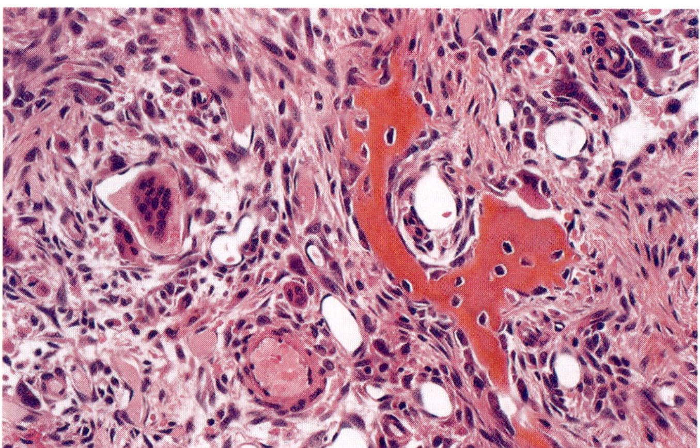

Fig. 29.36

Figs 29.35, 29.36 Peripheral reactive bone formation with osteoblastic rim in giant cell tumors.

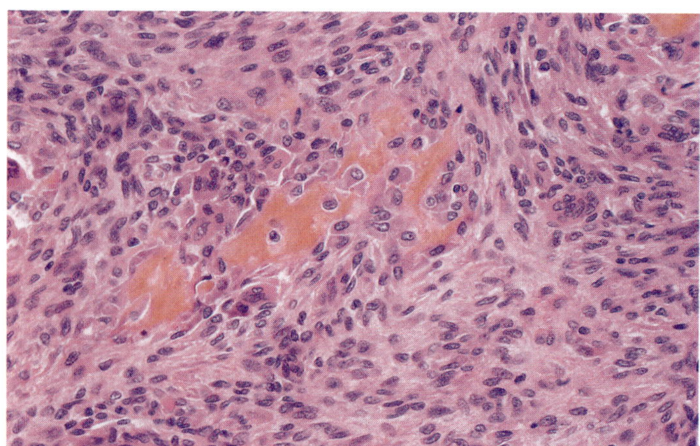

Fig. 29.37

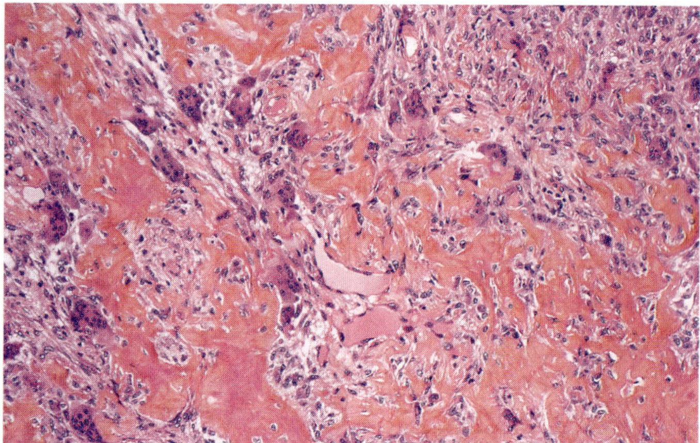

Fig. 29.38

Figs 29.37, 29.38 Seams of reactive bone in giant cell tumors.

Reactive bone formation is usually peripherally located; osteoid and woven bone are present in as many as 55% of tumors.[71] An osteoblastic rim can be found but usually tumor cells appear in close contact with the bone (Figs 29.35–29.42).

It has been assumed that a lymphocytic infiltration is related to an immunologic response[72] but usually it is not prominent, being composed of mature small lymphocytes of B and T type.[73]

In active tumors, the soft tissue extension is covered by a fibrous capsule or a shell of reactive periosteal bone shell. In aggressive tumors, these structures are permeated by tumoral tongues and in the metaphyseal bone area, the tumor may also demonstrate a permeative growth pattern.[74]

Intravascular invasion can be identified in about 5% of cases (Huvos 1991): the tumor distends the vascular lumen of small veins within or close to the tumoral tissue or is adherent to the vessel wall.[75] In our experience, intravascular invasion is found predominantly in tumors located in the axial skeleton and the lower end of the radius (Fig. 29.43).

The grading proposed in 1940 by Jaffe et al[76] has led to much debate about its real value. In grade I, the giant cells are numerous, mononuclear spindle or ovoid cells are few and mitotic activity is absent or very scarce. In grade II, mononuclear stromal cells are numerous, with moderate or marked atypia and mitotic activity is usually found. In grade III, giant cells are less numerous and smaller, mononuclear stromal cells exhibit obvious atypia and pleomorphism; mitotic activity is important, with abnormal forms.

This scheme has been modified by Sanerkin[75] and Huvos. For Sanerkin, grade I and II tumors represent the conventional giant cell tumors, aggressiveness being established on clinical and radiological findings; a grade II+, suggested by Lichtenstein, corresponds to borderline tumors with abnormal mitoses or vascular permeation. Grade III is a malignant tumor, showing frank sarcomatous changes. In the classification of Huvos, grade I represents conventional tumors, grade II borderline tumors and grade III are spindle cell sarcomas.

Image analyzer studies have been performed, evaluating

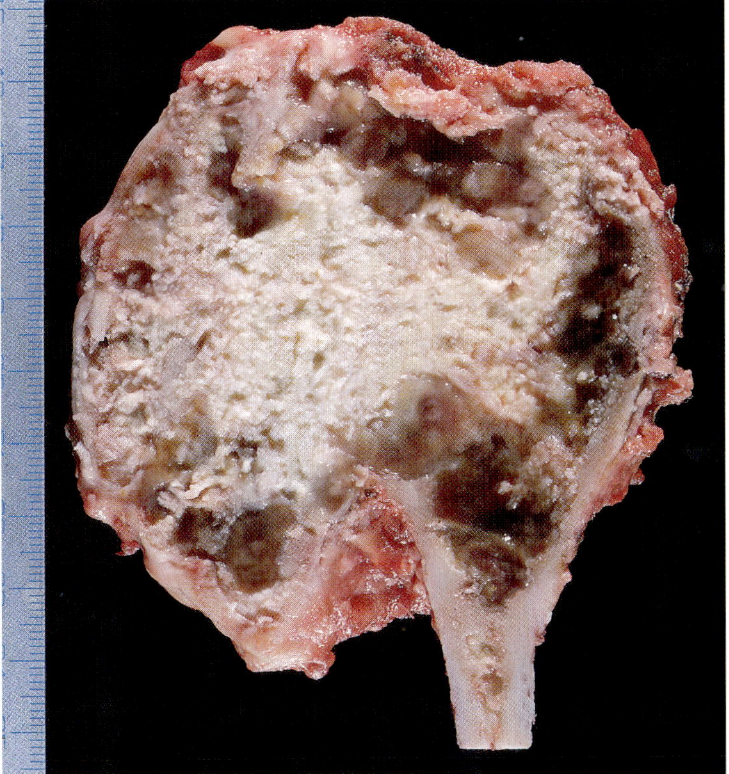

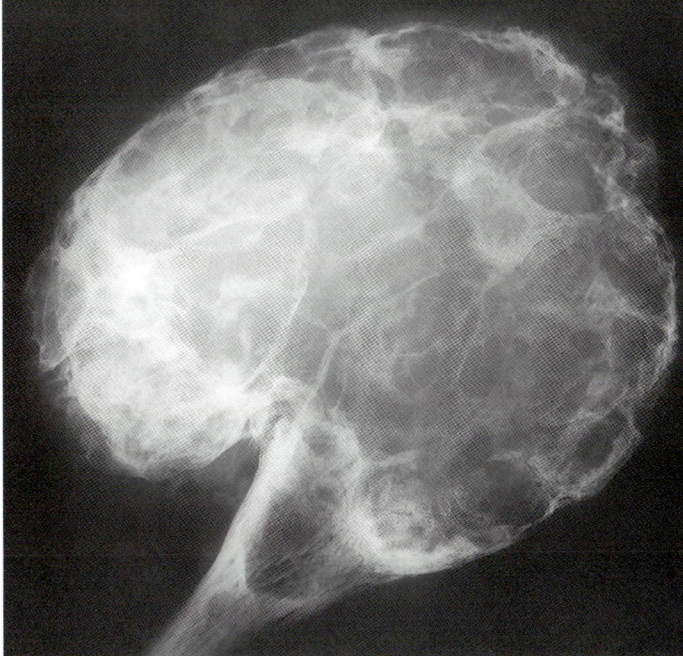

Fig. 29.40

Fig. 29.39

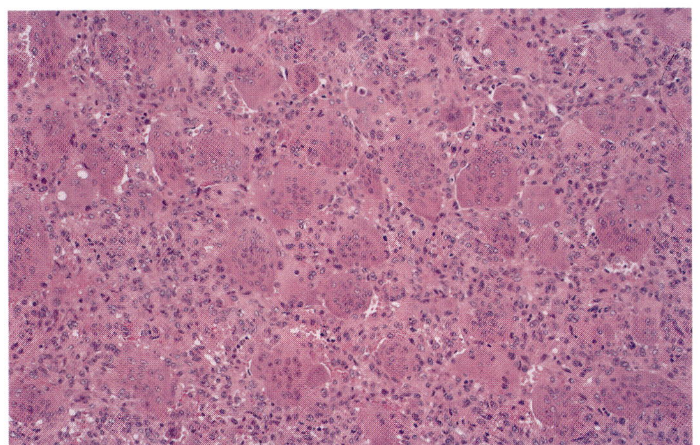

Fig. 29.41

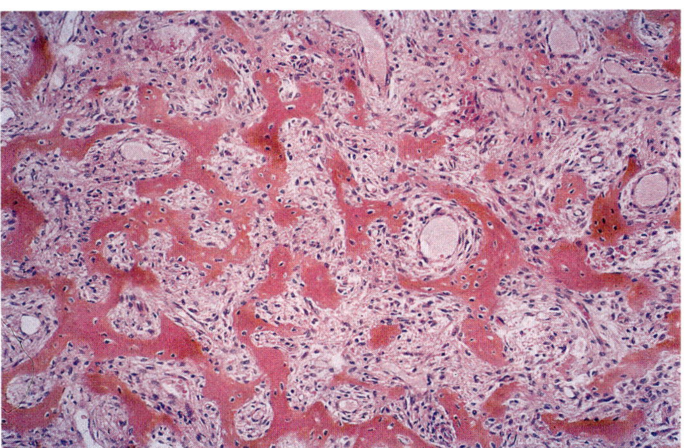

Fig. 29.42

Figs 29.39–29.42 Giant cell tumor of the fibula with massive expansion, infiltration by foamy macrophages, unusual reactive bone in the center of the lesion and a peripheral shell of mature reactive bone.

the cellularity, nuclear size and ratio of mononuclear stromal cells to giant cells,[77,78] as well as a texture analysis of the tumoral tissue.[79] In one report, the stromal cell atypia appears to be correlated significantly with the metastatic potential, but local recurrences cannot be predicted on the basis of the histological grading;[77] more clearcut features have to be found on morphometric studies.[78]

The mitotic count, advocated by some,[80] does not distinguish the three grades[75] and recurrences are only related to the inadequacy of treatment.

Most authors now believe that histopathological grading has no prognostic value and no correlation with the recurrence rate.[5,7,14,81,82] The only reliable histological findings may be the xanthomatous areas associated with an abundant fibrous tissue and scarce giant cells, in tumors exhibiting a thick sclerotic rim[5,14] (Mirra 1989); this form of tumor corresponds to latent or quiescent growths found in older patients and, according to Schajowicz, diagnosed erroneously as benign fibrous histiocytomas.[5]

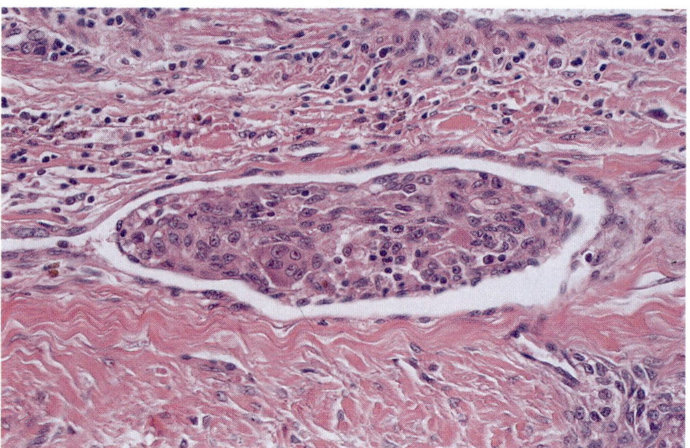

Fig. 29.43 Intravascular invasion in the soft tissues, close to a giant cell tumor of the radius.

CYTOPATHOLOGY

In the experience of some authors, fine-needle aspiration biopsy may be as accurate as a tissue needle biopsy in the diagnosis of giant cell tumors,[83] but cystic or aneurysmal bone cyst-like changes or massive necrosis may lead to an insufficient diagnosis. It should be stressed that imprint cytology is a very useful adjunctive tool, even if the final diagnosis relies on tissue sections[82] (Figs 29.44–29.47).

Mononuclear cells appear dispersed or in clusters; they are rounded, ovoid or spindle shaped with a moderate amount of well-defined cytoplasm. The nuclei have a slightly coarse chromatin pattern and usually a small nucleolus.[84] Giant cells may have from three to more than 50 nuclei.[82,85]

A cohesive cell grouping between the giant cells and the mononuclear cells has been described.[85]

IMMUNOHISTOCHEMISTRY, CELL CULTURE AND HISTOENZYMOLOGY

Many stromal mononuclear cells exhibit an immunoreac-

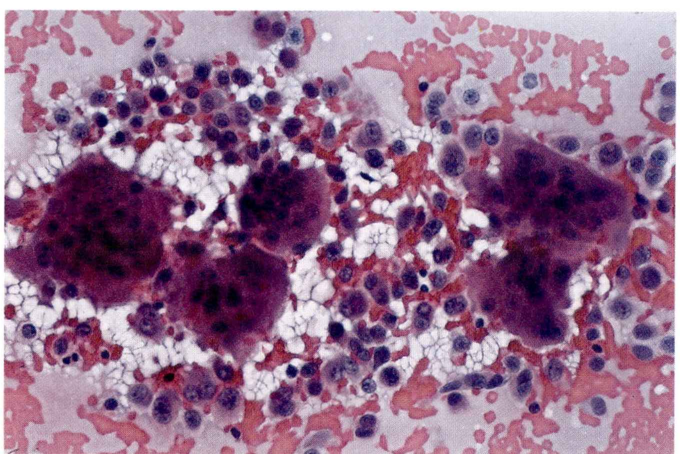

Fig. 29.44

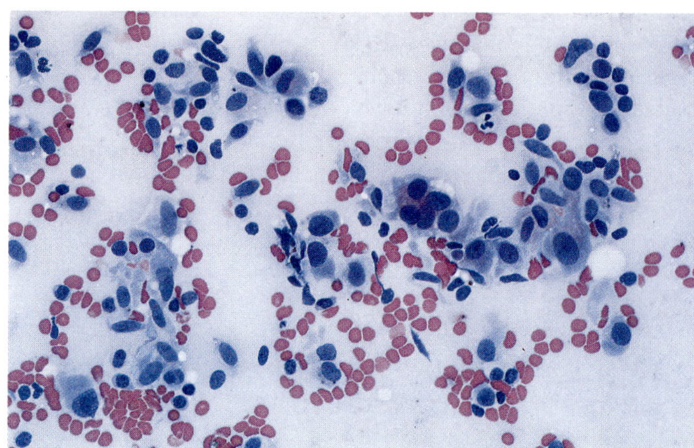

Fig. 29.46

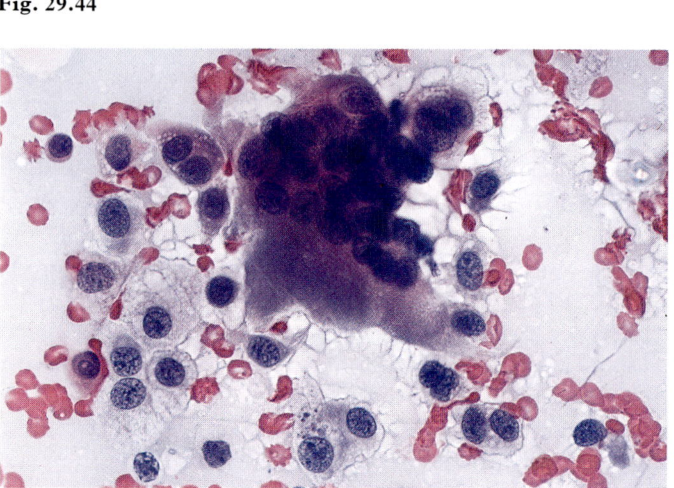

Fig. 29.45

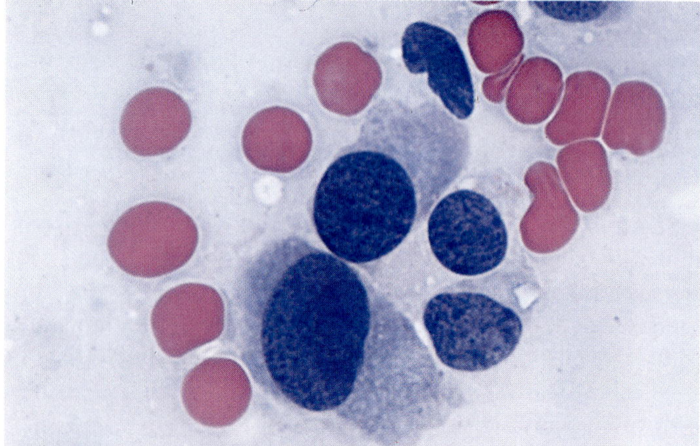

Fig. 29.47

Figs 29.44–29.47 Imprint cytology of giant cell tumors demonstrating the giant cells and the mononuclear cell component.

tivity with α1-antitrypsin, α1-antichymotrypsin and to a lesser extent with lysozyme.[86–89] More specific monoclonal antibodies against mature macrophages, 25-F-9 or factor XIIIa may be demonstrated.[89,90]

Many stromal mononuclear cells are also labeled with all the antibodies against the mononuclear phagocyte markers,[91] also in cultures.[92] L1 detected by the monoclonal antibody MAC387 is present in the macrophages[90] and a CD68 immunoreactivity is found mainly in the giant cells.[78] The considerable number of cells showing a monocyte-macrophage expression may reflect the particularly high infiltration by macrophages[70,73,89,93] or may be interpreted as an intrinsic part of the tumor.[92,94]

Spindle-shaped stromal cells may be labeled with vimentin,[95] laminin, fibronectin[86,95] and even α smooth muscle actin, osteocalcin and a very few with S-100 protein,[90,96] this last finding being important for the differential diagnosis with chondroblastoma.[86]

In cell culture systems, they produce types I and III collagen,[1,2,95] have receptors for parathyroid hormone and do not express macrophage markers.[1,2,71,89,95,97–100] The fibroblast-like stromal cell, according to double labeling immunohistochemical methods (PCNA, Ki-67), are the sole proliferating tumor cells.[89,90,95,100]

The stromal cells can express low levels of alkaline phosphatase activity and high levels of procollagen α1 and it has been suggested that these mesenchymal cells may express a phenotype similar to osteoblast-like cells.[73,78,87,90,101]

In cell culture systems, calcitonin receptors are found mostly on mononuclear cells of the monocyte-macrophage lineage,[102] which do not proliferate or survive in culture.[93,97]

The giant cells have many similarities with osteoclasts, expressing calcitonin receptors,[1,2,103] and their cell motility can be inhibited by calcitonin.[104] The antigenic phenotype is similar to that of osteoclasts isolated from bone,[1,2,98,104–110] with high levels of tartrate-resistant acid phosphatase. Moreover, MB1, a recently developed monoclonal antibody, reacts strongly with multinucleated giant cells and with osteoclasts of fetal bone,[111] as well as C22 and C35, osteoclast selective monoclonal antibodies.[112] Both cells exhibit a strongly positive membrane staining for LCA and CD68,[78,86,97,113] EBM11,[99] and are weakly positive with antibodies KB90 and UCHM1.[91]

Giant cells are viewed as arising from osteoclast precursor cells[1,2,70,73,97–99] or from stromal cells of the mononuclear phagocyte lineage, losing some of the mononuclear phagocyte-associated antigens.[91,97,100] Giant cells do not persist after immersion in culture,[97] fail to incorporate the tracer (3H) thymidine and are not detectable in tumor growth in nude mice; obviously, they are a non-neoplastic component.[92]

Transforming growth factor α produced by the giant cells and some stromal cells may play a role in the attraction and proliferation of the precursors of giant cells,[90,108] as may insulin-like growth factors.[109] Furthermore, in cultured tumor fluid, mononuclear cells produce cytokines that attract osteoclasts and their precursor in the tumor.[95,114]

Giant cells and stromal cells express IL-6 mRNA and IL-6 receptors.[115] IL-6 may act as both an autocrine and paracrine factor and may play an important role in the bone-resorbing capacities of the tumor cells.

IL-1 and TNFα produced by the giant cells may be responsible for the production of matrix metalloproteinases by stromal cells involved in the catabolism of extracellular matrix molecules.[116] A study of the bone resorptive factors has demonstrated the need for giant cells and mononuclear cells to express the original phenotype;[117] mononuclear cells are stimulated by IL-1, produced by the giant cells, to secrete prostaglandin E2 and matrix metalloproteinases.

Expression of matrix metalloproteinases in giant cells is the same as that in human osteoclasts.[118,119] Six proteinase activities have been purified from giant cell tumors and these enzymes are typical of cathepsins.[120,121] The role of the integrin expression of giant cells on different extracellular matrix proteins has also been investigated.[122]

Multinucleated giant cells have enzyme activities similar to osteoclasts.[123–125] Giant cells express tartrate-resistant and mononuclear cells tartrate-sensitive acid phosphate activity. Mannose receptor and platelet-derived growth factor, features of mature mononuclear phagocytes, are found only in mononuclear cells.[1,2,126] Enzyme activities, as well as CD68 immunoreactivity, are size dependent.[93,127]

Immunohistochemical, biochemical and histochemical studies have failed to identify estrogen receptors in giant cell tumors[128,129] but a more recent report shows evidence of estrogen receptors and a 66 kDa protein specific for human estrogen receptor, detected by immunoblot analysis[130] and recognized by a monoclonal antibody specific for human estrogen receptors.

The major points from the culture studies are the identification of three cell types.[1,2] A population of mononuclear cells with a fibroblastic morphology, resembling connective tissue stromal cells, produces types I and III collagen, has receptors for PTH and proliferates in cultures; this is the neoplastic component.[93,100] Mononuclear cells, lacking receptors for skeletal hormones, do not persist in culture and are probably of the monocyte-macrophage lineage. Large, multinucleated giant cells possess the phenotypic features of osteoclasts, including receptors for calcitonin.

The most important finding is that true tumor cells are the fibroblast-like cells having the capacity to recruit and interact with multinucleated giant cells.[1,2,89,93,95]

FLOW CYTOMETRY, DNA MICROSPECTROPHOTOMETRY AND AG-NORS

A definite aneuploidy has been found in clinically aggressive giant cell tumors[131] and in one study, using single cell DNA cytometry, there is a strong correlation between the nuclear DNA content and the clinical behavior.[132] Other studies show that the great majority of cases are diploid[133,134] and there is no significant correlation between DNA ploidy, histologic grade and the presence or absence of metastases.[134,135] In one report, most aneuploid giant cell tumors have shown a benign biologic behavior.[135]

However, aneuploidy in a benign giant cell tumor is a finding suggesting a thorough sampling of the tumor, to rule out an osteosarcoma or a malignant fibrous histiocytoma.[134,135]

On microspectrophotometric quantitation of DNA, there is a larger DNA content in mononuclear cells than in giant cells, without any irregular distribution.[136]

The nucleolar organizer region count after silver staining procedure cannot reliably differentiate borderline or intermediate lesions from benign or frankly malignant tumors.[137,138] In the same field, the staining of cell proliferation markers (MIB-1, monoclonal antibody against Ki-67) does not correlate with recurrences.[139]

CYTOGENETICS

Chromosomal abnormalities are found in 50% of tumors with an indolent course and in 97% of tumors which are locally aggressive or malignant.[140] The most common non-clonal abnormality is an unusual telomere-to-telomere chromosome translocation.[140–142] Chromosome 11 is predominantly involved in the telomeric fusion and the structural rearrangement.[142]

It has been suggested that telomeric reduction and telomeric activity may be the oncogenic events which maintain the transformed phenotype seen in giant cell tumors.[143–145] In culture, a karyotype presented a consistent translocation t(12;19)(q13q13) which may be related to the locally aggressive behavior of the tumor.[146] Other clonal, structural and/or numerical changes have recently been reported[147] but giant cell tumors lack the microsatellite instability found in some malignancies; that is, alterations or deletions within interspersed highly polymorphic tandem repeats of nucleotide base pairs.[148]

ELECTRON MICROSCOPY

Two distinct groups of mononuclear stroma cells have been delineated.[149–155]

Fibroblast-like cells have an oval or spindle shape. The rough endoplasmic reticulum is abundant and the Golgi apparatus well developed. The nucleus is irregularly shaped with a prominent nucleolus. Glycogen is found in small clusters. Cells are surrounded by bundles of collagen and are involved in the process of extracellular collagen deposition.[153,154]

Macrophage-like cells are small and round with many cell processes and a lysosome-rich cytoplasm.

Ultrastructural findings corroborate the view that one population of stromal cells may be derived from fibroblasts or undifferentiated mesenchymal cells of bone marrow, the other from the monocyte-macrophage osteoclast lineage. On autoradiographic findings, tritiated thymidine is incorporated only by the mononuclear cells and on electron microscopical autoradiography, only the fibroblast-like cells are found to proliferate.[150]

Giant cells have a smooth outer membrane or microvillous protrusions. Many organelles are found in the cytoplasm and the Golgi apparatus is well developed. On electron probe microanalysis, giant cells exhibit evidence of phagocytosis of Ca and Fe-containing particles.[149,156]

At least some giant cells undergo progressive degeneration, appearing as cells with closely packed spindle-shaped nuclei of high density.[82,155,156]

On tissue culture studies, it has been suggested that nuclei of giant cells are formed by amitotic division[123,157] but most authors believe that giant cells appear to arise by fusion of mononuclear tumor cells.[82,151,155,158]

A phosphatase activity located preferentially in the vesicles of the cytoplasmic membrane[159] is found mostly in giant cells.[151]

Giant cells cultured on devitalized bone slices remove the calcified bone matrix; the excavated resorption lacunae are similar to Howship's lacunae.[152] Two membrane modifications are specific: a ruffled border and a clear zone with cytoplasmic fine structures similar to those of osteoclasts.[152] Fluorescent F-actin dots called podosomes, identified by a rhodamine-conjugated phalloidin stain, are involved in bone resorption, determining the shape of the lacuna and the creation of an acidic microcompartment by substrate adhesion.[152,160]

So, giant cells having common structures for adhesion and resorption of bone can be regarded as osteoclasts.

Filamentous intranuclear inclusions bearing a very close resemblance to those in Paget's disease of bone have been described in the giant cells of the tumors associated with Paget's disease.[161–166]

Fibrils are packed in paracrystalline arrays and in cross-section, there is an electron-lucent core, suggesting a tubular structure. More rarely, they are located in the cytoplasm.[167] In our department, they are found in up to 49% of tumors not associated with Paget's disease. Their structure appears similar to that of paramyxovirus nucleocapsids.

Nuclear bodies have been encountered in the stromal mononuclear cells, appearing as a granular core enveloped by a multilayered coat.[167]

CLINICAL COURSE, TREATMENT AND PROGNOSIS

In 1–3.5% of cases, benign giant cell tumors may be complicated by lung metastases appearing as 'implants' with-

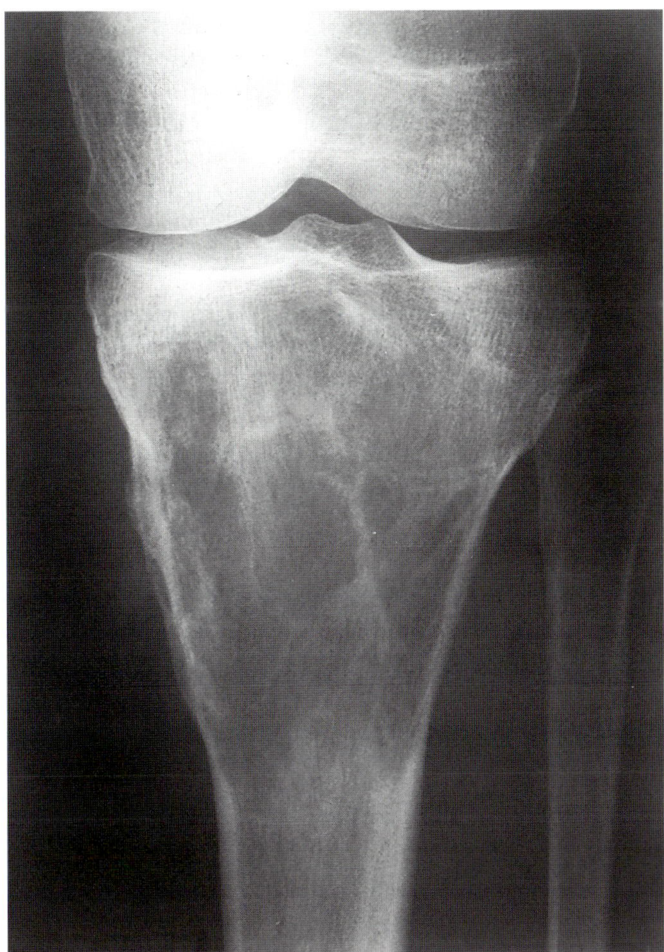

Fig. 29.48

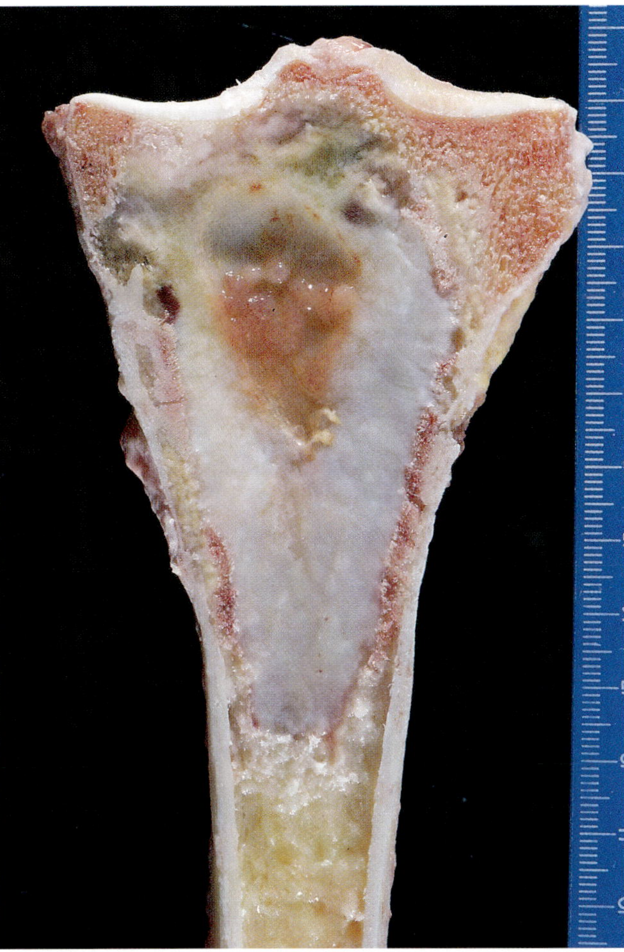

Fig. 29.49

Figs 29.48–29.50 Malignant giant cell tumor of the proximal part of the tibia.

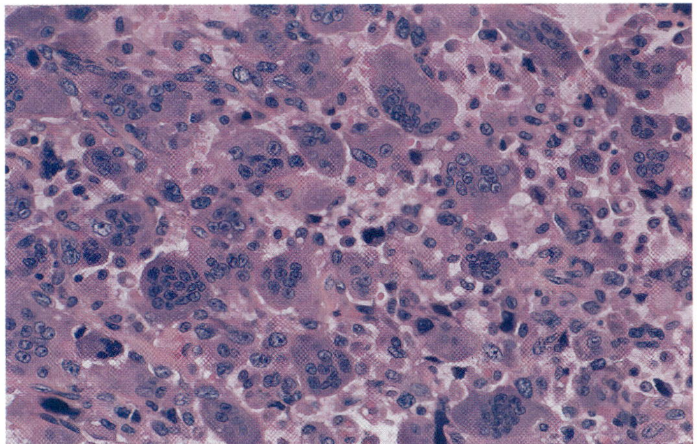

Fig. 29.50

out any malignant features, in the same way as some chondroblastomas.[69,168–179]

Lung metastases are more common in aggressive tumors with soft tissue extension or local recurrence.[172,175] They are rarely seen at initial presentation,[173,176] appearing on average 3.5 years after the diagnosis.[176] Even giant cell tumors of the phalanx and metacarpals can give rise to lung metastases,[180,181] but there is a high incidence of cases coming from the distal radius (38%[176]). A calcified rim may be detected in about 50% of cases, chiefly on CT scans, or they can calcify or ossify.

Tumor thrombi in venous channels or small to medium-sized arteries may be identified on the periphery of giant cell tumors.[172,177,178,182] but they are not necessarily predictive of pulmonary metastases.[69,75,173]

On flow cytometry, very few cases are aneuploid;[131,183,184] most cases are diploid on the primary tumors, the local recurrences and the systemic metastases.[174,185,186] The doubling time of pulmonary metastases correlates with a long survival time and by extrapolation, they begin to develop years before the primary tumor is diagnosed.[187]

They have a self-limiting behavior and some may regress spontaneously[171–173,177] or remain stationary.[170] Many respond favorably to wedge resection or lobectomy, even on recurrence; there is also some response to radiotherapy. The overall mortality ranges from 16% to 25% of cases, in part due to the immunosuppressive treatments or chemotherapy complications.

Very rarely, patients with local primary recurrences or, mostly, with lung metastases may present metastases in other sites such as the lymph nodes,[172,184,188,189] the skin,[190,191] the brain[191] or even bone.[172,181,192]

Many lesions diagnosed as *malignant giant cell tumors* are actually malignant fibrous histiocytomas, fibrosarcomas or osteosarcomas rich in multinucleated giant cells (Mirra 1989, Fechner & Mills 1993, Schajowicz 1994).[193,194] True malignant giant cell tumors (Figs 29.48–29.50) account for less than 5% of cases in most series and in 70% of cases are radiation-induced sarcomas.[24,195,196] The development of a sarcoma after external beam irradiation ranges from 7% to 25% of cases, with an average interval of about 12 years. Most patients die from pulmonary metastases.[193,195]

Rare primary malignant giant cell tumors are defined by Dahlin et al as sarcomas associated with a typical giant cell tumor at initial presentation or arising at the site of a pre-existing giant cell tumor.[195] The first proposition may be questionable, as the giant cell component can represent only a reactive phenomenon, even with a bimorphic histological pattern.[197]

Maybe the only true malignant giant cell tumors are those which show a progression or a dedifferentiation[198] of the initial benign tumor, leading to malignant fibrous histiocytomas,[198–200] fibrosarcomas[201] or osteosarcomas,[202,203] with an interval as long as 18[204] or even 30 years.[205]

Usual treatments of conventional giant cell tumors are curettage after exteriorization of the tumor, intralesional excision and reconstruction of the cavity by packing with bone chips, a resection followed by prosthetic devices with or without allografts or, less often, osteoarticular allografts.

Curettage is usually extended by chemical or physical means: cauterization by phenol, cryosurgery or local hyperthermia induced by the exothermic reaction of cement used to pack the cavity.

Radiation therapy has a poor control rate[206] and there is a well-known risk of radiation-induced sarcomas with a short latent period,[195] but with modern radiation tech-

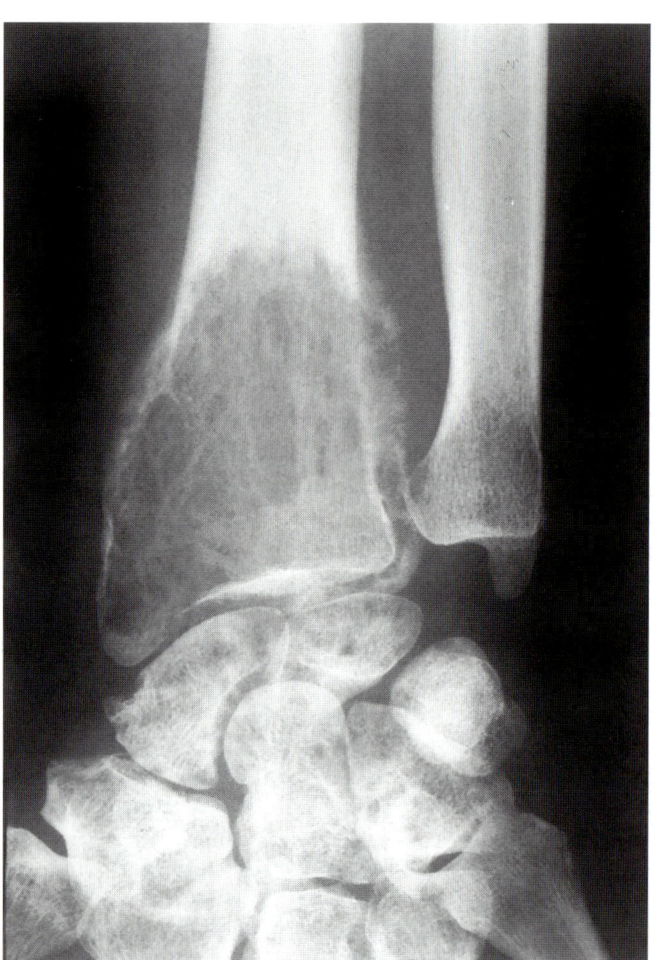

Fig. 29.51

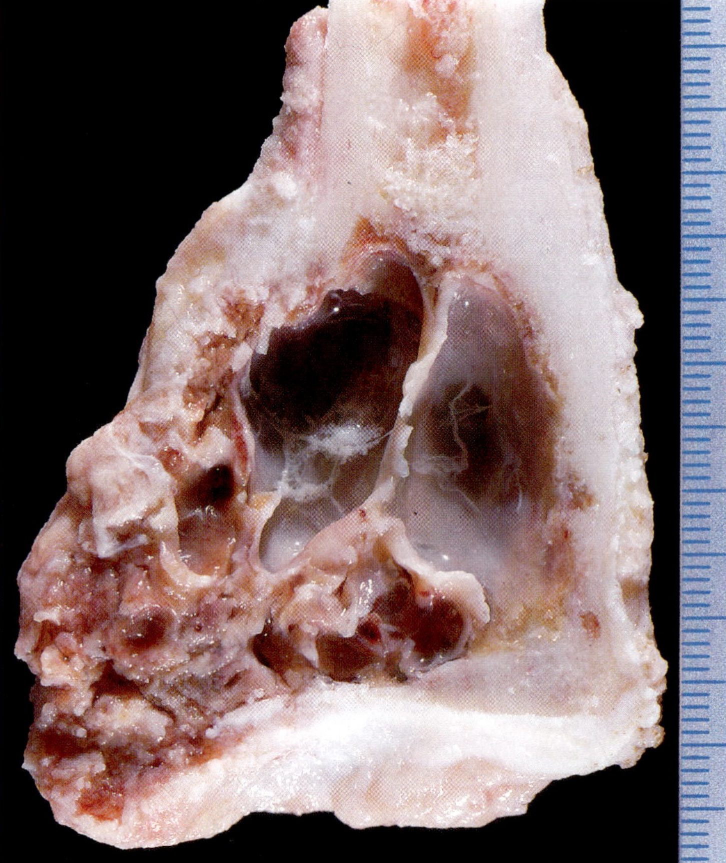

Fig. 29.52

Figs 29.51, 29.52 Recurrence of a giant cell tumor of the radius.

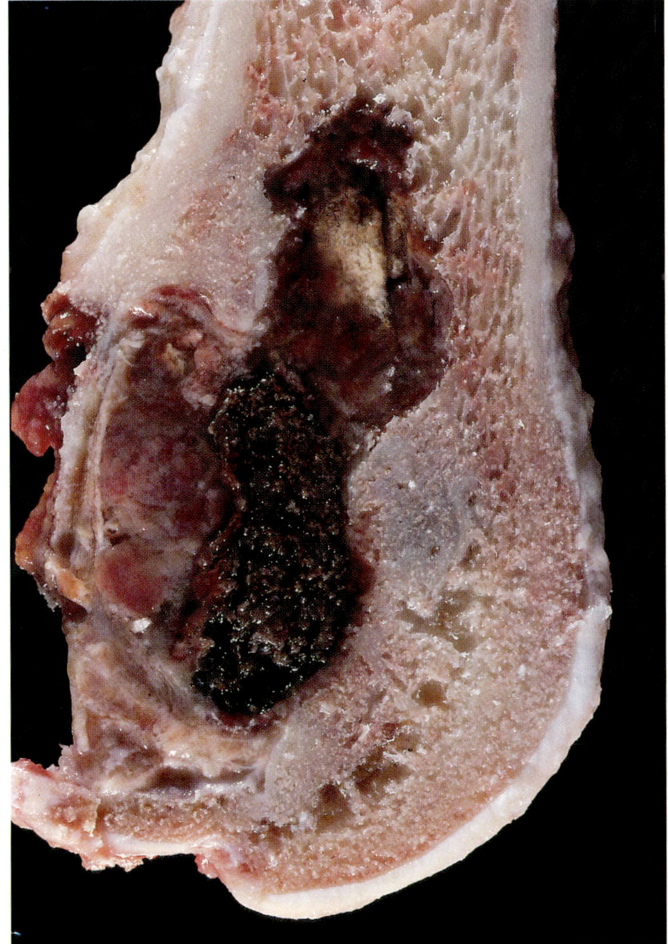

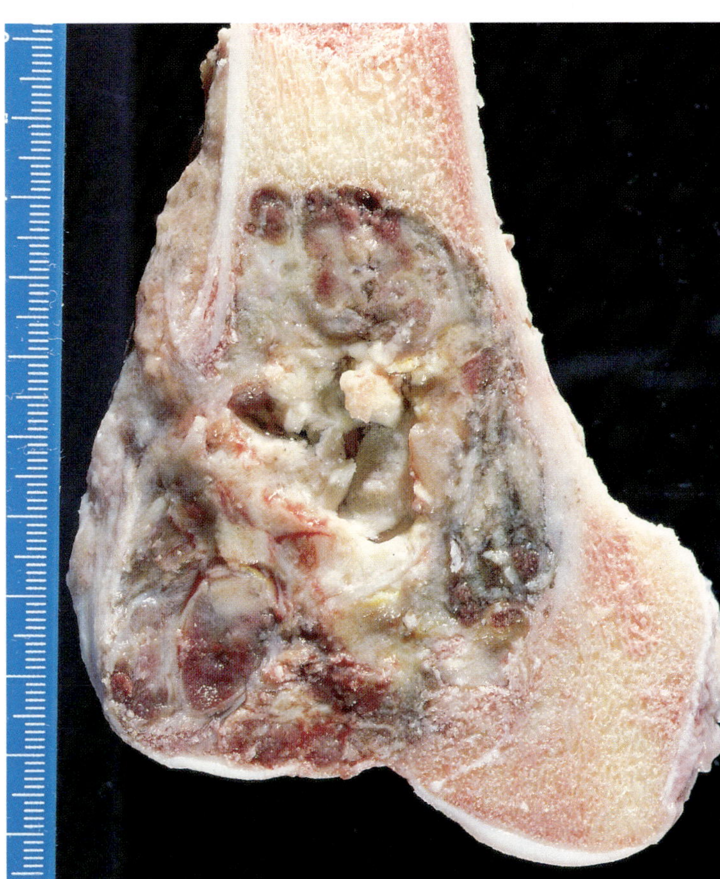

Fig. 29.53

Fig. 29.54

Figs 29.53, 29.54 Recurrences of giant cell tumors of the femur with resorption of the bone grafts.

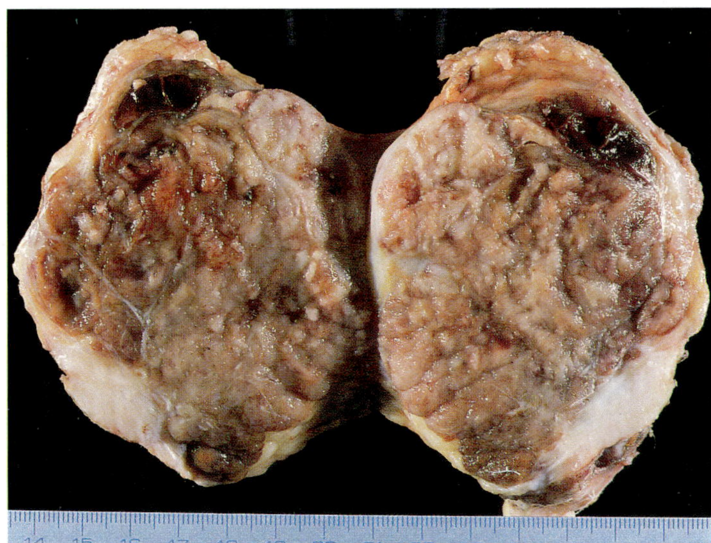

Fig. 29.55 Recurrence of a giant cell tumor of the femur in the popliteal region.

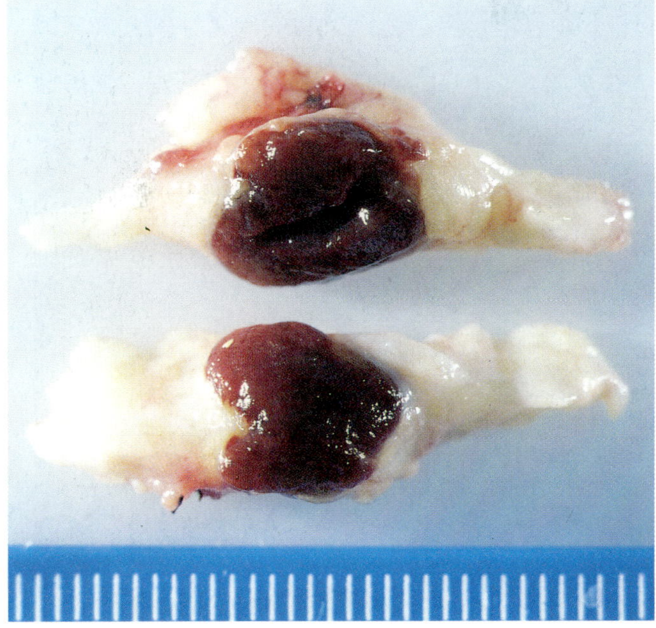

Fig. 29.56 Recurrence of a giant cell tumor of the tibia in the subcutaneous fat.

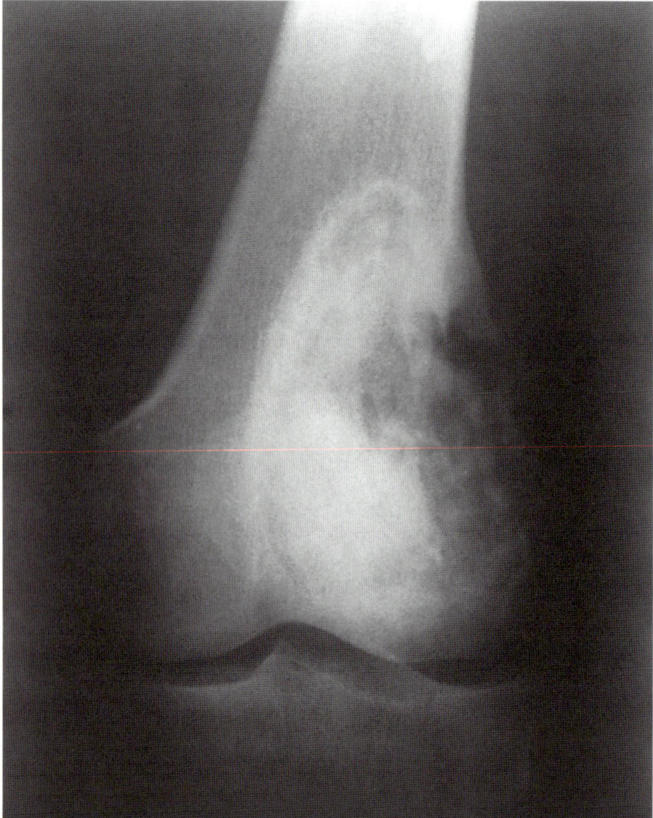

Fig. 29.57

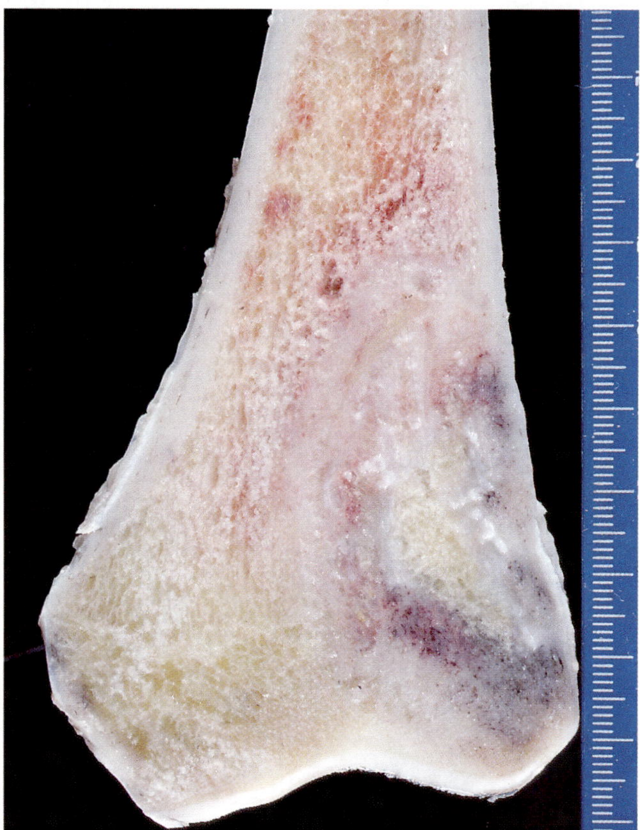

Fig. 29.58

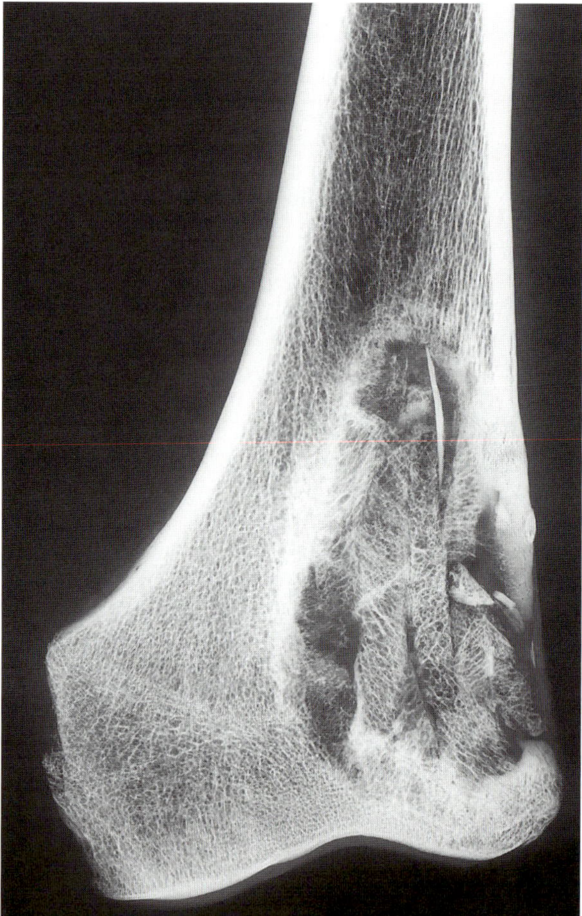

Fig. 29.59

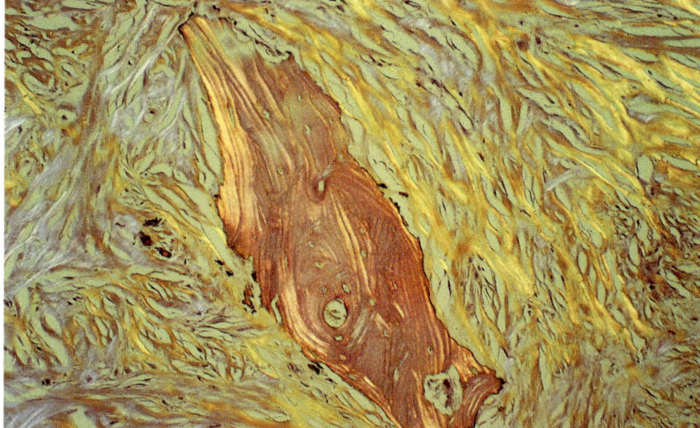

Fig. 29.60

Figs 29.57–29.60 Resorption of bone grafts in a curetted giant cell tumor of the femur misdiagnosed, on imaging, as a tumor recurrence.

niques, long-term control has been achieved in 70–85% of patients with spinal or sacral tumors.[206,207] Embolization is also used for unresectable giant cell tumors of the sacrum or vertebrae.[208]

There are no recognizable effects of chemotherapy.[208]

Recurrences after curettage occur in 30–60% of cases,

the lower incidence being for stage I–II tumors (Figs 29.51–29.56). A higher rate is found in stage III tumors, after pathologic fracture, in tumors of the hands and feet and the distal end of the radius.[209,210] Most recurrences occur within the first 2 years; late recurrences account for 1% of cases.[211]

After curettage and cement packing, the overall recurrence rate is 25%[212] but in some series, it is comparable to that of patients treated by resection, at about 7–15%.

Physiological resorption of the bone graft occurs in the first year[11] (Figs 29.57–29.60); after that time, osteolysis corresponds to a recurrence, but the physiological process may simulate a relapse.[213] Recurrence may appear in an apparently healed lesion.[11] In the same way, the radiolucent bone–cement interface may be confused with a recurrence,[208] but the tumor induces wider osteolysis, with local resorption of the peripheral sclerotic rim.[214,215]

Soft tissue recurrences (2% of cases) often exhibit a peripheral reactive rim of ossification,[216,217] which has also been described in synovial implants.[218] Xenogeneic transplantation of giant cell tumors into immunodeficient athymic mice has also shown the formation of a peripheral shell of new bone; the potential role of bone morphogenetic protein has been stressed.[219] More recently, it has been suggested that osteoinductive growth factors, such as transforming growth factors found in giant cell tumors by in situ hybridization, may stimulate the osteoblastic differentiation of mesenchymal progenitor cells in the extraosseous microenvironment.[220]

DIFFERENTIAL DIAGNOSIS

A brown tumor of hyperparathyroidism has to be excluded by biochemical investigations,[221] whatever the histologic findings. Classically, giant cells with fewer nuclei are irregularly distributed, most often close to frequent hemorrhages, inducing hemosiderin deposition. The stroma is richly vascularized and exhibits spindle cells with collagen production. The reactive new bone formation is more prominent. Giant cell reparative granulomas or 'solid'

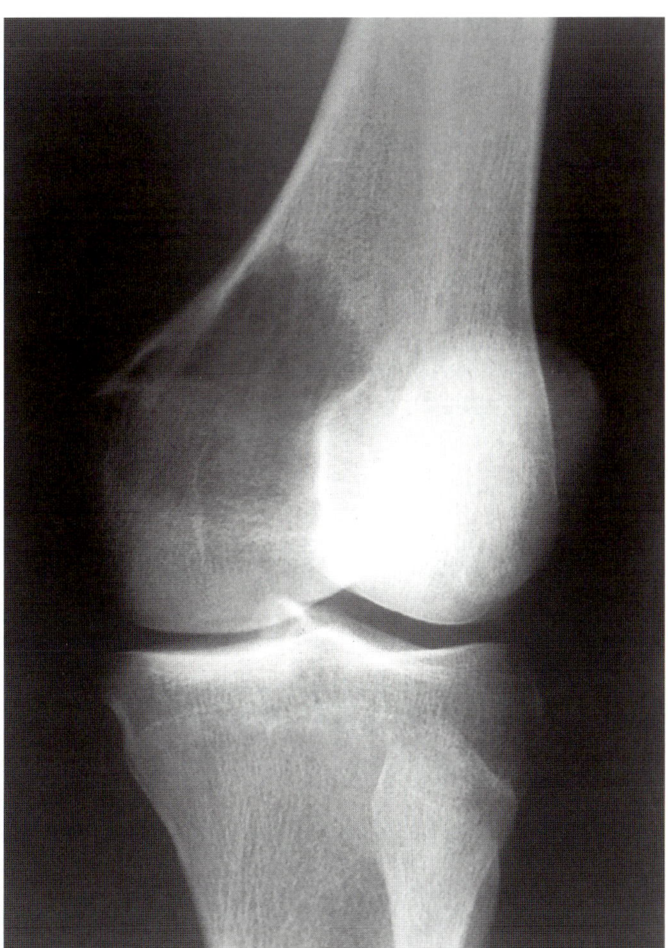

Fig. 29.61

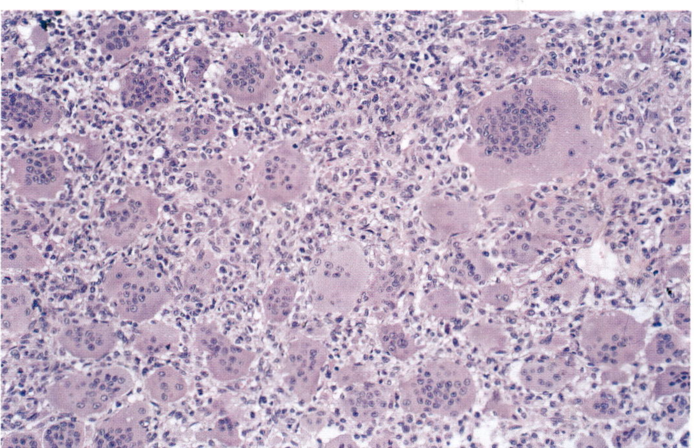

Fig. 29.62

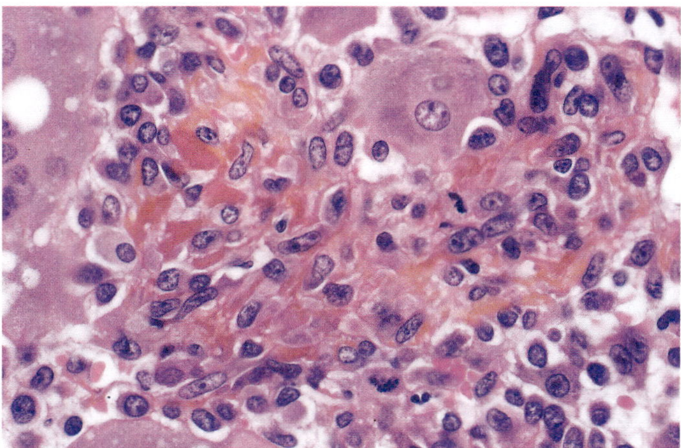

Fig. 29.63

Figs 29.61–29.63 Lytic metaphyseal lesion (19-year-old girl), combining areas of genuine giant cell tumor and areas of osteoblastic osteosarcoma.

areas of aneurysmal bone cysts are histologically similar (Fechner & Mills 1993).

In many cases, the differential diagnosis with an aneurysmal bone cyst is a problem of sampling as these lesions are frequently combined. A genuine aneurysmal bone cyst is devoid of large areas of mononuclear round or oval stromal cells; the cells are more spindle shaped and fewer giant cells are found, preferentially lining the fibrous septae.

The round or oval cells of chondroblastomas have a high nuclear–cytoplasmic ratio; the nuclei are frequently cleaved and the well-defined cytoplasm is rich in glycogen granules. Acidic sulfate glycosaminoglycans are found in the stroma[222] but the best indication is the immunopositivity for S-100 protein and in some cases for NSE and cytokeratins.

Areas of spindle stromal cells in a storiform pattern and sheets of foam cells in giant cell tumors may lead to a diagnosis of non-ossifying fibroma or benign fibrous histiocytoma; one has to rely on the finding of areas of close-packed mononuclear cells with diffusely distributed giant cells.

Osteosarcomas with a huge reactive giant cell component have to be excluded (Figs 29.61–29.63), as well as giant cell-rich fibrosarcomas, malignant fibrous histiocytomas and some forms of dedifferentiated chondrosarcomas.

Immunohistochemistry and electron microscopy are useful to rule out metastatic carcinomas with a prominent giant cell component from various primary sites such as breast, pancreas,[223] liver, thyroid, parotid gland and lung.[224] Metastatic amelanotic melanomas may be rich in giant cells.[225]

REFERENCES

1. Goldring S R, Schiller A L, Mankin H J, Dayer J M, Krane S M. Characterization of cells from human giant cell tumor of bone. Clin Orthop 1986: 204: 59–75
2. Goldring S R, Roelke M S, Petrison K K, Bhan A K. Human giant cell tumors of bone. Identification and characterization of cell types. J Clin Invest 1987: 79: 483–491
3. Joyner C J, Quinn J M, Triffitt J T, Owen M E, Athanasou N A. Phenotypic characterization of mononuclear and multinucleated cells of giant cell tumour of bone. Bone Miner 1992: 16: 37–48
4. Moser R P Jr, Kransdorf M J, Gilkey F W, Manaster B J. From the archives of the AFIP. Giant cell tumor of the upper extremity. Radiographics 1990: 10: 83–102
5. Schajowicz F, Granato D B, McDonald D J, Sundaram M. Clinical and radiological features of atypical giant cell tumours of bone. Br J Radiol 1991: 64: 877–889
6. Sung H W, Kuo D P, Shu W P, Chai Y B, Liu C C, Li S M. Giant cell tumor of bones: analysis of two hundred and eighty cases in Chinese patients. J Bone Joint Surg (Am) 1982: 64: 755–761
7. Frassica F J, Sanjay B K, Unni K K, McLeod R A, Sim F H. Benign giant cell tumor. Orthopedics 1993: 16: 1179–1183
8. Picci P, Manfrini M, Zucchi V et al. Giant cell tumor of bone in skeletally immature patients. J Bone Joint Surg (Am) 1983: 65: 486–490
9. Kransdorf M J, Sweet D E, Buetow P C, Giudici M A I, Moser R P Jr. Giant cell tumor in skeletally immature patients. Radiology 1992: 184: 233–237
10. Schutte H E, Taconis W K. Giant cell tumor in children and adolescents. Skeletal Radiol 1993: 22: 173–176
11. McInerney D P, Middlemiss J H. Giant cell tumour of bone. Skeletal Radiol 1978: 2: 195–204
12. Hudson T M, Schiebler M, Springfield D S, Enneking W F, Hawkins I F Jr, Spanier S S. Radiology of giant cell tumors of bone: computed tomography, arthro-tomography, and scintigraphy. Skeletal Radiol 1984: 11: 85–95
13. McDonald D J, Sim F H, McLeod R A, Dahlin D C. Giant cell tumor of bone. J Bone Joint Surg (Am) 1986: 68: 235–242
14. Campanacci M, Baldini N, Boriani S, Sudanese A. Giant cell tumor of bone. J Bone Joint Surg (Am) 1987: 69: 106–114
15. Hutter R V, Foote F W, Frazell E L, Francis K C. Giant cell tumors complicating Paget's disease of bone. Cancer 1963: 16: 1044–1056
16. Schajowicz F, Slullitel I. Giant cell tumor associated with Paget's disease of bone. J Bone Joint Surg (Am) 1966: 48: 1340–1349
17. Nusbacher N, Sclafani S J, Birla S R. Case report 155. Polyostotic Paget disease complicated by benign giant cell tumor of left clavicle. Skeletal Radiol 1981: 6: 233–235
18. Song I S, Chan K F, Tey P H, Choi H H. Case report 159. Giant cell tumor affecting L2 and L3 and Paget disease of bone. Skeletal Radiol 1981: 6: 299–301
19. Potter H G, Schneider R, Ghelman B, Healey J H, Lane J M. Multiple giant cell tumors and Paget disease of bone: radiographic and clinical correlations. Radiology 1991: 180: 261–264
20. Mirra J M, Bauer F C, Grant T T. Giant cell tumor with viral-like intranuclear inclusions associated with Paget's disease. Clin Orthop 1981: 158: 243–251
21. Pazzaglia U E, Barbieri D, Ceciliani L. An epiphyseal giant cell tumor associated with early Paget's disease. Clin Orthop 1988: 234: 217–220
22. Jacobs T P, Michelsen J, Polay J S, D'Amado A C, Canfield R E. Giant cell tumor in Paget's disease of bone. Familial and geographic clustering. Cancer 1979: 44: 742–747
23. Ruckstuhl H J, Morscher E, Remagen W, Ganz R, Beffa X. Giant cell tumors in combination with other primary bone tumors. Arch Orthop Trauma Surg 1981: 98: 1–6
24. Dahlin D C. Caldwell lecture. Giant cell tumor of bone: highlights of 407 cases. AJR 1985: 144: 955–960
25. Larsson S E, Lorentzon R, Boquist L. Giant-cell tumor of bone. J Bone Joint Surg (Am) 1975: 57: 167–173
26. Manaster B J, Doyle A J. Giant cell tumors of bone. Radiol Clin North Am 1993: 31: 299–323
27. Dahlin D C. Giant cell tumor of vertebrae above the sacrum. Cancer 1977: 39: 1350–1356
28. Shankman S, Greenspan A, Klein M J, Lewis M M. Giant cell tumor of the ischium. Skeletal Radiol 1988: 17: 46–51
29. Sanjay B K, Sim F H, Unni K K, McLeod R A, Klassen R A. Giant-cell tumours of the spine. J Bone Joint Surg (Br) 1993: 75: 148–154
30. Aoki J, Moser R P Jr, Vinh T N. Giant cell tumor of the scapula. A review of 13 cases. Skeletal Radiol 1989: 18: 427–434
31. Averill R M, Smith R J, Campbell C J. Giant cell tumors of the bones of the hand. J Hand Surg (Am) 1980: 5: 39–50
32. Wold L E, Swee R G. Giant cell tumor of the small bones of the hands and feet. Semin Diagn Pathol 1984: 1: 173–184
33. Aaron A D, Kenan S, Klein M J, Hausman M R, Abdelwahab I F, Lewis M M. Case report 810. Giant cell tumor of the first metatarsal. Skeletal Radiol 1993: 22: 543–545
34. Yin Y, Gilula L A, Kyriakos M, Manske P. Giant cell tumor of the distal phalanx of the hand in a child. Clin Orthop 1995: 310: 200–207
35. Sybrandy S, De La Fuente A A. Multiple giant-cell tumour of bone. J Bone Joint Surg (Br) 1973: 55: 350–358
36. Tornberg D N, Dick H M, Johnston A D. Multicentric giant cell tumors of the long bones. J Bone Joint Surg (Am) 1975: 57: 420–422

37. Sim F H, Dahlin D C, Beabout J W. Multicentric giant cell tumor of bone. J Bone Joint Surg (Am) 1977: 59: 1052–1060
38. Bose K, Sinniah R. An unusual giant cell tumour of bone. Int Orthop 1981: 5: 233–236
39. Williams H T. Multicentric giant cell tumor of bone. Clin Nucl Med 1989: 14: 631–633
40. Cummins C A, Scarborough M T, Enneking W F. Multicentric giant cell tumor of bone. Clin Orthop 1996: 322: 245–252
41. Ogihara Y, Sudo A, Shiokawa Y, Takeda K, Kusano I. Case report 862. Multiple giant cell tumor of bone (symmetrical lesions in both humeral heads). Skeletal Radiol 1994: 23: 487–489
42. Peimer C A, Schiller A L, Mankin H J, Smith R J. Multicentric giant cell tumor of bone. J Bone Joint Surg (Am) 1980: 62: 652–656
43. Feldman F. Case report 115. Multicentric giant cell tumors of skeleton (benign). Skeletal Radiol 1980: 5: 119–126
44. Singson R, Feldman F. Case report 229. Multiple (multicentric) giant cell tumors of bone. Skeletal Radiol 1983: 9: 276–281
45. Hindman B W, Seeger L L, Stanley P, Forrester D M, Schwinn C P, Tan S Z. Multicentric giant cell tumor: report of five new cases. Skeletal Radiol 1994: 23: 187–190
46. Wuisman P, Roessner A, Härle A, Erlemann R, Reiser M, Schmidt M. Giant cell tumor of sacrum, fibrous histiocytoma of ischium (benign), fibrous histiocytoma of tibia (benign). Skeletal Radiol 1989: 17: 592–597
47. Sherman M, Fabricius R. Giant cell tumor in the metaphysis of a child. J Bone Joint Surg (Am) 1961: 43: 1225–1229
48. Campanacci M, Giunti A, Olmi R. La localizazzione meta-diafisaria del tumore a cellule giganti. Chir Organi Mov 1975: 62: 29–34
49. Peison B, Feigenbaum J. Metaphyseal giant cell tumor in a girl of 14. Radiology 1976: 118: 145–146
50. Rietveld L A, Mulder J D, Brûtel De La Riviere G, Van Rijssel T G. Giant cell tumour: metaphyseal or epiphyseal origin? Diagn Imaging 1981: 50: 289–293
51. Ogihara Y, Tsuruta T. A case of giant-cell tumour of femoral shaft origin. Australas Radiol 1982: 26: 79–82
52. Visscher D W, Alexander R W, Dempsey T R. Case report 472. Heretical giant cell tumor in the diaphysis of the ulna in a 7-month-old boy. Skeletal Radiol 1988: 17: 285–288
53. Wilkerson J A, Cracchiolo A. Giant-cell tumor of the tibial diaphysis. J Bone Joint Surg (Am) 1969: 51: 1205–1209
54. Fain J S, Unni K K, Beabout J W, Rock M G. Nonepiphyseal giant cell tumor of the long bones. Cancer 1993: 71: 3514–3519
55. Bogumill G P, Schulz M A, Johnson L C. Giant cell tumor. A metaphyseal lesion. J Bone Joint Surg (Am) 1972: 54: 1558
56. Levine E, De Smet A A, Neff J R. Role of radiologic imaging in management planning of giant cell tumor of bone. Skeletal Radiol 1984: 12: 79–89
57. De Santos L A, Murray J A. Evaluation of giant cell tumor by computerized tomography. Skeletal Radiol 1978: 2: 205–212
58. Hermann S D, Mesgarzadeh M, Bonakdarpour A, Dalinka M K. The role of magnetic resonance imaging in giant cell tumor of bone. Skeletal Radiol 1987: 16: 635–643
59. Aoki J, Moriya K, Yamashita K et al. Giant cell tumors containing large amounts of hemosiderin. MR pathologic correlation. J Comput Assist Tomogr 1991: 15: 1024–1027
60. Aoki J, Tanikawa H, Ishii K et al. MRI findings indicative of hemosiderin in giant-cell tumor of bone: frequency, cause, and diagnostic significance. AJR 1996: 166: 145–148
61. Resnik C S, Steffe J W, Wang S E. Case report 353. Giant cell tumor of distal end of the femur, containing a fluid level as demonstrated by computed tomography. Skeletal Radiol 1986: 15: 175–177
62. Kaplan P A, Murphey M, Greenway G, Resnick D, Sartoris D J, Harmo S. Fluid-fluid levels in giant cell tumors of bone. J Comput Tomogr 1987: 11: 151–155
63. Buetow P C, Newman S, Kransdorf M J. Giant cell tumor of the tibia presenting as an expansile metaphyseal lesion with fluid-fluid levels on M R. Magn Reson Imaging 1990: 8: 341–344
64. Abdelwahab I F, Kenan S, Hermann G, Klein M J, Lewis M M. Case report 845. Fluid-filling giant cell tumor with an aneurysmal bone cyst component. Skeletal Radiol 1994: 23: 317–319
65. Gunterberg B, Kindblom L G, Laurin L. Giant cell tumor of bone and aneurysmal bone cyst. A correlated histologic and angiographic study. Skeletal Radiol 1977: 2: 65–74
66. Prando A, DeSantos L A, Wallace S, Murray J A. Angiography in giant-cell bone tumors. Radiology 1979: 130: 323–331
67. Van Nostrand D, Madewell J E, McNiesh L M, Kyle R W, Sweet D. Radionuclide bone scanning in giant cell tumor. J Nucl Med 1986: 27: 329–338
68. Levine E, De Smet A A, Neff J R, Martin N L. Scintigraphic evaluation of giant cell tumor of bone. AJR 1984: 143: 343–348
69. Bertoni F, Present D, Enneking W F. Giant cell tumor of bone with pulmonary metastases. J Bone Joint Surg (Am) 1985: 67: 890–900
70. Wood G W, Neff J R, Gollahon K A, Gourley W K. Macrophages in giant cell tumours of bone. J Pathol 1978: 125: 53–58
71. Shuffstall R M, Gregory J E. Osteoid formation in giant cell tumor of bone. Am J Pathol 1953: 29: 1123–1131
72. Johnston J. Giant cell tumor of bone. The role of the giant cell in orthopedic pathology. Orthop Clin North Am 1977: 8: 751–770
73. Aqel N M, Pringle J A, Horton M A. Cellular heterogeneity in giant cell tumor of bone (osteoclastoma): an immunohistochemical study of 16 cases. Histopathology 1988: 13: 675–685
74. Present D, Bertoni F, Hudson T, Enneking W F. The correlation between the radiologic staging studies and histopathologic findings in aggressive stage 3 giant cell tumor of bone. Cancer 1986: 57: 237–244
75. Sanerkin N G. Malignancy, aggressiveness and recurrence in giant cell tumor of bone. Cancer 1980: 46: 1641–1649
76. Jaffe H L, Lichtenstein L, Portis R B. Giant cell tumor of bone. Its pathologic appearance, grading, supposed variants and treatment. Arch Pathol 1940: 30: 993–1031
77. Komiya S, Inoue A, Nakashima M, Ueno A, Fujikawa K, Ikuta H. Prognostic factors in giant cell tumor of bone. A modified biological grading system useful as a guide to prognosis. Arch Orthop Trauma Surg 1986: 105: 67–72
78. Fornasier V L, Protzner K, Zhang I, Mason L. The prognostic significance of histomorphometry and immunohistochemistry in giant cell tumors of bone. Hum Pathol 1996: 27: 754–760
79. Kuwahara H, Shimazaki M, Morikita I, Chanoki Y, Sakurai M. Texture analysis of histological images of giant cell tumor of bone. Pathol Res Pract 1992: 188: 565–569
80. Murphy W R, Ackerman L V. Benign and malignant giant cell tumors of bone. Cancer 1956: 9: 317–339
81. Goldenberg R R, Campbell C J, Bonfiglio M. Giant cell tumor of bone. J Bone Joint Surg (Am) 1970: 52: 619–664
82. Boquist L, Larsson S E, Lorentzon R. Genuine giant-cell tumour of bone: a combined cytological, histopathological and ultrastructural study. Pathol Eur 1976: 11: 117–127
83. Sneige N, Ayala A G, Carrasco C H, Murray J, Raymond A K. Giant cell tumor of bone. Diagn Cytopathol 1985: 1: 111–117
84. Rios-Martin J, Otal-Salaverri C, Vazquez-Ramirez F J, Gonzalez-Campora R, Davidson H G. Fine needle aspiration diagnosis of aggressive giant cell tumor of bone. Acta Cytol 1995: 39: 550–554
85. Vetrani A, Fulciniti F, Boschi R et al. Fine needle aspiration biopsy diagnosis of giant cell tumor of bone. Acta Cytol 1990: 34: 863–867
86. Bouropoulou V, Kontogeorgos G, Manika Z. A histological and immunoenzymatic study on the histogenesis of 'giant cell tumor of bones'. Pathol Res Pract 1985: 180: 61–67
87. Emura I, Inoue Y, Ohnishi Y, Morita T, Saito H, Tajima T. Histochemical, immunohistochemical and ultrastructural investigations of giant cell tumors of bone. Acta Pathol Jpn 1986: 36: 691–702
88. Ling L, Klein M J, Sissons H A, Steiner G C. Lysozyme and alpha 1 antitrypsin in giant cell tumor of bone and in other lesions that contain giant cells. Arch Pathol Lab Med 1986: 110: 713–718
89. Roessner A, Vassallo J, Vollmer E, Zwadlo G, Sorg C, Grundmann E. Biological characterization of human bone tumors. X. The proliferation behavior of macrophages as compared to fibroblastic cells in malignant fibrous histiocytoma and giant cell tumor of bone. J Cancer Res Clin Oncol 1987: 113: 559–562
90. Hasegawa T, Hirose T, Seki K, Sano T, Hizawa K. Transforming

growth-factor-alpha and CD68 immunoreactivity in giant cell tumours of bone. J Pathol 1993: 170: 305–310

91. Brecher M E, Franklin W A, Simon M A. Immunohistochemical study of mononuclear phagocyte antigens in giant cell tumor of bone. Am J Pathol 1986: 125: 252–257

92. Komiya S, Sasaguri Y, Inoue A et al. Characterization of cells cultured from human giant-cell tumors of bone. Phenotypic relationship to the monocyte-macrophage and osteoclast. Clin Orthop 1990: 258: 304–309

93. Kasahara K, Yamamuro T, Kasahara A. Giant cell tumor of bone: cytological studies. Br J Cancer 1979: 40: 201–209

94. Ling L, Klein M J, Sissons H A, Steiner G C, Winchester R J. Expression of Ia and monocyte-macrophage lineage antigens in giant cell tumor of bone and related lesions. Arch Pathol Lab Med 1988: 112: 65–69

95. Kito M. Identification of cytokines produced by cells cultured from human giant cell tumors of bone (in Japanese). Nippon Seikeigeka Gakkai Zasshi 1991: 65: 918–930

96. Liu T C, Ji Z M, Wang L T. Giant cell tumors of bone. An immunohistochemical study. Pathol Res Pract 1989: 185: 448–453

97. Burmester G R, Winchester R J, Dimitriu-Bona A, Klein M, Steiner G, Sissons H A. Delineation of four cell types comprising the giant cell tumor of bone. Expression of Ia and monocyte macrophage-lineage antigens. J Clin Invest 1983: 71: 1633–1648

98. Horton M A, Lewis D, McNulty K, Pringle J A, Chambers T J. Monoclonal antibodies to osteoclastomas (giant cell bone tumors). Definition of osteoclast-specific antigens. Cancer Res 1985: 45: 5663–5669

99. Athanasou N A, Bliss E, Gatter K C, Heryet A, Woods C G, McGee J O. An immunohistochemical study of giant cell tumour of bone. Evidence for an osteoclast origin of the giant cells. J Pathol 1985: 147: 153–158

100. Abe Y, Yonemura K, Nishida K, Takagi K. Giant cell tumor of bone: analysis of proliferative cells by double-labeling immunohistochemistry with anti-proliferating cell nuclear antigen antibody and culture procedure. Nippon Seikeigeka Gakkai Zasshi 1994: 68: 407–414

101. Robinson D, Einhorn T A. Giant cell tumor of bone: a unique paradigm of stromal-hematopoietic cellular interactions. J Cell Biochem 1994: 55: 300–303

102. Maeda A, Matsui H, Kanamori M, Yudoh K, Tsuji H. Calcitonin receptors on neoplastic mononuclear cells cultured from a human giant-cell tumor of the sacrum. J Cancer Res Clin Oncol 1994: 120: 272–278

103. Nicholson G C, Horton M A, Sexton P M et al. Calcitonin receptors of human osteoclastoma. Horm Metab Res 1987: 19: 585–589

104. Chambers T J, Fuller K, McSheehy P M J, Pringle J A. The effects of calcium regulating hormones on bone resorption by isolated human osteoclastoma cells. J Pathol 1985: 145: 297–305

105. Zhou L, Feng C H, Li H P. Contrast study on multinucleated giant cells in giant cell tumours of bone and other multinucleated cells. Chin Med J (Engl) 1989: 102: 584–590.

106. Campanacci M, Bagnara G P, Serra M et al. Giant cell tumor of bone: a model for the in vitro human osteoclast characterization. Tumori 1989: 75: 389–395

107. Toyasawa S, Ogawa Y, Chang C K et al. Histochemistry of tartrate-resistant acid phosphatase and carbonic anhydrase isoenzyme II in osteoclast-like giant cells in bone tumour. Virchows Arch Pathol Anat Histopathol 1991: 418: 255–261

108. Zheng M H, Fan Y, Wysocki S J et al. Gene expression of transforming growth factor-beta 1 and its type II receptor in giant cell tumors of bone. Am J Pathol 1994: 145: 1095–1104

109. Middleton J, Arnott N, Walsh S, Beresford J. The expression of mRNA for insulin-like growth factors and their receptor in giant cell tumors of bone. Clin Orthop 1996: 322: 224–231

110. Grano M, Colucci S, De Bellis M et al. New model for bone resorption study in vitro: human osteoclast-like cells from giant cell tumors of bone. J Bone Miner Res 1994: 9: 1013–1020

111. Chilosi M, Gilioli E, Lestani M, Menestrina F, Fiore-Donati L. Immunohistochemical characterization of osteoclastoma and osteoclast-like cells with monoclonal antibody MB1 on paraffin-embedded tissues. J Pathol 1988: 156: 251–254

112. James I E, Walsh S, Dodds R A, Gowen M. Production and characterization of osteoclast-selective monoclonal antibodies that distinguish between multinucleated cells derived from different human tissues. J Histochem Cytochem 1991: 39: 905–914

113. Doussis I A, Puddle B, Athanasou N A. Immunophenotype of multinucleated and mononuclear cells in giant cell lesions of bone and soft tissue. J Clin Pathol 1992: 45: 398–404

114. Oreffo R O C, Marshall G J, Kirchen M et al. Characterization of a cell line derived from a human giant cell tumor that stimulates osteoclastic bone resorption. Clin Orthop 1993: 296: 229–241

115. Ohsaki Y, Takahashi S, Scarcez T et al. Evidence of an autocrine/paracrine role for interleukin-6 in bone resorption by giant cells from giant cell tumors of bone. Endocrinology 1992: 131: 2229–2234

116. Sasaguri Y, Komiya S, Sugama K et al. Production of matrix metalloproteinase-2 and metalloproteinase 3 (stromelysin) by stromal cells of giant cell tumors of bone. Am J Pathol 1992: 141: 611–621

117. Komiya S, Minamitani K, Inoue A. The pathogenesis and etiology of giant cell tumor of bone from a viewpoint of bone resorptive factors. Nippon Seikeigeka Gakkai Zasshi 1992: 66: 485–492

118. Ueda Y, Imai K, Tsuchiya H et al. Matrix metalloproteinase 9 (gelatinase B) is expressed in multinucleated giant cells of human giant cell tumor of bone and is associated with vascular invasion. Am J Pathol 1996: 148: 611–622

119. Rao V H, Bridge J A, Neff JR et al. Expression of 72 kDa and 92 kDa type IV collagenases from human giant-cell tumor of bone. Clin Exp Metastasis 1995: 13: 420–426

120. Page A E, Warburton M J, Chambers T J, Pringle J A, Hayman A R. Human osteoclastomas contain multiple forms of cathepsin B. Biochim Biophys Acta 1992: 1116: 57–66

121. Li Y P, Alexander M, Wucherpfennig A L, Yelick K P, Chen W, Stashenko P. Cloning and complete coding sequence of a novel human cathepsin expressed in giant cells of osteoclastomas. J Bone Miner Res 1995: 10: 1197–1202

122. Grano M, Colucci S, Zigrino P et al. Integrin expression and adhesion property of osteoclast-like cells from giant cell tumours of bone. Boll Soc Ital Biol Sper 1992: 68: 255–258

123. Schajowicz F. Giant-cell tumors of bone (osteoclastoma): a pathological and histochemical study. J Bone Joint Surg (Am) 1961: 43: 1–29

124. Ores R, Ortiz J, Rosen P. Localisation of acid phosphatase activity in a giant cell tumor of bone. Arch Pathol 1969: 88: 54–57

125. Yoshida H, Akeho M, Yumoto T. Giant cell tumor of bone. Enzyme, histochemical, biochemical and tissue cultures studies. Virchows Arch A Pathol Anat Histol 1982: 395: 319–330

126. Clohisy D R, Vorlicky L, Oegema T R Jr, Snover D, Thompson R C Jr. Histochemical and immunohistochemical characterization of cells constituting the giant cell tumor of bone. Clin Orthop 1993: 287: 259–261

127. Metze K, Ciplea A G, Hettwer H, Barckhaus R H. Size dependent enzyme activities of multinucleated (osteoclastic) giant cells in bone tumors. Pathol Res Pract 1987: 182: 214–221

128. Wold L E, Spelsberg T, Jiang N, Sim F. Steroid receptors and giant cell tumor of bone. Curr Top Pathol 1989: 80: 153–164

129. Ishibe M, Ishibe Y, Ishibashi T et al. Low content of estrogen receptors in human giant cell tumors of bone. Arch Orthop Trauma Surg 1994: 113: 106–109

130. Oursler M J, Pederson L, Fitzpatrick L, Riggs B L, Spelsberg T. Human giant cell tumors of the bone (osteoclastomas) are oestrogen target cells. Proc Natl Acad Sci USA 1994: 91: 5227–5231

131. Xiang J H, Spanier S S, Benson N A, Braylan R C. Flow cytometric analysis of DNA in bone and soft-tissue tumors using nuclear suspensions. Cancer 1987: 59: 1951–1958

132. Sun D, Biesterfeld S, Adler C P, Böcking A. Prediction of recurrence in giant cell bone tumors by DNA cytometry. Anal Quant Cytol Histol 1992: 14: 341–346

133. Sara A S, Ayala A G, el-Naggar A, Ro J Y, Raymond A K, Murray J A. Giant cell tumor of bone. A clinicopathologic and DNA flow cytometric analysis. Cancer 1990: 66: 2186–2190

134. Helio H, Karaharju E, Böhling T, Nordling S. Giant cell tumours of bone. A DNA-flow cytometric study. Eur J Surg Oncol 1994: 20: 200–206

135. Fukunaga M, Nikaido T, Shimoda T, Ushigome S, Nakamori K. A flow cytometric DNA analysis of giant cell tumors of bone including two cases with malignant transformation. Cancer 1992: 70: 1886–1894

136. Schajowicz F, Cabrini R L, Gimenez I. Microspectrophotometric quantitation of DNA in bone tumors with giant cells (osteoclastoma, osteosarcoma and chondroblastoma). Clin Orthop 1981: 156: 91–97

137. Bouropoulou V, Malkaki S, Karameris A. Ag.-Nors in giant cell tumor of bones: are they useful in the estimation of tumor's behavior? Arch Anat Cytol Pathol 1991: 39: 42–46

138. Clohisy J C, Schajowicz F, Vaziri D M et al. Assessment of argyrophilic nucleolar organizer region quantification in benign and malignant bone tumors. Clin Orthop 1995: 310: 229–236

139. Sulh M, Alba Greco M, Jiang T, Goswami S B, Present D, Steiner G. Proliferation index and vascular density of giant cell tumors of bone. Are they prognostic markers? Cancer 1996: 77: 2044–2051

140. Bridge J A, Neff J R, Bhatia P S, Sanger W G, Murphey M D. Cytogenetic findings and biologic behavior of giant cell tumors of bone. Cancer 1990: 65: 2697–2703

141. Bardi G, Pandis N, Mandahl N et al. Chromosome abnormalities in giant cell tumors of bone. Cancer Genet Cytogenet 1991: 57: 161–167

142. Bridge J A, Neff J R, Mouron B J. Giant cell tumor of bone. Chromosomal analysis of 48 specimens and review of the literature. Cancer Genet Cytogenet 1992: 58: 2–13

143. Schwartz H S, Jenkins R B, Dahl R J, Dewald G W. Cytogenetic analyses on giant cell tumors of bone. Clin Orthop 1989: 240: 250–260

144. Schwartz H S, Butler M G, Jenkins R B, Miller D A, Moses H L. Telomeric associations and consistent growth factor overexpression detected in giant cell tumor of bone. Cancer Genet Cytogenet 1991: 56: 263–276

145. Schwartz H S, Juliao S F, Sciadini M F, Miller L K, Butler M G. Telomerase activity and oncogenesis in giant cell tumor of bone. Cancer 1995: 75: 1094–1099

146. Noguera R, Llombart-Bosch A, Lopez-Gines C, Carda C, Fernandez CI. Giant-cell tumor of bone, stage II, displaying translocation t(12;19)(q13q13). Virchows Arch A Pathol Anat Histopathol 1989: 415: 377–382

147. McComb E N, Johansson S L, Neff J R, Nelson M, Bridge J A. Chromosomal anomalies exclusive of telomeric associations in giant cell tumor of bone. Cancer Genet Cytogenet 1996: 88: 163–166

148. Schneiner M, Hedges L, Schwartz H S, Butler M G. Lack of microsatellite instability in giant cell tumor of bone. Cancer Genet Cytogenet 1996: 88: 35–38

149. Aparisi T. Giant cell tumor of bone. Electron microscopic and histochemical investigations. Acta Orthop Scand 1978: 173(suppl): 1–38

150. Roessner A, Von Bassewitz D B, Schlake W, Thorwesten G, Grundmann E. Biologic characterization of human bone tumors III. Giant cell tumor of bone. A combined electron microscopical, histochemical and autoradiographical study. Pathol Res Pract 1984: 178: 431–440

151. Mii Y, Miyauchi Y, Morishita T et al. Osteoclast origin of giant cells in giant cell tumors of bone. Ultrastructural and cytochemical study of six cases. Ultrastruct Pathol 1991: 15: 623–629

152. Kanehisa J, Izumo T, Takeuchi M, Yamanaka T, Fujii T, Takeuchi H. In vitro bone resorption by isolated multinucleated giant cells from giant cell tumour of bone: light and electron microscopic study. Virchows Arch A Pathol Anat Histopathol 1991: 419: 327–338

153. Aparisi T, Arborgh B, Ericsson J L. Giant cell tumor of bone. Detailed fine structural analysis of different cell components. Virchows Arch A Pathol Anat Histol 1977: 376: 273–298

154. Aparisi T, Arborgh B, Ericsson J L. Giant cell tumor of bone: variations in patterns of appearance of different cell types. Virchows Arch A Pathol Anat Histol 1979: 381: 159–178

155. Hanaoka H, Friedman B, Mack R P. Ultrastructure and histogenesis of giant cell tumor of bone. Cancer 1970: 25: 1408–1423

156. Metze K. Osteoclastic origin of giant cells in giant cell tumors of bone – ultrastructure and cytochemical study of six cases. Ultrastruct Pathol 1992: 16: 601–602

157. Troise G D, Lustig E S, Schajowicz F, Gallardo H. Mitosis in tissue cultures of human giant cell tumors of bone. Oncology 1973: 28: 193–203

158. Steiner G C, Ghosh L, Dorfman H D. Ultrastructure of giant cell tumors of bone. Hum Pathol 1972: 3: 569–586

159. McCarthy E F, Serrano J A, Wasserkrug H L, Dorfman H D. The ultrastructural localization of secretory acid phosphatase in giant-cell tumor of bone. Clin Orthop 1979: 141: 295–302

160. Zambonin-Zallone A, Teti A, Grano M et al. Immunocytochemical distribution of extracellular matrix receptors in human osteoclasts: a beta3 integrin is co-localized with vinculin and talin in the podosomes of osteoclastoma giant cells. Exp Cell Res 1989: 182: 645–652

161. Welsh R A, Meyer A T. Nuclear fragmentations and associated fibrils in giant cell tumor of bone. Lab Invest 1970: 22: 63–72

162. Mirra J M, Gold R H. Case report 186. Giant cell tumor containing viral-like intranuclear inclusions in association with Paget's disease. Skeletal Radiol 1982: 8: 67–70

163. El Labban N G. Ultrastructural study of intranuclear tubulo-filaments in a giant cell tumor of bone in a patient with Paget's disease. J Oral Pathol 1984: 13: 650–660

164. Fornasier V L, Flores L, Hastings D, Sharp T. Virus-like filamentous intranuclear inclusions in giant-cell tumor not associated with Paget's disease of bone. J Bone Joint Surg (Am) 1985: 67: 333–336

165. Schajowicz F, Ubios A M, Araujo E S, Cabrini R L. Virus-like inclusions in giant cell tumor of bone. Clin Orthop 1985: 201: 247–250

166. Abelanet R, Daudet-Monsac M, Laoussadi S, Forest M, Vacher-Lavenu M C. Frequency and diagnostic value of the virus-like filamentous intranuclear inclusions in giant cell tumor of bone, not associated with Paget's disease. A study of 43 cases. Virchows Arch A Pathol Anat Histopathol 1986: 410: 65–68

167. Negoescu A, Mandache E. The ultrastructure of nuclear inclusions in the giant cell tumor of bone. Pathol Res Pract 1989: 184: 410–417

168. Hall F M, Frank H A, Cohen R B. Ossified pulmonary metastases from giant cell tumor of bone. AJR 1976: 127: 1046–1047

169. Szyfelbein W M, Schiller A L. Cytologic diagnosis of giant cell tumor of bone metastatic to lung. Acta Cytol 1979: 23: 460–464

170. Mirra J M, Ulich T, Magidson J, Kaiser L, Eckardt J, Gold R. A case of probable benign pulmonary 'metastases' or implants arising from giant cell tumor of bone. Clin Orthop 1982: 162: 245–254

171. Vanel D, Contesso G, Rebibo G, Zafrani B, Masselot J. Benign giant cell tumours of bone with pulmonary metastases and favourable prognosis. Skeletal Radiol 1983: 10: 221–226

172. Rock M G, Pritchard D J, Unni K K. Metastases from histologically benign giant cell tumor of bone. J Bone Joint Surg (Am) 1984: 66: 269–274

173. Bertoni F, Present D, Sudanese A, Baldini N, Bacchini P, Campanacci M. Giant cell tumor of bone with pulmonary metastases. Clin Orthop 1988: 237: 275–285

174. Ladanyi M, Traganos F, Huvos A G. Benign metastasizing giant cell tumors of bone. A DNA flow cytometric study. Cancer 1989: 64: 1521–1526

175. Maloney W J, Vaughan L M, Jones H H, Ross J, Nagel D A. Benign metastasizing giant cell tumor of bone. Clin Orthop 1989: 243: 208–215

176. Tubbs W S, Brown L R, Beabout J W, Rock M G, Unni K K. Benign giant-cell tumor of bone with pulmonary metastases. AJR 1992: 158: 331–334

177. Nojima T, Takeda N, Matsuno T, Inoue K, Nagashima K. Case report 869. Benign metastasizing giant cell tumor of bone. Skeletal Radiol 1994: 23: 583–585

178. Kay R M, Eckardt J J, Seeger L L, Mirra J M, Hak D J. Pulmonary metastasis of benign giant cell tumor of bone. Clin Orthop 1994: 302: 219–230

179. Stargardter F L, Cooperman L R. Giant cell tumor of sacrum with multiple pulmonary metastases and long-term survival. Br J Radiol 1971: 44: 976–979

180. Lopez-Barea F, Rodriguez-Peralto J L, Garcia-Giron J, Guemes-Gordo F. Benign metastasizing giant cell tumor of the hand. Clin Orthop 1992: 274: 270–274

181. Sanjay B K, Younge D A. Giant cell tumor of metacarpal with pulmonary and skeletal metastases. J Hand Surg (Br) 1996: 21: 126–132

182. Caballes R L. The mechanism of metastasis in the so called 'benign giant cell tumor of bone'. Hum Pathol 1981: 12: 762–767

183. Mellin W, Roessner A, Grundmann E, Wormann B, Hiddemann W, Immenkamp M. Biological characterization of human bone tumors. VII Detection of malignancy in a giant cell tumor of bone by flow cytometric DNA analysis. Pathol Res Pract 1985: 180: 619–625

184. Present D A, Bertoni F, Springfield D, Braylan R, Enneking W F. Giant cell tumor of bone with pulmonary and lymph node metastases. Clin Orthop 1986: 209: 286–291

185. Scott S M, Pritchard D J, Unni K K, Rainwater L M, Lieber M M. 'Benign' metastasizing giant cell tumor of bone: evaluation of nuclear DNA patterns by flow cytometry. J Orthop Res 1989: 7: 463–467

186. Takanami I, Imamura T, Morota N, Kodaira S. Recurrent pulmonary metastases from benign giant cell tumors of the bone: report of two cases and analysis of nuclear DNA content by flow cytometry. Surg Today 1994: 24: 476–480

187. Katz E, Nyska M, Okon E, Zajicek G, Robin G. Growth rate analysis of lung metastases from histologically benign giant cell tumor of bone. Cancer 1987: 59: 1831–1836

188. Budzilovich G N, Truchly G, Wilens S L. Tumor giant cells in regional lymph nodes of a case of recurrent giant cell tumor of bone. Clin Orthop 1963: 30: 182–187

189. Lewis J J, Healey J H, Huvos A G, Burt M. Benign giant-cell tumor of bone with metastasis to mediastinal lymph nodes. J Bone Joint Surg (Am) 1996: 78: 106–110

190. Serra J M, Muirragui A, Tadjalli H. Extensive distal subcutaneous metastases of a 'benign' giant cell tumor of the radius. Plast Reconstr Surg 1985: 75: 263–267

191. Cerroni L, Soyer H P, Smolle J, Kerl H. Cutaneous metastases of a giant cell tumor of bone. J Cutan Pathol 1990: 17: 59–63

192. Wray C C, MacDonald A W, Richardson R A. Benign giant cell tumour with metastases to bone and lung. J Bone Joint Surg (Br) 1990: 72: 486–489

193. Nascimento A G, Huvos A G, Marcove R C. Primary malignant giant cell tumor of bone. Cancer 1979: 44: 1393–1402

194. Shamsuddin A K, Varma V A, Toker C, Edwards C C. Ultrastructural features of a malignant giant cell tumor of bone with areas of osteogenic sarcoma. Mt Sinai J Med 1979: 46: 297–308

195. Rock M G, Sim F H, Unni K K et al. Secondary malignant giant cell tumor of bone. J Bone Joint Surg (Am) 1986: 68: 1073–1079

196. Boriani S, Sudanese A, Baldini N, Picci P. Sarcomatous degeneration of giant cell tumours. Ital J Orthop Traumatol 1986: 12: 191–199

197. Kenan S, Abdelwahab I F, Klein M J, Lewis M M. Case report 863. Osteosarcoma associated with giant cell tumor. Skeletal Radiol 1995: 24: 55–58

198. Meis J M, Dorfman H D, Nathanson S D, Haggar A M, Wu K K. Primary malignant giant cell tumor of bone: 'dedifferentiated' giant cell tumor. Mod Pathol 1989: 2: 541–546

199. Zhu X Z, Steiner G C. Malignant giant cell tumor of bone: malignant transformation of a benign giant cell tumor treated by surgery. Bull Hosp Jt Dis Orthop Inst 1990: 50: 169–176

200. Brooks J P, Pascal R R. Malignant giant cell tumor of bone: ultrastructural and immunohistologic evidence of histiocytic origin. Hum Pathol 1984: 15: 1098–1100

201. Gitelis S, Wang J W, Quast M, Schajowicz F, Templeton A. Recurrence of a giant cell tumor with malignant transformation to a fibrosarcoma twenty five years after primary treatment. J Bone Joint Surg (Am) 1989: 71: 757–761

202. Sundaram M, Martin A S, Tayob A A. Case report 182. Osteosarcoma arising in giant cell tumor of tibia. Skeletal Radiol 1982: 7: 282–285

203. Hefti F L, Gachter A, Remagen W, Nidecker A. Recurrent giant-cell tumor with metaplasia and malignant change not associated with radiotherapy. J Bone Joint Surg (Am) 1992: 74: 930–934

204. Ortiz-Cruz E J, Quinn R H, Fanburg J C, Rosenberg A E, Mankin H J. Late development of a malignant fibrous histiocytoma at the site of a giant cell tumor. Clin Orthop 1995: 318: 199–204

205. Venturi R. Osteosarcoma del femore insorto su antico tumore giganto-cellulare. Chir Organi Mov 1986: 71: 411–415

206. Schwartz L H, Okunieff P G, Rosenberg A, Suit H D. Radiation therapy in the treatment of difficult giant cell tumors. Int J Radiat Oncol Biol Phys 1989: 17: 1085–1088

207. Bell R S, Harwood A R, Goodman S B, Fornasier V L. Supervoltage radiotherapy in the treatment of difficult giant cell tumors of bone. Clin Orthop 1983: 174: 208–216

208. Carrasco C H, Murray J A. Giant cell tumors. Orthop Clin North Am 1989: 20: 395–405

209. Joly M A, Vazquez J J, Martinez A, Guillen F J. Blood-borne spread of a benign giant cell tumor from the radius to the soft tissue of the hand. Cancer 1984: 54: 2564–2567

210. Vander Griend R A, Funderburk C H. The treatment of giant-cell tumors of the distal part of the radius. J Bone Joint Surg (Am) 1993: 75: 899–908

211. Scully S P, Mott M P, Temple H T, O'Keefe R J, O'Donnell R J, Mankin H J. Late recurrence of giant-cell tumor of bone. J Bone Joint Surg (Am) 1994: 76: 1231–1233

212. O'Donnell R J, Springfield D S, Motwani H K, Ready J E, Gebhardt M C, Mankin H J. Recurrence of giant-cell tumors of the long bones after curettage and packing with cement. J Bone Joint Surg (Am) 1994: 76: 1827–1833

213. Mund D F, Yao L, Fu Y S, Eckardt J J. Case report 826. Physiological resorption of allograft simulating recurrent giant cell tumor. Skeletal Radiol 1994: 23: 139–141

214. Pettersson H, Rydholm A, Persson B. Early radiologic detection of local recurrence after curettage and acrylic cementation of giant cell tumors. Eur J Radiol 1986: 6: 1–4

215. Kattapuram S V, Phillips W C, Mankin H J. Giant cell tumor of bone: radiographic changes following local excision and allograft replacement. Radiology 1986: 161: 493–498

216. Cooper K L, Beabout J W, Dahlin D C. Giant cell tumor: ossification in soft-tissue implants. Radiology 1984: 153: 597–602

217. Ehara S, Nishida J, Abe M, Kawata Y, Saitoh H, Kattapuram S V. Ossified soft tissue recurrence of giant cell tumor of bone. Clin Imaging 1992: 16: 168–171

218. Dahlin D C. Case report 9. Giant cell tumor distal end of tibia, with osteocartilaginous synovial implants. Skeletal Radiol 1976: 1: 117–118

219. Bauer F C, Urist M R. The reaction of giant cell tumors of bone to transplantation into athymic nude mice, including observations on osteoinduction in the host bed. Clin Orthop 1981: 159: 257–264

220. Teot L A, O'Keefe R J, Rosier R N, O'Connell J X, Fox E J, Hicks D G. Extraosseous primary and recurrent giant cell tumors: transforming growth factor-beta 1 and -beta 2 expression may explain metaplastic bone formation. Hum Pathol 1996: 27: 625–632

221. Schwinn C P. Differential diagnosis of giant cell lesions of bone. In: Ackerman L V, Spjut H J, Abell M R, Eds. Bones and joints. Monogr Pathol 1976: 17: 236–299

222. Karabela-Bouropoulou V, Markaki S, Prevedorou D, Vidali N. A combined immunohistochemical and histochemical approach on the differential diagnosis of giant cell epiphyseal neoplasms. Pathol Res Pract 1989: 184: 184–187

223. Rosai J. Carcinoma of the pancreas simulating giant cell tumor of bone. Electron microscopic evidence of its acinar cell origin. Cancer 1968: 22: 333–344

224. Love G L, Daroca P J Jr. Bronchogenic sarcomatoid squamous cell carcinoma with osteoclast-like giant cells. Hum Pathol 1983: 14: 1004–1006

225. Daroca P J Jr, Reed R J, Martin P C. Metastatic amelanotic melanoma simulating giant-cell tumor of bone. Hum Pathol 1990: 21: 978–980

Ewing's sarcoma

J. M. Coindre

INTRODUCTION AND CLINICAL DATA

Ewing's sarcoma is a primitive malignant tumor of bone, composed of small round cells corresponding to the poorly differentiated form of a Primitive Neuroectodermal Tumor (PNET).

This highly malignant bone tumor was first recognized by Lucke in 1866,[1] but was popularized by Ewing in 1921.[2]

The histogenesis has been debated for a long time.[3] In his original report, Ewing proposed an endothelial origin but a hematopoietic origin was then suggested. However, the most important controversy was over whether Ewing's sarcoma was a specific entity or a metastatic neuroblastoma. A derivation from bone marrow reticular cells was also considered.

It is now widely accepted that Ewing's sarcoma belongs to the group of primitive neuroectodermal tumors (PNET). This group is composed of Ewing's sarcoma of bone and soft tissue, neuroepithelioma or primitive neuroectodermal tumor of bone and soft tissue. Askin's tumor arising in the thoracic wall is also a PNET. In the literature, two general terms are used to refer to these tumors: Ewing family of tumors or PNET family of tumors. These tumors have several common features: presence or induction of neural differentiation in cultured cells,[4] overexpression of the pseudoautosomal gene MIC2[5] and especially a t(11;22) (q24;q12) chromosomal translocation with a fusion transcript involving the EWS–FLI 1 or EWS–ERG genes.[6] Ewing's sarcoma can be considered as the most undifferentiated form and neuroepithelioma as the most differentiated form of the PNET family, with intermediate forms between these two extremes.[7] This is detailed in the next chapter.

Ewing's sarcoma represents approximately 5–15% of the primary malignant bone tumors. It is the fourth most common primary bone malignancy, following myeloma, osteosarcoma and chondrosarcoma, and the second most common malignant bone tumor in children (Huvos 1991, Unni 1996).

Approximately 90% of cases occur between the ages of 5 and 30 years and the highest frequency of this tumour occurs in patients between 10 and 15 years (Huvos 1991, Unni 1996).[8,9] Before accepting the diagnosis of Ewing's sarcoma, metastatic neuroblastoma should be considered in children under 5 and lymphoma and metastatic carcinoma in patients over 30. Ewing's sarcoma has a male predominance (1.5:1) and is uncommon in Blacks and Chinese.

Localized pain and swelling are the most common symptoms. Most patients complain of pain for several months prior to the presence of a visible or palpable swelling. Pathologic fracture is unusual. Location-related symptoms may be observed including neurologic symptoms, pleural effusion and monoarthritis. Generalized symptoms such as fever, anemia, leukocytosis and increased sedimentation rate usually indicate disseminated disease.

SKELETAL DISTRIBUTION

The long tubular bones are those most often affected, with the femur as the single most common site, followed by the tibia and fibula and the humerus (Huvos 1991, Unni 1996).[8] The femur is affected in 20–27% of tumors, the tibia and fibula in 15–23% and the humerus in 8–11%. Ewing's sarcoma is typically metadiaphyseal, with a predominant diaphyseal extension in some cases.

Among the flat bones, the pelvis and ribs are the most common sites (Huvos 1991, Unni 1996).[8] The pelvic girdle accounts for 20–26% of the tumors and the ribs 7–11%. Any portion of any bone may be affected, but epiphyseal locations of the long bones, hand, foot, skull, sternum or ulna are rarely noted. Overall, from 72% to 76% of tumors are central or proximal (Huvos 1991, Unni 1996).[8,9]

IMAGING

The radiographic features are non-specific and reflect the aggressive nature of the tumor (Resnick 1995). Typically, the lesion is obviously malignant (Figs 30.1–30.5), showing osteolysis, cortical destruction, periosteal reaction and a soft tissue mass. The bone destruction is usually permeative or moth-eaten and poorly marginated. Radiographic changes may suggest a small lesion although most of the bone is involved.

The periosteal reaction is frequently exuberant with parallel layers of new bone ('onion-skin') or, less often, may be spiculated ('sunburst'). A gradual elevation of the periosteum with minimal radiographic changes may be the only periosteal modification.

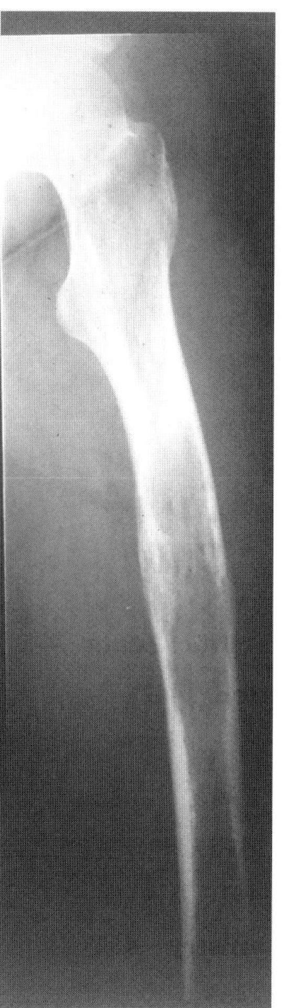

Fig. 30.1 Ewing's sarcoma of the femur.

Some degree of osteosclerosis may be seen (Figs 30.6, 30.7). Pure osteolysis (Figs 30.8, 30.9), pathologic fracture and osseous expansion are uncommon. A soft tissue mass with ill-defined borders and no calcification is often associated.

Rarely Ewing's sarcomas are almost completely juxtaosseous with no medullary component.[10] These periosteal Ewing's sarcomas may produce a 'saucerization' of the external cortex (Fig. 30.10).

Ewing's sarcoma can mimic most malignant lesions, especially osteosarcoma, lymphoma and metastatic carcinoma, and a few benign ones (Fig. 30.11), such as osteomyelitis, eosinophilic granuloma and aneurysmal bone cyst. Therefore, histologic confirmation is required in all cases (Huvos 1991).

CT scan can help to distinguish Ewing's sarcoma from other tumors such as osteosarcoma in difficult cases. It is also useful to define the extraosseous extent of the tumor, particularly in the pelvis (Figs 30.8, 30.9) and ribs.[12]

MRI is better and tends nowadays to replace CT except for the ribs. This technique must be performed to evaluate

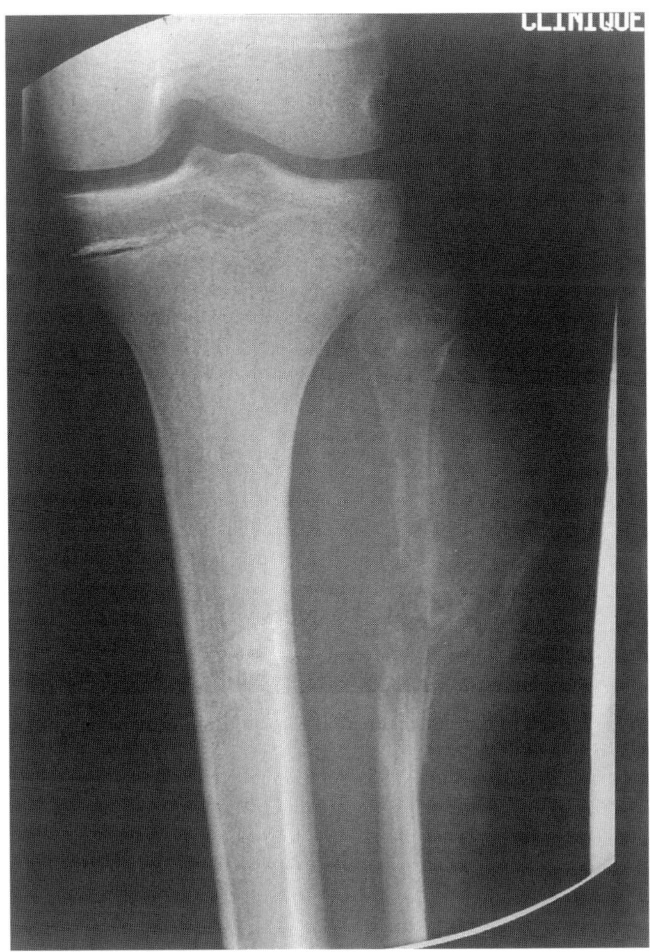

Fig. 30.2 Ewing's sarcoma of the proximal fibula with a soft tissue mass.

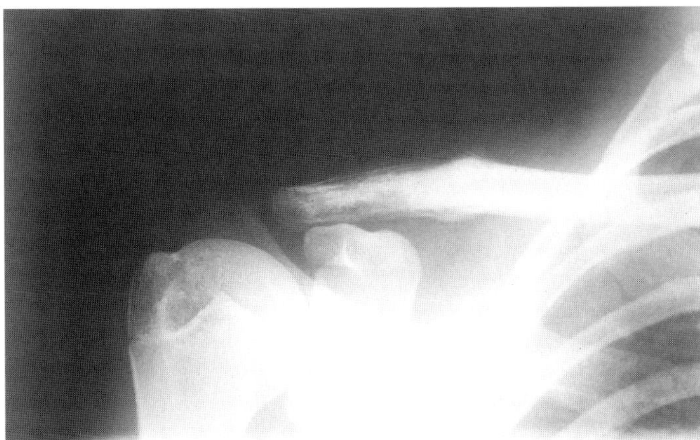

Fig. 30.3 Ewing's sarcoma of the distal clavicle.

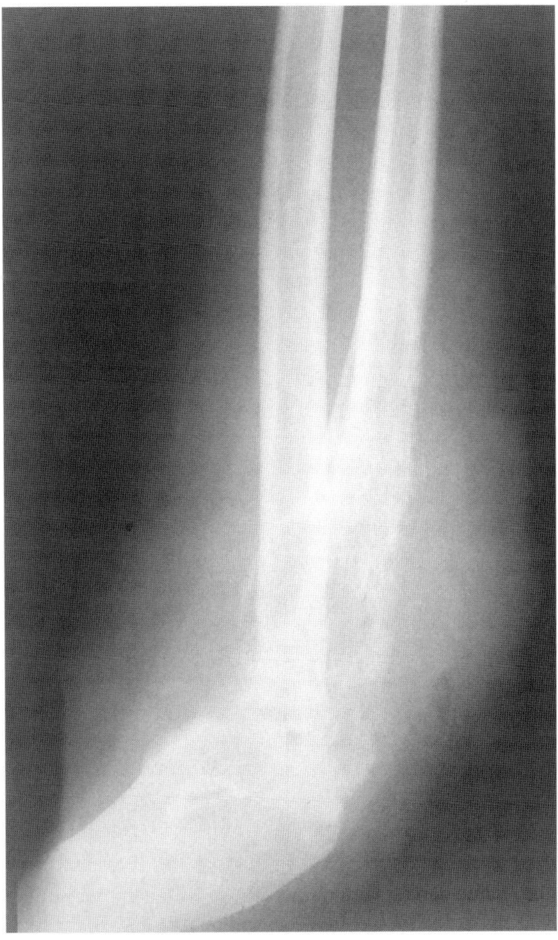

Fig. 30.4 Ewing's sarcoma of the cubitus in a black patient. (Courtesy of M. Forest MD.)

GROSS PATHOLOGY

The intraosseous component is firm, whitish gray, moist and glistens and frequently has an obvious diffuse involvement of the medullary cavity beyond the limits indicated on X-ray (Figs 30.12–30.17). Cortical breakthrough with a soft tissue mass is usually seen (Fig. 30.18). The latter is soft and friable, with necrotic, hemorrhagic and cystic areas (Fig. 30.19).

Nowadays, most specimens are modified by chemotherapy and/or radiotherapy and often show extensive necrosis and fibrosis.

HISTOPATHOLOGY

The typical form of Ewing's sarcoma is remarkably cellular with little or no intercellular stroma and several patterns are observed, either alone or in association (Huvos 1991, Unni 1996).[8,9,11] The most common pattern, described as diffuse or cohesive, consists of broad sheets of uniform small round cells (Fig. 30.20). The lobular pattern consists of clusters of cells separated by fibrovascular

tumor extent. It shows the extent of intraosseous and soft tissue involvement and can reveal bone changes not seen on X-ray (Figs 30.6, 30.7). The role of MRI in the assessment of tumor response to chemotherapy is still being evaluated (Resnick 1995).

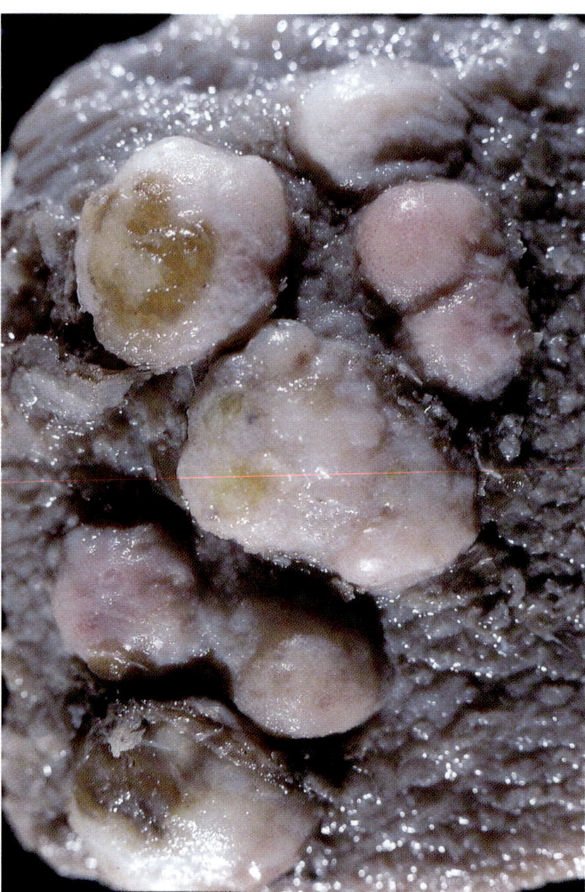

Fig. 30.5 Same patient with numerous cutaneous tumor nodules. (Courtesy of M. Forest M D.)

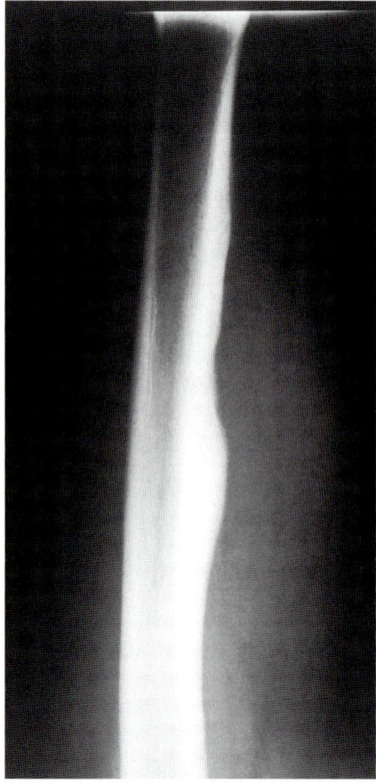

Fig. 30.6 Sclerotic Ewing's sarcoma of the femoral diaphysis.

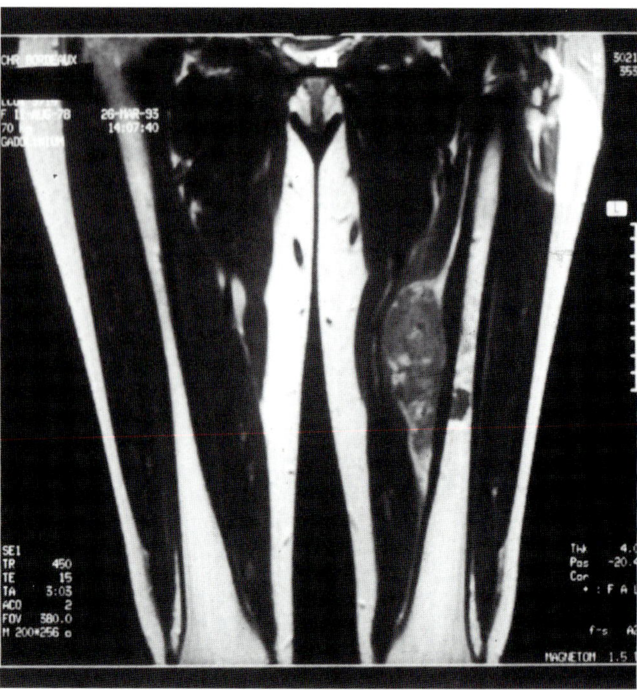

Fig. 30.7 MRI in the same patient as Fig. 30.6, showing osteolysis and a soft tissue mass.

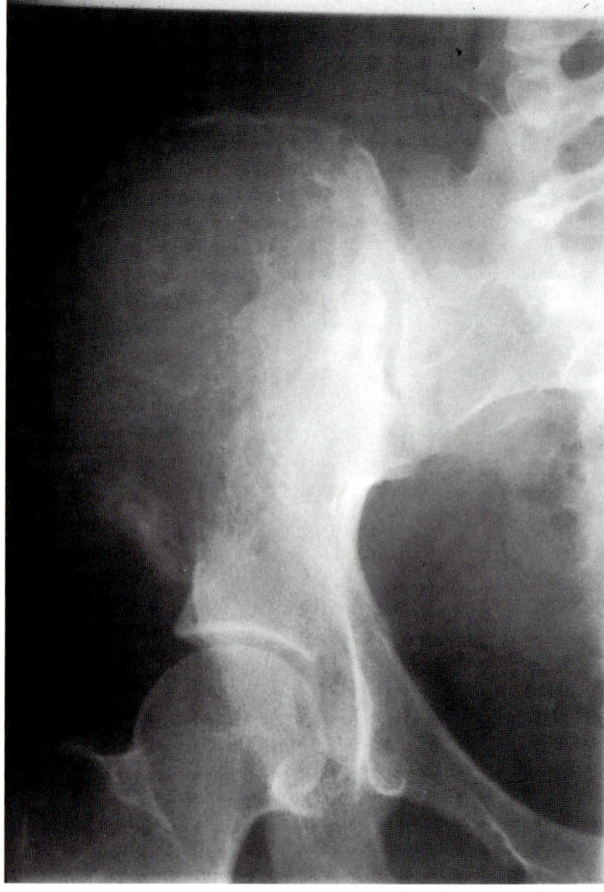

Fig. 30.8 Predominantly osteolytic Ewing's sarcoma of the ilium.

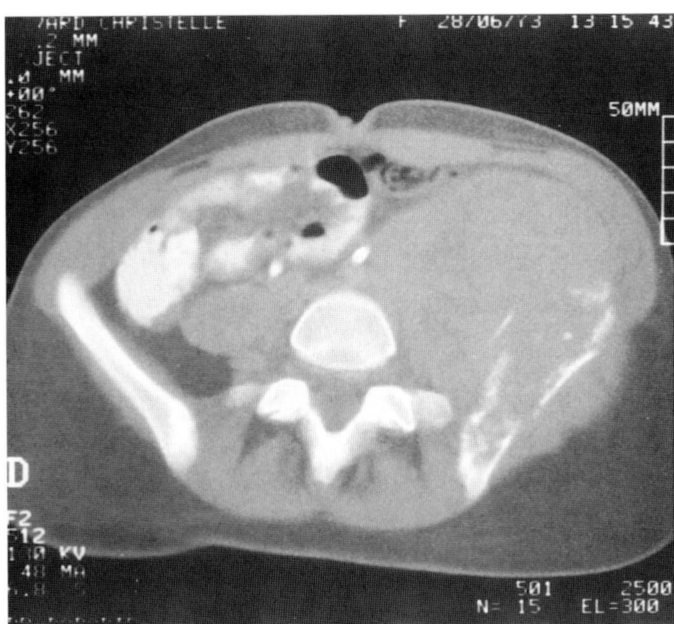

Fig. 30.9 CT scan in the same patient as Fig. 30.8, showing a huge extent in the pelvis.

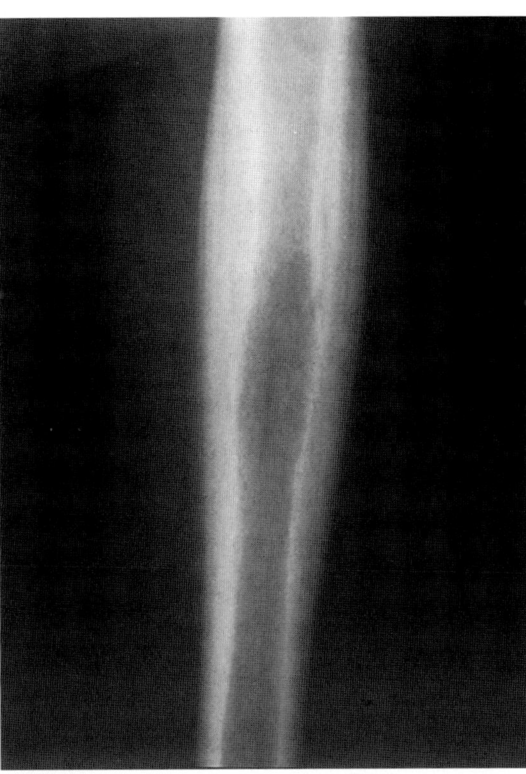

Fig. 30.11 Ewing's sarcoma of the proximal femur with regular periosteal new bone formation that could suggest a benign lesion.

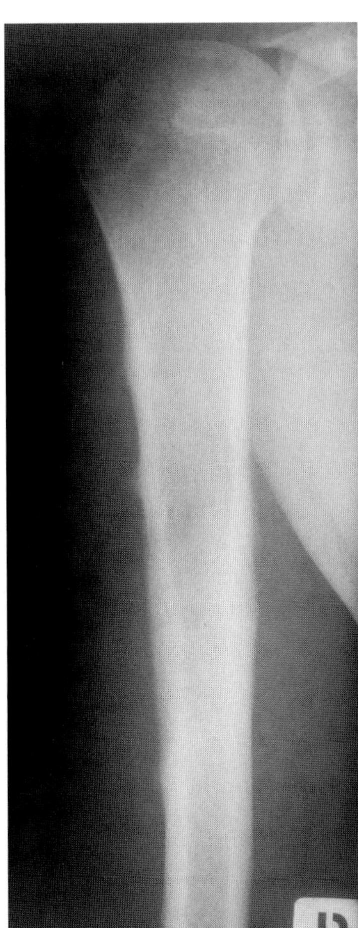

Fig. 30.10 Ewing's sarcoma of the proximal humerus with saucerization of the cortex.

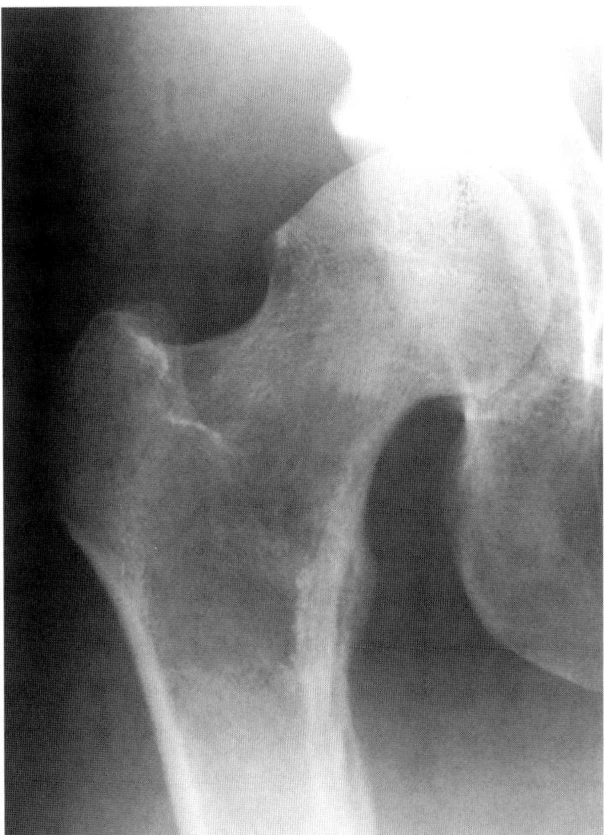

Fig. 30.12 Ewing's sarcoma of the proximal femoral metaphysis. (Courtesy of M. Forest MD.)

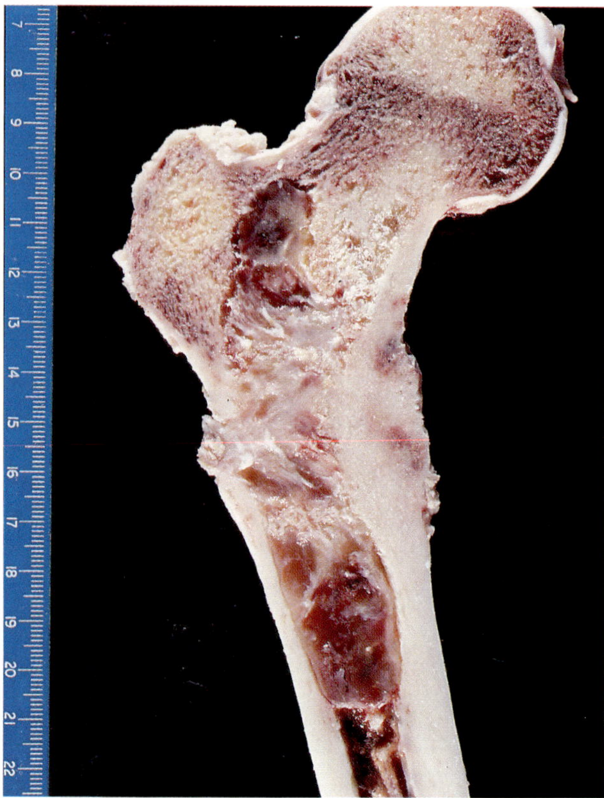

Fig. 30.13 Same patient: gross pathology. (Courtesy of M. Forest MD.)

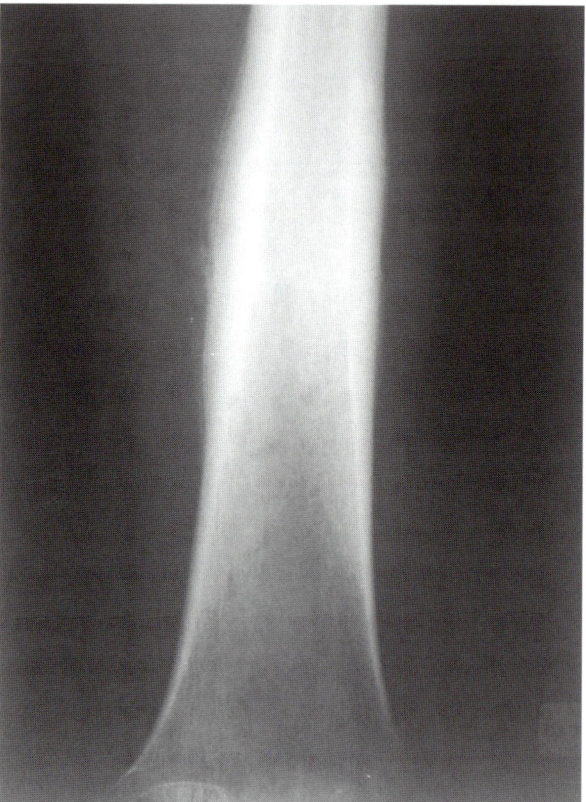

Fig. 30.14 Ewing's sarcoma of the distal femoral metadiaphysis. (Courtesy of M. Forest MD.)

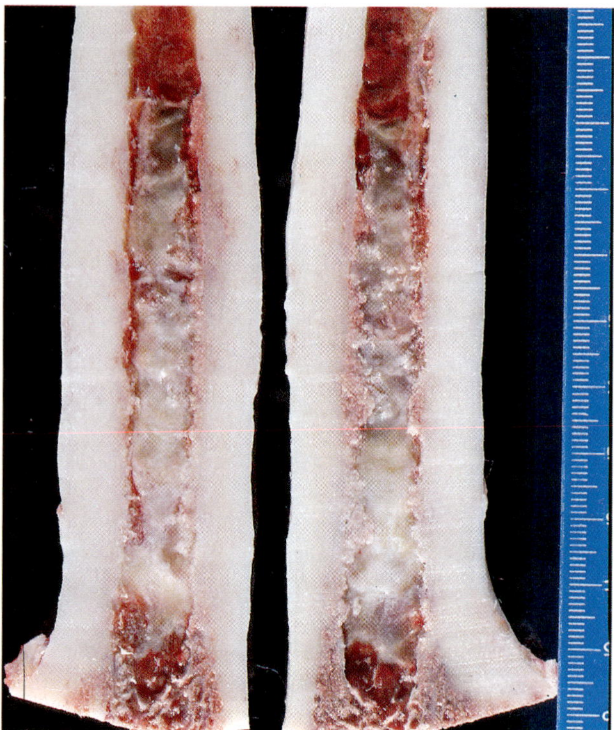

Fig. 30.15 Same patient: gross pathology. (Courtesy of M. Forest MD.)

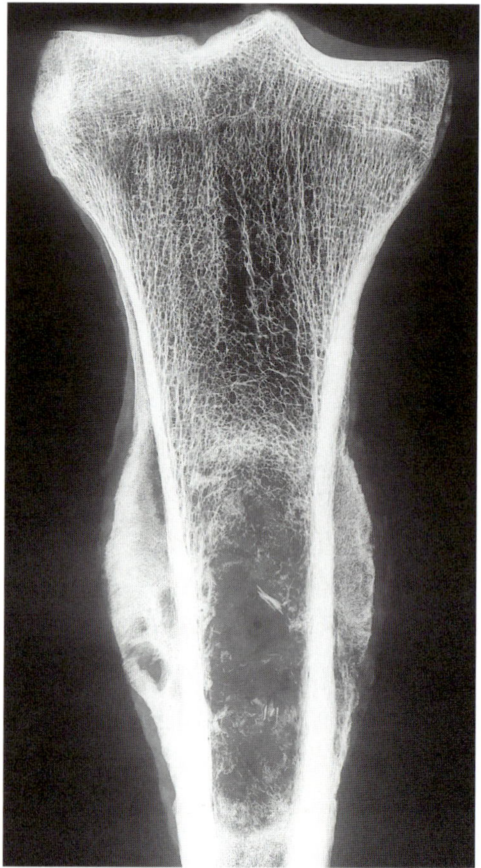

Fig. 30.16 Ewing's sarcoma of the proximal tibial metadiaphysis: X-ray of the specimen. (Courtesy of M. Forest MD.)

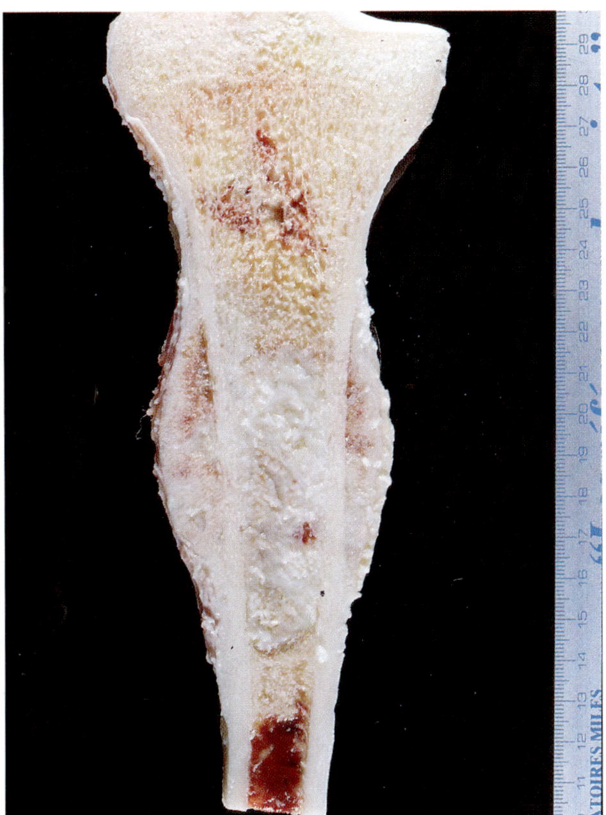

Fig. 30.17 Same patient: gross pathology. (Courtesy of M. Forest MD.)

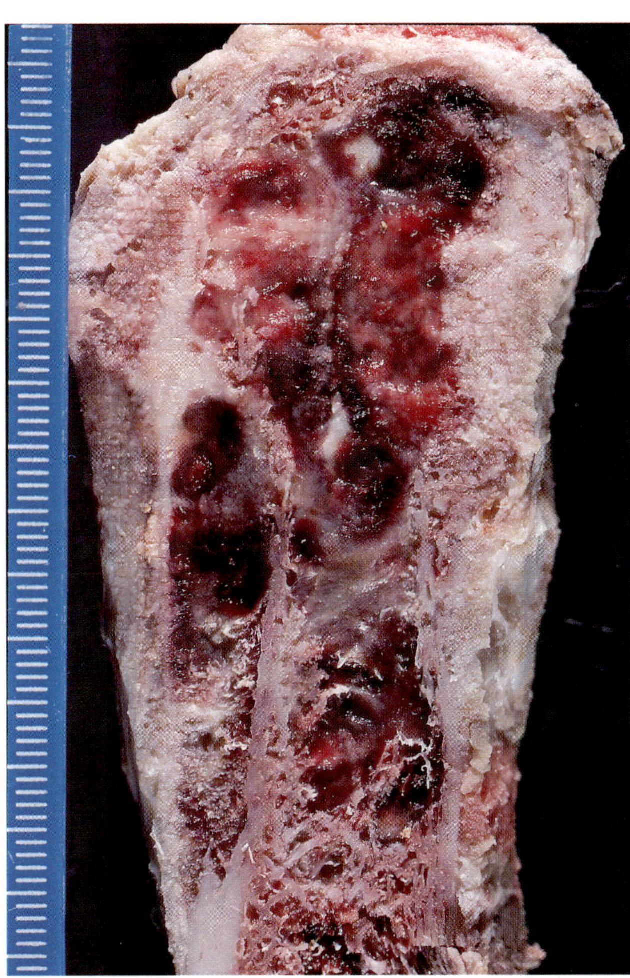

Fig. 30.19 Ewing's sarcomas of the iliac bone: necrotic, hemorrhagic and cystic areas after chemotherapy. (Courtesy of M. Forest MD.)

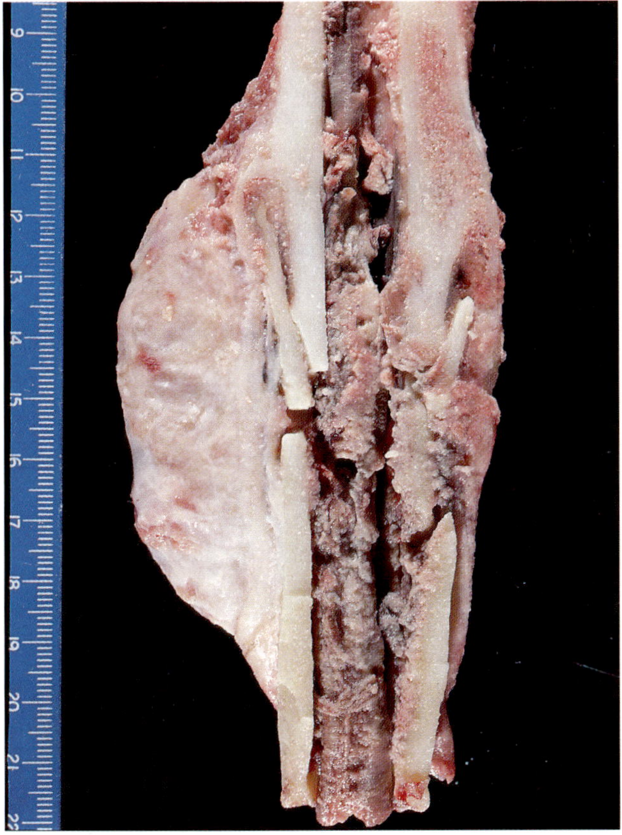

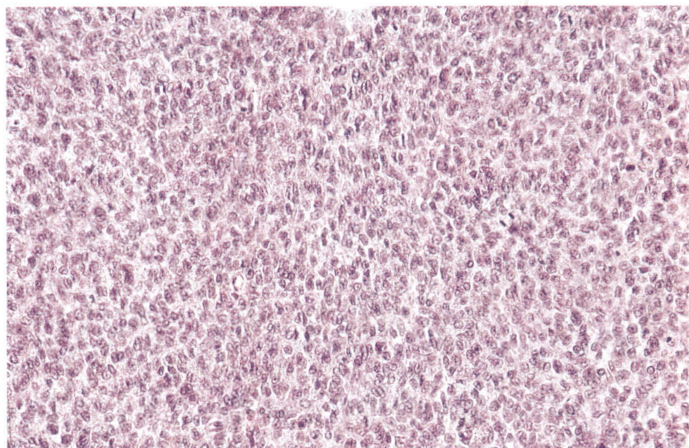

Fig. 30.20 Ewing's sarcoma of bone: diffuse or cohesive pattern.

Fig. 30.18 Ewing's sarcoma of the femoral diaphysis: massive involvement of bone with cortical breakthrough and a soft tissue mass. (Courtesy of M. Forest MD.)

septa (Fig. 30.21). A dissociated lobular pattern or alveolar pattern may be seen (Fig. 30.22). The filigree or chessboard pattern consists of strands of tumor cells separated by filigree fibrovascular stroma[8,9] (Fig. 30.23). This pattern represents an infiltrative invasion of surrounding normal tissue and is observed at the periphery of the tumor.

Pseudorosettes secondary to focal necrotic cell may be seen (Fechner & Mills 1993) Homer–Wright rosettes have been described in Ewing's sarcoma but are usually considered as a feature of PNET or neuroepithelioma.

The cell population consists of small round cells and dark cells.[9,12] Small round cells are the most characteristic and are 12–14 μu in diameter on average. They have a round nucleus with frequent indentations, a finely dispersed chromatin and one or two small nucleoli (Figs 30.24, 30.25). The cytoplasm is scant, pale or vacuolated (glycogen) (Fig. 30.26), with indistinct borders, so that the cytoplasm of several cells seems to form a syncytium with several nuclei inside.

Mitotic activity is variable but usually brisk.

Dark cells show denser and more elongated nuclei and

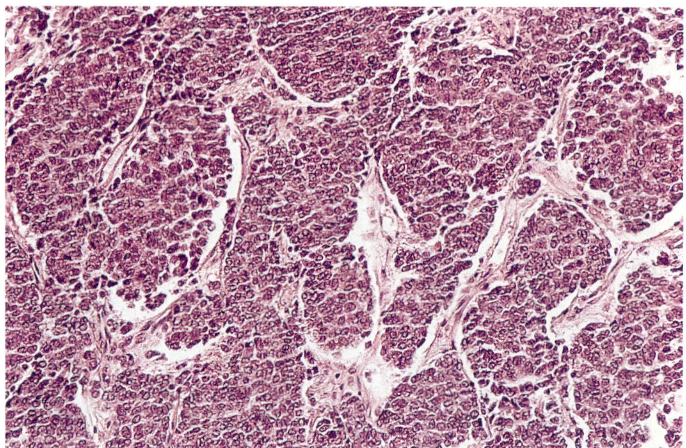

Fig. 30.21 Ewing's sarcoma of bone: lobular pattern.

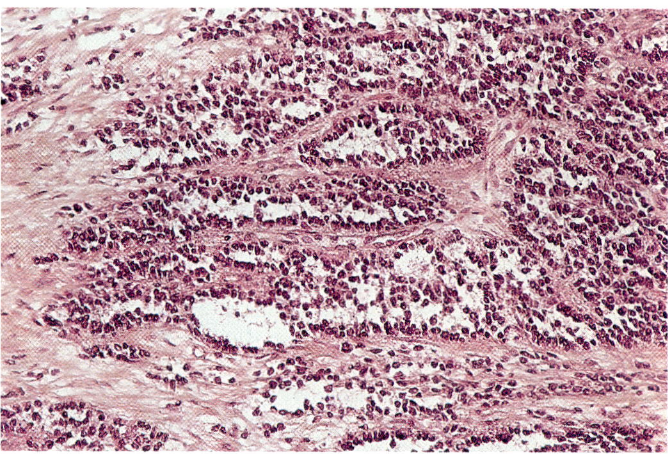

Fig. 30.22 Ewing's sarcoma of bone: alveolar pattern.

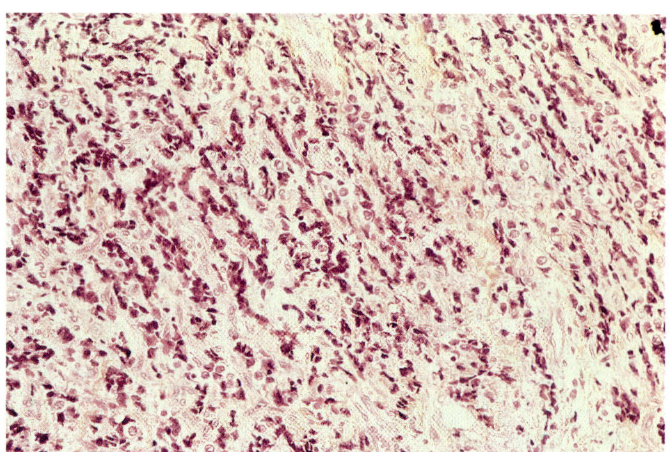

Fig. 30.23 Ewing's sarcoma of bone: filigree pattern.

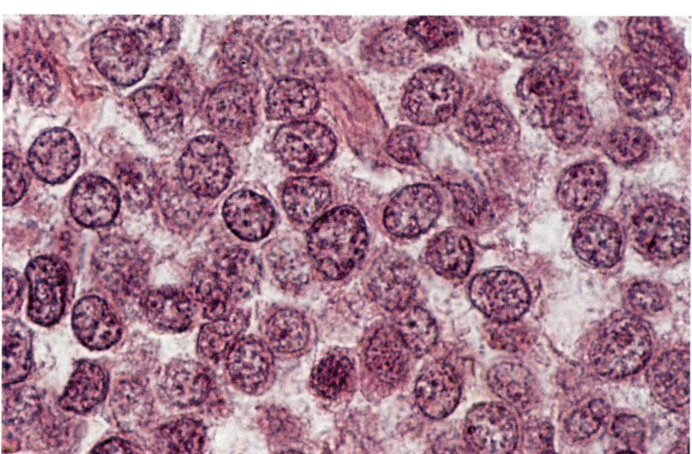

Fig. 30.24 Ewing's sarcoma of bone: monomorphic small round cells with regular round nuclei and scant cytoplasm.

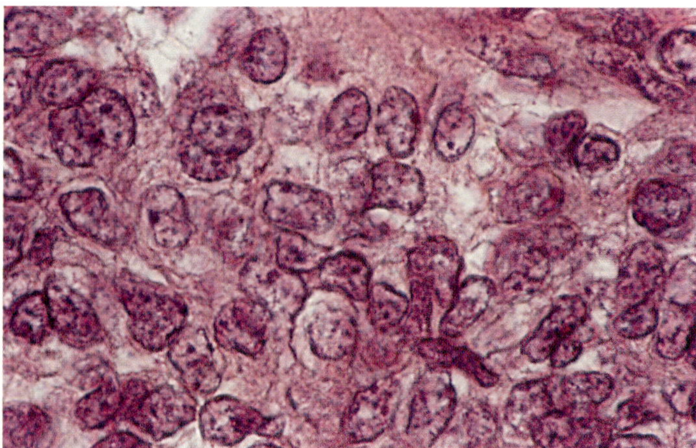

Fig. 30.25 Ewing's sarcoma of bone: small round cells with irregular nuclei showing indentations.

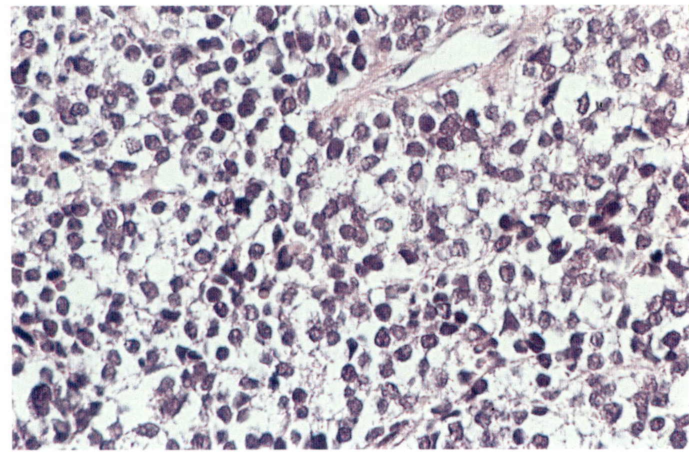

Fig. 30.26 Ewing's sarcoma of bone: small round cells with a clear and vacuolated cytoplasm.

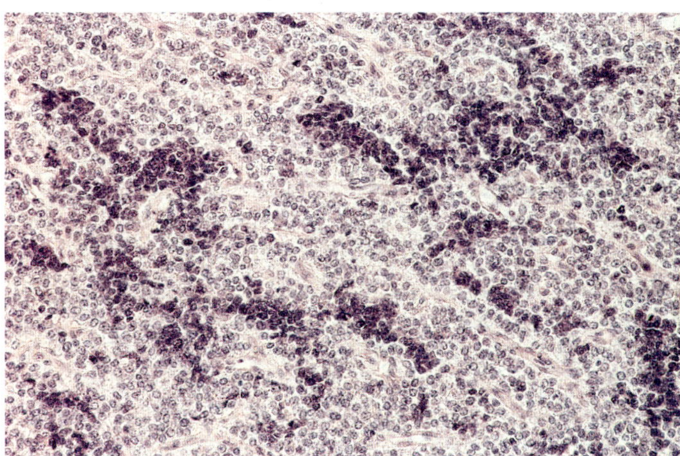

Fig. 30.28 Ewing's sarcoma of bone: biphasic pattern.

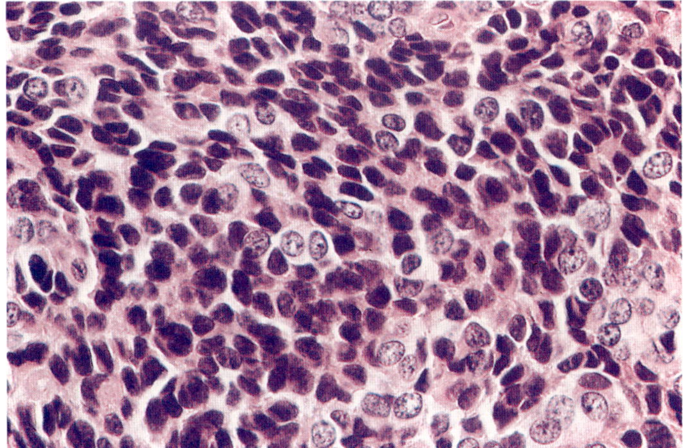

Fig. 30.27 Ewing's sarcoma of bone: dark cells.

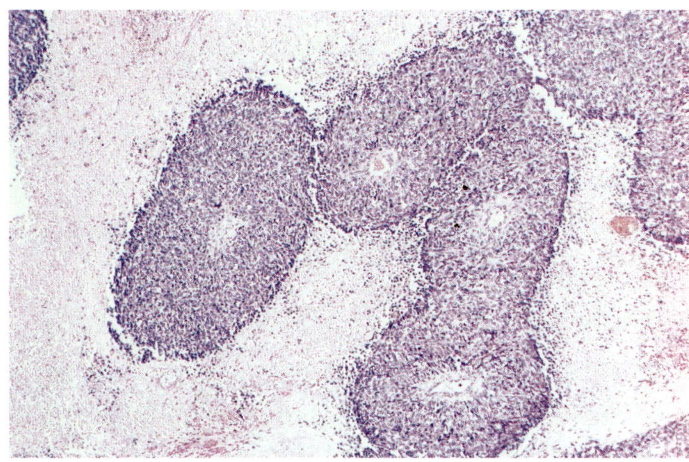

Fig. 30.29 Ewing's sarcoma of bone: necrosis with 'perithelial' arrangement.

tend to aggregate (Fig. 30.27). These cells are considered degenerative and transitional forms between these and the small round cells can be observed. A mixture of the two cell types produces a biphasic pattern, which is highly characteristic of Ewing's sarcomas, but not specific (Fig. 30.28). For Unni,[9] true spindling of the nuclei is incompatible with the diagnosis of Ewing's sarcoma, but artifactual spindling produced by crushing at the time of biopsy is not rare.

A well-developed vascular network is often present.

Coagulative necrosis is common (about 50% of cases) and may be massive or localized, often with a surviving cuff of tumor cells around larger blood vessels, creating a 'perithelial' arrangement (Fig. 30.29). Intramyofibrillar colonization by tumor cells may be seen.[10] Reactive bone formation (fig. 30.30) and fibroblastic tissue, especially in the subperiosteal area, may be present.

Histologic interpretation of the biopsy may be obscured by the poor quality of the sample, especially if there is

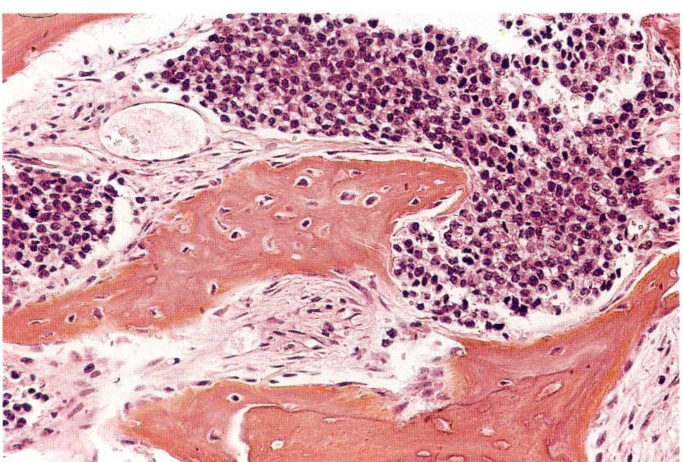

Fig. 30.30 Ewing's sarcoma of bone: reactive bone formation.

widespread tumor necrosis or poor preservation of tumor cells. Thus, an open, incisional biopsy is better than a needle biopsy (Huvos 1991).

The term 'atypical Ewing's sarcoma' or 'large cell variant' has been used to describe tumors with larger cells (19–24 μu in size), with larger and pleomorphic nuclei, prominent nucleoli and often acidophilic cytoplasm with better delineated borders[13] (Figs 30.31, 30.32). This variant represents 5–15% of all Ewing's sarcomas and is not associated with particular clinical characteristics, except that tumor location in one recent large series showed that the atypical variant presents with significantly fewer distal sites than the classic type.[9] Prognosis for the atypical variant is similar to that of classic Ewing's sarcomas.[9] An endothelial-like cell has been described and included in the category of atypical Ewing's sarcoma.[9,12]

Special stains, primarily reticulin stains and PAS, have traditionally been used to assist in the diagnosis of Ewing's sarcoma. This tumor characteristically contains very few reticulin fibers, except around the blood vessels, with no penetration of cell groups (Fig. 30.33), in contrast to lymphomas and rhabdomyosarcomas (Huvos 1991). PAS with and without diastase digestion shows large amounts of cytoplasmic glycogen in about 75% of cases (Fig. 30.34). This represents an important feature for the differential diagnosis with other small round cell tumors, but about 10% of Ewing's sarcomas are negative for PAS and variable amounts of glycogen can be demonstrated in neuroblastomas and lymphomas occasionally and in rhabdomyosarcomas commonly (Huvos 1991, Fechner & Mills 1993).

Pathologic examination with histologic mapping of the tumor resected after chemotherapy makes it possible to assess the quality of surgical margins and the effect of chemotherapy. Persistent tumor cells may be found in the subperiosteal region (Fig. 30.35), the soft tissue mass

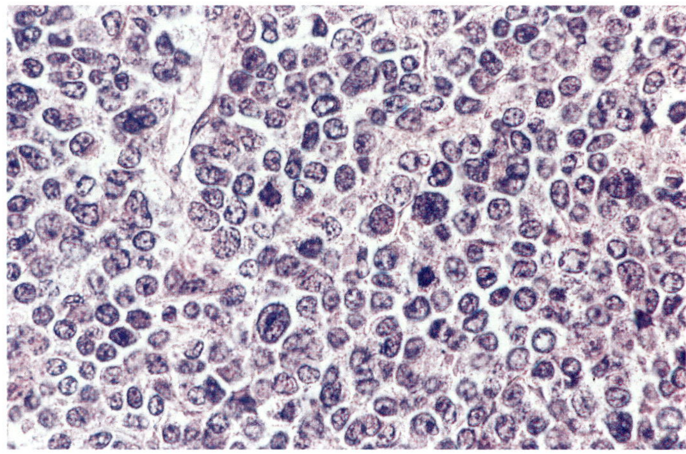

Fig. 30.31 Atypical Ewing's sarcoma of bone: tumor cells show larger and more pleomorphic nuclei than in conventional Ewing's sarcoma.

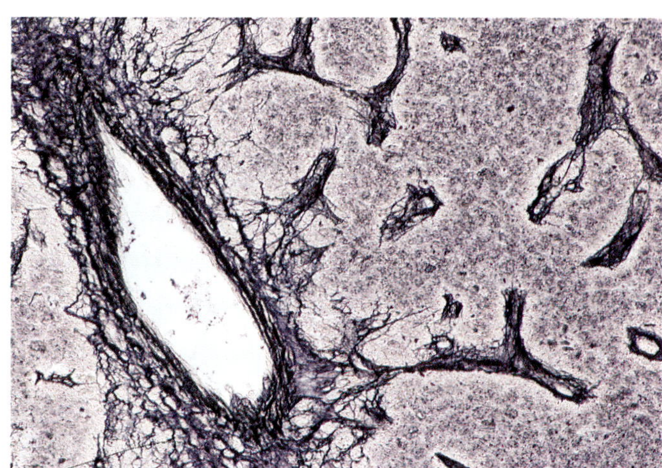

Fig. 30.33 Ewing's sarcoma of bone: reticulin fibers around blood vessels, but with no penetration of cell groups (reticulin stain).

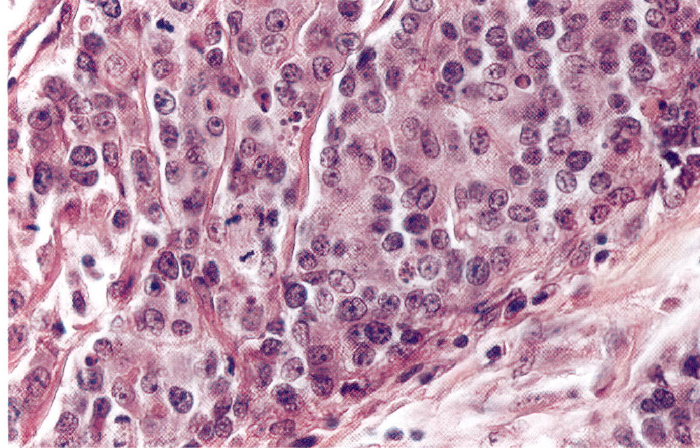

Fig. 30.32 Atypical Ewing's sarcoma of bone: tumor cells show pleomorphic nuclei and acidophilic cytoplasm.

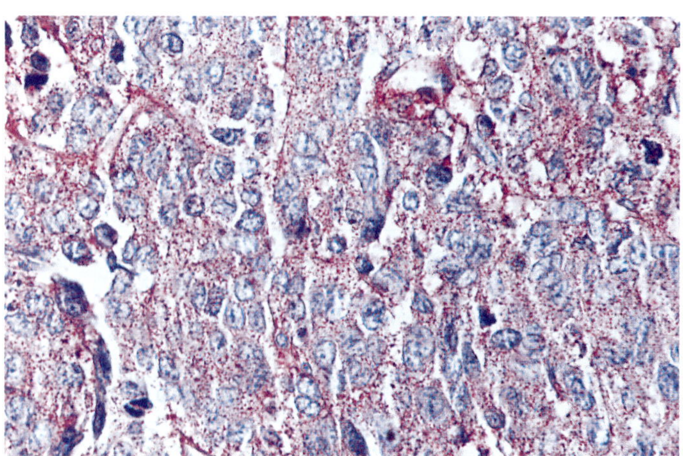

Fig. 30.34 Ewing's sarcoma of bone: large amounts of cytoplasmic glycogen (PAS).

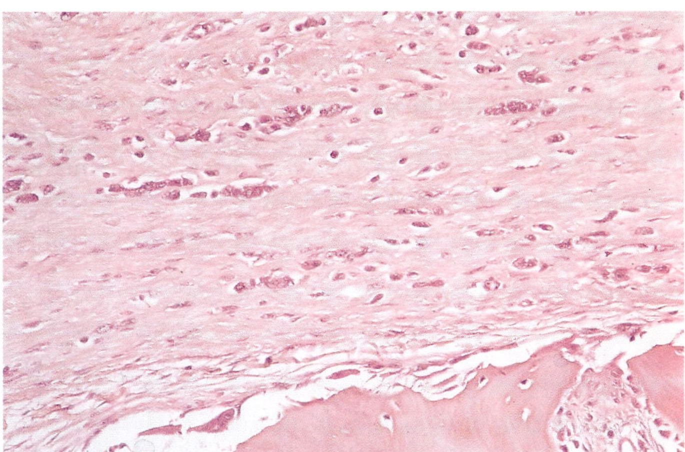

Fig. 30.35 Ewing's sarcoma of bone after chemotherapy: persistent scattered tumor cells in the subperiosteal region.

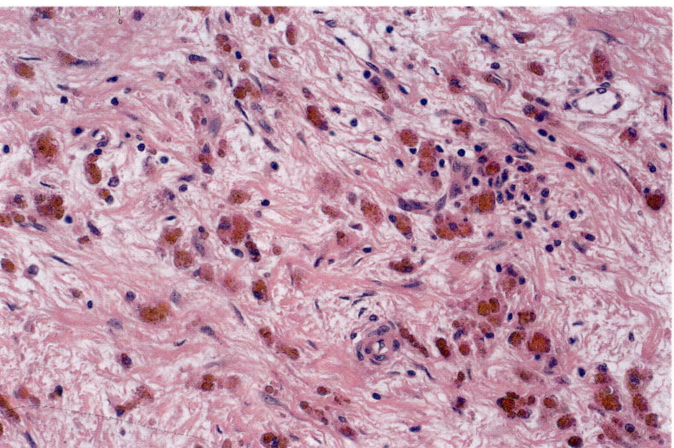

Fig. 30.37 Ewing's sarcoma of bone after chemotherapy: fibrosis with scattered chronic inflammatory cells and hemosiderin.

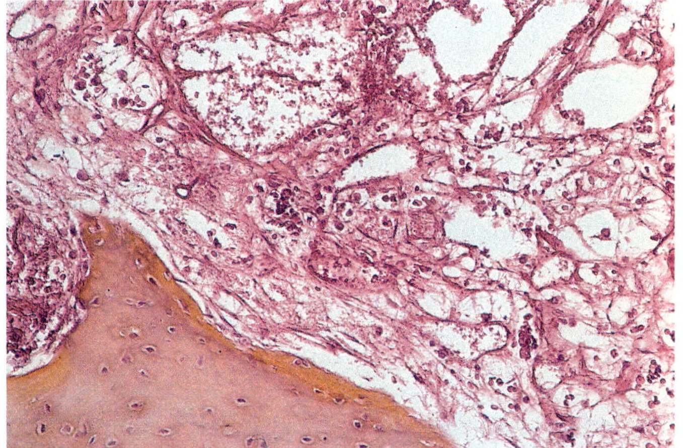

Fig. 30.36 Ewing's sarcoma of bone after chemotherapy: area of necrosis in association with hemorrhage.

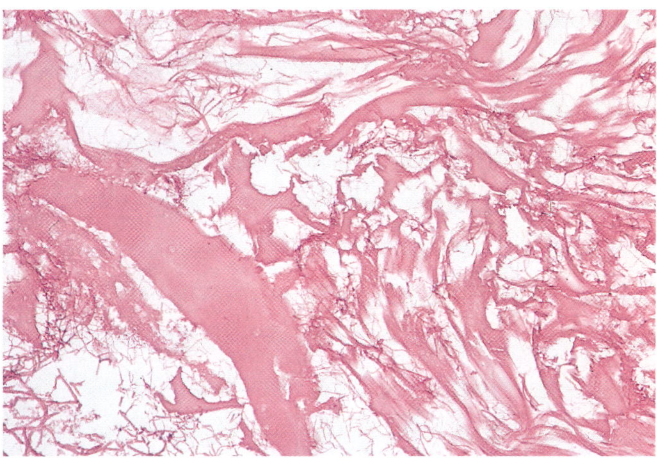

Fig. 30.38 Ewing's sarcoma of bone after chemotherapy: collagenization with new bone formation.

peripheral to the periosteum, the medullary space and in any area of hemorrhage.[14] These could be macroscopic nodules, small clumps of tumor cells or scattered individual tumor cells visible only at microscopy. Areas of necrotic tumor are frequently seen in association with reactive changes such as hemorrhage, edema, regenerative fibrovascular proliferation, scattered chronic inflammatory cells, hemosiderin and pseudocysts (Figs 30.36, 30.37). Varying degrees of collagenization with new bone formation are the final effects of chemotherapy (Fig. 30.38).

CYTOPATHOLOGY

Some authors suggest that fine-needle aspiration cytology can be used in the primary diagnosis for Ewing's sarcoma and that the diagnosis can be established when the clinical and radiographic findings are consistent with Ewing's sar-

coma.[15] This method can now be combined successfully with molecular biology tools such as RT-PCR and FISH (see Cytogenetics, chapter 4).

Touch imprint from biopsy should be performed systematically. It can be useful in determining whether the specimen is adequate for further examination, as opposed to necrotic tissue. In typical cases,[15–17] the cytological appearance is distinctive.

Smears are usually very cellular and the cells are fragile with frequent naked nuclei. A mixture of two types of cells is observed with a predominance of large cells containing a round nuclei with finely granular chromatin, one to three small nucleoli and a pale vacuolated cytoplasm and also a few small dark cells with a dense, irregular nucleus and a scanty cytoplasm (Figs 30.39, 30.40). PAS is more often positive on cytology preparations than on biopsies (Fig. 30.41).

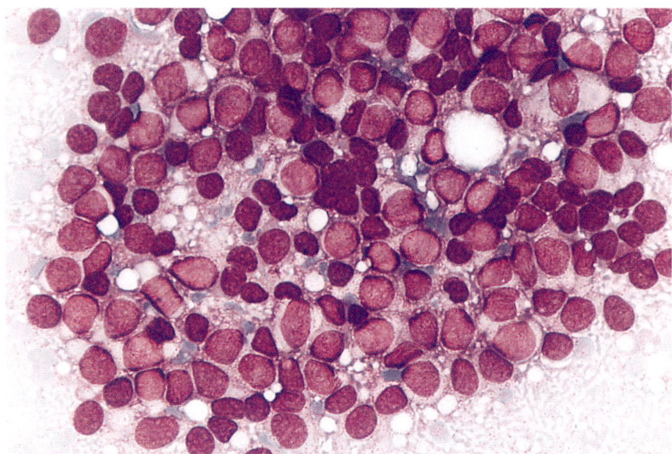

Fig. 30.39 Fine-needle aspiration cytology in Ewing's sarcoma of bone: mixture of large light and small dark cells (MGG).

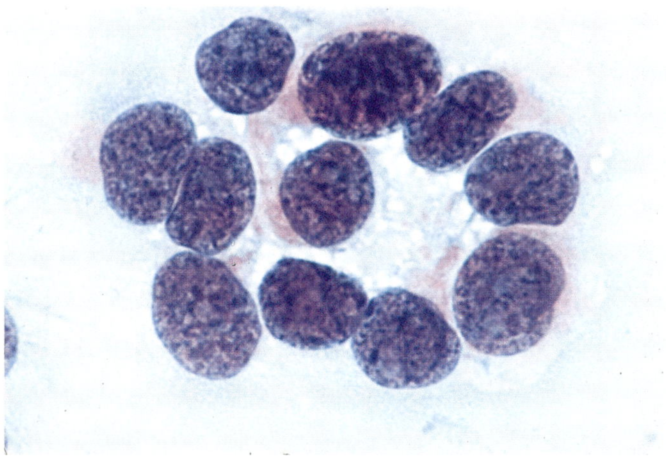

Fig. 30.40 Fine-needle aspiration cytology in Ewing's sarcoma of bone: tumor cells with a regular round nuclei with finely granular chromatin. (Courtesy of M. Forest MD.)

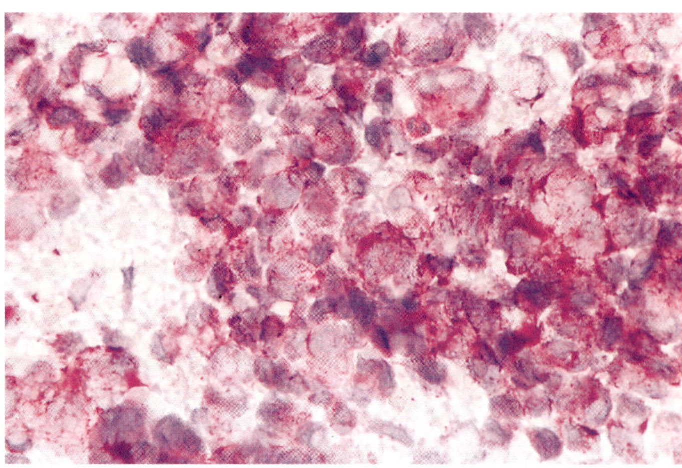

Fig. 30.41 Fine-needle aspiration cytology in Ewing's sarcoma of bone: large amounts of cytoplasmic glycogen (PAS).

IMMUNOHISTOCHEMISTRY

Until recently there was no specific marker for Ewing's sarcoma and immunohistochemistry was useful mainly for excluding other small round cell neoplasms such as malignant lymphoma, metastatic carcinoma and embryonal rhabdomyosarcoma. Currently, the use of antibodies to detect the MIC2 gene product is a valuable tool for diagnosing Ewing's sarcoma and related tumors. The MIC2 gene is a pseudoautosomal gene located on the short arms of the sex chromosomes. It codes for a transmembrane glycoprotein of relative molecular weight 30 000–32 000 kDa (p30/32), defined by the cluster of CD99.[22] The function of this protein is not known but it seems to be involved in cell adhesion processes.[19] The MIC2 gene appears to be expressed at various levels in virtually all human tissues, with significant overexpression in T cells, Ewing's sarcoma and related tumors.[20–22]

This protein is detected on formalin-fixed, paraffin-embedded tissue by a number of monoclonal antibodies including HBA-71, 12E7 and the commercially available O13 antibody. These antibodies benefit from heat-induced epitope retrieval but not from enzyme digestion. Immunoreactivity appears to be preserved after decalcification.

The literature shows a membrane immunoreactivity of Ewing's sarcoma and related tumors with the available antibodies in 87–100% of cases[18,20–25] (Fig. 30.42). Unfortunately, this immunoreactivity for CD99 is not specific and has been reported in most cases of lymphoblastic T cell lymphomas[26] and focally in some embryonal or alveolar rhabdomyosarcomas,[18,21–23] desmoplastic small round cell tumors,[22] small cell osteosarcomas[22] and Wilms' tumors.[22,24] On the other hand, neuroblastoma, ganglioneuroblastoma and medulloblastoma are uniformly negative.[18,20–23,25,27] A CD99 immunoreactivity has also

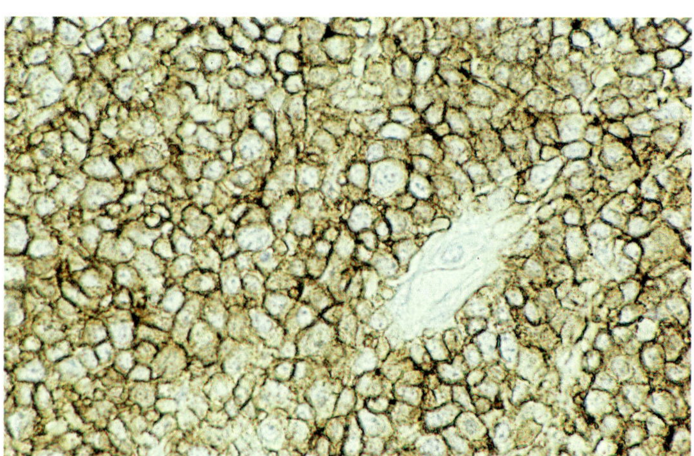

Fig. 30.42 Ewing's sarcoma of bone: strong and diffuse membrane positivity for the MIC2 gene product (immunohistochemistry – O13 antibody).

been reported with central nervous system tumors (ependymomas, glioblastomas, astrocytomas and meningiomas),[18,20,22,25] endocrine and neuroendocrine tumors (pancreatic islet cell tumors, gastrointestinal carcinoid and small cell carcinomas of the lung),[18,22,25] carcinomas[22] and spindle cell tumors such as synovial sarcomas.[28,29] In most of these tumors, positivity is cytoplasmic, granular or globular or focal or faint.

Thus, CD99 immunoreactivity is sensitive but not specific for Ewing's sarcoma and should be interpreted with caution: one must only admit diffusely strong membrane positivity after having used a panel of antibodies and ruled out a lymphoblastic T cell lymphoma.

Neural markers show variable results according to antibodies and techniques (Fechner & Mills 1993). Neuron-specific enolase and leu-7 are observed in a significant number of cases with the most sensitive techniques.[11,28–33] S-100 protein and synaptophysin are positive in a few cases.[32] Chromogranin and neurofilaments are not typically positive.

Vimentin is usually positive[30] and cytokeratin may be expressed in a few cases, usually in a minority of cells[22] (Fig. 30.43). Ewing's sarcoma cells are negative for leukocyte common antigen, L26 and CD3, desmin, myoglobin and factor VIII-related antigen.

FLOW CYTOMETRY

Flow cytometry studies on Ewing's sarcoma are few and only report on small series.[34,35] They show a low rate of DNA aneuploidy in comparison to the high malignant potential of these tumors. They are controversial regarding the prognostic value of DNA ploidy: Kowal-Vern et al[34] found no correlation between DNA ploidy and survival in a series of 21 cases, whereas Dierick et al[35] reported a significant relationship between DNA pattern and survival, with a poor prognosis in patients with aneuploid tumors in a series of 37 cases.

ELECTRON MICROSCOPY

Typical cells of Ewing's sarcoma have a rather primitive appearance. They are small, round or ovoid and bordered by occasional desmosome-like primitive intercellular junctions.[36] The most characteristic ultrastructural feature is the presence of varying amounts of cytoplasmic glycogen.[37,38] Many tumors show large amounts of glycogen particles of varying sizes. Cell organelles are usually sparse and cell processes and dense-core granules are absent. The nuclei are slightly irregular with finely granular chromatin and small nucleoli. In atypical Ewing's sarcoma, nuclei show marked grooving with prominent nucleoli.[39]

CYTOGENETICS

The high consistency of specific cytogenetic and molecular abnormalities in Ewing's sarcoma is remarkable and has enabled a greater understanding of the histogenesis of these tumors. These changes constitute a highly reliable marker for the diagnosis of Ewing's sarcoma and related tumors.

In 1983, cytogenetic analysis of Ewing's sarcoma demonstrated a consistent primary chromosome abnormality, the reciprocal translocation t(11;22) (q24;q12) which was reported by two independent groups[40,41] (Fig. 30.44). This finding was confirmed by others and was subsequently described in peripheral neuroepithelioma, Askin's

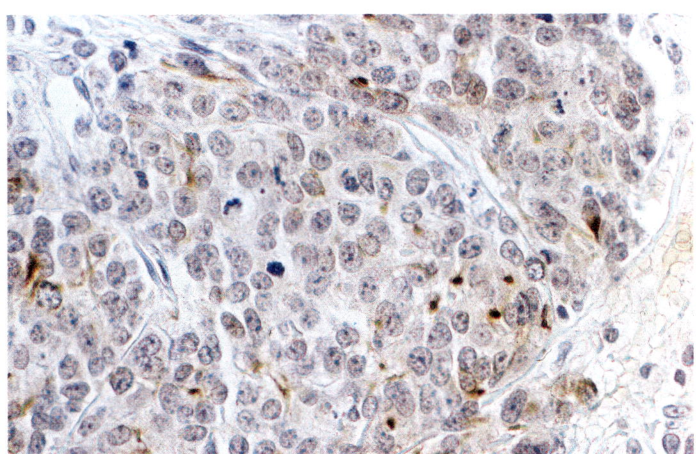

Fig. 30.43 Ewing's sarcoma of bone: a few tumor cells show a dot positivity for cytokeratin (immunohistochemistry – K11 antibody).

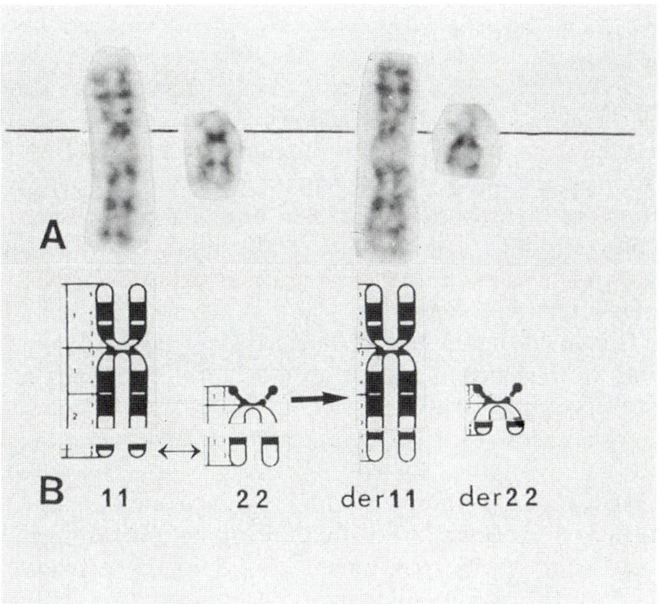

Fig. 30.44 Ewing's sarcoma of bone: partial karyotype showing the characteristic translocation t(11;22). (Courtesy of C. Turk-Carel MD.)

tumor and extraskeletal Ewing's sarcoma.[42–44] It has also been found in an esthesioneuroblastoma,[45] a neuroendocrine tumor of the small intestine[46] and a small cell osteosarcoma.[47] This change has never been reported in neuroblastomas, rhabdomyosarcomas or non-Hodgkin's lymphomas.[48]

Turc-Carel et al[49] evaluated the chromosome changes in 85 Ewing's sarcoma cases. The standard t(11;22) (q24;q12) was present in 83% of cases. The breakpoint on chromosome 22q12 occurred in 92% and on chromosome 11q24 in 88%. Five percent of the cases showed complex translocations involving a third chromosome in addition to chromosomes 11 and 22. Variant translocations involving 22q12 but with a chromosome other than 11 were observed in 4% of cases.

Additional secondary and non-specific changes have also been described.[48] They may be numerical, including both gains and losses, or structural, including translocations, deletions, inversions or duplications.

The translocation t(11;22) is highly consistent and specific in Ewing's sarcoma and cytogenetic analysis is a reliable tool for its diagnosis. It has been shown that this technique can be performed on tissue obtained by percutaneous biopsy.[50] However, limitations exist in the ability to karyotype these tumors, including the requirement for fresh tumor material, difficult and time-consuming techniques and frequent overgrowth of normal stromal cells during culture. Consequently, successful cytogenetic analysis is obtained in less than 50% of cases of Ewing's sarcoma.[51]

The recent cloning of the specific chromosome translocation t(11;22) (q24;q12) showed that this alteration results in a chimeric gene by juxtaposing the EWS gene on chromosome 22 and the FLI-1 gene on chromosome 11.[52,53] Two variant translocations have been described: t(21;22) (q12;q12) involving the ERG gene on chromosome 21 and t(7;22) (p22;q12) involving the ETV1 gene on chromosome 17.[54,55] EWS is a novel putative RNA-binding gene whose normal function is unknown. FLI-1, ERG and ETV1 are members of the ETS oncogene superfamily of transcriptional factors. The resulting chimeric genes encode a fusion protein. The EWS-FLI-1 fusion protein has transforming capabilities and has been implicated in pathogenesis.[56]

This molecular genetic characterization has led to novel tools for translocation detection. FISH (fluorescent in situ hybridization) makes it possible to detect translocation in interphase cells by using DNA probes specific to the chromosomal regions of interest[57,58] (see Ch. 4). This rapid, reliable and non-isotopic technique can be used as a diagnostic tool in Ewing's sarcoma on tumor touch imprints made from fresh or frozen material.[59]

The FISH technique shows chromosome rearrangements at the single cell level and allows morphological correlations. Rearrangements of the EWS gene have been

demonstrated by Southern blotting in almost all cases tested, but RT-PCR (reverse transcription-polymerase chain reaction) is currently the most useful technique for detecting the specific translocation in Ewing's sarcoma. In this tumor, the chromosome translocation results in a chimeric transcript (RNA). RNA from fresh or frozen material is copied by the reverse transcriptase into cDNA. The use of appropriate primer from each of the two genes involved in the translocation allows amplification of the specific chimeric cDNA by PCR. This specific positive PCR amplification can be visualized as a band of defined size on an agarose gel (Fig. 30.45).

RT-PCR has been used successfully on primary tumors, blood samples, bone marrow aspirates and peripheral stem cell harvests.[6,52,60–64] This technique is specific and highly sensitive, allowing the detection of one cell per million nucleated cells. It is rapid, reliable and efficient and can be used on small specimens obtained by fine-needle biopsies.[6]

In a series of 114 sarcomas, Delattre et al[6] showed a positive RT-PCR in 95% of cases of Ewing's sarcoma or related tumors; they proposed that the Ewing family of tumors should be redefined as the group of tumors that possess a chimeric transcript involving the EWS-FLI-1 or EWS-ERG genes. So far, 14 different chimeric transcripts have been identified.[65] No association between the type of

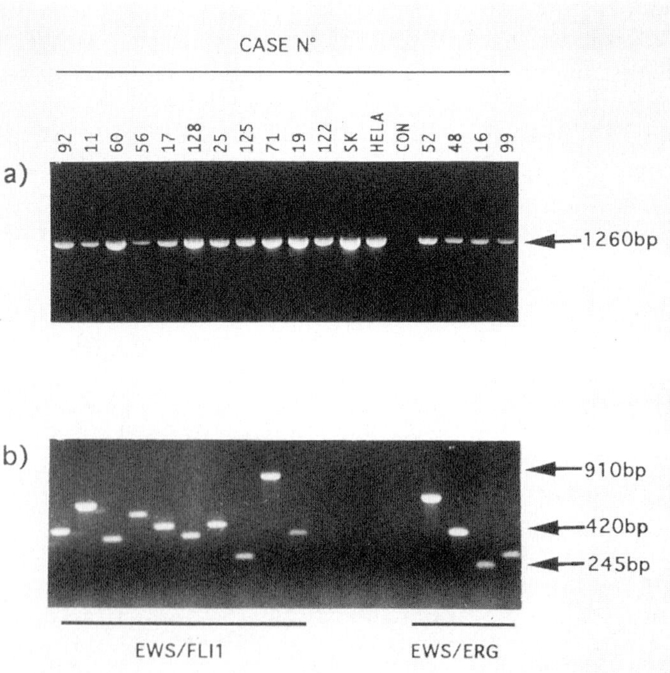

Fig. 30.45 Gel electrophoresis of RT-PCR from tumors of 15 patients with Ewing's sarcoma or primitive neuroectodermal tumor. The upper panel shows an internal control and the lower panel the amplified EWS-FLI1 fusion transcripts and EWS-ERG fusion transcripts. Case 122 shows no fusion transcript. (Courtesy of the New England Journal of Medicine; see ref[6].)

chimeric transcript and clinical features or histopathology has been observed,[62,64] but a possible prognostic advantage has been suggested for patients with localized disease and fusion type I transcripts.[64] Type of chimeric transcript is identical in primary and metastatic sites[60] and RT-PCR allows a more accurate clinical assessment of the dissemination of Ewing's sarcoma by demonstrating circulating tumor cells or occult bone marrow metastasis.

The clinical implications of these findings require further evaluation.[60,61,63]

The advantages and limits of MIC2 expression by immunohistochemistry and EWS gene rearrangement by RT-PCR have been compared.[66,67] These studies underline the lack of specificity of MIC2 expression and suggest the adoption of RT-PCR as a gold standard. Moreover, RNA extracted from paraffin-embedded samples has been shown to be suitable for RT-PCR analysis.[68]

Mutations of the p53 gene and amplification of the MDM2 gene have been reported in about 10% of Ewing's sarcomas.[69] An association of MDM2 amplification with advanced disease stage has been suggested.[69]

CLINICAL COURSE

Modern combined modality therapies with multiagent chemotherapy have made a significant improvement in the prognosis of Ewing's sarcoma of bone. The long-term disease-free survival rate has increased from less than 10%[70] to more than 40%.[71–75]

Prognosis is mainly determined by metastatic outcome. The incidence of metastatic disease at the time of diagnosis ranges from 15% to 35%.[9,72,76,77] Distant metastases will eventually occur in 40–50% of cases, with a localized tumor. Metastases are predominantly hematogenous and equally located in the lung and bone.[9,78] Local recurrence is observed in 15–30% of cases and is more frequent in pelvic locations.[75,79] The incidence of local recurrence also depends on the type of local treatment. Most patients relapse and die of disease within 5 years of treatment, but a few metastases and local recurrences may be seen later.[77]

With the improved survival following combined therapy, an increasing number of patients are now at risk of late effects, mainly growth defects and deformations related to radiotherapy and/or surgery and secondary cancers. Patients with Ewing's sarcoma are at a significantly increased risk of secondary cancers. A recent study has estimated an 8.5-fold risk of all cancers following Ewing's sarcoma, with a 100-fold risk for bone and soft tissue sarcomas.[80] Most of the tumors are located within the irradiated fields.

TREATMENT

The treatment of Ewing's sarcoma of bone is currently based on combined therapy with neoadjuvant chemotherapy, radiation therapy and surgical resection of the primary tumor.[71–75,77]

The complexity of this treatment requires close coordination among surgeons, chemotherapists, radiotherapists and pathologists to insure the best outcome with local and distant tumor control, preservation of function and as few adverse late effects as possible.

The demonstration of efficacy of adjuvant chemotherapy has been a major breakthrough in the treatment of Ewing's sarcoma. The use of active drugs in combination (vincristine, actinomycin-D, cyclophosphamide, adriamycin) has dramatically changed the prognosis of this tumor with a 5-year disease-free survival rate of 50–60%,[71–75] but with possible late relapses.[77]

Primary or neoadjuvant chemotherapy is currently given in order to make surgical excision easier, to treat the potential metastatic disease early and to allow postsurgical adjustment of chemotherapy according to histopathologic response.

Clinical trials during the past two decades have focused on identifying new effective drugs (ifosfamide, etoposide, cisplatin), more effective regimens and intensification of chemotherapy with autologous bone marrow transplantation in patients with metastatic disease or a poor prognosis localized tumor.[81]

With the improvement of overall survival, more local recurrences after radiation therapy alone and late adverse effects of the radiation therapy are being seen, leading to changes in local treatment, with more surgery and lower doses of irradiation. Currently, conservative surgery is recommended when possible, but the indications for surgery are still being evaluated for central locations such as pelvic tumors.[82,83]

Radiation therapy is highly effective in Ewing's sarcoma, but a meticulous technique is required to obtain the best effect, to maintain function and to minimize complications.[73,84,85]

Outstanding questions concern the possibility of improving prognosis and treatment of severe forms such as metastatic disease and large tumors.

PROGNOSIS

Several clinical and pathologic factors have been shown to have prognostic value in Ewing's sarcoma.

The presence of metastases at the time of diagnosis is obviously correlated with poor survival, with a 5-year survival rate of less than 10–35%[76–78,86] as compared to 54–74% for patients with localized disease at presentation.[71–73,75,87] The site and volume of the primary tumor have been repeatedly reported as being independent prognostic factors. Patients with a distal disease have a better prognosis than those with a proximal one. Patients with a pelvic tumor have the worst prognosis, with an overall survival rate of 15–35% as compared to 30–77% in patients with a non-pelvic tumor.[72,75,77] In fact, the prognostic value of tumor location could be directly linked to tumor volume. This parameter is difficult to evaluate but in the few studies reporting it, it is an important prognostic factor.[73,88] As a result of large size, gross soft tissue extension has also been associated with poor prognosis.[89]

Histologically, a filigree growth pattern has been associated with a worsened prognosis. In the large study by Terrier et al,[9] it is an independent prognostic factor in non-metastatic patients treated with modern therapy. Tumor necrosis has been associated with a poor prognosis in some studies[11,90] but not all.[9] The presence of atypical large cells does not have adverse prognostic importance.[9]

Treatment and response to treatment are important prognostic factors. The use of modern combined treatment with multiagent neoadjuvant chemotherapy has been associated with an improved prognosis.[9]

Surgical resection of the primary tumor has also been reported to be a good prognostic factor.[72,91]

Histologic response to preoperative chemotherapy has been shown to be one of the most important prognostic predictors.[14,73,92] In patients with less than 10% residual tumor cells, the 3-year survival rate is 79% as compared to 31% in the others.[73] However, estimation of residual cells per unit area of tumor is more difficult than in osteosarcomas, because in Ewing's sarcoma there is no osseous or cartilaginous framework. Picci et al[14] proposed a simple three-grade system in which grade I is defined by residual macroscopic tumor nodule, grade II by isolated microscopic nodules and grade III by no residual tumor cells. The 5-year disease-free survival rate was respectively 32%, 53% and 90%.

Pleotropic drug resistance mediated by MDR1 expression of P-glycoprotein has been evaluated before and after chemotherapy in Ewing's sarcoma.[93,94] A high incidence of elevated P-glycoprotein expression has been noted in about half of the cases, but apparently with no relationship with clinical chemoresistance and survival.

DIFFERENTIAL DIAGNOSIS

Non-Hodgkin's lymphoma of bone has to be excluded. More often, this tumor occurs in older patients but the radiologic features can be similar to those observed in Ewing's sarcoma. Histologically, lymphomas usually show a permeative growth pattern leaving intact bony trabeculae and a mixture of small and large tumor cells, with prominent nuclear convolutions and clefts. Special stains demonstrate little or no glycogen and an abundant network of reticulin fibers.

Immunohistochemistry is in practice the most useful tool for distinguishing lymphoma and Ewing's sarcoma. Leukocyte common antigen (CD45) is strongly positive in the former and B cell (CD20) and T cell (CD3) markers could also be useful. These markers are always negative in Ewing's sarcoma. However, one should keep in mind the positivity of O13 in most cases of lymphoblastic T cell lymphomas.[26]

Today, molecular biology techniques, particularly RT-PCR, represent the gold standard in solving the most difficult cases by demonstrating gene rearrangement in lymphomas and the specific fusion transcript in Ewing's sarcomas.

Small cell osteosarcoma may mimic a Ewing's sarcoma when osteoid production is inconspicuous or missing in a small biopsy. In these cases, radiographic features can be useful to demonstrate osteoid production by the tumor. Immunohistochemistry and molecular biology techniques could be useful, but focal O13 positivity[26] and translocation t(11;22)[51] have been reported in small cell osteosarcomas.

The differential diagnosis with a mesenchymal chondrosarcoma is a problem of sampling, when the chondroid component is missing on the biopsy. X-rays usually show the conventional features of chondrosarcoma with calcifications. Histologically, a hemangiopericytoma-like pattern with some spindle cells should suggest the diagnosis of mesenchymal chondrosarcoma and urge the pathologist to look for a chondroid component.

A metastatic neuroblastoma from an occult primary site should be considered in children under 5 years. The diagnosis can usually be confirmed by demonstration of elevated urinary levels of catecholamine metabolites. Histologically, Homer–Wright rosettes are usually present with a fibrillary intercellular background. Immunohistochemistry shows a strong positivity for neuron-specific enolase and a constant negativity for O13.[31] Cytogenetics show a deletion of the short arm of chromosome 1 and molecular biology a frequent amplification of the proto-oncogene N-myc.[95]

A metastatic small cell carcinoma has to be excluded in patients over 30 years. Usually, clinical history and immunohistochemistry provide the best clues for the diagnosis.

Poorly differentiated embryonal rhabdomyosarcoma and alveolar rhabdomyosarcoma involving bone by a metastatic process or, rarely, by direct extension can be mistaken for an atypical Ewing's sarcoma. Primary rhabdomyosarcoma has also been reported.[96] Immunohistochemistry, particularly with muscular markers, is usually the best tool to solve this problem. Alveolar rhabdomyosarcoma consistently shows a translocation t(2;13) which can be demonstrated by RT-PCR.[95]

Monophasic synovial sarcoma involving bone by direct extension can be deceptive, particularly when it is composed of small round cells. Histologically, the presence of fibrous tissue, calcifications, a hemangiopericytoma-like pattern and spindle cells should suggest the diagnosis. Special stains show a dense network of reticulin fibers and immunohistochemistry usually shows a positivity for epithelial markers. However, O13 positivity has been reported in synovial sarcomas[29] and positivity for epithelioid markers can be seen in Ewing's sarcomas.[22] Again, cytogenetic and molecular biology techniques represent good tools to solve difficult cases. A translocation t(X;18) which can be demonstrated by RT-PCR has been consistently reported in synovial sarcomas.[97]

COMMENTS FOR THE SURGICAL PATHOLOGIST

Ewing's sarcoma belongs to the group of primitive neu-

roectodermal tumors (PNET) and is characterized by a chimeric transcript involving the EWS-FLI-1 or EWS-ERG gene. RT-PCR tends to be the gold standard for detecting this transcript and for the diagnosis of Ewing's sarcoma. Detection of MIC2 expression by immunohistochemistry is useful but non-specific.

Modern combined modality therapies with multiagent chemotherapy have made a significant improvement in the prognosis of Ewing's sarcoma.

REFERENCES

1. Lucke A. Beitrage zur geschwulsthehre. Virchows Arch 1866: 35: 524–539
2. Ewing J. Diffuse endothelioma of bone. Proc NY Pathol Soc 1921: 21: 17–24
3. Dehner L P. Primitive neuroectodermal tumor and Ewing's sarcoma. Am J Surg Pathol 1993: 17: 1–13
4. Cavazzana A O, Miser J S, Jefferson J, Triche T J. Experimental evidence for a neural origin of Ewing's sarcoma of bone. Am J Pathol 1987: 127: 507–518
5. Fellinger E J, Garin Chesa P, Triche T, Huvos A G, Rettig W J. Immunohistochemical analysis of Ewing's sarcoma cell surface antigen p30/32^{MIC2}. Am J Pathol 1991: 139: 317–325
6. Delattre O, Zucman J, Melot T et al. The Ewing family of tumors – a subgroup of small-round-cell tumors defined by specific chimeric transcripts. N Engl J Med 1994: 331: 294–299
7. Ewing's sarcoma and its congeners: an interim appraisal (editorial). Lancet 1992: 339: 99–100
8. Kissane J M, Askin F B, Foulkes M, Stratton L B, Shirley S F. Ewing's sarcoma of bone: clinicopathologic aspects of 303 cases from the intergroup Ewing's sarcoma study. Hum Pathol 1983: 14: 773–779
9. Terrier P, Henry Amar M, Triche T J et al. Is neuroectodermal differentiation of Ewing's sarcoma of bone associated with an unfavourable prognosis? Eur J Cancer 1995: 31A: 307–314
10. Bator S M, Bauer T W, Marks K E, Norris D G. Periosteal Ewing's sarcoma. Cancer 1986: 58: 1781–1784
11. Daugaard S, Kamby C, Sunde L M, Myhre Jensen O, Schiodt T. Ewing's sarcoma. A retrospective study of histological and immunohistochemical factors and their relation to prognosis. Virchows Arch 1989: 414: 243–251
12. Llombart Bosch A, Contesso G, Henry-Amar M et al. Histopathological predictive factors in Ewing's sarcoma of bone and clinicopathological correlations. A retrospective study of 261 cases. Virchows Arch 1986: 409: 627–640
13. Nascimento A G, Cooper K L, Unni K K, Dahlin D C, Pritchard D J. A clinicopathologic study of 20 cases of large-cell (atypical) Ewing's sarcomas of bone. Am J Surg Pathol 1980: 4: 29–36
14. Picci P, Rougraff B T, Bacci G et al. Prognostic significance of histopathologic response to chemotherapy in nonmetastatic Ewing's sarcoma of the extremities. J Clin Oncol 1993: 11: 1763–1769
15. Dahl I, Akerman M, Angervall L. Ewing's sarcoma of bone. A correlative cytological and histological study of 14 cases. Acta Pathol Microbiol Immunol Scand A 1986: 94: 363–369
16. Akhtar M, Ali M A, Sabbah R. Aspiration cytology of Ewing's sarcoma. Light and electron microscopic correlations. Cancer 1985: 56: 2051–2060
17. Akerman M. Supporting tissues. In: Orell S R, Sterrett G F, Walters M N I, Whitaker D, Eds. Manual and atlas of fine needle aspiration cytology. Edinburgh: Churchill Livingstone, 1992, pp 299–334
18. Fellinger E J, Garin-Chesa P, Su S L, De Angelis P, Lane J M,

Rettig W J. Biochemical and genetic characterization of the HBA71 Ewing's sarcoma cell surface antigen. Cancer Res 1991: 51: 336–340
19. Gelin C, Aubrit T, Phalipan A. The E2 antigen, a 32 kd glycoprotein involved in T-cell adhesion processes, is the MIC2 gene product. EMBO J 1989: 8: 3253–3259
20. Ambros I M, Ambros P F, Strehl S, Kovar H, Gadner H, Salzer Kuntschik M. MIC2 is a specific marker for Ewing's sarcoma and peripheral primitive neuroectodermal tumors. Evidence for a common histogenesis of Ewing's sarcoma and peripheral primitive neuroectodermal tumors from MIC2 expression and specific chromosome aberration. Cancer 1991: 67: 1886–1893
21. Fellinger E J, Garin Chesa P, Glasser D B, Huvos A G, Rettig W J. Comparison of cell surface antigen HBA71 (p30/32MIC2), neuron-specific enolase, and vimentin in the immunohistochemical analysis of Ewing's sarcoma of bone. Am J Surg Pathol 1992: 16: 746–755
22. Stevenson A J, Chatten J, Bertoni F, Miettinen M. CD99(p30/32^{MIC2}) Neuroectodermal/Ewing's sarcoma antigen as an immunohistochemical marker. Review of more than 600 tumors and the literature experience. Appl Immunohistochem 1994: 2: 231–244
23. Ramani P, Rampling D, Link M. Immunocytochemical study of 12E7 in small round-cell tumours of childhood: an assessment of its sensitivity and specificity. Histopathology 1993: 23: 557–561
24. Perlman E J, Dickman P S, Askin F B, Grier H E, Miser J S, Link M P. Ewing's sarcoma–routine diagnostic utilization of MIC2 analysis: a Pediatric Oncology Group/Children's Cancer Group Intergroup study. Hum Pathol 1994: 25: 304–307
25. Weidner N, Tjoe J. Immunohistochemical profile of monoclonal antibody O13: antibody that recognizes glycoprotein p30/32MIC2 and is useful in diagnosing Ewing's sarcoma and peripheral neuroepithelioma. Am J Surg Pathol 1994: 18: 486–494
26. Riopel M, Dickman P S, Link M P, Perlman E J. MIC2 analysis in pediatric lymphomas and leukemias. Hum Pathol 1994: 25: 396–399
27. Pappo A S, Douglass E C, Meyer W H, Marina N, Parham D M. Use of HBA71 and anti-B2-microglobulin to distinguish peripheral neuroepithelioma from neuroblastoma. Hum Pathol 1993: 24: 880–885
28. Renshaw A A. O13 (CD99) in spindle cell tumors – reactivity with hemangiopericytoma, solitary fibrous tumor, synovial sarcoma, and meningioma but rarely with sarcomatoid mesothelioma. Appl Immunohistochem 1995: 3: 250–256
29. Dei Tos A P, Wadden C, Calonje E et al. Immunohistochemical demonstration of glycoprotein p30/32(MIC2) (CD99) in synovial sarcoma – a potential cause of diagnostic confusion. Appl Immunohistochem 1995: 3: 168–173
30. Moll R, Lee I, Gould V E, Berndt R, Roessner A, Franke W W. Immunocytochemical analysis of Ewing's tumors. Patterns of expressions of intermediate filaments and desmosomal proteins indicate cell type heterogeneity and pluripotential differentiation. Am J Pathol 1987: 127: 288–304
31. Pinto A, Grant L H, Hayes D F A, Schell M J, Parham D M.

Immunohistochemical expression of neuron-specific enolase and leu 7 in Ewing's sarcoma of bone. Cancer 1989: 64: 1266–1273

32. Tsuneyoshi M, Yokoyama R, Hashimoto H, Enjoji M. Comparative study of neuroectodermal tumor and Ewing's sarcoma of the bone. Histopathologic, immunohistochemical and ultrastructural features. Acta Pathol Jpn 1989: 39: 573–581

33. Carter R L, Al-Sam S Z, Corbett R P, Clinton S. A comparative study of immunohistochemical staining for neuron-specific enolase, protein gene product 9.5 and S-100 protein in neuroblastoma, Ewing's sarcoma and other round cell tumours in children. Histopathology 1990: 16: 461–467

34. Kowal-Vern A, Walloch J, Chon P E. Flow and image cytometric DNA analysis in Ewing's sarcoma. Mod Pathol 1992: 5: 56–60

35. Dierick A M, Langlois M, Oostveldt P V, Roels H. The prognostic significance of the DNA content in Ewing's sarcoma: a retrospective cytophotometric and flow cytometric study. Histopathology 1993: 23: 333–339

36. Navas Palacios J J, Aparicio Duque R, Valdes M D. On the histogenesis of Ewing's sarcoma. An ultrastructural, immunohistochemical, and cytochemical study. Cancer 1984: 53: 1882–1901

37. Mahoney J P, Alexander R W. Ewing's sarcoma. A light and electron-microscopy study of 21 cases. Am J Surg Pathol 1978: 2: 283–298

38. Llombart Bosch A, Blache R, Peydro Olaya A. Round-cell sarcomas of bone and their differential diagnosis with particular emphasis on Ewing's sarcoma and reticulosarcoma. A study of 233 tumors with optical and electron microscopic techniques. Pathol Annu 1982: 17 pt 2: 113–145

39. Llombart Bosch A, Blache R, Peydro Olaya A. Ultrastructural study of 28 cases of Ewing's sarcoma: typical and atypical forms. Cancer 1978: 41: 1362–1373

40. Aurias A, Rimbaut C, Buffe D, Dubousset J, Mazabraud A. Chromosomal translocations in Ewing's sarcoma. N Engl J Med 1983: 309: 496–497

41. Turc Carel C, Philip I, Berger M P, Philip T, Lenoir G M. Chromosomal translocations in Ewing's sarcoma. N Engl J Med 1983: 309: 497–498

42. Whang Peng J, Triche T J, Knutsen T, Miser J, Douglass E C, Israel M A. Chromosome translocation in peripheral neuroepithelioma. N Engl J Med 1984: 311: 584–585

43. De Chadarevian J P, Vekemans M, Seemayer T A. Reciprocal translocation in small-cell sarcomas. N Engl J Med 1984: 311: 1702–1703

44. Becroft D M, Pearson A, Shaw R L, Zwi L J. Chromosome translocation in extraskeletal Ewing's tumour. Lancet 1984: 2: 400

45. Whang Peng J, Freter C E, Knutsen T, Nanfro J J, Gazdar A. Translocation t(11;22) in esthesioneuroblastoma. Cancer Genet Cytogenet 1987: 29: 155–157

46. Vigfusson N V, Allen L J, Phillips J H, Alschibaja T, Riches W G. A neuroendocrine tumor of the small intestine with a karyotype of 46,XY,t(11;22). Cancer Genet Cytogenet 1986: 22: 211–218

47. Noguera R, Navarro S, Triche T J. Translocation (11;22) in small cell osteosarcoma. Cancer Genet Cytogenet 1990: 45: 121–124

48. Stephenson C F, Bridge J A, Sandberg A A. Cytogenetic and pathologic aspects of Ewing's sarcoma and neuroectodermal tumors. Hum Pathol 1992: 23: 1270–1277

49. Turc Carel C, Aurias A, Mugneret F et al. Chromosomes in Ewing's sarcoma. I. An evaluation of 85 cases of remarkable consistency of t(11;22)(q24;q12). Cancer Genet Cytogenet 1988: 32: 229–238

50. Hoffer F A, Gianturco L E, Fletcher J A, Grier H E. Percutaneous biopsy of peripheral primitive neuroectodermal tumors and Ewing's sarcomas for cytogenetic analysis. AJR 1994: 162: 1141–1142

51. Douglass E C. Chromosomal rearrangements in Ewing's sarcoma and peripheral neuroectodermal tumor (PNET). Semin Dev Biol 1990: 1: 393–396

52. Delattre O, Zucman J, Plougastel B et al. Gene fusion with an ETS DNA-binding domain caused by chromosome translocation in human tumours. Nature 1992: 359: 162–165

53. Zucman J, Delattre O, Desmaze C et al. Cloning and characterization of the Ewing's sarcoma and peripheral

neuroepithelioma t(11;22) translocation breakpoints. Genes Chromosomes Cancer 1992: 5: 271–277

54. Zucman J, Melot T, Desmaze C et al. Combinatorial generation of variable fusion proteins in the Ewing family of tumours. EMBO J 1993: 12: 4481–4487

55. Jeon I S, Davis J N, Braun B S et al. A variant Ewing's sarcoma translocation (7;22) fuses the EWS gene to the ETS gene ETV1. Oncogene 1995: 10: 1229–1234

56. May W A, Gishizky M L, Lessnick S L et al. Ewing sarcoma 11;22 translocation produces a chimeric transcription factor that requires the DNA-binding domain encoded by FLI1 for transformation. Proc Natl Acad Sci USA 1993: 90: 5752–5756

57. Desmaze C, Zucman J, Delattre O, Melot T, Thomas G, Aurias A. Interphase molecular cytogenetics of Ewing's sarcoma and peripheral neuroepithelioma t(11;22) with flanking and overlapping cosmid probes. Cancer Genet Cytogenet 1994: 74: 13–18

58. Taylor C, Patel K, Jones T, Kiely F, De Stavola B L, Sheer D. Diagnosis of Ewing's sarcoma and peripheral neuroectodermal tumour based on the detection of t(11;22) using fluorescence in situ hybridisation. Br J Cancer 1993: 67: 128–133

59. McManus A P, Gusterson B A, Pinkerton C R, Shipley J M. Diagnosis of Ewing's sarcoma and related tumours by detection of chromosome 22q12 translocations using fluorescence in situ hybridization on tumour touch imprints. J Pathol 1995: 176: 137–142

60. Peter M, Magdelenat H, Michon J et al. Sensitive detection of occult Ewing's cells by the reverse transcriptase-polymerase chain reaction. Br J Cancer 1995: 72: 96–100

61. Pfleiderer C, Zoubek A, Gruber B et al. Detection of tumour cells in peripheral blood and bone marrow from Ewing tumour patients by RT-PCR. Int J Cancer 1995: 64: 135–139

62. Ida K, Kobayashi S, Taki T et al. EWS-FLI-1 and EWS-ERG chimeric mRNAs in Ewing's sarcoma and primitive neuroectodermal tumor. Int J Cancer 1995: 63: 500–504.

63. Toretsky J A, Neckers L, Wexler L H. Detection of (11;22)(q24;q12) translocation-bearing cells in peripheral blood progenitor cells of patients with Ewing's sarcoma family of tumors. J Natl Cancer Inst 1995: 87: 385–386

64. Downing J R, Head D R, Parham D M et al. Detection of the (11;22)(q24;q12) translocation of Ewing's sarcoma and peripheral neuroectodermal tumor by reverse transcription polymerase chain reaction. Am J Pathol 1993: 143: 1294–1300

65. Zoubek A, Bockhorn Dworniczak B, Delattre O et al. Does expression of different EWS chimeric transcripts define clinically distinct risk groups of Ewing tumor patients? J Clin Oncol 1996: 14: 1245–1251

66. Ladanyi M, Lewis R, Garin Chesa P et al. EWS rearrangement in Ewing's sarcoma and peripheral neuroectodermal tumor. Molecular detection and correlation with cytogenetic analysis and MIC2 expression. Diagn Mol Pathol 1993: 2: 141–146

67. Scotlandi K, Serra M, Manara M C et al. Immunostaining of the p30/32(MIC2) antigen and molecular detection of EWS rearrangements for the diagnosis of Ewing's sarcoma and peripheral neuroectodermal tumor. Hum Pathol 1996: 27: 408–416

68. Adams V, Hany M A, Schmid M, Hassam S, Briner J, Niggli F K. Detection of t(11;22)(q24;q12) translocation breakpoint in paraffin-embedded tissue of the Ewing's sarcoma family by nested reverse transcription-polymerase chain reaction. Diagn Mol Pathol 1996: 5: 107–113

69. Ladanyi M, Lewis R, Jhanwar S C, Gerald W, Huvos A G, Healey J H. MDM2 and CDK4 gene amplification in Ewing's sarcoma. J Pathol 1995: 175: 211–217

70. Phillips R F, Higinbotham N L. The curability of Ewing's endothelioma of bone in children. J Pediatr 1967: 70: 391–397

71. Rosen G, Caparros B, Nirenberg A et al. Ewing's sarcoma: ten-year experience with adjuvant chemotherapy. Cancer 1981: 47: 2204–2213

72. Wilkins R M, Pritchard D J, Burgert E O Jr, Unni K K. Ewing's sarcoma of bone. Experience with 140 patients. Cancer 1986: 58: 2551–2555

73. Jurgens H, Exner U, Gadner H et al. Multidisciplinary treatment of primary Ewing's sarcoma of bone. A 6-year experience of a European Cooperative Trial. Cancer 1988: 61: 23–32.

74. Barbieri E, Emiliani E, Zini G et al. Combined therapy of localized Ewing's sarcoma of bone: analysis of results in 100 patients. Int J Radiat Oncol Biol Phys 1990: 19: 1165–1170

75. Nesbit M E Jr, Gehan E A, Burgert E O et al. Multimodal therapy for the management of primary, nonmetastatic Ewing's sarcoma of bone: a long-term follow-up of the First Intergroup study. J Clin Oncol 1990: 8: 1664–1674

76. Hayes F A, Thompson E I, Parvey L et al. Metastatic Ewing's sarcoma: remission induction and survival. J Clin Oncol 1987: 5: 1199–1204

77. Kinsella T J, Miser J S, Waller B et al. Long-term follow-up of Ewing's sarcoma of bone treated with combined modality therapy. Int J Radiat Oncol Biol Phys 1991: 20: 389–395

78. Cangir A, Vietti T J, Gehan E A et al. Ewing's sarcoma metastatic at diagnosis. Results and comparisons of two intergroup Ewing's sarcoma studies. Cancer 1990: 66: 887–893

79. Evans R, Nesbit M, Askin F et al. Local recurrence, rate and sites of metastases, and time to relapse as a function of treatment regimen, size of primary and surgical history in 62 patients presenting with non-metastatic Ewing's sarcoma of the pelvic bones. Int J Radiat Oncol Biol Phys 1985: 11: 129–136

80. Travis L B, Curtis R E, Hankey B F, Fraumeni J F Jr. Second cancers in patients with Ewing's sarcoma. Med Pediatr Oncol 1994: 22: 296–297

81. Hartmann O. New strategies for the application of high-dose chemotherapy with haematopoietic support in paediatric solid tumours. Ann Oncol 1995: 6(suppl 4): S13–16

82. Yang R S, Eckardt J J, Eilber F R et al. Surgical indications for Ewing's sarcoma of the pelvis. Cancer 1995: 76: 1388–1397

83. Scully S P, Temple H T, Okeeffe R J, Scarborough M T, Mankin H J, Gebhardt M C. Role of surgical resection in pelvic Ewing's sarcoma. J Clin Oncol 1995: 13: 2336–2341

84. Razek A, Perez C A, Tefft M et al. Intergroup Ewing's sarcoma study. Local control related to radiation dose, volume, and site of primary lesion in Ewing's sarcoma. Cancer 1980: 46: 516–521

85. Dunst J, Sauer R, Burgers J M V. Results of the cooperative Ewing's sarcoma studies CESS81 and CESS86. Cancer 1991: 67: 2818–2825

86. Wessalowski R, Jürgens H, Bodenstein A E. Results of treatment of primary metastatic Ewing's sarcoma. A retrospective analysis of 48 patients. Klin Pädiatr 1989: 200: 253–260

87. Burgert E O Jr, Nesbit M E, Garnsey L A et al. Multimodal therapy for the management of nonpelvic, localized Ewing's sarcoma of bone: intergroup study IESS-II. J Clin Oncol 1990: 8: 1514–1524.

88. Hayes F A, Thompson E I, Meyer W H et al. Therapy for localized Ewing's sarcoma of bone. J Clin Oncol 1989: 7: 208–213

89. Mendenhall C M, Marcus R B J, Enneking W F, Springfield D S, Thar T L, Million R R. The prognostic significance of soft tissue extension in Ewing's sarcoma. Cancer 1983: 51: 913–917

90. De Stefani E, Carzoglio J, Deneo Pellegrini H, Olivera L, Cendan M, Kasdorf H. Ewing's sarcoma: value of tumor necrosis as a predictive factor. Bull Cancer Paris 1984: 71: 16–21

91. Bacci G, Toni A, Avella M et al. Long-term results in 144 localized Ewing's sarcoma patients treated with combined therapy. Cancer 1989: 63: 1477–1486

92. Oberlin O, Patte C, Demeocq F et al. The response to initial chemotherapy as a prognostic factor in localized Ewing's sarcoma. Eur J Cancer Clin Oncol 1985: 21: 463–467

93. Roessner A, Ueda Y, Bockhorn Dworniczak B et al. Prognostic implication of immunodetection of P glycoprotein in Ewing's sarcoma. J Cancer Res Clin Oncol 1993: 119: 185–189

94. Hijazi Y M, Axiotis C A, Navarro S, Steinberg S M, Horowitz M E, Tsokos M. Immunohistochemical detection of P-glycoprotein in Ewing's sarcoma and peripheral primitive neuroectodermal tumors before and after chemotherapy. Am J Clin Pathol 1994: 102: 61–67

95. McManus A P, Gusterson B A, Pinkerton C R, Shipley J M. The molecular pathology of small round-cell tumours – relevance to diagnosis, prognosis, and classification. J Pathol 1996: 178: 116–121

96. Lucas D R, Ryan J R, Zalupski M M, Gross M L, Ravindranath Y, Ortman B. Primary embryonal rhabdomyosarcoma of long bone. Case report and review of the literature. Am J Surg Pathol 1996: 20: 239–244

97. Ladanyi M. The emerging molecular genetics of sarcoma translocations. Diagn Mol Pathol 1995: 4: 162–173

31

Primitive neuroectodermal tumor

J. M. Coindre

INTRODUCTION AND CLINICAL DATA

This is a primary malignant bone tumor belonging to the Ewing family of tumors, which presents clearcut neural differentiation. This definition is simple, but the exact criteria to be used to define neural differentiation vary from author to author.

The history of primary neuroectodermal tumor (PNET) has recently been detailed by Dehner.[1] PNET of bone was first described by Jaffe et al in 1984,[2] who suggested that some small round cell tumors which present as Ewing's sarcoma are neuroectodermal in nature. In fact, the first case of PNET was reported by Stout in 1918 in soft tissue.[3] Several cases of PNET were then reported in soft tissues, often in association with a major nerve. The term 'primitive neuroectodermal tumor' was proposed in 1973 by Hart & Earle for a group of brain tumors in children.[4] In 1975, Seemayer et al described cases of peripheral neuroectodermal tumors arising in the soft tissues.[5] The concept of Ewing's sarcoma arising only in bone and PNET only in soft tissue was weakened by the report of extraosseous Ewing's sarcoma by Angervall & Enzinger in 1975[6] and the report of PNET of bone by Jaffe et al in 1984.[2] A possible relationship between these two tumors then became apparent and today there is controversy over whether PNET is distinctly different from Ewing's sarcoma.

Moreover, the terms PNET, Askin's tumor and peripheral neuroepithelioma are used interchangeably, thus creating a confused nosology. In fact, Ewing's sarcoma and PNET share similar microscopic, ultrastructural, immunohistochemical and particularly cytogenetic and molecular features. Indeed, the modern concept is to consider these tumors as a single group of bone and soft tissue tumors called the Ewing family of tumors or the PNET family of tumors, in which typical Ewing's sarcoma represents the most undifferentiated end of a spectrum and PNET the most differentiated end.[1,7]

""

Clinical features of patients with PNET of bone are similar to those of patients with Ewing's sarcoma, with a median age of 15 years, a male preponderance and the same symptoms. A high rate of clinically detectable metastases at the time of initial diagnosis has previously been reported,[8,9] but this was not confirmed in a recent large series.[10]

SKELETAL DISTRIBUTION

Location of tumors is similar in PNET and Ewing's sarcoma.

Many, if not most, Askin's tumors are said to represent PNET (Figs 31.1, 31.2). In the initial report,[11] this tumor arising in the chest wall tended to recur locally rather than to disseminate distantly. A subsequent study[12] showed no major differences between the so-called Askin's tumor and Ewing's bone tumor located outside the thoracic wall.

IMAGING AND GROSS PATHOLOGY

These tumors are indistinguishable from Ewing's sarcoma.

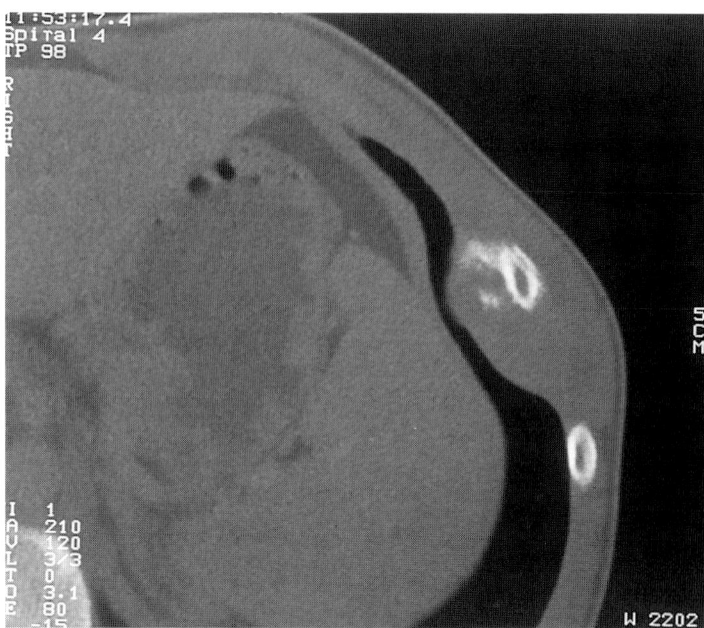

Fig. 31.2 Primitive neuroectodermal tumor of the rib (same patient as Fig. 31.1): computed tomographic scan showing the extraosseous extent of the tumor (Askin's tumor).

HISTOPATHOLOGY

Rosette formation is a necessary feature for the diagnosis of PNET for most authors, but there is no agreement on the type and number of rosettes required. Schmidt et al[13] insisted on the presence of Homer–Wright rosettes (Fig. 31.3), but Terrier et al[10] accepted both Homer–Wright rosettes and pseudorosettes.

For Tsuneyoshi et al[14] pseudorosettes may be encountered in Ewing's sarcoma. Cases of initially conventional Ewing's sarcoma without rosettes eventually proved to be PNET with typical Homer–Wright rosettes in the recurrence or metastases.[15] Intermediate forms have been reported as 'atypical Ewing's sarcoma with neuroectodermal features'.[16]

Rosettes are occasionally associated with a fibrillary intercellular background.

A lobular architecture and atypical large cells are more frequent in PNET than Ewing's sarcoma.[10] Ganglion cell differentiation may be present. Glycogen was said to be less than in Ewing's sarcoma, but this was not confirmed by a recent large series.[10]

IMMUNOHISTOCHEMISTRY

Most immunohistochemical studies have shown more similarities than differences between PNET and Ewing's sarcoma.

Both tumors are strongly and diffusely positive for antibodies detecting MIC2 expression[17–22] (Fig. 31.4). They are also positive for vimentin.

Fig. 31.1 Primitive neuroectodermal tumor of the rib: X-ray showing cortical destruction and periosteal new bone formation (Askin's tumor).

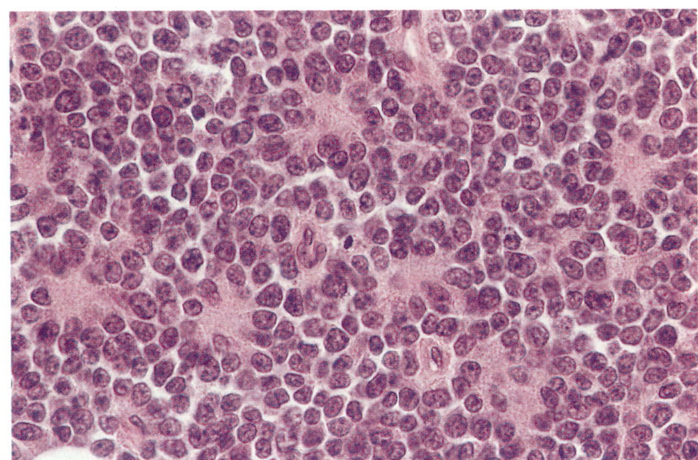

Fig. 31.3 Primitive neuroectodermal bone tumor: Homer–Wright rosettes.

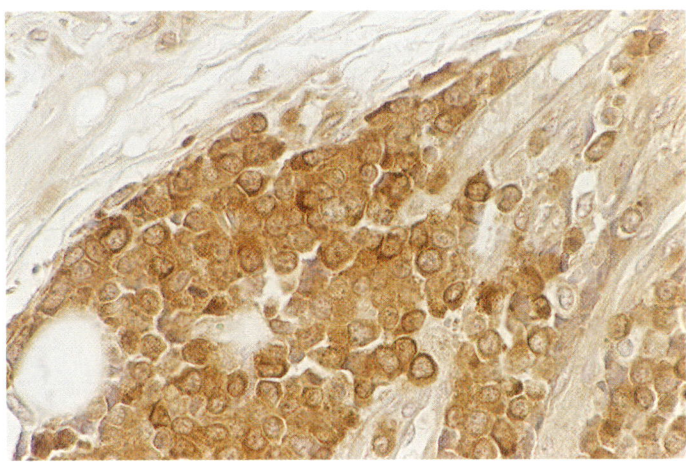

Fig. 31.5 Primitive neuroectodermal bone tumor: strong positivity for neuron-specific enolase (immunohistochemistry – NSE).

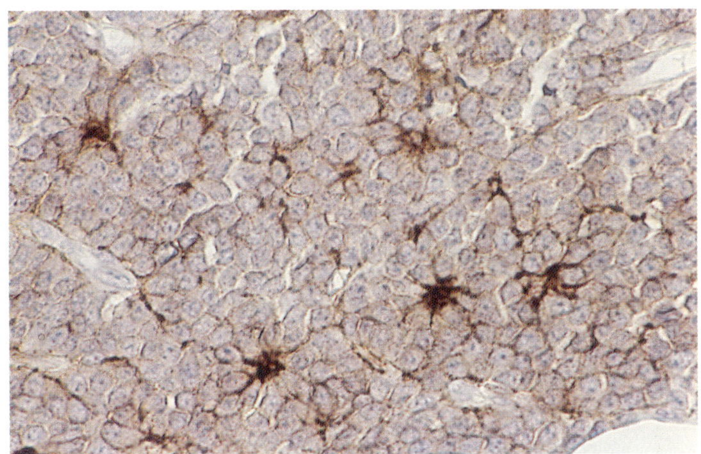

Fig. 31.4 Primitive neuroectodermal bone tumor: positivity for the MIC2 gene product (immunohistochemistry – 013 antibody).

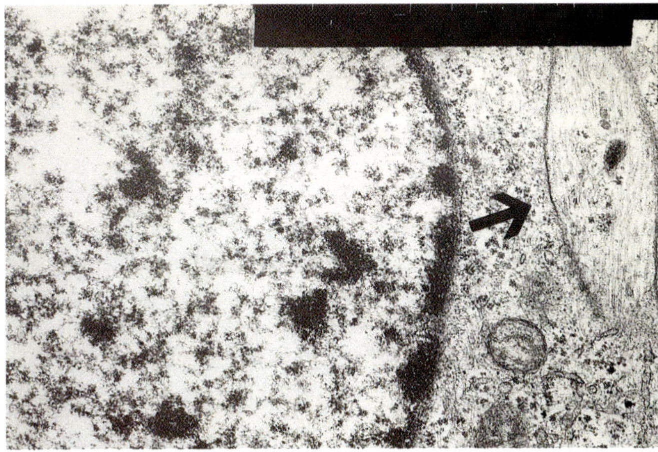

Fig. 31.6 Primitive neuroectodermal bone tumor: electron microscopy showing a cellular process (arrow) with numerous microtubules and neurosecretory granules (×8000). (Courtesy of L. Boccon-Gibod MD.)

Neural markers such as neuron-specific enolase (Fig. 31.5), S-100 protein, leu-7, synaptophysin, chromogranin and neurofilaments may be positive in PNET, but results have been variable.[2,9,14,23,24] These markers have been used in the definition of PNET in conjunction with Homer–Wright rosettes: neuron-specific enolase by Jürgens et al,[19] synaptophysin or neurofilaments by Fechner & Mills and at least two positive neural markers by Schmidt et al.[13] In fact, with the progress of immunohistochemical techniques, an increasing number of conventional Ewing's sarcomas have shown positive cells for the same neural markers.

CYTOGENETICS

Cytogenetic and molecular studies have clearly shown the same abnormalities in PNET, Askin's tumor and Ewing's sarcoma.[25–27] Identification of these specific abnormalities

has been one of the most important observations for supporting the hypothesis that these tumors belong to the same family, the so-called Ewing or PNET family of tumors.

ELECTRON MICROSCOPY

Electron microscopy retains an important role in the identification of neural differentiation in the field of small round cell malignant tumors.[28] In addition to undifferentiated areas with sometimes prominent clumps[23,29] of glycogen as seen in Ewing's sarcoma, elongated or interdigitating cellular processes with filaments and microtubules should be present for the diagnosis of PNET1 (Fig. 31.6, 31.7). Scattered dense-core granules in the cytoplasm[30] and a basal lamina surrounding the cells[23] may also be present.

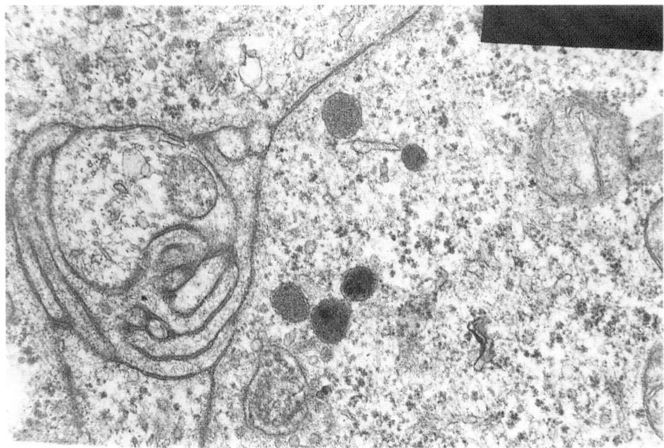

Fig. 31.7 Primitive neuroectodermal bone tumor: electron microscopy showing interdigitating cellular processes with neurosecretory granules (×20 000). (Courtesy of L. Boccon–Gibod MD.)

CLINICAL COURSE, TREATMENT AND PROGNOSIS

Treatment of bone PNET is similar to treatment of Ewing's bone sarcoma.

Several studies have suggested a poorer prognosis for bone PNET as compared to Ewing's bone sarcoma, thus justifying a distinction between these tumors.[8,13,14,23] However, most of these studies reported small series. In the Kiel series[13] more PNETs were central axial in location than were Ewing's sarcomas and the poorer prognosis of PNETs could be related to anatomical location rather than neuroectodermal differentiation.

In contrast to these studies, in a recent large series Terrier et al[10] reported no difference in prognosis in Ewing's bone sarcoma with or without neuroectodermal differentiation.

DIFFERENTIAL DIAGNOSIS

As for Ewing's bone sarcoma, bone PNET should be differentiated from non-Hodgkin's lymphoma, small cell osteosarcoma, mesenchymal chondrosarcoma, bone involvement by direct extension of a synovial sarcoma, metastatic rhabdomyosarcoma, small cell carcinoma and neuroblastoma. The same distinguishing criteria described in the chapter on Ewing's sarcoma can be applied to PNET.

The most challenging differential diagnosis of PNET is metastatic neuroblastoma, owing to neural differentiation in these two malignant small cell tumors. Metastatic neuroblastoma tends to occur in children less than 5 years old, is associated with high levels of urinary catecholamine metabolites, deletion of the short arm of chromosome 1, amplification of the protooncogene N-myc and is always immunohistochemically negative for O13 antibody.

As previously discussed, PNET and Ewing's sarcoma are closely related and are currently considered to be the two extremes of the spectrum of a single group of tumors called the Ewing family of tumors. Therefore, these two tumors are not clearly and reproducibly separable and should no longer be considered as separate entities.

REFERENCES

1. Dehner L P. Primitive neuroectodermal tumor and Ewing's sarcoma. Am J Surg Pathol 1993: 17: 1–13
2. Jaffe R, Santamaria M, Yunis E J et al. The neuroectodermal tumor of bone. Am J Surg Pathol 1984: 8: 885–898
3. Stout A P. A tumor of the ulnar nerve. Proc NY Pathol Soc 1918: 12: 2–12
4. Hart M N, Earle K M. Primitive neuroectodermal tumors of the brain in children. Cancer 1973: 32: 890–897
5. Seemayer T A, Thelmo W L, Bolande R P, Wiglesworth F W. Peripheral neuroectodermal tumors. Perspect Pediatr Pathol 1975: 2: 151–172
6. Angervall L, Enzinger F M. Extraskeletal neoplasm resembling Ewing's sarcoma. Cancer 1975: 36: 240–251
7. Ewing's sarcoma and its congeners: an interim appraisal (editorial). Lancet 1992: 339: 99–100
8. Rousselin B, Vanel D, Terrier-Lacombe M J, Istria B J, Spielman M, Masselot J. Clinical and radiologic analysis of 13 cases of primary neuroectodermal tumors of bone. Skeletal Radiol 1989: 18: 115–120
9. Jürgens H, Bier V, Harms D et al. Malignant peripheral neuroectodermal tumors. A retrospective analysis of 42 patients. Cancer 1988: 61: 349–357
10. Terrier Ph, Henry-Amar M, Triche T J et al. Is neuro-ectodermal differentiation of Ewing's sarcoma of bone associated with an unfavourable prognosis? Eur J Cancer 1995: 31A: 307–314
11. Askin F B, Rosai J, Sibley R K, Dehner L P, McAlister W H. Malignant small cell tumor of the thoracopulmonary region in childhood. A distinctive clinicopathologic entity of uncertain histogenesis. Cancer 1979: 43: 2438–2451
12. Contesso G, Llombart-Bosch A, Terrier Ph et al. Does malignant small round cell tumor of the thoracopulmonary region (Askin tumor) constitute a clinicopathologic entity? An analysis of 30 cases with immunohistochemical and electron-microscopic support treated at the Institute Gustave Roussy. Cancer 1992: 69: 1012–1020
13. Schmidt D, Herrmann C, Jürgens H, Harms D. Malignant peripheral neuroectodermal tumor and its necessary distinction from Ewing's sarcoma. A report from the Kiel pediatric tumor registry. Cancer 1991: 68: 2251–2259
14. Tsuneyoshi M, Yokoyama R, Hashimoto H, Enjoji M. Comparative study of neuroectodermal tumor and Ewing's sarcoma of bone. Histopathologic, immunohistochemical and ultrastructural features. Acta Pathol Jpn 1989: 39: 573–581
15. Ushigome S, Shimoda T, Nikaido T et al. Primitive neuroectodermal tumors of bone and soft tissue with reference to histologic differentiation in primary and metastatic foci. Acta Pathol Jpn 1992: 42: 483–493
16. Llombart-Bosch A, Lacombe M J, Contesso G, Peydro-Olaya A. Small round blue cell sarcoma of bone mimicking atypical Ewing's sarcoma with neuroectodermal features. An analysis of five cases with immunohistochemical and electron microscopic support. Cancer 1987: 69: 1570–1582
17. Ambros I M, Ambros P F, Strehl S, Kovar H, Gadner H, Salzer-Kuntschik M. MIC2 is a specific marker for Ewing's sarcoma and

peripheral primitive neuroectodermal tumors. Evidence for a common histogenesis of Ewing's sarcoma and peripheral primitive neuroectodermal tumors from MIC2 expression and specific chromosome aberration. Cancer 1991: 67: 1886–1893

18. Fellinger E J, Garin-Chesa P, Triche T J, Huvos A G, Rettig W J. Immunohistochemical analysis of Ewing's sarcoma cell surface antigen p30/32^{MIC2}. Am J Pathol 1991: 139: 317–325

19. Pappo A S, Douglass E C, Meyer W H, Marina N, Parham D M. Use of HBA71 and anti-β2 microglobin to distinguish peripheral neuroepithelioma from neuroblastoma. Hum Pathol 1993: 24: 880–885

20. Ramani P, Rampling D, Link M. Immunocytochemical study of 12E7 in small round-cell tumorus of childhood: an assessment of its sensitivity and specificity. Histopathology 1993: 23: 557–561

21. Perlman E J, Dickman P S, Askin F B, Grier H E, Miser J S, Link M P. Ewing's sarcoma. Routine diagnostic utilization of MIC2 analysis: a Pediatric Oncology Group/Children's Cancer Group intergroup study. Hum Pathol 1994: 25: 304–307

22. Weidner N, Tjoe J. Immunohistochemical profile of monoclonal antibody O13: antibody that recognizes glycoprotein p30/32^{MIC2} and is useful in diagnosing Ewing's sarcoma and peripheral neuroepithelioma. Am J Surg Pathol 1994: 18: 486–494

23. Llombart-Bosch A, Lacombe M J, Peydro-Olaya A, Perez-Bacete M, Contesso G. Malignant peripheral neuroectodermal tumours of bone other than Askin's neoplasm: characterization of 14 new cases with immunohistochemistry and electron microscopy. Virchows Arch (A) 1988: 412: 421–430

24. Shishikura A, Ushigome S, Shimoda T. Primitive neuroectodermal tumors of bone and soft tissue: histological subclassification and clinicopathologic correlations. Acta Pathol Jpn 1993: 43: 176–186

25. Whang-Peng J, Triche T J, Knutsen T, Miser J, Douglass E C, Israel M A. Chromosome translocation in peripheral neuroepithelioma. N Engl J Med 1984: 311: 584–585

26. Stephenson C F, Bridge J A, Sandberg A A. Cytogenetic and pathologic aspects of Ewing's sarcoma and neuroectodermal tumors. Hum Pathol 1992: 23: 1270–1277

27. Delattre O, Zucman J, Melot T et al. The Ewing family of tumors. A subgroup of small-round-cell tumors defined by specific chimeric transcripts. N Eng J Med 1994: 331: 294–299

28. Triche T. Neuroblastoma and other childhood neural tumors: a review. Pediatr Pathol 1990: 10: 175–193

29. Steiner G C, Graham S, Lewis M M. Malignant round cell tumor of bone with neural differentiation (neuroectodermal tumor). Ultrastruct Pathol 1988: 12: 505–512

30. Schmidt D, Mackay B, Ayala A G. Ewing's sarcoma with neuroblastoma-like features. Ultrastruct Pathol 1982: 3: 143–151

Primary lymphoma of bone

J. Diebold

INTRODUCTION

Malignant lymphomas (ML) represent the uncontrolled malignant proliferation of lymphoid cells. The clinical presentation may be an acute or chronic leukemia or a solid tumor, with one or multiple localizations. Bone can be involved at a microscopic level only, disclosed by a trephine bone marrow biopsy. Solid localized tumors of bone may also be observed, some of them presenting as primary lymphoma of bone.

DIFFERENT TYPES OF ML CLASSIFICATION

In tumor pathology, the basic principle for classifying different types of tumors is that they should be defined according to the tissue or cells from which they originate.

The lymphomatous cells are compared to normal lymphoid cells, precursors and mature, and to all the types of cells appearing during an immune reaction: centroblasts and centrocytes in the active germinal centers, immunoblasts, lymphoplasmocytoid cells, plasma cells, etc.[1]

In the Kiel classification,[1,2,3] ML are first divided in two groups, called low grade and high grade. This distinction is not based on clinical or evolutive data but on morphology. ML composed of a predominance of small cells ('cytes') with a nucleus showing dark blocks of chromatin and only small nucleoli are called 'low grade'. ML composed of a predominance of large cells ('blasts') with large pale nuclei and big nucleoli are called 'high grade'. This morphology is more or less correlated with the cell dividing capacity.

This has been confirmed by the results of a study using the monoclonal antibody Ki67. This antibody discloses a protein present in the nucleus of cells engaged in the mitotic cycle. Low-grade ML contain less than 10% positive cells while high-grade ML contain more than 30% positive cells and sometimes up to 60% or 90%.[4]

Low-grade ML have a long evolution but are often not

completely cured by treatment. High-grade ML have a more aggressive course but are often sensitive to chemotherapy and some may be completely cured. High-grade ML can occur at any moment during the course of a low-grade ML.

A second important distinction is based on the B or T cell origin. T cell ML are, in the majority of the cases, more aggressive than B cell ML.[4] The Kiel classification[1,2,3] was the first based on physiologic and immunologic data. This classification was mainly used for nodal ML. More recently, an international group of pathologists proposed a new nomenclature called REAL (Revised European American Lymphoma). This nomenclature is mainly based on the Kiel classification, but lists in addition new entities mainly of extranodal site.[5] The WHO has also organized a large international working group with the aim of proposing a classification of malignant proliferation of hematopoietic cells which can be used all over the world.

The entities which are currently recognized are listed briefly below.

Low-grade B cell ML

B-CLL, immunocytoma, hairy cell leukemia, plasmacytic lymphoma, centrocytic (mantle zone) ML, centroblastic-centrocytic ML, mucosa-associated B cell (Malt type) ML, monocytoid B cell ML.

High-grade B cell ML

Centroblastic ML, immunoblastic ML, Burkitt's ML, B-lymphoblastic ML/acute leukemia, anaplastic large cell ML, mediastinal large B cell ML with fibrosis, intravascular large B cell ML, T cell-rich (histiocyte-rich) B cell ML.

Low-grade T cell ML

T-CLL, small cerebriform ML (mycosis fungoides, Sézary's syndrome), lymphoepithelioid ML (Lennert's lymphoma), AILD type T cell ML, T-zone ML, pleomorphic T cell ML small cell predominance.

High-grade T cell ML

Pleomorphic T cell ML, medium and large cell predominance, including primary intestinal T cell ML and nasal T or NK ML/acute leukemia, anaplastic large cell ML, hepatosplenic γ-δ T cell ML

PRIMARY LYMPHOMA OF BONE

Definition

At any point in the evolution of one of the ML listed, a microscopic bone marrow involvement can be disclosed by a trephine bone marrow biopsy.[6] In some rare cases, for example T cell ML, such microscopic involvement may be the first sign of the disease, but it is not regarded as a primary lymphoma of bone.

A primary lymphoma of bone is a very rare condition which can be defined as a lymphoma showing a solitary bone tumor with possible extension to the regional lymph node but without involvement of other osseous or non-osseous sites within 6 months after the onset of symptoms[6-8] (Schajowicz 1994). With this definition, many of the primary lymphomas of the bone reported in the older literature cannot be considered as such. So a primary lymphoma of the bone seems to be extremely rare, comprising about 3–7% of malignant bone tumors[9-13] (Huvos 1991, Schajowicz 1994) and 1–3% of extranodal ML.[14]

Clinical symptoms

A primary bone lymphoma may appear at any age, with a median age between 30 and 40 years but it is rare before 10–15[15-18] (Huvos 1991, Schajowicz 1994). Both sexes can be involved, with a predominance for males in the majority of series[10,15] (Schajowicz 1994, Huvos 1991).

The description of reticulosarcoma by Oberling[19] and Parker & Jackson[20] emphasized that the most striking feature is the contrast between the general good condition of the patient and the painful, extensive, destructive bone lesion.

The most important symptom is pain of variable intensity. Swelling of the involved bone with a palpable mass and local tenderness are frequently associated. The onset is slow and often insidious. In cases of vertebral locations, neurologic symptoms do occur. Pathologic fracture seems to be observed relatively frequently and can reveal the bone lymphoma.

The majority of cases present as a monostotic lesion with extension to the soft tissue (stage I EA) or with a regional lymph node involvement (stage II EA).[10,15,21-23] In secondary bone involvement, with a tumor pattern corresponding to disseminated lymphoma, the patients also complain of weight loss, asthenia, poor general condition and fever.

Skeletal location

Any bone may be involved, but primary lymphoma occurs most commonly in the ilium, vertebrae and scapula and also long tubular bones, mainly the femur, tibia and humerus[15] (Huvos 1991, Schajowicz 1994). Skull and mandibular involvement have also been described.[10]

Biology

Apart from routine basic hematological examination, laboratory investigations include the study of lactic acid dehydrogenase (LDH) and β2-microglobulin.

Work-up

The initial work-up consists of a chest X-ray, bone scan, gallium scan, CT of the chest and abdomen to detect adenopathies, liver or spleen involvement. Bone marrow biopsy is also needed. The results allow determination of the stage of extension.[14,24]

Imaging

The presence of small areas of bone destruction in the medullary cavity of the metaphysis (Figs 32.1–32.5) or diaphysis of tubular bones is the most frequent initial radiologic change[10,15] (Schajowicz 1994). Rarely, they arise in the epiphysis of a long bone (Fig. 32.6) or in flat bone.

When the tumor is larger, the radiolucent lesions form large extensive areas, destroying the normal architecture of

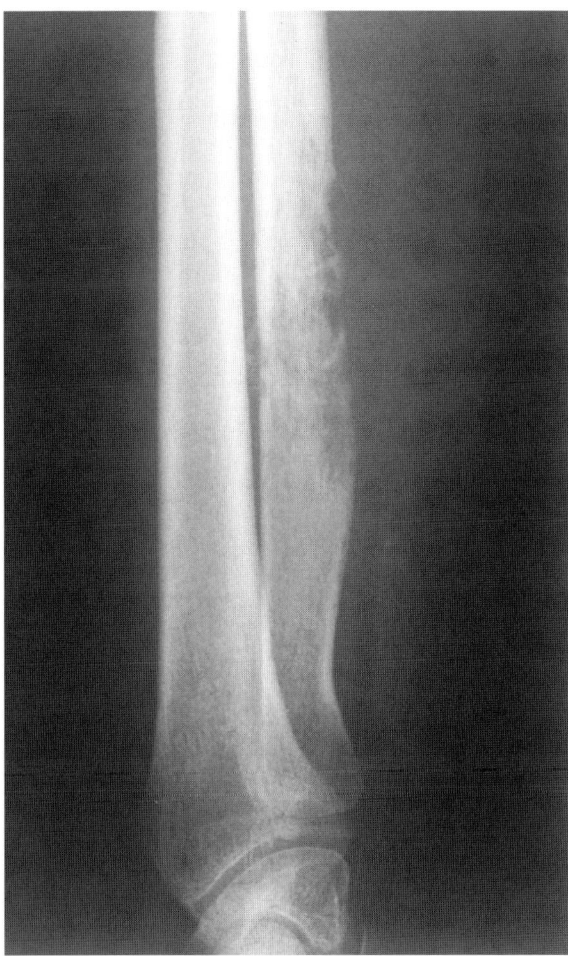

Fig. 32.2 High-grade B cell lymphoma. Involvement of the ulna. (Courtesy of M. Forest MD.)

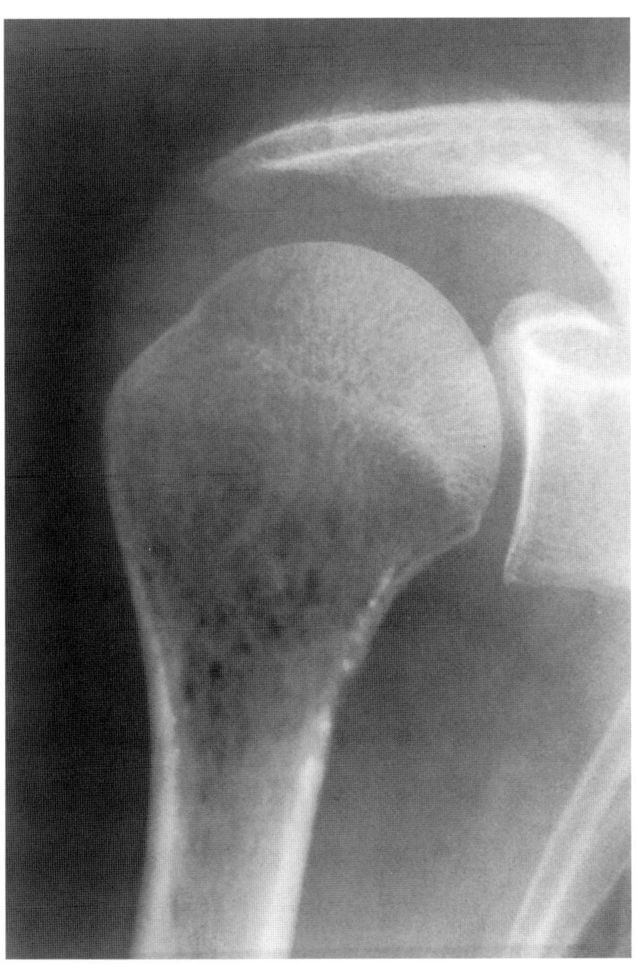

Fig. 32.1 High-grade B cell lymphoma. Humeral involvement. (Courtesy of M. Forest MD.)

the medulla and reaching the cortical bone which is partially or completely destroyed.

Periosteal new bone formation can be present but is often limited.[15] When the cortex is completely destroyed, a large soft tissue extension is always present. Radiologic evidence of a pathologic fracture may be seen.[15]

Technetium bone scanning can demonstrate an increased uptake at the periphery of the lesion and a decreased uptake in the center. Gallium scan shows a diffuse increased uptake throughout the tumor but little or no uptake at the periphery.

MRI can identify the lymphoma involvement on the findings of a low signal on T1-weighted images. It can also be useful for follow-up, but is not able to differentiate between healing bone and persistent disease.[15,25]

Gross pathology

The study of a resected tumor shows a wide area of bone destruction in the metadiaphyseal and/or diaphyseal areas.

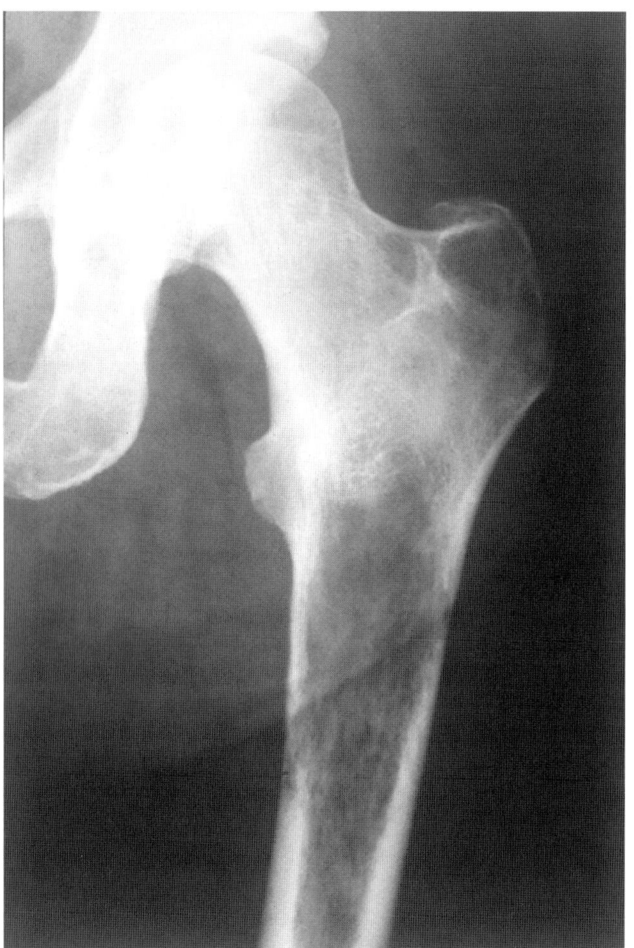

Fig. 32.3

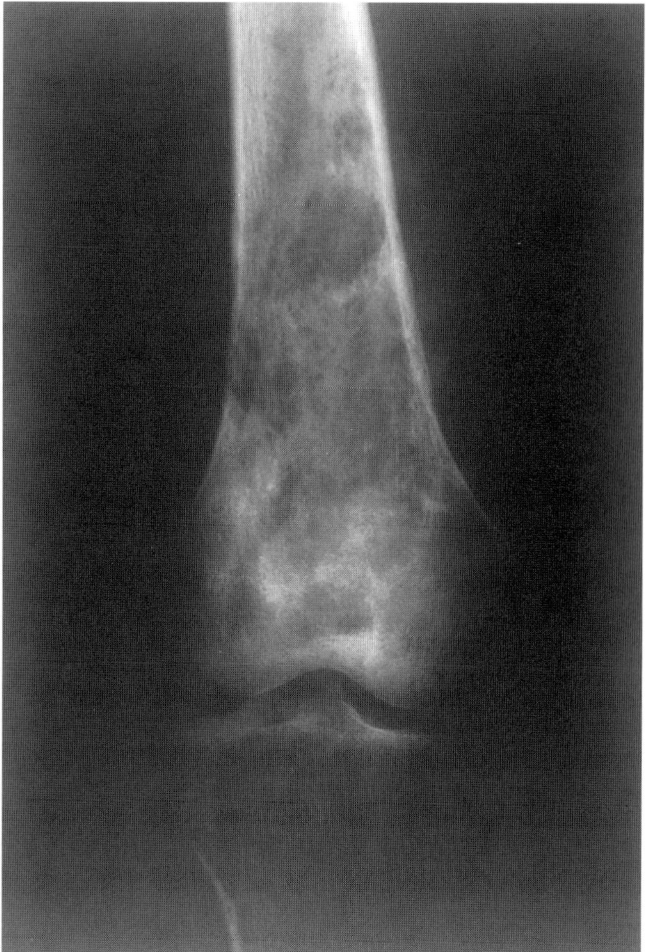

Fig. 32.4

Figs 32.3, 32.4 High-grade B cell lymphoma. Femoral involvement. (Courtesy of M. Forest MD.)

The cortical bone is thinned or distended, sometimes perforated or completely destroyed by the lymphomatous tissue. This tumoral tissue is whitish or grayish, firm, sometimes friable (fish flesh), with hemorrhagic or necrotic areas. Soft tissues around the bony lesion are destroyed and invaded by this lymphomatous tissue. There is often no periosteal reaction (Schajowicz 1994).

Histopathology

The diagnosis is based on a good large biopsy of the tumor. Imprints should be performed for cytopathologic study. The fresh biopsy should be sent immediately to the laboratory and divided into two parts, one for histopathology, fixed in a formalin solution, the other deeply frozen in liquid nitrogen and kept at −80°C for immunohistochemistry and, if needed, molecular biology (rearrangement of genes coding for T cell receptors or immunoglobulins, translocations, oncogenes, etc.). If possible, a cytogenetic study should also be done.

PRIMARY LARGE CELL LYMPHOMA OF BONE

It would appear that the majority of such primary bone lymphomas are composed of large B cells.[15,21,26–33] They correspond to the former 'reticulosarcoma'[19,20] or histiocytic sarcoma.[33]

Two main types of large B cell ML can be observed: centroblastic (large non-cleaved), which appears to be the most frequent,[15,21,22,23,30] and immunoblastic.[29]

Centroblastic ML

This type of lymphoma is composed of large cells with a round pale nucleus, delimitated by a sharp thin membrane and containing two or three medium-sized basophilic nucleoli. These nucleoli are symmetrically disposed, often in close contact with the nuclear membrane. The cytoplasm is amphophilic with hematein-eosin and basophilic with Giemsa stain.

Three subtypes of centroblastic ML can be recognized.

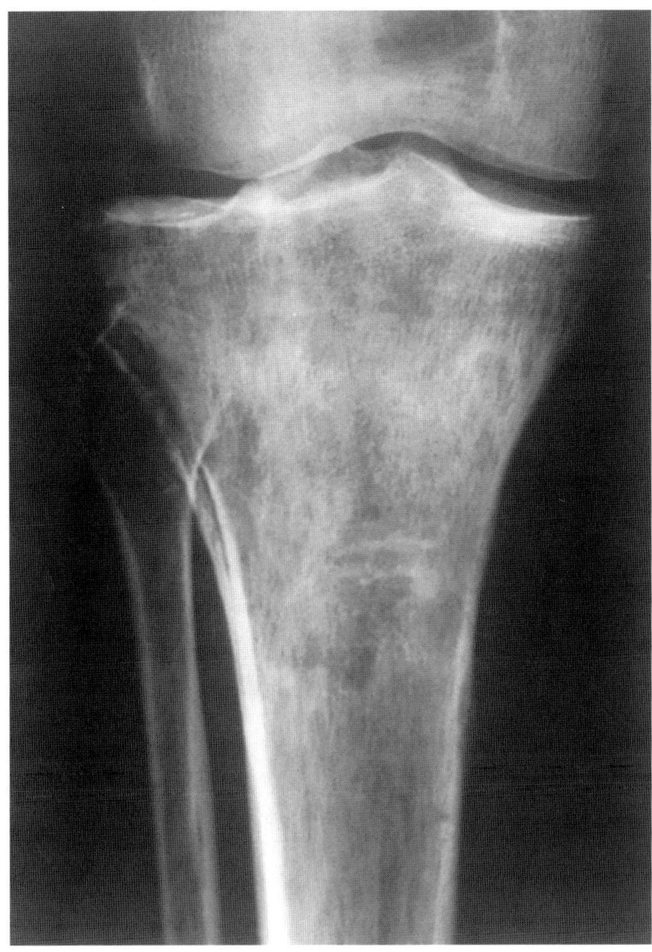

Fig. 32.5

Fig. 32.6

Figs 32.5, 32.6 Low-grade B cell lymphomas of centroblastic centrocytic type involving the tibia. (Courtesy of M. Forest MD.)

Monomorphic

The majority of the cells, up to 90%, present the morphology of typical centroblasts. Some smaller cells with the same morphology can be associated. It is possible to recognize rare cells with multilobated or cleaved nuclei.

Polymorphic

Typical centroblasts are associated with immunoblasts. The quantity of each type of cells is highly variable. The number of immunoblasts can be very high, up to 80–90%. At least 10% of centroblasts should be present for this diagnosis.

Multilobated

Typical centroblasts and immunoblasts are present in variable quantity, but the majority of the tumor cells exhibit a multilobated nucleus. Such big nuclei contain 3–5 lobes.[34] Immunohistochemistry demonstrates the following phenotype: expression of CD45, CD19, CD20 and surface monoclonal immunoglobulin with a predominance of the μ heavy chain.

Immunoblastic ML

The cells in these ML contain only immunoblasts; they have a large, round, pale nucleus, thick nuclear membrane, one single big basophilic nucleolus or sometimes one big centrally situated nucleolus with one or two smaller ones and extensive deeply basophilic cytoplasm (Fig. 32.7). In addition, some lymphomatous cells can show plasmacytic differentiation. Some immunoblasts show the morphology of plasmablasts with several medium-sized nucleoli in the center of the pale nucleus, an eccentric nucleus in the cytoplasm and hypertrophic Golgi apparatus showing as a pale area in the cytoplasm near the nucleus. Other cells are smaller, with the morphology of proplasma cells. Centroblasts are absent or very rare, representing less than 10%. So two types of B-immunoblastic ML can be described: one with plasma cell differentiation and one without.

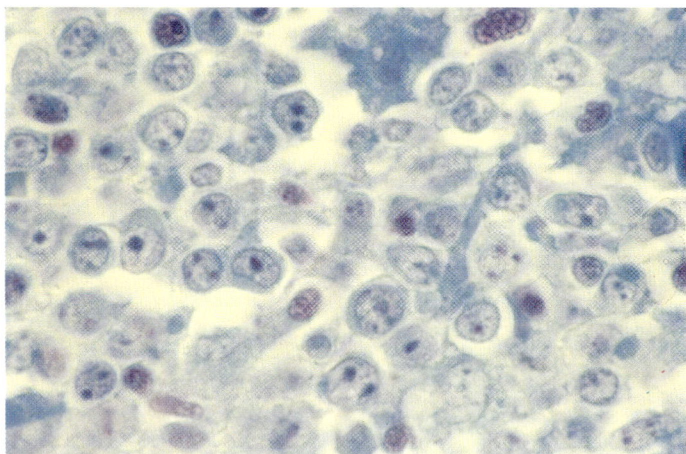

Fig. 32.7 Primary high-grade B cell lymphoma of the tibia. The lymphoma is composed of large cells with a round pale nucleus, a single big nucleolus and an abundant basophilic cytoplasm. (Giemsa.)

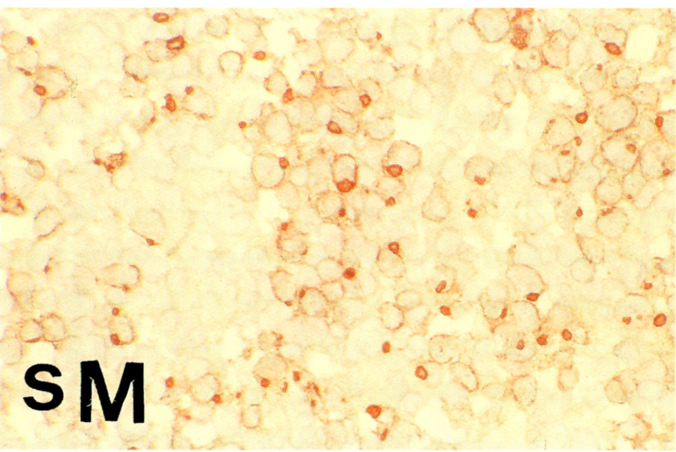

Fig. 32.8 Same case. The majority of the immunoblasts contain an inclusion made of monoclonal immunoglobulin (μ κ) occupying the Golgi area. Immunoperoxidase ABC amplification, with a polyclonal antibody against the heavy chain μ.

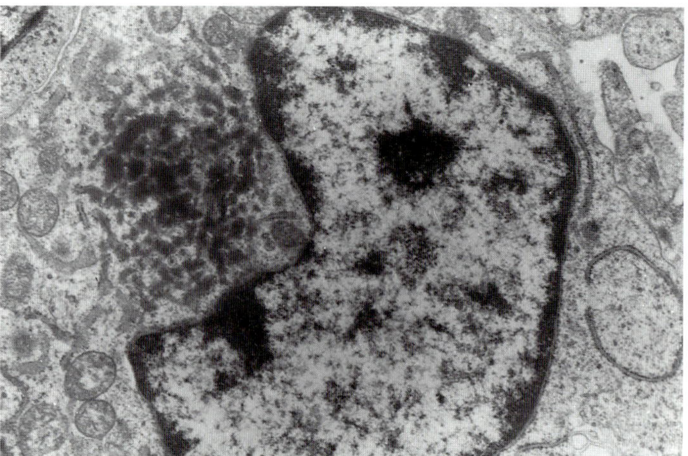

Fig. 32.9 Same case. Primary high-grade B cell lymphoma, immunoblastic type (updated Kiel classification). Concentration of immunoglobulins in the Golgi apparatus producing an electron-dense inclusion. Epon embedded tissue, electron microscopic study.

Immunohistochemistry confirms the B origin (CD19, CD20 positivity). The cells are also positive for EMA. They contain intracytoplasmic monoclonal immunoglobulin (Fig. 32.8), sometimes in the form of round dense inclusions,[29] recognized at the ultrastructural level (Fig. 32.9).

In both types of large B cell ML, the tumor cells are organized in large sheets, replacing and destroying the normal bone marrow tissue. Necrotic areas may be observed.

In many cases, numerous small lymphocytes infiltrate the sheets of tumor cells or produce clusters of small cells in close contact with or at a distance from the tumor cells. These lymphocytes are of T type and represent reactive cells. In the past, ML with such reactive small lympho-cytes were classified as diffuse mixed.[15] In addition, many histiocytes and macrophages can be seen inside or outside the tumor masses, as well as nests of polyclonal reactive plasma cells. Resorption of bone trabeculae by osteoclasts is frequently seen. It has been demonstrated that tumor cells in primary bone lymphoma produce cytokines (IL-1, IL-6, TNFα), stimulating osteoclasts.[35] Large collagenous bands can be observed around lymphoma cell sheets or penetrating the sheets, particularly in centroblastic ML.

Differential diagnosis

The cells of large B cell ML are larger than the cells of Ewing's sarcoma. The morphology of both the nucleus and the cytoplasm is also different: no 'ground glass' appear-ance of the nuclei, distinct cell border. The PAS reaction and the neuron-specific enolase research are negative.

A metastatic undifferentiated carcinoma can also be difficult to distinguish and immunohistochemistry is then very important. The neoplastic cells are cytokeratin positive and negative for CD45 (leukocyte common antigen) and for the B markers.

But the most important differential diagnosis is repre-sented by multiple myeloma composed of large cells: immunoblastic or plasmablastic variants. The only way to make a clearcut distinction between the two diseases is the clinical data: presence of typical multiple bone lesions on the X-rays, monoclonal immunoglobulin and electrophoretic serum peak.

A granulocytic sarcoma is sometimes difficult to distin-guish from some large B cell or lymphoblastic ML.[36] A careful study of imprints and Giemsa-stained paraffin sec-tions allows the diagnosis, based on the presence of exten-sive cytoplasm containing neutrophil or eosinophilic granules. The demonstration of a naphthol ASD chlorac-etate esterase activity and immunohistochemistry of myeloperoxidase or lysozyme confirms the diagnosis. The cells can also express CD15, CD4 and CD68.

Treatment and prognosis

Radiotherapy alone (40–50 Gy, 10 Gy per week) seems to be unable to cure completely all the primary bone lymphoma. In the published series, the majority of patients are now treated with combined radiotherapy and multidrug chemotherapy according to protocols used in nodal and extranodal ML (anthracyclin–containing regimen).[15,37]

Another strategy is based on wide excision of the tumor (en bloc resection) preceded and followed by a multidrug chemotherapy regimen[18,26,29] (Schajowicz 1994).

The prognosis is based more on the local extension and absence of dissemination than on histologic type. Clayton et al[21] report on a series of 26 large cell lymphomas: 17 were long-term survivors. In patients with the morphology of large cleaved cells, 67% were long-term survivors, but in patients with large non-cleaved cells, only 20% survived. Another publication reports the same results,[27] while another was unable to demonstrate the value of histologic type for the prognosis.[30] In this series, 55% of patients with localized disease had a 5-year survival rate against 9% in patients with disseminated disease. The site of primary involvement is also important. Involvement of pelvis and vertebrae seems to have a poor diagnosis (Schajowicz 1994).

ANAPLASTIC LARGE CELL ML

This recently described type of ML only rarely displays a primary bone lymphoma. As far as we know, 15 cases have been published.[38,39] Clinical presentation, radiologic changes and bone localization are the same as for large B cell ML.

At the histological level, the bone tissue is destroyed by sheets of large cells with an abundant cytoplasm, which is basophilic or with areas of variable basophilia. The big nucleus is roundish, ovoid or irregular, sometimes polylobed, with multiple medium to large nucleoli (Fig. 32.10).

This type of lymphoma corresponds to the majority of histiocytic sarcomas published in the past. Some Reed–Sternberg cells may be observed and mitosis is frequent. Bands of collagenous fibrosis surround or penetrate the sheets of tumor cells. At a distance from the tumor, single cell dissemination can occur (Fig. 32.11). Small reactive lymphocytes and macrophages are often associated.

Immunohistochemistry confirms the diagnosis, showing a positivity for CD45, CD30 and often for EMA and BNH9 but no expression of CD15 and cytokeratin. In some cases the tumor cells express T antigens (CD3, CD4) and this type seems to be the most frequent in bone.[39] Other anaplastic large cell lymphomas suggest a B cell origin (CD20 positive). Others are of null type, expressing neither B nor T cell-associated antigens.

The differential diagnosis with Hodgkin's disease can be difficult. Recently a translocation t(2–5) was described in about half of the anaplastic large cell ML. This translocation is responsible for fusion of the nucleophosmin (NPH) gene and a novel anaplastic lymphoma kinase (ALK) gene. The deregulated NPM-ALK products can be demonstrated by immunohistochemistry. It seems that this translocation is predominantly found in anaplastic large cell lymphomas and not in Hodgkin's disease. At the present time, there is no information about the presence of this translocation in primary bone presentation of this lymphoma. The prognosis seems to be favourable but in a few cases, a rapidly lethal course has been observed. Due to the rarity of this lymphoma, more data are needed.

OTHER TYPES

Diffuse centroblastic-centrocytic ML have also been observed.[15,21–23,27,30] They are composed of sheets of small to medium-sized centrocytes with a variable number of large centrocytes and centroblasts (Figs 32.12, 32.13).

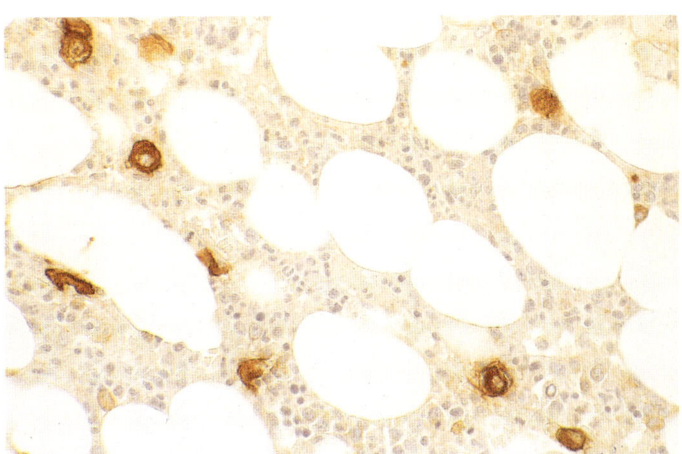

Fig. 32.10 Trephine biopsy of the iliac crest. Primary lymphoma, large anaplastic type with a null phenotype.

Fig. 32.11 Same case, distant from the main focus. Single cell dissemination of large anaplastic cells. Immunoperoxidase, ABC amplification with an anti-EMA polyclonal antibody.

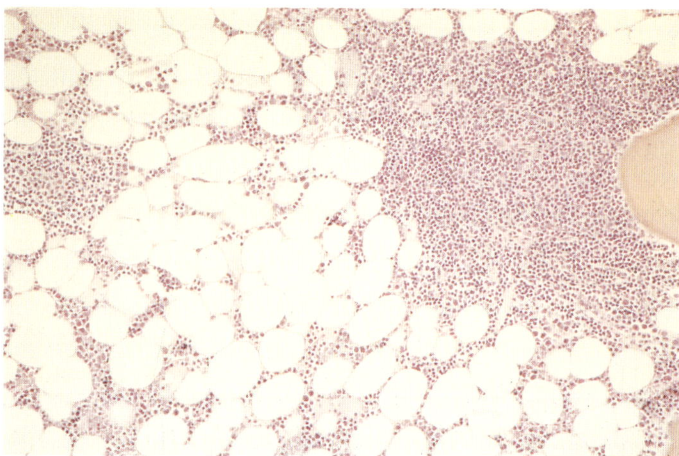

Fig. 32.12 Trephine biopsy of the iliac crest. Juxtatrabecular nodule corresponding to a centroblastic-centrocytic follicular lymphoma (low grade malignancy in the updated Kiel classification).

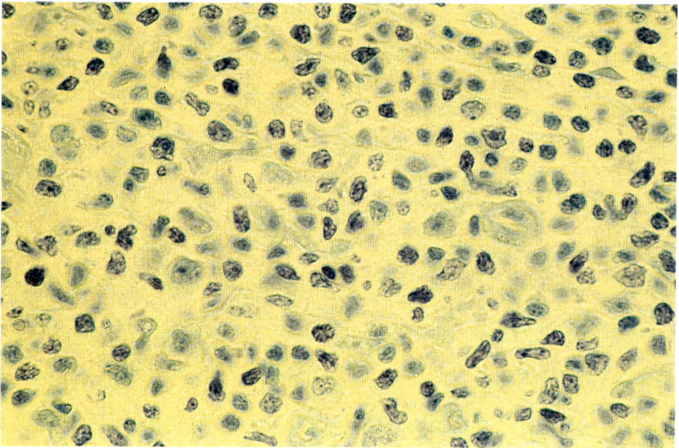

Fig. 32.13 Same case. In the follicle, the lymphoma population is composed of centrocytes (small and medium), also called cleaved nucleus cells, and centroblasts (large non-cleaved cells). (Giemsa.)

Extensive fibrosis and infiltration along the bone trabeculae are frequent. A typical follicular organization is not seen. Reactive lymphocytes, mainly of T phenotype, numerous histiocytes and nests of plasma cells are often present.[29,35] The outcome seems to be better than for large B cell ML.[27]

Burkitt's ML is seen only in facial bones (inferior and superior maxilla) and will not be described further.

Lymphoblastic ML have been described, as well as *centrocytic ML* (mantle cell ML). Currently we cannot be sure that these types of ML can really present as a primary bone tumor. In the majority of cases, lymphoblastic and mantle cell ML are disseminated diseases, appearing even as an acute leukemia for the lymphoblastic proliferation.

Small B cell ML

B-CLL and immunocytoma (lymphoplasmacytoid/cytic ML) do not produce large tumors. The infiltrate is interstitial with focal reinforcement or is packed, and massive. The cells in B-CLL are small with small, round nuclei showing dark areas of chromatin. Proliferative centers composed of prolymphocytes and immunoblasts appear as roundish pale areas. In immunocytoma, the cells show a plasmacytic differentiation and PAS-positive vacuoles can be present in the nuclei.

In a few cases severe osteopenia occurs, probably due to osteoclast stimulation by cytokines. Osteosclerosis is much rarer.[40,41]

In *hairy cell leukemia*, the bone marrow spaces are partially or totally infiltrated by small cells with a large pale cytoplasm, regularly surrounding a kidney-shaped or roundish nucleus. A systematic reticulinic myelofibrosis is always present. In about 10% of cases, this infiltrate is responsible for osteolytic destructive lesions, marked osteoporosis and aseptic necrosis of the femoral head.[5,42–46] Patients with such radiologic lesions suffer persistent bone pain, leading to the diagnosis. Sometimes a fracture can be the first symptom. In the majority of cases, solitary bone lesions are observed. They develop during the course of the disease, often many months after the diagnosis.[47] In more than 90% of cases the head and neck of the femur are involved, mostly on one side but very rarely on both sides. Other sites have also been described, in decreasing order of frequency: vertebrae, pelvis, skull, tibia, humerus and femur.[47]

T cell ML

Predominant bone marrow involvement in peripheral T cell ML is well known but until now no true primary bone ML of this type has been described.[48] In the past, many cases with multilobed nuclei were considered to be of T origin, but immunochemistry demonstrates that all these cases in fact exhibit a B phenotype and correspond to multilobed centroblastic ML.

Many older publications stressed the point that numerous cases remained unclassifiable[24,27,35,49] and the classification used does not allow us to determine how these lymphomas should be classified today.

REFERENCES

1. Lennert K, Feller A C. Histopathology of non-Hodgkin's lymphomas. 2nd ed. Berlin: Springer Verlag, 1992
2. Lennert K. Conceptual basis of the classification of malignant lymphomas. Med J Kagoshima Univ 1995: 47 (suppl 2): 7–31
3. Stansfeld A G, Diebold J, Kapanci Y et al. Updated Kiel classification for lymphomas. Lancet 1988: 1: 292–293, 372
4. Caulet S, Lesty C, Raphael M et al. Comparative quantitative study of Ki67 antibody staining in 78 B and T cell malignant lymphoma using 2 image analyser systems. Path Res Pract 1992: 188: 490–496
5. Harris N L, Jaffe E S, Stein H et al. A revised European-American classification of lymphoid neoplasms: a proposal from the international lymphoma study group. Blood 1994: 84: 1361–1392
6. Brunning R D, McKenna R W. Tumors of the bone marrow. Atlas for tumor pathology. 3rd series, fasc 9. Washington: AFIP, 1994, pp 380–408
7. Boston H C, Dahlin D C, Ivins J C, Cupps R E. Malignant lymphoma (so-called reticulum cell sarcoma) of bone. Cancer 1974: 34: 1131–1137
8. Wendling D, Hagenmüller I, Carbillet J P, Bosset J F. Les manifestations osseuses révélatrices des lymphomes malins non hodgkiniens. Sem Hôp Paris 1990: 66: 609–616
9. Blasius S, Edel G, Vestring T, Ueda Y, Wuisman P, Böcker W, Roessner A. Non-Hodgkin Lymphome mit primär ossärer Manifestation Erfahrungen aus dem Knochengeschwulstregister Westfalen. Verh Dtsch Ges Path 1992: 76: 146–150
10. Dahlin D C, Unni K K. Bone tumors: general aspects and data on 8542 cases. Springfield, Il: CC Thomas, 1986
11. Schmidt A G, Kohn D, Bernhards J, Braitinger S. Solitary skeletal lesions as primary manifestations of non-Hodgkin's lymphoma. Report of 2 cases and review of the literature. Arch Orthop Trauma Surg 1994: 113: 121–128
12. Spjut H, Dorfman H, Fechner R, Ackerman L. Tumours and tumor-like lesions of marrow origin in tumor of bone and cartilage. 2nd series, fasc 5. Washington: AFIP, 1983, pp 230–241
13. Ueda T, Aozasa K, Ohsawa M, Yoshikawa H, Uchida A, Ono K, Matsumoto K. Malignant lymphomas of bone in Japan. Cancer 1989: 64: 2387–2392
14. Dumont J, Mazabraud A. Primary lymphomas of bone (so-called 'Parker and Jackson's reticulum cell sarcoma'). Histological review of 75 cases according to the new classifications of non-Hodgkin's lymphomas. Biomedicine 1979: 31: 271–275
15. Baar J, Burkes R L, Bell R, Blackstein M E, Fernandes B, Langer F. Primary non Hodgkin's lymphoma of bone. A clinicopathologic study. Cancer 1994: 73: 1194–1199
16. Furman W L, Fitch S, Hustu O, Callihan T, Murphy S B. Primary lymphoma of bone in children. J Clin Oncol 1989: 7: 1275–1280
17. Howat J A, Thomas H, Waters K D, Campbell P E. Malignant lymphoma of bone in children. Cancer 1987: 59: 335–339
18. Limb D, Dreghorn C, Murphy J K, Mannion R. Primary lymphoma of bone. Int Orthop 1994: 18: 180–183
19. Oberling C. Les réticulosarcomes et les réticuloendothéliosarcomes de la moëlle osseuse (sarcomes d'Ewing). Bull Cancer 1928: 17: 259–296
20. Parker F Jr, Jackson J Jr. primary reticulum cell sarcoma of bone. Surg Gynecol Obstet 1939: 68: 45–53
21. Clayton F, Butler J J, Ayala A G, Ro J, Zornoza J. Non-Hodgkin's lymphoma in bone: pathologic and radiologic features with clinical correlates. Cancer 1987: 60: 2494–2501
22. Vassalo J, Roessner A, Vollmer E, Grundmann E. Malignant lymphomas with primary bone manifestations. Pathol Res Pract 1987: 182: 381–389
23. Vassalo J, Assuncao M C G A, Machado J C. Primitive malignant lymphoma of bone. Study of 14 cases. Ann Pathol 1988: 8: 44–48
24. Wollner N, Lane J M, Marcove R C et al. Primary skeletal non-Hodgkin's lymphomas in the pediatric age group. Med Pediatr Oncol 1992: 20: 506–513
25. Stiglbauer R, Augustini I, Kramer J, Schurawitzki H, Immof H, Radaszkiewicz T. MRI in the diagnosis of primary lymphoma of bone. Correlation with histopathology. J Comput Assist Tomogr 1992: 16: 248–253
26. Desai S, Jambhekar N A, Soman C S, Advani S H. Primary lymphoma of bone. A clinico-pathologic study of 25 cases reported over 10 years. J Surg Oncol 1991: 46: 265–269
27. Dosoretz D E, Raymond A K, Murphy G F et al. Primary lymphoma of bone. The relationship of morphologic diversity to clinical behavior. Cancer 1982: 50: 1009–1014
28. Falini B, Binazzi R, Pileri S et al. Large cell lymphoma of bone: a report of 3 cases of B-cell origin. Histopathology 1988: 12: 177–190
29. Fiche M, Le Tourneau A, Audouin J, Touzard R C, Diebold J. A case of primary osseous malignant immunoblastic B cell lymphoma with intracytoplasmic mu lambda immunoglobulin inclusions. Histopathology 1990: 16: 167–172
30. Ostrowski M L, Unni K K, Banks P M et al. Malignant lymphoma of bone. Cancer 1986: 58: 2646–2655
31. Radaszkiewicz T, Hansmann M L. Primary high grade malignant lymphomas of bone. Virchows Arch A Pathol Anat Histopathol 1988: 413: 269–274
32. Vassalo J, Mellin W, Pill C, Roessner A, Grundmann E. Flow cytometric DNA analysis of malignant lymphomas with primary bone manifestations. J Cancer Res Clin Oncol 1987: 113: 249–252
33. Mahoney P, Alexander R W. Primary histiocytic lymphoma of bone. A light and ultrastructural study of 4 cases. Am J Surg Pathol 1980: 4: 149–161
34. Pettit C K, Zukerberg R, Gray M H et al. Primary lymphoma of bone. A B-cell neoplasm with a high frequency of multilobated cells. Am J Surg Pathol 1990: 14: 329–334
35. Hicks D G, Gokan T, O'Keefe R J et al. Primary lymphoma of bone. Correlation of magnetic resonance imaging features with cytokine production by tumor cells. Cancer 1995: 75: 973–980
36. Neiman R S, Barcos M, Berard C et al. Granulocytic sarcoma. A clinico-pathologic study of 61 biopsied cases. Cancer 1981: 48: 1426–1437
37. Bacci G, Jaffe N, Emiliani E et al. Therapy for primary non-Hodgkin's lymphoma of bone and a comparison of results with Ewing's sarcoma. Ten years experience at the Istituto Ortopedico Rizzoli. Cancer 1986: 57: 1468–1472
38. Chan J K, Ng C S, Hui P K et al. Anaplastic large cell Ki-1 lymphoma of bone. Cancer 1991: 68: 2186–2191
39. Ishizawa M, Okabe H, Matsumoto K, Hukuda S, Hodohara K, Ota S. Anaplastic large cell Kil lymphoma with bone involvement. Report of 2 cases. Virchows Arch 1995: 427: 105–110
40. Marcelli C, Chappard D, Rossi J F et al. Histologic evidence of an abnormal bone remodeling in B-cell malignancies other than multiple myeloma. Cancer 1988: 62: 1163–1170
41. Rossi J F, Bataille R, Chappard D, Alexandre C, Janbon C. B cell malignancies presenting with unusual bone involvement and mimicking multiple myeloma. Am J Med 1987: 83: 10–16
42. Arkel Y S, Lake-Lewin D, Savopoulos A A. Bone lesions in hairy cell leukemia. A case report and response of bone pains to steroids. Cancer 1984: 53: 2401–2403
43. Demanes J, Lane N, Beckstead J H. Bone involvement in hairy-cell leukemia. Cancer 1982: 49: 1697–1701
44. Huaux J P, Noël H, Bastien P. Bony lesions in hairy cell leukemia. Various therapeutic considerations à propos of a case report. Acta Clin Belg 1984: 39: 339–351
45. Quesada J R, Keating M J, Libshitz H I. Bone involvement in hairy cell leukemia. Am J Med 1983: 74: 228–231
46. Rhyner K, Streuli R, Kistler G S. Haarzell-Leukaemie (hairy cell leukemia) mit Knochenveränderungen. Schweiz Med Wochenschr 1977: 107: 863–871
47. Herold C J, Wittich G R, Schwarzinger I. Skeletal involvement in hairy cell leukemia. Skeletal Radiol 1988: 17: 171–175
48. Colon-Otero G, McClure S P, Phyliky R L, White W L, Banks P M. Peripheral T cell lymphoma simulating Hodgkin's disease with initial bone marrow involvement. Mayo Clinic Proc 1986: 61: 68–71
49. Limb D, Dreghorn C, Murphy J K, Mannion R. Primary lymphoma of bone. Int Orthop 1994: 18: 180–183

Bone involvement in Hodgkin's lymphoma, leukemias, myeloproliferative disorders and mastocytosis

J. Diebold

CHAPTER CONTENTS

BONE INVOLVEMENT IN HODGKIN'S LYMPHOMA

Hodgkin's disease (HD) is now thought to be due to the proliferation of a lymphoid cell and the use of the term 'Hodgkin's lymphoma (HL)' is recommended. Two main types of HL have been described. The nodular paragranuloma (nodular lymphocyte-predominant HL) only rarely involves bone so only classic HL will be described. This has two subtypes: nodular sclerosing HL (NSHL) and diffuse HL (DHL).[1,2]

Incidence and clinical data

In 1988 in the USA, the incidence was 2.8 cases per 100 000 persons, with a preponderance of males over females and whites over blacks.[3] Rare in children less than 10 years of age, HL shows a peak between 20 and 30, declines until 50, then increases again. HL is more frequent in females only in the late teens and early 20s.[3,4]

Two types of bone involvement by HL have been described.

Firstly, microscopic bone marrow involvement is disclosed by trephine bone biopsy.[1,5,3,6,7–13] Such involvement is secondary to a hematogenous dissemination in patients with initial stage I or II, transforming to stage IV, but in patients with a clinical stage IV, bone marrow involvement seems to have no clinical relevance or prognostic value.[10]

Bone marrow involvement is discovered at the time of diagnosis in about 3–15% of cases.[2,5,10,11,14] The incidence increases during the evolution of the disease, reaching an average of more than 50% at autopsy.[2,3,5] Patients have constitutional symptoms and are often older than average, with a median age of 45–50 years.

Secondly, in a few patients (less than 30 published cases), initial presentation is that of bone tumor, often solitary and sometimes apparently primary.[15–29] Most frequently, in approximately 60% of these cases,[29] the bone tumor is discovered as a relapse during the evolution of treated HL.

Pain at the site of involvement is the most common symptom. Pain is deep, localized, unremitting and often nocturnal, with exacerbation after alcohol consumption. In patients with multiple sites of involvement, often only one site is painful, the others being discovered by systematic radiography.[29] Constitutional symptoms are often present, as are neurologic deficits, particularly with vertebral or skull localization.[29]

Skeletal distribution is as follows: vertebrae (lumbar or thoracic), ilium, rib, sternum, clavicle, femur, humerus, skull.[23,29–35]

Imaging

Radiologic evidence of bone involvement occurs, according to earlier studies, in 10–15% of HL,[29] but it seems to be very rare at initial presentation. Small localized lytic lesions are the most frequent changes.

In bone lesions presenting as bone tumors, the lesions, single or multiple, can be sclerotic, lytic or mixed. The majority are lytic, representing 75% of the cases in one series,[30] while in the same series only 14% of cases were sclerotic and 18% mixed. In other publications[36–38] the mixed form is more frequent (Figs 33.1–33.3). This discrepancy probably reflects a difference in criteria. An ivory vertebra is thought to be induced by a periosteal reaction secondary to adjacent lymph node involvement by contiguous spread of the disease.[30] In relapsing patients, single or multiple lesions are found with the same frequency.[29] Bone scanning can reveal additional lesions in negative radiographic areas in 33% of patients.[29]

Gross pathology

This lesion is known mainly from necropsy studies. Tumor nodules of variable size (from 1 mm to 10 cm or

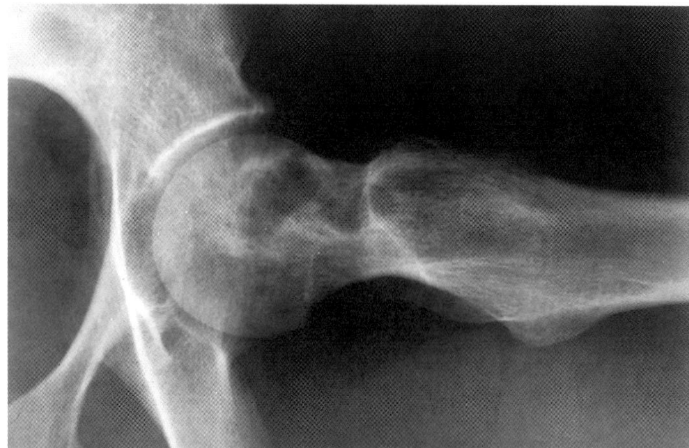

Fig. 33.1 Hodgkin's disease. Femoral involvement (Courtesy of M. Forest MD.)

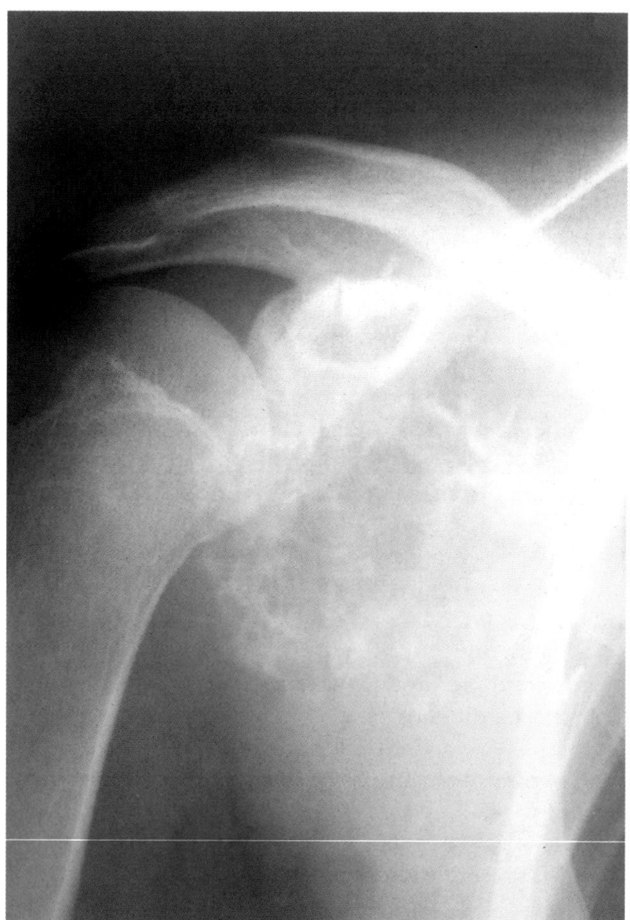

Fig. 33.2 Hodgkin's disease. Humeral involvement. (Courtesy of M. Forest MD.)

more) are seen in the bone with bone destruction. Extraosseous extension may be observed. The tumor tissue is whitish to yellowish with hemorrhagic and necrotic areas. In the rare, so-called primary HL of the bone, a

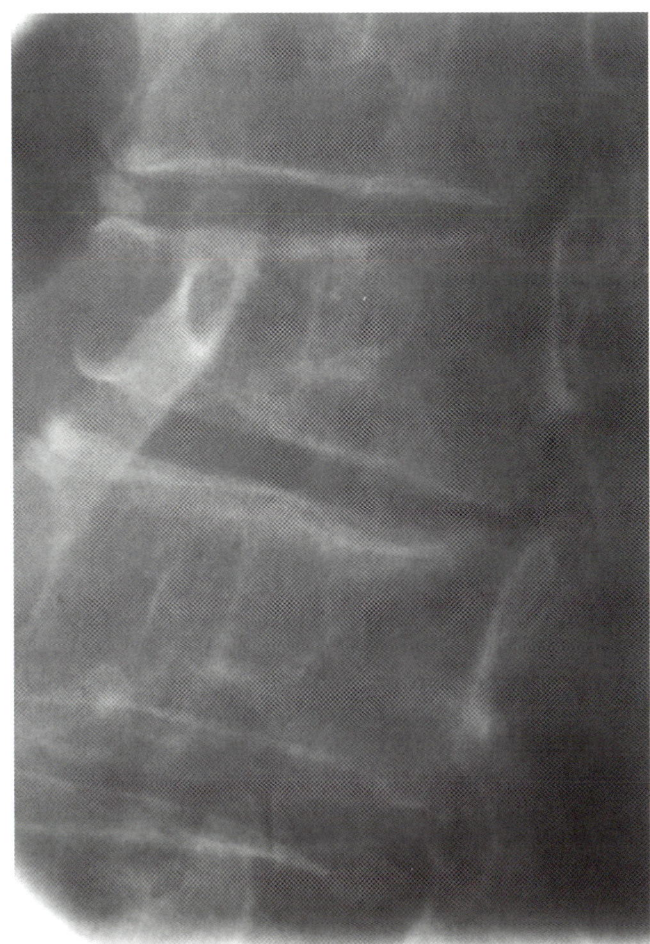

Fig. 33.3 Hodgkin's disease. Vertebral location (T11 level). (Courtesy of M. Forest MD.)

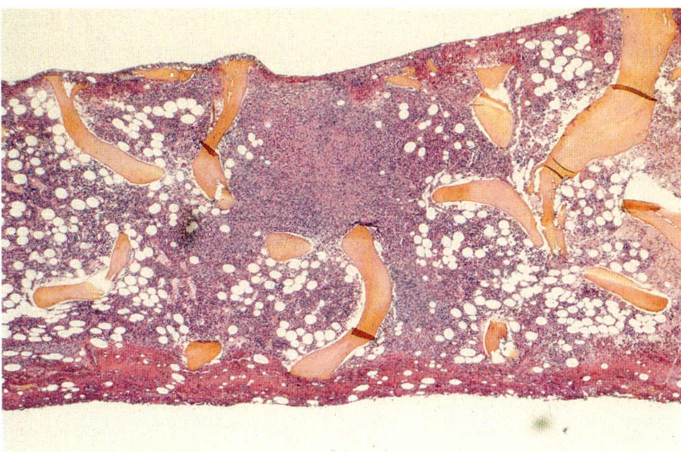

Fig. 33.4 Hodgkin's disease. Trephine biopsy of the iliac crest. Massive infiltration of a medullary space with extension into the neighboring area.

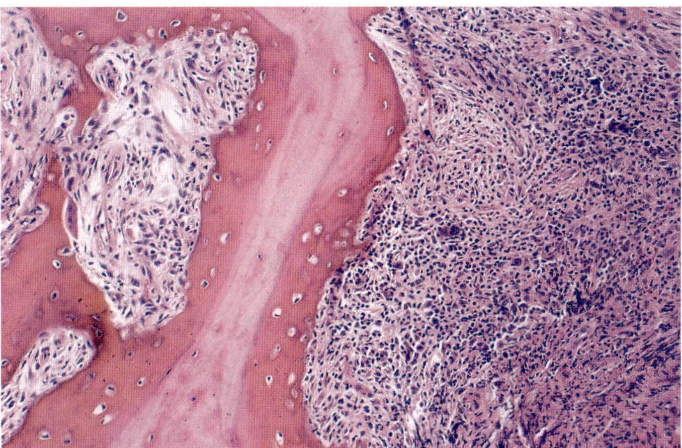

Fig. 33.5 Vertebral location of Hodgkin's disease. Near the tumor infiltrate, there is modification of the bone trabeculae (thickening due to endosteal bone formation).

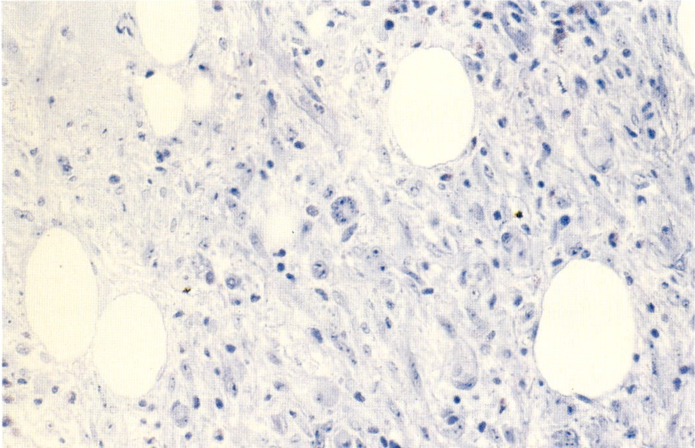

Fig. 33.6 Bone involvement in Hodgkin's disease. Classic Hodgkin's disease with fibrosis, various reactive cells and a typical Reed–Sternberg cell. (Giemsa.)

massive tumor destroys the bone with extension to the soft tissue.

Histopathology

The lesions are characterized by a fibrosis developing in bone marrow spaces, replacing the normal tissue, surrounding bone marrow trabeculae which can be normal, destroyed by osteoclast hyperplasia or thickened by new bone formation (Figs 33.4, 33.5).

In the fibrosis, a variable quantity of lymphocytes, plasma cells, histiocytes, eosinophil and neutrophil granulocytes exhibit diffuse or nodular infiltrates (Fig. 33.6). Typical Reed–Sternberg cells (RS), lacunar cells and Hodgkin's cells are dispersed in the reactive infiltrate. Areas of acidophilic necrosis are often observed.

Due to the fact that differentiation between NSHL and diffuse HL mixed cellularity can be difficult in a lymph node and almost impossible in extranodal sites, it was recommended in the past that HL in histologic subtypes outside lymph nodes should not be classified.[1,2,39] For these reasons, it is almost impossible to collect useful data from the existing literature. It seems that such tumorous bone involvement is particularly frequent in patients with NSHL.[2] The discovery of lacunar cells prompts the diagnosis of a NSHL.

In some cases, fibrosis is the main feature. RS and lacunar cells can be rare and difficult to recognize. Numerous sections should be studied. Immunohistochemistry is then very useful. In the absence of typical RS or lacunar cells, caution is recommended before proposing the diagnosis of HL in a patient with diffuse myelofibrosis, even if HL has been demonstrated in another site. Myelofibrosis of other origin, particularly iatrogenic (X-rays!), can be seen in the absence of tumor involvement. The non-involved bone marrow shows hyperplasia of one or all the main myeloid series with eosinophilia and sometimes a pseudomyeloproliferative disorder appearance. Plasma cell hyperplasia is also frequent.

Immunohistochemistry

The RS and lacunar cells express CD30 and CD15 (Fig. 33.7) but neither CD45 nor EMA.[1] A few express CD20, but not all. In rare cases, CD3 can be demonstrated in the cytoplasm. They contain granzym, perforin and Tia 1 as NK or cytotoxic lymphocytes. CD3-positive lymphocytes are present around the tumor cells, in a rosette pattern. CD68 demonstrates the presence of a variable number of histiocytes. A few CD20-positive B cells are present, often in small nests. Plasma cells are polyclonal. Tumor cells are associated with EBV in about 35% of cases, the RS cells being positive for LMP-1 and EBER 1, respectively demonstrated by immunohistochemistry and in situ hybridization.

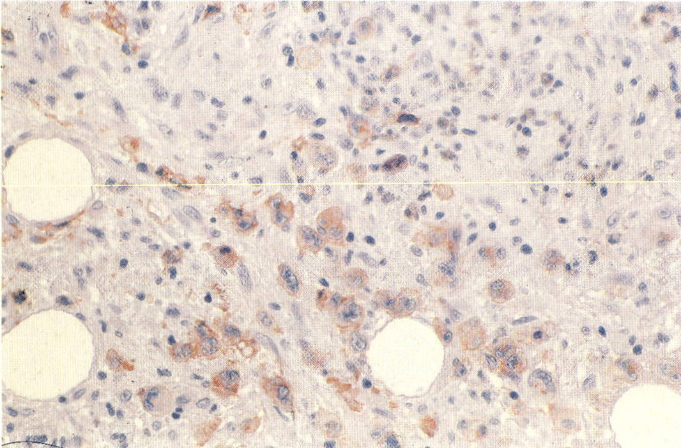

Fig. 33.7 Same case. Many Reed–Sternberg cells express CD15. The same picture was obtained with CD30. Immunoperoxidase, ABC amplification technique, with a monoclonal antibody recognizing CD15.

Differential diagnosis

HL should not be confused with:

- Langerhans cell histiocytosis (eosinophilic granuloma of the bone): the morphology of the typical histiocytes is completely different from RS or lacunar cells;
- peripheral T cell malignant lymphoma: RS cells can be present but the surrounding population is tumorous and immunohistochemistry is helpful;
- myelofibrosis secondary to fracture, radiotherapy, chemotherapy, etc.

Treatment

A microscopic bone marrow involvement represents the result of a hematogenous extension corresponding to stage IV of the Ann Arbor staging system. Lytic bone tumors are also interpreted as being the result of hematogenous extension. In fact, it seems that the majority of so-called primary HL of the bone are secondary to direct invasion from an adjacent lymph node, leading to a local bony lesion corresponding to a stage IE with the same prognosis as a local nodal disease.[15,25] According to the clinical/surgical staging, patients should be treated with radiotherapy and chemotherapy or chemotherapy alone. Bone marrow allograft is also often used.

Disease course and prognosis

In the past the 5-year survival was estimated to be generally less than 10%.[30,40] It is difficult to judge the effects of modern treatment on bone involvement in HL. This condition is rare and only small series have been published.[15,16] It seems that such a tumorous presentation does not affect the survival curve if the treatment is correct.[13,15]

Avascular necrosis of bone was an infrequent complication which occurred in the past in HL patients treated with combination chemotherapy including steroids, often in conjunction with radiotherapy. Osteonecrosis was often localized in the femoral and/or humoral heads[41] or in sternum and ribs.[42] A swelling of the sternum was the first symptom. Only tomography revealed lesions presenting as irregularly shaped areas of decreased density. A biopsy was performed showing pieces of living and necrotic bone surrounded by fibrosis with an inflammatory infiltrate comprising granulocytes but also lymphocytes and plasma cells. No remaining tumorous infiltrate could be recognized.

Comments for the surgical pathologist

A diagnosis of HL should not be made in the absence of typical RS or lacunar cells. The study of multiple sections is mandatory and immunohistochemistry should always be performed.

BONE INVOLVEMENT IN ACUTE LEUKEMIA

Frequency

Bone pain occurs in about 60% of these patients, representing one of the initial symptoms in 25% of cases.[3,43,44] In almost all cases, bone involvement is disclosed by imaging.[43]

Clinical presentation

Bone pain can be the first clinical symptom of an acute leukemia, particularly in a child. The onset is often sudden, with fever. The pain can be either intermittent or constant. Bone pain can appear after trauma. The pain is frequently sharp, severe and well localized, with exquisite tenderness[3,43] (Schajowicz 1994), but it can also be mild and poorly defined.

Various long bones may be the site of pain. Bones in the lower extremity are involved twice as frequently as those in the upper extremity.[43] The vertebral column as well as pelvis and ribs can also be affected. Pain localized to joints is also frequent, causing migratory arthralgia[43–46] which simulates rheumatic fever or rheumatoid arthritis. Such pain involves mainly the knees, but also the shoulders and hands. Commonly both hands and knees are involved simultaneously. At variable intervals, successive joint involvement may be observed. The joints are sometimes swollen and tender to touch. Erythema may be present. A tumorous presentation has also been described.[47–50]

Skeletal distribution

The lesions are observed preferentially in tubular bones, in the proximal end of the humerus, in the femur and the tibia, mainly near the knee (Huvos 1991, Schajowicz 1994). In addition, vertebrae, ribs and pelvis may also be involved.

Imaging[50–55] (Huvos 1991, Schajowicz 1994)

Clinical symptoms may be present and even severe without radiographic lesions. On the other hand, roentgenographic modifications can often exist in the absence of clinical symptoms, for example without pain.[43,50,53]

Mild radiographic alterations, listed below, can be observed in the majority of patients with leukemia independently from the histologic type, whether acute myeloblastic, myelomonoblastic or lymphoblastic (Fig. 33.8). More extensive lesions are present in about 50% of cases.

1. *Metaphyseal radiolucent bands.* The earliest changes in children are represented by slender transverse radiolu-

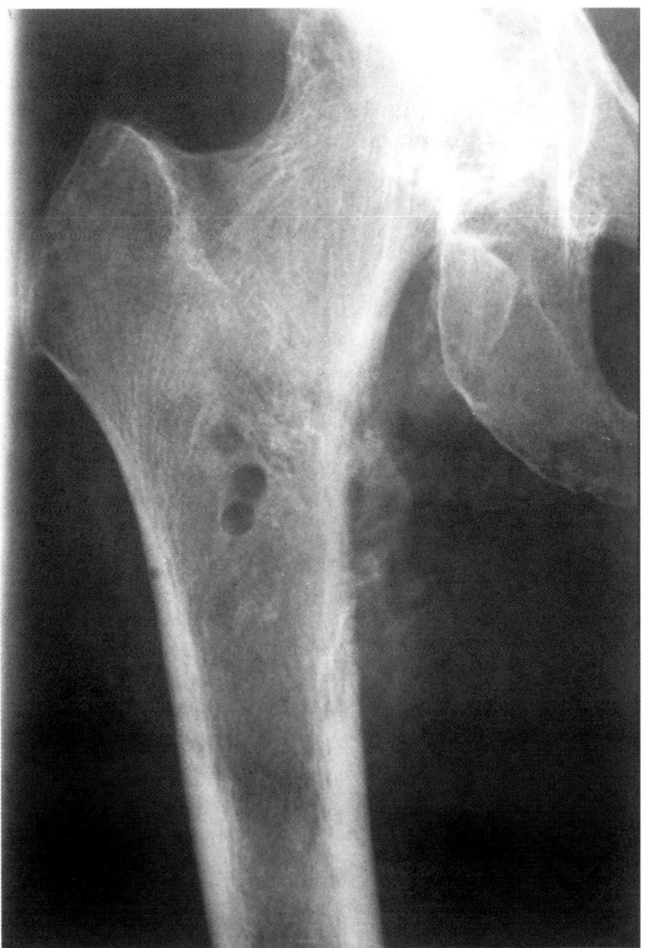

Fig. 33.8 Femoral location of an acute myeloblastic leukemia. (Courtesy of M. Forest MD.)

cent zones in the epiphyseal-diaphyseal areas. These lesions are discovered in long tubular bones. They are rarely observed in adults due to epiphyseal fusion. In flat bones, ilium and ischium, they are seen beneath the cortex.

The bands measure between 2 and 15 mm in width and are often bilateral. These lesions are nonspecific and are also seen in malnutrition and in diverse other diseases. They are more suggestive of acute leukemia after 2 years of age.[43] The radiolucent bands seem to be the result of decreased bone formation.

2. *Spontaneous fractures.* These can occur at the site of radiolucent bands, involving mainly the capital femoral epiphyses and the proximal humeral epiphyses.

3. *'Growth arrest' lines.* In the metaphysis of tubular bones, particularly in children, transverse lines of increased density are often seen. In these dense lines, the bone spicules are larger than the spicules in adjacent areas and comprise unabsorbed calcified cartilaginous matrix.

4. *Osteolytic lesions.* The earliest lesions of this type are responsible for punctate areas, one of the most character-

istic radiographic patterns observed in patients with acute leukemia. They show a moth-eaten appearance in long bone metaphyses.[47,51,52] The punctate lesions can coalesce, forming a diffuse or confluent radiolucency, often with a striated appearance. In advanced disease, confluent destruction can be observed, corresponding to lysis and necrosis of the trabecular bone with areas of hemorrhage.

Solitary leukemic pseudotumorous nodules totally replacing bone trabeculae and extending to the adjacent soft tissue are responsible for so-called geographic lesions. This radiographic pattern corresponds to granulocytic sarcoma.[47,48,50,52]

5. *Cortical and periosteal lesions*. Half of leukemic children present with destructive cortical lesions, with or without periosteal reaction, located mostly in the metaphysis of the femur. These lesions seem to be particularly painful.

Periosteal reaction with new bone formation is seen mainly along the diaphysis of the tibia and fibula but also along the lateral sides of the ilium, superior margin of the ischium and inferior margin of the pubis.

6. *Osteosclerotic lesions*. In some cases, increased radiopacity can occur. Such focal or diffuse osteosclerotic changes are often isolated. They may also be associated with radiolucent modifications or periosteal osteogenesis.

Histopathology

General pattern

In all cases, the bone marrow spaces are heavily infiltrated by leukemic cells, replacing the normal fat tissue and the hematopoietic cells. Bony trabeculae are often thin with irregular outlines.[58] Cortical destruction and subperiosteal new bone formation are also often observed. In some cases, bony trabeculae are thickened, surrounded by fibrosis with some osteoclasts corresponding to the so-called osteosclerosis.

Lymphoblastic acute leukemia (Fig. 33.9)

The bone marrow spaces are diffusely infiltrated by small to medium lymphoid cells with an ovoid, often convoluted nucleus, one or two small nucleoli and a pale cytoplasm. Mitosis is frequent. Many dispersed macrophages sometimes cause a starry-sky pattern. Large necrotic areas may be seen in some spaces. Only immunohistochemistry allows distinction of B or T origin by demonstrating that the leukemic cells express the phenotype of an immature T cell (thymocyte) or B cell (B, pre-B, pre-pre-B). The demonstration of a tdt expression allows clearcut distinction from some other types of B or T cell malignant lymphomas.

Myeloblastic, monoblastic or myelomonoblastic acute leukemia

Myeloblasts are large cells with ovoid or kidney-shaped

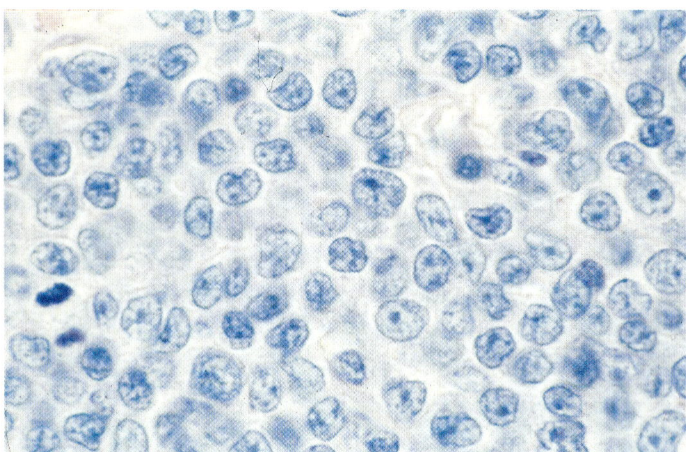

Fig. 33.9 Acute lymphoblastic-leukemia. Medium-sized cells with roundish, more or less irregular nuclei (convoluted), with small nucleoli and pale cytoplasm. Mitoses can be numerous. (Giemsa.)

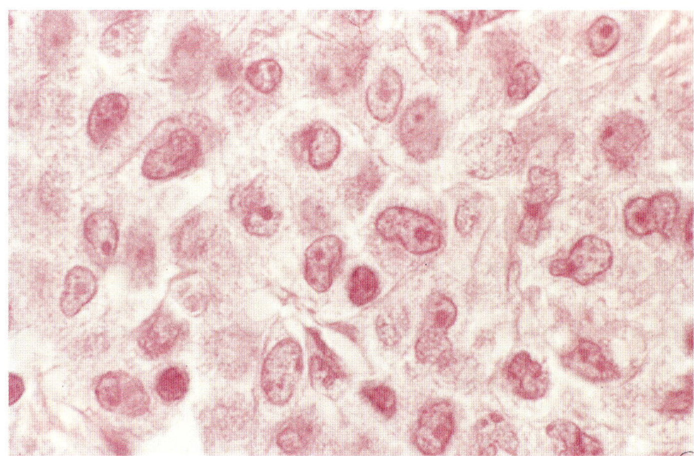

Fig. 33.10 Acute myeloblastic-leukemia. Large, ovoid, often kidney-shaped nucleus and a large granular cytoplasm.

nuclei (Fig. 33.10), one or two small nucleoli and azurophilic or neutrophilic granules in the extensive cytoplasm (Fig. 33.11). In these cells, a naphthol ASD chloracetate esterase can be demonstrated by the Leder reaction on paraffin sections. They contain myeloperoxidase, lysozyme and elastase demonstrable by immunohistochemistry. These blasts are also CD15 and CD34 positive.

Monoblasts are sometimes round with an ovoid or kidney-shaped nucleus, surrounded by a pale gray cytoplasm without granules (Fig. 33.12). Sometimes the nucleus can be very irregular. These cells are CD68 positive and they contain lysozyme but no myeloperoxidase.

Granulocytic sarcoma

This is a solid tumor composed of myelo and/or monoblasts destroying the bone architecture and responsible for large

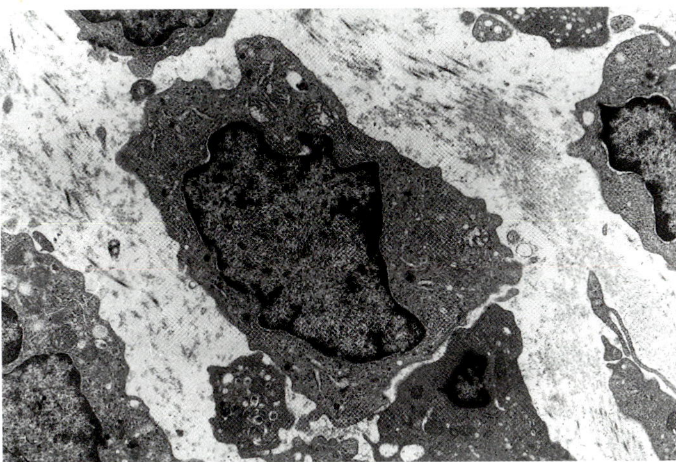

Fig. 33.11 Acute myeloblastic leukemia. Presence of granulations in the cytoplasm of the malignant cells. (Epon-embedded tissue.)

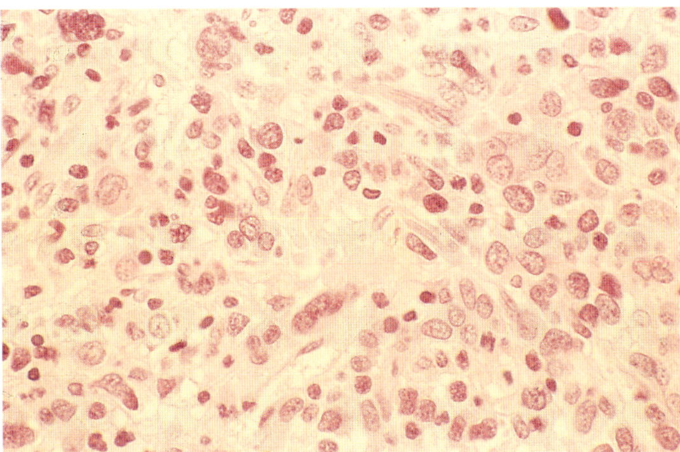

Fig. 33.13 Acute megakaryoblastic leukemia with diffuse collagenous fibrosis. Note the medium and large cells corresponding to immature cells.

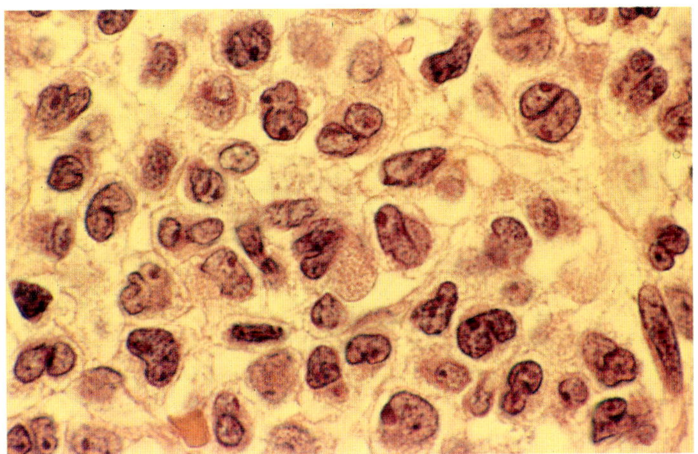

Fig. 33.12 Acute monoblastic leukemia. The leukemic cells show irregular, twisted nuclei and large pale cytoplasm.

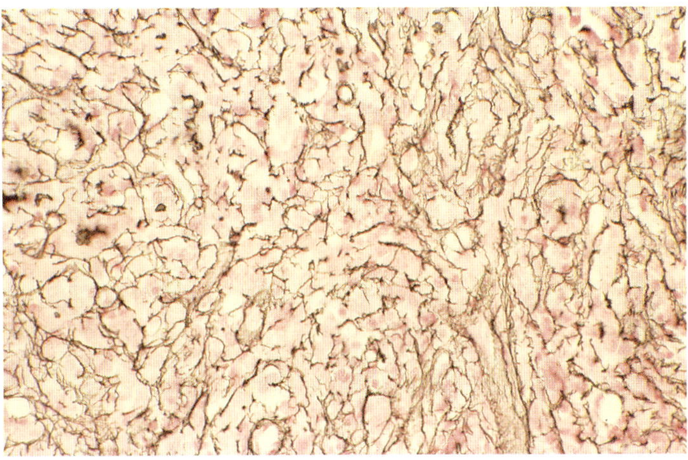

Fig. 33.14 Same case. Diffuse fibrosis. (Silver impregnation according to Gordon-Sweet.)

lytic lesions of bone.[3,47,49,50–53,58–60] This tumor mainly occurs in the skull, ribs, spine and sternum and more often in children. It was called chloroma in the past due to a transitory greenish color visible on macroscopic study, secondary to the presence of a green myeloperoxidase pigment. Such a tumor may occur in patients with chronic myeloproliferative disorders such as CML or primary myelofibrosis.

Acute megakaryoblastic leukemia (Fig. 33.13)

Some of these are associated with a diffuse severe collagen myelofibrosis (Fig. 33.14) destroying the hematopoietic tissue.[61] The blastic cells are small and difficult to distinguish from blastic cells of other origin. In other cases, atypical megakaryocytes can be observed, some of which can be labeled with antibodies recognizing factor VIII-related antigen, H and Y blood groups (BNH9) and platelet glycoprotein II b/III. New bone formation can be

responsible for sclerotic lesions of bone at the radiographic level. In some cases, the development of large localized megakaryocytic or megakaryoblastic proliferation can be responsible for localized osteolytic lesions.[52]

Bone infarction

In about 15% of patients with acute lymphoblastic leukemia, bone infarction can be disclosed either during life or at autopsy. Such ischemic necrosis occurs at any time during the disease. Two mechanisms have been suggested: invasion of the vessel wall and occlusion of periosteal arteries or insufficiency of oxygen supply to the large leukemic cell masses. Such infarction shows no specific radiographic changes, but is often the major cause of severe bone pain. Extensive areas of ischemic necrosis destroy the densely infiltrated bone marrow tissue with bone necrosis. Myelofibrosis is often present in the adjacent bone marrow spaces. This myelofibrosis is probably secondary to fibroblast stimulation by cytokines produced by either the leukemic cells or stimulated adjacent reactive cells.

Course and prognosis

The degree of bone involvement in leukemia has no prognostic significance.[43,62,63] All the radiologic and clinical symptoms disappear with treatment. During relapse, the location and character of bone pain are similar to those at the time of initial diagnosis and radiologic changes reappear.

Methotrexate induces bone changes. This drug is responsible for severe bone pain in the lower extremities, osteoporosis and fracture. Pain increases progressively. The role of methotrexate may be suspected when blood and sternal puncture smears and bone marrow biopsy do not disclose leukaemic infiltrate. Withdrawal of methotrexate is usually followed by disappearance of pain.

Patients with bone infarction seem to have a shorter survival. The prognostic value of myelofibrosis is controversial. In some series, it is regarded as having a bad influence on survival while in other series, its presence does not seems to indicate a bad prognosis.

Differential diagnosis

The clinical presentation can mimic rheumatic fever, rheumatoid arthritis, septic arthritis or osteomyelitis. Some radiographic changes are not specific and radiolucent bands can be observed in other diseases, for example in malnutrition.

At the histopathologic level, the main differential diagnosis is represented by malignant lymphomas, for example B-CLL, Burkitt's lymphoma and even centroblastic lymphoma or diverse T cell malignant lymphoma. One of the most difficult diagnosis is represented by a blastic transformation of a mantle zone lymphoma with bone marrow involvement; demonstration of an expression of bcl-1 can be very useful here.

BONE INVOLVEMENT IN CHRONIC MYELOPROLIFERATIVE DISORDERS

Frequency

Bone marrow is always modified in the chronic myeloproliferative disorders but bone lesions are induced only in certain cases and in some types of myeloproliferative disorder, particularly during transformation. Such lesions remain rare[64-66] (Schajowicz 1994).

Clinical presentation

Bone pain in extremities[64,67] (Huvos 1991) and sternal tenderness or tumor formation[69] have been reported as the initial manifestations of acute blastic transformation of CML and idiopathic myelofibrosis.[51]

Spontaneous fracture and arthralgias simulating rheumatoid arthritis have also been reported. In addition, clinical symptoms and biological modifications typical of such chronic myeloproliferative disorders can be found.

Imaging

In CML, rare bone lesions are of the osteolytic type.[67,69-73] Extensive destruction of the head of the femur has been described. In idiopathic myelofibrosis, diffuse areas of sclerosis are found in long bones and ilium.[72,74]

Histopathology

A bone marrow trephine biopsy allows distinction between the different types of chronic myeloproliferative disorder and helps to establish a precise diagnosis.[3,75-77]

In CML, the marrow appears densely packed, due to the proliferation of the granulocytic series. Large sheets of immature myeloid precursors with the morphology of myelocytes, promyelocytes and some metamyelocytes are seen surrounding the bone trabeculae and often the arteries. Granulocytes accumulate in the central regions of the medullary spaces, around the sinuses. The number of eosinophils is increased. Erythropoiesis is reduced, comprising normal, mainly mature erythroblasts. Megakaryocytes can be rare or numerous, with some heterotopia and a few small forms. Macrophages are present, containing vacuoles or hemosiderin. Some may contain lipofuscin stained blue by Giemsa's solution (sea-blue histiocytes). In rare cases, macrophages resemble Gaucher cells.

Bone trabeculae can be normal or may show rarefaction. The reticulum framework is often normal. A slight systematized myelofibrosis may be observed.

Two subtypes have been described according to the presence or absence of associated proliferation of the megakaryocytic series. The unilinear granulocytic type may transform in blastic crisis.[50] The bilinear granulocytic-megakaryocytic type may transform to myelofibrosis or osteomyelofibrosis which decreases the risk of developing blastic crisis.[50,75] There are no morphologic differences between Ph1 chromosome-positive or negative cases.

Myelofibrosis/osteomyelofibrosis[3,74-76] can be secondary to previous chronic myeloproliferative disorders or to other diseases (metastasis, bone disease, drugs, etc.), or may be primary (agnogenic myeloid metaplasia). Three grades can be distinguished:

1. diffuse reticulum fibers increase with thickening of the normal network;
2. fine and coarse fibrosis develop around megakaryocyte clusters and vessels;

3. diffuse coarse collagenous fibrosis destroying the bone marrow tissue.

Numerous elongated megakaryocytes are present between the collagen bundles and in the lumen of the dilated sinuses.

Primitive bone production also shows great variation from one case to another. Three grades can be defined[3,74–77] (Schajowicz 1994):

1. small foci of new bone formation;
2. thickening of the trabeculae by endosteal new bone associated with metaplastic bone arising from myelofibrosis (Fig. 33.15);
3. complete replacement of the trabeculae by a network of primitive bone with reduction of the size of the bone marrow spaces (Fig. 33.16).

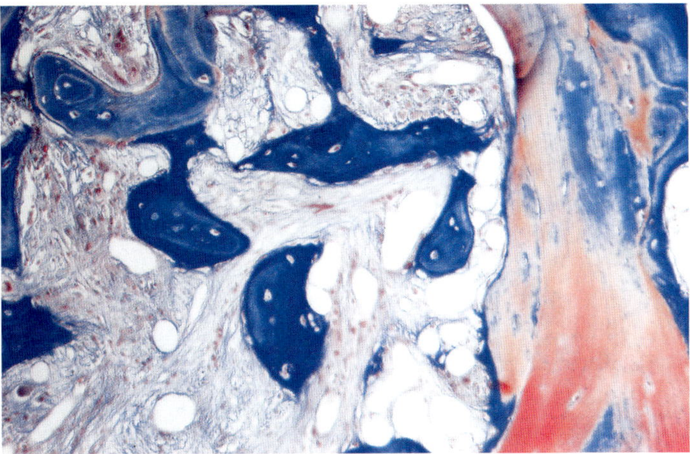

Fig. 33.15 Agnogenic myeloid metaplasia. Typical osteomyelosclerosis with metaplastic osteogenesis arising from the collagenous myelofibrosis. (Masson's trichrome stain.)

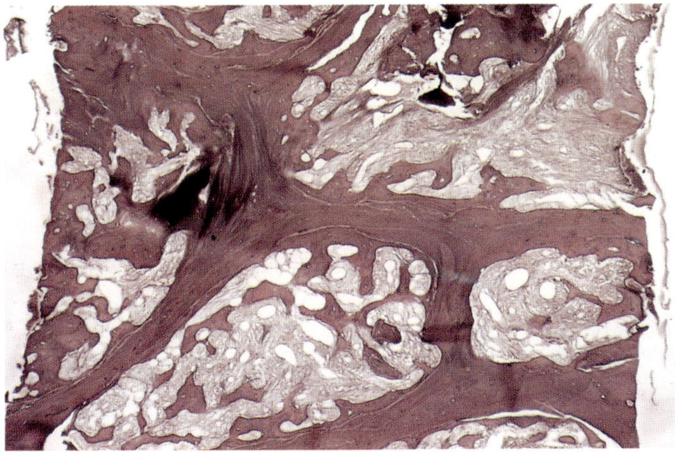

Fig. 33.16 Agnogenic myeloid metaplasia. This low magnification demonstrates the importance of diffuse myelofibrosis and of new bone formation, progressively reducing the active bone marrow. (Silver impregnation according to Gordon-Sweet.)

Prognosis

Bone lesions have prognostic value only when they reflect a blastic crisis. The symptoms and the lesions disappear under treatment, but reappear during relapses.

As in acute leukemia, methotrexate can be responsible for painful bone lesions (Schajowicz 1994).

BONE INVOLVEMENT IN SYSTEMIC MASTOCYTOSIS

Introduction and clinical data

Mastocytosis represents an abnormal proliferation of mast cells in one or more organs. Bone is involved particularly in systemic mastocytosis, which represents approximately 10% of mastocytosis cases. Such multivisceral mastocytosis can be observed at any age from young adults to advanced age (median age ranging from 48 to 71 years in different series).[3]

Patients with skin localization are younger than those without. Both sexes can be involved, with a slight predominance of males.

Two main types of systemic mastocytosis can be distinguished:[78–81]

1. a *benign or indolent type*, characterized by skin involvement, associated with hepatosplenomegaly but without constitutional symptoms;
2. an *aggressive or malignant type*, with multiorgan involvement but without skin localization.
   Constitutional symptoms vary greatly between patients but include fatigue, fever, night sweats and weight loss.

In both types, symptoms due to the release of chemical mediators produced by mast cells, particularly histamine, can be observed. Flush syndrome, generalized pruritis, headache, tachycardia, hypotension and syncope can be experienced. These symptoms are much more important in patients with aggressive mastocytosis. Drugs or other factors can be responsible for eliciting these symptoms. Many other symptoms have been described: abdominal pain, nausea, vomiting, diarrhea, gastrointestinal bleeding, bronchospasm, arthralgia, diverse neurologic and psychiatric manifestations.

Among laboratory findings, one of the most important is represented by serum elevation of histamine, prostaglandin D2 or their metabolites, heparin and particularly tryptase. Hematologic abnormalities are frequent. A bone tumor presentation revealed by radiography or spontaneous fracture has been reported in a few cases.

Skeletal distribution

The bones most frequently involved are the ilium and tubular bones, particularly the femur and the humerus.

Imaging

Several radiographic changes have been described. Such modifications are found in about 70% of cases of systemic mastocytosis.[82–84] These changes include:

1. *circumscribed osteolytic areas*: roundish small osteolytic zones can be seen in the diaphysis or metaphysis of tubular bones (femur, tibia) or in the skull;
2. *circumscribed sclerotic areas*: dense roundish or rectangular areas are observed in tubular bones or vertebrae;
3. *generalized osteoporosis*: these changes often predominate in the vertebrae[82,83,85] but can also be observed in the ribs and ilium. Spontaneous fractures may be observed, particularly vertebral compression fractures;[83,85–87]
4. *generalized osteosclerosis*: bones of the thorax, pelvis, spine, skull and particularly long bones (humerus, femur, radius) show diffuse dense modifications with thickening of the cortex and narrowing of the medulla;
5. an association of different types of lesions is frequently seen, comprising mixed osteosclerotic and osteoporotic processes.

Histopathology[3,78–81]

In *indolent systemic mastocytosis*, the bone marrow shows multiple nodular lesions. These lesions are composed of small nests of large, roundish, ovoid or fusiform cells with a pale cytoplasm showing a faint eosinophilic granular pattern on H & E stain (Fig. 33.17). Staining with Giemsa or toluidine blue solutions reveals the presence of densely packed metachromatic granules obscuring the nucleus (Fig. 33.18). A few mast cells show degranulation.

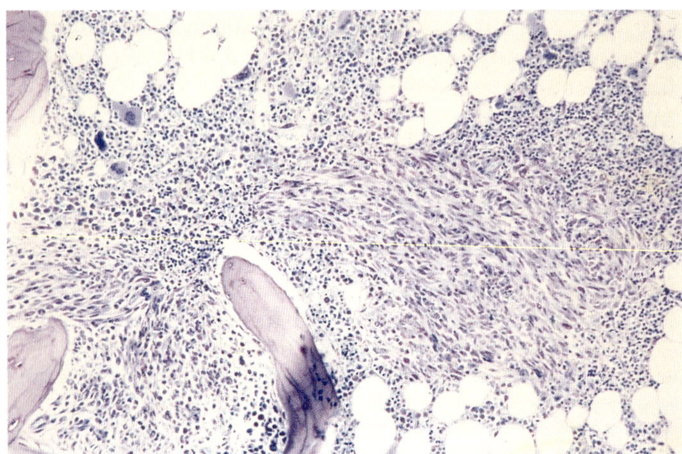

Fig. 33.17 Systemic mastocytosis, associated with primary thrombocytemia. Two nodules composed of fusiform cells (mast cells) are recognizable, surrounded by lymphoid cells. Note the presence of numerous giant megakaryocytes in the bone marrow as seen in thrombocytemia. (Giemsa.)

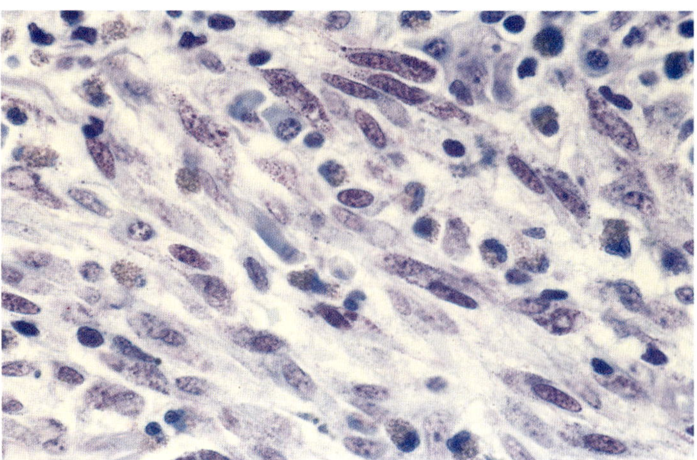

Fig. 33.18 Same case. This higher magnification allows recognition of the presence of metachromatic granules typical of mast cells in the majority of fusiform cells. Note also the numerous lymphocytes and plasma cells. (Giemsa.)

Around these nests of mast cells, fibroblasts and collagen bundles produce a more or less extended fibrosis. Numerous small lymphocytes surround these nodules. Nests of mature plasma cells are frequently observed as well as iron-laden macrophages. Foci of eosinophils are also frequent.

The mast cells are all of the same size with a single regular nucleus, elongated, roundish or reniform, and a small nucleolus. Due to their shape mast cells can be confused with fibroblasts, histiocytes or plasma cells. The nodules show either peritrabecular or perivascular localization. They are dispersed in the bone marrow spaces. The adjacent bone marrow is normocellular or hyperplastic. Sometimes a chronic myeloproliferative disorder, a myelodysplastic syndrome or even a malignant lymphoma may be found.

In *aggressive malignant mastocytosis*, diffuse infiltrates of the bone marrow spaces are seen. The mast cells are often large with irregular nuclei and big nucleoli. They are often binucleated. Mitoses are frequent. The extensive cytoplasm contains a variable number of metachromatin granules. Some cells are more or less degranulated. These cells form large sheets, destroying and replacing the normal bone marrow (Fig. 33.19). A few eosinophils are dispersed between the mast cells. Fibrotic bands of variable thickness are observed throughout or around the tumorous sheets.

Bone trabeculae show important modifications due to accelerated bone remodeling. The trabeculae are thickened by endosteal and metamorphic bone formation and they are surrounded by a collagenous fibrosis. There are greater numbers of osteoblasts and osteoclasts, with an increase in osteoclastic resorbing surface.[86]

Cytology

Imprints or smears exhibit numerous mast cells. The copi-

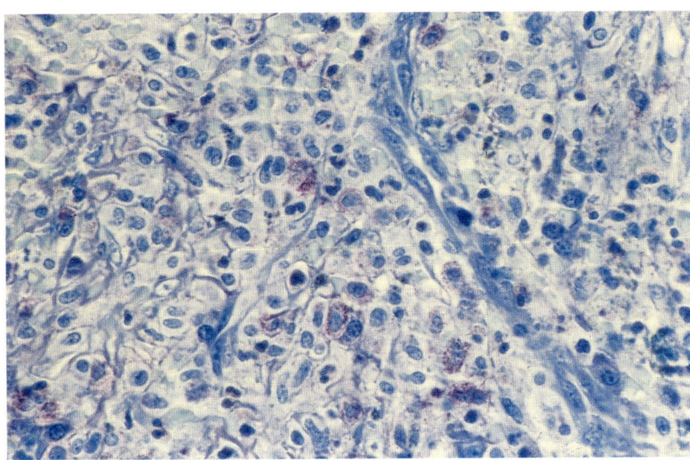

Fig. 33.19 Malignant systemic mastocytosis. The bone marrow is diffusely invaded and destroyed by roundish cells with a large pale cytoplasm and an ovoid or kidney-shaped, sometimes bilobed nucleus. A variable number of metachromatic granules can be seen in the cytoplasm of these cells. Collagen fibers are increased (myelofibrosis). (Giemsa.)

ous cytoplasm of the cells is filled by many violet metachromatic coarse granules. The cells are round or ovoid, resembling plasma cells or fusiform fibroblasts.

Histo- and cytoenzymology and immunohistochemistry[3,78–81]

The granules are well stained by Giemsa and toluidine blue, showing metachromasia, and are alcian blue positive. They exhibit a spontaneous fluorescence after acridin orange staining. On frozen section, tryptase activity can be demonstrated. On formalin-fixed undecalcified tissue, the cells are positive with the Leder reaction, corresponding to the activity of a naphthol ASD chloracetate esterase, but this reaction is not positive after decalcification. Peroxidases are negative.

Immunohistochemistry is not really useful. Most cells contain vimentin, lysozyme and elastase. They are positive for CD68 as histiomonocytes.

Cytogenetics

Abnormalities have been found, comparable to those seen in chronic myeloproliferative disorders (5q-, 11q-). No specific chromosomal abnormality has been shown.

Ultrastructural findings

The mast cells in systemic mastocytosis exhibit typical granules, small or medium, containing dense material with scrolls or lamellae. Degranulation is observed in many cells with empty vacuoles replacing the granules.

Differential diagnosis

The radiologic changes seen in systemic mastocytosis may suggest many diseases: carcinomatous metastases, Paget's disease, multiple myeloma, lymphomas, Hodgkin's lymphoma, chronic myeloproliferative disorders (mainly idiopathic myelofibrosis) or fluorosis. An iliac crest bone marrow trephine biopsy is very useful, allowing easy diagnosis.

At the histological level, a Giemsa stain allows elimination of lymphomas, myeloid cell proliferations and carcinomatous metastasis.

Course

A benign systemic mastocytosis can exist for many years and patients often die from unrelated causes.[3] The evolution is shorter in malignant systemic mastocytosis. The following factors are associated with a poor prognosis: old age, constitutional symptoms, abnormal liver function tests, anemia, thrombocytopenia, diffuse bone marrow infiltrate, anisokaryosis, binucleated cells, association with chronic myeloproliferative disorders, acute myeloid leukemia, myelodysplasia, malignant lymphoma.[3,78–81]

Treatment

No curative treatment is currently known. The treatment is largely supportive. H1 and/or H2 histamine receptor antagonists are used. Substances inhibiting degranulation have also been used, as well as inhibitors of bone resorption. Chemotherapy associated with steroids and/or radiotherapy is indicated in aggressive malignant mastocytosis.

REFERENCES

1. Diebold J, Jungman P, Molina T, Audouin J. Recent advances in Hodgkin's disease: an overview and review of the literature. Curr Diagn Pathol 1995: 2: 153–162
2. Dorfman R F. Relationship of histology to site in Hodgkin's disease. Cancer Res 1971: 31: 1786–1793
3. Brunning R D, McKenna R W. Tumors of the bone marrow. Atlas of tumor pathology, 3rd series, fasc 9. Washington: AFIP, 1994, pp 369–379
4. Gross S B, Robertson W W Jr, Lange B J, Bunin N J, Drummond D S. Primary Hodgkin's disease of bone. A report of 2 cases in adolescents and review of the literature. Clin Orthop 1992: 283: 276–280
5. Diebold J, Temmim L, Bernadou A. La biopsie médullaire osseuse au cours de la maladie de Hodgkin. Sem Hop Paris 1977: 53: 103–111
6. Duhamel G, Najman A, André R. Les localisations à la moëlle osseuse de la maladie de Hodgkin. Leur place dans l'évolution de la maladie. Etude par biopsie médullaire de 100 observations. Nouv Presse Med 1971: 79: 2305–2308
7. Han T, Stutzman L, Rogue A L. Bone marrow biopsy in Hodgkin's

disease and other neoplastic diseases. JAMA 1971: 217: 1239–1241

8. Horan F T. Bone marrow involvement in Hodgkin's disease. Br J Surg 1969: 56: 277–281

9. Kaplan H S. Hodgkin's disease. 2nd ed. Cambridge: Harvard University Press, 1980, pp 220–222

10. Munker R, Hasenclever D, Brosteanu O, Hiller E, Diehl V. Bone marrow involvement in Hodgkin's disease: an analysis of 135 consecutive cases. J Clin Oncol 1995: 13: 403–409

11. O'Carroll D I, McKenna R W, Brunning R D. Bone marrow manifestations of Hodgkin's disease. Cancer 1976: 38: 1717–1728

12. Pris J, Fabre J, Corberand J et al. Biopsies de moëlle et maladie de Hodgkin. Nouv Rev Fr Hemat 1973: 13: 410–415

13. Webb D I, Ubogy G, Silver R T. Importance of bone marrow biopsy in the clinical staging of Hodgkin's disease. Cancer 1970: 26: 313–317

14. Rosenberg S A. Hodgkin's disease of the bone marrow. Cancer Res 1971: 31: 1733–1736

15. Abbondanzo S L, Devaney K. Hodgkin's disease involving bone and adjacent soft tissue in adults. A clinicopathologic and immunophenotypic study of 7 cases. Int J Surg Pathol 1996: 3: 147–154

16. Arnold H S, Meese E H, D'Amato N A, Maughon J S. Localized Hodgkin's disease presenting as a sternal tumor and treated by total sternectomy. Ann Thorac Surg 1966: 2: 87–93

17. Borg M F, Chowdhury A D, Bhoopal S, Benjamin C S. Bone involvement in Hodgkin's disease. Australas Radiol 1993: 37: 63–66

18. Chan K W, Rosen G, Miller D P, Tan C T. Hodgkin's disease in adolescents presenting as a primary bone lesion. A report of 4 cases and review of the literature. Am J Pediatr Hematol Oncol 1982: 4: 11–17

19. Eustace S, O'Regan R, Graham D, Carney D. Primary multifocal skeletal Hodgkin's disease confined to bone. Skeletal Radiol 1995: 24: 61–63

20. Fried G, Ben Arieh Y, Haim N, Dale J, Stein M. Primary Hodgkin's disease of the bone. Med Pediatr Oncol 1995: 24: 204–207

21. Gold R H, Mirra J M. Case report 101. Primary Hodgkin disease of humerus. Skeletal Radiol 1979: 4: 233–235

22. Kooreman P J, Haex A J. Hodgkin's disease of the skeleton. Acta Med Scand 1943: 115: 177–196

23. MacCormick R, Covert A, Gross M. Primary bony involvement in Hodgkin's disease. Can Med Assoc J 1989: 140: 1059–1060

24. Ozdemirli M, Mankin H J, Aisenberg A C, Harris N L. Hodgkin's disease presenting as a solitary bone tumor. A report of 4 cases and review of the literature. Cancer 1996: 77: 79–88

25. Parker B R, Marglin S, Castellino R A. Skeletal manifestations of leukemia, Hodgkin's disease and non Hodgkin's lymphoma. Semin Roentgenol 1980: 15: 302–315

26. Spencer J, Dresser R. Lymphoblastoma (Hodgkin's and sarcoma type) of bone. N Engl J Med 1936: 214: 877–879

27. Sullivan W T, Solonick D M. Case report 414. Nodular sclerosing Hodgkin disease involving sternum and chest wall. Skeletal Radiol 1987: 16: 166–169

28. Vassalo J, Roessner A, Vollmer E, Grundmann E. Malignant lymphomas with primary bone manifestation. Pathol Res Pract 1987: 182: 381–389

29. Newcomer L N, Silverstein M B, Cadman E C, Farber L R, Bertino J R, Prosnitz I R. Bone involvement in Hodgkin's disease. Cancer 1982: 49: 338–342

30. Granger W, Whitaker P. Hodgkin's disease in bone with special reference to periosteal reaction. Br J Radiol 1967: 40: 939–948

31. Lecanet D, Bernageux J, Basch A, Goguel A, Bismuth V. Localisations osseuses de la maladie de Hodgkin. Ann Radiol 1971: 14: 845–861

32. Manoli A 2nd, Blaustein J C, Pedersen H E. Sternal Hodgkin's disease. Report of 2 cases. Clin Orthop 1988: 228: 20–25

33. Meher-Homji D R, De Souza L J, Mohanty B, Calcuttawalla T F. Unusual sternal mass in Hodgkin's disease. A case report. J Bone Joint Surg (Am) 1972: 54: 402–404

34. Vieta J O, Friedell H L, Craver L F. A survey of Hodgkin's disease and lymphosarcoma in bone. Radiology 1942: 39: 1–15

35. Zenni J C, Alm D, Grenier P H, Bernard J F, Nahum H. Les localisations sternales de la maladie de Hodgkin. A propos de 2 cas. J Radiol 1980: 61: 281–283

36. Beachley M D, Lau B P, King E R. Bone involvement in Hodgkin's disease. Am J Roentgenol Radium Ther Nucl Med 1972: 114: 559–563

37. Fucilla I S, Hamman A. Hodgkin's disease in bone. Radiology 1961: 77: 53–59

38. Hustu H O, Pinkel D. Lymphosarcoma, Hodgkin's disease and leukemia in bone. Clin Orthop 1967: 52: 83–93

39. Braustein E M. Hodgkin's disease of bone: radiographic correlation with the histologic classification. Radiology 1980: 137: 643–646

40. Pertella Y, Kijanen I. Roentgenologic bone lesions in lymphogranulomatosis maligna: analysis of 453 cases. Ann Clin Gynaecol Fenn 1965: 54: 414–424

41. Timothy A R, Park W M, Cannell L B. Osteonecrosis in Hodgkin's disease. Br J Radiol 1978: 51: 328–332

42. Blijham G H, Vermeulen A, Mendes De Leon D E. Osteonecrosis of sternum and rib in a patient treated for Hodgkin's disease. Cancer 1985: 56: 2292–2294

43. Lascari A D. Leukemia in childhood. Springfield: Charles C Thomas, 1970, pp 163–170

44. Rogalsky R J, Black G B, Reed M H. Orthopaedic manifestations of leukemia in children. J Bone Joint Surg (Am) 1986: 68: 494–501

45. Evans T I, Nercessian B M, Sanders K M. Leukemic arthritis. Semin Arthritis Rheum 1994: 24: 48–56

46. Marsh W L Jr, Bylund D, Heath V C, Anderson M J. Osteoarticular and pulmonary manifestations of acute leukemia. Case report and review of the literature. Cancer 1986: 57: 385–390

47. Fayemi A O, Gerber M A, Cohen I, Davis S, Rubina D. Myeloid sarcoma. Review of the literature and report of a case. Cancer 1973: 32: 253–258

48. Healey J H, Lane J M, Erlandson R A, Bullough P G. Solid leukemia tumor. An uncommon presentation of common disease. Clin Orthop 1985: 194: 248–251

49. Miller L P, Steinhertz P G, Miller D R. Granulocytic sarcoma of the clavicle. Am J Pediatr Hematol Oncol 1982: 4: 425–427

50. Neiman R S, Barcos M, Berard C et al. Granulocytic sarcoma: a clinico-pathologic study of 61 biopsied cases. Cancer 1981: 48: 1426–1437

51. Akber J, Gallagher M T, Mathew L, Ayoub D, Miale T D. Destructive skeletal lesions as the primary initial manifestation of acute childhood leukemia. Am J Pediatr Hematol Oncol 1988: 10: 258–260

52. Dharmasena F, Wickham N, McHugh P J, Catovsky D, Galton D A. Osteolytic tumors in acute megakaryoblastic leukemia. Cancer 1986: 58: 2273–2277

53. Hermann G, Feldman F, Abdelwahab F. Skeletal manifestations of granulocytic sarcoma (chloroma). Skeletal Radiol 1991: 20: 509–512

54. Hughes R G, Kay H E M. Major bone lesions in acute lymphoblastic leukemia. Med Pediat Oncol 1982: 10: 67–70

55. Kushner D C, Weinstein H J, Kirkpatrick J A. The radiologic diagnosis of leukemia and lymphoma in children. Semin Roentgenol 1980: 15: 316–334

56. Thoms L B, Forkner C E, Frei E, Besse B E, Stabenau J R. The skeletal lesions of acute leukemia. Cancer 1961: 14: 608–621

57. Koeffler H P, Mundy G R, Golde D W, Cline M J. Production of bone resorbing activity in poorly differentiated monocytic malignancy. Cancer 1978: 41: 2438–2443

58. Pomeranz S, Hawkins H, Towbin R, Lisberg W N, Clark R A. Granulocytic sarcoma (chloroma): C T manifestations. Radiology 1983: 155: 167–170

59. Welch P, Grossi C, Carrol A et al. Granulocytic sarcoma with an indolent course and destructive skeletal disease. Tumour characterization by immunologic markers, electron microscopy, cytochemistry and cytogenetic studies. Cancer 1986: 57: 1005–1010

60. Wiernik P, Serpick A. Granulocytic sarcoma (chloroma). Blood 1970: 35: 361–369

61. Karsick S, Karasic D, Schilling J. Acute megakaryoblastic leukemia (acute 'malignant' myelofibrosis). An unusual cause of osteosclerosis. Skeletal Radiol 1982: 9: 45–46

62. Mancini A F, Rosito P, Vitelli A et al. I1 significato prognostico delle lesioni ossee nella leucemia acuta linfoblastica del bambino. Pediatr Med Chir 1983: 5: 547–549

63. Pastore G, Miniero R, Cordero Di Montezemolo L et al. Significato prognostico delle lesioni ossee nei bambini con leucemia linfoblastica acuta. Haematologica 1981: 66: 750–755

64. Rudorf I, Seidel R. Knochenbeteiligung bei chronisch-myeloischer Leukämie. Z Gesamte Inn Med 1980: 22: 830–831

65. Schabel S I, Tyminski L, Holland R D, Rittemberg G M. The skeletal manifestations of chronic myelogenous leukemia. Skeletal Radiol 1980: 5: 145–149

66. Valimaki M, Vuopio P, Liewendahl K. Bone lesions in chronic myelogenous leukemia. Acta Med Scand 1981: 210: 403–408

67. Campbell E Jr, Maldonado W, Suhrland G. Painful lytic bone lesion in an adult with chronic myelogenous leukemia. Cancer 1975: 35: 1354–1356

68. Longo D L, Whang-Peng J, Jaffe E, Triche T J, Young R C. Myeloproliferative syndromes: a unique presentation of chronic myelogenous leukemia (CML) as a primary tumor of bone. Blood 1978: 52: 793–801

69. Crain S M, Choudhury A M, Molnar Z, Jablokow V R. Destructive osteolytic bone lesions in chronic granulocytic leukemia. III Med J 1982: 162: 213–217

70. Frydecka I, Bieniek J, Brodzka W. Osteolytic lesion in chronic myelogenous leukemia. Folia Haematol Int Mag Klin Morphol Blutforsch 1984: 111: 610–613

71. Junca Piera J, Duran Suarez J R, Triginer Boixeda J. Lesiones osteoliticas en la leucemia mieloide cronica. Med Clin (Barc) 1981: 76: 259–261

72. Moseley J E. Patterns of bone change in the leukemias and myelosclerosis. J Mt Sinai Hosp 1961: 18: 1–31

73. Nesbitt J, Roth R E. Solitary lytic bone marrow in an adult with chronic myelogenous leukemia. Radiology 1955: 64: 724–726

74. Smith R E, Chelmowski M K, Szabo E J. Myelofibrosis: a concise review of clinical and pathologic features and treatment. Am J Hematol 1988: 29: 174–180

75. Bartl R, Frisch B, Wilmanns W. Potential of bone marrow biopsy in chronic myeloproliferative disorders (MPD). Eur J Haematol 1993: 50: 41–52

76. Georgii A, Vykoupil K F, Thiele J. Classification of chronic myeloproliferative diseases by bone marrow biopsies. Hematological and cytogenetic findings and clinical course. In: Frish B, Bartl R, Eds. Bone marrow biopsies up-dated. New prospects for clinical diagnosis. Basel: Karger, 1984, pp 41–56

77. Thiele J, Simon K G, Fischer R, Zankovich R. Follow-up studies with sequential bone marrow biopsies in chronic myeloid leukemia and so-called (idiopathic) osteomyelofibrosis. Evolution of histopathological lesions and clinical course in 40 patients. Pathol Res Pract 1988: 183: 434–445

78. Lennert K, Parwaresch M R. Mast cells and mast cell neoplasia. A review. Histopathology 1979: 3: 349–365

79. Lortholary O, Audouin J, Le Tourneau A, Diebold J. Le mastocyte et sa pathologie. 2ème partie: histopathologie des mastocytoses. Ann Pathol 1991: 11: 92–100

80. Parwaresch M R, Horny H P, Lennert K. Tissue mast cell in health and disease. Pathol Res Pract 1985: 179: 439–461

81. Travis W D, Li C Y, Bergstrahl E J, Yam L T, Swee R G. Systemic mast cell disease. Analysis of 58 cases and literature review. Medicine 1988: 67: 345–368

82. Deshayes P, Arinal P, Dreyfus P et al. Les localisations osseuses de la mastocytose. Sem Hôp 1969: 45: 524–530

83. Sagher F, Even-Paz Z. Mastocytosis and the mast cell. Chicago: Year Book Medical, 1967

84. Schweiter M E, Irwin G A. Case report 561. Systemic mastocytosis. Skeletal Radiol 1989: 18: 411–413

85. Andrew S M, Freemont A J. Skeletal mastocytosis. J Clin Pathol 1996: 46: 1033–1035

86. Fallon M D, Whyte M P, Teitelbaum S L. Systemic mastocytosis associated with generalized osteopenia. Hum Pathol 1981: 12: 813–820

87. Raffi M, Firooznia H, Golimbu C, Balthazar E. Pathologic fracture in systemic mastocytosis. Radiographic spectrum and review of the literature. Clin Orthop 1983: 120: 260–267

Myeloma

J. Diebold

FREQUENCY

This neoplastic disease is defined as a proliferation of plasma cells with varying degrees of immaturity, inducing atypical forms and showing multiple or diffuse bone involvement. These plasma cell proliferations are often associated with the presence of abnormal proteins in the blood and urine and occasionally with the presence of amyloid in the tumor tissue and other organs[1,7,3] (Schajowicz 1994).

Myeloma is an example of immunoglobulin producing monoclonal gammopathies. It accounts for 20–50% of primary bone tumors (Schajowicz 1994). In the USA, the incidence is 2–3.9 cases per 100 000 people, with a higher incidence among black Americans[1,5] (Schajowicz 1994). Myeloma accounts for about 1% of malignant tumors and 10% of hematologic malignancies.[3] The incidence also varies from one part of the world to another. The sex ratio shows a male predominance of 3:2. The disease develops in adults over 35 and the incidence increases with age.

Myeloma represents one of the entities called plasma cell dyscrasias[2] (Schajowicz 1994), which are produced by the proliferation of a single clone of immunoglobulin-secreting cells. Plasma cell dyscrasias comprise not only plasma cell myeloma, but also monoclonal gammopathy of undetermined significance, Waldenström macroglobulinemia, heavy chain diseases and primary amyloidosis.

MULTIPLE MYELOMA (KAHLER'S DISEASE)

Clinical data[1,2,3] (Schajowicz 1994)

Localized or diffuse bone pain is present in more than 80% of these patients. Sciatica or cruralgia may be observed in patients with vertebral locations.

A bone tumor (rib, sternum, head) may be the first symptom in about 10% of patients. Spontaneous fracture is the presenting feature in about 5% of cases. In addition, fever and loss of weight are often seen. Symptoms of hyperviscosity syndrome, hypercalcemic syndrome or amyloidosis may also be observed.

Biological data

Immunoelectrophoresis discloses the presence in the blood of a monoclonal immunoglobulin component (IgG in 50–60%, IgA in 20–35%, rarely IgD or IgE or only one light chain). κ or γ light chains are present in the urine. For the diagnosis, sternal puncture smears and iliac crest trephine biopsy are both necessary.

Sites of involvement[1,2,3] (Schajowicz 1994)

Bones involved are those containing red marrow: vertebrae, ribs, skull and pelvis in about 60–75% and long bones, scapula, sternum and mandible in 40–50%.

Imaging[1,2] (Schajowicz 1994)

The typical appearance is caused by the presence of numerous round osteolytic lesions without sclerotic margins (Figs 34.1–34.7). They may increase in size and coalesce, destroying the bone and the overlying cortex. Growth of the tumor can cause expansion of the thinned cortex in long bones, sternum or rib.

Pathologic fractures can occur in different bones, ribs or vertebrae with collapse of the vertebral bodies.

A rare type of myeloma is represented by the development of sclerotic bone lesions showing a nodular or diffuse pattern.

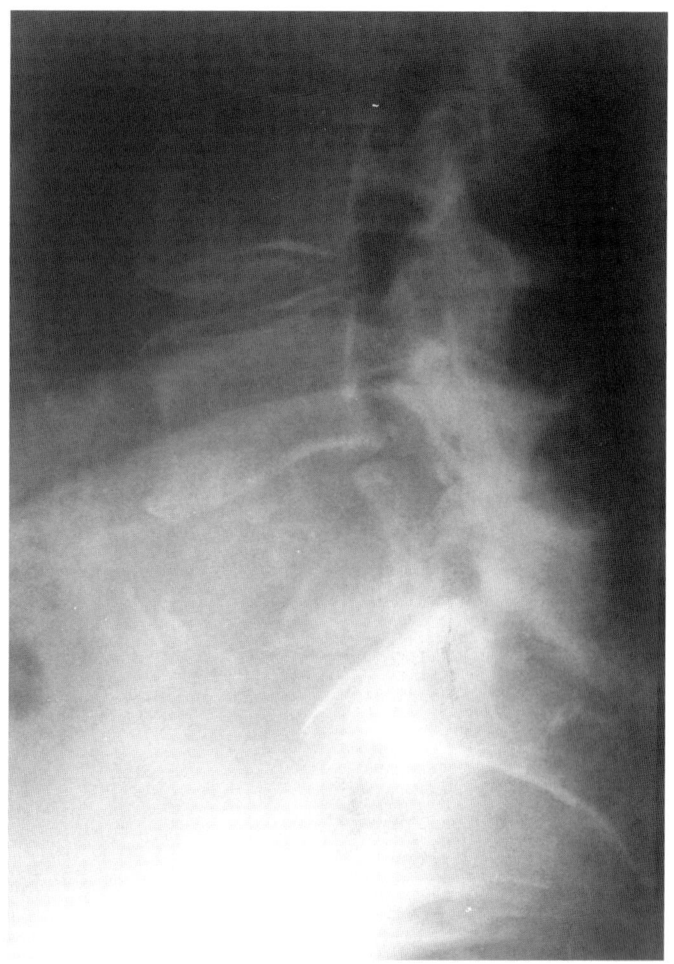

Fig. 34.1 Myeloma: vertebral location. (Courtesy of M. Forest MD.)

Cytopathology[1,3,6,7,8]

In sternal aspirates, a diagnosis of myeloma can be considered when the average plasma cell content is over 10%. It is also important to determine the morphology of the neoplastic cells due to the fact that plasma cell hyperplasia, occurring in infectious diseases (pneumonia, septicemia) or in immune disorders (Castleman's disease), can be as frequent as 40%. In some cases, immunohistochemistry is mandatory, demonstrating the mono- or polyclonality of the plasma cell population. In typical plasma cell myeloma, the average plasma cell count is 20–36%.[2,3,8,9]

The neoplastic cells express variable morphology:

1. Some resemble mature plasma cells (Marschalko type).

2. Some are more lymphoid, with a dark nucleus resembling a lymphocyte and a basophilic ovoid cytoplasm producing cells which can be named 'lymphoplasmacytoid' cells or 'lymphoid plasma' cells. Myeloma with such a morphology represents 5% of cases.

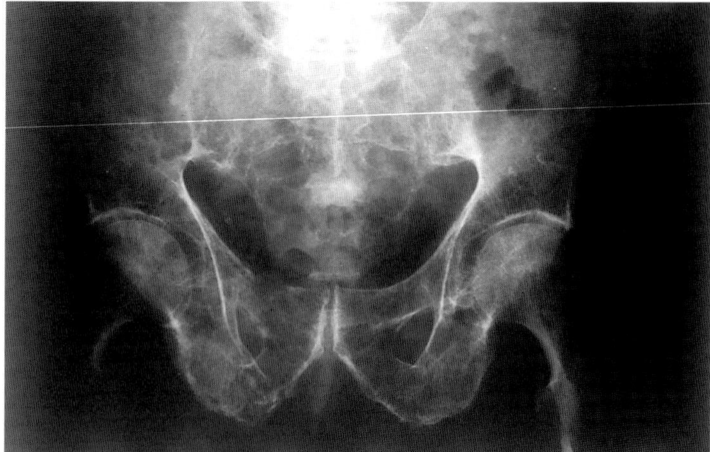

Fig. 34.2 Myeloma: pelvic involvement. (Courtesy of M. Forest MD.)

3. Plasma cells with a more blastic appearance may also be seen and are often larger than reactive plasma cells. Variable cytoplasmic changes have been described:[2] fraying of the cytoplasmic borders, cytoplasmic shedding,

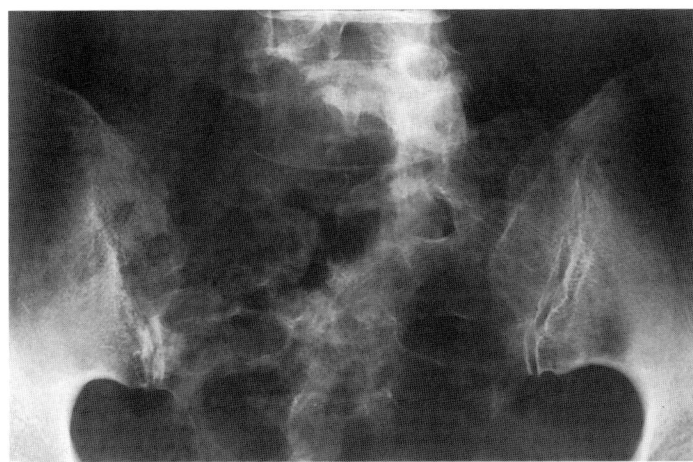

Fig. 34.3 Myeloma: pelvic involvement. (Courtesy of M. Forest MD.)

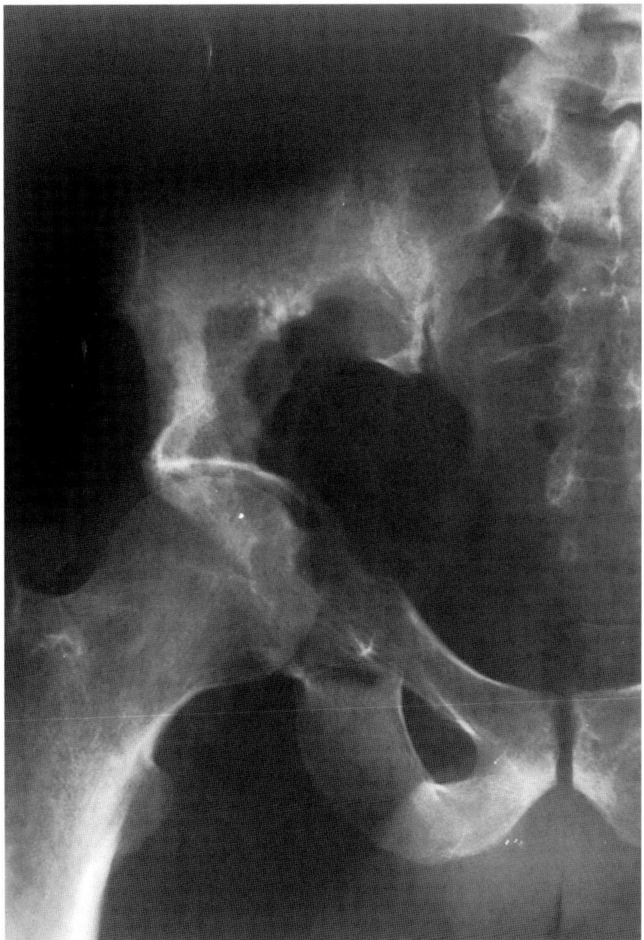

Fig. 34.4 Myeloma: acetabular location. (Courtesy of M. Forest MD.)

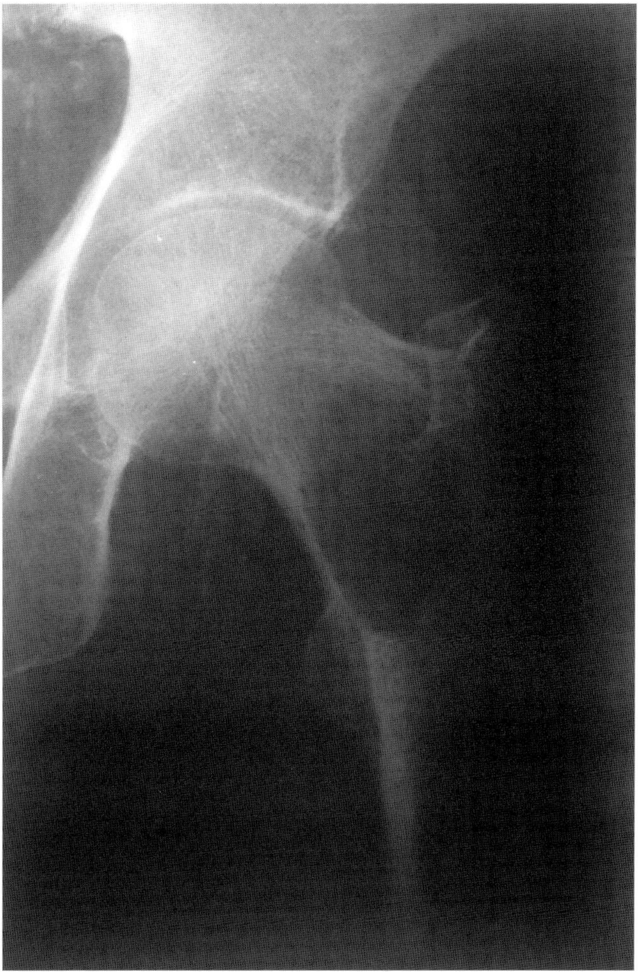

Fig. 34.5 Myeloma: femoral involvement. (Courtesy of M. Forest MD.)

or intranuclear inclusions with hyaline appearance are frequent.[2] Occasionally neoplastic plasma cells may develop erythrophagocytosis.[2] The nucleus is also larger with a less condensed chromatin, a paler appearance and variably prominent nucleoli.

4. Some larger cells resembling plasmablasts and immunoblasts may be observed.

5. In a few cases (2%), many tumor cells have notched nuclei with marked lobulation, exhibiting a more or less monocytoid configuration.[9,10] These bizarre plasma cells can represent the majority of the tumor cells. The diagnosis is then very difficult.

Gross pathology

Small nodules measuring around 1 cm or less are found in the bones, destroying and replacing the bone marrow. The nodules are composed of a soft grayish tissue (Fig. 34.8). Coalescence of nodules produces a large multilobular tumor which destroys the bone architecture and the cortex, with extension into adjacent soft tissues.

presence of vacuoles, granules, hyaline inclusions, small or large crystalline inclusions. The cytoplasmic inclusions may be composed of multiple small amphophilic granules or vacuoles with inclusions resembling Chinese characters.[2] Multiple, small Russell body-type intracytoplasmic

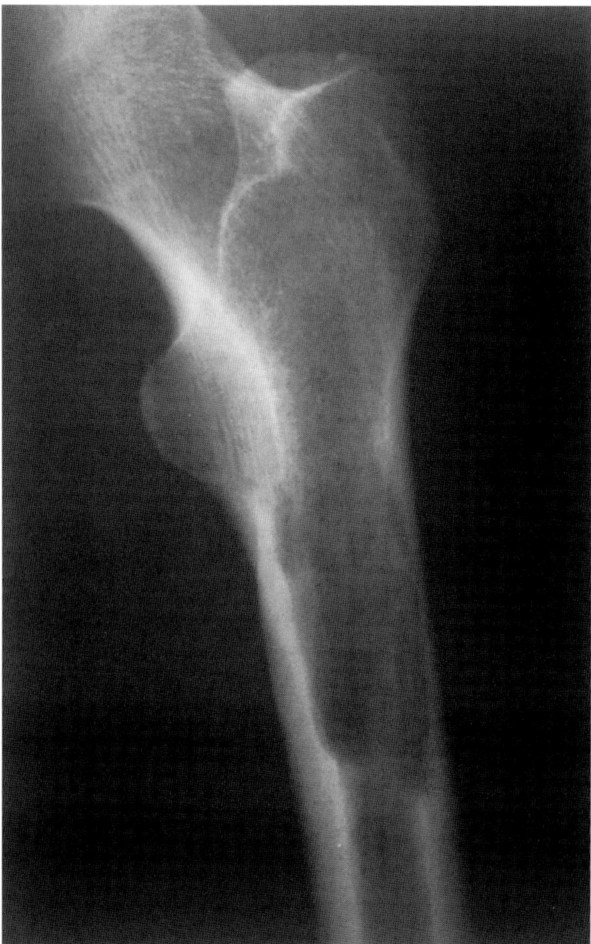

Fig. 34.6 Myeloma: femoral involvement. (Courtesy of M. Forest MD.)

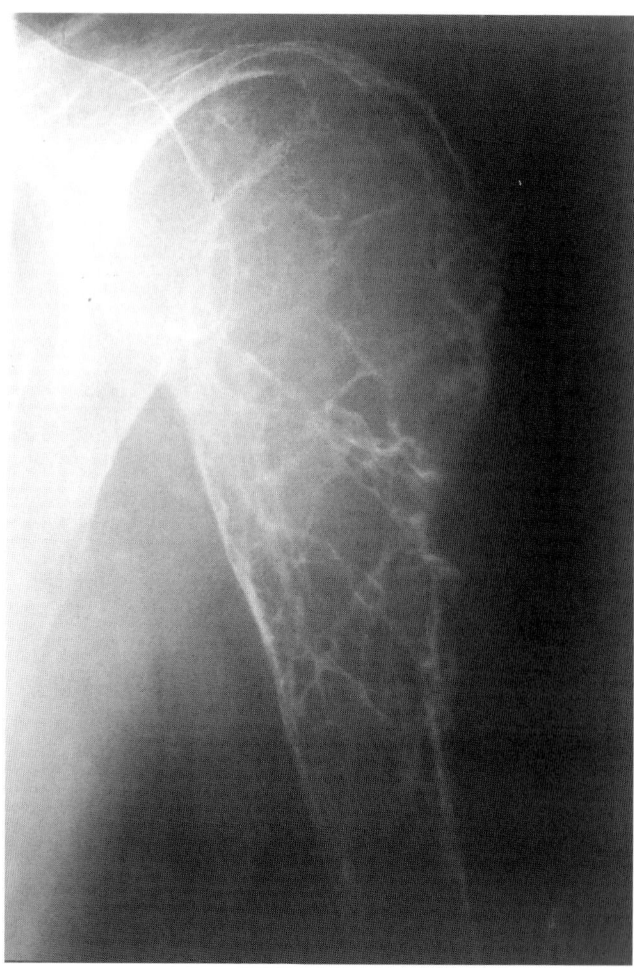

Fig. 34.7 Myeloma: humeral involvement. (Courtesy of M. Forest MD.)

Such coalescent tumors in short bones are responsible for fracture. Collapse of vertebral bodies can occur with spinal cord nerve root or spinal nerve compression. Metastatic calcium deposits, due to hypercalcemia secondary to bone destruction, can be found in lung and kidney parenchyma.

Histopathology[1,3,6,7,8,9,11,24] (Schajowicz 1994)

The tumor nodules are made of densely packed plasma cells, with absent or rare fibrous bands. The hematopoietic and fatty marrow are destroyed. A massive involvement is evidenced.

In some cases, the tumor cells are arranged in lobules and strands separated by bands of collagen surrounding capillaries and small vessels. This pattern may appear in multiple focal lesions or in scanty rare irregularly distributed focal lesions.

In other cases, early lesions only comprise small nests of tumor cells dispersed between the adipose cells, more or less intermingled with hematopoietic cells (Fig. 34.9). These foci are always at a distance from the arteries and capillaries which are surrounded only by reactive plasma cells. Nests of tumor cells can develop along the bone trabeculae (Fig. 34.10). This form indicates interstitial involvement which can be minimal and difficult to diagnose.

The trabeculae can be normal, particularly in early lesions. In massive tumors, destruction of bone trabeculae can be recognized as due to osteoclastic hyperplasia (Fig. 34.11). In rare cases, thick collagen bands surround vessels and bone trabeculae, which show reactive osteoblastic bone formation. Such changes are seen in the rare manifestation of the disease known as osteosclerotic myeloma[1-3] (Schajowicz 1994).

Seven types of tumor cells can be recognized:

1. *Mature plasma cells, Marschalko's type* (Fig. 34.9). These cells resemble reactive plasma cells: around eccentric nucleus with a 'cartwheel' pattern of thick chromatin, absent or small nucleolus, a large ovoid or triangular basophilic cytoplasm, with a clear juxtanuclear halo corresponding to a huge Golgi apparatus. Some giant forms can also be observed.

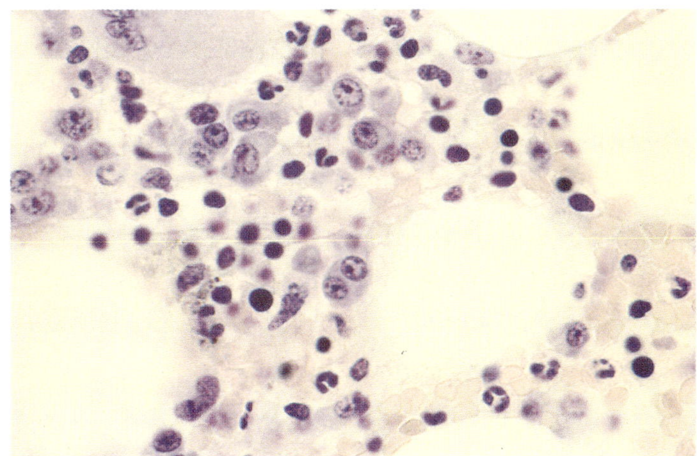

Fig. 34.8 Myeloma: sternal involvement.

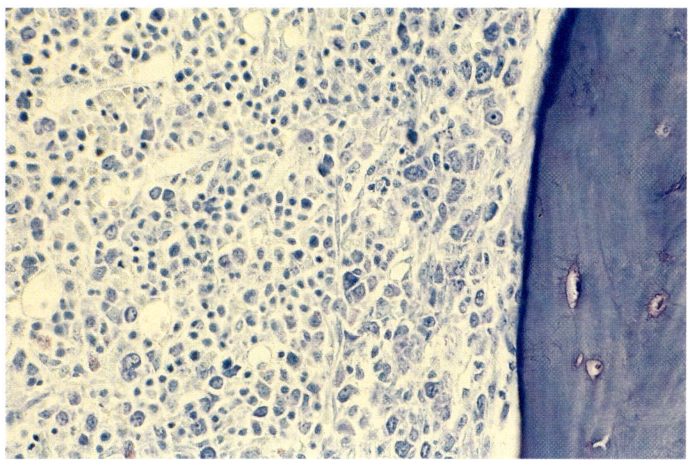

Fig. 34.10 Myeloma, small juxtatrabecular infiltrate. (Giemsa.)

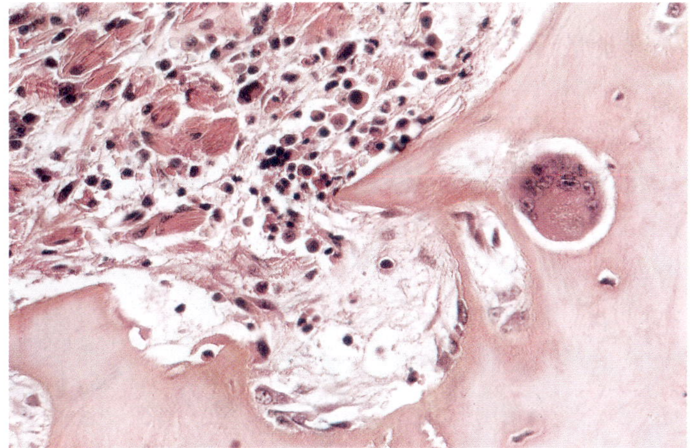

Fig. 34.11 Myeloma. Osteoclastic resorption of bone.

Fig. 34.9 Myeloma, early interstitial infiltrate, Marschalko type. (Giemsa.)

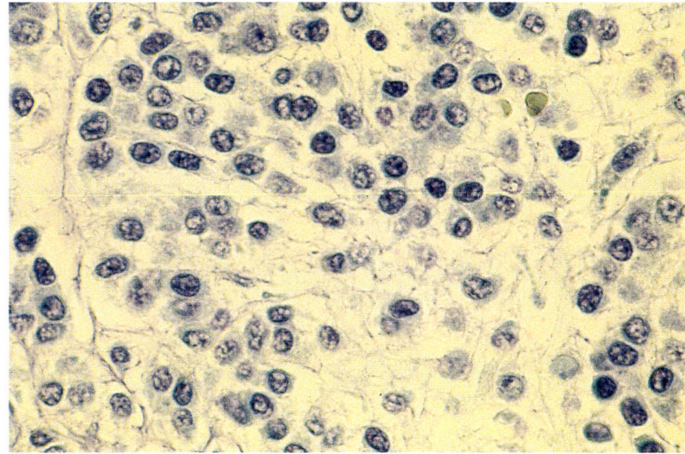

Fig. 34.12 Myeloma. Small lymphoid plasma cell type. (Giemsa.)

2. *Lymphoid plasma cells* (Fig. 34.12). These cells are smaller with scanty cytoplasm and a round nucleus with broader chromatin blocks.

3. *Proplasmocytes* (Figs 34.13, 34.14). The cells are larger with a paler nucleus and a medium-sized, centrally situated nucleolus.

4. Plasma cells with *irregular 'cleaved' nuclei or notched plasma cells*[1,2,6,7,10,11] (Fig. 34.15).

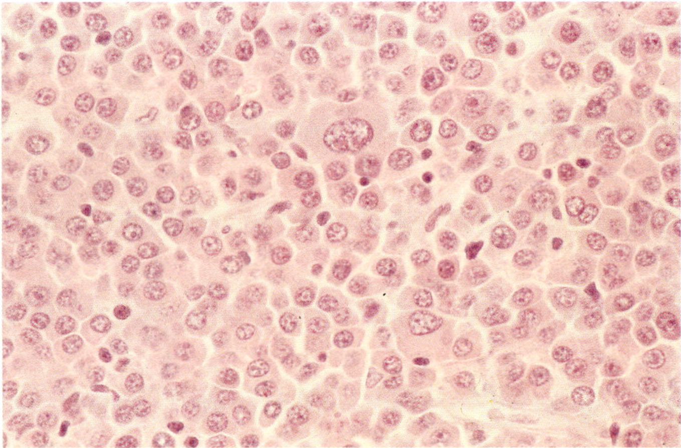

Fig. 34.13 Myeloma, intermediate type with giant cell.

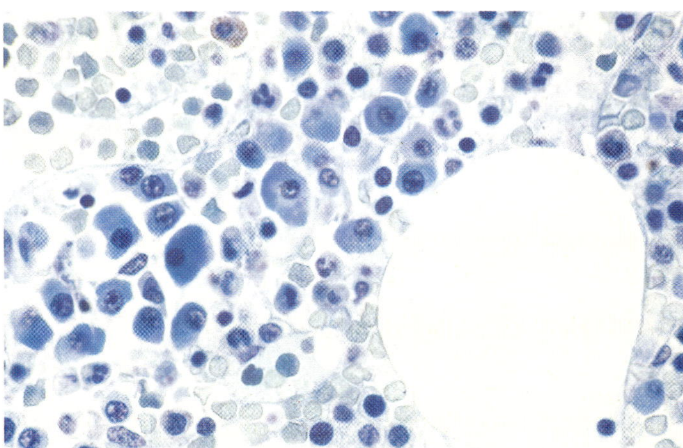

Fig. 34.14 Myeloma, intermediate type. (Giemsa.)

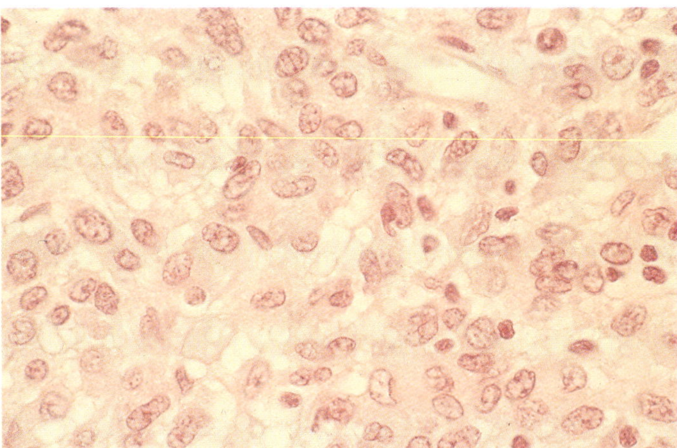

Fig. 34.15 Myeloma. Plasma cells with notched nuclei.

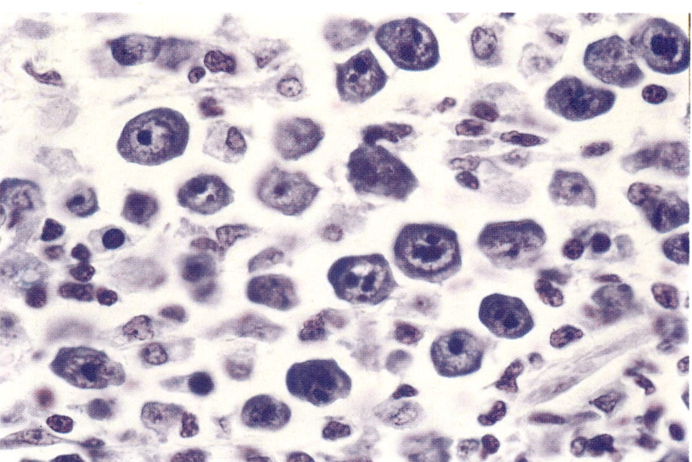

Fig. 34.16 Myeloma, immunoblastic type. (Giemsa.)

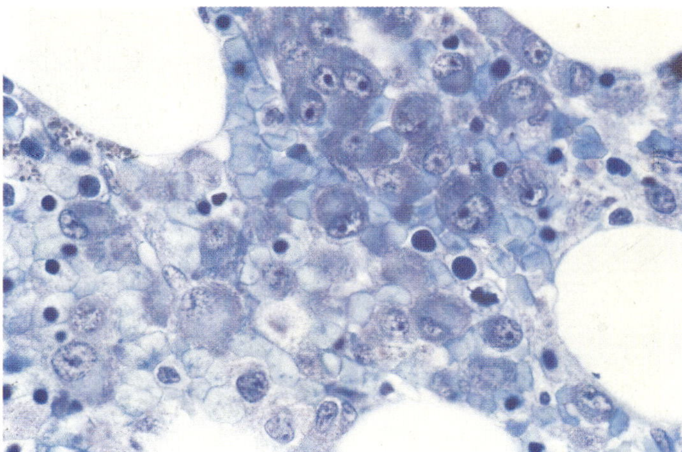

Fig. 34.17 Myeloma, plasmablastic type. (Giemsa.)

5. *Immunoblasts* (Fig. 34.16). These large cells are round with a big, roundish pale nucleus containing a big centrally situated nucleolus. The surrounding cytoplasm is abundant and deeply basophilic.[13]

6. *Plasmablasts* (Fig. 34.17). These cells have the morphology of immunoblasts with a large eccentric basophilic cytoplasm and a pale juxtanuclear halo representing a hypertrophic Golgi apparatus. In the center of the nucleus, 2–3 medium-sized nucleoli can be recognized.[13]

7. *Giant cells* (Fig. 34.14). Often multinucleated, these giant cells can sometimes mimic Reed–Sternberg cells.

In the same patients, successive biopsies can demonstrate an evolution from minimal to interstitial and focal and then massive involvement.[2,3,6,7]

Intranuclear vacuoles or minute vacuoles on the nuclear membrane can be recognized. They are PAS positive when they contain IgA. Sometimes immunoglobulin crystals can be seen in the cytoplasm of tumor cells, particularly in rare IgD myeloma.[14]

In a small number of cases, many histiocytes can be seen. They can contain immunoglobulin crystals.[14]

Classification of myeloma

According to the morphology of the tumor cells, myelomas have been divided into four cytologic types:[11,12] mature, intermediate, immature and plasmablastic. This classification has prognostic value: the plasmablastic type shows a median survival period of 10 months, while the three other types have a 35-month survival period.[11,13] This is a simplification of the classification into six types proposed by Bartl et al.[6,7]

To define more precisely the total amount of plasma cells in the bone marrow, a histologic staging system has been proposed:[6,7,11]

stage I: less than 10% of the bone marrow is involved;
stage II: 20–50% is involved;
stage III: more than 50% involved.

A good correlation can be demonstrated between the size of the tumor mass, the clinical stage and the prognosis.[6,7]

Immunohistochemistry

Plasma cells are positive for non-specific esterase and acid phosphatase on imprints and frozen sections. On paraffin sections, demonstration of light chains shows whether the tumorous cells are producing mono- or polytypic light chains.[15]

Monotypic plasma cells are considered monoclonal and monoclonality is correlated with malignant proliferation. Positivity is granular in the cytoplasm. The perinuclear cisterna is also positive, occasionally with a few small dots or large intranuclear vacuoles (Figs 34.18–34.21).

The majority of myelomas express IgA or IgG. A few cases produce IgD or IgE. In some cases, only κ or γ light chains are present.

B cell antigens (CD19, CD20, CD10), myeloid antigens (CD13, CD33) and also HLD DR, CD45 and some adhesion molecules (CD11b, CD11c) may exist.[16]

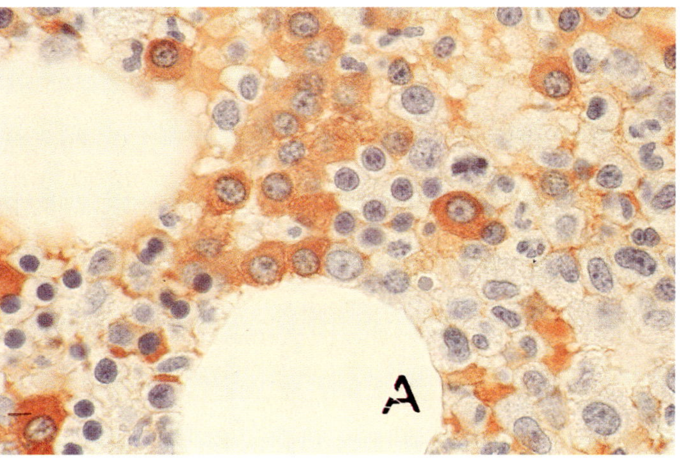

Fig. 34.19 Myeloma, intermediate type. Demonstration of IgA secretion. Immunoperoxidase, ABC technique on paraffin section.

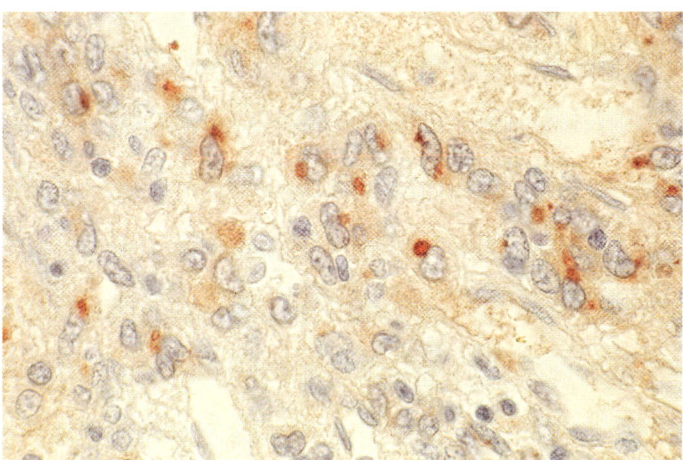

Fig. 34.20 Myeloma, notched plasma cell type. Expression of λ chain production as small dots on the perinuclear cisterna and of a large single round dot probably corresponding to the Golgi apparatus. Immunoperoxidase, ABC technique, λ light chain demonstration.

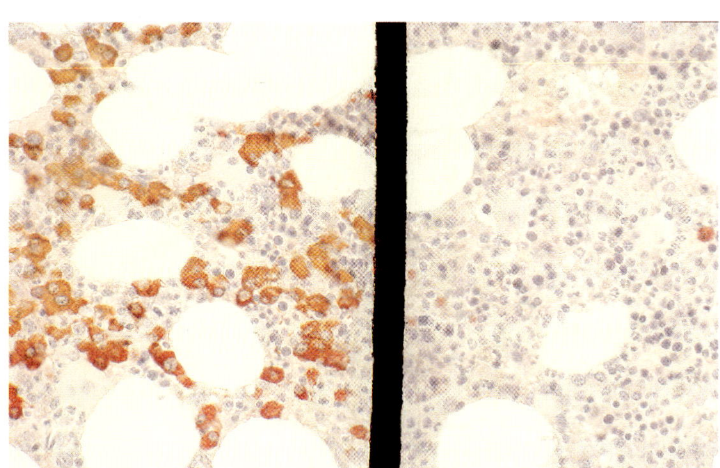

Fig. 34.18 Myeloma. Demonstration of monotypy for κ light chain. Immunoperoxidase, ABC technique on paraffin section. *Left*: κ; *right*: λ.

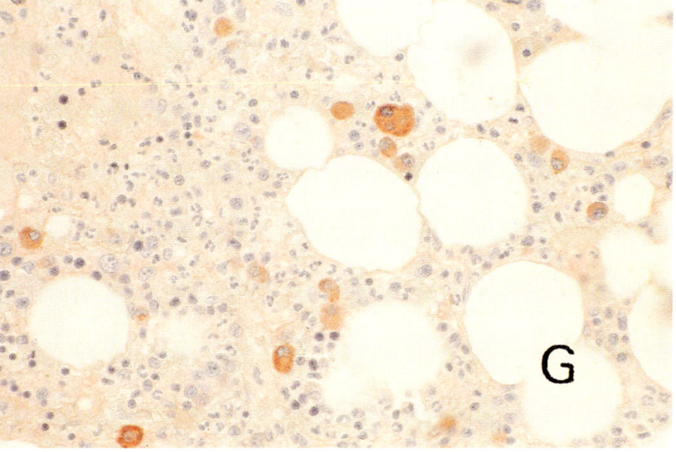

Fig. 34.21 Myeloma, early interstitial infiltrate. Immunohistochemistry is useful to detect monoclonal plasma cells, here secreting a γ heavy chain, with an abnormal morphology and topography. Immunoperoxidase, ABC technique.

In addition, myeloma cells are CD54 positive, this being an adhesion molecule allowing cell aggregation.[16]

Cytogenetics[16,17]

Cytogenetic abnormalities, if present, are complex, with structural changes (translocations, deletions) in 90% of cases and numerical abnormalities in 85%.[16] No specific changes characteristic of myeloma have been discovered.[16]

Alterations of the immunoglobulin in many chain loci on chromosome 14 seem to be common while alterations of the light chain genes on chromosomes 2 and 22 are rare.[14] A t(11–14) has been described in some cases, but this is different from the translocation found in mantle zone lymphoma, without bcl-1 rearrangement.[16]

The presence of cytogenetic modifications suggests a poor prognosis.

Correlation between morphology and immunoglobulin secretion

There is no direct relation between morphology and monoclonal immunoglobulin type, in the majority of the cases.[2] Only a few cases of IgA myeloma show marked pleomorphism of the plasma cell, with the presence of giant multinucleated plasma cells, flame plasma cells and cells exhibiting a pale, fragmented cytoplasm.

In one study,[9] 20% of cases distinguished by 'lymphoid plasma cells' were IgD myeloma.

Pale staining intranuclear inclusions can be observed in all types of myeloma in hematoxylin and eosin. They are more frequent in IgA myelomas (about 20%).[9] In addition, in this type of myeloma, the content of the intranuclear vacuoles is PAS positive.

Intracytoplasmic crystalline inclusions constituted by κ light chains are characteristic of myeloma occurring in Fanconi's disease.

DIFFUSE DECALCIFYING MYELOMATOSIS[1,2,3,6,7] (Schajowicz 1994)

The marrow of many bones is completely replaced by a grayish tissue, diffusely infiltrating the bone, sometimes with small nodules. Grossly, bone destruction is less evident. Microscopic study demonstrates a bone rarefaction (osteoporosis) and a diffuse infiltration by plasma cells.

SOLITARY MYELOMA[1,2,3,6,7,16,18,19,20,21] (Schajowicz 1994)

This type is characterized by a single tumor destroying the central part of a short bone (vertebrae, rib) or long bones. The cortex is thinned, without expansion into the surrounding tissue. In some cases, destruction of the cortex can be seen.

PLASMA CELL LEUKEMIA[1,2,3,22,23]

Neoplastic plasma cells represent more than 20% of peripheral blood cells. Such leukemias can be diagnosed before multiple myeloma. Bone marrow is diffusely infiltrated. Hepatosplenomegaly is also frequent with accumulation of plasma cells in the lumen of the spleen sinuses or the liver sinusoids.

The patients have a high tumor mass with extraosseous involvement. Thrombocytopenia and high serum LDH are frequent, as well as hypodiploid plasma cells and complex cytogenetic abnormalities.

This leukemia results from the proliferation of immature plasma cells, requiring prompt chemotherapy. The median survival is about 20 months.[22]

ASSOCIATED AMYLOIDOSIS

Amyloidosis occurs in 10–25% of cases of myeloma (Schajowicz 1994). Generalized amyloidosis is frequent with involvement of kidneys, spleen, adrenal glands and liver. Localized amyloidosis can originate in the bone. At the microscopic level, amyloid deposits cause small, more or less confluent nodules between the sheets of plasma cells (Fig. 34.22) or small perivascular infiltrations (Fig. 34.23). Amyloid material is homogeneous, eosinophilic and Congo red positive with green polarization (Fig. 34.24), metachromatic with crystal violet and fluorescent with thioflavine. Giant cell reaction is often observed around aggregates of amyloid (Fig. 34.22).

ASSOCIATED DISEASES

Castleman's disease, which may be uni- or multicentric, may be associated mainly with solitary plasmacytoma or with osteosclerotic myeloma. Multiple symptoms can also be seen corresponding to the POEMS syndrome: polyneu-

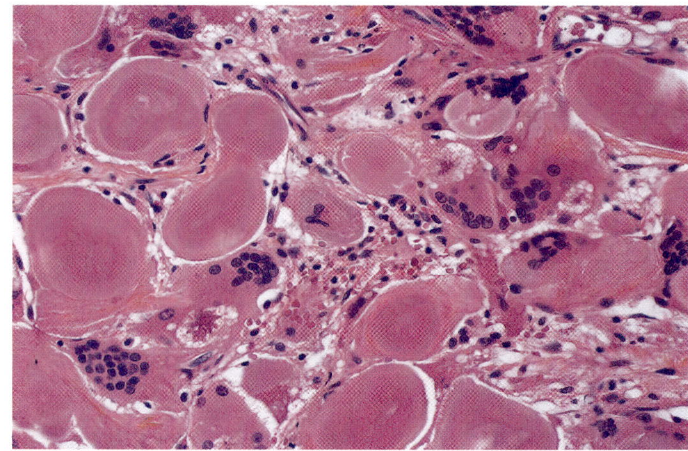

Fig. 34.22 Myeloma. Interstitial amyloid deposit, with giant cell reaction. (Courtesy of M. Forest MD.)

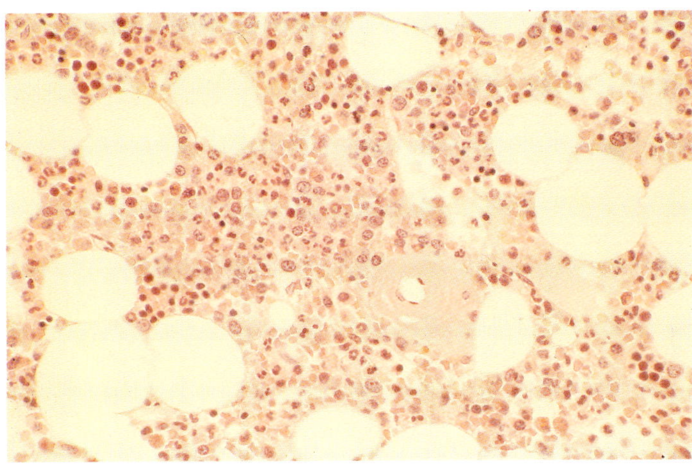

Fig. 34.23 Myeloma, vascular amyloidosis.

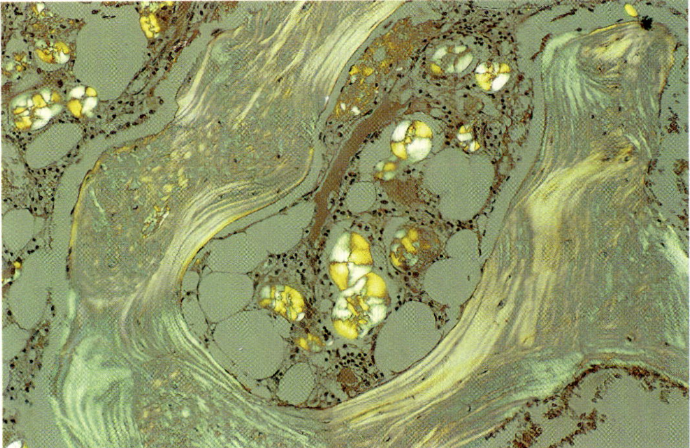

Fig. 34.24 Myeloma. Congo red staining studied in polarized light. (Courtesy of M. Forest MD.)

ropathy, organomegaly, endocrine disease, monoclonal immunoglobulin and skin lesions.[24] POEMS syndrome is probably due to the hyperproduction of cytokines. Cytokines like IL-6 seem to play an important role in the development of myeloma.[25]

TREATMENT

The treatment of myeloma is mainly based on poly- chemotherapy,[5] with regimens including either melphalan, cyclophosphamide and prednisone or adriamycin, vincristine, cyclophosphamide and prednisone.[1,2] A careful follow-up should avoid hypercalcemic syndrome.

Relapses are treated according to the same scheme.[2,5] Radiotherapy can also be used, for example on isolated tumors. Surgery is sometimes needed for spontaneous fracture or vertebral collapses with compression. Total excision represents the best treatment for solitary plasmacytoma.

PROGNOSIS AND COURSE[1,2,3,8]

A complete remission is never achieved. Multiple myeloma is always fatal, about 50% of the patients dying within 2 years of diagnosis (Schajowicz 1994). IgG myeloma has the best prognosis with a 35% survival rate at 5 years. IgA and other types of myeloma have a worse prognosis. Only solitary plasmacytoma has a better prognosis.

DIFFERENTIAL DIAGNOSIS

A proliferation of mature plasma cells must be differentiated from severe reactive plasmacytosis, which can occur during infectious diseases or immune disorders like Castleman's disease. Chronic osteomyelitis in the form of the central abscess described by Brodie can be very difficult to distinguish. Clinical data and the polyclonality of the plasma cell population help to determine the diagnosis.

The rare lymphoid plasma cell type can be confused with B-CLL or lymphoplasmacytoid immunocytoma. The diagnosis is based on clinical presentation and on the demonstration of IgM secretion.

The diagnosis in pleomorphic plasma cell myeloma can be very difficult, with bone marrow localization of other lymphomas of B type (centroblastic, centrocytic) or of T type. The clinical presentation and immunohistochemistry aid the diagnosis.

Myeloma with a predominance of large cells of immunoblastic and/or plasmablastic type cannot be distinguished from immunoblastic ML by morphology or immunohistochemistry. Only clinical data and imaging can provide the right diagnosis.

REFERENCES

1. Azar H A, Potter M. Multiple myeloma and related disorders. New York: Harper and Row, 1973
2. Brunning R D, McKenna R W. Tumors of the bone marrow. Atlas of tumor pathology. Washington: AFIP, 1994, pp 323–350
3. Kyle R A. Multiple myeloma: review of 869 cases. Mayo Clin Proc 1975: 50: 29–40
4. Ries L A, Hankey B F, Miller B A, Hartman A M, Edwards B K. Cancer statistics review 1973–1988. National Cancer Institute NIH Pub. No. 91–2789, 1991
5. Alexanian R, Dimopoulos M A. Management of multiple myeloma. Semin Hematol 1995: 32: 20–30
6. Bartl R, Frisch B, Fatem-Moghadam A, Kettner G, Jaeger K, Sommerfeld W. Histologic classification and staging of multiple myeloma. A retrospective and prospective study of 674 cases. Am J Clin Pathol 1987: 87: 342–355
7. Bartl R, Frisch B, Wilmanns N. Morphology of multiple myeloma. In: Malpas J S, Bergsagel D E, Kyle R A, Eds. Myeloma: biology and management. Oxford: Oxford University Press, 1995, pp 82–123

8. Kyle R A. Diagnostic criteria of multiple myeloma. Hematol Oncol Clin North Am 1992: 6: 347–358

9. Reed M, McKenna R W, Bridges R, Parkins J, Frizzera G, Brunning RD. Morphologic manifestations of monoclonal gammopathies. Am J Clin Pathol 1981: 76: 8–23

10. Zukerberg L R, Ferry J A, Conlon M, Harris N L. Plasma cell myeloma with cleaved multilobated and monocytoid nuclei. Am J Clin Pathol 1990: 93: 657–661

11. Sailer M, Vykoupil K F, Peest D, Cordewey R, Deicher H, Georgii A. Prognostic relevance of a histologic classification system applied in bone marrow biopsies from patients with multiple myeloma. A histopathological evaluation of biopsies from 153 untreated patients. Eur J Haematol 1995: 54: 137–146

12. Sukpanichnant S, Cousar J B, Leesasiri A, Graber S E, Greer J P, Collins R D. Diagnostic criteria and histologic grading in multiple myeloma: histologic and immunohistologic analysis of 176 cases with clinical correlation. Hum Pathol 1994: 25: 308–318

13. Greipp P R, Raymond N M, Kyle R A, O'Fallon W M. Multiple myeloma: significance of plasmablastic subtype in morphological classification. Blood 1985: 65: 305–310

14. Gabriel L, Escribano L, Perales J, Bellas C, Odriozola J, Navarro J L. Multiple myeloma with crystalline inclusions in most hematopoietic cells. Am J Hematol 1985: 18: 405–411

15. Wolf B C, Brady K, O'Murchadha M T, Neiman R S. An evaluation of immunohistologic stains for immunoglobulin light chains in bone marrow biopsies in benign and malignant plasma cell proliferations. Am J Clin Pathol 1990: 94: 742–746

16. Moscinski L C, Ballester O F. Recent progress in multiple myeloma. Hematol Oncol 1994: 12: 111–123

17. Laï J L, Zandecki M, Mary J Y et al. Improved cytogenetics in multiple myeloma: a study of 151 patients including 117 patients at diagnosis. Blood 1995: 85: 2490–2997

18. Bacci G, Calderoni P, Cervellati C, Zambaldi A. Solitary plasmacytoma of bone: a report of 19 cases. Ital J Orthop Traumatol 1982: 8: 469–478

19. Bataille R, Sany J. Solitary myeloma: clinical and prognostic features of a review of 114 cases. Cancer 1981: 48: 845–851

20. Guida M, Casamassima A, Abbate I et al. Solitary plasmacytoma of bone and extramedullary plasmacytoma: 2 different nosological entities? Tumori 1994: 80: 370–377

21. Meis J M, Butler J J, Osborne B M, Ordonez N G. Solitary plasmacytoma of bone and extramedullary plasmacytomas. A clinico-pathologic and immunohistochemical study. Cancer 1987: 59: 1475–1485

22. Dimopoulos M A, Palumbo A, Delasalle K B, Alexanian R. Primary plasma cell leukemia. Br J Haematol 1994: 88: 754–759

23. Kyle R A, Maldonado J E, Bayrd E D. Plasma cell leukemia. Report of 17 cases. Arch Intern Med 1974: 133: 813–818

24. Miralles G D, O'Fallon J R, Talley N J. Plasma-cell dyscrasia with polyneuropathy. The spectrum of POEMS syndrome. N Engl J Med 1992: 327: 1919–1923

25. Klein B. Cytokine, cytokine receptors, transduction signals, and oncogenes in human multiple myeloma. Semin Hematol 1995: 32: 4–19

35

Bone metastases

M. Forest

GENERAL CONSIDERATIONS

Metastatic cancer is the most common malignant bone tumor, but the reported frequency varies greatly, depending on the stage of the disease, the imaging techniques and the extent of morphological sampling. The overall incidence of bone metastases in cancer is approximately 30%.[1,2]

Any malignant tumor can metastasize to the skeleton but carcinomas of the breast, prostate, lung, kidney and gastrointestinal tract account for about 80% of all metastases.[2] There is a high frequency of adenocarcinomas[3] but the incidence may be influenced by the histological subtype of the tumor and in bronchial cancers, oat cell carcinomas metastasize more frequently than other histological types.[4]

Soft tissue and bone sarcomas metastasize frequently to bone,[5] with a clinical incidence of 18%, the axial skeleton being most commonly involved.

In children, by far the most common metastatic cancer is the neuroblastoma, often with a diffuse skeletal involvement, followed by Ewing's sarcomas, osteosarcomas, embryonal rhabdomyosarcomas, teratocarcinomas and Wilms' tumors.[6,7] In 80% of cases they are located in the spine, ribs, skull, femur and pelvis. In long bones, metaphyses are involved, with a bilateral and symmetrical distribution in many cases.[6,8]

Metastases have been reported in bones involved by *Paget's disease*,[9–11] with a possible role for hypervascularity, but in practice the association is unusual[12] (Fig. 35.1).

Bone metastases as a *first manifestation of a tumor* are located in the spine in 80% of cases;[13,14] in 3–4% of patients, the site of the cancer remains unknown.[15] Most occult carcinomas involve the lung, kidney and pancreas.[15,16]

For the pathologist, the *search for the primary tumor* employs the usual immunohistochemical techniques. In some cases, the haphazardly distributed osteoid produc-

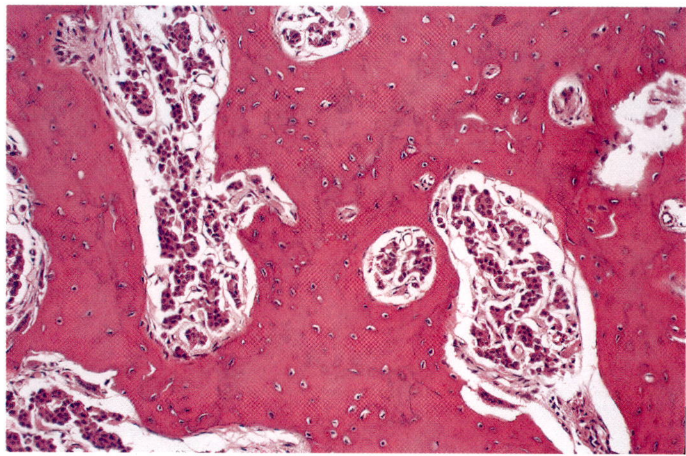

Fig. 35.1 Metastasis of a breast carcinoma involving Paget's disease of the pelvis.

tion found in osteoblastic metastases may lead to a diagnosis of osteosarcoma (Fechner & Mills 1993). More usually, spindle cell carcinomas and especially sarcomatoid renal carcinomas produce some diagnostic problems with an overlap of immunohistochemical reactions; the differential diagnosis between anaplastic carcinomatous metastases and undifferentiated sarcomas remains unsettled, despite extensive immunohistochemical and ultrastructural investigations.[17]

The usefulness of cytopathological techniques is obvious when one has only to confirm the presence of a known malignancy with adequate material and in many cases, a carcinoma may be diagnosed or differentiated from a sarcoma.[18,19]

Systematic iliac crest bone biopsies can document tumor dissemination, even when the X-rays are negative. In one series, 20% of the biopsies were positive with normal bone scans, 30% positive with normal X-rays (Bartl & Frisch 1993), tumor appearing as intrasinusoidal emboli or micrometastases.

Bone marrow aspirates and biopsies are now performed to enable accurate staging of the malignant disease.[20] *Micrometastases* are detected by immunofluorescent antibody analysis, double immunohistochemical labeling techniques,[21] marrow cultures or PCR,[22] if the histological findings are negative.

Micrometastatic seeding of bone marrow occurs early in the natural course of cancer. In breast cancer, it is correlated with vascular and lymphatic invasion, a tumor size greater than 5 cm, the presence of axillary node involvement and a trend toward negative receptor expression.[20,23,24] Cancer cells are found on bone marrow aspirates in 35% of cases with immunohistochemistry.[23,24]

Micrometastases are found in 20–33% of patients with a prostatic cancer at N0M0 stage[21,22] and in 65% of patients with extraprostatic disease.[22] There is also a correlation with established risk factors such as local tumor

extent, lymph node involvement and tumor differentiation.[21]

In colorectal cancers and lung carcinomas, micrometastases are found with an incidence of 21–32%; in neuroblastomas, micrometastases are detected in 50–67% of cases, correlating with a poor prognosis.[20]

BASIC MECHANISMS OF CANCER CELL ADHESION, OSTEOLYSIS, DESTRUCTION OF CARTILAGE AND REACTIVE BONE FORMATION

The initial steps of bone colonization, cancer cell attachment to endothelial cells and to matrix proteins such as laminin and fibronectin,[25] are probably mediated by integrins.

The invasive properties are related to proteolytic enzymes, matrix metalloproteinases produced by tumor cells which degrade the basement membrane collagen as well as the bone extracellular matrix.[25]

Tumor cells, macrophages and osteoclasts may be involved in bone resorption. Tumor cells are frequently found adjacent to resorbed bone margins; on ultrastructural examination, they have been demonstrated resorbing bone (Bartl & Frisch 1993) and experimentally, breast cancer cells have been shown to induce mineral release and stimulate matrix resorption in coculture experiments.[26] More recently, murine melanoma cells have been identified directly in contact with the resorbing bone surfaces and have been able to degrade an osteoid-like matrix.

In this mechanism of bone resorption, two phases have been suggested: a predominent osteoclastic activity, followed by a cancer cell-mediated degradation.[27] However, direct evidence of bone resorption by tumor cells is not clearly demonstrated[28] and cancer cells play a minor role in osteolysis.

On scanning electron microscopy, resorption pits are made by osteoclasts[25] and morphological studies on metastases of lung cancer demonstrate clearly that the tumor grows in the osteolytic defects produced by activated osteoclasts.[29] Moreover, extension of tumor into resorption lacunae still populated by osteoclasts is often observed.[29]

In metastatic breast cancer, quantitative histomorphometric measurements have shown that the number of osteoclasts is significantly increased[30] and the major mechanism of bone resorption is osteoclast mediated; in bone metastases from renal carcinoma, osteoclasts also play a major role.[31]

Human tumor-associated macrophages, isolated from primary lung carcinomas, induce resorption lacunae in vitro and it seems that a minor population of tumor-associated macrophages are capable of differentiating into bone-resorbing cells in the presence of marrow stromal cells.[28]

The main consequence of metastatic tumor invading

bone is an activation of both osteoblast and osteoclast activities and the osteoclastic effect predominates in most tumors.[29,30,32]

Cancer cells stimulate osteoclastic activity by secreting transforming growth factors, interleukins, prostaglandins and parathyroid hormone-related proteins.[33] Powerful osteoclast cytokines are released, such as tumor necrosis factor and interleukin 1.[34] Interleukin 6 is produced by osteoclasts in response to stimulation by interleukin 1 and a parathyroid hormone-related peptide by cancer cell lines, increasing the recruitment of osteoclasts.

Transforming growth factor α is also a powerful stimulator of osteoclast formation and of osteoclastic bone resorption in vivo and in vitro; TGFβ may inhibit or stimulate osteoclastic bone resorption.

The role of prostaglandins of the E series produced by cancer cells is unclear;[34] they may increase osteoclast formation in culture or inhibit the activities of isolated osteoclasts. The levels of prostaglandin production within tumors do not predict later metastases in bone or the grade of malignancy.[32]

Parathyroid hormone-related protein (PTH-rP) is produced frequently by breast cancer cells.[34] PTH-rP stimulates osteoclastic bone resorption in vivo and in vitro and stimulates renal tubular calcium reabsorption. It can be identified by immunohistochemistry and in situ hybridization chiefly for tumors that produce hypercalcemia by a humoral mechanism; 90% of breast cancers that metastasize to bone express PTH-rP and it is identified in 60% of tumor tissues of normocalcemic breast cancer patients.[35]

Procathepsin-D is a precursor of a lysosomal proteinase, cathepsin D, secreted by a number of human breast cancer cell lines; it activates osteoclasts directly.[34]

The role of *proteinases*, particularly type I collagenase, remains undetermined; its secretion by osteoblasts may facilitate the removal of the non-mineralized layer of bone, allowing osteoclasts access to the underlying mineralized bone.[32]

Resorption of bone near a tumor may help to provide an environment favorable for the development of metastases; matrix factors released may be chemotactic for tumor cells and also promote tumor growth.[35] Extracellular matrix components can regulate the synthesis, secretion and activity of matrix metalloproteinases in cancer cells;[36] type I collagen promotes tumor cell growth, chemotaxis and adhesion,[33,34] as well as α HS glycoprotein, osteocalcin, synthetic peptides and TGFβ.[33] The local ambient concentration of calcium in the extracellular fluid may also influence the production of osteotropic factors such as PTH-rP.[34]

The *resistance of cartilage* to neoplastic invasion is not absolute, in spite of some experimental work demonstrating extractable cartilage factors which inhibit tumor-associated collagenase and angiogenesis. Morphological studies in squamous cancers of the head and neck demonstrate that the cartilage undergoing focal metaplastic ossification is destroyed by osteoclasts, but the destructive cartilage process is thought to be mediated principally by lysosomal hydrolases derived from tumor cells or from chondrocytes themselves.[37]

Reactive immature woven bone is present in 40% of metastases, irrespective of the primary site of the tumor.[38]

In culture, prostatic cancer cells can produce osteoblast-stimulating factors[39] and mRNA extracted from tumor cells codes for a factor with osteoblast-stimulating activity. Bone morphogenetic proteins, urokinase type plasminogen activator and basic fibroblastic growth factor are also produced.[25]

In breast cancer, cancer cell lines produce TGFβ which can stimulate in vitro osteoblasts to produce collagen, osteocalcin and alkaline phosphatases. Osteoblastic metastases are mediated by osteoblasts stimulated by factors derived from the osseous stroma or by cytokines produced by tumor cells.

New bone is laid down directly on trabecular bone surfaces or is found in the marrow cavity as primitive woven bone; branches of osteoid may extend from the trabecular surfaces into the central marrow areas, forming lacy networks.[40] The reactive bone formation may be associated with capillary and fibroblast proliferation as well as with infiltration by inflammatory cells and macrophages.

Changes in the cancellous bone have been termed 'carcinomatous osteodysplasia'.[41]

After tetracycline labeling, undecalcified bone biopsies from osteosclerotic metastases from prostatic cancer have shown an increased trabecular bone volume and in 50% of cases, morphologic and dynamic evidence of osteomalacia, defined by the increase in osteoid seam thickness and decrease in the calcification rate.[42] For other investigators, those findings are only related to the high bone turnover state and the thick seams of poorly mineralized osteoid characteristic of osteomalacia are not identified.[43]

THE SPREAD OF CANCER CELLS

Tumor cells may spread to the periosteum by lymphatic channels and then directly extend to the adjacent bone, but usually they metastasize to bone almost exclusively by the hematogeneous route.

The arterial circulation may be involved and it has been demonstrated experimentally that tumor cells may invade bone by the systemic arterial circulation.[44] Tumor colonization of vertebrae is predominantly located in the hematopoietic bone marrow adjacent to the cartilaginous growth plate of the vertebral bodies where tortuous loops and arcades of arterioles behave functionally as end arteries[44] (Figs 35.2, 35.3).

However, skeletal metastases, especially in the axial skeleton, occur most frequently as a result of spread in the vertebral venous system which consists of a network of

flow in the incidence of lumbar, spinal and pelvic metastases of cancers of the prostate, of spinal and humeral metastases of breast and colorectal cancers[46] and in part in metastases of hepatocellular carcinomas.[47] In autopsied cases, 70% of metastases from prostatic carcinomas are found in the pelvis, sacrum and lower vertebral column.

SKELETAL DISTRIBUTION

Irrespective of the primary tumor involved, the most frequently affected regions are the vertebral column, particularly the lumbosacral region,[48,49] the pelvis, the proximal femur, skull, ribs and proximal humerus.[50]

The distribution of *skeletal metastases* is closely related to the distribution of the red marrow in adults, demonstrated by the fact that more than 80% of bone metastases are in

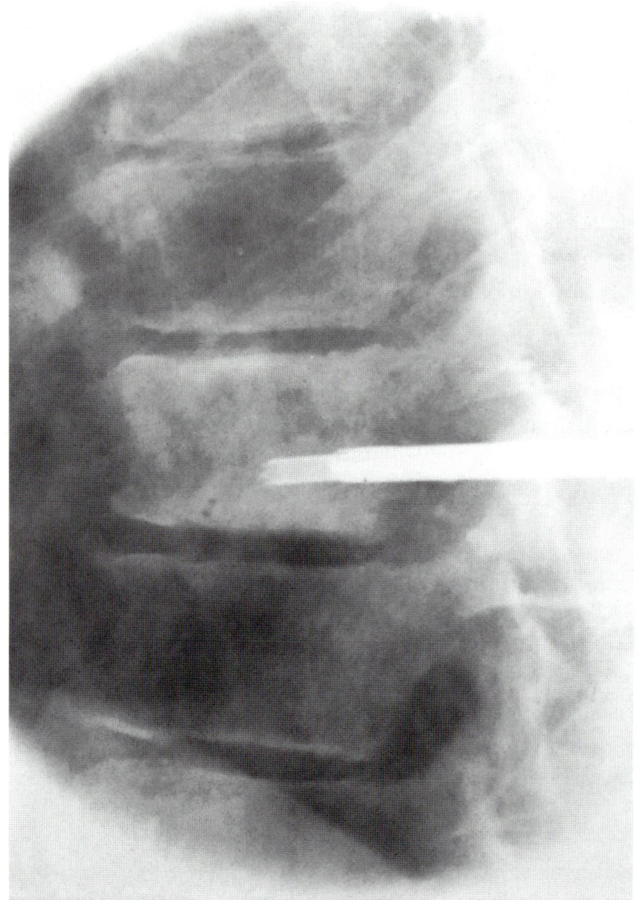

Fig. 35.2

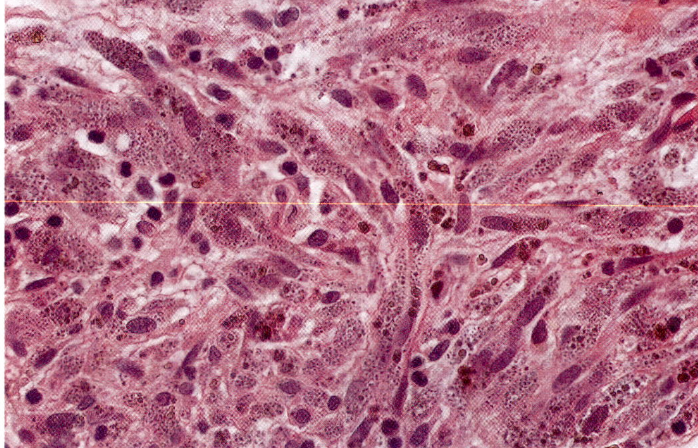

Fig. 35.3

Figs 35.2, 35.3 Vertebral metastasis of a melanoma (T8 level).

valveless veins surrounding the lumbar vertebrae with extensive connections with the inferior and superior vena cava, the prostatic venous complex, the pelvic, thoracic, mammary veins and brain.[45]

This vertebral venous plexus is implicated by retrograde

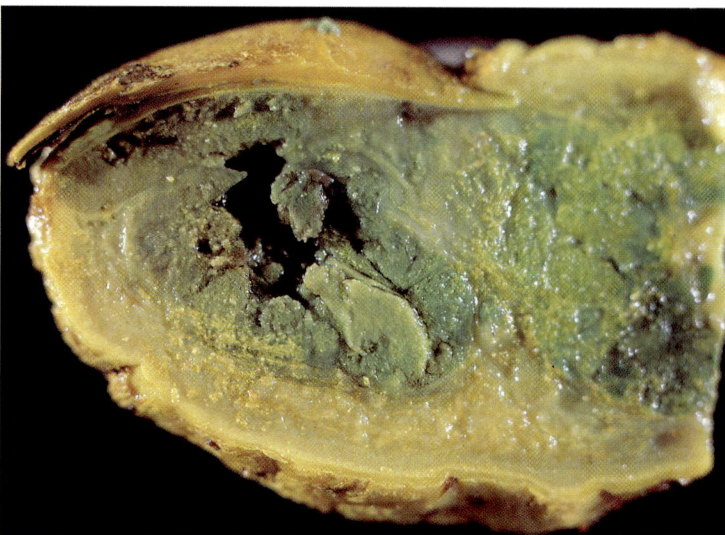

Fig. 35.4 Metastasis of a hepatocarcinoma involving the great toe.

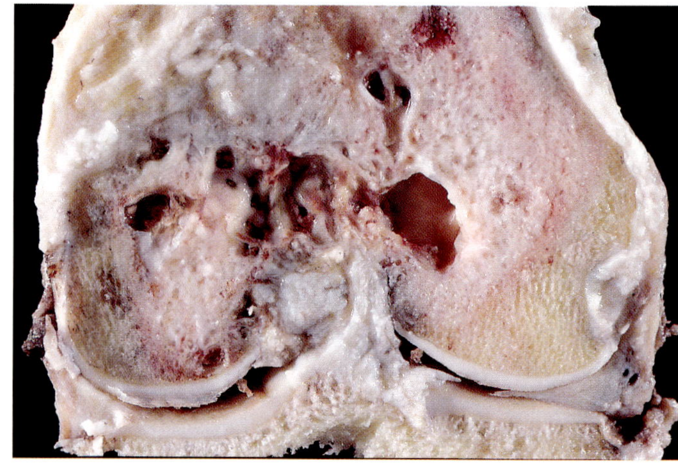

Fig. 35.5 Femoral metastasis of a squamous carcinoma of the cervix, with involvement of the knee joint.

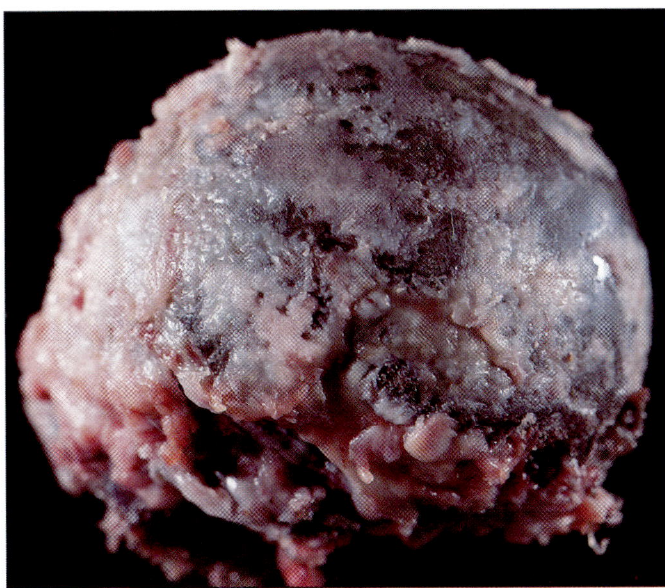

Fig. 35.6 Metastasis of a melanoma in the hip joint, with black staining of the femoral cartilage.

the axial skeleton.[51] In cases of a pathological distribution of red marrow, metastases follow the altered pattern of red marrow,[50] confirming the much-quoted words of Paget on the 'dependence of the seed upon the soil'.

The slow blood flow and the histological aspects of the large capillaries and sinusoidal networks communicating with central veins are implicated in the frequency of tumor clusters in the paratrabecular sinusoids; marrow sinusoids are lined by endothelial cells displaying 60 angstrom fenestrae and lacking basement membranes.[52]

Vertebral metastases are most frequently found in the lumbar part of the spine, followed by thoracic, cervical and sacral portions.[52–54]

Neoplastic spread by way of Batson's plexus to the basivertebral veins has been demonstrated on CT scans[55] and the position of the mestastases is correlated with the site of entry of the vertebral vessels, that is, the posterior portion of the vertebral body.[54,56]

If an absent pedicle is the first radiological sign of metastatic disease, the vertebral body is the most frequent

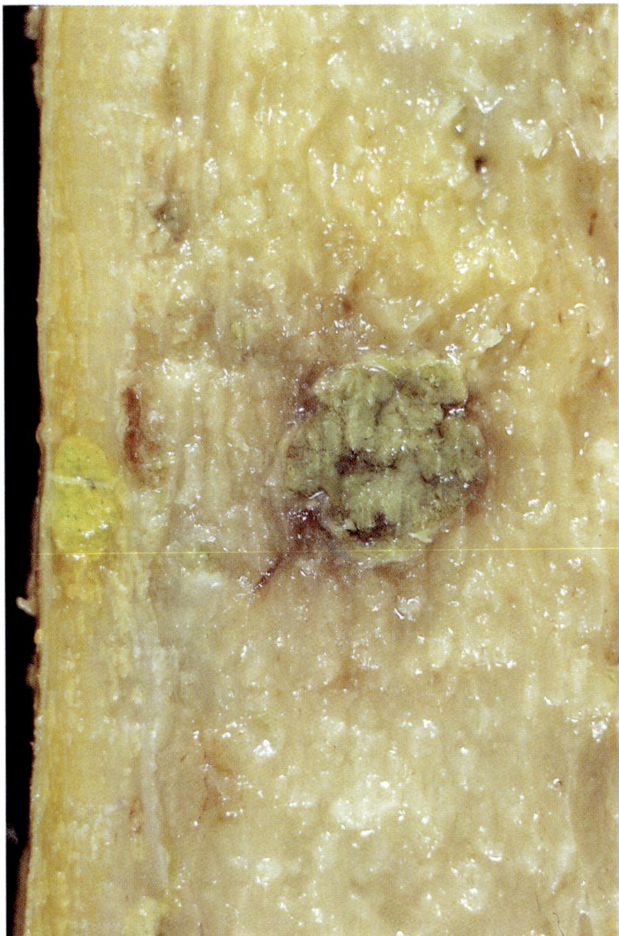

Fig. 35.7

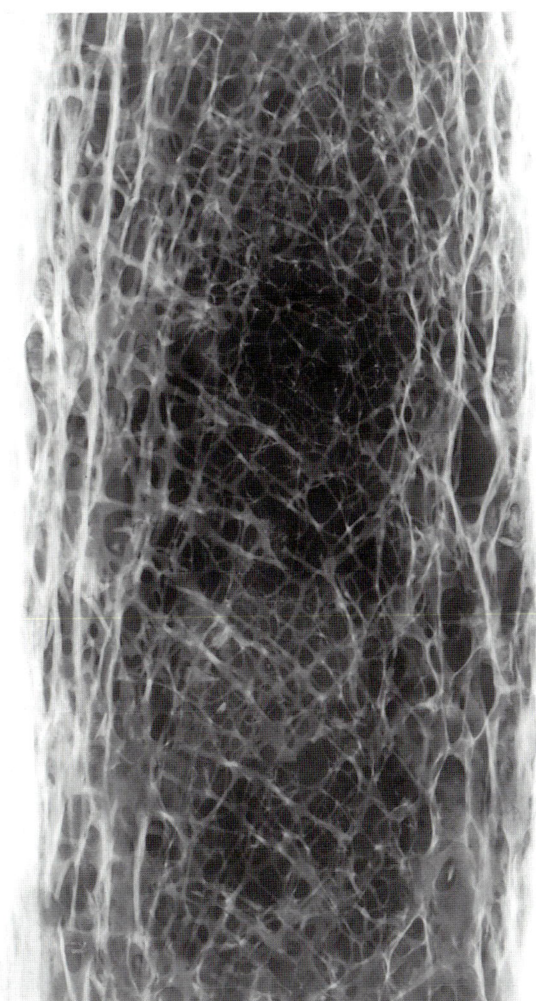

Fig. 35.8

Figs 35.7, 35.8 Tibial metastasis from an occult hepatocarcinoma.

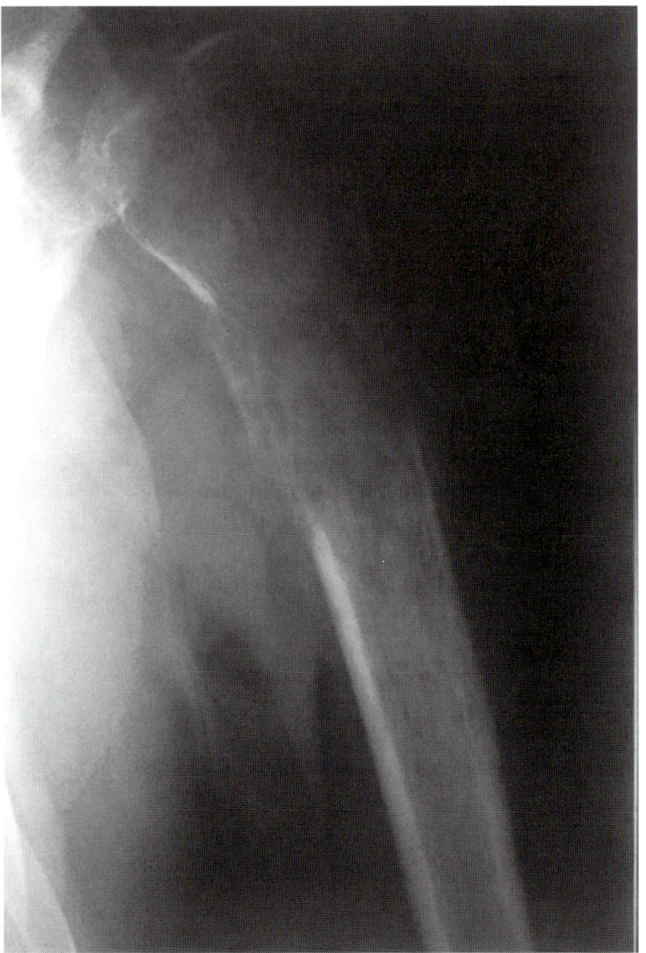

Fig. 35.9

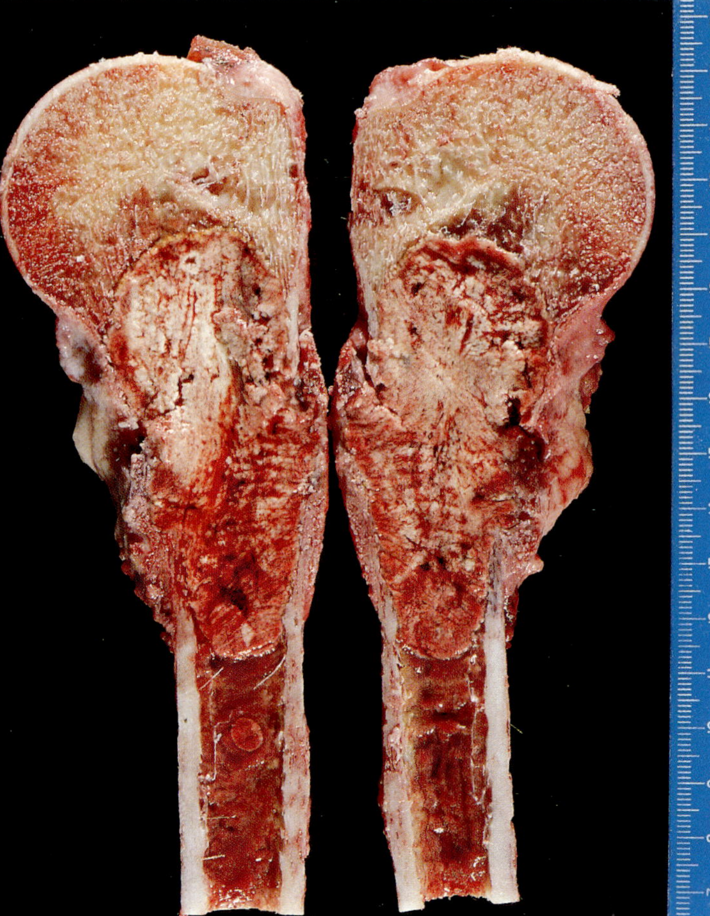

Fig. 35.10

Figs 35.9, 35.10 Humeral metastasis from an occult renal adenocarcinoma.

initial site, with involvement of the pedicle by direct extension or from the posterior elements.[56]

Cancer cells invade the spinal canal through the foramina of the vertebral veins rather than destroying the cortical bone, which is a late event.[44]

Metastases or tumoral extension to the disc are rare events[57] and presumably the high intradiscal pressure acts as a barrier;[58] it may be associated with degenerative changes or cartilaginous (Schmorl's) node formation. The tumor may infiltrate the disc from the rim of the vertebral body not covered by the cartilaginous plate, through the space beneath the longitudinal ligament or by hematogenous invasion via small vessels.[58]

Metastases to the hands are unusual, with an incidence of 0.1%,[59] occurring in patients with widespread metastases;[60] less commonly, acrometastases are the initial presentation of malignancy.[60–62] Bronchial carcinoma is the most common neoplasm metastasizing to the hand,[63] followed by breast and kidney carcinomas. Other primaries have been

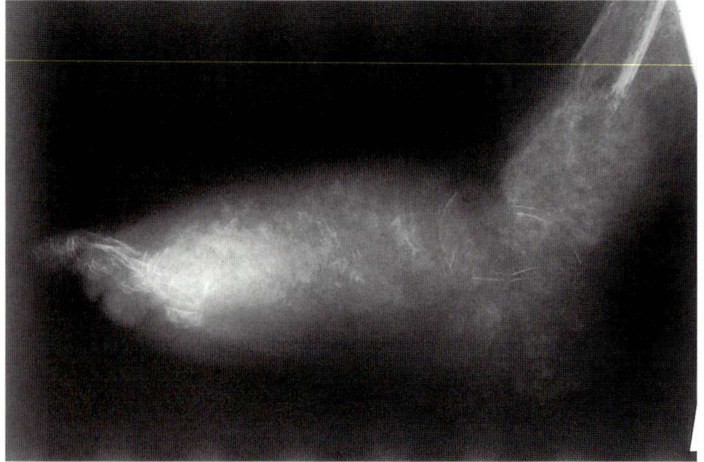

Fig. 35.11 Tumoral osteolysis of the foot: metastasis of a lung carcinoma.

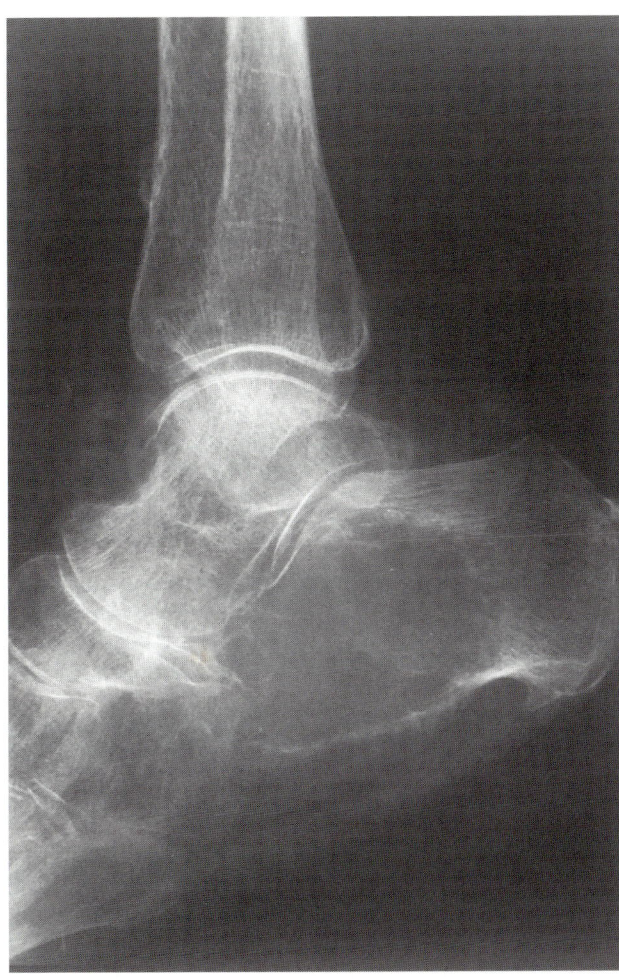

Fig. 35.12 Lytic metastasis of a renal adenocarcinoma involving the calcaneus.

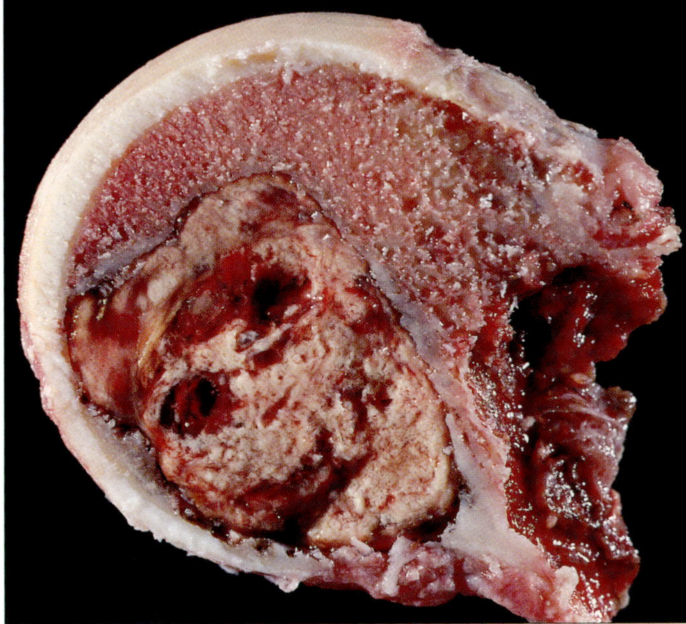

Fig. 35.13 Lytic metastasis of a renal adenocarcinoma involving the femoral head.

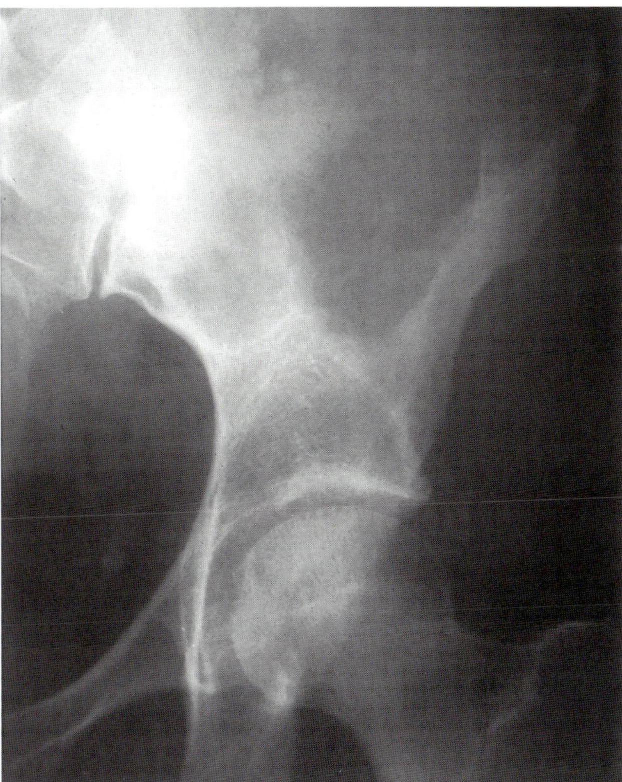

Fig. 35.14

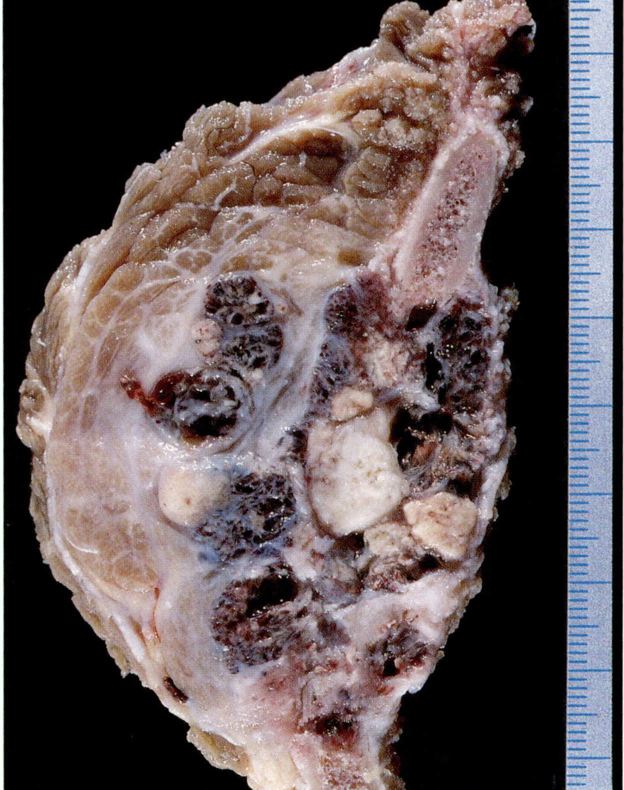

Fig. 35.15

Figs 35.14, 35.15 Expansile and lytic metastasis of a renal adenocarcinoma in the iliac wing, treated by embolization and resection.

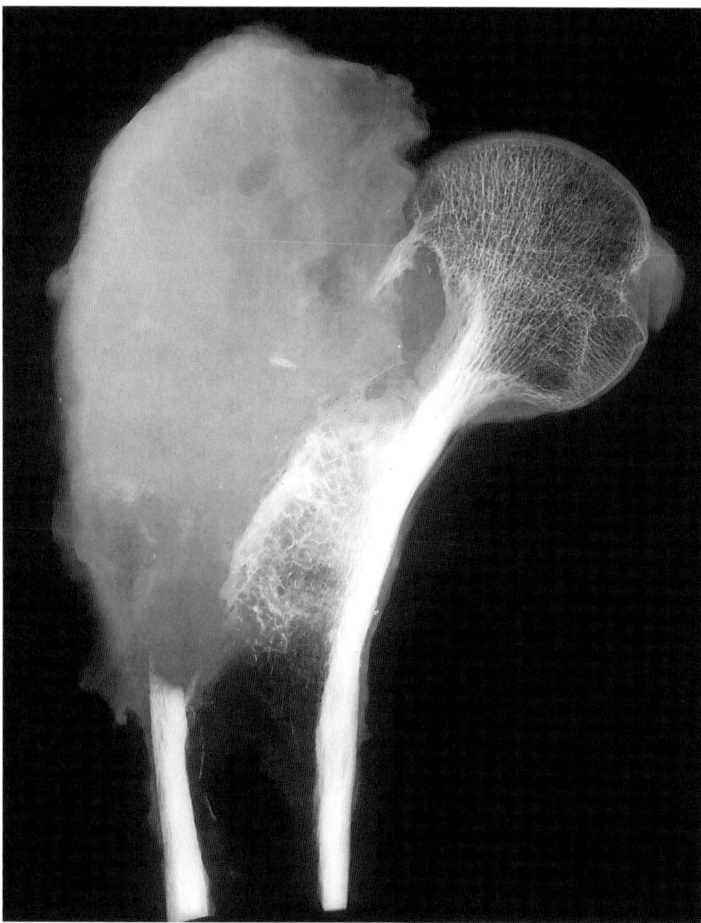

Fig. 35.16 Expansile and lytic femoral metastasis from a renal adenocarcinoma.

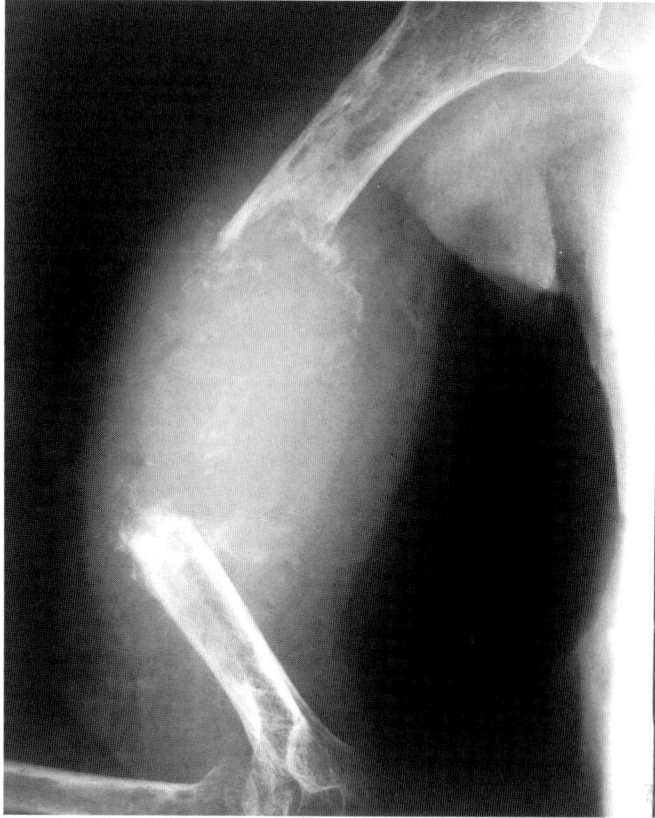

Fig. 35.17

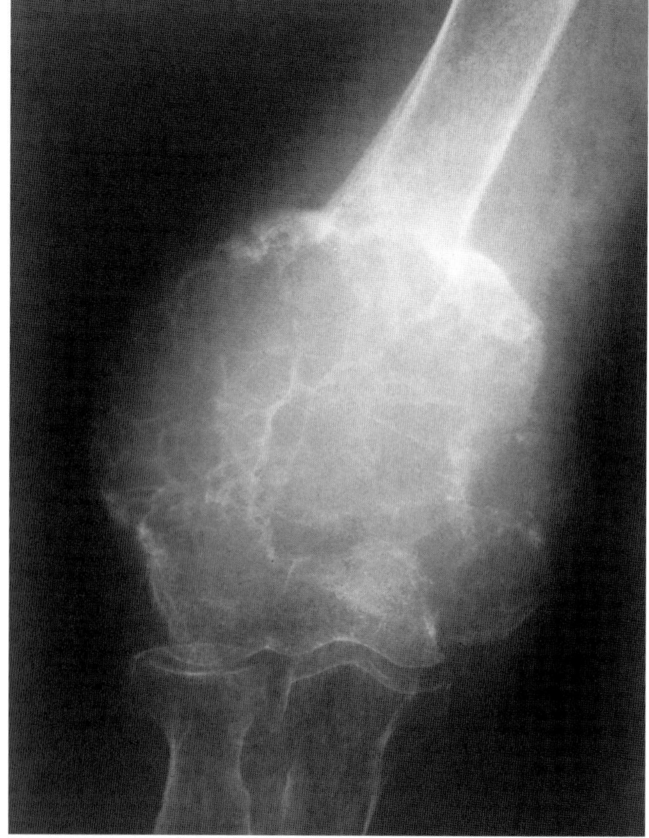

Fig. 35.18

reported: carcinomas of the esophagus, colon and rectum, prostate and uterus and even sarcomas such as osteosarcomas.[60]

The distal phalanges are most commonly affected and the role of their greater arterial flow has been implicated. Multiple lesions may be present, most frequently osteolytic with a soft tissue component; they may mimic infection.

Subdiaphragmatic tumors metastasize more frequently to *the foot*[60,61,64] (Fig. 35.4). Tumors of the bladder have a remarkable tendency to involve the foot, presumably by communication between the spinal veins of the lumbar region and the iliofemoral venous system.[61]

Skeletal metastases to periarticular bone may result in *intraarticular invasion* and the knee is the predominant site of joint involvement[65] (Fig. 35.5). Examination of synovial fluid may demonstrate a non-inflammatory bloody effusion or tumoral cells in half the cases.[65] The most common primary tumors are lung and breast carcinomas.

Very rarely, a *hematogenous spread to the synovium* occurs

Figs 35.17, 35.18 Expansile and lytic metastases from thyroid adenocarcinomas.

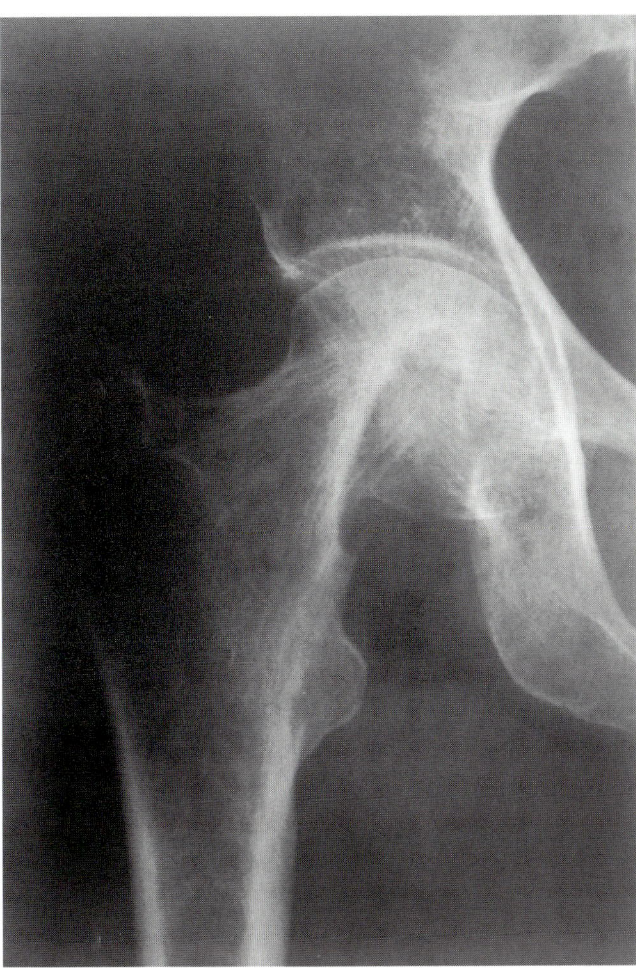

Fig. 35.19

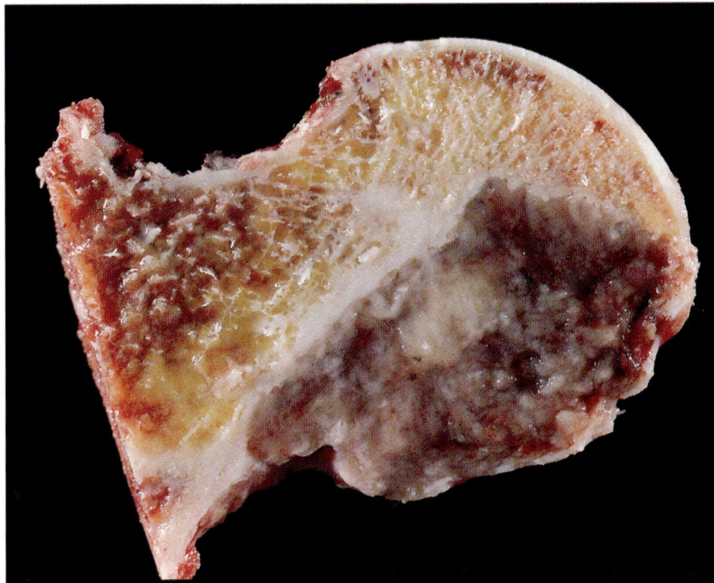

Fig. 35.20

Figs 35.19, 35.20 Lytic femoral metastasis from a thyroid adenocarcinoma.

without bone involvement,[66–69] appearing as a monoarticular arthritis (Fig. 35.6). The synovium may exhibit only reactive inflammatory changes in the proximity of metastatic tumors, with hypervascularity and a cellular infiltration with lymphocytes and plasma cells.[70,71]

IMAGING

If the multiplicity of lesions is the hallmark of metastatic disease, solitary lesions are relatively frequent and may be the initial presentation of occult carcinomas, such as some hepatocellular or renal carcinomas.[31]

The majority of metastases are *osteolytic and destructive* (Figs 35.7–35.26), with well-defined lucent defects (geographic bone destruction); the multiple lucent areas may also have a tendency to coalesce (moth-eaten destruction) or may be associated with a cortical lysis (permeative bone destruction). These patterns, as defined by Lodwick, reflect the rate of tumoral growth and may be combined.

Osteolytic metastases originate from tumors of the lung, breast, kidney, thyroid and gastrointestinal tract but also from the cervix, uterus, bladder, oral cavity and larynx. Carcinomas of the thyroid and kidney may exhibit large, expansile metastatic lesions, but expansion of bone is found also in metastases from tumors of the breast,[72] lung and malignant melanomas.

Osteoblastic metastases (Figs 35.27–35.36) may be so extensive that the entire skeleton appears uniformly dense. Ivory vertebrae of metastatic prostatic carcinomas are well known. Osteosclerotic metastases can be found in breast cancers, oat cell carcinomas[4] or adenocarcinomas of the lung, bronchial and gastrointestinal carcinoids,[73] carcinomas of the stomach, colon, pancreas, medulloblastomas, seminomas and even medullary carcinomas of the thyroid.

Dystrophic punctate or annular calcifications, frequently found in mucin-producing adenocarcinomas, may mimic the mineralized chondroid matrix of a primary bone tumor.[74]

Mixed osteolytic-osteoblastic changes are common in breast carcinomas (Figs 35.37, 35.38).

In a *long bone*, any portion may be involved, but there is a special predilection for the metaphysis and the midshaft in the region supplied by the nutrient vessels (Wilner 1982).

Cortical metastases (Fig. 35.39) may be the only evidence of metastatic disease,[75] appearing as intracortical focal lesions, large osteolytic lesions, cortical saucerized lesions with defined periosteal reaction or tumors extending into the soft tissues and medullary cavity.[76–78] They are located in the diaphysis or the metadiaphysis, close to a nutrient artery, and mostly involve the femoral bones, in some cases with a symmetrical distribution.[79]

Carcinomas of the lung are the primary tumors in most cases, but cases have been reported involving metastases from tumors of the breast, kidney, pancreas, larynx and

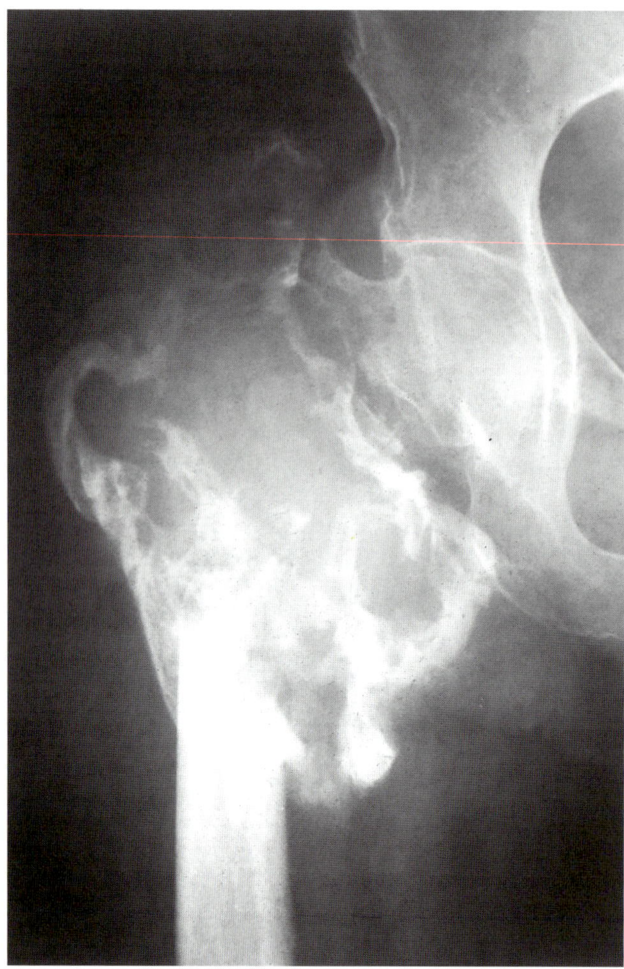

Fig. 35.21

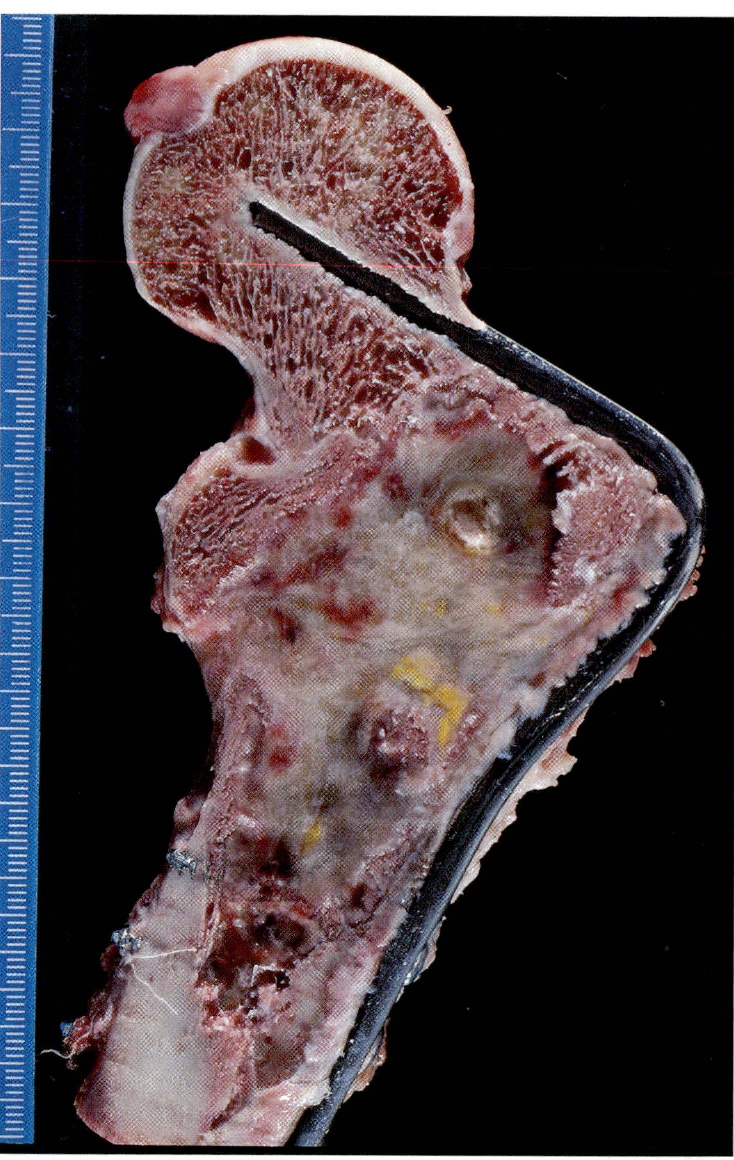

Fig. 35.22

Figs 35.21, 35.22 Extensive lytic femoral metastases from thyroid carcinomas.

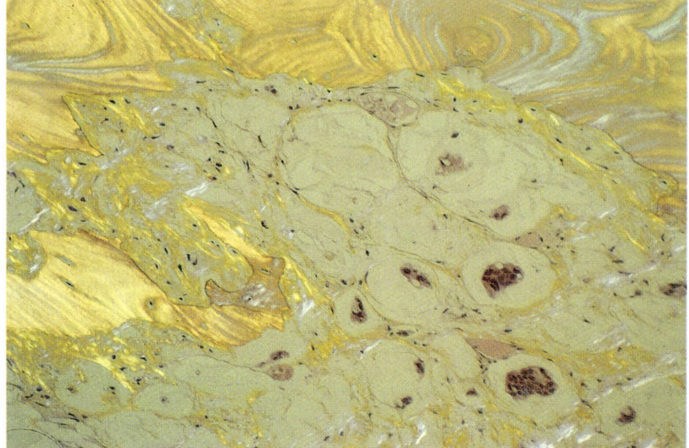

Fig. 35.23

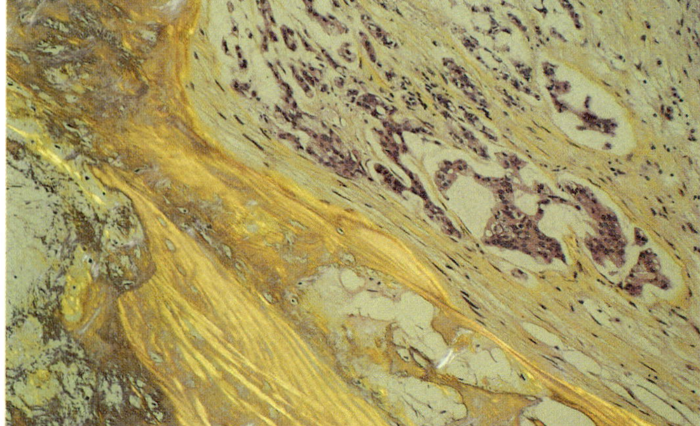

Fig. 35.24

Figs 35.23, 35.24 Lytic vertebral metastasis from a breast mucinous adenocarcinoma (polarized light).

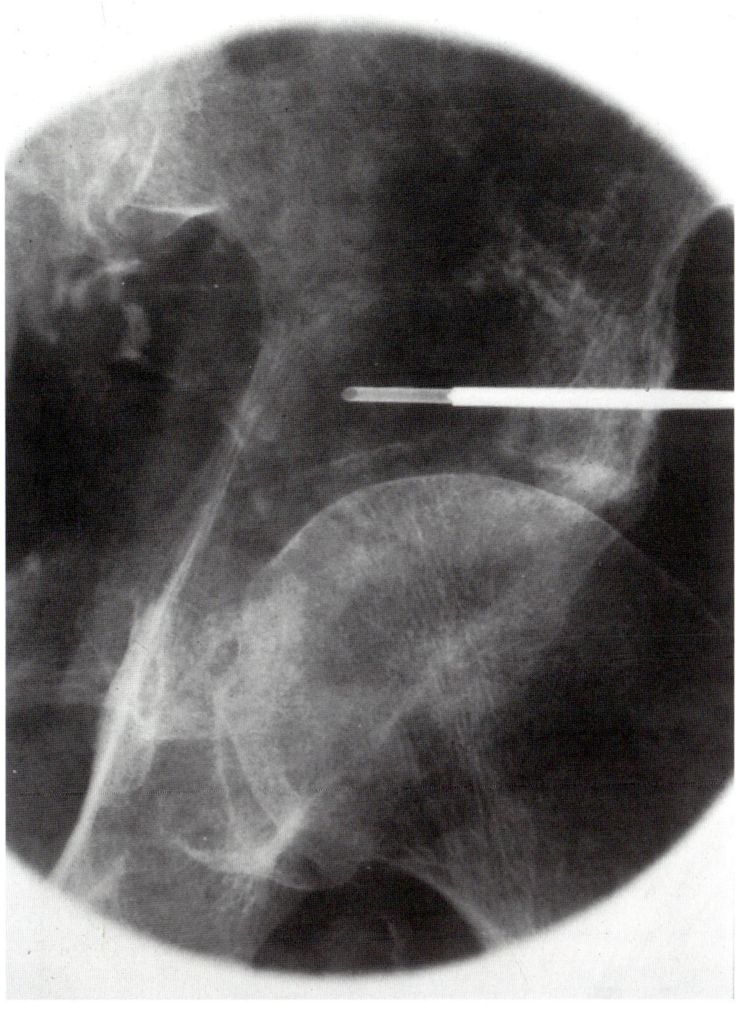

Fig. 35.25

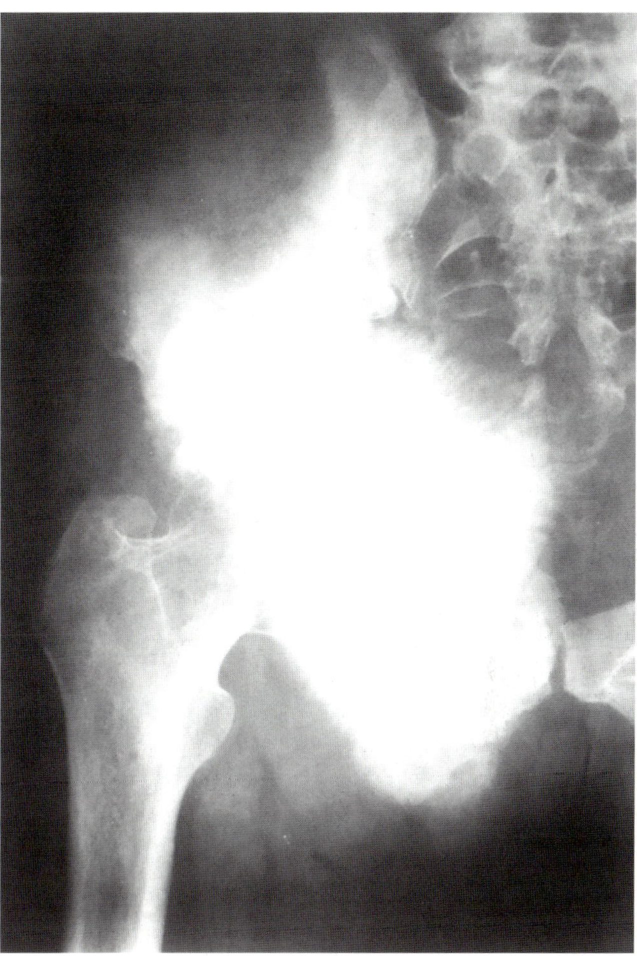

Fig. 35.27 Widespread osteoblastic metastasis from a prostatic adenocarcinoma involving the pelvis.

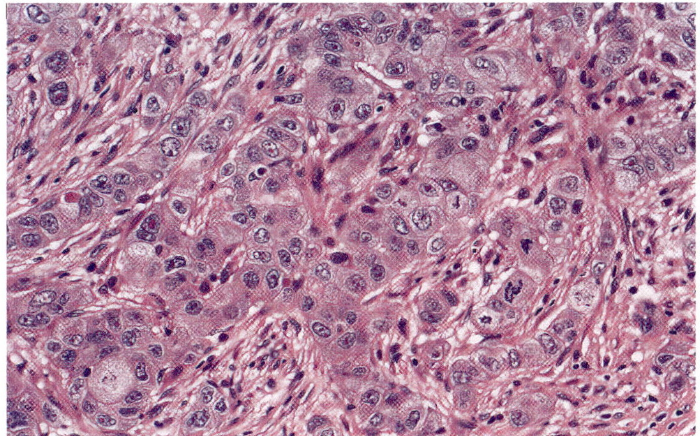

Fig. 35.26

Figs 35.25, 35.26 Lytic acetabular metastasis of a bladder carcinoma.

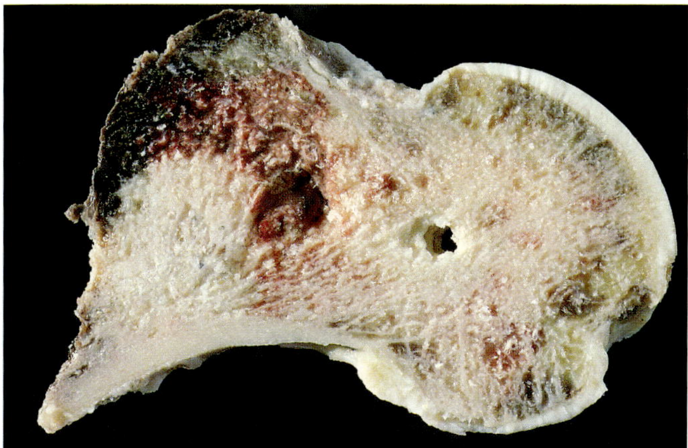

Fig. 35.28 Osteoblastic metastasis from a prostatic adenocarcinoma involving the femur.

uterus. The role of the distinct intracortical network of intercommunicating capillaries has been suggested, the capillaries being supplied by anastomotic branches from periosteal, medullary and nutrient arterial vessels.[75]

Periosteal bone formation in metastatic disease may mimic osteosarcoma (Fig. 35.40). In some cases, it may correspond to a pathologic fracture. It is an uncommon response to metastatic tumors (1–2% of cases[80,81]) and

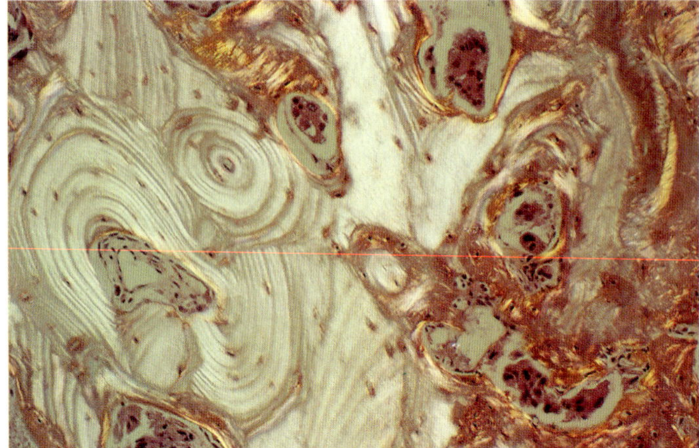

Fig. 35.29

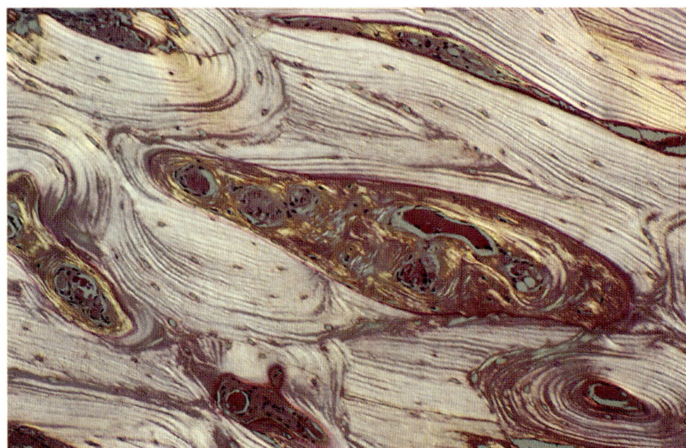

Fig. 35.30

Figs 35.29, 35.30 Bone formation in a vertebral metastasis from a prostatic adenocarcinoma (polarized light).

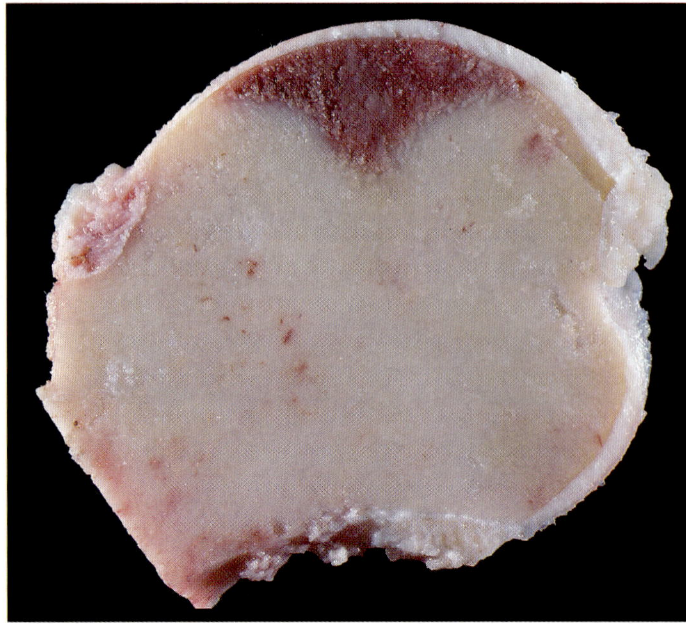

Fig. 35.31

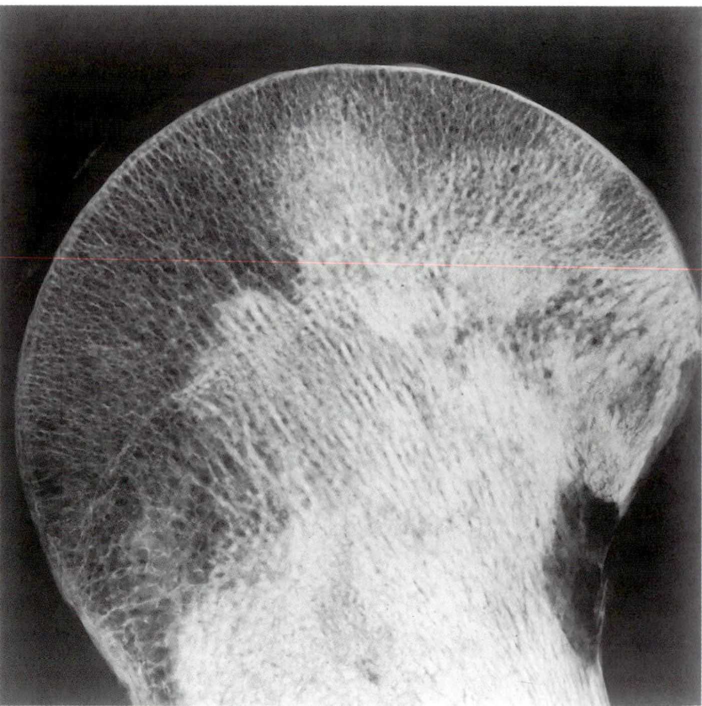

Fig. 35.32

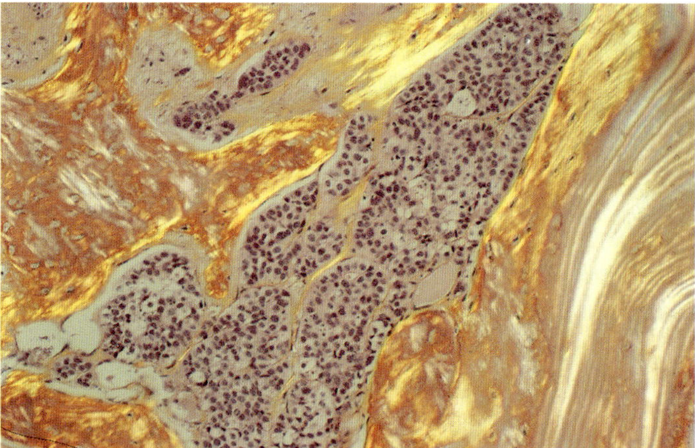

Fig. 35.33

Figs 35.31–35.33 Osteoblastic metastasis from a breast adenocarcinoma in the femoral head; massive bone formation (polarized light).

the majority of cases are associated with osteoblastic metastases.

Dense periosteal reactions, Codman triangles, lamellated reactions and sunburst spiculated reactions have been reported.[82–84] The periosteal reaction does not form in the area of rapid and maximal bone destruction.[84] Various sites are involved: pelvis, femur, scapula, humerus,[85] tibia, fibula,[83] skull and, in a few cases, vertebrae.[80,81] The most frequent primary tumors are prostatic cancers,[85,86] followed by gastrointestinal[81,87] and bronchial tumours and neuroblastomas.[80,83,84] They have been reported in metastases from retinoblastomas, carcinoid tumors, bladder

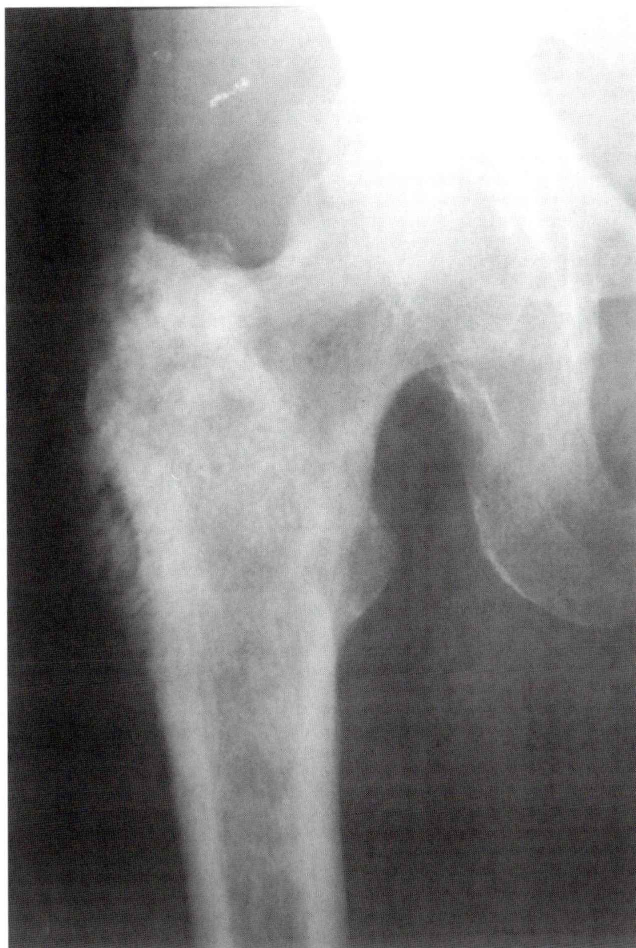

Figs 35.34

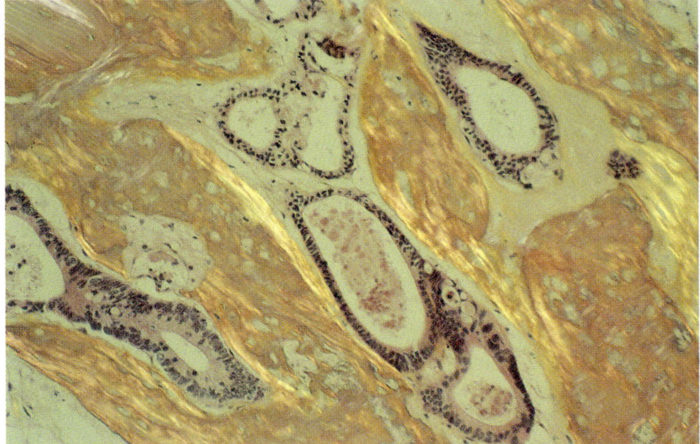

Figs 35.35

Figs 35.34, 35.35 Periosteal reaction and osteoblastic changes in a femoral metastasis from an adenocarcinoma of the colon (polarized light).

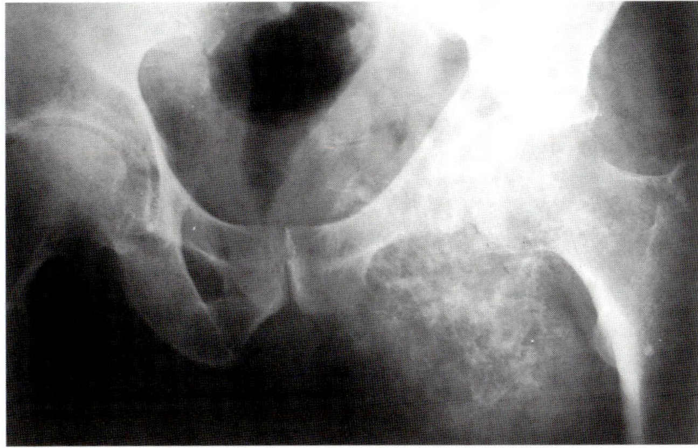

Fig. 35.36 Ischiatic metastasis from a bladder carcinoma mimicking a chondrosarcoma on imaging.

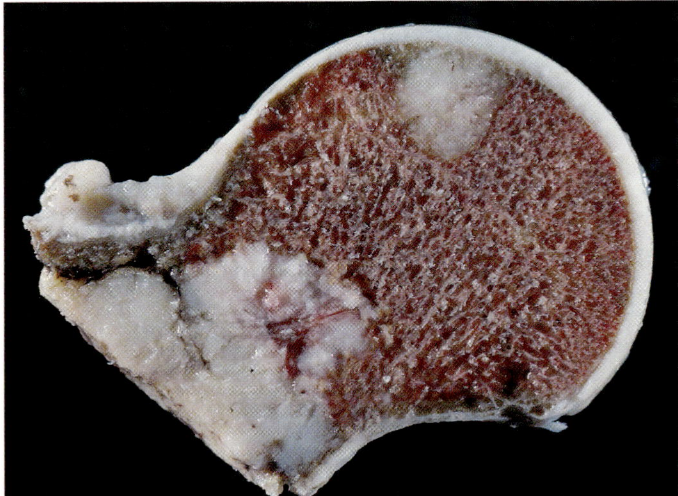

Figs 35.37

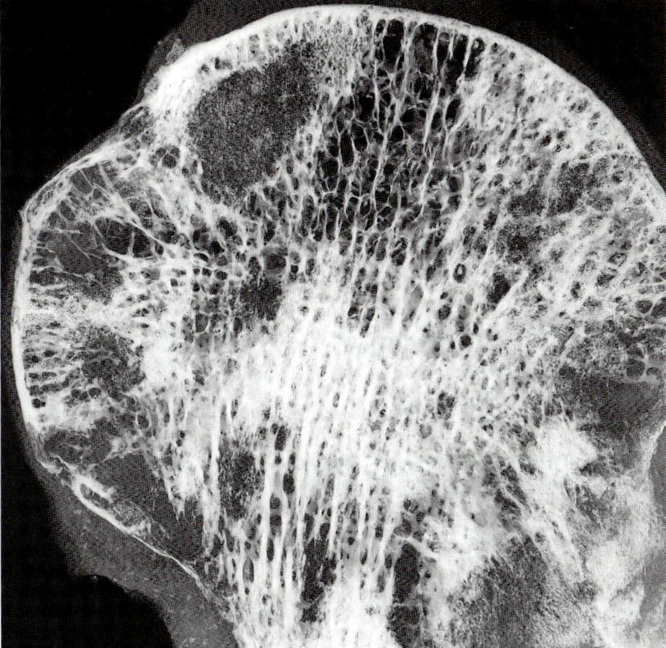

Figs 35.38

Figs 35.37, 35.38 Mixed osteolytic and osteoblastic changes in femoral metastases from breast adenocarcinomas.

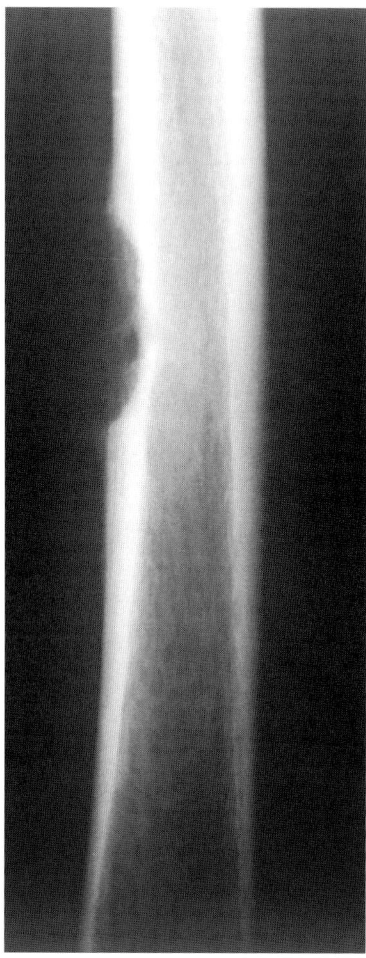

Fig. 35.39 Cortical metastasis from a lung carcinoma in femoral location.

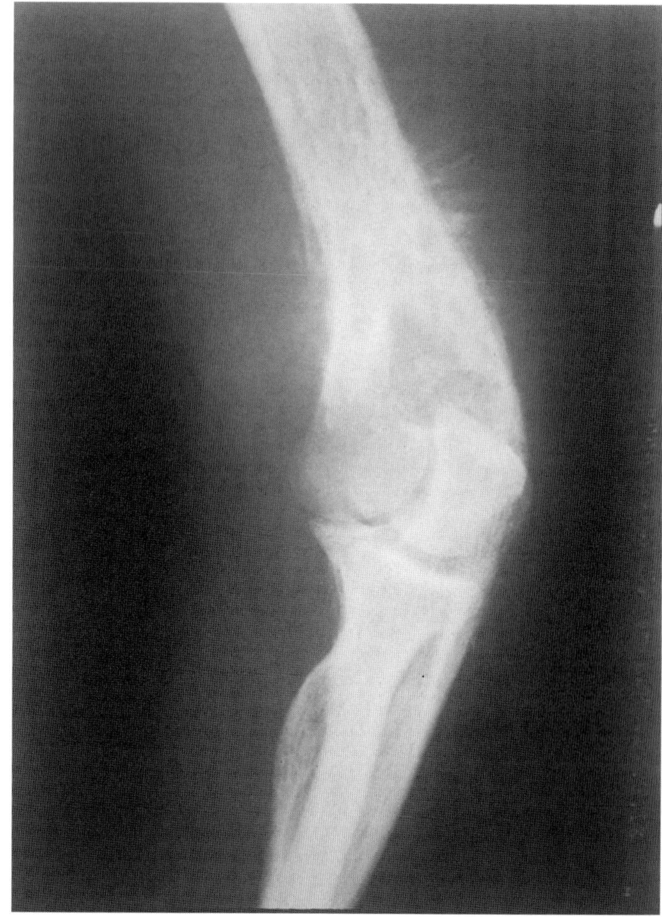

Fig. 35.40 Sunburst spiculated reaction in a humeral metastasis from an adenocarcinoma of the colon.

tumors, thyroid and adrenal gland tumors[88] and even rhabdomyosarcomas.[84] They are rarely found in metastatic breast cancers.[83]

PRIMARY BONE TUMORS OR METASTASES?

Sporadic and perplexing cases without identification of a primary lesion[89] have been reported, including an extensive sacral carcinoid tumor, an extrarenal juxtaglomerular cell tumor in bone,[90] intraosseous chondroid syringomas,[91,92] a multicentric mixed tumor of bone,[93] an extrapulmonary small cell carcinoma in bone[94] and a clear cell sarcoma.[95]

REFERENCES

1. Abrams H L, Spiro R, Goldstein N. Metastases in carcinoma. Analysis of 1000 autopsied cases. Cancer 1950: 3: 74–85
2. Johnston A D. Pathology of metastatic tumors in bone. Clin Orthop 1970: 73: 8–32
3. Schmid C, Marocolo D, Tombesi V, Beretta G. Bone marrow biopsy in the staging of malignant epithelial tumors. Appl Pathol 1983: 1: 343–347
4. Muggia F M, Hansen H H. Osteoblastic metastases in small-cell (oat-cell) carcinoma of the lung. Cancer 1972: 30: 801–805
5. Wong W S, Kaiser L R, Gold R H, Fon G T. Radiographic features of osseous metastases of soft-tissue sarcomas. Radiology 1982: 143: 71–74
6. Leeson M C, Makley J T, Carter J R. Metastatic skeletal disease in the pediatric population. J Pediatr Orthop 1985: 5: 261–267
7. O'Connor M T, Currier B L. Metastatic disease of the spine. Orthopedics 1992: 15: 611–620
8. Ogden J A, Ogden D A. Skeletal metastasis: the effect on the immature skeleton. Skeletal Radiol 1982: 9: 73–82
9. Kalinowski D T, Goodwin C A. Case report 179. Metastatic disease developing in Paget disease in the distal end of the femur. Skeletal Radiol 1981: 7: 229–231
10. Powell N. Metastatic carcinoma in association with Paget's disease of bone. Br J Radiol 1983: 56: 582–585
11. Nicholas J J, Srodes C H, Herbert D, Hoy R J, Peel R L, Goodman M A. Metastatic cancer in Paget's disease of bone. Orthopedics 1987: 10: 725–729
12. Schajowicz F, Velan O, Santini Araujo E et al. Metastases of carcinoma in the pagetic bone. Clin Orthop 1988: 228: 290–296

13. Nottebaert M, Exner G U, Von Hoschtetter A R, Schreiber A. Metastatic bone disease from occult carcinoma: a profile. Int Orthop 1989: 13: 119–123

14. Baron M G, De La Gandara I, Espinosa E, De Paredes M L G, Zamora P, Mondejar J L. Bone metastases as the first manifestation of a tumour. Int Orthop 1991: 15: 373–376

15. Simon M A, Bartucci E J. The search for the primary tumor in patients with skeletal metastases of unknown origin. Cancer 1986: 58: 1088–1095

16. Rougraff B T, Kneisl J S, Simon M A. Skeletal metastases of unknown origin. J Bone Joint Surg (Am) 1993: 75: 1276–1281

17. McCartney D K, Euliano J J Jr. Undifferentiated sarcoma of bone versus undifferentiated metastatic carcinoma – a diagnostic dilemma. Orthopedics 1994: 17: 636–640

18. Knapp D, Abdul-Karim F W. Fine needle aspiration cytology of acrometastasis. Acta Cytol 1994: 38: 589–591

19. Singh H K, Silverman J F, Balance W A Jr, Parle H K. Unusual small bone metastases from epithelial malignancies: diagnosis by fine-needle aspiration cytology with histologic confirmation. Diagn Cytopathol 1995: 13: 192–195

20. Papac R J. Bone marrow metastases. Cancer 1994: 74: 2403–2413

21. Oberneder R, Riesenberg R, Kriegmair M et al. Immunocytochemical detection and phenotypic characterization of micrometastatic tumour cells in bone marrow of patients with prostate cancer. Urol Res 1994: 22: 3–8

22. Wood D P Jr, Banks E R, Humphreys S, McRoberts J W, Rangnekar V M. Identification of bone marrow micrometastases in patients with prostate cancer. Cancer 1994: 74: 2533–2540

23. Cote R J, Rosen P P, Hakes T B et al. Monoclonal antibodies detect occult breast carcinoma metastases in the bone marrow of patients with early stage disease. Am J Surg Pathol 1988: 12: 333–340

24. Cote R J, Rosen P P, Lesser M L, Old L J, Osborne M P. Prediction of early relapse in patients with operable breast cancer by detection of occult bone marrow micrometastases. J Clin Oncol 1991: 9: 1749–1756

25. Mundy G R, Yoneda T. Facilitation and suppression of bone metastasis. Clin Orthop 1995: 312: 34–44

26. Eilon G, Mundy G R. Direct resorption of bone by human breast cancer cells in vitro. Nature 1978: 276: 726–728

27. Galasko C S. Skeletal metastases. Clin Orthop 1986: 210: 18–30

28. Athanasou N A, Quinn J M. Human tumour-associated macrophages are capable of bone resorption. Br J Cancer 1992: 65: 523–526

29. Cramer S F, Fried L, Carter K J. The cellular basis of metastatic bone disease in patients with lung cancer. Cancer 1981: 48: 2649–2660

30. Taube T, Elomaa I, Blomqvist C, Beneton M N, Kanis J A. Histomorphometric evidence for osteoclast-mediated resorption in metastatic breast cancer. Bone 1994: 15: 161–166

31. Aoki J, Yamamoto I, Hino M et al. Osteoclast-mediated osteolysis in bone metastasis from renal cell carcinoma. Cancer 1988: 62: 98–104

32. Dodwell D J. Malignant bone resorption: cellular and biochemical mechanisms. Ann Oncol 1992: 3: 257–267

33. Orr F W, Sanchez-Sweatman O H, Kostenuik P, Singh G. Tumor-bone interactions in skeletal metastasis. Clin Orthop 1995: 312: 19–33

34. Mundy G R. Mechanisms of osteolytic bone destruction. Bone 1991: 12 (suppl 1): S1–S6

35. Orr F W, Kostenuik P, Sanchez-Sweatman O H, Singh G. Mechanisms involved in the metastasis of cancer to bone. Breast Cancer Res Treat 1993: 25: 151–163

36. Manishen W J, Sivananthan K, Orr F W. Resorbing bone stimulates tumor cell growth. Am J Pathol 1986: 123: 39–45

37. Carter R L. A role for local osteoclasts in determining the differential susceptibility of human cartilage and bone to invasion by carcinoma. Diagn Histopathol 1982: 5: 213–217

38. Galasko C S. Mechanisms of lytic and blastic metastatic disease of bone. Clin Orthop 1982: 169: 20–27

39. Jacobs S C, Pikna D, Lawson R K. Prostatic osteoblastic factor. Invest Urol 1979: 17: 195–198

40. Aoki J, Yamamoto I, Hino M et al. Sclerotic bone metastasis: radiologic-pathologic correlation. Radiology 1986: 159: 127–132

41. Burkhardt R, Frisch B, Schlag R, Sommerfeld W. Carcinomatous osteodysplasia. Skeletal Radiol 1982: 8: 169–178

42. Charhon S A, Chapuy M C, Delvin E E, Valentin-Opran A, Edouard C M, Meunier P J. Histomorphometric analysis of sclerotic bone metastases from prostatic carcinoma with special reference to osteomalacia. Cancer 1983: 51: 918–924

43. Clarke N W, McClure J, George N J. Osteoblast function and osteomalacia in metastatic prostate cancer. Eur Urol 1993: 24: 286–290

44. Arguello F, Baggs R B, Duerst R E, Johnstone L, McQueen K, Frantz C N. Pathogenesis of vertebral metastasis and epidural spinal cord compression. Cancer 1990: 65: 98–106

45. Batson O V. The function of the vertebral veins and their role in the spread of metastases. Ann Surg 1940: 112: 138–149

46. Vider M, Maruyama Y, Narvaez R. Significance of the vertebral venous (Batson's) plexus in metastatic spread in colorectal carcinoma. Cancer 1977: 40: 67–71

47. Okazaki N, Yoshino M, Yoshida T, Hirohashi S, Kishi K, Shimosato Y. Bone metastasis in hepatocellular carcinoma. Cancer 1985: 55: 1991–1994

48. Boland P J, Lane J M, Sundaresan N. Metastatic disease of the spine. Clin Orthop 1982: 169: 95–102

49. Drury R A B, Palmer P H, Higman W J. Carcinomatous metastasis to the vertebral bodies. J Clin Pathol 1964: 17: 448–457

50. Galasco C S. Skeletal metastases. Clin Orthop 1986: 210: 18–30

51. Thrall J H, Ellis B I. Skeletal metastases. Radiol Clin North Am 1987: 25: 1155–1170

52. Berrettoni B A, Carter J R. Mechanisms of cancer metastasis to bone. J Bone Joint Surg (Am) 1986: 68: 308–312

53. Fornasier V L, Horne J G. Metastases to the vertebral column. Cancer 1975: 36: 590–594

54. Algra P R, Heimans J J, Valk J, Nauta J J, Lachniet M, Van Kooten B. Do metastases in vertebrae begin in the body or the pedicles? AJR 1992: 158: 1275–1279

55. Sartoris D J, Resnick D, Guerra J Jr. Vertebral venous channels: CT appearances and differential considerations. Radiology 1985: 155: 745–749

56. Asdourian P L, Weidenbaum M, DeWald R L, Hammerberg K W, Ramsey R G. The pattern of vertebral involvement in metastatic vertebral breast cancer. Clin Orthop 1990: 250: 164–170

57. Resnick D, Niwayama G. Intervertebral disc abnormalities associated with vertebral metastasis. Observations in patients and cadavers with prostatic cancer. Invest Radiol 1978: 13: 182–190

58. Yasuma T, Yamauchi Y, Arai K, Makino E. Histopathologic study on tumor infiltration into the intervertebral disc. Spine 1989: 14: 1245–1248

59. Gottlieb P D, Parikh S J, Singh J K. Case report 295. Metastatic disease of the carpus (primary site: bronchogenic carcinoma). Skeletal Radiol 1985: 13: 154–158

60. Healey J H, Turnbull A D, Miedema B, Lane J M. Acrometastases. J Bone Joint Surg (Am) 1986: 68: 743–746

61. Libson E, Bloom R A, Husband J E, Stoker D J. Metastatic tumours of bones of the hand and foot. Skeletal Radiol 1987: 16: 387–392

62. Abrahams T G. Occult malignancy presenting as metastatic disease to the hand and wrist. Skeletal Radiol 1995: 24: 135–137

63. Nagendran T, Patel M N, Gaillard W E, Imm F, Walker M. Metastatic bronchogenic carcinoma to the bones of the hand. Cancer 1980: 45: 824–828

64. Gall R J, Sim F H, Pritchard D J. Metastatic tumors to the bones of the foot. Cancer 1976: 37: 1492–1495

65. Munn R K, Pierce S T, Sloan D, Weeks J A. Malignant joint effusions secondary to solid tumor metastasis. J Rheumatol 1995: 22: 973–975

66. Goldenberg D L, Kelley W, Gibbons R B. Metastatic adenocarcinoma of synovium presenting as an acute arthritis. Arthritis Rheum 1975: 18: 107–110

67. Fam A G, Kolin A, Lewis A J. Metastatic carcinomatous arthritis and carcinoma of the lung: a report of two cases diagnosed by synovial fluid cytology. J Rheumatol 1980: 7: 98–104

68. Murray G C, Persellin R H. Metastatic carcinoma presenting as monoarticular arthritis. Arthritis Rheum 1980: 23: 95–100

69. Ritch P S, Hansen R M, Collier B D. Metastatic renal cell

carcinoma presenting as shoulder arthritis. Cancer 1983: 51: 968–972

70. Gerster J C, Jaquier E, Ribaux C. Nonspecific inflammatory monoarthritis in the vicinity of bony metastases. J Rheumatol 1987: 14: 844–847

71. Lagier R. Synovial reaction caused by adjacent malignant tumors. J Rheumatol 1977: 4: 65–72

72. Mootoosamy I M, Anchor S C, Dacie J E. Expanding osteolytic bone metastases from carcinoma of the breast: an unusual appearance. Skeletal Radiol 1985: 14: 188–190

73. Johnson D G, Osborne D, Bossen E H. Case report 185. Metastasis to the femur from a bronchial carcinoid tumor. Skeletal Radiol 1982: 7: 293–295

74. Ribalta T, Shannon R L, Ro J Y, Carrasco C H, Ayala A G. Case report 645. Metastatic mucin-producing adenocarcinoma consistent with urachal origin. Skeletal Radiol 1990: 19: 616–619

75. Hendrix R W, Rogers L F, Davis T M Jr. Cortical bone metastases. Radiology 1991: 181: 409–413

76. Greenspan A, Klein M J, Lewis M M. Case report 272. Skeletal (predominantly) cortical metastases in the left femur arising from a bronchogenic carcinoma. Skeletal Radiol 1984: 11: 297–301

77. Greenspan A, Klein M J, Lewis M M. Case report 284. Osteolytic cortical metastasis in the femur from bronchogenic carcinoma. Skeletal Radiol 1984: 12: 146–150

78. Greenspan A, Norman A. Osteolytic cortical destruction: an unusual pattern of skeletal metastases. Skeletal Radiol 1988: 17: 402–406

79. Deutsch A, Resnick D, Niwayama G. Case report 145. Bilateral, almost symmetrical skeletal metastases (both femora) from bronchogenic carcinoma. Skeletal Radiol 1981: 6: 144–148

80. Bloom R A, Libson E, Husband J E, Stocker D J. The periosteal sunburst reaction to bone metastases. Skeletal Radiol 1987: 16: 629–634

81. Sanzari R, Paton P, Boutet O, Guasch F, Charhon A, Tete R. Metastases osseuses pseudo-sarcomateuses des cancers recto-sigmoido-coliques. Sem Hôp Paris 1992: 68: 1369–1373

82. Penn M B, Schnier G J. Metastatic prostatic carcinoma simulating primary osteogenic sarcoma. J Coll Radiol Aust 1964: 8: 160–165

83. Norman A, Ulin R. A comparative study of periosteal new bone response in metastatic bone tumors (solitary) and primary bone sarcomas. Radiology 1969: 92: 705–708

84. Wyche L D, De Santos L A. Spiculated periosteal reaction in metastatic disease resembling osteosarcoma. Orthopedics 1978: 1: 215–221

85. Legier J F, Tauber L N. Solitary metastasis of occult prostatic carcinoma simulating osteogenic sarcoma. Cancer 1968: 22: 168–172

86. Lehrer H Z, Maxfield W S, Nice C M. The periosteal 'sunburst' pattern in metastatic bone tumors. Am J Roentgenol Radium Ther Nucl Med 1970: 108: 154–161

87. Pope T L Jr, Paling M, Renner J B, Kruse B. Exuberant periosteal reaction in solitary skeletal metastases: a mimic of primary skeletal neoplasms. Orthopedics 1990: 13: 261–264

88. Vilar J, Lezana A H, Pedroza C S. Spiculated periosteal reaction in metastatic lesions of bone. Skeletal Radiol 1979: 3: 230–233

89. Schnee C L, Hurst R W, Curtis M T, Friedman E D. Carcinoid tumor of the sacrum: case report. Neurosurgery 1994: 35: 1163–1167

90. Chen W S, Chang J W. Extrarenal juxtaglomerular cell tumor in bone. Chin Med J (Engl) 1987: 100: 78–82

91. Wagoner W L, Spencer R B, Ramos R P. Chondroid syringoma. A rare occurrence in the hallux. J Am Podiatr Med Assoc 1993: 83: 424–425

92. Barreto C A, Lipton M N, Smith H B, Potter G K. Intraosseous chondroid syringoma of the hallux. J Am Acad Dermatol 1994: 30: 374–378

93. Rose A G, Heselson N G, Marks R K, Kranold D. Multicentric mixed tumor of bone with pulmonary involvement. Skeletal Radiol 1992: 21: 140–145

94. Raina V, Milroy R, Al-Dawoud A, Dunlop D, Soukop M. Extrapulmonary small cell carcinoma of bone. Postgrad Med J 1992: 68: 147–148

95. Yokoyama R, Mukai K, Hirota T, Beppu Y, Fukuma H. Primary malignant melanoma (clear cell sarcoma) of bone. Cancer 1996: 77: 2471–2475

Pathology of pseudotumoral lesions

36

Solitary bone cyst

M. Forest

CHAPTER CONTENTS

INTRODUCTION AND CLINICAL DATA

Solitary, simple, unicameral or juvenile bone cyst is an intramedullary cavity lined by a thin connective tissue membrane and usually filled with a clear fluid.

The incidence, among the biopsied primary bone tumors, is about 3%, but it appears to be a more common lesion in orthopedic practice, with an equal sex ratio in some series[1] or a male predominance of 2:1.

More than 90% of the cases are diagnosed in the first two decades of life (Schajowicz 1994), with a peak incidence between 3 and 14 years. Cysts of the pelvis and calcaneus are more frequent in patients older than 20 years,[2] but this finding is debated.[3]

Clinical symptoms are local tenderness, pain and swelling or joint stiffness. Solitary bone cysts may attain a large size without symptoms, as in the scapula.[4] In most cases (60%), pain is related to a fracture. Occasionally, growth retardation or premature closure of the growth plate is found in long bones.

PATHOGENESIS

Many theories have been suggested for the formation of a solitary bone cyst, including local disturbance in bone growth,[4] role of preexisting lesions,[5–7] small nests of synovial cells trapped in an intraosseous position[8] or intramedullary hemorrhages as some posttraumatic cysts may have the same histologic features.[9,10]

The most favored mechanism is an alteration in the pattern of venous drainage;[5,11–13] internal pressure is slightly higher than the normal pressure of bone marrow and the PO_2 of the cyst fluid is lower than that of the venous or arterial blood, suggesting a venous obstruction.[13] Bone resorption may be due to a developmental anomaly occurring in the veins, with venous stasis, elevated internal pressure and fluid accumulation.[14]

Biochemical analyses have shown that the cyst fluid

resembles serum, but values of alkaline and acid phosphastases are higher and the total protein content is smaller.[11,15,16] The cyst fluid contains bone resorptive factors: prostaglandins, interleukin 1 and proteolytic enzymes.[14,16,17] Degeneration of cell membranes and breakdown of the matrix may also be caused by oxygen-free radicals produced by localized ischemia due to the elevated internal pressure.[15] Further microcirculatory disturbances may be induced by the elevated activity of lysosomal enzymes, increasing the osmotic pressure of the fluid with water accumulation and higher hydrostatic pressure.[18]

SKELETAL DISTRIBUTION

The most common locations are the proximal humerus and proximal femur (80%) (Figs 36.1–36.4), followed by the proximal tibia and calcaneus[19–22] (Figs 36.5, 36.6). Other locations have been reported including the pelvis, the sacrum,[23] the spine,[24–27] the scapula,[28–30] the clavicle,

the ribs,[31] phalanx,[32] metatarsals,[33] and even the patella.[34] In the pelvis, the most common location is the wing of the innominate bone[3,35] (Figs 36.7–36.13). Occasionally, multiple cysts may be found in one bone or different bones[36–40] (Figs 36.14, 36.15).

IMAGING

In long bones, the lucent well-defined lesion with a narrow zone of transition is centrally located, with a mild symmetrical expansion of bone. The cortex is thinned but remains intact; there is no periosteal reaction in the absence of fracture. The cyst may appear trabeculated or multiloculated due to ridges on the inner surface of the cortex.

The cyst involves the metaphysis, abutting the epiphyseal plate; involvement of the epiphysis is a rare occurrence.[41,42] In patients with immature skeletons, it may cross the cartilage plate and penetrate into the epiphysis or apophysis.[43]

The total length is variable, but the cyst may involve the

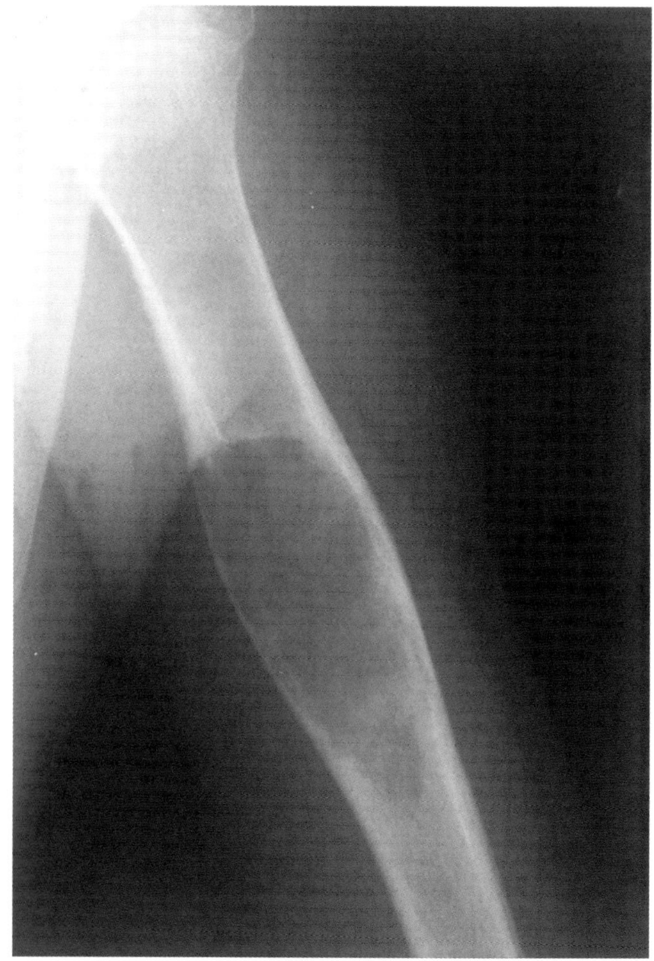

Fig. 36.1

Fig. 36.2

Figs 36.1, 36.2 Solitary bone cysts of the humerus.

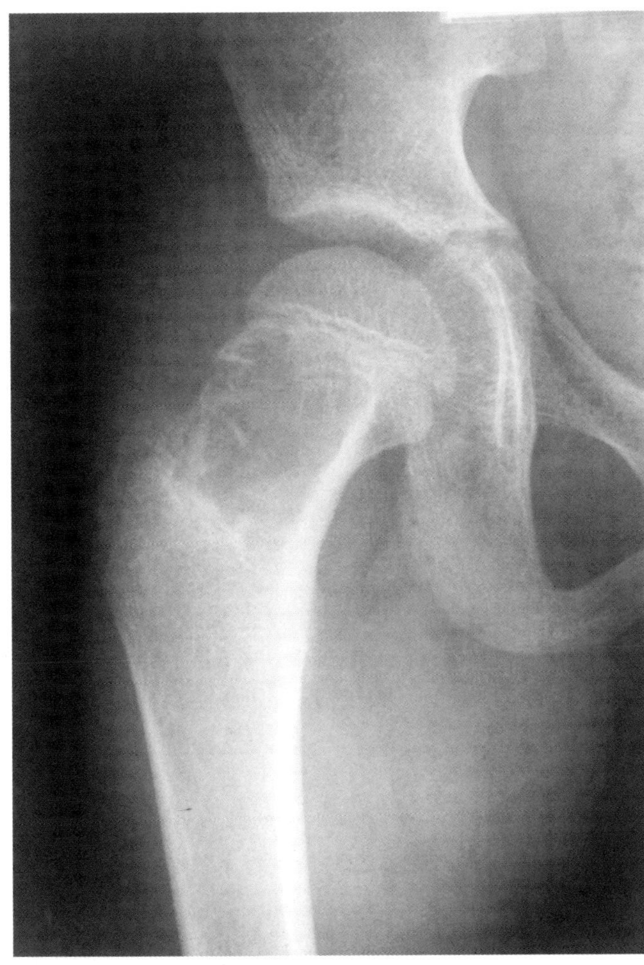

Fig. 36.3

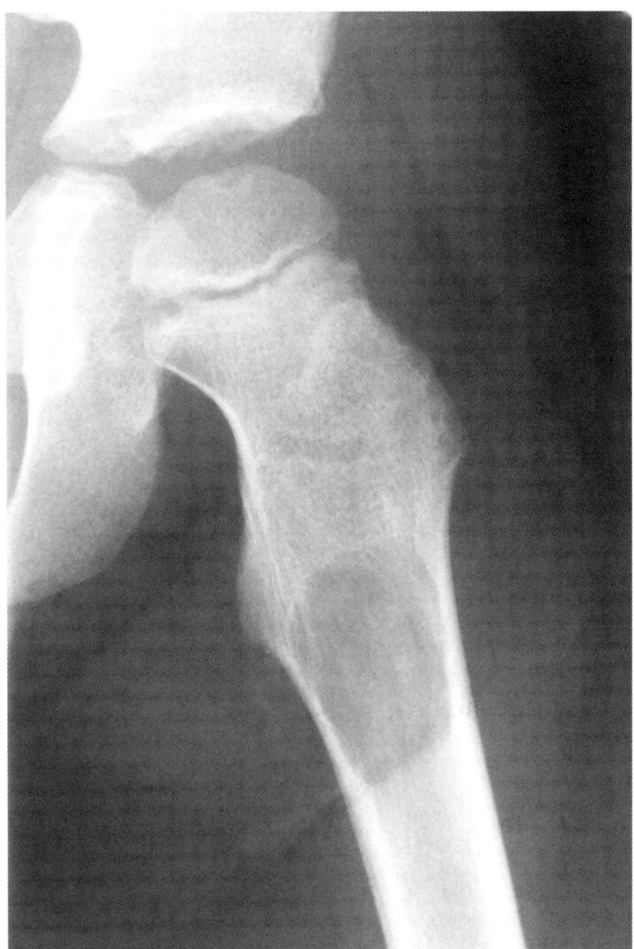

Fig. 36.4

Figs 36.3, 36.4 Solitary bone cysts of the femur.

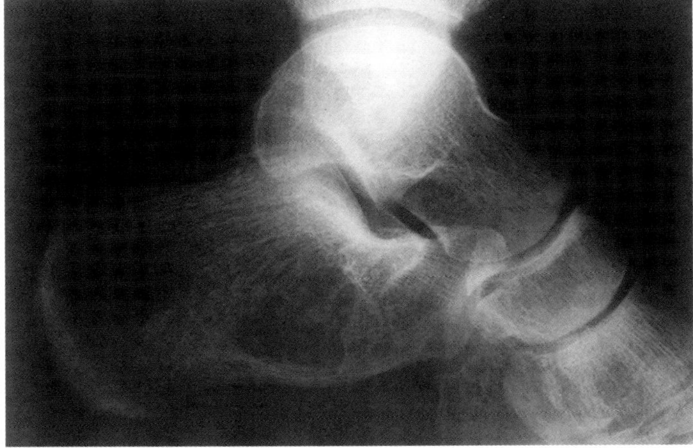

Fig. 36.5

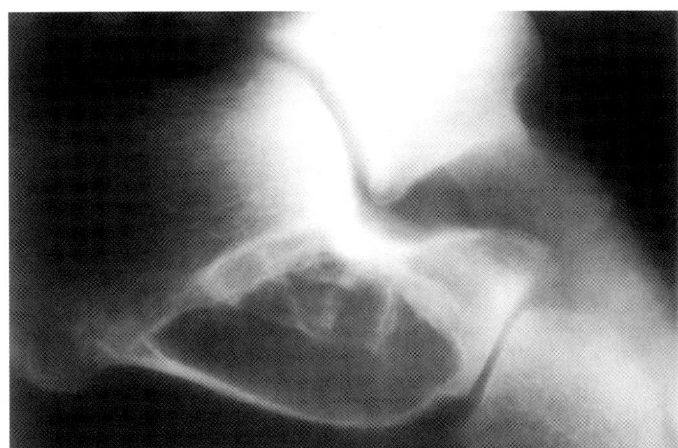

Fig. 36.6

Figs 36.5, 36.6 Solitary bone cysts of the calcaneus.

entire shaft. With growth the lesion moves shaftward, away from the metaphysis, becoming a latent form, according to Jaffe but this view is debated.

The fallen fragment sign, found in 26% of cases, is a prominent radiologic feature.[44,45] Single or multiple fragments of the cyst wall, associated with a pathologic frac-

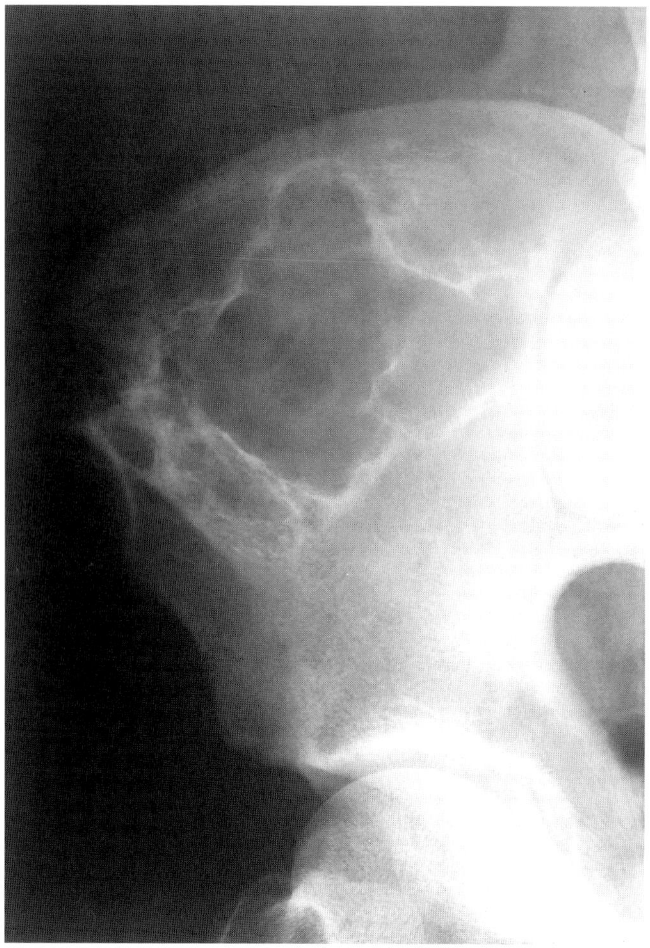

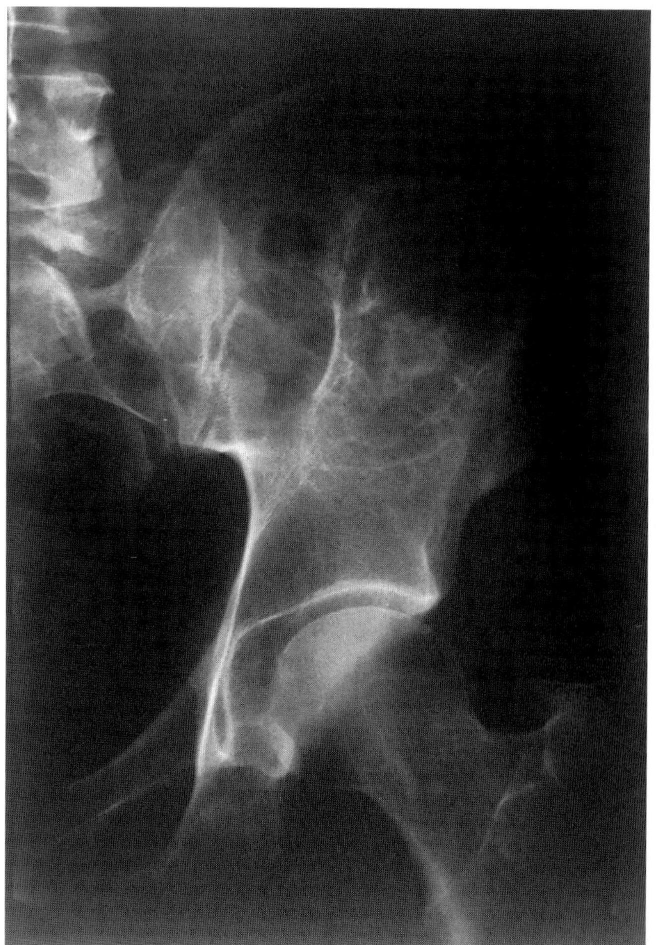

Fig. 36.7 Solitary bone cyst of the ilium with peripheral reactive sclerosis.

Fig. 36.8

ture, are found intramedullary, confirming the cystic character of the lesion.

The radionuclide bone scan may be normal or exhibit decreased activity in the center of the cyst.

CT scan can demonstrate gas–fluid or fluid–fluid levels.[46–48] Intracystic fibrous septa have been demonstrated in some cases, following local injection of radiopaque medium.[49] On MRI examination, the cysts exhibit a low signal intensity on T1 and a high signal intensity on T2-weighted images; a fluid–fluid level may be demonstrated.[48]

In the calcaneus, the cyst develops in the mid to anterior part of the bone, in an inferior location; the shape of the purely lytic, well-marginated lesion is characteristic, with usually no expansion of bone,[21] or pathologic fractures. On imaging, it has to be differentiated from lipomas, which are more lucent, and from simulated cysts which demonstrate a nutrient foramen[50] are never symptomatic. Pseudocysts are also found in the proximal humerus, appearing as cyst-like rarefactions of bone.[51,52]

In flat bones such as the ilium or the scapula,[3,29,53] the cysts may be quite large, with a multitrabeculated appearance.

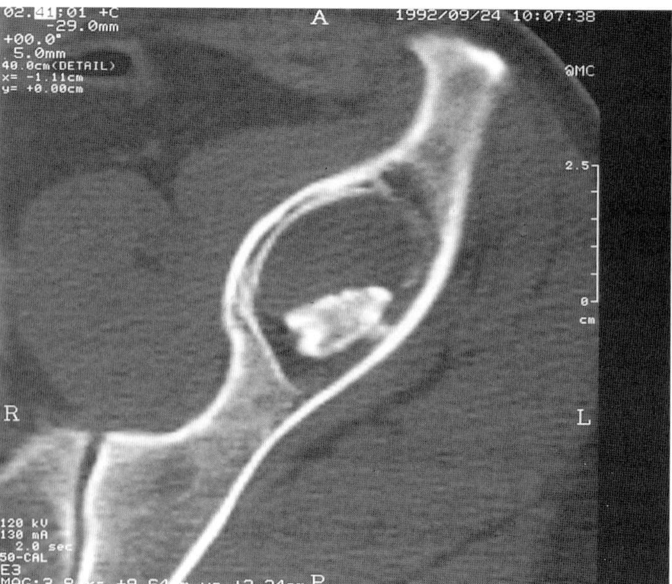

Fig. 36.9

Figs 36.8, 36.9 Solitary bone cyst of the ilium with a core of necrotic bone lying free in the cavity.

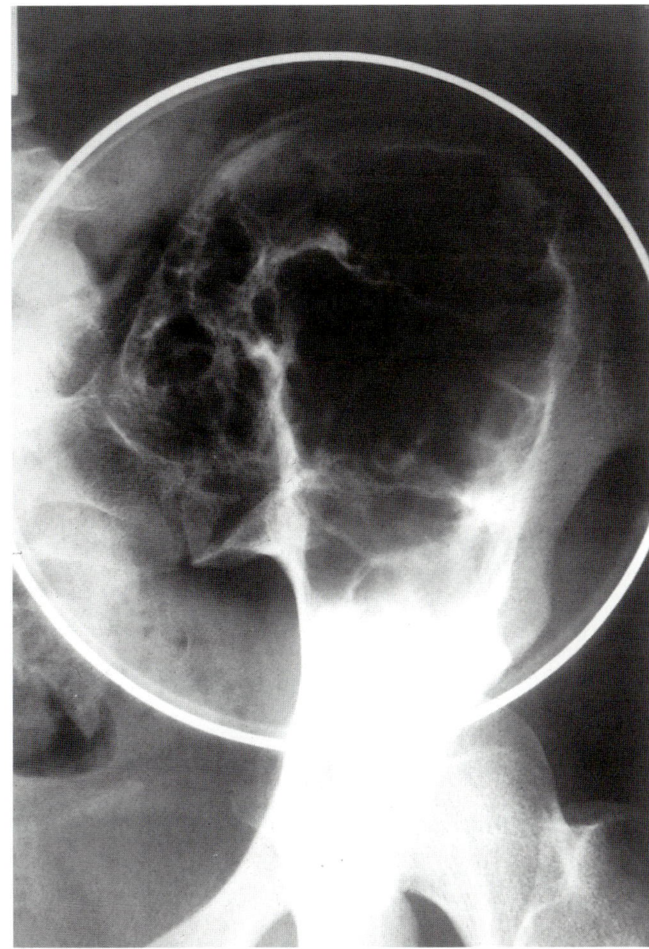

Fig. 36.10

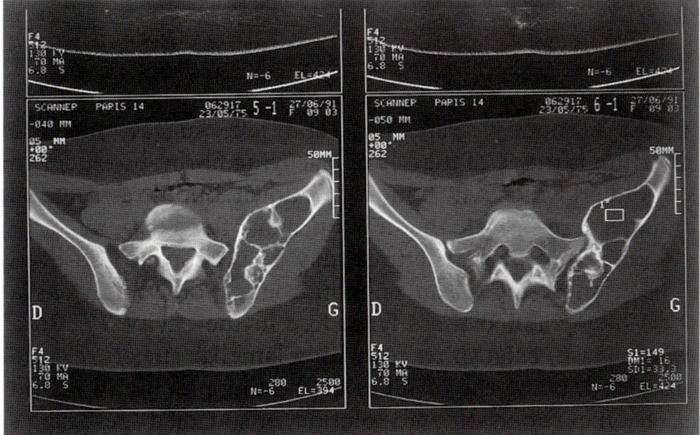

Fig. 36.11

Figs 36.10, 36.11 Solitary bone cyst of the ilium with few septae.

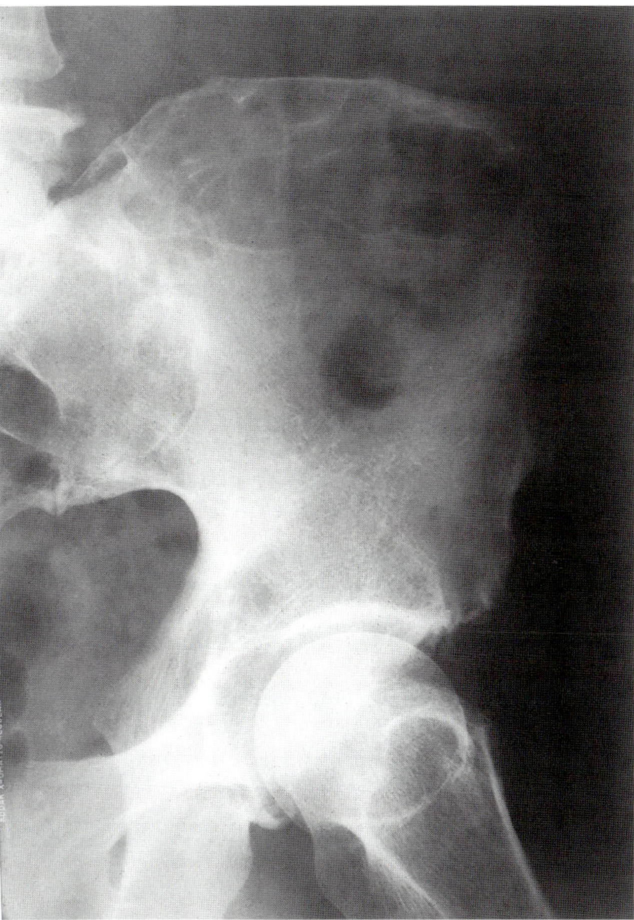

Fig. 36.12

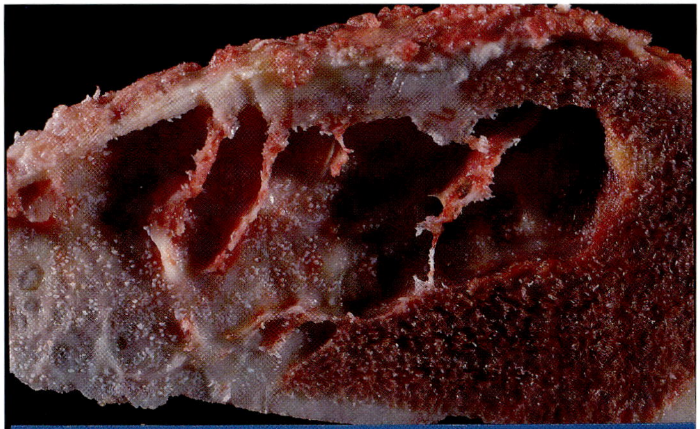

Fig. 36.13

Figs 36.12, 36.13 Solitary bone cyst of the iliac crest with a multiloculated appearance.

GROSS PATHOLOGY

The cortex appears very thin, as does the inner smooth membrane. The cyst fluid is clear or yellowish and the cavity may be empty. After a fracture, the cyst is filled with blood or clots, the membrane is thicker and fibrinous or fibrous membranes may be responsible for a multilocular appearance.

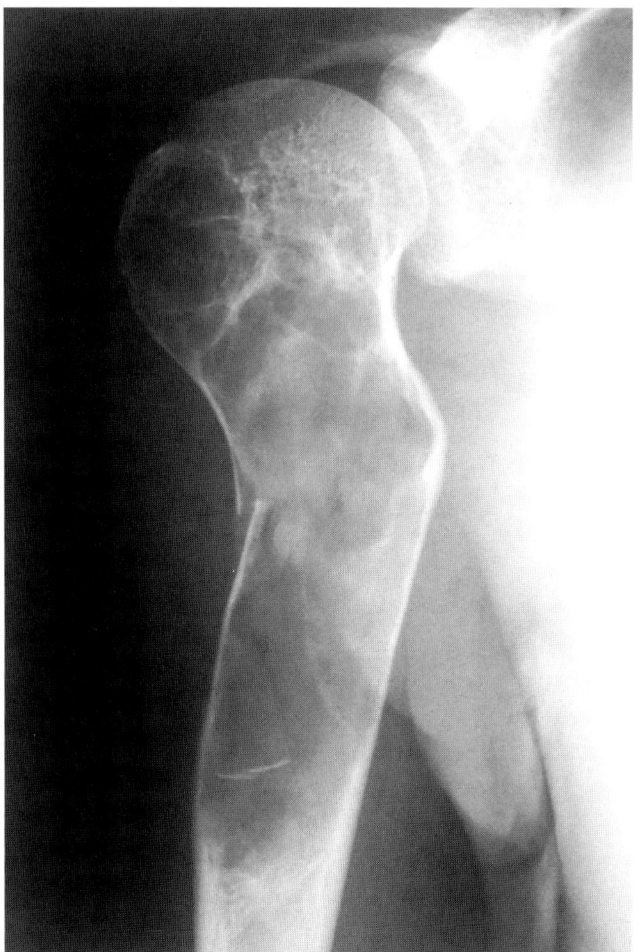

Fig. 36.14

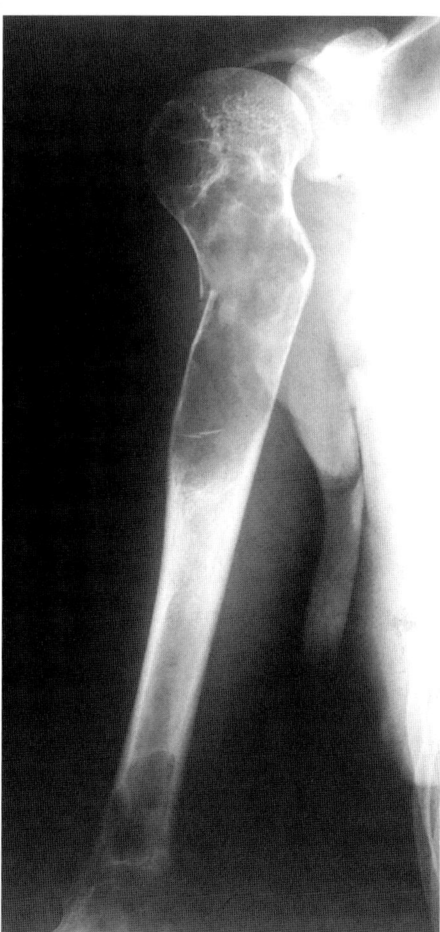

Fig. 36.15

Figs 36.14, 36.15 Fractured solitary bone cyst of the humerus with fallen fragments of the cortex and a second lesion in the distal part of the bone.

HISTOPATHOLOGY

The wall of the cyst is well-vascularized new bone produced by the periosteum. The lining membrane is loose connective tissue; immature bone or osteoid trabeculae with a rim of osteoblasts can be detected even in the absence of fracture (Figs 36.16–36.18). The membrane is usually composed of layers of flattened cells.

Following a fracture, hemorrhages are associated with hemosiderin deposition, cholesterol clefts, granulation tissue and osteoclast-like giant cells.

In 9–70% of cases,[8,54,55] cementum-like structures of varying size, isolated or confluent, are found in the wall of the cyst (Figs 36.19–36.26). This strongly eosinophilic and irregularly calcified material is devoid of cells, lamellar layers or peripheral Sharpey's fibers.[8,54] It may be surrounded by osteoid or immature bone with a rim of osteoblasts.[8,54,56,57]

This cementum-like structure appears quite characteristic of solitary bone cysts; it is not found in other cystic conditions of bone.[57] Sanerkin[57] and Jaffe suggest that the structure is made of masses of calcifying fibrin, producing a scaffold on which new bone is laid down, but ultrastructural findings demonstrate that it is a peculiar form of bone.

Cementum-like structures may be numerous and even appear on X-ray as an enchondroma[56] or, grossly, as a coral-like calcified mass lying free in the cavity.[56,57] In a unique case, calcospherites with a lamellar structure were described, being the result of alternating precipitation and diffusion of supersaturated solution, or so-called Liesegang's rings.[58]

DNA CONTENT

DNA cytophotometry shows a DNA diploid distribution.[55]

CYTOGENETICS

In a case of a femoral solitary bone cyst, 11.6% of cells

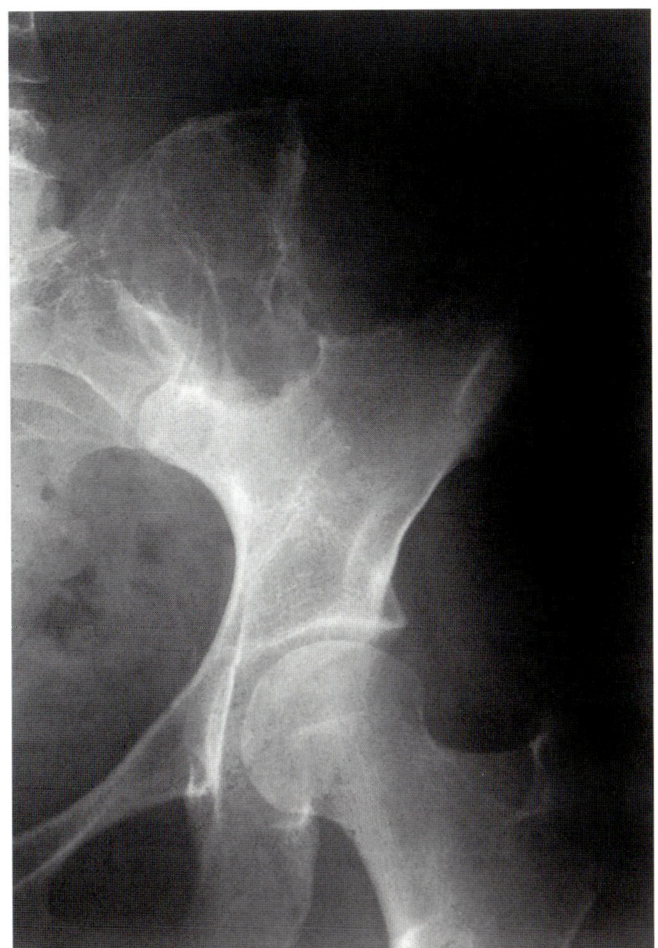

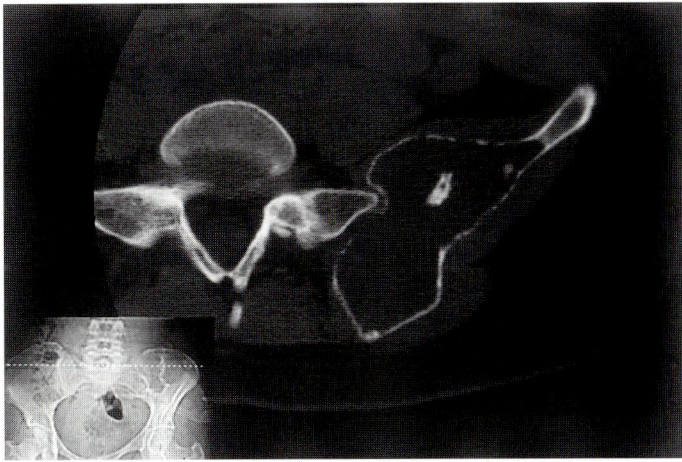

Fig. 36.17

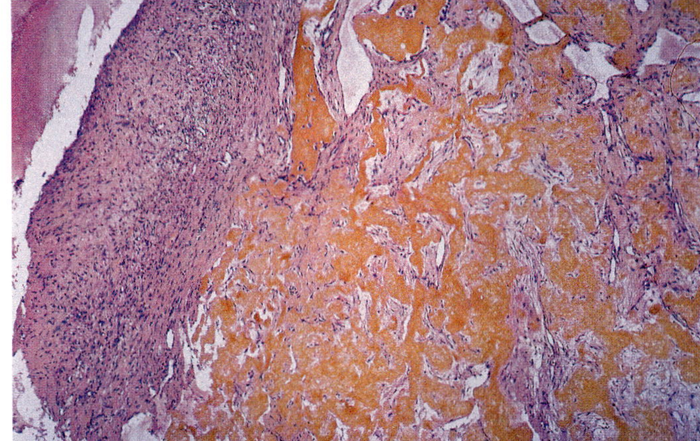

Fig. 36.16

Fig. 36.18

Figs 36.16–36.18 Solitary bone cyst of the ilium: the cavity is bordered by fibrous tissue covering immature bone production.

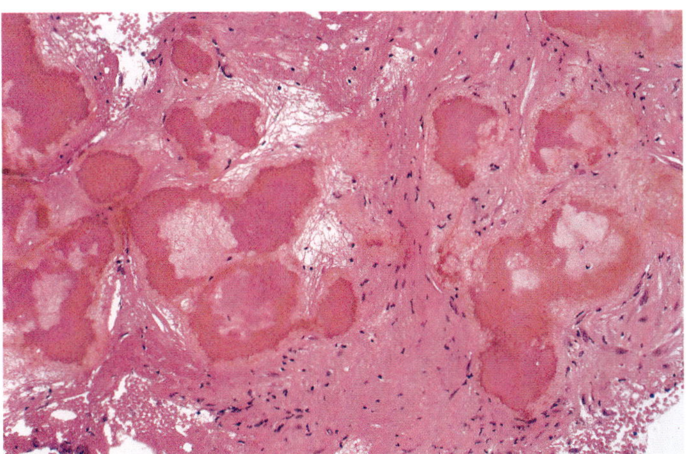

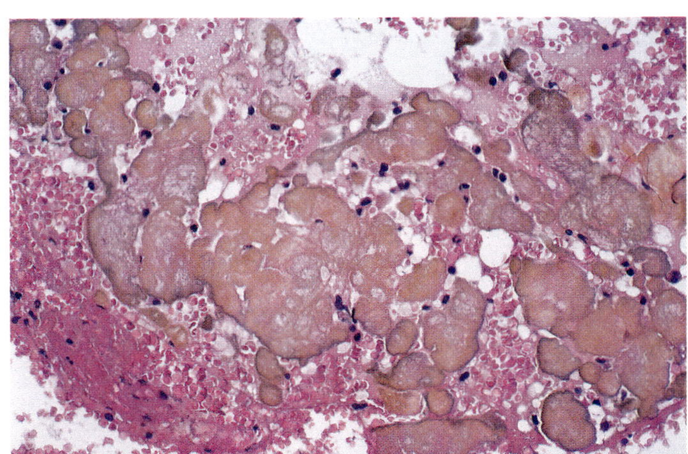

Fig. 36.19

Fig. 36.20

Figs 36.19, 36.20 Solitary bone cysts: cementum-like structures, some of them lying free in the cavity.

presented a complex clonal structural rearrangement involving chromosomes 4, 6, 8, 16 and 21 and both chromosomes 22.[59]

ELECTRON MICROSCOPY

The membrane has a cellular component of fibroblasts

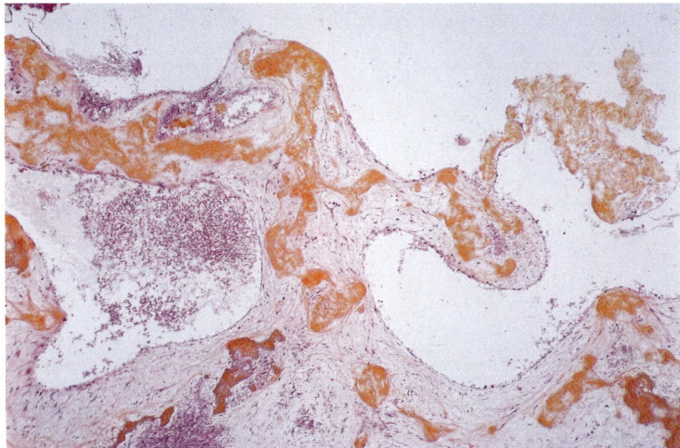

Fig. 36.21

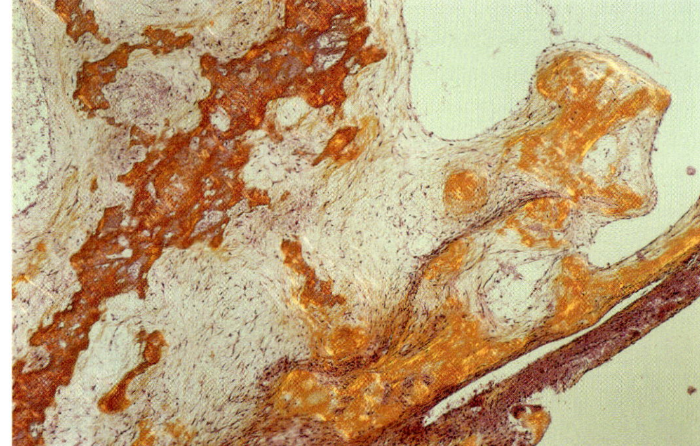

Fig. 36.23

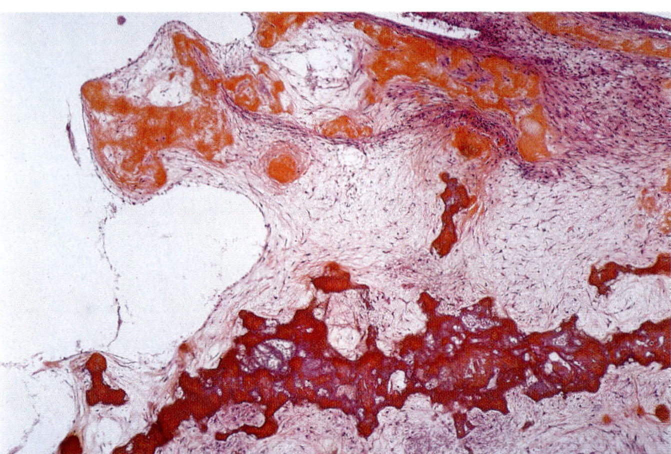

Fig. 36.22

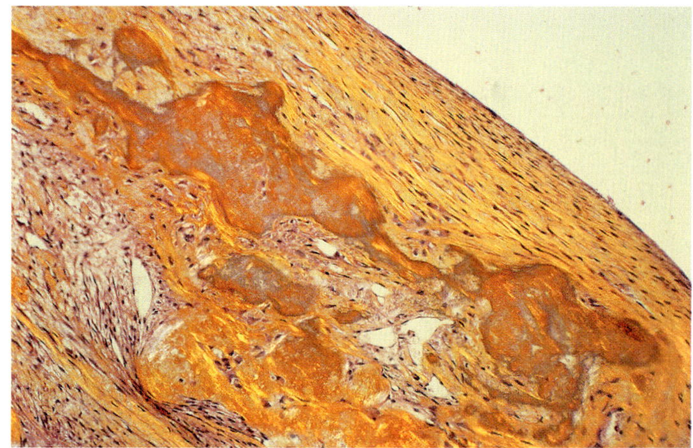

Fig. 36.24

Figs 36.21–36.24 Overviews of the distribution of the eosinophilic and irregularly calcified material in the membranes of solitary bone cysts (Figs 36.21 and 36.24 polarized light).

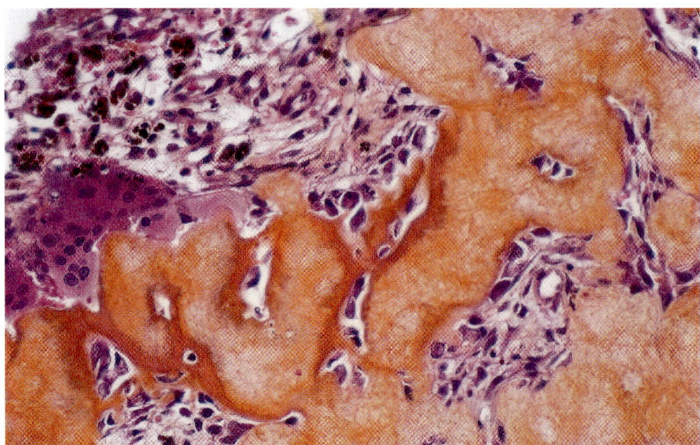
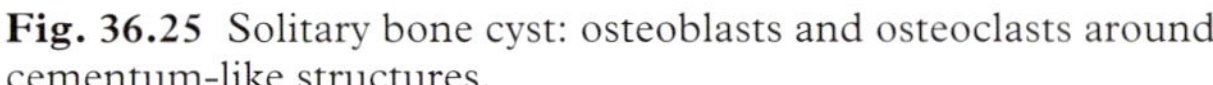

Fig. 36.25 Solitary bone cyst: osteoblasts and osteoclasts around cementum-like structures.

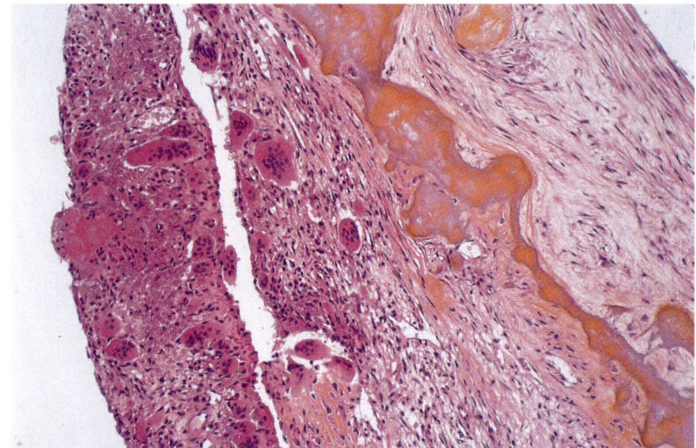

Fig. 36.26 Fractured solitary bone cyst of the humerus: the lining is more cellular with many reactive giant cells.

and myofibroblasts.[8] The lining cells of one case showed the ultrastructural features of synovial cells.[8] In the cementum-like areas, the numerous membrane-bound structures are matrix vesicles derived from osteoblasts, leading to the identification of a peculiar form of bone; this material is not derived from calcified fibrin or blood clots.[8]

Ultrastructurally, the growth plate may present slits, an appreciable number of vessels in the hyaline and proliferative zones and a reduced number of chondrocytes with pronounced cellular degenerative changes.[60]

CLINICAL COURSE, TREATMENT AND PROGNOSIS

Rarely, spontaneous regression has been reported, even after a fracture and even in a calcaneal location.[19] Even more rarely, sarcomas have been described occurring in bone cysts.[61–63]

Curettage of the cyst and packing with bone chips is followed by a recurrence rate of 15–40%, particularly in children under 10 years of age.[2] Since 1974, local injections of steroids, after aspiration of the cyst fluid, have given similar results.[64,65] Drainage of the cyst fluid is also obtained by drilling holes in the cyst wall.[14]

DIFFERENTIAL DIAGNOSIS

In a few cases, especially after a fracture, a solitary bone cyst may be histologically quite similar to an aneurysmal bone cyst[66] (Figs 36.27–36.30); one has to rely for the diagnosis on the X-rays or on the finding of the cementum-like material.[57]

In 1969, the name 'cementoma of long bones' was proposed for two cases suggesting solitary bone cysts on imaging.[67] Many authors now believe that this lesion is a genuine solitary bone cyst, the cyst being completely filled

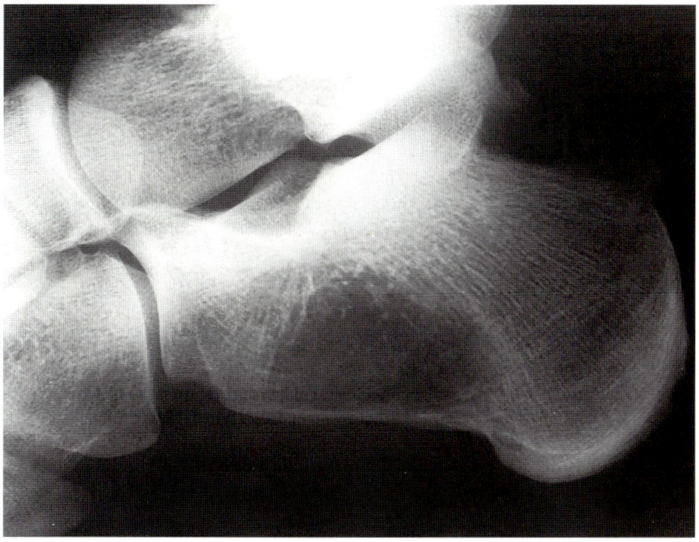

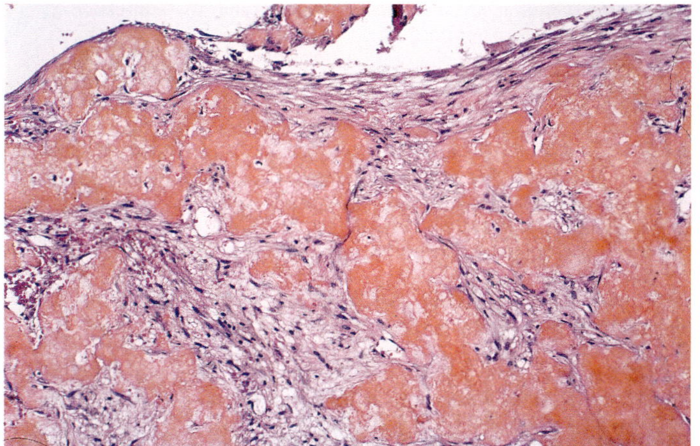

Fig. 36.27

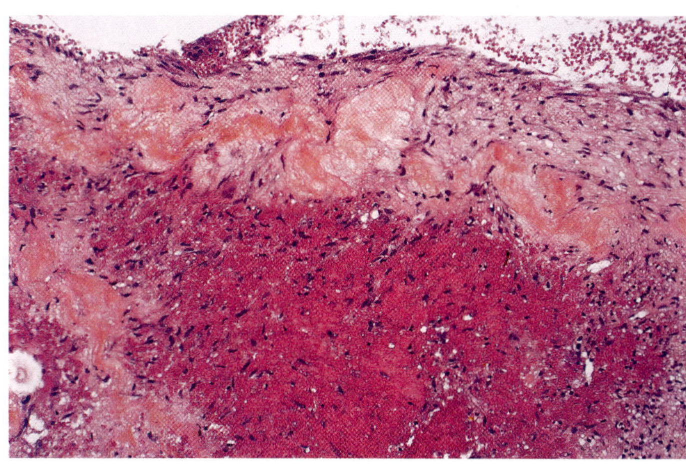

Fig. 36.29

Fig. 36.28

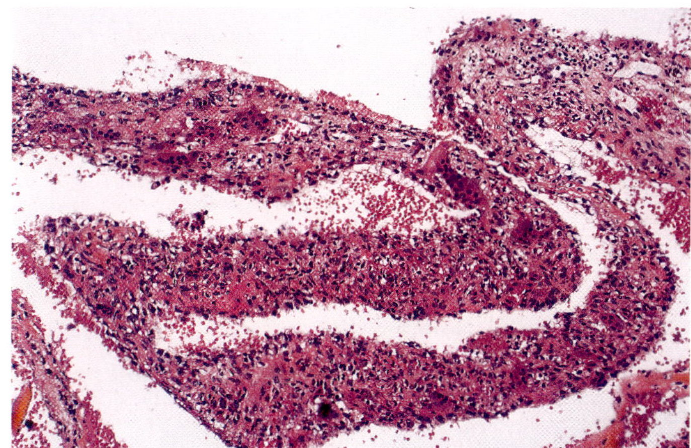

Fig. 36.30

Figs 36.27–36.30 Solitary bone cyst of the calcaneus with hemorrhage and aneurysmal bone cyst transformation.

by the mineralized component.[8, 54–56] The new term of 'calcifying solitary bone cyst' has recently been suggested.[55]

The lesions are found in older patients in various locations, including humerus, femur, tibia, pelvis and scapula.[55] The metaphyseal sclerotic lesion has cloudy dense opacities reminiscent of the popcorn pattern of enchondromas.[55,56] Histologically, a calcified cementum-like material is found, devoid of any cells.[54,55]

Rare, so-called cementoma-like bone fibromas have been reported,[68,69] exhibiting cement-like globular structures in a dense fibrous stroma. The name 'cementofibrous dysplasia' has been proposed,[70] as these peculiar lesions are not at all similar to calcifying bone cysts but are more like bone lesions described as ossifying fibromas or fibroosseous lesions of bone,[55,70,71] very closely related to fibrous dysplasia.

REFERENCES

1. Makley J T, Joyce M J. Unicameral bone cyst (simple bone cyst). Orthop Clin North Am 1989: 20: 407–415
2. Norman A, Schiffman M. Simple bone cysts: factors of age dependency. Radiology 1977: 124: 779–782
3. Abdelwahab I F, Hermann G, Norton K I, Kenan S, Lewis M M, Klein M J. Simple bone cysts of the pelvis in adolescents. J Bone Joint Surg (Am) 1991: 73: 1090–1094
4. Jaffe H L, Lichtenstein L. Unicameral bone cyst, with emphasis on the roentgen picture, pathologic appearance and pathogenesis. Arch Surg 1942: 44: 1004–1025
5. Broder H M. Possible precursor of unicameral bone cysts. J Bone Joint Surg (Am) 1968: 50: 503–507
6. Weisel A, Hecht H L. Development of a unicameral bone cyst. J Bone Joint Surg (Am) 1980: 62: 664–666
7. Watanabe H, Arita S, Chigira M. Aetiology of a simple bone cyst. Int Orthop 1994: 18: 16–19
8. Mirra J M, Bernard G W, Bullough P G, Johnston W, Mink G. Cementum-like bone production in solitary bone cysts (so-called 'cementoma' of long bones). Clin Orthop 1978: 135: 295–307
9. Phillips C D, Keats T E. The development of post-traumatic cyst-like lesions in bone. Skeletal Radiol 1986: 15: 631–634
10. Moore T E, King A R, Travis R C, Allen B C. Post-traumatic cysts and cyst-like lesions of bone. Skeletal Radiol 1989: 18: 93–97
11. Cohen J. Etiology of simple bone cyst. J Bone and Joint Surg (Am) 1970: 52: 1493–1497
12. Cohen J. Unicameral bone cysts: a current synthesis of reported cases. Orthop Clin North Am 1977: 8: 715–736
13. Chigira M, Maehara S, Arita S, Udagawa E. The aetiology and treatment of simple bone cysts. J Bone Joint Surg (Br) 1983: 65: 633–637
14. Komiya S, Minamitani K, Sasaguri Y, Hashimoto S, Morimatsu M, Inoue A. Simple bone cyst. Treatment by trepanation and studies on bone resorptive factors in cyst fluid with a theory of its pathogenesis. Clin Orthop 1993: 287: 204–211
15. Komiya S, Tsuzuki K, Mangham D C, Sugiyama M, Inoue A. Oxygen scavengers in simple bone cysts. Clin Orthop 1994: 308: 199–206
16. Markovic B, Cvijetic A, Karakasevic J. Acid and alkaline phosphatase activity in bone-cyst fluid. J Bone Joint Surg (Br) 1988: 70: 27–28
17. Shindell R, Connolly J F, Lippiello L. Prostaglandin levels in a unicameral bone cyst treated by corticosteroid injection. J Pediatr Orthop 1987: 7: 210–212
18. Gerasimov A M, Toporova S M, Furtseva L N, Berezhnoy A P, Vilensky E V, Alekseeva R I. The role of lysosomes in the pathogenesis of unicameral bone cysts. Clin Orthop 1991: 266: 53–63
19. Smith R W, Smith C F. Solitary unicameral bone cyst of the calcaneus. J Bone Joint Surg (Am) 1974: 56: 49–56
20. Van Linthoudt D, Lagier R. Calcaneal cysts. Acta Orthop Scand 1978: 49: 310–316
21. Abdelwahab I F, Lewis M M, Klein M J, Barbera C. Case report 515. Simple (solitary) bone cyst of the calcaneus. Skeletal Radiol 1989: 17: 607–610
22. Moreau G, Letts M. Unicameral bone cyst of the calcaneus in children. J Pediatr Orthop 1994: 14: 101–104
23. Ehara S, Rosenberg A E, El-Khoury G Y. Sacral cysts with exophytic components. Skeletal Radiol 1990: 19: 117–119
24. Dawson E G, Mirra J M, Yuhl E T, Lasser K. Solitary bone cyst of the cervical spine. Clin Orthop 1976: 119: 141–143
25. Wu K K, Guise E R. Unicameral bone cyst of the spine. J Bone Joint Surg (Am) 1981: 63: 324–326
26. Brodsky A E, Khalil M, Van Deventer L. Unicameral bone cyst of a lumbar vertebra. J Bone Joint Surg (Am) 1986: 68: 1283–1285
27. Matsumoto K, Fujii S, Mochizuki T, Hukuda S. Solitary bone cyst of a lumbar vertebra. Spine 1990: 15: 605–607
28. Prietto C, Orofino C F, Waugh T R. Unicameral bone cyst in the scapula. Clin Orthop 1977: 125: 183–184
29. Ruggieri P, Biagini R, Picci P. Case report 437. Solitary (unicameral, simple) bone cyst of the scapula. Skeletal Radiol 1987: 16: 493–497
30. Hresko M T, Miele J F, Goldberg M J. Unicameral bone cyst in the scapula of an adolescent. Clin Orthop 1988: 236: 141–144
31. Shulman H S, Wilson S R, Harvie J N, Cruickshank B. Unicameral bone cyst in a rib of a child. AJR 1977: 128: 1058–1060
32. Ewald F C. Bone cyst in a phalanx of a two-and-half year-old child. J Bone Joint Surg (Am) 1972: 54: 399–401
33. Perlmann M D, Maiocco J L, Rybczynski J M. Unicameral bone cyst of the first metatarsal. J Foot Surg 1989: 28: 38–41
34. Wientroub S, Salama R, Baratz M, Papo I, Weissman S L. Unicameral bone cyst of the patella. Clin Orthop 1979: 140: 159–161
35. Abdelwahab I F, Hermann G, Lewis M M, Klein M J. Case report 534. Simple bone cyst of the acetabulum and ischium. Skeletal Radiol 1989: 18: 157–159
36. Christman R O, Kopell H P. Bilateral benign bone cyst of the os calcis. Am J Roentgenol Radium Ther Clin Med 1961: 86: 318–320
37. Sadler A H, Rosenhaim F. Occurrence of two unicameral bone cysts in the same patient. J Bone Joint Surg (Am) 1964: 46: 1557–1560
38. Horibe K, Furuya K. Report of two cases of polyostotic bone cyst, occurring symmetrically in the bilateral humerus and femur shafts, respectively. Rinsho Sekei Geka 1976: 11: 965–972
39. Keret D, Kumar S J. Unicameral bone cysts in the humerus and femur in the same child. J Pediatr Orthop 1987: 7: 712–715
40. Chigira M, Takehi Y, Nagase M, Arita S, Shimizu T, Shinozaki T. A case of multiple simple bone cysts. Arch Orthop Trauma Surg 1987: 106: 390–393
41. Nelson J P, Foster R J. Solitary bone cyst with epiphyseal involvement. Clin Orthop 1976: 118: 147–150
42. Malawer M M, Markle B. Unicameral bone cyst with epiphyseal involvement. J Pediatr Orthop 1982: 2: 71–79
43. Capanna R, Van Horn J, Ruggieri P, Biagini R. Epiphyseal involvement in unicameral bone cysts. Skeletal Radiol 1986: 15: 428–432
44. McGlynn F J, Mickelson M R, EI-Khoury G Y. The fallen fragment sign in unicameral bone cyst. Clin Orthop 1981: 156: 157–159
45. Struhl S, Edelson C, Pritzker H, Seimon L P, Dorfman H D. Solitary (unicameral) bone cyst. The fallen fragment sign revisited. Skeletal Radiol 1989: 18: 261–265
46. Hahn P F, Rosenthal D I, Ehrlich M G. Case report 286. Gas within a solitary bone cyst of the proximal end of the left humerus. Skeletal Radiol 1984: 12: 214–217
47. Tsai J C, Dalinka M K, Fallon M D, Zlatkin M B, Kressel H Y.

Fluid–fluid level: a non-specific finding in tumors of bone and soft tissue. Radiology 1990: 175: 779–782

48. Burr B A, Resnick D, Syklawer R, Haghighi P. Fluid–fluid levels in a unicameral bone cyst: CT and MR findings. J Comput Assist Tomogr 1993: 17: 134–136

49. Capanna R, Albisinni U, Caroli G C, Campanacci M. Contrast examination as a prognostic factor in the treatment of solitary bone cyst by cortisone injection. Skeletal Radiol 1984: 12: 97–102

50. Keats T E, Harrison R B. The calcaneal nutrient foramen: a useful sign in the differentiation of true from simulated cysts. Skeletal Radiol 1979: 3: 239–240

51. Helms C A. Pseudocysts of the humerus. AJR 1978: 131: 287–288

52. Resnick D, Conne R O 3rd. The nature of humeral pseudocysts. Radiology 1984: 150: 27–28

53. Goldberg R P, Genant H K. Case report 67. Solitary bone cyst right ilium. Skeletal Radiol 1978: 3: 118–121

54. Adler C P. Tumour-like lesions in the femur with cementum-like material. Does a 'cementoma' of long bone exist? Skeletal Radiol 1985: 14: 26–37

55. Amling M, Werner M, Pösl M, Maas R, Korn U, Delling G. Calcifying solitary bone cyst: morphological aspects and differential diagnosis of sclerotic bone tumours. Virchows Arch 1995: 426: 235–242

56. Stelling C B, Martin W, Fechner R E, Alford B A, Strider D V. Case report 150. Solitary bone cyst with cementum-like bone production. Skeletal Radiol 1981: 6: 213–215

57. Sanerkin N G. Old fibrin coagula and their ossification in simple bone cysts. J Bone Joint Surg (Br) 1979: 61: 194–199

58. Kragel P J, Williams J, Garvin D F, Goral A B. Solitary bone cyst of the radius containing Liesegang's rings. Am J Clin Pathol 1989: 92: 831–833

59. Vayego S A, De Conti O J, Varolla-Garcia M. Complex cytogenetic rearrangement in a case of unicameral bone cyst. Cancer Genet Cytogenet 1996: 86: 46–49

60. Vasilev V, Andreeff I, Sokolov T, Vidinov N. Clinical-morphological and electron microscopic studies of the growth plate in solitary bone cysts. Arch Orthop Trauma Surg 1987: 106: 232–237

61. Johnson L C, Vetter H, Putschar W G. Sarcomas arising in bone cysts. Virchows Arch Pathol Anat 1962: 335: 428–451

62. Grabias S, Mankin H J. Chondrosarcoma arising in histologically proved unicameral bone cyst. J Bone Joint Surg (Am) 1974: 56: 1501–1509

63. Steinberg G G. Ewing's sarcoma arising in bone cyst. J Pediatr Orthop 1985: 5: 97–100

64. Bourne M H, Beabout J W, Wold L E, Sim F H. Simple bone cysts. Orthopedics 1986: 9: 1285–1289

65. Campanacci M, Capanna R, Picci P. Unicameral and aneurysmal bone cysts. Clin Orthop 1986: 204: 25–36

66. Johnston C E 2nd, Fletcher R R. Traumatic transformation of unicameral bone cyst into aneurysmal bone cyst. Orthopedics 1986: 9: 1441–1447

67. Friedman N B, Goldman R L. Cementoma of long bones. Clin Orthop 1969: 67: 243–248

68. Kolar J J, Horn V, Zidkova H, Sprindrich J. Cementifying fibroma (so-called 'cementoma') of tibia. Br J Radiol 1981: 54: 989–992

69. Horn V, Bozdech Z, Macek M, Foukal T, Kolar J, Zidkova H. Cementoma-like tumours of bone. Arch Orthop Trauma Surg 1982: 100: 267–272

70. Black D L, De Smet A A, Neff J R, Bhatia P. Case report 695. Cementifying fibroma of the proximal end of the tibia. Skeletal Radiol 1991: 20: 543–546

71. Sissons H A, Steiner G C, Dorfman H D. Calcified spherules in fibro-osseous lesions of bone. Arch Pathol Lab Med 1993: 117: 284–290

37

Aneurysmal bone cyst

M. Forest

INTRODUCTION AND CLINICAL DATA

An aneurysmal bone cyst or, more exactly, a multilocular hematic bone cyst (Schajowicz 1994) is a non-neoplastic expansile and locally destructive bone lesion characterized by channels or spaces filled with blood and separated by fibrous septa.

The lesion was established as a clinicopathological entity by Jaffe and Lichtenstein, in 1950, in two separate studies.[1–4] It accounts for approximately 2% of all primary bone tumors[5,6] and there is a slight female predominance of about 60% of cases.[5,7,8]

The majority of cases are diagnosed between 10 and 20 years of age. Aneurysmal bone cyst is very rare in children less than 5 years of age.[9] A few cases with a familial incidence have been reported.[10,11,12]

The clinical course is rapid: local pain and swelling of from several weeks to less than 6 months duration.[6,7] Occasionally, the lesion may grow slowly or may even be asymptomatic. Spinal cord or nerve compression, scoliosis and kyphosis may occur in vertebral locations. In patients with an immature skeleton, the invasion of the adjacent growth plate in some cases may induce abnormality of growth by premature fusion.

Pathologic fractures with an incidence of 8–25% of cases predominate in some series in the femur and humerus or the short tubular bones.

In 25% of cases, the initial symptoms are related to local trauma.[7] In about one-third of cases, aneurysmal bone cysts are associated with a coexistent lesion, either benign or, less often, malignant.

The concept of secondary aneurysmal bone cysts is well established[13–17] but some authors feel that the name of the principal lesion should be used.[7,18] The clinical presentation is that of the associated and primary lesion;[18] the aneurysmal bone cyst component may completely obliterate the first lesion.

The most common primary lesion is a giant cell tumor,

especially in skeletally immature patients.[18] Other common primary lesions are chondroblastomas ('cystic chondroblastomas', Schajowicz 1994), osteoblastomas and osteosarcomas. Various other entities have been reported: fibrous dysplasia,[19–21] chondromyxoid fibromas, non-ossifying fibromas, fibrosarcomas, malignant fibrous histiocytomas, hamartomas of the chest wall[22] and even metastases.[15]

It appears necessary to identify a substantial amount of tissue exhibiting the histological pattern of an aneurysmal bone cyst and to exclude common and non-specific cystic changes found in many benign and malignant tumors.[15]

PATHOGENESIS

Many authors have found that a local vascular change occurs,[1,2] evidenced by the rapid and marked extension and the elevation of pressure to arteriolar levels in manometric studies.[13] The arteriographic findings also suggest a local vascular disturbance of venous drainage leading to the development of an arteriovenous shunt, with subsequent dilatation of sinusoidal blood spaces. In fact, the reality of an arteriovenous fistula is not quite established.[23] The sinusoidal capillaries lack a basal membrane; the rupture of their walls may induce blood extravasations and secondary aneurysmal bone-cyst formation.[24] Aneurysmal bone cysts may well be the result of local hemorrhages.[25,26] Primary aneurysmal bone cysts are frequently encountered, but some may be induced by trauma[27–32] or by preexisting lesions.

Whatever the triggering event, the cyst fluid has a high fibrinolytic activity and a very low concentration of fibrinogen and plasminogen.[33] Fibrinolysis appears to be an important factor in the maintenance and expansion of aneurysmal bone cysts.[33]

SKELETAL DISTRIBUTION

Almost any bone may be involved, even the patella,[34] but 50–60% of cases are found in long bones, chiefly

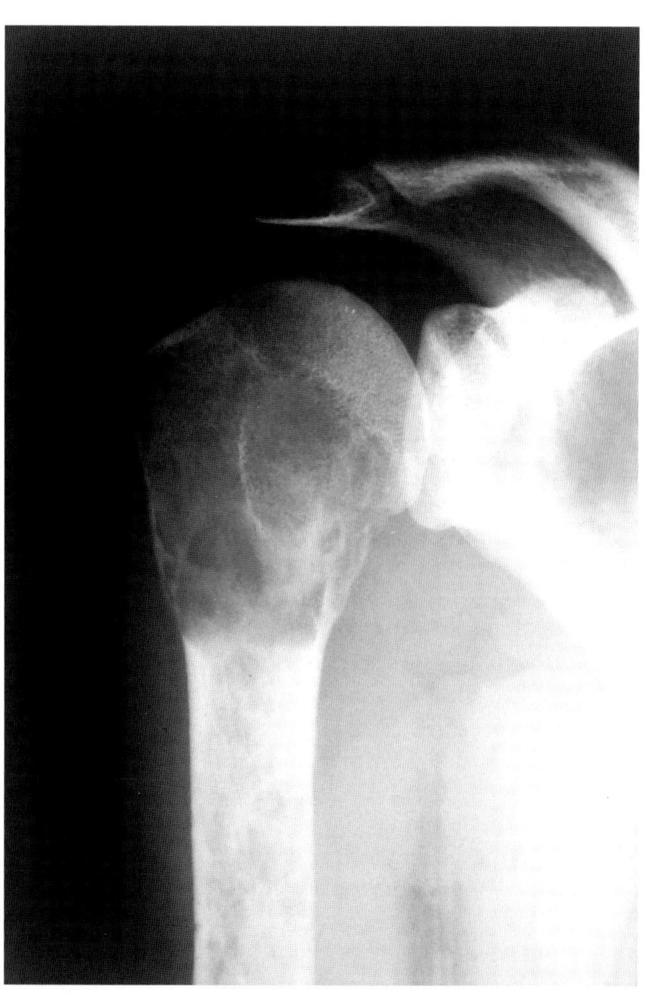

Fig. 37.1

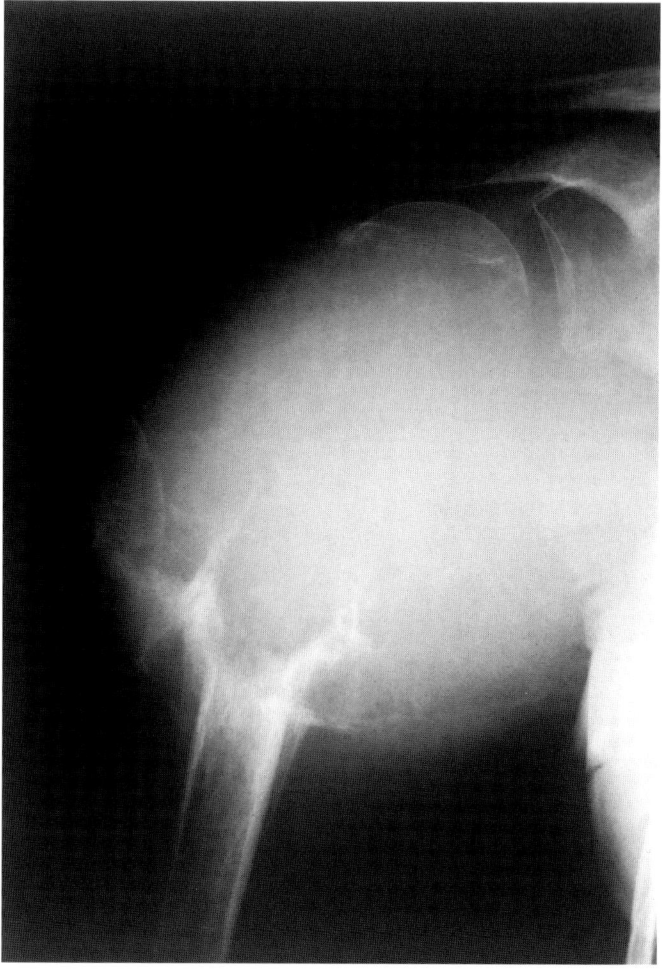

Fig. 37.2

Figs 37.1, 37.2 Aneurysmal bone cysts of the humerus.

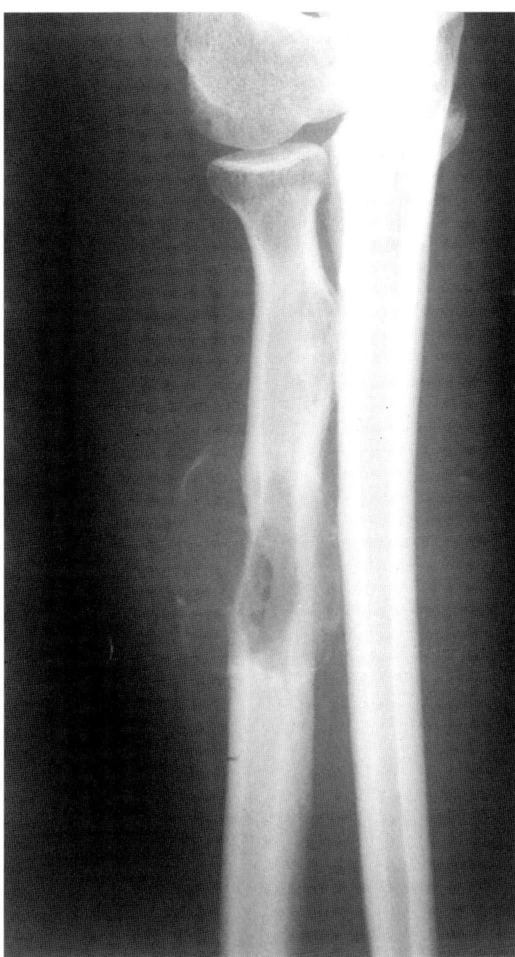

Fig. 37.3 Aneurysmal bone cyst of the radius.

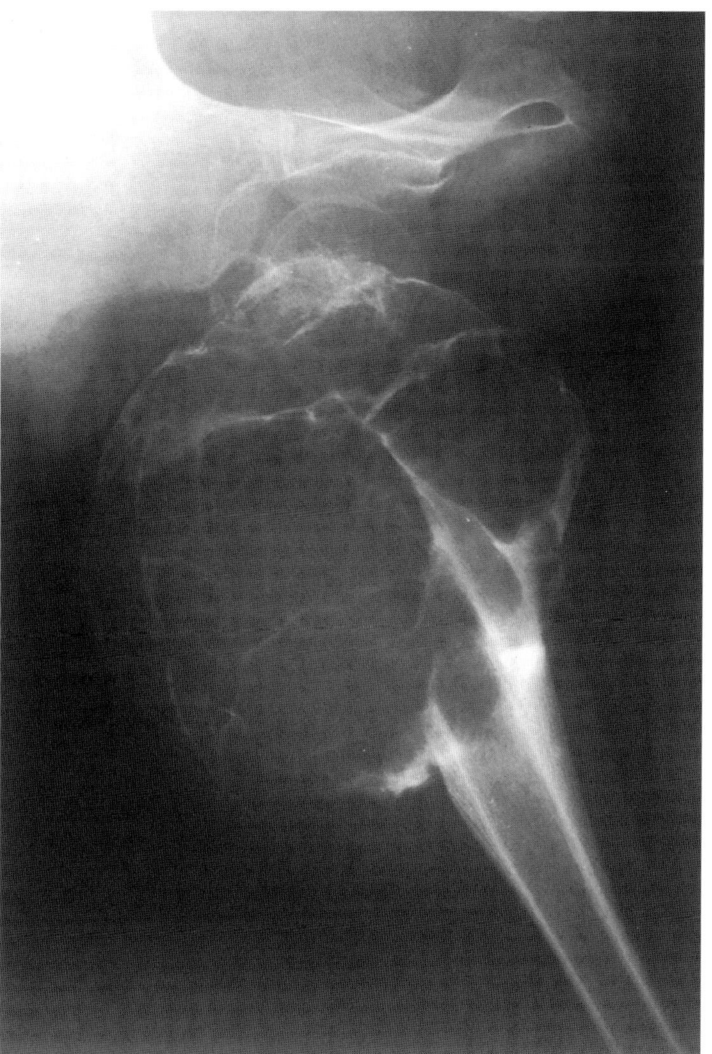

Fig. 37.4 Aneurysmal bone cyst of the proximal femur.

the distal femur, proximal tibia and proximal humerus (Figs 37.1–37.4), 12–30% in the spine (Figs 37.5, 37.6) and 18% in flat and short tubular bones (Figs 32.7–32.14).

In the spine, the lumbar and cervical areas are most often involved; a location in the sacrum is rare.[35,36] Pelvic location accounts for half of the cases involving the flat bones.[6]

Approximately 5% of cases are located in the hand[37] and the metacarpals are mostly involved; in the foot, location in the tarsal bones predominates.[6]

A bilateral and symmetrical involvement of bones is rare.[38,39] Multiple locations in ribs have been reported.[40] More common are contiguous spinal lesions by direct extension.[6]

Some most unusual aneurysmal bone cyst-like lesions have been reported involving the carotid artery with no underlying condition,[41] the central part of myositis ossificans[42] and the soft tissues of the shoulder.[43]

IMAGING

In long bones, most lesions are located in the metaphysis and involvement of the diaphysis occurs in only 10% of cases.[6] In adults, the epiphyseal part may be involved by direct extension (Fig. 37.15). In skeletally immature patients, direct extension across the epiphyseal cartilage is rare, but the growth plate may be invaded in about 10% of cases.[44–46]

More than half of the lesions are eccentrically located; less often they are cortical or central or may appear as a surface lesion in 7–8% of cases.[6,47] An eccentric involvement is more common in the large tubular bones; the subperiosteal type is mostly found in the diaphysis[47,48] (Figs 37.16, 37.17). Rare small cystic lesions restricted to the cortical bone have been reported[49,50] (Figs 37.18, 37.19).

The usual appearance is of a blown-out bone by a purely lytic lesion eventually producing a honeycomb pattern, internal trabeculations being related to ridges of the periosteal bone shell.

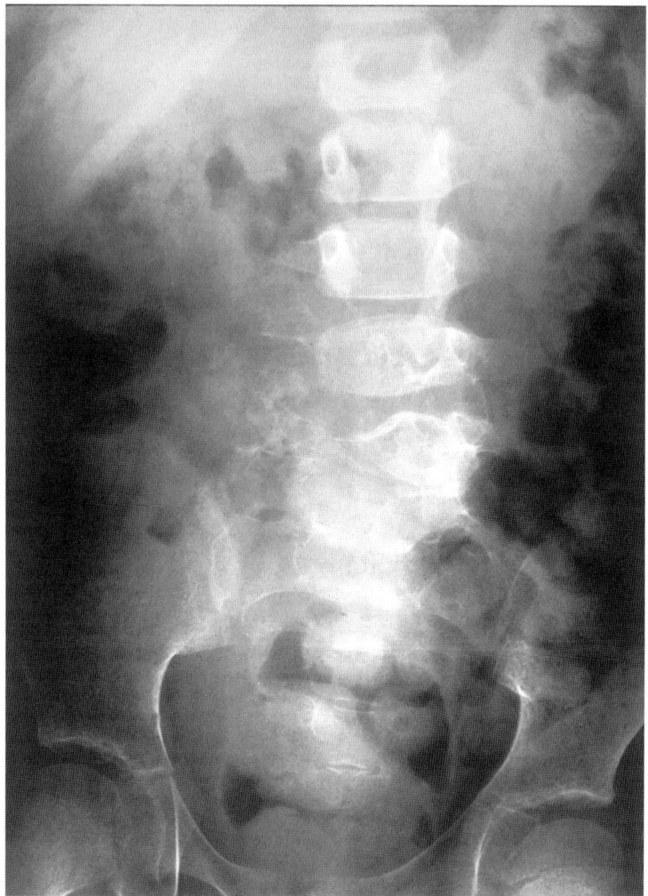

Fig. 37.5 Huge aneurysmal bone cyst of the lumbar spine.

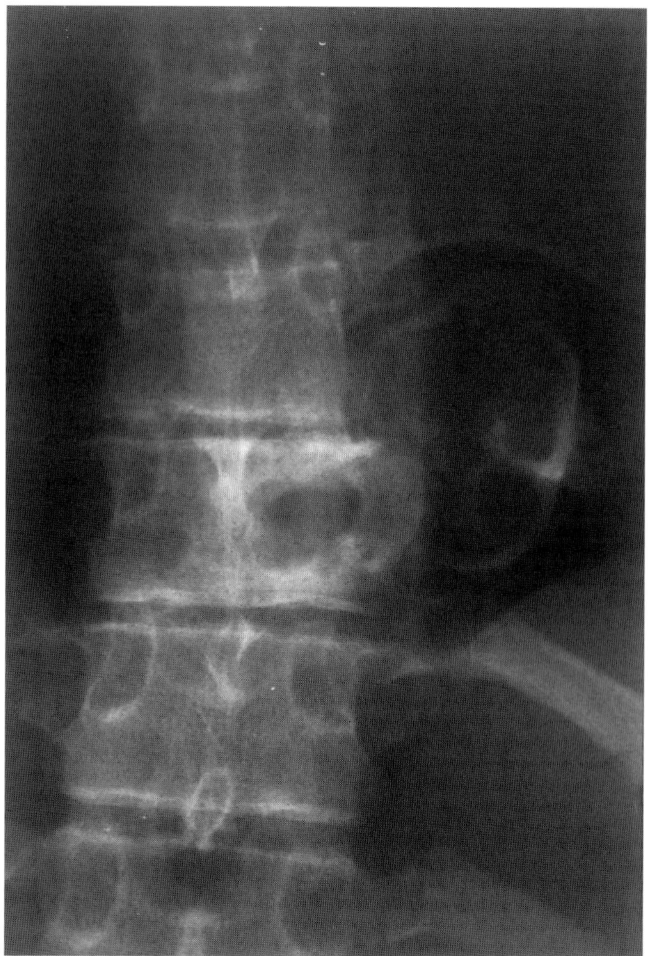

Fig. 37.6 Involuted aneurysmal bone cyst of the spine (T9 level).

The internal margins are well defined and geographic, with peripheral sclerosis in one-third of cases, but they may be poorly defined. In all cases, the cortex is thinned, with a periosteal reaction in more than half of the cases.[47,51]

Very rarely, some intralesional amorphous speckled calcifications are found, resembling an enchondroma.[52,53]

On imaging, four stages of development have been delineated: an initial lytic phase with permeative growth, a growth phase with a blown-out appearance and eventual prominent Codman's triangles, a stable phase with a soap bubble appearance, the expanded bone exhibiting trabeculations and being covered by a periosteal shell, and finally a healing phase with progressive ossification.[51,54]

On arteriography, an aneurysmal bone cyst is almost always hypovascular, with a peripheral thin hyperemic zone. Hypovascularization is due to the very slow blood flow and the arteriovenous shunting at the periphery.[55–57]

On scintigraphy, there is an increased uptake of radionuclide, mostly at the periphery.[58]

CT scans are useful to delineate the size and location of the lesion, especially in the spine and pelvis, and may demonstrate fluid levels[59] as well as the thin shell of periph-

eral reactive bone. Fluid levels are more easily demonstrated on MRI,[60,61] detecting uncoagulated blood[62] as well as internal septations.[63–65]

In the spine, the posterior arch and spinous process are involved in all cases, with direct extension to the adjacent vertebrae or ribs.[5,47,66] In up to 40% of cases, the lesion passes across the intervertebral space to another vertebra.[35] An isolated involvement of the vertebral body is very rare.

In flat bones, expansion of bone may be quite prominent.

In the hand, aneurysmal bone cyst usually involves the whole width of bone. The expansion is often asymmetrical and it may mimic a giant cell tumor or a giant cell reaction.[37]

Secondary aneurysmal bone cysts in 80% of cases have the radiologic appearance of the primary lesion[15] and 70% of aneurysmal bone cysts in epiphyseal locations are secondary forms (giant cell tumors, chondroblastomas).[13]

The so-called 'solid' aneurysmal bone cysts have similar radiographic features,[67,68] even with diaphyseal locations,[69] and in some series, a predilection for axial involvement.[67]

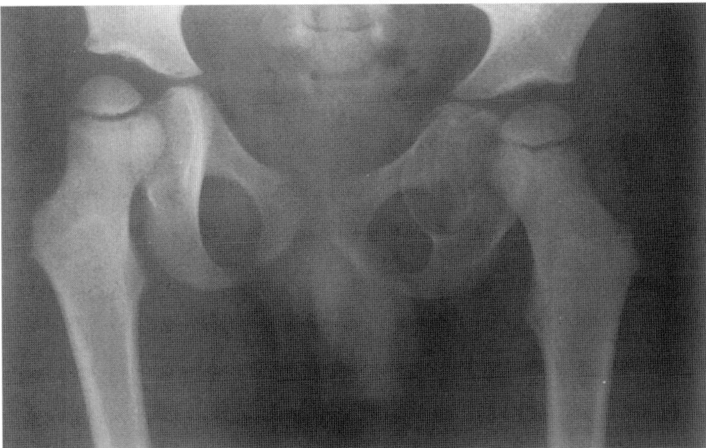

Fig. 37.7

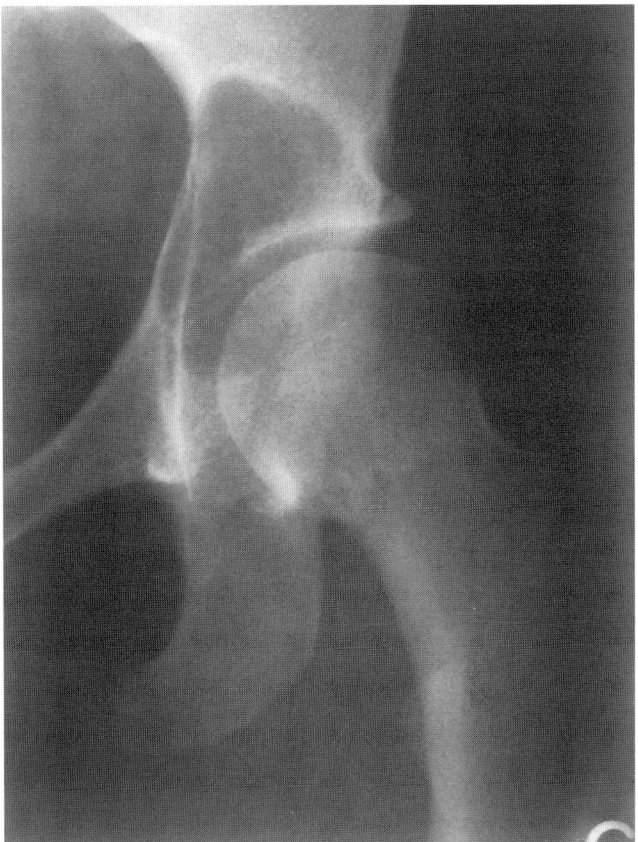

Fig. 37.9

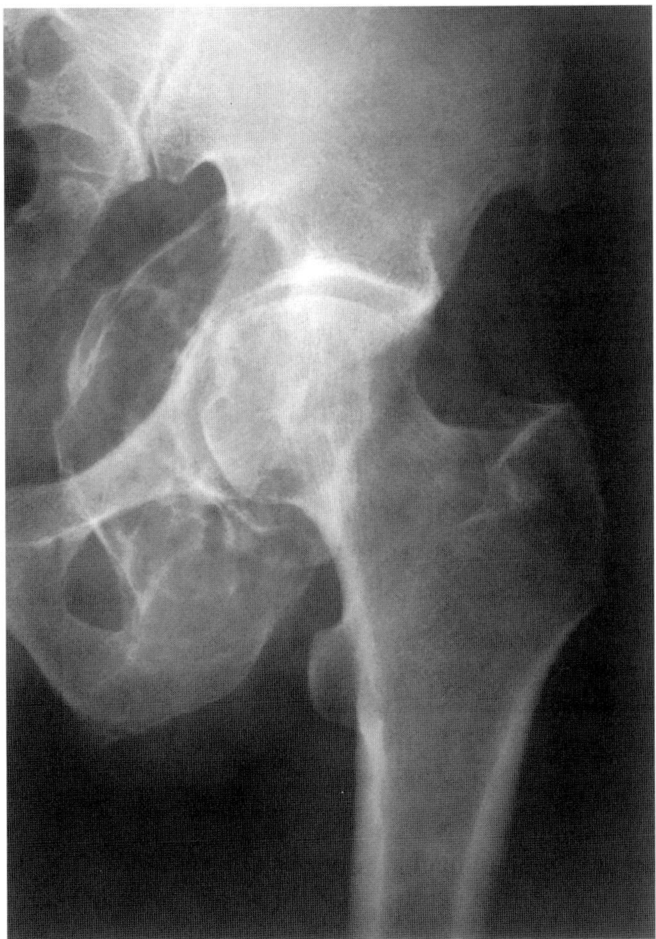

Fig. 37.8

Figs 37.7–37.10 Aneurysmal bone cysts of the pelvis.

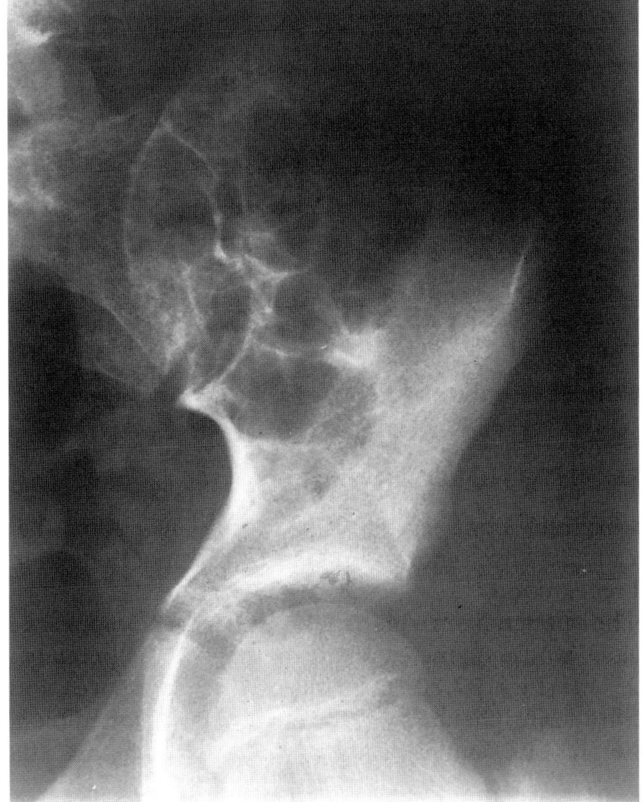

Fig. 37.10

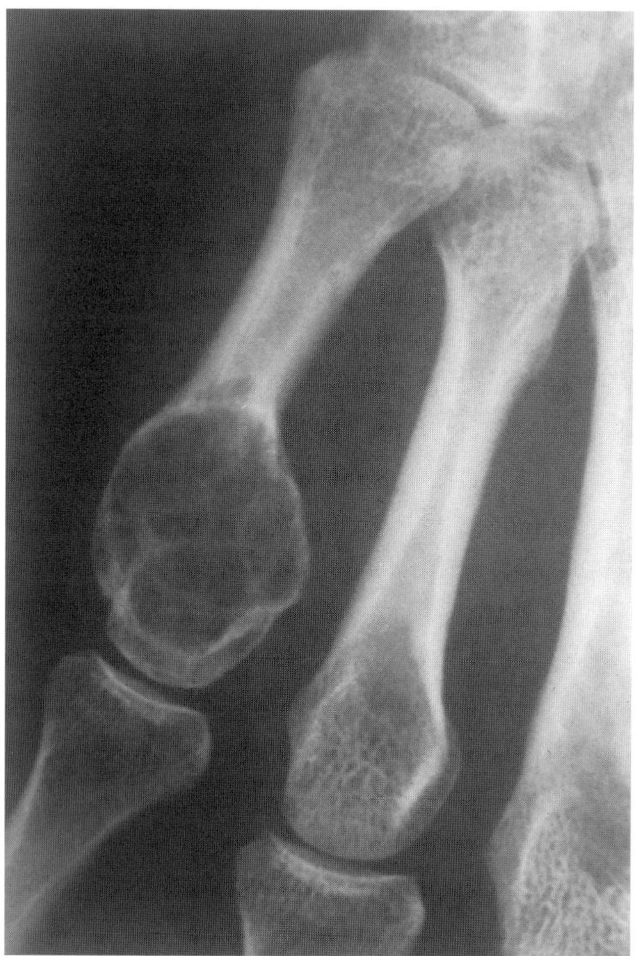

Fig. 37.11 **Fig. 37.12**

Figs 37.11, 37.12 Aneurysmal bone cysts in metacarpal locations.

GROSS PATHOLOGY

Aneurysmal bone cysts grow rapidly and most have already destroyed more than half the width of bone at initial recognition.[17]

The sponge-like tissue (Lichtenstein 1977) appears as cavities whose diameter ranges from a few millimeters to 1–2 cm (Figs 37.20–37.25); the vascular spaces form anastomosing channels usually filled with unclotted blood. Older lesions contain a serous or serosanguinous fluid. The cavities are surrounded by a gray or brownish tissue in which an osseous component may be identified.

The largest lesions are found in flat bones,[6] such as the ilium or scapula. Small aneurysmal bone cysts are usually more solid. A thin eggshell layer of periosteal bone covers the lesion. In the initial lytic phase, infiltration of the soft tissues is not an ominous finding.

'Solid' aneurysmal bone cysts are made of a fleshy, friable, fibrous or granular tissue with focal hemorrhages, covered by a layer of reactive bone.[68]

HISTOPATHOLOGY

Cavernous spaces are filled with blood. Thin or thick fibrous septa are lined by flattened fibroblastic cells or

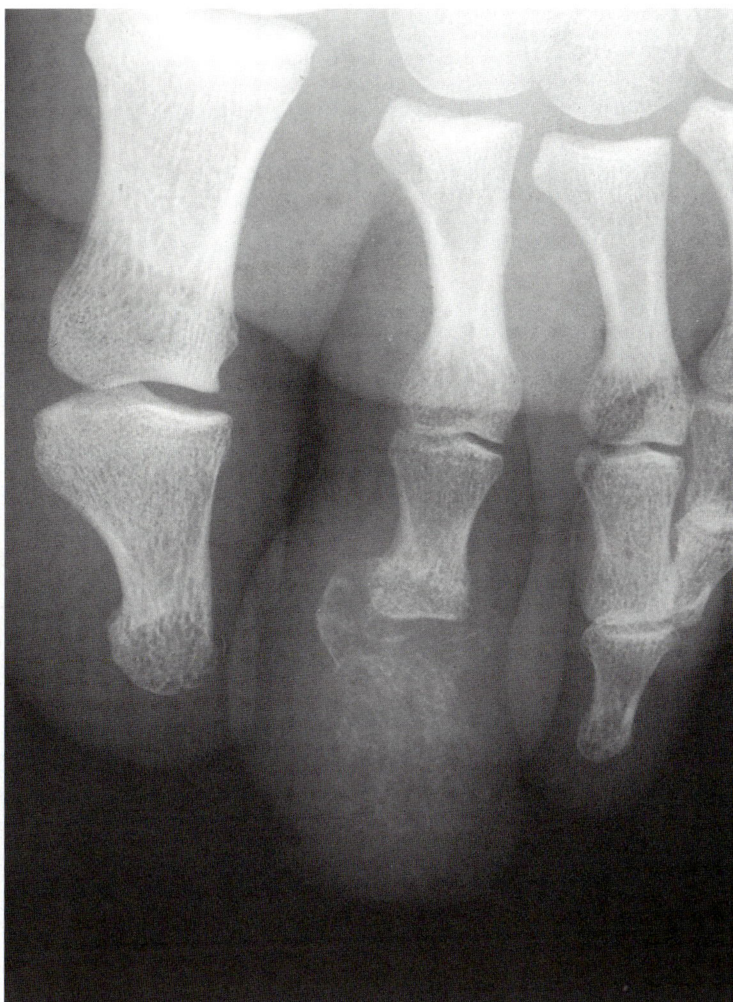

Fig. 37.13

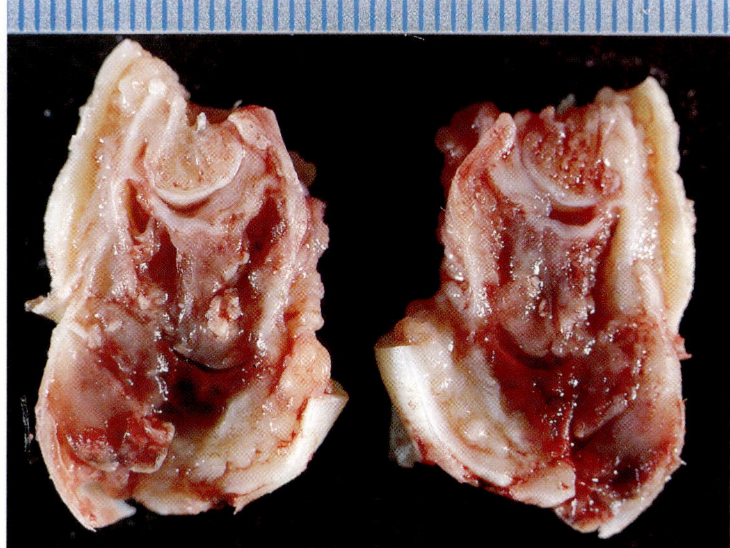

Fig. 37.14

Figs 37.13, 37.14 Aneurysmal bone cyst destroying the terminal phalanx of a toe.

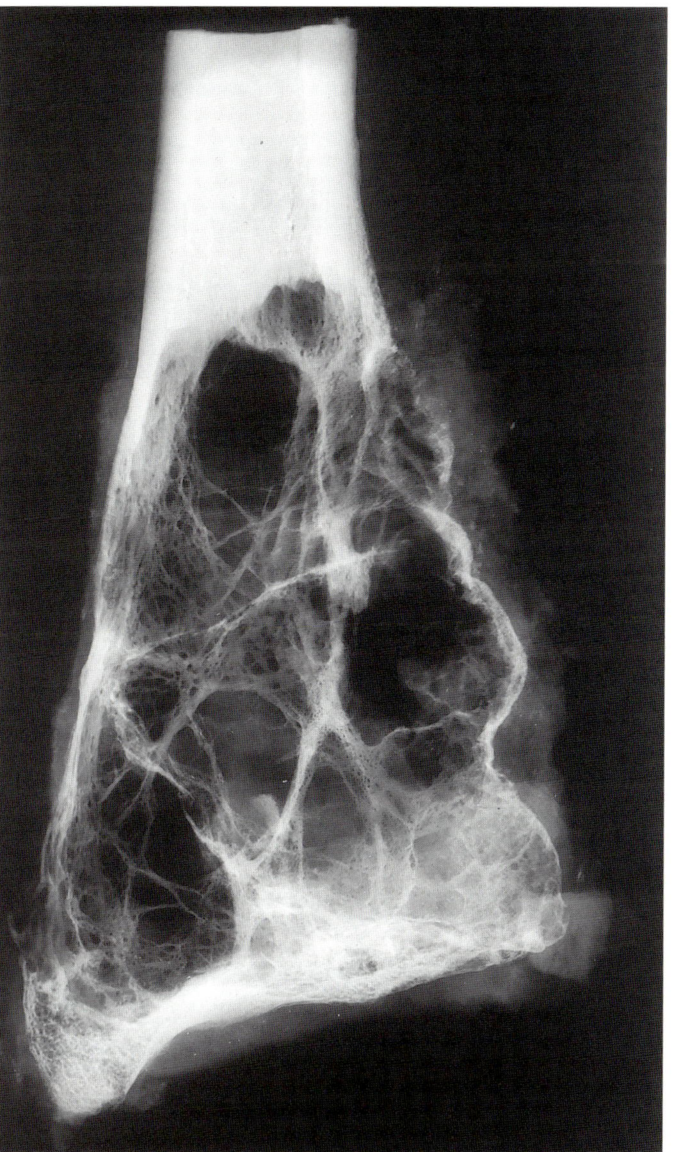

Fig. 37.15 Aneurysmal bone cyst of the radius extending to the epiphysis.

osteoclast-like giant cells, with no smooth muscle walls or elastic fibers[6,8,13,47,54] (Figs 37.26–37.36). The fibrous walls contain fibroblasts, histiocytes and osteoclast-like giant cells often concentrated around stromal hemorrhages and hemosiderin deposits. Mitotic figures, without atypical forms, may be numerous. Bulging vessels are found in the septa, mostly capillaries and vascular spaces probably originating from inflated capillaries[54] or small foci of dilated vascular sinusoids. In one series, a layered architecture was described, the deeper zone being less cellular.[70]

In the fibrous septa, bone is found in a lace-like or filigree pattern in some cases, but more often in a trabecular pattern with a prominent osteoblastic rim.[6]

Heavily calcified mineralized deposits or calcified matrix

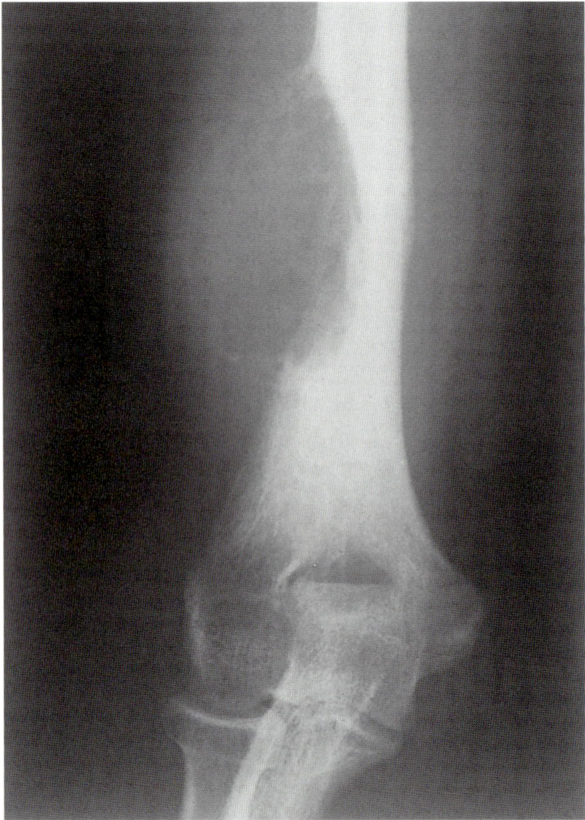

Fig. 37.16 Subperiosteal aneurysmal bone cyst of the humerus.

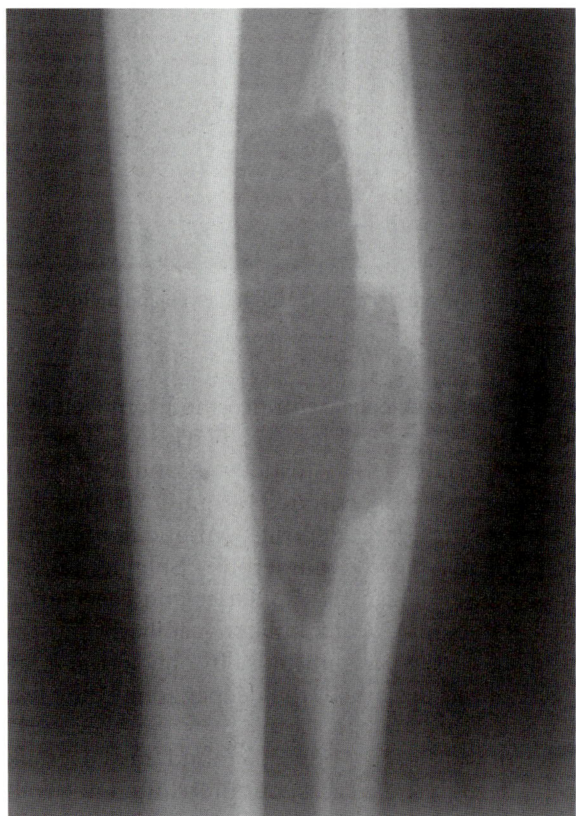

Fig. 37.17 Subperiosteal aneurysmal bone cyst of the fibula.

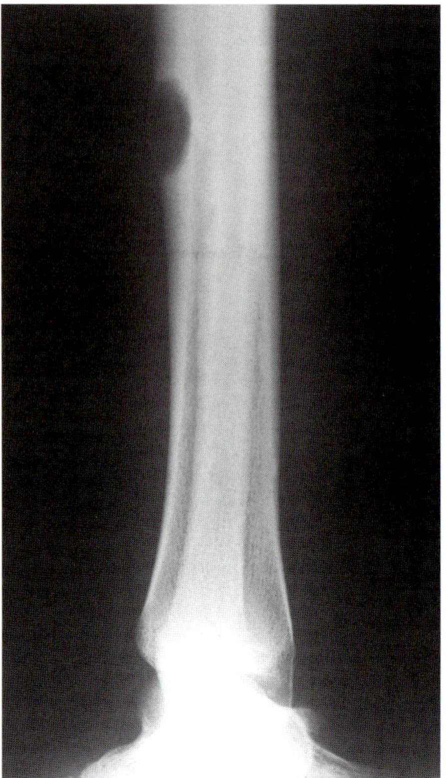

Fig. 37.18

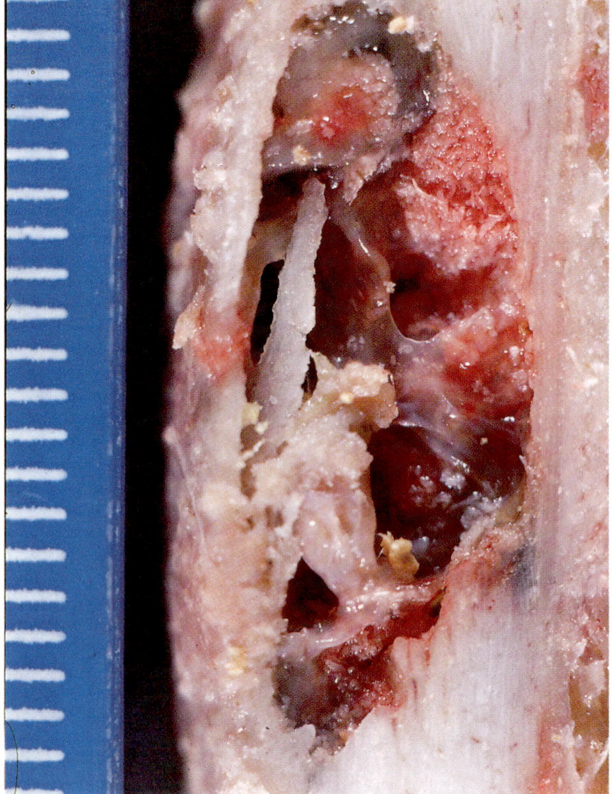

Fig. 37.19

Figs 37.18, 37.19 Rare intracortical aneurysmal bone cyst of the tibia shaft.

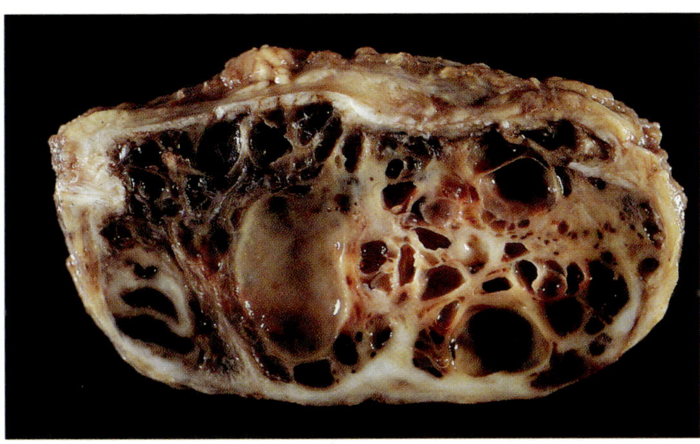

Fig. 37.20 Aneurysmal bone cyst arising from the acromion.

with a chondroid aura[6,8] or chondroid (Mirra 1989) are found in more than 35% of cases, lining the vascular spaces. They are characteristic of aneurysmal bone cysts[6,71] (Mirra 1989). They may appear also as hematoxyphilic foci of fibromyxoid tissue, with degenerative changes and calcification and rarely can even be demonstrated on X-ray as flocculent densities.[52]

The lesion is contained by the periosteal connective tissue or muscle or by a periosteal shell of bone; some foci of reactive cartilage may be found.[6] In bone, the lesional tissue can permeate between adjacent trabeculae.[8]

The so-called *'solid' variant* has been described by Sanerkin et al[71] and this form of aneurysmal bone cyst has gained wide acceptance,[26,68,72] accounting for 5–7.5% of all cases.[6,68] The age, sex predominance and clinical pre-

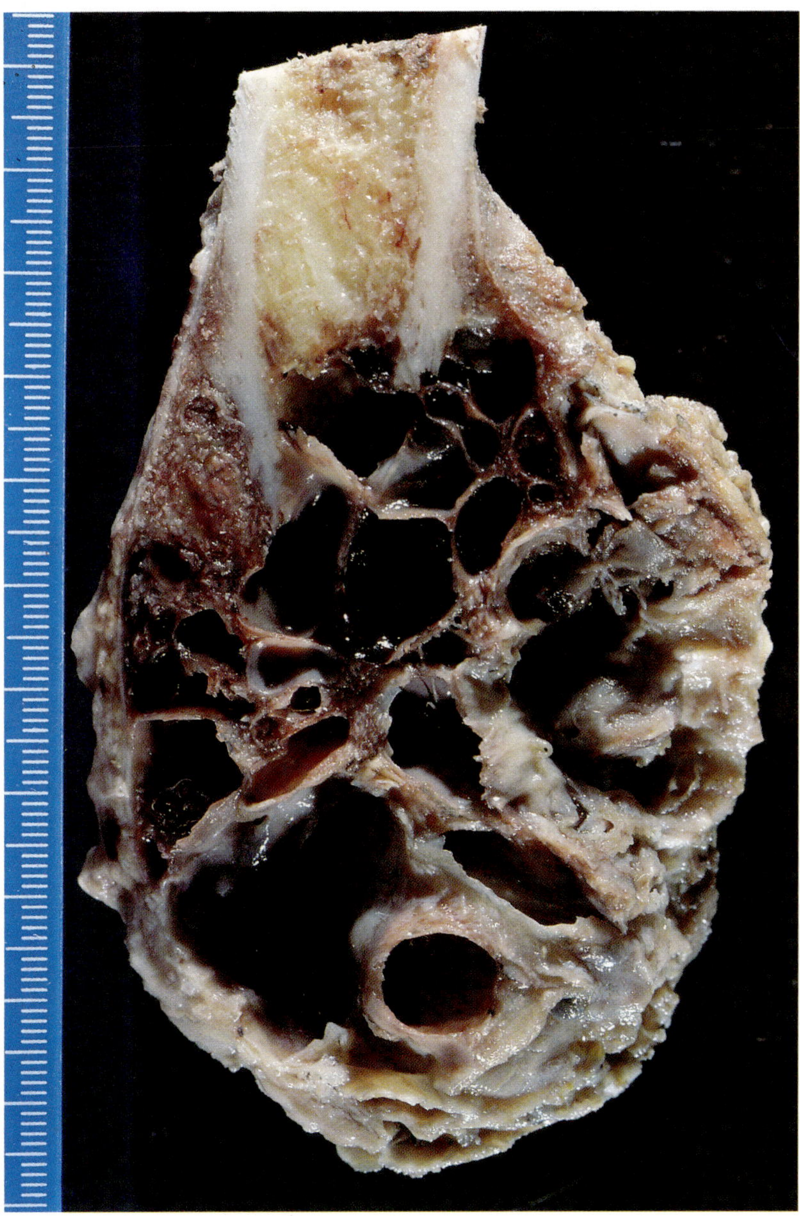

Fig. 37.21 Aneurysmal bone cyst destroying the distal femur.

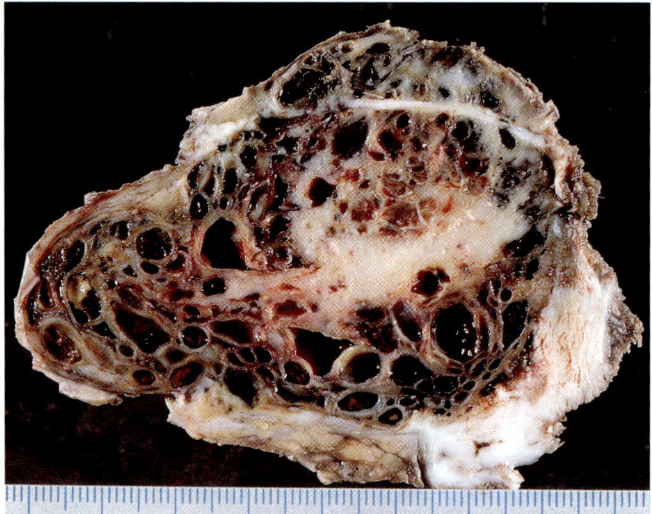

Fig. 37.22

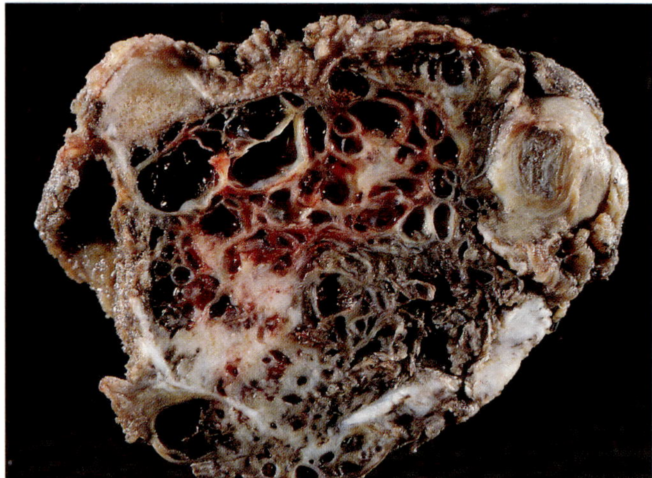

Fig. 37.23

Figs 37.22, 37.23 Aneurysmal bone cyst developing from the iliopubic ramus.

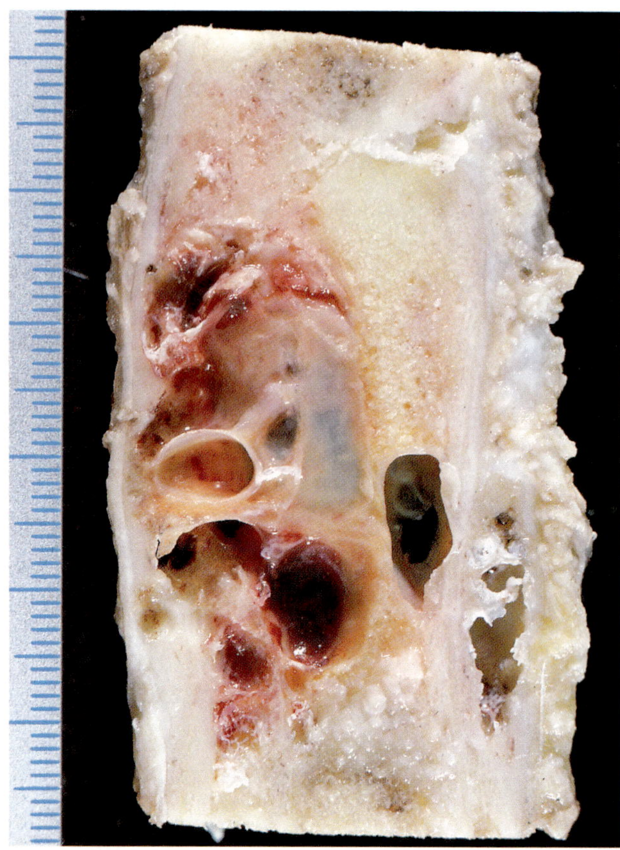

Fig. 37.24 Recurrence of an aneurysmal bone cyst of the humerus, with resorption of the bone grafts.

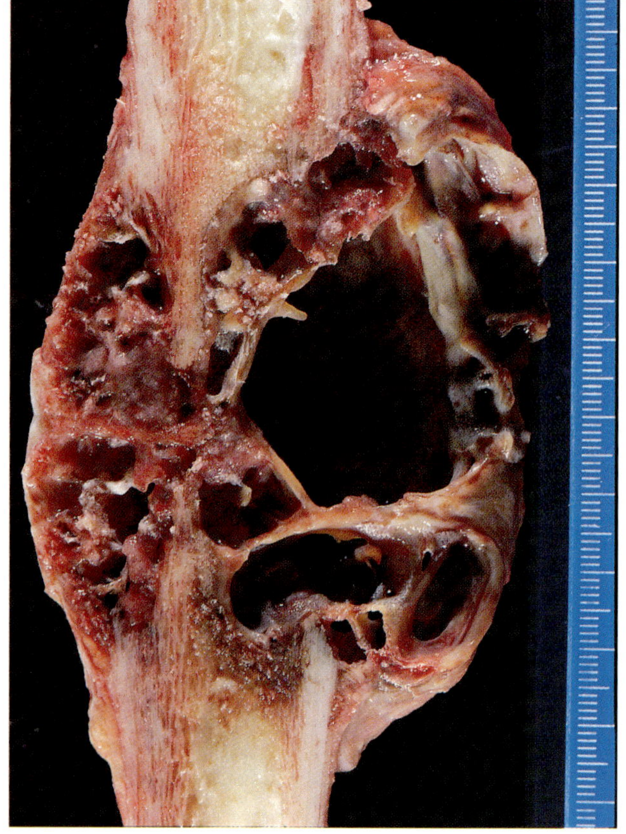

sentation are similar to the usual form.[26,67,68] Some lesions described in the sacrum may be similar to the 'solid' variant.[73]

There are no qualitative histologic differences from the usual form, but this is a non-cystic intraosseous lesion (Figs 37.37–37.40); histologically, aneurysmal dilated sinusoids are found lined by a fibrovascular tissue and giant cells, as well as by characteristic fibromyxoid areas with minimal or extensive calcifications in 60% of cases.[68]

The predominant fibroblastic or fibrohistiocytic cells are arranged in a whorled or storiform pattern,[26,72] appearing as a florid fibroblastic proliferation with a brisk mitotic activity, but there is no cellular pleomorphism. Osteoclast-like giant cells are distributed around areas of

Fig. 37.25 Aneurysmal bone cyst-like structures in a tibial metastasis of a thyroid adenocarcinoma.

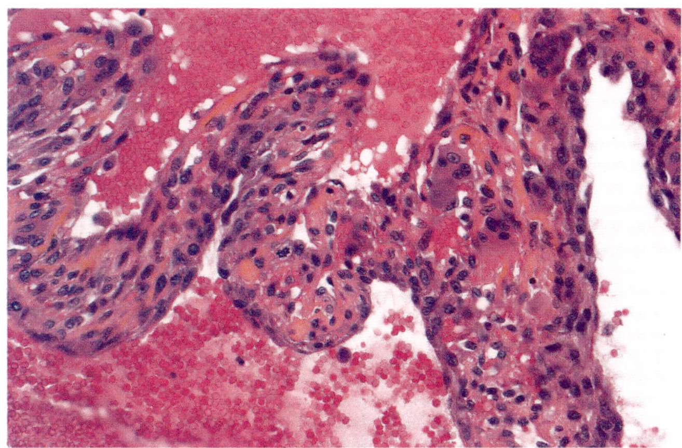

Fig. 37.26

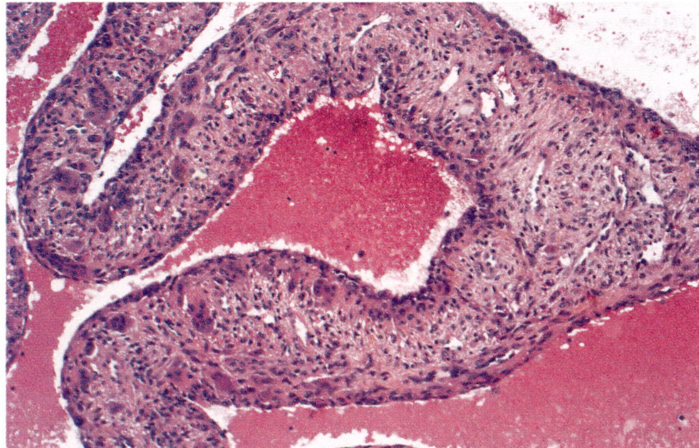

Fig. 37.27

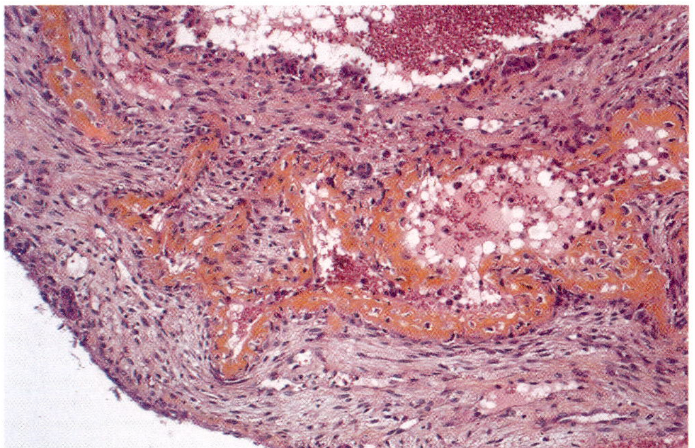

Fig. 37.28

Figs 37.26–37.28 Aneurysmal bone cyst: fibrous walls with fibroblasts, giant cells and reactive bone formation.

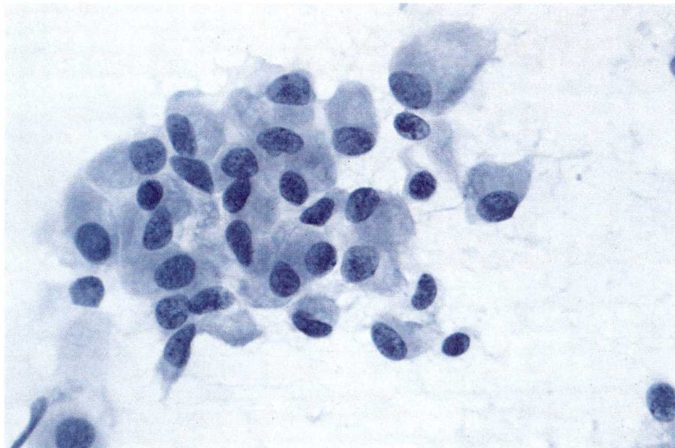

Fig. 37.29

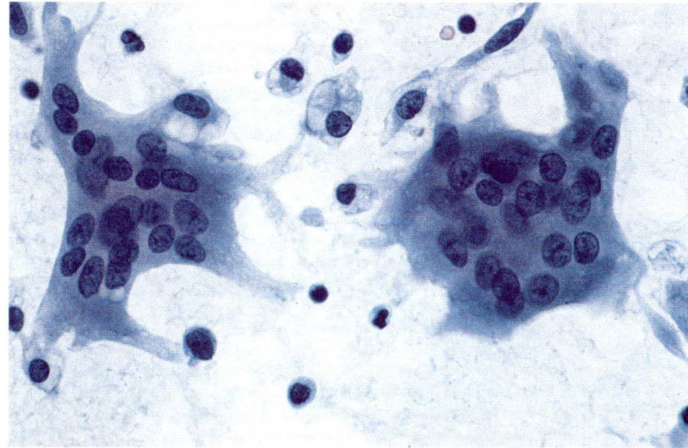

Fig. 37.30

Figs 37.29, 37.30 Imprint cytology of an aneurysmal bone cyst demonstrating only osteoblasts and osteoclast-like giant cells.

hemorrhage which can be prominent. The newly formed bone or osteoid may be quite extensive, even without osteoblastic rimming.[26,68,71]

IMMUNOHISTOCHEMISTRY

In the fibrous septa, stromal cells stain for acid phosphatase, lysozyme, α1-antitrypsin, α1-antichymotrypsin and factor XIIIa; myofibroblasts stain with muscle-specific actin.[24–26,39,74,75] In solid areas, the dilated blood vessels resemble aneurysmal spaces and are surrounded by a layer of collagen types IV and V; endothelial cells are positive for factor VIII-related antigen and express a strongly positive immunostaining for CD31.[39,74] Only alkaline phosphatase is present in the lining of aneurysmal spaces, which is devoid of collagen types IV and V and negative for factor VIII-related antigen, lectin, Ulex Europaeus and I agglutinin as well as for MAB-BW20, a monoclonal antibody directed against endothelial cells.[24,26,74,75] So, endothelial cells are definitely not identified in the lining.

CYTOGENETICS

Eight aneurysmal bone cysts have been investigated; all were karyotypically normal.[76] In selected cases, cytogenetic examination may be useful to exclude a telangiectatic osteosarcoma or a giant cell tumour which exhibits telomeric associations.[76]

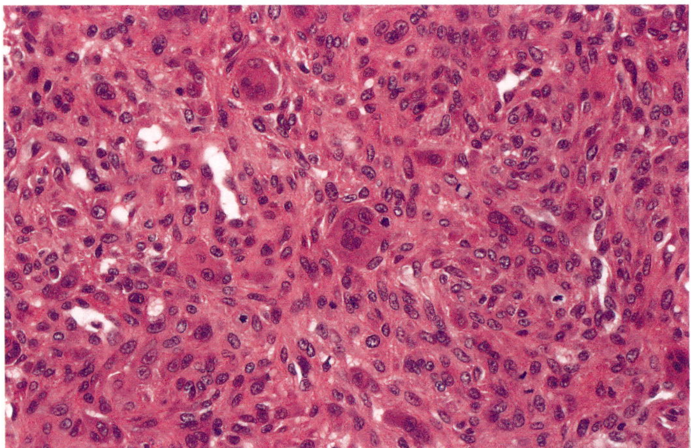

Fig. 37.31

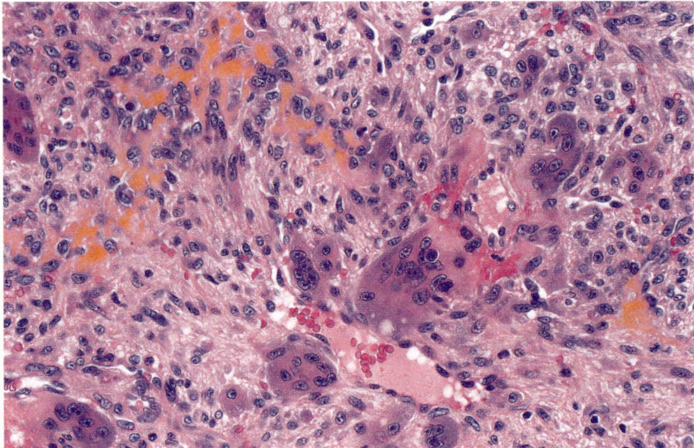

Fig. 37.32

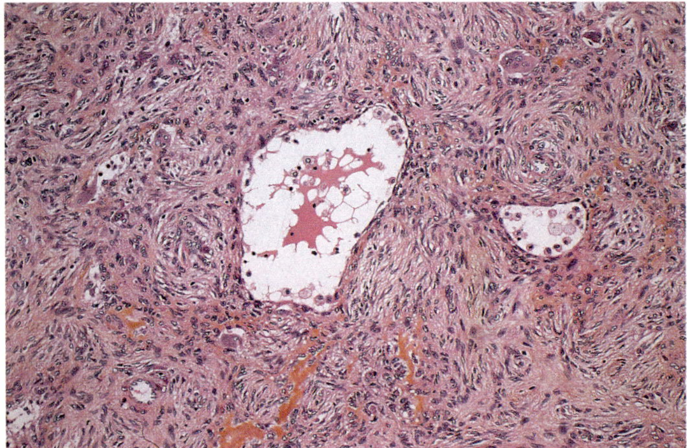

Fig. 37.33

Figs 37.31–37.33 Aneurysmal bone cysts: more cellular areas, with fibroblasts, reactive giant cells, normal mitotic figures, focal bone production and vascular spaces.

ELECTRON MICROSCOPY

The stromal cells have the fine structural features of fibroblasts, myofibroblasts, histiocytes and osteoblasts, associated with osteoclast-like multinucleated giant cells.[24,25,74,75,77,78] Siderosomes found in some cells are related to the extravasation of erythrocytes.[25]

The large aneurysmal spaces are devoid of basement membrane, Weibel–Palade bodies and pericytes; they are lined by spindle-shaped fibroblasts at various stages of differentiation, histiocytic cells or bundles of collagen. There is no fine structural feature of a specialized endothelium.

CLINICAL COURSE, TREATMENT AND PROGNOSIS

Despite the highly lytic character of the lesion, the prognosis is good and spontaneous cases of regression and healing as an ossified mass have been reported,[51,54,79,80] after biopsy,[5,7,81,82] after biopsy and embolization[83] or after incomplete removal.[26]

Few cases of malignant transformation have been described.[84,85] Most are radiation-induced osteosarcomas or fibrosarcomas[25] or telangiectatic osteosarcomas misdiagnosed as aneurysmal bone cysts;[86,87] only two cases presumably represent a malignant transformation.[85,88] A highly malignant surface-based osteosarcoma has been reported on the site of a previously treated aneurysmal bone cyst and viewed as the coexistence of two independent lesions.[89]

Curettage and bone grafting or cryosurgery are followed by a recurrence rate of 19–35%. Recurrences occur within the 2 years following treatment in 90% of cases.[8] Factors influencing the recurrence rate include the size,[13] the location in bone,[47] peripheral forms having a recurrence rate of only 5%, and the mitotic index of the initial lesion,[70] although this finding is debated.[9] The most important factor is age, more than 90% of recurrences occurring in patients younger than 20 years of age.[6,8,79] In young children, recurrences appear rapidly in radiographically aggressive or active aneurysmal bone cysts.[9]

Radiation therapy is used only in inoperable cases and there is a risk of radiation-induced sarcomas.[6,8,25]

In the pelvis, sacrum, spine or long bones when the subchondral bone is destroyed, selective arterial embolization is useful alone or in combination with surgery.[17,83,90,91]

DIFFERENTIAL DIAGNOSIS

Although a set of radiographic features can be defined on plain films,[92] in 14% of cases in one series, the differential diagnosis between giant cell tumor and aneurysmal bone cyst was radiologically impossible.[93] The differential diagnosis may be even more difficult in children, giant cell tumors being located in the metaphysis with prominent cystic changes. Histologically, difficulties may be caused by sampling, true giant cell tumors having a frequent secondary aneurysmal bone cyst component. Aneurysmal bone cysts have a predominantly fibroblastic cell

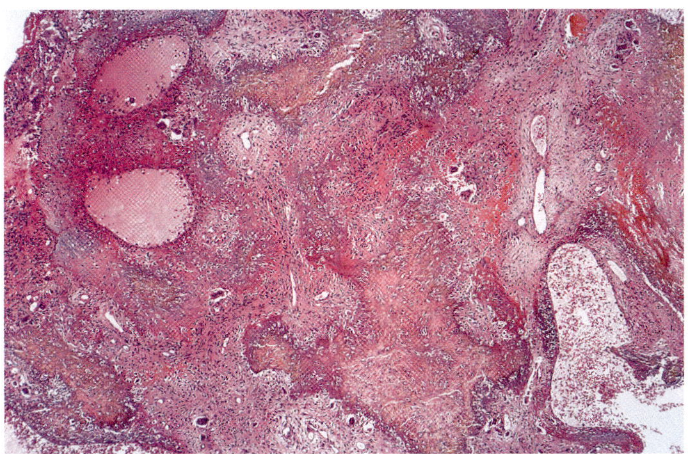

Fig. 37.34

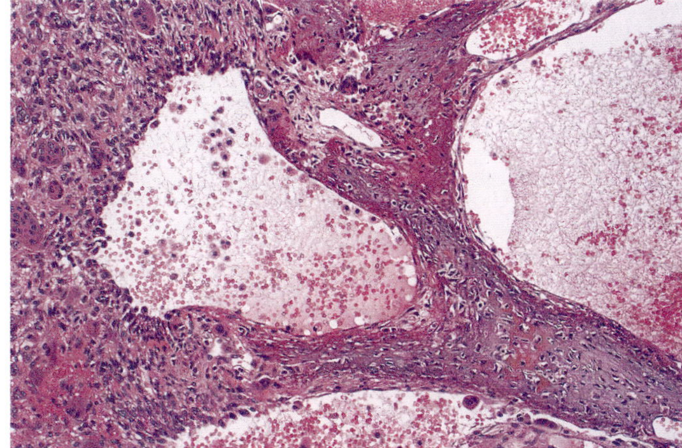

Fig. 37.35

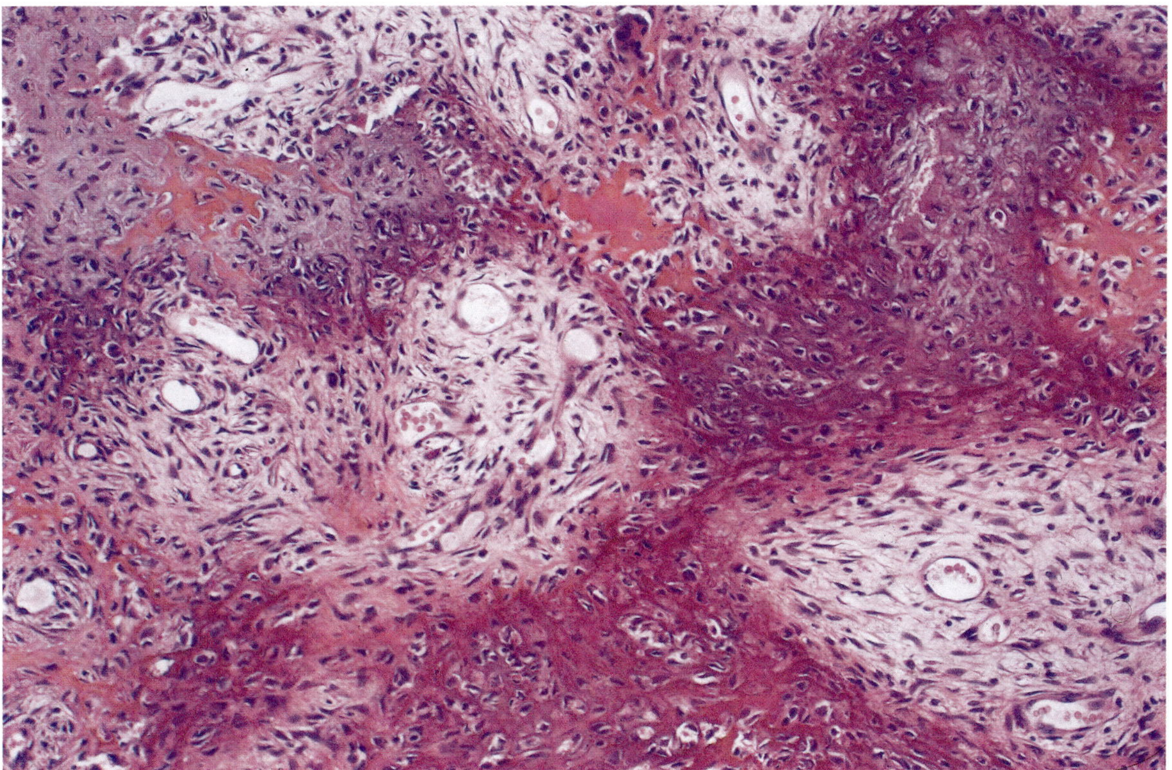

Fig. 37.36

Figs 37.34–37.36 Calcified matrix in the solid parts or the fibrous walls of aneurysmal bone cysts.

component, a focal distribution of giant cells, more re-active bone formation and characteristic calcifying fibro-myxoid areas. Occasionally, the two lesions may be indistinguishable[16,18]

Solitary bone cysts are unilocular lesions with little expansion of bone, the fluid being clear or serosanguinous, but in some cases, especially after a fracture,[94] the differential diagnosis with an aneurysmal bone cyst may be impossible.[5,18]

Solid aneurysmal bone cysts are histologically similar to giant cell reparative granulomas and the two lesions are related; there is no difference in the clinical and radiologic presentation.[5,26,68,71,72] Both lesions are also indistinguishable from the brown tumors of hyperparathyroidism.[5,26]

The differential diagnosis between solid aneurysmal bone cysts and well-differentiated osteosarcomas is easier, the former lesions being paradoxically much more cellular, with mitotic activity and reactive bone with osteoblastic rimming.

The initial stages of aneurysmal bone cysts may mimic a

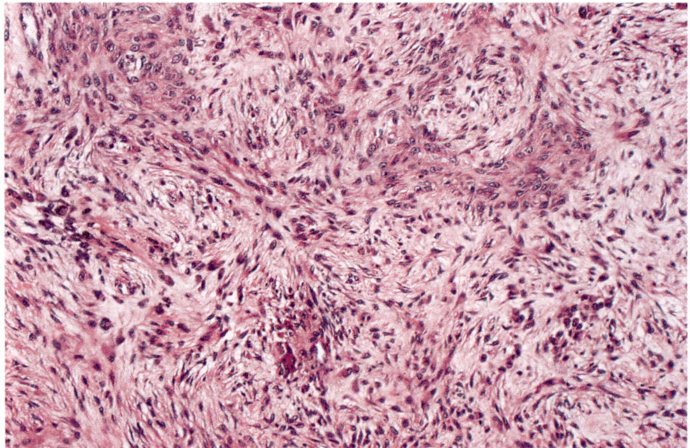

Fig. 37.37

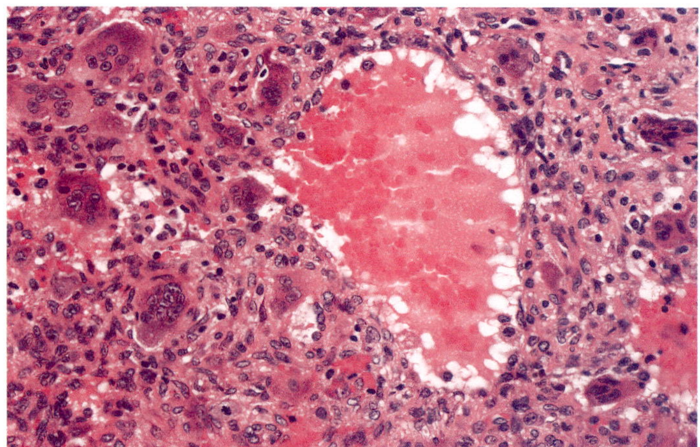

Fig. 37.39

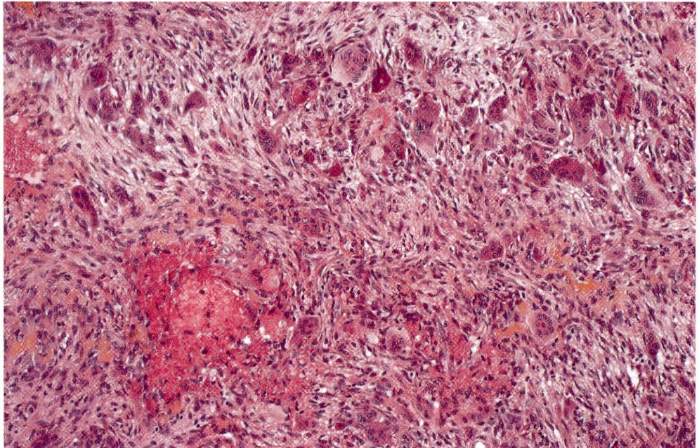

Fig. 37.38

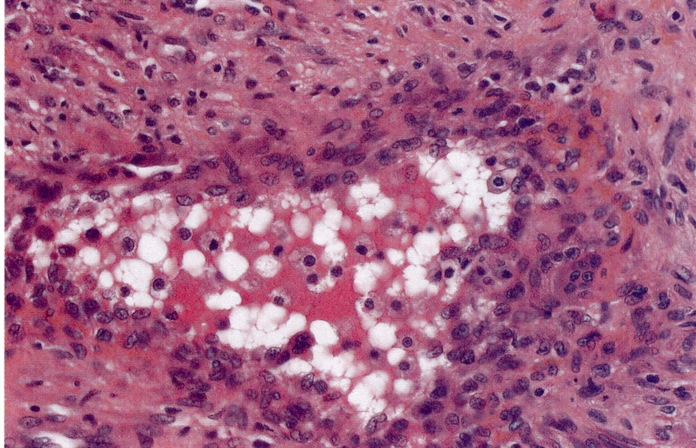

Fig. 37.40

Figs 37.37, 37.38 Aneurysmal bone cyst of the acetabulum, 'solid' variant: florid fibroblastic areas with giant cells and minute flecks of reactive bone.

Figs 37.39, 37.40 Aneurysmal bone cyst of the scapula, 'solid' variant: small dilated vascular spaces without endothelial lining.

malignant tumor radiographically and early stages of telangiectatic osteosarcomas may also resemble an aneurysmal bone cyst.[95] Furthermore, histologically, typical high-grade osteosarcomas may have an aneurysmal bone cyst-like component.[96] Telangiectatic osteosarcomas are diagnosed on the anaplastic cell component, with atypical mitoses and a more irregular bone formation. The differential diagnosis may be quite difficult[97] and a morphometric study has demonstrated that the most important characteristic of telangiectatic osteosarcomas is the nuclear size and, to a lesser extent, mitotic activity and cellularity.[98]

REFERENCES

1. Jaffe H L. Aneurysmal bone cyst. Bull Hosp Jt Dis 1950: 11: 3–13
2. Lichtenstein L. Aneurysmal bone cysts, a pathological entity commonly mistaken for giant-cell tumor, and occasionally for hemangioma and osteogenic sarcoma. Cancer 1950: 3: 279–289
3. Lichtenstein L. Aneurysmal bone cyst; further observations. Cancer 1953: 6: 1228–1237
4. Lichtenstein L. Aneurysmal bone cysts; observations on 50 cases. J Bone Joint Surg (Am) 1957: 39: 873–882
5. Dahlin D C, McLeod R A. Aneurysmal bone cysts and other non neoplastic conditions. Skeletal Radiol 1982: 8: 243–250
6. Vergel De Dios A M, Bond J R, Shives T C, McLeod R A, Unni K K. Aneurysmal bone cyst. A clinicopathologic study of 238 cases. Cancer 1992: 69: 2921–2931
7. Campanacci M, Capanna R, Picci P. Unicameral and aneurysmal bone cysts. Clin Orthop 1986: 204: 25–36
8. Tillman B P, Dahlin D C, Lipscomb P R, Stewart J R. Aneurysmal bone cyst: an analysis of ninety-five cases. Mayo Clin Proc 1968: 43: 478–495
9. Freiberg A A, Loder R T, Heidelberger K P, Hensinger R N. Aneurysmal bone cysts in young children. J Pediatr Orthop 1994: 14: 86–91
10. Vicenzi G. Familial incidence in two cases of aneurysmal bone cyst. Ital J Orthop Traumatol 1981: 7: 251–253
11. Greco F, De Palma L, Coletti V. A familial case of aneurysmal bone cyst. Arch Putti Chir Organi Mov 1983: 33: 441–446
12. Power R A, Robbins P D, Wood D J. Aneurysmal bone cyst in

monozygotic twins: a case report. J Bone Joint Surg (Br) 1996: 78: 323–324

13. Biesecker J L, Marcove R C, Huvos A G, Miké V. Aneurysmal bone cysts. Cancer 1970: 26: 615–625

14. Levy W M, Miller A S, Bonakdarpour A, Aegerter E. Aneurysmal bone cyst secondary to other osseous lesions. Report of 57 cases. Am J Clin Pathol 1975: 63: 1–8

15. Bonakdarpour A, Levy W M, Aegerter E. Primary and secondary aneurysmal bone cyst: a radiological study of 75 cases. Radiology 1978: 126: 75–83

16. Martinez V, Sissons H A. Aneurysmal bone cyst. Cancer 1988: 61: 2291–2304

17. Szendröi M, Cser I, Konya A, Renyi-Vamos A M. Aneurysmal bone cyst. Arch Orthop Trauma Surg 1992: 116: 318–322

18. Kransdorf M J, Sweet D E. Aneurysmal bone cyst: concept, controversy, clinical presentation, and imaging. AJR 1995: 164: 573–580

19. Buraczewski J, Dabska M. Pathogenesis of aneurysmal bone cyst. Relationship between aneurysmal bone cyst and fibrous dysplasia of bone. Cancer 1971: 28: 597–604

20. Diercks R L, Sauter A J, Mallens W M. Aneurysmal bone cyst in association with fibrous dysplasia. J Bone Joint Surg (Br) 1986: 68: 144–146

21. Mintz M C, Dalinka M K, Schmidt G R. Aneurysmal bone cyst arising in fibrous dysplasia during pregnancy. Radiology 1987: 165: 549–550

22. McCarthy E F, Dorfman H D. Vascular and cartilaginous hamartoma of the ribs in infancy with secondary aneurysmal bone cyst formation. Am J Surg Pathol 1980: 4: 247–253

23. Campanacci M, Zanoli S. Osservazioni morfologiche ed istomeccaniche sulla cisti aneurismatica dello scheletro. Arch Ital Anat Istol Patol 1962: 36: 251–273

24. Alles J U, Schulz A. Immunohistochemical markers (endothelial and histiocytic) and ultrastructure of primary aneurysmal bone cysts. Hum Pathol 1986: 17: 39–45

25. Aho H J, Aho A J, Einola S. Aneurysmal bone cyst, a study of ultrastructure and malignant transformation. Virchows Arch A Pathol Anat Histol 1982: 395: 169–179

26. Oda Y, Tsuneyoshi M, Shinohara N. 'Solid' variant of aneurysmal bone cyst (extragnathic giant cell reparative granuloma) in the axial skeleton and long bones. Cancer 1992: 70: 2642–2649

27. Ginsburg L D. Congenital aneurysmal bone cyst. Radiology 1974: 110: 175–176

28. Kushner D C, Vance Z, Kirkpatrick J A Jr. Case report 103. Post-traumatic aneurysmal bone cyst affecting third and fourth ribs. Skeletal Radiol 1979: 4: 240–243

29. Dabezies E J, D'Ambrosia R D, Chuinard R G, Ferguson A B Jr. Aneurysmal bone cyst after fracture. J Bone Joint Surg (Am) 1982: 64: 617–621

30. Johnston C E 2nd, Fletcher R R. Traumatic transformation of unicameral bone cyst into aneurysmal bone cyst. Orthopedics 1986: 9: 1441–1447

31. Dagher A P, Magid D, Johnson C A, McCarthy E F Jr, Fishman E K. Aneurysmal bone cyst developing after anterior cruciate ligament tear and repair. AJR 1992: 158: 1289–1291

32. Ratcliffe P J, Grimer R J. Aneurysmal bone cyst arising after tibial fracture. J Bone Joint Surg (Am) 1993: 75: 1225–1227

33. Ruiter D J, Lindeman J, Haverkate F, Hegt V N. Fibrinolytic activity in aneurysmal bone cysts. Am J Clin Pathol 1975: 64: 810–816

34. Pevny T, Rooney R J. Case report 876. Aneurysmal bone cyst of the patella. Skeletal Radiol 1994: 23: 664–667

35. Hay M C, Patterson D, Taylor T K. Aneurysmal bone cyst of the spine. J Bone Joint Surg (Br) 1978: 60: 406–411

36. Capanna R, Van Horn J R, Biagini R, Ruggieri P. Aneurysmal bone cyst of the sacrum. Skeletal Radiol 1989: 18: 109–113

37. Frassica F J, Amadio P C, Wold L E, Beabout J W. Aneurysmal bone cyst: clinicopathologic features and treatment of ten cases involving the hand. J Hand Surg (Am) 1988: 13: 676–683

38. Yadav S S, Aurora A L, Sharma S, Thomas S, Rajagopal N. Multicentric aneurysmal bone cyst. Indian J Cancer 1982: 19: 116–119

39. Karabela-Bouropoulou V, Liapi-Avgeri G, Paxinos O, Antoniou D.

Solid variant of aneurysmal bone cyst: a case report with bilateral involvement of the distal femoral metaphyses. Virchows Arch 1994: 425: 531–535

40. Von Huttig G, Rittmeyer K. Multiple aneurysmatische Knochenzysten bei 3 Monate altem Säugling. RÖFO 1978: 129: 796–797

41. Petrik P K, Findlay J M, Sherlock R A. Aneurysmal cyst, bone type, primary in an artery. Am J Surg Pathol 1993: 17: 1062–1066

42. Amir G, Mogle P, Sucher E. Case report 729. Myositis ossificans and aneurysmal bone cyst. Skeletal Radiol 1992: 21: 257–259

43. Rodriguez-Peralto J L, Lopez-Barea F, Sanchez-Herrera S, Atienza M. Primary aneurysmal cyst of soft tissues (extraosseous aneurysmal cyst). Am J Surg Pathol 1994: 18: 632–636

44. Dyer R, Stelling C B, Fechner R E. Epiphyseal extension of an aneurysmal bone cyst. AJR 1981: 137: 172–173

45. McCarthy S M, Ogden J A. Epiphyseal extension of an aneurysmal bone cyst. J Pediatr Orthop 1982: 2: 171–175

46. Capanna R, Springfield D S, Biagini R, Ruggieri P, Giunti A. Juxtaepiphyseal aneurysmal bone cyst. Skeletal Radiol 1985: 13: 21–25

47. Capanna R, Bettelli G, Biagini R, Ruggieri P, Bertoni F, Campanacci M. Aneurysmal cysts of long bones. Ital J Orthop Traumatol 1985: 11: 409–417

48. Burnstein M I, De Smet A A, Hafez G R, Heiner J P. Case report 611. Subperiosteal aneurysmal bone cyst of tibia. Skeletal Radiol 1990: 19: 294–297

49. Okada K, Masuda H, Shozawa T, Arai M. A small aneurysmal bone cyst restricted to the cortical bone of the femur resembling so-called subperiosteal giant cell tumor or subperiosteal osteoclasia. Acta Pathol Jpn 1989: 39: 539–544

50. Schoedel K, Shankman S, Desai P. Intracortical and subperiosteal aneurysmal bone cysts: a report of three cases. Skeletal Radiol 1996: 25: 455–459

51. Sherman R S, Soong K Y. Aneurysmal bone cyst: its roentgen diagnosis. Radiology 1957: 68: 54–64

52. Gold R H, Mirra J M. Case report 234. Aneurysmal bone cyst of left scapula with intramural calcified chondroid. Skeletal Radiol 1983: 10: 57–60

53. Sharma P, Elangovan S, Ratnakar C. Case report: calcification within aneurysmal bone cyst. Br J Radiol 1994: 67: 306–308

54. Dabska M, Buraczewski J. Aneurysmal bone cyst. Pathology, clinical course and radiologic appearances. Cancer 1969: 23: 371–389

55. Lindbom A, Soderberg G, Spjut H J, Sunnqvist O. Angiography of aneurysmal bone cyst. Acta Radiol 1961: 55: 12–16

56. Gunterberg B, Kindblom L G, Laurin S. Giant-cell tumor of bone and aneurysmal bone cyst. A correlated histologic and angiographic study. Skeletal Radiol 1977: 2: 65–74

57. De Santos L A, Murray J A. The value of arteriography in the management of aneurysmal bone cyst. Skeletal Radiol 1978: 2: 137–141

58. Hudson T M. Scintigraphy of aneurysmal bone cysts. AJR 1984: 142: 761–765

59. Hudson T M. Fluid levels in aneurysmal bone cysts: CT feature. AJR 1984: 142: 1001–1004

60. Tsai J C, Dalinka M K, Fallon M D, Zlatkin M B, Kressel H Y. Fluid–fluid level: a nonspecific finding in tumors of bone and soft tissue. Radiology 1990: 175: 779–782

61. Apaydin A, Orkaynak C, Yilmaz S et al. Aneurysmal bone cyst of metacarpal. Skeletal Radiol 1996: 25: 76–78

62. Hudson T M, Hamlin D J, Fitzsimmons J R. Magnetic resonance imaging in fluid levels in an aneurysmal bone cyst and in anticoagulated blood. Skeletal Radiol 1985: 13: 267–270

63. Zimmer W D, Berquist T H, Sim F H et al. Magnetic resonance imaging of aneurysmal bone cyst. Mayo Clin Proc 1984: 59: 633–636

64. Beltran J, Simon D C, Levy M, Herman L, Weis L, Mueller C F. Aneurysmal bone cysts: MR imaging at 1.5 T. Radiology 1986: 158: 689–690

65. Munk P L, Helms C A, Holt R G, Johnston J, Steinbach L, Neumann C. MR imaging of aneurysmal bone cysts. AJR 1989: 153: 99–101

66. Capanna R, Albisinni U, Picci P, Calderoni P, Campanacci M,

Springfield D S. Aneurysmal bone cyst of the spine. J Bone Joint Surg (Am) 1985: 67 : 527–531

67. Buirski G, Watt I. The radiological features of 'solid' aneurysmal bone cyst. Br J Radiol 1984: 57: 1057–1065

68. Bertoni F, Bacchini P, Capanna R et al. Solid variant of aneurysmal bone cyst. Cancer 1993: 71: 729–734

69. Gipple J R, Pritchard D J, Unni K K. Solid aneurysmal bone cyst. Orthopedics 1992: 15 : 1433–1436

70. Ruiter D J, Van Rijssel T G, Van Der Velde E A. Aneurysmal bone cysts. Cancer 1977: 39: 2231–2239

71. Sanerkin N G, Mott M G, Roylance J. An unusual intraosseous lesion with fibroblastic, osteoclastic, osteoblastic, aneurysmal and fibromyxoid elements. 'Solid' variant of aneurysmal bone cyst. Cancer 1983: 51: 2278–2286

72. Edel G, Roessner A, Blasius S, Erlemann R. 'Solid' variant of aneurysmal bone cyst. Pathol Res Pract 1992: 188: 791–796, 796–798

73. Dehner L P, Risdall R J, L'Heureux P. Giant-cell containing 'fibrous' lesion of the sacrum. Am J Surg Pathol 1978: 2: 55–70

74. Aho H J, Aho A J, Pelliniemi L J, Ekfors T O, Foidart J M. Endothelium in aneurysmal bone cyst. Histopathology 1985: 9: 381–387

75. Vollmer E, Roessner A, Lipecki K H, Zwadlo G, Hagemeier H H, Grundmann E. Biologic characterization of human bone tumors. VI The aneurysmal bone cyst: an enzyme histochemical, electron microscopical and immunohistochemical study. Virchows Arch B Cell Pathol Incl Mol Pathol 1987: 53: 58–65

76. Pfeifer F M, Bridge J A, Neff J R, Mouron B J. Cytogenetic findings in aneurysmal bone cyst. Genes Chromosomes Cancer 1991: 3: 416–419

77. Steiner G C, Kantor E B. Ultrastructure of aneurysmal bone cyst. Cancer 1977: 40: 2967–2978

78. Llombart-Bosch A, Peydro-Olaya A, Pellin A. Ultrastructure of vascular neoplasms. Pathol Res Pract 1982: 174: 1–41

79. Malghem J, Maldague B, Esselinckx W, Noel H, De Nayer P, Vincent A. Spontaneous healing of aneurysmal bone cysts. J Bone Joint Surg (Br) 1989: 71: 645–650

80. Saglik Y, Kapicioglu M I, Güzel B. Spontaneous regression of aneurysmal bone cyst. Arch Orthop Trauma Surg 1993: 112: 203–204

81. McQueen M M, Chalmers J, Smith G D. Spontaneous healing of an aneurysmal bone cyst. J Bone Joint Surg (Br) 1985: 67: 310–312

82. Scott I, Connell D G, Duncan C P. Regression of aneurysmal bone cyst following open biopsy. Can Assoc Radiol J 1986: 37: 198–200

83. Murphy W A, Strecker E B, Schoenecker P L. Transcatheter embolization therapy of an ischial aneurysmal bone cyst. J Bone Joint Surg (Br) 1982: 64: 166–168

84. Cremer H, Munzenberg K J. Aneurysmatische Knochenzyste mit malignem Verlauf. Z Orthop Ihre Grenzgeb 1980: 118: 225–235

85. Kyriakos M, Hardy D. Malignant transformation of aneurysmal bone cyst, with analysis of the literature. Cancer 1991: 68: 1770–1780

86. Gomes H, Menanteau B, Gaillard D, Behar C. Telangiectatic osteosarcoma. Pediatr Radiol 1986: 16: 140–143

87. Reed R J, Rothenberg M. Lesions of bone that may be confused with aneurysmal bone cyst. Clin Orthop 1964: 35: 150–162

88. Adler C P. Case report 111. Telangiectatic osteosarcoma of the femur with features of an aggressive aneurysmal bone cyst. Skeletal Radiol 1980: 5: 56–60

89. Wuisman P, Roessner A, Blasius S, Grünert J, Vestering T, Winkelmann W. High malignant surface osteosarcoma arising at the site of a previously treated aneurysmal bone cyst. J Cancer Res Clin Oncol 1993: 119: 375–378

90. De Cristofaro R, Biagini R, Boriani S et al. Selective arterial embolization in the treatment of aneurysmal bone cyst and angioma of bone. Skeletal Radiol 1992: 21: 523–527

91. Konya A, Szendroï M. Aneurysmal bone cysts treated by superselective embolization. Skeletal Radiol 1992: 21: 167–173

92. Freeby J A, Reinus W R, Wilson A J. Quantitative analysis of the plain radiographic appearance of aneurysmal bone cysts. Invest Radiol 1995: 30: 433–439

93. Erlemann R, Picker S, Müller-Miny H, Wuisman P, Edel G. Aneurysmatische knochenzyste oder riezenzelltumor. Wertigkeit der röntgendiagnostik zur differentialdiagnose. RÖFO 1993: 158: 343–347

94. Johnston C E 2nd, Fletcher R R. Traumatic transformation of unicameral bone cyst into aneurysmal bone cyst. Orthopedics 1986: 9: 1441–1447

95. Kaufman R A, Towbin R B. Telangiectatic osteosarcoma simulating the appearance of an aneurysmal bone cyst. Pediatr Radiol 1981: 11: 102–104

96. Funk D A, Unni K K. Case report 318. Grade 2 osteoblastic osteosarcoma with elements of aneurysmal bone cyst. Skeletal Radiol 1985: 14: 61–64

97. Vigliani F, Campailla E. Mimicry in osteogenic sarcoma: clinical considerations and report of two cases. Ital J Orthop Traumatol 1981: 7: 425–436

98. Ruiter D J, Cornelisse C J, Van Rijssel T G, Van Der Velde E A. Aneurysmal bone cyst and telangiectatic osteosarcoma. A histopathological and morphometric study. Virchows Arch A Pathol Anat Histol 1977: 373: 311–325

Ganglion and epidermoid cyst

M. Forest

INTRAOSSEOUS GANGLION

Introduction and clinical data

An intraosseous ganglion,[1] also called subchondral bone cyst[2] or juxtaarticular bone cyst, is a cystic lesion not associated with degenerative osteoarthritic changes and usually without direct communication with the joint cavity.

Intraosseous ganglions are more frequent in adults, between the second to six decades of life, with a slight male predominance.[3]

Clinical symptoms of long duration include a mild intermittent localized pain [3-6] or a painless swelling. Some lesions may be asymptomatic.

They are similar to their soft tissue counterparts[4,7] and the etiology of the bone lesions is still unsettled.[8] Some may be due to the penetration of an extraosseous ganglion into bone, with secondary cortical remodeling.[9-11] In rare cases, a channel communicating with the joint cavity has been described.[12] Various etiological factors have been suggested: synovial herniation or synovial nests, mechanical factors or minor trauma[2,3] or a fibroblastic proliferation with secondary degenerative changes and mucoid secretion.[5,6,8,13]

Skeletal distribution

The most common locations are in bones adjacent to the ankle, the hip and the knee joints;[3] in 33% of cases, the epiphyseal-metaphyseal portion of the tibia is involved[4,14] (Wilner 1982) (Figs 38.1–38.6) and 20% of the lesions are in carpal and tarsal bones[15,16] (Wilner 1982) (Fig. 38.7). Intraosseous ganglions have been reported in the humerus,[17,18-19] the radius (Fig. 38.8), the ulna,[20] the scapula,[21] the ilium[22] and phalanx[23] (Fig. 38.9).

Rarely, the lesion may appear as a cortical bone defect.[23,24]

Subperiosteal ganglion cysts are more frequent[25-36] in the diaphyseal or metaphyseal areas of the femur, tibia and radius. The most common site is the anteromedial aspect

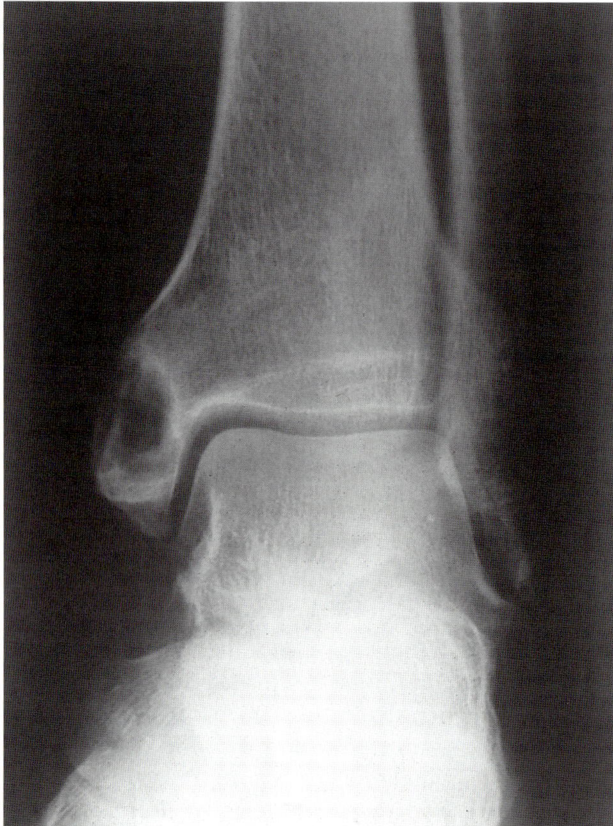

Fig. 38.1 Intraosseous ganglion of the tibia.

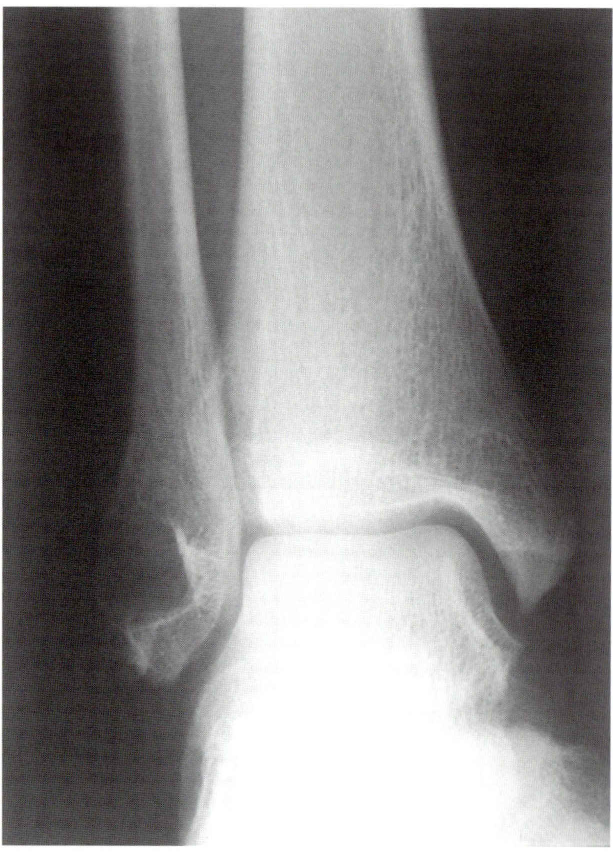

Fig. 38.2 Intraosseous ganglion of the fibula.

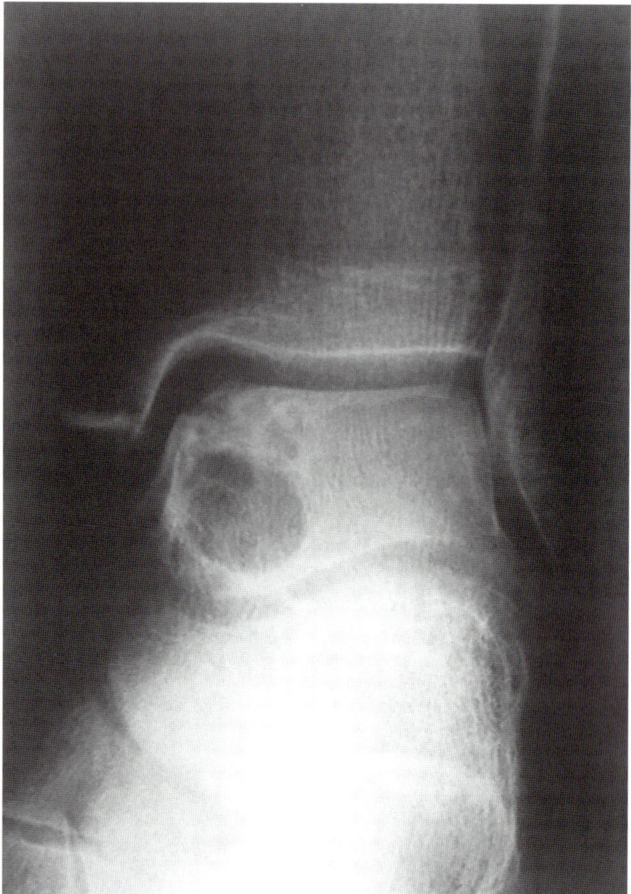

Fig. 38.3

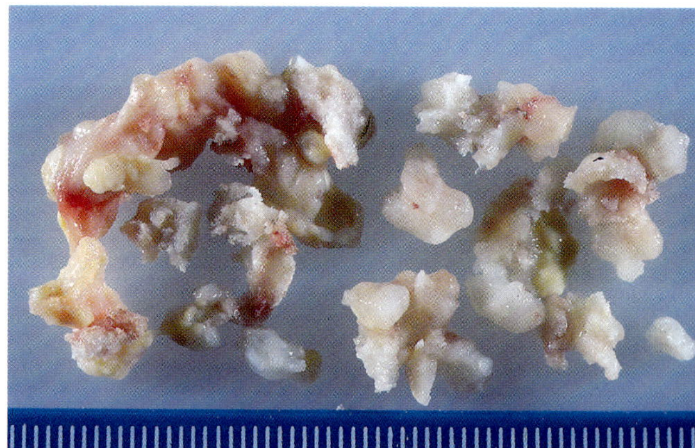

Fig. 38.4

Figs 38.3, 38.4 Intraosseous ganglion of the talus.

of the proximal tibia;[30–32] the cystic mass is well defined, with a slight erosion or scalloping of the cortex and reactive bone formation.

Multiple, bilateral and symmetrical lesions have been reported.[3–6,35–40]

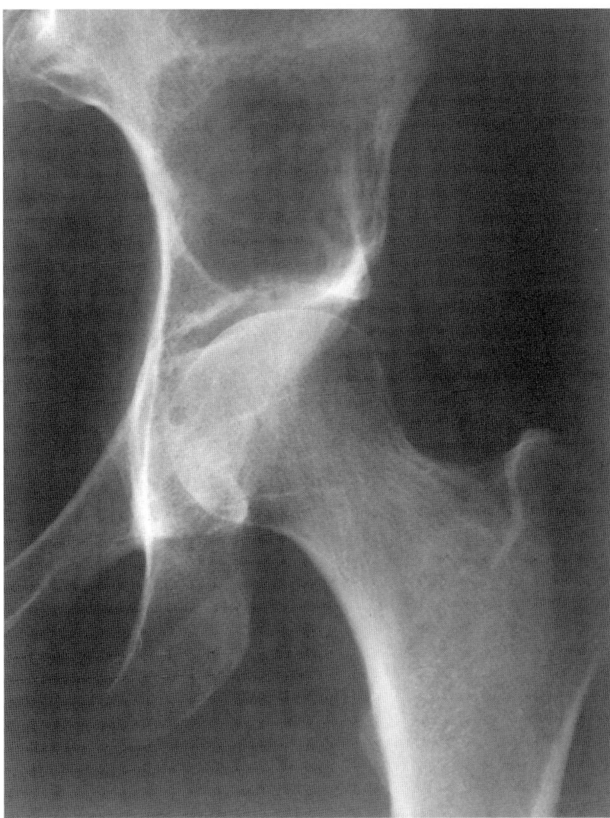

Fig. 38.5 Intraosseous ganglion of the ilium.

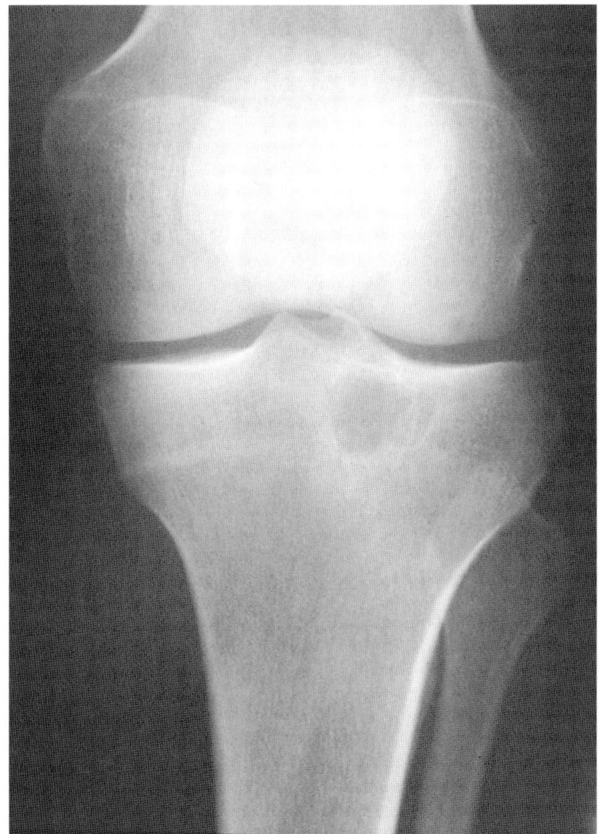

Fig. 38.6 Intraosseous ganglion of the tibia.

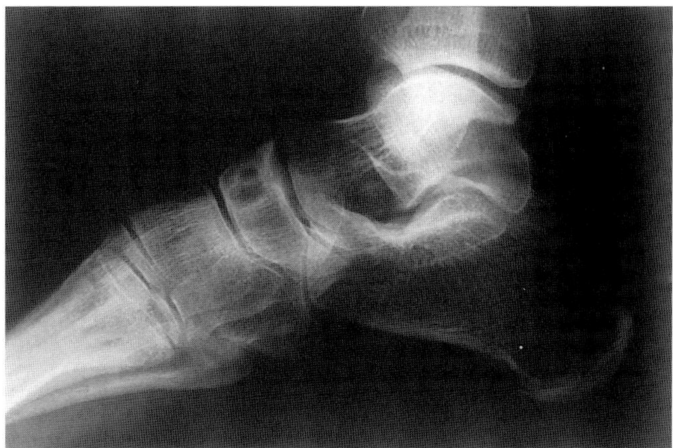

Fig. 38.7 Intraosseous ganglion: tarsal location.

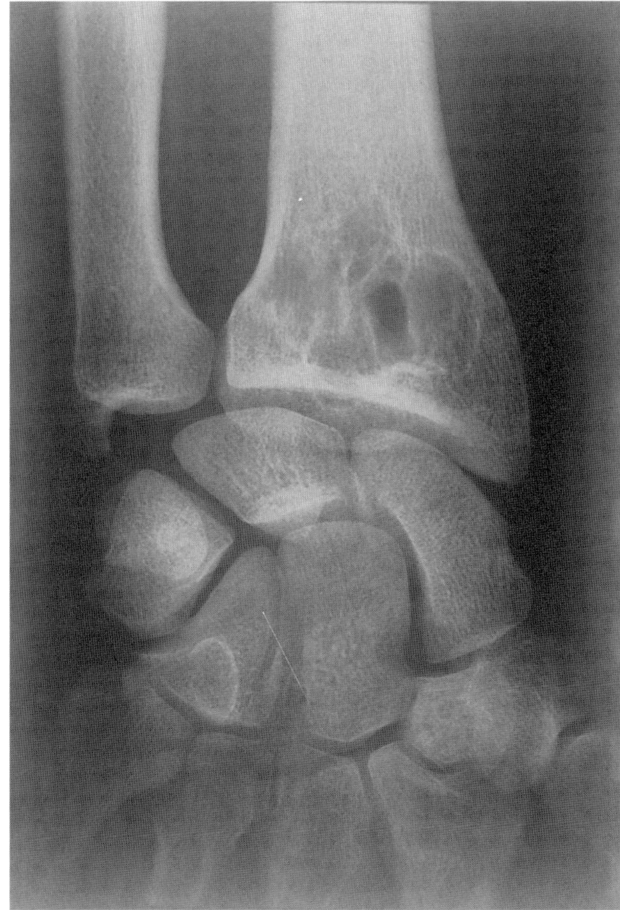

Fig. 38.8 Intraosseous ganglion of the radius.

Imaging

An intraosseous ganglion appears as a well-defined, oval or round, uni- or multilocular osteolytic area with a thin rim of sclerotic bone. The majority are eccentrically located.[8] The cortex may be thinned or expanded but, the adjacent articular surface is normal.

On MRI, there is low or intermediate signal intensity

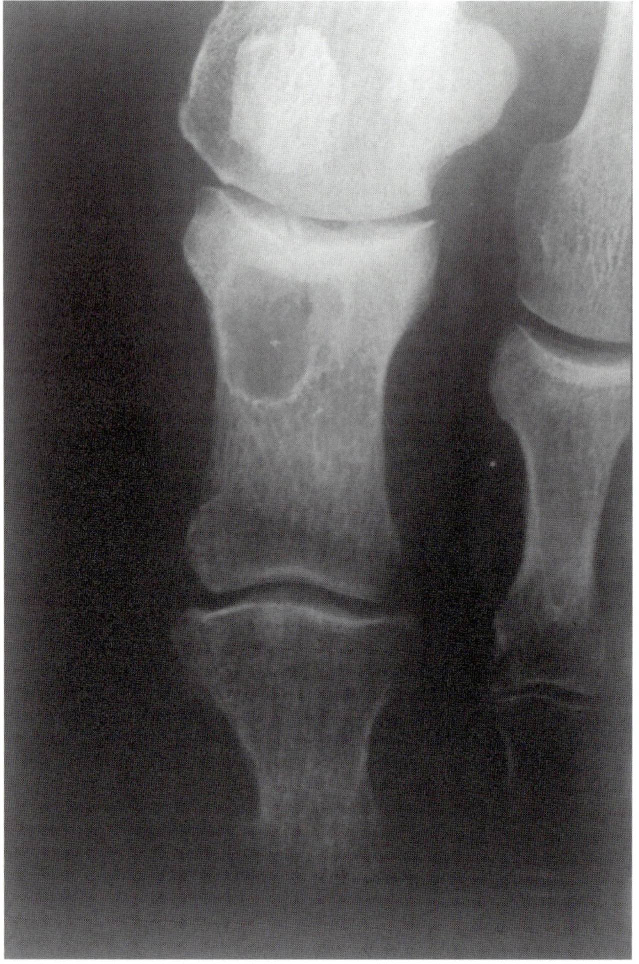

Fig. 38.9 Intraosseous ganglion: location in the proximal phalanx of the great toe.

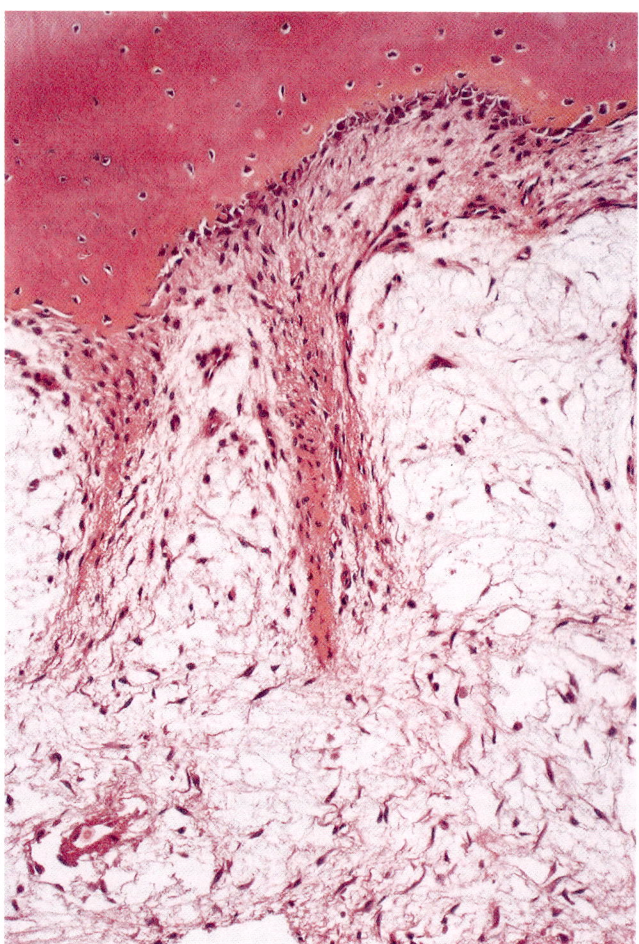

Fig. 38.10 Intraosseous ganglion: stellate or fibroblast-like cells in a mucoid ground substance.

on T1 and high signal intensity on T2-weighted images.[31,33,34,39,40] On CT or MRI, gas–fluid levels or gas bubbles may be found.[17,18,20,41]

Gross pathology

An intraosseous ganglion is usually small, 1–2 cm,[3] but the size ranges from a few millimeters to 7 cm.[24] A yellowish, viscous, mucoid, jelly-like material is surrounded by a white fibrous capsule.

Histopathology

An intraosseous ganglion is not a synovial cyst[42–46] and there is no synovial lining.[2,4,7,9] Histological features are similar to those of soft tissue lesions.[7] Stellate or fibroblast-like cells produce a large amount of mucoid ground substance (Figs 38.10, 38.11). Some cells may exhibit a vacuolar cytoplasm with mucoid production[3] and occasionally, foam cells are found.[4]

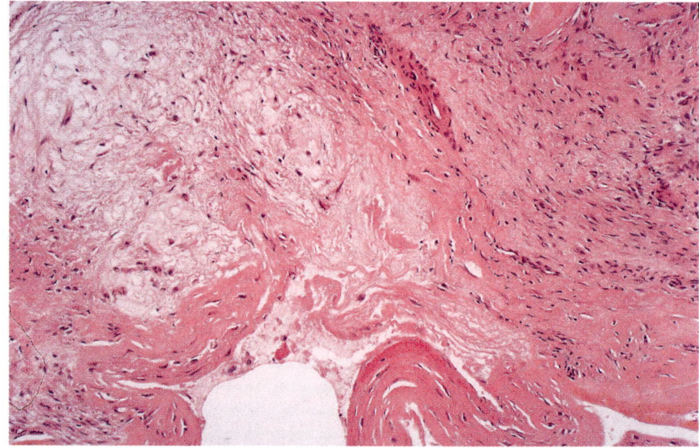

Fig. 38.11 Intraosseous ganglion: fibrous area with some mucoid ground substance.

Electron microscopy

The cells are fibroblasts and macrophages distributed in a myxoid connective tissue.[47]

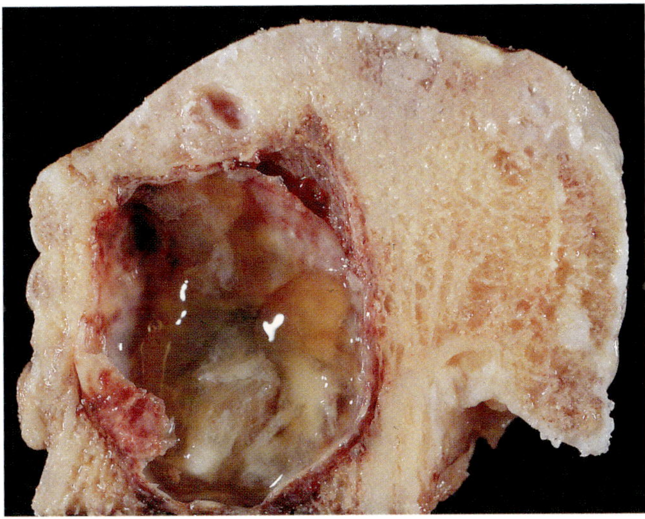

Fig. 38.12

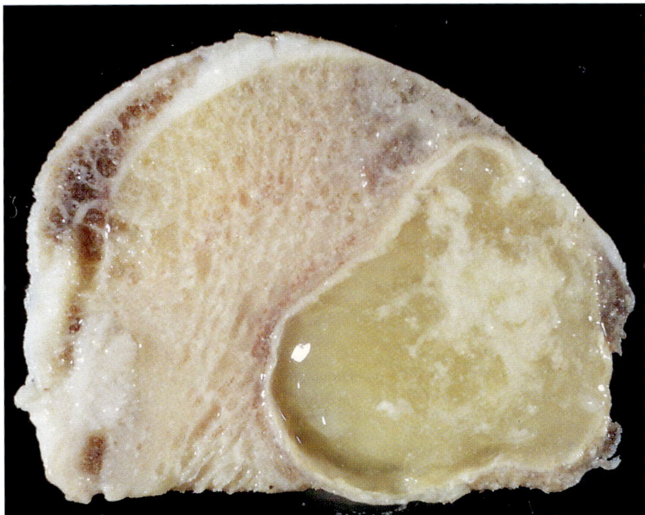

Fig. 38.13

Figs 38.12, 38.13 Huge osteoarthritic cysts of the femoral head.

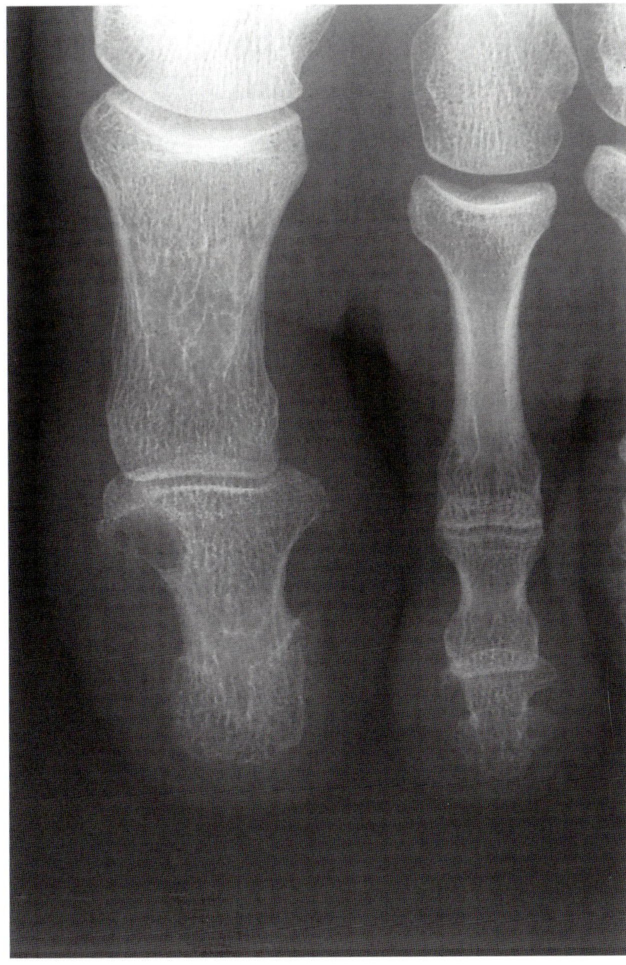

Fig. 38.14

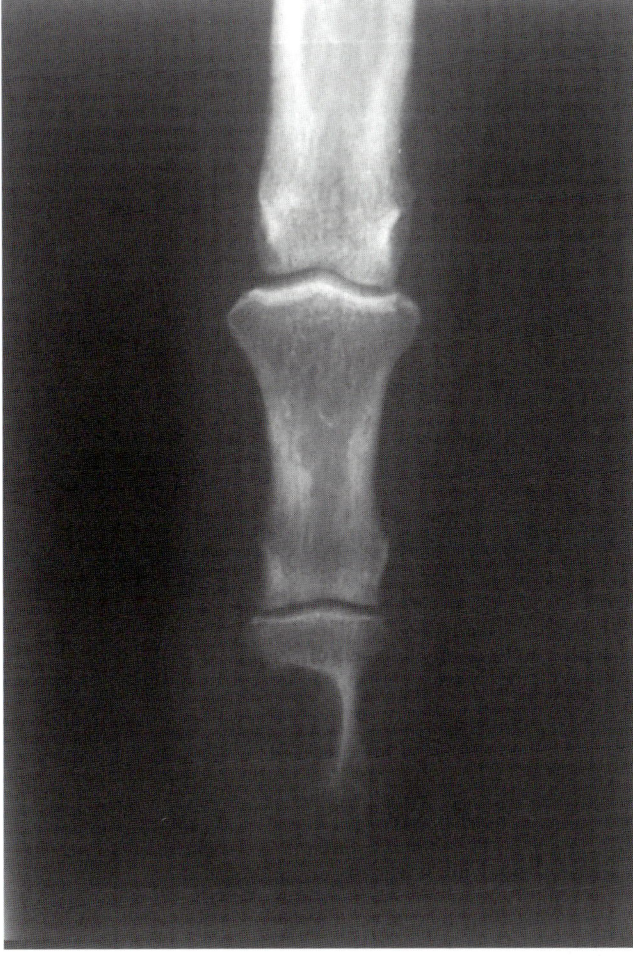

Fig. 38.15

Figs 38.14, 38.15 Intraosseous epidermoid cysts of phalanges.

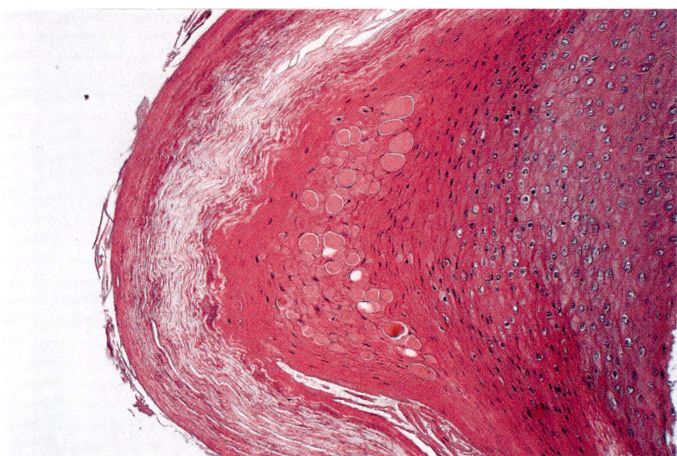

Fig. 38.16 Typical squamous epithelium of an intraosseous epidermoid cyst.

Treatment

Curettage with or without bone grafting is performed, with no recurrences in some series[8] but a few in others.[3,15]

Differential diagnosis

Asymptomatic cysts associated with osteoarthritis may be very difficult to differentiate from intraosseous ganglia, without the clinical and radiological findings, especially in the hip and the knee joint[48] (Figs 38.12, 38.13). Osteoarthritic cysts are the result of the blow-out of synovial fluid through cartilaginous defects into the subchondral bone. They appear also as sharply circumscribed lytic defects filled with a yellow gelatinous fluid. Some may expand.[49] In contrast to intraosseous ganglia, they are more centrally located, rarely solitary,[25] have a smaller size and are associated with articular degenerative changes.[20] Histologically, the fibroblasts and the myxoid material are sometimes associated with necrotic bone, cartilage debris or cartilaginous metaplasia.[3]

INTRAOSSEOUS EPIDERMOID CYSTS

Epidermal inclusion cysts or epidermoid cysts are located predominantly in the calvarium and in the tufts of the terminal finger phalanges[50–52] (Figs 38.14, 38.15); in this latter location, a posttraumatic cause is likely and there is a distinct relationship with trauma.[53,54] They are mostly found in male patients[54] and multiple lesions have been reported.

Unusual locations are the hallux,[52,54] metacarpal bones,[55] the ulna,[53] the femur,[56] the tibia,[57] the sacrum[58] and the sternum (Mirra 1989).

In the phalanges, they appear on X-ray as a roundish osteolytic area located in the tuft; the lesion is sharply demarcated, sometimes with sclerotic margins. The cortex is thinned, expanded or broken.

Grossly, the cavity is empty or filled with caseous material.[54]

Histologically, the typical thin squamous epithelium is surrounded by a dense fibrous stroma (Fig. 38.16). Rupture of the cyst with spread of keratinized debris and fat material may induce a foreign body reaction and cholesterol granulomas.

Excision is curative.

REFERENCES

1. Crabbe W A. Intraosseous ganglia of bone. Br J Surg 1966: 53: 15–17
2. Woods C G. Subchondral bone cysts. J Bone Joint Surg (Br) 1961: 43: 758–766
3. Schajowicz F, Clavel Sainz M, Slullitel J A. Juxtaarticular bone cysts (intraosseous ganglia). J Bone Joint Surg (Br) 1979: 61: 107–116
4. Bauer T W, Dorfman H D. Intra osseous ganglion. Am J Surg Pathol 1982: 6: 207–213
5. Feldman F, Johnston A. Intra osseous ganglion. Am J Roentgenol Radium Ther Nucl Med 1973: 118: 328–343
6. Feldmann F. Ganglia of bone: theories, manifestations and presentations. CRC Crit Rev Clin Radiol Nucl Med 1973: 4: 303–332
7. Pope T L Jr, Fechner R E, Keats T E. Intra-osseous ganglion. Skeletal Radiol 1989: 18: 185–187
8. Helwig U, Lang S, Baczynski M, Windhager R. The intraosseous ganglion. A clinico-pathological report on 42 cases. Arch Orthop Trauma Surg 1994: 114: 14–17
9. Kambolis C, Bullough P G, Jaffe H L. Ganglionic cystic defects of bone. J Bone Joint Surg (Am) 1973: 55: 496–505
10. McBeath A A, Neidhart D A. Acetabular cyst with communicating ganglion. J Bone Joint Surg (Am) 1976: 58: 267–269
11. Bowers W H, Hurst L C. An intraarticular-intraosseous carpal ganglion. J Hand Surg (Am) 1979: 4: 375–377
12. Salzer M, Salzer-Kuntschik M. Ganglein mit Knochenbeteiligung. Arch Orthop Unfall Chir 1968: 64: 87–99
13. Menges V, Prager P, Cserhati M D, Becker W, Griss P, Wurster K. Das intraossäre Ganglion. Z Orthop Ihre Grenzgeb 1977: 115: 67–75
14. Goldman R L, Friedman N B. Ganglia ('synovial cysts') arising in unusual locations. Clin Orthop 1969: 63: 184–189
15. Sim F H, Dahlin D C. Ganglion cysts of bone. Mayo Clin Proc 1971: 46: 484–488
16. Thornton D, Farrer A K. Intraosseous ganglion of the cuboid bone. J Foot Ankle Surg 1993: 32: 443–452
17. Brown D M, Young V L, Groner J P, Higgs P E, Gilula L A. Intraosseous ganglion of the trapezoid. J Hand Surg (Am) 1994: 19: 607–608
18. Hahn P F, Rosenthal D I, Ehrlich M G. Case report 286. Gas within a solitary bone cyst of the proximal end of the left humerus. Skeletal Radiol 1984: 12: 214–217
19. Ehara S, Kattapuram S V, Khurana J S, Rosenberg A E. Case report 551. Intraosseous ganglion of the olecranon with vacuum phenomenon. Skeletal Radiol 1989: 18: 329–330
20. Yaghmai I, Foster W C. Case report 404. Intraosseous ganglion of the distal end of the ulna with a pathologic fracture. Skeletal Radiol 1987: 16: 153–156
21. Yamato M, Saotome K, Tamai K, Yamaguchi T. Case report 783. Intraosseous ganglion of scapula. Skeletal Radiol 1993: 22: 227–228
22. Weinberg S, Schneider H. Case report 211. Intra osseous ganglion of the ilium. Skeletal Radiol 1982: 9: 61–63
23. Posner M A, Green S M. Intraosseous ganglion of a phalanx. J Hand Surg (Am) 1984: 9: 280–282

24. Menendez L R, Chandler D R, Moore T M, Schwinn C P. Diaphyseal intra osseous ganglion. Clin Orthop 1988: 227: 310–312

25. Dungan D H, Seeger L L, Mirra J M. Case report 555. Intraosseous ganglion cyst of the distal end of tibia. Skeletal Radiol 1989: 18: 385–388

26. Byers P D, Wadsworth T G. Periosteal ganglion. J Bone Joint Surg (Br) 1970: 52: 290–295

27. Campanacci M, Cervellati C. Cisti mucose periostee e intraossee. Chir Organi Mov 1971: 60: 221–232

28. Kay N R. Sub-periosteal ganglia. Acta Orthop Scand 1971: 42: 173–177

29. Grange W J. Subperiosteal ganglion. J Bone Joint Surg (Br) 1978: 60: 124–125

30. Heyse-Moore G H, Grange W J. Case report 82. Subperiosteal ganglion. Skeletal Radiol 1979: 3: 255–256

31. McCarthy E F, Matz S, Steiner G C, Dorfman H D. Periosteal ganglion: a cause of periosteal erosion. Skeletal Radiol 1983: 10: 243–246

32. Kenan S, Mobley K, Steiner G C, Lewis M M. Periosteal ganglion. Bull Hosp Jt Dis Orthop Inst 1987: 47: 46–51

33. Kenan S, Abdelwahab I F, Klein M J, Hermann G, Lewis M M. Lesions of juxtacortical origin (surface lesions of bone). Skeletal Radiol 1993: 22: 337–357

34. Abdelwahab I F, Kenan S, Hermann G, Klein M J, Lewis M M. Periosteal ganglia. CT and MR imaging features. Radiology 1993: 188: 245–248

35. Nadas S, Landry M, Duvoisin B, Richoz B, Maire P. Subperiosteal ganglionic cyst of the iliac wing. Skeletal Radiol 1995: 24: 541–542

36. Kobayashi H, Kotoura Y, Hosono M, Tsuboyama T, Sakahara H, Konishi J. Periosteal ganglion of the tibia. Skeletal Radiol 1996: 25: 381–383

37. Pellegrino E A Jr, Olson J R. Bilateral carpal lunate ganglia. Clin Orthop 1972: 87: 225–227

38. Campanacci M, Gulino G. Cisti mucosa intraossea bilaterale. Chir Organi Mov 1974: 61: 367–370

39. Logan S E, Gilula L A, Kyriakos M. Bilateral scaphoid ganglion cysts in an adolescent. J Hand Surg (Am) 1992: 17: 490–495

40. Lorente R, Moreno M, Quiles M. Bilateral intraosseous ganglia of the lunate: a case report. J Hand Surg (Am) 1992: 17: 1084–1085

41. Tanaka H, Araki Y, Yamamoto H, Yamamoto T, Tsukaguchi I. Intraosseous ganglion. Skeletal Radiol 1995: 24: 155–157

42. Okada K, Unoki E, Kubota H et al. Periosteal ganglion. Skeletal Radiol 1996: 25: 153–157

43. Rosenthal D I, Schwartz A N, Schiller A L. Case report 170. Subperiosteal synovial cyst of knee. Skeletal Radiol 1981: 7: 142–145

44. Hicks J D. Synovial cysts in bone. Aust NZ J Surg 1956: 26: 138–143

45. Crane A R, Scarano J J. Synovial cysts (ganglia) of bone. J Bone Joint Surg (Am) 1967: 49: 355–361

46. Graf L, Freyschmidt J. Die subchondrale Synovialzyste (intraossäre Ganglion). RÖFO 1988: 148: 398–402

47. De Santis E. I gangli dell'osso. Arch Putti Chir Organi Mov 1978: 29: 257–276

48. Ostlere S J, Seeger L L, Eckardt J J. Subchondral cysts of the tibia secondary to osteoarthritis of the knee. Skeletal Radiol 1990: 19: 287–289

49. Glass T A, Dyer R, Fisher L, Fechner R E. Expansile subchondral bone cyst. AJR 1982: 139: 1210–1211

50. Byers P, Mantle J, Salm R. Epidermal cysts of phalanges. J Bone Joint Surg (Am) 1966: 48: 577–581

51. Fisher E R, Gruhn J, Skerrett P. Epidermal cyst in bone. Cancer 1958: 11: 643–648

52. Roth S I. Squamous cysts involving the skull and phalanges. J Bone Joint Surg (Am) 1964: 46: 1442–1450

53. Mollan R A, Wray A R, Hayes D. Traumatic epidermoid cyst of ulna. J Bone Joint Surg (Br) 1982: 64: 456–457

54. Schajowicz F, Aiello C L, Slullitel I. Cystic and pseudo cystic lesions of the terminal phalanx with special reference to epidermoid cysts. Clin Orthop 1970: 68: 84–92

55. Oda Y, Hashimoto H, Tsuneyoshi M, Ono N. Case report 742. Intra osseous epidermoid cyst arising in the fifth metacarpal bone. Skeletal Radiol 1992: 21: 343–345

56. Maritz N G, De Bruin B. Epidermal cysts of the femur. S Afr Med J 1980: 58: 779–780

57. Exner G, Hort W, Böger A. Epidermoidzyste der Tibia. Z Orthop Ihre Grenzgeb 1978: 116: 362–368

58. Adachi H, Yoshida H, Yumoto T et al. Intraosseous epidermal cyst of the sacrum. Acta Pathol Jpn 1988: 38: 1561–1564

39

Eosinophilic granuloma

M. Forest

INTRODUCTION AND CLINICAL DATA

Eosinophilic granuloma, first described by Jaffe & Lichtenstein in 1940,[1] is a proliferation of Langerhans cells which constitute a subpopulation belonging to the mononuclear phagocyte system.[2–4]

The term 'histiocytosis X' was proposed by Lichtenstein in 1953[5] to cover a spectrum of diseases including Hand–Schuller–Christian disease, Letterer–Siwe disease and eosinophilic granuloma. Some authors believe that, on clinical grounds, Letterer–Siwe disease should not be classified in the same syndrome.[6] More recently, the terms 'Langerhans cell histiocytosis'[7,8] or 'Langerhans cell granulomatosis'[9] have been suggested as a more accurate pathological description for a disease which may be a disorder of immunoregulation or a neoplastic process (demonstration of clonality and of an aberrant phenotype[10,11]).

This chapter is restricted to eosinophilic granuloma as a solitary or multiple bone lesion, which accounts for 70% of cases of Langerhans cell histiocytosis and fewer than 1% of all bone tumor-like lesions.[12]

Two-thirds of cases are diagnosed in the first and second decades of life, with a peak incidence between 5 and 10 years; it is not infrequent in adults and sometimes multiple lesions may occur.[13] Males are affected twice as often as females.

The most common complaint is pain, often worse at night,[14] or tenderness or a localized swelling. Eosinophilic granuloma may be asymptomatic. Pathologic fractures occur, with an incidence of 17%, half the cases involving the spine.[14]

SKELETAL DISTRIBUTION

Solitary lesions predominate over multiple lesions, but 10% of patients will develop a multifocal disease.[15] Eosinophilic granuloma may be found in any bone, but the skull (calvarium) is the most common site in adults

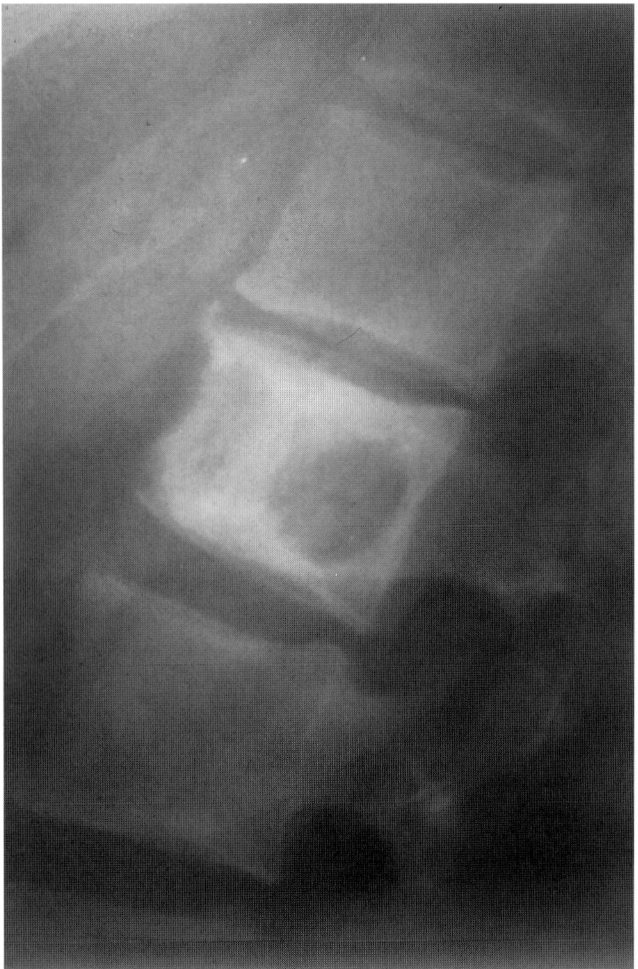

Fig. 39.1 Eosinophilic granuloma: punched-out lesion of a vertebral body.

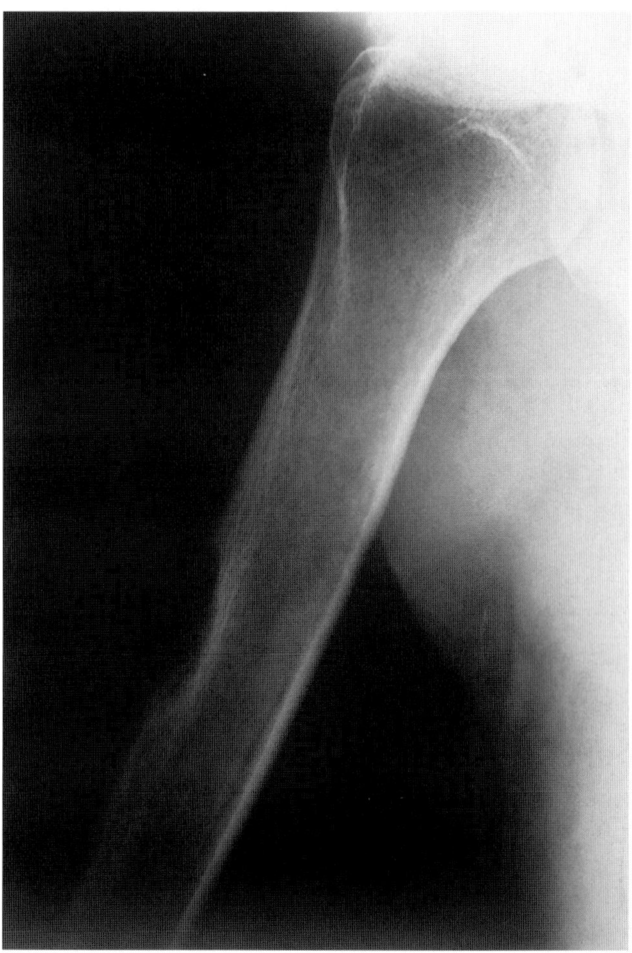

Fig. 39.2 Eosinophilic granuloma: erosion of the cortex of the humeral shaft.

and children[14] with a reported incidence as high as 50%, followed by vertebral bodies and long tubular bones (Figs 39.1–39.6). Skull, ribs and pelvic bones (ilium) (Figs 39.7, 39.8) are predominantly involved in adults[13] and skull and long tubular bones (proximal end of femur and humerus), in children.[14] Small bones of the hands and feet are rarely affected.[16]

IMAGING

Radiological findings depend on the location.[17]

In flat bones, eosinophilic granuloma is usually a well-defined, punched-out lesion with a beveled appearance due to the various degrees of destruction of the cortical walls.[18]

In the spine, the vertebral body is involved in 90% of cases, leading to a variable degree of collapse. Chiefly in children, the entire height of the vertebral body may be lost (vertebra plana). Less often, the lesion is bubbly and expansile, involving the spinous processes without significant collapse.[19] Thoracic and lumbar spinal loca-

tions predominate. Adjacent vertebrae may be involved in some cases, with a normal height of the intervertebral disc.

In long bones, eosinophilic granuloma is located in the diaphysis in two-thirds of cases.[15] Epiphyseal involvement is unusual,[20–23] as are cortical locations.[24]

Eosinophilic granuloma is a lytic medullary lesion with sharply defined margins or, less often, a permeative pattern.[14] The scalloping of the cortex is due to endosteal erosions, eventually followed by breakthrough and a soft tissue mass.[18] The bone may be expanded.[25]

Periosteal reactions are found in one-third of cases,[14,18] with or without fractures. Periosteal bone formation and bone expansion are unusual in adults. The lesion and the bone destruction may be quite extensive,[26] mimicking Ewing's sarcoma,[15,27,28] especially in children.

On bone scans, there is a mild radionuclide accumulation which is increased at the margins of the osteolytic process.[29] Cold lesions predominate in the pelvis and vertebral column. False-negative bone scintigrams are found in up to 35% of cases.[15,30]

CT scans are useful to demonstrate the extent of bone

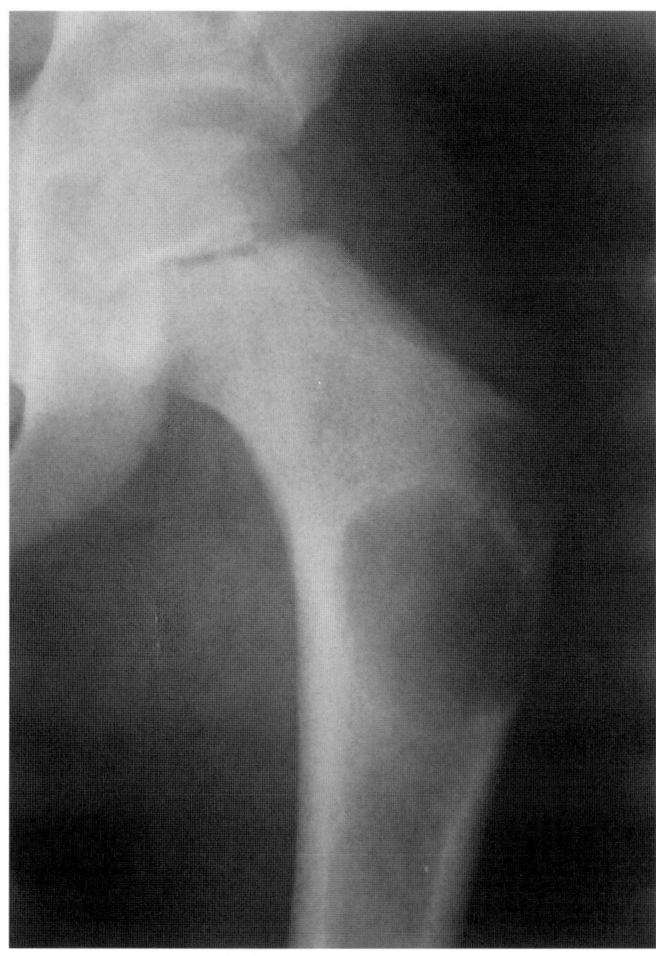

Fig. 39.3

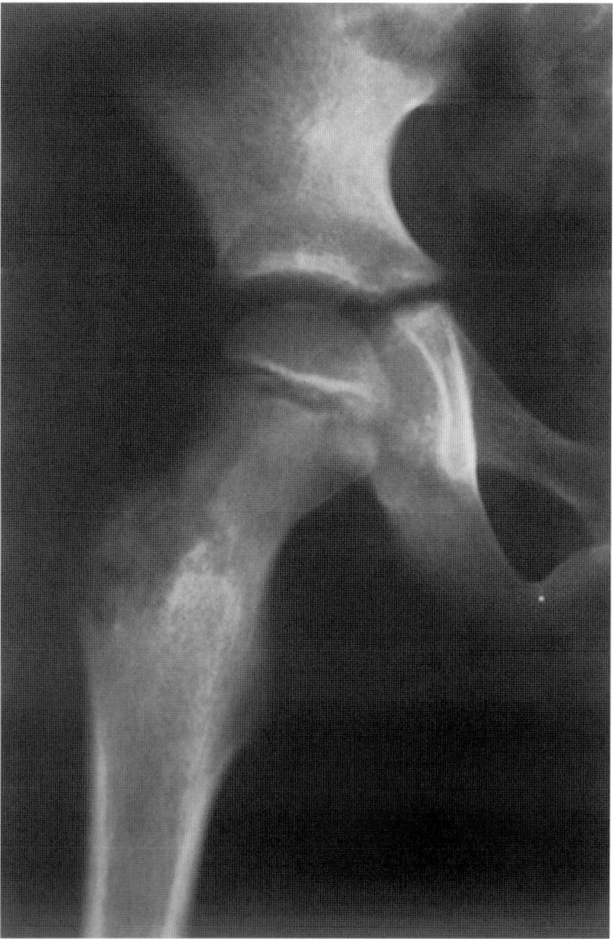

Fig. 39.4

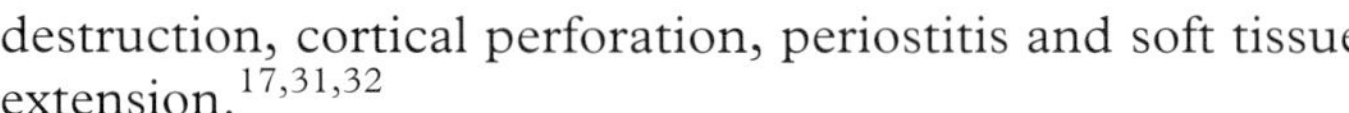

Figs 39.3, 39.4 Eosinophilic granulomas in femoral location.

destruction, cortical perforation, periostitis and soft tissue extension.[17,31,32]

On MRI, the signal intensity is intermediate or high on T1 and high on T2-weighted images, with enhanced contrast after injection of contrast medium.[15,33,34] In the early phases, extensive and ill-defined bone marrow and soft tissue edema may appear as a flare phenomenon, simulating osteomyelitis, Ewing's sarcoma or lymphoma, like some cases of chondroblastomas or osteoblastomas.[34] A low signal endosteal rim may be an early feature of healing.[35] MRI may identify lesions not found on plain films.[36]

GROSS PATHOLOGY

The tissue is soft, brown or yellow, with hemorrhage, necrotic areas or cyst formation.

HISTOPATHOLOGY

Langerhans cells are the pathognomonic cytologic component (Figs 39.9, 39.10), appearing as mononuclear

elements averaging 12 μu at the largest diameter.[37] Binucleated or multinucleated cells are usual.

The pale or acidophilic cytoplasm is well demarcated and cytoplasmic vacuoles may be found. The signs of phagocytic activity are reduced[38] or absent,[4,39] but Langerhans cells are capable of lipid accumulation.

Characteristically, the nucleus is bean shaped, folded, grooved, indented or polylobulated, with a granular chromatin pattern and one or few nucleoli which may be inconspicuous or prominent. Multinucleated Langerhans cells have the same nuclear profile.[39] Mitotic figures are found in variable number.[40]

Langerhans cells are distributed in sheets or small clusters or are isolated within a granuloma; numbers vary from case to case[41,42] and they may be quite sparse.

Associated mononuclear or multinucleated typical histiocytes have phagocytic activity, ingesting hemosiderin or lipids with the appearance of foamy macrophages or xanthomatous histiocytes (Figs 39.11, 39.12). Eosinophils may be numerous (Figs 39.13–39.15), but in less than 10% of cases, they are not found.[40] The so-called

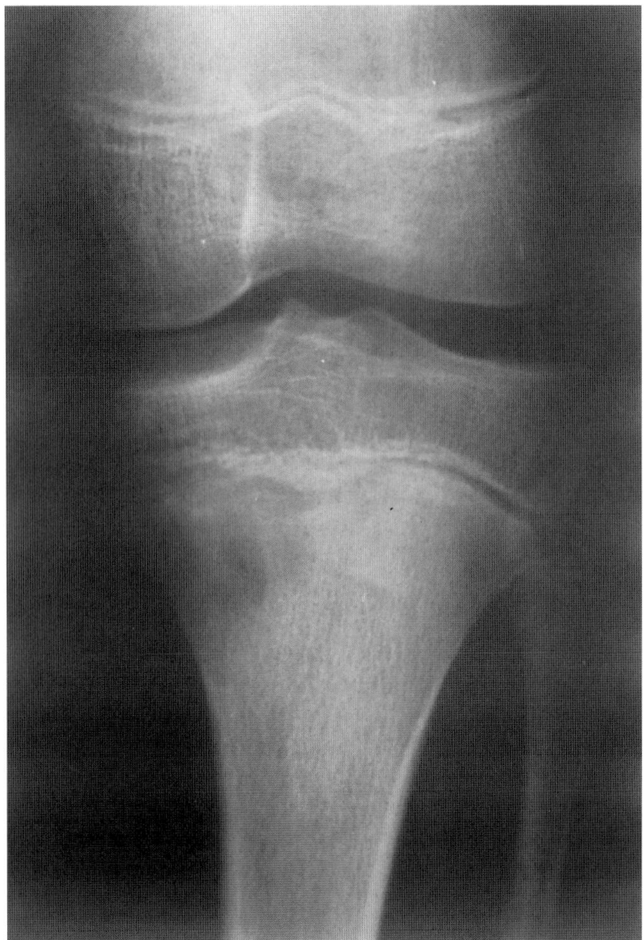

Fig. 39.5 Eosinophilic granuloma in the metaphysis of the tibia.

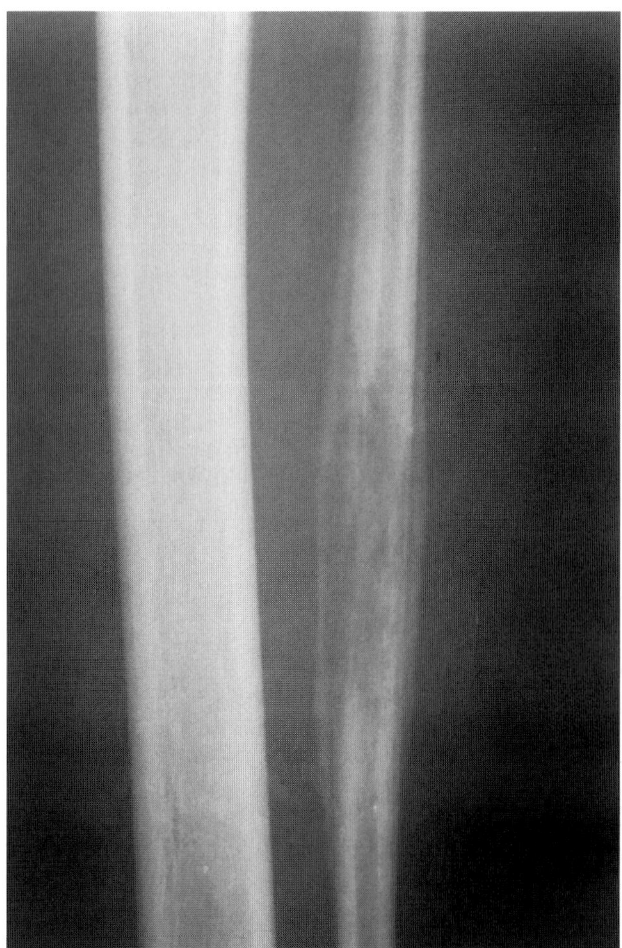

Fig. 39.6 Permeative pattern of bone destruction and periosteal reaction of an eosinophilic granuloma of the fibula, mimicking a Ewing's sarcoma.

'eosinophilic' abscesses reflect the aggregation of cells with necrosis in some lesions. A lymphocytic infiltrate can be prominent (Fig. 39.16), eventually associated with plasma cells and neutrophils. Numerous osteoclast-like giant cells are not unusual. A capillary network is easily found.

Secondary changes include hemorrhage, areas of coagulative necrosis with Charcot–Leyden crystals[43] due to the lysis of eosinophils and, in the later stages, massive fibrosis.

In most cases, the peripheral osteolysis is obvious, with numerous osteoclasts and entrapment of lamellar bone[14] (Figs 39.17–39.19); the resorption of bone has been related to interleukin 1 and prostaglandin production.[44,45]

Some authors have suggested that stages of evolution can be delineated: a proliferative stage with predominantly Langerhans cells, a granulomatous stage with eosinophils, lymphocytes, plasma cells, neutrophils and necrosis, a xanthomatous stage with foam cells followed by the disappearance of the granuloma and replacement by increased amounts of collagen[2,40,46] (Fig. 39.20). In fact, lipidization and xanthomatous formation are not

necessary for gradual resolution and fibrosis[47] (Jaffe 1972, Huvos 1991).

CYTOPATHOLOGY

On smears (Figs 39.21–39.24), Langerhans cells and all the cytologic components of the granuloma are easily characterized if the material is representative.[48–54] Even Charcot–Leyden crystals may be found. Immunocytochemical studies can be performed and if the diagnosis is certain, immediate intralesional injection of methylprednisolone can induce a progressive and even complete healing.[54]

However, some lesions may necessitate a Tru-cut biopsy, immunohistochemistry and ultrastructural examination. Smears are not always a substitute for histological sections[50] and some misdiagnosed cases have been reported as Ewing's sarcoma, osteomyelitis or even metastatic carcinoma. Cytologically the main differential diagnosis is chondroblastoma, cells showing nuclear grooving and

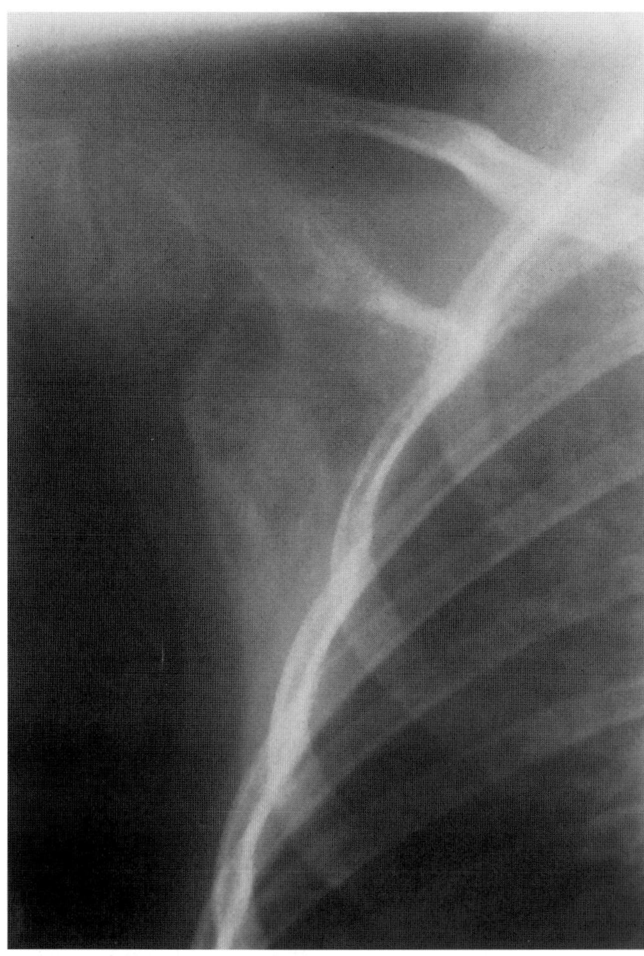

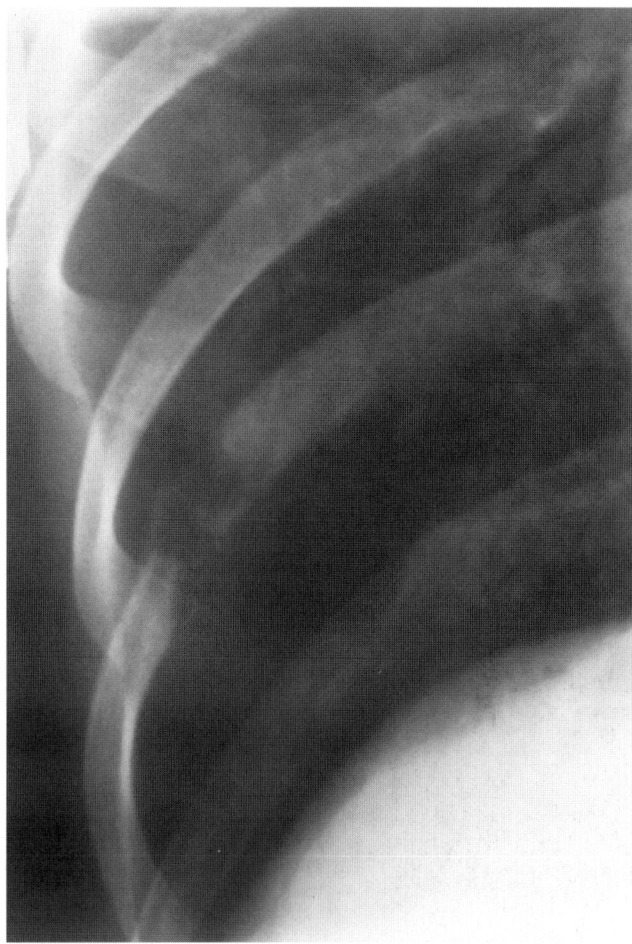

Fig. 39.7 Eosinophilic granuloma of the scapula appearing as a poorly defined osteolytic lesion.

Fig. 39.8 Eosinophilic granuloma of a rib appearing as a destructive lytic lesion.

S-100 positivity, but negative for CD1 and lacking Birbeck granules.[53]

ENZYME-HISTOCHEMICAL STUDIES AND IMMUNOHISTOCHEMISTRY

Enzymatic activities of Langerhans cells and histiocytosis X cells are shown by the presence of non-specific esterase, acid phosphatase and adenosine triphosphatase.[3] In an eosinophilic granuloma, one set of cells with 'dot-like' acid phosphatase staining is often positive for leucyl-β-naphthylamidase, negative for naphthyl-acetate esterase and lysozyme and corresponds to Langerhans cells. The other set, with diffuse positivity for acid phosphatase and lysozyme, shows obvious phagocytosis and corresponds to reactive macrophages.[39]

Histiocytosis X cells and Langerhans cells exhibit a cell surface membrane and perinuclear staining with peanut agglutinin,[55,56] in contrast to macrophages which react with CD68, lysozyme, α1-antitypsin, α1-antichymotrypsin and immunoglobulins.[4,56,57]

Histiocytosis X cells and Langerhans cells react with antibodies directed against leukocyte antigens, with CD1 (OKT6) on frozen sections, CD1a on paraffin-embedded material[3,4,7,59-61] (Fig. 39.25), leu-M3, OKT4 and CD68 with a granular cytoplasmic pattern.[11,57,58] CD2 and CD3 cytoplasmic reactions are considered as an aberrant phenotype, as is the unexpected finding of placental alkaline phosphatase.[11] Leu-M1 negativity is useful in the differential diagnosis with Reed–Sternberg cells.[62]

Immunoelectron microscopy has shown that the majority of cells containing Birbeck granules express CD1;[59] cytoplasmic expression of CD1-CD1a and the identification of Birbeck granules are viewed as definitive criteria for the diagnosis of Langerhans cell histiocytosis.[7,8,59]

Histiocytosis X cells and Langerhans cells exhibit S-100 protein cytoplasmic and nuclear staining[3,4,7,11,42,57,60] (Fig. 39.26), but CD1 and CD1a are more specific markers;[4,59] 2–70% of Langerhans cells are positive for S-100 protein and CD1a.[42,60] Giant cells with the nuclear characteristics of Langerhans cells also stain with S-100 protein and CD68.[11,26]

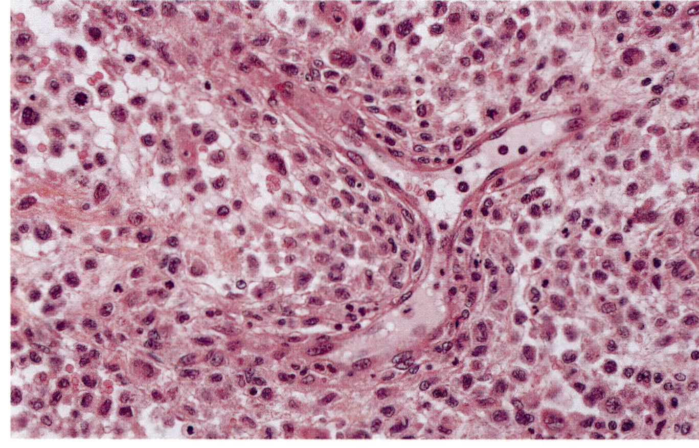

Fig. 39.9

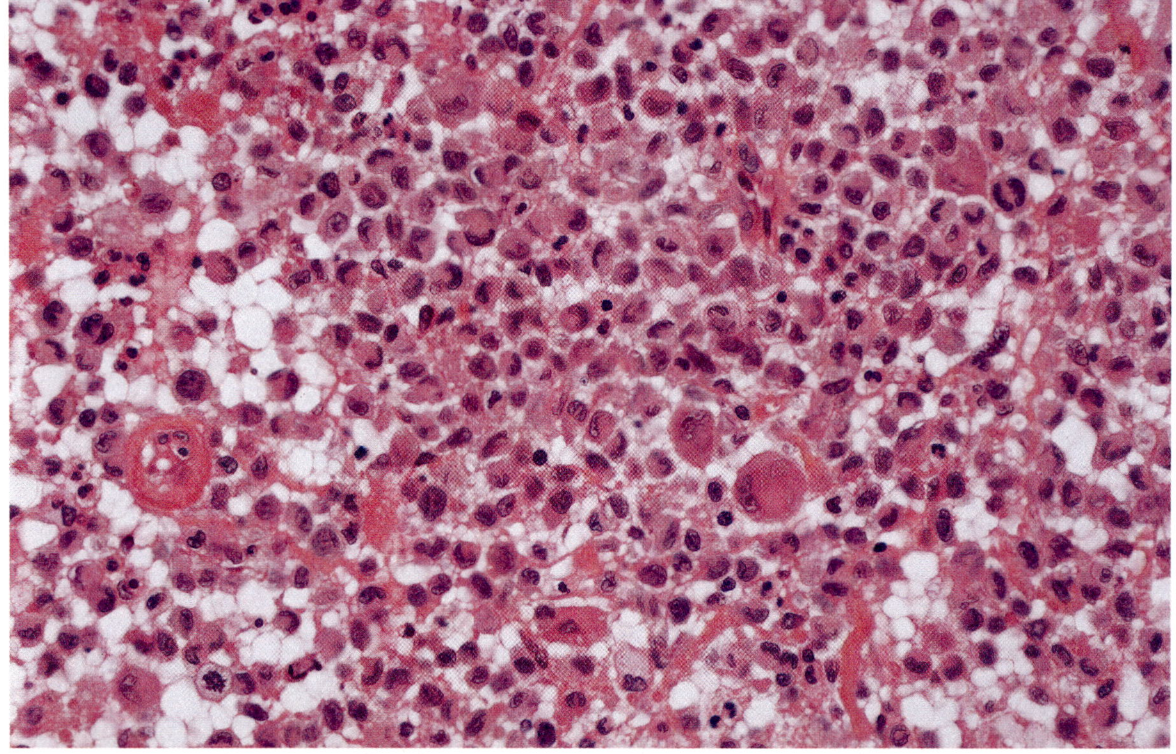

Fig. 39.10

Figs 39.9, 39.10 Eosinophilic granuloma: sheets of mono- or multinucleated Langerhans cells with folded or grooved nuclei and acidophilic cytoplasm.

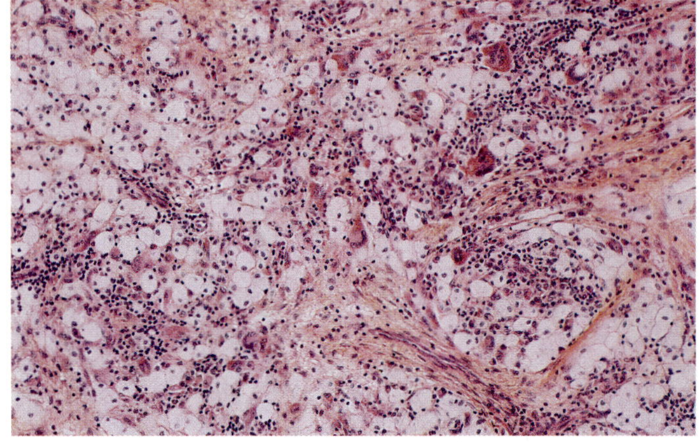

Fig. 39.11

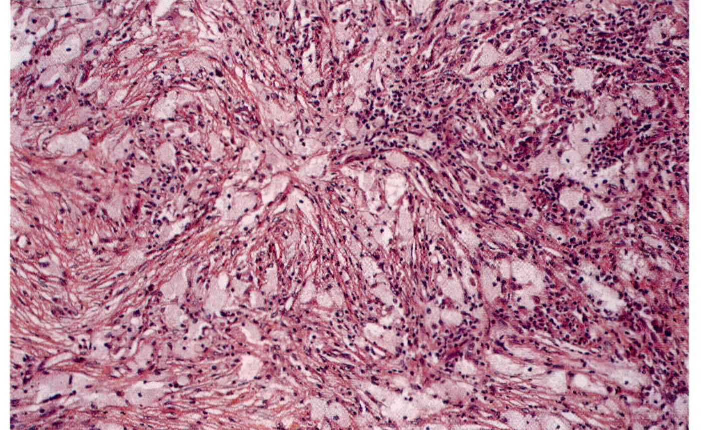

Fig. 39.12

Figs 39.11, 39.12 Eosinophilic granuloma: associated xanthomatous cells.

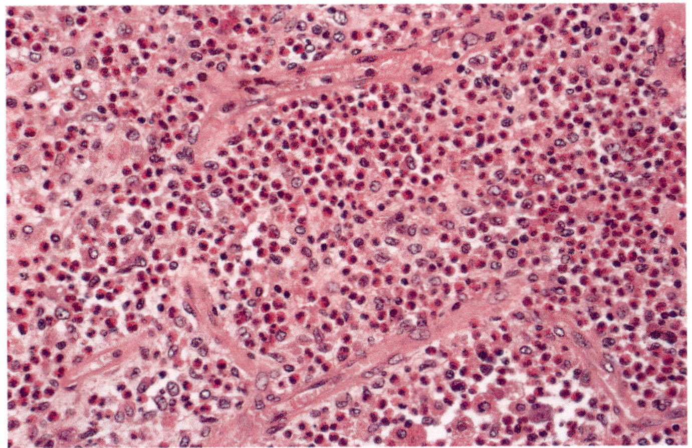

Fig. 39.13

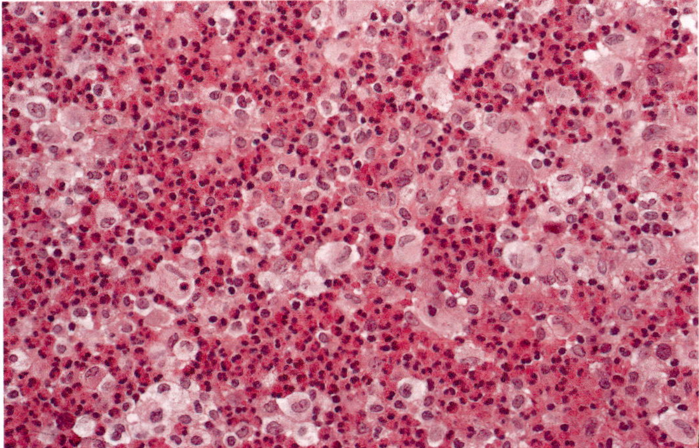

Fig. 39.14

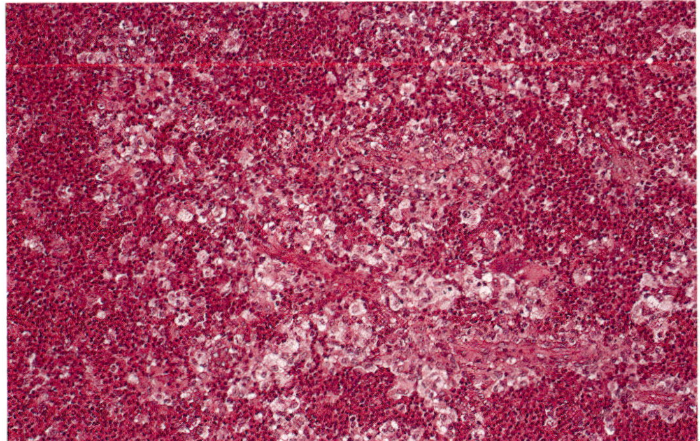

Fig. 39.15

Figs 39.13–39.15 Eosinophilic granuloma: various degrees of eosinophilic cell infiltrates.

Positivity with vimentin has been reported.[62]

The growth fraction has been investigated and a significant proportion of cells stain with PCNA antibody, Ki51 and Ki67.[11]

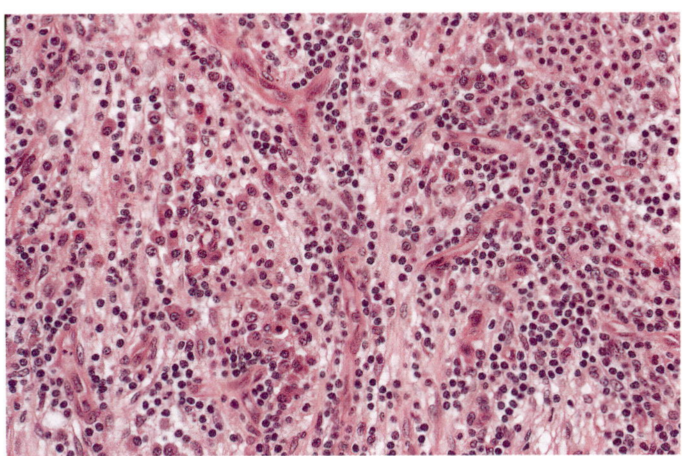

Fig. 39.16 Eosinophilic granuloma: infiltration by lymphocytes.

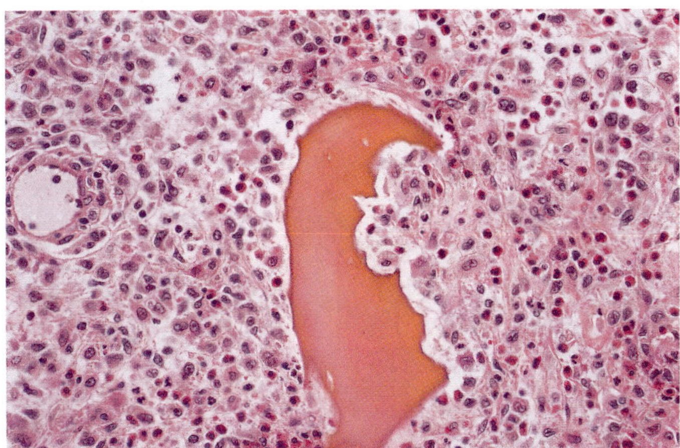

Fig. 39.17

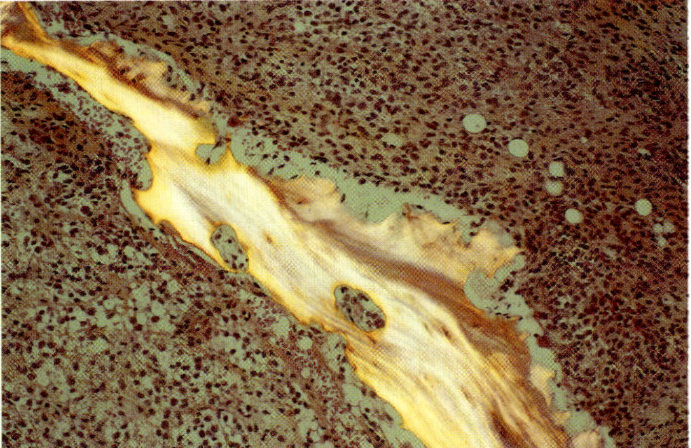

Fig. 39.18

Figs 39.17–39.19 Eosinophilic granuloma: osteolysis is obvious with entrapment of bone and marks of osteoclastic resorption of the cancellous and cortical bone (polarized light).

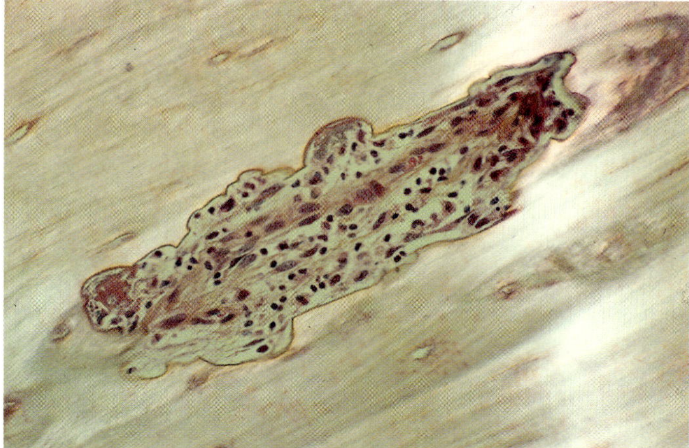

Fig. 39.19

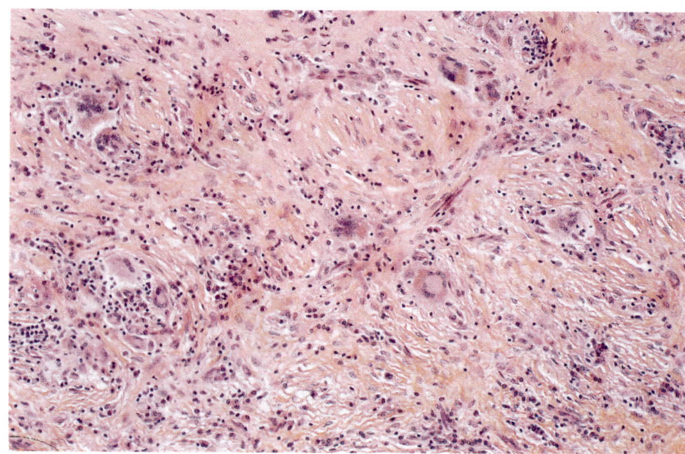

Fig. 39.20 Late stage of an eosinophilic granuloma with fibrosis, sparse giant cells and few lymphocytes.

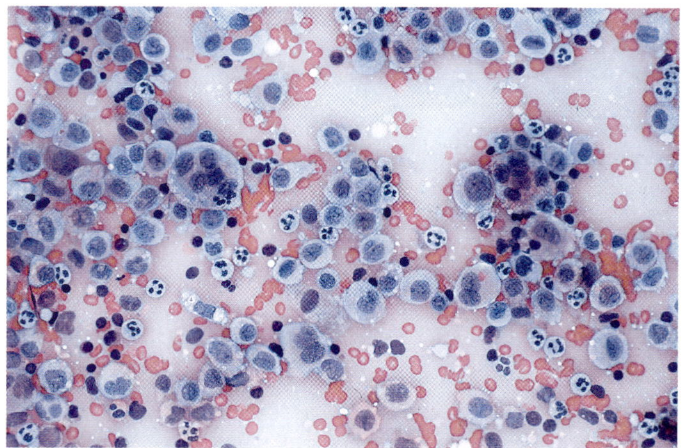

Fig. 39.21

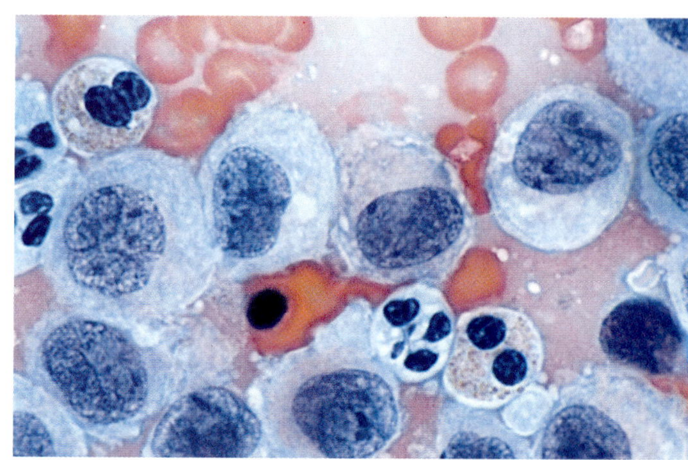

Fig. 39.23

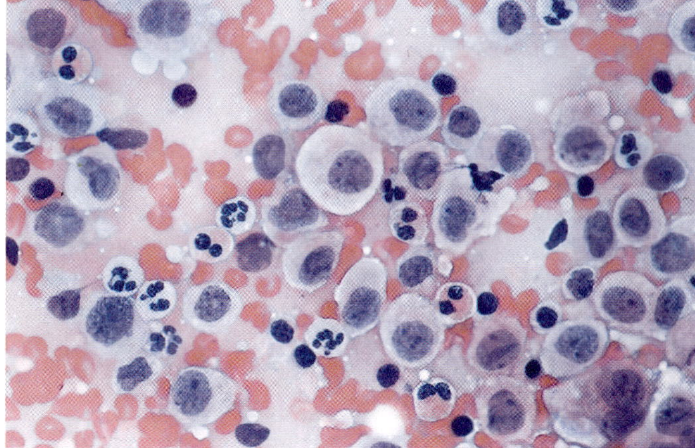

Fig. 39.22

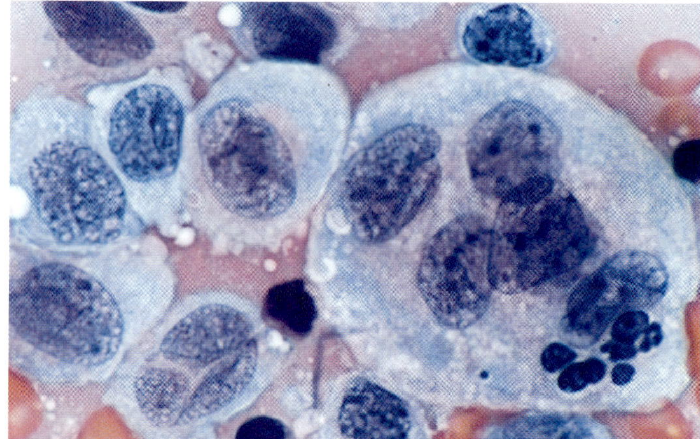

Fig. 39.24

Figs 39.21–39.24 Hallmarks of an eosinophilic granuloma on imprint cytology: nuclear folding or grooving of the Langerhans cells, mono- or multinucleated cells, eosinophils, neutrophils and lymphocytes.

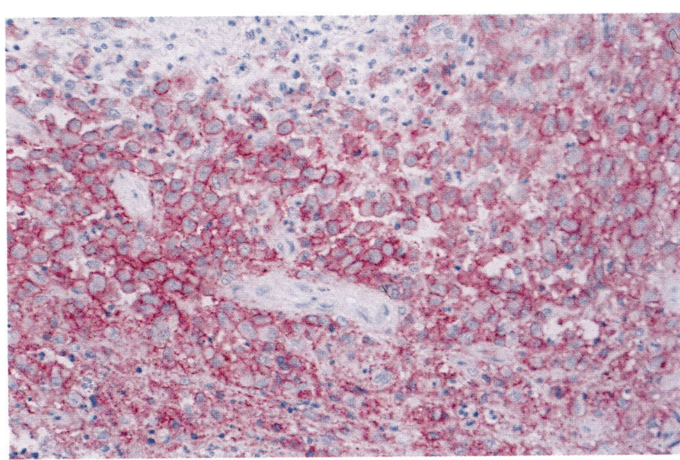

Fig. 39.25 Eosinophilic granuloma of a rib: CD1a immunostaining.

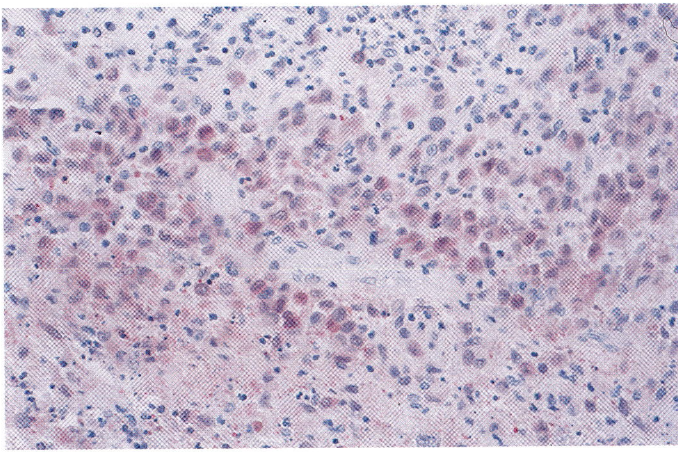

Fig. 39.26 Eosinophilic granuloma of a rib: S-100 protein immunostaining.

Histiocytosis X cells present some distinct immunophenotypic properties not usually expressed by Langerhans cells: a significant CD4 staining, immunoreactivity for complement receptors, Fc-IgG receptors, IL-2 receptors and transferrin receptors and a weak reaction with myelomonocytic antigens.[57]

FLOW CYTOMETRY

Except for one report with aneuploidy but with the clinical features of malignant histiocytosis,[63] most cases with solitary or multiple bone lesions demonstrate no aneuploid cell subpopulations.[64,65]

ELECTRON MICROSCOPY

Langerhans cells share many of the ultrastructural features of histiocytes: a very irregular border with pseudopods, a variable number of lysosomes, phagosomes, lysosomal granules, lipid and glycogen[37,42] and an irregularly shaped, deeply indented nucleus with abundant euchromatin and peripheral condensed heterochromatin. Nucleoli are present in most cells.[37]

A constant and characteristic feature,[66,67] but one not specific to Langerhans cell histiocytosis, is a cytoplasmic organelle identified by Birbeck in 1961, known as a Birbeck granule, Langerhans cell granule, X-body or X-granule.[68] Langerhans cell granules may be found in relatively few cells, even in proliferative lesions,[37] but they can be identified in suboptimally preserved material.[42,67] They are difficult to find in cells where the number of lysosomes and phagocytic bodies increases or in healing lesions.[67] They are not seen in phagocytic histiocytes.[4,39] Langerhans cell granules are mostly found in the peripheral zone, close to the plasma membrane.[69] They appear as complex invaginations of the cell membrane,[68] with a rod-shaped structure of variable length but constant width of about 33 nm;[42] the long, straight or incurved rod structure has five membrane layers[70,71] and it may appear to be dumbbell or racquet-shaped. These zipper-like structures can also be seen connecting Langerhans cells.[39,42,68,69]

Lamellar bodies[72] are membrane-bound cytoplasmic inclusions containing curved or straight trilamellar membranes, mostly found around the Golgi zone[39] and connected with the granular endoplasmic reticulum. They do not appear to be specific.[73]

COURSE, TREATMENT AND PROGNOSIS

In about half of cases, a mild cytological atypia usually associated with the mitotic rate may be found[40] but there is no relationship with the clinical course and recurrence.[14,40] In the same way, the presence or absence of eosinophils or lymphocytes is not a valuable criterion[40] and there is no histologic finding which reliably predicts the course, despite some reports.[74,75]

The extreme variation in progression, regression or even spontaneous healing appears to be related to age, the number of lesions and eventual visceral involvement.[42,76] Adult patients with more than three osseous lesions are likely to have visceral involvement.[13]

Solitary lesions are cured by simple curettage, or intralesional injections of steroids, even in cases of marked bone destruction[18,77] or by low-dose radiation therapy or chemotherapy in cases of non-cured lesions although a radiation-induced osteosarcoma has been reported.[78]

Healing is characterized by a trabecular pattern of bone,[79] while irradiated lesions resolve with sclerosis.[80]

Recurrences are rare; additional lesions usually develop within 1 or 2 years after initial presentation.

Malignant lymphomas, Hodgkin's disease, leukemia and even solid tumors (including lung carcinomas) have been reported in the clinical course of Langerhans cell histiocytosis, with an incidence of 3.5%,[81,82] presumably indicating two distinct processes: a reactive focal Langerhans cell proliferation or a therapy-related tumor.

DIFFERENTIAL DIAGNOSIS

In current practice, osteomyelitis is the most difficult diagnosis, as Langerhans cell histiocytosis may have many lymphocytes and neutrophils with scattered Langerhans cells. An eosinophic infiltration is unusual in osteomyelitis and in xanthogranulomatous osteomyelitis, comprising only foamy histiocytes and neutrophils.[83]

In the healing stage, Langerhans cell histiocytosis with a prominent xanthomatous component may resemble a fibrous cortical defect or a non-ossifying fibroma, but there is no storiform pattern (Huvos 1991).

Malignant lymphomas are ruled out by immunohistochemistry.

Hodgkin's disease in bone locations exhibits fibrosis, sheets of inflammatory cells including histiocytes and only infrequent cells suggestive of Reed–Sternberg cells.[84] The classic immunophenotype for nodular sclerosis, mixed cellularity and lymphocyte-depleted Hodgkin's disease in bone, is the expression of CD15 and CD30 and the lack of CD45 and T cell and B cell markers.[84]

Localized eosinophilic fibrohistiocytic lesion of bone is a form of mastocytosis showing aggregates or nodules of fibrohistiocytic cells, numerous eosinophils, plasma cells and only a few mast cells.[85,86]

Sinus histiocytosis with massive lymphadenopathy may present as a solitary osseous lesion.[87–91] Histiocytic cells lack the irregular contours, grooves or indentations of Langerhans cells; they express S-100 protein but contain lysozyme, α1-antitrypsin, α1-antichymotrypsin and stain for mac-387 and leu-22.[90] They may demonstrate lymphophagocytosis.[91]

Erdheim–Chester disease or lipid granulomatosis symmetrically affects the distal lower extremities with a diffuse diaphyseal-metaphyseal sclerosis,[92–94] sparing the axial skeleton; rarely, ribs and sternum may be involved.[95] The disorder may be found in the heart, lung, kidney and retroperitoneum, but the spleen is usually spared.[96,97] Histologically, Erdheim–Chester disease may mimic Langerhans cell histiocytosis[98] and there may be a link between the two entities.[94,98,99] An irregular bone thickening[92] is associated with filling of the marrow spaces and Haversian canals with lipid-laden histiocytes, lymphocytes, plasma cells and occasional eosinophils. S-100 protein immunostaining is positive[100] but Langerhans cell granules are not detected.

COMMENTS FOR THE SURGICAL PATHOLOGIST

The definitive diagnosis of Langerhans cell histiocytosis has to be established by the detection of Birbeck granules or CD1 or CD1a expression by immunohistochemistry, if one follows the official rules of the Histiocyte Society. In practice, the diagnosis in many cases is established on crude histologic sections[13,14] or even on cytopathological findings alone.[54]

REFERENCES

1. Jaffe H L, Lichtenstein L. Eosinophilic granuloma of bone. Arch Pathol 1944: 37: 99–118
2. Nezelof C. Histiocytosis X: a histological and histogenetic study. Perspect Pediatr Pathol 1979: 5: 153–178
3. Beckstead J H, Wood G S, Turner R R. Histiocytosis X and Langerhans cells: enzyme histochemical and immunologic similarities. Hum Pathol 1984: 15: 826–833
4. Ide F, Iwase T, Saito I, Uememura S, Nakajima T. Immunohistochemical and ultrastructural analysis of the proliferating cells in histiocytosis X. Cancer 1984: 53: 917–921
5. Lichtenstein L. Histiocytosis X. Integration of eosinophilic granuloma of bone, 'Letterer–Siwe disease' and 'Schüller–Christian' disease as related manifestations of a single nosologic entity. Arch Pathol 1953: 56: 84–102
6. Lieberman P H, Jones C R, Dargeon H W, Begg C F. A reappraisal of eosinophilic granuloma of bone, Hand–Schuller–Christian syndrome and Letterer–Siwe syndrome. Medicine (Baltimore) 1969: 48: 375–400
7. Favara B E, Jaffe R. Pathology of Langerhans cell histiocytosis. Hematol Oncol Clin North Am 1987: 1: 75–97
8. Chu T, D'Angio G J, Favara B E, Ladisch S, Nesbit M, Pritchard J. Histiocytosis syndromes in children. Lancet 1987: 2: 41–42
9. Lieberman P H, Jones C R, Steinman R M et al. Langerhans cell (eosinophilic) granulomatosis. Am J Surg Pathol 1996: 20: 519–552
10. Wilman C L, Busque L, Griffith B B et al. Langerhans' cell histiocytosis (histiocytosis X). A clonal proliferative disease. N Engl J Med 1994: 331: 154–160
11. Hage C, Wilman C L, Favara B E, Isaacson P G. Langerhans cell histiocytosis (Histiocytosis X): immunophenotype and growth fraction. Hum Pathol 1993: 24: 840–845
12. Makley J T, Carter J R. Eosinophilic granuloma of bone. Clin Orthop 1986: 204: 37–44
13. Wester S M, Beabout J W, Unni K K, Dahlin D C. Langerhans cell granulomatosis (histiocytosis X) of bone in adults. Am J Surg Pathol 1982: 6: 413–426
14. Kilpatrick S E, Wenger D E, Gilchrist G S, Shives T C, Wollan P C, Unni K K. Langerhans' cell histiocytosis (Histiocytosis X) of bone. Cancer 1995: 76: 2471–2484
15. Stull M A, Kransdorf M J, Devaney K O. Langerhans cell histiocytosis of bone. Radiographics 1992: 12: 801–823
16. Jennings C D, Stelling C B, Powell D E. Case report 199. Eosinophilic granuloma of the right third metacarpal. Skeletal Radiol 1982: 8: 229–231
17. David R, Oria R A, Kumar R et al. Radiologic features of eosinophilic granuloma of bone. AJR 1989: 153: 1021–1026
18. Nauert C, Zornoza J, Ayala A, Harle T S. Eosinophilic granuloma of bone: diagnosis and management. Skeletal Radiol 1983: 10: 227–235
19. Johnson S, Klostermeier T, Weinstein A. Case report 768. Eosinophilic granuloma of the cervical spine. Skeletal Radiol 1993: 22: 63–65
20. Stern M B, Cassidy R, Mirra J. Eosinophilic granuloma of the proximal tibia epiphysis. Clin Orthop 1976: 118: 153–156

21. Usui M, Matsuno T, Kobayashi M, Yagi T, Sasaki T, Ishii S. Eosinophilic granuloma of the growing epiphysis. Clin Orthop 1983: 176: 201–205

22. Leeson M C, Smith A, Carter J R, Makley J T. Eosinophilic granuloma of bone in the growing epiphysis. J Pediatr Orthop 1985: 5: 147–150

23. David D, Oria R A, Kumar R et al. Radiologic features of eosinophilic granuloma of bone. AJR 1989: 153: 1021–1026

24. Mayo-Smith W, Rosenthal D I, Kattapuram S V, Rosenberg A E. Case report 542. Eosinophilic granuloma of femur. Skeletal Radiol 1989: 18: 245–247

25. Thijn C J, Martijn A, Postma A, Molenaar W M. Case report 615. Histiocytosis X (eosinophilic granuloma of the fibula). Skeletal Radiol 1990: 19: 309–311

26. Adler C P, Schaefer H E. Case report 508. Histiocytosis X of the left femur-proximal segment. Skeletal Radiol 1988: 17: 531–535

27. McKenzie A H, Day F G. Eosinophilic granuloma of the femoral shaft simulating Ewing's sarcoma. J Bone Joint Surg (Am) 1957: 39: 408–413

28. Biswal B M, Lal P, Uppal R, Mallik S. Unifocal Langerhans cell histiocytosis (eosinophilic granuloma) resembling Ewing's sarcoma. Australas Radiol 1994: 38: 313–314

29. Crone-Münzebrock W, Brassow F. A comparison of radiographic and bone scan findings in histiocytosis X. Skeletal Radiol 1983: 9: 170–173

30. Kumar R, Balachandran S. Relative roles of radionuclide scanning and radiographic imaging in eosinophilic granuloma. Clin Nucl Med 1980: 5: 538–542

31. Mitnik J S, Pinto R S. Computed tomography in the diagnosis of eosinophilic granuloma. J Comput Assist Tomogr 1980: 4: 791–793

32. Jabra A A, Fishman E K. Eosinophilic granuloma simulating an aggressive rib neoplasm: CT evaluation. Pediatr Radiol 1992: 22: 447–448

33. De Schepper A M, Ramon F, Van Marck E. MR imaging of eosinophilic granuloma. Skeletal Radiol 1993: 22: 163–166

34. Beltran J, Aparisi F, Bonmati L M, Rosenberg Z S, Present D, Steiner G C. Eosinophilic granuloma: MRI manifestations. Skeletal Radiol 1993: 22: 157–161

35. Davies A M, Pikoulas C, Griffith J. MRI of eosinophilic granuloma. Eur J Radiol 1994: 18: 205–209

36. George J C, Buckwalter K A, Cohen M D, Edwards M K, Smith R R. Langerhans cell histiocytosis of bone: MR imaging. Pediatr Radiol 1994: 24: 29–32

37. Favara B E. The pathology of 'histiocytosis'. Am J Pediatr Hematol Oncol 1981: 3: 45–56

38. Basset F, Nezelof C, Ferrans V J. The histiocytoses. Pathol Annu 1983: 18 Pt 2: 27–78

39. Elema J D, Atmosoerodjo-Briggs J E. Langerhans cell and macrophages in eosinophilic granuloma: an enzyme histochemical, enzyme-cytochemical study. Cancer 1984: 54: 2174–2181

40. Risdall R J, Dehner L P, Duray P, Kobrinsky N, Robison L, Nesbit M E Jr. Histiocytosis X (Langerhans cell histiocytosis). Prognostic role of histopathology. Arch Pathol Lab Med 1983: 107: 59–63

41. Mickelson M R, Bonfiglio M. Eosinophilic granuloma and its variations. Orthop Clin North Am 1977: 8: 933–945

42. Favara B E, McCarthy R C, Mierau G W. Histiocytosis X. Hum Pathol 1983: 14: 663–676

43. Ayres W W, Silliphant W M. Charcot–Leyden cristals in eosinophilic granuloma of bone. Am J Clin Pathol 1958: 30: 323–327

44. Gonzalez-Crussi F, Hsueh W, Wiederhold M D. Prostaglandins in histiocytosis-X. PG synthesis by histiocytosis-X cells. Am J Clin Pathol 1981: 75: 243–253

45. Arenzana-Seisdedos F, Barbey S, Virelizier J L, Kornprobst M, Nezelof C. Histiocytosis X: purified (T6+) cells from eosinophilic bone granuloma produce interleukin 1 and prostaglandin E2 in culture. J Clin Invest 1986: 77: 326–329

46. Green W T, Farber S. 'Eosinophilic or solitary' granuloma of bone. J Bone Joint Surg 1942: 24: 499–526

47. Schajowicz F, Slullitel J. Eosinophilic granuloma of bone and its relationship to Hand–Schuller–Christian and Letterer–Siwe syndromes. J Bone Joint Surg (Br) 1973: 55: 545–565

48. Franzen S, Stenkvist B. Cytologic diagnosis of eosinophilic granuloma reticuloendotheliosis. Acta Pathol Microbiol Scand 1968: 72: 385–390

49. Thommesen P, Frederiksen P, Löwhagen T, Willems J S. Needle aspiration biopsy in the diagnosis of lytic lesions in histiocytosis X, Ewing's sarcoma and neuroblastoma. Acta Radiol Oncol Radiat Phys Biol 1978: 17: 145–149

50. Katz R L, Silva E G, De Santos L A, Lukeman J M. Diagnosis of eosinophilic granuloma of bone by cytology, histology and electron microscopy of transcutaneous bone aspiration biopsy. J Bone Joint Surg (Am) 1980: 62: 1284–1290

51. Musy J P, Ruf L, Ernerup I, Baltisser-Bielecka I. Cytopathologic diagnosis of an eosinophilic granuloma of bone by needle aspiration biopsy. Acta Cytol 1989: 33: 683–685

52. Van Heerde P, Maarten Egeler R. The cytology of Langerhans cell histiocytosis (histiocytosis X). Cytopathology 1991: 2: 149–158

53. Elsheikh T, Silverman J F, Wakely P E Jr, Holbrook C T, Joshi V V. Fine needle aspiration cytology of Langerhans' cell histiocytosis (eosinophilic granuloma) of bone in children. Diagn Cytopathol 1991: 7: 261–266

54. Shabb N, Fanning C V, Carrasco C H et al. Diagnosis of eosinophilic granuloma of bone by fine-needle aspiration with concurrent institution of therapy. Diagn Cytopathol 1993: 9: 3–12

55. Ree H J, Kadin M E. Peanut agglutinin: a useful marker for histiocytosis X and interdigitating reticulum cells. Cancer 1986: 57: 282–287

56. Hajdu I, Zhang W, Gordon G B. Peanut agglutinin binding as a histochemical tool for diagnosis of eosinophilic granuloma. Arch Pathol Lab Med 1986: 110: 719–721

57. Ruco L P, Pulford K A, Mason D Y et al. Expression of macrophage-associated antigens in tissues involved by Langerhans' cell histiocytosis (Histiocytosis X). Am J Clin Pathol 1989: 92: 273–279

58. Ornvold K, Ralfkaier E, Carstensen H. Immunohistochemical study of the abnormal cells in Langerhans cell histiocytosis (histiocytosis X). Virchows Arch A Pathol Anat Histopathol 1990: 416: 403–410

59. Murphy G F. Cell membrane glycoproteins and Langerhans cells. Hum Pathol 1985: 16: 103–112

60. Malone M. The histiocytoses of childhood. Histopathology 1991: 19: 105–119

61. Emile J F, Wechsler J, Brousse N et al. Langerhans' cell histiocytosis. Definite diagnosis with the use of monoclonal antibody O10 on routinely paraffin-embedded samples. Am J Surg Pathol 1995: 19: 636–641

62. Azumi N, Sheibani K, Swartz W G, Stroup R M, Rappaport H. Antigenic phenotype of Langerhans cell histiocytosis. Hum Pathol 1988: 19: 1376–1382

63. Goldberg N S, Bauer K, Rosen S T et al. Histiocytosis X. Flow cytometric DNA-content and immunohistochemical and ultrastructural analysis. Arch Dermatol 1986: 122: 446–450

64. Rabkin M S, Wittwer C T, Kjeldsberg C R, Piepkorn M W. Flow-cytometric DNA content of histiocytosis X (Langerhans cell histiocytosis). Am J Pathol 1988: 131: 283–289

65. Ornvold K, Carstensen H, Larsen J K, Christensen I J, Ralfkaier E. Flow cytometric DNA analysis of lesions from 18 children with Langerhans cell histiocytosis (Histiocytosis X). Am J Pathol 1990: 136: 1301–1307

66. Hamoudi A B, Little M, Newton W A et al. Significance of X granules in histiocytosis X: an ultrastructural study. Pediatr Pathol 1985: 3: 93–102

67. Mierau G W, Favara B E. S-100 protein immunohistochemistry and electron microscopy in the diagnosis of Langerhans cell proliferative disorders. A comparative assessment. Ultrastruct Pathol 1986: 10: 303–309

68. Hammar S. Langerhans cells. Pathol Annu 1988: 23 Pt 2: 293–328

69. Robb I A, Jimenez C L, Carpenter B F. Birbeck granules or Birbeck junctions? Intercellular 'zipperlike' lattice junctions in eosinophilic granuloma of bone. Ultrastruct Pathol 1992: 16: 423–428

70. Sagebiel R W, Reed T H. Serial reconstruction of the characteristic granule of the Langerhans cell. J Cell Biol 1968: 36: 595–602

71. Friedman B, Hanaoka H. Langerhans cell granules in eosinophilic granuloma of bone. J Bone Joint Surg (Am) 1969: 51: 367–374

72. Basset F, Escaig J, Le Crom M. A cytoplasmic membranous complex in histiocytosis X. Cancer 1972: 29: 1380–1386

73. Mierau G W, Favara B E, Brenman J M. Electron microscopy in histiocytosis X. Ultrastruct Pathol 1982: 3: 137–142

74. Newton W A Jr, Hamoudi A B. Histiocytosis: a histologic classification with clinical correlation. Perspect Pediatr Pathol 1973: 1: 251–283

75. Frederiksen P, Thommesen P. Histiocytosis X. Histologic appearance correlated to prognosis and extent of disease. Acta Radiol Oncol Radiat Phys Biol 1978: 17: 10–16

76. Bollini G, Jouve J L, Gentet J C, Jacquemier M, Boulaya J M. Bone lesions in histiocytosis X. J Pediatr Radiol 1991: 1: 469–477

77. Ruff S, Chapman G K, Taylor T K, Ryan M D. The evolution of eosinophilic granuloma of bone: a case report. Skeletal Radiol 1983: 10: 37–39

78. Komp D M. Long-term sequelae of histiocytosis X. Am J Pediatr Hematol Oncol 1981: 3: 163–168

79. Alexander J E, Seibert J J, Berry D H, Glasier C M, Williamson S L, Murphy J. Prognostic factors for healing of bone lesions in histiocytosis X. Pediatr Radiol 1988: 18: 326–332

80. Sartoris D J, Parker B R. Histiocytosis X: rate and pattern of resolution of osseous lesions. Radiology 1984: 152: 679–684

81. Kjeldsberg C R, Kim H. Eosinophilic granuloma as an incidental finding in malignant lymphoma. Arch Pathol Lab Med 1980: 104: 137–140

82. Egeler R M, Neglia J P, Puccetti D M, Brennan C A, Nesbit M E. Association of Langerhans cell histiocytosis with malignant neoplasms. Cancer 1993: 71: 865–873

83. Cozzutto C. Xanthogranulomatous osteomyelitis. Arch Pathol Lab Med 1984: 108: 973–976

84. Ozdemirli M, Mankin H J, Aisenberg A C, Harris N L. Hodgkin's disease presenting as a solitary bone tumor. Cancer 1996: 77: 79–88

85. Rywlin A M, Hoffman E P, Ortega R S. Eosinophilic fibrohistiocytic lesion of bone marrow: a distinctive new morphologic finding, probably related to drug hypersensitivity. Blood 1972: 40: 464–470

86. Brinkley A B Jr, O'Brien M W. Case report 320. Localized eosinophilic fibro-histiocytic lesion of bone (tibia) – a localized form of mastocytosis. Skeletal Radiol 1985: 14: 68–72

87. Lewin J R, Das S K, Blumenthal B I, D'Cruz C, Patel R B, Howell G E. Osseous pseudotumor: the sole manifestation of sinus histiocytosis with massive lymphadenopathy. Am J Clin Pathol 1985: 84: 547–550

88. Unni K K. Case report 457. Sinus histiocytosis with massive lymphadenopathy (Rosai–Dorfman disease) presenting as lesion in the sacrum. Skeletal Radiol 1988: 17: 129–132

89. Allegranza A, Barbareschi M, Solero C L, Fornari M, Lasio G. Primary lymphohistiocytic tumour of bone: a primary osseous localization of Rosai–Dorfman disease. Histopathology 1991: 18: 83–86

90. Eisen R N, Buckley P J, Rosai J. Immunophenotypic characterization of sinus histiocytosis with massive lymphadenopathy (Rosai–Dorfman disease). Semin Diagn Pathol 1990: 7: 74–82

91. Walker P D, Rosai J, Dorfman R F. The osseous manifestations of sinus histiocytosis with massive lymphadenopathy. Am J Clin Pathol 1981: 75: 131–139

92. Bohne W H O, Goldman A B, Bullough P G. Case report 96. Chester–Erdheim disease (lipogranulomatosis). Skeletal Radiol 1979: 4: 164–167

93. Martin W 3rd, Klein A, Buss D. Case report 213. Erdheim–Chester disease. Skeletal Radiol 1982: 9: 69–71

94. Brower A C, Worsham G F, Dudley A H. Erdheim–Chester disease: a distinct lipoidosis or part of the spectrum of histiocytosis? Radiology 1984: 151: 35–38

95. Dalinka M K, Turner M L, Thompson J J, Lee R E. Lipid granulomatosis of ribs. Focal Erdheim–Chester disease. Radiology 1982: 142: 297–299

96. Resnick D, Greenway G, Genant H, Brower A, Haghighi P, Emmett M. Erdheim–Chester disease. Radiology 1982: 142: 289–295

97. Freyschmidt J, Ostertag H, Lang W. Case report 365. Erdheim–Chester disease. Skeletal Radiol 1986: 15: 316–322

98. Waite R J, Doherty P W, Liepman M, Woda B. Langerhans cell histiocytosis with the radiographic findings of Erdheim–Chester disease. AJR 1988: 150: 869–871

99. Strouse P J, Ellis B I, Shifrin L Z, Shah A R. Case report 710. Symmetrical eosinophilic granuloma of the lower extremities (proven) and Erdheim–Chester disease (probable). Skeletal Radiol 1992: 21: 64–67

100. Ono K, Oshiro M, Uemura K et al. Erdheim–Chester disease: a case report with immunohistochemical and biochemical examination. Hum Pathol 1996: 27: 91–95

Hyperparathyroidism

J. Amouroux

INTRODUCTION AND CLINICAL DATA

The increased level of parathyroid hormone in blood, which defines hyperparathyroidism, results from several causes corresponding to different clinical and biological conditions.[1,2]

Primary hyperparathyroidism (HPT I) is characterized by excessive parathyroid hormone secretion, as a result of autonomous functioning of the parathyroid glands, which are not controlled by serum calcium levels. This results from single (50–80%) or multiple (10%) adenomas, diffuse hyperplasia (10–40%) or, rarely, carcinoma. There is a persistent or intermittent hypercalcemia.

Secondary hyperparathyroidism (HPT II) consists of a response of the parathyroid glands to hypocalcemia. The latter usually results from chronic renal failure but sometimes from malabsorption. It is caused by hyperplasia of the glands and is associated with normal or low serum calcium levels. During renal osteodystrophy, its commonest cause is the absence of renal 1-hydroxylase which blocks the synthesis of 1–25(OH)2D3 and interferes with intestinal absorption of calcium.

Tertiary hyperparathyroidism (HPT III) occurs after a long-standing history of secondary hyperparathyroidism due to hyperplasia and autonomous functioning of the parathyroid glands, uncontrolled by calcemia. It results in hypercalcemia which requires surgical excision of parathyroid tissue.

Osteoclastic resorption, induced by excessive levels of parathyroid hormone, leads to diffuse demineralization of the skeleton. Resorption, which is particularly intense in some areas, may produce cystic radiographic lesions that can mimic primary bone tumors. This condition, described in 1891 by von Recklinghausen, was attributed to hyperfunctioning of the parathyroid glands by Mandl in 1926. More recently, precise knowledge of the clinical and biological features of the disease has allowed early diagnosis, before the occurrence of the osseous abnormalities.

There are many clinical symptoms of HPT I; they are not very specific but they are valuable signs as they may lead to suspicion of the diagnosis which can be confirmed by biological investigations.

The main signs are urinary calcium lithiasis, gastric or duodenal ulcer, pancreatitis, behavioral disturbance, polyuria associated with polydipsia and articular or osseous pains.

Biological data demonstrate hypercalcemia associated with hypophosphatemia, hypercalciuria and hyperphosphaturia. Blood levels of parathyroid hormone are increased, which confirms the diagnosis.

Diagnosis of HPT II and III is based on surveillance of biological data during the course of chronic renal failure.

Bone lesions are symptomatic in only 10–25% of cases and severe forms where bone tumor is suspected are much less common.

IMAGING

The essential lesion, caused by excessive levels of parathyroid hormone, is increased osteoclastic bone resorption. Its demonstration requires high quality radiographic examination with macroradiography or digitized radiography of the bones, where abnormalities are best seen. The earliest changes are observed especially in the hands (Fig. 40.1).

The most suggestive lesion is subperiosteal bone resorption. It may be seen in multiple skeletal sites but is particularly conspicuous on the radial aspect of the phalanges, especially the middle phalanx of the index and middle fingers.[3] It is best demonstrated using fine-grain film and optical or radiographic magnification.

Another site where resorption is easily observed is the phalangeal tufts, which may be completely resorbed.[4] Additional sites include the metaphyses of long bones (Fig. 40.2), the acromioclavicular, sternoclavicular and sacroiliac joints and symphysis pubis. These images may be associated with endosteal resorption, especially in the hands, and subchondral bone resorption. The latter most often lies in the joints mentioned above and results in destruction of the trabeculae beneath the surface of carti-

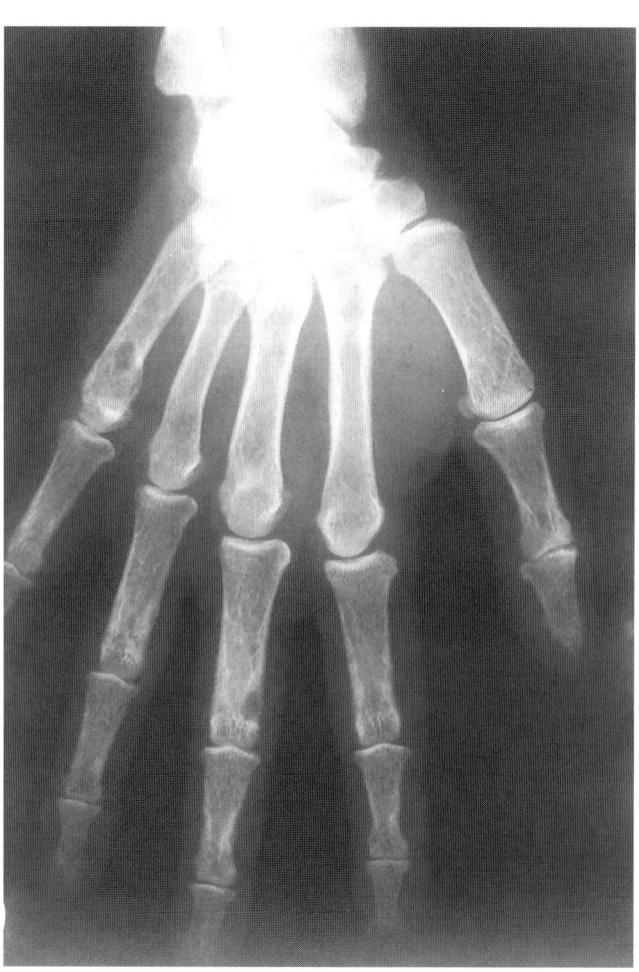

Fig. 40.1 Lytic lesions and resorption of the phalangeal tufts in primary hyperparathyroidism. (Courtesy of M. Forest MD.)

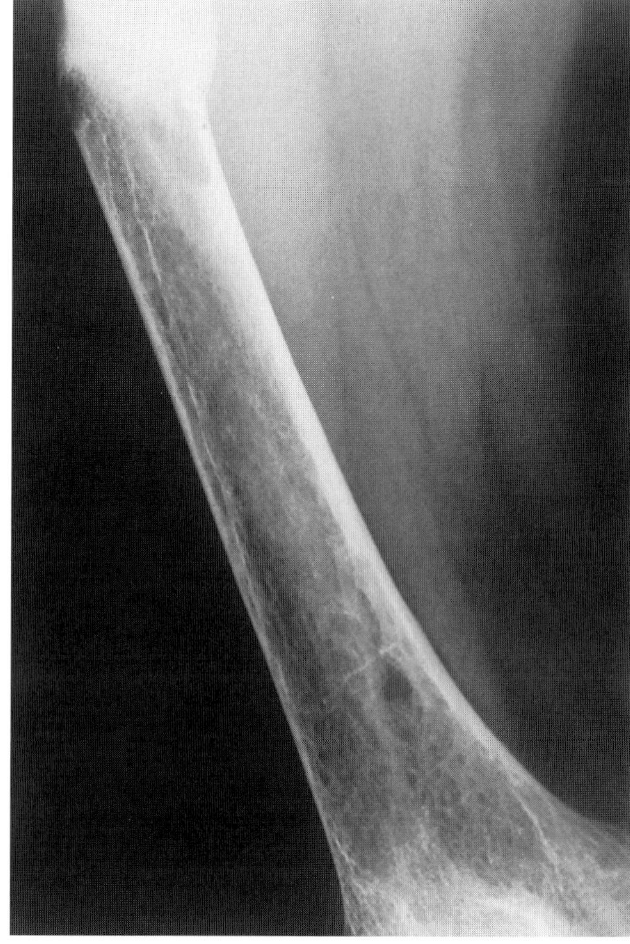

Fig. 40.2 Lytic lesions in the femoral shaft, primary hyperparathyroidism. (Courtesy of M. Forest MD.)

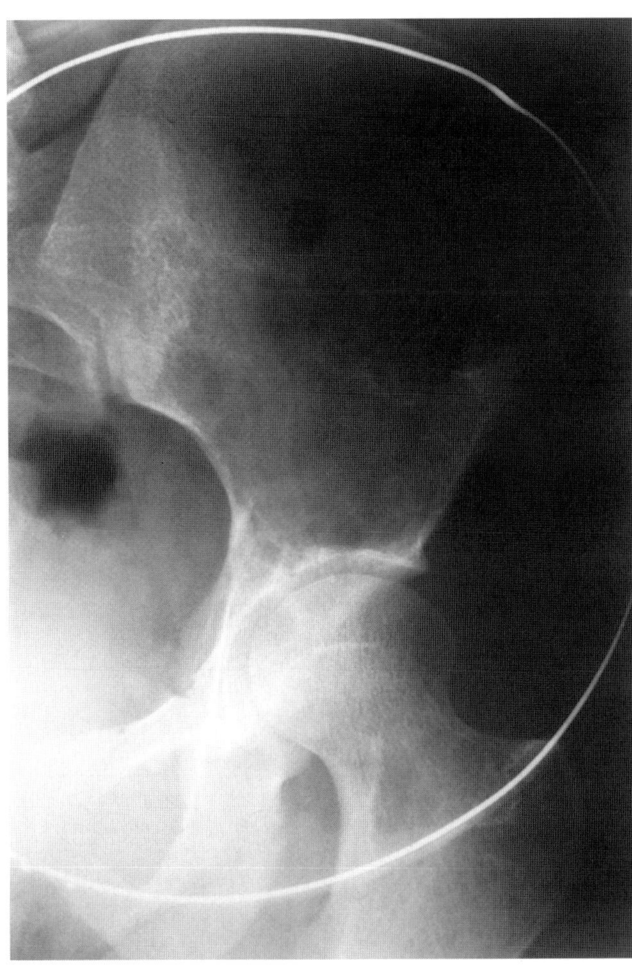

Fig. 40.3 Osteolysis of the iliac wing, primary hyperparathyroidism. (Courtesy of L. M. Patricot MD.)

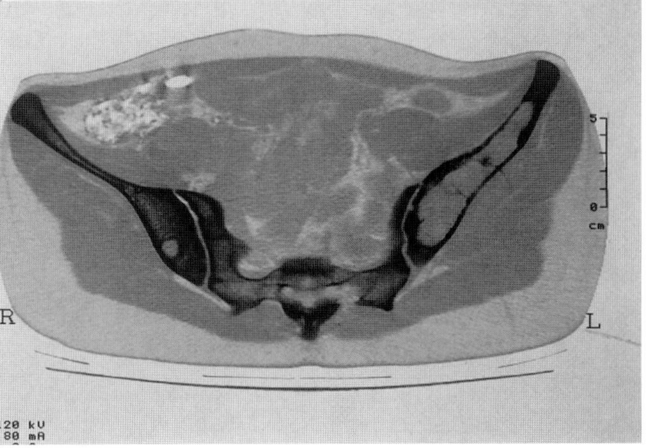

Fig. 40.4 Same case: CT scan. (Courtesy of L. M. Patricot MD.)

lage. Bone is then replaced by fibrous tissue and newly formed bone trabeculae. This may sometimes lead to subchondral microfractures and epiphyseal collapse. This increased remodeling may result in osteosclerosis.[5,6] The latter is particularly observed in the skull, where it forms round patches that may display pseudopagetic changes, and in the vertebrae where the margins are lined by a large radiodense band (rugger-jersey spine).

More severe involvement of bone results in the lacunar and geodic form termed 'osteitis fibrosa cystica' which is found in both HPT I and HPT II[7,8] (Figs 40.3, 40.4). It accounts for the brown tumors localized in the axial or appendicular skeleton which appear as eccentric cortical osteolysis localized especially in the facial bones, pelvis, ribs and femurs. In long bones, pathologic foci, frequently multiple, mostly involve the diaphyses. Vertebral involvement is uncommon[9] and may be complicated by spinal cord compression or even paraplegia.[10]

GROSS PATHOLOGY

Brown tumors, uncommon pseudotumoral manifestations of HPT, are the only lesions induced by HPT that display macroscopic changes. They present as highly vascularized fibrous areas, containing cystic cavities which are filled with lipid or hemorrhagic fluid. Elsewhere, medullary fibrosis forms round brownish masses that deform bone and displace periosteum. The color of these brown tumors results from the accumulation of hemosiderin released by interstitial hemorrhage.

HISTOPATHOLOGY

A biopsy of an osteolytic lesion due to HPT demonstrates no characteristic features. Resorbed bone trabeculae are replaced by loose fibrous tissue containing scattered osteoclastic giant cells. These may be numerous enough to suggest a diagnosis of giant cell tumor (Figs 40.5–40.8). Fibrous tissue contains hemosiderin in variable amounts. It is commonly hollowed by cavities without proper walls, suggesting solitary or aneurysmal cyst.[11]

Biopsy at a distance from a pseudotumoral lesion displays aspects of osteoclastic bone resorption with multiple resorption lacunae containing osteoclasts or undergoing repair, showing fibrous tissue and osteoclasts. This feature indicates a metabolic disorder involving the entire bone tissue and should lead to radiography of the whole skeleton and phosphocalcic investigations, if not already performed.

COURSE AND TREATMENT

The natural course of either HPT I or II is towards worsening of the lesions. Bone lesions extend and multiply, resulting in increasing functional disturbance. The worst danger during HPT I is the occurrence of malignant hypercalcemia that may lead to death.

Treatment of HPT I requires surgical excision of

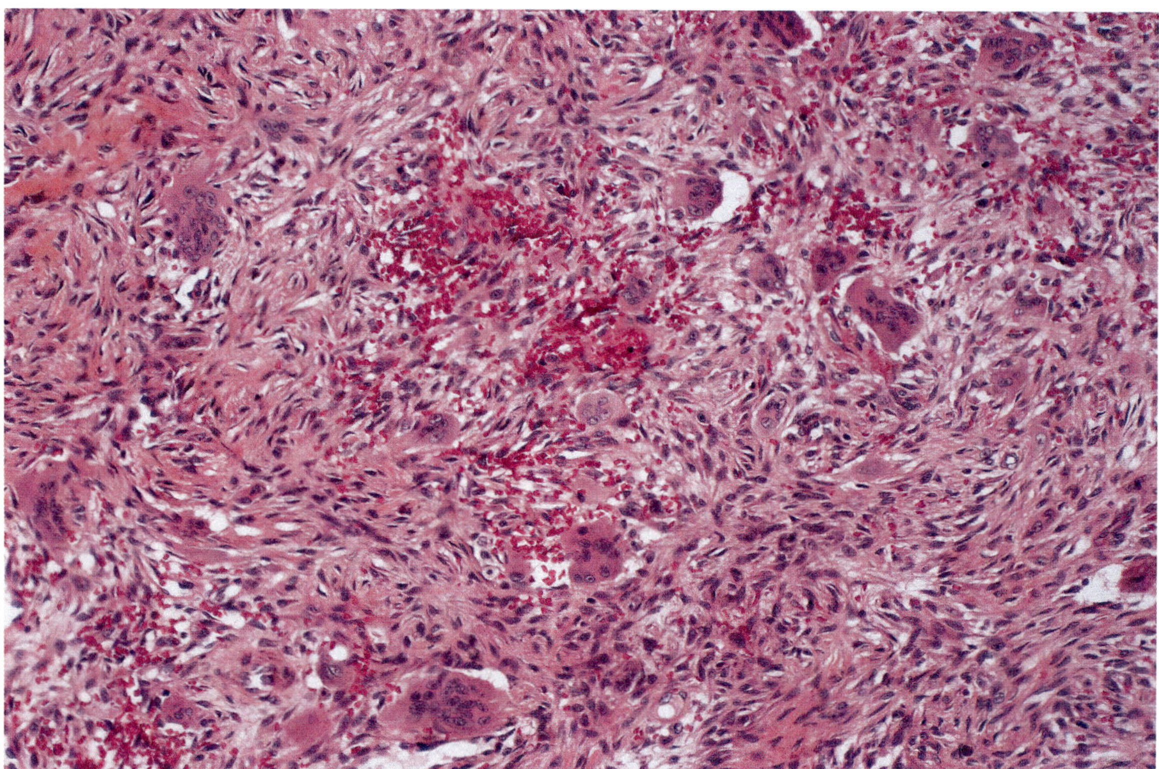

Fig. 40.5

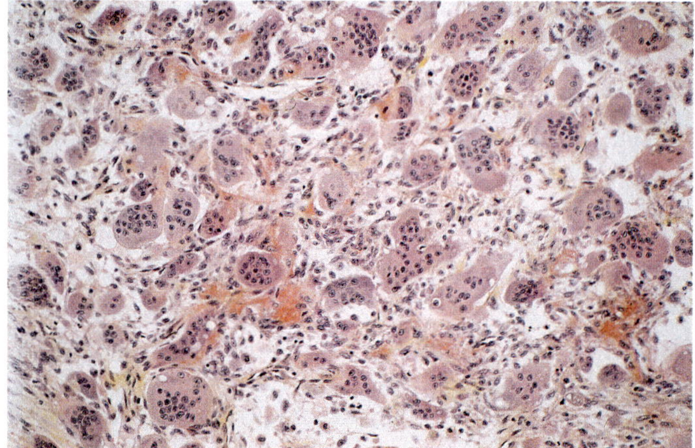

Fig. 40.6

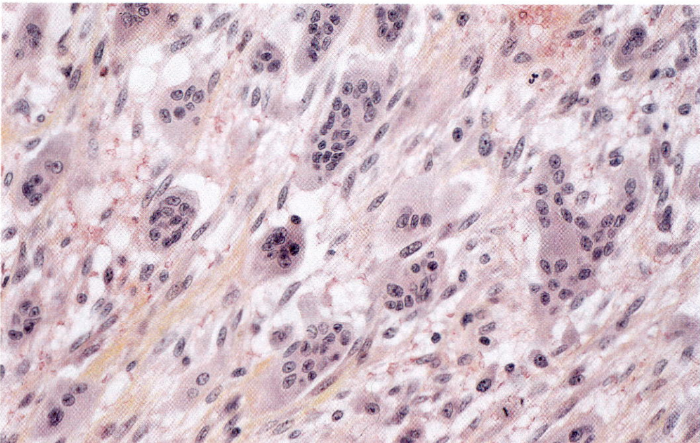

Fig. 40.8

Figs 40.5–40.8 Histological features of brown tumors: fibrous tissue with scattered giant cells. (Courtesy of M. Forest MD.)

Fig. 40.7

parathyroid tissue, either tumoral or hyperplastic. Finding it is not always easy and, after negative cervicotomy, sometimes requires sternotomy and careful search for tumor in the mediastinum. Excision of adenoma results in a normalization of the biological data. Osseous pain disappears and lesions undergo slow healing.

In HPT II, the treatment consists of correction of calcemia. Excision of the parathyroid glands is only necessary in cases of autonomous functioning.

DIFFERENTIAL DIAGNOSIS

Radiographic appearances in bones, commonly multiple and extensive, may suggest a metastatic process.[7,12]

On histology, diagnostic problems are mostly represented by localized areas of bone resorption, which suggest a variety of neoplastic or neoplastic-like diseases, particularly giant cell tumor and aneurysmal or simple cyst. Among these diagnoses, the most frequent is a low-grade giant cell tumor. The pathologist must be aware of some unusual features (Mirra 1989):

- the site of involvement is most often diaphyseal or metaphyseal, rarely epiphyseal;
- the lesion is sometimes multiple;
- it contains focal or extensive hemorrhages and large bands of fibrous tissue;
- foci of bone formation may be found, so that the appearance is very similar to that of giant cell reparative granuloma (Unni 1996).

In questionable cases, these features justify exploration of blood levels of calcium, phosphorus and parathyroid hormone, allowing the diagnosis of HPT. Any cystic lesion of the skeleton, single or multiple, requires the same approach.

The finding of increased osteoclastic resorption within a bone biopsy, with no pseudotumoral lesion or at a distance from one, requires a search for a neighboring lesion that can explain it (infection, bone tumor, arthropathy). If the result is negative and there is still doubt, the same biological investigations must be carried out for it is the most reliable diagnostic feature of HPT.

REFERENCES

1. Potts J T, Deftos L J. Parathyroid hormone, calcitonine, vitamine D, bone and bone mineral metabolism. In: Bondy P K, Rosenberg L E, Eds. Duncan's disease of metabolism. Vol II. Endocrinology. 7th ed. Philadelphia: Saunders, 1974
2. Avioli L V, Raisz L G. Bone metabolism and disease. In: Bondy P K, Rosenberg L E, Eds. Metabolic control and disease. 8th ed. Philadelphia: Saunders, 1980
3. Meema H E, Meema S, Oreopoulos D G. Periosteal resorption of finger phalanges: radial versus ulnar surfaces. J Can Assoc Radiol 1978: 29: 175–182
4. Sundaram M, Philipp S R, Wolferson M K, Riaz M A, Rao B J. Ungual tufts in the follow-up of patients on maintenance dialysis. Skeletal Radiol 1980: 5: 247–249
5. Genant H K, Baron J M, Strauss F H II, Jowsey J. Osteosclerosis in primary hyperparathyroidism. Am J Med 1975: 59: 104–113
6. Lachman M, Kricun M E, Schwartz E E. Primary hyperthyroidism with patchy diffuse osteosclerosis at multiple skeletal sites. Skeletal Radiol 1985: 13: 248–252
7. Bassler T, Bong E T, Brynes R K. Osteitis fibrosa cystica simulating metastatic tumor. An almost-forgotten relationship. Am J Clin Pathol 1993: 100: 697–700
8. Idelson B A, Rudikoff J, Smith G W. Renal osteodystrophy. Unusual roentgenologic manifestations. JAMA 1974: 230: 870–872
9. Barlow I W, Archer I A. Brown tumor of the cervical spine. Spine 1993: 18: 936–937
10. Sundaram M, Scholz C. Primary hyperparathyroidism presenting with acute paraplegia. AJR 1977: 128: 674–681
11. Jaffe H L. Hyperparathyroidism (Recklinghausen's disease of bone). Arch Pathol 1933: 16: 63–112, 236–258
12. Joyce J M, Idea R J, Grossman S J, Liss R G, Lyons J B. Multiple brown tumors in unsuspected primary hyperparathyroidism mimicking metastatic disease on radiograph and bone scan. Clin Nucl Med 1994: 19: 630–635

Osteomyelitis

M. Forest

For the pathologist, osteomyelitis is in most cases a straightforward diagnosis but clinically, radiographically and less often histologically it may mimic many bone tumors or other pseudotumoral conditions.

The differential diagnosis between subacute or chronic forms of osteomyelitis, now more frequent, is difficult due to the lack of acute symptoms, the insidious onset and the finding of a lytic process with some degree of sclerosis.[1–7] The most usual clinical misdiagnoses are osteoid osteoma,[8] osteosarcoma[9] and Ewing's sarcoma.[10]

UNCOMMON FORMS OF OSTEOMYELITIS ON RADIOLOGICAL AND HISTOLOGICAL FINDINGS OR CLINICAL COURSE

Brodie's abscess is typically a metaphyseal lesion in a long bone, first reported by Brodie in 1832 as a small, eccentric, lytic lesion with reactive sclerosis[11] (Figs 41.1, 41.2). It accounts for 2–5% of all forms of osteomyelitis.

The most usual location is on long bones, involving the tibia in 50% of cases, but unusual locations have been reported, ranging from the femoral neck to the patella.[12] Diaphyseal locations are not uncommon, as well as periosteal reactions and sequestrae.[12]

The size of the lesion is 1–4 cm, with a fluid, mucoid or purulent content. The abscess is lined by granulation tissue and limited by a fibrous reaction. In one series, half of the cases were confused with eosinophilic granulomas, enchondromas, chondrosarcomas and even metastases[12] on radiological examination.

Cystic osteomyelitis is a peculiar form not generally known to clinicians and pathologists (Bogumill & Schwamm 1984). It may appear as an incidental finding or represent an osteomyelitis partially cured by treatment. It is located in the epiphysis and may mimic a solitary bone cyst. The cavity may be filled with some neutrophils.

Chronic sclerosing osteomyelitis involves mostly children and young adults.[13] The onset is insidious, with local pain.

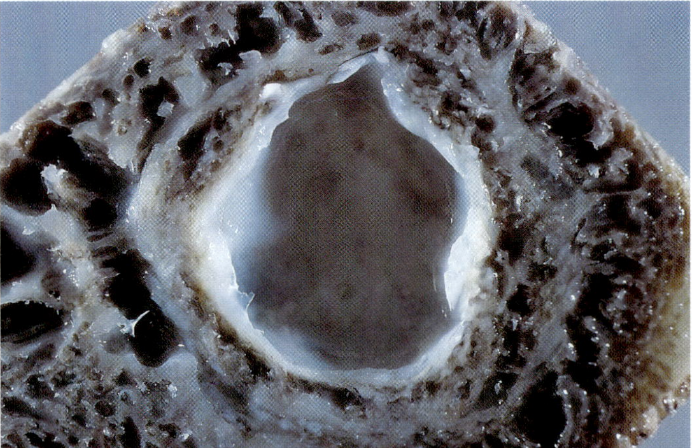

Fig. 41.1

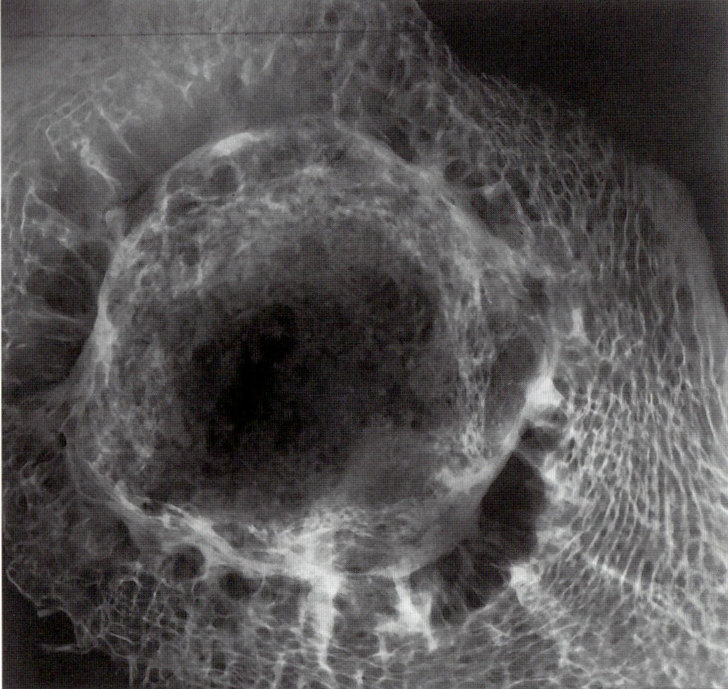

Fig. 41.2

Figs 41.1, 41.2 Chronic abscess of the iliac wing misdiagnosed, on imaging, as a bone tumor.

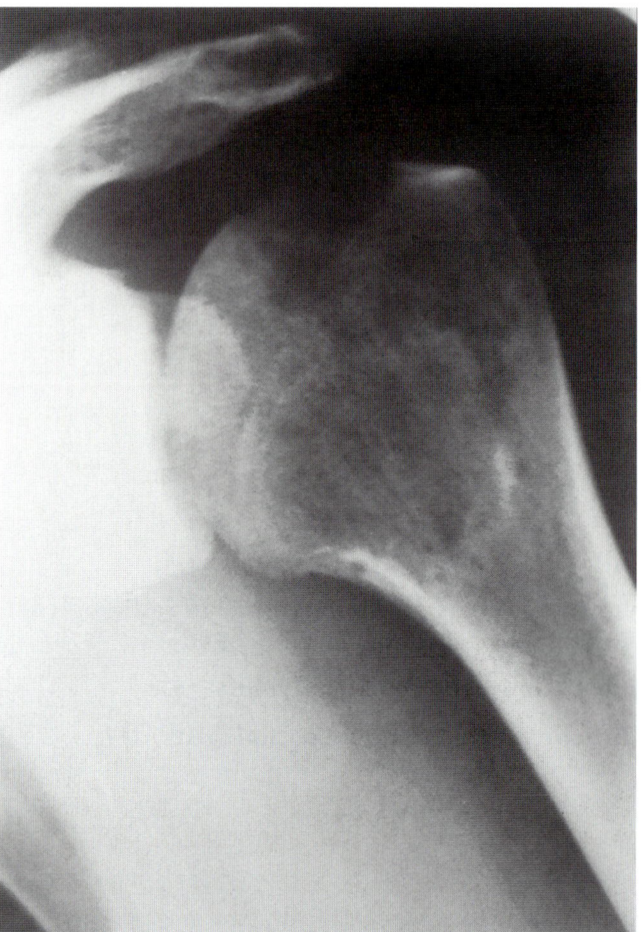

Fig. 41.3

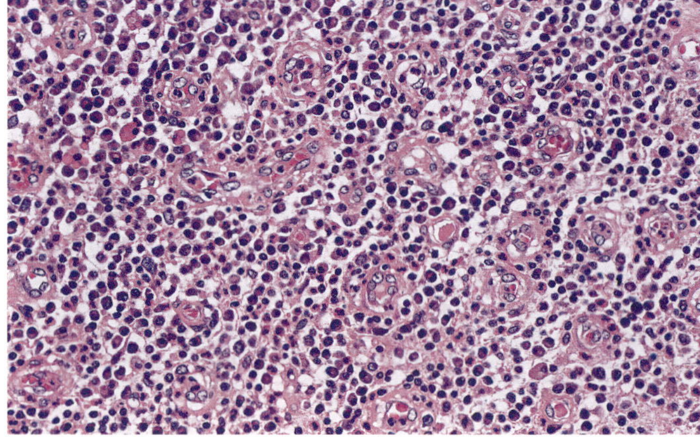

Fig. 41.4

Figs 41.3, 41.4 Plasma cell osteomyelitis of the proximal humerus.

On X-ray, there are cystic areas surrounded by a varying degree of sclerosis, often pronounced which may be confused with osteoid osteomas, osteoblastomas, osteosarcomas, Paget's disease or fibrous dysplasia.[13] Shafts of long bones or the mandible are frequently involved; bone is distended and thickened, without suppuration, sequestration or fistulization. Infection may be caused by a low-virulence anaerobic bacteria[13] but often cultures are sterile.

Plasma cell osteomyelitis is a special form of primary chronic hematogenous osteomyelitis, sometimes confused with tumors[14–21] (Figs 41.3–41.6).

Metaphyses or epiphyses of long bones are involved, as well as vertebral bodies. On X-ray, the osteolytic area is limited by peripheral sclerosis without sequestration. Histologically, three zones may be delineated: a huge infiltration of plasma cells associated with distinct capillar-

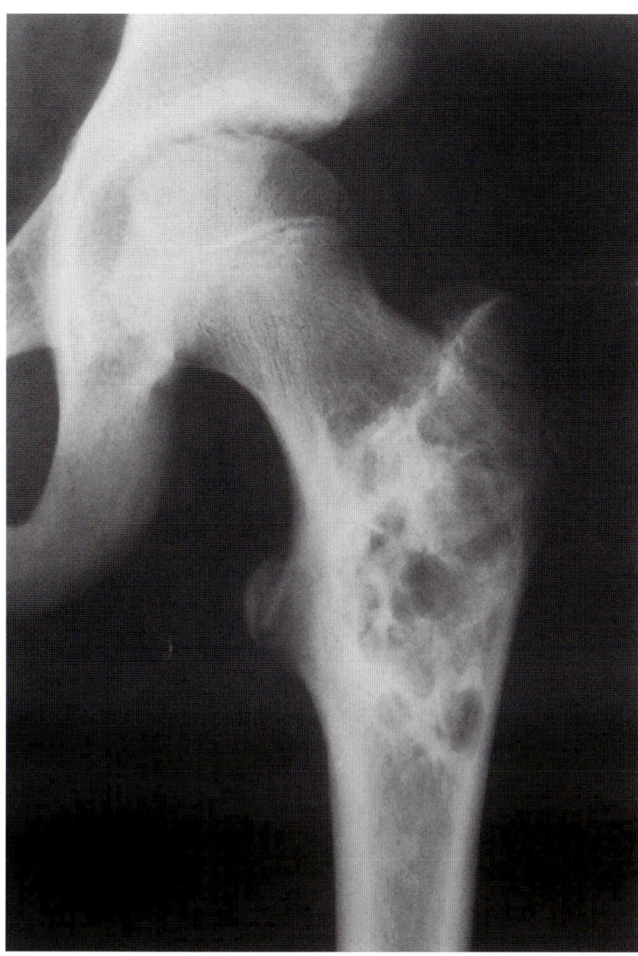

Fig. 41.5

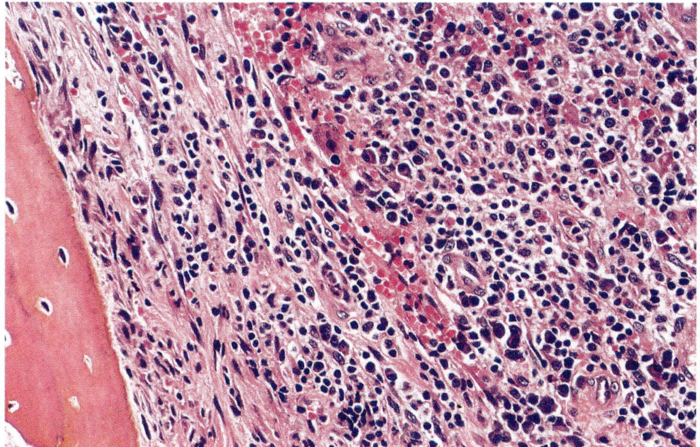

Fig. 41.6

Figs 41.5, 41.6 Plasma cell osteomyelitis of the femoral metaphysis.

ies, a peripheral reactive fibrous tissue and a more peripheral fibrosis and edema of bone marrow tissue. Cultures are positive for *Staphylococcus Aureus*[17,19] in less than 25% of cases.

Xanthomatous osteomyelitis[22] is unusual in having a prominent cellular component of foamy macrophages associated with numerous neutrophils, plasma cells with Russell bodies, fibrin precipitates, necrosis, hemorrhage and peripheral sclerosis. The lesion may be confused with Langerhans cell histiocytosis, Erdheim–Chester disease, Rosai–Dorfman disease, lipogranulomas or bone xanthomas.

Malakoplakia, a disorder involving a unique abnormal histiocytic response, is rarely found in bone[23–27] but it may be radiologically confused with a tumoral process. Sheets of histiocytes are associated with scattered lymphocytes and fibroblasts. Within histiocytes, Michaelis–Gutmann bodies are stained with PAS and von Kossa techniques. Ultrastructurally, Michaelis–Gutmann bodies appear as phagolysosomes with layers around a central core of dense granular material, engulfing whorls or loops of membrane fragments and occasionally bacilli.

Recurrent multifocal osteomyelitis[28,29] involves different bones at different times and the clinical course may be prolonged for years. Radiologically, it may be confused with Ewing's sarcoma or eosinophilic granuloma.[30] Histological findings are non-specific: an acute inflammatory process forming occasional abscesses and in the later stages, lymphocytes and reactive bone formation. Cultures are usually negative and in some cases, there is a relationship with palmoplantar pustulosis.

Condensing osteitis of the clavicle[31–33] is an enlargement and sclerosis of the medial aspect of the clavicle, sometimes bilateral, appearing most often in women. The lesion shows an increased uptake of radioisotope and may be confused with osteoblastic metastases. Periosteal reaction may occur. Histologically, cancellous bone is increased in amount and thickened. The process is thought to be a response to mechanical stress or a low-grade staphylococcal osteomyelitis.[33]

Chronic vertebral osteomyelitis involves predominantly the vertebral bodies, at the lower thoracic and lumbar levels. Periosteal reactions are unusual. Through the disc, infection can involve the adjacent vertebra. Vertebral osteomyelitis may coexist with or mimic a vertebral metastasis,[34] especially in the lumbar spine, with similar osteoblastic and osteolytic lesions. In metastatic disease, the disc space is usually spared.

TUMORS COMPLICATING OSTEOMYELITIS

These are unusual, with an incidence ranging from 0.2% to 1.7% of all cases of osteomyelitis[35–37] (Figs 41.7–41.12). There is a male predominance. Some tumors may appear early in the course of osteomyelitis (1.5–2 years) but in most cases, the duration of symptoms is decades, with an average of 32 years.[38,39]

The sites most affected are the lower extremities and especially the tibia, the femur and the bones of the foot.[36,38]

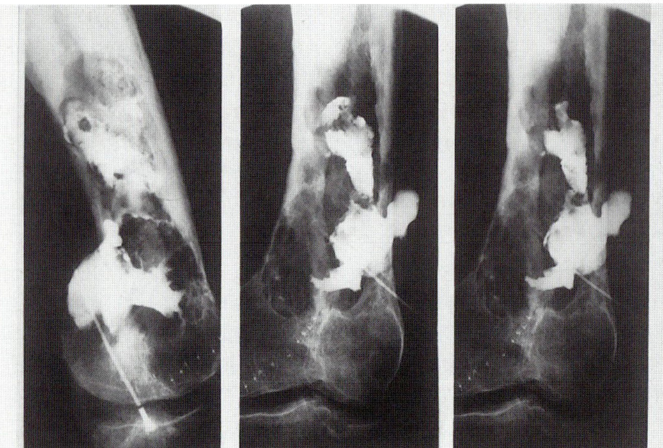

Fig. 41.7

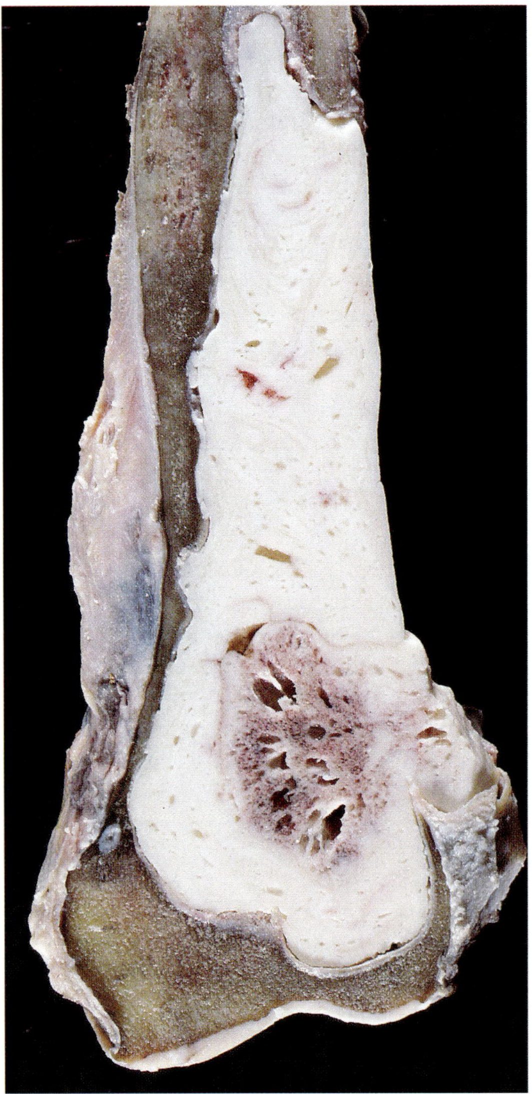

Fig. 41.8

Figs 41.7, 41.8 Osteomyelitis of the femur (clinical course of 35 years), complicated by an epidermoid carcinoma extending into the bone cavity which has been excised and packed with cement.

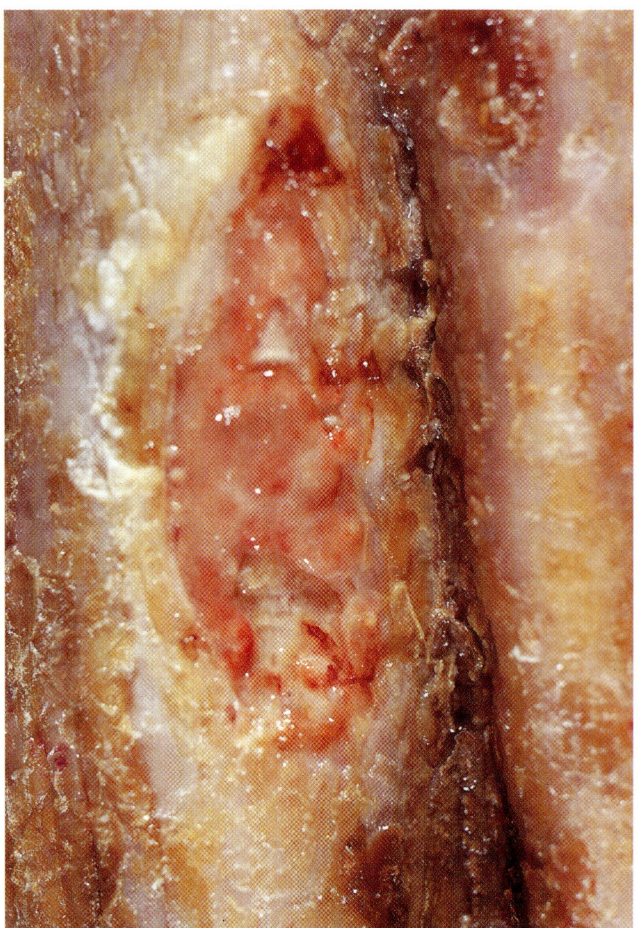

Fig. 41.9 Epidermoid carcinoma complicating a Brodie's abscess of the tibia.

Frequently, there is a change in the bacterial flora, *Staphylococcus aureus* being replaced by a predominantly Gram-negative flora.[40,41]

Most patients have epidermoid carcinomas developing in the orifice of the fistula, less often in the walls of the fistula or even deep in the bone.[35–37,42–50]

Histologically, carcinomas are usually well-differentiated squamous cell tumors with a low grade of malignancy; in many cases, they may be difficult to differentiate from pseudocarcinomatous hyperplasia, in the absence of obvious bone or lymphatic involvement.[35,43] Rare cases may exhibit a spindle cell component (Milgram 1990).

Late metastases involve regional lymph nodes or more distant sites in 14–30% of cases,[36–38] even if the carcinoma is extremely well differentiated.[35]

Sarcomas are much rarer than carcinomas, also located along the draining sinus or deeper in bone. Fibrosarcomas have been reported,[51–55] as well as malignant fibrous histiocytomas,[56–58] angiosarcomas[59–62] and rhabdomyosarcomas.[60] Osteosarcomas are most unusual.[63]

Sarcomas have a mean incidence of metastases of 56%,[36] in some cases with a very aggressive course.[57,60]

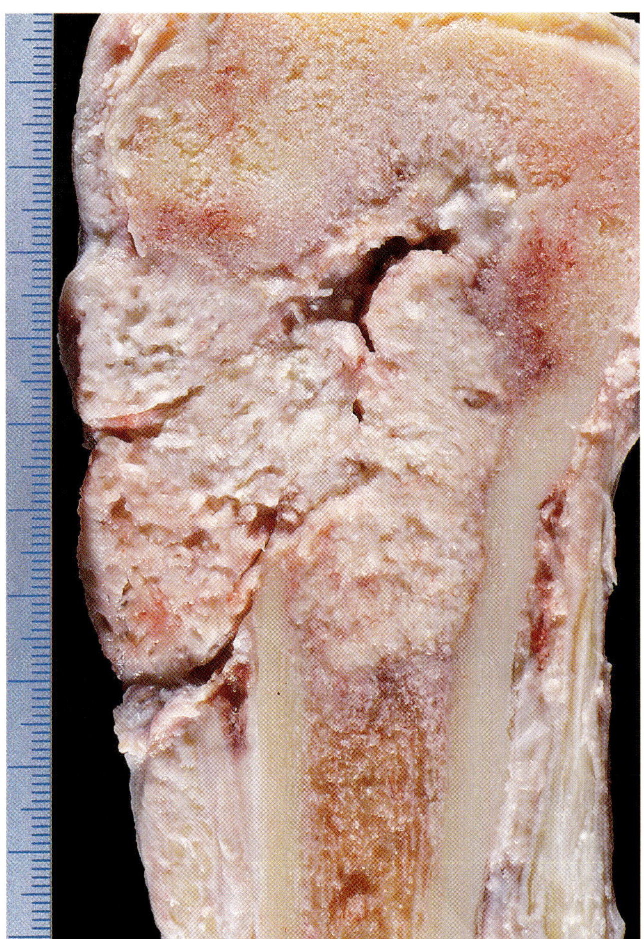

Fig. 41.10

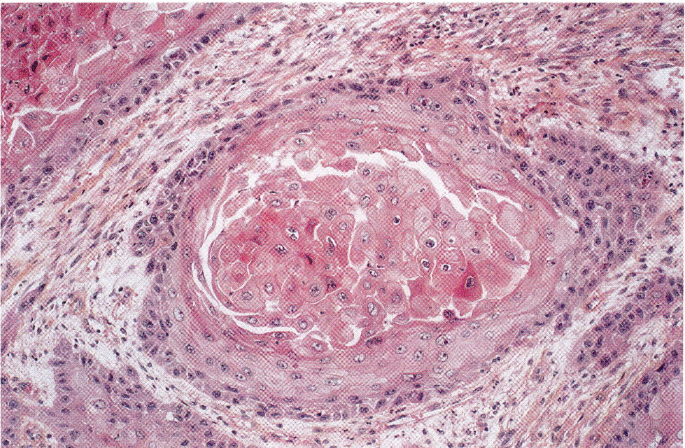

Fig. 41.11

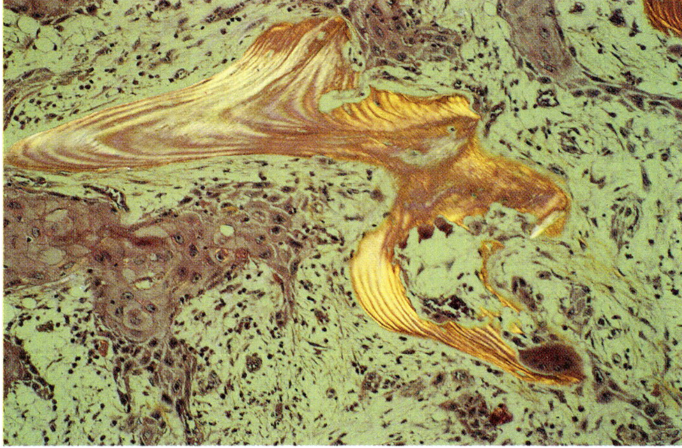

Fig. 41.12

Figs 41.10–41.12 Well-differentiated squamous cell carcinoma complicating an osteomyelitis of the tibia and extending into the bone shaft.

Myelomas have been described,[64–67] as well as rare lymphomas.[68]

COMMENTS FOR THE SURGICAL PATHOLOGIST

Immunohistochemistry can now reduce the frequency of misdiagnoses of such lesions as Langerhans cell histiocytosis, Ewing's sarcoma,[69] lymphomas, Hodgkin's disease in bone, metastases of carcinomas and malignant fibrous histiocytomas with profuse inflammatory infiltrates.

Differential diagnosis is more difficult when the sclerotic and hypervascularized bone may represent a low-grade infection or a trauma-related bone formation or be a part of an osteoid osteoma.

REFERENCES

1. Cabanela M E, Sim F H, Beabout J W, Dahlin D C. Osteomyelitis appearing as neoplasms. A diagnostic problem. Arch Surg 1974: 109: 68–72
2. Unni K K, McLeod R A, Dahlin D C. Conditions that simulate primary neoplasms of bone. Pathol Annu 1980: 15 Pt 1: 91–131
3. Kozlowski K, Anderson R J, Hochberger O, Sacher M. Tumorous osteomyelitis. Pediatr Radiol 1984: 14: 404–406
4. Lindenbaum S, Alexander H. Infections simulating bone tumors. A review of subacute osteomyelitis. Clin Orthop 1984: 184: 193–203
5. Rebmann K, Friedel B. Tumorsimulierende entzündliche Knochenveränderungen. Beitr Orthop Traumatol 1986: 33: 359–362
6. Juhn A, Healey J H, Ghelman B, Lane J M. Subacute osteomyelitis presenting as bone tumors. Orthopedics 1989: 12: 245–248
7. Willis R B, Rozencwaig R. Pediatric osteomyelitis masquerading as skeletal neoplasia. Orthop Clin North Am 1996: 27: 625–634
8. Kandel S N, Mankin H J. Pyogenic abscess of the long bones in children. Clin Orthop 1973: 96: 108–117
9. Bretagne M C, Jolly A, Mouton J N, Metaizeau J P, Beau A, Tréheux A. Osteomyelite pseudo sarcomateuse de l'enfant. J Radiol Electrol Med Nucl 1977: 58: 1–4
10. Cserhati M D. Zur Differentialdiagnose von Geschwulskrankheinten: Plasmazelluläre Osteomyelitis–Ewing–Sarkom. Z Orthop Ihre Grenzgeb 1978: 116: 749–752

11. Bonfiglio M. Case report 791. Bone abscess, chronic osteomyelitis. Skeletal Radiol 1993: 22: 367–370
12. Miller W B Jr, Murphy W A, Gilula L A. Brodie abscess: reappraisal. Radiology 1979: 132: 15–23
13. Collert S, Isaacson J. Chronic sclerosing osteomyelitis (Garré). Clin Orthop 1982: 164: 136–140
14. Exner G U. Die plasmazelluläre osteomyelitis. Langenbecks Arch Chir 1970: 326: 165–185
15. Cserhati M D. Die Plasmazelluläre Osteomyelitis als tumorvortäuschendeknochenläsion. Orthop Praxis 1976: 12: 1010–1013
16. Uehlinger E. Plasmazelluläre Osteomyelitis der distalen Tibia metaphyse (Osteomyelitis subacuta). Arch Orthop Unfallchir 1977: 88: 249–253
17. Yasuma T, Nakajima Y. Clinicopathologic study on plasma cell osteomyelitis. Acta Pathol Jpn 1981: 31: 835–844
18. Ewers A, Kuhne W, Grasshoff H. Plasmazelluläre osteomyelitis. Zentralbl Chir 1982: 107: 863–866
19. Zahran M H, Kaufmann H J. Case report 336. Plasmacellular osteomyelitis of the iliac bone organized partially calcified hematoma of the sacrum. Skeletal Radiol 1985: 14: 296–300
20. Varzos P N, Galinski A W, Gandhi V H, Graziano T A, Snider D W. Chronic plasma cell osteomyelitis. J Am Podiatr Med Assoc 1985: 75: 258–261
21. Dohler J R, Hansmann M L. Plasmacellulare und sklerosierende Osteomyelitis. Chirurg 1993: 64: 190–194
22. Cozzutto C. Xanthogranulomatous osteomyelitis. Arch Pathol Lab Med 1984: 108: 973–976
23. Gupta R K, Schuster R A, Christian W D. Autopsy findings in a unique case of malacoplakia. Arch Pathol 1972: 93: 42–48
24. Colby T V. Malakoplakia. Am J Surg Pathol 1978: 2: 377–382
25. Van Den Bout A H, Dreyer L. Malacoplakia of bone. J Bone Joint Surg (Br) 1981: 63: 254–256
26. Anastasiades K D, Otis J B, Campbell W G Jr. Vertebral malakoplakia. J Bone Joint Surg (Am) 1987: 69: 458–462
27. Tyagi N, Sherwani R, Sadiq S A, Maheshwari V, Abbas M, Tyagi S P. Malakoplakia of bone presenting as a pathological fracture. Postgrad Med J 1994: 70: 461–462
28. Björksten B, Boquist L. Histopathological aspects of chronic recurrent multifocal osteomyelitis. J Bone Joint Surg (Br) 1980: 62: 376–380
29. Gamble J G, Rinsky L A. Chronic recurrent multifocal osteomyelitis: a distinct clinical entity. J Pediatr Orthop 1986: 6: 579–584
30. Albrechtsen J, Jurik A G. Malignant osteosclerotic lesions of the pelvis. RÖFO 1994: 160: 183–185
31. Brower A C, Sweet D E, Keats T E. Condensing osteitis of the clavicle: a new entity. Am J Roentgenol Radium Ther Nucl Med 1974: 121: 17–21
32. Kruger G D, Rock M G, Munro T G. Condensing osteitis of the clavicle. J Bone Joint Surg (Am) 1987: 69: 550–557
33. Jones M W, Carty H, Taylor J F, Ibrahim S K. Condensing osteitis of the clavicle: does it exist? J Bone Joint Surg (Br) 1990: 72: 464–467
34. Voravud N, Theriault R, Hortobagyi G. Vertebral osteomyelitis mimicking bone metastases in breast cancer patients. Am J Clin Oncol 1992: 15: 428–432
35. Fitzgerald R H Jr, Brewer N S, Dahlin D C. Squamous cell carcinoma complicating chronic osteomyelitis. J Bone Joint Surg (Am) 1976: 58: 1146–1148
36. Giunti A, Laus M. Malignant tumours in chronic osteomyelitis. Ital J Orthop Traumatol 1978: 4: 171–182
37. Gebhart M, Fabeck L, Müller C. Transformation maligne des ostéomyélites chroniques et des escarres. Acta Orthop Belg 1993: 59: 327–332
38. Sedlin E D, Fleming J L. Epidermoid carcinoma arising in chronic osteomyelitis foci. J Bone Joint Surg (Am) 1963: 45: 827–838
39. Sankaran-Kutty M, Corea J R, Ali M S, Kutty M K. Squamous cell carcinoma in chronic osteomyelitis. Clin Orthop 1985: 198: 264–267
40. Manale B L, Brower T D. The significance of bacterial flora in carcinoma in chronic osteomyelitis. Surg Gynecol Obstet 1973: 136: 63–64
41. Blidi M, Gatefosse M, Barjonnet G, Bedoucha J S, Wajcner G. Epidermoid carcinoma complicating chronic osteomyelitis of the femur. Rev Rhum (Engl.Ed.) 1996: 63: 62–64
42. Hejna W F. Squamous-cell carcinoma developing in the chronic draining sinuses of osteomyelitis. Cancer 1965: 18: 128–132
43. Johnson L L, Kempson R L. Epidermoid carcinoma in chronic osteomyelitis: diagnostic problems and management. J Bone Joint Surg (Am) 1965: 47: 133–145
44. Greenspan A, Norman A, Steiner G. Case report 146. Squamous cell carcinoma arising in chronic draining sinus tract secondary to osteomyelitis of right tibia. Skeletal Radiol 1981: 6: 149–151
45. Ziets R J, Evanski P N, Lusskin R, Lee M. Squamous-cell carcinoma complicating chronic osteomyelitis in a toe. Foot Ankle 1991: 12: 178–181
46. Bartnicke B J. Imaging rounds: 107. Squamous cell carcinoma arising in chronic osteomyelitis. Orthop Rev 1991: 20: 625–628
47. Dereure O, Guillot B, Bonnel F, Barneon G, Montpoint S, Guilhou J J. Dégénérescence carcinomateuse des fistules d'ostéomyélite chronique. Ann Dermatol Vénéreol 1993: 120: 675–678
48. Jorgensen S, Nurnberg B M, Torholm C. Planocellulaert karcinom udviklet i krosnik fistulerende osteomyelitis. Ugeskr Laeger 1993: 155: 2277–2278
49. Noonan K J, Goetz D D, Marsh J L, Peterson K K. Rapidly destructive squamous cell carcinoma as a complication of chronic osteomyelitis. Orthopedics 1993: 16: 1140–1144
50. Leis S B, Bayne O, Karlin J M, Scurran B L, Reiner M. Squamous cell carcinoma: an unusual early complication of postoperative osteomyelitis. J Foot Ankle Surg 1994: 33: 21–27
51. Kirshbaum J D. Fibrosarcoma of the tibia following chronic osteomyelitis. J Bone Joint Surg (Am) 1949: 31: 413–416
52. Waugh W. Fibrosarcoma occurring in chronic bone sinus. J Bone Joint Surg (Br) 1952: 34: 642–645
53. Denham R H, Dingley A F. Fibrosarcoma occurring in a draining sinus. J Bone Joint Surg (Am) 1963: 45: 32–39
54. Morris J M, Lucas D B. Fibrosarcoma within a sinus tract of chronic draining osteomyelitis. J Bone Joint Surg (Am) 1964: 46: 853–857
55. Akbarnia B A, Wirth C R, Colman N. Fibrosarcoma arising from chronic osteomyelitis. J Bone Joint Surg (Am) 1976: 58: 123–125
56. Kennedy C, Stoker D J. Malignant fibrous histiocytoma complicating chronic osteomyelitis. Clin Radiol 1990: 41: 435–436
57. Czerwinski E, Skolarczyk A, Frasik W. Malignant fibrous histiocytoma in the course of chronic osteomyelitis. Arch Orthop Trauma Surg 1991: 111: 58–60
58. Helio H, Kivioja A, Karaharju E O, Elomaa I, Knuutila S. Malignant fibrous histiocytoma arising in a previous site of fracture and osteomyelitis. Eur J Surg Oncol 1993: 19: 479–484
59. Gualtieri G, Montina S. Angiosarcoma in processo osteomielitico. Minerva Ortop 1970: 21: 585–588
60. Johnston R M, Miles J S. Sarcomas arising from chronic osteomyelitis sinuses. J Bone Joint Surg (Am) 1973: 55: 162–168
61. Olmi R, Rubbini L. Angiosarcoma in osteomielite cronica. Chir Organi Mov 1975: 61: 765–768
62. Bacchini P, Calderoni P, Gherlinzoni F, Gualtieri G. Angiosarcoma in chronic osteomyelitis. Ital J Orthop Traumatol 1984: 10: 393–398
63. Sirikulchayanonta V, Sathaphatayavongs B, Dhaphasut N. Parosteal osteogenic sarcoma arising from a chronic draining sinus. J Med Assoc Thai 1978: 61: 602–607
64. Baitz T, Kyle R A. Solitary myeloma in chronic osteomyelitis. Arch Intern Med 1964: 113: 872–876
65. Schiemer H G, Wohlenberg H. Chronische Osteomyelitis und Plasmozytom. Verh Dtsch Ges Pathol 1970: 54: 402–408
66. Parsons S W, Downey T. Solitary myeloma in chronic osteomyelitis presenting as a lower femoral fracture. Injury 1984: 16: 17–18
67. Roger D J, Bono J V, Singh J K. Plasmacytoma arising from a focus of chronic osteomyelitis. J Bone Joint Surg (Am) 1992: 74: 619–623
68. Mittelmeier H, Schmitt O. Hochmalignes T-Zell-Lymphom unter dem Bild einer Femur-Osteomyelitis. Arch Orthop Trauma Surg 1980: 96: 291–294
69. Howard C B, Einhorn M, Dagan R, Yagupski P, Porat S. Fine-needle bone biopsy to diagnose osteomyelitis. J Bone Joint Surg (Br) 1994: 76: 311–314

Hydatid disease and tuberculosis

M. Forest

OSSEOUS HYDATIDOSIS

In hydatid disease, man is an intermediate host, via fecal contamination of food or water, and the dog is the definitive host. The disease is endemic in sheep-raising areas.[1,2]

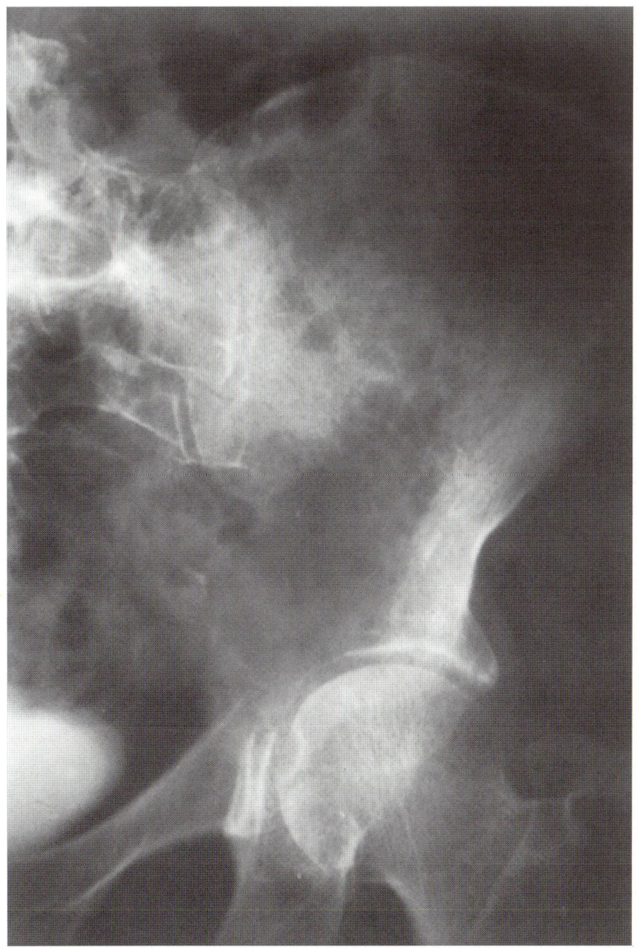

Fig. 42.1 Hydatid disease of the pelvis.

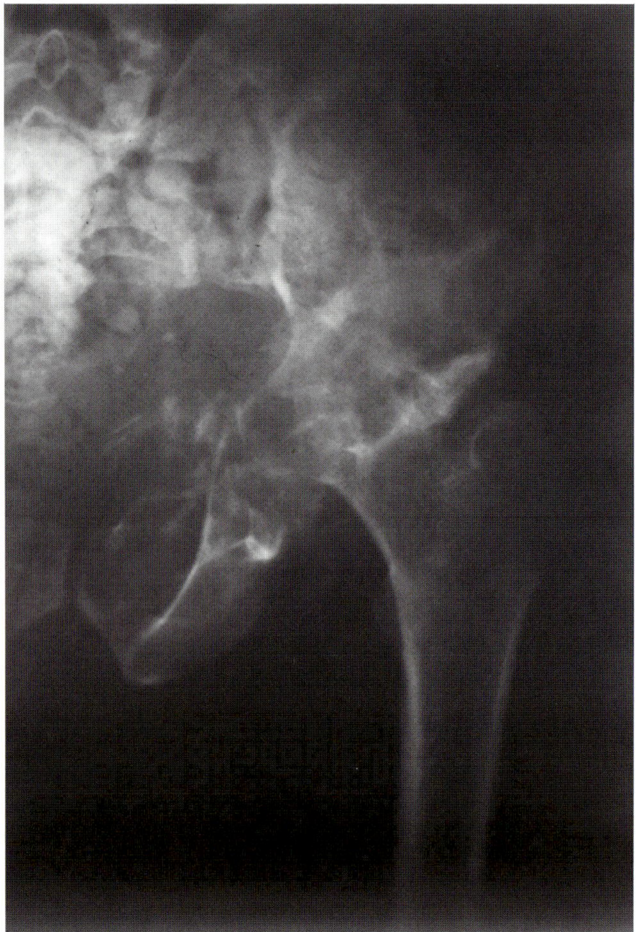

Fig. 42.2

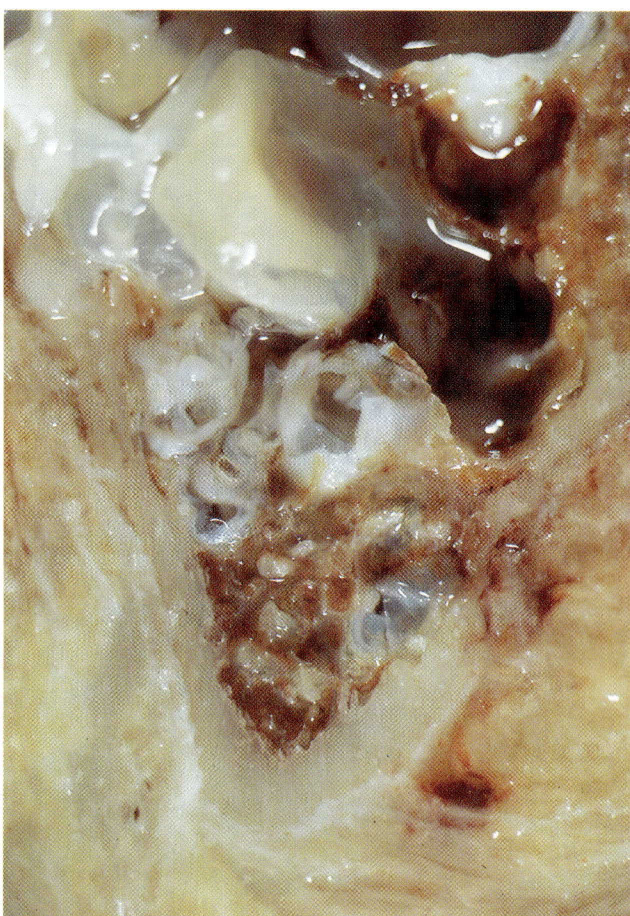

Fig. 42.3

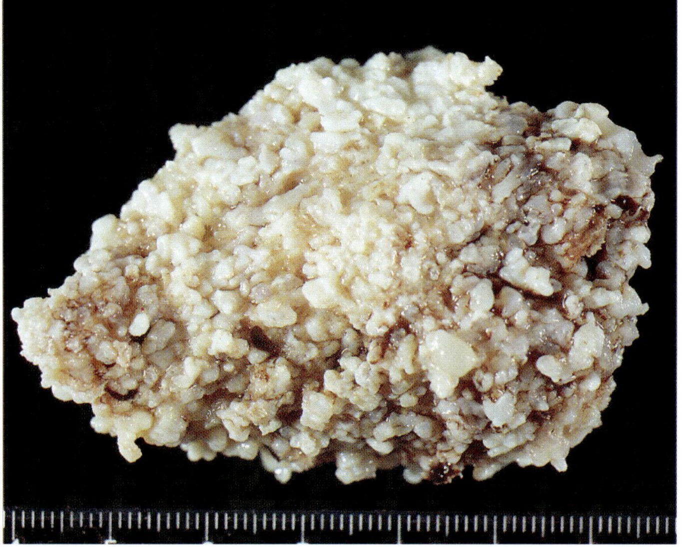

Fig. 42.4

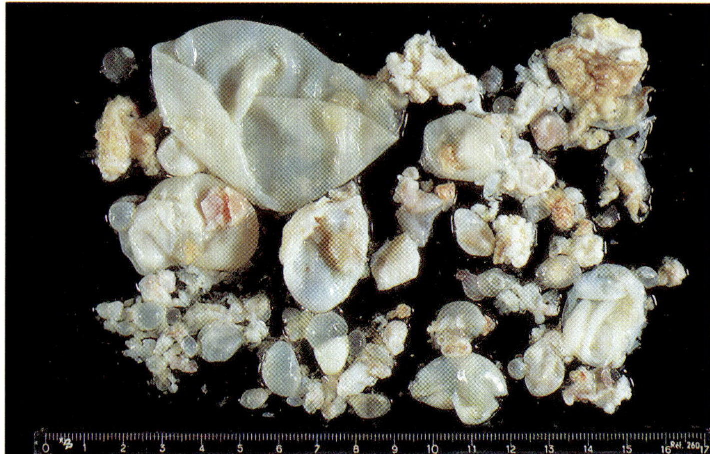

Fig. 42.5

Figs 42.2–42.5 Hydatid disease of the pelvis: a sequestrum is covered by numerous vesicles. Many are fertile.

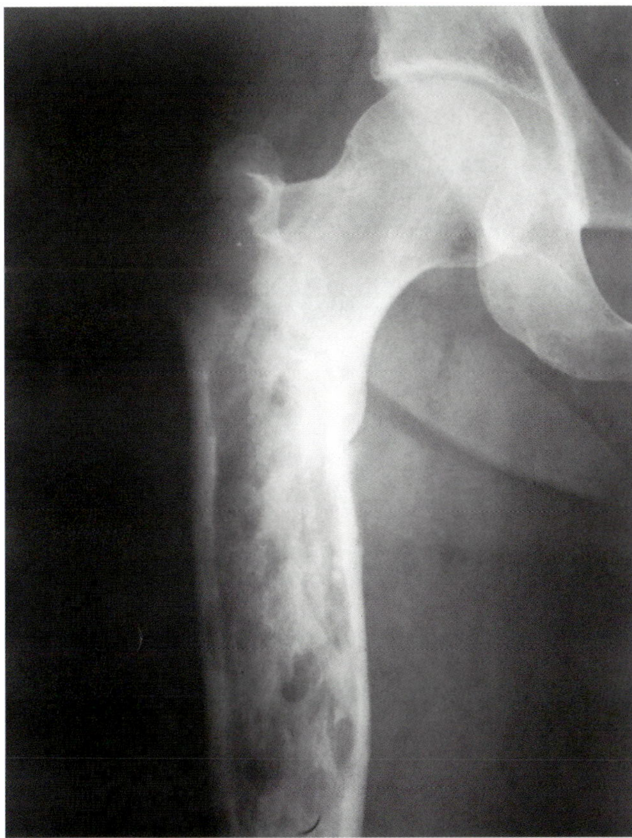

Fig. 42.6

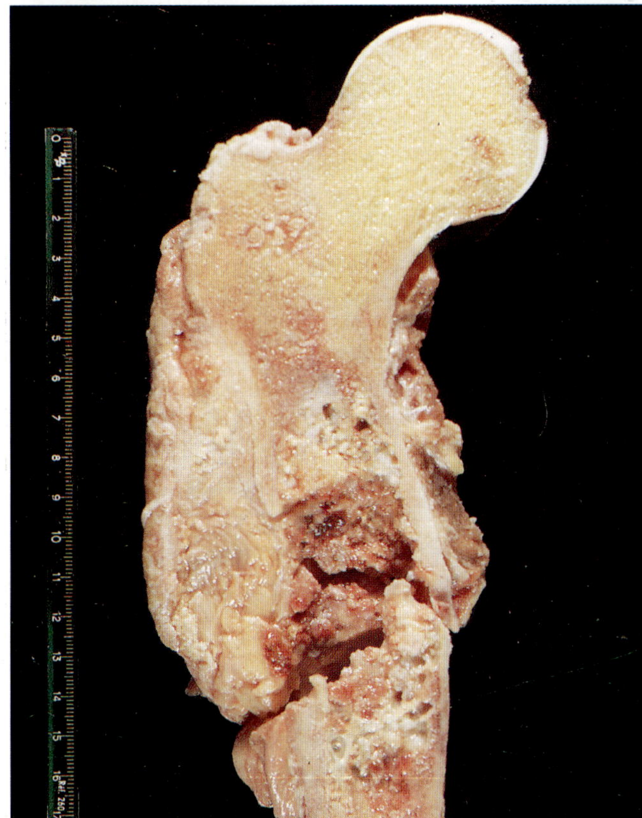

Fig. 42.7

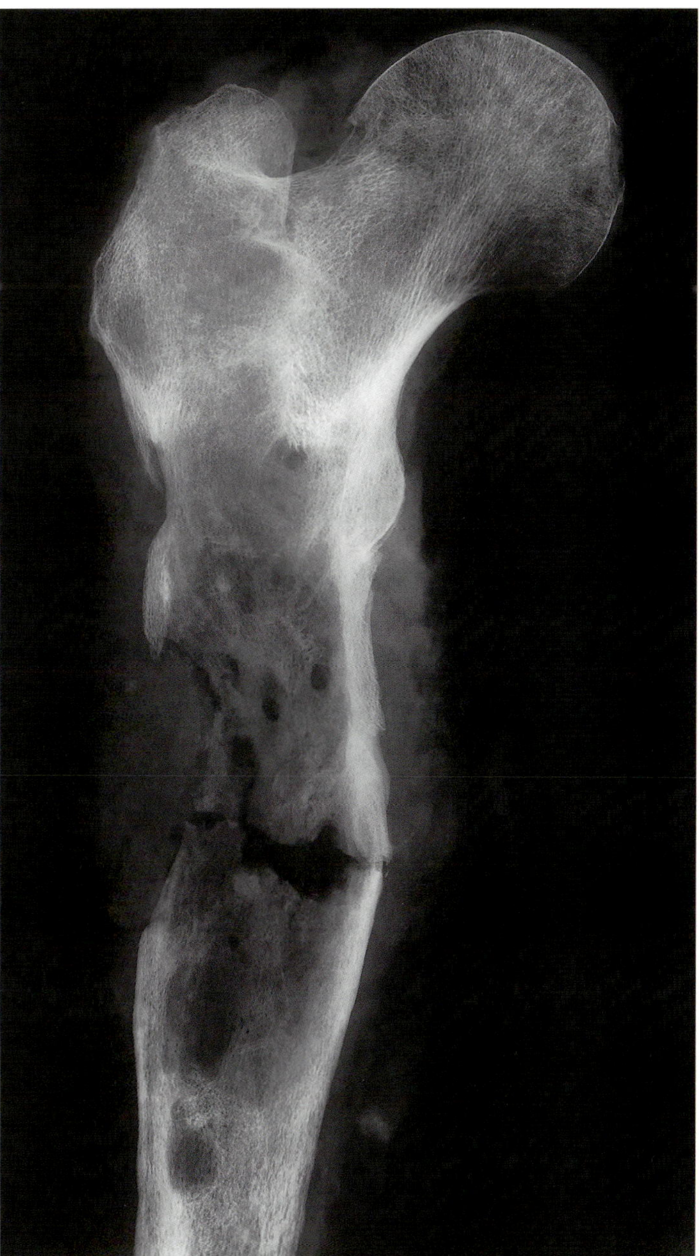

Fig. 42.8

Figs 42.6–42.8 Wide spread involvement of a femur by hydatid disease: pathologic fracture.

Echinococcus granulosus is the most common osseous form in man, echinococcus multilocularis being exceptional in bone.[3–5]

Embryos from the ingested eggs migrate through the intestinal wall and by venous and lymphatic spread, most commonly involve the lung and the liver with the development of the larval form.

Any part of the body may be involved but primary bone lesions are unusual (1–2% of cases[6–9]). Bone lesions may be associated with visceral involvement.[10]

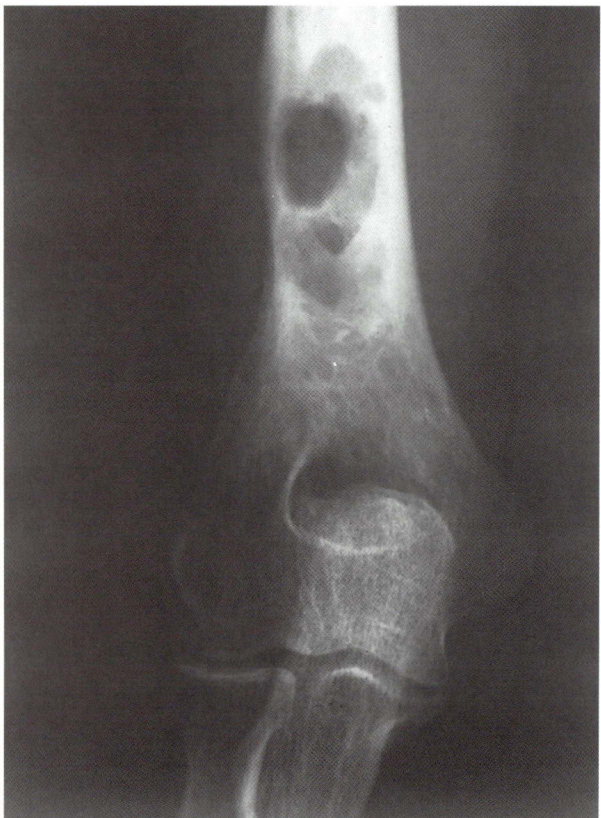

Fig. 42.9 Hydatid disease of the humerus.

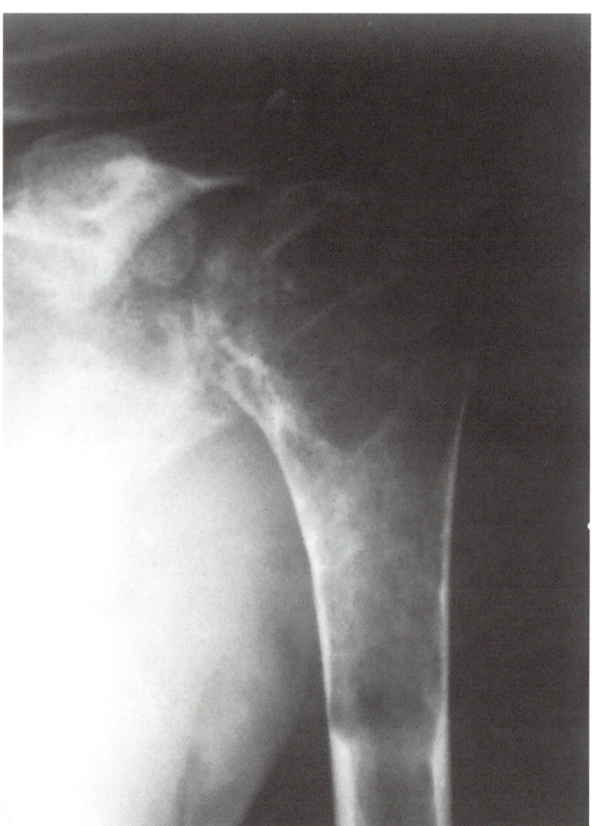

Fig. 42.10

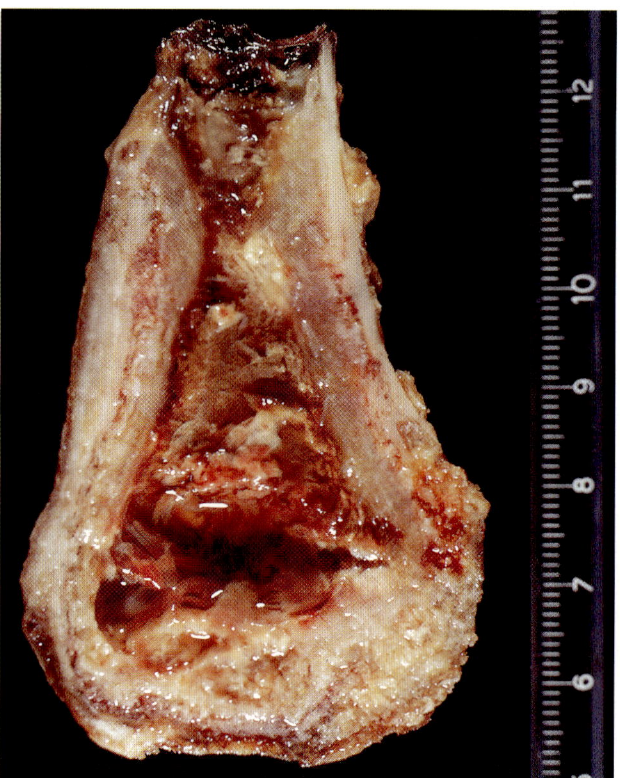

Fig. 42.11

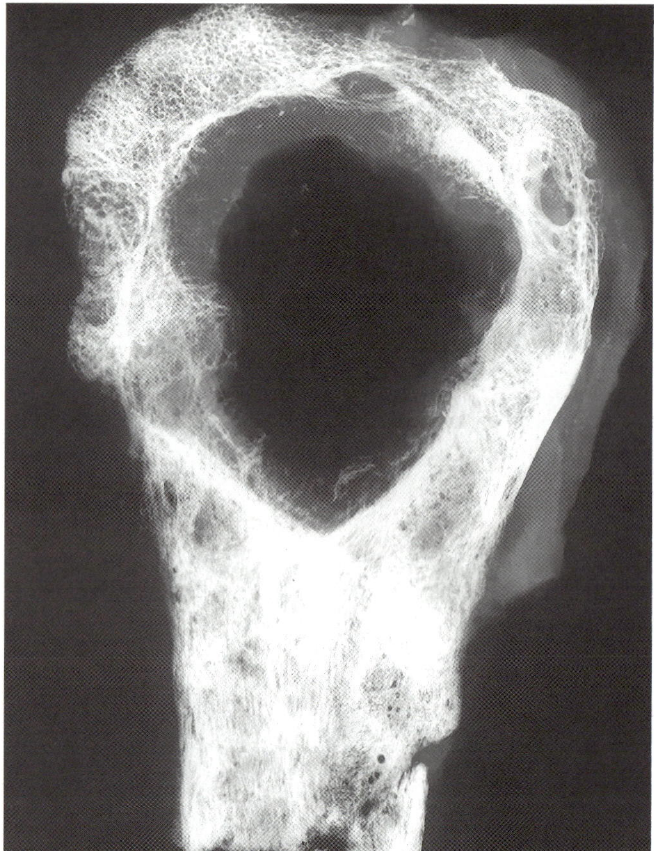

Fig. 42.12

Figs 42.10–42.12 Hydatid disease of the proximal humerus.

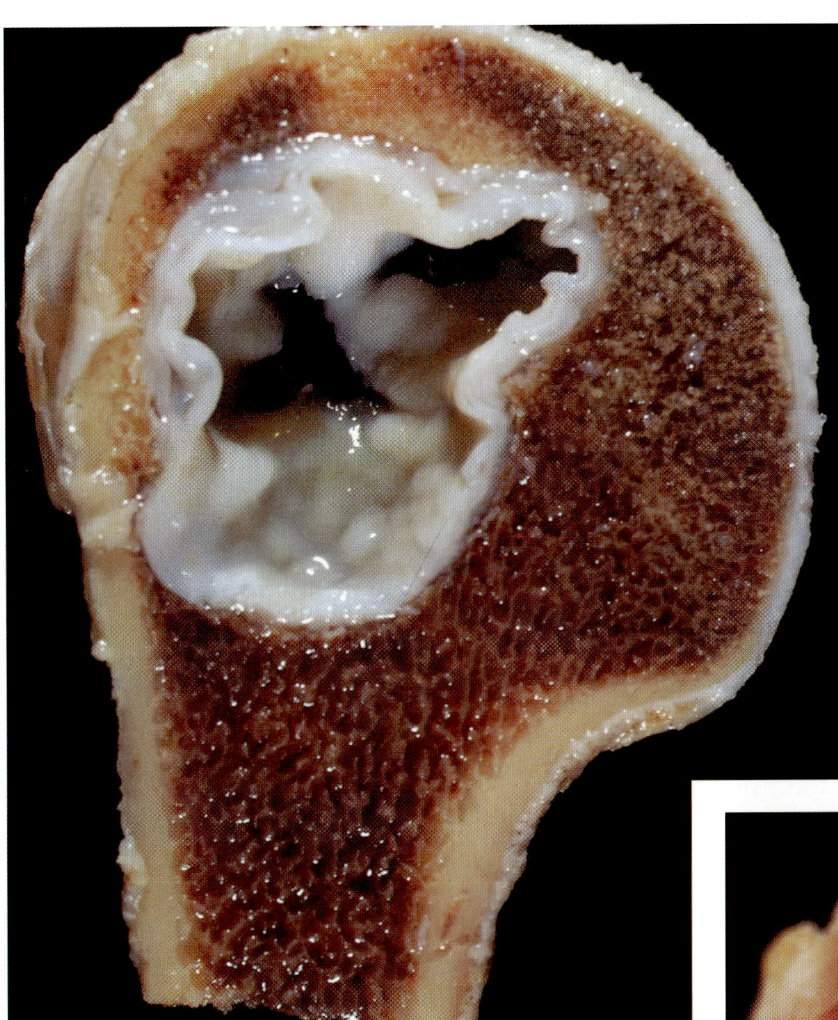

Figs 42.13–42.15 Hydatid disease of the shoulder involving the humeral head and the scapula.

Fig. 42.13

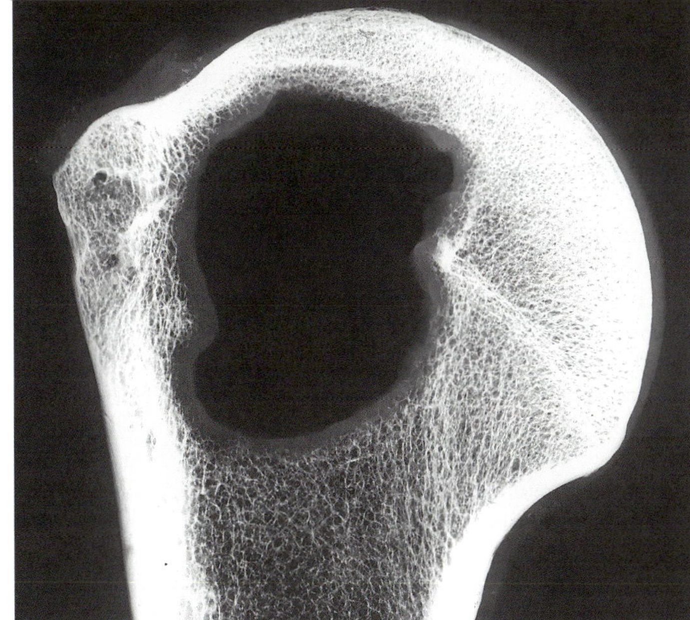

Fig. 42.14

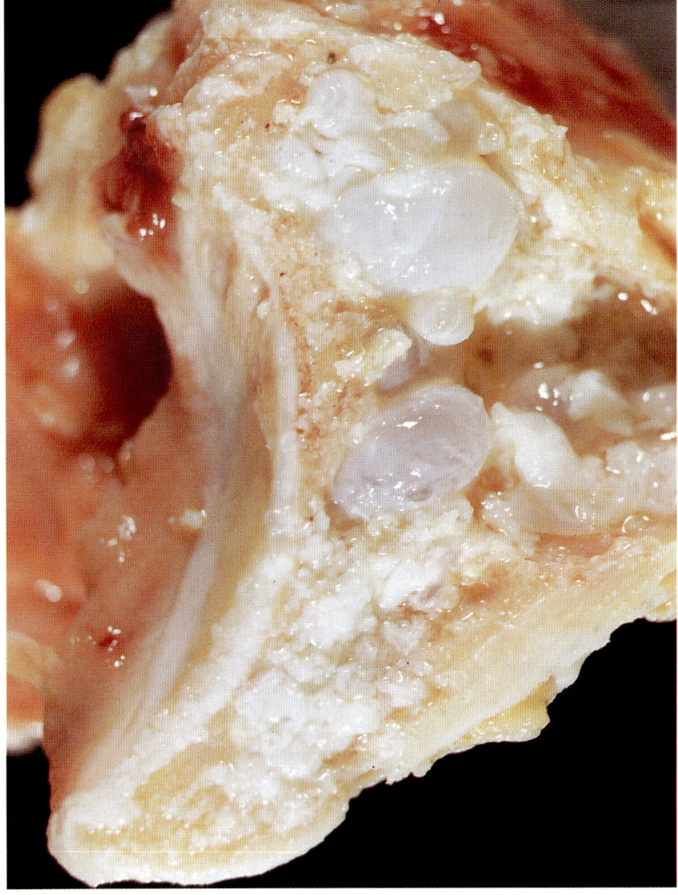

Fig. 42.15

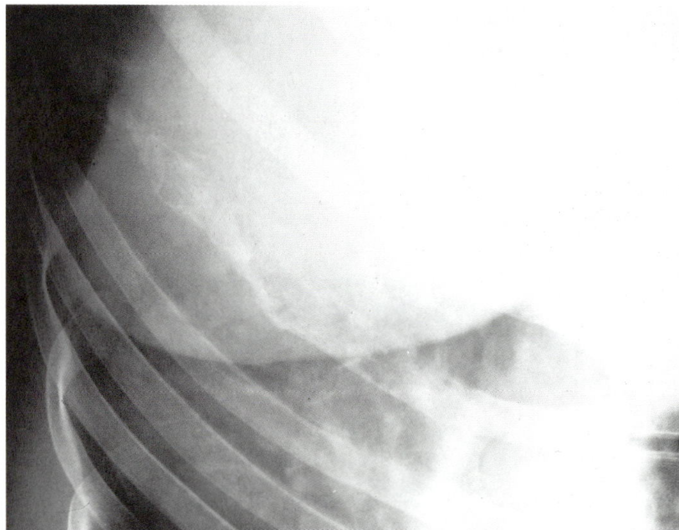

Fig. 42.16

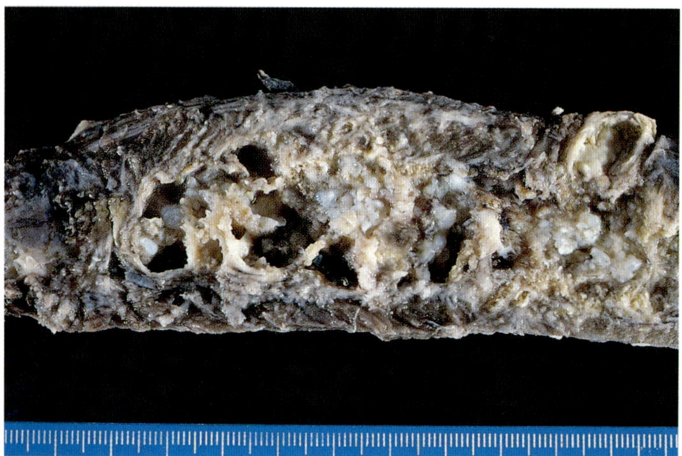

Fig. 42.17

Figs 42.16, 42.17 Hydatid disease of the ninth rib.

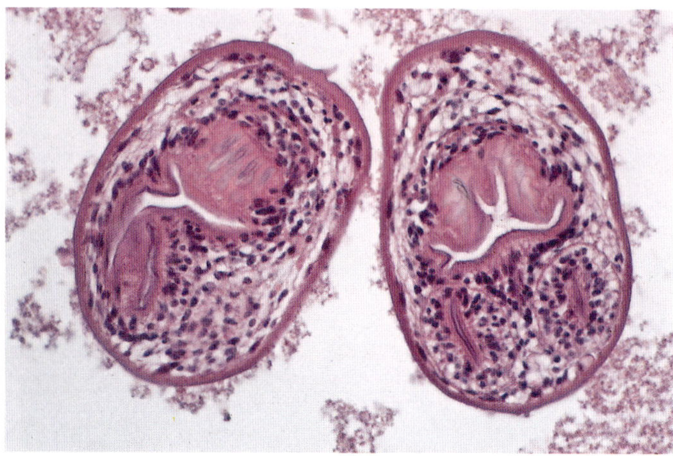

Fig. 42.18 Hydatid disease of the humerus: scolices and hooks in the fluid of the cyst.

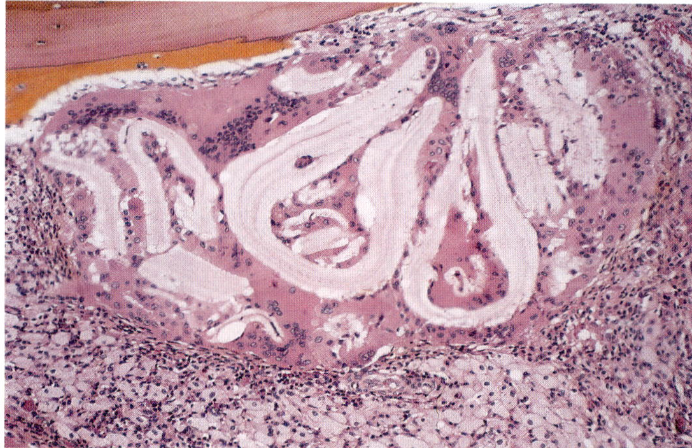

Fig. 42.19

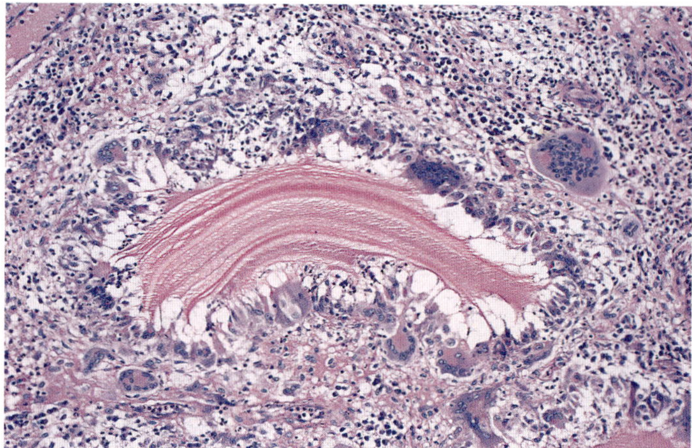

Fig. 42.20

Figs 42.19, 42.20 Hydatid disease of a rib: extensive foreign body reaction induced by ruptured membranes.

The parasitic disease is usually diagnosed in the 30–50-year-old age group.[9] The clinical course is protracted, with pain, pathologic fractures, transarticular extension, secondary infection or rupture in the spinal canal in vertebral locations. Some patients are asymptomatic.

Among serologic tests, the indirect hemagglutination test seems to be the most effective.[9]

The spine, pelvis (ilium) and hip are involved in 60% of cases[11] (Figs 42.1–42.5). Of axial lesions, 50% are found in the thoracic area, 20% in the lumbar area, 10% in the cervical area and 20% in the sacrum.[11,12] Primary hydatid disease of the spine may be due to the embolization of embryos via the arterial spinal circulation and via the paravertebral plexus of Batson.[13] Lesions arise in the vertebral body and spread to the neural arch and ribs, with eventual extraosseous extension into the paraspinal space.[13]

Long bones are involved in 28% of cases (Figs 42.6–42.14), ribs[14] and scapula in 8% (Figs 42.15–42.17), skull and phalanges in 4%.[6,8]

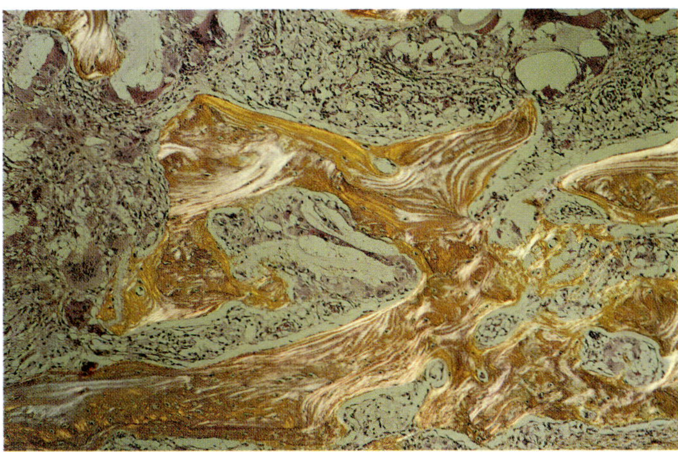

Fig. 42.21

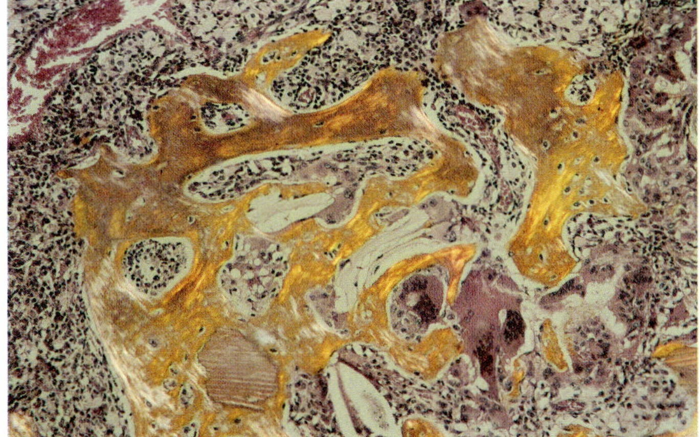

Fig. 42.22

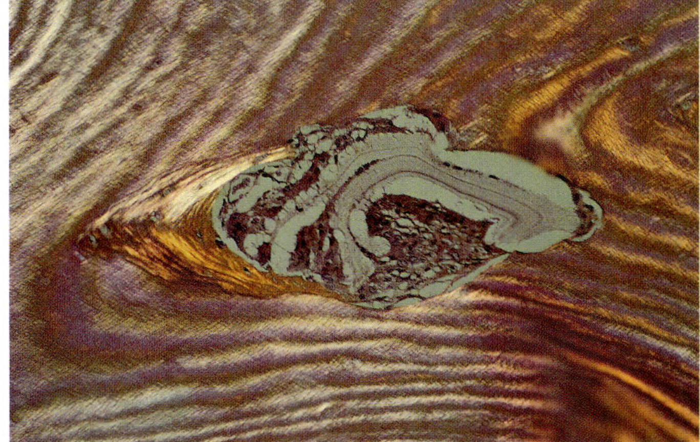

Fig. 42.23

Figs 42.21–42.23 Hydatid disease of a rib: bone remodeling (polarized light). Fragments of laminated membrane are even found in the cortex.

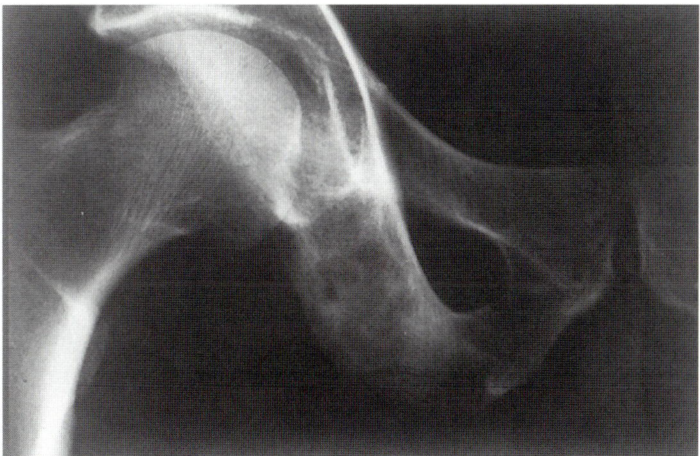

Fig. 42.24

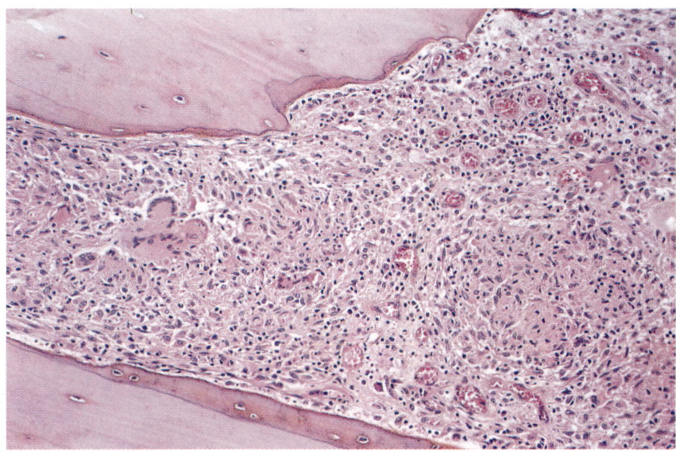

Fig. 42.25

Figs 42.24, 42.25 Tuberculosis of the ischium.

Usually, bone hydatidosis is monostotic, but frequently adjacent skeletal sites and muscles are invaded.[15]

On imaging, areas of osteolysis may be large and often appear multilocular, with sharp, slightly sclerotic or blurred margins.[4] Single or multiple lesions may induce an expansion of bone without any periosteal reaction.[4,16,17] Reactive sclerosis is usually associated with secondary infection.[17]

CT scans and MRI are useful for the evaluation of the cystic lesions, intralesional fluid or extraosseous spread but findings are not specific for the disease[4,5,8,18] and only in 50% is the disease diagnosed before operation.[19]

Histologically (Figs 42.18–42.23), due to the mechanical resistance of bone, a single large cyst is not found and the dense fibrous outer adventitial layer is not formed, except in some very rare cases.[20]

Medullary spaces are infiltrated by minute, thin-walled cysts and microvesicles are produced by exogenous budding. The cysts may be sterile (Jaffe 1972), with no germinal layer,[13,17] or may be fertile with brood capsules, scolices and hooks developing from the germinal layer. Rupture of the laminated membrane usually induces an extensive foreign body reaction, with reactive giant cells, lymphocytes and, more rarely, eosinophils.[17]

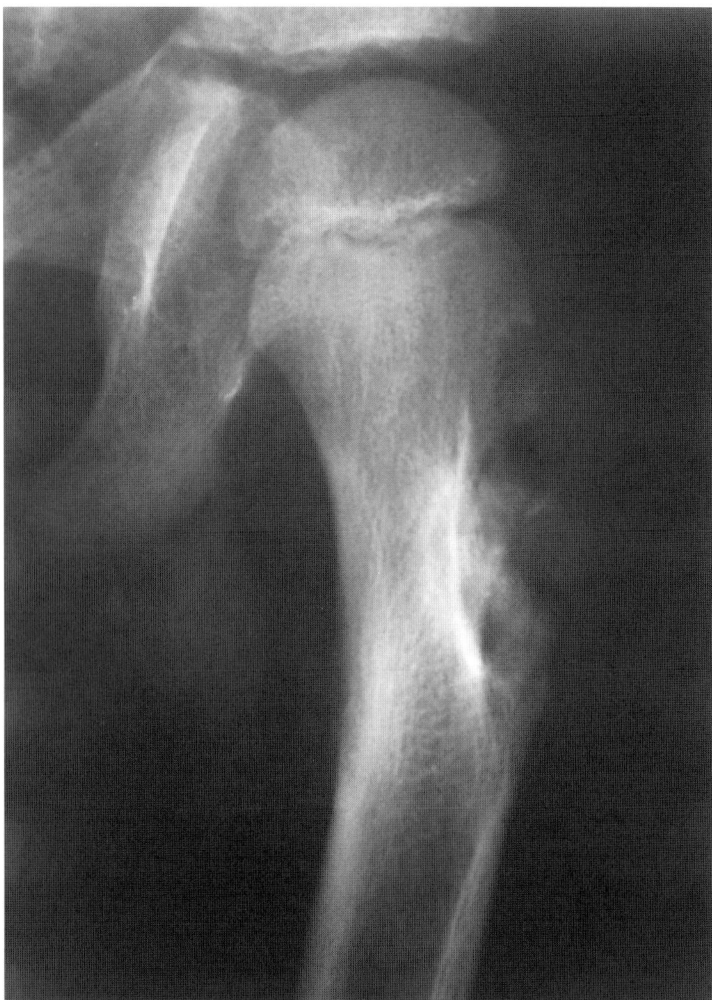

Fig. 42.26 Tuberculosis of the proximal femur.

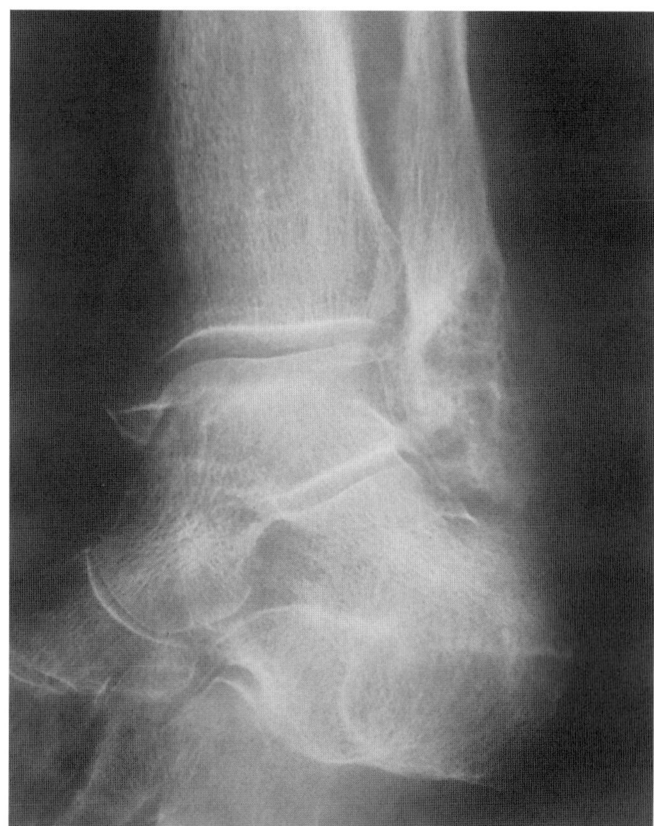

Fig. 42.27 Tuberculosis of the fibula.

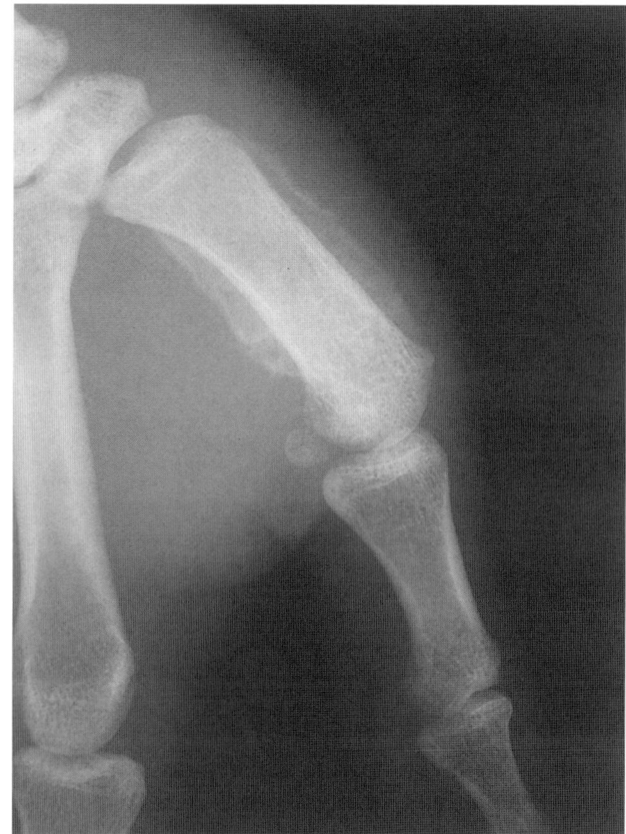

Fig. 42.28 Tuberculosis of a metacarpal.

The extremely unusual alveolar echinococcosis of bone exhibits communicating cavities with a PAS-positive layered cell-free cuticle, containing a necrotic gelatinous material.[3] The inflammatory reaction produces granulomatous or epithelioid changes, plasma cells, lymphocytes, macrophages and histiocytic giant cells.[3] Scolices are rare.

The treatment is surgery with or without formalin, hypotonic salines, chemotherapy and antihelminthic drugs, over a period of up to 2 years.[21] Recurrences or extension of the disease are frequent (70–80%), especially in vertebral locations.[2]

OSSEOUS TUBERCULOSIS

Obviously, the differential diagnosis of osseous tuberculosis with tumors has to be considered only on clinical and radiological findings (Figs 42.24–42.28). Unusual radiological presentations include solitary lytic lesions involving the subarticular areas of large joints with preservation of articular cartilage[22] and in the spine, involvement of a single vertebral body or separate skip lesions with preservation of the intervertebral disc.[23,24] Healing of vertebral lesions may even lead to an ivory vertebra.[25,26]

Punched-out radiolucent foci in the flat bones of the pelvis or skull may mimic a metastatic process[27] (Milgram 1990) or may resemble Ewing's sarcoma, eosinophilic granuloma or osteomyelitis.

Expansion of a bone in the hand or foot with mild or florid periostitis, usually found in children ('spina ventosa'), should not be confused with a tumor.[28]

Cystic tuberculosis is a solitary or multiple bone lesion involving the diaphyses and metaphyses of long bones, with a tendency to symmetrical distribution.[29-31] The cortex may be thinned and in the early stages, there is no periosteal reaction.

REFERENCES

1. Alldred A J, Nisbet N N. Hydatid disease in bone in Australasia. J Bone Joint Surg (Br) 1964: 46: 260–267
2. Markaki P, Markaki S, Prevedorou D, Bouropoulou V. Echinococcosis of bone: clinicolaboratory findings and differential diagnostic problems. Arch Anat Cytol Pathol 1990: 38: 92–94
3. Dorn R, Küsswetter W, Wünsch P. Alveolar echinococcosis of the femur. Acta Orthop Scand 1984: 55: 371–374
4. Torricelli P, Martinelli C, Biagini R, Ruggieri P, De Cristofaro R. Radiographic and computed tomographic findings in hydatid disease of bone. Skeletal Radiol 1990: 19: 435–439
5. Hayasaka K, Aburano T, Tanaka Y. MR imaging in alveolar echinococcosis of bone. Radiat Med 1995: 13: 179–182
6. Hooper J, McLean J. Hydatid disease of the femur. J Bone Joint Surg (Am) 1977: 59: 974–976
7. Ferrandez H D, Gomez-Castresena F, Lopez-Duran L, Mata P, Brandau D, Sanchez-Barba A. Osseous hydatidosis. J Bone Joint Surg (Am) 1978: 60: 685–690
8. Bouras A, Lardé D, Mathieu D, Delepine G, Benameur C, Ferrané J. The value of computed tomography in osseous hydatid disease (echinococcosis). Skeletal Radiol 1984: 12: 192–195
9. Agarwal S, Shah A, Kadhi S K, Rooney R J. Hydatid bone disease of the pelvis. Clin Orthop 1992: 280: 251–255
10. Jlidi R, Yaakoubi M T, Ladeb M F, Ben Ayeche M L, Ghannouchi G, Moula T. L'hydatidose osseuse. Ann Pathol 1992: 12: 98–101
11. Braithwaite P A, Lees R F. Vertebral hydatid disease: radiological assessment. Radiology 1981: 140: 763–766
12. Yegen C, Ozer A F, Aktan A O, Yalin R. Sacrococcygeal hydatid cyst: another entity in the differential diagnosis of sacrococcygeal chordoma. Paraplegia 1993: 31: 479–481
13. Von Sinner W N, Akhtar M. Case report 833. Primary spinal echinococcosis (Echinococcus granulosus) of lumbosacral spine. Skeletal Radiol 1994: 23: 220–223
14. Bonakdarpour A, Zadeh Y F, Maghssoudi H, Sharied S, Levy W. Costal echinococcosis. AJR 1973: 118: 371–377
15. De Cristofaro R, Ruggieri P, Biagini R, Picci P. Osseous hydatidosis. Case report 629. Skeletal Radiol 1990: 19: 461–464
16. Beggs I. The radiology of hydatid disease. AJR 1985: 145: 639–648
17. Von Sinner W N. Case report 616. Hydatid disease (HD) involving multiple bones and soft tissue. Skeletal Radiol 1990: 19: 312–316
18. Giordano G B, Cerisoli M, Bernardi B. Hydatid cysts of the spine. J Comput Assist Tomogr 1982: 6: 408–409
19. Booz M Y. The value of plain films in hydatid disease of bone. Clin Radiol 1993: 47: 265–268
20. Abelanet R, Forest M, Palangié A, Meary R, Tomeno B, Languepin A. L'echinococcose osseuse. Ann Anat Pathol (Paris) 1975: 20: 133–148
21. Wirbel R J, Mues P E, Mutschler W E, Salomon-Looijen M. Hydatid disease of the pelvis and the femur. Acta Orthop Scand 1995: 66: 440–442
22. Abdelwahab I F, Present D A, Klein M J. Case report 390. Tuberculous pseudotumor of the proximal end of the right tibia without obvious synovial involvement. Skeletal Radiol 1986: 15: 652–656
23. Weaver P, Lifeso R M. The radiological diagnosis of tuberculosis of the adult spine. Skeletal Radiol 1984: 12: 178–186
24. Marom E M, Porter A, Gornish M, Cohen M, Russo I. Atypical skeletal tuberculosis. Skeletal Radiol 1995: 24: 620–622
25. Naim-ur-Rahman V. Atypical forms of spinal tuberculosis. J Bone Joint Surg (Br) 1980: 62: 162–165
26. Ahmadi J, Bajaj A, Segall H D, Zee C S. Spinal tuberculosis: atypical observations at MR imaging. Radiology 1993: 189: 489–493
27. Tsay M H, Chen M C, Jaung G Y, Pang K K, Chen B F. Atypical skeletal tuberculosis mimicking tumor metastases: report of a case. J Formos Med Assoc 1995: 94: 428–431
28. Abdelwahab I F, Lewis M M, Klein M J, Hermann G. Case report 528. Tuberculous dactylitis (right great toe). Skeletal Radiol 1989: 18: 133–135
29. Shannon F B, Moore M, Houkom J A, Waecker N J Jr. Multifocal cystic tuberculosis of bone. J Bone Joint Surg (Am) 1990: 72: 1089–1092
30. Mazas-Artasona L, Led A, Espinosa H, Sufrate D, Gil M. Case report 737. Cystic tuberculosis of femur. Skeletal Radiol 1992: 21: 323–325
31. Rasool M N, Govender S, Naidoo K S. Cystic tuberculosis of bone in children. J Bone Joint Surg (Br) 1994: 76: 113–117

43

Paget's disease

J. Amouroux

INTRODUCTION AND CLINICAL DATA

Paget's disease affects 3% of adults over the age of 40. Its frequency increases with age and reaches 10% of the population over the age of 80.[1] It is characterized by excessive and abnormal remodeling of bone tissue but its etiology remains unknown. A genetic cause probably exists, as familial forms and disease in identical twins have been reported.[2,3] A viral cause has been suggested by identification of inclusion bodies in osteoclasts, which resemble paramyxovirus, but the role of this as an etiological factor has not been proved.[4]

Paget's disease affects males more often and earlier than females.

Asymptomatic forms represent about 20% of the cases. Disease is then revealed by radiography.

The most frequent symptoms are pain or tenderness of the affected skeletal sites. Enlargement of bones may result in an increased size of the skull, its progressive deformation with accentuation of the frontal eminences, kyphosis or changes of long bones of the limbs. Pathological fractures may occur. Neurologic complications are rather common, resulting from spinal cord compression. Involvement of the base of the skull can also be accompanied by compression of cranial nerves and may result in deafness. Congestive heart failure is possible, due more to hyperemia and increased blood flow in pagetic bone than to the presence of arteriovenous shunts.

Elevation of alkaline phosphatase levels in the serum and hydroxyproline levels in the urine reflects increased bone formation by osteoblasts and its resorption by osteoclasts, respectively. These biological markers are useful to assess the activity of the disease.

SKELETAL DISTRIBUTION

In monostotic or polyostotic forms, the lesions of Paget's disease are most common in the axial skeleton. The pelvis

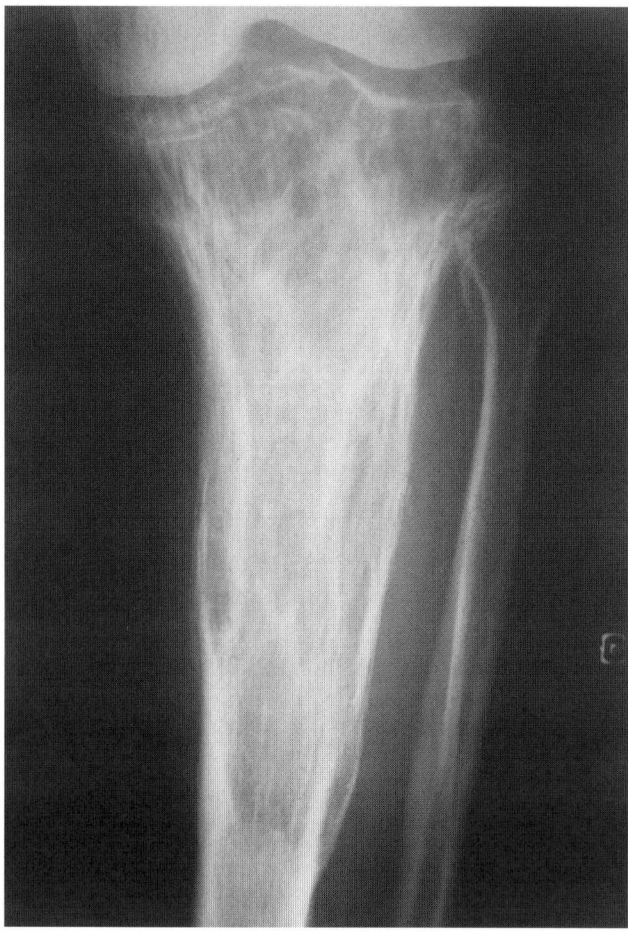

Fig. 43.1 Paget's disease: lytic and sclerotic lesions involving the tibia. (Courtesy of M. Forest MD.)

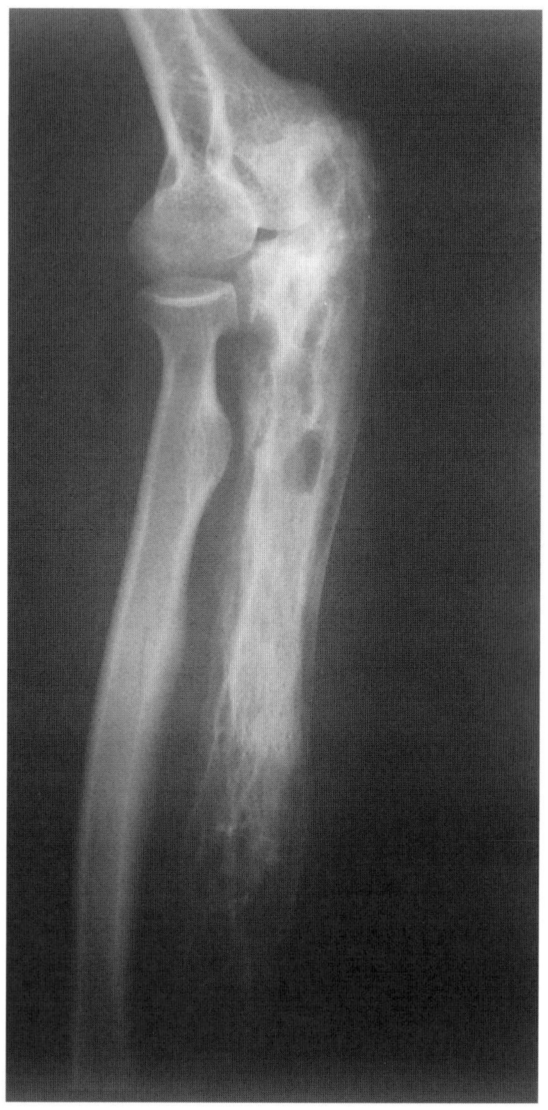

Fig. 43.2 Paget's disease: lytic and sclerotic lesions involving the ulna. (Courtesy of M. Forest MD.)

is affected in 30–75% of cases, sacrum in 30–60% and the spine, particularly the lumbar segment, in 30–75% (Resnick 1995). The proximal part of long bones, especially the femur, is frequently involved (25–35% of the cases). Radiography of the lumbar spine, the pelvis and the femoral heads allows recognition of the disease in 90% of cases.

These sites are the most commonly involved but any bone may be affected by the disease.

IMAGING

The initial phase of osteoclastic hyperactivity results in osteolytic lesions, occurring usually in the skull but also in the pelvis or long bones of the extremities, presenting as osteolytic areas termed 'osteoporosis circumscripta'. This osteolytic phase may be apparent in the whole skeleton[5,6] (Figs 43.1–43.5). In tubular bones, osteolysis almost exclusively arises in the epiphyseal subchondral bone and then progresses towards the metaphysis and diaphysis. The average rate of progression of lesions is about 1 cm a year.[7]

During the course of disease, osteoblastic reaction results in areas of radiodensity and the global density of bone increases.[8] Bone density of vertebral bodies may increase to such a point that it produces aspects of ivory vertebrae. Involvement of the pelvis is seldom diffuse; it predominates in or affects one side exclusively.

Bone scintigraphy is employed in the evaluation of the extent of Paget's disease.[9] Scintigraphic abnormalities may precede radiographic signs. However, lesions are more easily detected by radiography than scintigraphy in the quiescent or inactive forms of the disease.

Computed tomography scanning is helpful to detect complications such as articular abnormalities, especially in the hip, occurrence of malignant change or vertebral involvement with neurologic symptoms.

Magnetic resonance imaging is also used in the evaluation of complications. It defines changes and hypervascularization of the bone marrow.[8,10]

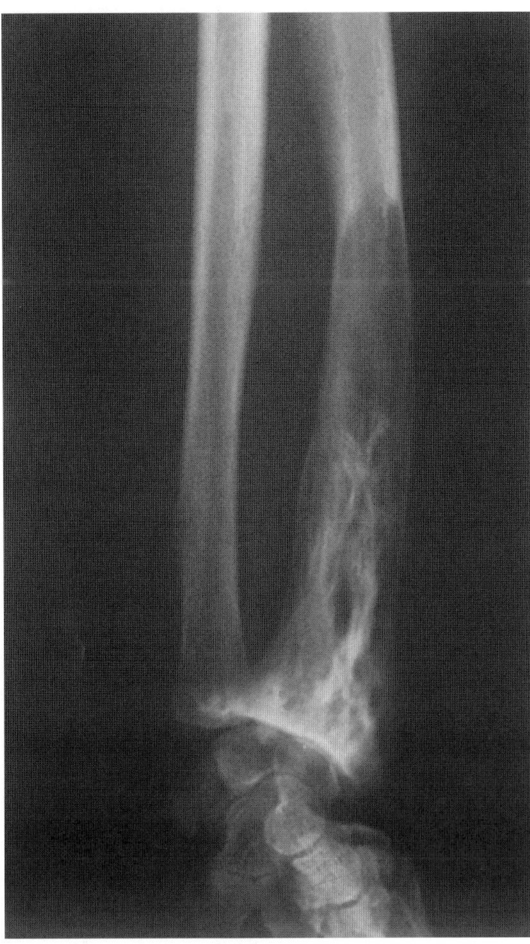

Fig. 43.3 Paget's disease: lytic form in the radius. (Courtesy of M. Forest MD.)

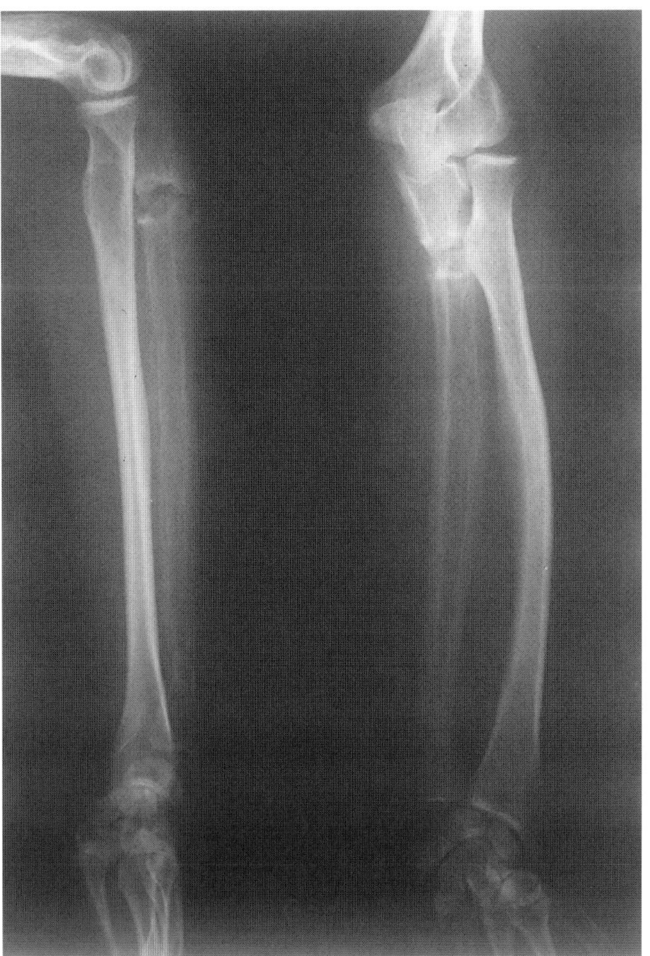

Fig. 43.4 Paget's disease: lytic form in the ulna. (Courtesy of M. Forest MD.)

GROSS PATHOLOGY

Pagetic bone is broader, heavier and more irregular than normal bone. It is heterogeneous on cut section. Distinction between Haversian and cancellous bone vanishes. Cortical bone is often thick but curved, especially in the lower limbs. The medullary canal is made of bone and fibrous tissue arranged without any precise architecture, containing large cyst-like areas devoid of bone trabeculae. When the latter remain, they are scanty, broad and coarse, with a fibrillar aspect. Bone marrow appears fibrous and highly vascularized. Large and numerous vessels are also found in the periosteum.

HISTOPATHOLOGY

Paget's disease is characterized by an excessive and abnormal remodeling of bone. It results in a considerable increase of osteoclastic resorption followed by a marked osteoblastic reaction that produces immature primary bone (woven bone) (Figs 43.6–43.9). This acceleration of bone remodeling leads to severe architectural abnormali-ties, with an abnormally dense bone made of trabeculae separated by fibrous and highly vascularized bone marrow.

Bone trabeculae display a mosaic or puzzle pattern (Figs 43.10, 43.11), with elements separated from each other by irregular basophilic lines termed 'cement lines'. The latter separate small areas of bone with lamellar structure and with collagen fibers that are discontinuous with those of neighboring units (the collagen fibers end at the cement lines).

Osteoclastic hyperactivity and the subsequent osteoblastic response evolve through active phases followed by stages during which pagetic bone is locally inactive or quiescent. The process periodically starts again and disease extends to further areas of the skeleton. Increased remodeling may be evaluated by scintigraphy or biological markers (serum alkaline phosphatase and urine hydroxyproline).

ELECTRON MICROSCOPY

Ultrastructural study of osteoclasts in Paget's disease allowed Mills and Rebel to identify intranuclear inclusions

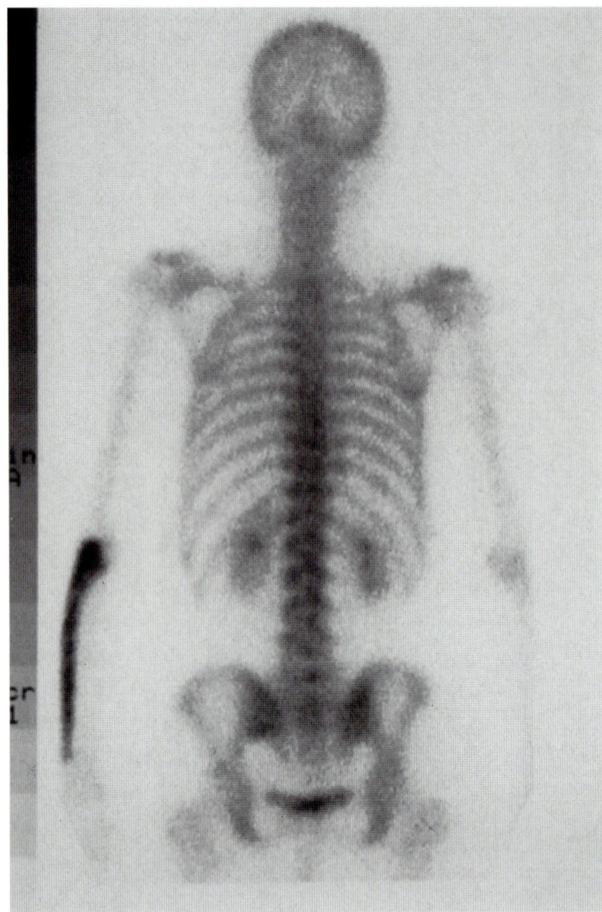

Fig. 43.5 Same case as Fig. 43.4: increased uptake on bone scan. (Courtesy of M. Forest MD.)

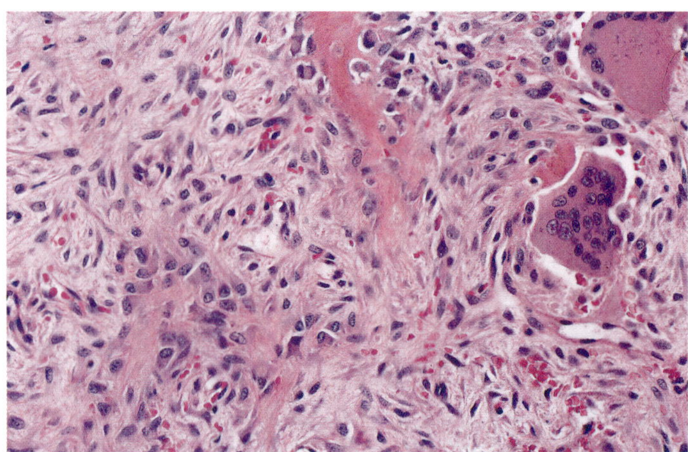

Fig. 43.7

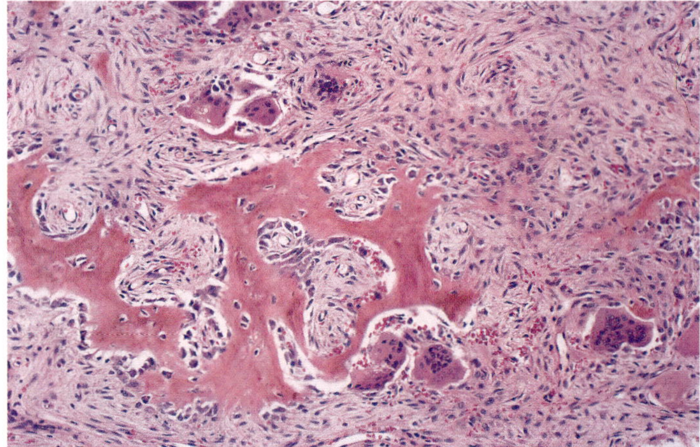

Fig. 43.8

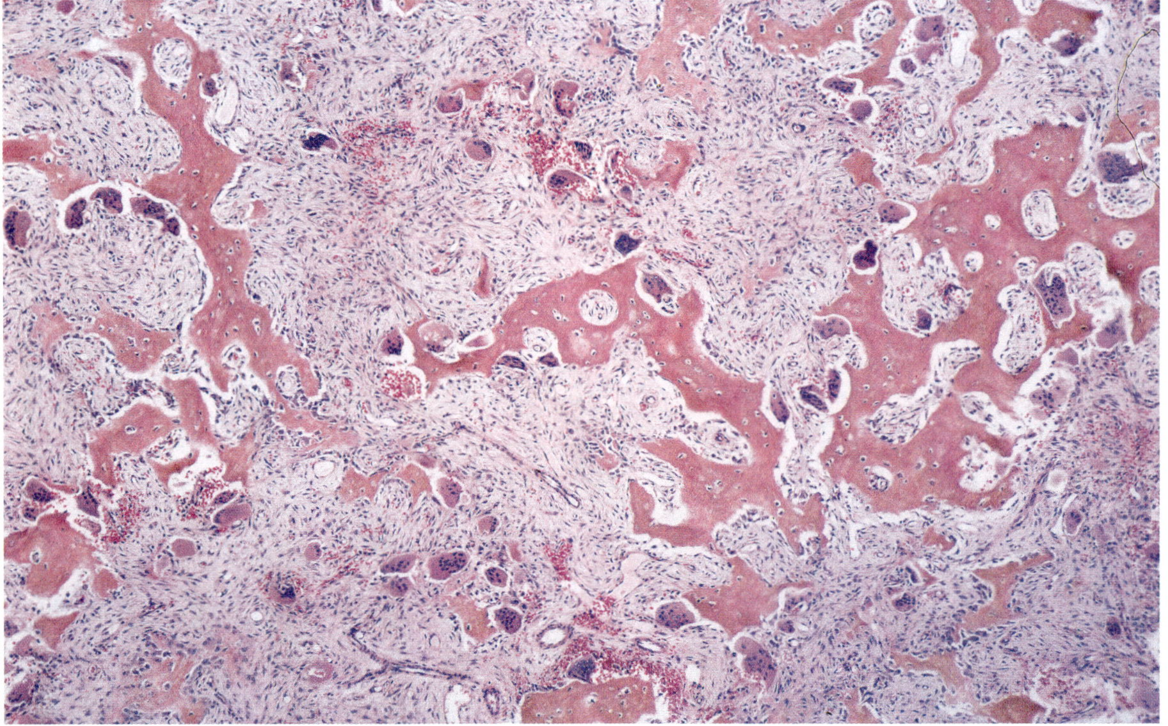

Fig. 43.6

Figs 43.6–43.9 Lytic forms of Paget's disease demonstrating new bone formation, osteoclastic and osteoblastic activity. (Courtesy of M. Forest MD.)

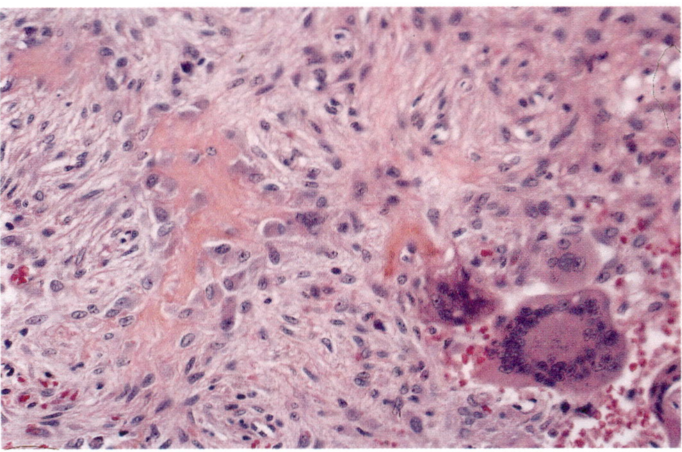

Fig. 43.9

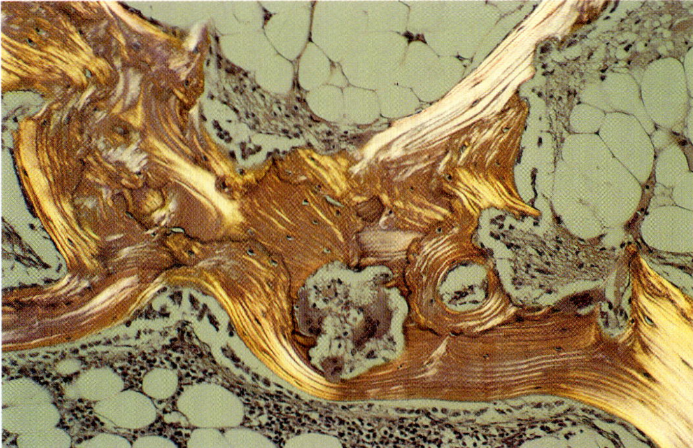

Fig. 43.10

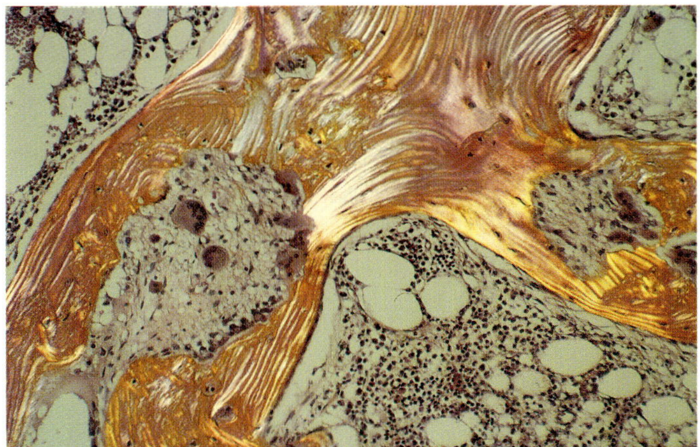

Fig. 43.11

Figs 43.10, 43.11 Paget's disease: active lesions already exhibiting a mosaic pattern (polarized light). (Courtesy of M. Forest MD.)

peculiar to these cells and never found in normal osseous tissue. The appearance of inclusions points to a paramyxovirus of the measles group. Such intranuclear filamen-

tous inclusions have also been reported within giant cells of giant cell tumor of bone, with or without Paget's disease. Their role in the pathogenesis of Paget's disease remains hypothetical.[4,11]

COURSE

Multiple complications may occur during the course of Paget's disease: long bone, spine or skull deformations, neurologic disorders, arthropathies, cortical fissuring in diaphyseal convex parts of long bones. However, the most severe complication is the occurrence of tumor in pagetic bone. It may be a sarcoma, a giant cell tumor or preferential localization of another tumor, such as metastasis, myeloma or malignant lymphoma.[12,13]

Sarcomatous degeneration, reported in some of the first described cases of Paget's disease, affects 1% of patients.[14–16] In patients whose pagetic skeletal involvement is very extensive, sarcomatous transformation may occur in 5–10% of cases. Most often, the tumor develops in pagetic bone as a single focus. In some patients, multiple foci represent either a multicentric tumor or dissemination of an initial tumoral focus to pagetic bone.[17]

Sarcomatous transformation usually occurs in patients between 55 and 80 years old, earlier in males. It results in increased pain and soft tissue swelling. Sites usually affected are femur, pelvis and humerus. Other sites may be involved, such as skull or spine. Sarcoma sometimes arises in the site of a previous healed fracture.[18] Histological types vary: the commonest is osteosarcoma (60–80%), followed by fibrosarcoma (20–25%), chondrosarcoma (10%), malignant fibrous histiocytoma and hemangiosarcoma. Extensive osteolysis is the most frequent radiographic feature, with cortical disruption and tumoral invasion into the soft tissues. Prognosis is bleak, especially in patients with multiple tumoral foci.[19]

Giant cell tumor is a rare complication, mostly occurring in the skull or facial bones. The pagetic involvement, usually polyostotic, is not always obvious radiographically and may sometimes only be demonstrated histologically. The tumor shows a lytic image with a tumoral mass developing in the soft tissues. Usually giant cell tumor is benign with a good prognosis.[20–22]

Paget's disease may be associated with myeloma, Hodgkin's disease, other malignant lymphomas or leukemias.[23,24]

Hypervascularization of the pagetic bone probably plays some part in the preferential localization of metastases in these bones.[25] Usual sites of primary tumors are breast, kidney, lung, prostate and colon. The diagnosis of metastasis complicating Paget's disease is often suggested because of increased pain.

Whatever their nature, these tumoral complications are usually revealed by increased pain and soft tissue mass. These features are accompanied by radiographic lytic lesions. Some tumors may be revealed by a pathologic fracture. Bone formation is rare except in osteosarcomas. An excessive bone density may indicate the metastasis of a prostatic carcinoma.

TREATMENT

The therapeutic agents include calcitonin and diphosphonates, which improve biological and histological data but not radiographic features or the long-term course of the disease.

DIFFERENTIAL DIAGNOSIS

In the osteolytic initial phase of Paget's disease, all aspects of bone radiolucencies may present a problem, particularly osteoporosis, lytic metastases and myeloma (multiple or solitary).

In the more frequent, predominantly osteosclerotic forms, with cancellous bone abnormalities, all causes of increased bone density must be considered: metastases, especially of prostatic origin, myelofibrosis, fluorosis, mastocytosis and renal osteodystrophy.

REFERENCES

1. Harris E D Jr, Krane S M. Paget's disease of bone. Bull Rheum Dis 1968: 18: 506–511
2. Jones J V, Reed M F. Paget's disease. A family with six cases. Br Med J 1967: 4: 90–91
3. Wu R K. Familial incidence of Paget's disease and secondary osteogenic sarcoma. A report of three cases from a single family. Clin Orthop 1991: 265: 306–309
4. Rebel A, Baslé M, Pouplard A, Malkani K, Filmon R, Lepatezour A. Bone tissue in Paget's disease of bone. Ultrastructure and immunocytology. Arthritis Rheum 1980: 23: 1104–1114
5. Eisman J A, Martin T J. Osteolytic Paget's disease. Recognition and risks of biopsy. J Bone Joint Surg (Am) 1986: 68: 112–117
6. Jacobs P. Osteolytic Paget's disease. Clin Radiol 1974: 25: 137–144
7. Zadek R E, Milgram J W. Progression of Paget's disease in the tibia. J Bone Joint Surg (Am) 1976: 58: 876–878
8. Mirra J M, Brien E W, Tehranzadeh J. Paget's disease of bone: review with emphasis on radiologic features. Skeletal Radiol 1995: 24: 163–184
9. Wellman H N, Schauwecker D, Robb J A, Khairi M R, Johnston C C. Skeletal scintimaging and radiography in the diagnosis and management of Paget's disease. Clin Orthop 1977: 127: 55–62
10. Kaufmann G A, Sundaram M, McDonald D J. Magnetic resonance imaging in symptomatic Paget's disease. Skeletal Radiol 1991: 20: 413–418
11. Mills B G, Singer F R, Weiner L P, Suffen S C, Stabile E, Holst P. Evidence of both respiratory syncytial virus and measles virus antigens in the osteoclasts of patients with Paget's disease of bone. Clin Orthop 1984: 183: 303–311
12. Haibach H, Farrell C, Dittrich F J. Neoplasm arising in Paget's disease of bone: a study of 82 cases. Am J Clin Pathol 1985: 83: 594–600
13. Hadjipavlou A, Lander P, Srolovitz H, Enker J P. Malignant transformation in Paget's disease of bone. Cancer 1992: 70: 2802–2808
14. Wick M R, Siegal G P, Unni K K, McLeod R A, Gredtizer H G. Sarcoma of bone complicating osteitis deformans (Paget's disease): fifty years' experience. Am J Surg Pathol 1981: 5: 47–59
15. Huvos A G, Butler A, Bretsky S S. Osteogenic sarcoma associated with Paget's disease of bone. A clinicopathologic study of 65 patients. Cancer 1983: 52: 1489–1495
16. Price C H G, Goldie W. Paget's sarcoma of bone. A study of 80 cases from the Bristol and the Leeds bone tumour registries. J Bone Joint Surg (Br) 1969: 51: 205–224
17. Choquette D, Haraoui B, Altman R D. Simultaneous multifocal sarcomatous degeneration in Paget's disease of bone. Clin Orthop 1983: 179: 308–311
18. Bessler W, Bloch J. Sarcoma formation in Paget's osteitis deformans after fractures. Schweiz Med Vschr 1962: 92: 205–209
19. Smith J, Botet J F, Yeh S D J. Bone sarcoma in Paget's disease. A study of 85 patients. Radiology 1984: 152: 583–590
20. Jacobs T P, Michelsen J, Polay J S, D'Amado A C, Canfield R E. Giant cell tumors in Paget's disease of bone. Familial and geographic clustering. Cancer 1979: 44: 742–747
21. Nusbacher N, Sclafani S J, Birla S R. Polyostotic Paget's disease complicated by benign giant cell tumor of left clavicle. Skeletal Radiol 1981: 6: 233–235
22. Potter H G, Schneider R, Ghelman B, Healey J H, Lane J M. Multiple giant cell tumors and Paget's disease of bone: radiographic and clinical correlations. Radiology 1991: 180: 261–264
23. Stehens G C, Lennington W J, Schwartz H S. Primary lymphoma and Paget's disease of the femur. Am J Clin Pathol 1994: 101: 783–786
24. Price C H G. Myeloma occurring with Paget's disease of bone. Skeletal Radiol 1976: 1: 15–19
25. Schajowicz F, Velan O, Araujo E S et al. Metastases of carcinoma in the pagetic bone. A report of two cases. Clin Orthop 1988: 228: 290–296

Fibrous dysplasia

M. Forest

INTRODUCTION AND CLINICAL DATA

Fibrous dysplasia[1,2] is a developmental disorder in which bone is replaced by islands of metaplastic woven bone in a background of spindle cell stroma. This distinct entity is viewed as a developmental anomaly of the bone-forming mesenchyme with an arrest of maturation at the woven bone stage.[1,3]

The disease may involve one bone (monostotic form, 85% of cases) or multiple bones (polyostotic form, 15% of cases). Lesions may be clustered in one or two anatomic regions of the upper or lower extremity (monomelic form) or exhibit a widespread involvement of the skeleton.

It accounts for approximately 7% of all bone tumors and tumor-like lesions. Males and females are affected about equally and 75% of cases are diagnosed before the age of 30 years.[4]

Most monostotic lesions, especially in ribs or pelvic locations, are asymptomatic; chief complaints are a slight pain, tenderness, swelling or deformity. The disease may be revealed by a pathologic fracture. In the polyostotic form, two-thirds of patients have symptoms before the age of 10;[4] symptoms begin early in life and include multiple pathologic fractures in long bones, leading to 'shepherd's crook' deformities. Pathologic fractures usually heal well, but may be followed by pseudarthrosis (Huvos 1991); their incidence is high (85% of cases[4]).

An abnormal cutaneous pigmentation is found in about 50% of polyostotic cases; it is rarely found in solitary lesions. The McCune–Albright syndrome, accounting for 3% of polyostotic forms, is characterized by the association of polyostotic fibrous dysplasia with areas of pigmentation, differing from neurofibromatosis by irregular, dented borders and endocrine disorders (acromegaly, hyperthyroidism, hyperparathyroidism, Cushing's syndrome and precocious puberty in females[5]).

A rise in serum alkaline phosphatase is found in one-third of patients, but is not correlated with the extent of

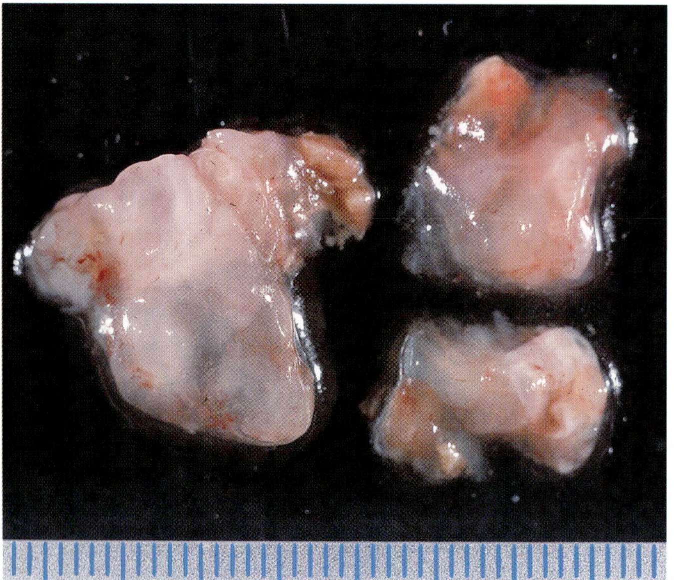

Fig. 44.1

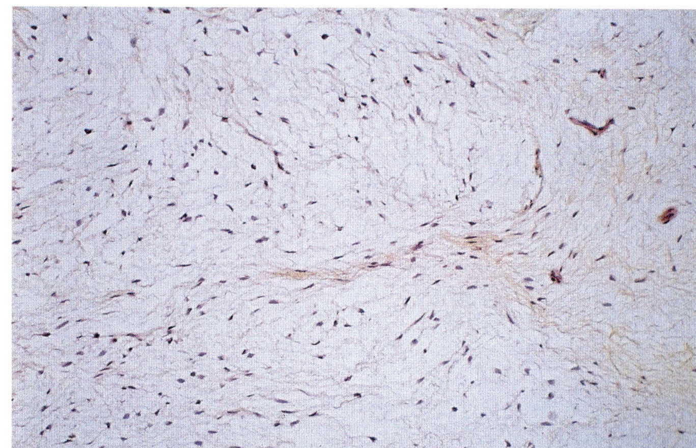

Fig. 44.2

Figs 44.1, 44.2 Intramuscular myxoma of the thigh close to a polyostotic fibrous dysplasia.

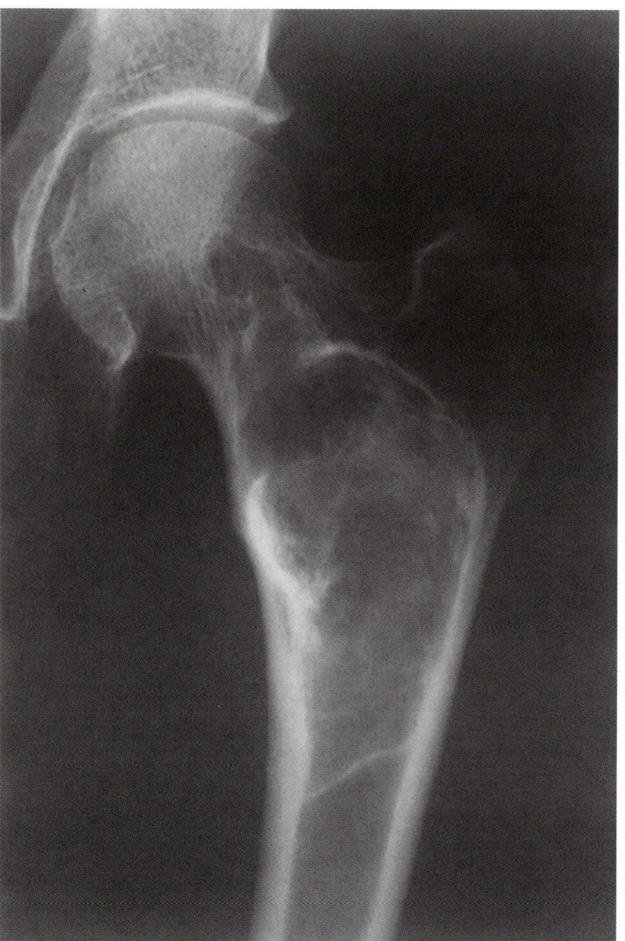

Fig. 44.3

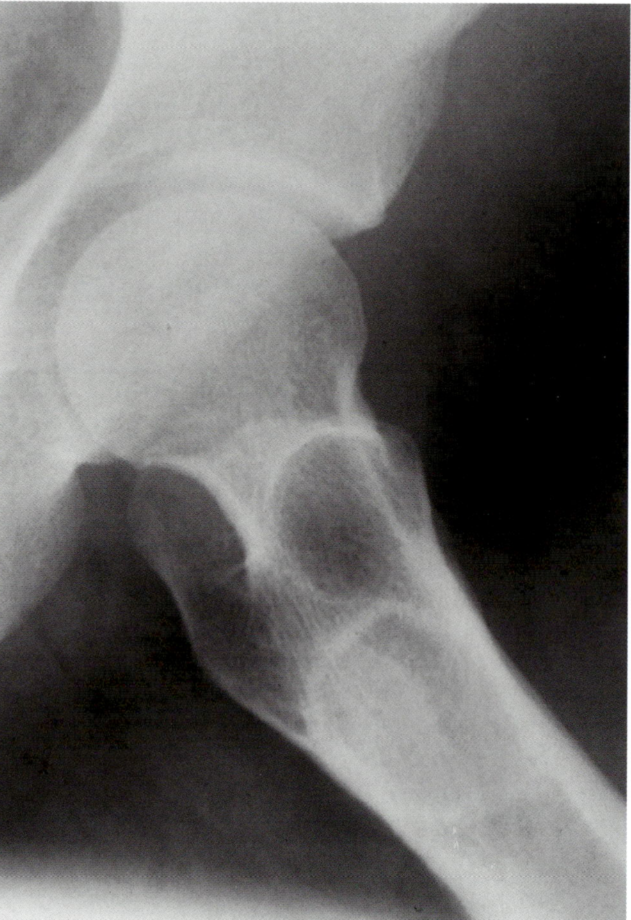

Fig. 44.4

Figs 44.3, 44.4 Fibrous dysplasia involving proximal femur (monostotic forms).

the disease. Hypophosphatemic rickets has been reported, chiefly with McCune–Albright syndrome.[6–9]

Various associated diseases have been described: desmoplastic fibroma,[10,11] eosinophilic granuloma,[12] giant cell reparative granuloma,[13] secondary aneurysmal bone cysts,[14,15] but chiefly intramuscular myxomas, first reported in 1926[16–33] (Figs 44.1, 44.2). They are more frequent in polyostotic forms and have been reported with McCune–Albright syndrome.[6,24]

Intramuscular myxomas appear considerably later after the diagnosis of fibrous dysplasia, occurring in groups or clusters in the vicinity of the most severely involved bone. Distinct from the bone lesion, they are located within striated muscles, predominantly in the lower extremities and on the right side. Increasing rapidly in size, they may be very large and often multiple.

SKELETAL DISTRIBUTION

Any bone may be involved, but in the monostotic form, the most common sites are the femur (upper third),[34,35] the ribs[36] and craniofacial bones,[4] followed by the tibia, humerus and pelvis (Figs 44.3–44.12). Spinal involvement is unusual (Figs 44.13, 44.14) as well as location in the small bones of the hand and foot.[37–49]

In polyostotic forms, the femur, tibia, humerus, pelvic bones, ribs, bones of the hand and foot are frequent locations. Spinal involvement usually involves the lumbar spine.[50]

The monostotic form does not progress to a polyostotic form (Huvos 1991).

IMAGING

Radiographic findings are the same in monostotic or polyostotic disease, but solitary lesions are usually smaller.

In long bones, fibrous dysplasia appears as an osteolytic lesion at the end of the diaphysis, less often at the metaphysis (Fig. 44.15); isolated epiphyseal involvement is rare, but fibrous dysplasia may extend to the epiphysis after clo-

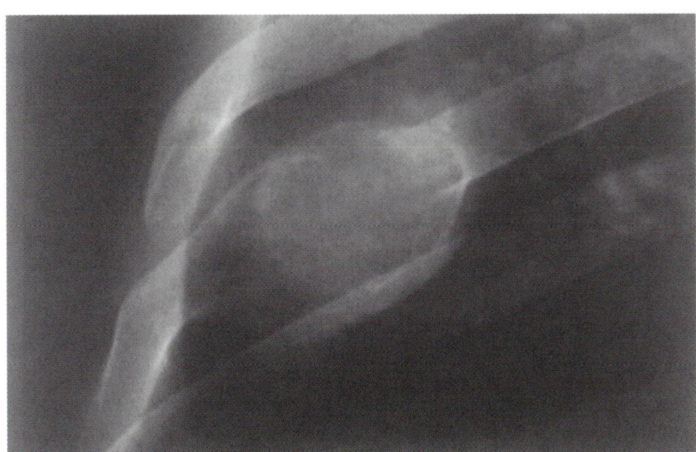

Fig. 44.5

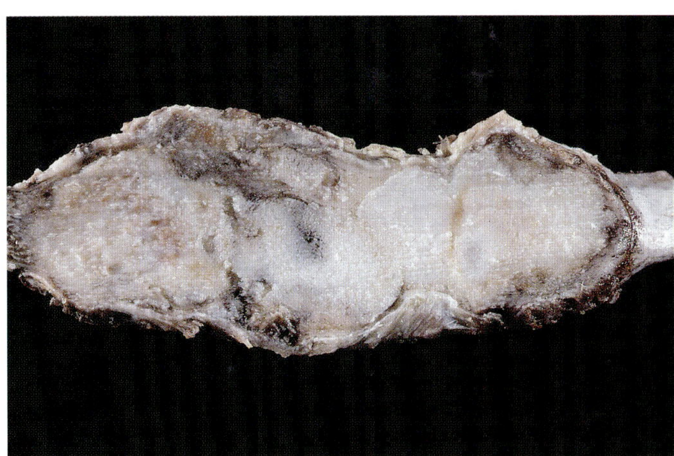

Fig. 44.6

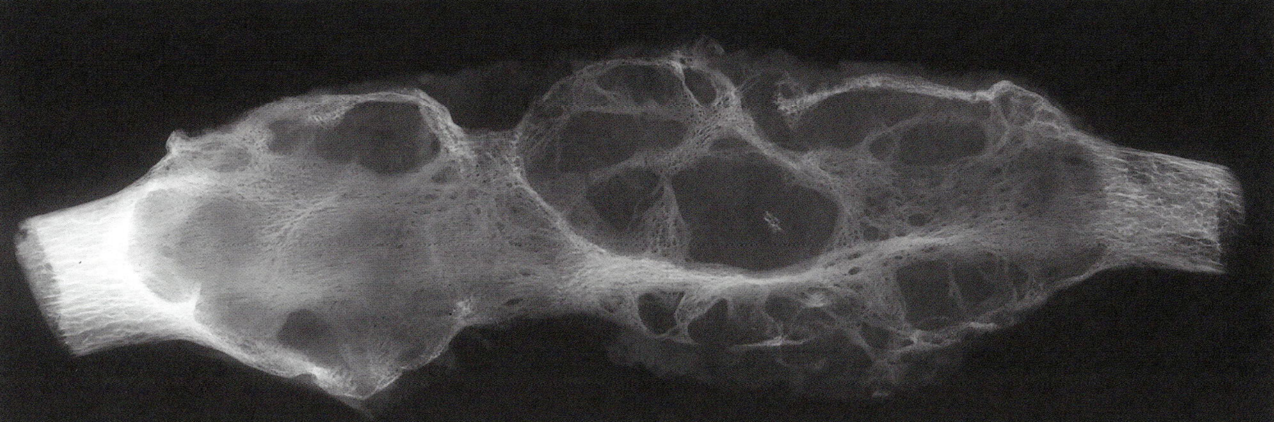

Fig. 44.7

Figs 44.5–44.7 Monostotic fibrous dysplasia of a rib with marked expansion of bone.

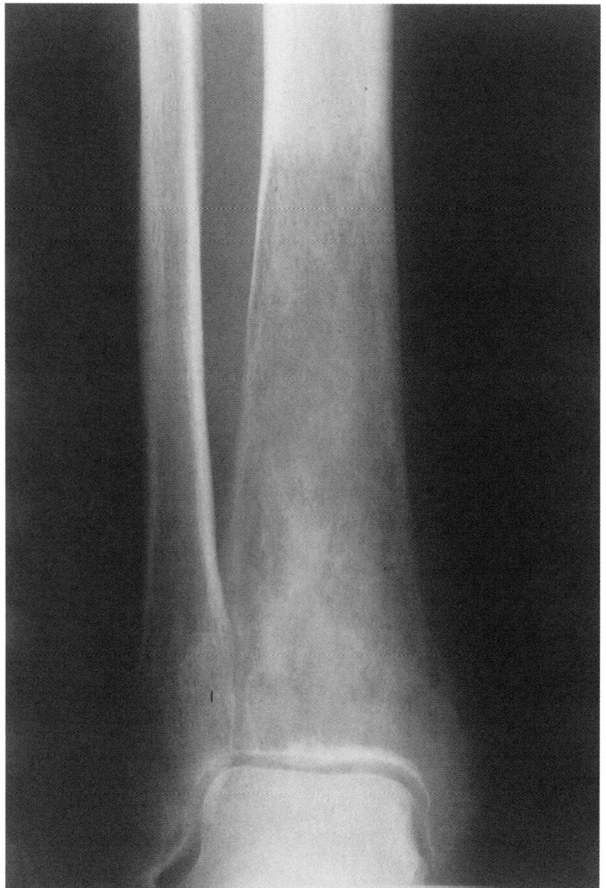

Fig. 44.8 Fibrous dysplasia of the tibia with atypical, poorly defined upper margins.

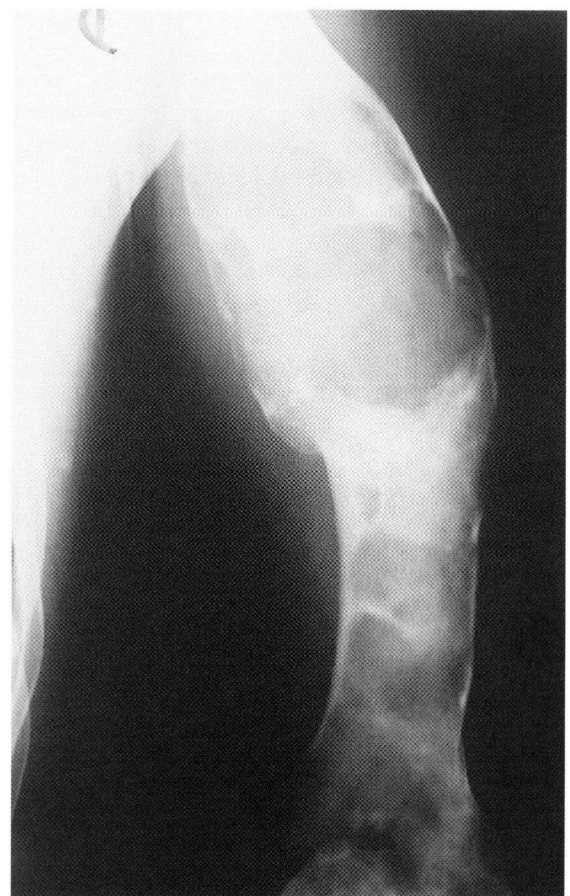

Fig. 44.9

sure of the growth plate.[51,52] In the most typical location, the upper end of the femur (Fig. 44.16), the lesion is rarely confined to the femoral neck[34] and is mostly found in intertrochanteric, juxtametaphyseal or diametaphyseal regions.[35]

Usually centrally located, the lesion is round, elongated and often expansile; it may involve the entire shaft of the bone. It may be entirely radiolucent or have an amorphous, hazy 'ground glass' appearance due to the fine component of woven bone or exihibit increased density depending on the amount of bone formation and calcification (Figs 44.17–44.20). Punctate or flocculent calcifications correspond to a cartilaginous component (Fig. 44.21). Rarely, a sequestrum may be found within the lesion.[53]

In some cases, a trabeculated multiloculated aspect is due to a scalloped pattern of endosteal erosion. The margins are sharply defined or sclerotic; in old lesions, a thick layer of reactive bone is called a 'rind' (Fig. 44.22). In other cases, the cortex is thinned and eroded.

Figs 44.9, 44.10 Fibrous dysplasia of humerus (monostotic and polyostotic forms), both cases partially cystic.

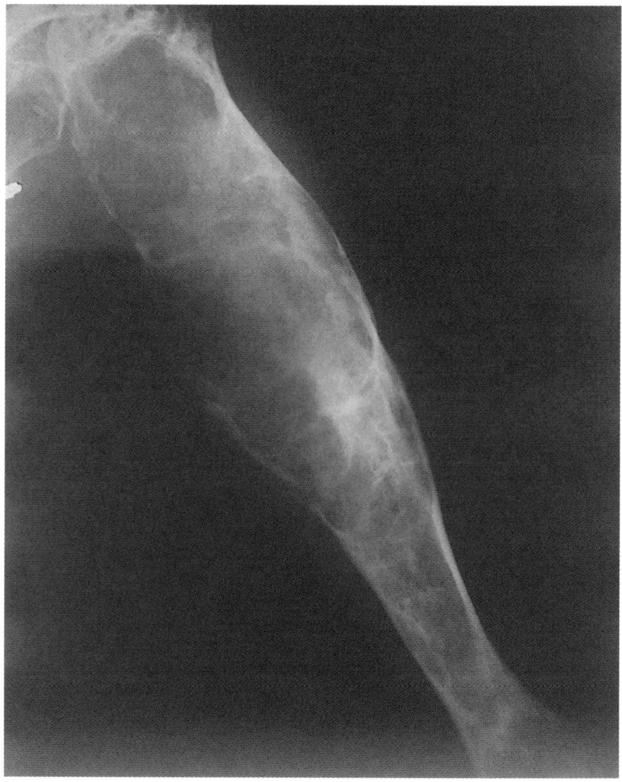

Fig. 44.10

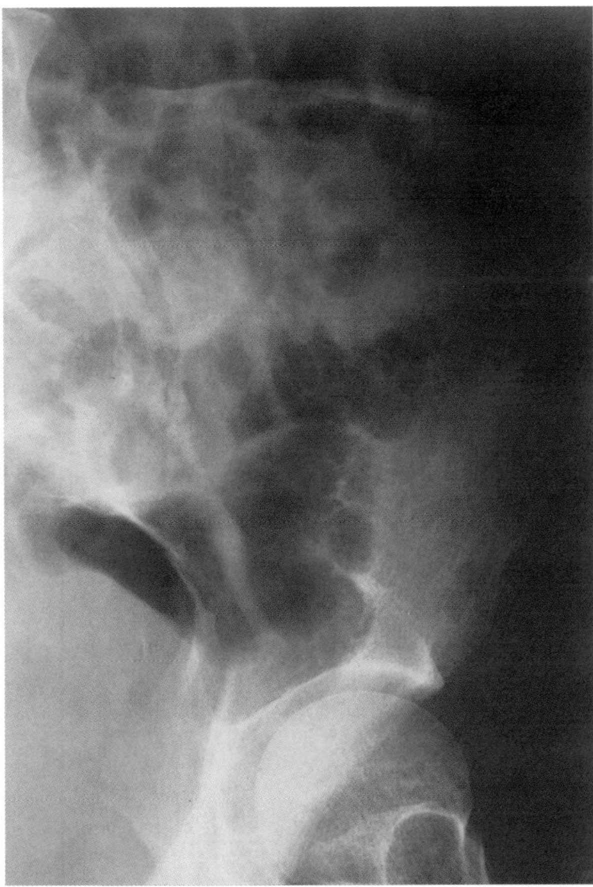

Fig. 44.11

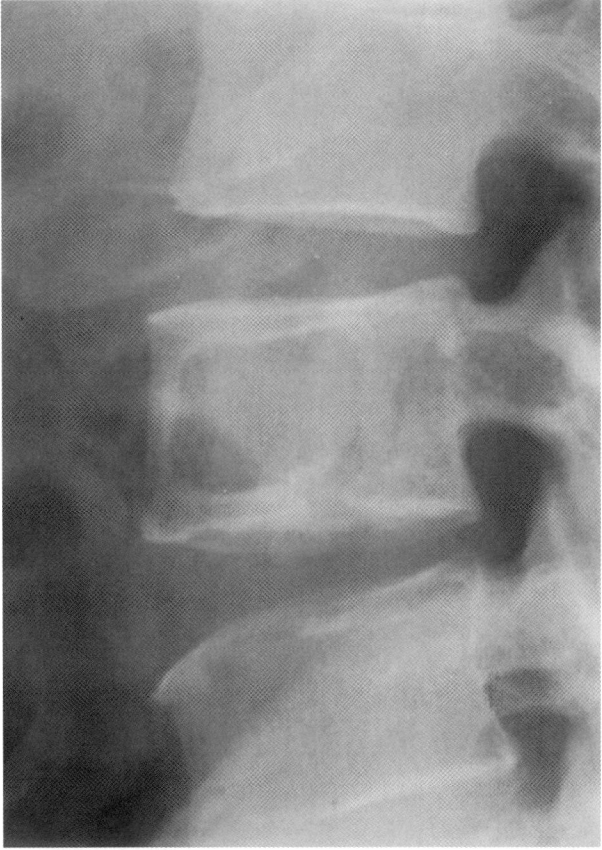

Fig. 44.13

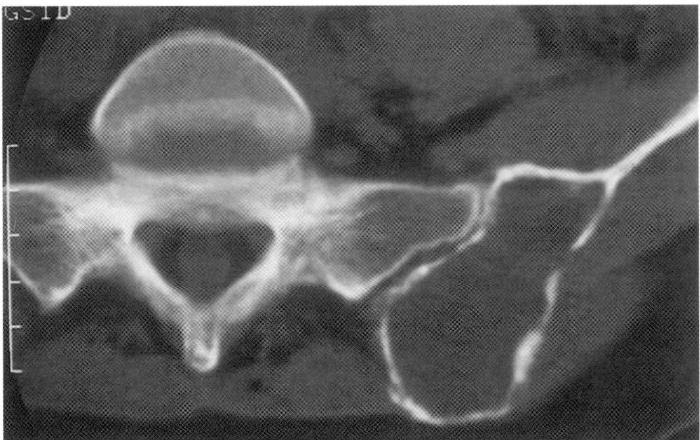

Fig. 44.12

Figs 44.11, 44.12 Cystic monostotic fibrous dysplasia of the pelvis.

Associated findings are deformities due to pathologic fractures and abnormal tubulation (Figs 44.23–44.26).

Bone scintigraphy shows an increased uptake of radioisotope[54–55] in 90% of cases, and arteriography demonstrates an intense diffuse capillary blush (Hudson 1987).

Figs 44.13, 44.14 Monostotic fibrous dysplasias of the lumbar spine.

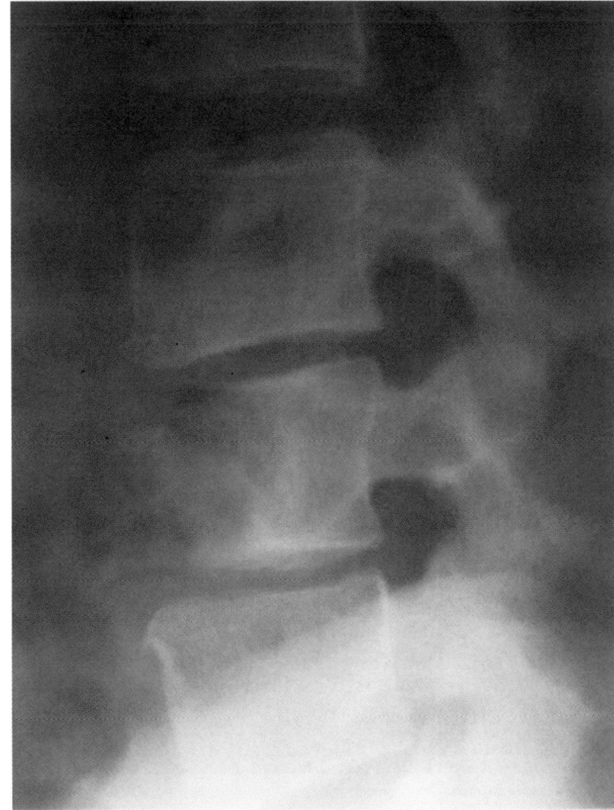

Fig. 44.14

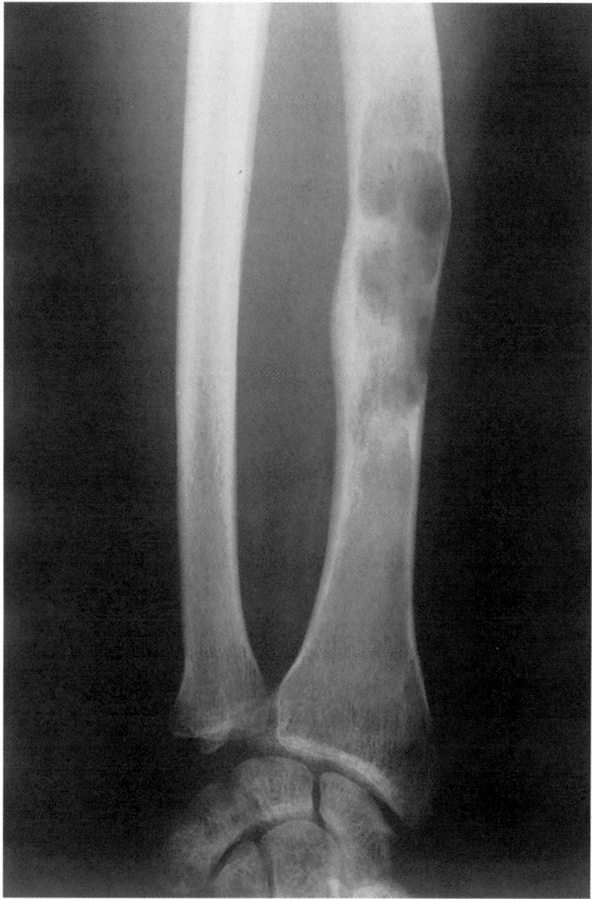

Fig. 44.15 Radiolucent monostotic fibrous dysplasia of the radius.

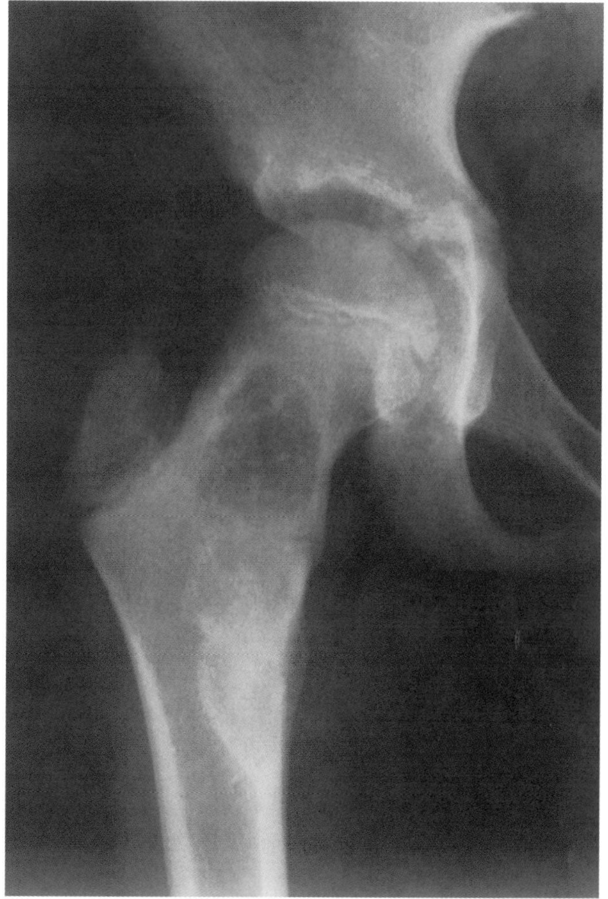

Fig. 44.16 Monostotic fibrous dysplasia of the femur: lucent area associated with a calcified part.

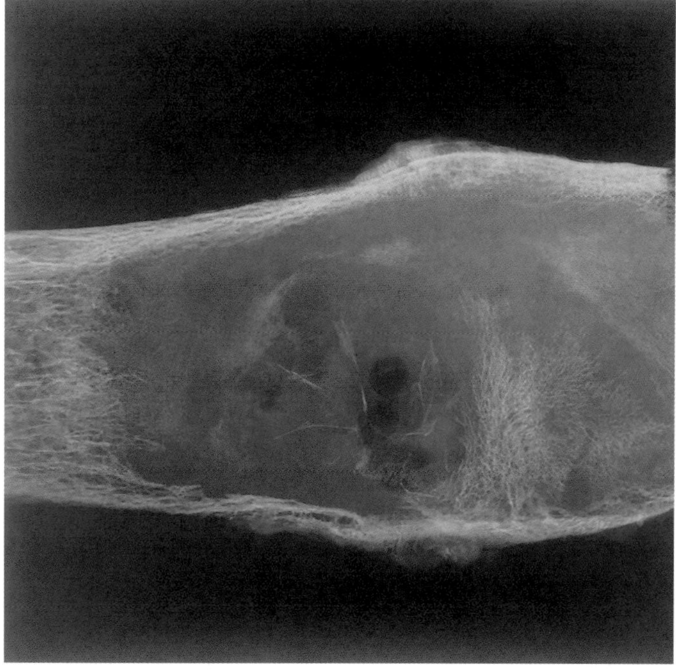

Fig. 44.17

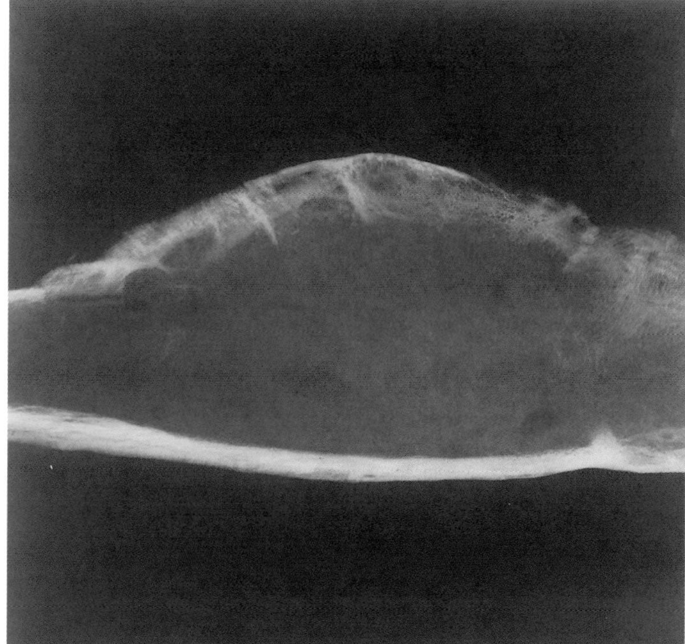

Fig. 44.18

Figs 44.17, 44.18 Monostotic fibrous dysplasia of ribs: X-rays of slabs demonstrating fine lesional bone formation.

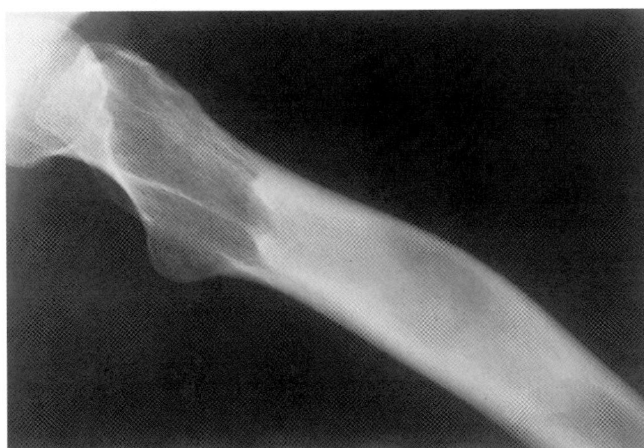

Fig. 44.19 Monostotic fibrous dysplasia of the tibia: 'ground glass' appearance.

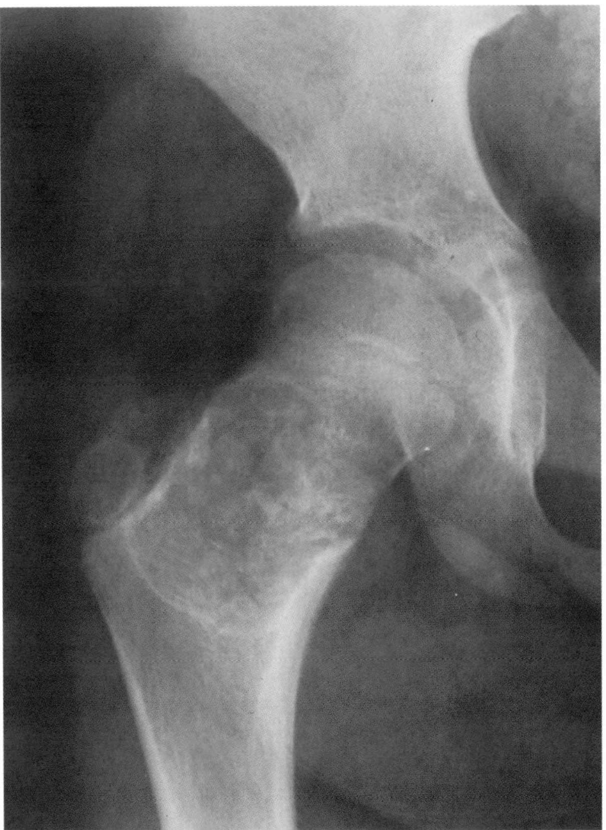

Fig. 44.21 Punctate calcifications in a monostotic fibrous dysplasia of the femur with a cartilaginous component.

Fig. 44.20 Monostotic fibrous dysplasia of the femur: huge calcification and sharply defined margins.

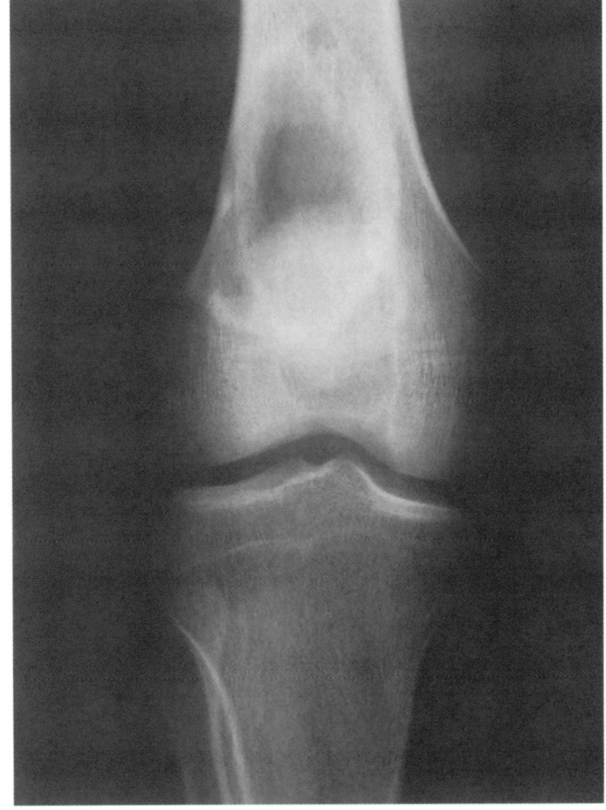

Fig. 44.22 Monostotic fibrous dysplasia of the femur: thick peripheral layer of reactive bone.

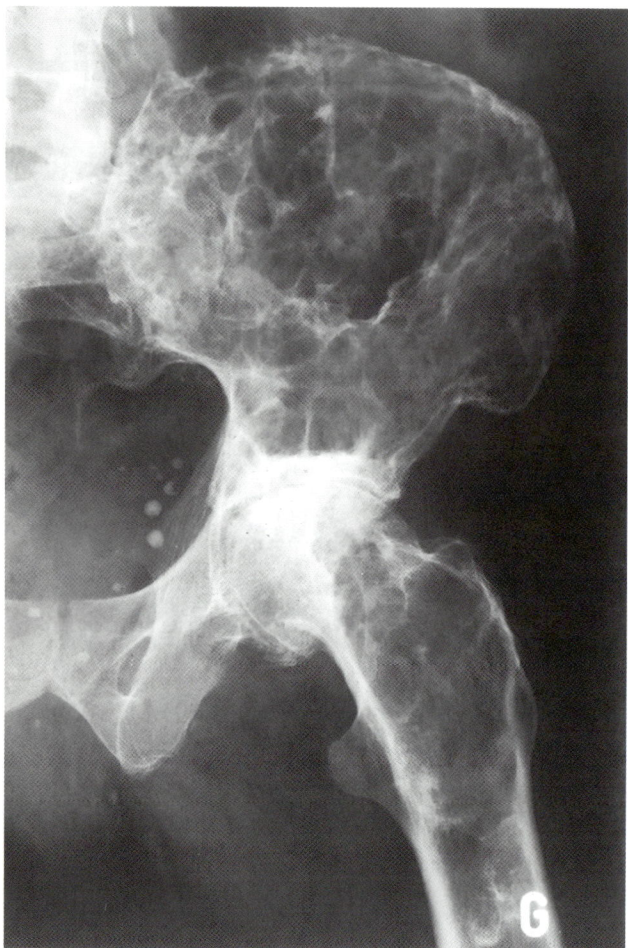

Fig. 44.23

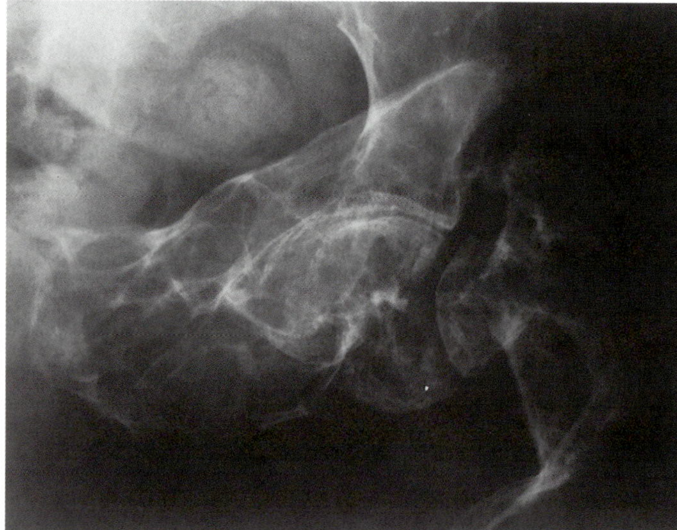

Fig. 44.24

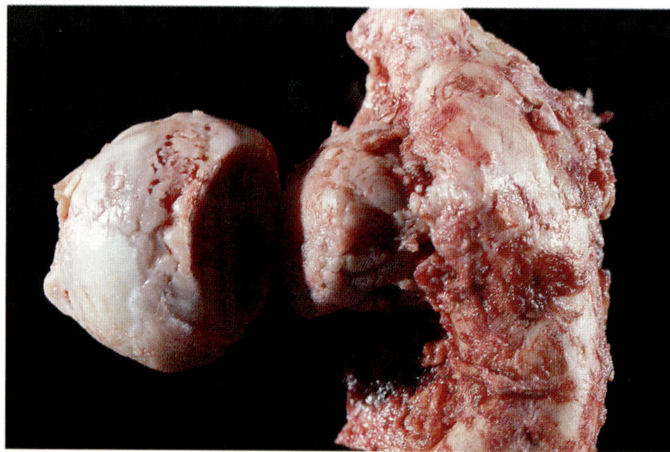

Fig. 44.25

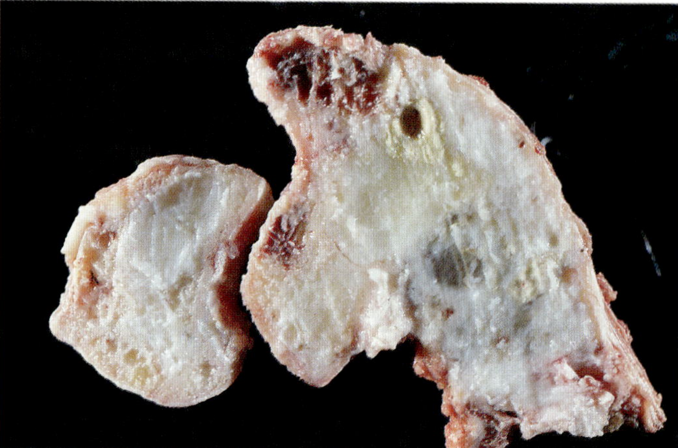

Fig. 44.26

Figs 44.23–44.26 Widespread involvement of the pelvis and femur in a case of polyostotic fibrous dysplasia, with deformities and pseudarthrosis.

CT scan is useful, demonstrating the 'ground glass' structure and the extent of bone involvement.[56]

On MRI, the signal intensity is variable, being low in T1, intermediate or high in T2-weighted images.[4,50,57] Fluid–fluid levels can be demonstrated on MRI or CT, corresponding to cystic degeneration with serous fluid and clot or to secondary aneurysmal bone formation.[58–61] Cystic changes, particularly frequent in rib locations,[62] may induce a rapid enlargement, mimicking malignant changes.[58,63] Rare cases may exhibit cortical bony destruction and a soft tissue mass well demonstrated on CT scans and MRI.[64]

GROSS PATHOLOGY

Bone is replaced by a grayish-white, firm, fibrous tissue, more or less gritty (Figs 44.25–44.28). Small or large cystic cavities filled with a serous fluid may be found. Cartilage foci are occasionally present, more often in the polyostotic form and especially in the proximal femur.[4] The cortex is thickened and expanded and exhibits internal ridges or is thinned and eroded but with intact periosteum.

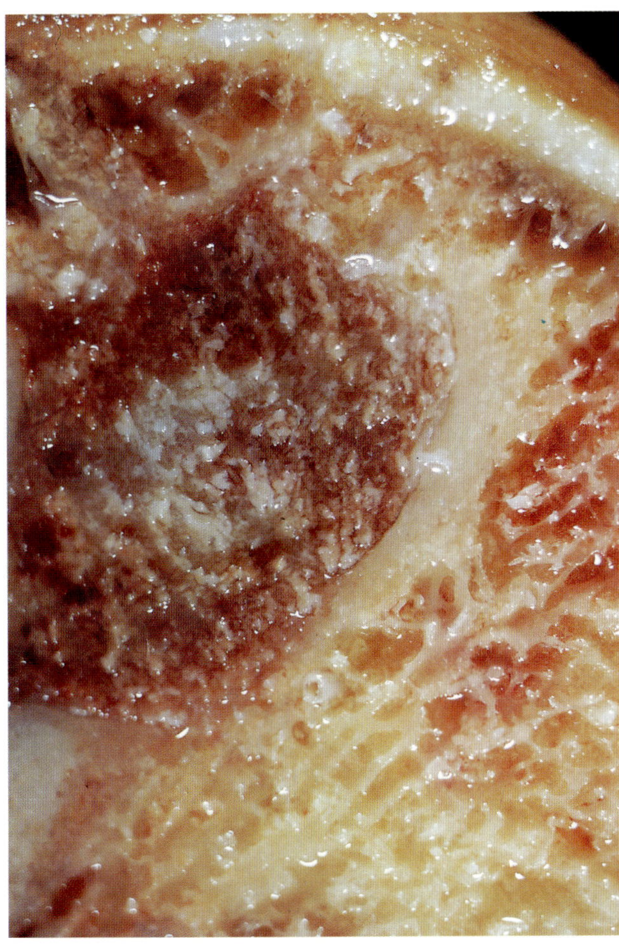

Fig. 44.27

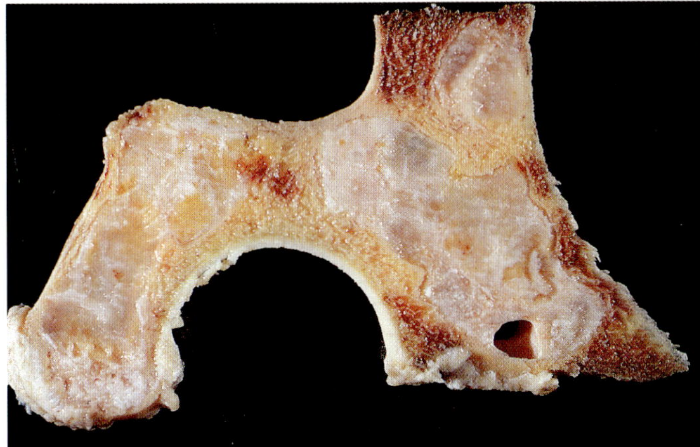

Fig. 44.28

Figs 44.27, 44.28 Polyostotic fibrous dysplasia (femur and ilium).

HISTOPATHOLOGY

The fibrous stroma is composed of small spindle cells with an oval nucleus and indistinct cytoplasmic borders. In younger patients, it may be quite cellular, but there is no mitotic activity. Cells may be arranged in bundles, but there is no real pattern of organization of the fibrous tissue. In some areas, it may be loose, with plump, stellate cells (Schajowicz 1994).

In the fibrous stroma, newly formed trabeculae of immature bone or osteoid of different sizes are irregularly distributed, appearing as round islands, curved or slender serpiginous forms or irregular networks, described as Chinese characters or 'alphabet soup' (Figs 44.29–44.37).

Immature bone appears to arise directly out of the connective tissue stroma. Osteoblastic rimming is not a feature of fibrous dysplasia, but osteoblasts can frequently be seen on the surface of trabeculae, in limited areas.[4,65] Trabeculae may be bordered by wide osteoid seams (Milgram 1990), but do not mature entirely to lamellar bone; even if some degree of lamellar bone formation is found (Huvos 1991), the architecture is never that of normal lamellar bone.[4] Some trabeculae may be partially resorbed by osteoclasts. In different cases, bone production may be very important or the fibrous tissue may predominate.

The fibrous stroma can exhibit a pinwheel or storiform pattern,[4,65] myxoid change, especially near cyst formation, small groups of foam cells or giant cells, usually associated with hemorrhage (Figs 44.38–44.42).

Older lesions show a more dense and sometimes hyalinized tissue, much less cellular, with prominent cement lines or even a mosaic pattern in bone (Fig. 44.43).

Foci of hyaline cartilage are found mostly in polyostotic forms (10–15% of cases) (Figs 44.44, 44.45). In a lesion complicated by a pathologic fracture, reactive new bone trabeculae have prominent osteoblastic rimming; the periosteal callus is usually normal, but there is poor endosteal callus formation.

HISTOCHEMISTRY

Alkaline phosphatase activity has been found in fibrocytic cells, mostly in the regions of bone formation.[66–69] Acid phosphatase is restricted to the very few osteoclasts.[69]

CYTOGENETICS

Cytogenetic analysis of short-term cultures has shown multiple clonal structural rearrangements with evidence of clonal evolution, suggesting a tumoral process resulting from somatic mutations,[70] but other studies demonstrate only numerical changes. The significance of chromosomal findings is unclear.[71,72]

ELECTRON MICROSCOPY

The cells of the fibrous stroma resemble fibroblasts and

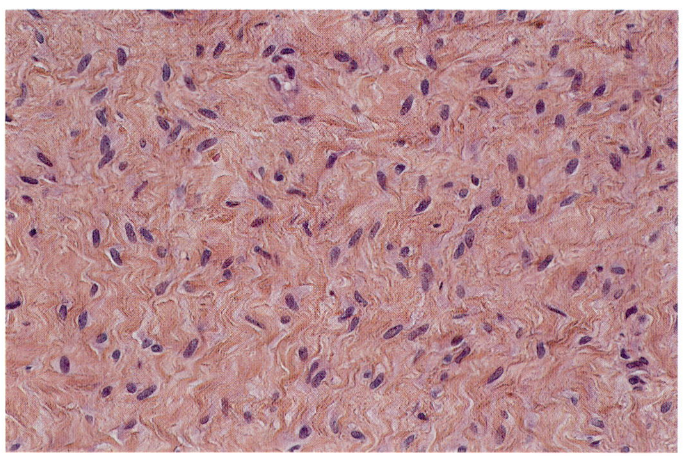

Fig. 44.29

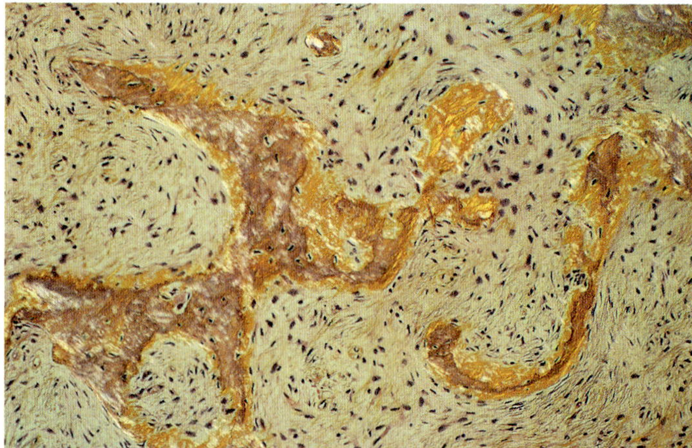

Fig. 44.31

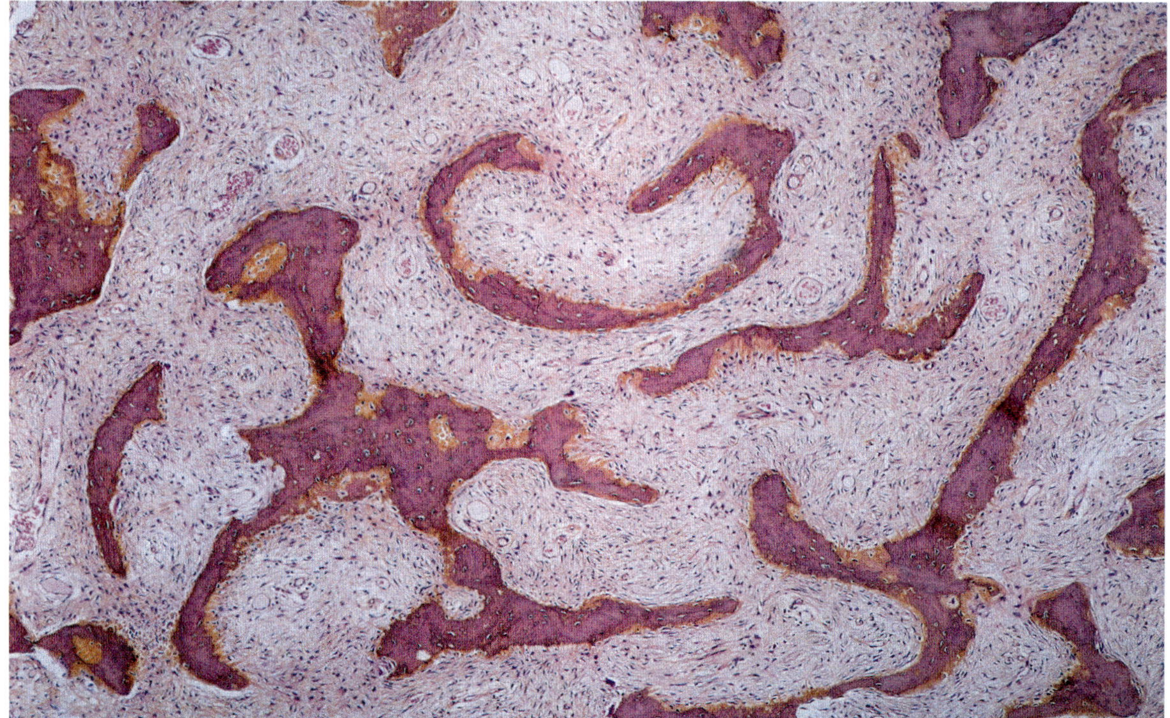

Fig. 44.30

Figs 44.29–44.37
Fibrous dysplasia:
fibrous stroma made of
regular small spindle
cells with aspects of the
bone trabeculae
appearing as irregular
networks or round
islands (Figs 44.31 and
44.33: polarized light).

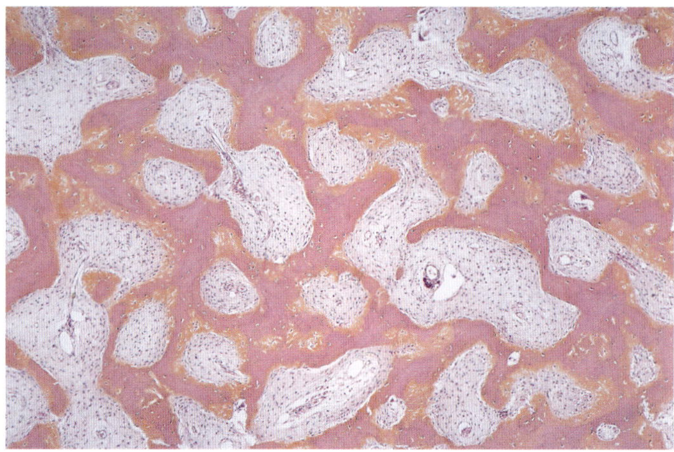

Fig. 44.32

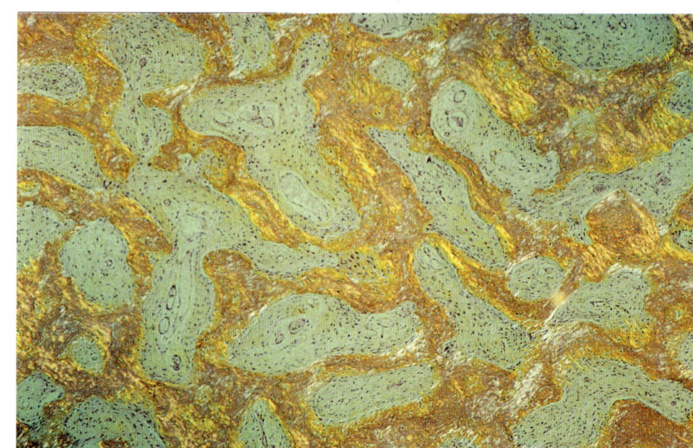

Fig. 44.33

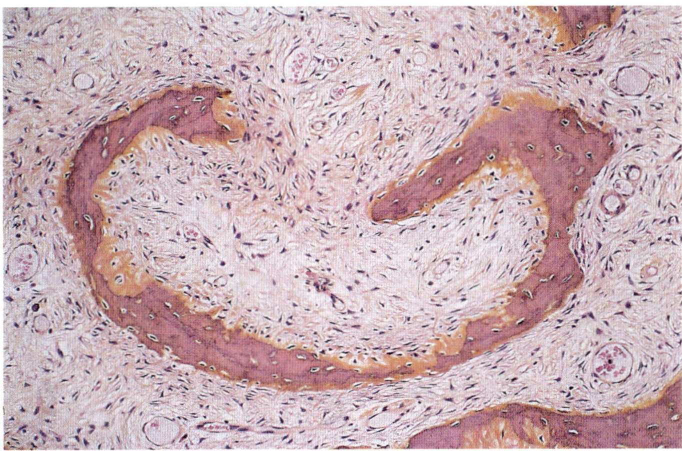

Fig. 44.34

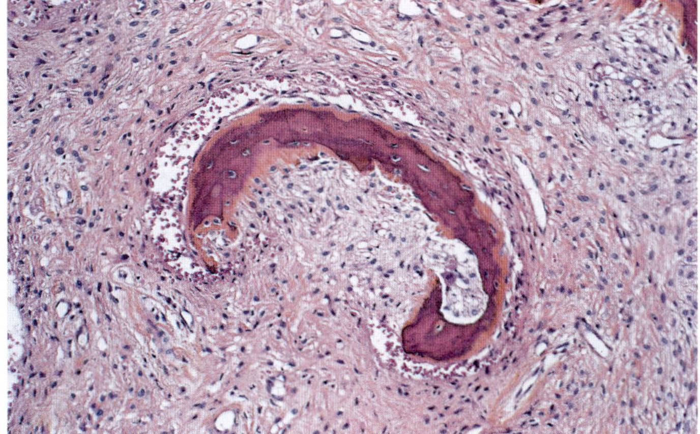

Fig. 44.35

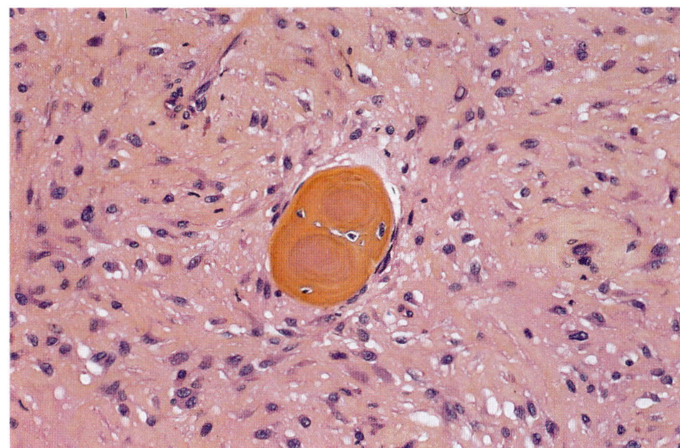

Fig. 44.36

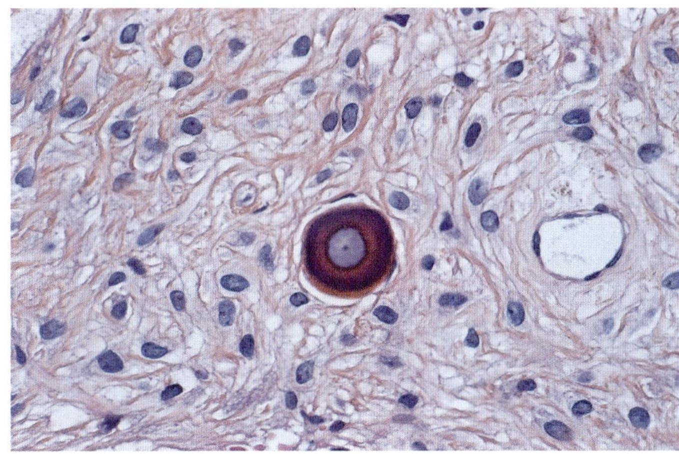

Fig. 44.37

myofibroblasts, with many intermediate cells. Some of them contain intracytoplasmic collagen.[73,74]

Besides normal collagen fibers, densely packed, very fine fibrillar structures without clearcut periodical crossbanding may indicate retardation of collagen maturation.[69]

The cells lining osteoid resemble fibroblasts, but are involved in the process of bone formation.[74,75] The immature woven bone mineralization is mediated by matrix vesicles.[74]

Ultrastructural findings corroborate the views of Lichtenstein, fibrous dysplasia being an anomaly of the bone-forming mesenchyme with formation of abnormal osteoblasts, resembling the early stages of membranous ossification.[74]

VARIANTS OF FIBROUS DYSPLASIA

'Fibrous dysplasia protuberans' is the term recently proposed for some lesions which erode the cortex and protrude beyond the normal bone, mimicking a surface lesion of bone.[76] The rare cases reported involve the tibia,

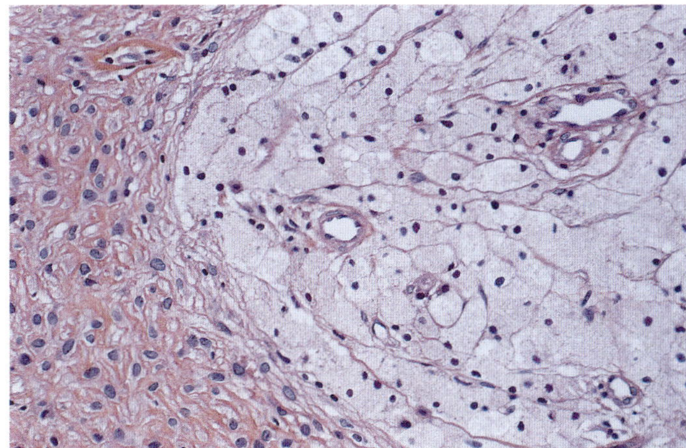

Fig. 44.38 Monostotic fibrous dysplasia of the femur: infiltration by foam cells.

rib and phalanx[48,76] (Fig. 44.46). The periphery of the exophytic mass may be covered by a fibrocartilaginous cap-like structure.[76]

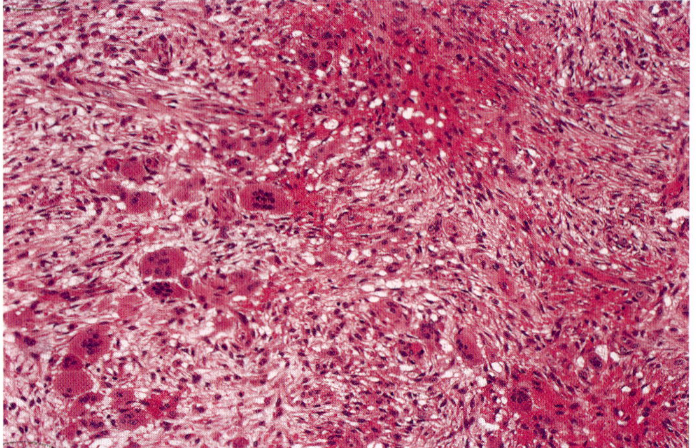

Fig. 44.39

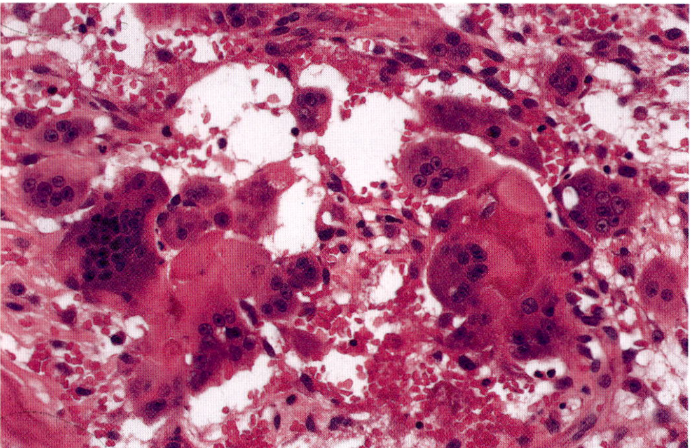

Fig. 44.40

Figs 44.39, 44.40 Giant cells in fibrous dysplasia.

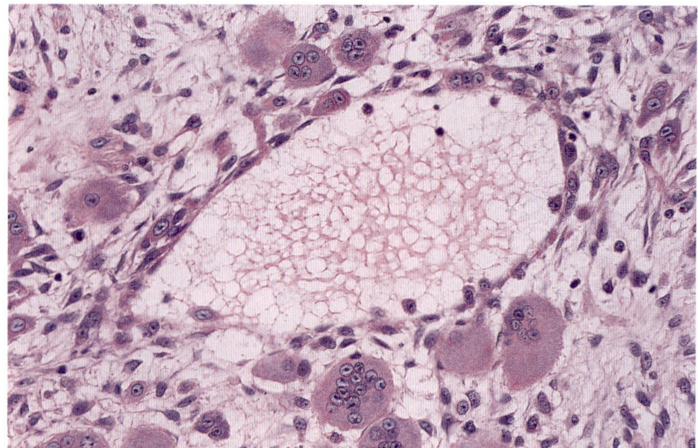

Fig. 44.41

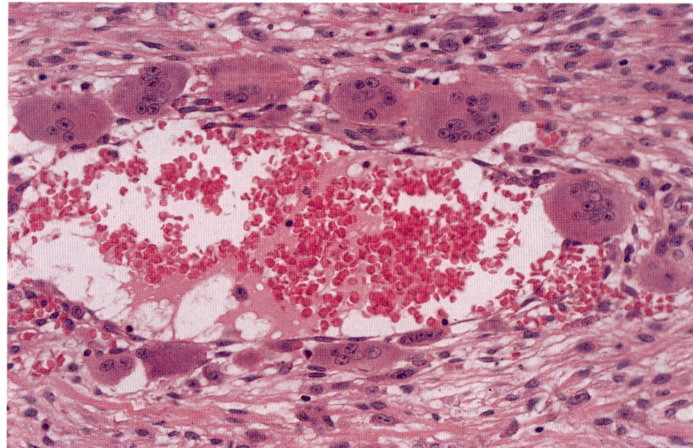

Fig. 44.42

Figs 44.41, 44.42 Fibrous dysplasia: giant cells around vascular spaces, presumably corresponding to early aneurysmal bone cyst-like changes.

Some fibroosseous lesions of the proximal femur, most often asymptomatic, have been termed '*liposclerosing myxofibrous tumors*'.[77] Some of the histological findings are similar to fibrous dysplasia – 'ground glass' structure, sclerotic borders and cystic changes – but aspects include non-ossifying fibroma-like areas, lipomatous territories, pseudo-Paget bone, necrotic fat with ischemic woven bone and foci of hyaline cartilage.[77]

Cartilage islands are common in fibrous dysplasia, particularly in polyostotic forms;[78] some cases may present extensive cartilage formation[78–80] and grossly the tissue of fibrous dysplasia may be entirely cartilaginous.[65]

Fibrous dysplasia with a massive cartilaginous component has been named *fibrocartilaginous dysplasia* (Unni 1996) or fibrochondrodysplasia[79–82] and is mostly found in the proximal femur and tibia.[83] Histologically, the hyaline cartilage islands may present a columnar arrangement of cartilage cells like the pattern of a growth plate, with enchondral ossification.[78,83] Cartilage islands arise as developmental 'rests' from the epiphyseal cartilage[78] and

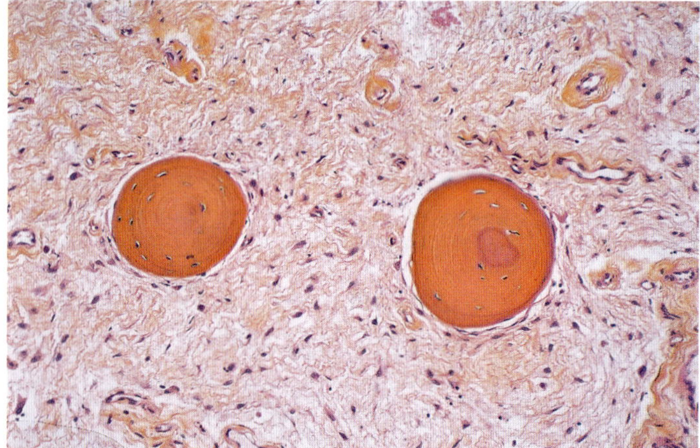

Fig. 44.43 Monostotic fibrous dysplasia of the femur: old lesion with a lesser cellularity of the fibrous stroma.

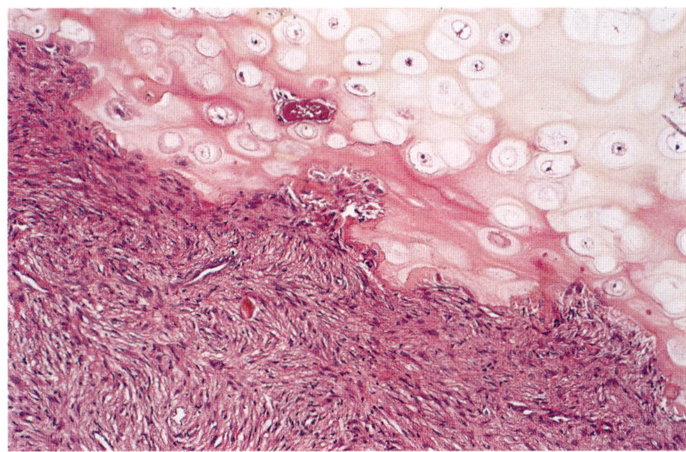

Fig. 44.44

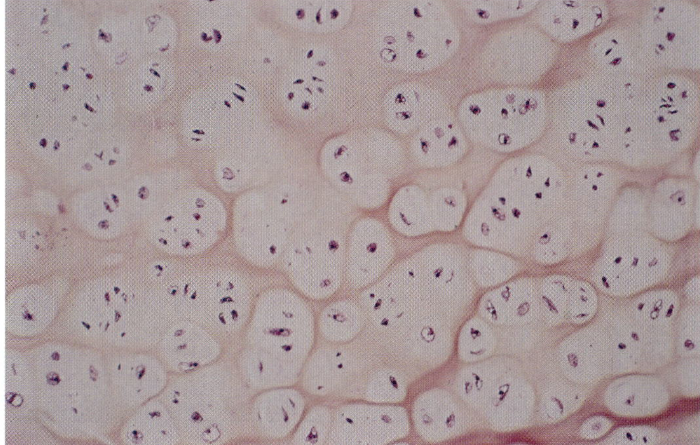

Fig. 44.45

Figs 44.44, 44.45 Monostotic fibrous dysplasia of the femur with a cartilaginous component.

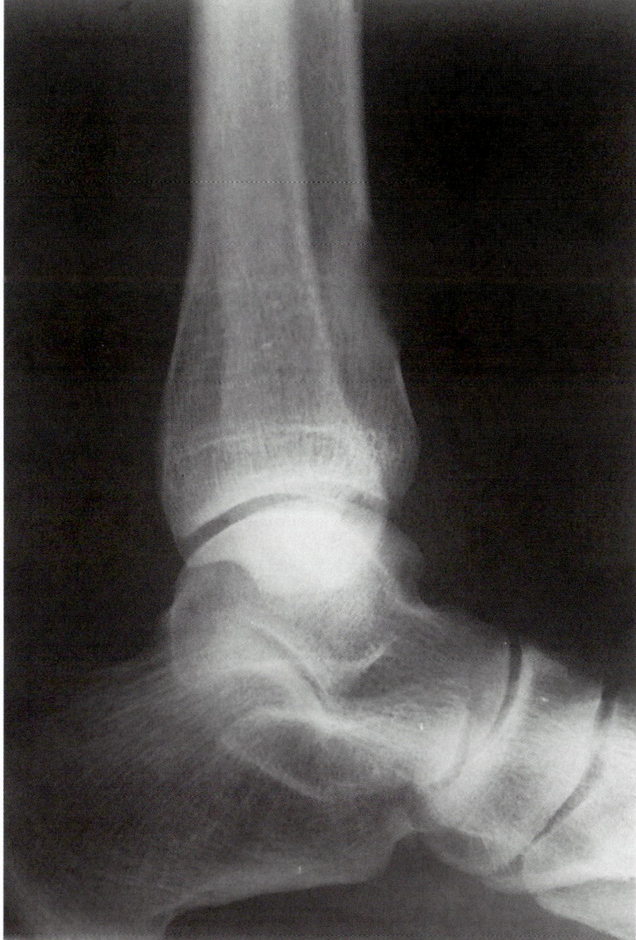

Fig. 44.46 Monostotic fibrous dysplasia of the tibia protruding on the surface of bone.

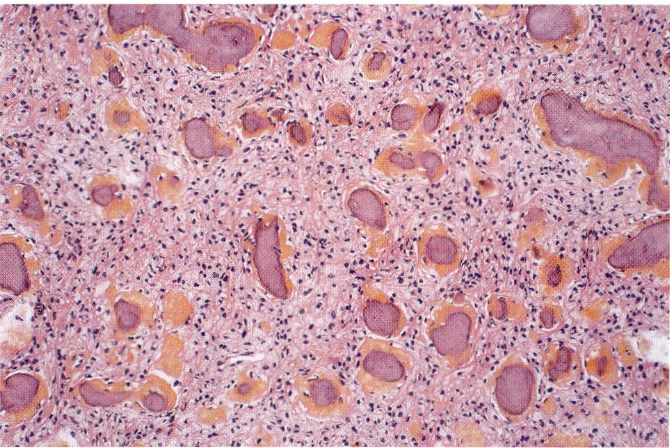

Fig. 44.47 Typical monostotic fibrous dysplasia of the femur exhibiting, in some fields, numerous calcified spherules.

similar appearances have been reported in patients with osteogenesis imperfecta.[84]

The cartilage formation has to be differentiated from fracture callus and from rare chondrosarcomas arising in fibrous dysplasia.[85,86]

Calcified spherules exhibiting concentric lamellations may be found in some areas of fibrous dysplasia[87] (Fig. 44.47). Lesions with an overwhelming number of calcified spherules have been reported under the names of ossifying fibroma,[88] cementifying fibroma or cementoma,[89,90] cementifying fibroma-like lesions,[91] cementofibrous dysplasia,[92] fibroosseous lesions[93] and cementoossifying fibromas[94] (Figs 44.48–44.53).

Most patients are adolescents or young adults, with no sex predominance.[93,94] The lesions may be asymptomatic or painful, being reported in the shafts of long bones, craniofacial bones, spine and pelvis; clinical and radiographic findings are very similar to fibrous dysplasia.[94]

Histologically, a dense fibrous stroma is made of spindle-shaped cells without nuclear pleomorphism or mitotic activity. Many cement-like globular structures are isolated or aggregated in clusters, without osteoblastic rimming. Many are at least partially calcified and some may merge

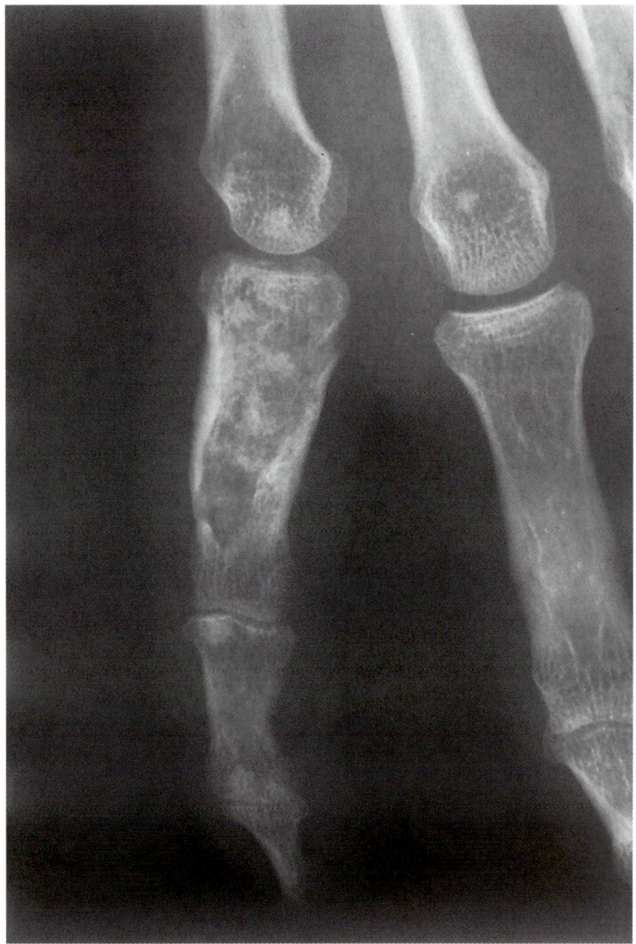

Fig. 44.48

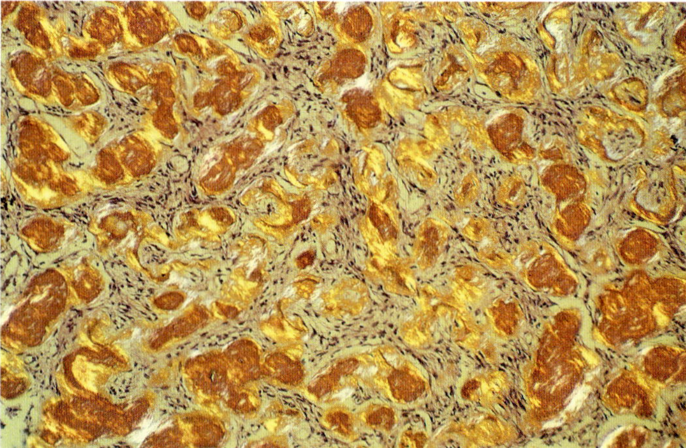

Fig. 44.50

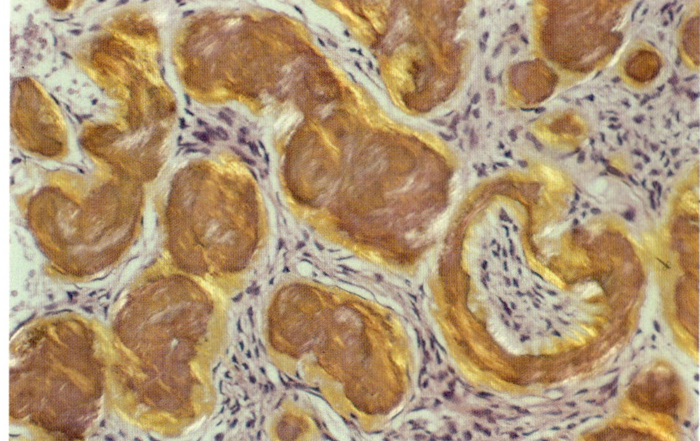

Fig. 44.51

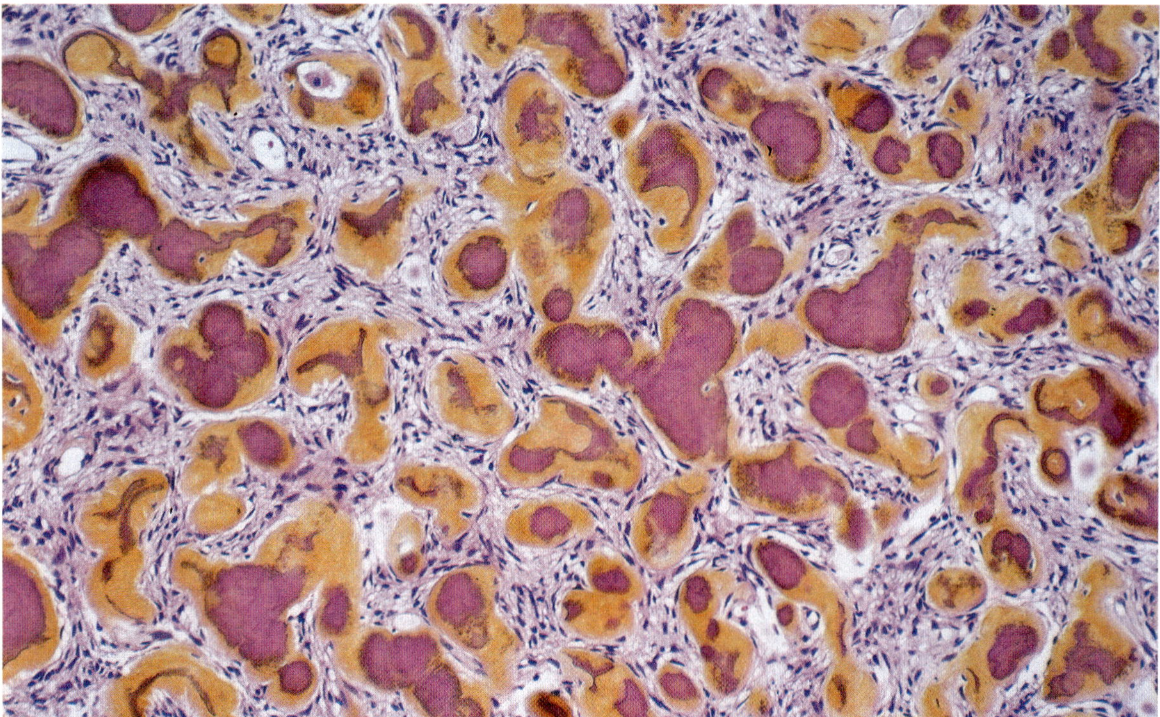

Fig. 44.49

Figs 44.48–44.51 Cementifying fibroma-like lesion of a phalanx (Figs 44.50 and 44.51: polarized light).

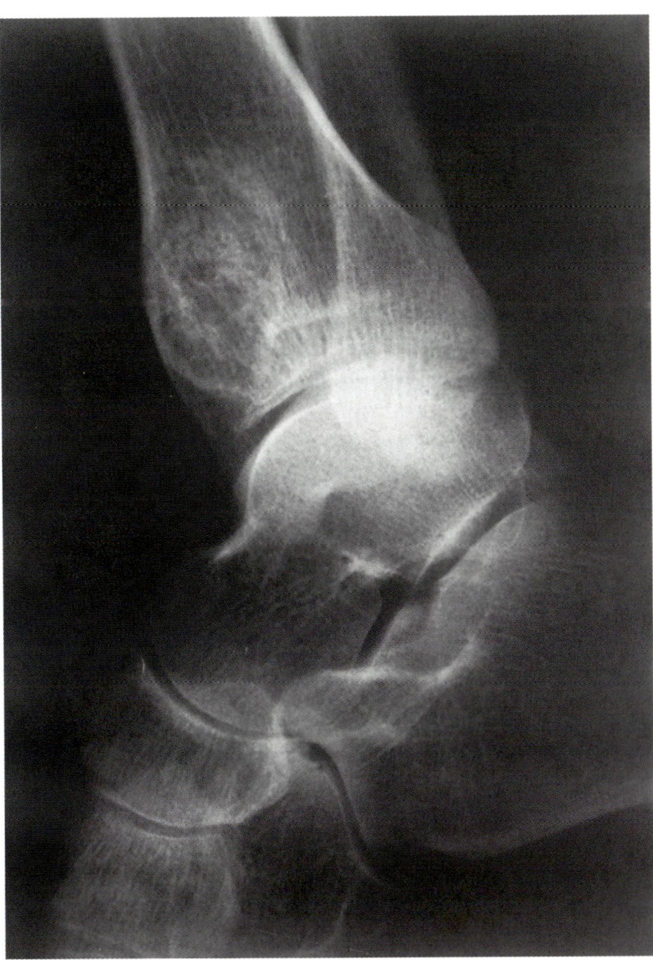

Fig. 44.52

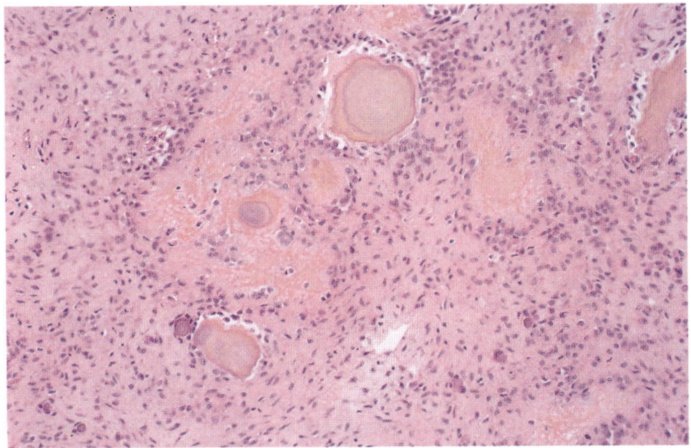

Fig. 44.53

Figs 44.52, 44.53 Cementifying fibroma-like lesion of the distal tibia.

with more elongated trabeculae of bone having the pattern of fibrous dysplasia.[93,94] Ultrastructural findings are also very similar to those of fibrous dysplasia.[91,93] This peculiar form of fibrous dysplasia with spherules having the histo-

logical features of bone should not be regarded as cementoma or cementifying fibroma.[94]

The treatment is curettage and bone grafting.

CLINICAL COURSE, TREATMENT AND PROGNOSIS

The clinical course is variable and some monostotic lesions may heal spontaneously.[95] In most cases, there is a progression up to the age of puberty, followed by stabilization or progression at a slower rate.

Surgical treatment is performed to prevent or treat pathologic fractures or to correct deformities. Segmental resection may be performed in some monostotic lesions. Radiation therapy increases the risk of malignant transformation (Schajowicz 1994).

The incidence of malignant transformation is about 0.4–0.5% of cases,[96–98] the highest incidence of 4% being related to Albright's syndrome;[96,98] sarcomatous degeneration is found more commonly in the polyostotic form.[96,99] Malignancy may occur without prior irradiation,[100] but in half the cases radiation therapy is implicated.

The mean interval from the time of initial diagnosis is 13.5 years.[96] The sites of malignancy reflect the distribution of bones involved by fibrous dysplasia.[26,101] Clinical symptoms are pain, swelling, a soft tissue mass or a pathologic fracture.[97,102]

Reported forms of tumors are mostly osteosarcomas and fibrosarcomas, followed by chondrosarcomas, malignant fibrous histiocytomas,[102,103] giant cell sarcomas (presumably osteosarcomas) and rhabdomyosarcomas. Rare cases of clear cell chondrosarcoma[101] and mesenchymal chondrosarcoma[104] have been described. Chondrosarcomas[105–107] have to be differentiated from the large amounts of cartilage found in extensive fibrochondrodysplasia.[65,81,108]

Unusual presentations are the occurrence of osteosarcomas at an exceptionally early age[109] or in bony regeneration, following Ilizarov femoral lengthening through fibrous dysplasia.[110]

In situ hybridization has shown that fibroblastic cells of fibrous dysplasia express high levels of c-fos protooncogene,[111] which may be the first step in the carcinogenesis of bone sarcomas.

DIFFERENTIAL DIAGNOSIS

A desmoplastic fibroma usually has a greater spindle cell component with bundles of collagen and is devoid of metaplastic bone formation.

Some fields of fibrous dysplasia may resemble a non-ossifying fibroma[112] and a misdiagnosis of malignant fibrous histiocytoma has been reported;[113] both lesions have no characteristic bone formation.

Intraosseous, well-differentiated osteosarcoma may present small, round islands of tumoral bone production, as in parosteal osteosarcoma, but tumor cells are elongated, with focal nuclear pleomorphism and long arrays of tumoral bone distributed in a parallel fashion.

Some authors believed osteofibrous dysplasia was only a different expression of fibrous dysplasia,[114] but it is now viewed as a separate entity. Histologically, the woven bone formation is associated with a prominent osteoblastic rimming and a zonal pattern with maturation to lamellar bone in peripheral areas.

In tibial locations, on imaging and also histologically, fibrous dysplasia has to be differentiated from adamantinoma. Fibrous dysplasia occurs in younger patients, with anterior bowing and a 'ground glass' appearance of the matrix;[115] there is no moth-eaten destruction. Histological-

ly, in adamantinoma, separate foci made of fibrous tissue with osteoid and bone formation have been considered as areas of fibrous dysplasia;[112,116,117] more recently, they have been viewed as an integral part of the adamantinoma,[118,119] maybe reflecting a mesenchymal differentiation of the tumor.[120] This component may predominate over the epithelial islands and necessitates a thorough histological sampling of the lesion.[113,114]

In ribs, some symmetrical lesions named fibroosseous dysplasias may present as fusiform expansions with a variable degree of calcification.[121] Exhibiting xanthomatous macrophages, hemosiderin deposits, cholesterol crystals and trabeculae of woven bone with peripheral maturation, they presumably correspond to a healing process following intramedullary hemorrhage due to subclinical trauma.[121]

REFERENCES

1. Lichtenstein L. Polyostotic fibrous dysplasia. Arch Surg 1938: 36: 874–898
2. Lichtenstein L, Jaffe H L. Fibrous dysplasia of bone. Arch Pathol 1942: 33: 777–816
3. Reed R J. Fibrous dysplasia of bone: a review of 25 cases. Arch Pathol 1963: 75: 480–495
4. Kransdorf M J, Moser R P Jr, Gilkey F W. Fibrous dysplasia. Radiographics 1990: 10: 519–537
5. MacMahon H E. Albright's syndrome – thirty years later (polyostotic fibrous dysplasia). Pathol Annu 1971: 6: 81–146
6. Lever E G, Pettingale K W. Albright's syndrome associated with a soft-tissue myxoma and hypophosphataemic osteomalacia. J Bone Joint Surg (Br) 1983: 65: 621–626
7. Dent C E, Gertner J M. Hypophosphataemic osteomalacia in fibrous dysplasia. Q J Med 1976: 45: 411–420
8. McArthur R G, Hayles A B, Lambert P W. Albright's syndrome with rickets. Mayo Clin Proc 1979: 54: 313–320
9. Park Y K, Unni K K, Beabout J W, Hodgson S F. Oncogenic osteomalacia: a clinicopathologic study of 17 bone lesions. J Korean Med Sci 1994: 9: 289–298
10. West R, Huvos A G, Lane J M. Desmoplastic fibroma of bone arising in fibrous dysplasia. Am J Clin Pathol 1983: 79: 630–633
11. Bridge J A, Rosenthal H, Sanger W G, Neff J R. Desmoplastic fibroma arising in fibrous dysplasia. Chromosomal analysis and review of the literature. Clin Orthop 1989: 247: 272–278
12. Gatwood C M B, Besterly J R. Coexistent polyostotic fibrous dysplasia and eosinophilic granuloma of bone. Am J Roentgenol Radium Ther Nucl Med 1966: 97: 110–117
13. De Smet A A, Travers H, Neff J R. Case report 207. Giant cell reparative granuloma of left femur arising in polyostotic fibrous dysplasia. Skeletal Radiol 1982: 8: 314–318
14. Diercks R L, Sauter A J, Mallens W M. Aneurysmal bone cyst in association with fibrous dysplasia. J Bone Joint Surg (Br) 1986: 68: 144–148
15. Mintz M C, Dalinka M K, Schmidt R. Aneurysmal bone cyst arising in fibrous dysplasia during pregnancy. Radiology 1987: 165: 549–550
16. Henschen F. Fall von ostitis fibrosa mit multiplen tumoren in der umgebenden muskulatur. Vehr Dtsch Ges Pathol 1926: 21: 93–97
17. Krogius A. Ein fall von ostitis fibrosa mit multiplen fibromyxomatosen muskeltumoren. Acta Chir Scand 1928: 64: 465–472
18. Uehlinger E. Osteofibrosis deformans juvenilis (Polyostotische fibröse Dysplasie Jaffe-Lichtenstein). Virchows Arch Pathol Anat 1940: 306: 255–299
19. Braunwarth K. Gleidizeltiges Aufreten von fibröser Dysplasie (Jaffé-Lichtenstein) und extraosalen fibromyxomen. Fortschr Roentgenstrahl 1953: 78: 589–593
20. Mazabraud A, Semat P, Roze R. A propos de l'association des fibromyxomes des tissus mous à la dysplasie fibreuse des os. Presse Med 1967: 75: 2223–2228
21. Leung T K, Vauzelle J L, Patricot L M, Lejeune E, Queneau P. Etude ultrastructurale et cytochimique d'un myxome musculaire associé à une dysplasie fibreuse. Ann Anat Pathol (Paris) 1971: 16: 417–428
22. Wirth W A, Leavitt D, Enzinger F M. Multiple intramuscular myxomas. Another extraskeletal manifestation of fibrous dysplasia. Cancer 1971: 27: 1167–1173
23. Ireland D C, Soule E H, Ivins J C. Myxoma of somatic soft tissues. Mayo Clin Proc 1973: 48: 401–410
24. Logel R J. Recurrent intramuscular myxoma associated with Albright syndrome. J Bone Joint Surg (Am) 1976: 58: 565–568
25. Blasier R D, Ryan J R, Schaldenbrand M F. Multiple myxomata of soft tissue associated with polyostotic fibrous dysplasia. Clin Orthop 1986: 206: 211–214
26. Witkin G B, Guilford W B, Siegal G P. Osteogenic sarcoma and soft tissue myxoma in a patient with fibrous dysplasia and hemoglobins. J Baltimore S Clin Orthop 1986: 204: 245–252
27. Biagini R, Ruggieri P, Boriani S, Picci P. The Mazabraud syndrome: case report and review of the literature. Ital J Orthop Traumatol 1987: 13: 105–111
28. Glass-Royal M C, Nelson M C, Albert F, Lack E E, Bogumill G P. Case report 557. Solitary intramuscular myxoma in a patient with polyostotic fibrous dysplasia. Skeletal Radiol 1989: 18: 392–398
29. Sundaram M, McDonald D J, Merenda G. Intramuscular myxoma: a rare but important association with fibrous dysplasia of bone. AJR 1989: 153: 107–108
30. Gianoutsos M P, Thompson J F, Marsden F W. Mazabraud's syndrome: intramuscular myxoma associated with fibrous dysplasia of bone. Aust NZ J Surg 1990: 60: 825–828
31. Gober G A, Nicholas R W. Case report 800. Skeletal fibrous dysplasia associated with intramuscular myxoma (Mazabraud's syndrome). Skeletal Radiol 1993: 22: 452–455
32. Prayson M A, Leeson M C. Soft-tissue myxomas and fibrous dysplasia of bone. Clin Orthop 1993: 291: 222–228
33. Aoki T, Kouho H, Hisaoka M, Hashimoto H, Nakata H, Sakai A. Intramuscular myxoma with fibrous dysplasia. Pathol Int 1995: 45: 165–171
34. Savage P E, Stoker D J. Fibrous dysplasia of the femoral neck. Skeletal Radiol 1984: 11: 119–123
35. Nakashima Y, Kotoura Y, Nagashima T, Yamamuro T, Hamashima Y. Monostotic fibrous dysplasia in the femoral neck. Clin Orthop 1984: 191: 242–248
36. Zimmer J F, Dahlin D C, Clough D G, Clagett O T. Fibrous dysplasia of bone. Analysis of 15 cases of surgically verified costal fibrous dysplasia. J Thorac Surg 1956: 31: 488–496
37. Resnik C S, Lininger J R. Monostotic fibrous dysplasia of the cervical spine. Radiology 1984: 151: 49–50

38. Hayter R G, Becton J L. Fibrous dysplasia of a metacarpal. J Hand Surg (Am) 1984: 9: 587–589

39. Gropper P T, Mah J Y, Gelfant B M, Bell H M. Monostotic fibrous dysplasia of the hand. J Hand Surg (Br) 1985: 10: 404–406

40. Rosenblum B, Overby C, Levine M, Handler M, Sprecher S. Monostotic fibrous dysplasia of the thoracic spine. Spine 1987: 12: 939–942

41. Nigrisoli M. Monostotic fibrous dysplasia of the spine. Ital J Orthop Traumatol 1987: 13: 273–278

42. Kahn A 3rd, Rosenberg P S. Monostotic fibrous dysplasia of the thoracic spine. Spine 1988: 13: 592–593

43. Troop J K, Herring J A. Monostotic fibrous dysplasia of the lumbar spine. J Pediatr Orthop 1988: 8: 599–601

44. Stirrat A N, Fyfe I S, Fisher C J. Fibrous dysplasia of the axis. Spine 1989: 14: 243–245

45. Hu S S, Healey J H, Huvos A G. Fibrous dysplasia of the second cervical vertebra. J Bone Joint Surg (Am) 1990: 72: 781–783

46. Smith M D, Bohlman H H, Gideonse N. Fibrous dysplasia of the cervical spine. J Bone Joint Surg (Am) 1990: 72: 1254–1258

47. Ehara S, Kattapuram S V, Rosenberg A E. Fibrous dysplasia of the spine. Spine 1992: 17: 977–979

48. Vigorita V, D'Ambrosio F, Verde R, Kauderer C, Bryk E. Case report 784. Fibrous dysplasia of the second pedal digit. Skeletal Radiol 1993: 22: 441–443

49. Nabarro M N, Giblin P E. Monostotic fibrous dysplasia of the thoracic spine. Spine 1994: 19: 463–465

50. Hoffman K L, Bergman A G, Kohler S. Polyostotic fibrous dysplasia with severe pathologic compression fracture of L2. Skeletal Radiol 1995: 24: 160–162

51. Nixon G W, Condon V R. Epiphyseal involvement in polyostotic fibrous dysplasia. Radiology 1973: 106: 167–170

52. Heaston D K, Gelman M I. Case report 37. Fibrous dysplasia of the humerus. Skeletal Radiol 1977: 2: 61–64

53. Pratt A D, Felson B, Wiot J F, Paige M. Sequestrum formation in fibrous dysplasia. Am J Roentgenol Radium Ther Nucl Med 1969: 106: 162–165

54. Machida K, Makita K, Nishikawa J, Ohtake T, Ilio M. Scintigraphic manifestation of fibrous dysplasia. Clin Nucl Med 1986: 11: 426–429

55. Johns W D, Gupta S M, Kayani N. Scintigraphic evaluation of polyostotic fibrous dysplasia. Clin Nucl Med 1987: 12: 627–631

56. Daffner R H, Kirks D R, Gehweiler J A Jr, Heaston D K. Computed tomography of fibrous dysplasia. AJR 1982: 139: 943–948

57. Utz J A, Kransdorf M J, Jelinek J S, Moser R P Jr, Berrey B H. MR appearance of fibrous dysplasia. J Comput Assist Tomogr 1989: 13: 845–851

58. Simpson A H, Creasy T S, Williamson D M, Wilson D J, Spivey J S. Cystic degeneration of fibrous dysplasia masquerading as sarcoma. J Bone Joint Surg (Br) 1989: 71: 434–436

59. Tsai J C, Dalinka M K, Fallon M D, Zlatkin M B, Kressel H Y. Fluid–fluid level: a nonspecific finding in tumors of bone and soft tissue. Radiology 1990: 175: 779–782

60. Fisher A J, Totty W G, Kyriakos M. MR appearance of cystic fibrous dysplasia. J Comput Assist Tomogr 1994: 18: 315–318

61. Nguyen B D, Lugo-Olivieri C H, McCarthy E F, Frassica F J, Ma L D, Zerhouni E A. Fibrous dysplasia secondary aneurysmal bone cyst. Skeletal Radiol 1996: 25: 88–91

62. Malloy P C, Scott W W Jr, Hruban R H. Case report 769. Fibrous dysplasia. Skeletal Radiol 1993: 22: 66–69

63. De Iure F, Campanacci L. Clinical and radiographic progression of fibrous dysplasia: cystic change or sarcoma? Chir Organi Mov 1995: 80: 85–89

64. Yao L, Eckardt J J, Seeger L L. Fibrous dysplasia associated with cortical bony destruction: CT and MR findings. J Comput Assist Tomogr 1994: 18: 91–94

65. Unni K K, McLeod R A, Dahlin D C. Conditions that simulate primary neoplasms of bone. Pathol Annu 1980: 15 Pt 1: 91–131

66. Schajowicz F, Cabrini R L. Histochemical studies of bone in normal and pathological conditions. J Bone Joint Surg (Br) 1954: 36: 474–489

67. Changus G W. Osteoblastic hyperplasia of bone: histochemical appraisal of fibrous dysplasia of bone. Cancer 1957: 10: 1157–1161

68. Jeffree G M. Enzymes in fibroblastic lesions. J Bone Joint Surg (Br) 1972: 54: 535–546

69. Remagen W, Gudat F, Heitz P. Histochemical and electron-microscopic aspects of bone tumor diagnosis. Recent Results Cancer Res 1976: 54: 157–165

70. Mertens F, Albert A, Heim S et al. Clonal structural chromosome aberrations in fibrous dysplasia. Genes Chromosomes Cancer 1994: 11: 271–272

71. Tarkkanen M, Kaipainen A, Karaharju E et al. Cytogenetic study of 249 consecutive patients examined for a bone tumor. Cancer Genet Cytogenet 1993: 68: 1–21

72. Dal Cin P, Sciot R, Speleman F et al. Chromosome aberrations in fibrous dysplasia. Cancer Genet Cytogenet 1994: 77: 114–117

73. Ohira O. Electron microscopic studies of fibrous dysplasia. Nippon Seikeigeka Gakkai Zasshi 1981: 55: 497–507

74. Greco M A, Steiner G C. Ultrastructure of fibrous dysplasia of bone: a study of its fibrous, osseous and cartilaginous components. Ultrastruct Pathol 1986: 10: 55–66

75. Bertrand G, Minard M F, Simard C, Rebel A. Etude ultrastructurale d'un cas de dysplasie fibreuse monostotique. Ann Anat Pathol (Paris) 1978: 23: 81–89

76. Dorfman H D, Ishida T, Tsuneyoshi M. Exophytic variant of fibrous dysplasia (fibrous dysplasia protuberans). Hum Pathol 1994: 25: 1234–1237

77. Ragsdale B D. Polymorphic fibro-osseous lesions of bone: an almost site-specific diagnostic problem of the proximal femur. Hum Pathol 1993: 24: 505–512

78. Sanerkin N G, Watt I. Enchondromata with annular calcification in association with fibrous dysplasia. Br J Radiol 1981: 54: 1027–1033

79. Drolshagen L F, Reynolds W A, Marcus N W. Fibrocartilaginous dysplasia of bone. Radiology 1985: 156: 32

80. Hermann G, Klein M, Abdelwahab I F, Kenan S. Fibrocartilaginous dysplasia. Skeletal Radiol 1996: 25: 509–511

81. Pelzmann K S, Nagel D Z, Salyer W R. Case report 114. Polyostotic fibrous dysplasia and fibrochondrodysplasia. Skeletal Radiol 1980: 5: 116–118

82. Fauré C, Guichard J P, Ligerot A, Sirinelli D. Les formes cartilagineuses de la dysplasie fibreuse de Jaffé-Lichtenstein. J Radiol 1987: 68: 657–663

83. Ishida T, Dorfman H D. Massive chondroid differentiation in fibrous dysplasia of bone (fibrocartilaginous dysplasia). Am J Surg Pathol 1993: 17: 924–930

84. Goldman A B, Davidson D, Pavlov H, Bullough P G. 'Popcorn' calcifications: a prognostic sign in osteogenesis imperfecta. Radiology 1980: 136: 351–358

85. Huvos A G, Higinbotham N L, Miller T R. Bone sarcomas arising in fibrous dysplasia of bone. J Bone Joint Surg (Am) 1972: 54: 1047–1056

86. Dabska M, Buraczewski J. On malignant transformation in fibrous dysplasia of bone. Oncology 1972: 26: 369–383

87. Van Horn P E, Dahlin D C, Bickel W H. Fibrous dysplasia: a clinical pathologic study of orthopedic surgical cases. Proc Staff Meet Mayo Clin 1963: 38: 175–189

88. Sissons H A, Kancherla P L, Lehman W B. Ossifying fibroma of bone: report of two cases. Bull Hosp Jt Dis Orthop Inst 1983: 43: 1–13

89. Kolar J J, Horn V, Zidkova H, Sprindrich J. Cementifying fibroma (so-called 'cementoma') of tibia. Br J Radiol 1981: 54: 989–992

90. Horn V, Bozdech Z, Macek M, Foukal T, Kolar J, Zidkova H. Cementoma like tumours of bone. Arch Orthop Trauma Surg 1982: 100: 267–272

91. Povysil C, Matejovsky Z. Fibro-osseous lesion with calcified spherules (cementifying fibroma like lesion) of the tibia. Ultrastruct Pathol 1993: 17: 25–34

92. Black D L, De Smet A A, Neff J R, Bhatia P. Case report 695. Cementifying fibroma of the proximal end of the tibia. Skeletal Radiol 1991: 20: 543–546

93. Sissons H A, Steiner G C, Dorfman H D. Calcified spherules in fibro-osseous lesions of bone. Arch Pathol Lab Med 1993: 117: 284–290

94. Voytek T M, Ro J Y, Edeiken J, Ayala A G. Fibrous dysplasia and cementoossifying fibroma. A histologic spectrum. Am J Surg Pathol 1995: 19: 775–781

95. Grabias S L, Campbell C J. Fibrous dysplasia. Orthop Clin North Am 1977: 8: 771–783

96. Schwartz D T, Alpert M. The malignant transformation of fibrous dysplasia. Am J Med Sci 1964: 247: 1–20

97. Taconis W K. Osteosarcoma in fibrous dysplasia. Skeletal Radiol 1988: 17: 163–170

98. Ruggieri P, Sim F H, Bond J R, Unni K K. Osteosarcoma in a patient with polyostotic fibrous dysplasia and Albright's syndrome. Orthopedics 1995: 18: 71–75

99. Campanacci M, Bertoni F, Capanna R. Malignant degeneration in fibrous dysplasia. Ital J Orthop Traumatol 1979: 5: 373–381

100. Unni K K, Dahlin D C. Premalignant tumors and conditions of bone. Am J Surg Pathol 1979: 3: 47–60

101. Ruggieri P, Sim F H, Bond J R, Unni K K. Malignancies in fibrous dysplasia. Cancer 1994: 73: 1411–1424

102. Ishida T, Machinami R, Kojima T, Kikuchi F. Malignant fibrous histiocytoma and osteosarcoma in association with fibrous dysplasia of bone. Pathol Res Pract 1992: 188: 757–763

103. Amin R, Ling R. Case report: malignant fibrous histiocytoma following radiation therapy of fibrous dysplasia. Br J Radiol 1995: 68: 1119–1122

104. Blackwell J B. Mesenchymal chondrosarcoma arising in fibrous dysplasia of the femur. J Clin Pathol 1993: 46: 961–962

105. Maeyama I, Iribe K, Takeshima Y, Ushigome S. Chondrosarcoma arising in fibrous dysplasia (in Japanese). Clin Orthop Surg 1970: 5: 183–186

106. Feintuch T A. Chondrosarcoma arising in a cartilaginous area of previously irradiated fibrous dysplasia. Cancer 1973: 31: 877–881

107. De Smet A A, Travers H, Neff J R. Chondrosarcoma occurring in a patient with polyostotic fibrous dysplasia. Skeletal Radiol 1981: 7: 197–201

108. Halawa M, Aziz A A. Chondrosarcoma in fibrous dysplasia of the pelvis. J Bone Joint Surg (Br) 1984: 66: 760–764

109. Brodeur G M, Caces J, Williams D L, Look A T, Pratt C B. Osteosarcoma, fibrous dysplasia, and a chromosomal abnormality in a 3-year-old child. Cancer 1980: 46: 1197–1201

110. Harris N L, Eilert R E, Davino N, Ruyle S, Edwardson M, Wilson V. Osteogenic sarcoma arising from bony regenerate following Ilizarov femoral lengthening through fibrous dysplasia. J Pediatr Orthop 1994: 14: 123–129

111. Candeliere G A, Glorieux F H, Prud'Homme J, St-Arnaud R. Increased expression of the c-fos proto-oncogene in bone from patients with fibrous dysplasia. N Engl J Med 1995: 332: 1546–1551

112. Cohen D M, Dahlin D C, Pugh D G. Fibrous dysplasia associated with adamantinoma of the long bones. Cancer 1962: 15: 515–521

113. Levack B, Revell P A, Roper B A. Adamantinoma associated with fibrous dysplasia. Int Orthop 1986: 10: 253–259

114. Schajowicz F, Santini-Araujo E. Adamantinoma of the tibia masked by fibrous dysplasia. Clin Orthop 1989: 238: 294–301

115. Bloem J L, Van Der Heul R O, Schuttevaer H M, Kuipers D. Fibrous dysplasia vs adamantinoma of the tibia: differentiation base on discriminant analysis of clinical and plain film findings. AJR 1991: 156: 1017–1023

116. Baker P L, Dockerty M B, Coventry M B. Adamantinoma (so-called) of long bones. J Bone Joint Surg (Am) 1954: 35: 704–720

117. Delarue J, Chomette G, Brocheriou C. Adamantinome du tibia et 'dysplasie fibreuse'. Ann Anat Pathol (Paris) 1964: 9: 373–378

118. Unni K K, Dahlin D C, Beabout J W, Ivins J C. Adamantinomas of long bones. Cancer 1974: 34: 1796–1805

119. Keeney G L, Unni K K, Beabout J W, Pritchard D J. Adamantinoma of long bones. Cancer 1989: 64: 730–737

120. Weiss S W, Dorfman H D. Adamantinoma of long bone. Hum Pathol 1977: 8: 141–153

121. Kandel R A, Pritzker K P, Bedard Y C. Symmetrical fibro-osseous dysplasia of rib – post-traumatic dysplasia? Histopathology 1981: 5: 651–658

Osteofibrous dysplasia

M. Forest

INTRODUCTION AND CLINICAL DATA

Cortical osteofibrous dysplasia[1] is a fibrosseous lesion occurring mostly in the tibia, found usually in young children and containing scattered bone trabeculae with a margin of active osteoblasts.

The condition was described by Franghenheim in 1921[2] and later under various names including congenital fibrous defect or pseudarthrosis,[3] intracortical fibrous dysplasia,[4] ossifying fibromas of long bone[5–7] and more recently, osteofibrous dysplasia of the tibia and fibula.[8] Cortical osteofibrous dysplasia seems to be the best term; it has been advocated by Schajowicz and by the pathologists of the AFIP.[1]

In some cases, a 'maturation' of osteofibrous dysplasia to fibrous dysplasia has been demonstrated[9] and the two lesions may be related or even identical processes, differing in location (cortical or medullary), age and activity (osteoblastic rimming).[9,10–13]

The age range is from newborns[1,8,14,15,16] to 39 years.[1] More than 60% of patients are younger than 5 years of age.[17] The male:female ratio is about 6:5.[18–20]

The disease usually runs a protracted course. The symptoms appear in the first decade of life:[3,8,21] bowing of the tibia or pain related to pathologic fractures. One case has been complicated by a presumably unrelated synovial sarcoma.[22]

SKELETAL DISTRIBUTION

The specific location is the cortex of the tibia. In one-fifth of cases, the adjacent fibula is involved.[1,8,11,18,23] Isolated fibular lesions can occur,[20] as well as bilateral tibial lesions. Rare cases may involve the femur (Huvos 1991), the humerus, radius and ulna[12,24] and possibly the thoracolumbar spine.[25]

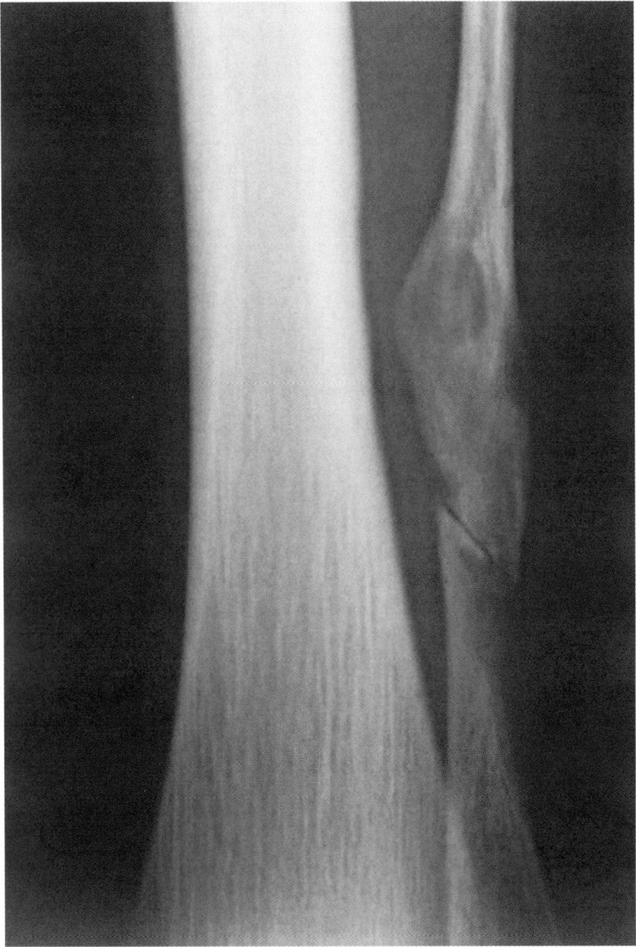

Fig. 45.1 Cortical osteofibrous dysplasia: isolated fibular involvement.

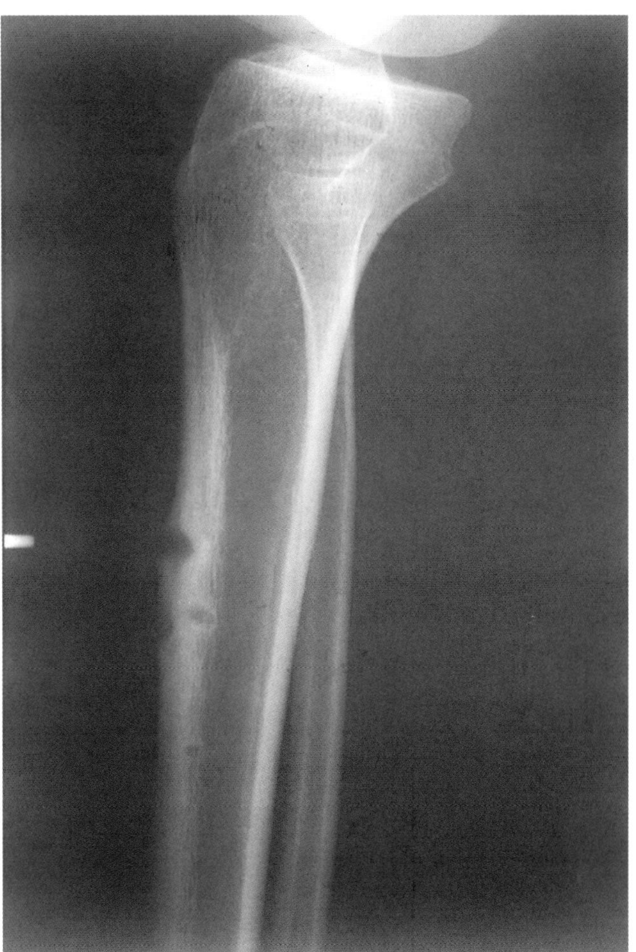

Fig. 45.2 Cortical osteofibrous dysplasia of the tibia.

IMAGING

In 70% of cases, osteofibrous dysplasia appears as multifocal cortical osteolytic areas, eccentrically and anteriorally located, with an osteosclerotic margin[1,18,21,23] (Figs 45.1–45.5). Less often, the lesion may be a single lytic area (Figs 45.6, 45.7) or may extend to the majority of the diaphysis. Some cases exhibit a 'ground glass' appearance in the matrix.[8] Most lesions are located in the middle third of the tibia shaft and the distal third of the fibula. An anterior bowing of the tibia is found in many cases.

CT scans demonstrate the absence of medullary involvement[18,19,26] and high attenuation values. On MRI, increased signals on T1 and T2-weighted images have been reported, in contrast to fibrous dysplasia.[27]

There is an increased uptake on isotope scans.[18,19]

GROSS PATHOLOGY

The lesional tissue is firm and gritty, pale white, yellowish-white or gray-tan.[28] The cortex is usually thinned and expanded.

HISTOPATHOLOGY

Osteoid and bone trabeculae have varying shapes, sizes and degrees of calcification;[28] the newly formed bone is characterized by a prominent osteoblastic margin[1,8,23,28] and few osteoclasts (Figs 45.8–45.18).

The fibrous stroma is less cellular than that of fibrous dysplasia[8,29] and is devoid of mitotic activity.[1,30] Some myxoid changes or a focal storiform pattern may be found.[1]

A zonal architecture is detected in significant measure;[1,8,23] the center is predominantly fibrous, with thin immature woven bone in the peripheral territories, and bone trabeculae are wider, more mature and lamellar, merging with the cortex.

IMMUNOHISTOCHEMISTRY

The spindle cells of the stroma exhibit immunopositivity for vimentin.[1,23,30] Cytokeratin-positive cells, indistinguishable from other cells in HE staining, are found in the majority of cases and not in fibrous dysplasia[1,23,30,31]

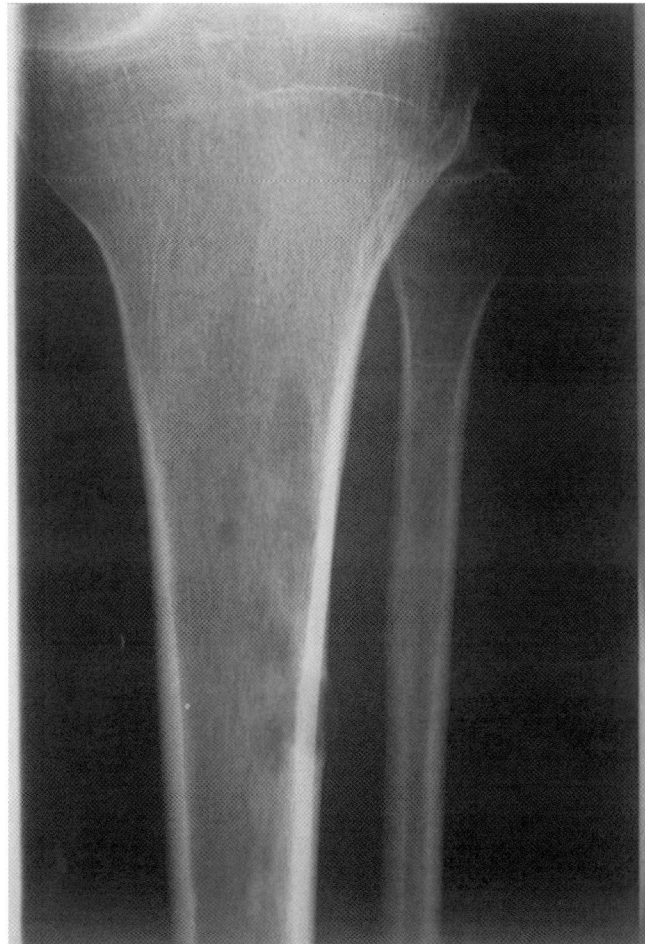

Fig. 45.3

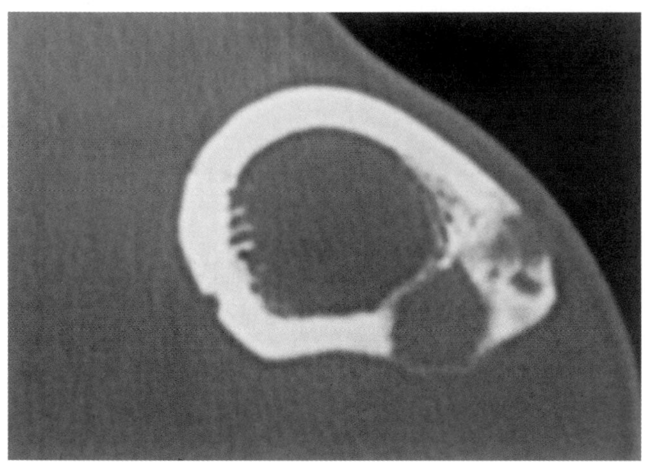

Fig. 45.4

Figs 45.3, 45.4 Cortical osteofibrous dysplasia of the tibia: absence of medullary involvement demonstrated on CT scan.

(Fig. 45.19). With monoclonal antibodies, the expression and distribution of the cytokeratin subtypes are similar to that of adamantinomas.[30,31]

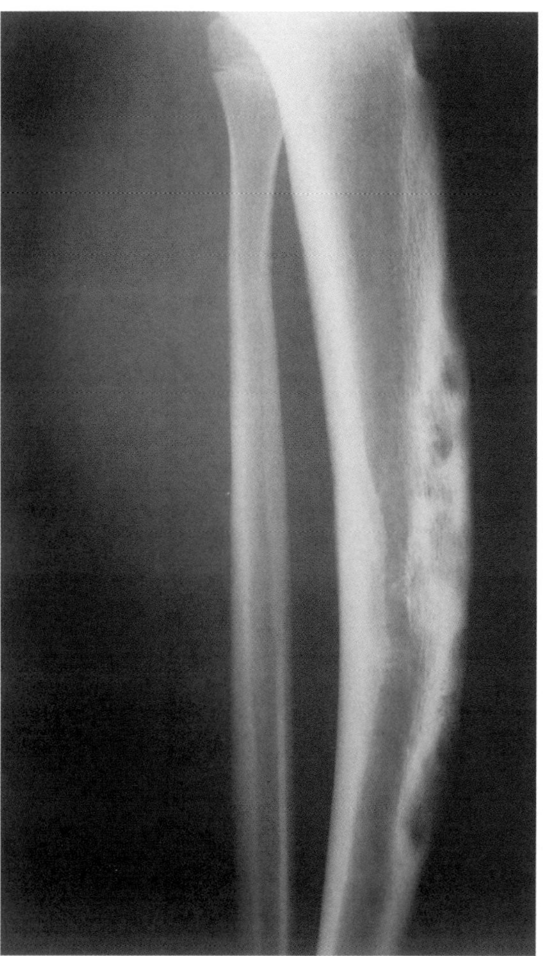

Fig. 45.5 Cortical osteofibrous dysplasia of the tibia with anterior bowing.

CYTOGENETICS

Cytogenetic and fluorescent in situ hybridization studies have demonstrated a trisomy 12 and trisomy for chromosomes 7,8 and 22. Trisomy 7 and 12 have also been found in adamantinomas. These common chromosomal anomalies are further support for a potential link between the two lesions.[32]

ELECTRON MICROSCOPY

Osteoblasts, osteocytes and osteoclasts are similar to those in reactive lesions.[5] The cells near active bone formation have the features of both osteoblasts and fibroblasts. The stromal cells are viewed as preosteoblasts, with a dilated rough endoplasmic reticulum, abundant cytoplasmic organelles, cytoplasmic filaments and glycogen.[29]

COURSE, TREATMENT AND PROGNOSIS

The clinical course is slowly progressive but some lesions

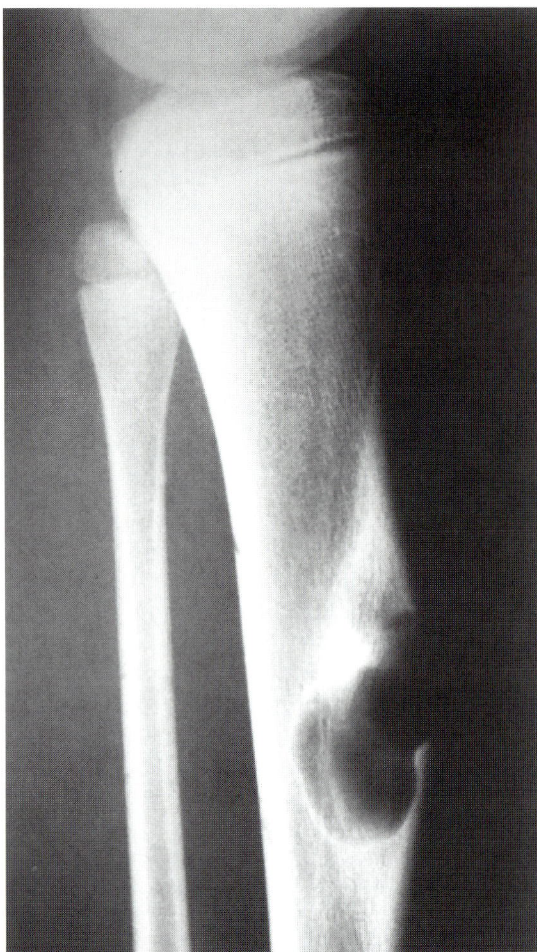

Fig. 45.6

Figs 45.6, 45.7 Cortical osteofibrous dysplasia of the tibia: single lytic area.

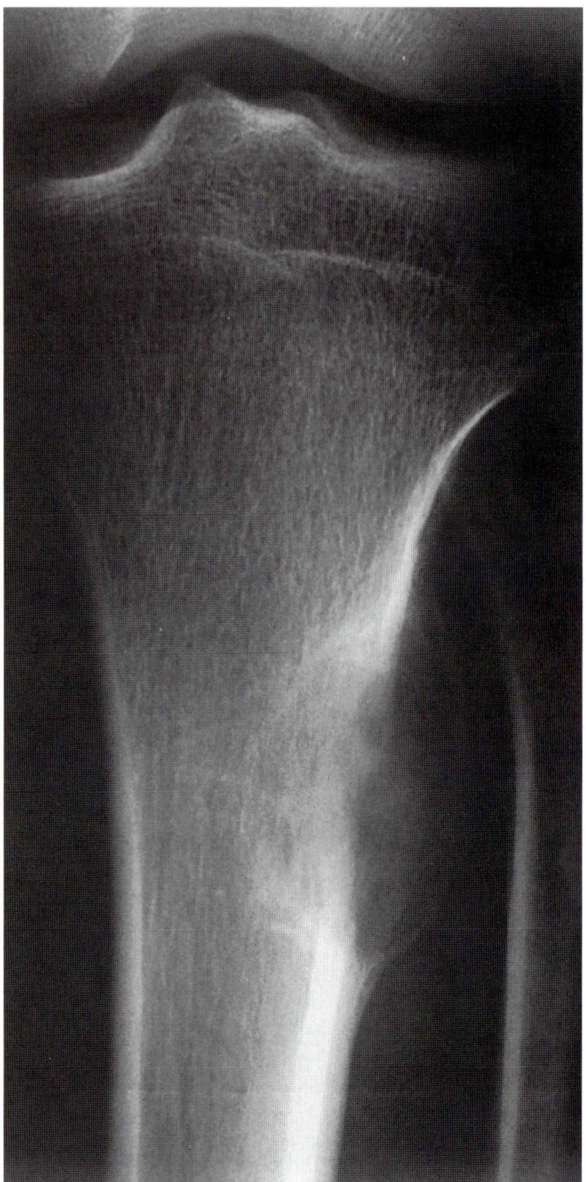

Fig. 45.7

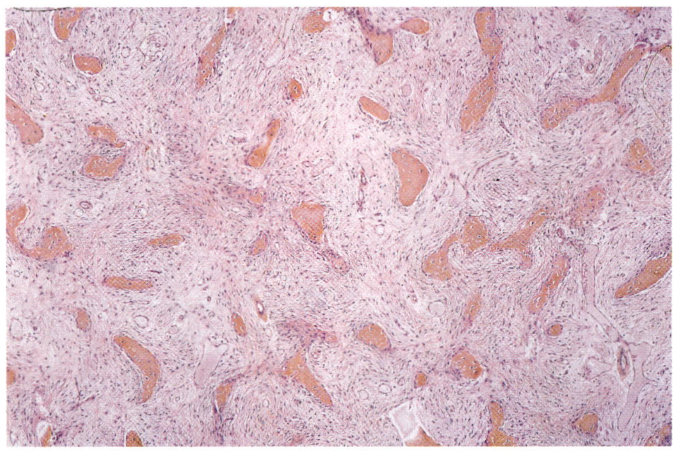

Fig. 45.8 Cortical osteofibrous dysplasia of the tibia: overview of the architectural pattern.

may regress spontaneously in early infancy. Those discovered later in life may regress or progress until adolescence and then stabilize.[8] However, a more aggressive course has also been reported.[12,33,34]

With surgery performed before 15 years of age, there is a high recurrence rate.[5,18,19,21,24,28,33,35] Surgical treatment should be restricted to extensive lesions or if there is a risk of fracture. After 15 years of age, definitive surgery is a marginal excision with bone grafting[24] or a conservative curettage with cryosurgery and bone grafting (Huvos 1991).

DIFFERENTIAL DIAGNOSIS

Osteofibrous dysplasia has to be differentiated from

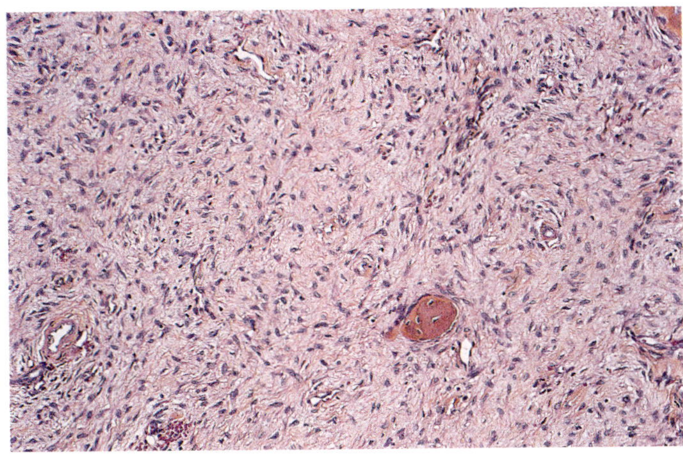

Fig. 45.9

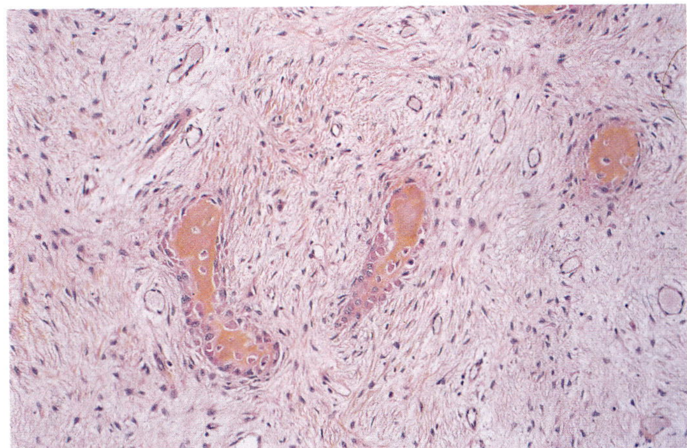

Fig. 45.10

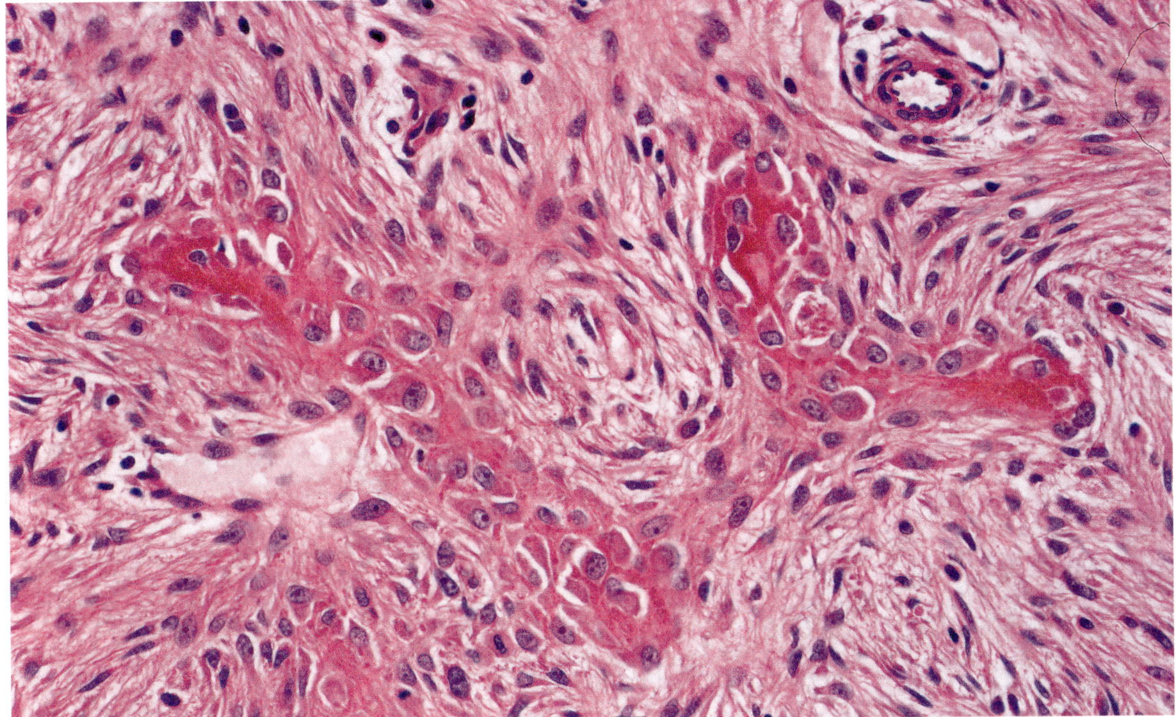

Fig. 45.12

Figs 45.9–45.13
Histological hallmark of cortical osteofibrous dysplasia: bone trabeculae with an osteoblastic margin in fibrous stroma.

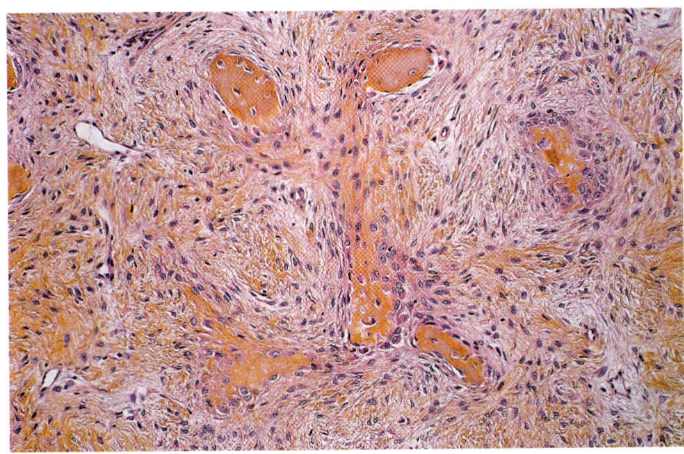

Fig. 45.11

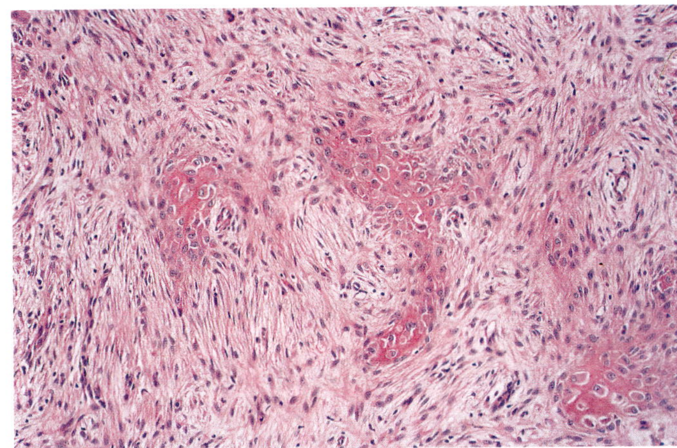

Fig. 45.13

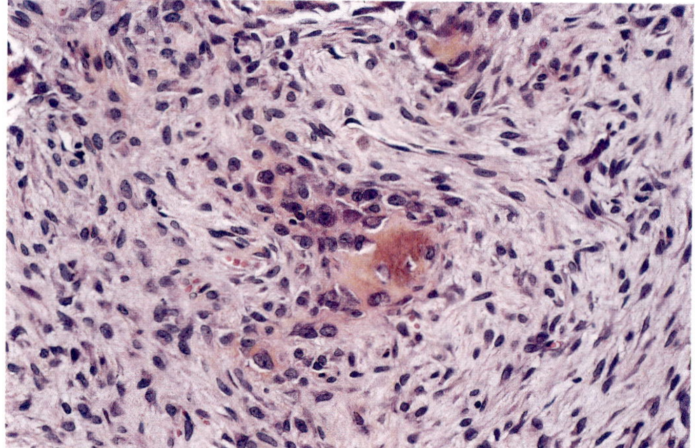

Fig. 45.14

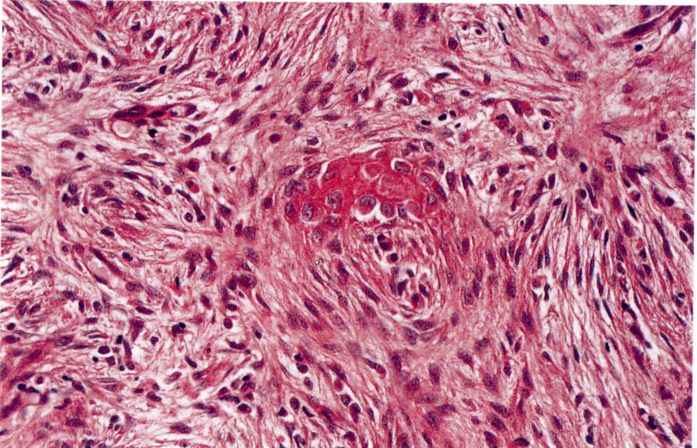

Fig. 45.15

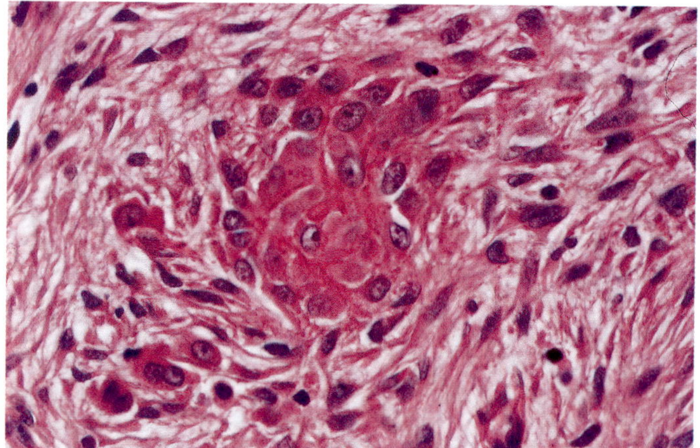

Fig. 45.16

Figs 45.14–45.16 Cortical osteofibrous dysplasia: details of the fibrous stroma with osteoblastic differentiation and bone formation.

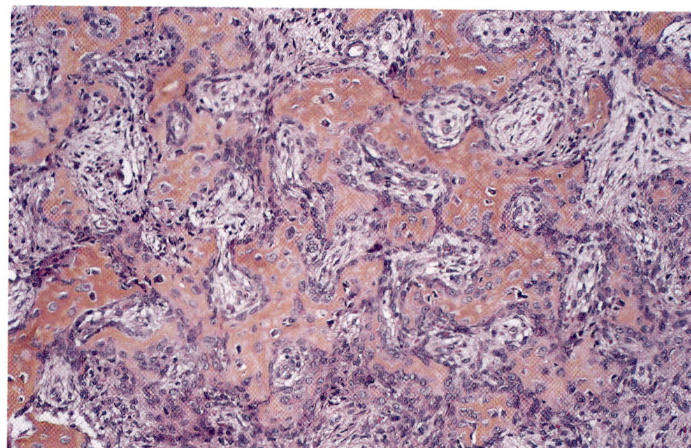

Fig. 45.17

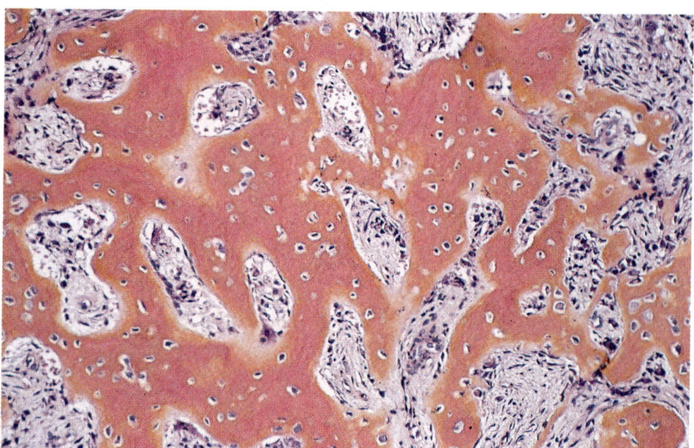

Fig. 45.18

Figs 45.17, 45.18 Cortical osteofibrous dysplasia: wider and more mature bone trabeculae at the periphery of the lesion.

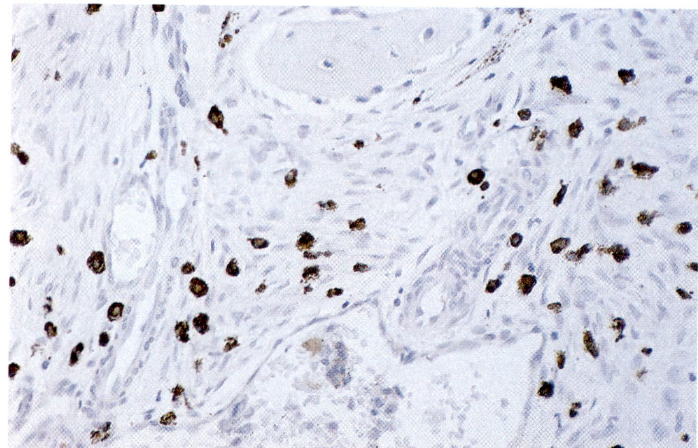

Fig. 45.19 Cortical osteofibrous dysplasia of the tibia: scattered cytokeratin-positive cells.

fibrous dysplasia following trauma, with reactive bone formation.

The so-called 'differentiated' adamantinomas, osteo-fibrous dysplasia-like adamantinomas or 'juvenile adaman-

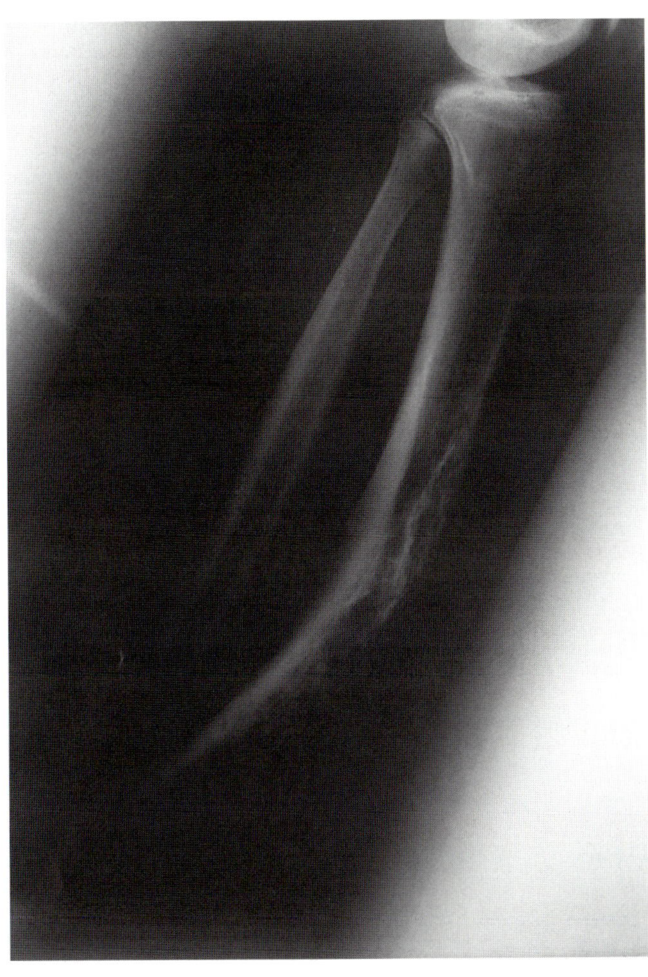

Fig. 45.20

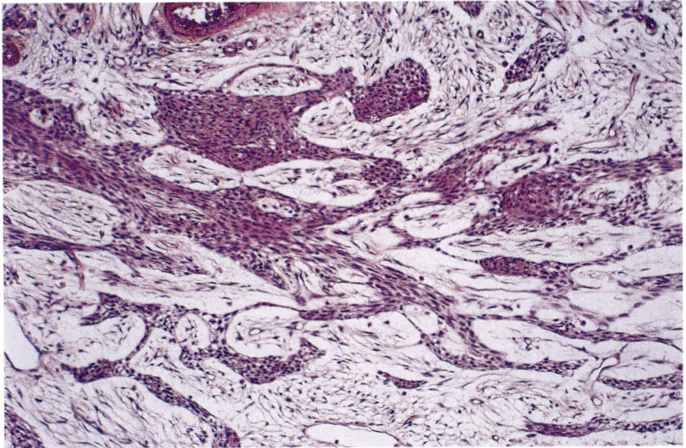

Fig. 45.21

Figs 45.20, 45.21 Osteofibrous dysplasia associated with adamantinoma of the tibia.

tinomas' exhibit scattered epithelial cells, small islands with occasional squamous differentiation and small tubular structures, especially in the central areas.

COMMENTS FOR THE SURGICAL PATHOLOGIST

Single, scattered cytokeratin-immunoreactive cells should not lead to an overdiagnosis of adamantinoma.[1,31] Conversely, although osteofibrous dysplasia does not necessarily give rise to an adamantinoma, a thorough sampling of all the excision material is necessary to find the typical epithelial islands of adamantinoma which are sometimes underdiagnosed[12,13,36,37] (Figs 45.20, 45.21).

REFERENCES

1. Sweet D E, Vinh T N, Devaney K. Cortical osteofibrous dysplasia of long bones and its relationship to adamantinoma. Am J Surg Pathol 1992: 16: 282–290
2. Franghenheim P. Angeborene ostitis fibrosa als ursache einer intrauterinen unterschenkelfraktur. Arch Klin Chir 1921: 117: 22–29
3. Semian D W, Willis J B, Bove K E. Congenital fibrous defect of the tibia mimicking fibrous dysplasia. J Bone Joint Surg (Am) 1975: 57: 854–857
4. Johnson L C. Congenital pseudoarthrosis, adamantinoma of bone, and intracortical fibrous dysplasia of the tibia. J Bone Joint Surg (Am) 1972: 54: 1355
5. Kempson R L. Ossifying fibroma of long bones. A light and electron microscopic study. Arch Pathol Lab Med 1966: 82: 218–233
6. Goergen T G, Dickman P S, Resnick D, Saltzstein S L, O'Dell C W, Akeson W H. Long bone ossifying fibromas. Cancer 1977: 39: 2067–2072
7. Markel S F. Ossifying fibroma of long bone: its distinction from fibrous dysplasia and its association with adamantinoma of long bone. Am J Clin Pathol 1978: 69: 91–97
8. Campanacci M, Laus M. Osteofibrous dysplasia of the tibia and fibula. J Bone Joint Surg (Am) 1981: 63: 367–375
9. Park Y K, Unni K K, McLeod R A, Pritchard D J. Osteofibrous dysplasia: clinicopathologic study of 80 cases. Hum Pathol 1993: 24: 1339–1347
10. Grabias S L, Campbell C J. Fibrous dysplasia. Orthop Clin North Am 1977: 8: 771–783
11. Casputen B M, Rochon L, Rosman M A, Marton D. Osteofibrous dysplasia. J Can Assoc Radiol 1980: 31: 50–53
12. Campbell C J, Hawk T. A variant of fibrous dysplasia (osteofibrous dysplasia). J Bone Joint Surg (Am) 1982: 64: 231–236
13. Schajowicz F, Santini-Araujo E. Adamantinoma of the tibia masked by fibrous dysplasia. Clin Orthop 1989: 238: 294–301
14. Smith N M, Byard R W, Foster B, Morris L, Clark B, Bourne A J. Congenital ossifying fibroma (osteofibrous dysplasia) of the tibia. Pediatr Radiol 1991: 21: 449–451
15. Anderson M J, Townsend D R, Johnston J O, Bohay D R. Osteofibrous dysplasia in the newborn. J Bone Joint Surg (Am) 1993: 75: 265–167
16. Hindman B W, Bell S, Russo T, Zuppan C W. Neonatal osteofibrous dysplasia: report of two cases. Pediatr Radiol 1996: 26: 303–306
17. Abdelwahab I F, Hermann G, Zawin J, Lewis M M, Klein M J. Case report 543. Osteofibrous dysplasia of tibia. Skeletal Radiol 1989: 18: 249–251
18. Klein M, Becker M H, Genieser N B, Tzimas N. Case report 161. Ossifying fibroma of tibia (and fibula). Skeletal Radiol 1981: 6: 307–309
19. Blackwell J B, McCarthy S W, Xipell J M, Vernon-Roberts B, Duhig R E. Osteofibrous dysplasia of the tibia and fibula. Pathology 1988: 20: 227–233

20. Castellote A, Garcia-Pena P, Lucaya J, Lorenzo J. Osteofibrous dysplasia. Skeletal Radiol 1988: 17: 483–486

21. Resnik C S, Young J W, Levine A M, Aisner S C. Case report 604. Osteofibrous dysplasia (ossifying fibroma) of tibia. Skeletal Radiol 1990: 19: 217–219

22. Ben Arush M W, Ben Arieh Y, Bialik V, Goldsher D, Meller I, Berant M. Synovial sarcoma associated with osteofibrous dysplasia. Am J Pediatr Hematol Oncol 1992: 14: 261–264

23. Ishida T, Iijima T, Kikuchi F, Kitagawa T, Tanida T, Imamura T, Machinami R A. Clinicopathological and immunohistochemical study of osteofibrous dysplasia, differentiated adamantinoma, and adamantinoma of long bones. Skeletal Radiol 1992: 21: 493–502

24. Wang J W, Shih C H, Chen W J. Osteofibrous dysplasia (ossifying fibroma of long bones). Clin Orthop 1992: 278: 235–243

25. Ohyama T, Ohara S, Momma F, Moto A, Nakata Y. Ossifying fibroma of the thoracolumbar spine. Surg Neurol 1992: 37: 231–235

26. Zeanah W R, Hudson T M, Springfield D S. Computed tomography of ossifying fibroma of the tibia. J Comput Assist Tomogr 1983: 7: 688–691

27. Dominguez R, Saucedo J, Fenstermacher M. MRI findings in osteofibrous dysplasia. Magn Reson Imaging 1989: 7: 567–570

28. Nakashima Y, Yamamuro T, Fujiwara Y, Kotoura Y, Mori E, Hamashima Y. Osteofibrous dysplasia (ossifying fibroma of long bones). Cancer 1983: 52: 909–914

29. Komiya S, Inoue A. Aggressive bone tumorous lesion in infancy: osteofibrous dysplasia of the tibia and fibula. J Pediatr Orthop 1993: 13: 577–581

30. Benassi M S, Campanacci L, Gamberi G et al. Cytokeratin expression and distribution in adamantinoma of the long bones and osteofibrous dysplasia of tibia and fibula. An immunohistochemical study correlated to histogenesis. Histopathology 1994: 25: 71–76

31. Ueda Y, Blasius S, Edel G, Wuisman F, Böcker W, Roessner A. Osteofibrous dysplasia of long bones – a reactive process to adamantinomatous tissue. J Cancer Res Clin Oncol 1992: 118: 152–156

32. Bridge J A, Dembinski A, DeBoer J, Travis J, Neff J R. Clonal chromosomal abnormalities in osteofibrous dysplasia. Implications for histopathogenesis and its relationship with adamantinoma. Cancer 1994: 73: 1746–1752

33. Schoenecker P L, Swanson K, Sheridan J J. Ossifying fibroma of the tibia. J Bone Joint Surg (Am) 1981: 63: 483–488

34. Springfield D S, Rosenberg A E, Mankin H J, Mindell E R. Relationship between osteofibrous dysplasia and adamantinoma. Clin Orthop 1994: 309: 234–244

35. Bosse A, Niersert W, Wuisman P, Roessner A. Fibröse Dysplasie versus osteofibröse dysplasie. Z Orthop Ihre Grenzgeb 1993: 131: 42–50

36. Alguacil-Garcia A, Alonzo A, Pettigrew N M. Osteofibrous dysplasia (ossifying fibroma) of the tibia and fibula and adamantinoma. Am J Clin Pathol 1984: 82: 470–474

37. Ueda Y, Roessner A, Bosse A, Edel G, Bocker W, Wuisman P. Juvenile intracortical adamantinoma of the tibia with predominant osteofibrous dysplasia-like features. Pathol Res Pract 1991: 187: 1039–1043, 1043–1044

46

Giant cell reaction

M. Forest

CHAPTER CONTENTS

INTRODUCTION AND CLINICAL DATA

Giant cell reaction is a fibrous lesion with giant cells and reactive bone, found predominantly in the small bones of the extremities.

It was originally described by Jaffe in 1953 as a jaw lesion, with the name 'giant cell reparative granuloma', and by Ackerman & Spjut in the small tubular bones of the hands under the name 'giant cell reaction'.[1,2] 'Giant cell reparative granuloma of extragnathic sites' is another suggested term.[3]

The majority of patients are in the second or third decades of life,[4,5] with a slight male predominance[6] and in a few cases a history of minor trauma.[3,7] Clinical findings are pain, swelling or a pathologic fracture.[8] Some patients are asymptomatic.

Unusual multicentric lesions have been reported in the hand or the foot,[9–11] as well as an association with polyostotic fibrous dysplasia,[12] Paget's disease[13] and enchondromatosis.[14]

SKELETAL DISTRIBUTION

Most cases involve the phalanges, metacarpals and metatarsals (Figs 46.1–46.4). Less common sites are the wrist and the talus or tarsal bones[5] (Fig. 46.5). A few cases have been reported in the spine,[3,15] the ribs,[3] humerus,[16] femur[17] and tibia in a subperiosteal location.[18]

IMAGING

In short tubular bones, the purely lytic lesion is well defined and oriented along the long axis of bone,[9] with some expansion; it may be trabeculated.[6] The cortex is thinned but intact. Most lesions are metaphyseal but may involve the entire tubular bone. A giant cell reaction has been described crossing the growth plate.[19] A periosteal reaction is unusual.[8]

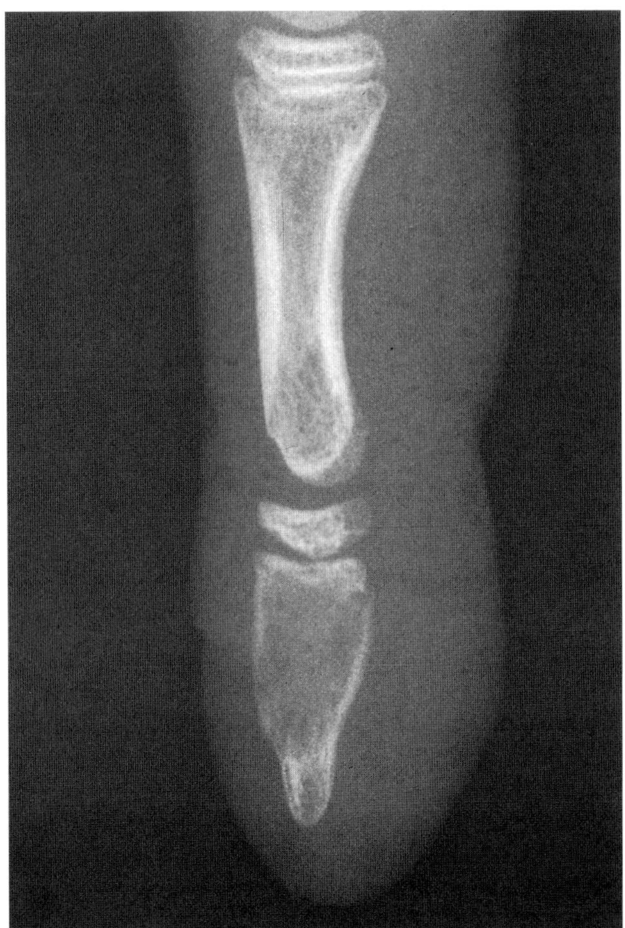

Fig. 46.1 Giant cell reaction of a phalanx.

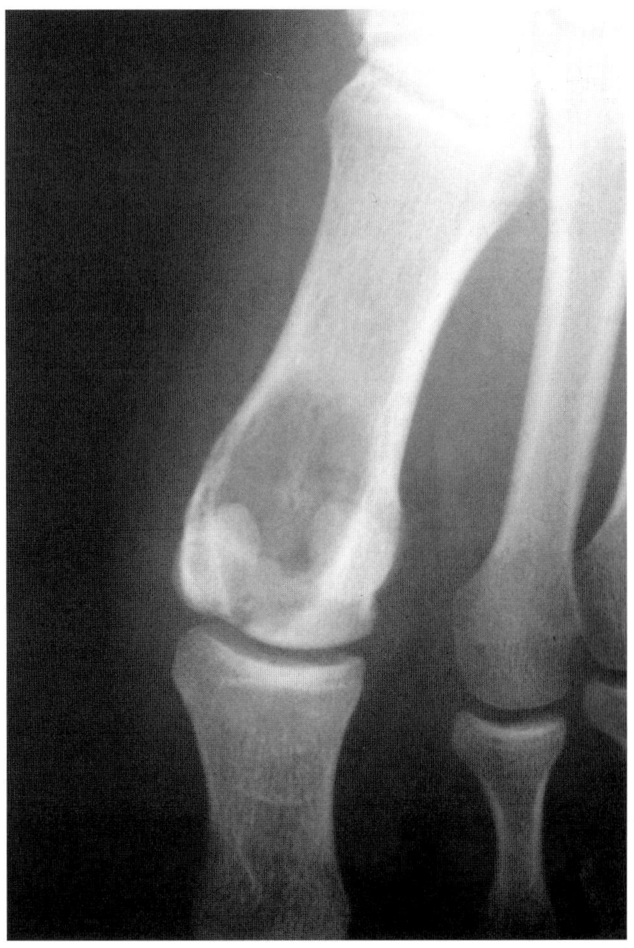

Fig. 46.2

Figs 46.2–46.4 Giant cell reaction of metacarpal.

GROSS PATHOLOGY

The tissue is brown or gray, friable and gritty, with eventual cystic spaces.[3] Extension into the soft tissues is infrequent.[5–7]

HISTOPATHOLOGY

The fibrous stroma, with bland or slightly hyperchromatic spindle cells, may be very cellular and highly vascularized[6,20] or may exhibit large amounts of collagen.[21] Mitotic figures are rare. Numerous or sparse osteoclast-like giant cells are focally aggregated or distributed around hemorrhages[5,9] (Figs 46.6, 46.7).

Trabeculae of newly formed bone or osteoid may be quite extensive;[21] some of them are lined by osteoblasts[3] (Figs 46.8, 46.9).

Hemosiderin deposits and hemosiderin-laden macrophages are related to stromal hemorrhages.

Histiocyte-like cells or infiltration by lymphocytes and plasma cells can occur, as well as a storiform pattern or myxoid changes.

Prominent cystic vascular spaces may be found in the primary lesion or in recurrences, resembling an aneurysmal bone cyst[3,8,9] (Fig. 46.10).

IMMUNOHISTOCHEMISTRY

The stromal cells stain for α1-antichymotrypsin, α1-antitrypsin and factor XIIIa.[22] A myofibroblastic phenotype has been identified, with expression of both vimentin and actin in the stromal cells.[20,22] Osteoclast-like cells show positive staining for CD68, vimentin and LCA.[20]

ELECTRON MICROSCOPY

The mononuclear stromal cells have the characteristic appearance of fibroblasts, containing collagen fibrils, aggregates of glycogen particles or iron pigment.[3,23]

CLINICAL COURSE, TREATMENT AND PROGNOSIS

Conservative treatment by curettage and bone grafting is

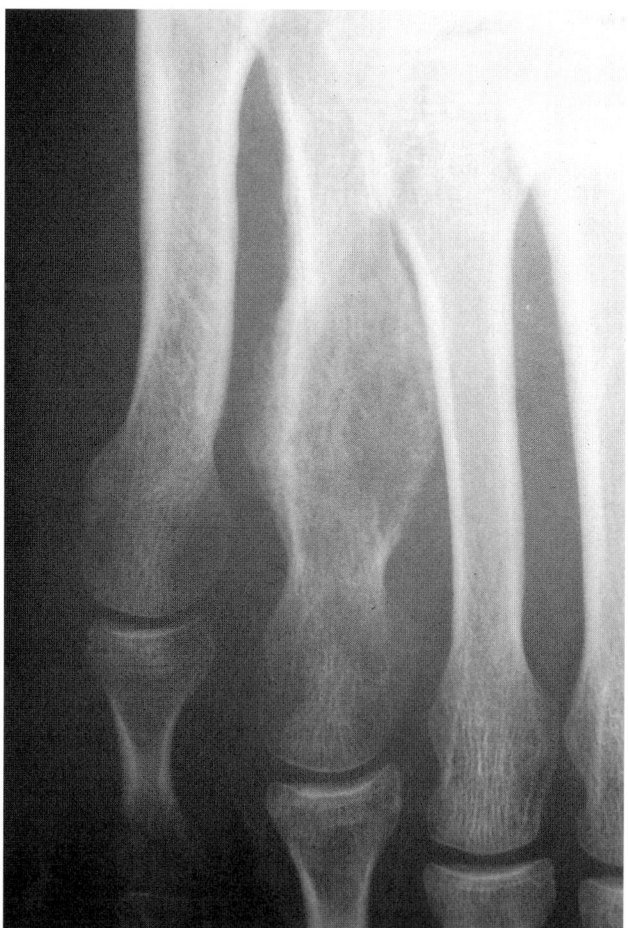

Fig. 46.3

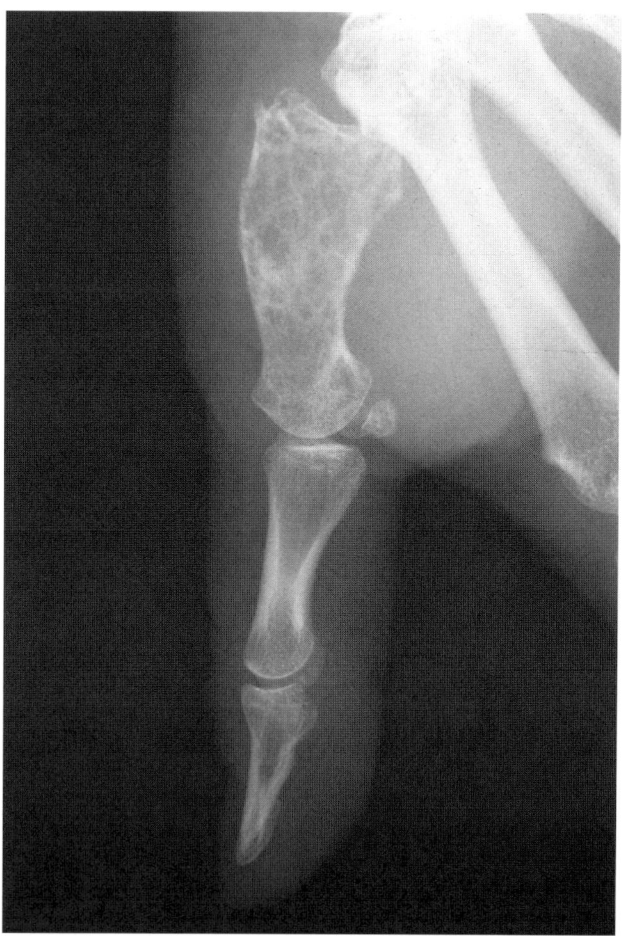

Fig. 46.4

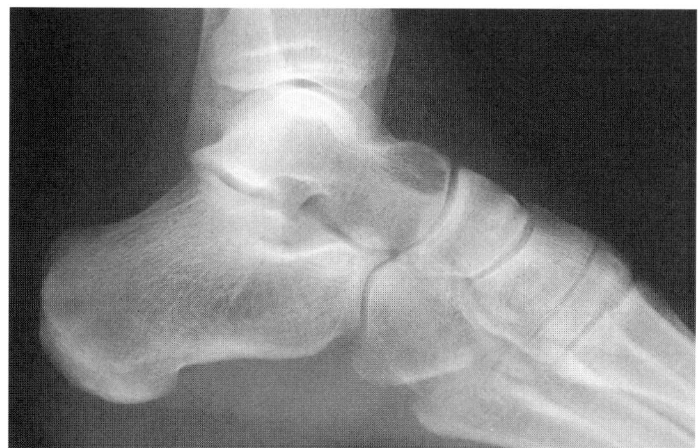

Fig. 46.5 Giant cell reaction of the talus.

curative for primary lesions and recurrences, which have a rate ranging from 36% to 50% of cases. Rare second recurrences have been reported.[3,24] The recurrence rate appears to be lower than that of giant cell tumors in the same location.[8] The few cases reported in long bones seem to have a better prognosis.[22]

DIFFERENTIAL DIAGNOSIS

A brown tumor of hyperparathyroidism is histologically indistinguishable from a giant cell reaction.[3,5,8,25] Serum calcium, phosphorus, alkaline phosphatase and parathyroid hormone levels have to be checked as well as the absence of radiographic generalized skeletal rarefaction.[5,26]

In small tubular bones, a giant cell tumor is usually an epiphyseal lesion, expanding bone,[5] but in many cases the distinction from a giant cell reaction is difficult radiologically and histologically.[6,8,27] Furthermore, a pathologic fracture through a giant cell tumor may induce reactive bone formation with an osteoblastic margin.[8] In a giant cell reaction, the stroma is more fibrous, with a high content of reticulin fibers,[6] without sheets of polygonal, spindle or plump mononuclear cells; giant cells with fewer nuclei[8] are clustered and trabecular osteoid with osteoblastic rimming is more prominent.

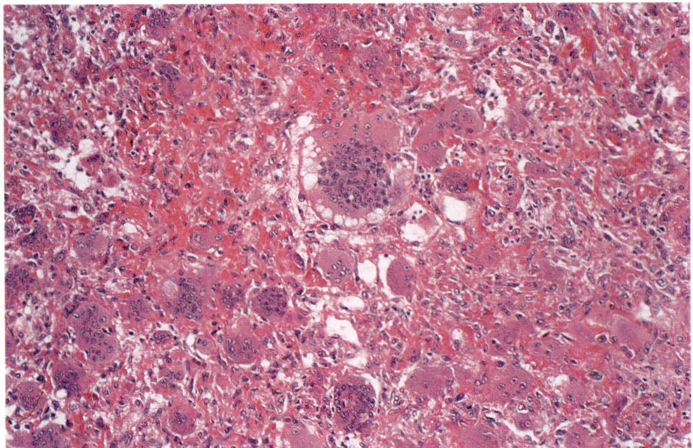

Fig. 46.6

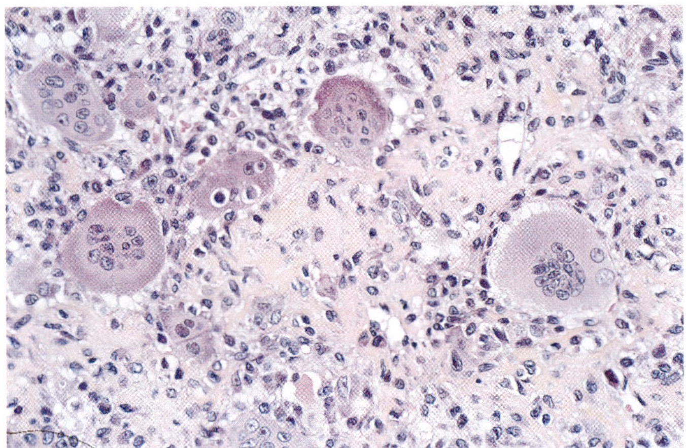

Fig. 46.7

Figs 46.6, 46.7 Giant cell reaction: giant cell component in hemorrhagic or collagenous areas.

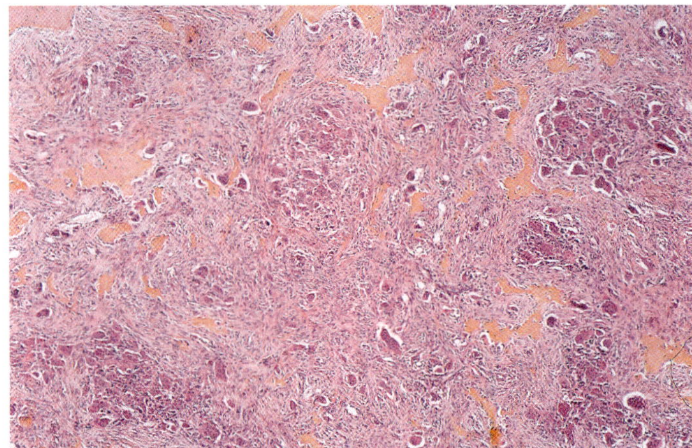

Fig. 46.8

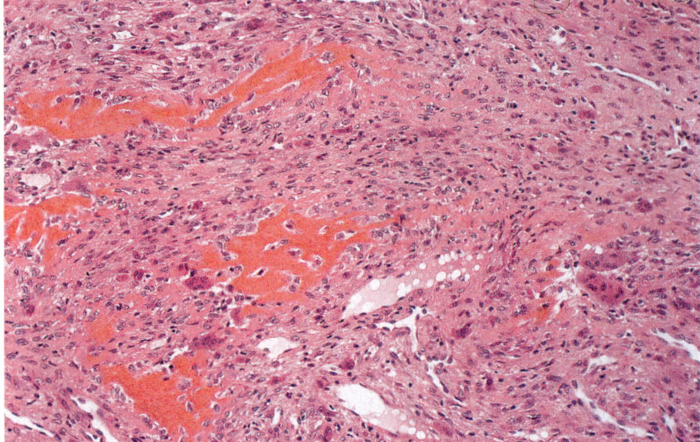

Fig. 46.9

Figs 46.8, 46.9 Giant cell reaction: reactive bone formation.

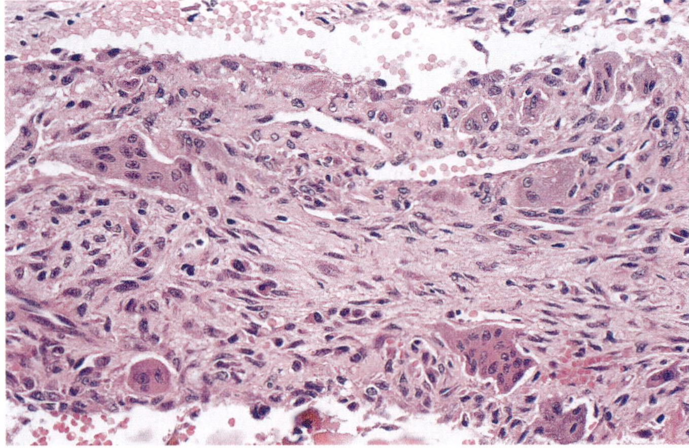

Fig. 46.10 Giant cell reaction: associated aneurysmal bone cyst component.

Foam cells and a storiform pattern of the spindle cells may in some cases resemble a non-ossifying fibroma.[8,21]

Many authors suggest that a giant cell reaction is histologically indistinguishable from the solid portions of an aneurysmal bone cyst, both presumably representing responses to intraosseous hemorrhages. A solid fibrohistiocytic/myofibroblastic proliferation may evolve into a typical aneurysmal bone cyst;[20] therefore, the skeletal distribution of giant cell reactions has to be determined, with more cases in the ribs, pelvic bones, vertebrae, humerus, femur, tibia and even the sacrum.[22,28]

REFERENCES

1. Ackerman L V, Spjut H J. Tumors of bone and cartilage. Atlas of tumor pathology, section II, fasc 4. Washington: AFIP, 1962, pp 282, 344–345
2. Jernstrom P, Stark H H. Giant cell reaction of a metacarpal. Am J Clin Pathol 1971: 55: 77–81
3. Lorenzo J C, Dorfman H D. Giant cell reparative granuloma of short tubular bones of the hands and feet. Am J Surg Pathol 1980: 4: 551–563
4. Capozzi J D, Green S, Levy R N, Schwartz I S. Giant cell reaction of small bones. Clin Orthop 1987: 214: 181–184
5. Ratner V, Dorfman H D. Giant cell reparative granuloma of the hand and foot bones. Clin Orthop 1990: 260: 251–258
6. Picci P, Baldini N, Sudanese A, Boriani S, Campanacci M. Giant cell reparative granuloma and other giant cell lesions of the bones of the hands and feet. Skeletal Radiol 1986: 15: 415–421
7. Merkow R L, Bansal M, Inglis A E. Giant cell reparative granuloma in the hand. J Hand Surg (Am) 1985: 10: 733–739
8. Wold L E, Dobyns J H, Swee R G, Dahlin D C. Giant cell reaction (giant cell reparative granuloma) of the small bones of the hands and feet (30 cases). Am J Surg Pathol 1986: 10: 491–496
9. Glass T A, Mills S E, Fechner R E, Dyer R, Martin W, Armstrong P. Giant cell reparative granuloma of the hands and feet. Radiology 1983: 149: 65–68
10. Caskey P M, Wolf M D, Fechner R E. Multicentric giant cell granuloma of the small bones of the hand. Clin Orthop 1985: 193: 199–205
11. Robinson D, Hendel D, Halperin N, Levin S. Multicentric giant-cell reparative granuloma. A case in the foot. Acta Orthop Scand 1989: 60: 232–234
12. De Smet A A, Travers H, Neff J R. Case report 207. Giant cell reparative granuloma of the left femur arising in polyostotic fibrous dysplasia. Skeletal Radiol 1982: 8: 314–318
13. Upchurch K S, Simon L S, Schiller A L, Rosenthal D I, Campion E W, Krane S M. Giant cell reparative granuloma of Paget's disease of bone: a unique clinical entity. Ann Intern Med 1983: 98: 35–40
14. Oda Y, Iwamoto Y, Ushijima M, Masuda S, Sugioka Y, Tsuneyoshi M. Case report 877. Giant cell reparative granuloma arising in enchondromatosis. Skeletal Radiol 1994: 23: 669–671
15. Inoue H, Tsuneyoshi M, Enjoji M, Shinohara N, Yokoyama K. Giant-cell reparative granuloma of the thoracic vertebra. Acta Pathol Jpn 1986: 36: 745–750
16. Thomas I H, Chow C W, Cole W G. Giant cell reparative granuloma of the humerus. J Pediatr Orthop 1988: 8: 596–598
17. Hermann G, Abdelwahab I F, Klein M J, Berson B D, Lewis M M. Case report 603. Giant cell reparative granuloma of the distal end of right femur. Skeletal Radiol 1990: 19: 367–369
18. Kenan S, Lewis M M, Abdelwahab I F, Klein M. Subperiosteal giant-cell reparative granuloma. J Bone Joint Surg (Br) 1994: 76: 810–813
19. Wenner S M, Johnson K. Giant cell reparative granuloma of the hand. J Hand Surg (Am) 1987: 12: 1097–1101
20. Panico L, Passeretti U, De Rosa N, D'Antonio A, De Rosa G. Giant cell reparative granuloma of the distal skeletal bones. Virchows Arch 1994: 425: 315–320
21. Schwinn C P. Differential diagnosis of giant cell lesions of bone. Monogr Pathol 1976: 17: 236–299
22. Oda Y, Tsuneyoshi M, Shinohara N. 'Solid' variant of aneurysmal bone cyst (extragnathic giant cell reparative granuloma) in the axial skeleton and long bones. Cancer 1992: 70: 2642–2649
23. Helpap B, Totovic V, Bechtelsheimer H. Giant cell reaction in the small tubular bones. A light and electron microscopic study. J Cancer Res Clin Oncol 1981: 101: 219–226
24. Bertheussen K J, Holck S, Schiodt T. Giant cell lesion of bone of the hand with particular emphasis on giant cell reparative granuloma. J Hand Surg (Am) 1983: 8: 46–49
25. Bertoni F, Laus M, Campanacci M. Giant cell reaction of bone. Ital J Orthop Traumatol 1980: 6: 239–247
26. Lingg G, Roessner A, Fiedler V, Lübbesmeyer H J, Peters P E, Grundmann E. Das Reparative riesenzellengranulom der Extremitäten. RÖFO 1985: 142: 185–188
27. D'Alonzo R T, Pitcock M D, Wilford L W. Giant cell reaction of bone. J Bone Joint Surg (Am) 1972: 54: 1267–1271
28. Bertoni F, Bacchini P, Capanna R et al. Solid variant of aneurysmal bone cyst. Cancer 1993: 71: 729–734

47

Osteopoikilosis and melorheostosis

M. Forest

OSTEOPOIKILOSIS

Introduction and clinical data

Osteopoikilosis, also called osteopathia condensans disseminata or spotted bone disease, is a sclerosing bone dysplasia appearing as sporadic cases or with an autosomal dominant pattern of genetic transmission.[1]

The condition is usually asymptomatic and may be diagnosed at any age; both sexes are equally affected. Bone lesions can increase or decrease in size or number or even disappear, especially in children.

In 25% of cases, bone lesions are associated with subcutaneous nodules, a predisposition to keloid formation and scleroderma-like lesions (the Buschke–Ollendorff syndrome). They may also be associated with other forms of sclerosing bone dysplasias, most commonly osteopathia striata and melorheostosis, in the so-called mixed sclerosing bone dystrophies[2–5] or 'overlap syndromes'.[6]

Skeletal distribution

The lesions are symmetrically[7] but unequally distributed, with a predilection for the epiphyses and metaphyses of long tubular bones and with frequent involvement of the pelvis,[6] the scapula, carpus, tarsus and small tubular bones of the hands and feet.[1] They are unusual in the skull, facial bones, ribs and spine.

Imaging

Numerous small foci of increased radiodensity are well defined, homogeneous, round or oval, usually 3–5 mm in diameter, the long axis being parallel to that of the involved bone trabeculae[8] (Figs 47.1–47.12). Some may be linked to the endosteal surface of the cortex in the metaphysis.[6]

Radiological findings are characteristic and similar to those of bone islands.

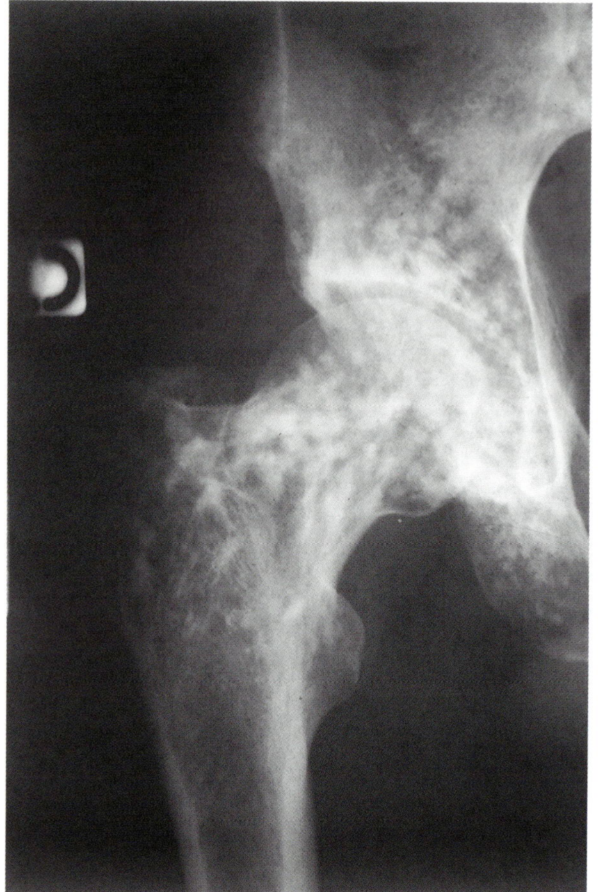

Fig. 47.1

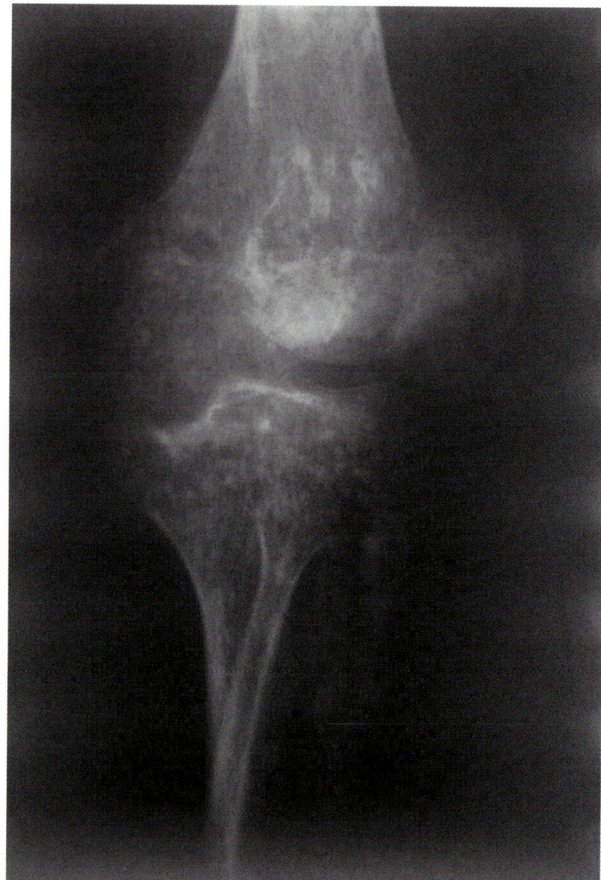

Fig. 47.2

Figs 47.1, 47.2 Widespread lesions of osteopoikilosis involving the pelvis, proximal and distal femurs, proximal humerus and scapulae.

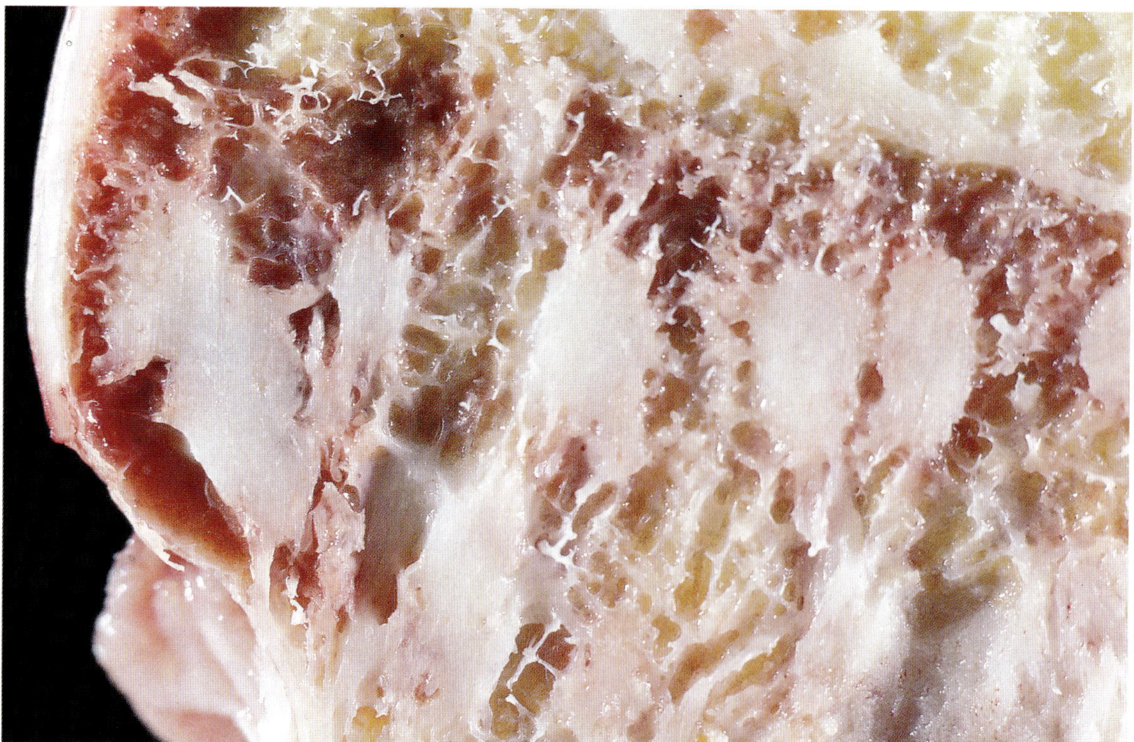

Fig. 47.3

Figs 47.3–47.10 Osteopoikilosis of a femoral head (same case as Fig. 47.1) with numerous round or oval foci of sclerotic bone; some of them are linked to the endosteal surface of the cortex.

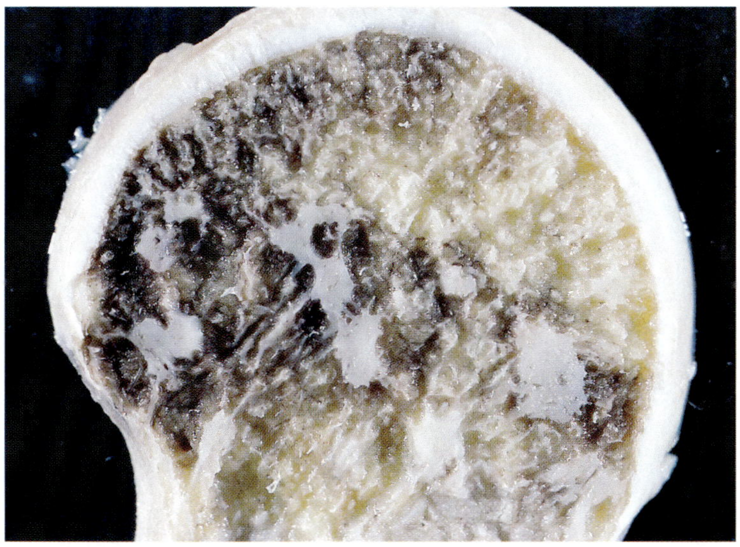

Fig. 47.4

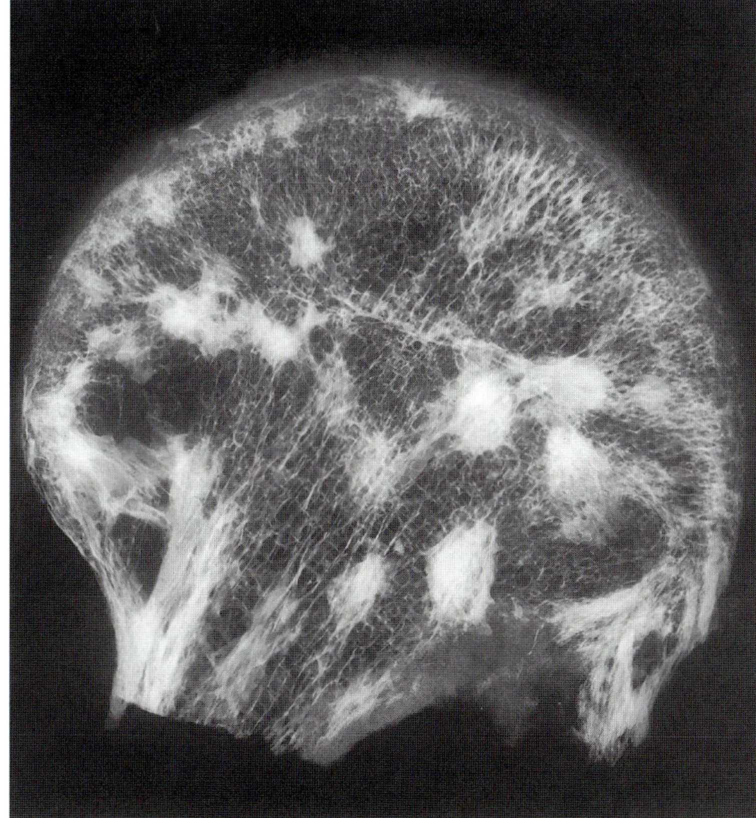

Fig. 47.5

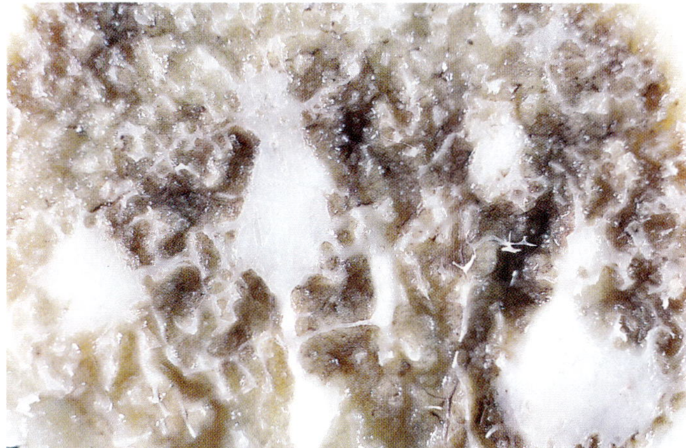

Fig. 47.6

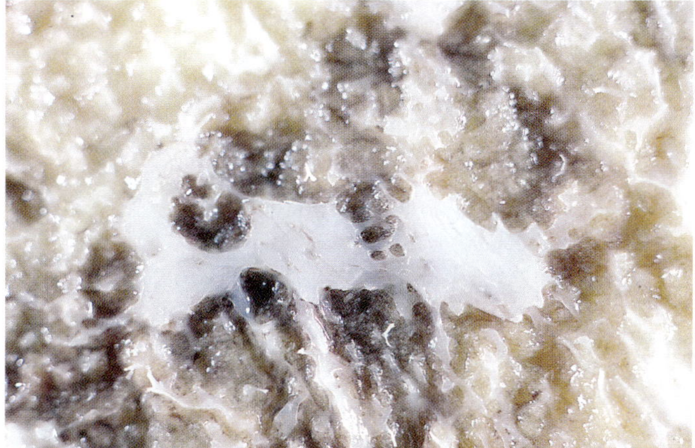

Fig. 47.7

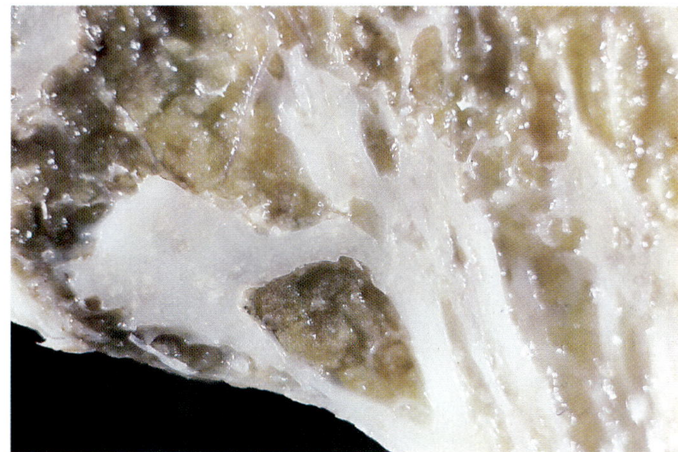

Fig. 47.8

On radionuclide bone scan, an increased activity has been reported in a young patient[9] but most lesions exhibit a lack of uptake.[10,11]

Histopathology

The histological structure is similar to that of bone islands: foci of sclerotic and lamellar compact bone, with some Haversian systems. The lesions are devoid of appositional remodeling, active resorption or a cartilaginous component.[8] The thickened trabeculae merge gradually into the surrounding cancellous bone, which is normal[6] (Figs 47.13–47.16).

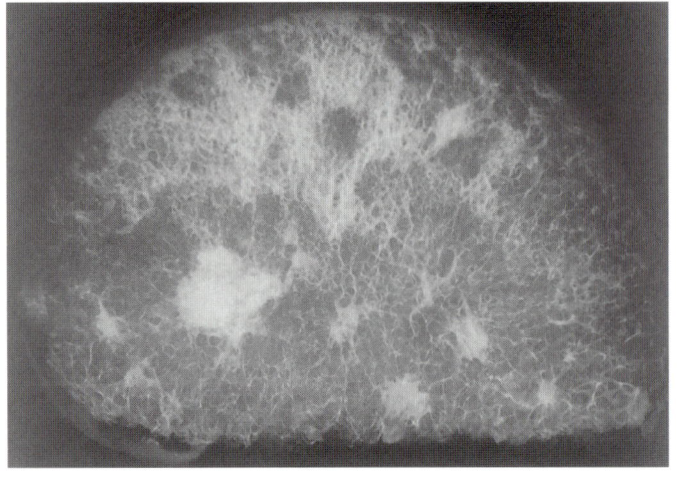

Fig. 47.9

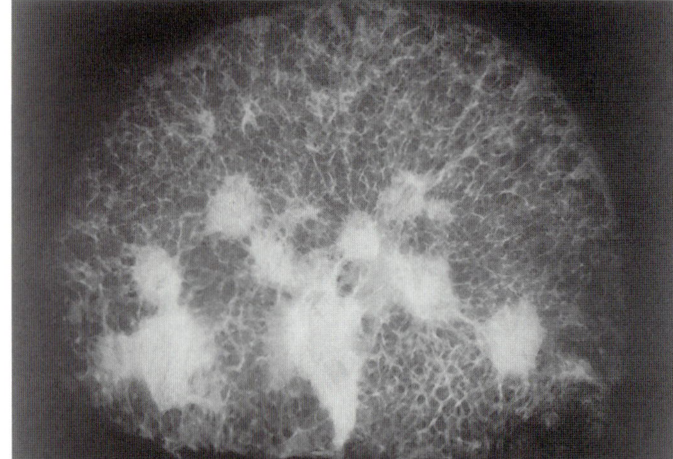

Fig. 47.10

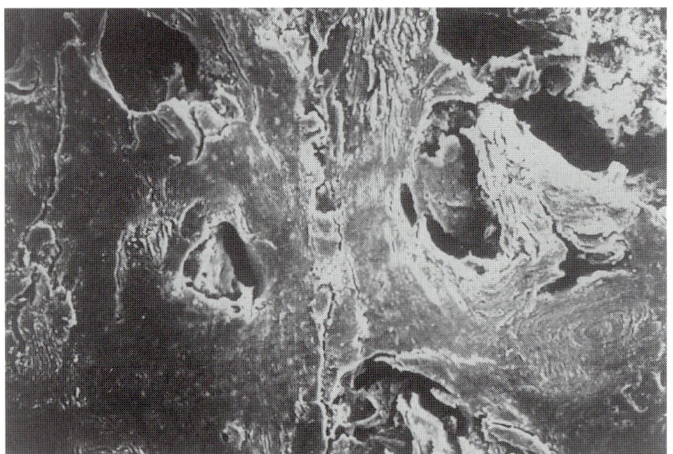

Fig. 47.11

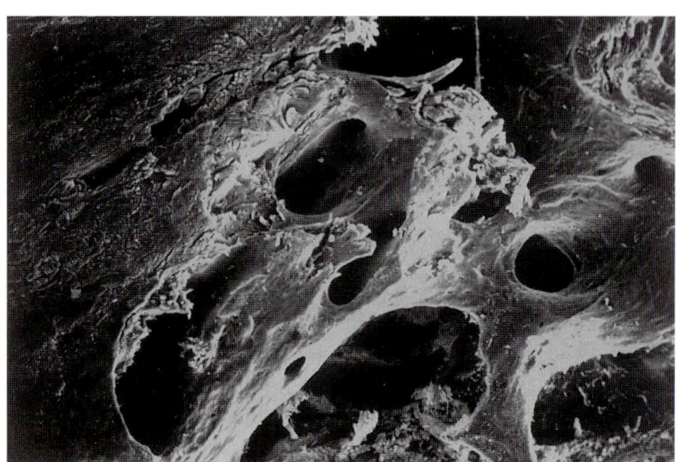

Fig. 47.12

Figs 47.11, 47.12 SEM study of osteopoikilosis demonstrating the relationship of the sclerotic foci with the adjacent trabeculae of bone.

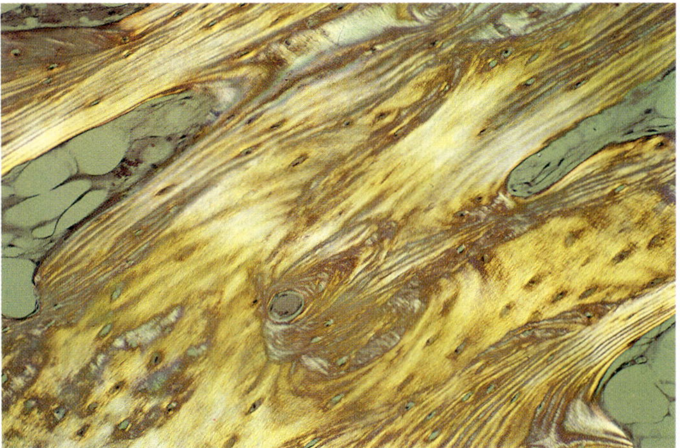

Fig. 47.13

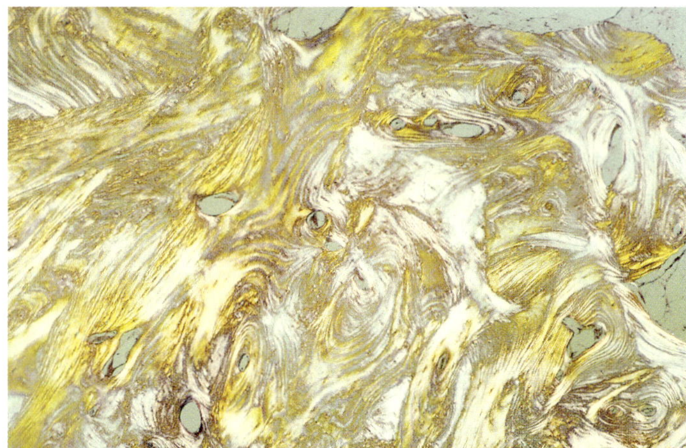

Fig. 47.14

Figs 47.13, 47.14 Osteopoikilotic bone has a lamellar and compact architecture (polarized light).

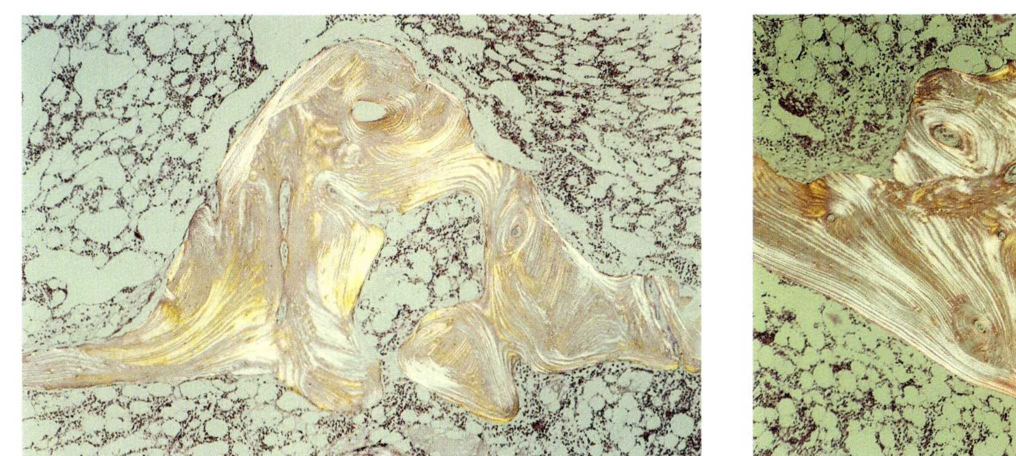

Fig. 47.15

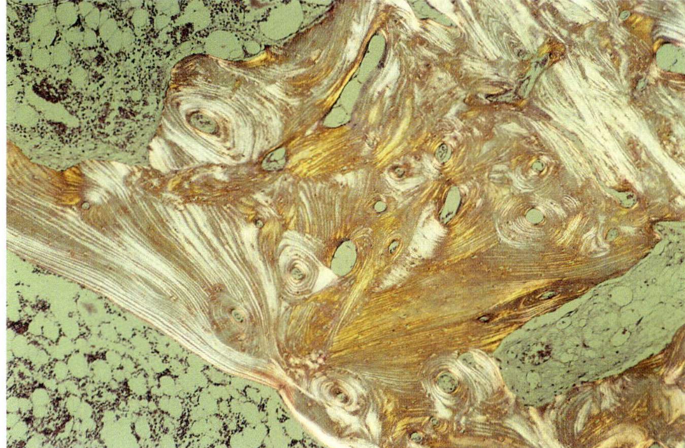

Fig. 47.16

Figs 47.15, 47.16 Foci of osteopoikilosis have the same structure as that of bone islands (polarized light).

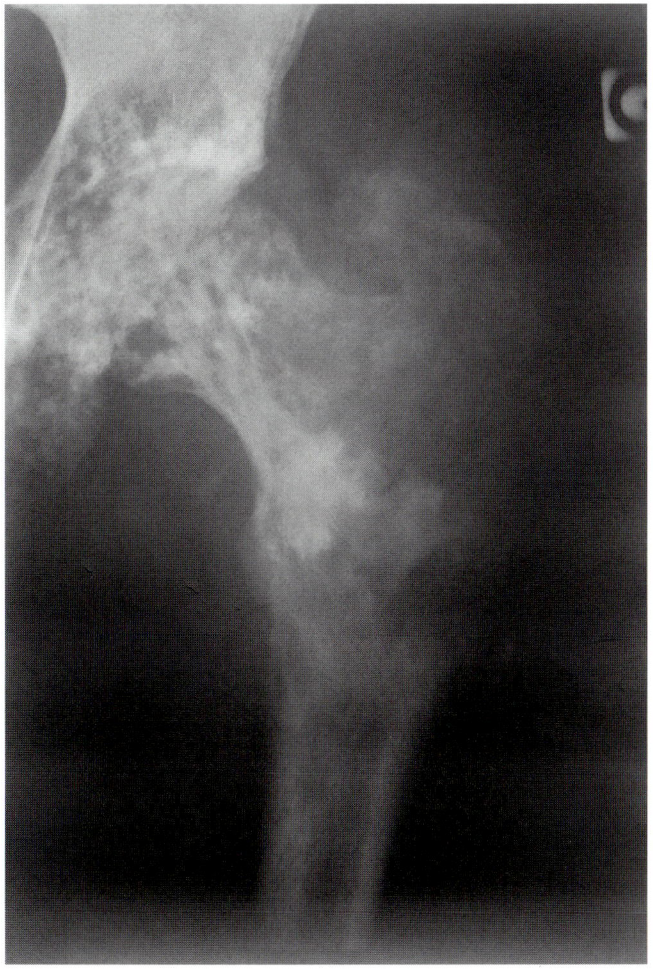

Fig. 47.17

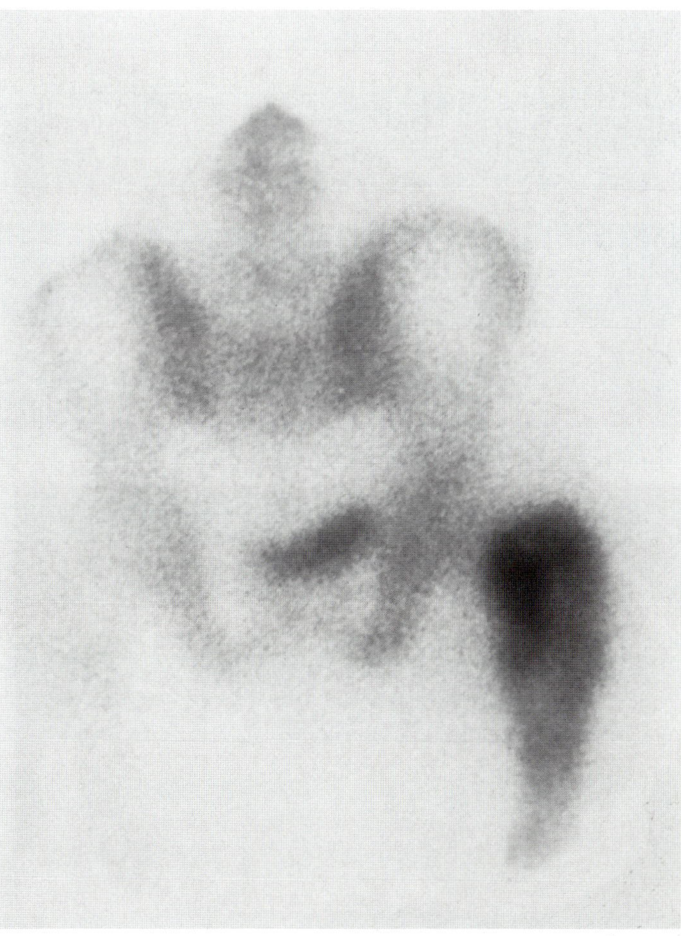

Fig. 47.18

Figs 47.17–47.22 Osteoblastic osteosarcoma arising in a femur with lesions of osteopoikilosis (same case as Fig. 47.1).

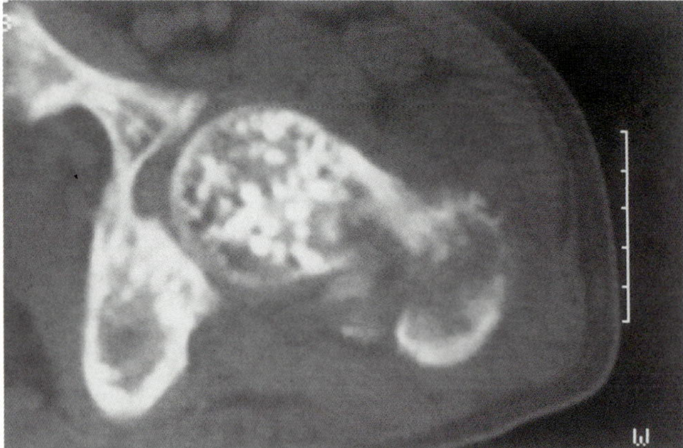

Fig. 47.19

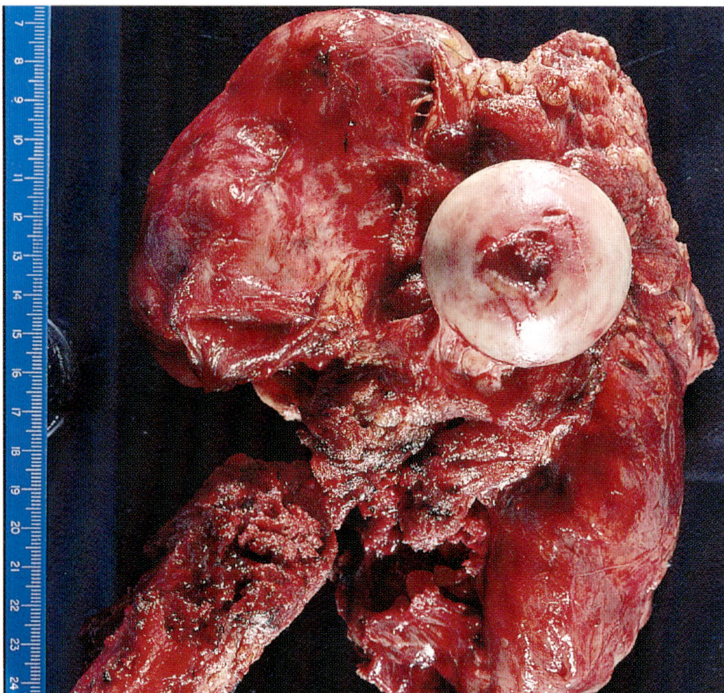

Fig. 47.20

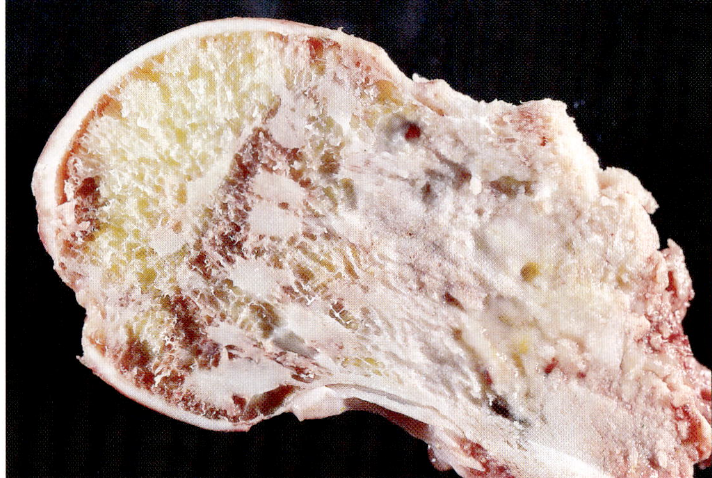

Fig. 47.21

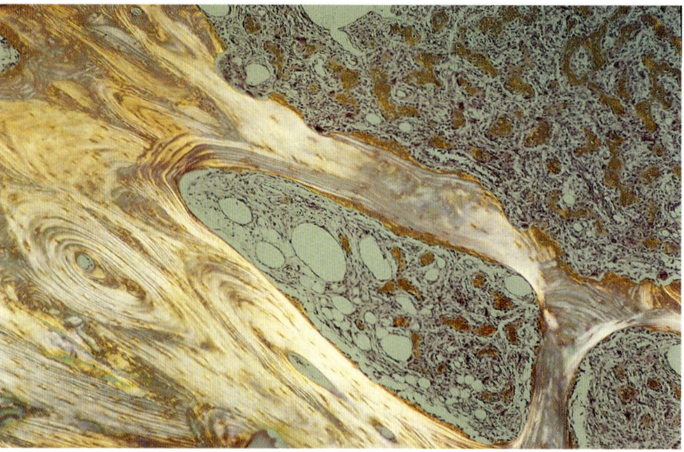

Fig. 47.22

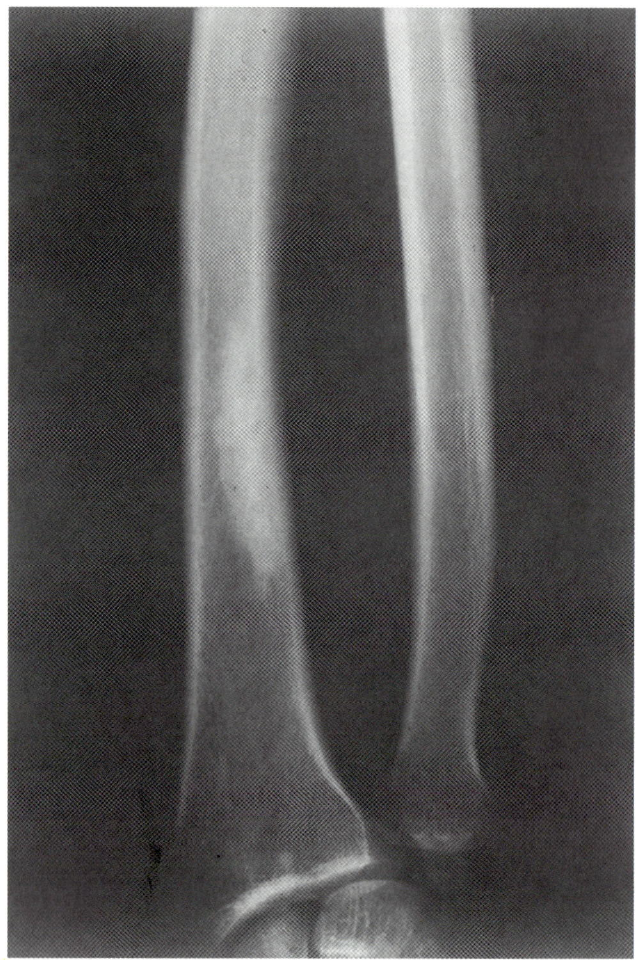

Fig. 47.23 Melorheostosis of the radius.

Osteopoikilosis and tumors

The few tumors reported should be viewed as coincidental events: giant cell tumor in the femur,[12] plasmacytoma,[13] humeral chondrosarcoma[14] and osteosarcoma of the tibia[15] (Figs 47.17–47.22).

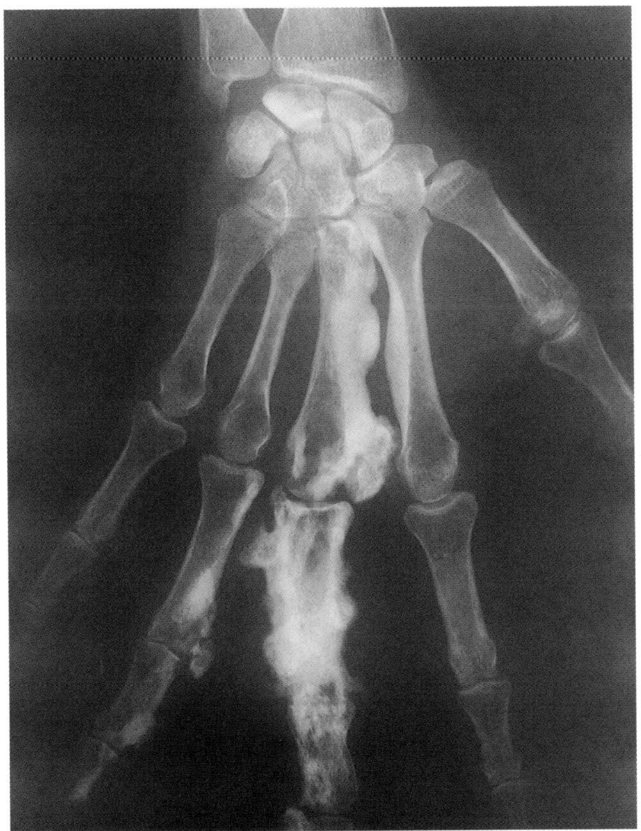

Fig. 47.24

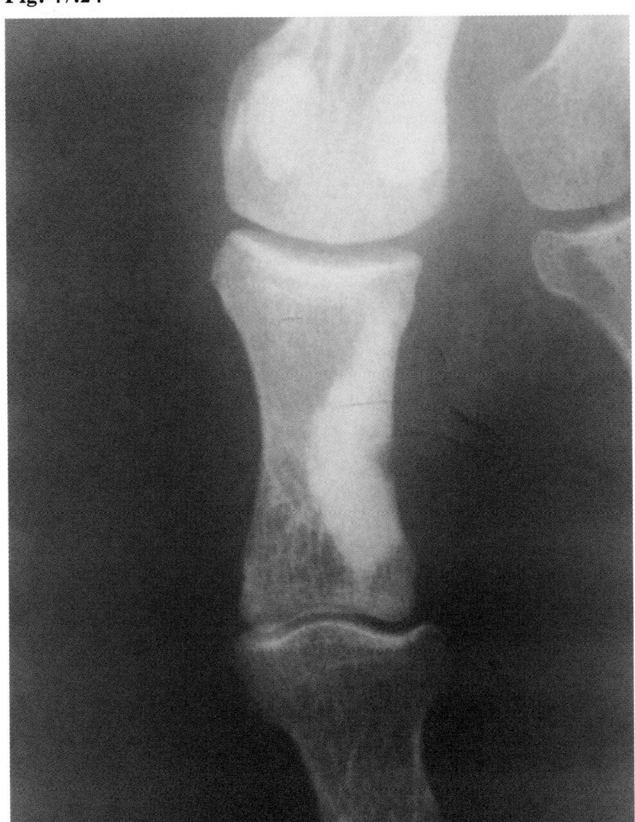

Fig. 47.25

Figs 47.24, 47.25 Melorheostosis of the hand.

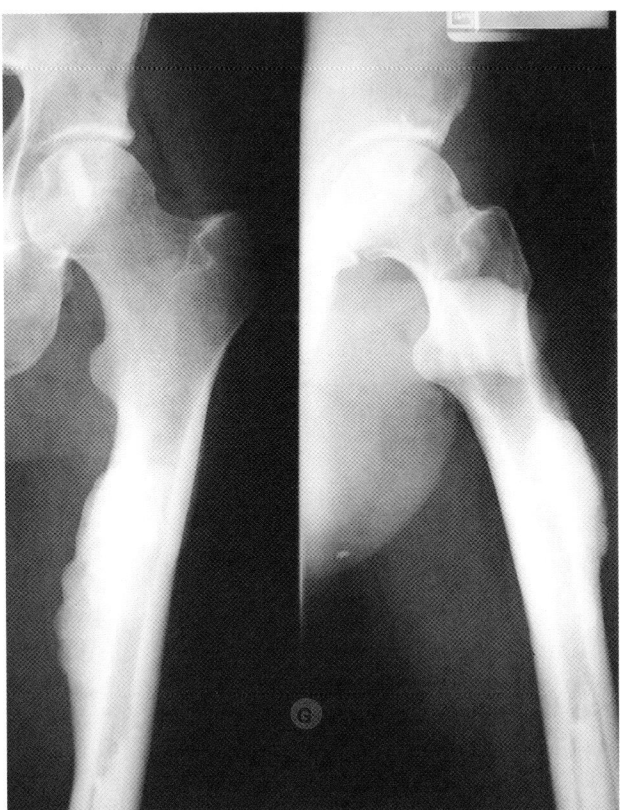

Fig. 47.26

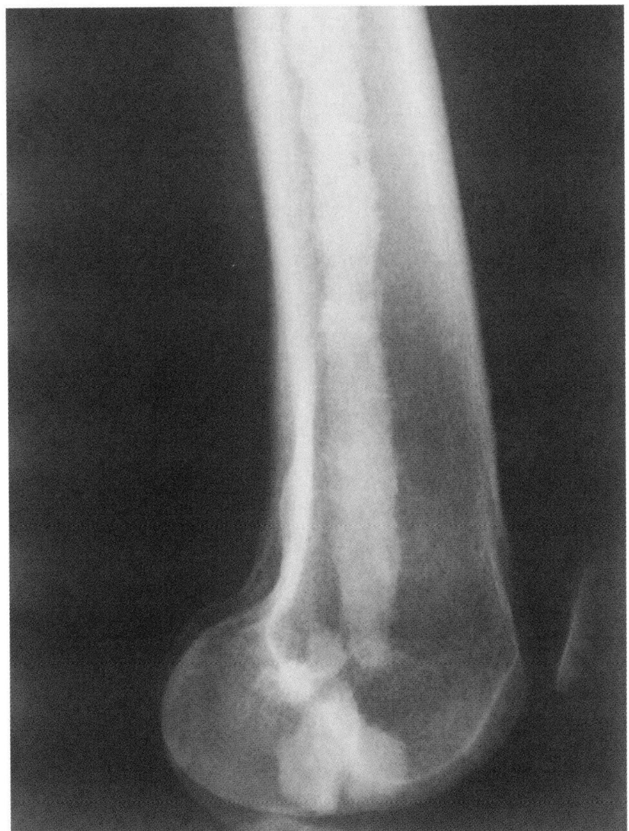

Fig. 47.27

Figs 47.26, 47.27 Melorheostosis of the femur.

Differential diagnosis

Some osteoblastic metastases from breast carcinoma may be cold on radionuclide bone scans and histologically, small strands of malignant cells may be overlooked,[16] but usually the uniform size and the symmetrical distribution of the lesions of osteopoikilosis are obvious.

MELORHEOSTOSIS

Introduction and clinical data

An irregular sclerotic thickening of the endosteal and periosteal surface of a tubular bone, resembling candle wax, is the hallmark of melorheostosis, a rare, non-heritable mesodermal disorder of bone and soft tissue.

The condition is most frequently diagnosed during childhood or in young adults and occasionally even at birth.[17] The sex distribution is equal.[18] Some patients may be asymptomatic but clinical symptoms are pain, deformity, joint contractures and limitation of motion, limb length discrepancy and atrophy of muscles.[19]

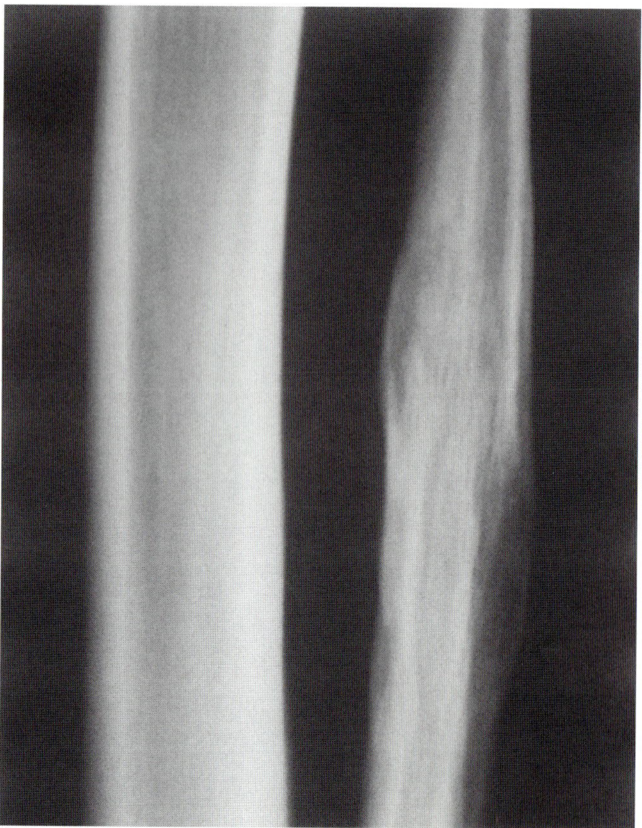

Fig. 47.29

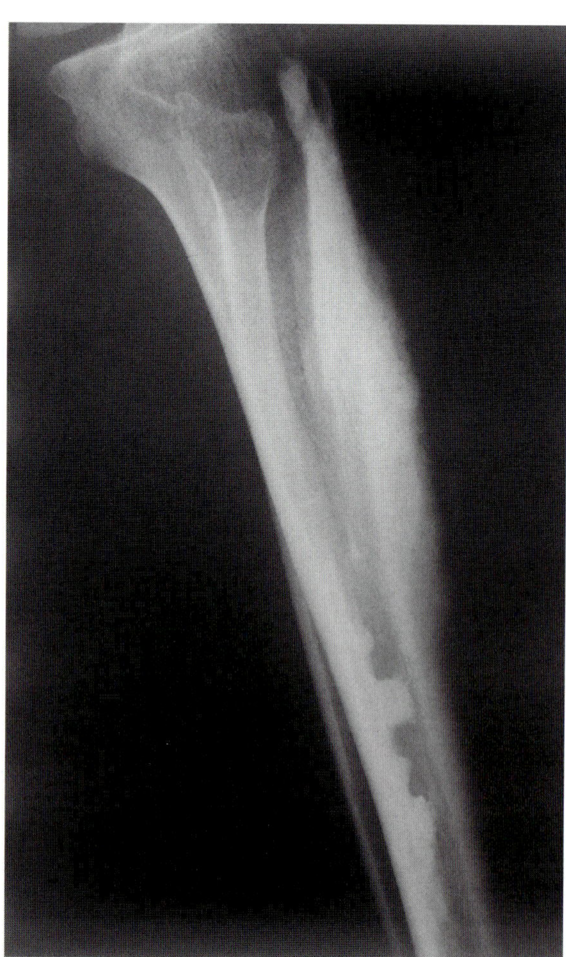

Fig. 47.28 Melorheostosis of the tibia.

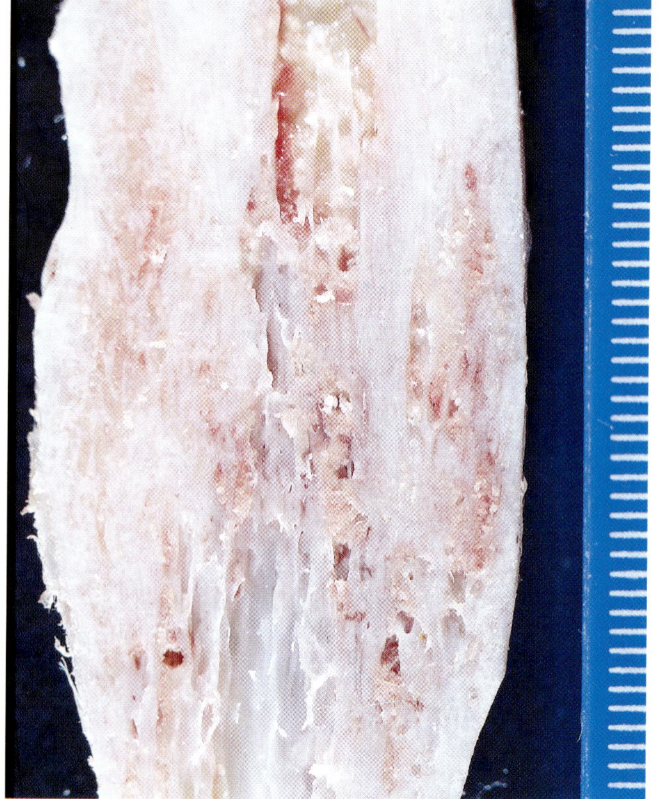

Fig. 47.30

Figs 47.29, 47.30 Melorheostosis of the fibula.

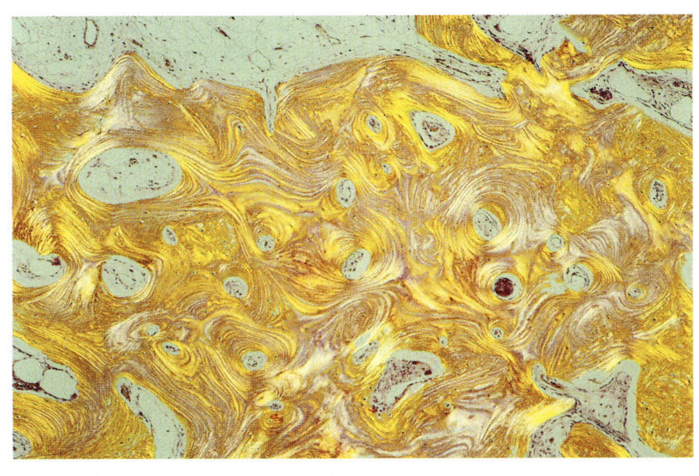

Fig. 47.31

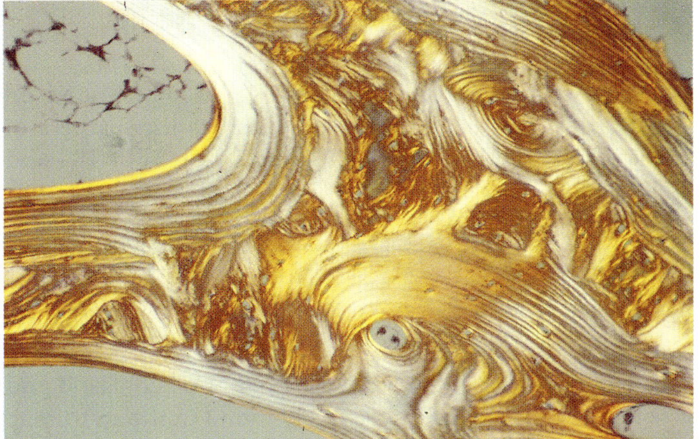

Fig. 47.32

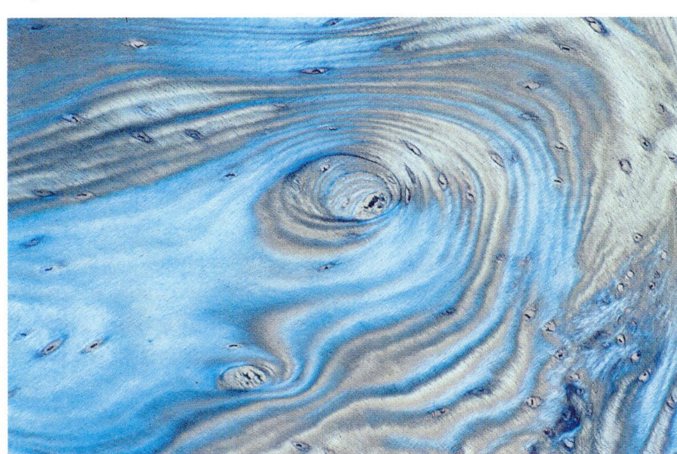

Fig. 47.33

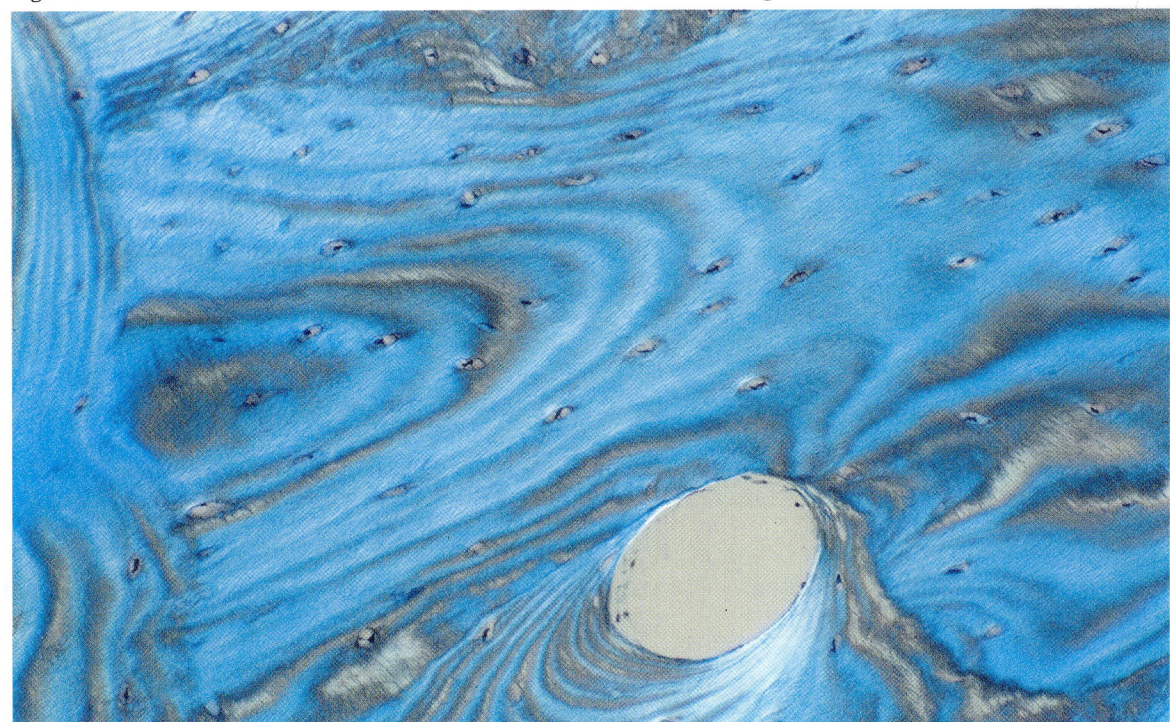

Fig. 47.34

Fig. 47.35

Figs 47.31–47.35
Melorheostosis:
thickened bone with a
lamellar architecture
(polarized light).

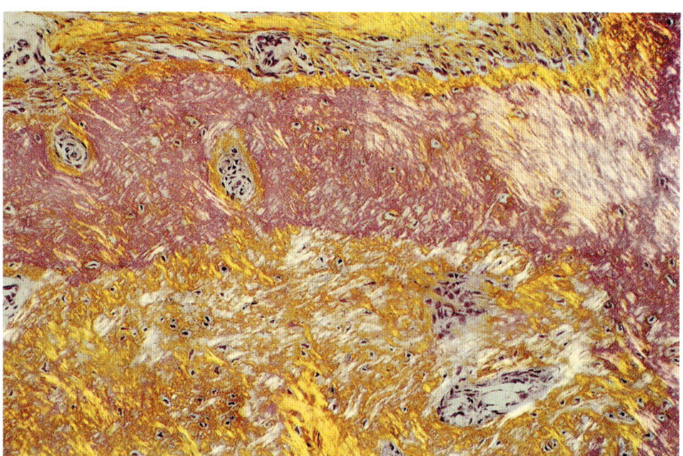

Fig. 47.36 Melorheostosis: immature bone in peripheral territories (polarized light).

Melorheostosis may be associated with scleroderma, lymphatic dysplasias, glomus tumor, arteriovenous aneurysms, hemangiomas[20] and aggressive fibromatosis.[21] Intrathecal lipoma or fibrolipomatous tissue has been identified in rare vertebral locations.[22,23]

A sclerotomal distribution of the lesions has been demonstrated.[24] Melorheostosis may be the result of a segmental sensory nerve lesion, the paraarticular ossifications of soft tissues being related to the involvement of a corresponding myotome.[24]

Skeletal distribution

Changes are usually limited to a single limb, chiefly the lower limb (monomelic distribution),[24] but may involve multiple bones (polyostotic form) or only one bone (monostotic form).[6]

Alterations of the limb are frequently associated with lesions in the pelvis and shoulder girdle[25] and may extend to the small bones of hands and feet.[19,24] Involvement of the skull, facial bones, ribs and vertebrae is unusual.[22–25]

Osteosclerotic lesions are progressive, spreading in a linear fashion,[26] and may cross an open epiphyseal plate or a joint space,[18] simulating osteochondromatosis.[27]

Symptomatic paraarticular soft tissue mineralized masses may be located around the hip, the knee, ankle, shoulder and wrist.[26–29]

Imaging

The exuberant hypertrophic subperiosteal and endosteal bone formation is well defined, with wavy contours and a linear pattern of distribution in the long axis of the limb (Figs 47.23–47.30).

The cortical hyperostosis is usually eccentric and endosteal hyperostosis may partially or completely obliterate the medullary cavity.

In some cases, linear streaks or punctate osteosclerotic foci resemble osteopathia striata or osteopoikilosis, especially in flat or irregular bones.[22]

Scintigraphy shows an increased uptake of radionuclides.[10]

The thickening of the cortex is well demonstrated on CT scans.[28] On MRI, melorheostosis has the features of cortical bone, with a low signal intensity on both T1- and T2-weighted images.[25,28]

Histopathology

Bony trabeculae are thickened with normal-appearing, irregularly distributed Haversian systems and a lamellar architecture (Figs 47.31–47.36). Foci of osteoblastic and osteoclastic activity are more easily found in the soft tissue masses, as well as immature bone within fibrous tissue and cartilage islands or caps undergoing ossification.[26,27,29]

Clinical course, treatment and prognosis

The slowly progressive course is marked by increasing pain and deformity.[19] The treatment is symptomatic.[17]

The relationship between the prolonged process of bone formation and the very few sarcomas reported is purely speculative. An osteosarcoma and a malignant fibrous histiocytoma have been described, both in the femur.[30,31]

REFERENCES

1. Benli I T, Akalin S, Boysan E, Mumcu E F, Kis M, Tûrkoglu D. Epidemiological, clinical and radiological aspects of osteopoikilosis. J Bone Joint Surg (Br) 1992: 74: 504–506
2. Walker G F. Mixed sclerosing bone dystrophies. J Bone Joint Surg (Br) 1964: 46: 546–552
3. Abrahamson M N. Disseminated asymptomatic osteosclerosis with features resembling melorheostosis, osteopoikilosis, and osteopathia striata. J Bone Joint Surg (Am) 1968: 50: 991–996
4. Whyte M P, Murphy W A, Fallon M D, Hahn T J. Mixed-sclerosing-bone dystrophy. Skeletal Radiol 1981: 6: 95–102
5. Cantatore F P, Carrozzo M, Loperfido M C. Mixed sclerosing bone dystrophy with features resembling osteopoikilosis and osteopathia striata. Clin Rheumatol 1991: 10: 191–195
6. Greenspan A. Sclerosing bone dysplasias – a target site approach. Skeletal Radiol 1991: 20: 561–583
7. Chigira M, Kato K, Mashio K, Shinozaki T. Symmetry of bone lesions in osteopoikilosis. Acta Orthop Scand 1991: 62: 495–496
8. Lagier R, Mbakop A, Bigler A. Osteopoikilosis: a radiological and pathological study. Skeletal Radiol 1984: 11: 161–168
9. Mungovan J A, Tung G A, Lambiase R E, Noto R B, Davis R P. Tc-99m MDP uptake in osteopoikilosis. Clin Nucl Med 1994: 19: 6–8
10. Whyte M P, Murphy W A, Siegel B A. 99mTc-pyrophosphate bone imaging in osteopoikilosis, osteopathia striata and melorheostosis. Radiology 1978: 127: 439–443

11. Tong E C, Samii M, Tchang F. Bone imaging as an aid for the diagnosis of osteopoikilosis. Clin Nucl Med 1988: 13: 816–819

12. Ayling R M, Evans P E. Giant cell tumor in a patient with osteopoikilosis. Acta Orthop Scand 1988: 59: 74–76

13. Bethge J F, Ridderbusch K E. Uber osteopoikilie und nas neue krankheitsbild hyperostose bei osteopoikilie. Ergebn Chir Orthop 1967: 49: 138–182

14. Grimer R J, Davies A M, Starkic C M, Sncath R S. Chondrosarcome chez un patient porteur d'ostéopoikilie. Rev Chir Orthop Reparatrice Appar Mot 1989: 75: 188–190

15. Mindell E R, Northup C S, Douglass H O. Osteosarcoma associated with osteopoikilosis. J Bone Joint Surg (Am) 1978: 60: 406–408

16. Ghandur-Mnaymneh L, Broder L E, Mnaymneh W A. Lobular carcinoma of the breast metastatic to bone with unusual clinical, radiologic, and pathologic features mimicking osteopoikilosis. Cancer 1984: 53: 1801–1803

17. Hove E, Sury B. Melorheostosis. Acta Orthop Scand 1971: 42: 315–319

18. Campbell C J, Papademetriou T, Bonfiglio M. Melorheostosis: a report of the clinical, roentgenographic and pathological findings in fourteen cases. J Bone Joint Surg (Am) 1968: 50: 1281–1304

19. Caudle R J, Stern P J. Melorheostosis of the hand. J Bone Joint Surg (Am) 1987: 69: 1229–1231

20. Kessler H B, Recht M P, Dalinka M K. Vascular anomalies in association with osteodystrophies – a spectrum. Skeletal Radiol 1983: 10: 95–101

21. Ippolito V, Mirra J M, Motta C, Chiodera P, Bonetti M F. Case report 771. Melorheostosis in association with desmoid tumor. Skeletal Radiol 1993: 22: 284–288

22. Garver P, Resnick D, Haghighi P, Guerra J. Melorheostosis of the axial skeleton with associated fibrolipomatous lesions. Skeletal Radiol 1982: 9: 41–44

23. Raby N, Vivian G. Case report 478. Melorheostosis of the axial skeleton with associated intrathecal lipoma. Skeletal Radiol 1988: 17: 216–219

24. Murray R O, McCredie J. Melorheostosis and the sclerotomes: a radiological correlation. Skeletal Radiol 1979: 4: 57–71

25. Isaacs P, Resnick D. MR appearance of axial melorheostosis. Skeletal Radiol 1993: 22: 47–48

26. Goldman A B, Schneider R, Huvos A S, Lane J. Melorheostosis presenting as two soft-tissue masses with osseous changes limited to the axial skeleton. Skeletal Radiol 1993: 22: 206–210

27. Gold R H, Mirra J M. Case report 35. Melorheostosis. Skeletal Radiol 1977: 2: 57–58

28. Yu J S, Resnick D, Vaughan L M, Haghighi P, Hughes T. Melorheostosis with an ossified soft tissue mass: MR features. Skeletal Radiol 1995: 24: 367–370

29. Khurana J S, Ehara S, Rosenberg A E, Rosenthal D I. Case report 510. Melorheostosis of ilium, femur, and adjacent soft tissues. Skeletal Radiol 1988: 17: 539–541

30. Böstman O M, Holmström T, Riska E B. Osteosarcoma arising in a melorheostotic femur. J Bone Joint Surg (Am) 1987: 69: 1232–1237

31. Baer S C, Ayala A G, Ro J Y, Yasko A W, Raymond A K, Edeiken J. Case report 843. Malignant fibrous histiocytoma of the femur arising in melorheostosis. Skeletal Radiol 1994: 23: 310–314

48

Membranous lipodystrophy

M. Forest

INTRODUCTION AND CLINICAL DATA

Membranous lipodystrophy is a rare disease, predominantly affecting the fatty tissues of bones and the brain.

Pathologic bone changes were first described in 1964 under the name 'polycystic lipomembranous osteodysplasia';[1,2] they were later associated with neuropsychiatric symptoms of a sclerosing leukoencephalopathy.[3]

More than 130 cases have been reported, most of them in Scandinavia and Japan, isolated cases coming from the United States, Italy, South Africa, Turkey and France. There is no sex predominance and the disease has a recessive mode of inheritance.[1,3,4]

Initial symptoms, in adolescence or around 20 years of age,[1] are pain, tenderness and swelling in joints or a pathologic fracture, occurring most frequently around the ankle or the knee. By the age of 30 years, almost all patients have pathologic features due to the skeletal changes.[1,5,6] Laboratory tests are within normal limits.[7]

Bone lesions remain unchanged or progress very slowly[1,6] but after 30 years of age neuropsychiatric symptoms increase, bearing a close resemblance to Alzheimer's disease. Death may occur at about 40–50 years of age.[3,6]

SKELETAL DISTRIBUTION

Bone lesions appear in the epiphyses and metaphyses of long bones, but are more conspiciuous in the carpal and tarsal bones, metacarpals, metatarsals and phalanges, with a symmetrical distribution[1] (Figs 48.1, 48.2). The axial skeleton is usually spared.[8]

IMAGING

Osteolytic multiloculated areas have poorly defined margins, with some expansion of bone but without peripheral sclerosis.[1] The cortex may be scalloped or thinned but is not interrupted. In the absence of fracture, there is no periosteal reaction.

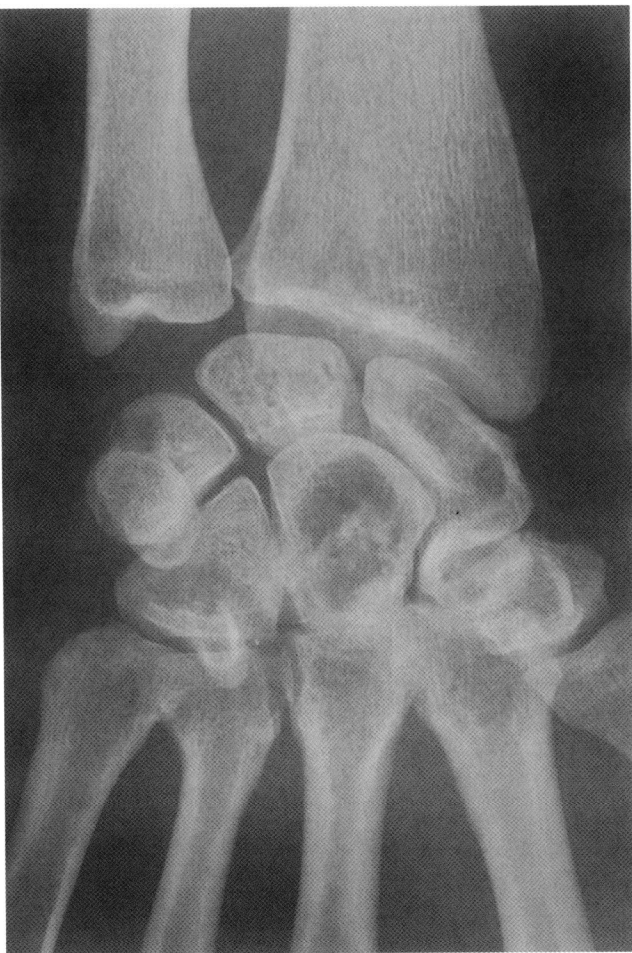

Fig. 48.1

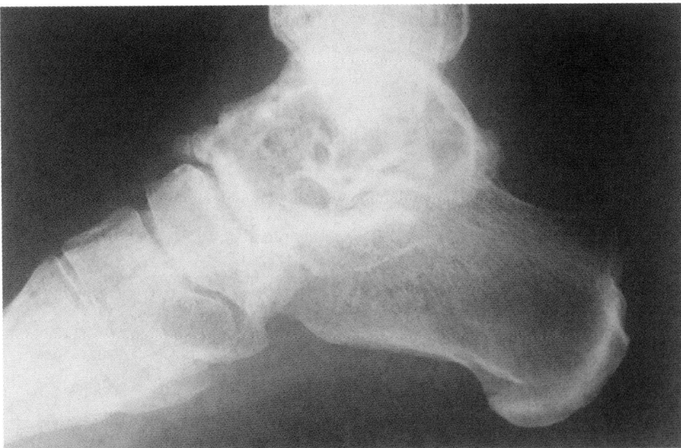

Fig. 48.2

Figs 48.1, 48.2 Membranous lipodystrophy involving carpal and tarsal bones, the talus and femoral heads in a 32-year-old man.

GROSS PATHOLOGY

The cortex is thinned. Cystic areas are filled with a yellow or grayish-white gelatinous or mucoid tissue, with no bone remnants.[9]

HISTOPATHOLOGY AND HISTOCHEMISTRY

The normal bone marrow is replaced by undulating membranes, also found on the periphery, among normal-appearing adipocytes.[10] The numerous hyaline, eosinophilic and refractile membranes surround single cells or larger cystic spaces[6,9] (Figs 48.3–48.10). In these areas, nuclei are not seen.[9]

Some lesions may be found in the synovial membrane, fatty tissue[6] or even in distant sites of the body.[11]

The membranous structures are strongly stained with PAS,[9] oil red O and Sudan black B, moderately with alcian blue and luxol fast blue and weakly with toluidine blue.[12,13]

The carbohydrate components of the membranes have been studied using marker-labeled lectins at light and electron microscopic levels, demonstrating α D-galactose residues.[13,14]

In the brain, a leukodystrophy of the sudanophilic type is associated with atrophy of the cortex, demyelinization of the white matter, proliferation of glial tissue and calcifications of the basal ganglia.[11]

ELECTRON MICROSCOPY

The undulating membranes exhibit two layers (Figs 48.11, 48.12). Numerous minute tubular structures are arranged perpendicular to the inner surface, which appears very dense.[4,5,6,8,9,13,15] The outer surface is poorly defined, merging with the interstitial connective tissue.[6,15] Thinner membranes may be devoid of tubular structures.[13]

These findings are viewed as terminal breakdown products of fat cell membranes[1] and degenerating adipose cells have been identified at the lipid–cytoplasmic interface.[13,14]

PATHOGENESIS

The etiopathogenesis of the wide range of degenerative changes in adipose cells is actually unknown. A disorder of lipid metabolism has been suggested[9,11] but there is no specific substance found on biochemical analysis,[6,15] nor any anomaly of the lipid metabolic enzymes[15] and the mucopolysaccharide metabolism also appears normal.[15]

Developmental anomalies of the blood vessels have been found and in autopsy studies, abnormal blood vessels have been described in bone and brain lesions, with a thickening of the basement membrane and extravasation of the plasma constituent.[2] However, the lesions are not associated with circulatory disturbances,[13] even though when they resemble lesions of fatty tissue found in protracted ischemic limb necrosis.[16,17] Similar lesions have been reported in various conditions, including fat tissue granulomas, lupus erythematosus, dermatomyositis, Farber's disease and rheumatoid arthritis treated by corticosteroids.[5]

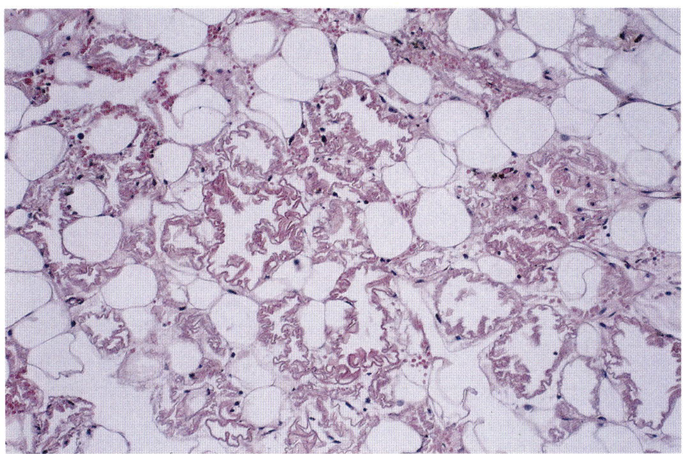

Fig. 48.3

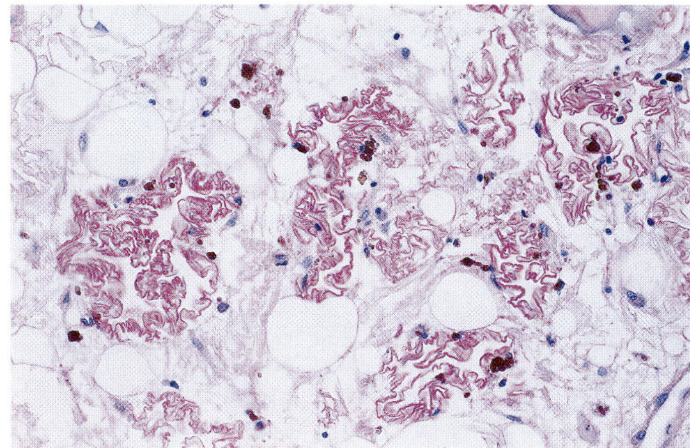

Fig. 48.5

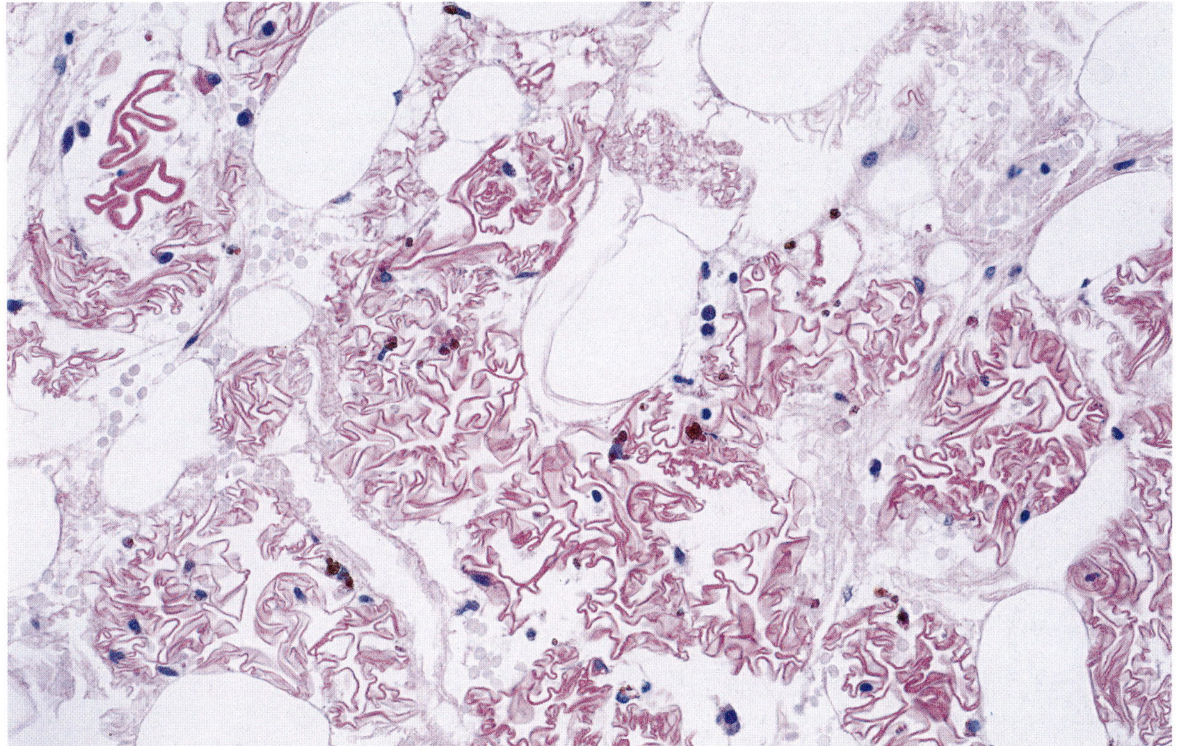

Fig. 48.4

Figs 48.3–48.6 Numerous undulating and eosinophilic membranes with some normal-appearing adipocytes. (PAS stain.)

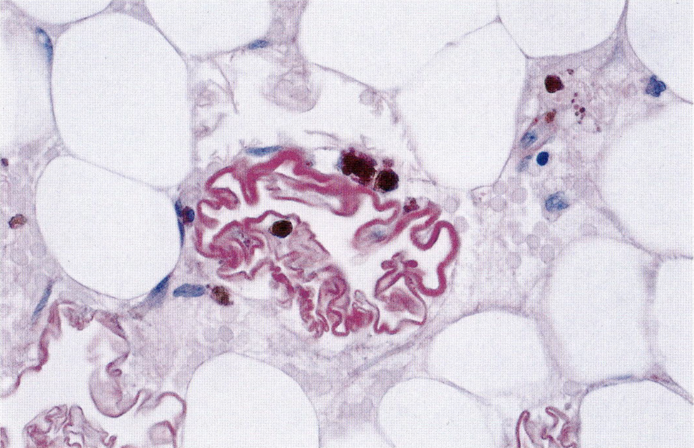

Fig. 48.6

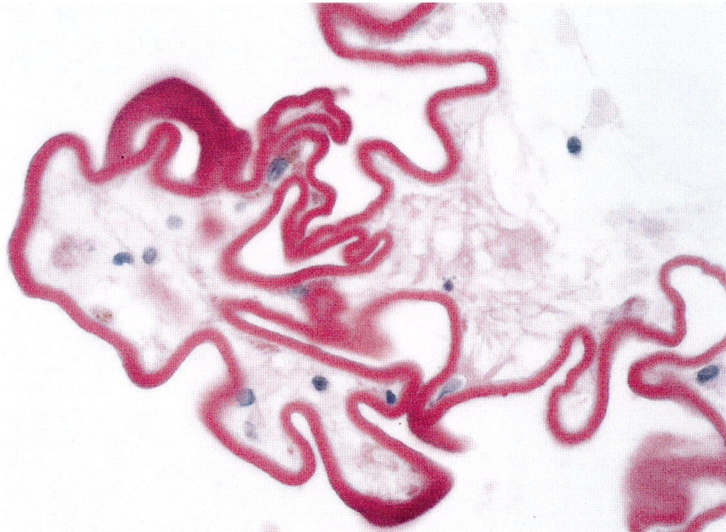

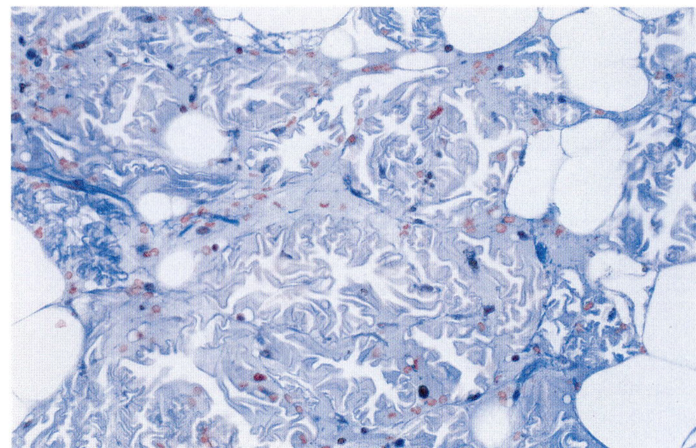

Fig. 48.7   **Fig. 48.8**

Figs 48.7, 48.8 Membranous lipodystrophy: highly refractile appearance of the membranes. (PAS and trichrome stain.)

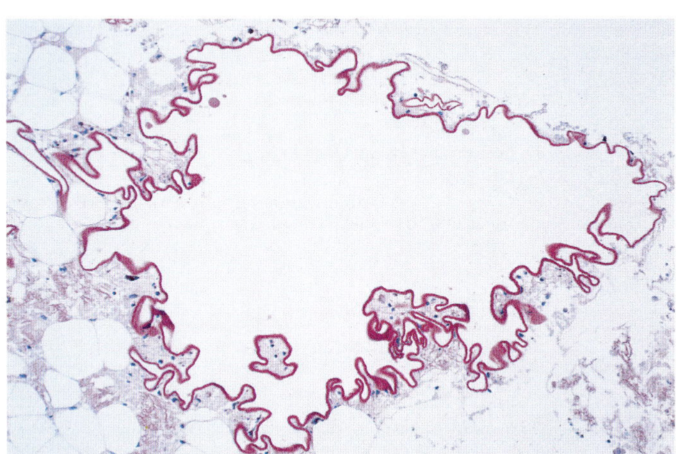

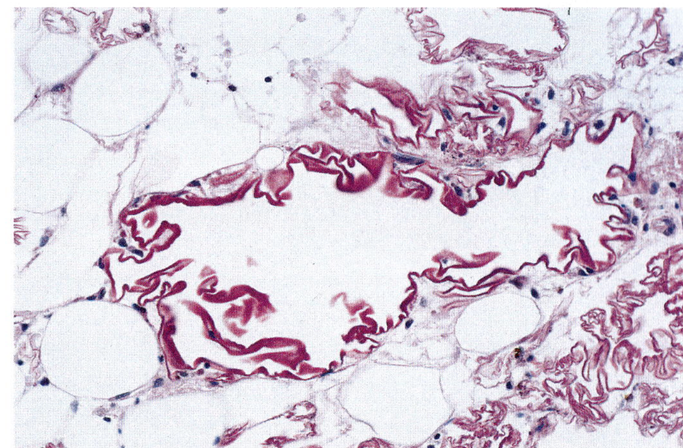

Fig. 48.9   **Fig. 48.10**

Figs 48.9, 48.10 Membranous lipodystrophy: cystic spaces lined by the membranes. (PAS stain.)

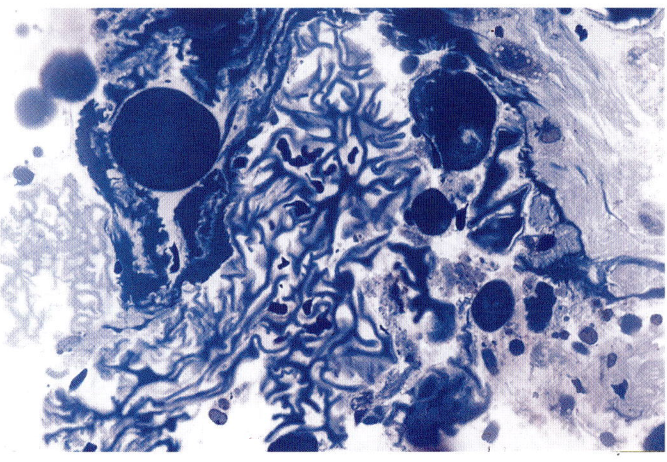

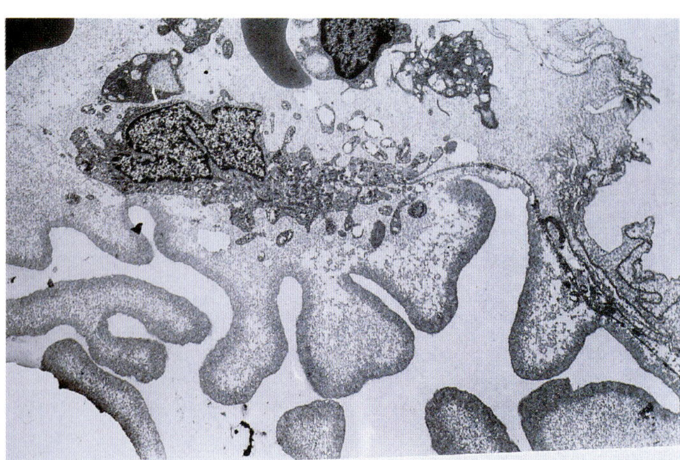

Fig. 48.11   **Fig. 48.12**

Figs 48.11, 48.12 Ultrastructure of membranous lipodystrophy: refractile aspect on semi-thin sections, two layers demonstrated on ultra-thin sections. (×4900.)

DIFFERENTIAL DIAGNOSIS

On imaging, bone lesions may be confused with cystic angiomatosis, lymphangiomatosis, fibrous dysplasia or hyperparathyroidism,[1] but there is a symmetrical distribution and associated mental changes.[7]

Some cases have been diagnosed, even histologically, as lipomatosis[18] but rare multiple lipomas with a symmetrical distribution have been reported only in Japan[6] and they are devoid of the characteristic undulating membranous structures.

REFERENCES

1. Mâkelâ P, Jârvi O, Hakola P, Virtama P. Radiologic bone changes of polycystic lipomembranous osteodysplasia with sclerosing leukoencephalopathy. Skeletal Radiol 1982: 8: 51–54
2. Kalimo H, Sourander P, Järvi O, Hakola P. Vascular changes and blood–brain barrier damage in the pathogenesis of polycystic lipomembranous osteodysplasia with sclerosing leukoencephalopathy (membranous lipodystrophy). Acta Neurol Scand 1994: 89: 353–361
3. Hakola H P. Neuropsychiatric and genetic aspects of a new hereditary disease characterized by progressive dementia and lipomembranous polycystic osteodysplasia. Acta Psychiatr Scand 1972: 232 (suppl): 1–173
4. Hasegawa Y, Inagaki Y. Membranous lipodystrophy (lipomembranous polycystic osteodysplasia). Clin Orthop 1983: 181: 229–232
5. Yaghishita S, Ito Y, Ikezaki R. Lipomembranous polycystic osteodysplasia. Virchows Arch A Pathol Anat Histol 1976: 372: 245–251
6. Akai M, Tateishi A, Cheng C H et al. Membranous lipodystrophy. J Bone Joint Surg (Am) 1977: 59: 802–809
7. Pazzaglia U E, Benazzo F, Castelli C, Boiocchi M, Beluffi G. Case report 381. Membranous lipodystrophy (MLD). Skeletal Radiol 1986: 15: 474–477
8. Edvardsen P, Halvorsen T B, Nesse O. Lipomembranous osteodysplasia. Int Orthop 1983: 7: 99–103
9. Wood C. Membranous lypodystrophy of bone. Arch Pathol Lab Med 1978: 102: 22–27
10. Kocer N, Dervisoglu S, Ersavasti G, Altug A, Cokyüksel O. Case report 867. Membranous lipodystrophy (polycystic lipomembranous osteodysplasia). Skeletal Radiol 1994: 23: 577–579
11. Nasu T, Tsukahara Y, Terayama K. A lipid metabolic disease 'membranous lipodystrophy'. Acta Pathol Jpn 1973: 23: 539–558
12. Fujiwara M. Histopathological and histochemical studies of membranocystic lesion (Nasu) (in Japanese). Shinshu Med J 1979: 27: 78–100
13. Kitajima I, Suganuma T, Murata F, Nagamatsu K. Ultrastructural demonstration of *Maclura pomifera* agglutinin binding sites in the membranocystic lesions of membranous lypodystrophy (Nasu Hakola disease). Virchows Arch A Pathol Anat Histopathol 1988: 413: 475–483
14. Suganuma T, Ihida K, Matsunaga S, Tsuyama S, Sakov T, Murata F. Glycoconjugate histochemistry and ultrastructural study of membranous lipodystrophy. Acta Histochem Cytochem 1987: 20: 21–30
15. Pazzaglia U E, Benazzo F, Byers P D, Riboni L, Ceciliani L. Pathogenesis of membranous lipodystrophy. Clin Orthop 1987: 225: 279–287
16. Machinami R. Membranous lipodystrophy-like changes in ischemic necrosis of the legs. Virchows Arch A Pathol Anat Histopathol 1983: 399: 191–205
17. Machinami R. Incidence of membranous lipodystrophy-like change among patients with limb necrosis caused by chronic arterial obstruction. Arch Pathol Lab Med 1984: 108: 823–826
18. Preziuso L, Muncibi F, Aglietti F G. A case of membranous lipodystrophy with skeletal involvement. Chir Organi Mov 1992: 77: 205–211

49

Callus and periosteal reactions

M. Forest

OSTEOBLASTIC AND OSTEOLYTIC PROCESSES FOLLOWING TRAUMA

In the first 3 weeks following a fracture, the brisk cellular activity of a *callus* may be confused with a malignant tumor (Figs 49.1–49.16): numerous spindle-shaped, stellate or ovoid cells with a high nuclear–cytoplasmic ratio infiltrate the surrounding tissues and prominent mitotic activity occurs. The first deposits of osteoid are devoid of osteoblastic rimming and may contribute to a misdiagnosis of osteosarcoma.[1]

Within 3–6 weeks, the new bone has acquired a trabecular pattern, with a regular osteoblastic margin and osteoblasts appearing as plump, active cells with a prominent Golgi zone (Mirra 1989). In some cases, bone forms regular arcades associated with thin-walled vessels. The absence of cellular pleomorphism and osteoid edged by a single layer of osteoblasts are important pointers to benignancy.[1] (Mirra 1989).

Patients with *osteogenesis imperfecta* may develop a markedly hypertrophic callus, even after minimal trauma or a surgical procedure, or may have no clinical evidence of fracture[2,3] (Figs 49.17–49.20).

The rapid enlargement over a few weeks with pain, elevation of sedimentation rate and serum alkaline phosphatase may simulate an aggressive lesion.[3–9] On X-ray, whorls of new bone formation are well circumscribed without a spiculated sunburst reaction and osteolysis.

Histologically, the callus is a primitive woven bone in lethal forms, woven and lamellar bone in adolescents and adults, and without a normal distribution of osteons. An irregularity in diameter of the collagen fibers and a splitting of their ends have been described in the non-callus tissue.[8,9]

A few cases of osteosarcoma have been reported in patients with osteogenesis imperfecta, appearing as sporadic entities not correlated with the underlying process.[10–14]

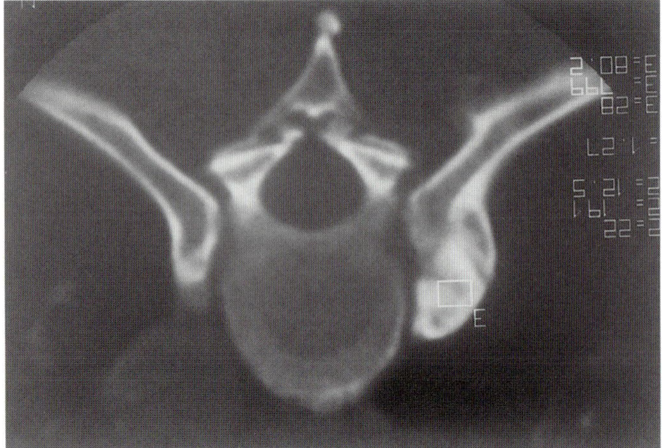

Fig. 49.1

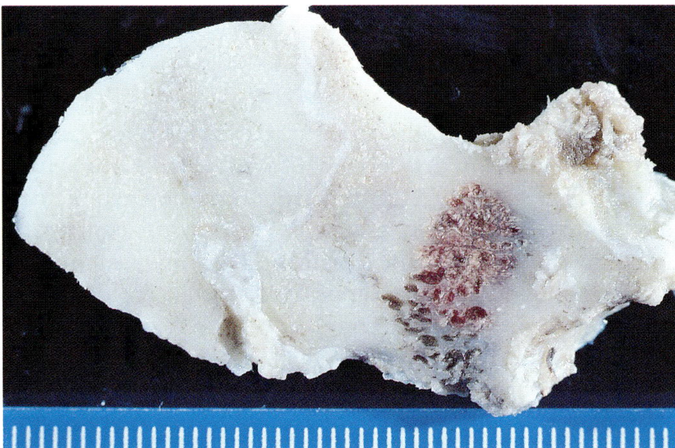

Fig. 49.2

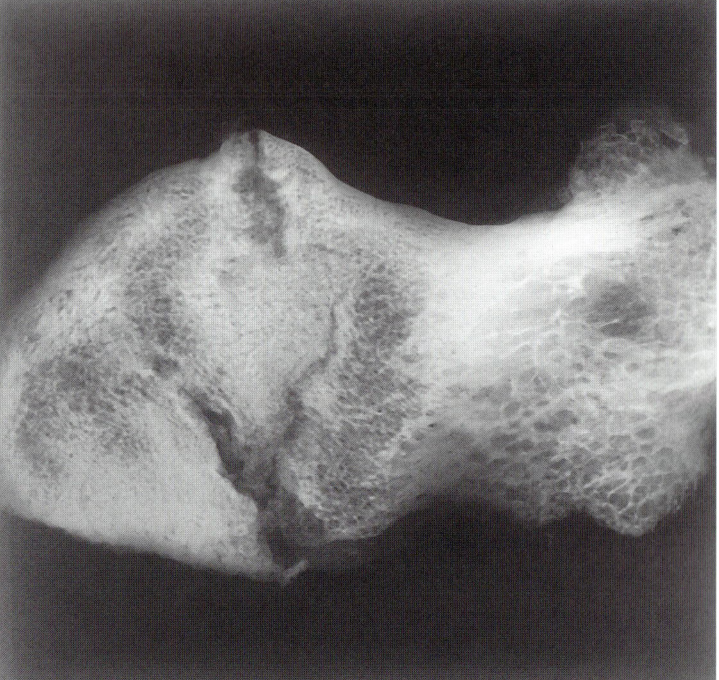

Fig. 49.3

Figs 49.1–49.3 Hypertrophic callus of a rib fracture suspected, on imaging, to be a tumor.

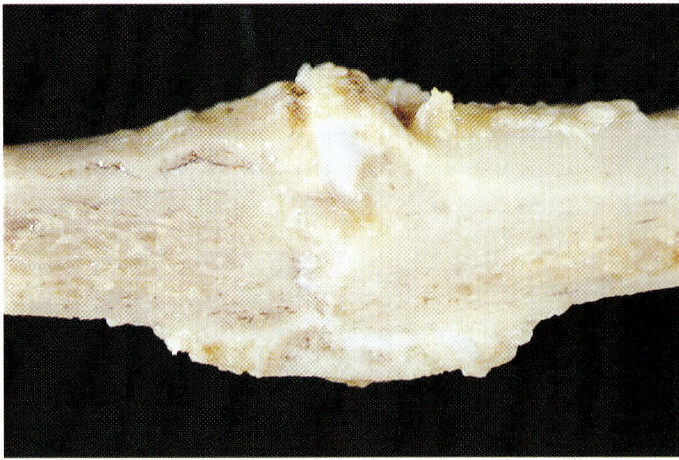

Fig. 49.4

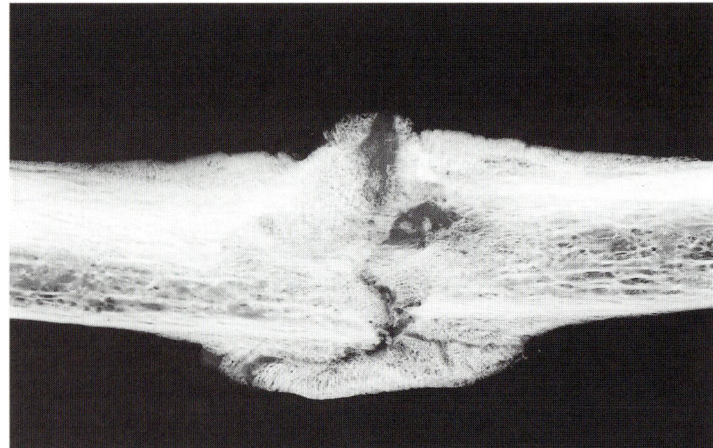

Fig. 49.5

Figs 49.4, 49.5 Painful fracture of a rib, with external periosteal bridging.

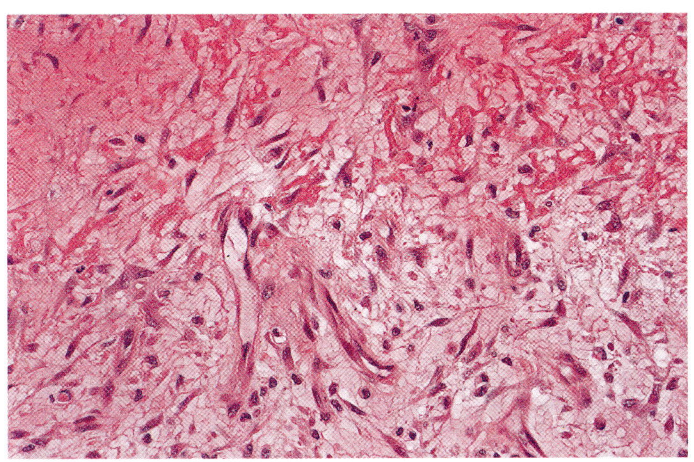

Fig. 49.6

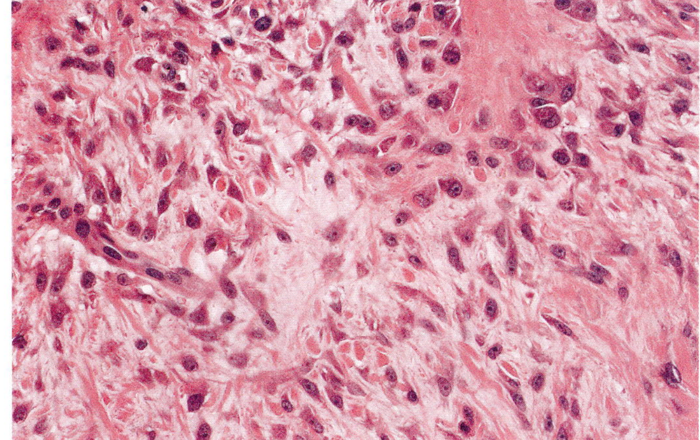

Fig. 49.7

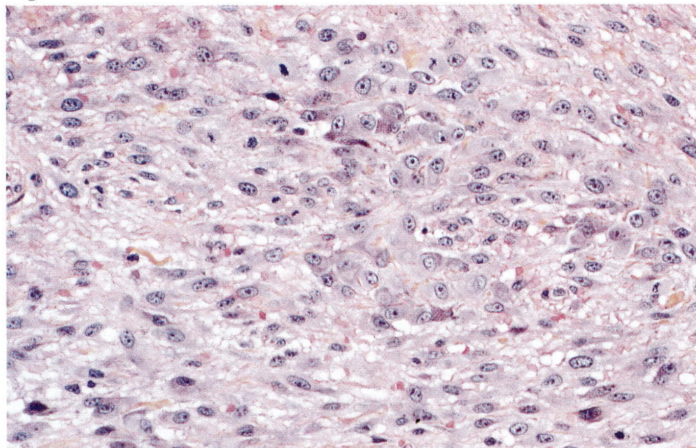

Fig. 49.8
Figs 49.6–49.8 Brisk cellular activity of a callus, in the first 15 days.

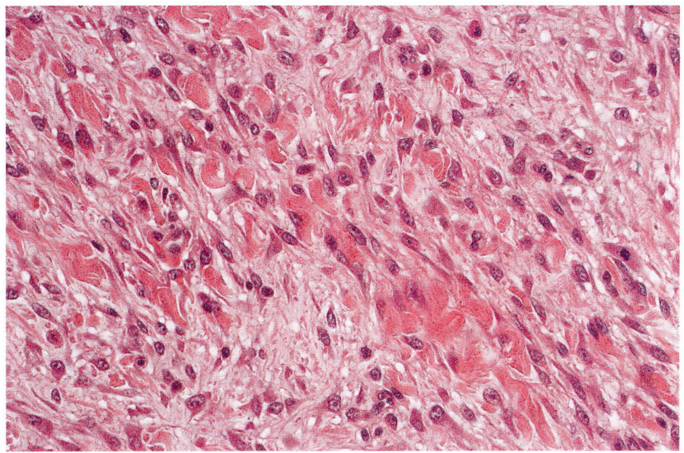

Fig. 49.9

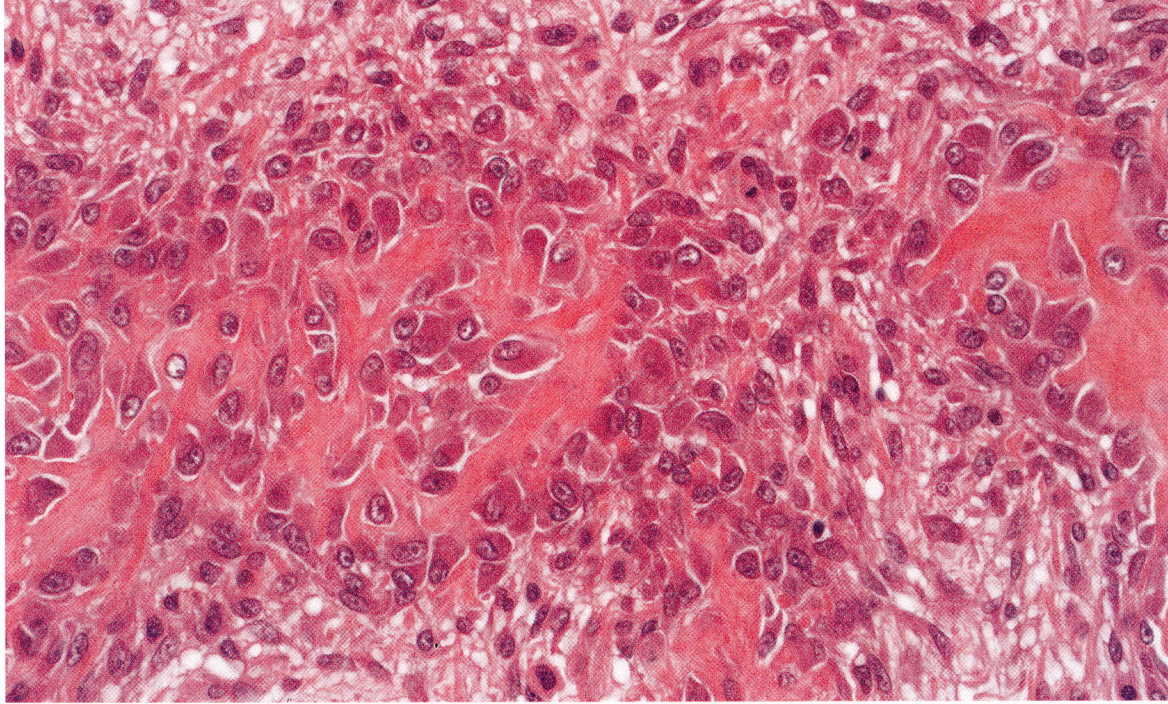

Figs 49.9, 49.10
Osteoblastic
differentiation in a
callus.

Fig. 49.10

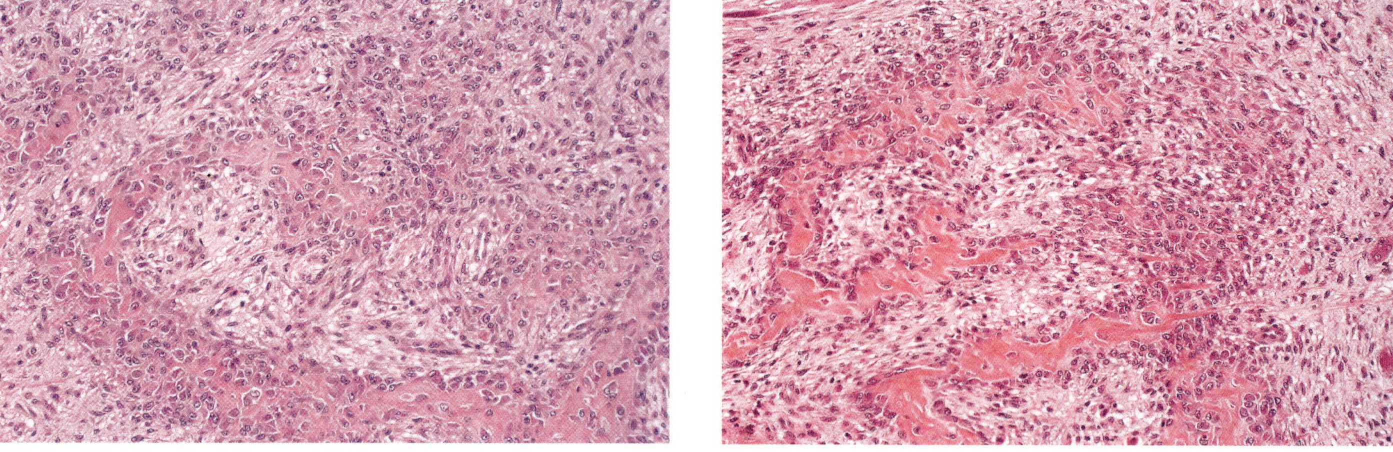

Fig. 49.11　　　　　　　　　　　　　　　**Fig. 49.12**

Figs 49.11, 49.12　Osteoblastic cellular component of a callus with osteoid production.

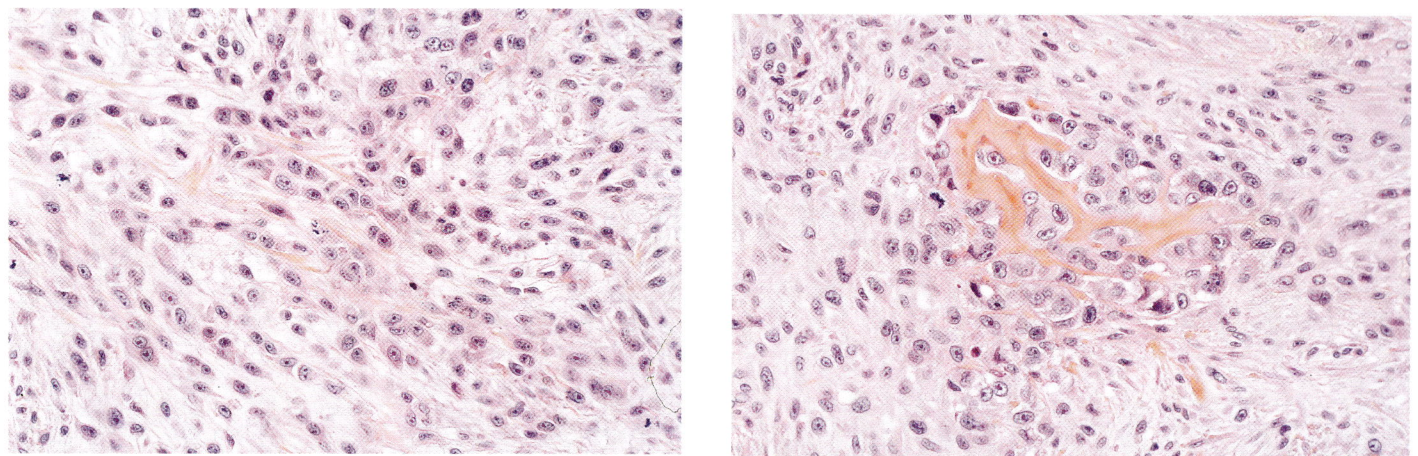

Fig. 49.13　　　　　　　　　　　　　　　**Fig. 49.14**

Figs 49.13, 49.14　Osteoblastic osteosarcoma versus a callus: nuclear abnormalities and abnormal mitotic figures are helpful for the differential diagnosis, apart from the absence of osteoblastic rimming.

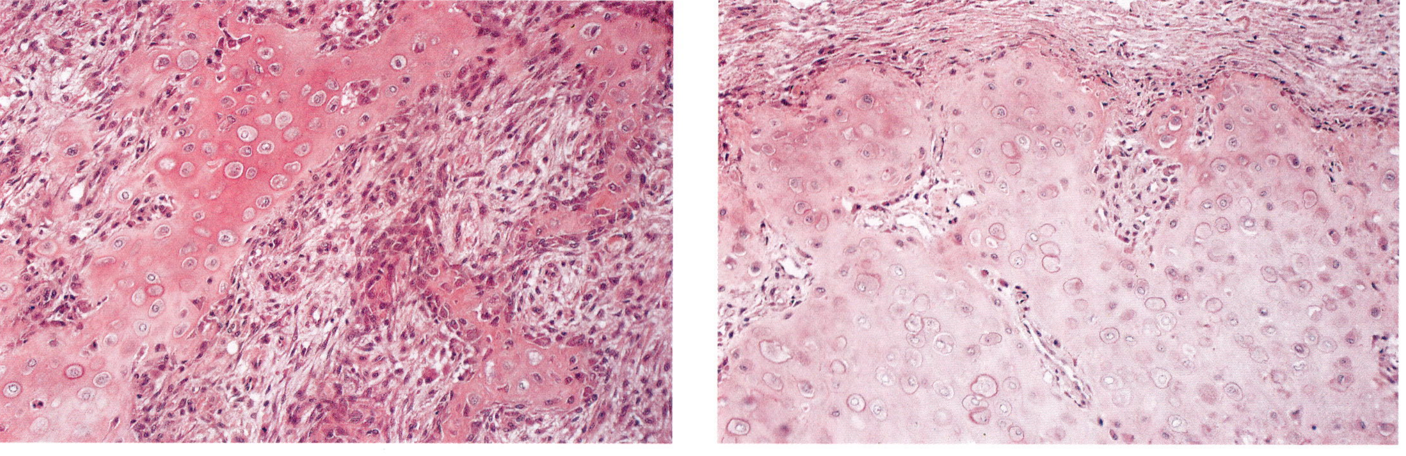

Fig. 49.15　　　　　　　　　　　　　　　**Fig. 49.16**

Figs 49.15, 49.16　Hypertrophic cartilage in a callus.

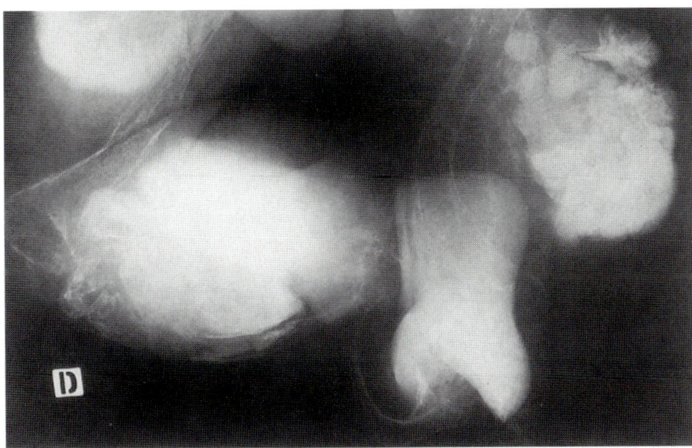

Fig. 49.17

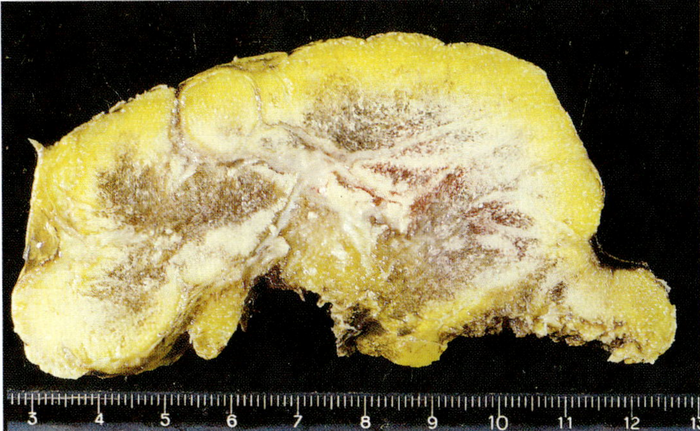

Fig. 49.18

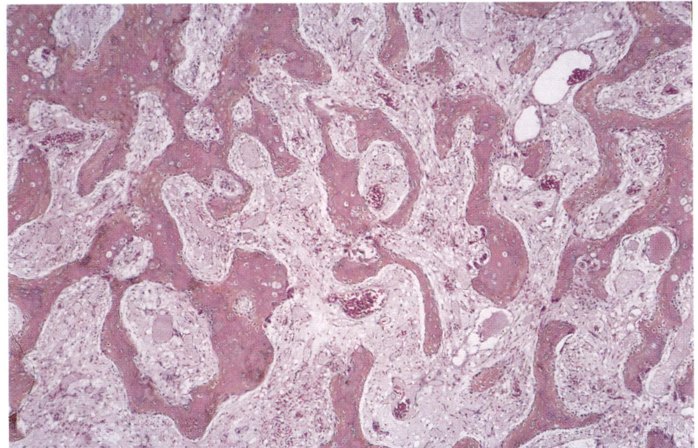

Fig. 49.20

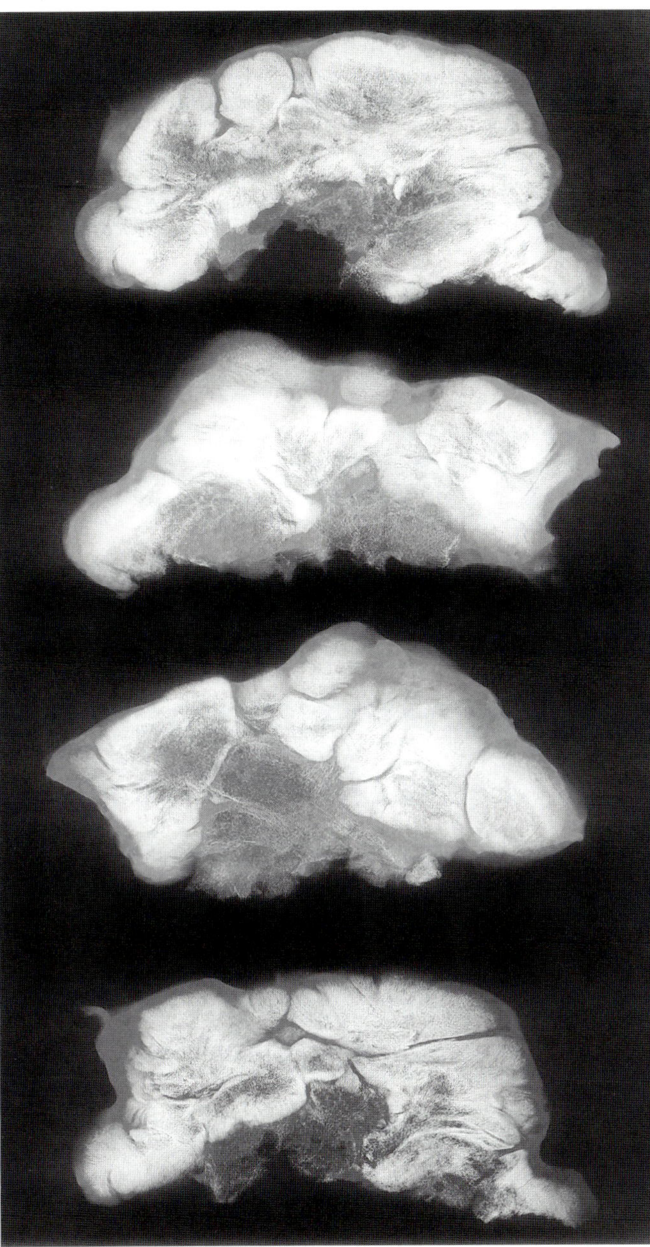

Fig. 49.19

Figs 49.17–49.20 Bilateral hypertrophic femoral callus in osteogenesis imperfecta.

On imaging, *periosteal reactions*[15] or *stress fractures* (Figs 49.21–49.23) may be confused with osteosarcomas, Ewing's sarcomas,[16] eosinophilic granulomas, osteo-myelitis,[17] osteoid osteomas,[18] periosteal desmoids[19] or even metastases.[20]

Abnormal stress on normal bone induces *fatigue frac-tures* while normal forces on bone with decreased elastic resistance induce *insufficiency fractures*.[17] Fatigue fractures are commonly seen in adolescents and young adult males;[21,22] in contrast to osteosarcomas, the pain is relieved by rest.[23]

The commonest site is the posterior cortex of the proxi-

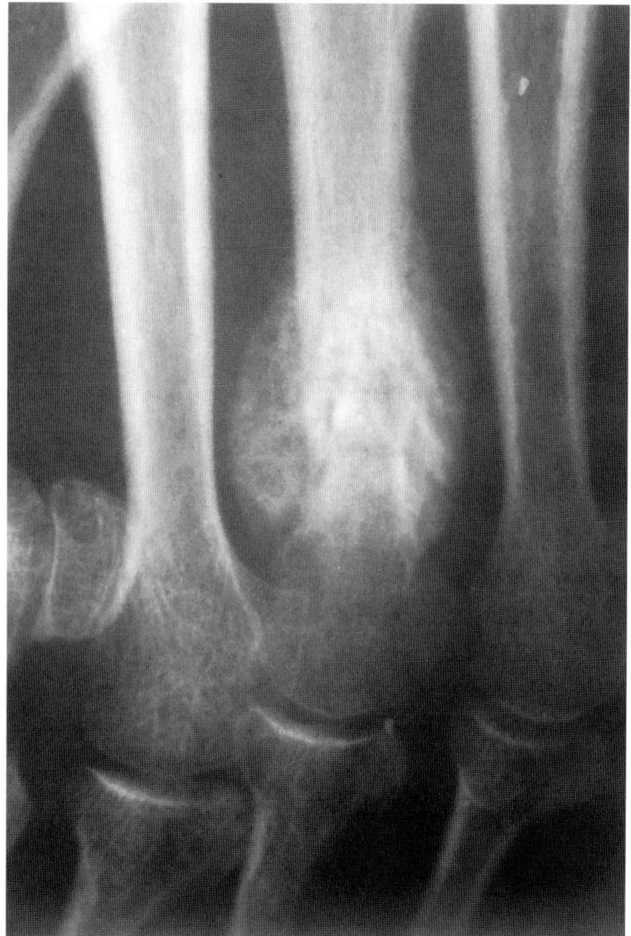

Fig. 49.21 Fatigue fracture of a metatarsal.

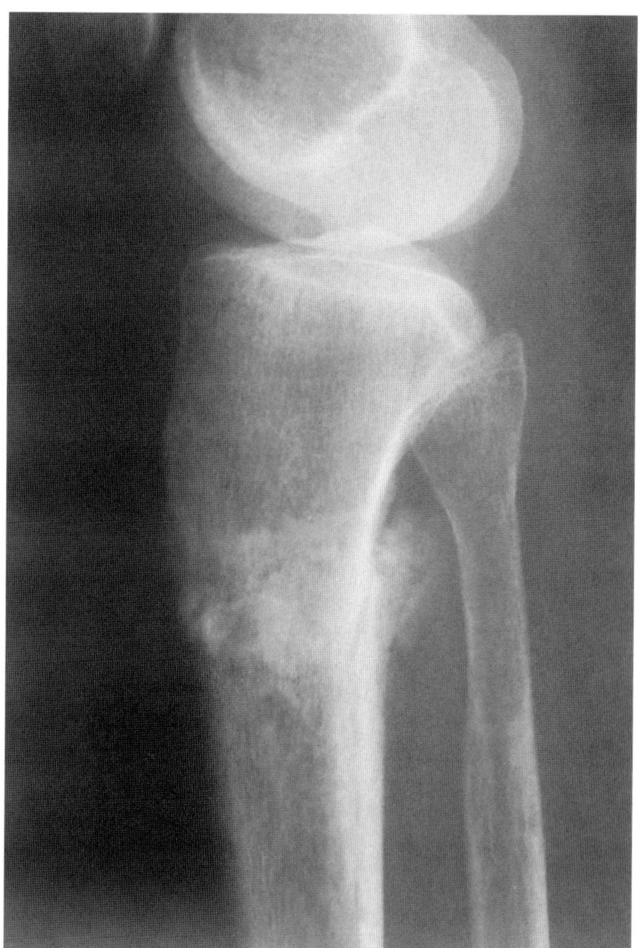

Fig. 49.22

mal third of the tibia[20–22] but the shaft of the femur may also be involved.[17,23] The cortical break is perpendicular to the shaft[18] and may be demonstrated on CT and MRI.

Clues to benignancy are the ininterrupted periosteal reaction, the absence of cortical destruction and a sharply marginated area of increased uptake on bone scanning;[22,24] the sensitivity of the latter technique approaches 100%.[25]

A *reactive endosteal bone formation* may also be confused with a tumor[26] (Figs 49.24–49.28), appearing as lamellar new bone deposited on preexisting trabecular surfaces or as woven bone forming new networks in medullary spaces.[26]

Trauma with extensive hemorrhage may induce *cyst-like lesions* which may even mimic a unicameral bone cyst.[27,28] Cortical lesions are found in children and more central, expanding lesions in adults.[27]

A *diffuse demineralization* of a limb bone immobilized after trauma may appear as multiple areas of radiolucency and scalloped defects of the cortex, with an unusual moth-eaten destruction simulating myeloma or metastatic disease.[29–31] These are rather prominent in the humeral

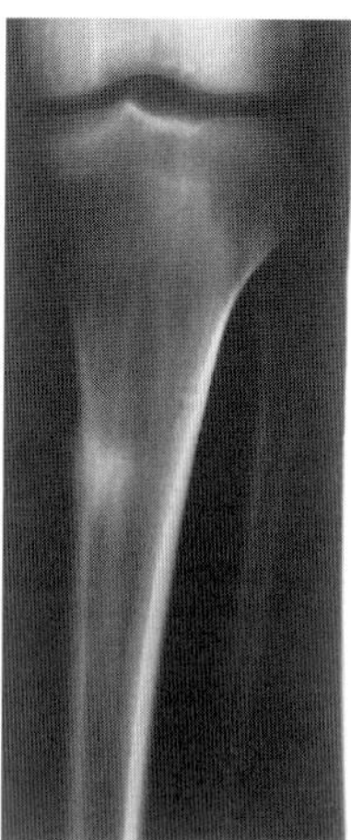
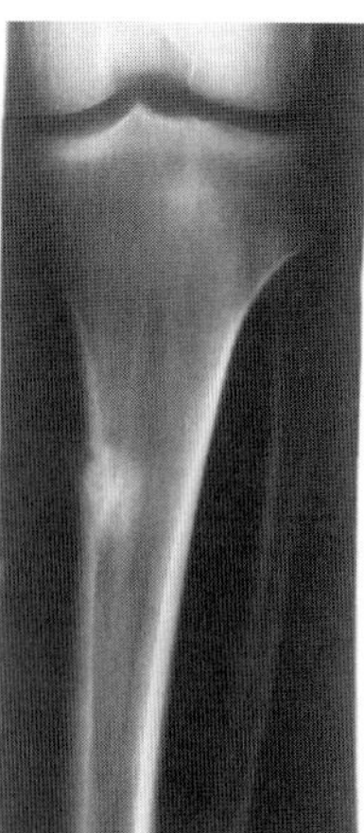
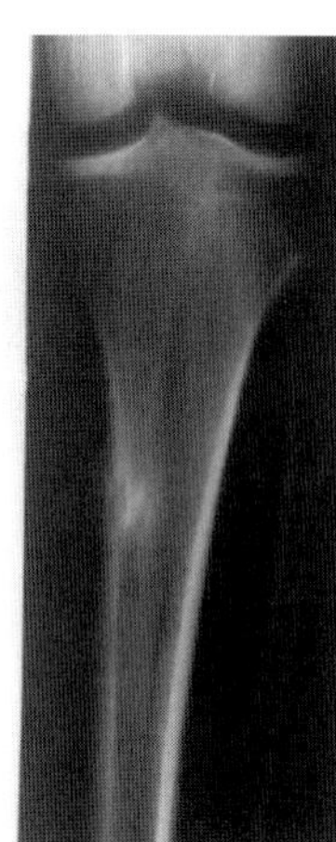

Fig. 49.23

Figs 49.22, 49.23 Fatigue fractures of the tibia.

diaphysis, showing a 'herring-bone' pattern of medullary trabeculation.[30,32]

The unusual healing pattern of *posttraumatic osteolysis* in the pubic bone or in the distal end of the clavicle may simulate a malignant tumor such as a chondrosarcoma.[33–35]

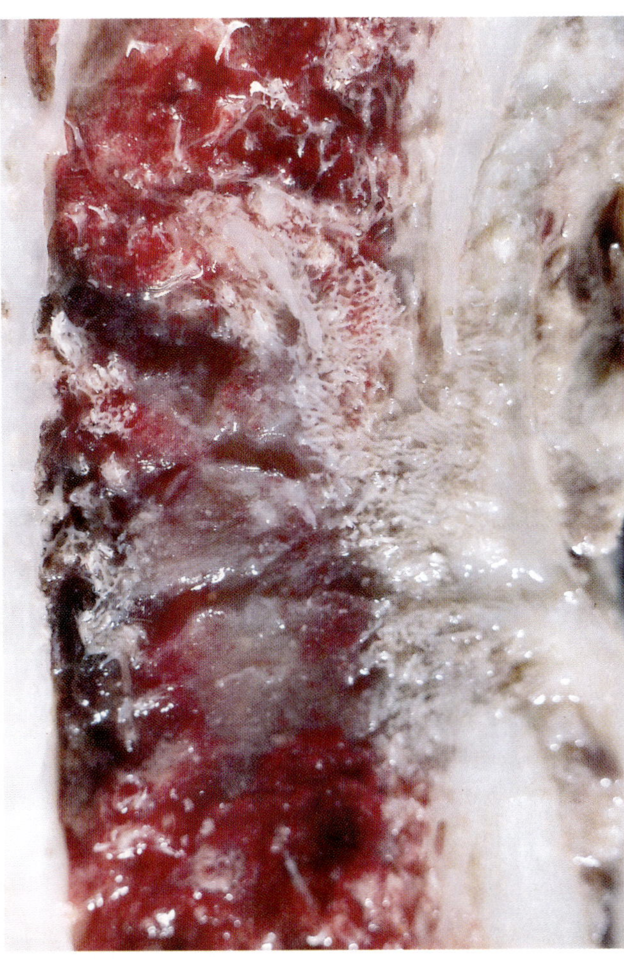

Fig. 49.24

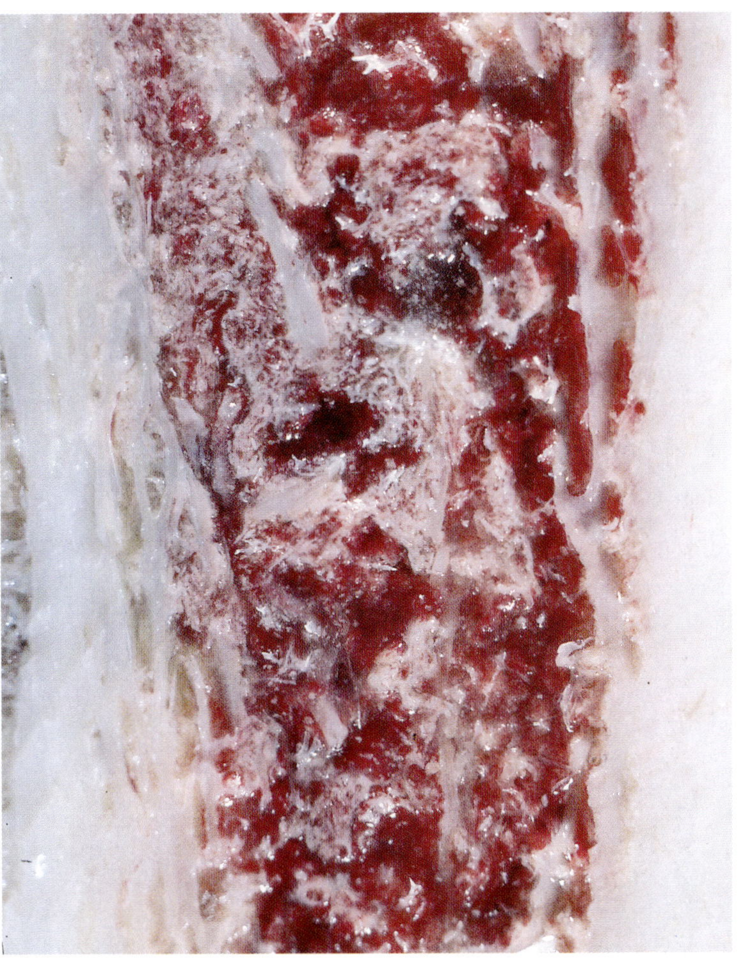

Fig. 49.25

Figs 49.24–49.26 Limited resection of the cortex of the tibia for a periosteal osteosarcoma; 6 months after, bone formation in the medullary cavity is diagnosed as a recurrence, although it is in fact an endosteal callus.

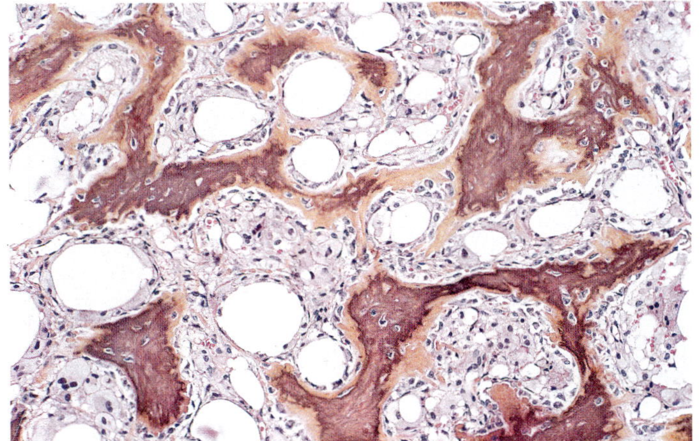

Fig. 49.26

In the same way, ischial apophyseolysis due to traumatic avulsion may simulate a chondrosarcoma or osteosarcoma by an exuberant callus formation.[36]

FLORID REACTIVE PERIOSTITIS

This reactive process predominantly involves the tubular bones of the hands and feet,[37,38] mostly in women with an average age of 25–30 years.

Clinical symptoms are a swelling, tenderness or pain, with a history of minor trauma in less than half the cases.[37]

On imaging, a soft tissue swelling is associated with a periosteal reaction; the cortex may be intact or eroded.[37]

Histologically, the fibrous tissue is composed of spindle cells with prominent nucleoli and normal mitotic activity; they are distributed in interlacing fascicles, in some cases with a myxoid appearance. The fibrous tissue is associated with cartilage and bone. Ossification is more pronounced at the periphery of the mass and may be a prominent feature.[39,40]

Excision is curative.

The differential diagnosis is myositis ossificans which exhibits a lucent zone between the cortex and the lesion,[38] but the two conditions may be related.[39] A parosteal osteosarcoma appears as a dense, lobulated, sclerotic mass, paradoxically much less cellular and with more mature bone formation.

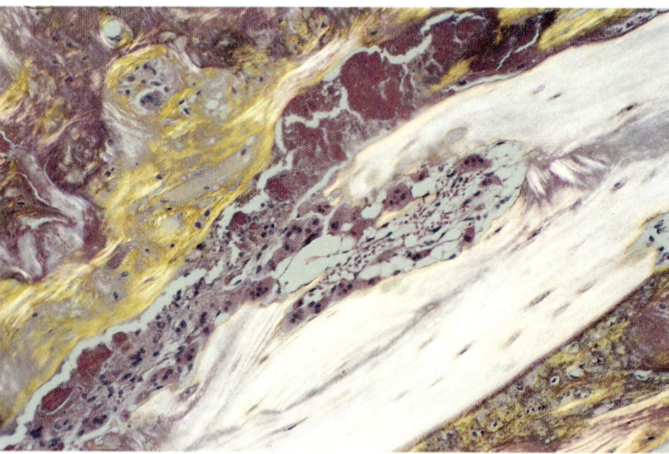

Fig. 49.27

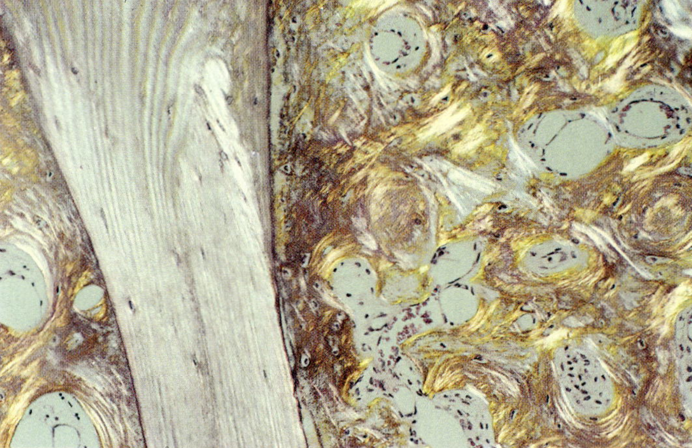

Fig. 49.28

Figs 49.27, 49.28 Endosteal callus of the tibia, after biopsy of a malignant fibrous histiocytoma (polarized light).

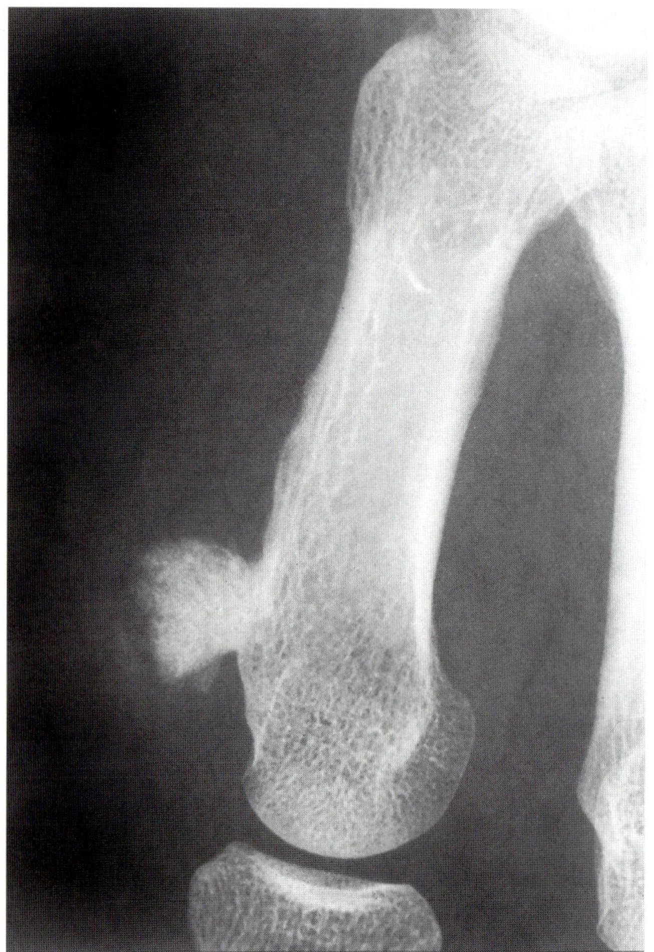

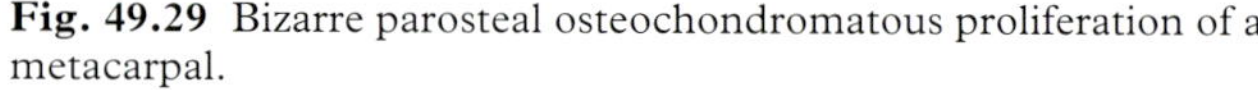

Fig. 49.29 Bizarre parosteal osteochondromatous proliferation of a metacarpal.

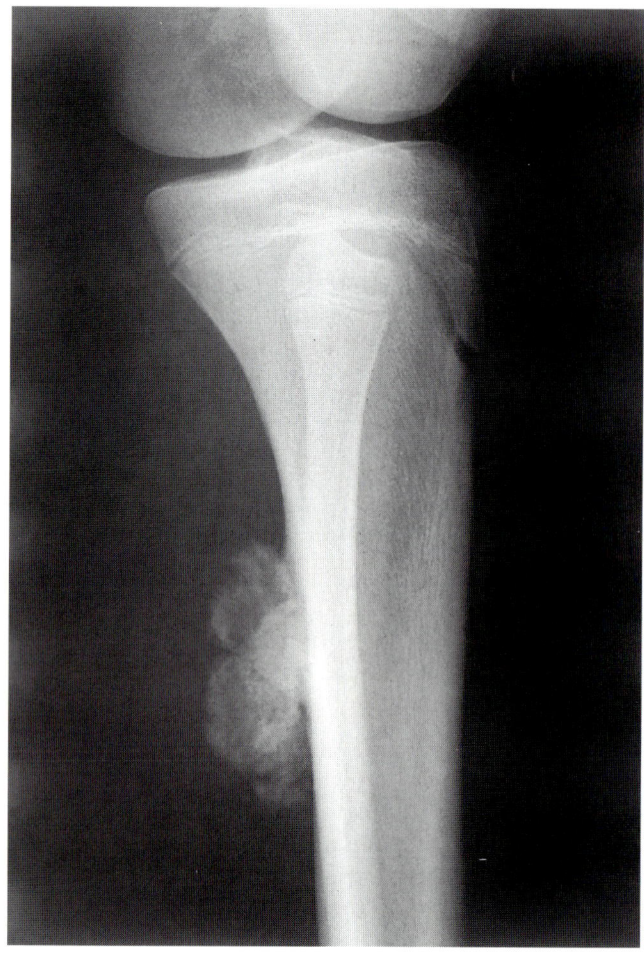

Fig. 49.30 Bizarre parosteal osteochondromatous proliferation of the tibia.

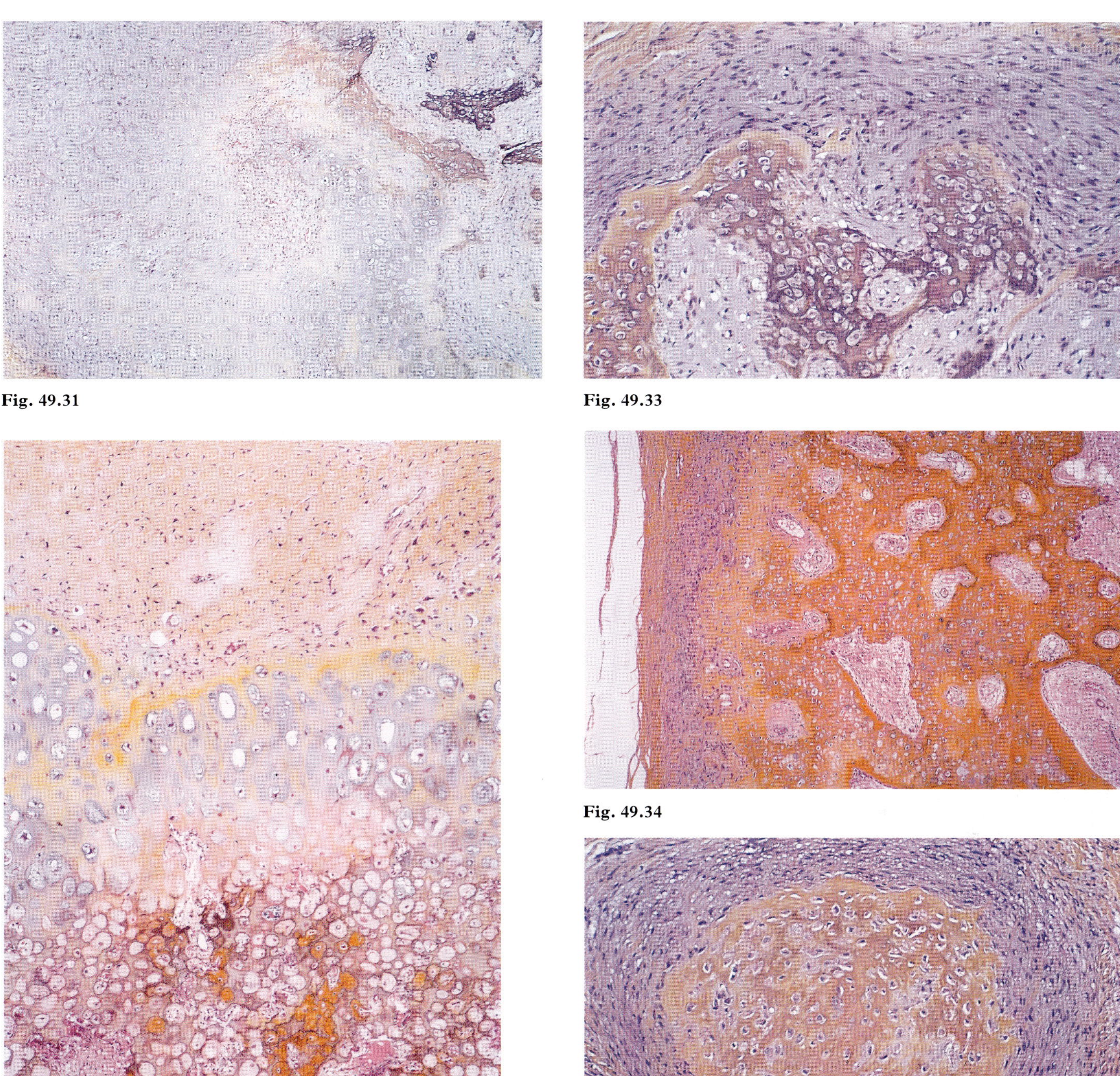

Fig. 49.31

Fig. 49.33

Fig. 49.32

Fig. 49.34

Fig. 49.35

Figs 49.31–49.36 Bizarre parosteal osteochondromatous proliferation: caps or lobules of cartilage with disordered growth and mineralization, irregularly calcified osteoid and dense proliferative fibrous tissue.

BIZARRE PAROSTEAL OSTEOCHONDROMATOUS PROLIFERATIONS OF BONE

Mushroom-shaped calcified masses 'stuck on' the cortex are rare lesions found predominantly in the hand.[41,42] Most patients are in their third or fourth decades[41] with a history of trauma in some cases.[43] Clinical symptoms are a tumefaction or a slight pain.[44]

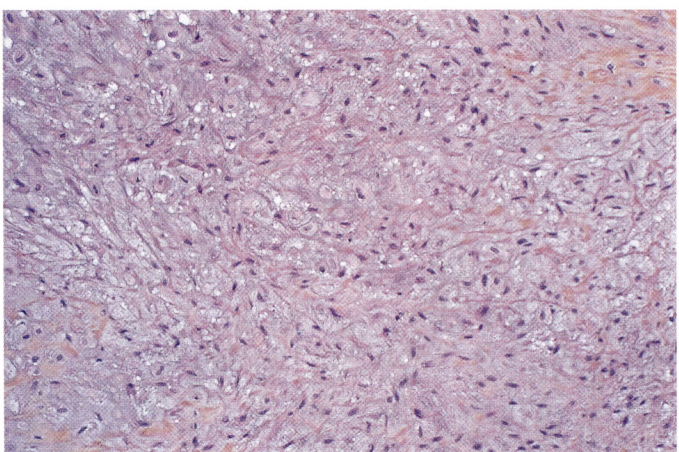

Fig. 49.36

Most lesions occur on proximal phalanges, metatarsals and metacarpals[41,44,45] (Fig. 49.29). A quarter of cases are on the long bones[41,42,46] (Fig. 49.30) or even on the skull.

On X-ray, a heavily calcified mass arises directly from the cortical surface which shows little or no alterations.[42]

Grossly, the lesion is pedunculated or sessile, looking like an osteochondroma, with a size ranging from 0.4 to 3 cm.[41]

Histologically, cartilage with bizarre, enlarged or binucleated nuclei forms a cap or lobules in a dense proliferative fibrous tissue. The maturation of cartilage to bone appears very irregular,[42,43,47] with disordered growth. Irregularly calcified osteoid or bone trabeculae are bordered by osteoblasts or spindle cells (Figs 49.31–49.36).

The treatment is excision, but there is an unusually high rate of recurrence (more than half of the cases[42]).

The differential diagnoses are osteochondroma, but the lesion arises directly from the cortical surface with continuity with the underlying osseous medulla, turret exostoses, which are smaller with more organized bone production,[44] and parosteal osteosarcomas, which are very rare in the small bones of hand and foot, exhibiting slender, short and irregular bone trabeculae.[44]

A single term of 'proliferative parosteal processes of phalanges' has been suggested, designating bizarre parosteal osteochondromatous proliferations, florid reactive periostosis and turret exostoses as lesions related to trauma, with various appearances depending on the maturation of the process, the breaching of the periosteum and the local anatomic features.[48]

REFERENCES

1. Kahn L B, Wood F W, Ackerman L V. Fracture callus associated with benign and malignant bone lesions and mimicking osteosarcoma. Am J Clin Pathol 1969: 52: 14–24
2. Fairbank H A, Baker S L. Hyperplastic callus formation with or without evidence of a fracture in osteogenesis imperfecta. Br J Surg 1948: 36: 1–16
3. Kutsumi K, Nojima T, Yamashiro K et al. Hyperplastic callus formation in both femurs in osteogenesis imperfecta. Skeletal Radiol 1996: 25: 384–387
4. Laurent L E, Salenius P. Hyperplastic callus formation in osteogenesis imperfecta. Acta Orthop Scand 1967: 38: 280–289
5. Banta J V, Schreiber R R, Kulik W J. Hyperplastic callus formation in osteogenesis imperfecta simulating osteosarcoma. J Bone Joint Surg (Am) 1971: 53: 115–122
6. Roberts J B. Bilateral hyperplastic callus formation in osteogenesis imperfecta. J Bone Joint Surg (Am) 1976: 58: 1164–1166
7. Lehmann H W, Nerlich A, Brenner R E, Bodo M, Müller P K. Hyperplastic callus formation in osteogenesis imperfecta. Eur J Pediatr Surg 1992: 2: 281–284
8. Stöss H, Freisinger P. Osteogenesis imperfecta mit hyperplastischer Kallusbildung. Pathologe 1993: 14: 112–116
9. Stöss H, Pontz B, Vetter U, Karbowski A, Brenner R, Spranger J. Osteogenesis imperfecta and hyperplastic callus formation: light and electron microscopic findings. Am J Med Genet 1993: 45: 260
10. Klenerman L, Ockenden B G, Townsend A C. Osteosarcoma occurring in osteogenesis imperfecta. J Bone Joint Surg (Br) 1967: 49: 314–323
11. Lasson U, Harms D, Wiedemann H R. Osteogenic sarcoma complicating osteogenesis imperfecta. Eur J Pediatr 1978: 129: 215–218
12. Reid B S, Hubbard J D. Osteosarcoma arising in osteogenesis imperfecta. Pediatr Radiol 1979: 8: 110–112
13. Rutkowski K, Resnick P, McMaster J H. Osteosarcoma occurring in osteogenesis imperfecta. J Bone Joint Surg (Am) 1979: 61: 606–608
14. Gagliardi J A, Evans E M, Chandnani V P, Myers J B, Pacheco C M. Osteogenesis imperfecta complicated by osteosarcoma. Skeletal Radiol 1995: 24: 308–310
15. Ragsdale B D, Madewell J E, Sweet D E. Radiologic and pathologic analysis of solitary bone lesions. part II: periosteal reactions. Radiol Clin North Am 1981: 19: 749–793
16. Linscheid R L, Coventry M B. Unrecognized fractures of long bones suggesting primary bone tumors. Proc Staff Meet Mayo Clin 1962: 37: 599–606
17. Meaney J E, Carty H. Femoral stress fractures in children. Skeletal Radiol 1992: 21: 173–176
18. Murcia M, Brennan R E, Edeiken J. Computed tomography of stress fracture. Skeletal Radiol 1982: 8: 193–195
19. Pistolesi G F, Caudana R, D'Attoma N, Residori E, Pregarz M. Case report 686. Stress fracture at the distal end of femur simulating 'periosteal desmoid'. Skeletal Radiol 1991: 20: 454–457
20. Tuite M J, De Smet A A, Gaynon P S. Tibial stress fracture mimicking neuroblastoma metastasis in two young children. Skeletal Radiol 1995: 24: 287–290
21. Solomon L. Stress fractures of the femur and tibia simulating malignant bone tumours. S Afr J Surg 1974: 12: 19–25
22. Davies A M, Evans N, Grimer R J. Fatigue fractures of the proximal tibia simulating malignancy. Br J Radiol 1988: 61: 903–908
23. Levin D C, Blazina M E, Levine E. Fatigue fractures of the shaft of the femur: simulation of malignant tumour. Radiology 1967: 89: 883–885
24. Davies A M, Carter S R, Grimer R J, Sneath R S. Fatigue fractures of the femoral diaphysis in the skeletally immature simulating malignancy. Br J Radiol 1989: 62: 893–896
25. Anderson M W, Greenspan A. Stress fractures. Radiology 1996: 199: 1–12
26. Aoki J, Yamamoto I, Hino M et al. Reactive endosteal bone formation. Skeletal Radiol 1987: 16: 545–551
27. Phillips C D, Keats T E. The development of post-traumatic cyst-like lesions in bone. Skeletal Radiol 1986: 15: 631–634
28. Moore T E, King A R, Travis R C, Allen B C. Post-traumatic cysts and cyst-like lesions of bone. Skeletal Radiol 1989: 18: 93–97

29. Jones G. Radiological appearances of disuse osteoporosis. Clin Radiol 1969: 20: 345–353
30. Keats T E, Harrison R B. A pattern of post-traumatic demineralization of bone simulating permeative neoplastic replacement: a potential source of misinterpretation. Skeletal Radiol 1978: 3: 113–116
31. Joyce J M, Keats T E. Disuse osteoporosis: mimic of neoplastic disease. Skeletal Radiol 1986: 15: 129–132
32. Kattapuram S V, Khurana J S, Ehara S, Ragozzino M. Aggressive posttraumatic osteoporosis of the humerus simulating a malignant neoplasm. Cancer 1988: 62: 2525–2527
33. Goergen T G, Resnick D, Riley R R. Post traumatic abnormalities of the public bone simulating malignancy. Radiology 1978: 126: 85–87
34. Hall F M, Goldberg R P, Kasdon E J, Glick H. Post-traumatic osteolysis of the pubic bone simulating a malignant lesion. J Bone Joint Surg (Am) 1984: 66: 121–126
35. McCarthy B, Dorfman H D. Pubic osteolysis. A benign lesion of the pelvis closely mimicking a malignant neoplasm. Clin Orthop 1990: 251: 300–307
36. Unni K K, McLeod R A, Dahlin D C. Conditions that may simulate primary neoplasms of bone. Pathol Annu 1980: 15 Pt 1: 91–131
37. Spjut H J, Dorfman H D. Florid reactive periostitis of the tubular bones of the hands and feet. A benign lesion which may simulate osteosarcoma. Am J Surg Pathol 1981: 5: 423–433
38. Kovach J C, Truong L, Kearns R J, Bennett J B. Florid reactive periostitis. J Hand Surg (Am) 1986: 11: 902–905
39. Jongeward R H Jr, Martel W, Louis D S, Okoye M I, Walter N. Case report 304. Florid reactive periostitis proximal phalange of the left 5th finger. Skeletal Radiol 1985: 13: 169–173
40. Kwittken J, Branche M. Fasciitis ossificans. Am J Clin Pathol 1969: 51: 251–255
41. Nora F E, Dahlin D C, Beabout J W. Bizarre parosteal osteochondromatous proliferations of the hands and feet. Am J Surg Pathol 1983: 7: 245–250
42. Meneses M F, Unni K K, Swee R G. Bizarre parosteal osteochondromatous proliferation of bone (Nora's lesion). Am J Surg Pathol 1993: 17: 691–697
43. Twiston Davies C W. Bizarre parosteal osteochondromatous proliferation in the hand. J Bone Joint Surg (Am) 1985: 67: 648–650
44. De Lange E E, Pope T L Jr, Fechner R E, Keats T E. Case report 428. Bizarre parosteal osteochondromatous proliferation (BPOP). Skeletal Radiol 1987: 16: 481–483
45. Kissel C G, McQuaid M, Lucas D R, Sundareson A S, Klimecki R S. Bizarre parosteal osteochondromatous proliferation. An unusual bone tumor. J Am Podiatr Med Assoc 1995: 85: 301–305
46. Cooper P N, Malcom A J. A bizarre parosteal osteochondromatous proliferation of the radius. Histopathology 1993: 22: 78–80
47. Teoh H H, Bethwaite P B, Thurston A J. Bizarre parosteal osteochondromatous proliferation of the hand in a young man. Pathology 1992: 24: 211–213
48. Yuen M, Friedman L, Orr W, Cockshott W P. Proliferative periosteal processes of phalanges: a unitary hypothesis. Skeletal Radiol 1992: 21: 301–303

50

Bone infarct

M. Forest

INTRODUCTION AND CLINICAL DATA

In the metaphysis of long tubular bones, ischemic death of the cellular constituents of bone and marrow may be idiopathic or associated with a wide variety of diseases: irradiation, caisson disease, storage diseases, occlusive vascular disease, collagen diseases, infection, lymphoproliferative disorders, corticosteroid therapy and even chemotherapy.[1,2]

Most bone infarcts are asymptomatic but some may be painful.[1,3,4] In many reports, there is a male predominance. In about 60% of cases, infarcts are multiple, symmetrically distributed and frequently associated with femoral head necrosis.[4]

SKELETAL DISTRIBUTION

Most cases are located in the lower part of the femur or the upper part of the tibia and humerus.

IMAGING

On plain films, the early changes are subtle, mottled, ill-defined radiolucencies in the diametaphyseal region of long bones, which may be misdiagnosed as aggressive lesions.[3]

Bone infarcts become visible by reactive changes along the borders, as the reactive peripheral sclerosis widens, with peripheral calcification of the marrow fat (Milgram 1990) leading to an irregular serrated shell separated from the cortex by a narrow band of cancellous bone (Wilner 1982) (Figs 50.1–50.6).

Bone infarcts appear as wedge-shaped densities running longitudinally in the shaft of the bone. Rarely, a periosteal thickening is associated.[4] They may remain unchanged for years or may undergo a partial resorption of the necrotic bone.

On MRI, early infarcts show a central area with a high

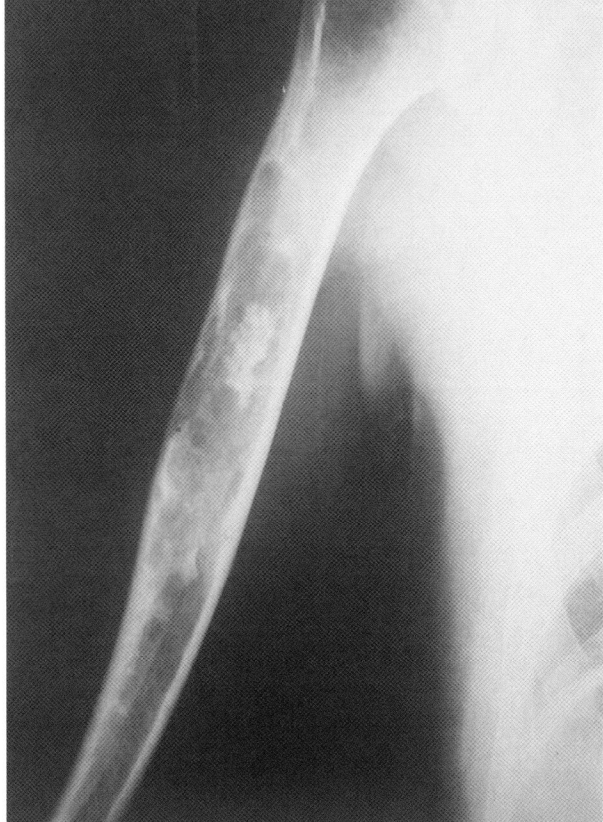

Fig. 50.1

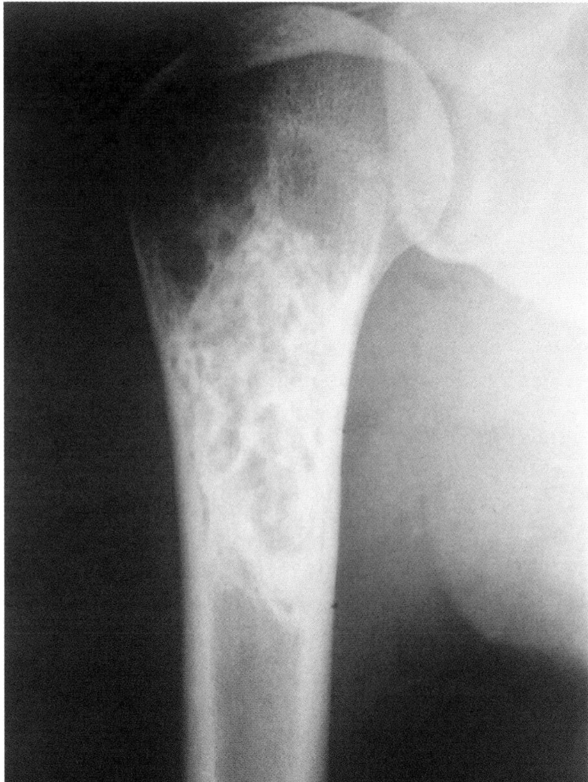

Fig. 50.2

Figs 50.1, 50.2 Bone infarcts in humeral location.

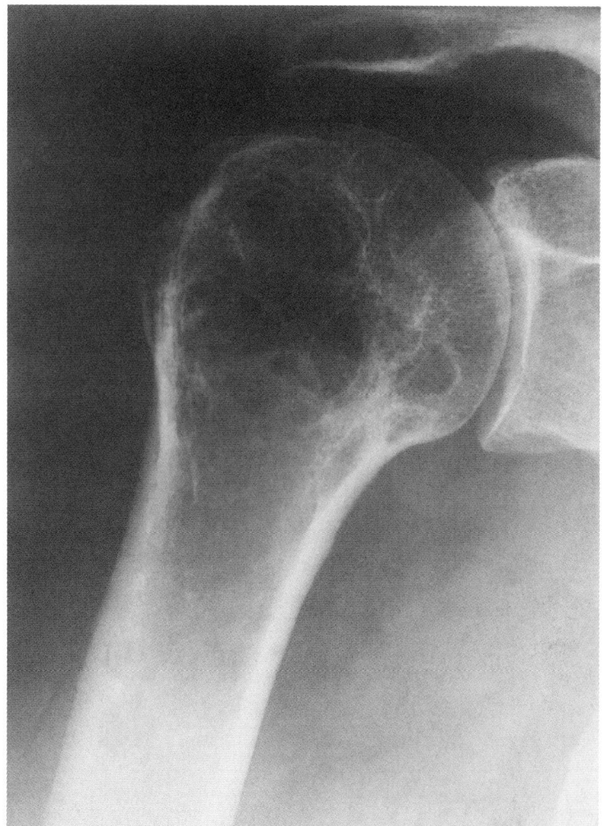

Fig. 50.3 Bone infarct of the humeral head, mainly cystized.

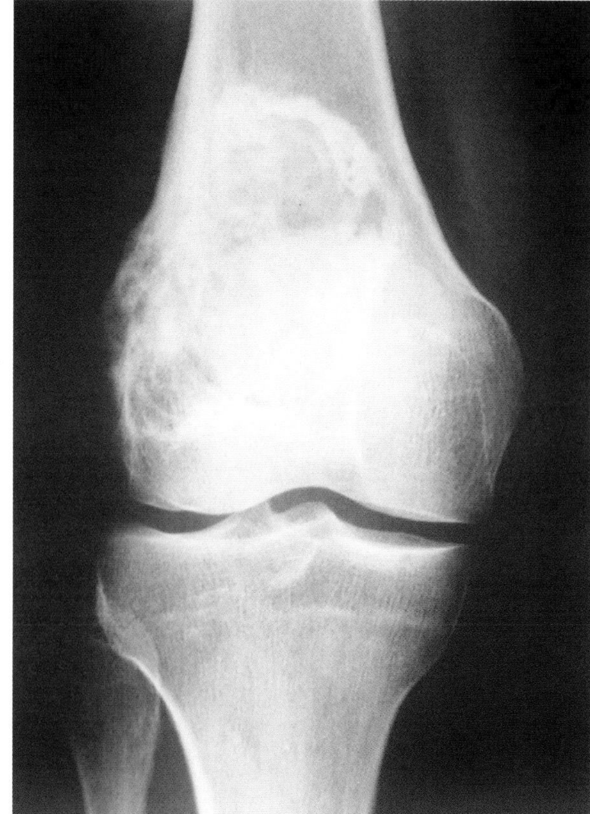

Fig. 50.4 Bone infarct of the distal femur.

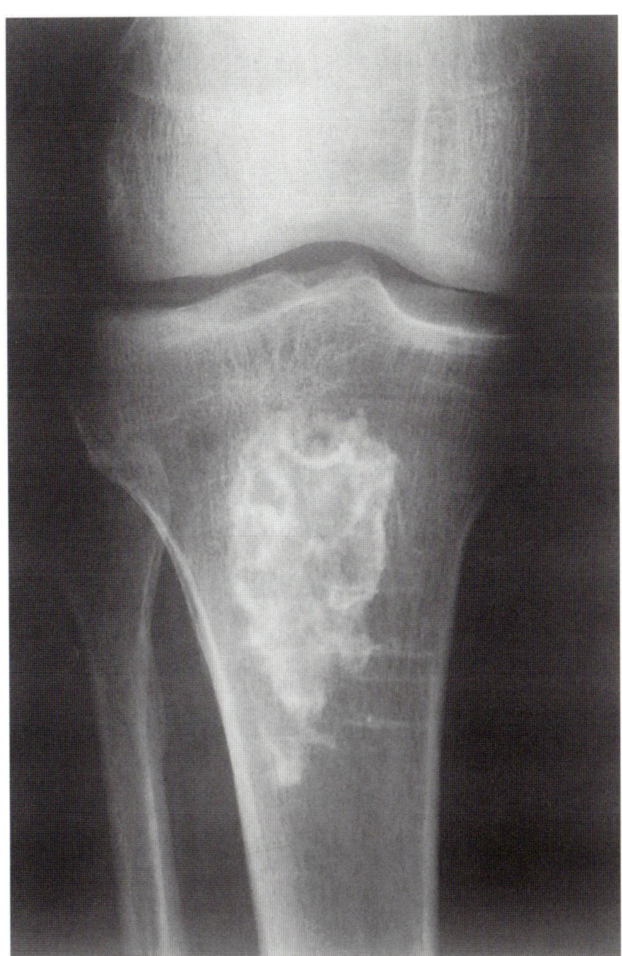

Fig. 50.5 Bone infarct of the proximal tibia.

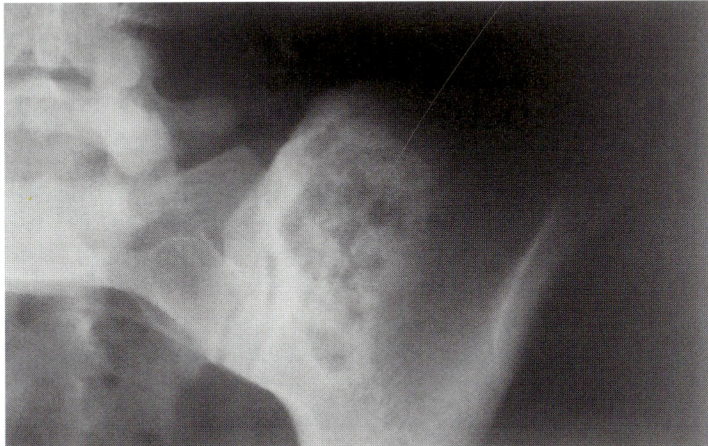

Fig. 50.6 Bone infarct of the iliac wing.

or intermediate signal on T1- and a high signal on T2-weighted images, reflecting the associated edema,[3,5] with a thin serpentine low signal border.[3] A low signal intensity on T1- and T2-weighted images is characteristic

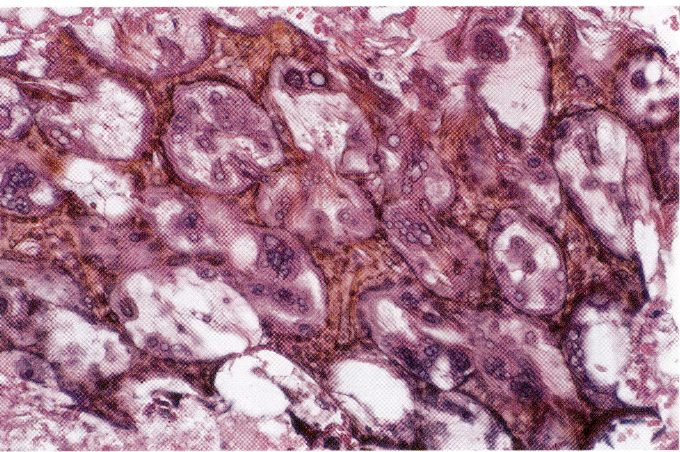

Fig. 50.7

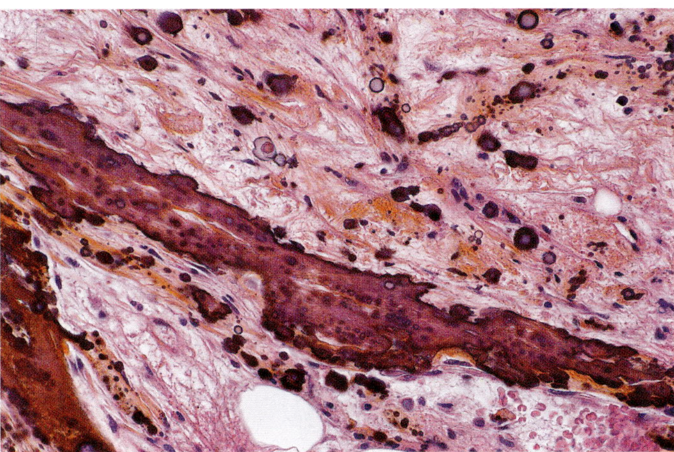

Fig. 50.8

Figs 50.7, 50.8 Bone infarct: necrosis of the fat marrow with dystrophic mineralization.

of mature bone marrow infarction.[3,6] Bone infarcts may in some cases only be visible on MRI.[4]

Cystic degeneration is rare[1] and predominates in the tibia and humerus[7] (Fig. 50.3).

HISTOPATHOLOGY

The earliest histological signs of bone infarction involve the fat marrow: necrotic fat cells are disrupted with degenerative changes and secondary calcification (Milgram 1990).

Later, the core of dead bone and marrow is embedded in scar tissue with few fibroblasts and hemosiderin-laden or foamy histiocytes. Atypical ischemic bone is found in the fibrous tissue or on the surface of the bone trabeculae. A progressive dystrophic mineralization appears as a deposition of calcium salts in degenerating or necrotic tissues (Figs 50.7–50.13).

Revascularization and formation of both lamellar and

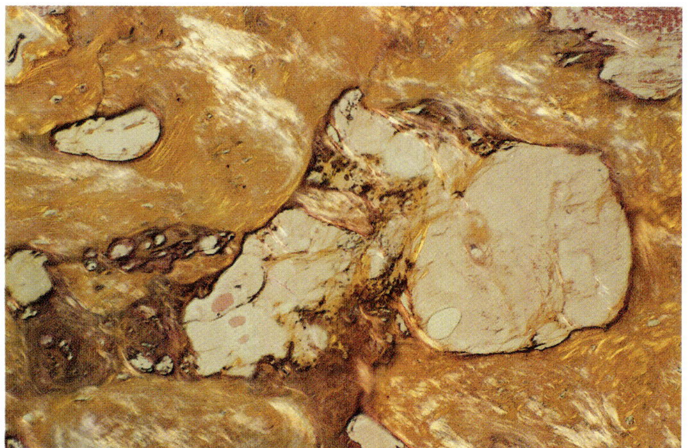

Fig. 50.9

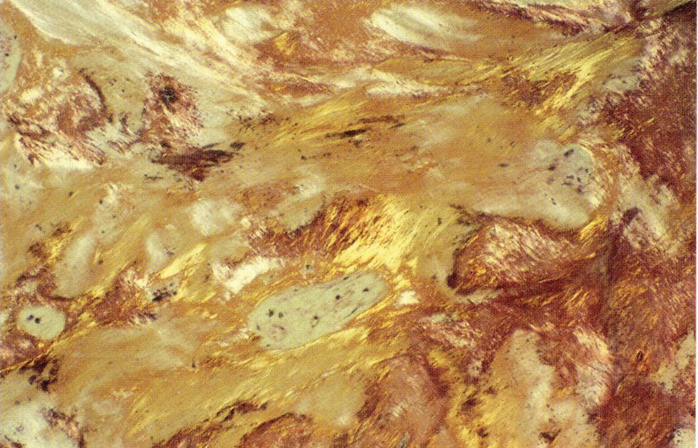

Fig. 50.10

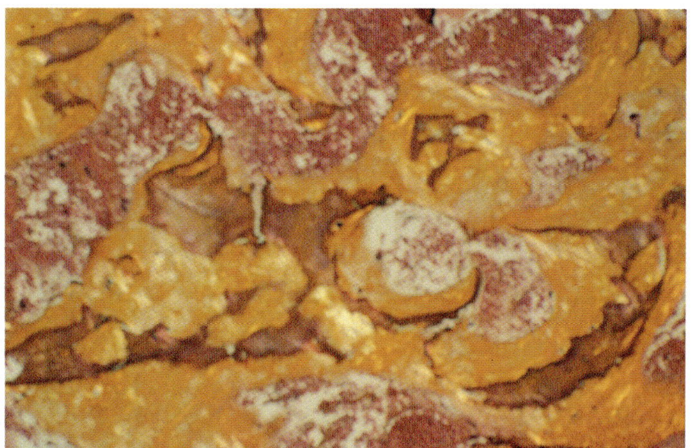

Fig. 50.11

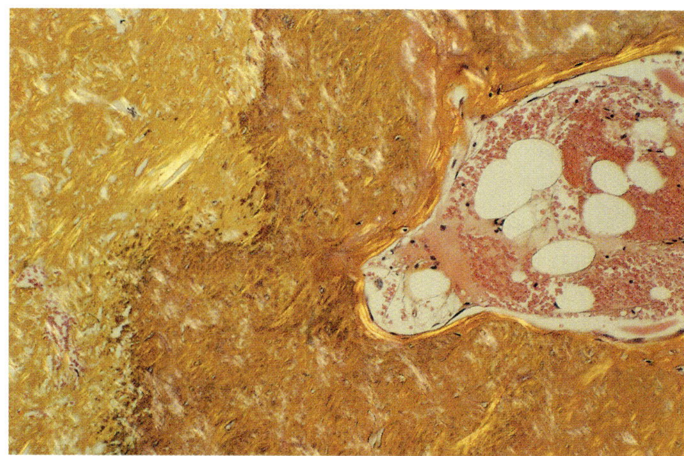

Fig. 50.12

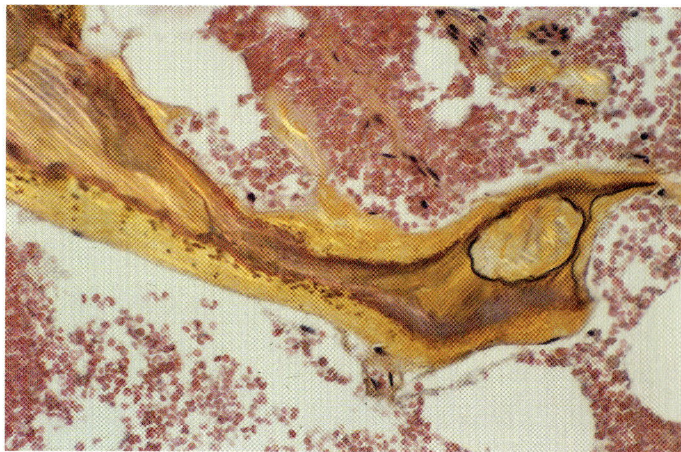

Fig. 50.13

Figs 50.9–50.13 Bone infarct: formation of ischemic bone (polarized light).

Bone infarcts with cyst formation exhibit a hyalinized fibrous wall with dystrophic calcifications[7] (Fig. 50.14).

BONE INFARCTS AND TUMORS

Cases of sarcomatous transformation from infarcts of bone in patients not exposed to radiation are very uncommon,[9] but it has been suggested that the underlying necrotic bone may be obliterated by the sarcomatous process.[10–12] About 50 instances have been documented[13] in idiopathic cases or cases related to caisson disease and other disorders.

Patients are in their fifth to seventh decades and men are more commonly affected.[9]

The clinical symptom is pain and, on imaging, a destructive area, a periosteal reaction and a soft tissue mass are found.[6,9] More than 75% of patients have large, multiple bone infarcts,[14] the distal end of the femur and proximal end of the tibia being the favored locations.

The sarcoma is found at the periphery or around the

ischemic bone predominates at the border of the bone infarct; the creeping substitution of the non-viable bone is only detected focally[1,8] and there is little histological change over a period of years, during gradual revascularization (Milgram 1990).

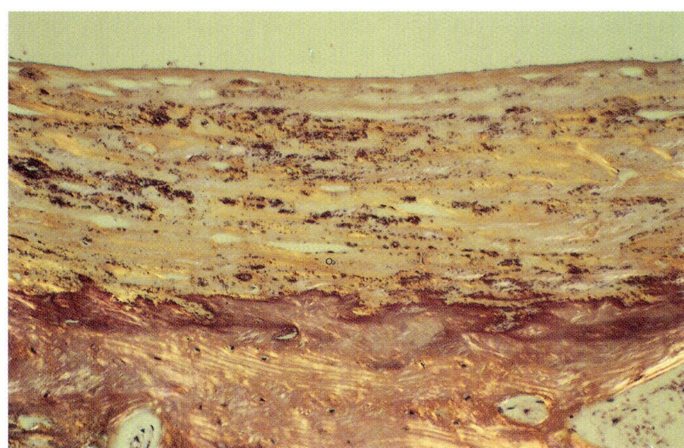

Fig. 50.14 Inner border of a cystized bone infarct, with dystrophic mineralization in the fibrous lining (polarized light).

bone infarct.[6,13] An unusual presentation is the existence of two tumors in separate bones.[15]

More than two-thirds of sarcomas are malignant fibrous histiocytomas,[6,9,11,12,14,15–21] with earlier reports involving fibrosarcomas.[10,22] Osteosarcomas are found in less than one-fifth of cases[11,13,21,23,24] (Figs 50.15, 50.16) and angiosarcomas are even rarer.[25–27]

Tumors appear to arise from the reactive fibroblastic borders (Milgram 1990) and Mirra[12] believed for a time that the reparative process may undergo a malignant transformation, sarcomas being viewed as 'scar sarcomas'. However, in most cases, large infarcts are not totally replaced by the reparative process, which may cease totally, and florid fibroblastic or histiocytic proliferations are difficult to find.[13,21]

DIFFERENTIAL DIAGNOSIS

On imaging, calcifying enchondromas have to be differentiated from bone infarcts, exhibiting clusters of flocculent calcifications with no serpiginous distribution.

On plain films, bone infarcts may mimic chondrosarcomas, especially the clear cell type,[28] osteosarcomas,

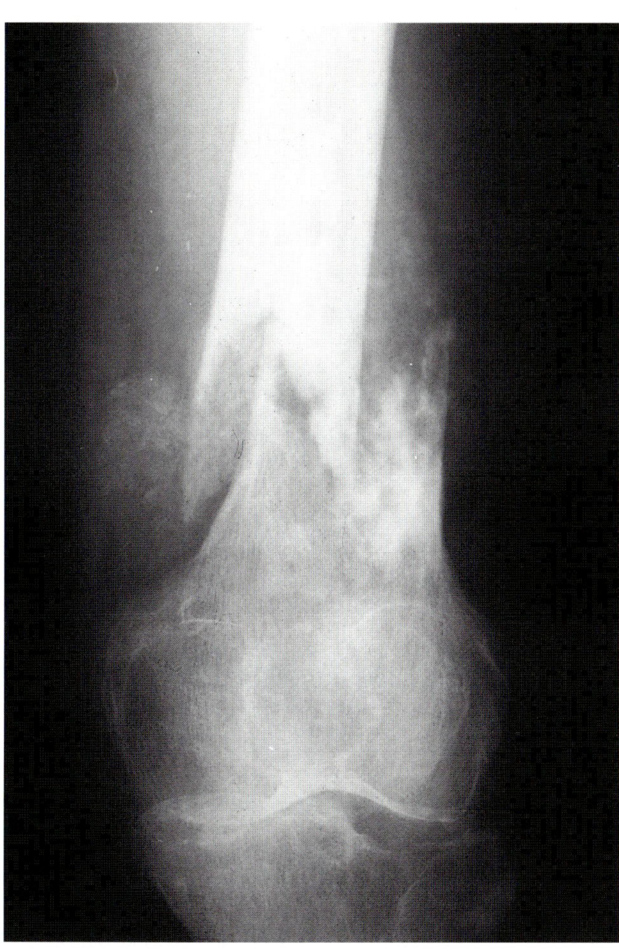

Fig. 50.15

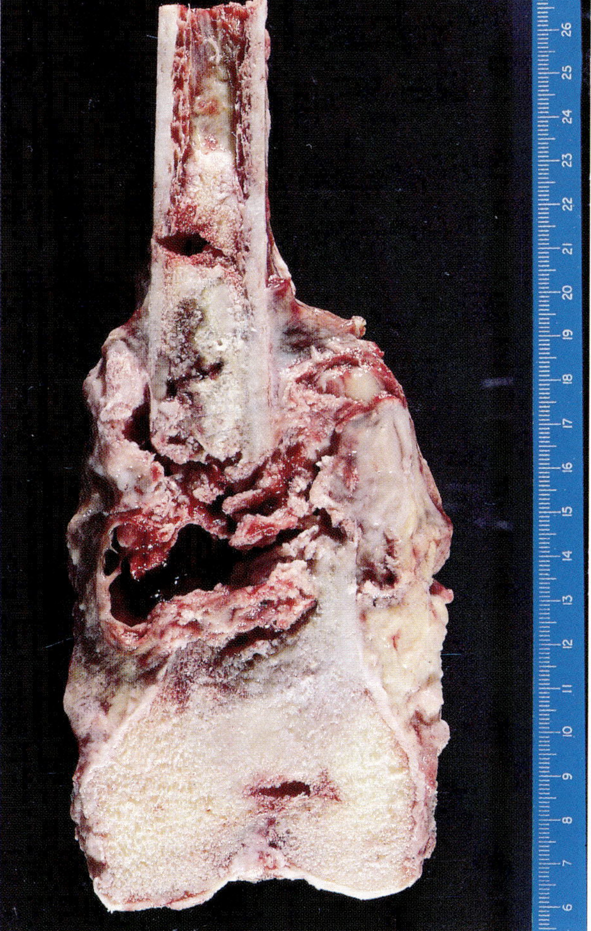

Fig. 50.16

Figs 50.15, 50.16 Osteosarcoma with a pathologic fracture associated with an old bone infarct in the femoral shaft, as an incidental finding.

although the bone scan is normal,[29] and even Ewing's sarcomas.[30-32]

Bone lipomas may present considerable calcification, reactive ossification and even cystic change, but bone infarcts contain the original bone trabeculae and do not induce any expansion of the cortex (Milgram 1990).

REFERENCES

1. Bullough P G, Kambolis C P, Marcove R C, Jaffe H L. Bone infarctions not associated with caisson disease. J Bone Joint Surg (Am) 1965: 47: 477–491
2. Ollivier L, Leclere J, Vanel D et al. Femoral infarction following intraarterial chemotherapy for osteosarcoma of the leg: a possible pitfall in magnetic resonance imaging. Skeletal Radiol 1991: 20: 329–332
3. Munk P L, Helms C A, Holt R G. Immature bone infarcts: findings on plain radiographs and MR scans. AJR 1989: 152: 547–549
4. Lafforgue P, Schiano A, Acquaviva P C. Les infarctus osseux, ou ostéonécroses aseptiques metaphysaires et diaphysaires 'idiopathiques' des os longs. Rev Rhum Mal Osteoartic 1990: 57: 359–366
5. Rajah R, Young J, Conway W F. Acute hemorrhagic infarct with edema. Skeletal Radiol 1995: 24: 158–159
6. Gaucher A A, Regent D M, Gillet P M, Pere P G, Aymard B M, Clement V. Case report 656. Malignant fibrous histiocytoma in a previous bone infarct. Skeletal Radiol 1991: 20: 137–140
7. Norman A, Steiner G. C. Radiographic and morphological features of cyst formation in idiopathic bone infarction. Radiology 1983: 146: 335–338
8. Kahlstrom S C, Phemister D B. Bone infarcts. Case report with autopsy findings. Am J Pathol 1946: 22: 947–963
9. Abrahams T G, Hull M. Case report 394. Malignant fibrous histiocytoma (MFH) arising in an infarct of bone. Skeletal Radiol 1986: 15: 578–583
10. Dorfman H D, Norman A, Wolff H. Fibrosarcoma complicating bone infarction in a caisson worker. J Bone Joint Surg (Am) 1966: 48: 528–532
11. Mirra J M, Bullough P G, Marcove R C, Jacobs B, Huvos A G. Malignant fibrous histiocytoma and osteosarcoma in association with bone infarcts. J Bone Joint Surg (Am) 1974: 56: 932–940
12. Mirra J M, Gold R H, Marafiote R. Malignant (fibrous) histiocytoma arising in association with a bone infarct in sickle-cell disease: coincidence or cause and effect? Cancer 1977: 39: 186–194
13. Torres F X, Kyriakos M. Bone infarct-associated osteosarcoma. Cancer 1992: 70: 2418–2430
14. Galli S J, Weintraub H P, Proppe K H. Malignant fibrous histiocytoma and pleomorphic sarcoma in association with medullary bone infarcts. Cancer 1978: 41: 607–619
15. Heselson N G, Price S K, Mills E E, Conway S S, Marks R K. Two malignant fibrous histiocytomas in bone infarcts. J Bone Joint Surg (Am) 1983: 65: 1166–1171
16. Michael R H, Dorfman H D. Malignant fibrous histiocytoma associated with bone infarcts. Clin Orthop 1976: 118: 180–183
17. Péré P, Adolphe J, Delgoffe C, Froment N, Gaucher A. Ostéonécroses epiphysaires, infarctus osseux multiples et histiocytofibrome malin. Rev Rhum Mal Osteoartic 1984: 51: 427–430
18. Breen T F, Healy W L. Malignant fibrous histiocytoma arising in medullary long bone infarct. Orthopedics 1987: 10: 1169–1173
19. Frierson H F Jr, Fechner R E, Stallings R G, Wang G J. Malignant fibrous histiocytoma in bone infarct. Cancer 1987: 59: 496–500
20. Abdelwahab I F, Hermann G, Lewis M M, Klein M J. Transformation of an idiopathic bone infarct into malignant fibrous histiocytoma in a female. Bull Hosp Jt Dis Orthop Inst 1988: 48: 197–203
21. Desai P, Perino G, Present D, Steiner G C. Sarcoma in association with bone infarcts. Report of five cases. Arch Pathol Lab Med 1996: 120: 482–489
22. Furey J G, Ferrer-Torrels M, Reagan J W. Fibrosarcoma arising at the site of bone infarcts. J Bone Joint Surg (Am) 1960: 42: 802–810
23. Heater K, Collins P A. Osteosarcoma in association with infarction of bone. J Bone Joint Surg (Am) 1987: 69: 300–302
24. Resnik C S, Aisner S G, Young J W, Levine A. Case report 767. Osteosarcoma arising in bone infarction. Skeletal Radiol 1993: 22: 58–61
25. Abdelwahab I F, Kenan S, Klein M J, Lewis M M. Case report: angiosarcoma occurring in a bone infarct. Clin Radiol 1992: 45: 412–414
26. Pins M R, Mankin H J, Xavier R J, Rosenthal D I, Dickersin G R, Rosenberg A E. Malignant epithelioid hemangioendothelioma of the tibia associated with a bone infarct in a patient who had Gaucher disease. J Bone Joint Surg (Am) 1995: 77: 777–781
27. Matsuno T, Kaneda K, Takeda N. Development of angiosarcoma at the site of a bone infarct. Clin Orthop 1996: 327: 259–263
28. Greenfield G B, Cardenas C, Dawson P J, Stenzler S. Case report 650. Grade II chondrosarcoma of the proximal end of the right femur. Skeletal Radiol 1991: 20: 67–70
29. Strecker W, Gilula L A, Kyriakos M. Case report 479. Idiopathic healing infarct of bone simulating osteosarcoma. Skeletal Radiol 1988: 17: 220–225
30. Cohen J, Brown K A, Grice D S. Ewing's tumor of the talus (astragalus) simulating aseptic necrosis. J Bone Joint Surg (Am) 1953: 35: 1008–1012
31. Weissman S L, Salama R, Papo Y, Loewenthal M. Ewing's tumor of the talus misdiagnosed as avascular necrosis. J Bone Joint Surg (Am) 1966: 48: 333–336
32. Wientroub S, Michels H, Baratz M, Shili R, Salama R. Ewing's tumor of the cuboid bone simulating avascular necrosis. J Bone Joint Surg (Am) 1979: 61: 951–952

51

Myositis ossificans

M. Forest

INTRODUCTION AND CLINICAL DATA

Myositis ossificans is a circumscribed heterotopic new bone formation. Some authors have rightly stressed that the term is inadequate, as inflammation is usually absent and the ossifying process is located between the muscle bundles.[1–3] The term 'posttraumatic mineralization' has been suggested,[2] although the lesion may occur without a history of trauma. The condition has also been described under the names of heterotopic ossification and pseudomalignant osseous tumor of soft tissues.[4]

Young adults, predominantly males, are affected; the condition is extremely rare in young children under 10 years of age[5] but a case has been reported with an onset soon after birth.[6] Clinical symptoms are pain, tenderness and soft tissue swelling and many cases, but not all, are related to minor trauma.[7]

LOCATION

In 80% of cases myositis ossificans is found in the large muscles of the extremities. In the hand, young females are usually affected, with a predilection for proximal phalanges and the hypothenar region.[8] The process has been documented in a number of other sites.[9]

IMAGING

On X-ray, amorphous calcifications appear within 2–6 weeks after the onset of symptoms.[1] In 6–8 weeks, the lesion is circumscribed by a calcified rim and separated from the cortex by a lucent line.[7,10] The sharply circumscribed mass becomes smaller and mature in 5–6 months (Figs 51.1–51.10).

A periosteal reaction may be observed in 40% of cases;[7,11] in rare cases, the adjacent surface of the periosteum is excavated.[2]

On bone scans, the lesion appears as an isolated and well-demarcated area of increased uptake.[7,13]

On arteriography, there is a diffuse blush and a fine neovascularization; mature lesions are avascular.[14]

CT scans demonstrate very well the rim of mineraliza-

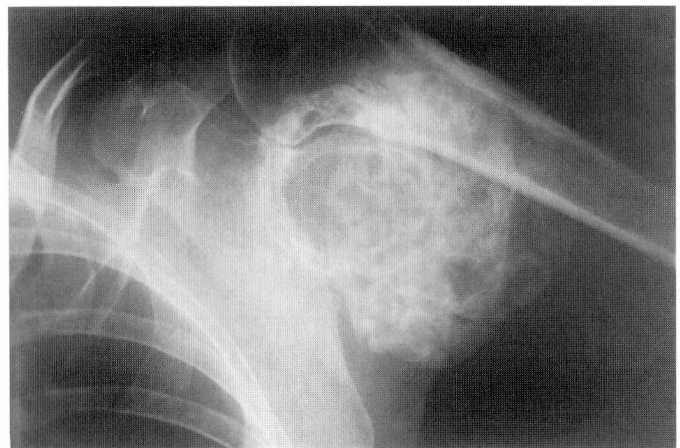

Fig. 51.1 Myositis ossificans located in the axilla.

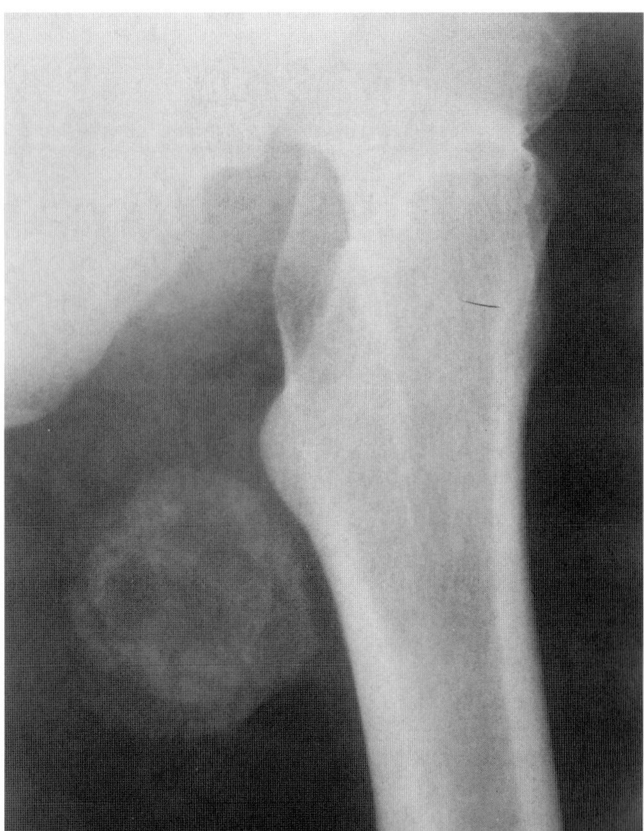

Fig. 51.3

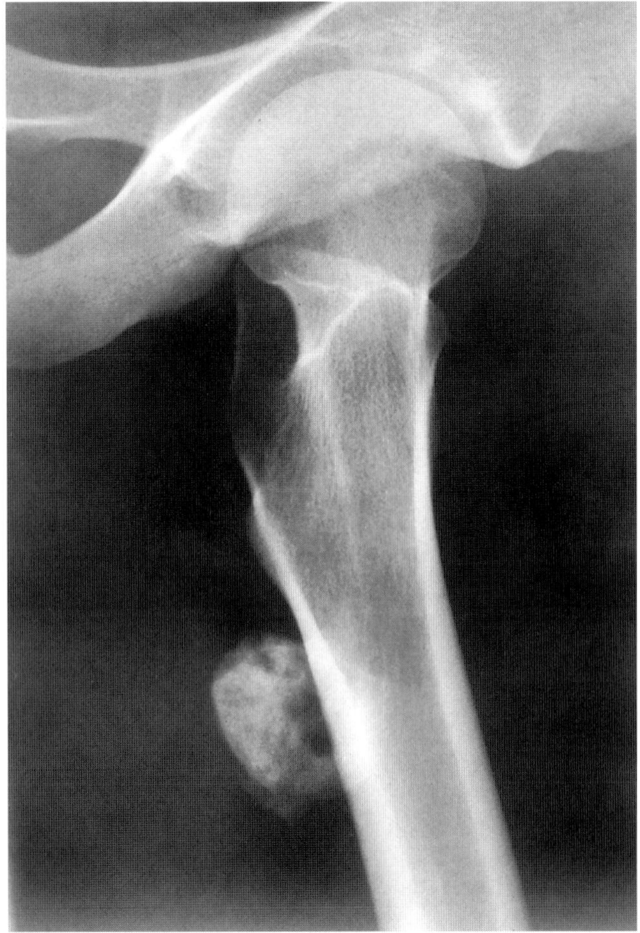

Fig. 51.2

Figs 51.2–51.4 Myositis ossificans in muscles of the thigh (Fig. 51.4: MRI).

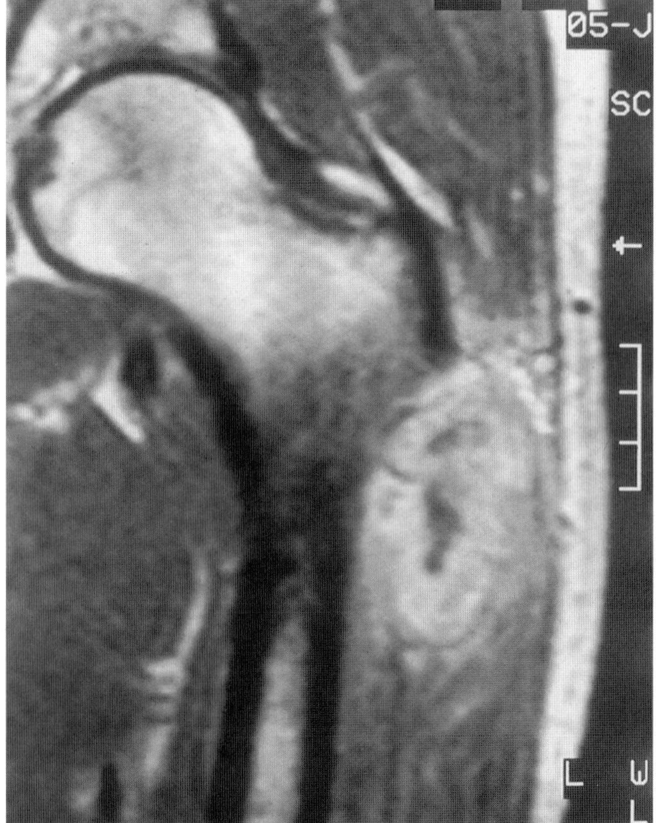

Fig. 51.4

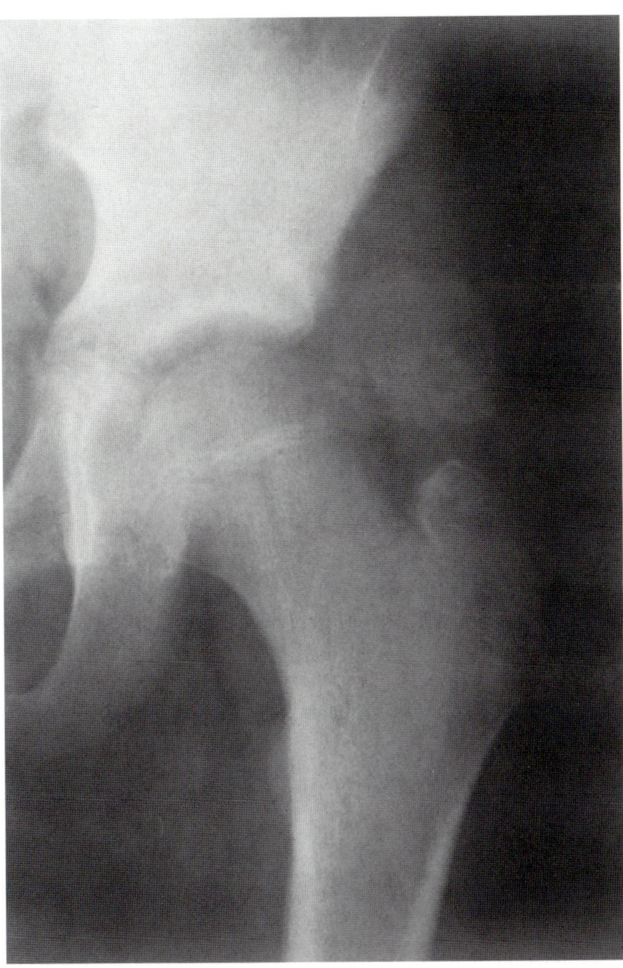

Fig. 51.5

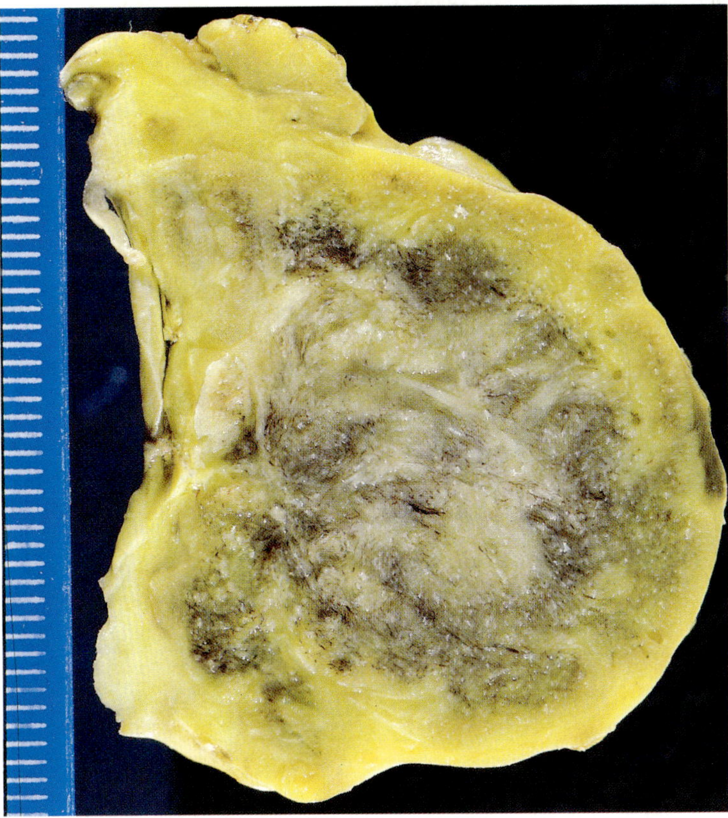

Fig. 51.6

Figs 51.5–51.7 Myositis ossificans in the muscles of the hip, with a faint peripheral shell of bone.

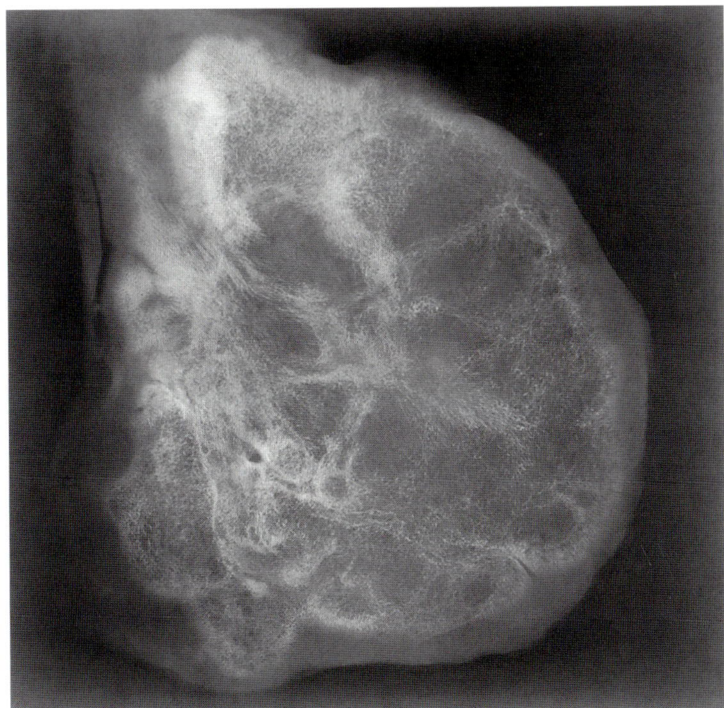

Fig. 51.7

tion around the lesion and the decreased CT tissue attenuation in the center.[15–18] Mature lesions exhibit a diffuse ossification.

On MRI, early lesions may mimic malignancy, with extensive edema in the soft tissues and bone marrow.[18,19] MR features of mature lesions are similar to those of mature bone.[20] On T2-weighted images, a thin hypointense rim is found in some cases, enhanced after administration of gadolinium.[20,21]

GROSS PATHOLOGY

The well-circumscribed mass is white, soft or gritty, gelatinous or hemorrhagic in the center. A bone network is located in the periphery; cystic changes have been reported with a yellowish clear fluid.[22] In half the cases, the lesion may be adherant to the periosteum.[3]

HISTOPATHOLOGY

Early lesions (2–3 weeks) appear as a central core of proliferating fibroblasts with numerous normal mitotic

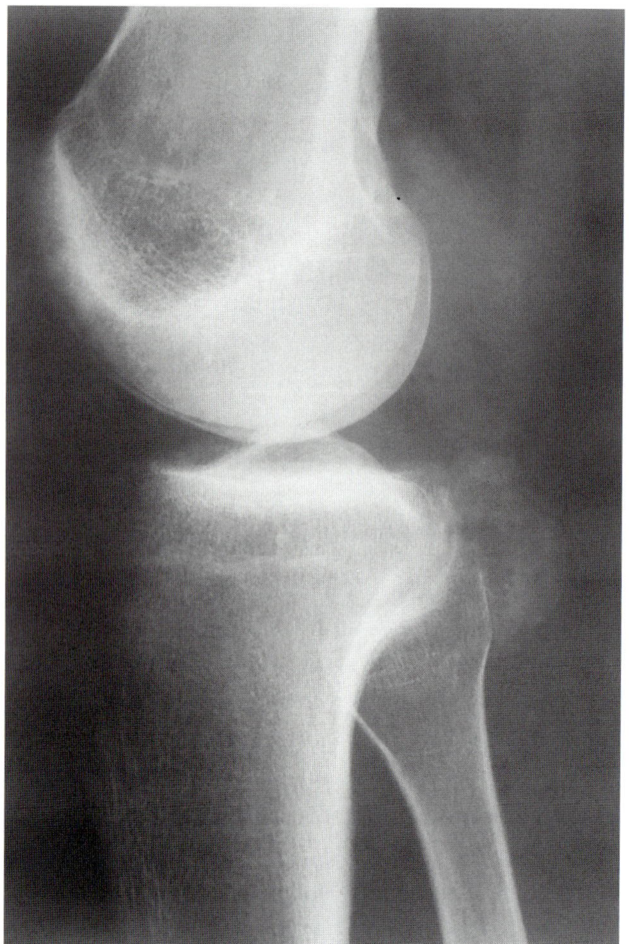

Fig. 51.8

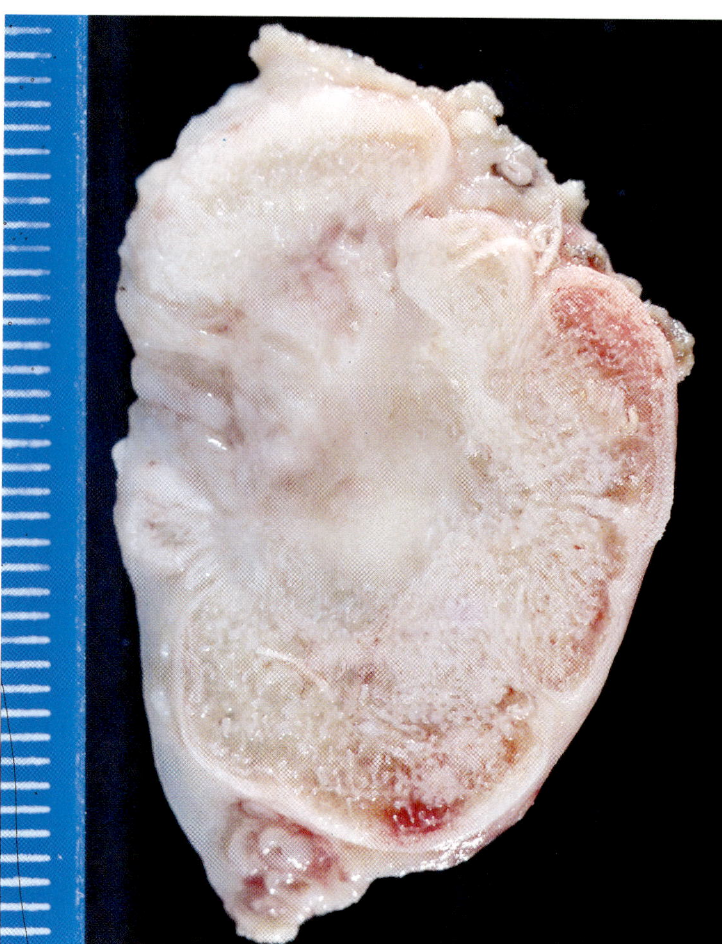

Fig. 51.9

Figs 51.8–51.10 Myositis ossificans with adherences to the periosteum of the tibia and massive peripheral bone formation.

figures. The process may be extremely cellular and in some cases, a prominent myxoid stroma may mimic a nodular fasciitis[18] (Figs 51.11, 51.12).

Intermediate lesions show peripheral bone formation, osteoid being rimmed by plump active osteoblasts. Cartilage may also be conspicuous, with endochondral ossification[7,22] as well as a prominent vascular proliferation (Figs 51.13–51.16).

Late lesions are characterized by a shell of mature lamellar bone (Figs 51.17, 51.18). A large number of osteoclasts may be found at the periphery. Bone is separated from muscle by a loose myxoid or compressed fibrous tissue.

The process is well characterized by a zoning pattern of peripheral bone maturation: a central undifferentiated zone, an intermediate zone with woven bone and an outer zone of maturing bone.

Cyst formation is sometimes seen, as are central hemorrhages or aneurysmal bone cyst-like changes.[23] The histological resemblances between the solid parts of aneurysmal bone cysts and a florid myositis ossificans have been stressed by Dahlin.[24]

CYTOPATHOLOGY

It is debatable whether a diagnosis can be made on smears.[8] Fine-needle aspiration may suggest a benign lesion, with clusters of proliferating fibroblasts, osteoblasts, osteoclast-like giant cells and immature mesenchymal cells.[5,25,26]

ELECTRON MICROSCOPY

Myofibroblasts are the main cell type at the earliest stage of the process.[3,27] A regular mineralizing front has been found, but with an abnormal collagen periodicity of 300 angstroms in early lesions.[7,28]

CLINICAL COURSE AND TREATMENT

The treatment is excision and recurrences are rare.[7] No convincing cases of malignant transformation have been reported, if one excepts the misdiagnoses with osteosarcoma. Spontaneous regression may even occur.[1]

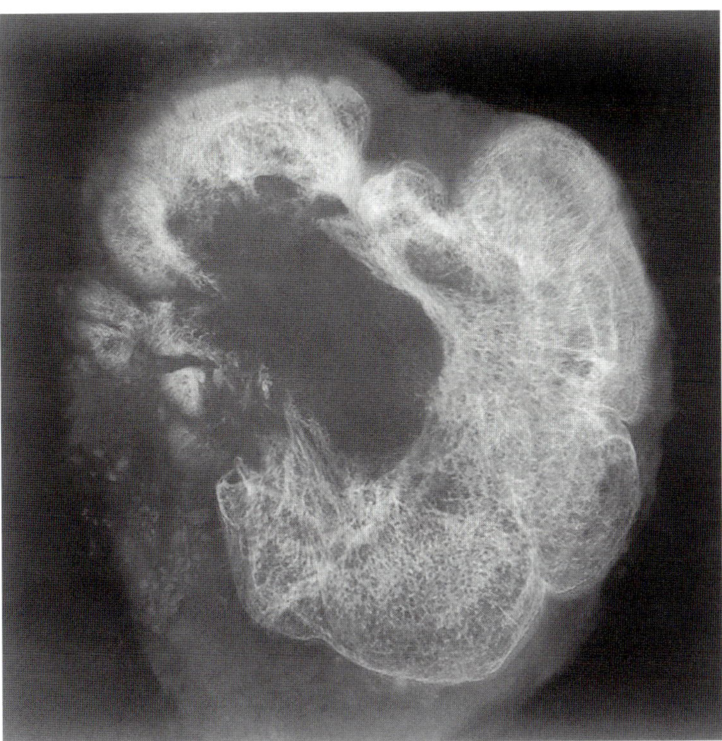

Fig. 51.10

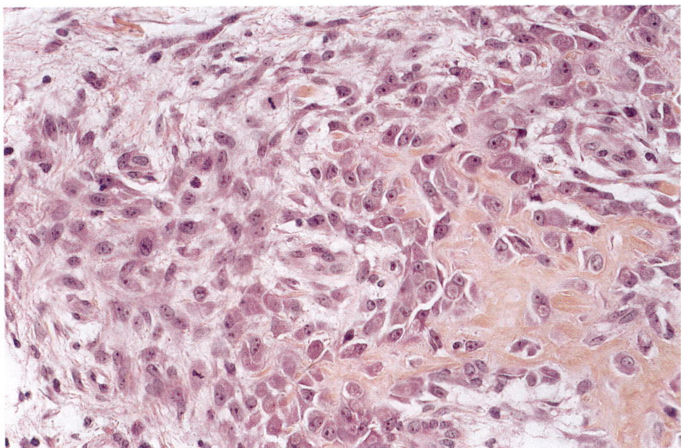

Fig. 51.12

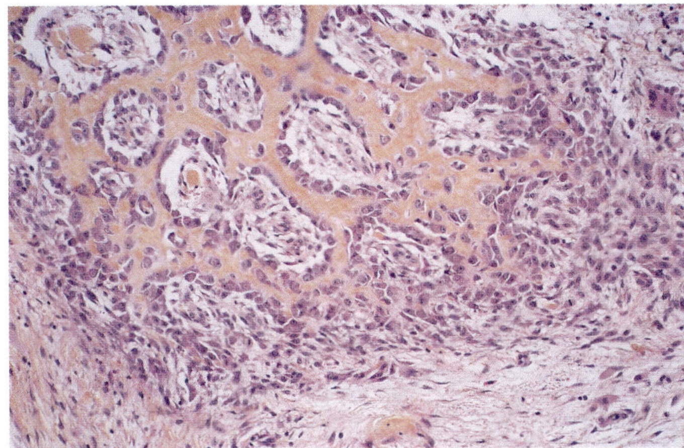

Fig. 51.13

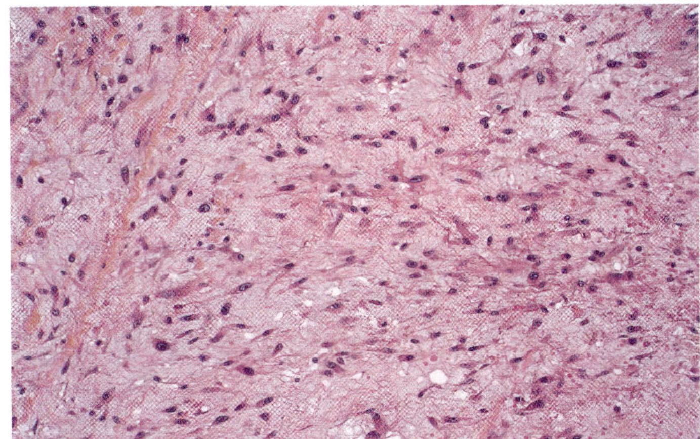

Fig. 51.11 Myositis ossificans: early lesion with proliferating fibroblasts.

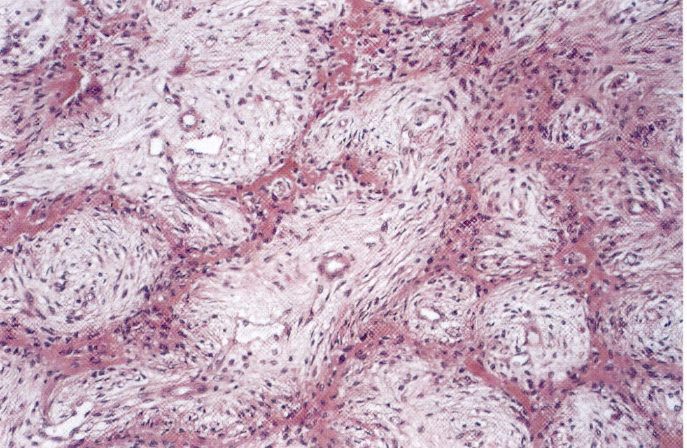

Fig. 51.14

DIFFERENTIAL DIAGNOSIS

Myositis ossificans may be confused, especially in the early stages, with parosteal or extraosseous osteosarcomas[3,7,12,15,22] and vice-versa (Figs 51.19–51.22).

Osteosarcomas, including rare, well-differentiated osteosarcomas of the soft tissues,[29] have a disorderly growth with a reverse zoning effect, that is, immature woven bone or osteoid is found in the periphery and mature osseous trabeculae are centrally located. In well-differentiated forms, elongated plump fibroblast-like spindle cells are

Figs 51.12–51.14 Myositis ossificans: osteoblastic differentiation, network of bone rimmed by osteoblasts and loose vascular stroma.

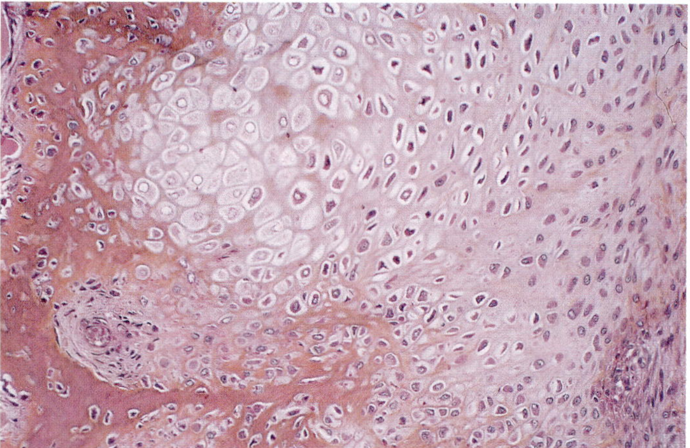

Fig. 51.15

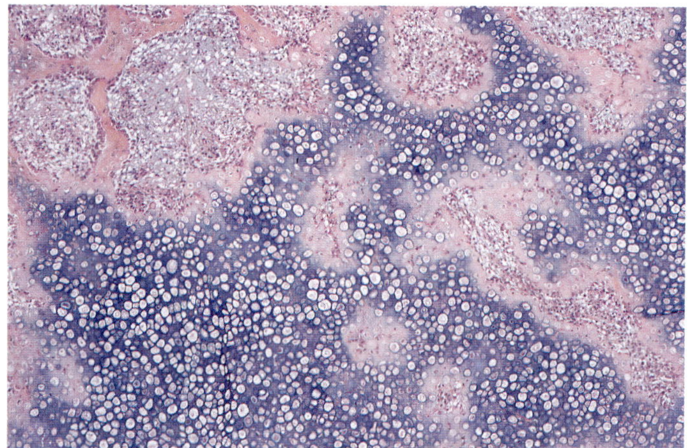

Fig. 51.16

Figs 51.15, 51.16 Myositis ossificans: cartilage component.

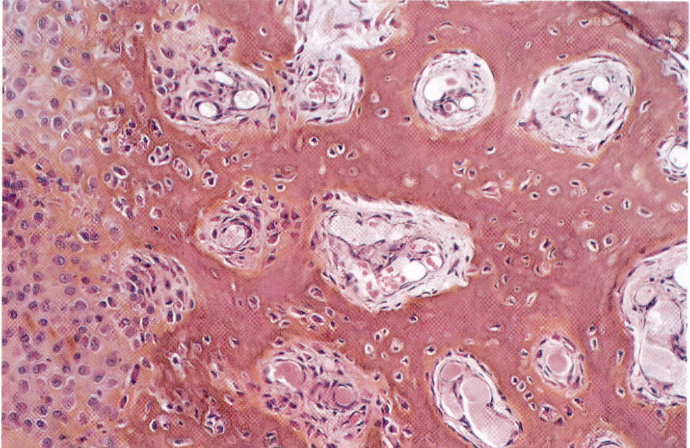

Fig. 51.17 Myositis ossificans: peripheral bone maturation.

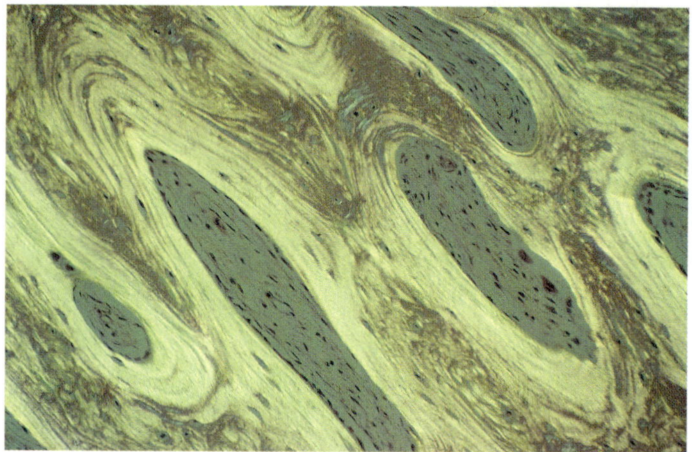

Fig. 51.18 Myositis ossificans: mature lesion with a shell of lamellar bone (polarized light).

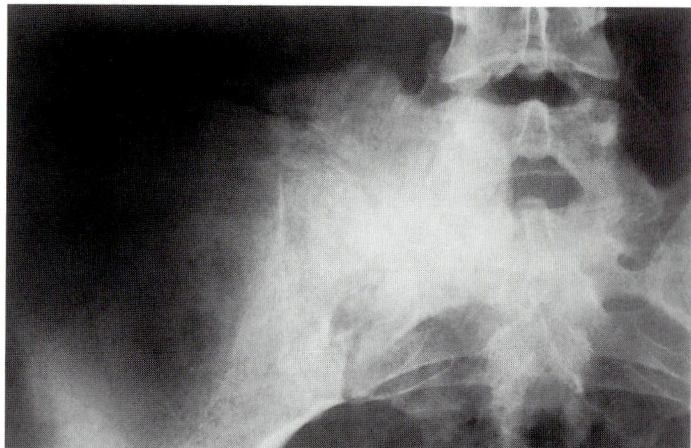

Fig. 51.19

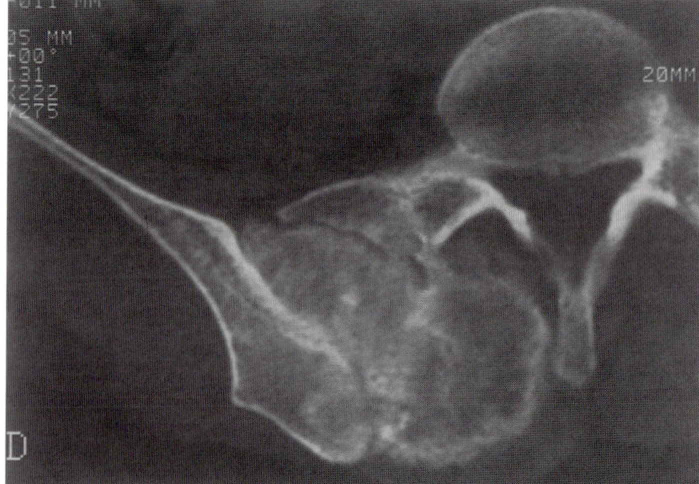

Fig. 51.20

Figs 51.19–51.22 Myositis ossificans is confused with osteosarcomas but the reverse may happen. Mass close to the sacroiliac joint with a peripheral bone maturation, initially diagnosed as myositis ossificans on imaging and on biopsy; early recurrence is an expanding tumor with the histology of an osteoblastic osteosarcoma (Fig. 51.22).

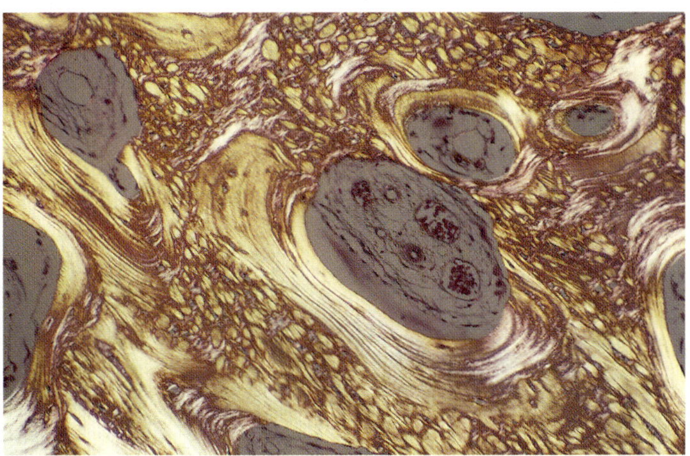

Fig. 51.21

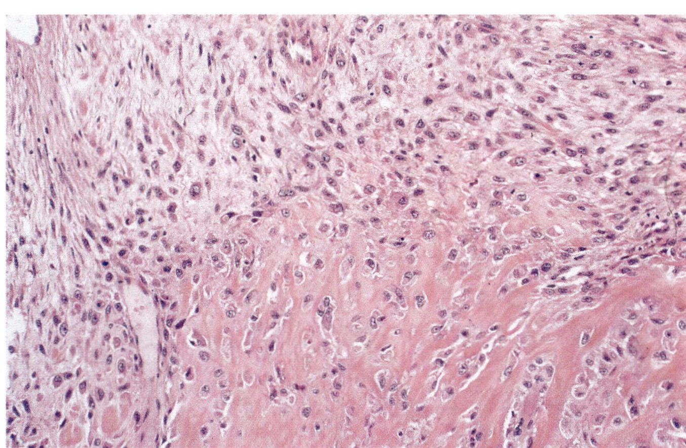

Fig. 51.22

distributed in a parallel arrangement, with mild nuclear atypia and rare mitoses; there is an infiltration of the neighboring tissues. An unusually rapid growth and pain are more suggestive of myositis ossificans.

Fibrodysplasia ossificans progressiva is an inherited dis-

order most often found in the first decade of life[30] and associated with a variety of skeletal abnormalities involving particularly the phalanges. Soft tissue lesions are multiple small nodules with low cellularity and a central progressive and marked ossification.[30]

REFERENCES

1. Ackerman L V. Extra-osseous localized non-neoplastic bone and cartilage formation (so-called myositis ossificans). Clinical and pathological confusion with malignant neoplasms. J Bone Joint Surg (Am) 1958: 40: 279–298
2. Gold R H, Mirra J M, Kaplan L, Grant S. Case report 68. Post-traumatic mineralization (myositis ossificans circumscripta), of the forearm with secondary erosion into the ulna. Skeletal Radiol 1978: 3: 123–126
3. Nuovo M A, Norman A, Chumas J, Ackerman L V. Myositis ossificans with atypical clinical, radiographic, or pathologic findings: a review of 23 cases. Skeletal Radiol 1992: 21: 87–101
4. Angervall L, Stener B, Stener I, Ahren C. Pseudomalignant osseous tumor of soft tissue. J Bone Joint Surg (Br) 1969: 51: 654–663
5. Clapton W K, James C L, Morris L L, Davey R B, Peacock M J, Byard R W. Myositis ossificans in childhood. Pathology 1992: 24: 311–314
6. Pazzaglia U E, Beluffi G, Columbo A, Marchi A, Coci A, Ceciliani L. Myositis ossificans in the newborn. J Bone Joint Surg (Am) 1986: 68: 456–458
7. Ogilvie-Harris D J, Fornasier V L. Pseudomalignant myositis ossificans; heterotopic new-bone formation without a history of trauma. J Bone Joint Surg (Am) 1980: 62: 1274–1283
8. De Smet L, Maes G, Fabry G. Fast-growing pseudomalignant myositis ossificans of the hand. Acta Orthop Belg 1994: 60: 101–105
9. Lopez Barea F, Rodriguez Peralto J L, Gonzales Lopez J, Sanchez Perez Grueso F. Case report 694. Cervical paravertebral circumscribed myositis ossificans. Skeletal Radiol 1991: 20: 539–542
10. Schütte H E, Van Der Heul R O. Pseudomalignant, nonneoplastic osseous soft tissue tumors of the hand and foot. Radiology 1990: 176: 149–153
11. Norman A, Dorfman H D. Juxta cortical circumscribed myositis ossificans: evolution and radiographic features. Radiology 1970: 96: 301–306
12. Goldman A B. Myositis ossificans circumscripta: a benign lesion with a malignant differential diagnosis. AJR 1976: 126: 32–40
13. Suzuki Y, Hisada K, Takeda M. Demonstration of myositis ossificans by 99m Tc pyrophosphate bone scanning. Radiology 1974: 111: 663–664
14. Yaghmai I. Myositis ossificans. Diagnostic value of arteriography. AJR 1977: 128: 811–816
15. Ackerman L V, Ramamurthy S, Jablokow V, Van Drunen M, Kaplan E. Case report 488. Post-traumatic myositis ossificans mimicking a soft tissue neoplasm. Skeletal Radiol 1988: 17: 310–314
16. Amendola M A, Glazer G M, Agha F P, Francis I R, Weatherbee L, Martel W. Myositis ossificans circumscripta: computed tomographic diagnosis. Radiology 1983: 149: 775–779
17. Zeanah W R, Hudson T M. Myositis ossificans: radiologic evaluation of two cases with diagnostic computed tomograms. Clin Orthop 1982: 168: 187–191
18. Kransdorf M J, Meis J M, Jelinek J S. Myositis ossificans. MR appearance with radiologic-pathologic corelation. AJR 1991: 157: 1243–1248
19. Ehara S, Nakasato T, Tamakawa Y, Yamataka H, Murakami H, Abe M. MRI of myositis ossificans circumscripta. Clin Imaging 1991: 15: 130–134
20. De Smet A A, Norris M A, Fisher D R. Magnetic resonance imaging of myositis ossificans: analysis of seven cases. Skeletal Radiol 1992: 21: 503–507
21. Cvitanic O, Sedlak J. Case report. Acute myositis ossificans. Skeletal Radiol 1995: 24: 139–141
22. Sumiyoshi K, Tsuneyoshi M, Enjoji M. Myositis ossificans. Acta Pathol Jpn 1985: 35: 1109–1122
23. Amir G, Mogle P, Sucher E. Case report 729. Myositis ossificans and aneurysmal bone cyst. Skeletal Radiol 1992: 21: 257–259
24. Dahlin D C, McLeod R A. Aneurysmal bone cyst and other nonneoplastic conditions. Skeletal Radiol 1982: 8: 243–250
25. Popok S M, Naib Z M. Fine-needle aspiration cytology of myositis ossificans. Diagn Cytopathol 1985: 1: 236–240
26. Rööser B, Herrlin K, Rydholm A, Akerman M. Pseudo-malignant myositis ossificans. Clinical, radiologic, and cytologic diagnosis in five cases. Acta Orthop Scand 1989: 60: 457–460
27. Povysil C, Matejovsky Z. Ultrastructural evidence of myofibroblasts

in pseudomalignant myositis ossificans. Virchows Arch A Pathol Anat Histol 1979: 381: 189–203

28. Caulet T, Adnet J, Pluot M, Gougeon J, Hopfner C. Myosite ossifiante circonscrite. Etude histochimique et ultrastructurale d'une observation. Virchows Arch A Pathol Anat 1969: 348: 16–35

29. Yi E S, Schmookler B M, Malawer M M, Sweet D E. Well-differentiated extraskeletal osteosarcoma. A soft-tissue homologue of parosteal osteosarcoma. Arch Pathol Lab Med 1991: 115: 906–909

30. Cramer S F, Ruehl A, Mandel M A. Fibrodysplasia ossificans progressiva: a distinctive bone-forming lesion of the soft tissue. Cancer 1981: 48: 1016–1021

Pathology of tumors and pseudotumoral lesions of the joints

52

Benign tumors and cysts of synovium

A. M. Bergemer

SYNOVIAL CYSTS AND GANGLIA

Synovial cysts and ganglion cysts (or ganglia) are cavities arising in the vicinity of joints and containing mucoid viscous fluid. Some authors believe they are distinct entities,[1] while others think they both belong to a spectrum of lesions.[2] The current theory is that ganglia are caused by degenerative changes in the connective tissue resulting in disintegrating cystic cavities, whereas synovial cysts are true synovial cavities. In clinical practice, the distinction between them seems to be of little importance.

Synovial cysts arise in the vicinity of numerous joints. They are often associated with articular abnormalities, such as rheumatoid arthritis, osteoarthritis, trauma and pigmented villonodular synovitis.[3,4] They occur at all ages but preferentially in young adults, with an average age of about 40.

Ganglion cysts develop in the connective tissue of joint capsules, tendon sheaths, menisci, ligaments and aponeuroses. Their etiology is unknown, although an unusual physical exercise of the involved joint or repeated microtrauma has been reported. In the spine, degenerative lesions of the facet joints and intervertebral discs are often present.[5] Sex ratio is 2–3 females:1 male. There is a predominance of young people.[1]

Symptoms due to synovial or ganglion cysts vary according to their location. The main clinical sign is the presence of a mass near the joint, painful or not, gradually increasing in size

Synovial cysts usually develop in the knee (Baker's cysts), then shoulder and hip, elbow, hand, ankle, wrist, foot and spine (apophyseal joints).[3,4]

Ganglion cysts essentially develop in the dorsum of the wrist (54–68% of cases) and less frequently in wrist flexors, fingers, dorsum of the foot, knee, spine (near facet joints or in the ligamentum flavum), ankle and other sites.[1,6]

Synovial and ganglion cysts are indistinguishable on diagnostic imaging.

Radiographs are often normal or may demonstrate pressure erosions of the underlying bone or a mass in the soft tissues near the joint.[1,7]

Ultrasonography is helpful to demonstrate precise connections of the cyst with the surrounding structures.[7] Ruptured cysts may be difficult to identify due to lack of fluid.[4]

CT scan and MRI give more precise analysis of the relations of the cyst with adjacent structures and of its extent.[4,7] They demonstrate well-defined walls, most often with a fluid content (but sometimes a gas content[8] or calcifications in some cysts of the spine[2]) or septa.[7]

Arthrography may complement ultrasound, CT or MRI, especially when rupture is suspected.[4,7] Synovial cysts communicate with the joint cavity, but ganglia usually do not, except in rare reported cases.[9]

Synovial cysts display various gross features (Figs 52.1, 52.2): thin or thick fibrous walls with a smooth or villous inner surface.[3] Some areas of hemosiderin pigmentation or cartilage formation may be seen. Cyst content is viscous, mucoid, fibrinous or hemorrhagic.[3]

Ganglion cysts (Fig. 52.3) consist of several interconnecting cavities: a 'main cyst' communicates via multiple 'pseudopodia' with several smaller capsular cysts.[1,9]

Histologically, synovial cysts are lined by flattened or cuboid synovial cells. Their walls consist of more or less dense fibrous tissue. The walls of ganglia consist of fibrous tissue, containing variable numbers of fibroblasts, without a true synovial cell lining.[1,10,11] The collagenous wall of ganglia may contain in variable proportions small foci of mucoid or myxoid degeneration, focal histiocytes, hemosiderin deposits, calcifications and thick-walled small vessels.[8,12,13] The ganglion cavity is often subdivided by septa.[13] There may be several mucin-filled clefts (capsular cysts) at the base of the ganglion, corresponding to areas of degenerative change in the connective tissue.[10,11,13]

Ultrastructural features favor the hypothesis of the degenerative nature of ganglia. The walls of ganglia consist of a fibrous and mucopolysaccharide matrix in which are embedded elongated cells, quite different from synoviocytes, described as degenerative non-secreting smooth muscle cells[12] or multifunctional mesenchymal cells.[14] Other cells observed are fibroblasts and occasionally macrophages.[12] Some authors suggest that the content of ganglia seems to be degenerative,[12] whereas others think that it is secreted by the mesenchymal cells of the wall.[14]

In both synovial cysts and ganglia, the treatment depends on clinical symptoms, location and evolution of the lesion. Aspiration of the cyst, alone or followed by intraarticular corticosteroid injections, may be sufficient and even repeated in most cases. When conservative therapy fails to avoid recurrences or in some particular locations, radical surgical therapy is indicated.[2,4,7,9,11,13]

Synovial cysts, even surgically treated, may recur in vari-

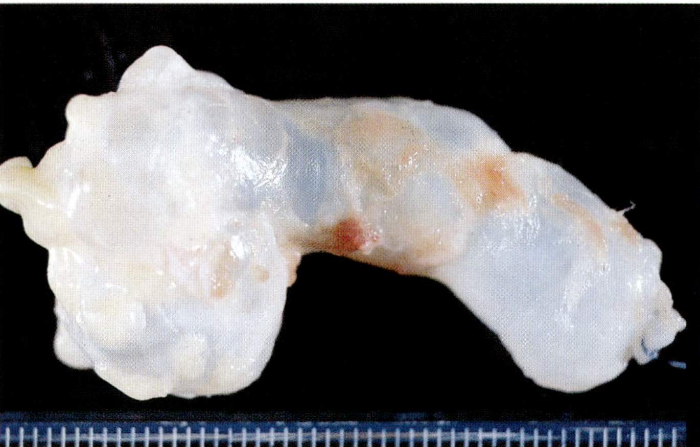

Fig. 52.1

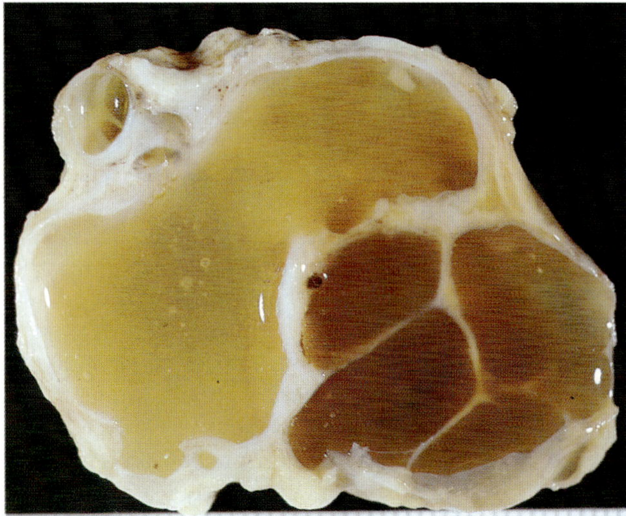

Fig. 52.2

Figs 52.1, 52.2 Synovial cysts of the knee joint. (Courtesy of M. Forest MD.)

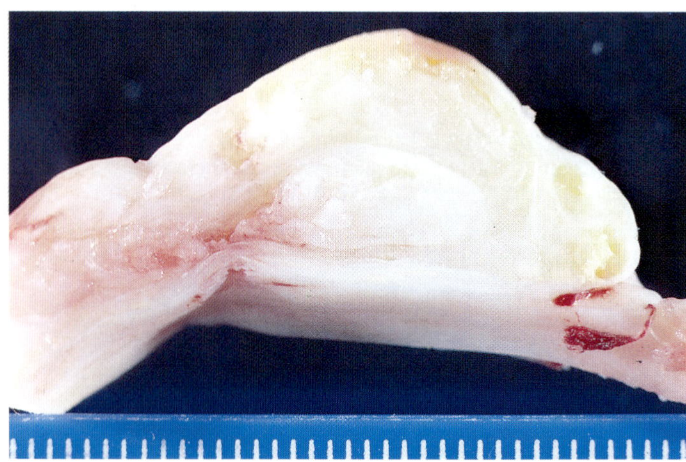

Fig. 52.3 Ganglion of the hip joint. (Courtesy of M. Forest MD.)

able proportions.[3] The prognosis is often that of the associated joint disease (e.g. rheumatoid arthritis). Sometimes, new synovial cysts arise in other articular sites, without recurrence at the primary one.[3]

The prognosis of ganglia is variable: some disappear, spontaneously or after conservative therapy, with or without recurrences.[1,13] Radical surgical excision may be followed by recurrences.

SYNOVIAL HEMANGIOMA

Synovial hemangiomas are usually localized in the synovium, occurring preferentially in children and young adults (average age 25 years).[15] Males are more frequently affected than females (65% vs 35%).[15] Symptoms are frequent in childhood (60% of cases) and raise the possibility of a congenital origin.

Clinical symptoms are variable and may be intermittent, usually including pain, alone or with swelling, soft paraarticular mass, articular effusions, hemorrhagic or not, and rare recurrent hemarthrosis.[15] Hemangiomas may also be encountered in the tendon sheaths, involving the tendon and its surrounding tissues.[15]

Synovial hemangiomas may be isolated or associated with angiomatosis of soft tissue (e.g. Klippel–Trenaunay and Parkes–Weber syndromes). These do not have the same course nor prognosis as isolated ones, so some authors distinguish them from pure synovial hemangiomas.[15] In this group of diseases, cutaneous hemangiomas may overlie the articular lesion.[16]

The sites of involvement are usually the knee (60%), then the elbow (30%) and fingers or other rare (10%) locations.[15] Articular hemangiomas may be intraarticular (pure synovial), juxtaarticular or mixed.[15,17] In the knee, the lesion is usually localized in the synovial cavity, but in 30% of cases lies in a bursal sac.[15] Hemangiomas of the tendon sheath occur preferentially in the hand, forearm and ankle.[15]

In most cases radiographic findings exhibit either no particular abnormality or an ill-defined intraarticular soft tissue mass with mild demineralization of adjacent bones; phleboliths may be encountered.[15] In children, advanced ossification of epiphyses may be seen.[18] Arthrography may be normal or reveal a non-specific, irregular filling defect.[15] CT scan, MRI and arteriography are very useful for diagnosis and study of distribution of the lesions.[15,19] At arthroscopy, the distinction may be difficult between a nodular hemangioma and a villonodular synovitis, since there have been reports describing a concurrence of these two lesions.[18]

Grossly, the lesion can be diffuse (30%) or localized (70%, nodular). Average size is about 4 cm. It may be pigmented in some cases and grossly exhibits a villous surface.[15] When nodular, it often arises in the infrapatellar fat pad.

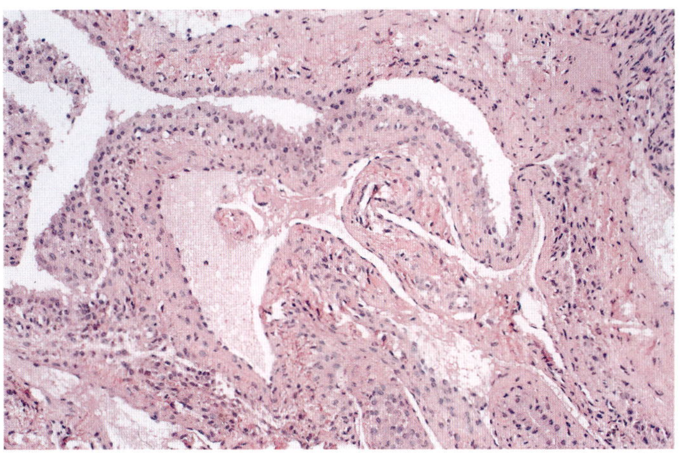

Fig. 52.4 Hemangioma of the synovium (knee joint). (Courtesy of M. Forest MD.)

Histologically, the most frequent pattern is that of a cavernous hemangioma (50% of cases) (Fig. 52.4). The next most frequent type is capillary (25%), then arteriovenous (20%) and venous hemangioma (5%).[15] Diffuse forms may involve adjacent muscles or soft tissue.[17] Some lesions may exhibit intravascular thrombosis, sometimes associated with areas of papillary endothelial hyperplasia, or be partially infarcted. Hemosiderin deposits are often present.

An early surgical excision or an arthroscopic ablation is easy when the lesion is localized[16] but difficult or impossible when it is extensive. A complete surgical excision is curative in pure synovial hemangiomas, while recurrences are frequent in extensive forms or angiomatosis.[15]

SYNOVIAL LIPOMA AND LIPOMATOUS LESIONS

These rare, benign synovial lesions consist of mature fat developing in the synovium, intraarticularly or in the tendon sheaths. Two main forms have been described: true lipoma, consisting of solid fatty masses occurring mainly within tendon sheaths,[20] and diffuse lipomatous involvement of the synovium, usually intraarticular, producing swollen villi, a condition known as lipoma arborescens[20–23] (Jaffe 1972).

Lipoma of tendon sheaths occurs in young adults. Clinical symptoms, usually present for several years, are pain of the involved articulation, sometimes associated with a swelling or occasionally inflammatory changes of the overlying soft tissues.[20]

The etiology of lipoma arborescens is unknown. Most cases arise de novo, but some have been reported in association with degenerative joint disease, trauma, rheumatoid arthritis or diabetes mellitus, so it has been suggested that this lesion is a reactive change.[21,22] It predominates in males. Clinical presentation is typically that of a joint swollen for many years, usually painless and

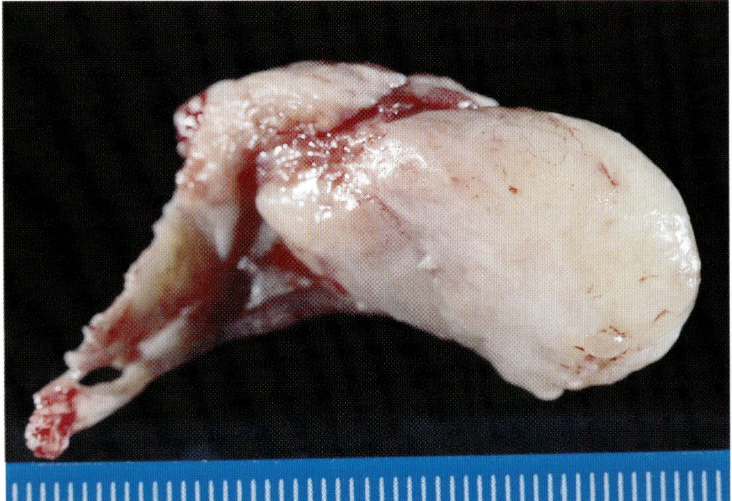

Fig. 52.5 Lipoma of the synovium (knee joint). (Courtesy of M. Forest MD.)

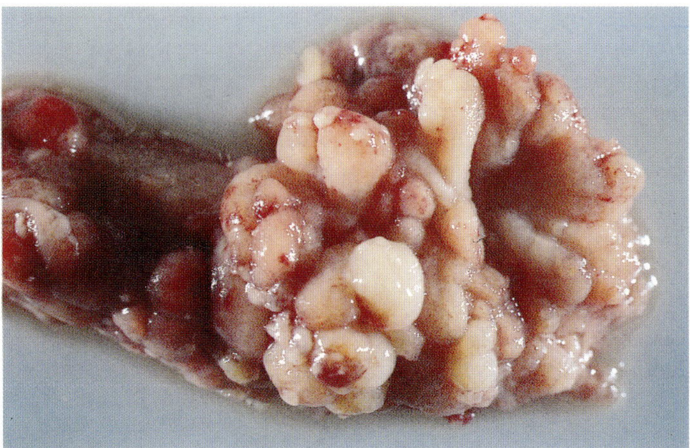

Fig. 52.6

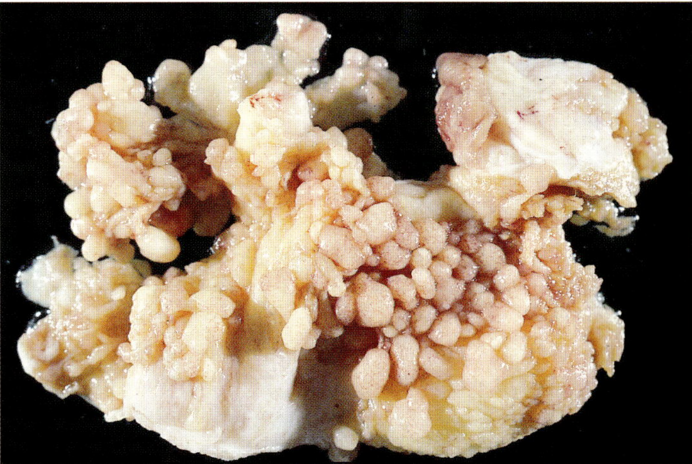

Fig. 52.7

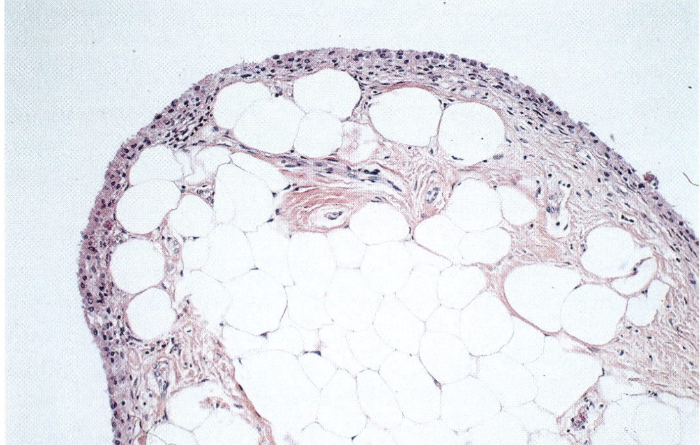

Fig. 52.8

Figs 52.6–52.8 Lipomatosis of the synovium (knee joint). (Courtesy of M. Forest MD.)

sometimes accompanied by intermittent articular effusions.[21,22]

True intraarticular lipoma is extremely rare and usually occurs in the knee as a solitary mass of adipose tissue (Fig. 52.5), with no known etiology[23] (Jaffé 1972).

Lipoma of tendon sheaths affects the wrist and hand in most cases, less commonly the ankle and foot. About half of the cases are bilateral.

Lipoma arborescens occurs most often in the knee joint and particularly in the suprapatellar pouch.[21,22,23–26] It can sometimes be bilateral in the knee.[22,27] Other articular locations have been rarely reported, such as ankle or wrist.[22]

Radiography exhibits images of lesser density than the soft tissues in the vicinity. Arthrography demonstrates non-specific intraarticular filling defects.[21]

Ultrasonography and CT scan are useful in assessing the synovial nature of the mass; the fronds of a lipoma arborescens are obvious, their hyperechoic appearance and density being suggestive of their fatty nature.[21,25,26] MRI is useful in the preoperative evaluation of the extent of the lesion and exhibits its specific features, especially a signal intensity similar to that of the fat on all pulse sequences.[24,25]

In lipoma arborescens, there is a gross extensive villous proliferation of the thickened synovium (Figs. 52.6, 52.7). The villi are yellowish-white or orange.[22,27]

Lipoma of tendon sheaths presents as a smooth, orange mass, which demonstrates its typical nodular or villous (lipoma arborescens) aspect when the sheath is opened.

Histologically, lipoma arborescens demonstrates typical villous proliferation of the thickened synovium. The subsynovial tissue is completely replaced by dense clusters of mature fat cells, between occasional vessels (Fig. 52.8). The synovial lining cells may exhibit mild hyperplasia.[22]

The very rare non-villous intraarticular lipoma demonstrates the characteristic architecture of a lipoma.

Lipomas of tendon sheaths, villous or nodular, exhibit the same histopathological patterns.[20]

The suggested treatment for lipoma arborescens is a complete synovectomy performed as an open procedure.[22,26] The functional prognosis of the joint depends on its previous status, since rare cases have been reported with progression of osteoarthritic changes after synovectomy.[22]

REFERENCES

1. Mc Everdy B. Simple ganglia. Br J Surg 1962: 49: 585–594
2. Hsu K Y, Zucherman J F, Shea W J, Jeffrey R A. Lumbar intraspinal synovial and ganglion cysts (facet cysts). Ten-year experience in evaluation and treatment. Spine 1995: 20: 80–89
3. Burleson R J, Bickel W H, Dahlin D C. Popliteal cyst. A clinicopathologic survey. J Bone Joint Surg (Am) 1956: 38: 1265–1274
4. Gullo G J, Venta L. Giant synovial cysts. Orthopedics 1993: 15: 110–116
5. Onofrio B, Mih A D. Synovial cysts of the spine. Neurosurgery 1988: 22: 642–647
6. Haase J. Extradural cyst of ligamentum flavum L4. A case. Acta Orthop Scand 1972: 43: 32–38
7. Treadwell E L. Synovial cysts and ganglia: the value of magnetic resonance imaging. Semin Arthritis Rheum 1994: 24: 61–70
8. Lin R M, Wey K L, Tzeng C C. Gas-containing 'ganglion' cyst of lumbar posterior longitudinal ligament at L3. Spine 1993: 18: 2528–2532
9. Angelides A C, Wallace P F. The dorsal ganglion of the wrist: its pathogenesis, gross and microscopic anatomy, and surgical treatment. J Hand Surg 1976: 1: 228–235
10. Lawson G M, Salter D M, Hooper G. The histopathology of fibrous flexor sheath ganglia. J Hand Surg (Br) 1994: 19: 258–260
11. Matthews P. Ganglia of the flexor tendon sheaths in the hand. J Bone Joint Surg (Br) 1973: 55: 612–617
12. Ghadially F N, Mehta P N. Multifunctional mesenchymal cells resembling smooth muscle cells in ganglia of the wrist. Ann Rheum Dis 1971: 30: 31–42
13. Soren A. Pathogenesis, clinic, and treatment of ganglion. Arch Orthop Trauma Surg 1982: 99: 247–252
14. Psaila J V, Mansel R E. The surface ultrastructure of ganglia. J Bone Joint Surg (Br) 1978: 60: 228–233
15. Devaney K, Vinh T N, Sweet D E. Synovial hemangioma: a report of 20 cases with differential diagnostic considerations. Hum Pathol 1993: 24: 737–745
16. Shapiro G S, Fanton G S. Intraarticular hemangioma of the knee. Arthroscopy 1993: 9: 464–466
17. Halborg A, Hansen H, Sneppen H O. Haemangioma of the knee joint. Acta Orthop Scand 1968: 39: 209–216
18. Bobechko W P, Kostuik J P. Childhood villonodular synovitis. Can J Surg 1968: 11: 480–486
19. Aalberg J R. Synovial hemangioma of the knee. A case report. Acta Orthop Scand 1990: 61: 88–89
20. Sullivan C R, Dahlin D C, Bryan R S. Lipoma of the tendon sheath. J Bone Joint Surg (Am) 1956: 38: 1275–1280
21. Armstrong S J, Watt I. Lipoma arborescens of the knee. Br J Radiol 1989: 62: 178–180
22. Hallel T, Lew S, Bansal M. Villous lipomatous proliferation of the synovial membrane (lipoma arborescens). J Bone Joint Surg (Am) 1988: 70: 264–270
23. Pudlowski R M, Gilula L A, Kyriakos M. Intraarticular lipoma with osseous metaplasia: radiographic pathologic correlation. AJR 1979: 132: 471–473
24. Feller J F, Rishi M, Hughes E C. Lipoma arborescens of the knee: MR demonstration. AJR 1994: 163: 162–164
25. Grieten M, Buckwalter K A, Cardinal E, Rougraff B. Case report 873. Lipoma arborescens. Skeletal Radiol 1994: 23: 652–655
26. Martinez D, Millner P A, Coral A, Newman R J, Hardy G J, Butt W P. Case report 745. Synovial lipoma arborescens. Skeletal Radiol 1992: 21: 393–395
27. Arzimanoglu A. Bilateral arborescent lipoma of the knee. A case report. J Bone Joint Surg (Am) 1957: 39: 976–979

Pigmented villonodular synovitis

J. Amouroux

INTRODUCTION AND CLINICAL DATA

In 1941 Jaffe assembled under the common term of pigmented villonodular synovitis[1] dissimilar lesions hitherto described by different names, i.e.:

- giant cell tumors of synovial tendon sheaths, which may be localized, most often occurring in fingers, flexor tendons or interphalangeal joints, or diffuse, usually arising in the vicinity of large joints;
- actual pigmented villonodular synovitis, developing in joint cavities, most often knee or hip;
- villonodular bursitis, with the same aspect, occurring in the bursae surrounding large joints, but with no connection with articular cavities.

These lesions, thought to be rare, are in fact the most frequent pseudotumoral or tumoral lesions arising in the synovium. Their nature remains uncertain. Among the possible origins, tumoral, inflammatory or metabolic, the first is more generally favored although it is impossible to exclude any other etiology.

The disease affects males and females equally and occurs mostly in the young adult: 50% of the patients are between 20 and 40 years old.[2] Children may also be affected.[3,4,5]

Clinical symptoms vary according to the type of the lesion. In localized tenosynovitis, there is painless swelling of tendon sheaths on the palmar or dorsal surface of the wrist or on palmar digital sheaths. Villonodular bursitis gives rise to a prominent and often worrying swelling of soft tissues. In intraarticular forms, there is moderate pain of mechanical type and an articular swelling due to the tumor itself and to the effusion that often accompanies it. Locking episodes may occur in cases of a pedunculated nodule.[6]

SKELETAL DISTRIBUTION

Pigmented villonodular synovitis mostly occurs in large

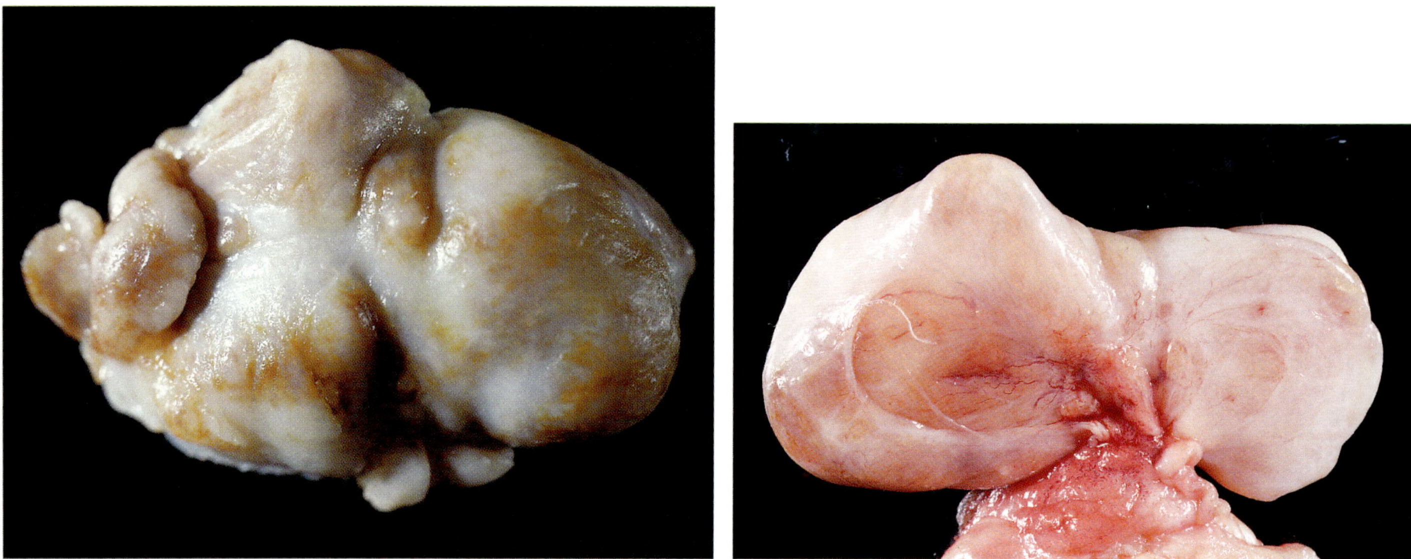

Fig. 53.1

Fig. 53.2

Figs 53.1, 53.2 Localized pigmented villonodular synovitis of the knee. (Courtesy of M. Forest MD.)

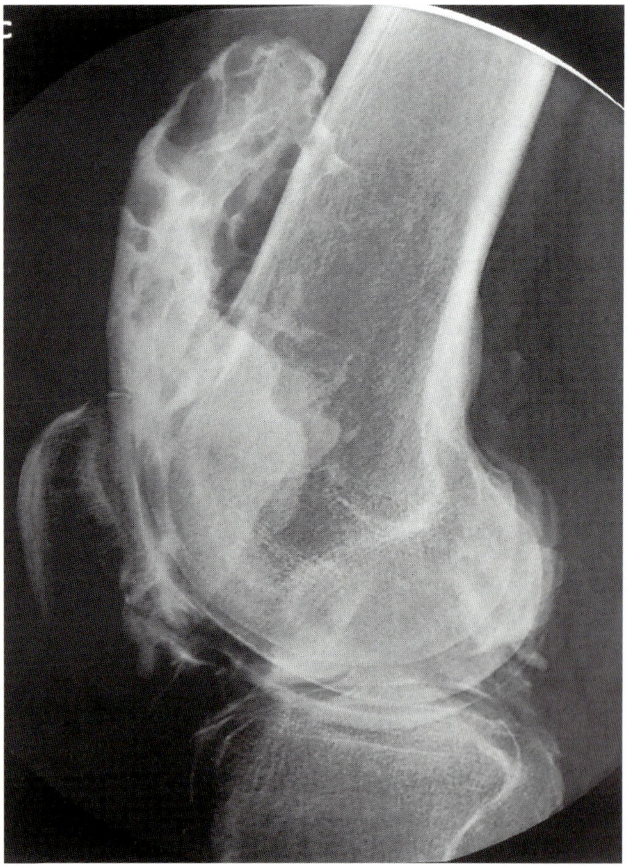

Fig. 53.3

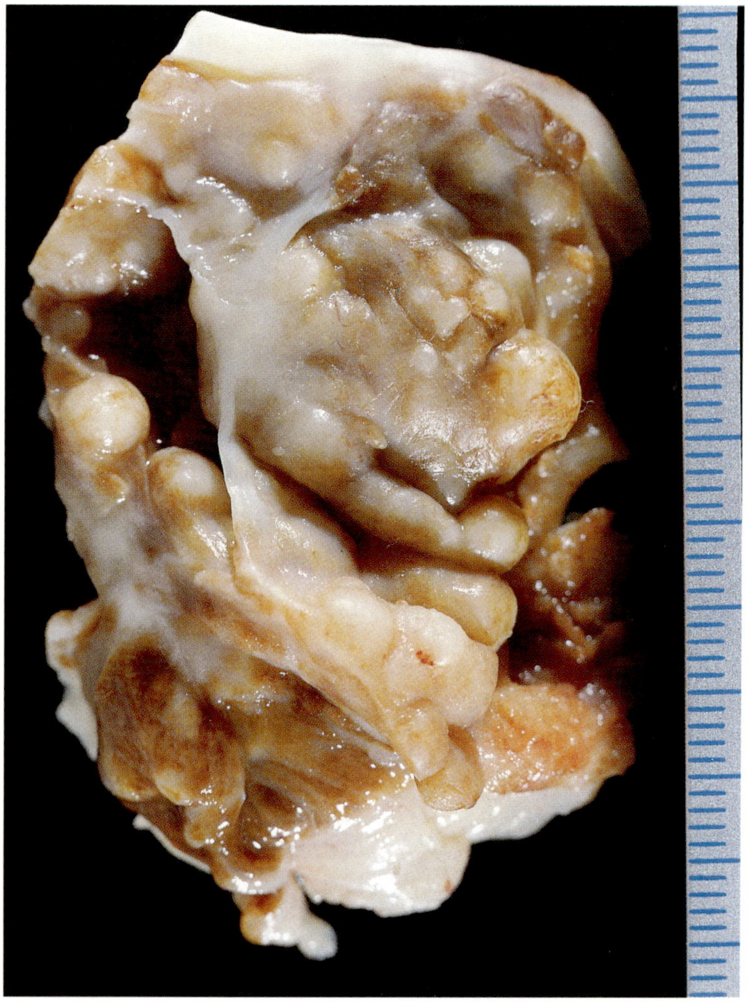

Fig. 53.4

Figs 53.3, 53.4 Pigmented villonodular synovitis located in the suprapatellar bursa: correlation of arthrography with gross findings. (Courtesy of M. Forest MD.)

joints: knee 70–80%, hip 13%, ankle 7%, shoulder, wrist and foot 2%. The elbow is rarely affected.[7]

Spinal involvement is also rare and the reported cases are most often located in the lumbar spine, rarely in the cervical spine.[8] The tumor forms an epidural mass arising near the facet joints.

Some exceptional locations have been reported such as the sacroiliac or temporomandibular joints. Lesions are rarely multifocal.[5]

IMAGING

In localized forms, radiographs are usually normal. In diffuse forms, bone erosions are often seen. They present as scratch erosions in the region of reflection of the synovium and especially as geodes. The latter are epiphyseal, peripheral, polycyclic, sometimes multiple, surrounded by a thin radiopaque border. They show a mirror development, for example in the intercondylar notch and below tibial spines. They may be located far from the articular space, in the femoral neck for example. Geodes are more frequent in narrow joints, such as hip, elbow and wrist. Calcifications are rare.

CT scan may give information on the hemosiderin content of the lesion.[9] MRI is currently the best diagnostic examination, for it shows intraarticular effusion, bone erosions and hemosiderin-laden tumoral mass. Hemosiderin is best demonstrated by gradient echo sequencing. MRI may allow diagnosis in some locations where radiography is often normal (pigmented villonodular synovitis of the posterior compartment of the knee).[10] It also gives very helpful information on extension of the lesions into the joint and surrounding soft tissues.[11]

GROSS PATHOLOGY

Localized pigmented villonodular synovitis is a nodular, diversely colored, gray, yellow or brown tumefaction, from several millimeters up to 3 or 4 cm in diameter (Figs 53.1, 53.2).

In diffuse forms (Figs 53.3–53.10), on a surgical specimen or during arthroscopy, the synovial membrane shows

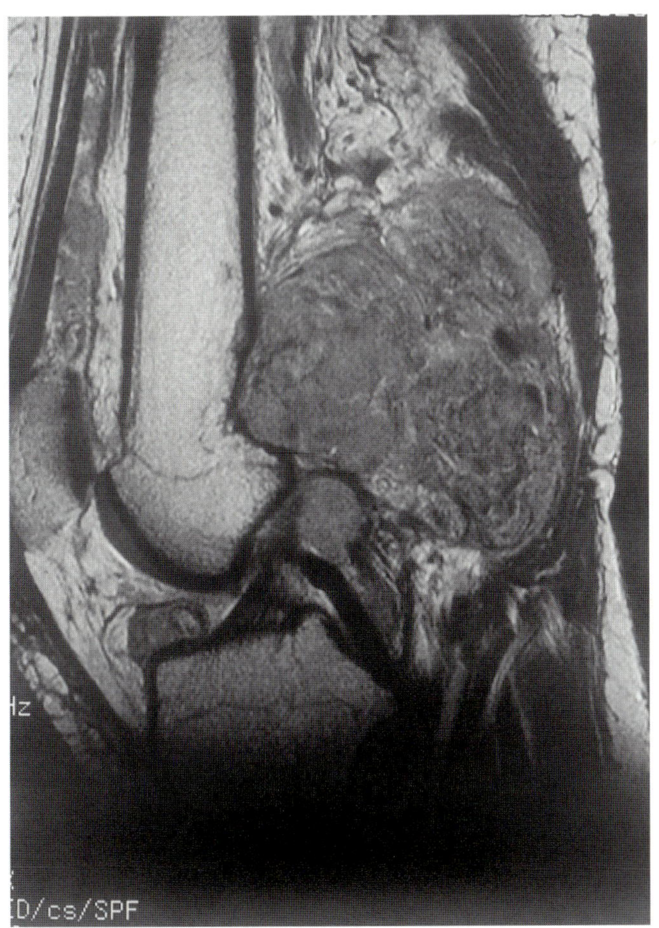

Fig. 53.5

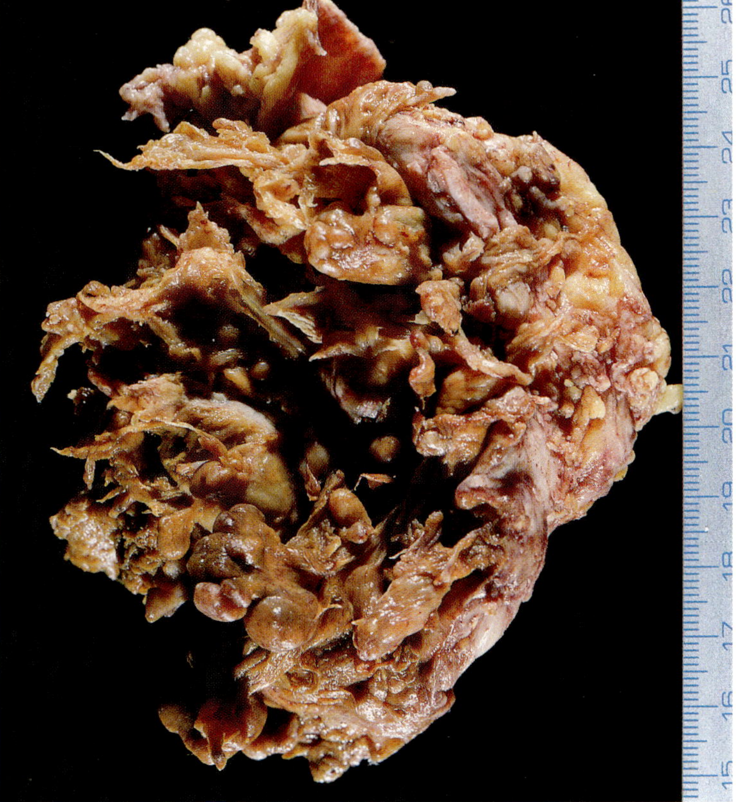

Fig. 53.6

Figs 53.5, 53.6 Pigmented villonodular synovitis of the knee: correlation of MRI with gross findings. (Courtesy of M. Forest MD.)

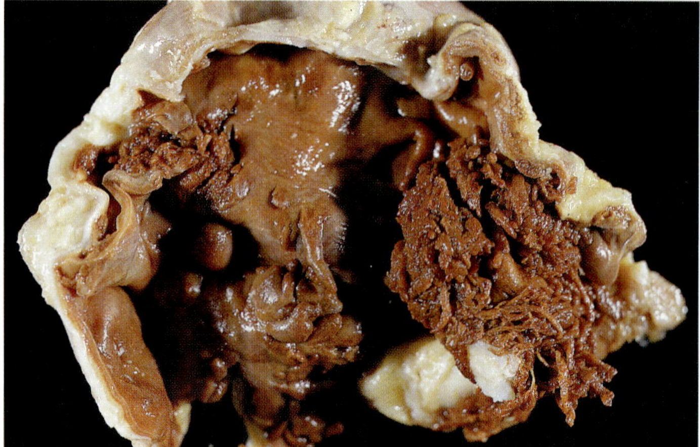

Fig. 53.7

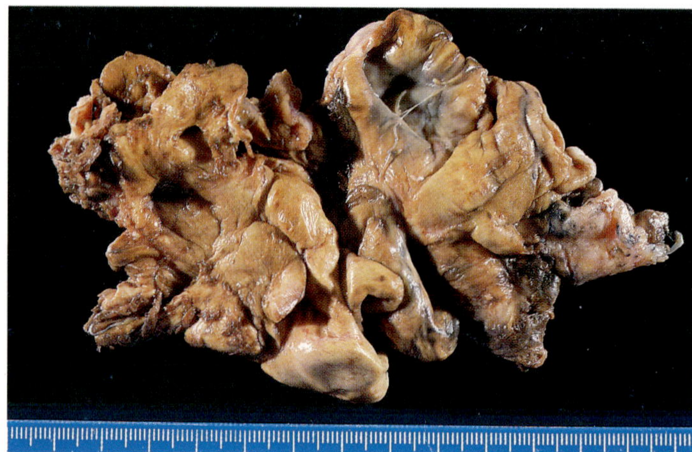

Fig. 53.8

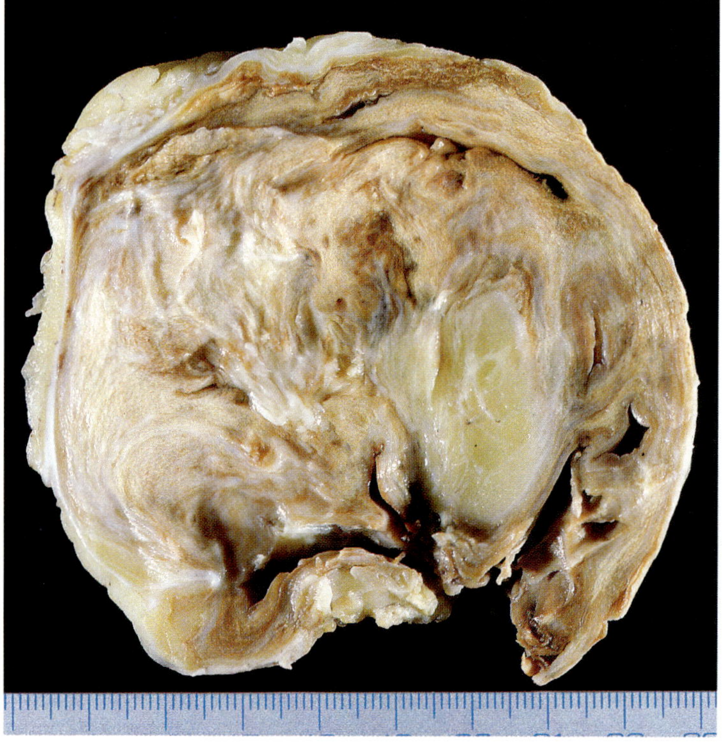

Fig. 53.9

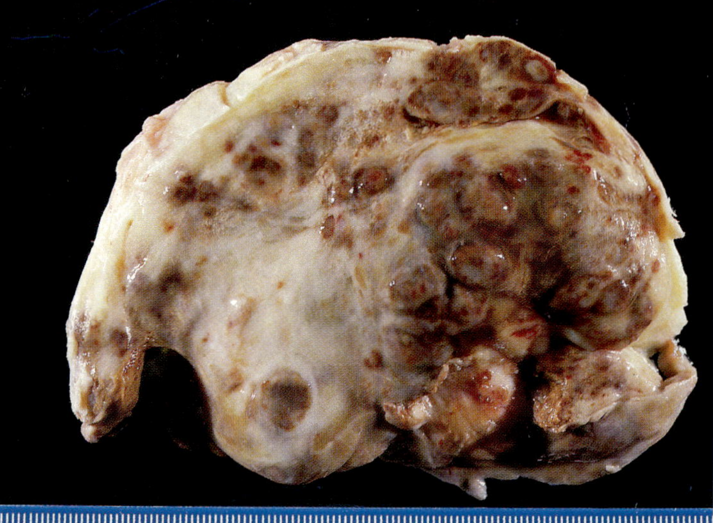

Fig. 53.10

Figs 53.7–53.10 Diffuse forms of pigmented villonodular synovitis of the knee. (Courtesy of M. Forest MD.)

a villous and nodular hyperplastic tissue. The nodules are sessile or pedunculated, often variegated, their color varying from one area to another according to iron and lipid content.

In aggressive forms, the tissue invades bone, through widening of the vascular foramins, articular capsule and even the surrounding soft parts, penetrating areas of lower resistance (Figs 53.11–53.27).

HISTOPATHOLOGY

In villous areás, the lesion is composed of thick synovial excrescences bulging into the articular cavity, where they often merge but are separated from one another by clefts lined by synovial cells (Figs 53.28, 53.29). Nodules form exophytic, usually well circumscribed, lobulated masses that are broadly attached to the synovium.

The lesion often exhibits a fibrous capsule from which collagenous septa divide vague nodules. This capsule is not always complete and the lesion merges into normal synovium or involves neighboring soft tissues, particularly fat and muscle, through the joint capsule.

The histological appearance varies considerably between different cases and, within the same lesion, from one area

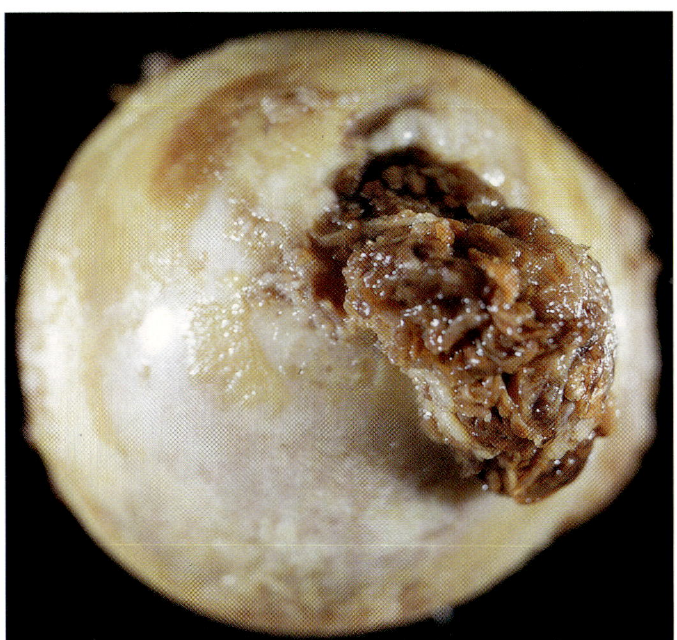

Fig. 53.11

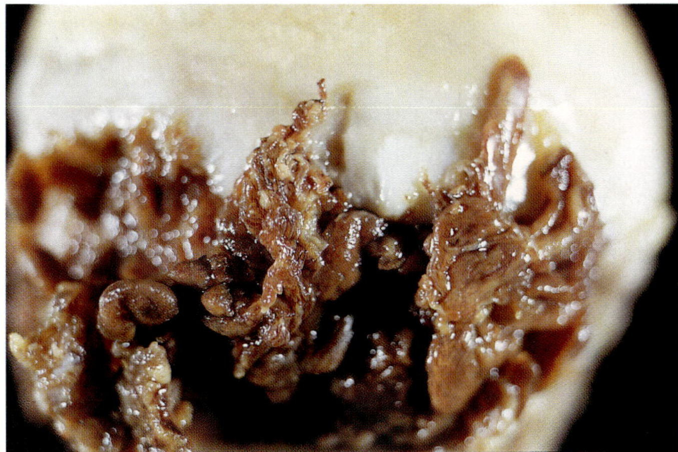

Fig. 53.12

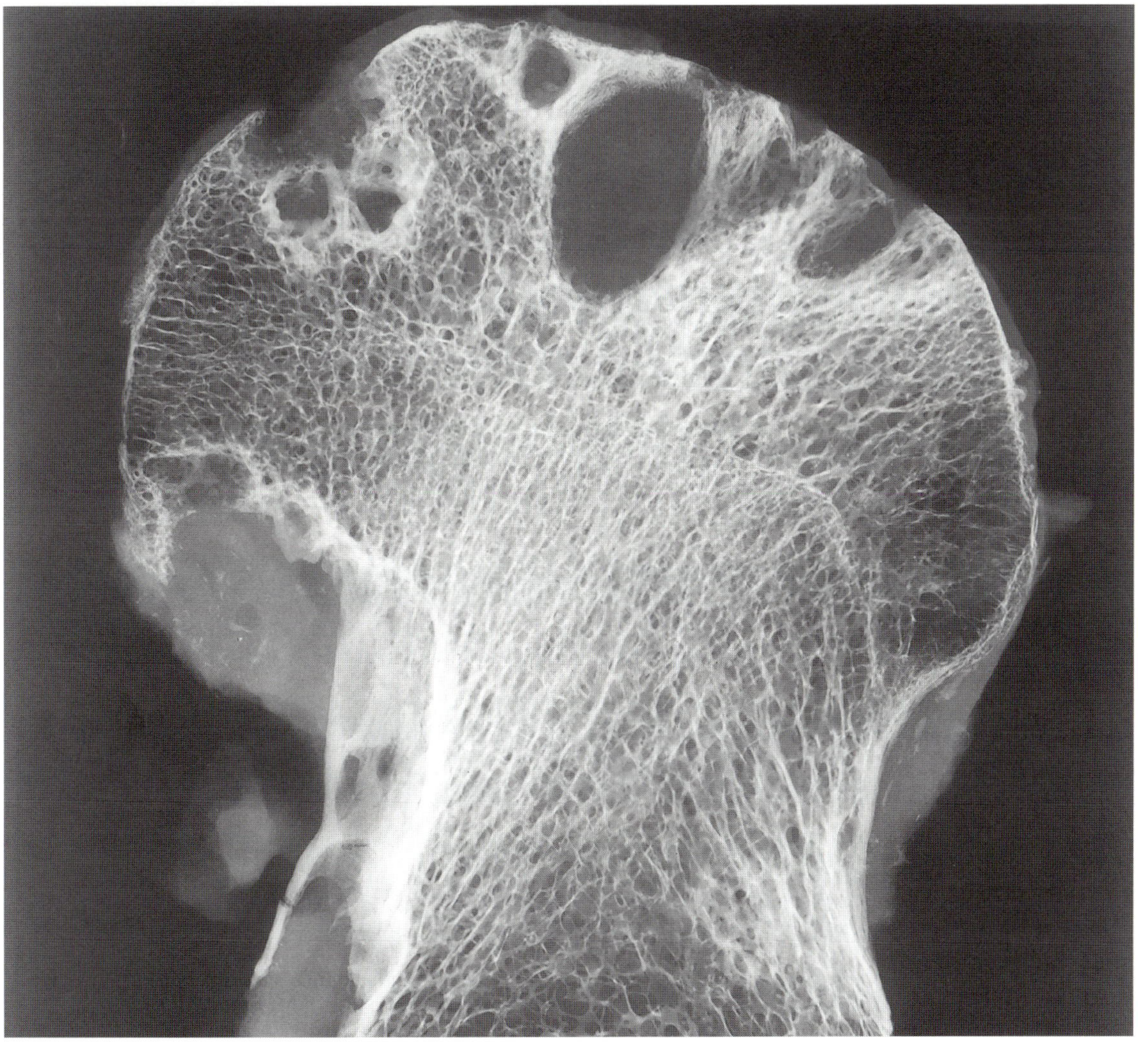

Fig. 53.13

Figs 53.11–53.14 Diffuse form of pigmented villonodular synovitis involving the hip joint. (Courtesy of M. Forest MD.)

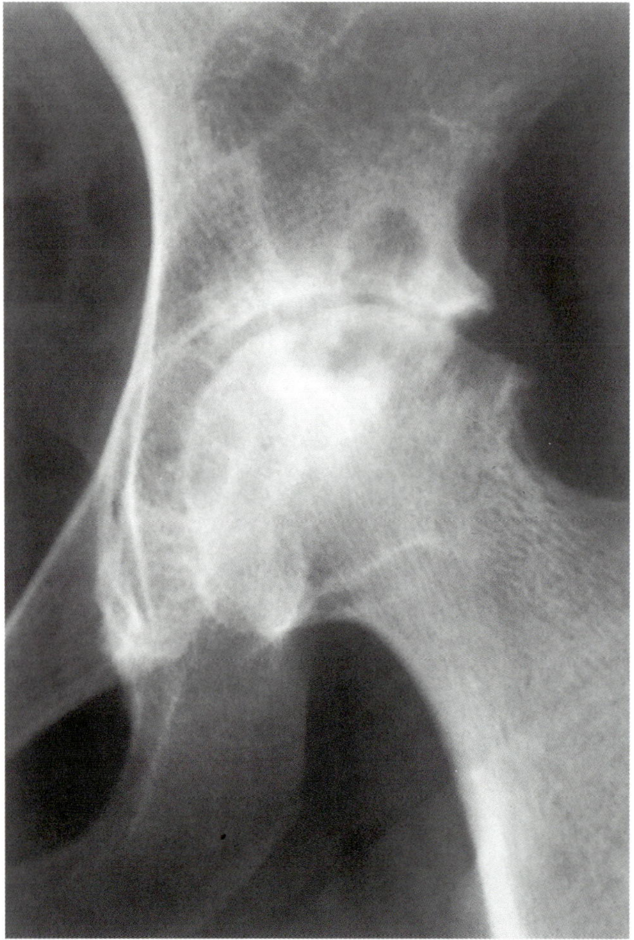

Fig. 53.14

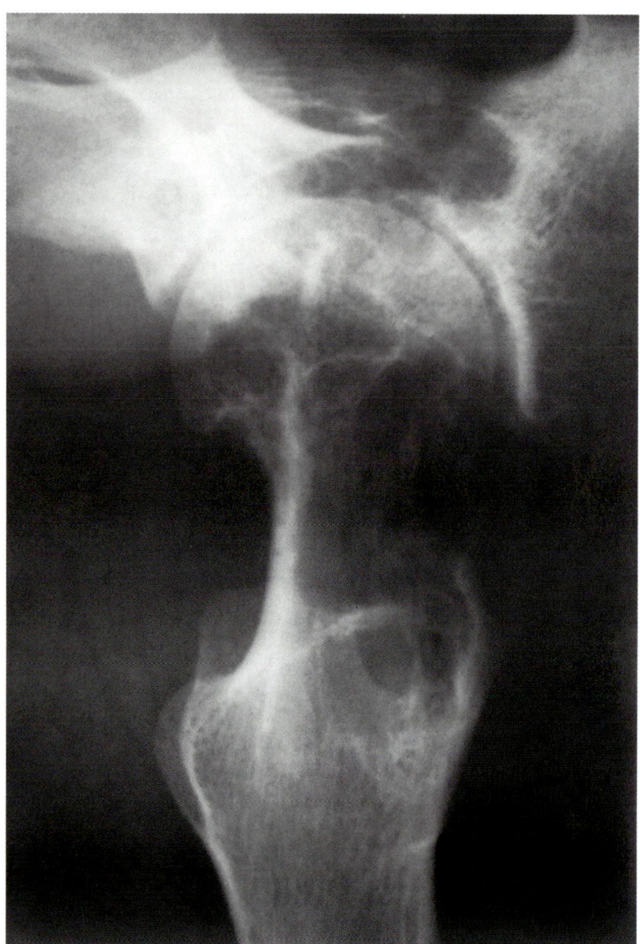

Fig. 53.15

to another. Appearance depends on the proportion of mononuclear cells, giant cells and xanthoma cells and the degree of collagenization (Figs 53.30–53.32). Hemosiderin pigmentation, also variable in different areas, is responsible for the brownish color of many lesions. When there are small amounts of hemosiderin, Perls' staining procedure can be helpful (Figs 53.33–53.35).

Most lesions contain an important mononuclear cell component, with round or polygonal elements that become spindle shaped in very fibrous areas. Cleftlike spaces may be seen, due either to recession of the joint space, lined by synovial cells, or to disintegration cavities caused by lack of cellular cohesion (Figs 53.36, 53.37).

Giant cells are a constant finding. Often numerous and randomly distributed, they may be less abundant in very cellular lesions, particularly in recurrences. These cells, formed by fusion of mononuclear cells, can exhibit many nuclei.

Foam or xanthomatous cells sometimes appear in great numbers in areas which appear grossly yellow or yellowish-white. Some of them show fine hemosiderin granules.

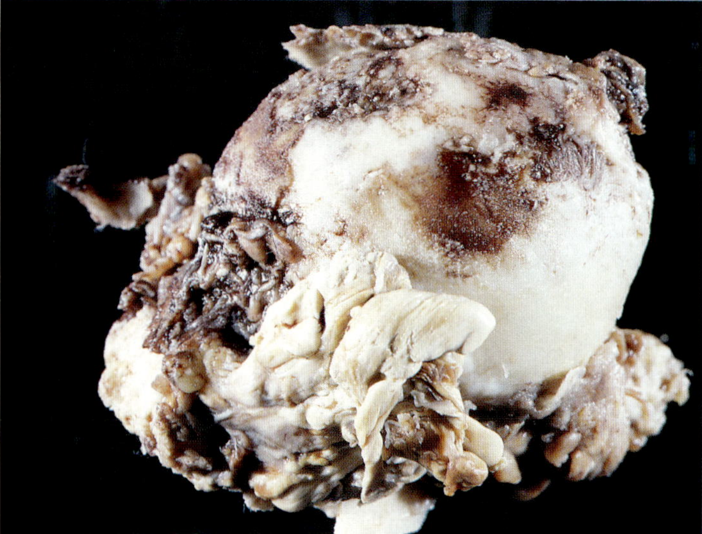

Fig. 53.16

Figs 53.15–53.18 Pigmented villonodular synovitis causing a massive erosion of the femoral neck. (Courtesy of M. Forest MD.)

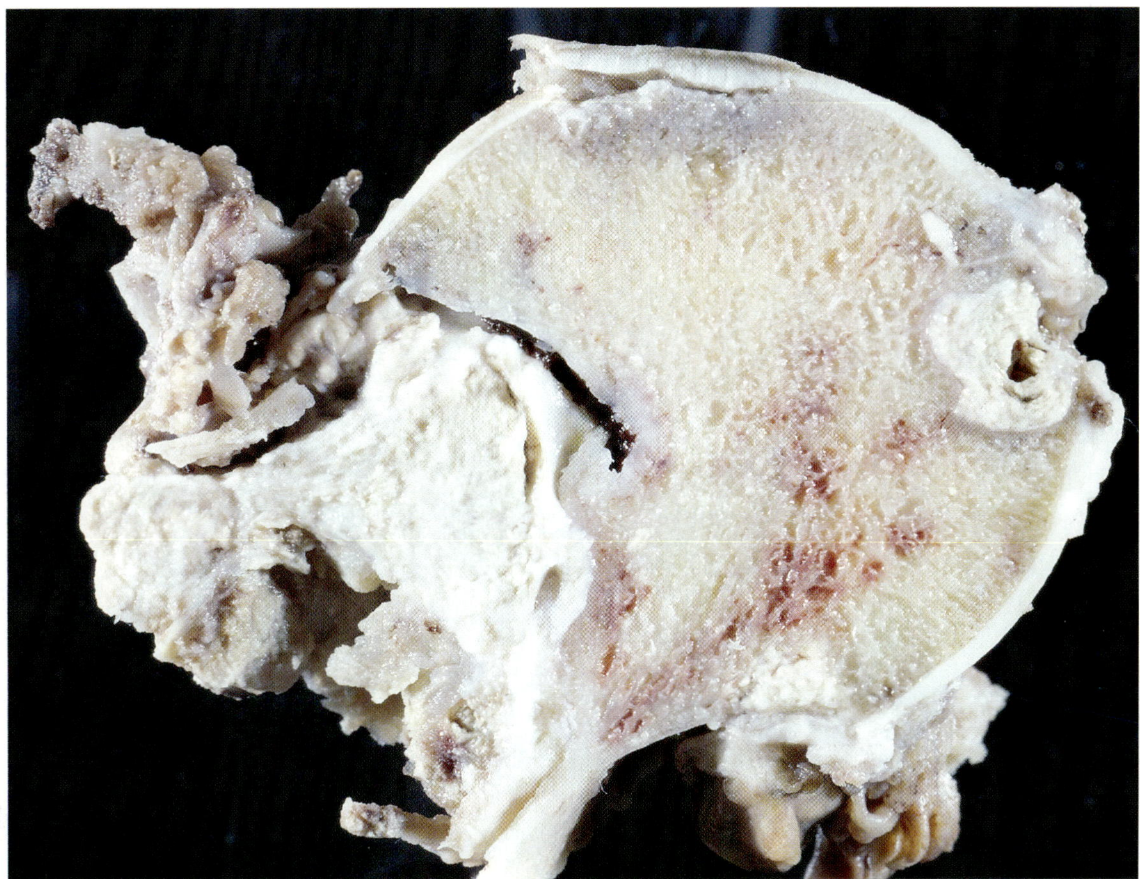

Fig. 53.17

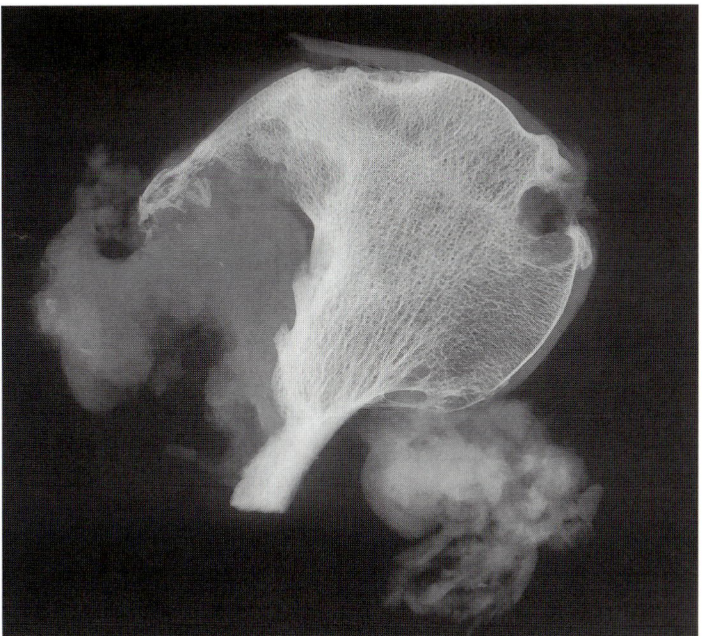

Fig. 53.18

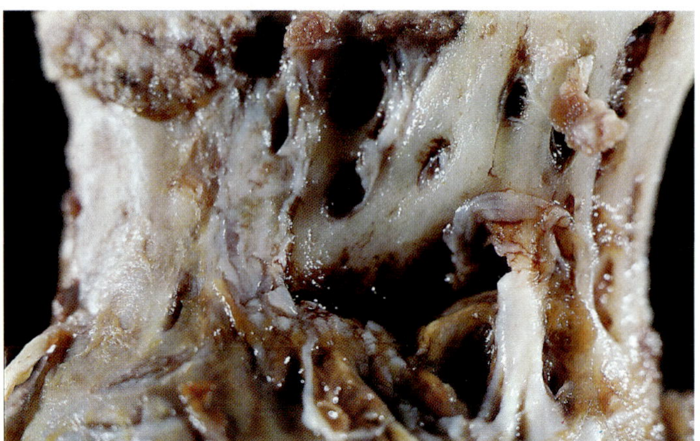

Fig. 53.19

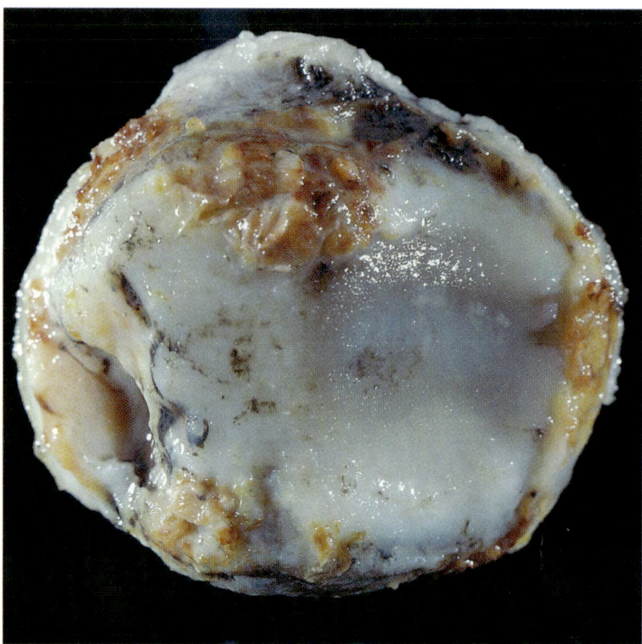

Fig. 53.21 Pigmented villonodular synovitis of the knee: involvement of the patella. (Courtesy of M. Forest MD.)

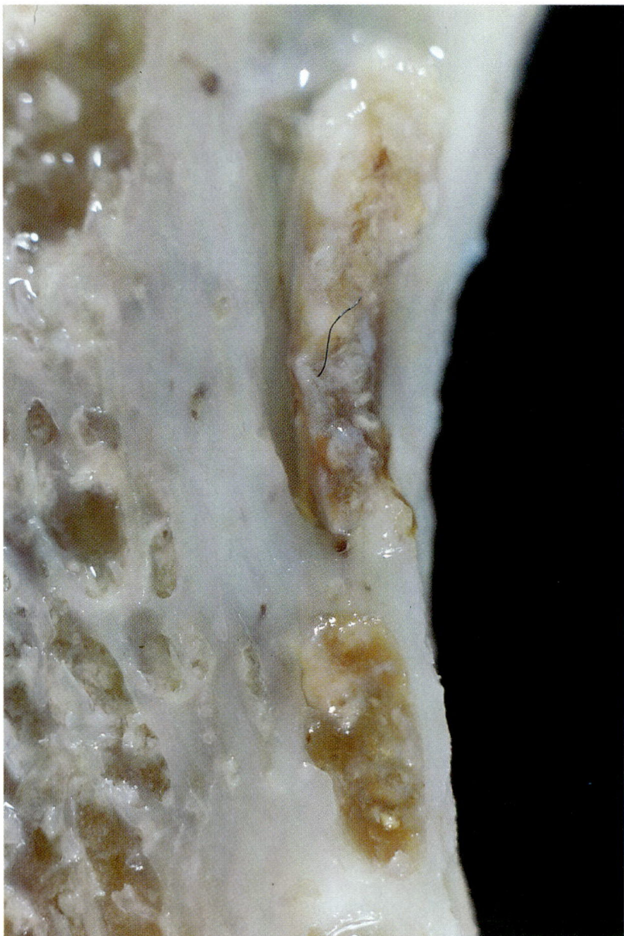

Fig. 53.20

Figs 53.19, 53.20 Pigmented villonodular synovitis of the hip extending to the femoral neck. (Courtesy of M. Forest MD.)

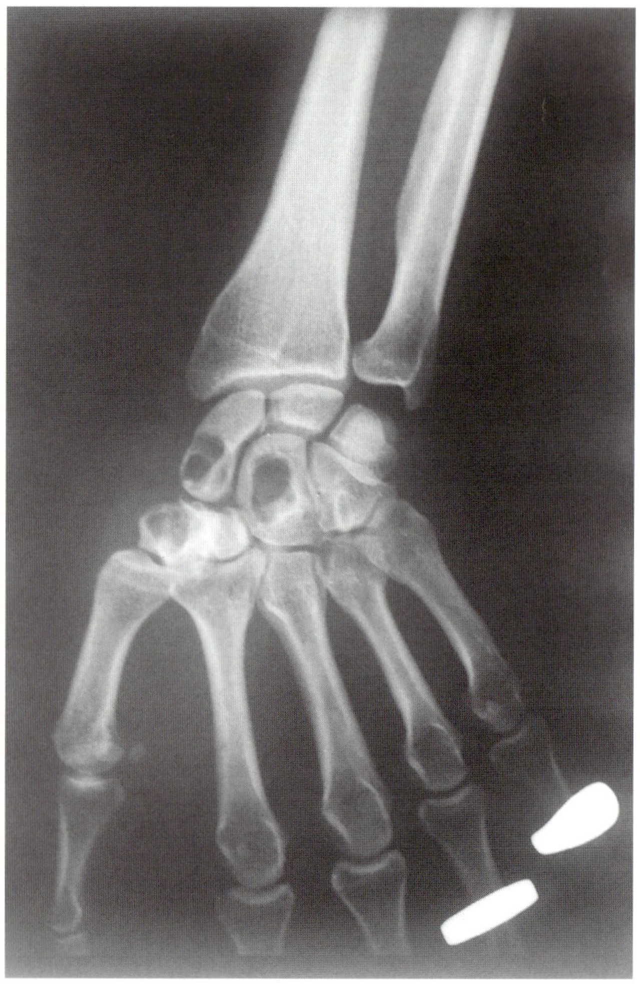

Fig. 53.22 Pigmented villonodular synovitis: involvement of carpal bones.

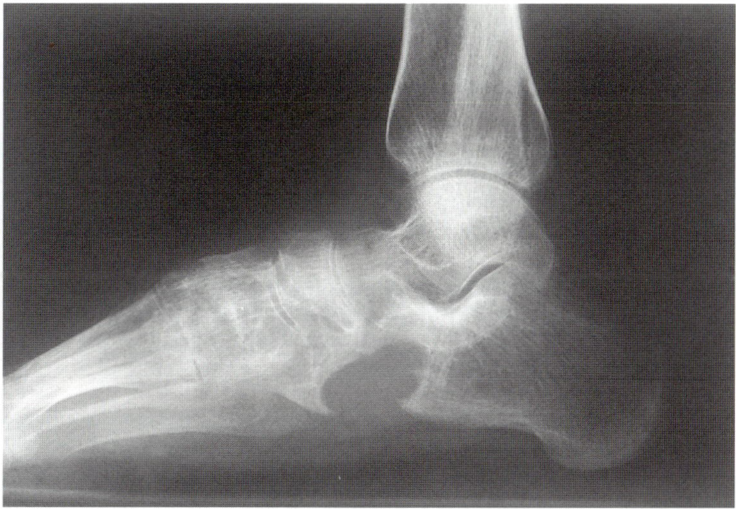

Fig. 53.23 Pigmented villonodular synovitis of the foot: involvement of the calcaneus and tarsal bones. (Courtesy of M. Forest MD.)

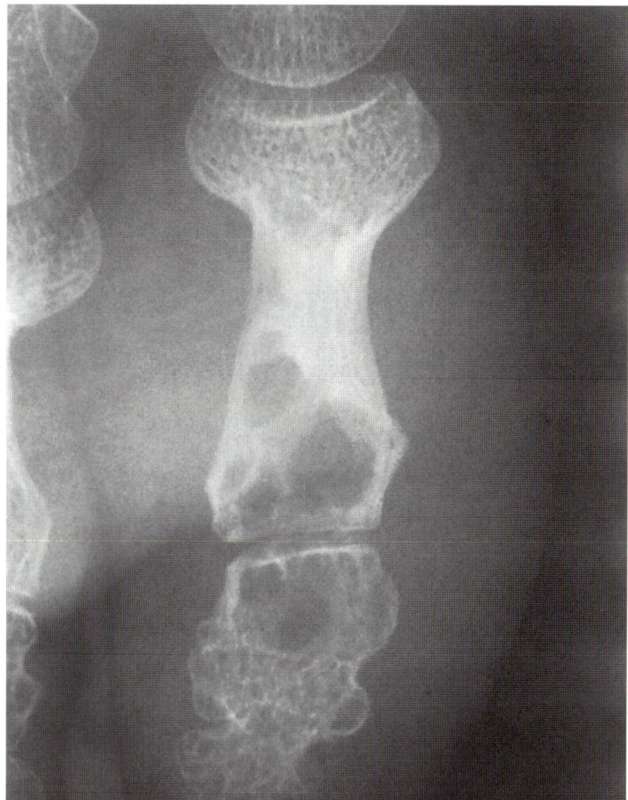

Fig. 53.25

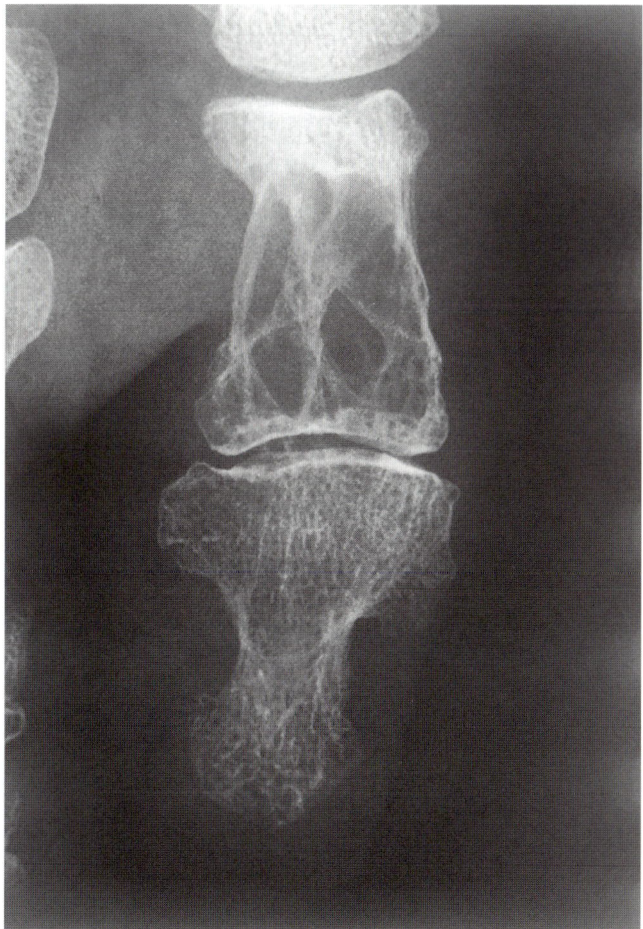

Fig. 53.24 Pigmented villonodular synovitis: involvement of the phalanx of a toe. (Courtesy of M. Forest MD.)

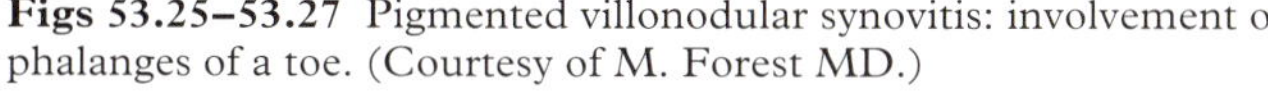

Figs 53.25–53.27 Pigmented villonodular synovitis: involvement of phalanges of a toe. (Courtesy of M. Forest MD.)

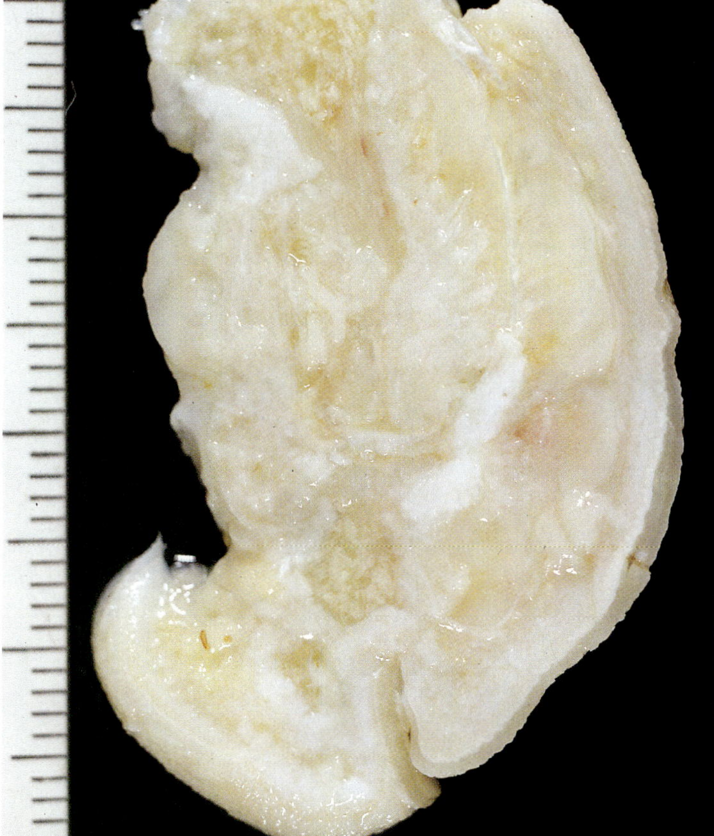

Fig. 53.26

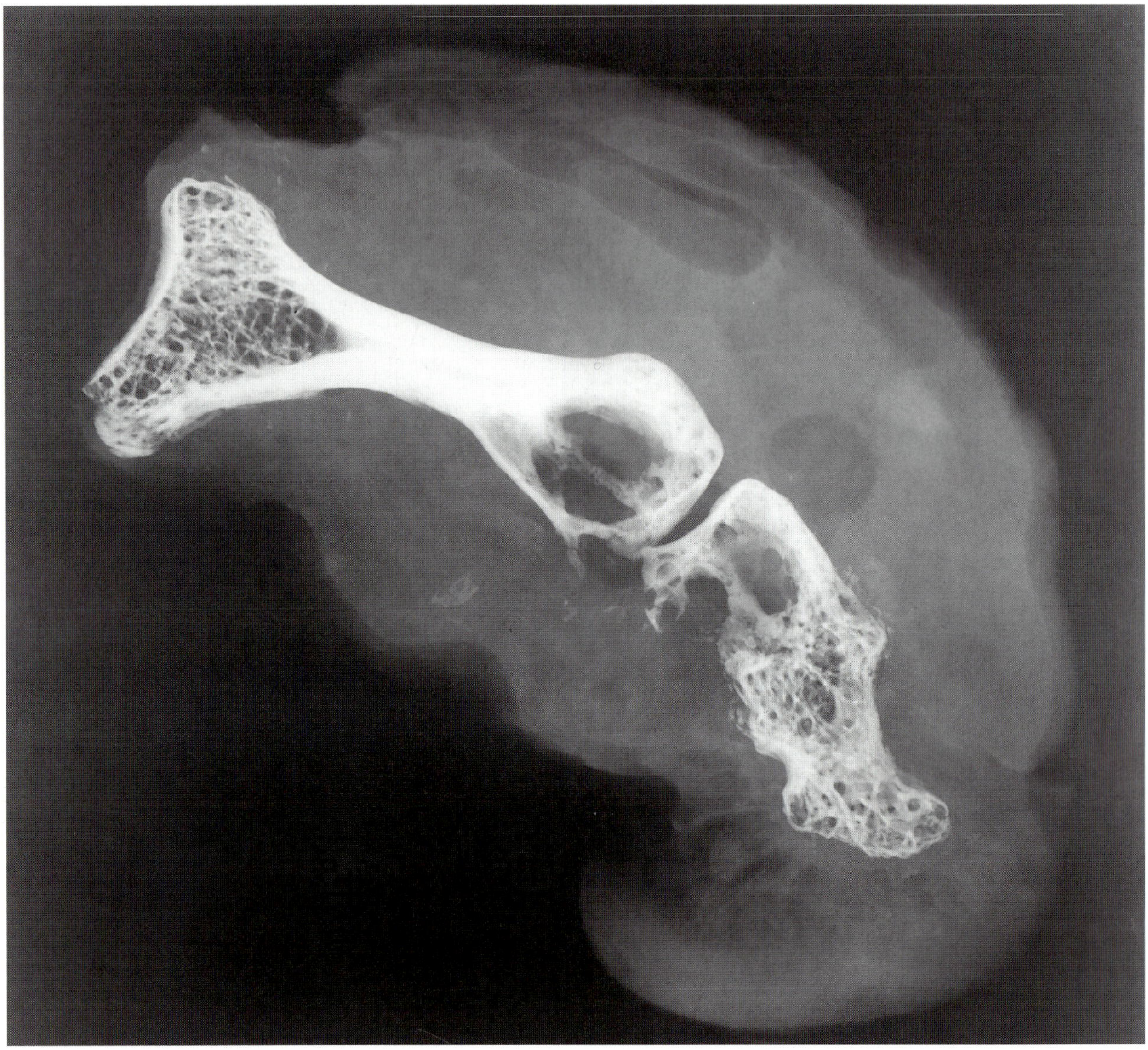

Fig. 53.27

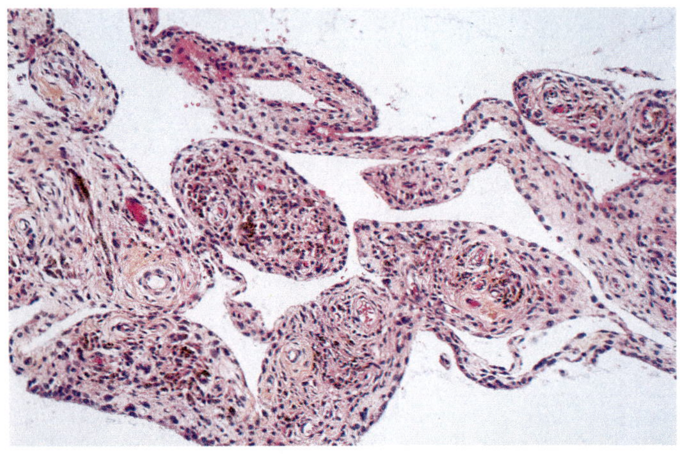

Fig. 53.28

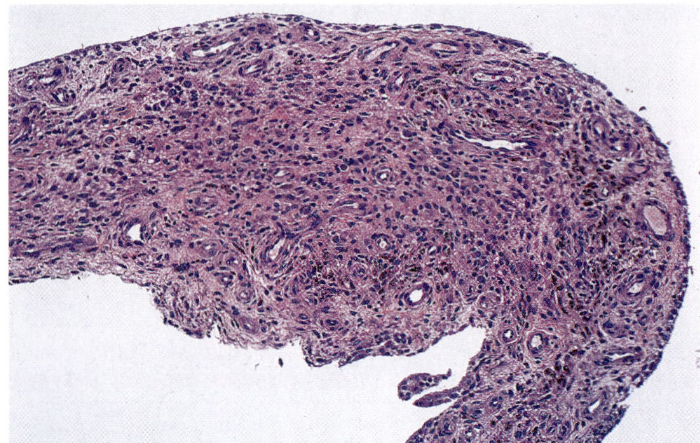

Fig. 53.29

Figs 53.28, 53.29 Villous areas of a pigmented villonodular synovitis of the knee. (Courtesy of M. Forest MD.)

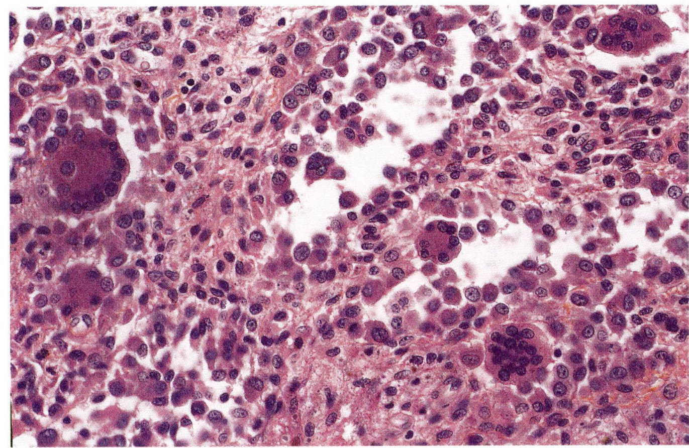

Fig. 53.30 Pigmented villonodular synovitis: mononuclear and giant cells. (Courtesy of M. Forest MD.)

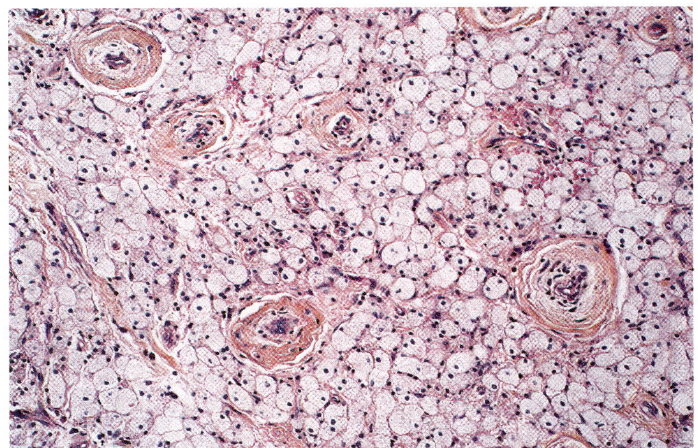

Fig. 53.31 Pigmented villonodular synovitis: xanthoma cells. (Courtesy of M. Forest MD.)

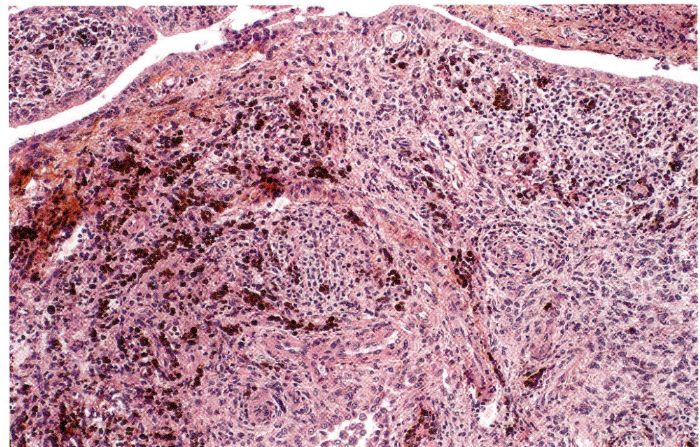

Fig. 53.32 Pigmented villonodular synovitis: hemosiderin deposits. (Courtesy of M. Forest MD.)

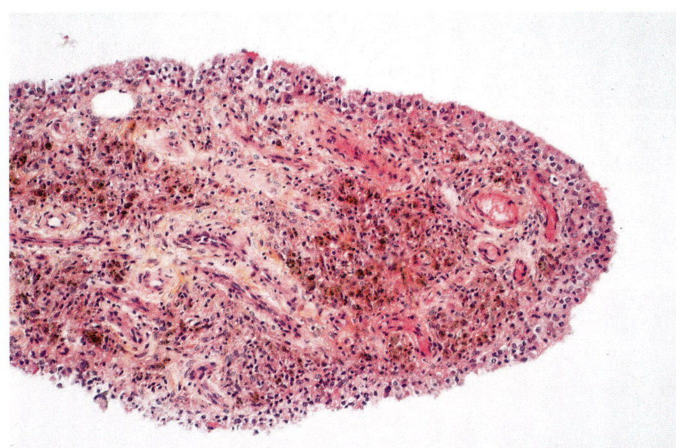

Fig. 53.33

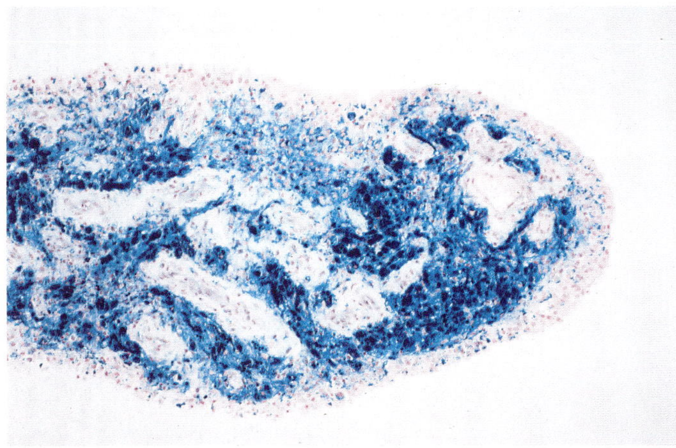

Fig. 53.34

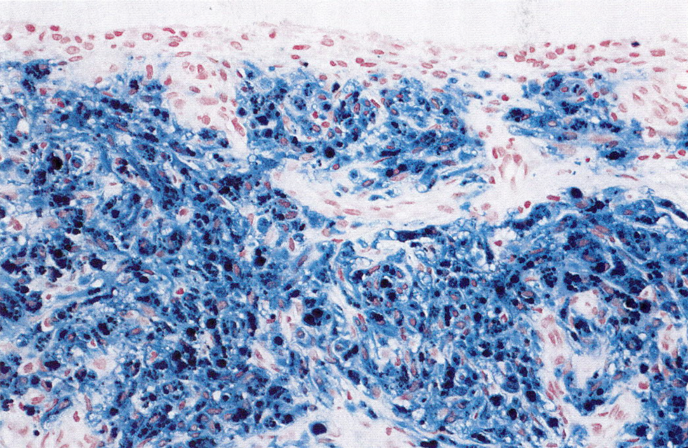

Fig. 53.35

Figs 53.33–53.35 Pigmented villonodular synovitis: Perls' stain. (Courtesy of M. Forest MD.)

Foci of osseous or cartilaginous metaplasia may be seen. A high mitotic rate suggests an actively growing lesion and may indicate recurrence.[6] In about 1–5% of cases tumoral embolus may be observed in small veins draining

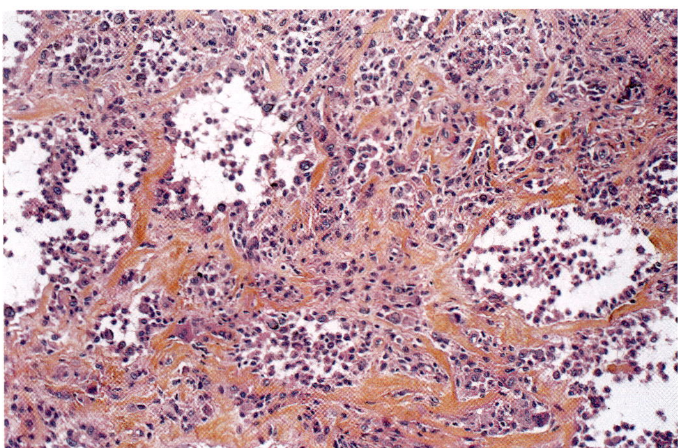

Fig. 53.36

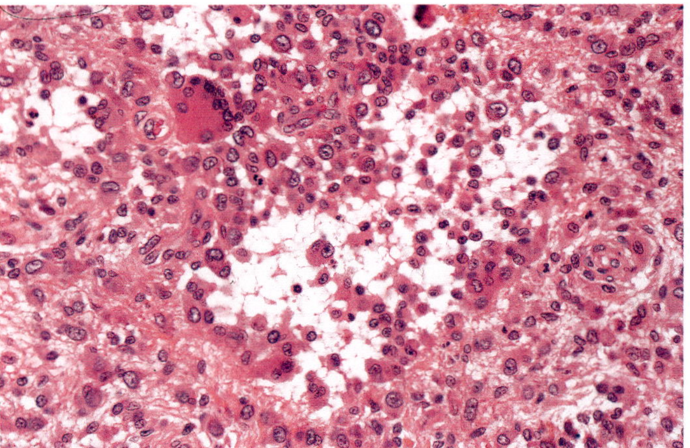

Fig. 53.37

Figs 53.36, 53.37 Pigmented villonodular synovitis: cleftlike spaces. (Courtesy of M. Forest MD.)

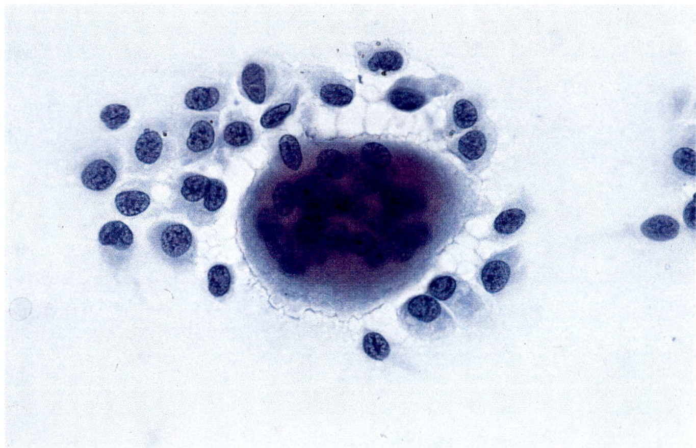

Fig. 53.38 Pigmented villonodular synovitis: mononuclear and giant cells on imprint material. (Courtesy of M. Forest MD.)

the lesion.[12] The finding of mitotic figures should not lead to the automatic assumption that the lesion is malignant.

Numerous pigmented villonodular lesions contain variable inflammatory infiltrates. Lymphocytes are the most common cellular type. Some lesions display collagenous sclerosis, probably due to their long duration. Other, usually nodular lesions are more or less necrotic, probably due to torsion of their pedicle. Diagnosis is usually possible, owing to the presence of giant cell outlines and small amounts of hemosiderin within areas of coagulation necrosis.

In aggressive forms which lead to bone erosions or infiltration into soft tissues, examination of specimens demonstrates lesional spread invading bone marrow spaces or muscle through the capsule. Locally aggressive behavior of some pigmented villonodular lesions may be explained by the presence of large amounts of metalloproteinases, collagenase and stromelysin, which can be the mediators of cartilage and bone tissue destruction.[13]

CYTOPATHOLOGY

Fine-needle aspiration may be helpful in diagnosing pigmented villonodular synovitis. Smears display giant and mononuclear cells in variable proportions, the association of which suggests the diagnosis. Anisokaryosis and mitotic figures are rare[14,15] (Fig. 53.38).

IMMUNOHISTOCHEMISTRY

Mononuclear cells express vimentin, lysozyme, α1-antitrypsin, α1-antichymotrypsin and CD68, all markers of histiomonocytic lineage. Giant cells react with the same antibodies, though expression of vimentin is inconstant.[16]

FLOW CYTOMETRY

Most of the cells are diploid in flow cytometry DNA studies. Among 25 cases of articular or tenosynovial pigmented villonodular synovitis studied by Abdul-Karim, three had an aneuploid population. One of these cases with anisokaryosis of the mononuclear and giant cells displayed signs of aggressive behavior and recurred 4 years after initial treatment. No malignant transformation was observed.[17]

CYTOGENETICS

A few studies have been performed which demonstrated variable single karyotypic abnormalities. The most frequent is a trisomy 5 and 7, the presence of which indicates the probable tumoral origin of the lesion. Fletcher has observed a trisomy 7 in 35% of metaphase cultured cells.[18,19]

COURSE

In most cases, pigmented villonodular synovitis is a benign

lesion, capable of local recurrence after treatment but unable to metastasize.

In localized forms, recurrences develop in 10–20% of the cases and seem to be more frequent in very cellular tumors with high mitotic rate. In diffuse forms, they are more frequent and may attain 40% of the cases in some series.[12] In recent reports, recurrences seem less frequent: 18–25%.[2,20]

Recurrence rate increases with follow-up data, some of them occurring very late. Thus the cumulative probability of recurrence for the knee increases from 15% at 5 years to 35% at 25 years.[20] In a case reported also in the knee, recurrence occurred 17 years after the initial excision.[21]

Some cases display a worse course,[22] such as a report with a late recurrence of pigmented villonodular synovitis of the knee accompanied by contralateral metastases in the thigh, which was composed of areas of fibroblastic and histiocytic proliferation displaying a high mitotic rate.[23] This was the same in the case reported by Enzinger, where a recurring pigmented villonodular synovitis of the foot was accompanied by pulmonary metastases.[12]

Cases of pigmented villonodular synovitis that may be considered malignant remain very exceptional and some reported as malignant pigmented villonodular synovitis are more likely to be soft tissue sarcomas with giant cells and do not exhibit the usual morphological features of pigmented villonodular synovitis.

TREATMENT

There are different possible treatments of pigmented villonodular synovitis:

- Synovectomy is the best treatment, done surgically or by arthroscopy. Surgical therapy allows excision of the synovial lesions and curettage of bone geodes. It may be followed by postoperative joint stiffness and does not prevent recurrences.[24] Arthroscopic synovectomy allows treatment of anterior lesions of the knee, subquadricipital space and condylar regions. It has a lower risk of joint stiffness than surgical synovectomy and may be repeated in cases of recurrence.
- Osmic acid or yttrium 90 synoviorthesis may be proposed first, but is most often complementary to surgical or arthroscopic synovectomy.
- Radiotherapy is seldom used. It should be kept for very aggressive forms, for which surgical therapy would imply severe functional sequelae or even amputation. It has also been used in particular vertebral locations or in recurrent lesions in elderly people.[25]
- Total arthroplasty is only used in very destructive forms, particularly of the hip. It gives excellent results but does not totally prevent recurrences. Its use should be exceptional in young patients.

Indications must take into consideration different para-meters such as location, diffuse or localized type and presence of a potentially aggressive component with tumoral extension into bone or soft tissues.

Nodular forms in tendon sheaths and intraarticular localized pigmented villonodular synovitis require surgical or arthroscopic excision. If the excision is adequate, there will usually be no need for complementary treatment. If the tumor is sessile and some tumoral residues persist in the synovium, complementary synoviorthesis may be considered.

Diffuse type of pigmented villonodular synovitis in the knee requires complete surgical or arthroscopic synovectomy.[24] Synoviorthesis using osmic acid or, in people older than 45 years, yttrium 90 may complete this intervention. The latter allows wide curettage of intraosseous lesions, if present. Arthroplasty should be reserved for severe bone lesions.

Therapeutic indications are similar in diffuse type pigmented villonodular synovitis of the hip.

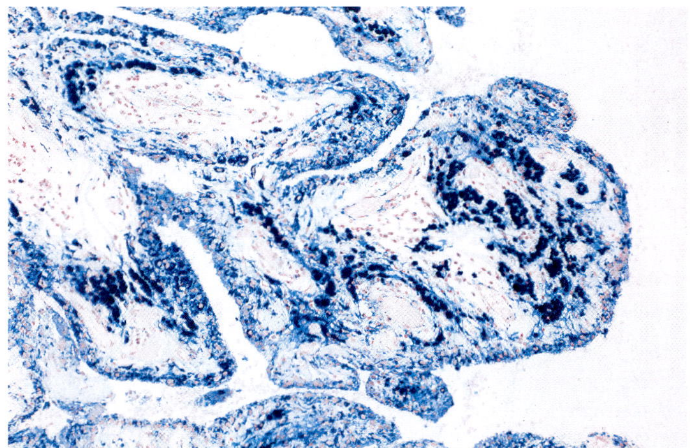

Fig. 53.39 Hemarthrosis of the knee joint: Perls' staining of the synovium. (Courtesy of M. Forest MD.)

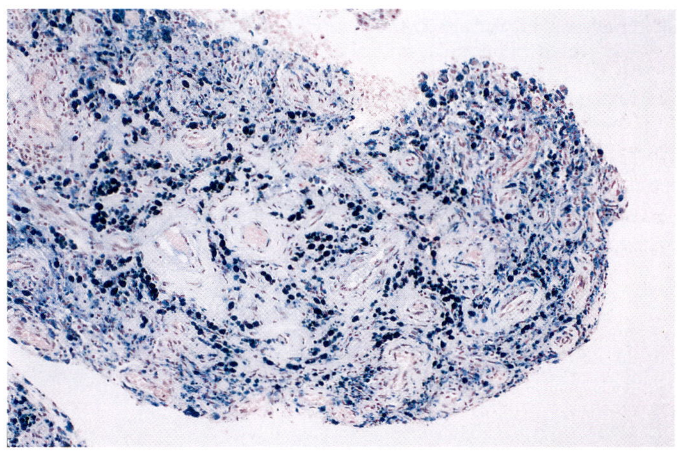

Fig. 53.40 Hemarthrosis of the knee joint (hemophilia): Perls' staining of the synovium. (Courtesy of M. Forest MD.)

DIFFERENTIAL DIAGNOSIS

The diagnosis may be difficult and the following must be borne in mind:

- Resorption of recurrent hemarthrosis, particularly in the course of hemophilia, gives rise to intense hyperplasia of the synovium with numerous long, thin, highly pigmented villi, but devoid of appreciable histiocytic proliferation (Figs 53.39, 53.40).
- Hemangioma also has a tumoral and pigmented aspect. Diagnosis is made on the vascular proliferation without histiocytic hyperplasia.[26]

- Detritic synovitis, due to resorption of prosthetic wear fragments, results in an important histiocytic and giant cell infiltration of the synovium, often hemosiderin pigmented. Presence of prosthetic debris, particularly under polarized light examination, suggests the diagnosis.

The remaining problem is that of malignant giant cell tumors. Except for some very rare and well-documented cases, every soft tissue tumor containing giant cells must be ruled out, such as clear cell sarcomas, fibrosarcomas, epithelioid sarcomas and chiefly malignant fibrous histiocytomas.

REFERENCES

1. Jaffe H L, Lichtenstein L, Sutro C J. Pigmented villonodular synovitis, bursitis and tenosynovitis. A discussion of the synovial and bursal equivalents of the tenosynovial lesion commonly denoted as xanthoma, xanthogranuloma, giant cell tumor or myeloplaxoma of the tendon sheath, with some consideration of this tendon sheath lesion itself. Arch Pathol 1941: 31: 731–765
2. Myers B W, Masi A T. Pigmented villonodular synovitis and tenosynovitis: a clinical, epidemiological study of 166 cases and literature review. Medicine (Balt) 1980: 59: 223–238
3. Soifer T, Guirguis S, Vigorita V J, Bryke E. Pigmented villonodular synovitis in a child. J Pediatr Surg 1993: 28: 1597–1600
4. Kang G H, Chi J G, Choi I H. Pigmented villonodular synovitis in the sacral joint with extensive bone destruction in a child. Pediatr Pathol 1992: 12: 725–730
5. Kay R M, Eckardt J J, Mirra J M. Multifocal pigmented villonodular synovitis in a child. A case report. Clin Orthop 1996: 322: 194–197
6. Rao A S, Vigorita V J. Pigmented villonodular synovitis (giant cell tumor of the tendon sheaths and synovial membrane). A review of eighty-one cases. J Bone Joint Surg (Am) 1984: 66: 76–94
7. Cotten A, Flipo R M, Chastanet P, Desvignes-Noulet M C, Duquesnoy B, Delcambre B. Pigmented villonodular synovitis of the hip: review of radiographic features in 58 patients. Skeletal Radiol 1995: 24: 1–6
8. Karnezis T A. Pigmented villonodular synovitis in a vertebra. A case report. J Bone Joint Surg (Am) 1990: 72: 927–930
9. Rosenthal D I, Aronow S, Murray W T. Iron content of pigmented villonodular synovitis detected by CT. Radiology 1979: 133: 409–411
10. Muscolo D L, Makino A, Costa-Paz M, Ayerza M A. Localized pigmented villonodular synovitis of the posterior compartment of the knee: diagnosis with magnetic resonance imaging. Arthroscopy 1995: 11: 482–485
11. Hughes T H, Sartoris D J, Schweitzer M E, Resnick D L. Pigmented villonodular synovitis: MRI characteristics. Skeletal Radiol 1995: 24: 7–12
12. Enzinger F M, Weiss S W. Soft tissue tumors. 3rd ed. St Louis: Mosby, 1995
13. Darling J M, Glimcher L H, Shortkroff S, Albano B, Gravalles E M. Expression of metalloproteinases in pigmented villonodular synovitis. Hum Pathol 1994: 25: 825–830
14. Wakely P E Jr, Frable W G. Fine-needle aspiration biopsy cytology of giant-cell tumor of tendon sheath. Am J Clin Pathol 1994: 102: 87–90
15. Gonzalez-Campora R, Herrero E S, Otal-Salaverri C et al. Diffuse tenosynovial giant cell of soft tissues: report of a case with cytologic and cytogenetic findings. Acta Cytol 1995: 39: 770–776
16. Jozsa L. Immunohistochemical characterization of pigmented villonodular synovitis. Zentralbl Pathol 1992: 138: 119–123
17. Abdul-Karim F W, El-Naggar A K, Joyce M J, Makley J T, Carter J R. Diffuse and localized tenosynovial giant cell tumor and pigmented villonodular synovitis. A clinicopathologic and flow cytometric DNA analysis. Hum Pathol 1992: 23: 729–735
18. Fletcher J A, Henkle C, Atkins L, Rosenberg A E, Morton C C. Trisomy-5 and trisomy-7 are non random aberrations in pigmented villonodular synovitis: confirmation of trisomy-7 in uncultured cells. Genes Chromosomes Cancer 1992: 4: 264–266
19. Mertens F, Orndal C, Mandahl N et al. Chromosome aberrations in tenosynovial giant cell tumors and nontumorous synovial tissue. Genes Chromosomes Cancer 1993: 6: 212–217
20. Schwartz H S, Unni K K, Pritchard D J. Pigmented villonodular synovitis. A retrospective review of the affected large joints. Clin Orthop 1989: 247: 243–255
21. Panagiotopoulos E, Tyllianakis M, Lambiris E, Siablis D. Recurrence of pigmented villonodular synovitis of the knee 17 years after the initial treatment. Clin Orthop 1993: 295: 179–182
22. Nielsen A L, Klaer T. Malignant giant cell tumor of synovium and locally destructive pigmented villonodular synovitis: ultrastructural and immunohistochemical study and review of the literature. Hum Pathol 1989: 20: 765–771
23. Choong P F, Willen H, Nilbert M et al. Pigmented villonodular synovitis. Monoclonality and metastasis. A case for neoplastic origin? Acta Scand Orthop 1995: 66: 64–68
24. Ogilvie-Harris D J, McLean J, Zarnett M E. Pigmented villonodular synovitis of the knee. The results of total arthroscopic synovectomy, partial arthroscopic synovectomy and arthroscopic local excision. J Bone Joint Surg (Am) 1992: 74: 119–123
25. O'Sullivan B, Cummings B, Catton B et al. Outcome following radiation treatment for high-risk pigmented villonodular synovitis. Int J Rad Oncol 1995: 32: 777–786
26. Devaney K, Vinh T N, Sweet D E. Synovial hemangioma. A report of 20 cases with differential diagnostic considerations. Hum Pathol 1993: 24: 737–745

54

Synovial chondromatosis

J. Amouroux

INTRODUCTION AND CLINICAL DATA

Synovial chondromatosis is a benign disease characterized by formation of multiple cartilaginous nodules in synovial tissue, which bulge into the joint space. They may become detached as intraarticular loose cartilaginous bodies.

The cartilage is frequently associated with osseous tissue, leading to the often used term of osteochondromatosis.

The pathogenesis remains unclear, possible hypotheses being a benign neoplasm or a metaplasia. It mostly follows a short course which sometimes spontaneously regresses.[1]

The disorder is rare in children, usually occurring in the third to fifth decades of life.[2] It is twice as frequent in males as in females.

Symptoms are usually mild and not very specific. Functional disturbance is as a rule minimal and late, with moderate pain, articular swelling due to joint effusion and limitation of motion. Locking of the joint is suggestive, but rare. Examination sometimes reveals the presence of loose bodies on palpation of the synovial recesses. After a course of several years, a painful functional disability may develop, due to secondary osteoarthritis.

SKELETAL DISTRIBUTION

Two-thirds of the cases of synovial chondromatosis affect the knee (Fig. 54.1). Other rather common sites are the hip and elbow (Fig. 54.2). More rarely, the disorder is located in the shoulder (Fig. 53.3), ankle, wrist or even small joints (Fig. 54.4) such as the acromioclavicular or temporomandibular joints. In the latter, association with pigmented villonodular synovitis may be found,[3,4] as well as in other locations (Figs 54.5, 54.6). There may be bilateral joint involvement in about 10% of the cases located in large joints. More diffuse forms are uncommon. Except for a case of bilateral location in the knee in two brothers,[5] no familial factor is known.

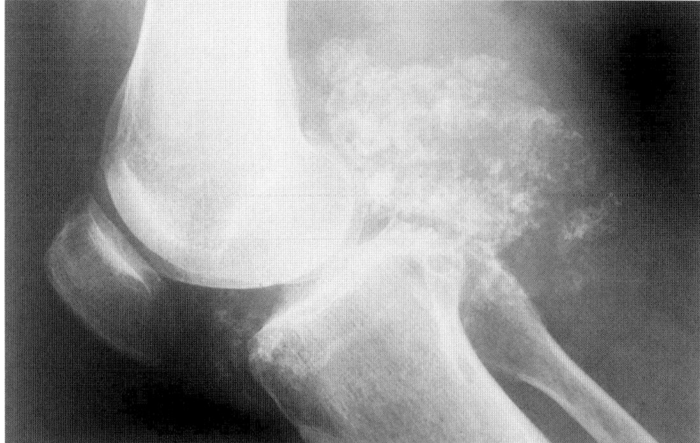

Fig. 54.1 Synovial chondromatosis of the knee joint. (Courtesy of M. Forest MD.)

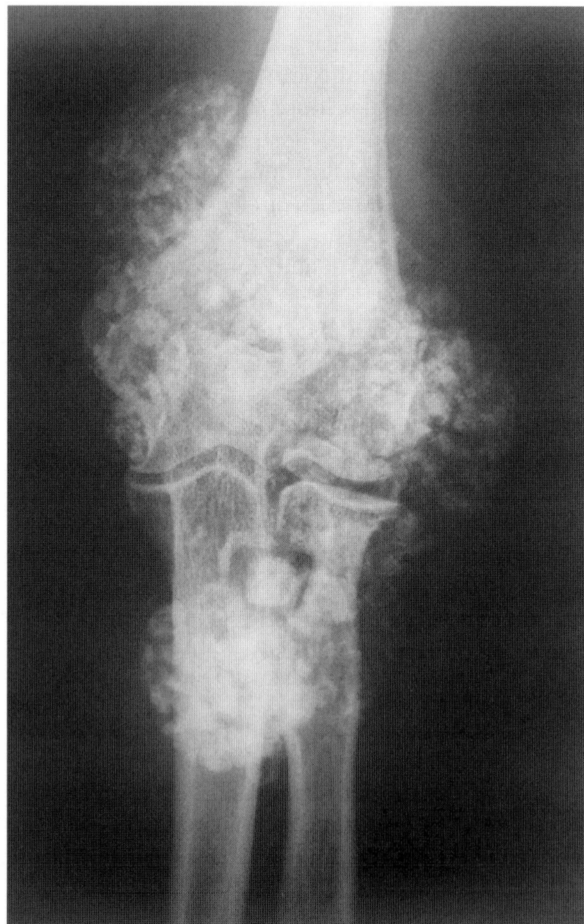

Fig. 54.2 Synovial chondromatosis of the elbow. (Courtesy of M. Forest MD.)

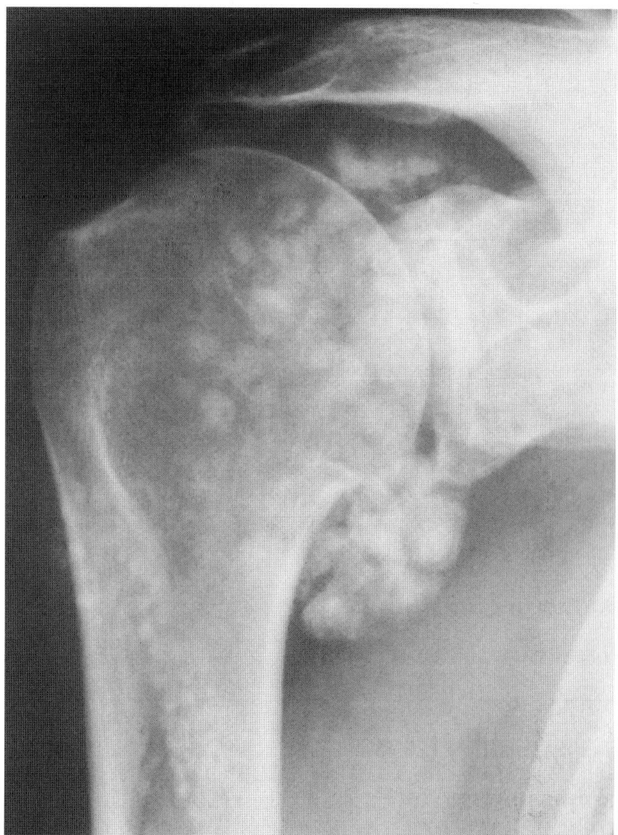

Fig. 54.3 Synovial chondromatosis of the shoulder. (Courtesy of M. Forest MD.)

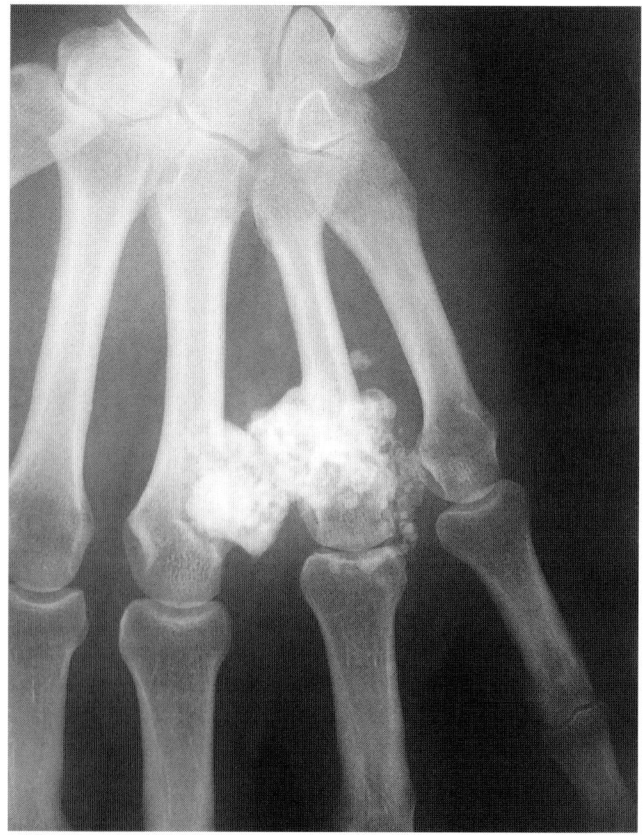

Fig. 54.4 Synovial chondromatosis of metacarpal joint. (Courtesy of M. Forest MD.)

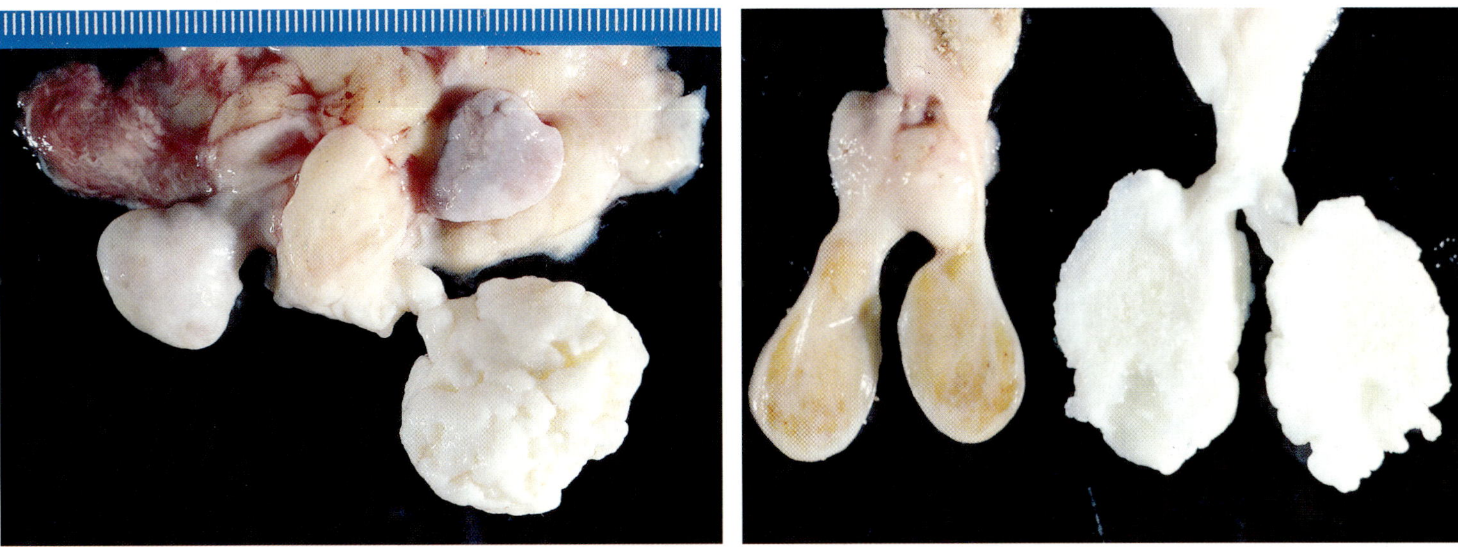

Fig. 54.5   **Fig. 54.6**

Figs 54.5, 54.6 Synovial chondromatosis of the knee associated with pigmented villonodular synovitis. (Courtesy of M. Forest MD.)

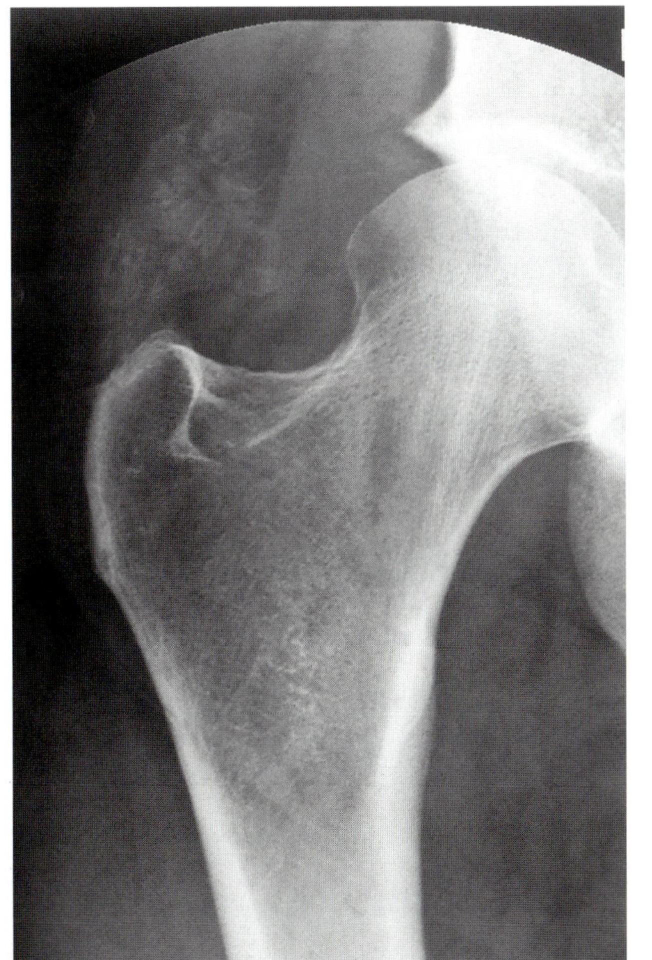

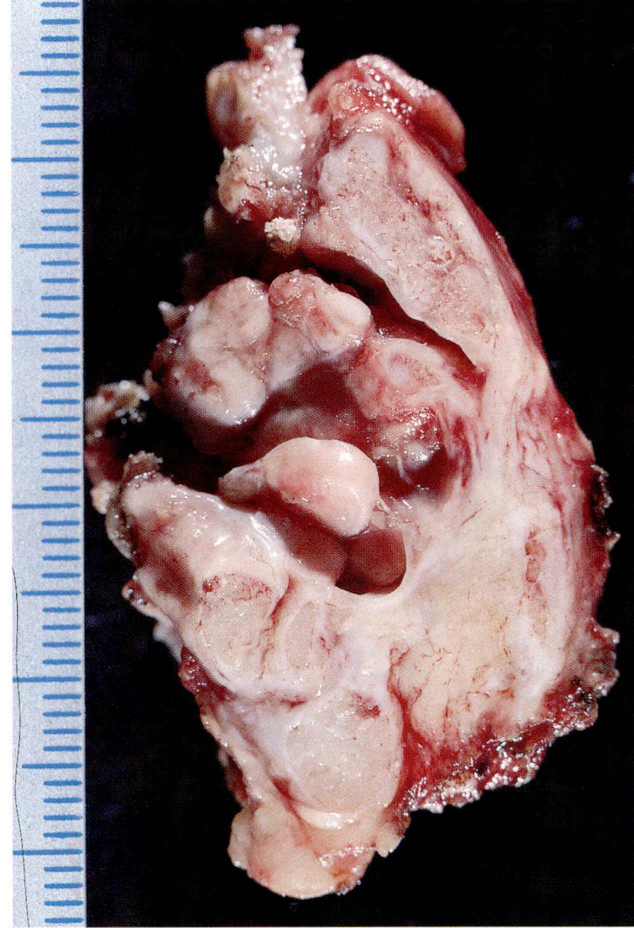

Fig. 54.7   **Fig. 54.8**

Figs 54.7, 54.8 Synovial chondromatosis located in a bursa of the hip. (Courtesy of M. Forest MD.)

Synovial chondromatosis may also develop in bursae and synovial tendon sheaths. It then results in juxtaarticular loose bodies (Figs 54.7, 54.8).

IMAGING

Usually radiography, demonstrating multiple osteocartilaginous loose bodies in a joint, allows an easy diagnosis. These are small radiopaque nodules, showing variable degrees of mineralization. The largest nodules are often limited by a dense peripheral line, whereas their centers are not very dense. Whole ossified loose bodies may display fine bony trabeculation.

Non-calcified and non-ossified loose bodies are revealed as filling defects by arthrography. CT scan, associated with arthrography if necessary, is helpful to locate loose intraarticular bodies and to demonstrate pressure bone erosions. The latter are mostly seen in the femoral neck (Fig. 54.9) and in the proximal end of humerus; they may be complicated by pathologic fractures.[6,7] In the late stages of the disorder, secondary osteoarthritic lesions may be found, with narrowing of the joint space, eburnation of the articular surfaces and osteophyte formation.

GROSS PATHOLOGY

Loose bodies are usually numerous (Figs 54.9–54.12), often over 1000. They range in size from 1 mm to 1 or 2 cm, are white, round or oval, sometimes polyhedral, mulberry-shaped or multilobar. They are sometimes free within the joint space, sometimes attached to the synovium by a thin pedicle. Others are embedded in the synovial membrane from which they form sessile bulges (Figs 54.13–54.18). The synovium may be massively affected by osteochondromatosis, but involvement is usu-

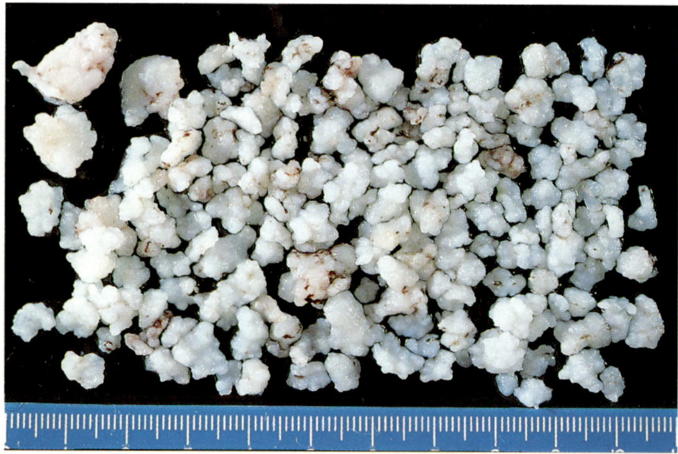

Fig. 54.10

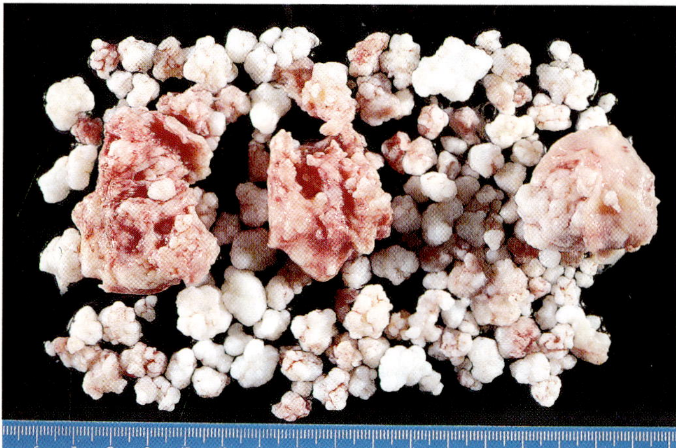

Fig. 54.11

Figs 54.10, 54.11 Synovial chondromatosis of the shoulder with recurrence. (Courtesy of M. Forest MD.)

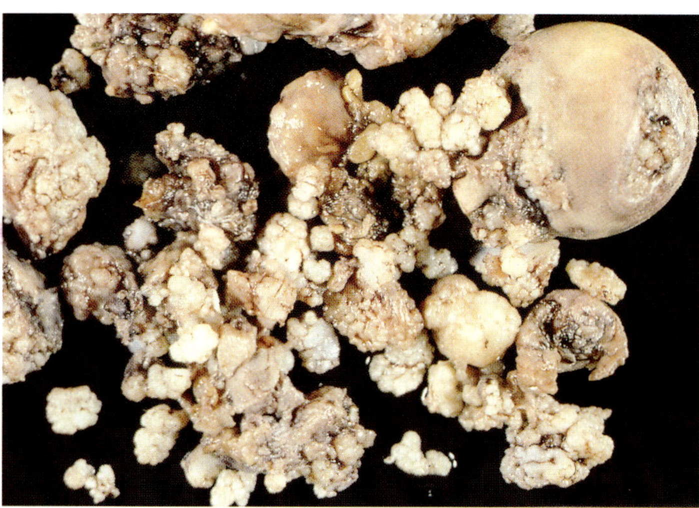

Fig. 54.9 Synovial chondromatosis of the hip joint.

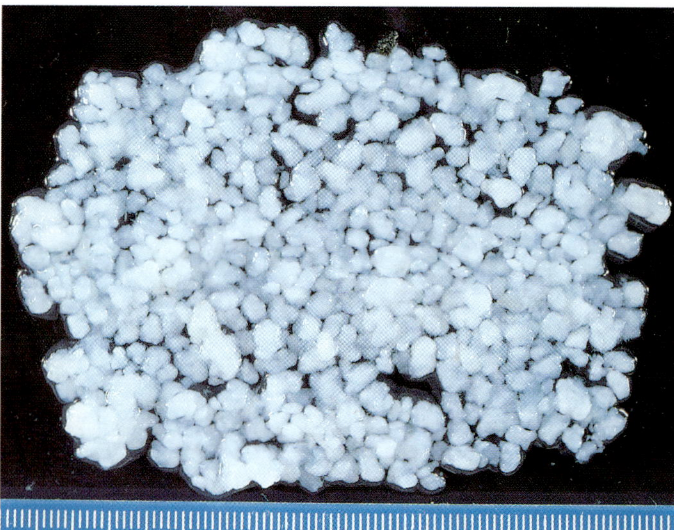

Fig. 54.12 So-called microchondromatosis of the knee joint. (Courtesy of M. Forest MD.)

Figs 54.13, 54.14 Synovial chondromatosis of the hip joint. (Courtesy of M. Forest MD.)

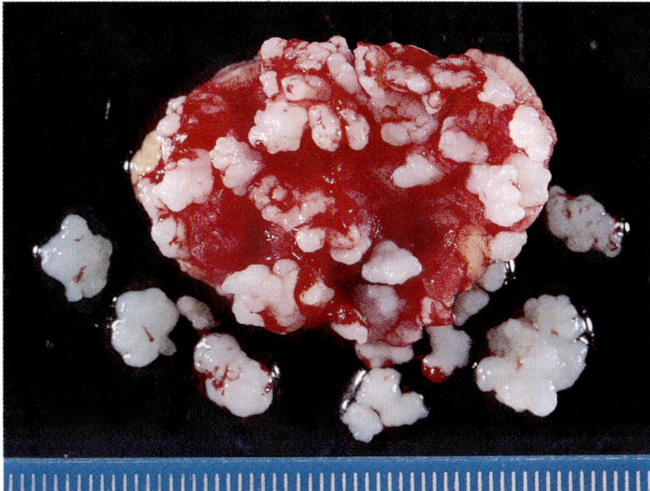

Fig. 54.13

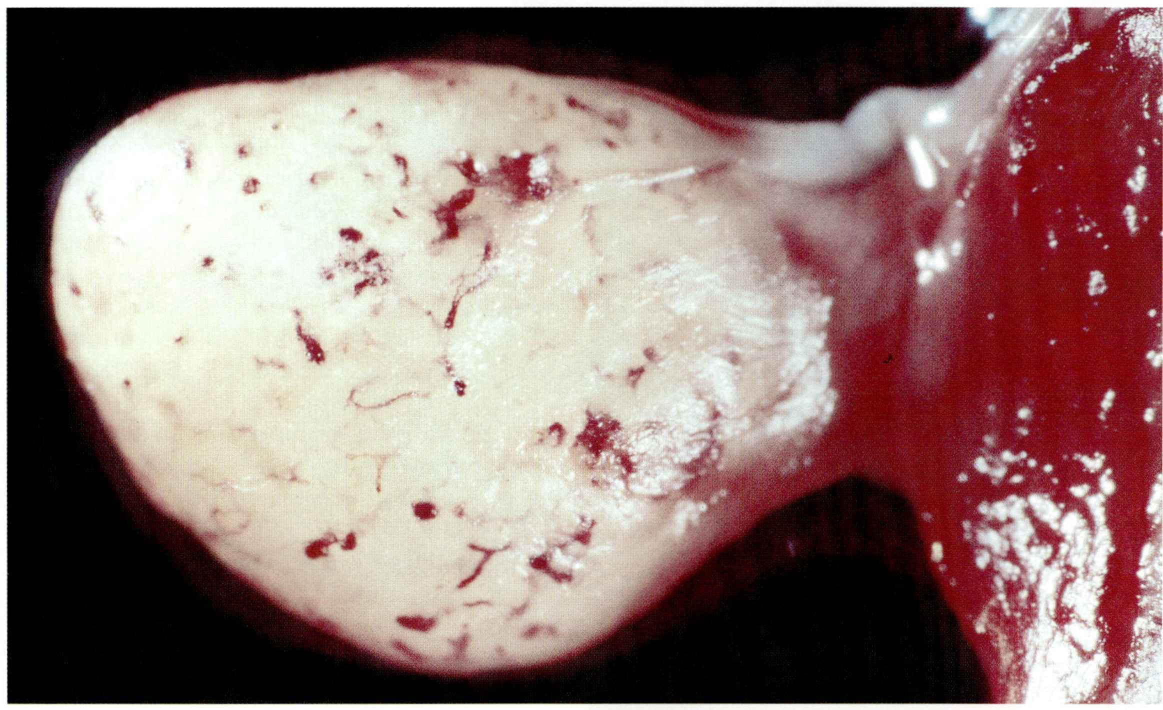

Fig. 54.14

ally confined to a small area.[8] The area of contact between synovium and cartilage is the surface usually affected.

HISTOPATHOLOGY

In the first stage of the disease small cartilaginous islands form within the subsynovial connective tissue (Fig. 54.19), without any lesion of the synovial cell lining. Ultrastructural studies have demonstrated a progressive transition between synovial fibrocytes and chondrocytes.[9] The cartilage is hyaline in type, rarely myxoid and may be altered by

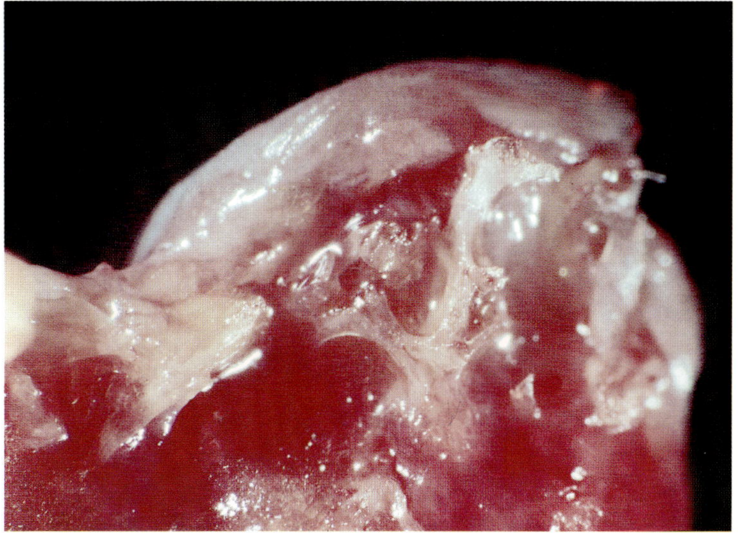

Fig. 54.15 Synovial chondromatosis of the hip joint: ossified nodule in the synovium. (Courtesy of M. Forest MD.)

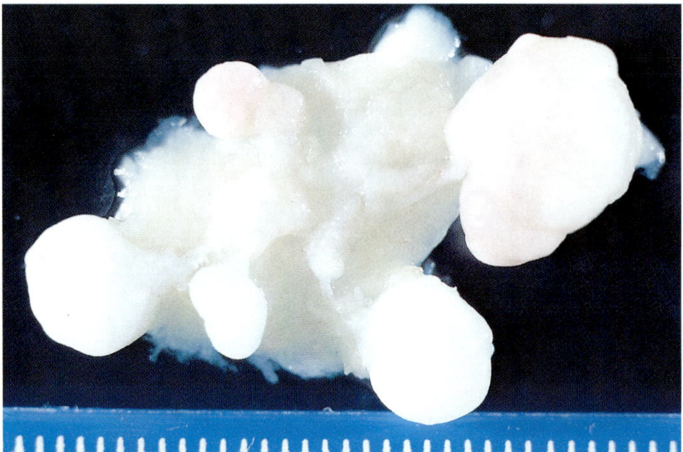

Fig. 54.16

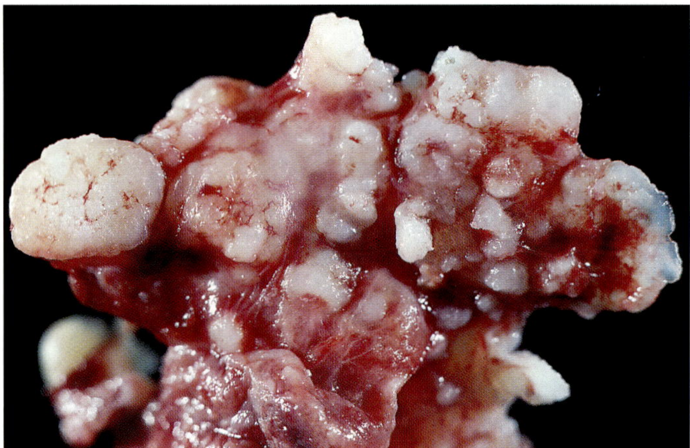

Fig. 54.17

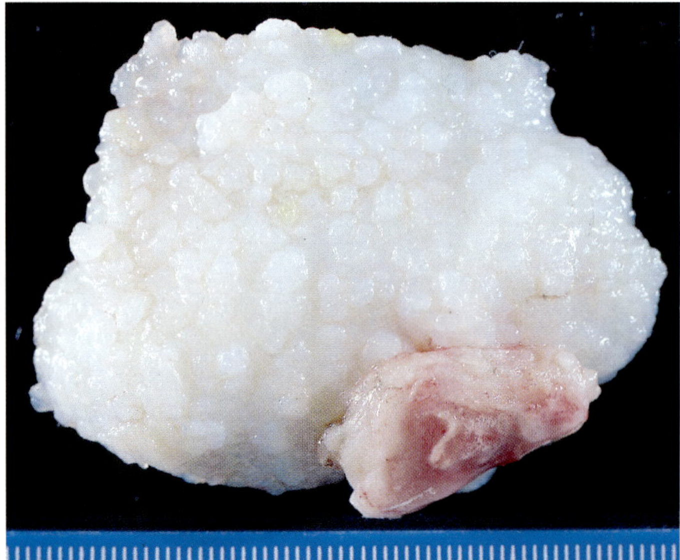

Fig. 54.18

Figs 54.16–54.18 Synovial chondromatosis of the knee joint. (Courtesy of M. Forest MD.)

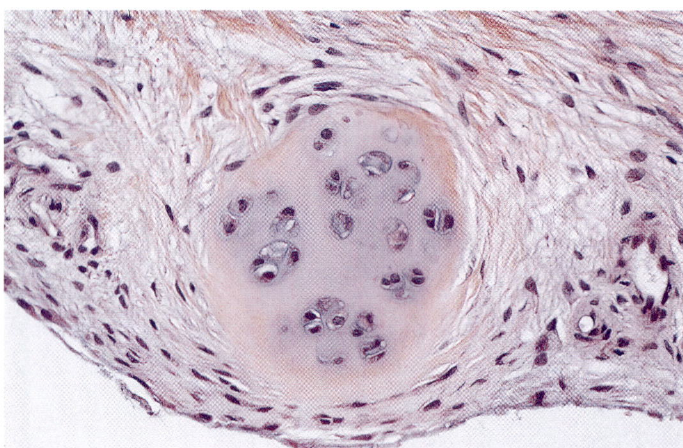

Fig. 54.19 Synovial chondromatosis: island of cartilage in the synovium. (Courtesy of M. Forest MD.)

calcification of its perilacunar matrix or, more often, by formation of fine osseous trabeculae (Figs 54.20–54.22). The latter are separated from each other by fatty, sometimes hematopoietic marrow. As a rule, loose bodies are purely cartilaginous. On the other hand, osteocartilaginous or osseous nodules require a vascular supply and are usually pedunculated. When they become detached, osseous tissue and marrow become necrotic, whereas loose cartilaginous bodies may continue to grow, as they are fed by synovial fluid (Fig. 54.23). Pedunculated loose bodies are covered with a fine layer of synovial tissue.

Chondrocytes, arranged in small clusters, are large and, in about two-thirds of cases, display a more or less atypical aspect, with irregular nuclei and binucleate cells[10] (Figs 54.24–54.27). These features are sometimes worrying enough to cause differential diagnostic problems with chondrosarcoma.[11]

COURSE

Synovial chondromatosis seems to progress in three steps:

1. multifocal cartilage metaplasia of subsynovial tissue;
2. growth, pedunculation of nodules and release of some as loose bodies;
3. resorption of some cartilaginous foci by synovial tissue which progressively resumes its normal morphologic features, whereas remodeling of loose bodies occurs.[12]

Another pathogenetic hypothesis has been proposed: fragments of cartilage could become detached by trauma, minor or otherwise, grow within the synovial fluid and possibly be taken up by the synovium.[13] This theory may explain synovial chondromatosis secondary to osteoarthritis but is not suitable for young patients with no traumatic history.

Most authors agree with the first hypothesis and all admit that the course of the disease does not exceed 5–10 years.

In the course of synovial chondromatosis, alteration of

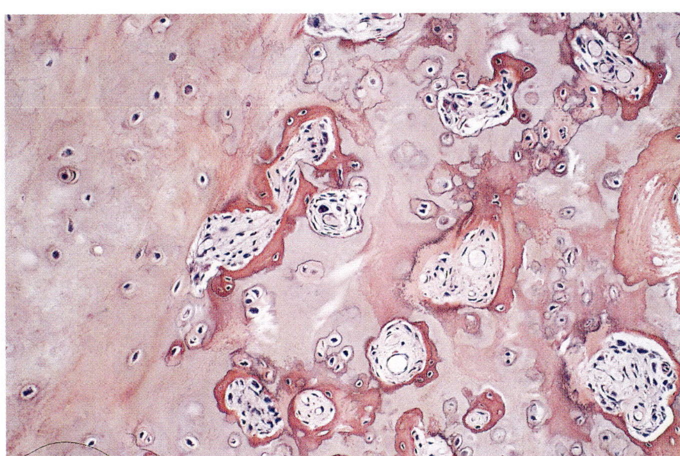

Fig. 54.20

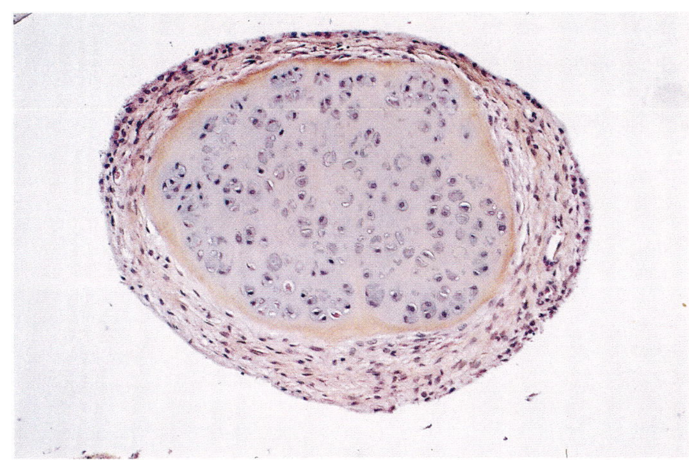

Fig. 54.23 Synovial chondromatosis: loose body covered by a synovial lining. (Courtesy of M. Forest MD.)

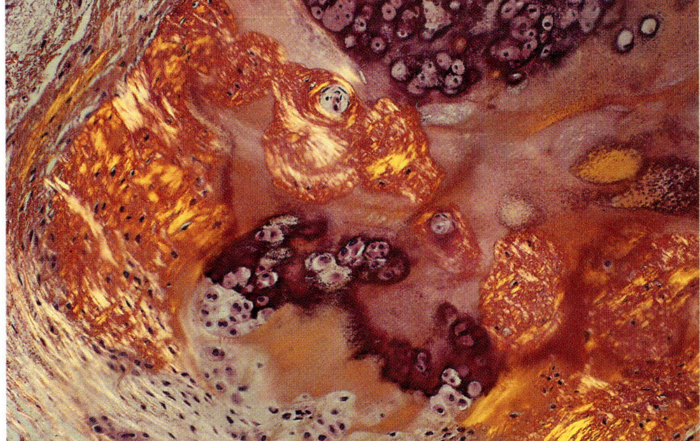

Fig. 54.21

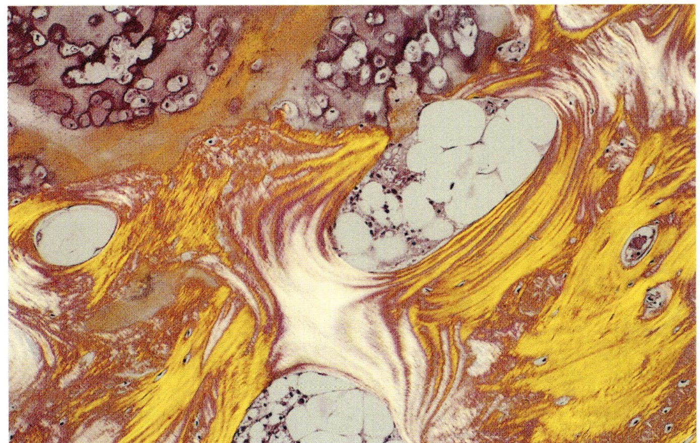

Fig. 54.22

Figs 54.20–54.22 Synovial chondromatosis: areas of calcification and ossification (Figs 54.21, 54.22: polarized light). (Courtesy of M. Forest MD.)

articular surfaces by hard intraarticular loose bodies often develops. It results in secondary osteoarthritis responsible for definitive functional disturbances.

A rare but severe complication is the occurrence of a synovial chondrosarcoma in the course of synovial chondromatosis. Synovial chondrosarcoma is a very rare tumor, with less than 30 reported cases. Half of the patients have a past history of synovial chondromatosis. A male predominance is found in two-thirds of the cases. The age of onset ranges from 28 to 70.

Symptomatology is limited to pain and swelling which have usually been present for several years. In two patients a synovial biopsy, done 24 and 25 years before, revealed synovial chondromatosis.[14,15] The usual site is the knee, but others have been reported, such as hip, elbow and ankle.

Radiographs disclose calcified loose bodies in a joint but especially in the periarticular soft parts.[16] Bone erosions may also be seen.[11]

Gross pathological aspects look like those of synovial chondromatosis, but are different because they extend into soft tissue or bone.[14,17]

Cartilage is usually more edematous than in synovial chondromatosis. Cartilaginous lobules are much more cellular and the most peripheral cells of each nodule are more spindle shaped than chondrocyte-like.[11] Chondrocytes are not arranged in islands but form large sheets often dissociated by myxoid changes. The histoprognostic grading system for intraosseous chondrosarcomas is used: tumors are classified in three grades.

The course resembles that of intraosseous chondrosarcomas with frequent occurrence of lung metastases.

TREATMENT

Therapeutic abstention is authorized as long as synovial chondromatosis remains asymptomatic. In symptomatic forms, excision of loose bodies is necessary and may be complemented by synovectomy. Arthroscopy is preferred to arthrotomy as it is less often followed by postoperative

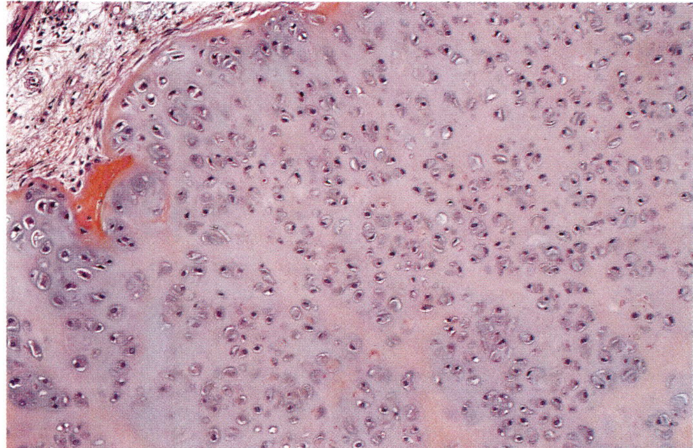

Fig. 54.24

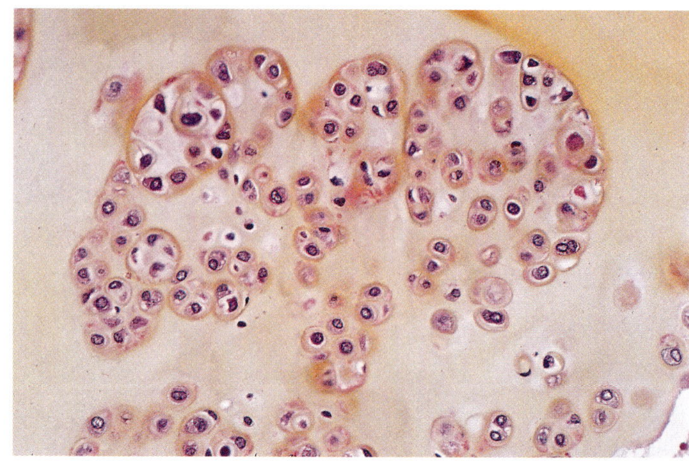

Fig. 54.26

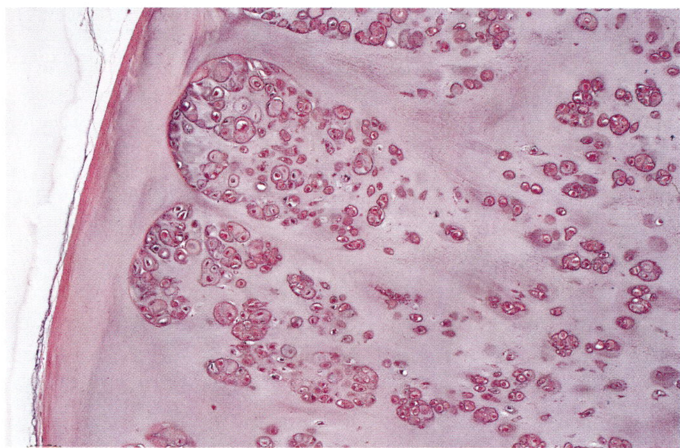

Fig. 54.25

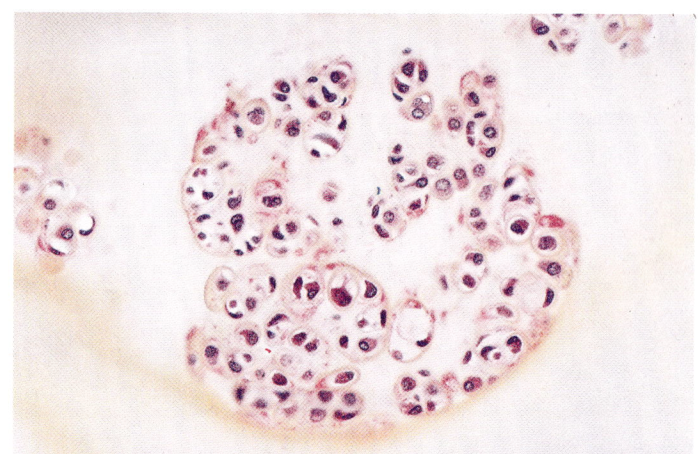

Fig. 54.27

Figs 54.24–54.27 Synovial chondromatosis of the knee: high cellularity and chondrocytes with plump nuclei distributed in clusters. (Courtesy of M. Forest MD.)

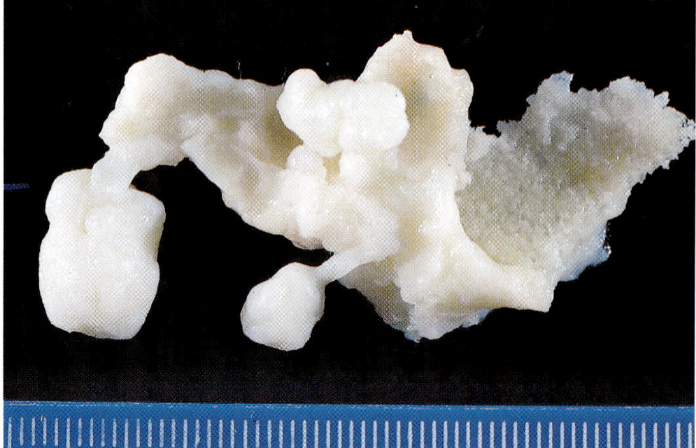

Fig. 54.28 Synovium of the knee with pedunculated nodules (osteoarthritis). (Courtesy of M. Forest MD.)

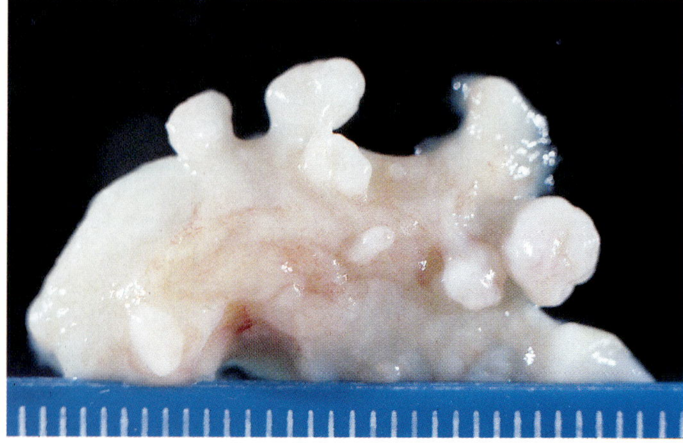

Fig. 54.29 Synovium of the elbow with pedunculated nodules (osteoarthritis). (Courtesy of M. Forest MD.)

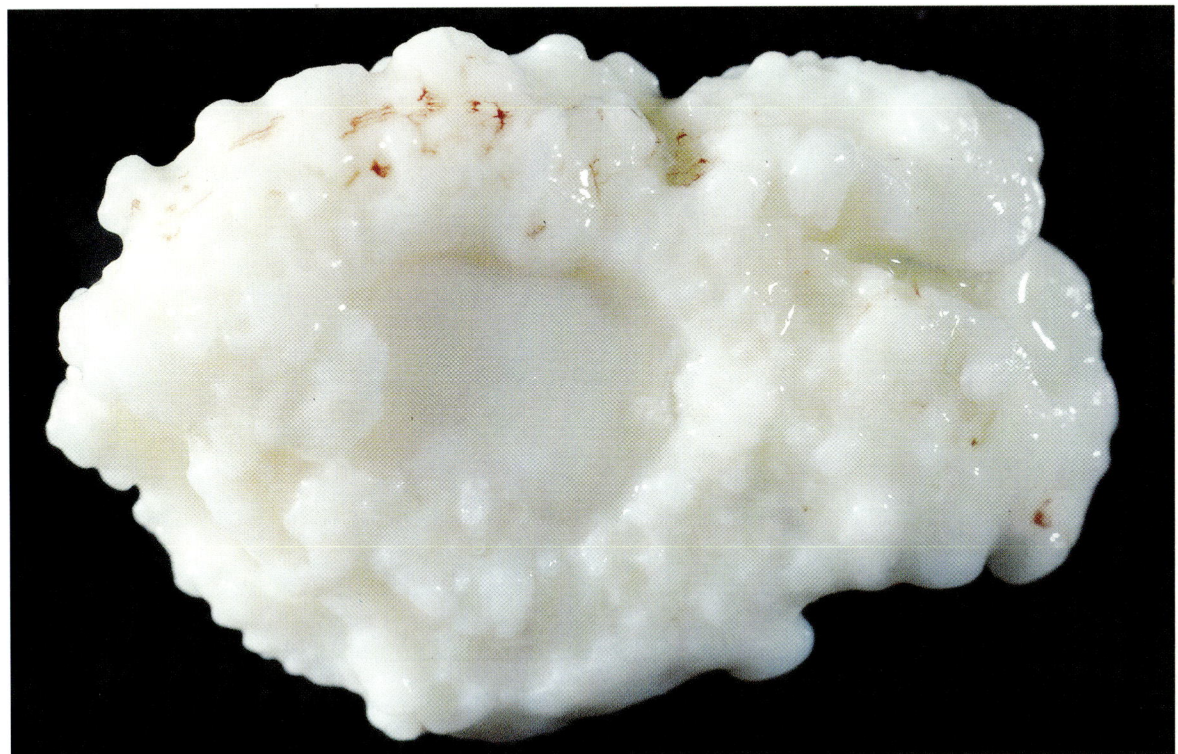

Fig. 54.30

Figs 54.30, 54.31 Loose bodies of osteochondritis dissecans (knee joint). (Courtesy of M. Forest MD.)

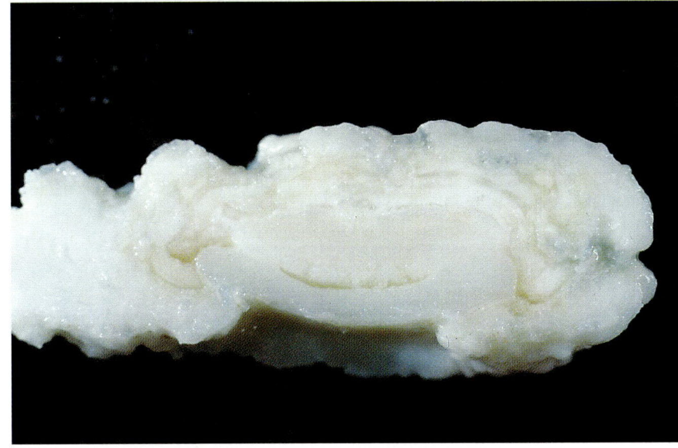

Fig. 54.31

stiffness. For the same reason, complete synovectomy should be avoided and excision confined to the pathologic area must be preferred.[18] Recurrence is rare and requires renewal of the initial treatment. Rare cases of synovial chondrosarcoma certainly require aggressive surgical therapy, such as amputation or, when possible, extraarticular resection followed by reconstruction.

DIFFERENTIAL DIAGNOSIS

The most important differential diagnosis, although rare, is synovial chondrosarcoma, primary or secondary to synovial chondromatosis. Cell abnormalities, rather frequent in synovial chondromatosis, have a poor diagnostic value. More important is the presence of spindle cells, myxoid changes and necrotic foci. Mitotic figures are uncommon. Extracapsular extent of cartilaginous nodules is suggestive of chondrosarcoma, though synovial chondromatosis may display the same course.[19]

The differential diagnosis is especially difficult with other conditions which release cartilaginous or osteocartilaginous fragments into the joint space: osteoarthritis, traumas, osteochondritis dissecans, aseptic epiphyseal necrosis, neurogenic (Charcot's) arthropathies (Figs 54.28–54.31). In all these conditions, fragments of cartilage and bone are progressively resorbed, sometimes surrounded by macrophages or even giant cells. Progressive transition between cartilage and synovial tissue, which exists in syn-

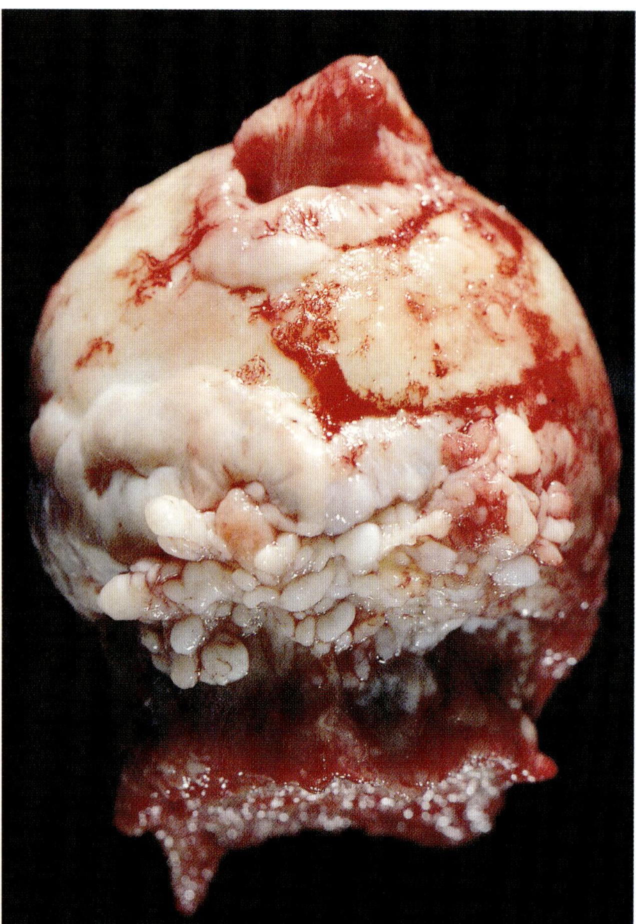

Fig. 54.32

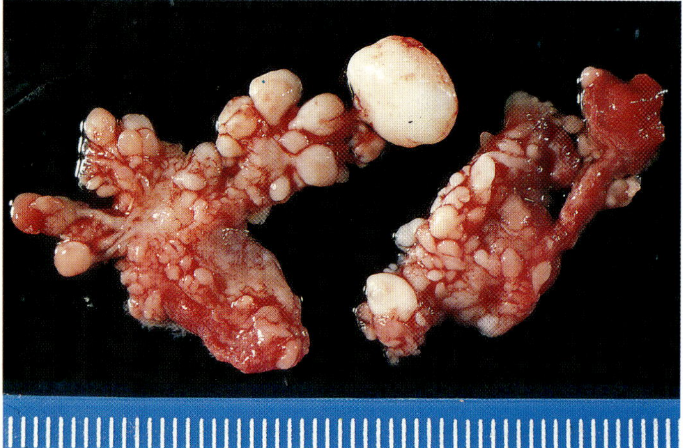

Fig. 54.33

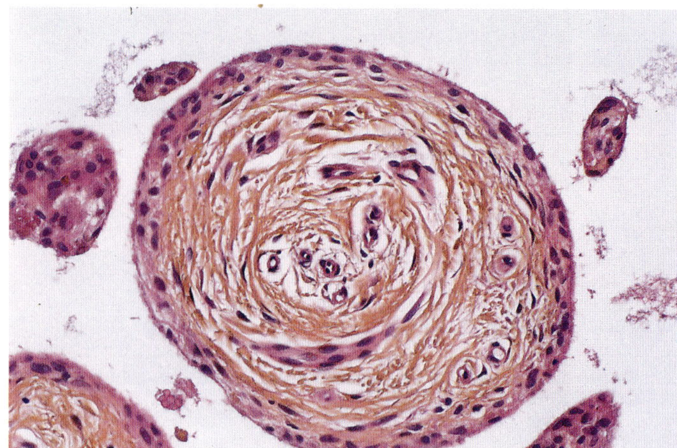

Fig. 54.34

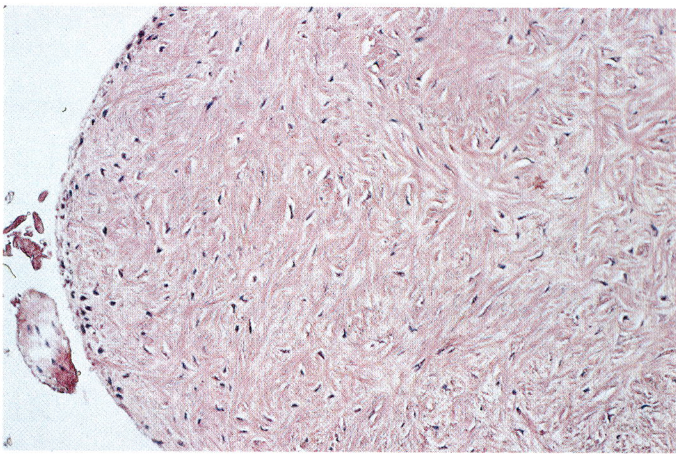

Fig. 54.35

Figs 54.32–54.35 Osteoarthritis of the hip joint: fibrous nodules in the synovium grossly mimicking a synovial chondromatosis. (Courtesy of M. Forest MD.)

ovial chondromatosis, is completely lacking here. Moreover, articular debris shows organoid structure and is devoid of nuclear atypia.[20]

The contrast is particularly obvious between a loose body of synovial chondromatosis and a loose body of osteochondritis dissecans, this being a frequent problem for the surgeon. In the latter condition, the osteochondral fragment or the dead subchondral bone is partly surrounded by rings of reactive cartilage and the articular surface is hollowed by a niche corresponding to the loose body, whereas in synovial chondromatosis, articular surfaces stay unchanged for a long time.

Finally, unusual lesions of the synovium may have a gross appearance mimicking synovial chondromatosis, but without any cartilage formation, as in the loose bodies made only of fibrous tissue (Figs 54.32–54.35).

REFERENCES

1. Milgram J W. Synovial osteochondromatosis. A histopathological study of thirty cases. J Bone Joint Surg (Am) 1977: 59: 792–801
2. Murphy F P, Dahlin D C, Sullivan C R. Articular synovial chondromatosis. J Bone Joint Surg (Am) 1962: 44: 77–86
3. Raibley S O. Villonodular synovitis with synovial chondromatosis. Oral Surg 1977: 44: 279–284
4. Takagi M, Ishikawa G. Simultaneous villonodular synovitis and synovial chondromatosis of the temporomandibular joint. Report of a case. J Oral Surg 1981: 39: 699–701
5. Trias A, Quintana O. Synovial chondrometaplasia: review of world literature and study of 18 Canadian cases. Can J Surg 1976: 19: 151–158
6. Norman A, Steiner G C. Bone erosion in synovial chondromatosis. Radiology 1986: 161: 749–752
7. Szypryt P, Twining P, Preston B J, Howell C J. Synovial chondromatosis of the hip joint presenting as a pathologic fracture. Br J Radiol 1986: 59: 339–401
8. Fechner R E. Neoplasms and neoplasm-like lesions of the synovium. In: Ackerman L V, Spjut H G, Abell M A, Eds. Bones and joints. Baltimore: Williams and Wilkins, 1976, pp 157–186
9. McCarty E F, Dorfman H D. Primary synovial chondromatosis. An ultrastructural study. Clin Orthop 1982: 168: 178–186
10. Leu J Z, Matsubara T, Hirohata K. Ultrastructural morphology of early cellular changes in the synovium of primary synovial chondromatosis. Clin Orthop 1992: 276: 299–306
11. Bertoni F, Unni K K, Beabout J W, Sim F H. Chondrosarcomas of the synovium. Cancer 1991: 67: 155–162
12. Milgram J W. The development of loose bodies in human joints. Clin Orthop 1977: 124: 292–303
13. Kay P R, Freemont A J, Davies D R A. The etiology of multiple loose bodies. J Bone Joint Surg (Br) 1989: 71: 501–504
14. Hamilton A, Davis R I, Hayes D, Mollan R A. Chondrosarcoma developing in synovial chondromatosis. A case report. J Bone Joint Surg 1987 (Br): 69: 137–140
15. Perry B E, McQueen D A, Lin J J. Synovial chondromatosis with malignant degeneration to chondrosarcoma. J Bone Joint Surg (Am) 1988: 70: 1259–1261
16. King J W, Spjut H J, Fechner R E, Vanderpool D W. Synovial chondrosarcoma of the knee joint. J Bone Joint Surg (Am) 1967: 49: 1389–1396
17. Dunn E J, McGavran M H, Nelson P, Greer R B. Synovial chondrosarcoma. Report of a case. J Bone Joint Surg (Am) 1974: 56: 811–813
18. Ogilvie-Harris D J, Saleh K. Generalized synovial chondromatosis of the knee: a comparison of removal of the loose bodies alone or with arthroscopic synovectomy. Arthroscopy 1994: 10: 166–170
19. Ontell F, Greenspan A. Chondrosarcoma complicating synovial chondromatosis: findings with magnetic resonance imaging. Can Assoc Radiol J 1994: 45: 318–323
20. Villacin A B, Brigham L N, Bullough P G. Primary and secondary synovial chondrometaplasia. Histopathologic and clinicoradiologic differences. Hum Pathol 1979: 10: 439–451

55

Synovial sarcoma

J. Amouroux

INTRODUCTION AND CLINICAL DATA

Synovial sarcoma is, clinically and morphologically, a well-defined entity, usually arising in the paraarticular regions of the extremities.

Its frequency is estimated as being between 6% and 10% of all soft tissue sarcomas. In Enzinger's series, it comes fourth, after malignant fibrous histiocytoma, liposarcoma and rhabdomyosarcoma.[1]

Its histogenesis remains uncertain. It may derive from poorly differentiated mesenchymal cells. However, its localization and its microscopic resemblance to normal synovium justify the use of the term 'synovial sarcoma', almost unanimously accepted.

This tumor primarily occurs in adolescents and young adults, between 15 and 40. In Enzinger's series (345 cases), the median age is 26.5 years. Seventy-two percent of affected patients are under 40 years old. Although it is rare under the age of 10 years, several series have been published including children and adolescents.[2,3]

Males are more often affected than females. The sex ratio is 1.2 males for 1 female.

The tumor presents as a deep-seated painful swelling. Pain alone, without any swelling, is more uncommon. There may be a moderate limitation of motion. Severe functional disturbance or weight loss is only encountered in poorly differentiated synovial sarcomas of long duration and large size.

Most often, the tumor grows slowly and insidiously so that in almost all cases, diagnosis occurs 2–4 years late. Trauma does not seem to play any role in its development.

SKELETAL DISTRIBUTION

Synovial sarcoma primarily occurs in the extremities near a large joint, especially the knee region. The tumor is closely related to tendons, tendon sheaths, bursae and joint capsule, less often to fasciae and aponeuroses. Growth of the

"

tumor within the joint cavity is rare and amounts to fewer than 5% of cases.[4] Eighty-five to 95% of the cases develop in the limbs, twice as often in the lower as the upper limbs. It occurs in the head and neck regions, thoracic or abdominal wall, retroperitoneum, mediastinum or mesentery in only 5–15% of cases.

IMAGING

Radiography is of considerable help in clinical diagnosis and preoperative assessment of synovial sarcoma. The tumor presents as a round or oval, more or less lobulated mass of moderate density, usually located close to a large joint. The adjacent bone is usually uninvolved. In 15–20% of cases, there is a periosteal reaction or a superficial bone erosion and even invasion with massive bone destruction in cases of big, poorly differentiated sarcomas.[5]

The most distinctive radiological feature, found in 20% of cases, is the presence of multiple small opacities caused by calcifications and, less frequently, by bone formation. In most cases, it consists of fine stippling and, less frequently, of large radiopaque masses, which may look like other tumors, especially osteosarcoma.[6]

CT and MRI are very helpful in determining the precise site of origin and extent of the tumor.[7] MRI shows that the tumor is well circumscribed in 91% of cases, is contiguous with bone in 50% and involves bone in 21%. The appearance in T2 sequences is suggestive if the image is heterogeneous, and associates liquid levels, adipose areas and areas that are iso-, hyper- or hypointensive relative to fat. However, in some instances, it may be homogeneous and look like a benign, even cystic lesion.

GROSS PATHOLOGY

The gross appearance of synovial sarcoma is very variable, depending on its localization and rate of growth (Fig. 55.1). The slow-growing tumors are well circumscribed, round or multinodular. Compression of adjacent tissues leads to the development of a pseudocapsule. Some tumors contain by one or more cystic cavities (Fig. 55.2). Most of the tumors are closely attached to tendons, tendon sheaths or joint capsules. Their consistency is more or less firm, depending on their collagen content. On section they appear yellow or grayish. Their average diameter is 3–5 cm but some tumors may exceed 15 cm. Calcifications, although frequent, are difficult to see with the naked eye. Poorly differentiated and rapidly growing lesions are ill defined and often altered by hemorrhage, necrosis or cystic areas.

HISTOPATHOLOGY

Synovial sarcoma, unlike most other sarcomas, is composed of two different cell types, combination of which has

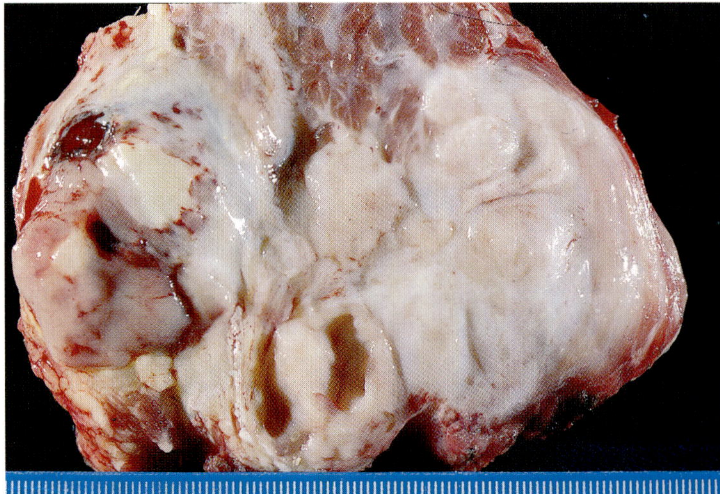

Fig. 55.1 Synovial sarcoma of the forearm. (Courtesy of M. Forest MD.)

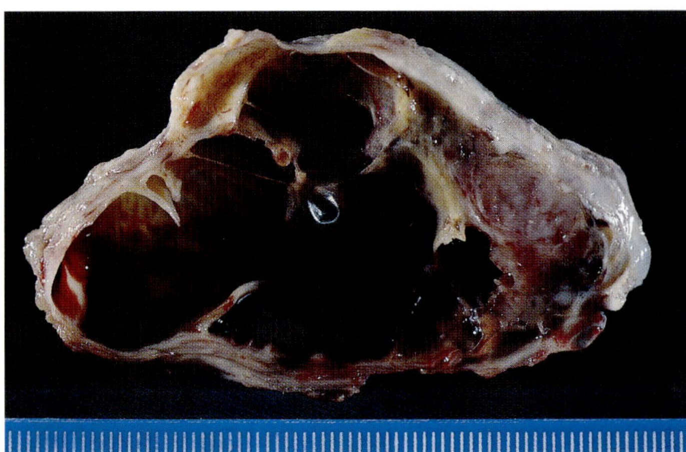

Fig. 55.2 Cystic synovial sarcoma in the popliteal fossa. (Courtesy of M. Forest MD.)

led to the description of several distinct histological varieties: on the one hand, epithelial-type cells, resembling those of a carcinoma, and on the other hand, spindle cells comparable to those of a fibrosarcoma.

The association of these two cell types allows recognition of the most usual biphasic synovial sarcoma, the less frequent monophasic spindle cell type, the very rare monophasic epithelial type and the poorly differentiated type.[8–12]

Biphasic synovial sarcoma

This is the most classic and easily recognizable type, due to the coexistence of the two basic cellular types of this tumor (Figs 55.3–55.5). The epithelial cells are characterized by large, round or oval nuclei, surrounded by a pale, abundant and sharply outlined cytoplasm. Cells are

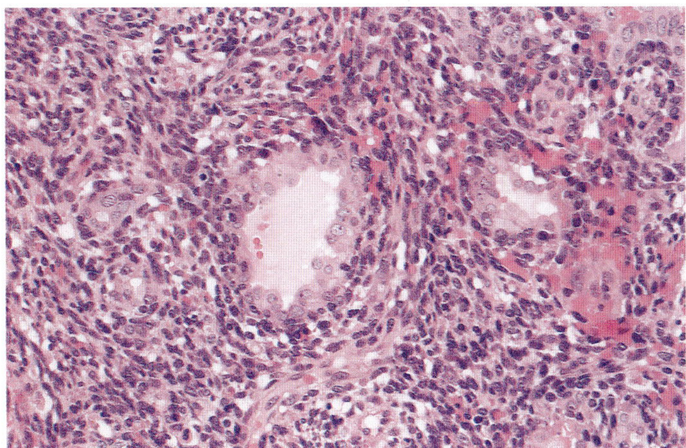

Fig. 55.3

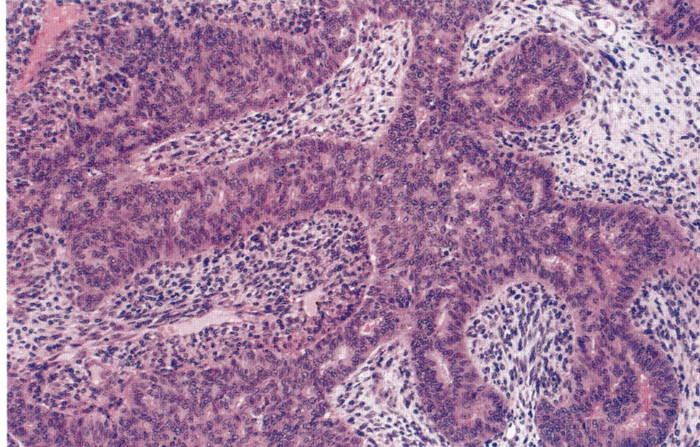

Fig. 55.4

Figs 55.3, 55.4 Biphasic synovial sarcoma. (Courtesy of M. Forest MD.)

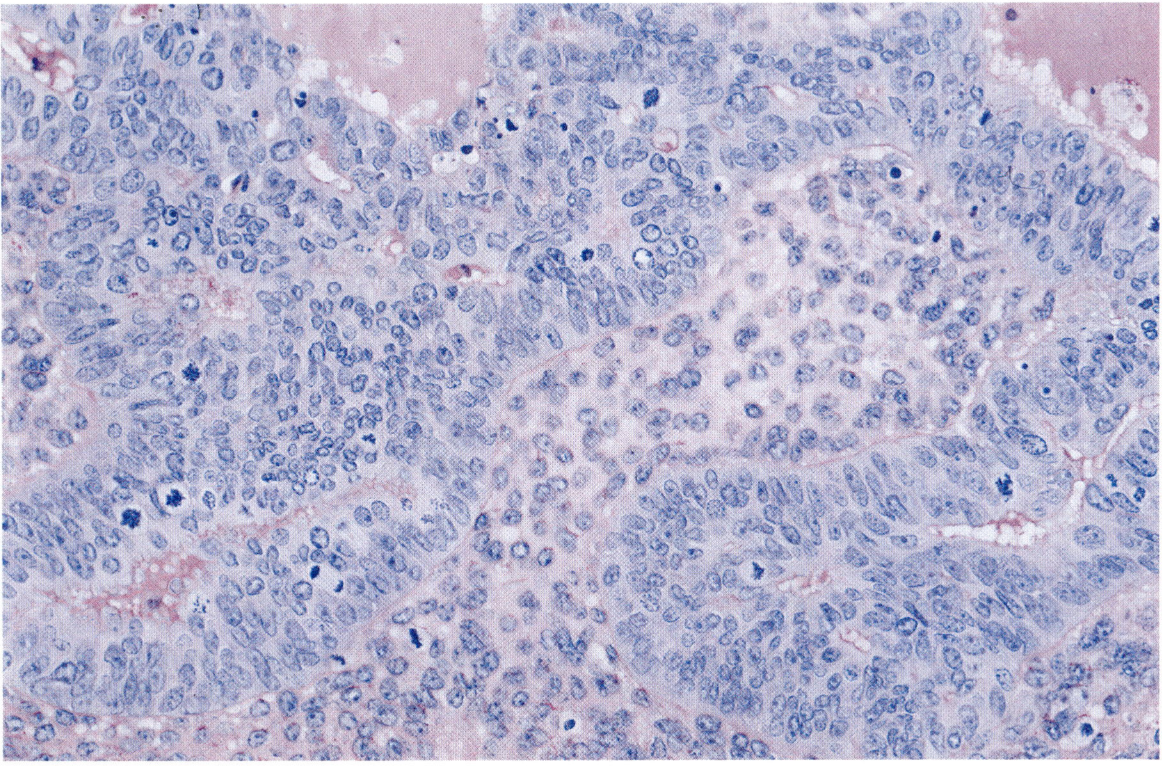

Fig. 55.5 Biphasic synovial sarcoma: PAS staining. (Courtesy of M. Forest MD.)

arranged in solid cords or nests and often line small irregular pseudoglandular cavities or clefts that may contain a homogeneous eosinophilic secretion. The presence of these cystic areas, that may extend outside the tumor boundaries and are often bordered by a cellular lining closely resembling normal synovium, suggests that sarcoma has developed within a bursa.

Epithelial proliferation may often exhibit a villous or papillary pattern similar to papillary carcinomas. In this component limited foci of squamous differentiation may be seen, occasionally associated with squamous pearls or keratohyaline granules.

The fibrous component consists of small, rather uniform, spindle-shaped cells, with indistinct cytoplasm and small nuclei. These cells are parallel with each other and grouped in interlacing fascicles, rather similar to those of a fibrosarcoma. Some peculiarities must be emphasized: shorter fascicles, no 'herring-bone' pattern, more irregular arrangement of the cells, darker nuclei and fewer mitotic figures. The latter occur equally in both epithelial and spindle-shaped components.

Cellular density often varies between different areas of the tumor, due to local edema, which can lead to a myxoid appearance, large amounts of collagen or calcification.

The presence of calcification or even ossification is an important diagnostic feature found in about 20% of synovial sarcomas. It may consist of irregularly distributed fine spherical calcifications or extensive, large calcifications or ossifications (Fig. 55.6) occupying an important part of the tumor. Calcification is more conspicuous at the periphery of the tumor than at its center.

Areas of chondroid metaplasia may be seen, mainly close to calcifications or ossifications.

The presence of mast cells is another frequent feature of synovial sarcomas, chiefly in the spindle cell areas of the tumor. Inflammatory or multinucleated giant cells are rare.

In some cases, vascularization is rich and the presence of dilated vessels within spindle cell areas may resemble hemangiopericytoma.

Involvement of the vascular walls by the tumor suggests a poor prognosis. Some changes, such as hemorrhages, are most prominent in poorly differentiated tumors.

Monophasic fibrous synovial sarcoma

This is the most frequently observed form of synovial sarcoma (Figs 55.7, 55.8). Its existence has been confirmed by the frequent association of the main spindle cell component with an epithelial element, even if very small. Immunostaining features of the cells, which often express typical epithelial cell antigens, and ultrastructural findings confirm the relationship between spindle and epithelial cells.

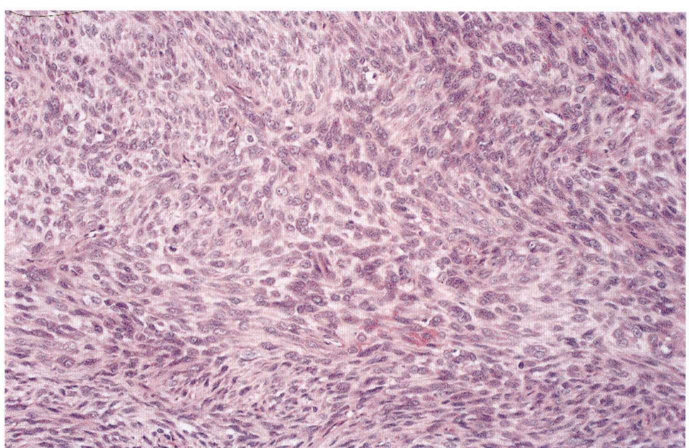

Fig. 55.7

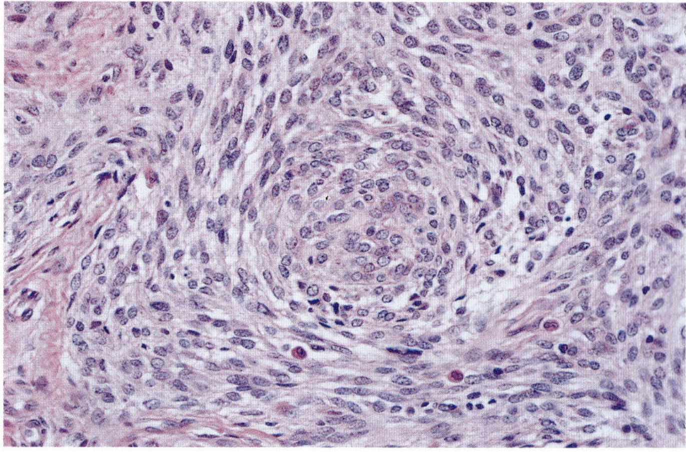

Fig. 55.8

Figs 55.7, 55.8 Monophasic fibrous synovial sarcoma. (Courtesy of M. Forest MD.)

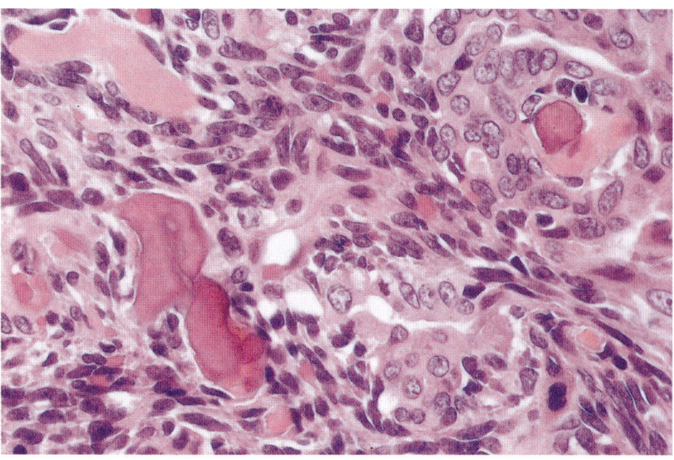

Fig. 55.6 Biphasic synovial sarcoma with ossified areas. (Courtesy of M. Forest MD.)

Cell proliferation is rather similar to the spindle component of the biphasic synovial sarcomas. The same features are found: fascicles of cells, myxoid changes, areas of hyalinization, presence of calcifications and mast cells. This type of synovial sarcoma may contain variable numbers of cells with rhabdoid aspects, the nuclei of which are displaced to the cytoplasmic membrane by an inclusion of intermediate filaments.[13] Symptomatology of this tumoral form is the same as the biphasic type.

Monophasic epithelial synovial sarcoma

This is a rare type, difficult to diagnose, often misinterpreted as a true epithelial tumor (Figs 55.9, 55.10). This has led to denial of the synovial origin of this kind of tumor and to the suggestion of such terms as 'soft tissue carcinoma' or 'carcinosarcoma'.

Before immunohistochemical data were available, these tumors were often considered as metastatic carcinomas,

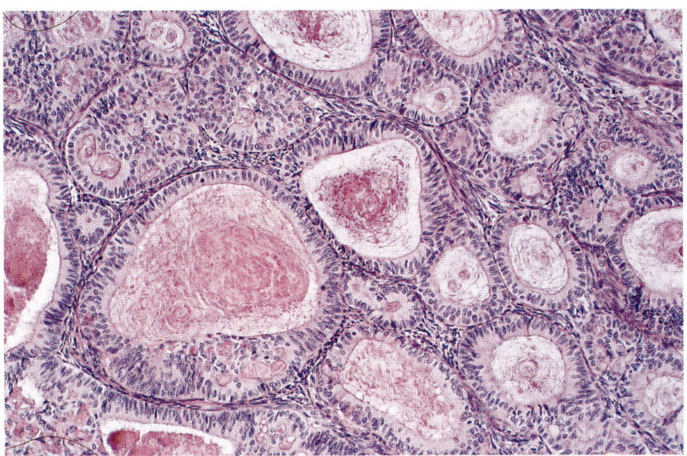

Fig. 55.9

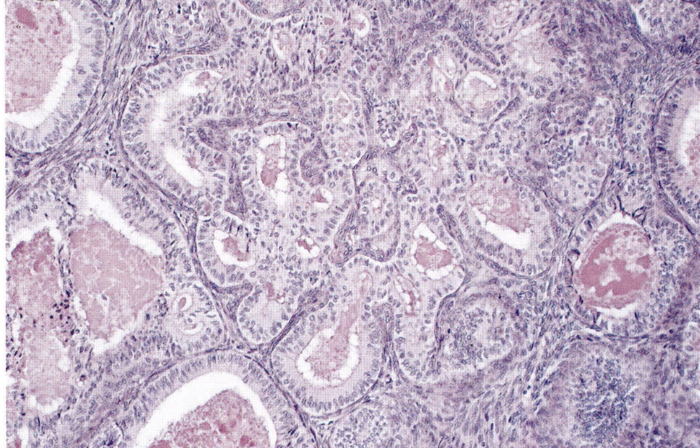

Fig. 55.10

Figs 55.9, 55.10 Monophasic epithelial synovial sarcoma. (Courtesy of M. Forest MD.)

adnexal carcinomas, malignant melanomas, epithelioid sarcomas or schwannomas.

Tumoral cells display the same features and the same architectural patterns as in the epithelial component of biphasic sarcomas. However, this tumor is very rarely composed of an epithelial pattern alone and careful screening of multiple sections most often reveals foci, although minute, of spindle-shaped cells. Helpful features for diagnosis are clinical data (young age of the patient, distal location of the tumor), presence of mast cells, calcifications and PAS-positive or alcianophilic material within intercellular spaces.

Poorly differentiated synovial sarcoma

Though it is difficult to separate the types of synovial sarcomas mentioned above, which may be considered the well-differentiated ones, from the frequent poorly differentiated forms, the latter must be recognized. As a matter of fact, their diagnosis is doubtful because their synovial origin is difficult to prove and their prognosis is poor: evolution is more aggressive, with earlier and more frequent invasion of the adjacent structures, particularly bone and a greater tendency to metastasize. The estimated incidence of this tumoral type is about 20% of all synovial sarcomas. The tumor is composed of small or intermediate-sized, oval or spindle-shaped cells, without any particular pattern. These tumoral cells simulate those of small cell carcinomas. Undifferentiated and well-differentiated areas are sometimes close together. In this tumoral type, vessels may be numerous and dilated, resembling features of malignant hemangiopericytoma.

HISTOCHEMISTRY

Special staining procedures are often helpful in the diag-

nosis of synovial sarcoma. Mucoid secretion is present within epithelial tumoral cells, intercellular clefts and pseudoglandular cavities. This secretion stains positively with PAS, colloidal iron, alcian blue and mucicarmine stains. These staining properties are not altered after treatment by amylase and hyaluronidase, but alcian blue is positive only at pH <5.7.[14] Mucoid material contains hyaluronic acid, chondroitin sulfate and sialic acid, the latter being present only in epithelial cells.

Another type of mucin is sometimes found in the tumor which is synthesized by the spindle cells and stains positively with alcian blue, but not with PAS. This mucin is rich in hyaluronic acid and positive staining disappears after treatment with hyaluronidase.

Reticulin stain may be helpful to display the biphasic epithelial and spindle cell pattern, reticulinic meshes being much thinner in epithelial than in spindle cell areas.

IMMUNOHISTOCHEMISTRY

Reactivity for low and high molecular weight cytokeratins may be present in both the epithelial and spindle cell components (Fig. 55.11). The latter also express EMA (Fig. 55.12). This immunostaining is positive in nearly all biphasic synovial sarcomas and in a majority of monophasic fibrous types. Amongst the different cytokeratins, the most specific for synovial sarcoma seem to be keratin 7 and 19. Anticytokeratin antibodies are the best markers of the epithelial differentiation of the tumor, but keratin is also expressed in about half of the cases by the spindle cell component of the biphasic or monophasic tumors.

Of course, expression of vimentin by spindle cells is almost constant. Thus coexpression of cytokeratin and vimentin, occurring in one-third of biphasic and about half of monophasic types, displays an immunohistochemical profile which is very suggestive of this tumoral type.

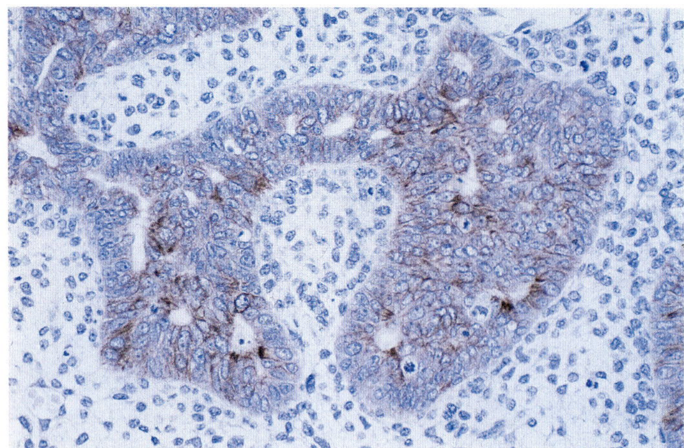

Fig. 55.11 Synovial sarcoma: cytokeratin immunostaining. (Courtesy of M. Forest MD.)

Fig. 55.12 Synovial sarcoma: EMA immunostaining. (Courtesy of M. Forest MD.)

Epithelial and to a lesser degree spindle-shaped cells may express EMA and sometimes CEA.[13]

Immunostaining may demonstrate collagen IV and laminin, which are two major components of basal lamina. These basal lamina-like structures occur continuously along the periphery of epithelial elements in biphasic tumors, but also in an intermittent pattern within some monophasic sarcomatous areas. This reaction may be helpful in more positively identifying epithelial differentiation, even incomplete or faint, in areas where it is difficult to find with usual staining procedures.[13,15,16]

Immunohistochemistry allows the evaluation of cell proliferative activity, with the help of antibodies such as PCNA or Ki67.[17,18]

ELECTRON MICROSCOPY

In biphasic tumors, lining cells of the glandular cavities are connected by tight junctions of moderate length and, further from the lumina, by desmosomes with short tonofilaments. Microvilli are present on the apical surfaces of the epithelial cells and as filopodia in intercellular spaces, often dilated. Glandular lumina and intercellular clefts often contain amorphous material corresponding to mucins. Epithelial cells contain organelles usually found in this kind of cell, with variable numbers of lysosomes and small glycogen aggregates. The cytoplasm contains intermediate filaments and rare tonofibrils. A continuous basal lamina, absent in the normal synovium, usually separates the epithelial islands and tubular gland-like structures from the surrounding spindle cell component.[19–21]

Ultrastructural features of monophasic fibrous synovial sarcomas are similar to those of the spindle cell component of the biphasic type.[22] Aspects of epithelial differentiation are often present, such as intercellular clefts of varying size lined by microvilli, as are also poorly differentiated intercellular junctions or desmosome-like structures. Distinct basal lamina are not found within these areas but there are sometimes basal lamina-like structures or condensed ground substance at the cell surfaces. There are usually no features of epithelial differentiation in the poorly differentiated monophasic synovial sarcomas.

CYTOPATHOLOGY

Cytopathological techniques allow experienced pathologists to diagnose a number of benign and malignant soft tissue tumors. The exact type of sarcoma is, however, more difficult to specify.[23] An accurate diagnosis can be done in the biphasic type of synovial sarcoma, particularly if cytokeratin and vimentin immunostaining procedures show positivity, even focal.[24]

The establishment, from a metastatic pleural effusion, of a cell line displaying morphological features of the monophasic spindle cell type of synovial sarcoma may be very useful in further investigations on synovial sarcoma.[25]

FLOW CYTOMETRY

Oda conducted a DNA flow cytometry study in 30 patients. The S+G2M phase fraction, although correlated with the extent of PCNA staining, was not a significant prognostic factor. The same can be said for ploidy.[17,26]

CYTOGENETICS

Cytogenetic studies of synovial sarcomas demonstrate the almost constant presence of a balanced translocation between chromosomes X and 18, t(X;18)(p11.2;q11.2) in tumors of both the biphasic and monophasic fibrous types, as well as in poorly differentiated synovial sarcomas.[27–29]

During recent years, different authors have reported two possible breakpoints, more specifically linked to the two main types of synovial sarcomas, biphasic and monophasic fibrous.[29-31] Fluorescent in situ hybridization (FISH) allows retrospective studies of this cytogenetic abnormality on paraffin-embedded specimens.[32,33]

COURSE

The course of synovial sarcoma is burdened by the occurrence of recurrences and metastases, responsible for a long-term prognosis that remains poor and depends largely on the type of therapy. Cases with the poorest outcome are those treated exclusively by limited excision with insufficient margins and with no complementary therapy. In these cases, the recurrence rate reaches 70–83%.[8]

With adequate surgical therapy and adjunctive radiotherapy, the recurrence rate falls as low as about 30%.[1] Multiple recurrences over a period of several years are not rare. Although recurrence usually develops within the first 2 years following surgery, late recurrences may be observed, sometimes beyond 10 years.

Metastases occur in about half of cases, often appearing late; their main sites are lungs (94%), followed by lymph nodes (10–20%) and bone marrow.[34] Lung metastases are very rarely present at the time of diagnosis of the original tumor. Histological features of the metastatic lesions are very similar to those of the primary tumor, although in biphasic types the spindle cell component is more prominent, as cell differentiation diminishes and mitotic activity increases.

TREATMENT

Local surgical excision without adjunctive therapy is insufficient for recovery. All authors agree with the necessity for rapid and radical surgery, including excision of the entire involved muscle or muscle group and possibly even limb amputation. These surgical indications depend mainly on tumor size and location. Radical excision is often impossible for tumors situated close to large joints: this justifies the use of radiotherapy in these cases.

Current therapeutic strategy includes preoperative radiotherapy and chemotherapy, often limited excision and postoperative chemotherapy.[35-37]

A complete surgical excision followed by radiotherapy seems to be the best treatment for small tumors while amputation may be best for very large or unresectable neoplasms. Radiation of regional lymph nodes is preferable to excision, but it should be limited to those cases with high suspicion of lymph node metastases.

The rather slow growth rate of the tumor justifies surgical therapy, even repeated, when lung metastasis occurs.[38] Indications for chemotherapy are tumors of unfavorable prognosis, in the hope of preventing or suppressing metastases. Chemotherapy does not seem to change the histological features of metastases.

PROGNOSIS

Synovial sarcoma is a prognostically unfavorable tumor. However, in recent series 5-year survival rates have improved and may exceed 60%. Ten-year survival rates are no better than 20%.[10] These two figures reflect the frequency of late metastasis, leading to death.

The following factors allow an estimation of the prognosis.

1. *Age.* Young age of the patient, under 15 years, is a feature of favorable prognosis in the 31 children of Ladenstein's series, the survival rate of which is 74.2%.[3]

2. *Tumor size.* Tumors up to 5 cm have a better prognosis than larger ones. Thus, in Oda's series, 11 of 14 patients with a tumoral size exceeding 5 cm died within the first year, whereas the eight patients whose tumor was smaller than or equal to 5 cm were alive at 10 years.[10] Pain seems to play a favorable role as it reveals small-sized tumors, thus allowing an earlier diagnosis. In the same way, distal location of the tumor seems to have a good prognosis. Superficial or deep location of the tumor does not influence prognosis.

3. *Histological type.* There is no agreement as to the prognostic significance according to different studies. Some of them conclude that monophasic spindle cell tumors have a poorer prognosis but very large series do not demonstrate significant differences between these tumoral types.[1,10] However, Oda attaches a negative value to the existence of rhabdoid cells in synovial sarcomas. Very poorly differentiated tumors always have an unfavorable prognosis.

4. *Existence of calcification and/or ossification* results in a better prognosis: 5-year and 10-year survival rates reach 82% and 66%, respectively, for Varela-Duran & Enzinger's 32 patients.[9] Recurrence rate is 34%.

5. *Proliferative activity.* This is a very important prognostic factor, most often evaluated by the number of mitotic figures in 10 high-power (×400) fields (10 hpf). Prognosis becomes frankly less favorable when there are more than 10 mitoses per 10 hpf. This proliferative activity may be estimated by flow cytometry[26] or immunostaining with Ki67 or PCNA.

6. *Nuclear grade.* Irregularity of the nuclear size, coarse chromatin and presence of one or more sometimes prominent nucleoli suggest a poor prognosis.

7. *Necrosis.* Extensive necrosis, more than 50% of the tumor surface area, is a negative feature.

8. *Rich vascularization.* As it may give rise to metastasis, this is also an unfavorable prognostic factor.

9. *Quality of surgical therapy* is of important prognostic

value: if excision is complete with wide margins, the outcome is much more favorable than if resection is limited.

DIFFERENTIAL DIAGNOSIS

Diagnosis of synovial sarcoma is usually easy in biphasic types. However, some tumors may cause difficult problems.

• *Epithelioid sarcoma.* There are such resemblances between these two neoplasms that epithelioid sarcoma has been considered as a variant of synovial sarcoma. In fact, differences, essentially clinical, separate them. Epithelioid sarcoma readily occurs in hand and forearm, often superficially with cutaneous ulcerations. Grossly, the tumor appears as a multinodular mass, often necrotic. There is never any mucin within the lesion. It is composed of spindle-shaped cells, which usually stain for both cytokeratin and vimentin.

• *Clear cell sarcoma* (malignant melanoma of soft tissues) develops in young adults from tendons and aponeuroses. It is composed of compact aggregates of round cells and fascicles of spindle-shaped cells, with pale-staining nuclei, prominent nucleoli and pale-staining cytoplasm with usually abundant glycogen. Tumoral cells do not stain for cytokeratin but there are in the majority of cases some cells that stain for S-100 protein and HMB45 antigen. Ultrastructurally, melanosomes or premelanosomes are usually demonstrable in the cytoplasm. When there is no staining for S-100 protein and no cytoplasmic melanosomes, the diagnosis of synovial sarcoma (mono- or biphasic type) or sarcoma of unknown histogenesis may be considered.

• *Malignant schwannomas* (malignant peripheral nerve sheath tumors) may give rise to a problem of differential diagnosis with synovial sarcoma, particularly in the 15% of cases in which spindle cells are intermingled with elements of other types, such as epithelial cells sometimes with distinct glandular differentiation. Tumor cells express S-100 protein, but this may be encountered in some synovial sarcomas.

• Monophasic fibrous synovial sarcomas may be difficult to distinguish from fibrosarcoma. The most helpful features suggesting the diagnosis of synovial sarcoma are the presence of calcifications and mast cells and particularly the expression of epithelial markers by tumoral cells.

• In the rare *epithelial type* of synovial sarcoma, the diagnostic problem is essentially to make the distinction with adnexal or metastatic carcinomas. This problem is virtually insoluble in the absence of a spindle cell component, even very focal, within the tumor.

REFERENCES

1. Enzinger F M, Weiss S W. Soft tissue tumors. 3rd ed. St Louis: Mosby, 1995
2. Pappo A S, Fontanesi J, Luo X et al. Synovial sarcoma in children and adolescents: the St Jude Children's Research Hospital experience. J Clin Pathol 1994: 12: 2360–2366
3. Ladenstein R, Treuner J, Koscielniak E et al. Synovial sarcoma of childhood and adolescence. Report of the German CWS-81 study. Cancer 1993: 71: 3647–3655
4. McKinney C D, Mills S E, Fechner R E. Intraarticular synovial sarcoma. Am J Surg Pathol 1992: 16: 1017–1020
5. Horowitz A L, Resnick D, Watson R C. The roentgen features of synovial sarcomas. Clin Radiol 1973: 24: 481–488
6. Milchgrub S, Ghandur-Mnaymneh L, Dorfman H D, Albores-Saavedra J. Synovial sarcoma with extensive osteoid and bone formation. Am J Surg Pathol 1993: 17: 357–363
7. Jones B C, Sundaram M, Kransdorf M J. Synovial sarcoma: MR imaging findings in 34 patients. AJR 1993: 161: 827–830
8. Menendez L R, Brien E, Brien W W. Synovial sarcoma: a clinico-pathologic study. Orthop Rev 1992: 21: 465–471
9. Varela-Duran J, Enzinger F M. Calcifying synovial sarcoma. Cancer 1982: 50: 345–352
10. Oda Y, Hashimoto H, Tsuneyoshi M, Takeshita S. Survival in synovial sarcoma. A multivariate study on prognostic factors with special emphasis on the comparison between early death and long-term survival. Am J Surg Pathol 1993: 17: 35–44
11. Majeste R M, Beckman E N. Synovial sarcoma with an overwhelming epithelial component. Cancer 1988: 61: 2527–2531
12. Weidner N, Goldman R, Johnston J. Epithelioid monophasic synovial sarcoma. Ultrastruct Pathol 1993: 17: 287–294
13. Ordóñez N G, Mahfouz S M, Mackay B. Synovial sarcoma. An immunohistochemical and ultrastructural study. Hum Pathol 1990: 21: 733–749
14. Katenkamp D, Stiller D. Synovial sarcoma of the abdominal wall: light microscopic, histochemical and electron microscopic investigations. Virchows Arch Pathol Anat 1980: 388: 349–360
15. Guarino M, Christensen L. Immunohistochemical analysis of extracellular matrix components in synovial sarcoma. J Pathol 1994: 172: 279–284
16. Lopes J M, Bjerkehagen B, Holm R, Bruland O, Sobrinho-Simoes M, Nesland J M. Immunohistochemical profile of synovial sarcoma with emphasis on the epithelial-type differentiation. A study of 49 primary tumours, recurrences and metastases. Pathol Res Pract 1994: 190: 168–177
17. Oda Y, Hashimoto H, Takeshita S, Tsuneyoshi M. The prognostic value of immunohistochemical staining for proliferating cell nuclear antigen in synovial sarcoma. Cancer 1993: 72: 478–485
18. Lopes J M, Bjerkehagen B, Holm R, Bruland O, Sobrinho-Simoes M, Nesland J M. Proliferative activity of synovial sarcoma: an immunohistochemical evaluation of Ki-67 labeling indices of 52 primary and recurrent tumors. Ultrastruct Pathol 1995: 19: 101–106
19. Mickelson M R, Brown G A, Maynard J A, Cooper R R, Bonfiglio M. Synovial sarcoma. An electron microscopic study of monophasic and biphasic forms. Cancer 1980: 45: 2109–2116
20. Dickersin G R. Synovial sarcoma: a review and update with emphasis on the ultrastructural characterization of the non glandular component. Ultrastruct Pathol 1991: 15: 379–402
21. Fischer C. Synovial sarcoma: ultrastructural and immunohistochemical features of epithelial differentiation in monophasic and biphasic tumors. Hum Pathol 1986: 17: 995–1008
22. Krall R A, Kostianosky M, Patchefsky A S. Synovial sarcoma. A clinical, pathological and ultrastructural study of 26 cases supporting the recognition of a monophasic variant. Am J Surg Pathol 1981: 5: 137–151
23. Bennert K W, Abdul-Karim F W. Fine needle aspiration cytology versus needle core biopsy of soft tissue tumor. A comparison. Acta Cytologica 1994: 38: 381–384
24. Aisner S C, Seidman J D, Burke K C, Young J W. Aspiration cytology of biphasic and monophasic synovial sarcoma. A report of two cases. Acta Cytologica 1993: 37: 413–417

25. Sonobe H, Manabe Y, Furihata M et al. Establishment and characterization of a new human synovial sarcoma cell line, HS-SY-II. Lab Invest 1992: 67: 498–504

26. EI-Naggar A K, Ayala A G, Abdul-Karim F W et al. Synovial sarcoma. A DNA flow cytometric study. Cancer 1990: 65: 2295–2300

27. Turc-Carel C, Dal Cin P, Limon J, Li F, Sandberg A A. Translocation X;18 in synovial sarcoma. Cancer Genet Cytogenet 1986: 23: 93

28. Dal Cin P, Rao U, Jani-Sait S, Karakousis C, Sandberg A A. Chromosomes in the diagnosis of soft tissue tumors. I. Synovial sarcoma. Mod Pathol 1992: 5: 357–362

29. De Leeuw B, Balemans M, Weghuis D O et al. Molecular cloning of the synovial sarcoma-specific translocation (X;18)(p11.2;q11.2) breakpoint. Hum Mol Genet 1994: 3: 745–749

30. Renwick P J, Reeves B R, Dal Cin P et al. Two categories of synovial sarcoma defined by divergent chromosome translocation breakpoints in Xp11.2, with implications for the histologic sub-classification of synovial sarcoma. Cytogenet Cell Genet 1995: 70: 58–63

31. Janz M, De Leeuw B, Weghuis D O et al. Interphase cytogenetic analysis of distinct X-chromosomal translocation breakpoints in synovial sarcoma. J Pathol 1995: 175: 391–396

32. Lee W, Han K, Harris C P, Shim S, Kim S, Meisner L F. Use of FISH to detect chromosomal translocations and deletions. Analysis of chromosome rearrangement in synovial sarcoma cells from paraffin-embedded specimens. Am J Pathol 1993: 143: 15–19

33. De Leeuw B, Suijkerbuijk R F, Weghuis D O et al. Distinct Xp11.2 breakpoint regions in synovial sarcoma revealed by metaphase and interphase FISH: relationship to histologic subtypes. Cancer Genet Cytogenet 1994: 73: 89–94

34. Ryan J R, Baker L H, Benjamin R S. The natural history of metastatic synovial sarcoma: experience of the Southwest Oncology group. Clin Orthop 1982: 164: 257–260

35. Kampe C E, Rosen G, Eilber F et al. Synovial sarcoma. A study of intensive chemotherapy in 14 patients with localized disease. Cancer 1993: 72: 2161–2169

36. Mullen J R, Zagars G K. Synovial sarcoma outcome following conservation surgery and radiotherapy. Radiotherapy and Oncology 1994: 33: 23–30

37. Wanebo H J, Temple W J, Popp M B, Constable W, Aron B, Cunningham S L. Preoperative regional therapy for extremity sarcoma. A tricenter update. Cancer 1995: 75: 2299–2306

38. Kawai A, Fukuma H, Beppu Y et al. Pulmonary resection for metastatic soft tissue sarcoma. Clin Orthop 1995: 310: 188–193

SECTION 5

Treatment

56

Orthopedic surgery of bone tumors

B. Tomeno   P. Anract

INTRODUCTION

In this chapter we discuss the different treatment possibilities available to the surgeon who has to deal with tumoral disorders of the locomotor system. These may involve the bone, the soft tissues or both.

These disorders may be benign and non-progressive (e.g. metaphyseal cortical defect) or benign and aggressive (like some giant cell tumors of bone). They may also be malignant and one must distinguish tumors of low malignancy (such as parosteal osteosarcoma) from those of high malignancy (such as classical osteosarcoma).

They occur at every anatomic site, each having its specific therapeutic limitations as regards tumoral resection and the repair of losses of substance. Hence there is an infinite range of situations, which we can only attempt to classify in this chapter; however, it is possible to lay down the main principles and general rules of treatment by defining methods and their limitations, advantages and disadvantages, together with their indications. These can be classed as follows:

1. procedures preserving the limb, which may be intratumoral (curettage and curettage + packing) or extratumoral (resections of various types: radical resection, wide resection, marginal resection, 'contaminated' resection);
2. procedures sacrificing the limb: amputation and disarticulation.

INTRATUMORAL PROCEDURES

These essentially apply to virtually all benign intraosseous tumors.

Curettage consists of evacuating the tumor from within, with particular attention to treating the walls of the cavity (scrupulous curettage and cauterization by various agents – liquid nitrogen, formol, diathermy – to minimize the risk of recurrence). Except for quite small tumors not weaken-

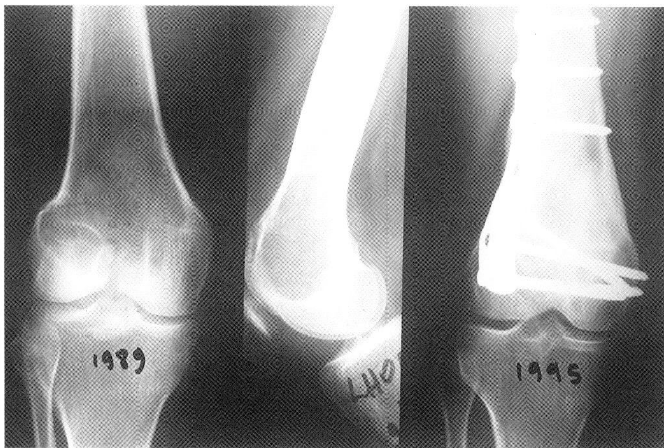

Fig. 56.1 Giant cell tumor of the lower femur. Late result (5 years) after curettage, filling with autogenous bone graft and osteosynthesis with a screwed plate.

ing the skeleton, it is rare for 'simple' curettage to prove satisfactory.

In the majority of cases, *curettage and packing*[1,2,3] are performed, both to restore a stronger skeleton and to decrease the incidence of recurrences. The packing material most often used is bone (Fig. 56.1): numerous small cancellous or corticocancellous fragments removed from the patient (autograft) or obtained from a bone back (allograft) or even a mixture of the two.

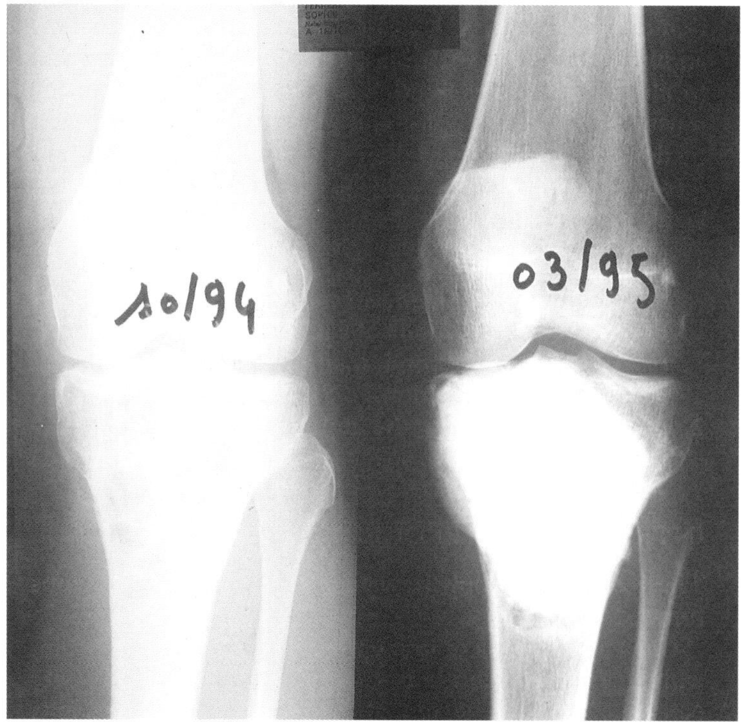

Fig. 56.2 Huge giant cell tumor of the upper tibia. After curettage, the cavity has been filled with surgical cement.

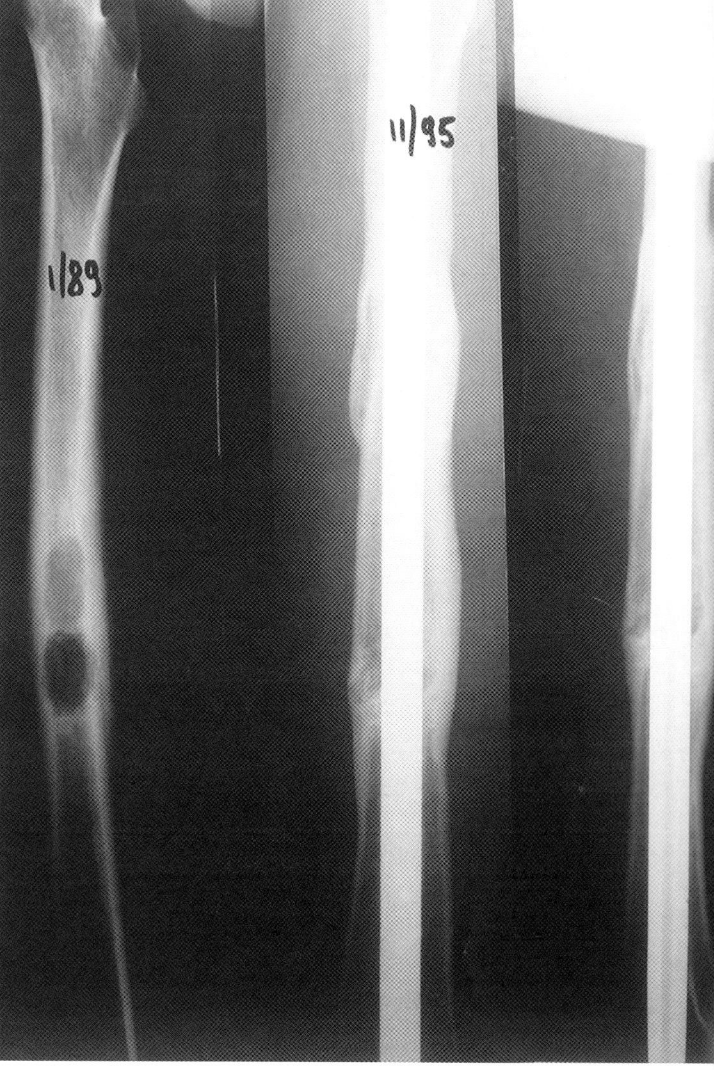

Fig. 56.3 Osteosarcoma of the middle part of the femur. Resection (12 cm), reconstruction with a bone bank allograft and an intramedullary nail.

Allografts are usually fragments of banked femoral heads (obtained during the insertion of hip prostheses). Their use avoids the problems of graft removal, which are far from negligible. For the purposes of curettage and packing, the results appear to be as good as when using autografts. Packing with bone derived from other animal species (xenografts) is little used.

Whatever the source of the packing, it must be complete and tight, with impacting by means of a graft punch to leave no crevice unfilled.

Trials of other materials are in progress (surgical cement, coral, alumina, hydroxyapatite), but these methods are still experimental. Cement (Fig. 56.2) seems to reduce the incidence of recurrences in giant cell tumors,[4] but apart from this special case it is only used in patients who have had repeated surgery with progressive loss of bone stock due to the taking of grafts, in benign tumors seen in the stage of infected recurrence (when the cement is combined with antibiotics) and in the palliative treatment of metastatic osteolytic defects (where it is very helpful).

When curettage has greatly weakened the bone (excision of more than a third of the peripheral cortex in the shaft or a very extensive cavity of the subchondral region of an epiphysis), it is essential to reinforce the packing by *osteosynthesis* with a plate and screws, a nail-plate or screw-plate to prevent the risk of postoperative fracture.

EXTRATUMORAL PROCEDURES PRESERVING THE LIMB

These are represented by different types of resection. The resection consists of removing the entire bony segment containing the tumor in a single block and without ever exposing the tumor, as well as any local invasion of the soft tissues. The approach should always be through healthy tissue at a distance from the lesion, excising in the process any preexisting scars including that of the biopsy.

After resection, it is usually necessary to complete the surgical procedure with a reconstruction stage.

The different types of resection

The term '*radical resection*' indicates an extremely wide resection passing outside the anatomic compartment where the disease has originated.

This is what Enneking[5,6] calls an 'extracompartmental' resection. For example, for an osteosarcoma of the lower

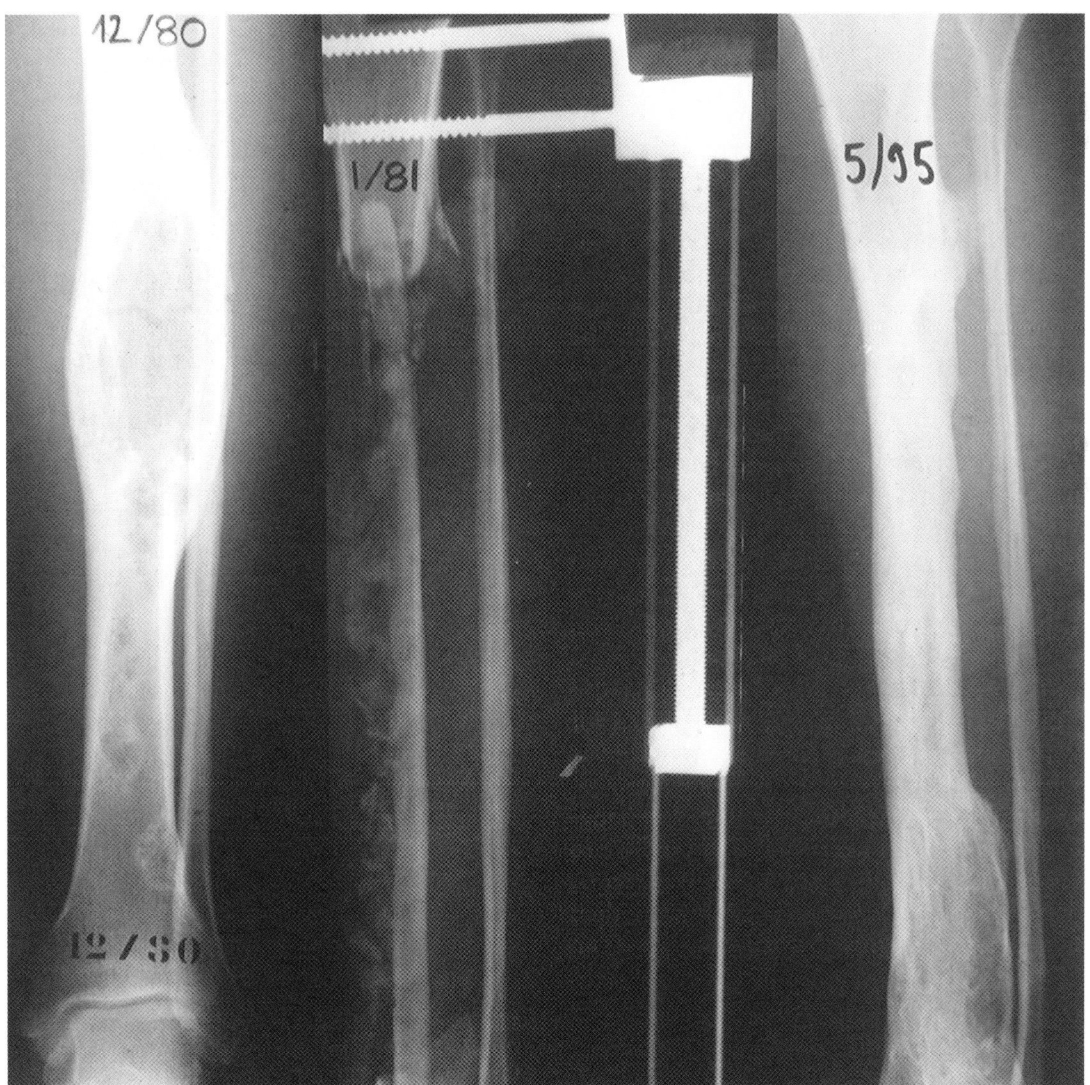

Fig. 56.4 Adamantinoma of the tibia. The reconstruction has been done with the contralateral vascularized fibula, anastomosed on the tibial anterior artery and surrounded by a lot of bone chips from the iliac crest. After 15 years one can see the progressive hypertrophy of the transplanted fibula.

part of the femur slightly invading the quadriceps, the femur is removed in its entirety with the whole of the anterior muscular compartment of the thigh, passing outside its aponeurotic septa. This 'Enneking' concept seems excessive to most authors[7,8,9] (including ourselves) as it does not provide any additional security compared with a simple wide resection.

Wide resection consists of passing a few cm from the tumor while remaining within its anatomic compartment. Such 'intracompartmental' surgery (to use Enneking's terminology) is much less mutilating functionally than the above. For an osteosarcoma of the lower end of the femur without much invasion of the soft tissues and without penetration of the joint, a wide resection removes all of the lower femur, all its capsuloligamentous attachments and a small layer of healthy muscle tissue with section of the diaphysis 3–5 cm above the upper intramedullary pole of the tumor.

If there is invasion of the joint (which is quite rare), it is also necessary to remove the entire articulation (but always in one piece and without ever opening it): this is a 'monoblock arthrectomy'.

It should be mentioned that in everyday practice the term 'resection' used by itself (i.e. not preceded by an adjective) indicates that the procedure is a 'wide' resection, as just described.

If the resection is made flush with the tumor boundaries, the term *'marginal resection'* is used. Marginal resection is indicated for benign lesions which are not intraosseous (osteochondromas) and may, if necessary, be used for tumors of low malignancy when a wide resection is impossible. For example, in a parosteal osteosarcoma developing behind the lower end of the femur and displacing the vascular bundle, one should pass between the tumor and the vessels while keeping a few mm from the lesion.

The term 'exeresis' is synonymous with resection but when employed alone without an adjective it signifies a marginal resection. In practice, it indicates a minimal removal of small benign bony lesions (osteochondroma, nidus of an osteoid osteoma). The term 'excision' is also synonymous with marginal resection, but is employed for tumors of the soft tissues (e.g. excision of a subcutaneous lipoma).

If at any time during the procedure the tumor is penetrated (because of clumsiness or because it is impossible to do otherwise) or if the tumor is removed in fragments, then the resection is said to be *'contaminated'*. It must then be considered as therapeutically inadequate, with an increased risk of local recurrence.

Reconstruction

Depending on the topography of the tumor, reconstruction (second stage of the procedure) relies on techniques of varying difficulty. These may be classified as follows.

1. *Cases where reconstruction is pointless*: the ribs, the upper three-quarters of the fibula, the obturator ring, the iliac wing, the blade of the scapula.

2. *Cases where simple continuity of the bone is to be restored* without reconstruction of the articulation (because the zone involved is non-articular or because loss of the joint is acceptable); this is the case in diaphysectomies and resection arthrodeses.

- *Diaphyseal reconstructions*[10] are made by combining

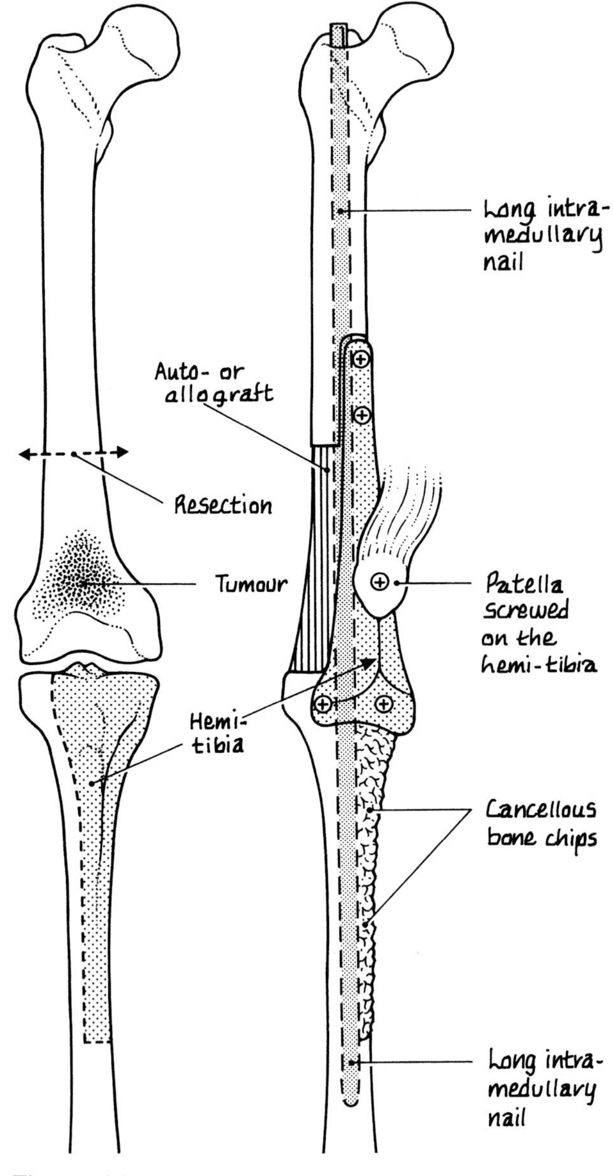

Fig. 56.6(a)

Fig. 56.5 (a) Resection arthrodesis of the knee (Juvara–Merle–d'Aubigne procedure): after removal of the lower femur the reconstruction is performed with a very long intramedullary nail; the defect is bridged by the ipsilateral hemitibia, a piece of allo- or autograft and some cancellous bone chips. (b) An example of this technique applied to a young woman with a multirecurrent giant cell tumor and the result after 11 years.

osteosynthesis and a bony contribution. Wherever technically possible, osteosynthesis by means of an intramedullary nail (Fig. 56.3) is to be preferred to other procedures (plate and screws, external fixators) as it provides an arrangement that is both stronger and better tolerated in the long term.

The bone element may be supplied by autografts or bank allografts or both. Difficulties of consolidation at either end of the assembly remain common; many patients need to be reoperated for pseudarthrosis or recurrent fracture, especially in cases where only allografts are used. When possible, autografts remain preferable, whether these are free bony transplants or, better, vascularized transplants[11,12] (transposition of a bony segment with its vessels (Fig. 56.4), which are anastomosed to the vessels of the receptor site).

- *Resection arthrodeses*[12,13,14] are used at the knee (where they are known by the name of Juvara's operation (Fig. 56.5)) and also at the wrist and ankle; elsewhere (shoulder, elbow, hip) they are little used because bony fusion is more difficult to obtain and joint stiffness is more difficult to tolerate. The choice between resection prosthesis (see 3 below) and resection arthrodesis is either a matter of personal choice or subject to technical limitations. If, in a resection of the knee, it is not possible to preserve or restore a proper extensor apparatus (quadriceps-patella-patellar tendon) it is preferable to get the patient to accept the disadvantages of an arthrodesed knee.

3. *Cases where an attempt is made to reconstruct an articulation* after having resected an epiphysis or a metaphysioepiphyseal zone. We shall not give an exhaustive review of the surgical techniques, which are numerous and still in the course of development. However, the following may be distinguished.

- Massive so-called *'conventional' prostheses*[15,16,17] where only metal and plastic replace the bone removed. Such

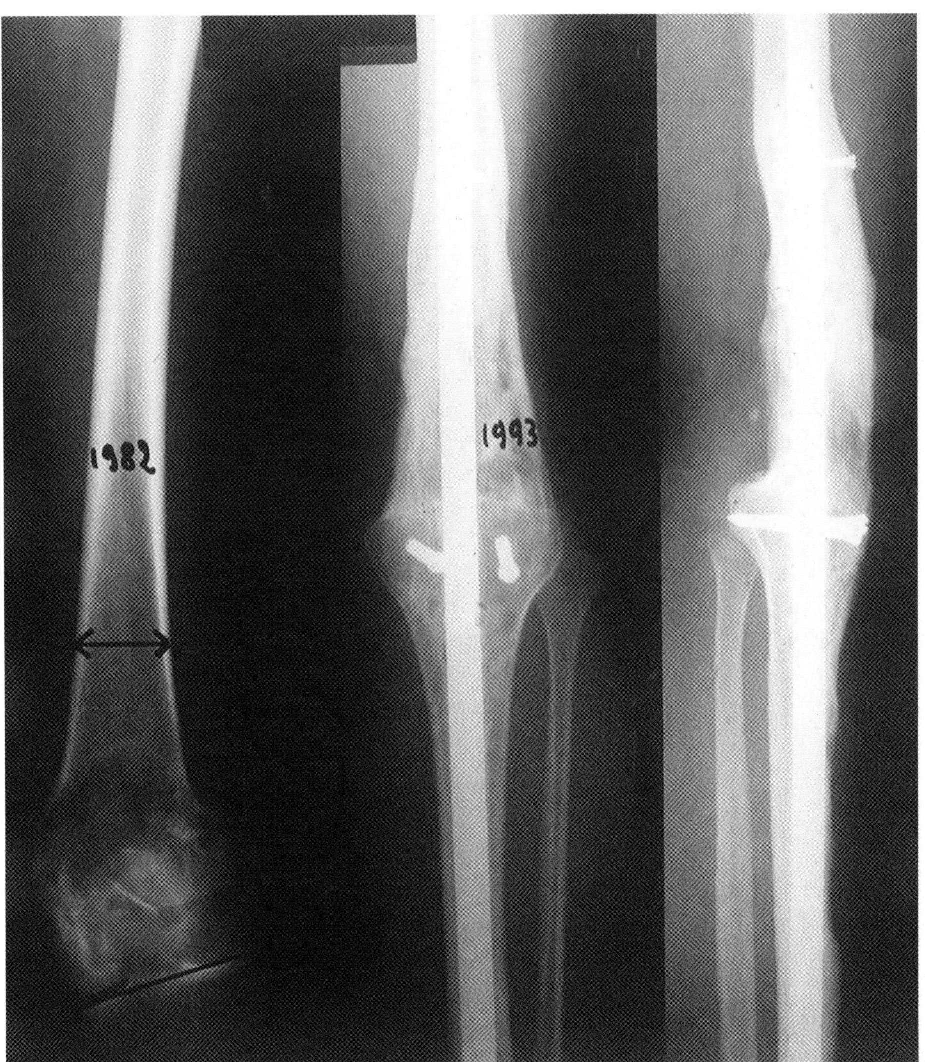

Fig. 56.5(b)

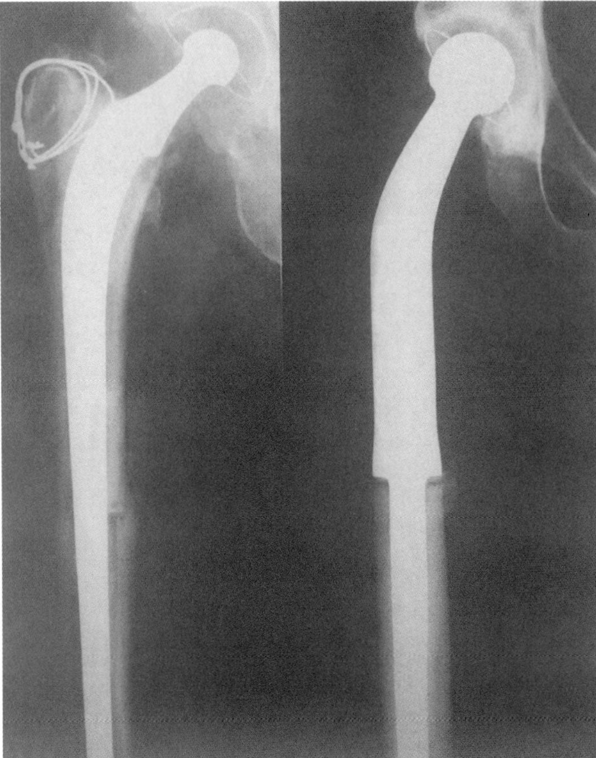

Fig. 56.6 Two types of massive hip reconstruction after resection of the proximal femur. Composite technique on the left (long stem prosthesis surrounded by a bone bank allograft); conventional massive hip prosthesis on the right.

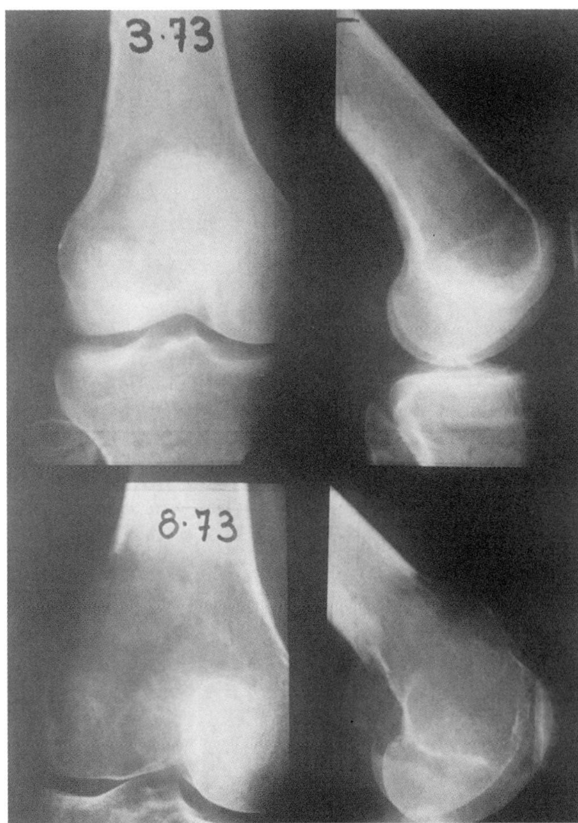

Fig. 56.7(a)

implants are currently used at the hip (Fig. 56.6 right), knee (Fig. 56.7) and shoulder (Fig. 56.8).

- Prostheses cuffed with *allografts*:[18,19] implants are used with stems of small diameter but these are surrounded by a bone cylinder obtained from a banked long bone. This procedure is very fashionable, but follow-up of operated patients after 5 or 6 years shows that quite often the allografts end by being absorbed or fragmenting (Fig. 56.9), causing loosening of the prosthesis and reoperations. It is only at the hip (Fig. 56.6 left) that the long-term functional results remain superior to those obtained by massive 'conventional' prostheses.

- *Massive simple allografts* (without an associated prosthesis) by transplantation of an entire banked articulation (or hemiarticulation) have a very uncertain future. Some

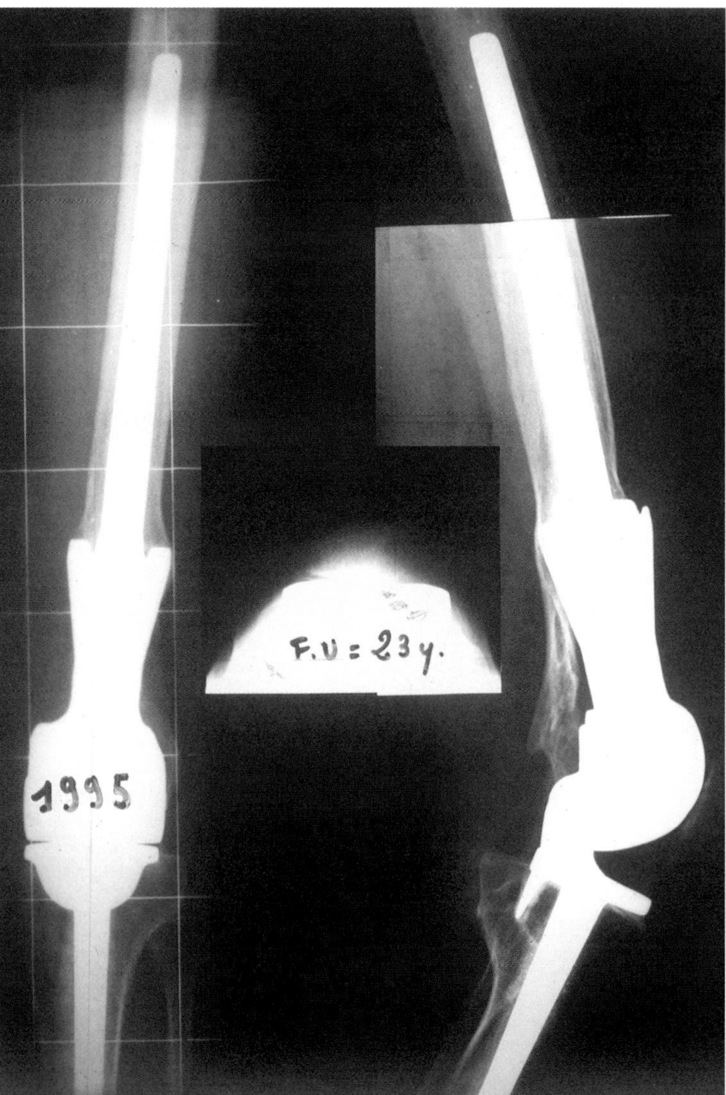

Fig. 56.7(b)

Fig. 56.7 (a) Aggressive giant cell tumor of the distal femur.
(b) Resection of the lower femur. Reconstruction with a conventional massive knee prosthesis. Excellent functional result more than 20 years later.

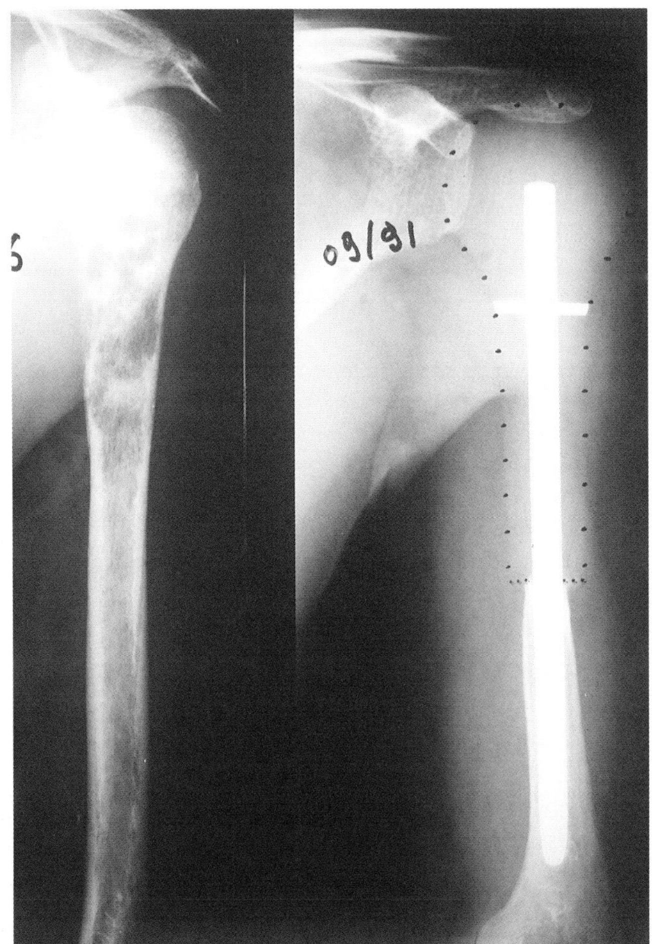

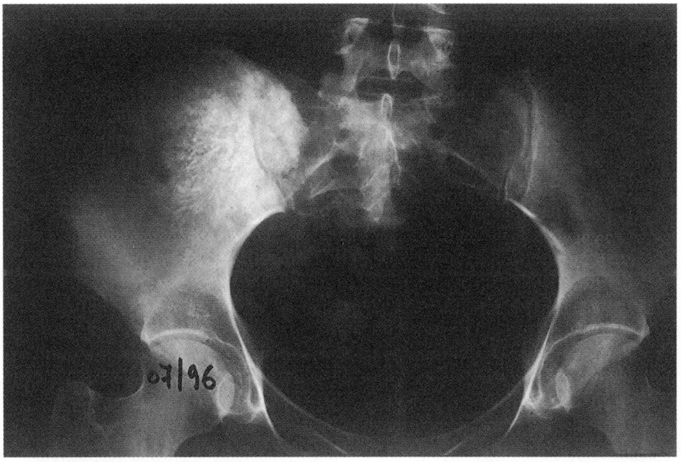

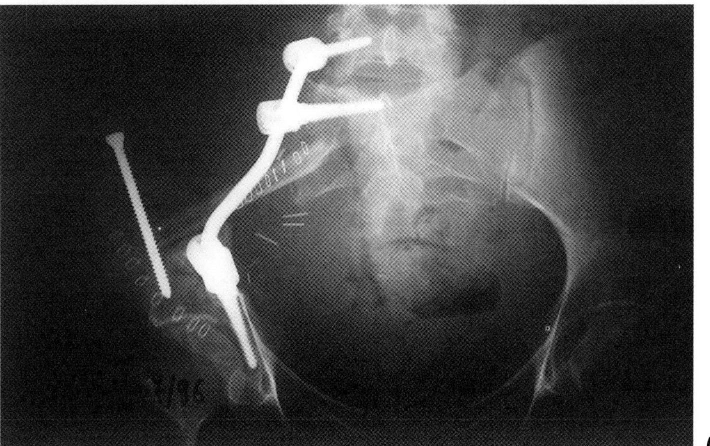

Fig. 56.8 After resection of the upper part of the humerus for osteosarcoma, the reconstruction is performed using a polyethylene prosthesis cuffing a metallic stem.

Fig. 56.10 (a) Osteosarcoma of the posterior part of the iliac wing. (b) Resection of this wing. Reconstruction between the sacrum and the acetabular top using osteosynthesis and autografts.

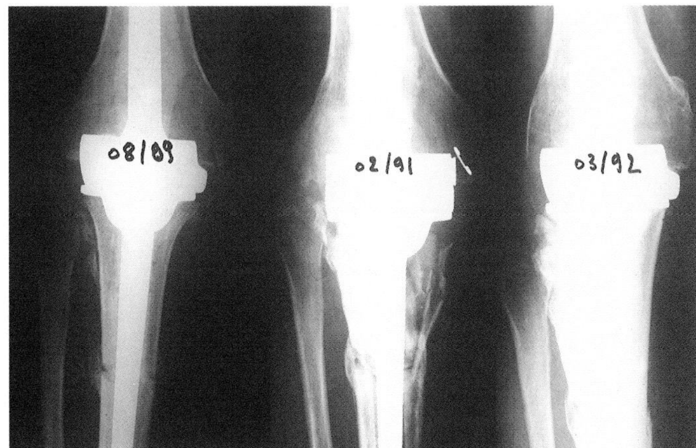

Fig. 56.9 Resection of the proximal tibia for osteosarcoma. The stem of the tibial component is surrounded by a massive bone bank allograft (on the left). In the middle, failure of the graft after 2 years by fragmentation and microfracture at the distal junction, shortening of the limb (note the fibula in contact with the condyle). The patient has been reoperated with a new allograft (on the right).

seem to be immediate successes but do not remain so in the long term because the transposed joint, deprived of all bony innervation, ends by behaving like a tabetic joint. They are therefore little used.

- *Longevity of prosthetic reconstructions*:[19,20] it would be naïve to believe that resection reconstructions allow life to continue indefinitely without serious problems. All prosthetic material is subject to wear, corrosion, loosening, even breakage, etc. As regards massive knee prostheses (as an example and considering this site only because it is by far the commonest), the chances that the prosthesis will still be in place (and in a functional condition) after 10 years are around 50%.

4. *Special cases of reconstruction of the trunk*

- In the *pelvis*,[21–26] reconstruction is pointless for isolated resections of the obturator ring. Isolated resections of the iliac wing are easily repaired by means of grafts interposed between the sacrum and the acetabular roof (Fig. 56.10).

Resection reconstructions of the acetabulum (either iso-

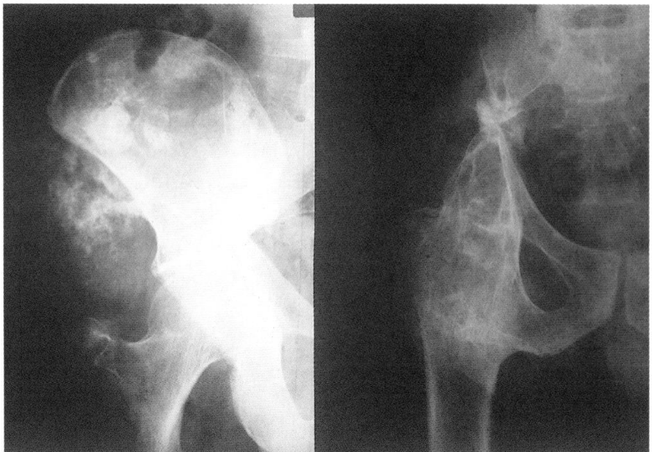

Fig. 56.11 Resection of the iliac wing and the acetabulum for chondrosarcoma. Reconstruction by arthrodesis between the upper femur and the obturator ring.

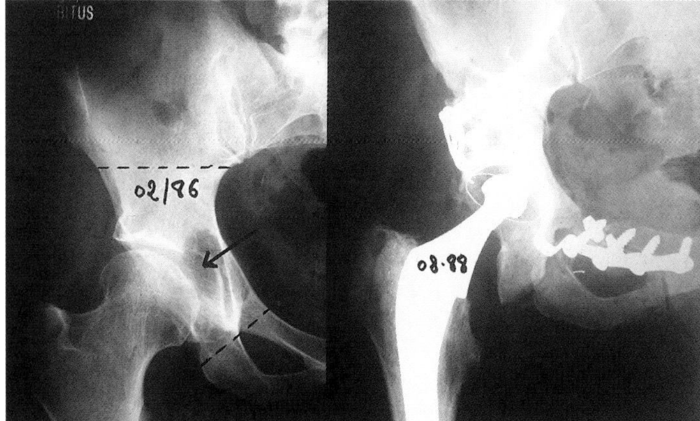

Fig. 56.12(a)

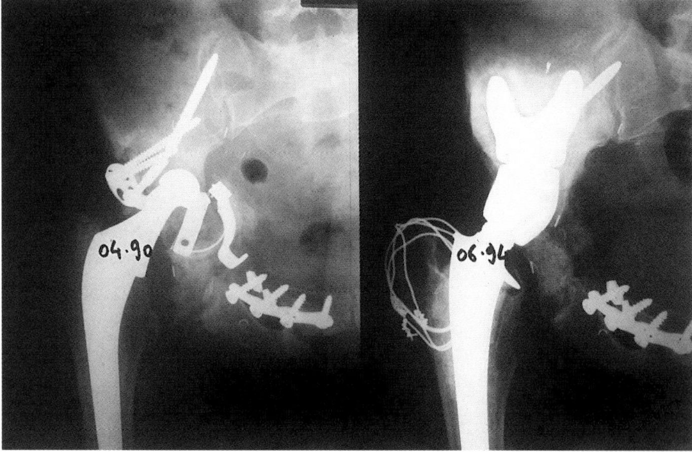

Fig. 56.12(b)

Fig. 56.12 (a) Resection (with monoblock arthrectomy) for an acetabular chondrosarcoma. The defect is filled with a pelvic bone bank allograft and a conventional hip prosthesis. (b) Some years later fracture of the allograft and loosening of the prosthesis occur (left). Secondary reconstruction (right) with a special prosthesis, the so-called 'saddle prosthesis'.[24] The remaining iliac wing is embedded in the concavity of the superior part (like an upside-down 'saddle') of the metallic component.

lated or combined with part of the iliac wing or obturator ring) are technically much more difficult. They rely on numerous and varied methods of repair which are not yet standardized. Theoretically, two methods are possible: to attempt an arthrodesis between the femur and what remains of the pelvis (Fig. 56.11) or else to try to reconstruct an articulation by bone grafts and/or a prosthesis (Figs 56.12a, 56.13). Postoperative complications are far from rare (Fig. 56.12b) and the functional outcome is often modest (or even debatable) and of uncertain duration.

• In the *mobile spine*, it is common to have to supplement the resection by a stage of stabilization (arthrodesis of several vertebrae). The different techniques of arthrodesis are now quite well mastered, whether these are posterior fusions (between the posterior arches) or anterior fusions (between the vertebral bodies). The resected vertebral bodies are usually reconstructed by means of bone

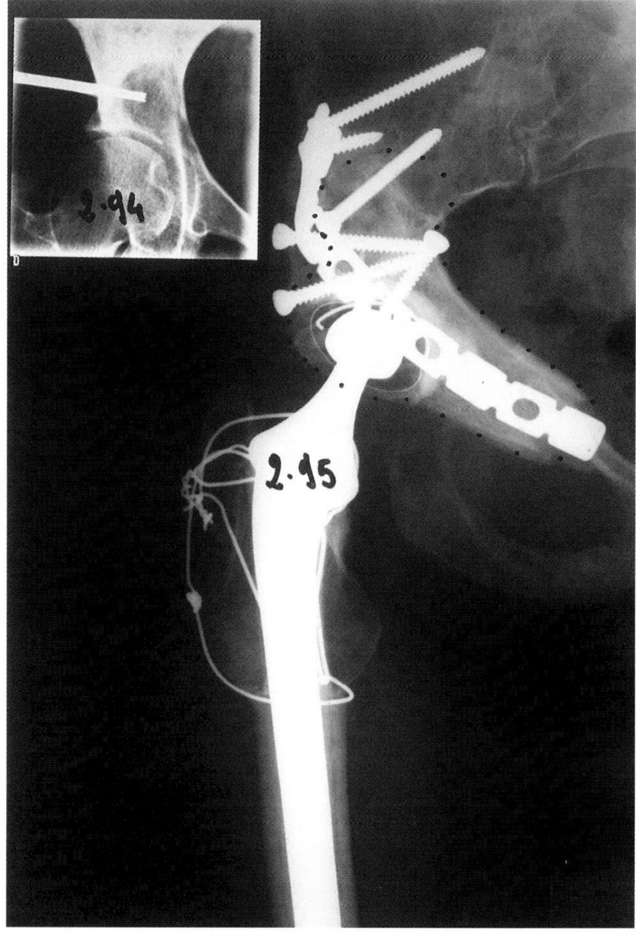

Fig. 56.13 Resection of the acetabulum for chondrosarcoma. The defect is bridged using the ipsilateral upper femur as an intercalary autograft between iliac wing and pubic ring (Puget's technique[25]). The cup of the total hip prosthesis is cemented into the trochanteric process of this graft. The proximal part of the femoral component is surrounded with a bone bank femoral head.

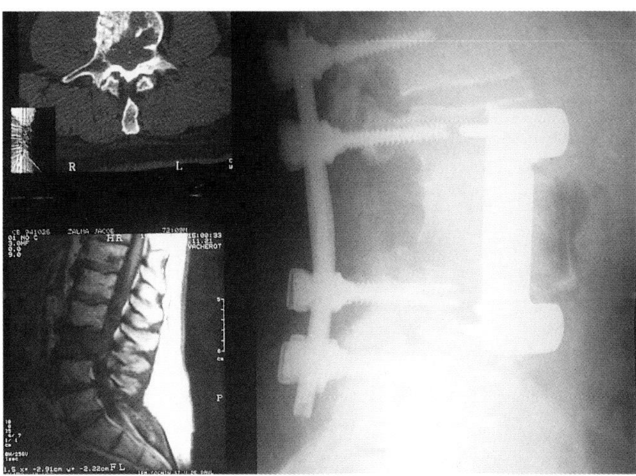

Fig. 56.14 Resection of the 3rd lumbar vertebra for chordoma. Using a posterior approach first, the posterior arch has been removed and an osteosynthesis performed, screwed into the vertebral pedicles. Using an anterolateral approach, the vertebral body has then been removed and replaced with a bone bank femoral head plus a screwed plate.

grafts (Fig. 56.14). In these spinal resections it is not uncommon to have to use a double approach, in one or two stages: one posterior (usual) and one anterior (by a lumbar approach or a thoracotomy). These procedures are usually quite formidable.

- *Malignant tumors of the sacrum*[27–29] (usually chordomas) are often treated by sacrectomy. Inferior partial sacrectomies (preserving only segments S1, S2 and sometimes S3) are simple enough procedures, which can be performed via a single posterior approach, do not require reconstruction and give rise to no orthopedic complications and few or no permanent genitourinary complications.

Total sacrectomies are quite another matter; the procedure is long and difficult and usually necessitates a double anterior and posterior approach and the collaboration of an orthopedic surgeon, a visceral and vascular surgeon and sometimes a urologist. Complications are common and neurologic sequelae are likely to be present, both in the lower limbs and in the genitovesicorectal complex: incontinence, impotence, iliac colostomy).

PROCEDURES SACRIFICING THE LIMB

Amputation and disarticulation are not necessarily synonymous with radical resection. An amputation may quite easily be marginal in relation to the disease (e.g. disarticulation of the hip for a large tumor of the entire proximal thigh) or even 'contaminated'. Conversely, amputation of the thigh for an osteosarcoma of the tibia is really a 'radical' procedure in Enneking's use of the term. Therefore, conservative surgery of the limb should not be routinely contrasted with its sacrifice.

Historically speaking, it is evident that amputation has become rare. Twenty-five years ago, sacrifice of the limb was considered obligatory for a primary malignant tumor in nine cases out of 10. Today, in at least nine cases out of 10, its preservation is possible. Resection without amputation, provided the lesion has been completely removed, in no way lessens the chances of cure.[30,31,32] What still sometimes compels us to consider the sacrifice of the limb is the state of the soft parts around the tumoral bone. In the bone itself, however extensive the tumor may be in length, we are always capable of resecting and replacing the skeletal segment more or less satisfactorily.

What compels us to amputate is what is happening around the bone:

- local infection (sometimes following biopsy) risks compromising the chances of reconstruction;
- preliminary irradiation may have led to sclerosis of the soft tissues, skin ulceration or joint stiffness in malposition such as severe flexion of the knee;
- the neurovascular axes are surrounded or invaded by the tumor (though it may still sometimes be possible to combine the resection with a vascular bypass or nerve graft);
- lastly, and most importantly, a very large extension into the soft tissues, although this may sometimes undergo considerable regression during preoperative chemotherapy; some patients considered for amputation at the time of initial diagnosis become resectable after 2–3 months of chemotherapy.

A special case is that of the young child who still has major potential for growth in length of the limbs. Resection reconstruction might be technically possible, but the healthy limb would grow independently ('extensible' prostheses[33,34] do exist but their performance is still limited). When the predicted inequality at the end of growth is too great it is unfortunately necessary to resort to amputation.

CONCLUSIONS: TREATMENT PROGRAMS RELATED TO DISEASES AND THEIR STAGE OF EVOLUTION

Benign tumors

1. *Benign and non-aggressive*:

- normally intraosseous tumors (chondroma, the 'quiet' form of giant cell tumor): curettage and packing;
- superficial bone tumors (osteochondromas, periosteal chondroma): marginal exeresis.

2. *Aggressive or multirecurrent benign tumors* (giant cell tumors of hyperactive type) and tumors whose benign nature has not been formally established: wide resection.

Malignant tumors

1. *Low malignancy*: in principle a wide resection, but this can be partly marginal if necessary (e.g. parosteal osteosarcoma).
2. *High malignancy*: wide resection (or radical for those who accept Enneking's principles); amputation (rare) is reserved for tumors with extensive local invasion, certain non-resectable recurrences and severe vascular or infective complications, as well as tumors in young children, as explained above in the paragraph dealing with amputation.
3. For *irretrievable cases* (tumors with metastases, lesions that are anatomically irremovable, secondary tumors, etc.): palliative surgery by partial resection, resection by fragmentation (= contaminated), curettage and packing with or without osteosynthesis.

Supplementary treatment

In this surgically oriented chapter, we have deliberately ignored the subject of complementary treatments of malignant lesions. Nevertheless, these are of cardinal importance.

Radiotherapy has lost ground in recent years but retains some indications: malignant tumors for which wide and complete exeresis is impossible because of the site of the lesion (axial skeleton), extensive local invasion, recurrences, etc. The indications for radiotherapy must also allow for the radiosensitivity of the tumor (Ewing's sarcoma is very radiosensitive, chondrosarcomas are usually radioresistant).

We note that for all highly malignant tumors of bone or soft tissues it is now customary to precede and follow the surgical procedure with several weeks of *chemotherapy*.

In fact, such so-called 'complementary' treatments have often become the principal treatments for these disorders thanks to which the prognosis has been considerably improved over the last 25 years. In very general terms, it may be argued that at the present time about two-thirds of primary malignant tumors of the locomotor system are curable, compared with a fifth a quarter of a century ago.

REFERENCES

1. Campanacci M, Baldini N, Boriani S, Sudanese A. Giant-cell tumor of bone. J Bone Joint Surg (Am) 1987: 69: 106–114
2. Gitelis S, Mallin B A, Piasecki P, Turner F. Intralesional excision compared with en bloc resection for giant-cell tumors of bone. J Bone Joint Surg (Am) 1993: 75: 1648–1654
3. Merle d'Aubigné R, Tomeno B. The treatment of giant-cell tumors. An analysis of 85 consecutive cases. Int Orthop 1977: 1: 159–164
4. O'Donnell R J, Springfield D S, Motwani H K et al. Recurrence of giant-cell tumors of the long bones after curettage and packing with cement. J Bone Joint Surg (Am) 1994: 76: 1827–1832
5. Enneking W F, Spanier S S, Goodman M A. A system for the surgical staging of musculoskeletal sarcoma. Clin Orthop 1980: 153: 106–120
6. Enneking W F. A system of staging musculoskeletal neoplasms. Clin Orthop 1986: 204: 9–24
7. Picci P, Bacci G, Ferrari S et al. Local recurrences after limb salvage procedures for osteosarcoma: correlation with margins and chemotherapy induced necrosis. Rev Chir Orthop 1993: 79: numero spécial (1er Congrés Europèen d'Orthopédie), abstract n°. 29
8. Rydho A, Rooser B. Surgical margins for soft-tissue sarcoma. J Bone Joint Surg (Am) 1987: 69: 1074–1078
9. Saddegh M K, Lindholm J, Lundberg A et al. Staging of soft-tissue sarcomas. Prognostic analysis of clinical and pathological features. J Bone Joint Surg (Br) 1992: 74: 495–500
10. Tomeno B, Gerber C. Les résections-reconstructions diaphysaires des grands os des membres. A propos de 23 cas. Rev Chir Orthop 1987: 73: 131–136
11. Gilbert A. Surgical technique. Vascularized transfer of the fibular shaft. Int J Microsurg 1979: 1: 100–106
12. Rasmussen M R, Bishop A T, Wood M B. Arthrodesis of the knee with a vascularized fibular rotatory graft. J Bone Joint Surg (Am) 1995: 77: 751–758
13. Juvara E. Procédé de résection de la partie supérieure du tibia. Presse Med 1921: 29: 241–243
14. Tomeno B, Istria R, Merle d'Aubigné R. La résection-arthrodèse du genou. Rev Chir Orthop 1978: 64: 323–332
15. Roberts P, Chan D, Grimer R J et al. Prosthetic replacement of the distal femur for primary bone tumours. J Bone Joint Surg (Br) 1991: 73: 762–769
16. Shih L, Sim F H, Pritchard D J, Rock M G, Chao E Y. Segmental total knee arthroplasty after distal femoral resection for tumor. Clin Orthop 1993: 292: 269–281
17. Bradish C F, Kemp H B, Scales J T et al. Distal femoral replacement by custom-made prosthesis. J Bone Joint Surg (Br) 1987: 69: 276–284
18. Dubousset J F, Missenard G. Allogreffes osseuses et résection pour tumeurs malignes au niveau des membres inférieurs. Acta Orthop Belg 1991 (suppl II): 90–97
19. Mankin H J, Gebhardt M C, Jennings L C, Springfield D S, Tomford W W. Long-term results of allograft replacement in the management of bone tumors. Clin Orthop 1996: 324: 86–97
20. Unwin P S, Cannon S R, Grimer R J et al. Aseptic loosening in cemented custom-made prosthetic replacements for bone tumors of the lower limb. J Bone Joint Surg (Br) 1996: 78: 5–13
21. Capanna R, Van Horn J R, Guernelli N. Complications of pelvic resections. Arch Orthop Trauma Surg 1987: 106: 71–77
22. Campanacci M, Capanna R. Pelvic resections. The Rizzoli Institute Experience. Orthop Clin North Am 1991: 22: 65–86
23. Enneking W F, Dunham W K. Resection and reconstruction for primary neoplasm involving the innominate bone. J Bone Joint Surg (Am) 1978: 60: 731–746
24. Nieder E, Elson R A, Engelbrecht E. The Saddle prosthesis for salvage of the destroyed acetabulum. J Bone Joint Surg (Br) 1990: 72: 1014–1022
25. Puget J, Utheza G. Reconstruction de l'os iliaque à l'aide du fémur homolatéral après résection pour tumeur pelvienne. Rev Chir Orthop 1986: 72: 151–155
26. Tomeno B. Procédés de reconstruction après résection totale ou partielle d'un hémibassin dans le traitement des tumeurs malignes de l'os iliaque. Rev Chir Orthop 1987: 77 (suppl 11): 95–98
27. Missenard G, Dubousset J, Genin J. Résection large de la sacro-iliaque. Technique, reconstruction, résultats anatomiques et fonctionnels. Rev Chir Orthop 1991: 77: 14–24
28. Samson I R, Springfield D S, Suit H D, Mankin H J. Operative treatment of sacrococcygeal chordoma. A review of twenty-one cases. J Bone Joint Surg (Am) 1993: 75: 1476–1484
29. Stener R, Gunterberg B. High amputation of the sacrum for extirpation of tumors. Principles and technique. Spine 1978: 3: 351–366
30. Stephenson R B, Kaufer H, Hankin F M. Partial pelvic resection as

an alternative to hindquarter amputation for skeletal neoplasms. Clin Orthop 1989: 242: 201–211

31. Dubousset J, Missenard G. Comparison of functional results of 26 patients with osteogenic sarcoma of the distal femur treated conservatively or by amputation. In: Enneking W F, Ed. Limb salvage in musculoskeletal oncology. New York: Churchill Livingstone, 1987, 435

32. Simon M A, Aschliman M A, Thomas N, Mankin H J. Limb salvage treatment versus amputation for osteosarcoma of the distal end of the femur. J Bone Joint Surg (Am) 1986: 68: 1331–1337

33. Gonzales-Herranz P, Burgos-Flores J, Ocete-Guzman J G et al. The management of limb-length discrepancies in children after treatment of osteosarcoma and Ewing's sarcoma. J Pediatr Orthop 1995: 561–565

34. Kenan S, Bloom N, Lewis M M. Limb-sparing surgery in skeletally immature patients with osteosarcoma. The use of an expandable prosthesis. Clin Orthop 1991: 270: 223–230

57

Surgical treatment of malignant bone tumors in children

H. Carlioz

INTRODUCTION

The treatment of malignant tumors of bone in children has made great strides over the last 20 years. The introduction of chemotherapy[1,2] has had two major consequences:

1. It has transformed the previously deplorable prognosis of osteosarcoma and Ewing's sarcoma, the two tumors of bone most common in childhood. Before the advent of chemotherapy, the 5-year cure rate in Ewing's sarcoma was less than 5%. In osteosarcoma it was of the order of 15–20%. These percentages have now increased to around 60%.[3]
2. By allowing tumor volume and soft tissue spread to be diminished, chemotherapy has also brought about a sea change in the outlook and methods of operative treatment.[4] Today, in the majority of cases, amputation has been superseded by excision of the tumor followed by reconstruction of the operated limb segment.[5,6]

Such conservative techniques had been developed for adult tumors before being used in children. In fact, the treatment of malignant tumors in adults and in children shares many common features.

In this pediatric chapter, we have limited ourselves to what is relevant in childhood alone. No details are given of aspects not specifically pediatric, including the basic principles of cancer surgery or the application of such principles, whenever this is identical to the management of adult cases. On the other hand, we emphasize whatever features of the treatment of childhood tumors are directly influenced by growth, by bone morphology in this age group, by the mechanical resistance of children's bones and by the presence of growth cartilage (GC).

Ewing's sarcoma sometimes affects very young children, whose slender diaphyses, with their low mechanical resistance, are ill suited to receiving a prosthesis.

Osteosarcomas, usually metaphyseal, often compromise the future development of the adjacent GC.[7]

The essential problems posed by malignant bone tumors in childhood therefore seem to us to be:

- a deficit in growth related to the unavoidable resection of one or two GCs because of their proximity to the tumor;
- the potential repercussions on growth cartilage of a prosthesis crossing it;
- the deterioration of joint prostheses, more rapid in children than in adults.

THE DEFICIT IN GROWTH DUE TO THE RESECTION OF GROWTH ZONES

Only the two surfaces of GC, epiphyseal and metaphyseal, are vascularized. No anastomoses between these two blood supplies cross the GC, which therefore acts as an ischemic barrier to invasion of the epiphysis by metaphyseal tumors.

It is important, in this context, to remember that none of the malignant bone tumors of childhood are of epiphyseal origin. When a tumor is excised, therefore, the epiphysis and the GC along with it should ideally be conserved. However, there are several potential reasons for including the GC and the adjoining epiphysis in the tumor resection:

1. The need to do so is obvious if the tumor has spread through the GC, the latter not being an absolute barrier despite its non-vascularity.
2. If the tumor extends to within 2 cm or less from the GC, it is best to include the GC in the resection.
3. Regardless of the tumor's spread within bone, if its soft tissue spread is extensive enough to straddle the periphery of the neighboring GC, it is wiser to sacrifice the latter. This is typically the case in an osteosarcoma of the distal end of the femur that remains at some distance from the GC within the bone but which spreads up to the top of the quadriceps bursa, making it necessary to remove the entire knee joint and the inferior femoral GC along with it.
4. Consequences of the absence of GC.[8]

Whatever the reason for which the GC has had to be removed, the consequence will be a predictable diminution of the length of the operated limb segment. The younger the child at the time of operation, the greater the discrepancy will be. The problem is thus more common in Ewing's sarcoma, which can affect very young children, than in osteosarcoma, which occurs more often in adolescence.

On the other hand, the commonest site of osteosarcoma is around the knee, in the distal metaphysis of the femur or the proximal metaphysis of the tibia. The two corresponding GCs are among the most active of those of long bones. The distal femoral cartilage contributes some 70% of the femur's residual growth and the proximal tibial cartilage some 55% of that of the tibia. If both have to be destroyed by the implant, a total knee prosthesis for example, less than 60% of the lower limb future growth will be lost.

Tables of long bone growth allow the degree of shortening that will result from resection of any particular GC to be forecast with adequate accuracy.[9,10,11] Thus, obliteration of the distal femoral GC in an 8-year-old boy will cause a discrepancy in length of 10 cm between the two lower limbs. If the proximal tibial GC also has to be destroyed, a discrepancy of 16–17 cm will have to be taken into account. At the same age, excising a tumor of the upper humerus together with the adjacent proximal GC (responsible for 80% of residual growth of the arm) will result in shortening of 8–10 cm.

In the lower limbs, a predicted discrepancy in length not exceeding 5–6 cm can be readily treated by means of contralateral epiphysiodesis, even if it means leaving a permanent but untroublesome difference of 1–2 cm. This is what happens in the majority of tumors in adolescents; the epiphysiodesis can be carried out immediately under the same anesthetic, or at least during the same hospital stay, as the operation for tumor resection and reconstruction. As we will see later, in the majority of cases reconstruction is achieved by means of an endoprosthesis.

When a greater discrepancy in length is predicted, it might, theoretically at least, necessitate later operative lengthening of the unaffected segment of the lower leg in the case of a femoral resection or the thigh in the case of a tibial tumor.

In practice, such a heavy program of surgical lengthening procedures takes 6 months out of a child's family life and school career and is rarely considered for a child already heavily burdened by the disease, chemotherapy, biopsy and operative resection. It is not even a possibility if the diaphyseal canal contains the stem of an endoprosthesis. The problem of length discrepancy therefore has to be tackled straight away, at the same time as the operation to excise the tumor.

One solution consists of reconstructing the resected region, not with a normal endoprosthesis comparable to that used in adults but with a special endoprosthesis that can be elongated little by little over the years following the resection reconstruction operation.

Such extendible prostheses were developed in the 1980s,[12,13] but, while no longer in the experimental phase, they are still subject to mechanical problems, jamming or breakage of the elongation system which, added to the complications common to all endoprostheses, restricts their use.

Lengthening of 19 cm has been achieved by means of these techniques,[21] but nevertheless, it seems wise to us to avoid their use for forecast discrepancies of more than 10 cm, even though the yield of contralateral epiphysiodesis should be taken into account.

The choice of reconstruction method following tumor excision thus becomes very difficult when the predicted discrepancy in length is as much as 10 or 15 cm. For example, resection of the distal end of the femur in a 5-year-old child with Ewing's sarcoma implies femoral shortening of around 15 cm, to which must be added a further 9 cm due to destruction of the proximal tibial GC if implantation of an endoprosthesis is planned. The same reasoning applies to a tumor of the proximal end of the tibia at the same age. A difference in length of this magnitude is intolerable. As we have just seen, this exceeds what can be considered a reasonable limit in the indications for reconstruction equalization using a prosthesis and epiphysiodesis. Amputation, once again, may have to be considered.

An external prosthesis allows normal social life and even some sporting activities to be pursued. This is especially true for a below-knee prosthesis in the case of a diaphyseal tumor of the tibia.

For femoral tumors, the stump of a thigh amputation is sometimes too short for a prosthesis to be fitted correctly. The stump needs to be almost the same length as the unaffected thigh for an external prosthesis with a flexible knee to be stable and well tolerated.

The extra length can be found in the lower leg below the resection of bone; it is preserved and brought up to the femoral section site, adjusting the heel to the right height for weight bearing in the prosthesis, just above the prosthetic knee joint. The forefoot, which now serves no purpose, is amputated to improve the appearance of the operated limb.

An improvement on this method consists of rotating the lower leg by 180° so that the heel is in front and the toes behind. The calf muscles, now anterior, take on the role of the quadriceps to move the knee joint of the prosthesis in extension; this is the Borggreve–Van Nes operation.[14] This rotation plasty gives patients an almost normal walking gait. Biodynamic studies have demonstrated better performances than those following classic amputation in terms of energy expenditure. The results of this procedure are comparable in both these aspects to those of a total knee endoprosthesis.[15]

The Borggreve–Van Nes operation carries a number of complications, including pseudarthrosis, compartment syndrome and late fracture, but one might expect its foremost disadvantage to be the unusual appearance it gives the lower limb, leading to harmful psychological consequences. In practice, this is not at all the case; the new orientation of the foot is well accepted and the result is not perceived as an amputation, as long as it has been properly explained and demonstrated prior to operation.

In summary, this is a suspended amputation which improves the external prosthesis and its use. The same principle has been extended to reconstructive surgery of

the hip after excision of tumor in the proximal part of the femur: the knee, brought up, turned around and fused to the pelvis, functions as a hip joint, while the foot replaces the knee, as in a Van Nes.[16]

REPERCUSSIONS ON GROWTH CARTILAGE OF A PROSTHESIS THAT CROSSES IT

When tumor excision and bone and joint reconstruction are possible, the ideal solution would be to use a graft of the same form and volume as that of the joint that has been removed. This could only be achieved by transplanting preserved cadaveric grafts.[17,18,19]

Unfortunately, the excellent short-term results cannot be maintained; osteoarticular transplants undergo gradual destruction and fragmentation and have to be replaced secondarily by endoprostheses.

Bone and joint reconstruction is therefore now only carried out using internal prostheses, custom made but essentially comparable to those used in adult degenerative disease.

In some tumor sites, prostheses can be implanted without requiring the sacrifice of GCs other than the one resected along with the tumor. Such is the case in tumors of the proximal end of the humerus and sometimes even in tumors of the femoral neck when it is deemed sufficient to replace the proximal end of the femur with a head and neck prosthesis without modifying the corresponding acetabular component.

Nevertheless, the majority of tumor excisions with joint reconstruction are carried out for tumors of the upper tibia or lower femur. The prosthetic replacement joint is fixed above and below the knee by stems which penetrate a long way into the medullary canal; the healthy GC is therefore crossed by the prosthesis which, if cemented in place, acts on it like a permanent epiphysiodesis. The final discrepancy in length is aggravated as a direct result; this problem was discussed in the first section of this chapter.

To avoid this harmful effect, it is possible to omit cementing the prosthesis in place on the healthy, non-tumor side of the joint. Harris lines, visible on follow-up radiographs over subsequent years, prove that it is possible in this way to preserve the growth function of a GC crossed by the prosthesis. However, it cannot be said that in the long term a GC crossed by a prosthesis, even without cement, will retain normal function. Furthermore, the absence of cement adversely affects the stability of the prosthesis. Further surgery may be necessary after some years, during which growth will have progressed; in this context, secondary cementing of the prosthesis will therefore have few consequences. Biological anchoring of the prosthesis, stimulated by giving it a porous surface texture, is not an alternative way of circumventing the 'epiphysiodesis' effect, as it will cause no less harm than cement.

SHORT LIFE OF TOTAL REPLACEMENT PROSTHESES IN CHILDREN

Children's higher level of activity, and probably also the poorer mechanical qualities of bone prior to completion of growth, may explain the high frequency of early aseptic loosening that their prostheses undergo compared to those of adults.[20]

When this occurs a revision operation is mandatory, either to change the prosthesis or to put the same prosthesis back into position, cementing it in place if it was not already cemented. For mechanical reasons aseptic loosening occurs more frequently in distal femoral or tibial prostheses than at any other site and unfortunately these are the prostheses most often used in pediatric oncology.

CONCLUSION

In children, as in adults, so-called 'radical' operations involving disarticulation and amputation have lost many of their indications in the treatment of malignant bone tumors.

Conservation of the limb is the usual solution and this means resection of the tumor using the principles of cancer surgery to dissect through healthy tissue and the replacement of lost structure by bone grafts or internal prostheses. There are few features of excision, grafting and implanting that are specific to children and we have therefore not dwelt on these techniques.

On the other hand, the anatomical conditions specific to childhood, the presence of active GCs and the small caliber of diaphyses, modify the indications for bone and joint reconstruction.

The difficulties involved in implanting endoprostheses in young children, their complications and the consequent paucity of indications for extendible prostheses, have already been sufficiently emphasized. The case of a prosthesis put in place at the age of 3 years is not, in our view, an example to be followed.[20]

Finally, here are some schematic indications for the treatment of malignant bone tumors in young children:

Lower limb

The GC of the proximal end of the femur (femoral head and neck) is not very active. Its obliteration, even at the age of 8 years, will result in a length discrepancy small enough to be corrected by epiphysiodesis. At this age and above, therefore, reconstruction using a femoral prosthesis is practicable. For a child considerably younger, a rotation operation would be preferable to disarticulation.

For tumors of the knee region,[21] if the length discrepancy resulting from resection and reconstructive surgery is likely to be as much as 15 cm, the Borggreve–Van Nes operation would be a more satisfactory solution. If the discrepancy is likely to be around 10 cm, an extendible prosthesis associated with a contralateral epiphysiodesis could be used. If it is likely to be less than 7–8 cm, a custommade endoprosthesis of the usual type, along with a contralateral epiphysiodesis, should suffice.[22]

At the distal end of the tibia, according to the patient age and the degree of local tumor spread, a below-knee amputation or excision followed by reconstruction using an autogenous vascularized fibular graft both yield an excellent functional outcome.

Upper limb

The final length of the operated limb is less important than in the lower limb; whenever possible, the hand is preserved.

Resection of a tumor of the proximal end of the humerus does not necessarily have to be followed by prosthetic reconstruction of the shoulder. The stability of this joint is of secondary importance. A medullary nail attached to the acromion can be enough to insure satisfactory use of the elbow and hand.

Diaphyseal tumors

These are treated by resection and reconstruction whenever the degree of regional spread permits. If the GCs at both ends of the bone are conserved, there will be no shortening of the operated limb and the conditions are close to those encountered in adults. A graft of diaphyseal bone from the bone bank,[23] or better still an autogenous vascularized fibular graft, will refashion good quality 'organic' bone.

Other sites

Some bones can be removed and left unreconstructed without disability: the scapula, the clavicle, the metacarpals and metatarsals, the upper 3/4 of the fibula.

In the pelvis, osteosarcoma is rare. Ewing's sarcomas are excised and reconstructive surgery, rather than being anatomical, should aim to restore the continuity of the pelvic ring, generally using autologous bone grafts.

Tumors of the vertebral column can rarely be resected satisfactorily in accordance with the principles of cancer surgery. Chemotherapy will be required, complemented by radiotherapy.

REFERENCES

1. Hudson M, Jaffe M R, Jaffe N, Ayala A. Pediatric osteosarcoma: therapeutic strategies, results and pronostic factors derived of a 10 years experience. J Clin Oncol 1990: 8: 1988–1997
2. Miser J S, Kinsella T J, Triche T J. Preliminary results of treatment of Ewing's sarcoma of bone in children and young adults: six months of intensive combined modality therapy without maintenance. J Clin Oncol 1988: 6: 484–490
3. Mercuri M, Capanna R, Manfrini M et al. The management of malignant bone tumors in children and adolescents. Clin Orthop 1991: 264: 156–168
4. Lawrence J A. Extremity osteosarcoma in childhood: prognostic value of radiologic imaging. Radiology 1993: 189: 43–47
5. Dubousset J, Missenard G, Genin J. Traitement chirurgical conservateur des sarcomes ostéogéniques des membres. Techniques et résultats fonctionnels. Rev Chir Orthop 1985: 71: 435–450
6. Dubousset J, Missenard G, Kalifa Ch. Management of osteogenic sarcoma in children and adolescents. Clin Orthop 1991: 270: 52–59
7. Canadell J, Forriol F, Cara J A. Removal of metaphyseal bone tumours with preservation of the epiphysis. J Bone Joint Surg (Br) 1994: 76: 127–132
8. Gonzales-Herranz P, Burgos-Flores J, Ocete-Guzman J G et al. The management of limb-length discrepancies in children after treatment of osteosarcoma and Ewing's sarcoma. J Pediatr Orthop 1995: 561–565
9. Anderson M, Green W T, Messner N B. Growth and prediction of growth in the lower extremities. J Bone Joint Surg (Am) 1963: 45: 1–14
10. Héchard P, Carlioz H. Méthode pratique de prévision des inégalités de longueur des membres inférieurs. Rev Chir Orthop 1978: 64: 81–87
11. Moseley C. A straight line graph for leg-length discrepancies. J Bone Joint Surg (Am) 1977: 59: 174–179
12. Kenan S, Bloom N, Lewis M M. Limb-sparing surgery in skeletally immature patients with osteosarcoma. The use of an expandible prosthesis. Clin Orthop 1991: 270: 223–230
13. Schiller C, Windhager S, Salzer-Kuntschik M, Kaider A, Kotz R. Extendable tumour endoprostheses for the leg in children. J Bone Joint Surg (Br) 1995: 77: 608–614
14. Kotz R, Salzer M. Rotation plasty for childhood osteosarcoma of the distal part of the femur. J Bone Joint Surg (Am) 1982: 64: 959–969
15. Cammisa F P, Glasser D B, Otis J C, Kroll M A, Lane J M, Healey J H. The Van Nes rotationplasty: a functionally viable reconstructive procedure in children who have a tumor of the distal end of the femur. J Bone Joint Surg (Am) 1990: 72: 1541–1547
16. Winkelman W W. Hip rotationplasty for malignant tumors of the proximal part of the femur. J Bone Joint Surg (Am) 1986: 68: 362–369
17. Delepine G, Delepine N. Résultats préliminaires de 79 allogreffes osseuses massives dans le traitement conservateur des tumeurs malignes de l'adulte et de l'enfant. Int Orthop 1988: 12: 21–29
18. Kohler R, Corge F, Brumafmentigny M, Moyer D, Paricot L. Massive bone allograft in children. Int Orthop 1990: 14: 249–254
19. Mankin H J, Doppelt S H, Sullivan R, Tomford W W. Osteoarticular and intercalary allograft transplantation in the management of malignant tumors of bone. Cancer 1982: 50: 613–630
20. Unwin P S, Cannon S R, Grimer R J, Kemp H B S, Sneath R S, Walker P S. Aseptic loosening in cemented custom-made prosthetic replacements for bone tumours of the lower limb. J Bone Joint Surg (Br) 1996: 78: 5–13
21. Finn H A, Simon M A. Limb salvage surgery in the treatment of osteosarcoma in skeletally immature individuals. Clin Orthop 1991: 262: 108–118
22. Kotz R, Schiller C, Windhager R, Ritschl P. Endoprostheses in children. First results. In: Langlais F, Tomeno B, Eds. Limb salvage. Berlin: Springer-Verlag, 1991, pp 591–599
23. Cara J L, Canadell J. Limb salvage for malignant bone tumors in young children. J Pediatr Orthop 1994: 14: 112–118

58

Pathology of bone and joints after orthopedic reconstructive surgery

M. Forest

GENERAL CONSIDERATIONS

Histological patterns of bone and joint tissues after orthopedic reconstructive surgery are now an expanding field for the surgical pathologist faced with factors ranging from reactions to plates or screws to the most intricate custom-made prostheses used for limb salvage surgery after tumor resection.

Some limitations arise from the fact that many of the morphological results come from orthopedic research laboratories using time-consuming technical methods to make sections with the implant still in place. With common histological techniques, the most intimate contact between the implant and the living bone is not well demonstrated and wear effects may be over looked or underestimated; however, the surgical pathologist has to complete his report and retrieval analysis is an invaluable opportunity to determine the characteristics of the implant's success or failure.[1]

The diagnosis of infection should not give rise to serious difficulties, with the use of frozen sections or touch imprints, the most reliable index being the population density of neutrophils.[2–8]

Over a longer period of time, late loosening is the most common reason for revision surgery.[9]

Some basic histological features can be deduced from the tissue reactions to screws and plates[10] (Figs 58.1–58.6).

The necrotic bone induced by surgical trauma is removed by osteoclasts and new woven or lamellar bone is formed, sometimes incorporating dead bone.

The fixation of all implants depends initially on the establishment of a mechanical interlock between the implant and the bone.[11] If the junctional tissue stresses are low and micromovements small, the most intimate contact between the implant and bone leads to osseointegration.[11] High junctional tissue strains or micromovements induce osteoclastic activity, fibrogenesis or chondrogenesis. Predominantly compressive strains enhance the amount of

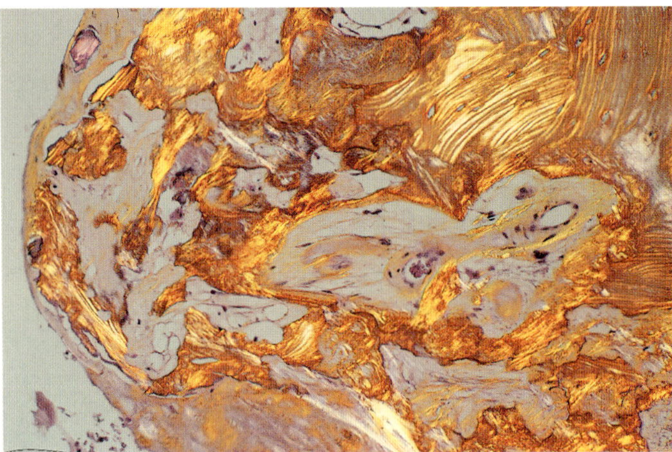

Fig. 58.1 Osteolysis and bone remodeling close to a compression screw (polarized light).

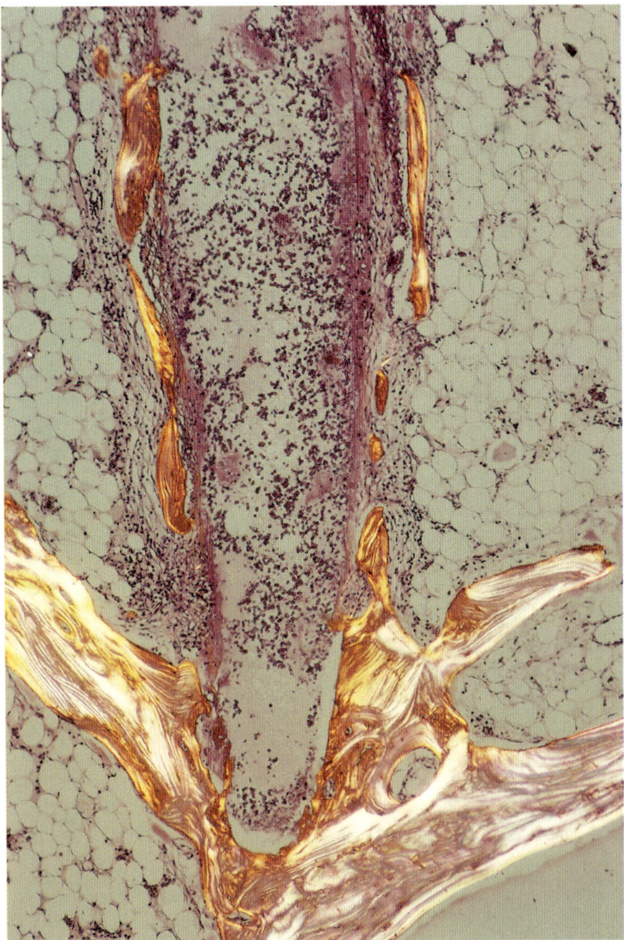

Fig. 58.2 Bone formation around the thread of a screw (polarized light).

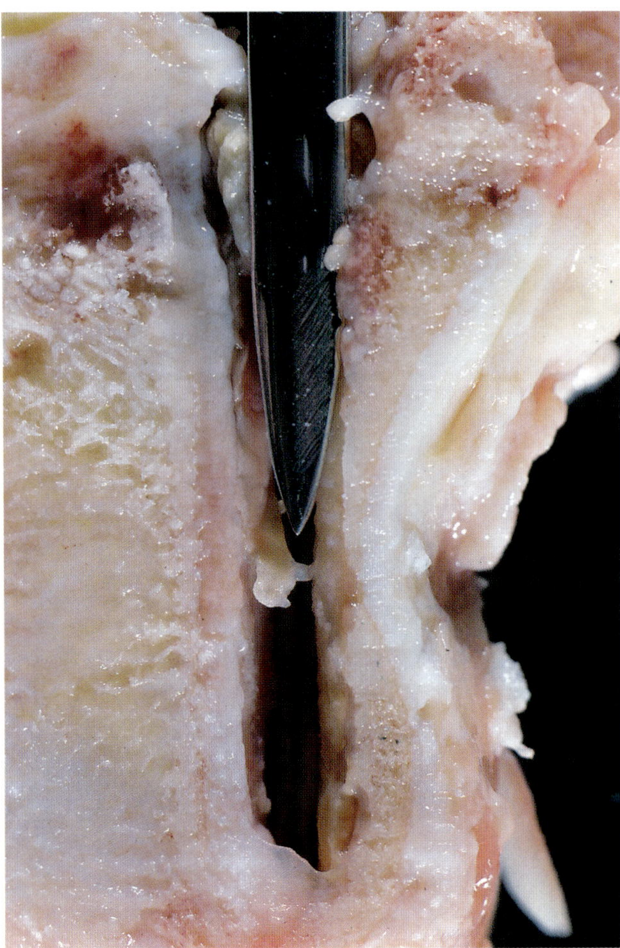

Fig. 58.3 Fibrous lining around a non-loosened plate in the femur.

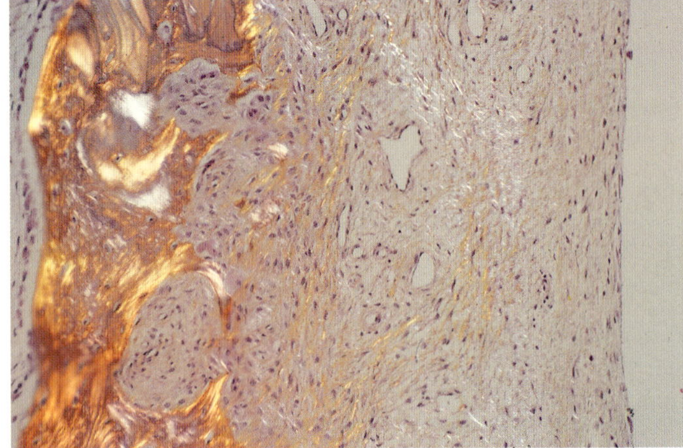

Fig. 58.4 Fibrous interface of a plate with peripheral remodeling of bone (polarized light).

fibrocartilage.[11] Inherent mechanical instability results in a replacement fibrosis following bone resorption, appearing as a fibrous encapsulation of the implant.[10]

TISSUES CLOSE TO WELL-FIXED ARTIFICIAL JOINT COMPONENTS

Repair following surgery in cemented total hip replace-

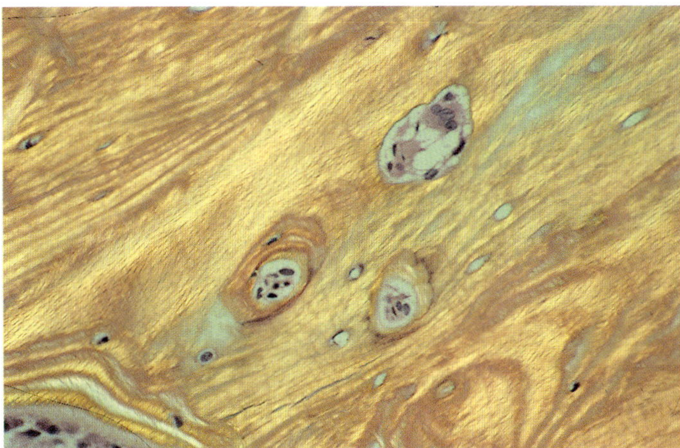

Fig. 58.5 Osteoblastic and osteoclastic activity in the cortex, close to a plate in the femur (polarized light).

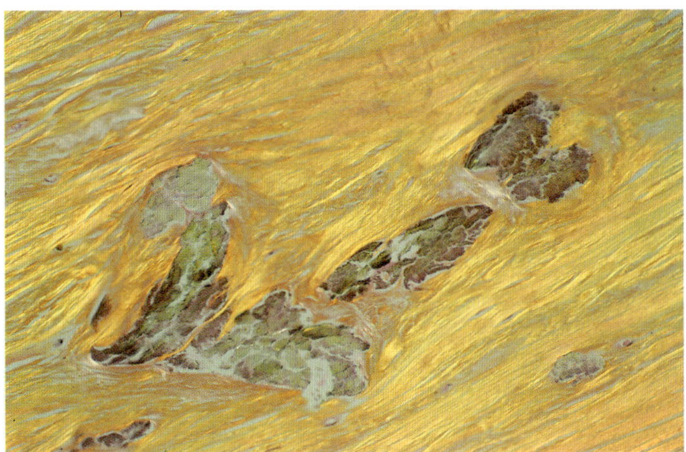

Fig. 58.6 Plate-like crystalline material due to corrosion, close to a screw plate (polarized light).

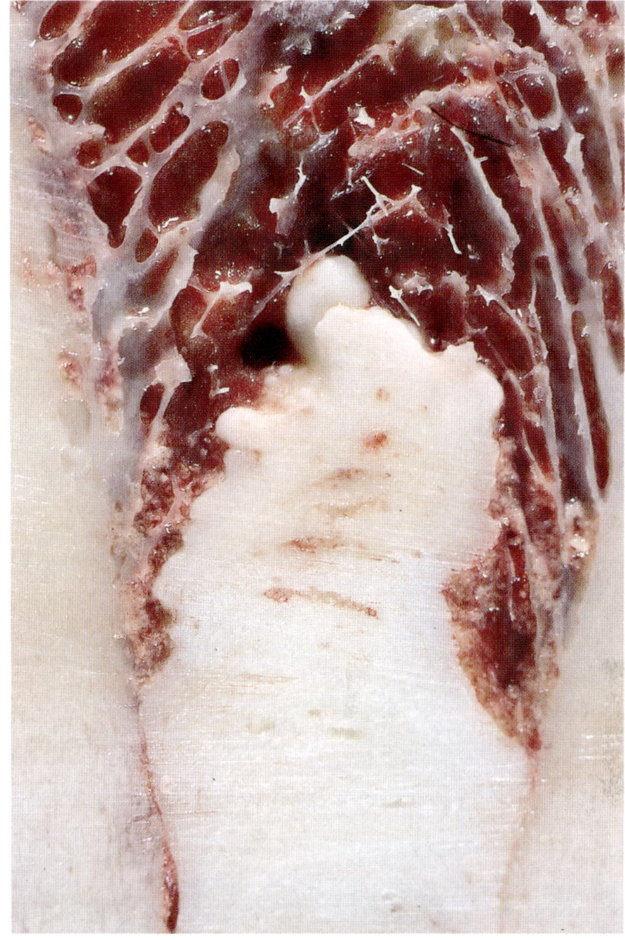

Fig. 58.7 Cement in the cancellous bone of the femur.

ments has been thoroughly investigated: bone necrosis is caused by the surgical reaming, heat of polymerization or toxicity of the unpolymerized monomer,[12] but the degree of tissue injury is limited, usually only a few millimeters.[13]

The implantation stage of the first weeks is followed by a healing process over several months, with removal of necrotic bone and new bone formation proceeding simultaneously.[9] Regeneration with bone remodeling and adaptation is completed in 2 years.[12,14]

A thin fibrous membrane develops between bone and cement[15,16] but bone can extend to the cement surface.[17] If there is initially a rigid fixation, osseointegration occurs; fibrous tissue is in fact rarely formed at the cement–bone interface.[18,19] An excellent interlock has been found even in specimens retrieved within the immediate postoperative period[16] (Figs 58.7–58.9).

On the ultrastructural level, cement may be in close contact with the living bone covered by a thin film of proteoglycans,[20] the markers of primary mineralization being extracellular matrix vesicles and calcifying nodules.[21]

The presence of reactive macrophages and giant cells at the bone–cement interface of stable prostheses has been repeatedly documented[9,12,22–26] and is viewed as a biologically unstable surface,[27] but this cellular component may be found without any obvious sign of bone resorption (Fig. 58.10).

The mechanical properties of the fibrous tissue at the interface have been evaluated experimentally; it has a mat-like structure and can resist compressive but not shearing stresses.[28]

Another membrane formation has been found between the femoral metal stem and the cement mantle in non-loosened as well as loosened components,[29] presumably induced by a shrinkage of the cement, thermal expansion of the stem, micromovements or organization of blood at the time of implantation[29] (Fig. 58.11).

The remodeling of bone results in an inner cortex around the cement mantle;[9,15,30] by a transfer of load, a secondary medullary canal is formed between the endo-

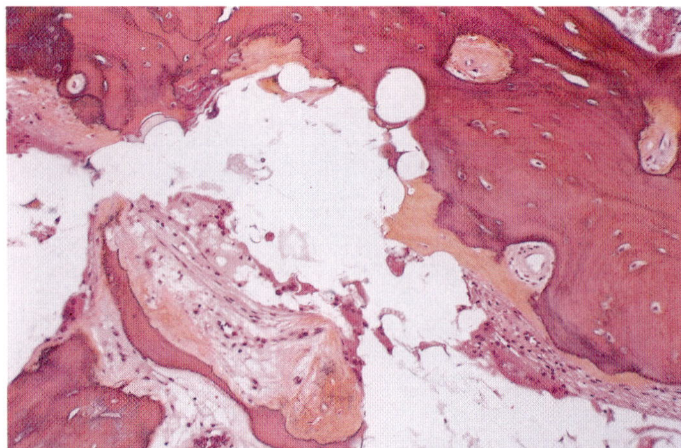

Fig. 58.8

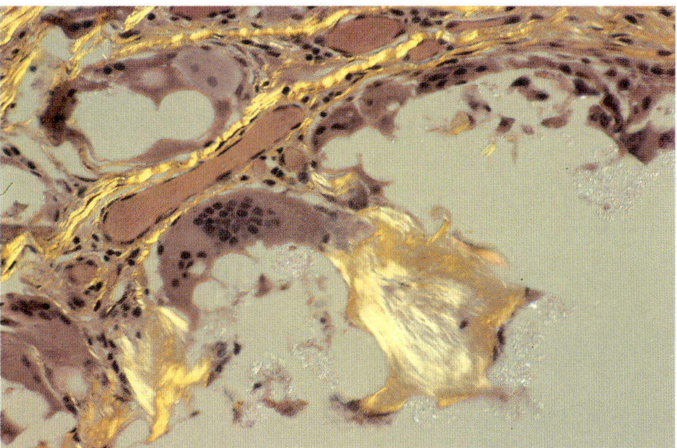

Fig. 58.9

Figs 58.8, 58.9 Hemispherical impressions in bone due to the dissolved cement with areas of osteoid production and some reactive giant cells, close to a well-fixed acetabular cup (Fig. 58.9: polarized light).

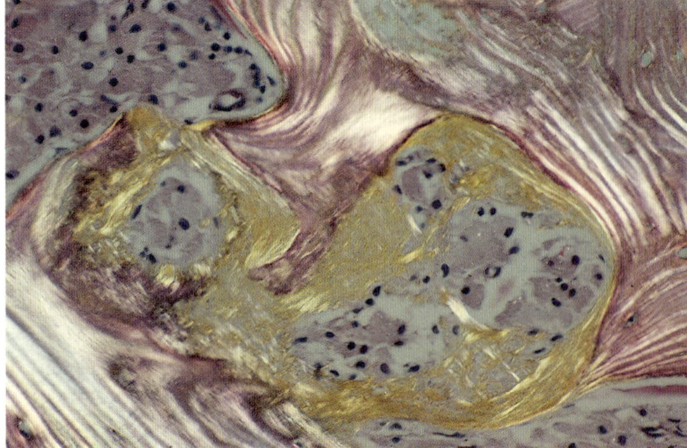

Fig. 58.10 Macrophages and woven bone in the metaphyseal area of a well-fixed total hip prosthesis.

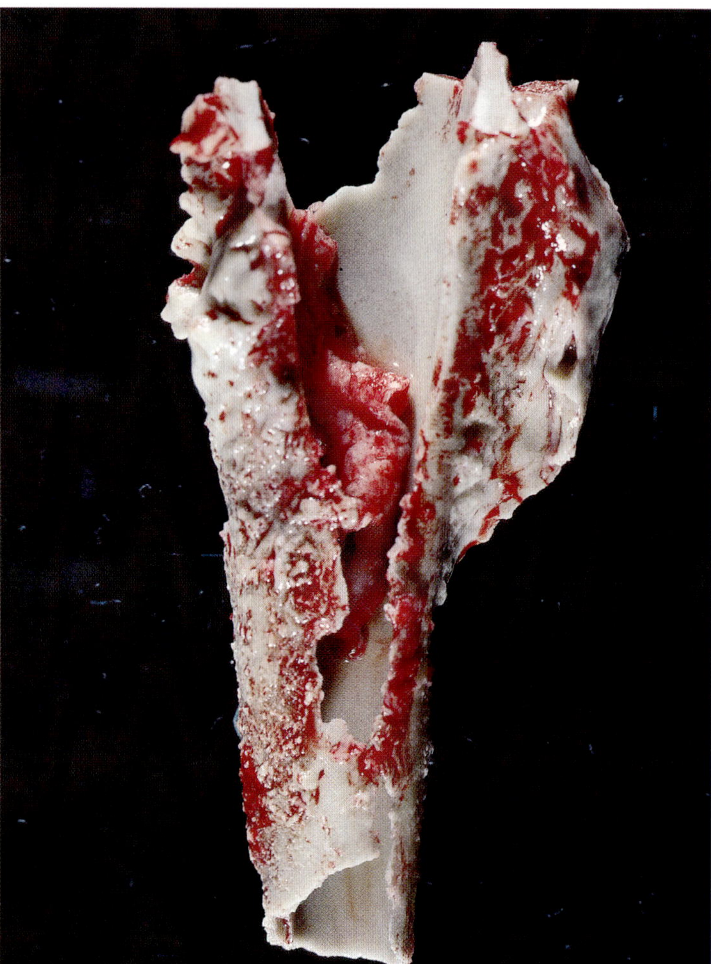

Fig. 58.11 Total hip prosthesis: mantle of cement with a membrane between the cement and the metal stem.

steal surface and the outer cortex. The endosteal remodeling is mainly responsible for the radiolucent lines.[30,31]

On retrieval specimens, there is a strong increase of osteoid at the bone–cement interface;[12,16,32,33] some ions released by the prosthesis (titanium, vanadium, aluminum) may interfere with the process of mineralization or act directly on the formation and growth of hydroxyapatite crystals.[34–36]

Non-loosened cementless femoral endoprostheses exhibit a thin fibrous lining, with fibrocartilage in the areas subjected to compressive load and a synovial-like lining depending on micromotion.[37–39]

Interfaces of non-loosened titanium hip prostheses may show a total osseointegration in the metaphysiodiaphyseal regions, whereas a membrane of connective tissue is interposed in the proximal areas. A secondary bone shell is also formed, with evidence of progressive bone remodeling.[40–42] Ultrastructurally, the new bone is in direct contact with the implant, the titanium being bordered by a layer of proteoglycans.[43]

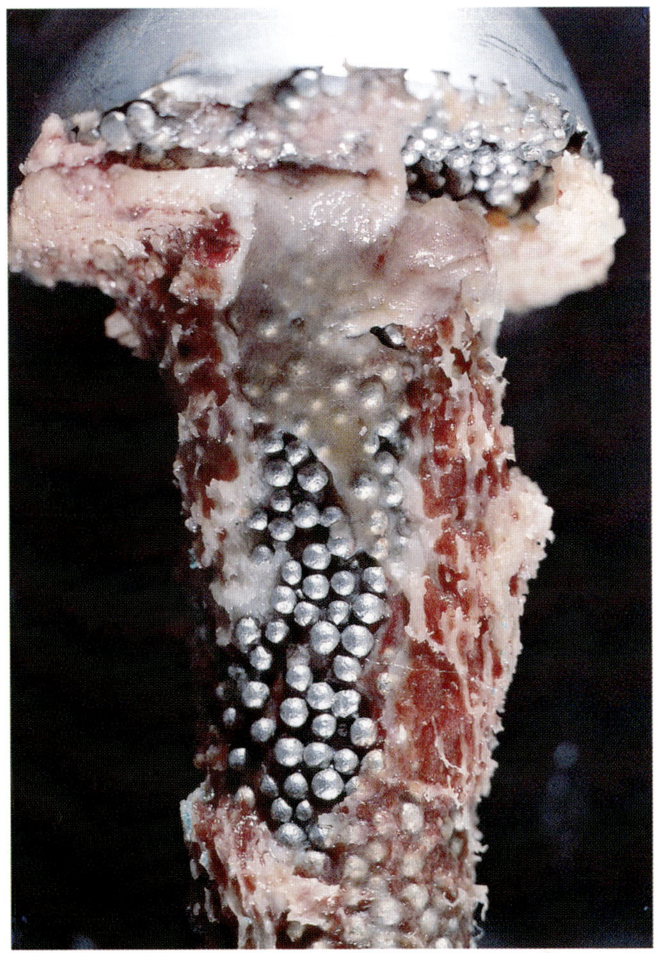

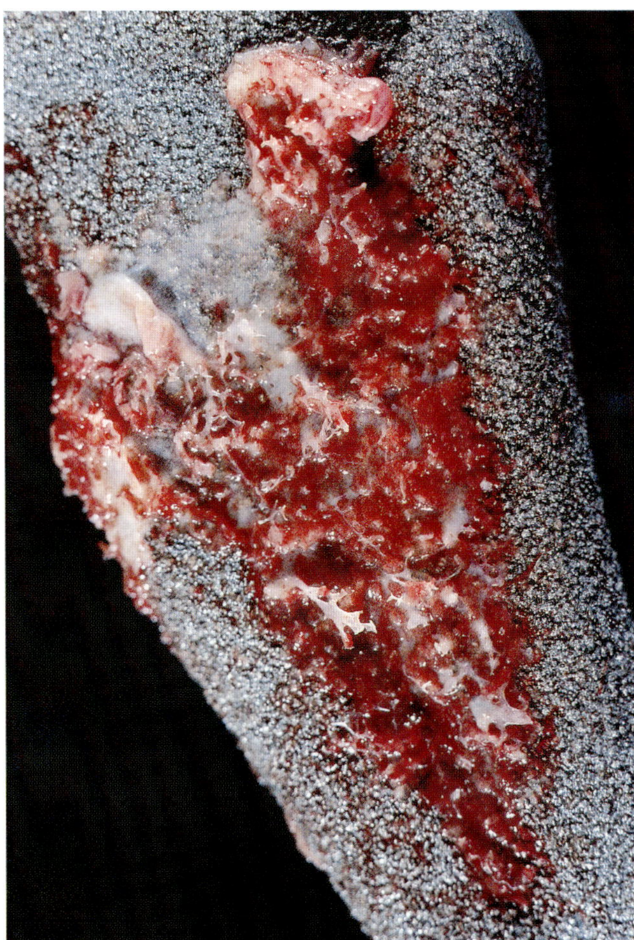

Fig. 58.12   **Fig. 58.13**

Figs 58.12, 58.13 Bone formation on femoral stems with macro- and microporosity (biologic ingrowth devices).

Numerous designs are used today as 'biologic ingrowth' prostheses, the macro- or microporosity of the stem providing a better biomechanical integration (Figs 58.12, 58.13). Bone ingrowth within a porous-coated implant is dependent on the pore size and the absence of initial implant micromovements;[44] it is primarily cortical and new endosteal bone forms a thin shell surrounding the implant[45] (Fig. 58.14).

A madreporic surface may be diffusely infiltrated by bone,[46] as well as porous-coated prostheses,[47] but in non-loosened prostheses, a large portion or even the whole of the porous surface can be devoid of any bone ingrowth, the bulk of the porous coating being covered by fibrous tissue[47–53] (Fig. 58.15). The limited degree of bone formation has been related to implant micromotion.[44]

A plasma-sprayed hydroxyapatite porous-coated implant increases the amount of bone ingrowth and skeletal attachment,[54,55] the space between the viable host bone and the prosthesis being rapidly bridged by new bone trabeculae.[56–59] Hydroxyapatite ceramics are osteoconductive, act-

ing as a scaffold for the ingrowth of new bone,[60] but the main problem is the strength of the coating–substrate interface.[60]

The articular capsule, usually completely removed during operation, regenerates within 6 months,[9] with a loose synovial tissue which is denser at the periphery and a flattened lining with cuboid or columnar cells.[9]

HISTOLOGICAL IDENTIFICATION OF WEAR DEBRIS

Most of the particles produced by wear or corrosion of implants are of submicron size and routine histological examination does not give a true estimate of their amount;[38,39,61,62] electron microscopy and spectroscopic techniques may be required.

Polymethylmethacrylate (self-curing bone cement) appears as single polymer spheres of approximately 30 μu in diameter,[63] or as large aggregates over 100 μu with a mulberry configuration[9,64] resulting from microfragmentation of the cement surface, abrasion or incomplete polymerization.

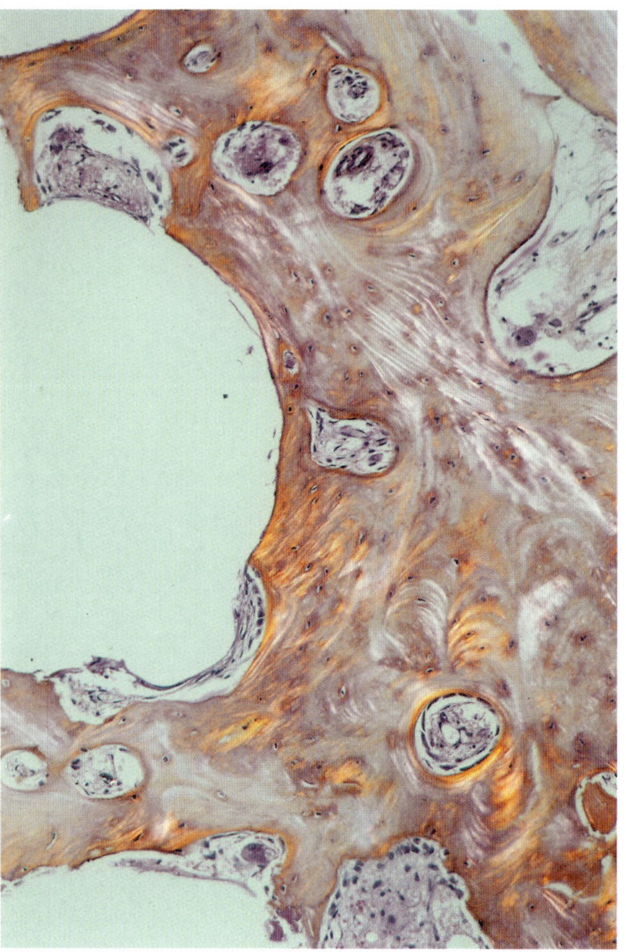

Fig. 58.14 Remodeling of bone in close contact with a bead of metal on a madreporic prosthesis (polarized light).

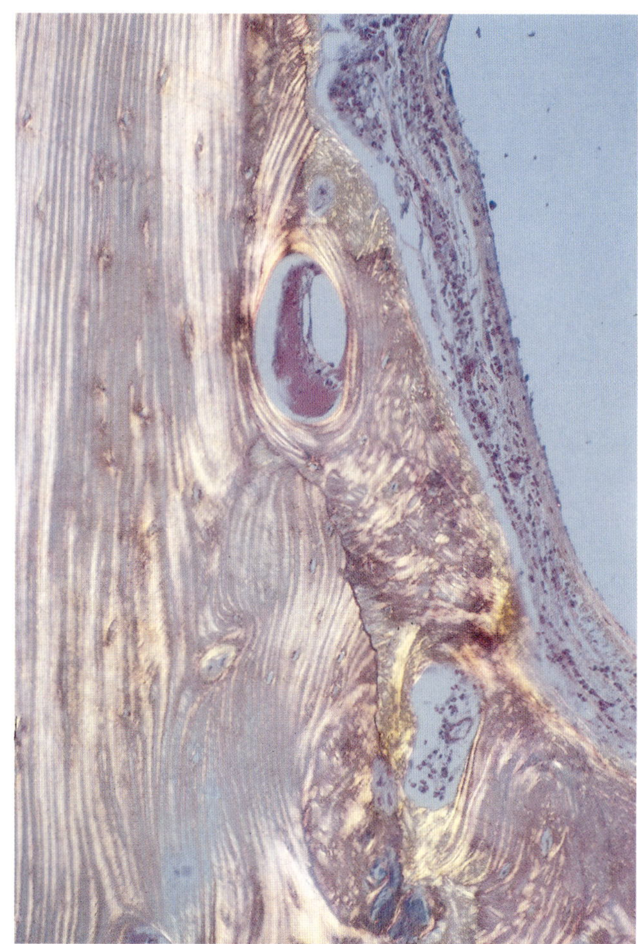

Fig. 58.15 Fibrous lining and new bone formation at the interface of a well-fixed non-cemented femoral stem (polarized light).

Smaller particles may be found in mononuclear macrophages.

Cement is dissolved in xylene and leaves round or oval spaces up to 80–100 μu or even larger, most of them being surrounded by a giant cell reaction producing a real syncytium (Figs 58.16–58.19). On frozen sections, cement appears as glassy and granular particles, non-birefringent in polarized light[14] and exhibiting a bright orange stain with Sudan III.

Cement is relatively inert, but some reports demonstrate an intracellular toxicity.[65–68] Its microstructure has been thoroughly studied on TEM and SEM.

Most bone cements are made radiopaque by the addition of barium sulfate or zirconium dioxide which are also very useful histological markers. The fine, round, gray-green particles of barium sulfate are about 5 μu, with little birefringence and strong refractility.[9,69] They may be inconspicuous in the cytoplasm on light microscopy,[69] away from the cement spaces or even in the lymph nodes.[67] Zirconium oxide particles are small, approximately 0.5 μu, but they can form larger aggregates,[9] appearing dark and exhibiting a flat birefringence on polarization. They may be detectable only by electron microscopy.[38,67]

Wear of ultra-high molecular weight *polyethylene* results from abrasion, fatigue, fusion defects or entrapped cement debris with three body wear[6,14,70–72] (Fig. 58.20); furthermore, metallic alloys can rub against polyethylene and metal ions or salts released by corrosion can accelerate chemical degradation.[6]

The size range and form are extremely variable: very fine dust, large flakes or fibers, filaments or shards looking transparent on histological examination and vividly birefringent on polarized light (Figs 58.21–58.24). The smallest particles, about 0.5 μu, are found in mononuclear macrophages,[72–75] exhibiting a diffuse cytoplasmic birefringence when viewed under polarized light.[76] They can stain positive with oil red O.[77] Large particles are partially or completely engulfed by giant cells, some of them exhibiting asteroid bodies which are viewed as a condensation of the cytoskeleton,[62] particularly in cases of high-grade wear.[9] Septate vacuolar phagosomes have been described enclosing polyethylene flakes.[78]

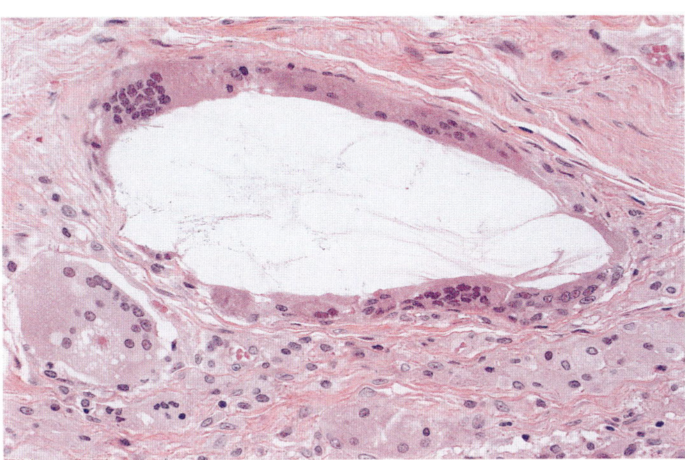

Fig. 58.16

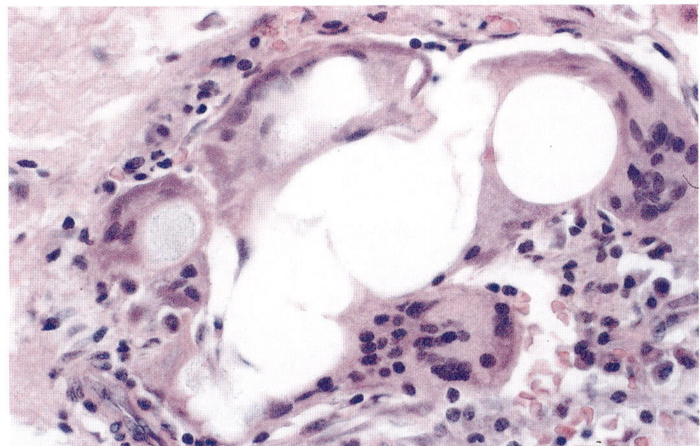

Fig. 58.17

Figs 58.16, 58.17 Cement debris surrounded by a giant cell reaction. The contrast medium appears as a grayish granular material.

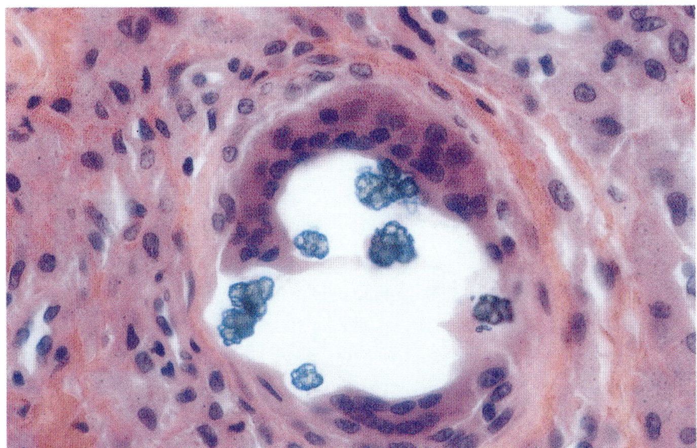

Fig. 58.18 Zirconium dioxide associated with cement.

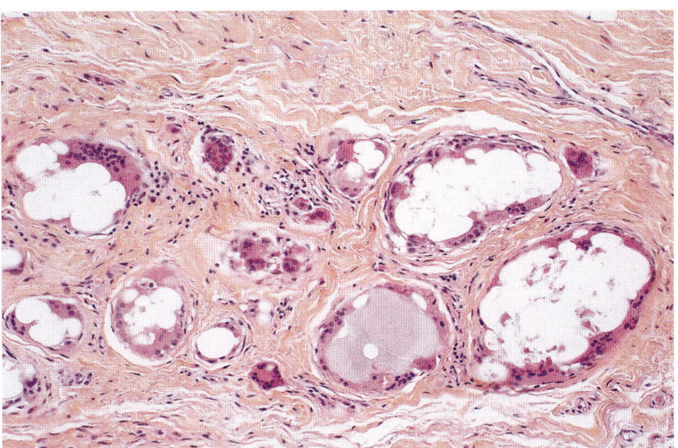

Fig. 58.19 Beads of cement located in the peripheral territories of a newly formed joint capsule.

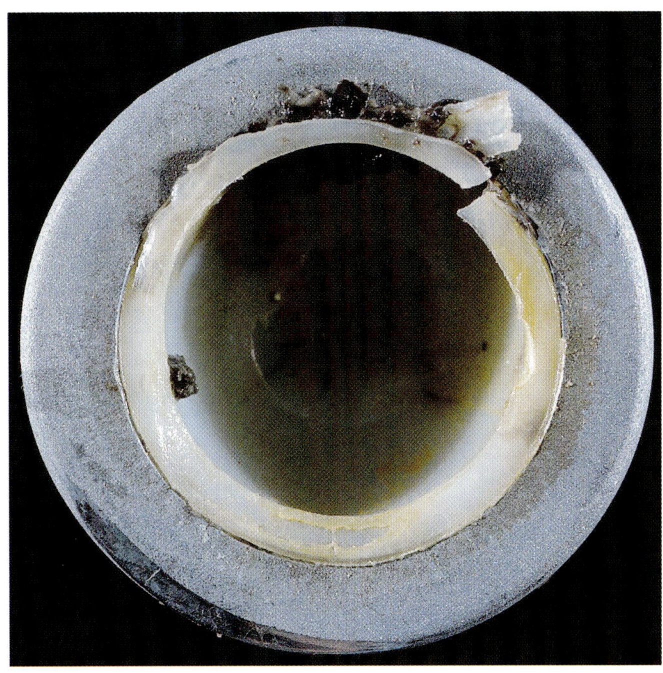

Fig. 58.20 Wear of a polyethylene cup, after 17 years of implantation.

Metallosis induces a grayish or black pigmentation of the soft tissues or even bone (Fig. 58.25). Metal is affected by chemical corrosion or predominantly released by abrasive or three body wear. Metal particles are both extra- and intracellular in mononuclear macrophages, appearing as small irregular black fragments of 1–5 μu although larger extracellular debris can be found[63] (Figs 58.26–58.29). The usual size is 0.7 μu but many of them are smaller than 0.1 μu, so special physical methods are needed for their identification.[9,14,35,75,79,80]

Under polarized light, there is a light scattering effect at the edges of the particles, presumably due to deposition of a metal proteinate.[22] Ultrastructurally, electron-dense par-

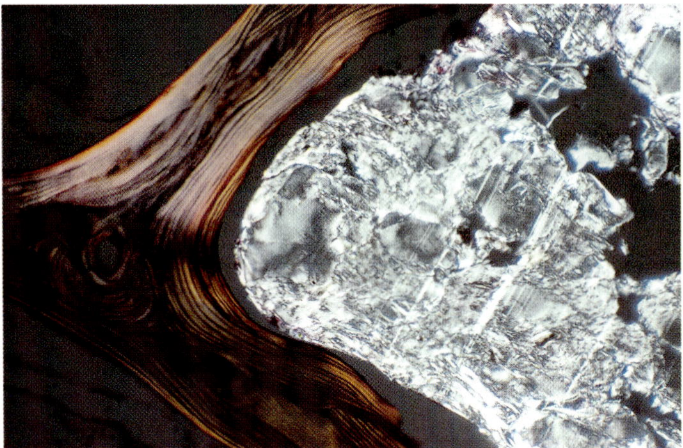

Fig. 58.21 Large fragment of polyethylene fitted in cancellous bone, without histiocytic reaction (polarized light).

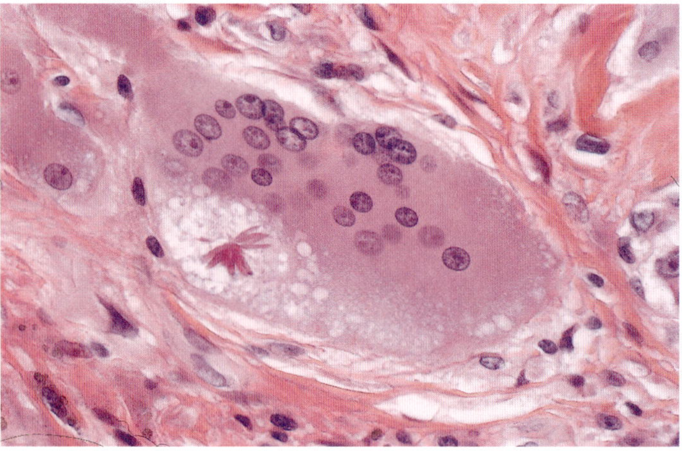

Fig. 58.24 Asteroid body in a reactive giant cell (polyethylene granuloma).

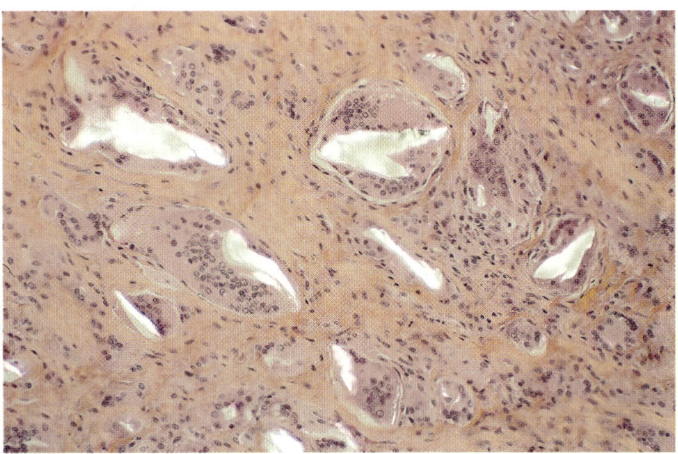

Fig. 58.22 Shards of polyethylene eliciting a giant cell reaction (polarized light).

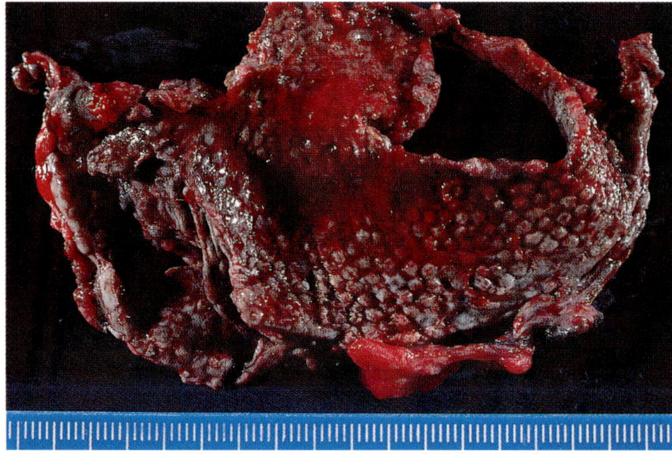

Fig. 58.25 Severe metallosis of the neocapsule of the hip joint (wear of titanium of a total hip prosthesis).

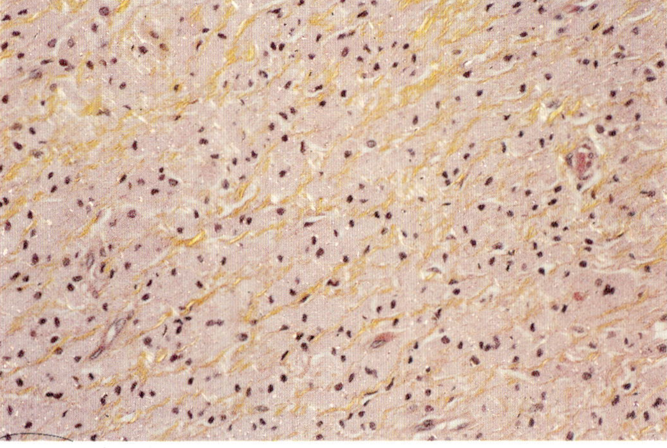

Fig. 58.23 Small polyethylene debris (polarized light).

ticles accumulate in phagolysosomes and the cells exhibit degenerative changes.[6,9,14,38,39,64,80,81]

Titanium metallosis may be found even in cases with no visible corrosion or fracture of the implant,[82,83] the particles being liberated most probably by wear rather than by corrosion and appearing as shard-shaped, angular debris.[14,80]

Metal particles can be associated with some lymphocytic infiltrates.[6,38]

The corrosion of metal may lead to microplate structures looking like closely packed, crystal-like deposits lying extracellularly in circumscribed light green or dark aggregates. This plate-like material is composed of a chromium compound containing iron and phosphorus.[10,84]

Ceramic wear particles of articulating parts appear as fragments of 5 µu or less in size; they may be stored in macrophages, the larger ones being extracellular[14,85] (Fig. 58.30). Usually, there is very little cellular response[14,38,39,85] but an intense histiocytic reaction has

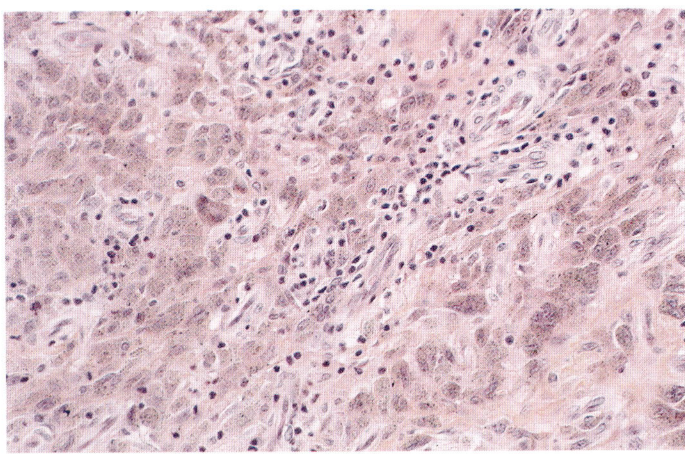

Fig. 58.26 Debris of metal in mononuclear macrophages, with a few lymphocytes (total hip prosthesis).

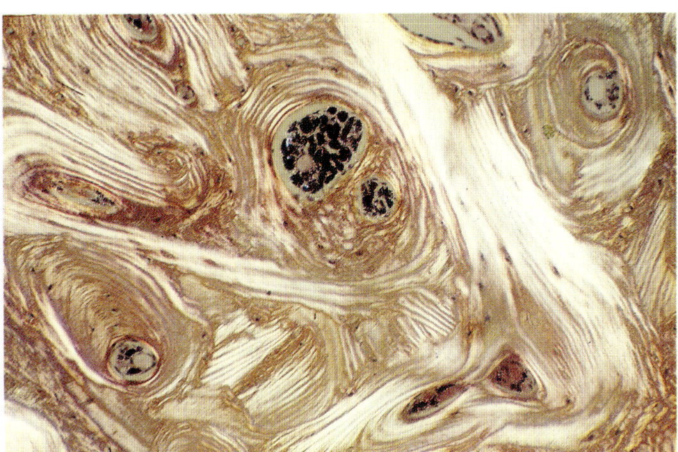

Fig. 58.29 Metallosis in Haversian canals (polarized light).

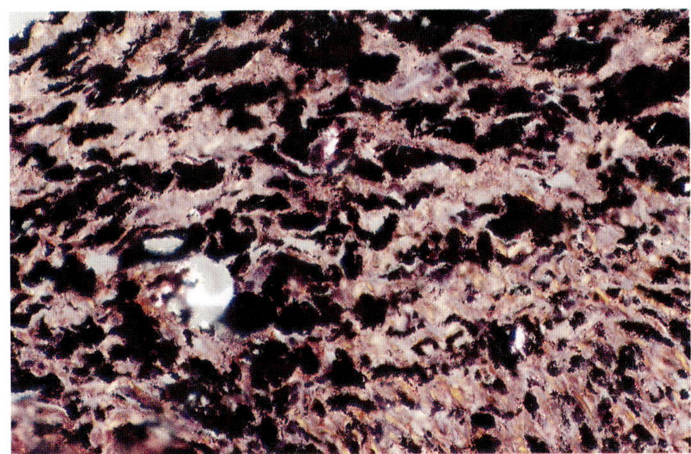

Fig. 58.27 Irregularly shaped particles of titanium with some polyethylene debris (polarized light).

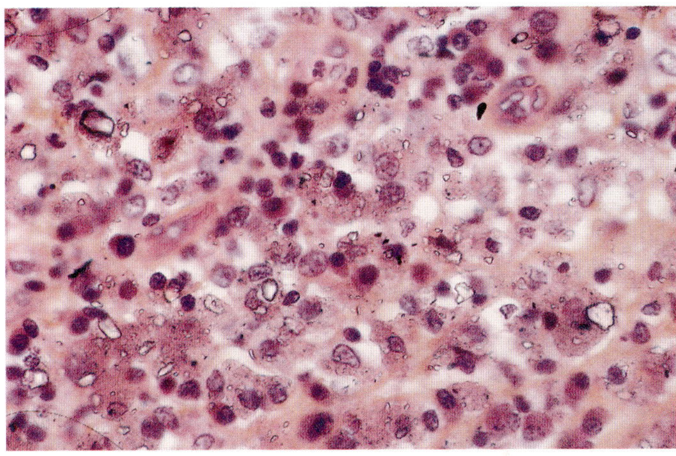

Fig. 58.30 Numerous particles of ceramic appearing as a glassy material (broken ceramic femoral head).

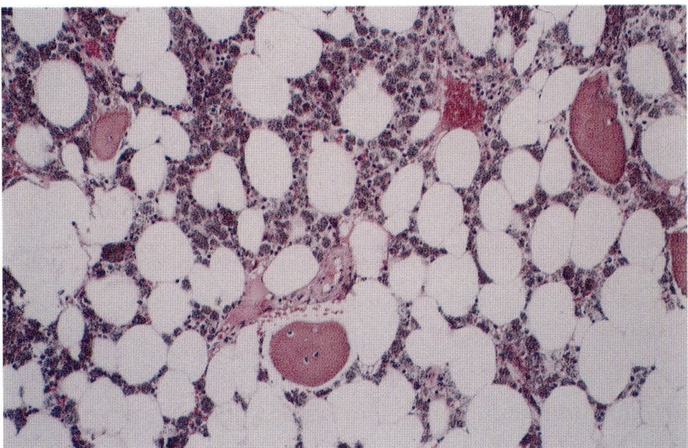

Fig. 58.28 Spread of metal particles in the bone marrow (total hip prosthesis).

been reported with submicron particles,[36] identified by electron microscopy.[9]

Carbon particles are bar-shaped, black, rectangular fragments from carbon-reinforced polyethylene components, with a variable size and diffraction at the edges on polarized light (Fig. 58.31). They may induce a gray or bluish-black discoloration of the tissues[14,86] and may be transported to lymph nodes. Carbon debris appear to be biologically inert, without foreign body giant cell reaction.[14,87]

HISTOLOGY OF ASEPTIC LOOSENING OF TOTAL JOINT REPLACEMENTS

The regenerating capsule presents as a fibrous scar tissue, old or recent fibrinous exudates or a fibrinoid-like material[5] lying close to the newly formed synovial lining, which is frequently hyperplastic (Figs 58.32, 58.33), but the main

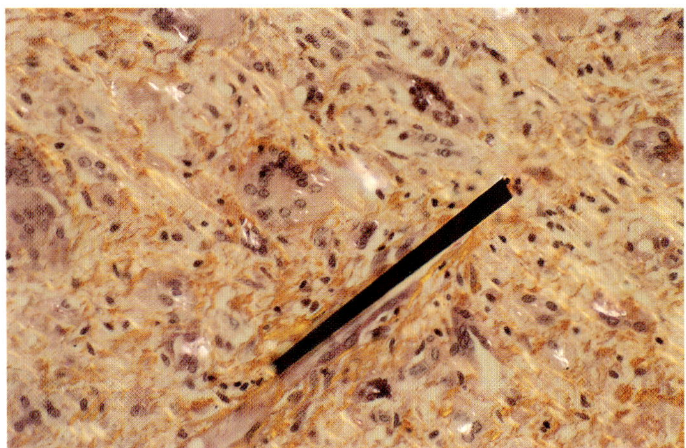

Fig. 58.31 Rod of carbon associated with a giant cell reaction to polyethylene, in a loosened total knee prosthesis (polarized light).

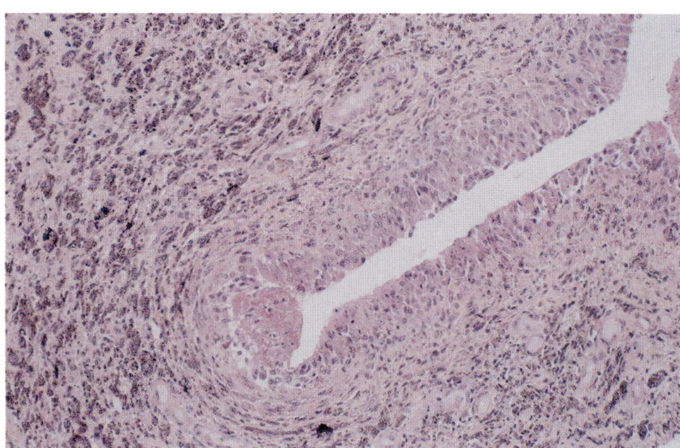

Fig. 58.33 Newly formed hyperplastic synovial lining associated with metallosis (loosened cemented total hip prosthesis).

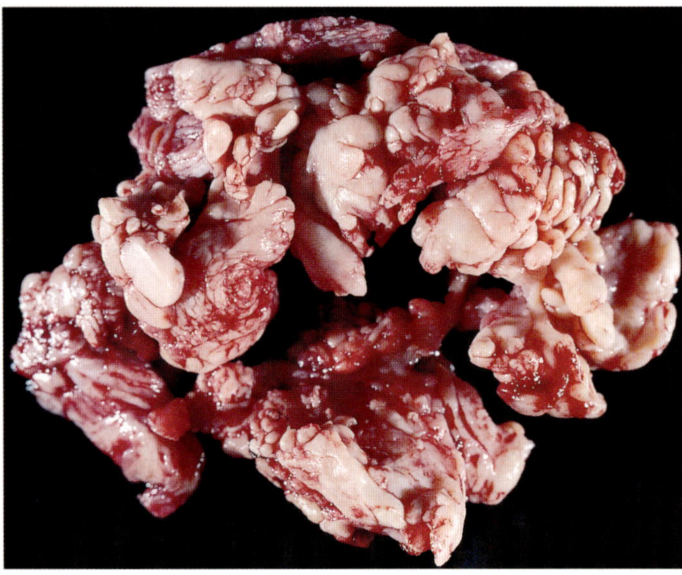

Fig. 58.32 Villous appearance of a hip neocapsule (loosened cemented total hip prosthesis).

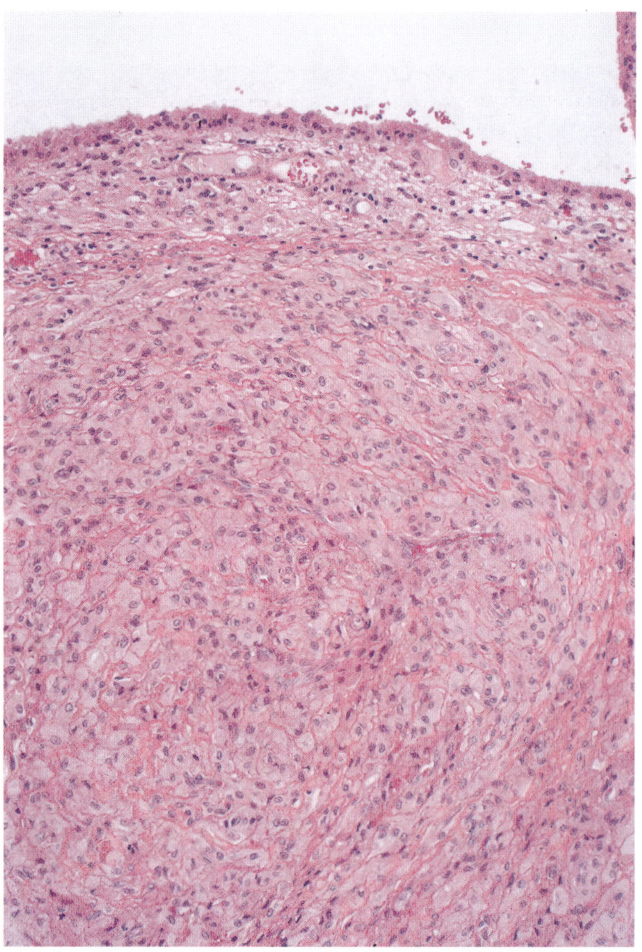

Fig. 58.34 Histiocytic granuloma of a neocapsule (cemented total hip prosthesis).

histological finding is the cellular reaction to wear debris (Fig. 58.34). The type and extent of this reaction depend on the rate of production of the particles, the form and surface of the debris and most of all on their size.[9,14,38,39,88] 1–5 μu particles are in the cytoplasm of mononuclear macrophages while, a giant cell reaction is elicited by the larger ones.

A large amount of intracellular debris is followed by cellular necrosis and subsequent release of lytic enzymes and undigested particles with further macrophagic recruitment.[26,64,80]

The sheets of macrophages may be devoid of any particles and the foamy cytoplasm is usually full of lipid material;[71] others may respond to altered methylmethacrylate, cement monomer, soluble ions from the stem or products of cell death only.[64,71]

The clinical picture can be dominated by a *prosthetic synovitis*[89] and wear debris is identified in the synovial fluid.

At the *implant–bone interface*, histology of the membrane has led to some topographic zoning[65,71,90–93] but a marked zonal distribution may not be recognizable[9,64,80,90] and in many cases, there is only a collagenous dense areolar tissue.

The prosthetic surface lining cells may have a synovial appearance[91,92] but these structures are inconstant and scattered; they are solely the consequence of motion or disruption of the connective tissue membrane,[26,63,65,90,94,95] and have been viewed as an 'implant bursitis'[88] (Figs 58.35, 58.36). The histiocytic granuloma is distributed in the middle zone and fibrosis is most prominent on the bone side.

Overall, the biochemical features of the membrane resemble granulation tissue.[96] Enzyme histochemical studies have shown a high level of acid phosphatase, non-specific esterase and NADH-diaphorase activity.[5,23,91,92]

In membranes of press-fit prostheses, the fibrous tissue is sparsely cellular and poorly vascularized;[37,65] membranes of biologic ingrowth prostheses are more vascular, exhibiting a loosely organized connective tissue with some islands of woven bone.[65]

Bone loss occurs with cemented or uncemented techniques[97] due to adaptive bone remodeling, with alterations in the stress distribution on the femur. Osteolysis may present as a diffuse femoral cortical thinning or as focal cystic lesions.[97] X-ray diffraction and microhardness studies have shown an increase of osteoid seams and poorly mineralized areas in the bone trabeculae at the interface.[98]

The mechanism of *femoral loosening* may initially involve micromotion, excessive stresses or uneven load distribution promoting osteoclastic activity.[63,90]

Initiation of failure on specimens retrieved from patients with stable components has been linked to a debonding of the cement from the metal stem,[30,99,100] with fragmentation or fracture of the mantle.[72,93]

Loosening of porous-coated femoral components may be related to the lack of bone growth into the porous coating, unsatisfactory porous coating, non-uniform contact or fatigue fractures of the ingrown bone.[101]

In hydroxyapatite-coated implants, the hydroxyapatite substrate can fail; particles may migrate and contribute to an excessive polyethylene wear.[102,103]

The *resorption of bone* is sometimes related to the histiocytic granuloma but histological findings are contradictory: sheets of histiocytes may be in close contact with the living bone without any sign of resorption, which appears to be due only to osteoclastic activity. Experimentally, conflicting results have also been reported: low-grade surface osteolysis[104–108] or no bone resorption.[109–111] These results may be related to the difficulties in distinguishing foreign body giant cells from osteoclasts in culture studies.[112]

During the last decade, many works have stressed the role of activated monocyte/macrophages in the increased

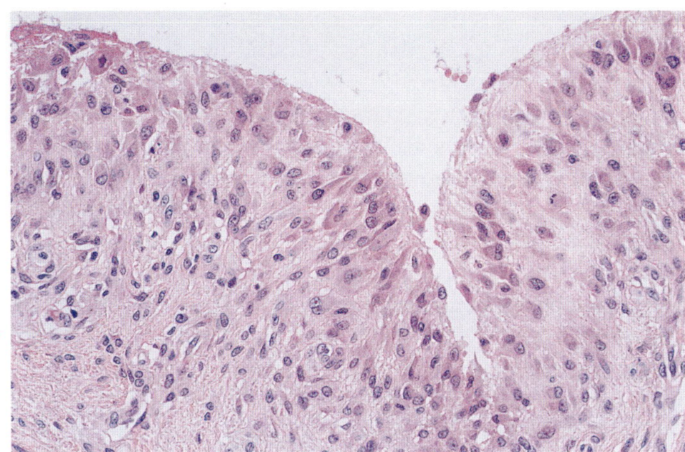

Fig. 58.35

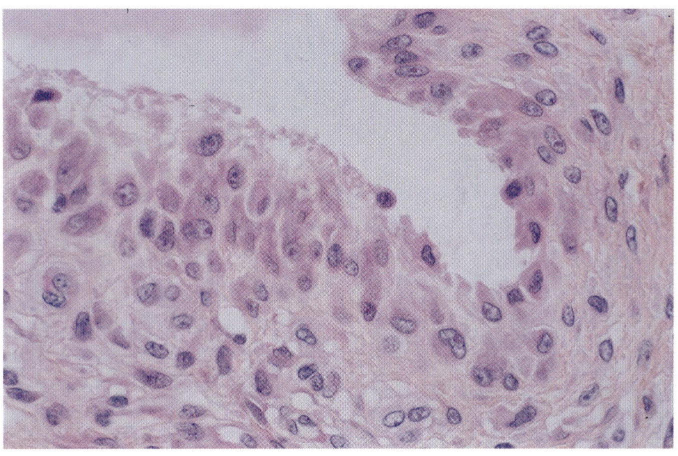

Fig. 58.36

Figs 58.35, 58.36 Synovial-like linings in the interface membranes of cemented (Fig. 58.35) and non-cemented (Fig. 58.36) femoral stems.

production of *cytokines*, *proteinases* and *prostanoids* presumably involved in the recruitment of osteoclasts and osteolysis, detected by tissue extracts of the interface, media of cultured cells, immunohistochemistry and in situ hybridization.[62,91,92,95,113–119]

More recently, the role of the macrophage has been restricted to the production of interleukin 1[120–122] or tumor necrosis factor and not prostaglandin E2 (PGE2), the osteoblasts being the cells leading to bone resorption, possibly through a PGE2–osteoclast-mediated mechanism.[123–125]

Macrophage-derived cytokines may also sustain the granulomatous reaction, by chemotaxis or by increasing the expression of adhesion molecules on endothelial cells.[118]

Collagenase and gelatinase B synthesized by the macrophages may presumably disclose the mineral fraction of bone, facilitating the action of osteoclasts,[36,107,126,127] as well as the lysosomal proteases, cathepsin B and G.[128–130]

The granulocyte-macrophage colony-stimulating factor

(GM-CSF) may induce the proliferation of macrophages and the early stages of fusion of multinucleated giant cells implicated in osteolysis.[131]

The dominating role of these products remains controversial as tissue levels are also elevated in stable prostheses;[16] PGE2 levels are even higher in synovial tissues from patients with osteoarthritis.[122]

The role of the few T lymphocyte infiltrates is also debatable; they are presumed to have some importance, secreting lymphokines which attract and activate additional macrophages,[115,132,133] but actually it appears that they are not required to initiate or sustain the host response to particulate debris.[93,134]

Similarly, the role of *mast cells* found in a degranulated state in the interface tissue remains to be settled.[135]

MASSIVE LIMB PROSTHESES

These are used as a salvage procedure for reconstruction after bone tumor resection, but also for failed total hip or knee prostheses.

The medullary reaming implies destruction of part of the vascular supply and also a remodeling of bone which depends on load adaptive formation or stress shielding. Studies of retrieval specimens in clinically stable prostheses have been reported.[136–138]

In *femoral prostheses*, a shell of bone is found adjacent to cement, predominantly in the diaphysis, by remodeling of the inner cortex; cortical remodeling results in a porous inner cortex (Fig. 58.37). At the plateau of the prosthesis, a pedicle of bone extends on the shaft, on the medial posterior side which is under compression.

In *upper limb prostheses* not subjected to loading, thick sclerotic bone is also found along the surface of the cement in retrieval specimens[139] or on radiographic studies.[140] The cortex is reduced by as much as half its original thickness by spongy substitution of the internal part (Figs 58.38–58.40). The adaptive process which creates a secondary canal, defined as 'spongeoizisation', has also been described in cases of cementless implantation[139] and has been reproduced experimentally.

Mega hip replacements give initially good results,[141] lasting 5 to 15 years; the severe cortical atrophy or spongy transformation is not correlated with loosening of the stem.[141] Approximately 25% of the prostheses become loose at 5 years, especially in the distal femur and proximal tibia, in young adults.[142,143]

MASSIVE OSTEOLYSIS IN TOTAL JOINT REPLACEMENTS

So-called 'aggressive granulomatosis'[144,145] is a condition of localized tumor-like bone resorption appearing on X-ray as ovoid cysts around the stem, without any infec-

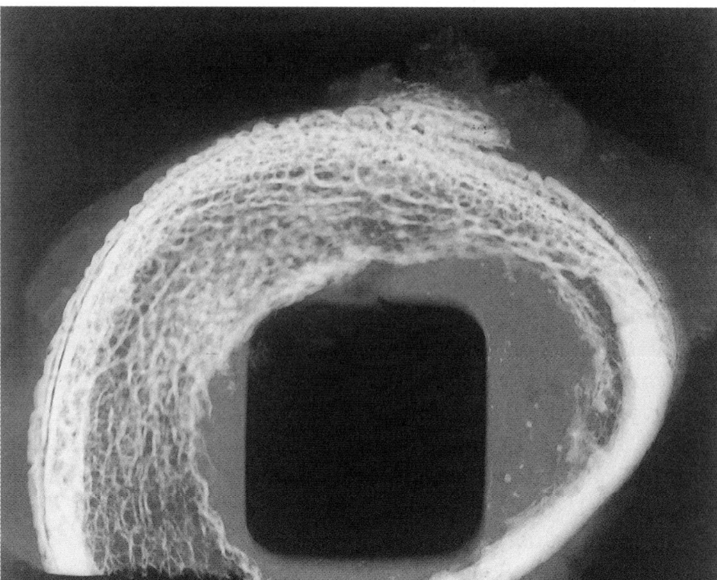

Fig. 58.37 Massive knee prosthesis inserted after tumor resection. X-ray of the metaphyseal area demonstrating a new shell of bone around the cement mantle.

tion.[146,147] It has been reported in stable or loosened, cemented or uncemented prostheses involving the hip or knee[148] and in prostheses used in limb-sparing procedures.[149]

In 90% of cases, increasing pain and radiographic evidence of loosening are found before the development of granulomatous pseudotumors;[150] the median time to appearance is 6 years[148] but it may be as short as a few months.[144,145,147,151]

The lesions may present as a cystic ballooning and resorption of bone with distension and elevation of the periosteum;[144,151] the rapid expansion can simulate hemophilic pseudotumors, aneurysmal bone cysts, tumors of bone, myeloma[152] or even lytic forms of Paget's disease (Figs 58.41, 58.42). Large acetabular lytic lesions have been reported[153–157] (Figs 58.43–58.46). Huge femoral lesions may induce a pathologic fracture.[158]

Paradoxically, histological findings are not remarkable: wear debris, histiocytic granulomas, collagenous tissue mixed with extensive fibrinoid necrosis[153] and hemorrhages. In some reports, more macrophages, more polyethylene debris and fewer activated fibroblasts have been found,[159] as well as greater activity levels of interleukin 1, interleukin 6 and tumor necrosis factor in culture supernatants,[160] but the term 'aggressive granulomatosis' has been disputed as only the distribution and bone lysis typify that complication.[9,16]

The cystic lesions have been attributed to high local stresses,[151] micromotion,[150,161] abrasion particles[99,151] and in well-fixed femoral components,[162] to local defects of the cement mantle, allowing the particulate debris to be trans-

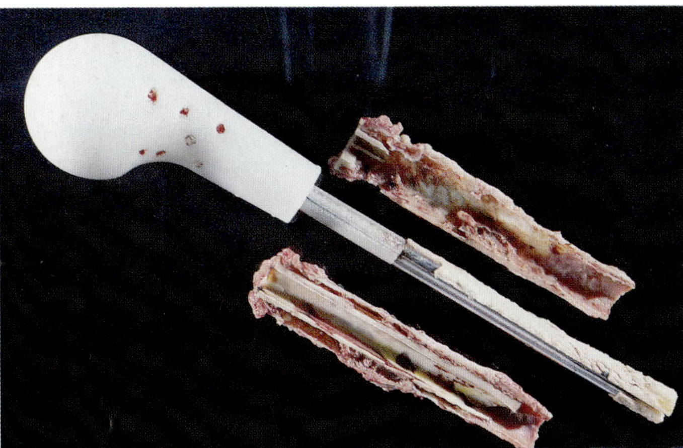

Fig. 58.38

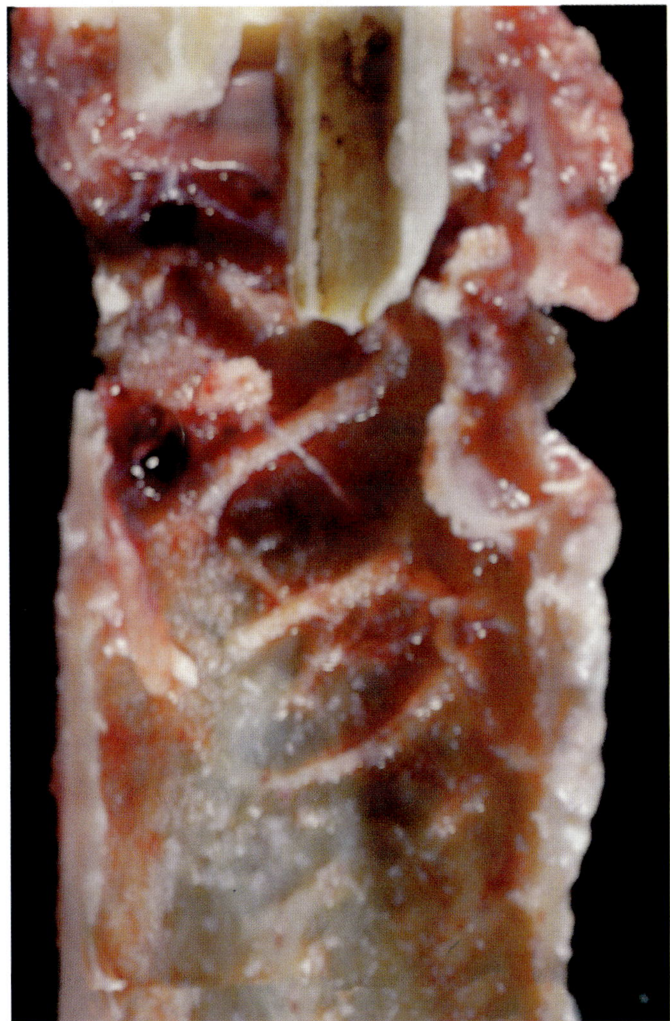

Fig. 58.39

Figs 58.38, 58.39 Massive cemented humeral prosthesis inserted after tumor resection. The prosthesis is well fixed, but there is considerable thinning of the cortex.

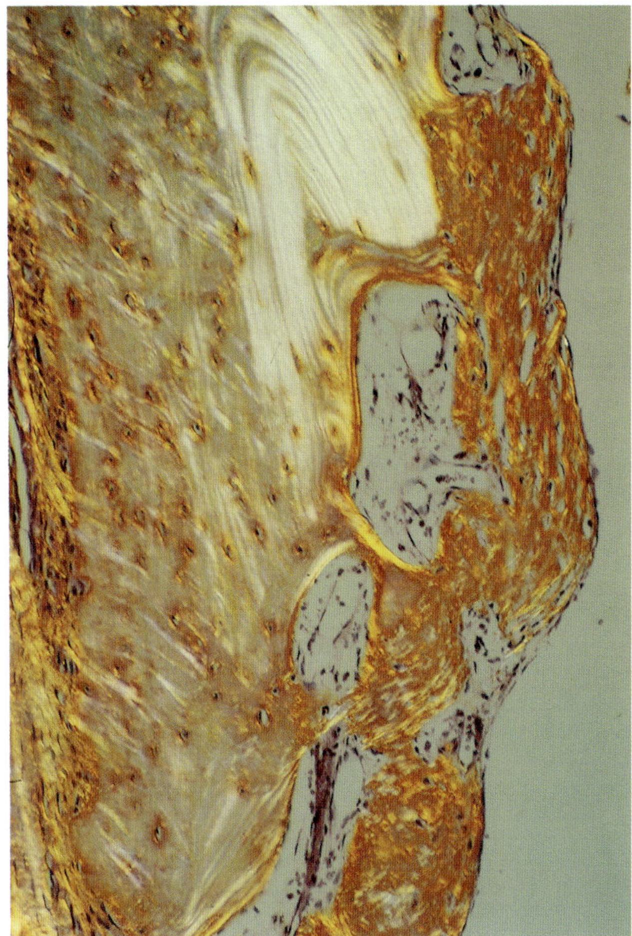

Fig. 58.40 Same case. New bone is separating cement from the very reduced cortex (polarized light).

ported from the joint cavity through a fibrous membrane between the stem and the cement.[29,163]

POSTPROSTHESIS LYMPH NODE HISTIOCYTOSIS[164]

Silicone lymphadenopathies are well-known complications of silicone prostheses used for the replacement of small joints; cases of reactive lymphadenopathies have been reported in patients with hip prostheses, but also with knee prostheses[165,166] or massive limb prostheses inserted after tumor surgery[167] (Figs 58.47, 58.48).

High levels of wear debris have been documented in periarticular tissues from patients with loose hip joint prostheses,[168–171] with further dissemination of debris, predominantly by lymphatic spread,[14,71] confirmed by electron microprobe analysis.[170]

The sinus histiocytosis seen in lymph nodes can resemble regional metastatic disease. Reactive lymphadenopathies have been found in patients with prostheses

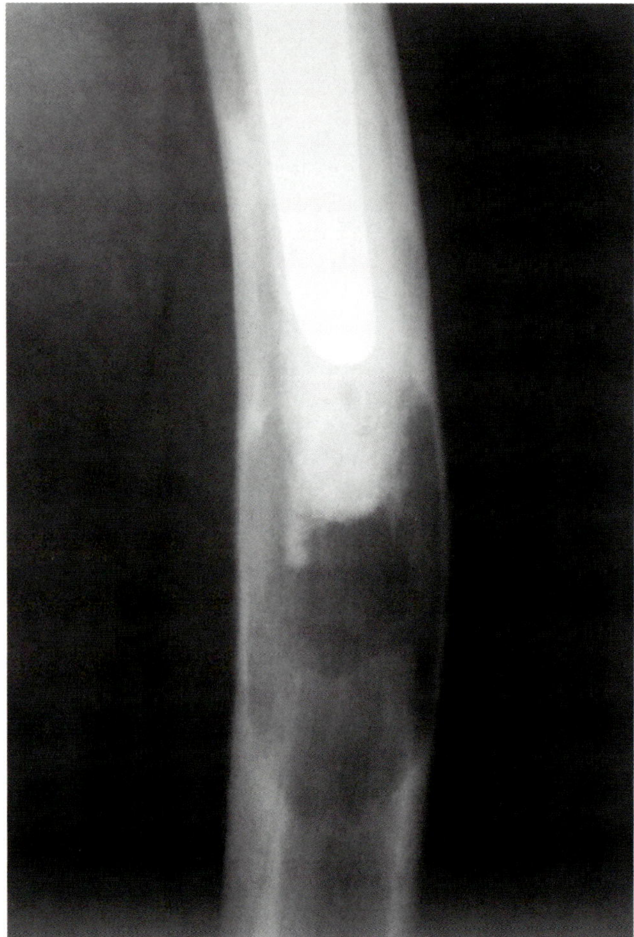

Fig. 58.41

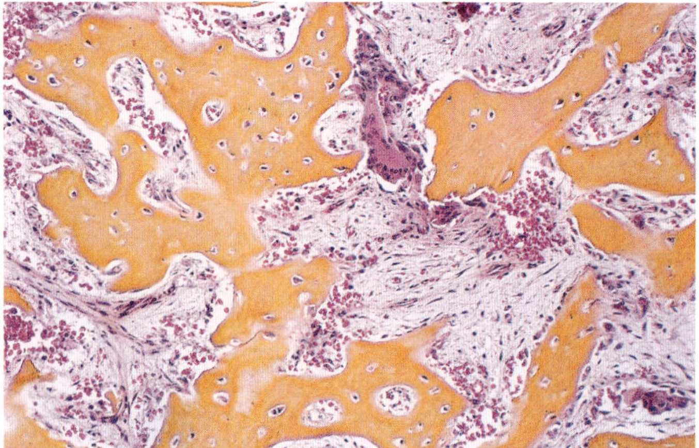

Fig. 58.42

Figs 58.41, 58.42 Lytic form of Paget's disease developing under the stem of a cemented total hip prosthesis.

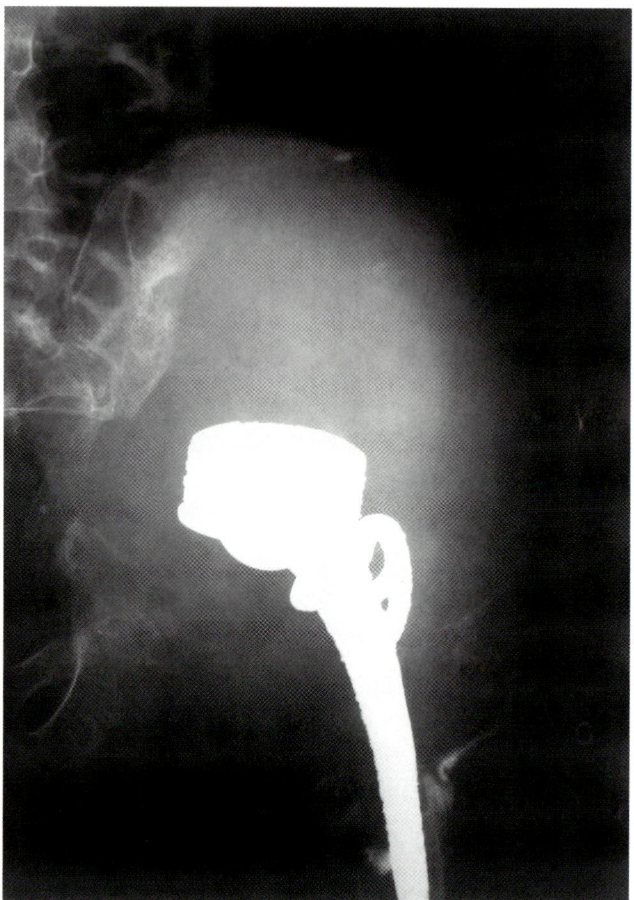

Fig. 58.43

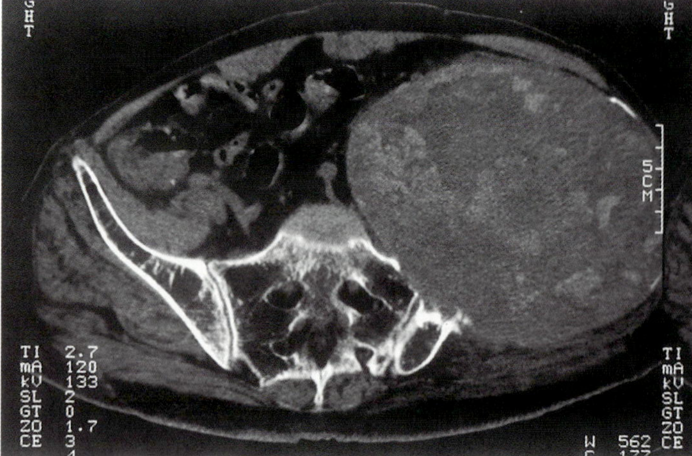

Fig. 58.44

Figs 58.43, 58.44 Pseudotumoral osteolysis of the pelvis around an uncemented total hip prosthesis inserted 11 years previously.

undergoing lymph node dissection in the pelvis for prostatic carcinoma,[164,172–175] carcinoma of the bladder,[173] endometrium[175] and ovary.[176] They have also been described in the axilla, during surgery for breast cancer[177] and melanoma.[178]

On autopsy studies, small amounts of wear debris are seen as soon as 1.5 years after surgery,[179] increasing with the duration of the implant, in solitary inguinal lymph nodes,[180] ipsilateral parailiac lymph nodes and bilaterally in paraaortic lymph nodes.[70,179]

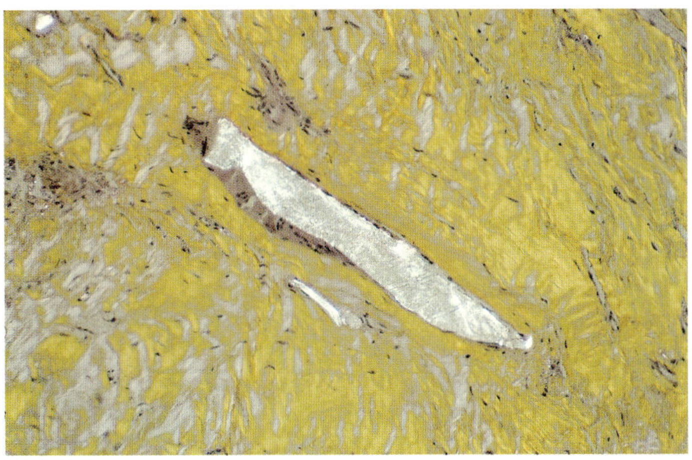

Fig. 58.45

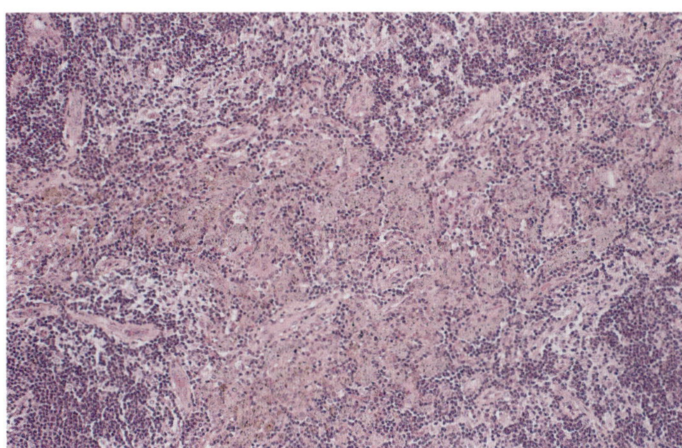

Fig. 58.47

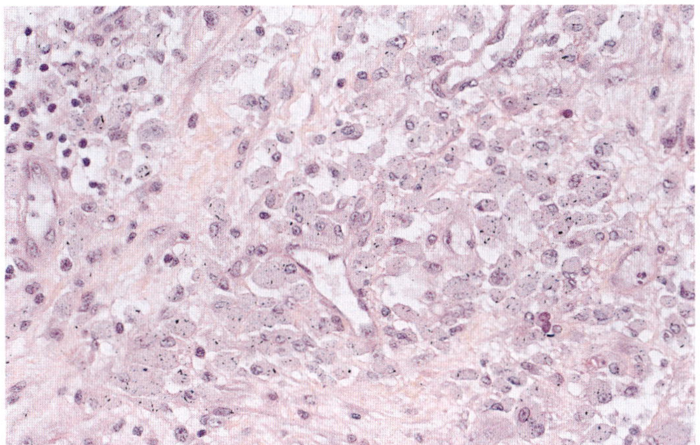

Fig. 58.46

Figs 58.45, 58.46 Same case. The mass is composed of a clot, fibrinoid-like material and a fibrous shell exhibiting polyethylene debris and a histiocytic reaction to metal.

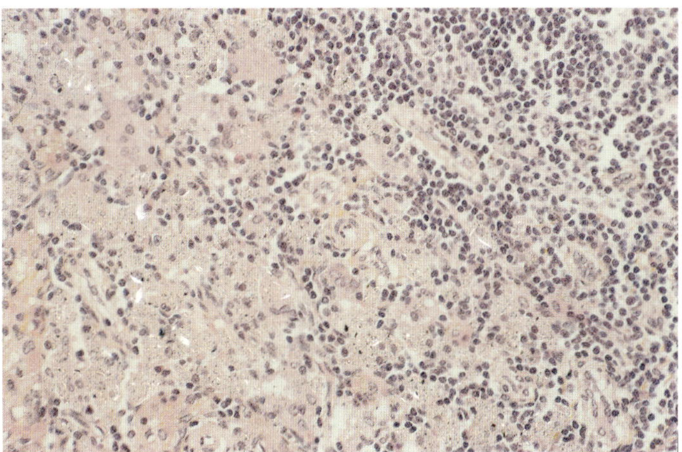

Fig. 58.48

Figs 58.47, 58.48 Inguinal lymphadenopathy close to a massive hip prosthesis inserted after resection of an osteosarcoma. Mononuclear macrophages are full of metal debris and small polyethylene fragments (Fig. 58.48: polarized light).

Histologically, the florid sinus histiocytosis[174] appears as large histiocytes filling and expanding the sinuses and interfollicular regions with various particles, but mostly polyethylene and metal. It has been stated that no reactive giant cells are found in lymph nodes as only small wear particles pass through the pseudocapsule,[179] but sarcoid-like features similar to the response to zirconium and beryllium have been reported in one case of soft tissue pseudotumor,[181] after total knee or hip replacement[181,182] and as an unusual systemic granulomatous reaction involving the abdominal lymph nodes, the spleen and the liver.[183]

An immunohistochemical study on lymph nodes has confirmed the macrophage differentiation and activation of several different cytokines.[175]

As for the differential diagnosis, the finding of birefringent material has to be viewed in the clinical context[184] as it may represent polyethylene or wear debris such as silica, talcum powder, or inhaled particles.[185]

TUMORS AND TOTAL JOINT REPLACEMENTS

Many animal experiments have demonstrated a direct correlation between sarcomas and injection of particulate metal debris, particularly cobalt, chromium and nickel, but also iron, lead, selenium, zinc and titanium.[14,186] Surgical polymers such as polyethylene and polymethylmethacrylate also induce local sarcomas experimentally.

A few cases of malignant tumors developing at the site of previous internal fixation have been reported, with a wide histological range from osteosarcoma to malignant lymphoma.[186–193]

With the widespread use of prostheses producing an increase in the total surface area available for metal ion release, there was some concern about the potential carcinogenicity of implants[194] after the first reports of tumors in man.[195–197] Up to now, about 30 cases have been quoted or reported, some of them without definite links with the prostheses, such as epidermoid carcinoma,[198] metastases[199,200] or malignant transformation in Maffucci's syndrome.[201]

The shortest time to diagnosis of malignancy after metal implantation was 5 months,[202] suggesting also that malignancy could be coincidental;[203] overall, the latent period of tumor presentation is about 7 years.

There is a predominance of malignant fibrous histiocytomas,[196,204–213] followed by osteosarcomas[14,195,210,214,215] (Figs 58.49–58.54), vascular tumors,[216,217] fibrosarcoma,[218] soft tissue sarcomas[196,219–221] and lymphoma.[218]

The incidence has been estimated as one case in 230 000, compared to one case in 100 000 for the development of a bone sarcoma and one case in 40 000 for a soft tissue sarcoma in the general population.[210] Incidence of tumors at remote sites in patients with joint replacement may also differ, with a greater incidence of leukemias and non-Hodgkin's lymphomas.[222]

BONE GRAFTS AND BONE SUBSTITUTES

In the field of bone grafting, some terms have to be defined for the pathological report.

When there is an intimate contact of the graft with the vascular host tissue, the necrotic bone is resorbed by osteoclastic activity; its gradual replacement by new bone is the process of *creeping substitution* which is dependent upon the speed of revascularization.

The promotion of osteogenic cells is *osteoinduction*.[223]

The ingrowth of capillaries and of osteoprogenitor cells from mesenchymal cells of the recipient in the scaffold of the graft is termed *osteoconduction*.

Incorporation is the envelopment of necrotic bone by the viable new bone.[224]

Incorporation of a *cancellous bone autograft* follows certain steps: necrosis of bone marrow and bone cells (but some of them are respected), ingrowth of granulation tissue and bone formation. Surface cells of the graft participate in early osteogenesis[225–227] and then primitive mesenchymal host cells differentiate into osteoblasts which produce seams of osteoid around the core of dead bone. The necrotic bone is further resorbed, with by 6 months a total replacement by viable bone.[228] The cancellous bone with a large surface area has the greatest potential for osteogenesis.[228]

Incorporation of a *cortical bone autograft* differs in the low rate of revascularization, the mechanism of creeping substitution and the completeness of repair.[224, 229]

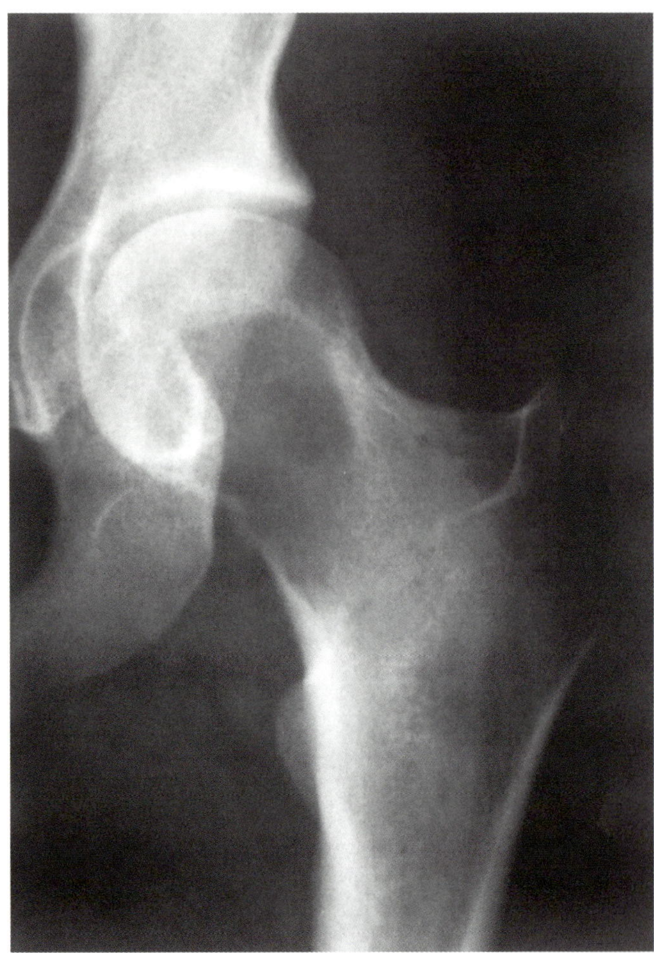

Fig. 58.49

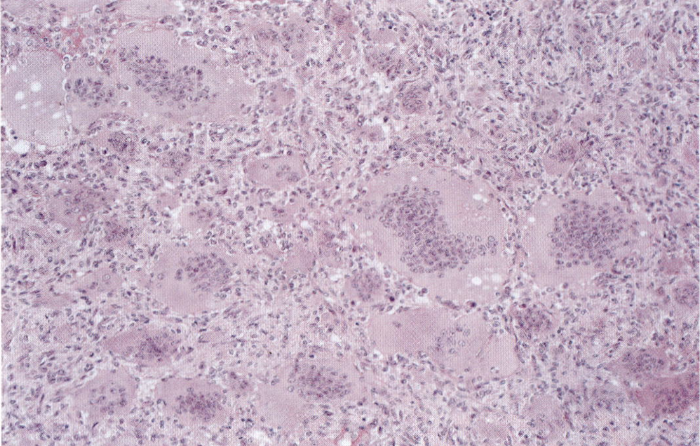

Fig. 58.50

Figs 58.49, 58.50 Benign giant cell tumor resected after a recurrence; reconstruction is performed with a massive hip prosthesis.

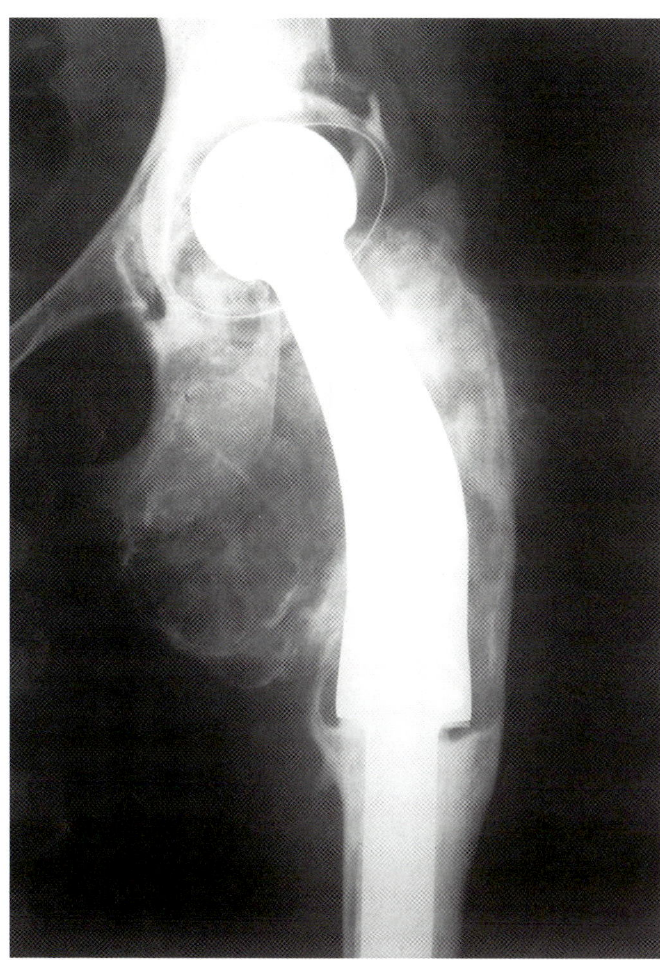

Fig. 58.51

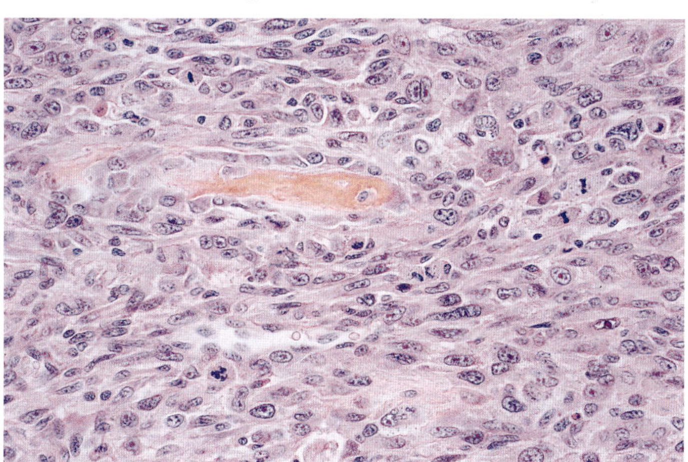

Fig. 58.52

Figs 58.51–58.53 Same case. Ten years after surgery, an osteosarcoma surrounds the prosthesis.

Fig. 58.53

Osteoclastic resorption, mainly peripheral, is the first event. The pattern of revascularization follows the preexisting Haversian canals, from the periphery to the interior of the graft. Incorporation is the function of the host cells, but also of the cambial layer of the graft periosteum and of some endosteal graft cells which have survived transplantation.[224,230]

Osteoconduction may take years in large cortical autografts.[228] Substantial amounts of necrotic bone can persist as interstitial lamellae,[230] the end result being an admixture of necrotic and viable bone.[228]

Large segmental autografts may be complicated by nonunion or fatigue fracture.

Allogenic bone evokes an immune response characterized

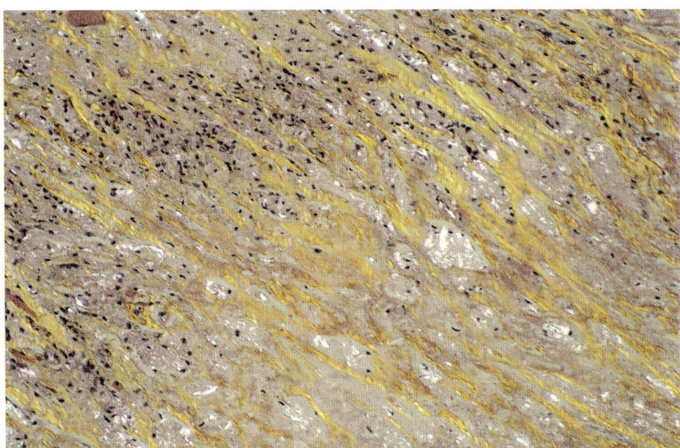

Fig. 58.54 Same case. The tumor is associated with fibrous tissue containing numerous polyethylene particles.

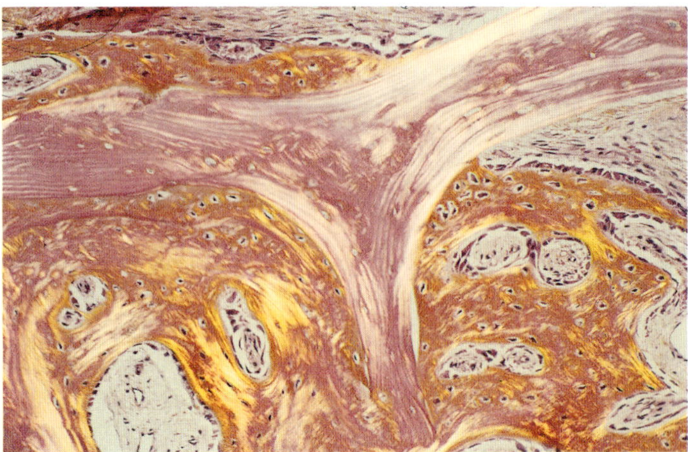

Fig. 58.55 New bone formation around a cancellous bone allograft.

by the appearance of activated lymphocytes, the major immunogenic component being the marrow and to a lesser extent the matrix components of bone.[224] However, satisfactory clinical results can be achieved with this procedure.

Cancellous allografts exhibit delayed sequences in all aspects of the repair process[225] and early fibrosis in the marrow predominates. The local inflammatory response, with a peak between the second and third weeks, produces a large number of infiltrating lymphocytes and may abate or persist for months, as the fibrovascular stroma eventually revascularizes the graft[231] (Figs 58.55, 58.56).

The successful incorporation of *cortical allografts* is based mainly on an external callus around the graft–host junction and only the ends of the graft are incorporated.[232] Internal repair is very limited and bone remodeling is only focal, if not absent.[233] If the graft is not frozen, some cells of the outer surface may remain viable, at a depth of 300 μu, and participate in osteogenesis.[231] Invasion of vascular buds through preexisting Haversian and Volkmann's canals, as well as their widening by osteoclastic resorption, occur only a few millimeters into the graft.[231]

Complications of cortical allografts are delayed union or non-union, fatigue fractures or even complete resorption of the graft material[224] but healing after a stress fracture may occur, the new host bone and periosteum encompassing the allograft.[224]

In massive *osseous* or *osteochondral allografts*, microradiographic[234] or histological studies[235] demonstrate that union takes place slowly at the cortical–cortical junction, the outer surface being the first site of osteogenesis.[234] Rehabitation also occurs a few millimeters under the surface[235,236] (Figs 58.57–58.60). In frozen massive osteochondral allografts, the cartilage is considered to be dead at the time of transplantation; the architecture is maintained, but it is almost acellular.[231,233] In some retrieved

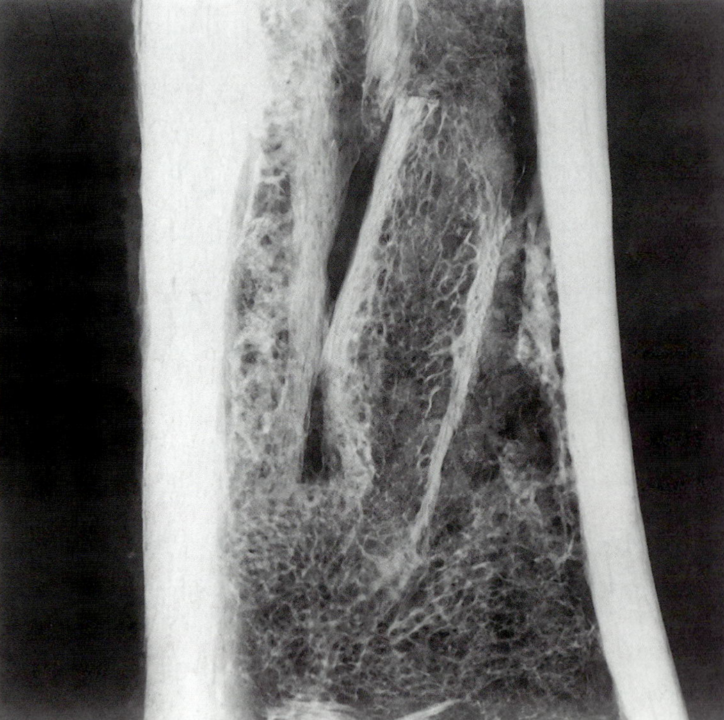

Fig. 58.56 Partial incorporation of bone allografts in the shaft of a humerus.

specimens it appears viable[236] but may show degenerative changes or an erosive pannus.[235,236] The subchondral plate remains necrotic.[235]

Graft failure within the first 3 years after transplantation is not due to immunologic rejection, but to the very sparse bone remodeling in the transplant.[232]

Mechanical factors are important in a bone graft incorporation for a successful bridging of the gap between the graft and host bone.[225,233] Compressive forces with an

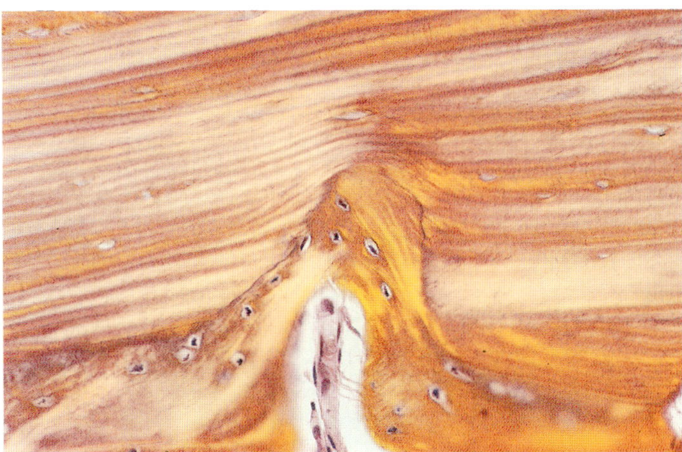

Fig. 58.57 Peripheral bone formation in a cortical bone allograft.

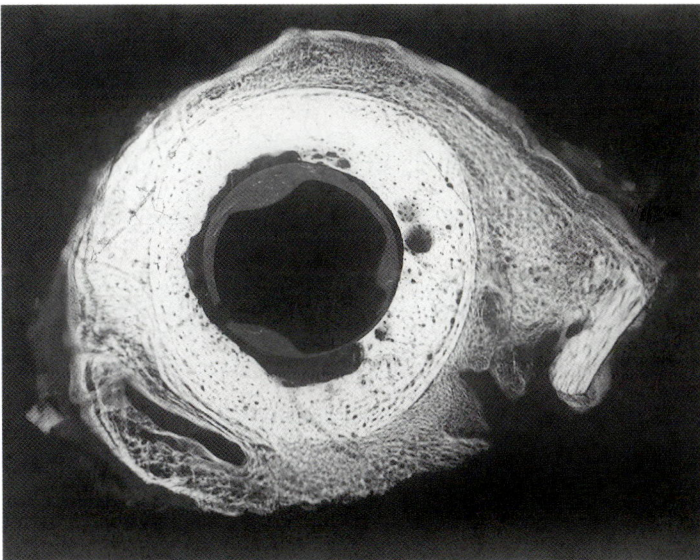

Fig. 58.60 Total knee prosthesis with a massive allograft which is surrounded by newly formed periosteal bone.

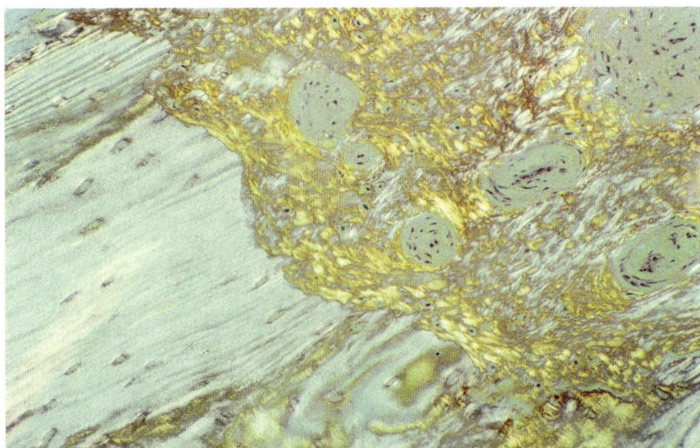

Fig. 58.58 Bone formation at the junction of a massive bone allograft and the host tissue (polarized light).

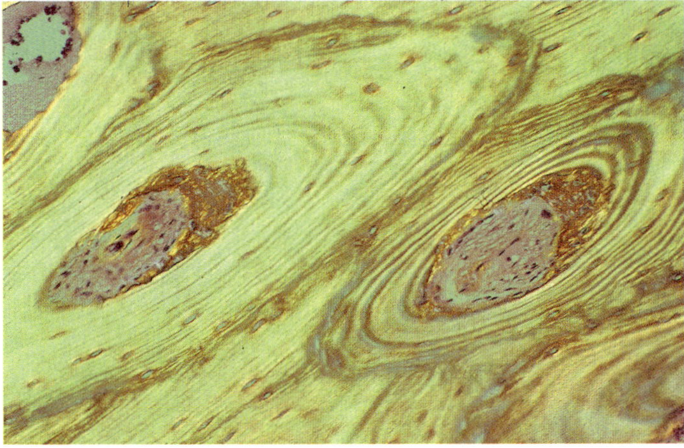

Fig. 58.59 Same case. Widening of the Haversian canals in the graft, with new bone deposition (polarized light).

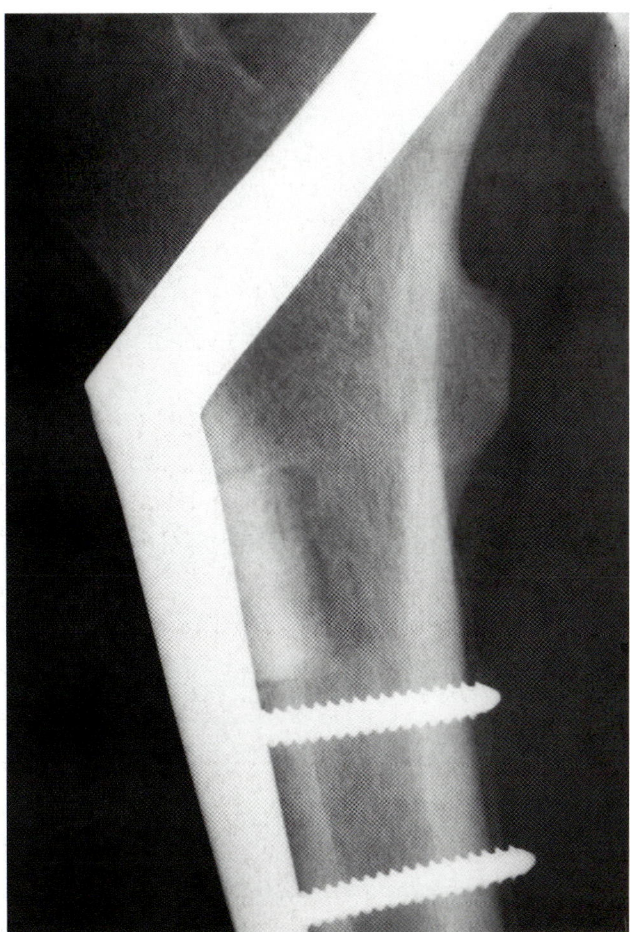

Fig. 58.61 Resection of an osteoid osteoma of the femur; the cavity is filled with a block of coral.

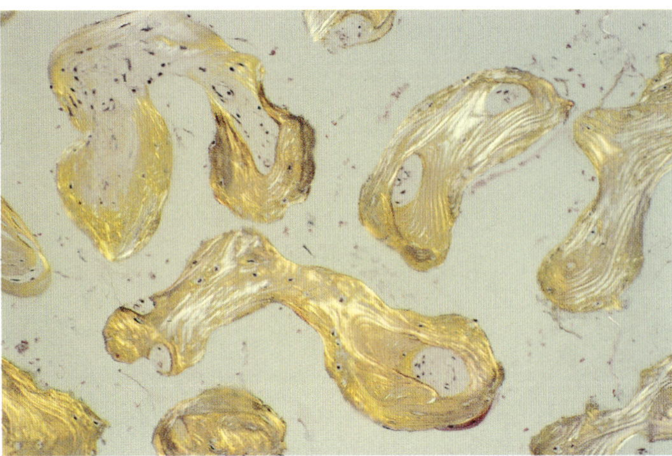

Fig. 58.62

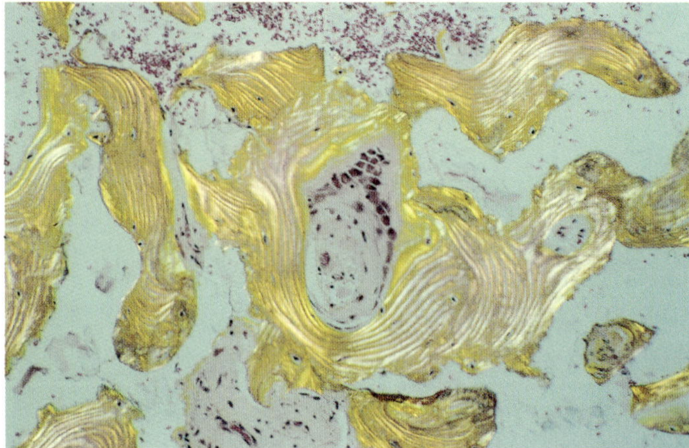

Fig. 58.63

Figs 58.62, 58.63 Same case. One year later, at the time of insert removal, a biopsy is performed at the periphery of the coral, demonstrating new bone formation in the pores of the material; the coral has been dissolved by the technique (polarized light).

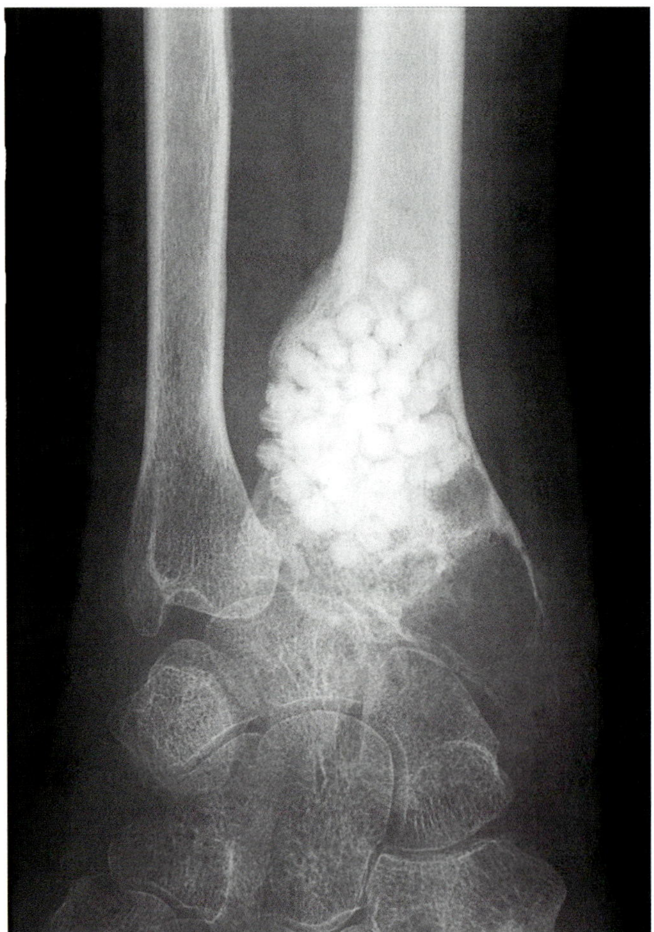

Fig. 58.64

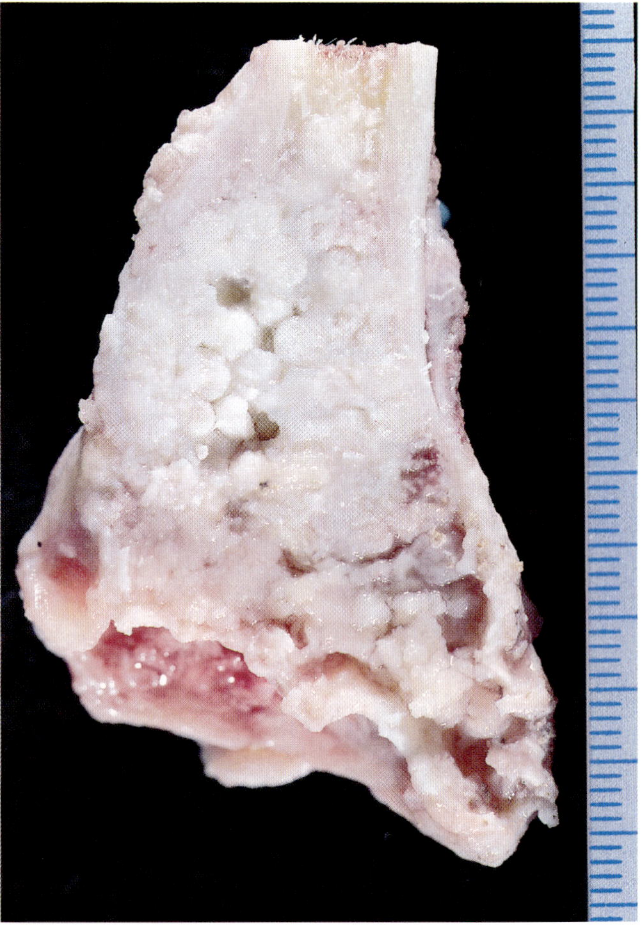

Fig. 58.65

Figs 58.64–58.66 Recurrence of a giant cell tumor of the radius. The tumor was initially curetted and the cavity packed with coral beads. There is no bone formation around the material, after a 2-year period.

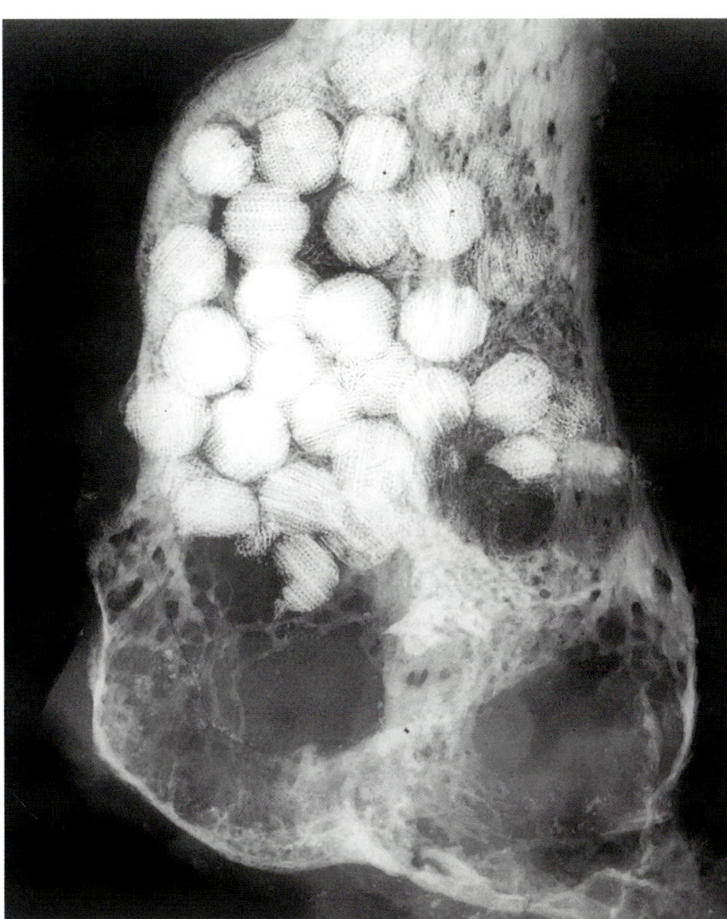

Fig. 58.66

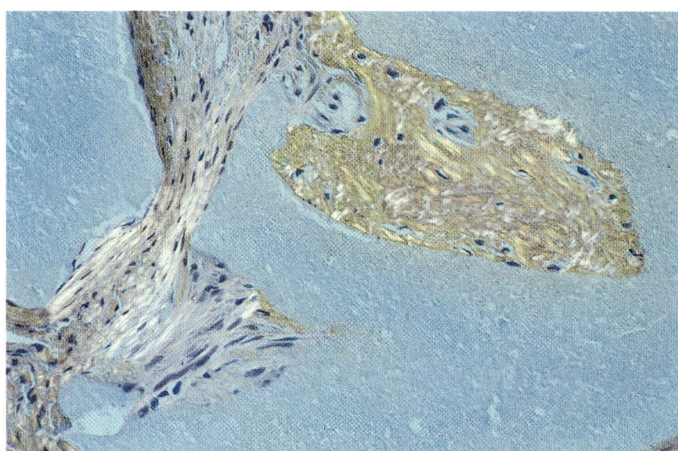

Fig. 58.67

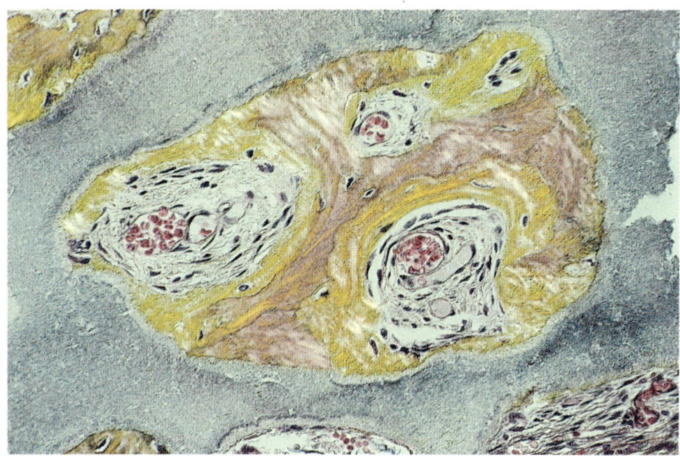

Fig. 58.68

Figs 58.67, 58.68 Bone cavity filled with a hydroxyapatite-tricalcium phosphate bone substitute. At 3 years, there is incomplete and peripheral bone formation (polarized light).

adequate amount of oxygen induce an osteoblastic differentiation, tension forces a fibroblastic differentiation while shear forces or a decreased amount of oxygen lead to differentiation into chondroblasts.[225,233]

Irradiation of the graft for sterilization and destruction of the antigens interferes with bone formation and the bone matrix fibrillar network is destroyed.[224] In *frozen allografts,* bone immunogenicity is partially retained, vascularization is delayed and osteogenesis is also lowered. *Freeze-dried bone grafts* follow the same patterns and the biomechanical properties are altered.[224] *Chemotherapy* may also interfere with the incorporation of bone grafts.[233]

Ceramics of different kinds, such as hydroxyapatite, tricalcium phosphate or a combination of both, are the most recent bone substitutes evaluated and are used for bone defects, cysts or benign tumors.[229,237]

Hydroxyapatite (coral) has a gross architecture similar to that of cancellous bone and biopsies have shown that new bone fills the hydroxyapatite pores when the trabeculae of bone are in close apposition to the hydroxyapatite pores, the optimal diameter of which ranges from 100 to 600 μu [237,238] (Figs 58.61–58.63).

Tricalcium phosphate biodegradation occurs at a slow rate, by passive dissolution and osteoclastic resorption,[237] while osteogenesis is developing. Both bone substitutes are brittle and are not used in load-bearing applications; they act mostly as a scaffold for incorporation of connective tissue and subsequent bone formation, which varies considerably from one case to another (Figs 58.64–58.70); moreover, individual particles often migrate from the implant site, before bone ingrowth.

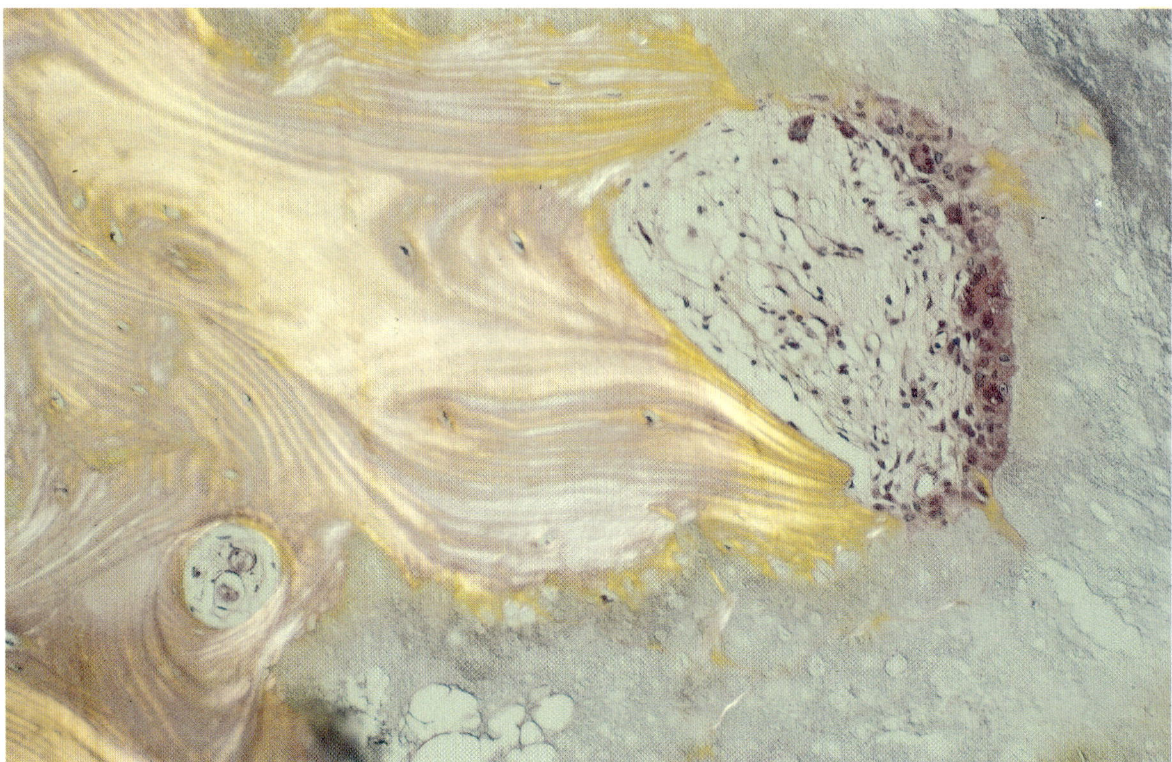

Fig. 58.69

Figs 58.69, 58.70 Hydroxyapatite bone substitute inserted in the femoral metaphysis. After a period of 1.5 years, osteoclastic and osteoblastic activities as well as woven bone formation are limited and peripherally located.

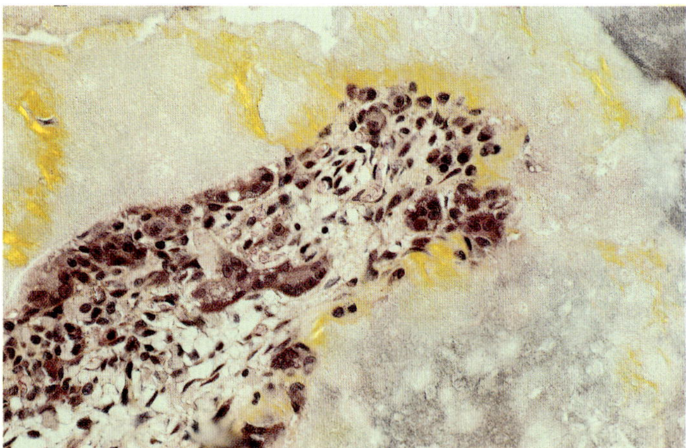

Fig. 58.70

REFERENCES

1. Kaplan S S. Biomaterial-host interactions: consequences, determined by implant retrieval analysis. Med Prog Technol 1994: 20: 209–230
2. Charosky C B, Bullough P G, Wilson P D Jr. Total hip replacement failures. A histological evaluation. J Bone Joint Surg (Am) 1973: 55: 49–58
3. Mirra J M, Amstutz H C, Matos M, Gold R. The pathology of the joint tissues and its clinical relevance in prosthesis failure. Clin Orthop 1976: 117: 221–240
4. Mirra J M, Marder R A, Amstutz H C. The pathology of failed total joint arthroplasty. Clin Orthop 1982: 170: 175–183
5. Eftekhar N S, Doty S B, Johnston A D, Parisien M V. Prosthetic synovitis. Hip 1985: 13: 169–183
6. Bullough P G, Di Carlo E F, Hansraj K K, Neves M C. Pathologic studies of total joint replacement. Orthop Clin North Am 1988: 19: 611–625
7. Pizzoferrato A, Savarino L, Stea S, Tarabusi C. Results of histological grading on 100 cases of hip prostheses. Biomaterials 1988: 9: 314–318
8. Feldman D S, Lonner J H, Desai P, Zuckerman J D. The role of intraoperative frozen sections in revision total joint arthroplasty. J Bone Joint Surg (Am) 1995: 77: 1807–1813
9. Löhrs U, Bos I. The pathology of artificial joints. Curr Top Pathol 1994: 86: 1–51
10. Sevitt S. Bone repair and fracture healing in Man. Edinburgh: Churchill Livingstone, 1981
11. Ling R S. Observations on the fixation of implants to the bony skeleton. Clin Orthop 1986: 210: 80–96

12. Willert H G, Ludwig J, Semlitsch M. Reaction of bone to methacrylate after hip arthroplasty (a long-term, gross, light-microscopic and scanning electron microscopic study). J Bone Joint Surg (Am) 1974: 56: 1368–1382

13. Jones L C, Hungerford D S. Cement disease. Clin Orthop 1987: 225: 192–206

14. Di Carlo E F, Bullough P G. The biologic responses to orthopedic implants and their wear debris. Clin Mater 1992: 9: 235–260

15. Charnley J. The reaction of bone to self-curing acrylic cement. A long-term histological study in man. J Bone Joint Surg (Br) 1970: 52: 340–353

16. Boss J H, Shajrawi I, Mendes D G. The nature of the bone-implant interface. Med Prog Technol 1994: 20: 119–142

17. Malcom A J. The bone-cement interface in long-standing prosthetic implants. In: Langlais F, Tomeno B, Eds. Limb salvage. Berlin: Springer-Verlag, 1991, pp 319–328

18. Jasty M, Maloney W J, Bragdon C R, Haire T, Harris W H. Histomorphological studies of the long-term skeletal responses to well fixed cemented femoral components. J Bone Joint Surg (Am) 1990: 72: 1220–1229

19. Schmalzried T P, Maloney W J, Jasty M, Kwong L M, Harris W H. Autopsy studies of the bone-cement interface in well-fixed cemented total hip arthroplasties. J Arthroplasty 1993: 8: 179–188

20. Linder L, Hansson H A. Ultrastructural aspects of the interface between bone and cement in man. J Bone Joint Surg (Br) 1983: 65: 646–649

21. Sela J, Bab I. The mechanism of 'primary mineralization' in the reaction of bone to injury and administration of implant. J Biomed Mater Res 1985: 19: 225–231

22. Revell P A. Tissue reactions to joint prostheses and the product of wear and corrosion. Curr Top Pathol 1982: 71: 73–101

23. Linder L, Carlsson A S. The bone-cement interface in hip arthroplasty. A histologic and enzyme histochemical study of stable components. Acta Orthop Scand 1986: 57: 495–500

24. Levack B, Revell P A, Freeman M A. Presence of macrophages at the bone-cement interface of stable hip arthroplasty components. Acta Orthop Scand 1987: 58: 384–387

25. Pazzaglia U E. Pathology of the bone-cement interface in loosening of total hip replacements. Arch Orthop Trauma Surg 1990: 109: 83–88

26. Fornasier V, Wright J, Seligman J. The histomorphologic and morphometric study of asymptomatic hip arthroplasty. Clin Orthop 1991: 271: 272–282

27. Freeman M A, Bradley G W, Revell P A. Observations upon the interface between bone and polymethylmethacrylate cement. J Bone Joint Surg (Br) 1982: 64: 489–493

28. Hori R Y, Lewis J L. Mechanical properties of the fibrous tissue found at the bone-cement cement interface following total joint replacement. J Biomed Mater Res 1982: 16: 911–927

29. Fornasier V L, Cameron H U. The femoral stem/cement interface in total hip replacement. Clin Orthop 1976: 116: 248–252

30. Maloney W J, Schmalzried T P, Jasty M, Kwong L M, Harris W H. The cement interface – retrieval studies. In: Morrey B F, Ed. Biological, material and mechanical considerations of joint replacement. New York: Raven Press, 1993, pp 51–69

31. Kwong L M, Jasty M, Mulroy R D, Maloney W J, Bragdon C, Harris W H. The histology of the radiolucent line. J Bone Joint Surg (Br) 1992: 74: 67–73

32. Draenert K, Rudigier J. Histomorphologie des Knochen-Zement-Kontaktes. Chirurg 1978: 49: 276–285

33. Lintner F, Bösch F, Brand G. Histologische Untersuchungen über Umbauvorgänge an der Zement-Knochengrenze bei Endoprothesen nach 3-bis 10 jähriger Implantation. Pathol Res Pract 1982: 173: 376–389

34. Stea S, Savarino L, Toni A, Sudanese A, Giunti A. Microradiographic and histochemical evaluation of mineralization inhibition at the bone-alumina interface. Biomaterials 1992: 13: 664–667

35. Buly R L, Huo M H, Salvati E, Brien W, Bansal M. Titanium wear debris in failed cemented total hip arthroplasty. J Arthroplasty 1992: 7: 315–323

36. Pizzoferrato A, Stea S, Savarino L, Granchi D, Ciapetti G. Histomorphometric evaluation and pathogenesis of prosthetic loosening. Chir Organi Mov 1994: 79: 245–255

37. Kozinn S C, Johanson N A, Bullough P G. The biologic interface between bone and cementless femoral endoprostheses. J Arthroplasty 1986: 1: 249–259

38. Howie D W. Tissue response in relation to type of wear particles around failed hip arthroplasties. J Arthroplasty 1990: 5: 337–348

39. Howie D W, Haynes D R, Rogers S D, McGee M A, Mearcy M J. The response to particulate debris. Orthop Clin North Am 1993: 24: 571–581

40. Lintner F, Zweymuller K, Böhm G, Brand G. Tissue reactions to titanium endoprostheses. J Arthroplasty 1986: 1: 183–195

41. Lintner F, Zweymuller K, Bôhm G, Brand G. Reactions of surrounding tissues to the cementless implant Ti 6AL 4V after an implantation period of several years. Arch Orthop Trauma Surg 1988: 107: 357–363

42. McCutchen J W, Collier J P, Mayor M B. Osteointegration of titanium implants in total hip arthroplasty. Clin Orthop 1990: 261: 114–125

43. Linder L, Albrektsson T, Bränemark P I et al. Electron microscopic analysis of the bone-titanium interface. Acta Orthop Scand 1983: 54: 45–52

44. Cameron H U, Pilliar R M, McNab I. The rate of bone ingrowth into porous material. J Biomed Mater Res 1976: 10: 295–302

45. Bobyn J D, Pilliar R M, Cameron H U, Weatherly G C. Osteogenic phenomena across endosteal bone-implant spaces with porous surfaced intramedullary implants. Acta Orthop Scand 1981: 52: 145–153

46. Portigliatti Barbos M. Bone ingrowth into madreporic prostheses. J Bone Joint Surg (Br) 1988: 70: 85–88

47. Engh C A, Bobyn J D, Glassman A H. Porous-coated hip replacement. The factors governing bone ingrowth, stress shielding and clinical results. J Bone Joint Surg (Br) 1987: 69: 45–55

48. Bobyn J D, Engh C A. Human histology of the bone-porous metal implant interface. Orthopedics 1984: 7: 1410–1421

49. Cook S D, Thomas K A, Haddad R J. Histologic analysis of retrieved human porous coated total joint components. Clin Orthop 1988: 234: 90–101

50. Collier J P, Mayor M B, Chae J C, Surprenant V A, Surprenant H P, Dauphinais L A. Macroscopic and microscopic evidence of prosthetic fixation with porous-coated materials. Clin Orthop 1988: 235: 173–180

51. Cook S D, Barrack R L, Thomas K A, Haddad R J. Quantitative histologic analysis of tissue growth into porous total knee components. J Arthroplasty 1989: 4(suppl): S33–S43

52. Collier J P, Bauer T W, Bloebaum R D et al. Results of implant retrieval from postmortem specimens in patients with well functioning long-term total hip replacement. Clin Orthop 1992: 274: 97–112

53. Jacobs J J, Sumner D R, Urban R M, Galante J O. Retrieval: successful uncemented implants. In: Morrey B F, Ed. Biological, material, and mechanical considerations of joint replacement. New York: Raven Press, 1993, pp 185–195

54. Bauer T W, Geesink R C, Zimmerman R, McMahon J T. Hydroxyapatite-coated femoral stems. J Bone Joint Surg (Am) 1991: 73: 1439–1452

55. Bloebaum R D, Bachus K N, Rubman M H, Dorr L D. Postmortem comparative analysis of titanium and hydroxyapatite porous-coated femoral implants retrieved from the same patient. J Arthroplasty 1993: 8: 203–211

56. Bloebaum R D, Merrell M, Gustke K, Simmons M. Retrieval analysis of a hydroxyapatite-coated hip prosthesis. Clin Orthop 1991: 269: 97–102

57. Furlong R J, Osborn J F. Fixation of hip prostheses by hydroxyapatite ceramic coatings. J Bone Joint Surg (Br) 1991: 73: 741–745

58. Hardy D C, Frayssinet P, Guilhem A, Lafontaine M A, Delince P E. Bonding of hydroxyapatite-coated femoral prostheses. J Bone Joint Surg (Br) 1991: 73: 732–740

59. Soballe K, Gotfredsen K, Brockstedt-Rasmussen H, Nielsen P T, Rechnagel K. Histologic analysis of a retrieved hydroxyapatite-coated femoral prosthesis. Clin Orthop 1991: 212: 255–258

60. Dhert W J. Retrieval studies on calcium phosphate-coated implants. Med Prog Technol 1994: 20: 143–154

61. Shanbhag A S, Jacobs J J, Glant T T, Gilbert J L, Black J, Galante J O. Composition and morphology of wear debris in failed uncemented total hip replacement. J Bone Joint Surg (Br) 1994: 76: 60–67

62. Chiba J, Schwendeman L J, Booth R E, Crossett L S, Rubash H E. A biochemical, histologic, and immunohistologic analysis of membranes obtained from failed cemented and cementless total knee arthroplasty. Clin Orthop 1994: 299: 114–124

63. Johanson N A, Bullough P G, Wilson P D, Salvati E A, Ranawat C S. The microscopic anatomy of the bone-cement interface in failed total hip arthroplasties. Clin Orthop 1987: 218: 123–135

64. Pazzaglia U E, Dell'Orbo C, Wilkinson M J. The foreign body reaction in total hip arthroplasties. A correlated light-microscopy, SEM, and TEM study. Arch Orthop Trauma Surg 1987: 106: 209–219

65. Lennox D W, Schofield B H, McDonald D F, Riley L H. A histologic comparison of aseptic loosening of cemented, press-fit, and biologic ingrowth prostheses. Clin Orthop 1987: 225: 171–191

66. Horowitz S M, Frondaza C G, Lennox D W. Effects of polymethylmethacrylate exposure upon macrophages. J Orthop Res 1988: 6: 827–832

67. Bos I, Lindner B, Seydel U et al. Untersuchungen über Lockerungsurchache bei Zementierten Hüftgelenkendoprothesen. Z Orthop 1990: 128: 73–82

68. Horowitz S M, Gautch T, Frondaza C M, Riley L. Macrophage exposure to polymethylmethacrylate leads to mediator release and injury. J Orthop Res 1991: 9: 406–413

69. Keen C E, Philip G, Brady K, Spencer J D, Levison D A. Histopathological and microanalytical study of zirconium dioxide and barium sulphate in bone cement. J Clin Pathol 1992: 45: 984–989

70. Walker P S, Bullough P G. The effect of friction and wear in artificial joints. Orthop Clin North Am 1973: 4: 273–293

71. Heilmann K, Diezel P B, Rossner J A, Brinkmann K A. Morphological studies in tissues surrounding alloarthroplastic joints. Virchows Arch A Pathol Anat Histol 1975: 366: 93–106

72. Willert H G, Buchhorn G H. Particle disease due to wear of ultrahigh molecular weight polyethylene. Findings from retrieval studies. In: Morrey B F, Ed. Biological, material, and mechanical considerations of joint replacement. New York: Raven Press, 1993, pp 87–102

73. Schmalzried T P, Jasty M, Harris W H. Periprosthetic bone loss in total hip arthroplasty. J Bone Joint Surg (Am) 1992: 74: 849–863

74. McKellop H A, Campbell P, Park S H et al. The origin of submicron polyethylene wear debris in total hip arthroplasty. Clin Orthop 1995: 311: 3–20

75. Hoene D, Rubash H. Isolation and characterization of wear particles generated in patients who have had failure of a hip arthroplasty without cement. J Bone Joint Surg (Am) 1995: 77: 1301–1310

76. Guttmann D, Schmalzried T P, Jasty M, Harris W H. Light microscopic identification of submicron polyethylene wear debris. J Appl Biomater 1993: 4: 303–307

77. Schmalzried T P, Jasty M, Rosenberg A, Harris W H. Histologic identification of polyethylene wear debris using Oil Red O stain. J Appl Biomater 1993: 4: 119–125

78. Hayashi T, Inoue H. Tissue reaction around loosened prostheses. A histological, X-ray microanalytic and immunological study. Acta Med Okayama 1986: 40: 229–241

79. Moran C A, Mullick F G, Ishak K G, Johnson F B, Hummer W B. Identification of titanium in human tissues: probable role in pathologic processes. Hum Pathol 1991: 22: 450–454

80. Lee J M, Salvati E A, Betts F, Di Carlo E F, Doty S B, Bullough P G. Size of metallic and polyethylene debris particles in failed cemented total hip replacements. J Bone Joint Surg (Br) 1992: 74: 380–384

81. Pazzaglia U E, Ceciliani L, Wilkinson M J, Dell'Orbo C. Involvement of metal particles in loosening of metal-plastic total hip prostheses. Arch Orthop Trauma Surg 1985: 104: 164–174

82. Agins H J, Alcock N W, Bansal W et al. Metallic wear in failed titanium-alloy total hip replacements. A histological and quantitative analysis. J Bone Joint Surg (Am) 1988: 70: 347–356

83. Nasser S, Campbell P A, Kilgus D, Kossovsky N, Amstutz H C. Cementless total joint arthroplasty prostheses with titanium-alloy articular surfaces. A human retrieval analysis. Clin Orthop 1990: 261: 171–185

84. Winter G D. Tissue reactions to metallic wear and corrosion products in human patients. J Biomed Mater Res 1974: 8: 11–26

85. Harms J, Mausle E. Tissue reaction to ceramic implant material. J Biomed Mater Res 1979: 13: 67–87

86. Groth H E, Shilling J M. Tissue response to carbon-reinforced polyethylene. J Orthop Res 1983: 1: 129–135

87. Parsons J R, Bhayani S, Alexander H, Weiss A B. Carbon fiber debris within synovial joint. A time-dependent mechanical and histologic study. Clin Orthop 1985: 198: 69–76

88. Galante J O, Lemons J, Spector M, Wilson P D Jr, Wright T M. The biologic effects of implant materials. J Orthop Res 1991: 9: 760–775

89. Kaufman R L, Tong I, Beardmore T D. Prosthetic synovitis: clinical and histological characteristics. J Rheumatol 1985: 12: 1066–1074

90. Linder L, Lindberg L, Carlsson A. Aseptic loosening of hip prostheses. A histologic and enzyme histochemical study. Clin Orthop 1983: 175: 93–104

91. Goldring S R, Schiller A L, Roelke M, Rourke C M, O'Neill D A, Harris W H. The synovial-like membrane at the bone-cement interface in loose total hip replacements and its proposed role in bone lysis. J Bone Joint Surg (Am) 1983: 65: 575–583

92. Goldring S R, Jasty M, Roelke M S, Rourke C M, Binghurst F R, Harris W H. Formation of a synovial-like membrane at the bone-cement interface. Its role in bone resorption and implant loosening after total hip replacement. Arthritis Rheum 1986: 29: 836–842

93. Jasty M, Jiranek W, Harris W H. Acrylic fragmentation in total hip replacements and its biological consequences. Clin Orthop 1992: 285: 116–128

94. Forest M, Carlioz A, Vacher Lavenu M C et al. Histological patterns of bone and articular tissues after orthopaedic reconstructive surgery (artificial joint implants). Pathol Res Pract 1991: 187: 963–977

95. Goodman S B, Chin R C, Chirn S S, Schurmann D J, Woalson S T, Masada M P. A clinical-pathologic-biochemical study of the membrane surrounding loosened and non loosened total hip arthroplasties. Clin Orthop 1989: 244: 182–187

96. Shoji H, Karube S, D'Ambrosia R D, Dabezies E J, Miller D R. Biochemical features of pseudomembrane at the bone-cement interface of loosened total hip prostheses. J Biomed Mater Res 1983: 17: 669–678

97. Jacobs J J, Sumner D R, Galante J O. Mechanisms of bone loss associated with total hip replacement. Orthop Clin North Am 1993: 24: 583–590

98. Savarino L, Stea S, Ciapetti G et al. Microstructural investigation of bone-cement interface. J Biomed Mater Res 1995: 29: 701–705

99. Jasty M J, Floyd W E, Schiller A L, Goldring S R, Harris W H. Localized osteolysis in stable non-septic total hip replacement. J Bone Joint Surg (Am) 1986: 68: 912–919

100. Jasty M, Maloney W J, Bragdon C R, O'Connor D O, Haire T, Harris W H. The initiation of failure in cemented femoral components of hip arthroplasties. J Bone Joint Surg (Br) 1991: 73: 551–558

101. Jasty M, Bragdon C R, Maloney W J, Haire T, Harris W H. Ingrowth of bone in failed fixation of porous-coated femoral components. J Bone Joint Surg (Am) 1991: 73: 1331–1337

102. Bloebaum R D, Dupont J A. Osteolysis from a press-fit hydroxyapatite-coated implant. J Arthroplasty 1993: 8: 195–202

103. Bloebaum R D, Beeks D, Dorr L D, Savory C, Dupont J A, Hofmann A A. Complications with hydroxyapatite particulate separation in total hip replacements. Clin Orthop 1994: 298: 19–26

104. Murray D W, Rushton N. Macrophages stimulate bone resorption when they phagocytose particles. J Bone Joint Surg (Br) 1990: 72: 988–992

105. Athanasou N A, Quinn J, Bulstrode C J. Resorption of bone by

inflammatory cells derived from the joint capsule of hip arthroplasties. J Bone Joint Surg (Br) 1992: 74: 57–62

106. Quinn J, Joyner C, Triffitt J T, Athanasou N A. Polymethylmethacrylate-induced inflammatory macrophages resorb bone. J Bone Joint Surg (Br) 1992: 74: 652–658

107. Yokohama Y, Matsumoto T, Hirakawa M et al. Production of matrix metalloproteinases at the bone-implant interface in loose total hip replacements. Lab Invest 1995: 72: 899–911

108. Pandey R, Quinn J, Joyner C, Murray D W, Triffitt J T, Athanasou N A. Arthroplasty implant biomaterial particle associated macrophages differentiate into lacunar bone resorbing cells. Ann Rheum Dis 1996: 55: 388–395

109. Chambers T J, Horton M A. Failure of cells of mononuclear phagocyte series to resorb bone. Calcif Tissue Int 1984: 36: 556–560

110. Pazzaglia U E, Pringle J A. The role of macrophages and giant cells in loosening of joint replacement. Arch Orthop Trauma Surg 1988: 107: 20–26

111. Pazzagia U E, Pringle J A. Bone resorption in vitro: macrophages and giant cells from failed total hip replacement versus osteoclasts. Biomaterials 1989: 10: 286–288

112. Kodaya Y, Al-Saffar N, Kobayashi A, Revell P A. The expression of osteoclast markers on foreign body giant cells. Bone Miner 1994: 27: 85–96

113. Herman J H, Sowder W G, Anderson D, Appell A M, Hopson C N. Polymethylmethacrylate-induced release of bone-resorbing factors. J Bone Joint Surg (Am) 1989: 71: 1530–1541

114. Ohlin A, Johnell O, Lerner U H. The pathogenesis of loosening of total hip arthroplasties. Clin Orthop 1990: 253: 287–296

115. Hopson C N, Herman J H. Prosthesis-associated pseudomembrane-induced bone resorption. Br J Rheumatol 1990: 29: 32–36

116. Jiranek W A, Machado M, Jasty M et al. Production of cytokines around loosened cementless acetabular components. J Bone Joint Surg (Am) 1993: 75: 863–879

117. Kim K J, Rubash H E, Wilson S C, D'Antonio J A, McClain E J. A histologic and biochemical comparison of the interface tissues in cementless and cemented hip prostheses. Clin Orthop 1993: 287: 142–152

118. Maloney W J, James R E, Smith R L. Human macrophage response to retrieved titanium alloy particles in vitro. Clin Orthop 1996: 322: 268–278

119. Perry M J, Mortuza F Y, Ponsford F M, Elson C J, Atkins R M. Analysis of cell types and mediator production from tissues around loosening joint implants. Br J Rheumatol 1995: 34: 1127–1134

120. Westacott C I, Taylor G, Atkins R, Elson C. Interleukin 1 alpha and beta production by cells isolated from membranes around aseptically loose total joint replacements. Ann Rheum Dis 1992: 51: 638–642

121. Al Saffar N, Revell P A. Interleukin-1 production by activated macrophages surrounding loosened orthopaedic implants: a potential role in osteolysis. Br J Rheumatol 1994: 33: 309–316

122. Shanbhag A S, Jacobs J J, Black J, Galante J O, Glant T T. Cellular mediators secreted by interfacial membranes obtained at revision total hip arthroplasty. J Arthroplasty 1995: 10: 498–506

123. Horowitz S M, Doty S B, Lane J M, Burstein A H. Studies of the mechanism by which the mechanical failure of polymethylmethacrylate leads to bone resorption. J Bone Joint Surg (Am) 1993: 75: 802–813

124. Horowitz S M, Rapuano B P, Lane J M, Burstein A H. The interaction of the macrophage and the osteoblast in the pathophysiology of aseptic loosening of joint replacements. Calcif Tissue Int 1994: 54: 320–324

125. Horowitz S M, Purdon M A. Mediator interactions in macrophage/particulate bone resorption. J Biomed Mater Res 1995: 29: 477–484

126. Santavirta S, Sorsa T, Konttinen Y T, Saari H, Eskola A, Eisen A Z. Role of the mesenchymal collagenase in the loosening of total hip prosthesis. Clin Orthop 1993: 290: 206–215

127. Hembry R M, Bagga M R, Reynolds J J, Hamblen D L. Stromelysin, gelatinase A and TIMP-1 in prosthetic interface tissue: a role for macrophages in tissue remodelling. Histopathology 1995: 27: 149–159

128. Schüller H M, Scholten P E, Lettinga K, Marti R K, Van Noorden C J. High cathepsin B activity in arthroplasty interface membranes. Acta Orthop Scand 1993: 64: 613–618

129. Takagi M, Konttinen Y T, Santavirta S et al. Extracellular matrix metalloproteinases around loose total hip prostheses. Acta Orthop Scand 1994: 65: 281–286

130. Takagi M, Konttinen Y T, Santavirta S, Kangaspunta P, Suda A, Rokkanen P. Cathepsin G and alpha 1-antichymotrypsin in the local host reaction to loosening of total hip prostheses. J Bone Joint Surg (Am) 1995: 77: 16–25

131. Al-Saffar N, Khwaja H A, Kadoya Y, Revell P A. Assessment of the role of GM-CSF in the cellular transformation and the development of erosive lesions around orthopaedic implants. Am J Clin Pathol 1996: 105: 628–639

132. Cook S D, McCluskey L C, Martin P C, Haddad R J. Inflammatory response in retrieved non cemented porous-coated implants. Clin Orthop 1991: 264: 209–221

133. Boynton E L, Henry M, Morton J, Waddell J P. The inflammatory response to particulate wear debris in total hip arthroplasty. Can J Surg 1995: 38: 507–515

134. Salter D M, Krajewski A S, Robertson S. Lymphocytes in pseudomembranes of late prosthetic joint failure. J Pathol 1992: 166: 271–275

135. Solovieva S A, Ceponis A, Konttinen Y T et al. Mast cells in loosening of totally replaced hips. Clin Orthop 1996: 322: 158–165

136. Blunn G W, Wait M E. Intramedullary cement fixation: a comparison of the fixation of custom-made prostheses with the fixation of standard joint replacements. In: Older J, Ed. Implant bone interface. London: Springer-Verlag, 1990, pp 151–163

137. Blunn G W, Wait M E, Scales J T. Intramedullary fixation of massive prostheses using acrylic cement: a retrieval study. In: Langlais F, Tomeno B, Eds. Limb salvage. Berlin: Springer-Verlag, 1991, pp 251–256

138. Blunn G W, Wait M E. Remodelling of bone around intramedullary stems in growing patients. J Orthop Res 1991: 9: 809–819

139. Gottsauner-Wolf F, Kotz R, Salzer M, Plenk H. Histomorphological findings in different cementless anchored humerus prostheses. In: Langlais F, Tomeno B, Eds. Limb salvage. Berlin: Springer-Verlag, 1991, pp 329–334

140. Capanna R, Van Horn J R, Ruggieri P et al. A study of the bone-cement interface in upper limb prostheses not subjected to loading. Ital J Orthop Traumatol 1987: 13: 89–97

141. Franzen H, Carlsson A, Johnsson R, Rydholm A, Onnerfält R. Bony atrophy after mega total hip replacements for bone tumors. Acta Orthop Scand 1994: 65: 513–516

142. Horowitz S M, Glasser D B, Lane J M, Healey J H. Prosthetic and extremity survivorship after limb salvage for sarcoma. Clin Orthop 1993: 293: 280–286

143. Urwin P S, Cannon S R, Grimer R J, Kemp H B, Sneath R S, Walker P S. Aseptic loosening in cemented custom-made prosthetic replacements for bone tumours of the lower limb. J Bone Joint Surg (Br) 1996: 78: 5–13

144. Tallroth K, Eskola A, Santavirta S, Konttinen Y T, Lindholm T S. Aggressive granulomatous lesions after hip arthroplasty. J Bone Joint Surg (Br) 1989: 71: 571–575

145. Paavilainen T, Tallroth K. Aggressive granulomatous lesions in cementless total hip arthroplasty. J Bone Joint Surg (Br) 1990: 72: 980–984

146. Harris W H, Schiller A L, Scholler J M, Freiberg R A, Scott R. Extensive localized bone resorption in the femur following total hip replacement. J Bone Joint Surg (Am) 1976: 58: 612–618

147. Scott W W Jr, Riley L H Jr, Dorfman H D. Focal lytic lesions associated with femoral stem loosening in total hip prosthesis. AJR 1985: 144: 977–982

148. Dannemaier W C, Haynes D W, Nelson C L. Granulomatous reaction and cystic bony destruction associated with high wear rate in a total knee prosthesis. Clin Orthop 1985: 198: 224–230

149. Kaste S C, Rao B N, Lynch M H, Parham D M, Meyer W H. Multifocal osteolysis following limb-sparing procedures: imaging findings and a review of the literature. Pediatr Radiol 1996: 26: 158–161

150. Griffiths H J, Burke J, Bonfiglio T A. Granulomatous pseudotumors in total joint replacement. Skeletal Radiol 1987: 16: 146–152

151. Huddleston H D. Femoral lysis after cemented hip arthroplasty. J Arthroplasty 1988: 3: 285–297

152. Shaw J A. Multiple myeloma. A differential consideration for osteolysis surrounding total hip arthroplasties. J Arthroplasty 1995: 10: 397–400

153. Bell R S, Ha'eri G B, Goodman S B, Fornasier V L. Case report 246. Osteolysis of the ilium associated with acetabular cup following total hip arthroplasty, secondary to foreign body reaction to polyethylene and methyl-methacrylate. Skeletal Radiol 1983: 10: 201–204

154. Mayo-Smith W, Rosenthal D I, Rosenberg A E, Harris W H. Case report 816. Rapid acceleration of osteolysis from loose cemented total hip replacement. Skeletal Radiol 1993: 22: 619–621

155. Hayek R J, Martinelli T J. Metallic wear debris in acetabular osteolysis in a mechanically stable cementless total hip replacement: report of a case. Orthopedics 1993: 16: 1277–1281

156. Maloney W J, Peters P, Engh C A, Chandler H. Severe osteolysis of the pelvis in association with acetabular replacement without cement. J Bone Joint Surg (Am) 1993: 75: 1627–1635

157. Pierson J L, Harris W H. Extensive osteolysis behind an acetabular component that was well fixed with cement. J Bone Joint Surg (Am) 1993: 75: 268–271

158. Pazzaglia U, Byers P D. Fractured femoral shaft through an osteolytic lesion resulting from the reaction to a prosthesis. J Bone Joint Surg (Br) 1984: 66: 337–339

159. Santavirta S, Konttinen Y T, Bergroth V, Eskola A, Tallroth K, Lindholm T S. Aggressive granulomatous lesions associated with hip arthroplasty. Immunopathological studies. J Bone Joint Surg (Am) 1990: 72: 252–258

160. Chiba J, Rubash H E, Kim K J, Iwaki Y. The characterization of cytokines in the interface tissues obtained from failed cementless total hip arthroplasty with and without femoral osteolysis. Clin Orthop 1994: 300: 304–312

161. Carlsson A S, Gentz C F, Linder L. Localized bone resorption in the femur in mechanical failure of cemented total hip arthroplasties. Acta Orthop Scand 1983: 54: 396–402

162. Maloney W J, Jasty M, Rosenberg A, Harris W H. Bone lysis in well-fixed cemented femoral components. J Bone Joint Surg (Br) 1990: 72: 966–970

163. Anthony P P, Gie G A, Howie C R, Ling R S. Localized endosteal bone lysis in relation to the femoral components of cemented total hip arthroplasties. J Bone Joint Surg (Br) 1990: 72: 971–979

164. Bjornsson B L, Truong L D, Cartwright J, Abrams J, Rutledge M L, Wheeler T M. Pelvic lymph node histiocytosis mimicking metastatic prostatic adenocarcinoma: association with hip prostheses. J Urol 1995: 154: 470–473

165. Bauer T W, Saltarelli M, McMahon J T, Wilde A H. Regional dissemination of wear debris from a total knee prosthesis. J Bone Joint Surg (Am) 1993: 75: 106–111

166. Benz E B, Sherburne B, Hayek J E, Falchuk K H, Sledge C B, Spector M. Lymphadenopathy associated with total joint prostheses. A report of two cases and a review of the literature. J Bone Joint Surg (Am) 1996: 78: 588–593

167. Shinto Y, Uchida A, Yoshikawa H, Araki N, Kato T, Ono K. Inguinal lymphadenopathy due to metal release from a prosthesis. J Bone Joint Surg (Br) 1993: 75: 266–269

168. Willert H G. Reactions of the articular capsule to wear products of artificial joint prostheses. J Biomed Mater Res 1977: 11: 157–164

169. Dorr L D, Bloebaum R, Emmanual J, Meldrum R. Histologic, biochemical, and ion analysis of tissue and fluids during total hip arthroplasty. Clin Orthop 1990: 261: 82–95

170. Langkamer V G, Case C P, Heap P et al. Systemic distribution of wear debris after hip replacement. J Bone Joint Surg (Br) 1992: 74: 831–839

171. Betts F, Wright T, Salvati E A, Beskey A, Bansal M. Cobalt-alloy metal debris in periarticular tissues from total hip revision arthroplasties. Clin Orthop 1992: 276: 75–82

172. Gray M H, Talbert M L, Talbert W M, Bansal M, Hsu A. Changes seen in lymph nodes draining the site of large joint prostheses. Am J Surg Pathol 1989: 13: 1050–1056

173. Albores-Saavedra J, Vuitch J, Delgado R, Wiley E, Hagler H. Sinus histiocytosis of pelvic lymph nodes after hip replacement. A histiocytic proliferation induced by cobalt-chromium and titanium. Am J Surg Pathol 1994: 18: 83–90

174. Morawski D R, Coutts R D, Handal E G, Luibel J, Santore R F, Ricci J L. Polyethylene debris in lymph nodes after a total hip arthroplasty. J Bone Joint Surg (Am) 1995: 77: 772–776

175. Hicks D G, Judkins A R, Sickel J Z, Rosier R N, Puzas J E, O'Keefe R J. Granular histiocytosis of pelvic lymph nodes following total hip arthroplasty. The presence of wear debris, cytokine production, and immunologically activated macrophages. J Bone Joint Surg (Am) 1996: 78: 482–496

176. Bertrand A F, Bertrand G, Dauver N, Richard M C. Une cause méconnue d'adénopathies profondes: histiocytose ganglionnaire au polyéthylène, satellite de prothèses articulaires. Ann Radiol 1993: 36: 114–117

177. O'Connell J X, Rosenberg A E. Histiocytic lymphadenitis associated with a large joint prosthesis. Am J Clin Pathol 1993: 99: 314–316

178. Charny C B, Jacobowitz G, Melamed J, Tata M, Harris M N. Sinus histiocytosis mimicking metastatic melanoma in lymph nodes of a patient with a large joint prosthesis: case report and review of the literature. J Surg Oncol 1995: 60: 128–130

179. Bos I, Johannisson R, Löhrs U, Lindner B, Seydel U. Comparative investigations of regional lymph nodes and pseudocapsules after implantation of joint endoprostheses. Pathol Res Pract 1990: 186: 707–716

180. Mohr W, Wessinghage D, Kogel H. 'Massive' chronische Sinushistiozytose inguinaler Lymphknoten bei Patienten mit Gelenkendoprothesen. Pathologe 1991: 12: 17–20

181. Jacobs J J, Urban R M, Wall J, Black J, Reid J D, Veneman L. Unusual foreign-body reaction to a failed total knee replacement: simulation of a sarcoma clinically, and a sarcoid histologically. J Bone Joint Surg (Am) 1995: 77A: 444–451

182. Svensson O, Mathiesen E B, Reinholt F P, Blomgren G. Formation of a fulminant soft-tissue pseudotumor after uncemented hip arthroplasty. J Bone Joint Surg (Am) 1988: 70: 1238–1242

183. Peoc'h M, Moulin C, Pasquier B. Systemic granulomatous reaction to a foreign body after hip replacement. N Engl J Med 1996: 335: 133–134

184. Bauer T W. Identification of orthopaedic wear debris (editorial, comment). J Bone Joint Surg (Am) 1996: 78: 479–483

185. Shea K G, Bloebaum R D, Avent J M, Birk T, Samuelson K A. Analysis of lymph nodes for polyethylene particles in patients who had a primary joint replacement. J Bone Joint Surg (Am) 1996: 78: 497–504

186. Ward J J, Thornbury D D, Lemons J E, Dunham W K. Metal-induced sarcoma. Clin Orthop 1990: 252: 299–306

187. McDougall A. Malignant tumor at site of bone plating. J Bone Joint Surg (Br) 1956: 38: 709–713

188. Dube V E, Fisher D E. Hemangioendothelioma of the leg following metallic fixation of the tibia. Cancer 1972: 30: 1260–1266

189. Tayton K J. Ewing's sarcoma at the site of a metal plate. Cancer 1980: 45: 413–415

190. McDonald I. Malignant lymphoma associated with internal fixation of a fractured tibia. Cancer 1981: 48: 1009–1011

191. Dodion P, Putz P, Amiri-Lamraski M H et al. Immunoblastic lymphoma at the site of an infected vitallium bone plate. Histopathology 1983: 6: 807–813

192. Lee Y S, Pho R W, Nather A. Malignant fibrous histiocytoma at site of metal implant. Cancer 1984: 54: 2286–2289

193. Hughes A W, Sherlock D A, Hamblen D L, Reid R. Sarcoma at the site of a single hip screw. J Bone Joint Surg (Br) 1987: 69: 470–472

194. Apley A G. Editorial: malignancy and joint replacement: the tip of an iceberg? J Bone Joint Surg (Br) 1989: 71: 1

195. Penman H G, Ring P A. Osteosarcoma in association with total hip replacement. J Bone Joint Surg (Br) 1984: 66: 632–634

196. Bago-Granell J, Aguire-Cayadell M, Nardi N, Tallada N. Malignant fibrous histiocytoma at the site of a total hip arthroplasty. J Bone Joint Surg (Br) 1984: 66: 38–40

197. Swann M. Malignant soft-tissue tumor at the site of a total hip replacement. J Bone Joint Surg (Br) 1984: 66B: 629–631

198. Mazabraud A, Florent J, Laurent M. Un cas de carcinome épidermoide développé au contact d'une prothèse articulaire de hanche. Bull Cancer 1989: 76: 573–581

199. Kolstad K, Högstorp H. Gastric carcinoma metastasis to a knee with a newly inserted prosthesis: a case report. Acta Orthop Scand 1990: 61: 369–370

200. Kahn D G, Blazina M E. Incidental metastatic mammary carcinoma in a total knee arthroplasty patient. Clin Orthop 1993: 295: 142–145

201. Harris W R. Chondrosarcoma complicating total hip arthroplasty in Maffucci's syndrome. Clin Orthop 1990: 260: 212–214

202. Jacobs J J, Rosenbaum D H, Hay R M, Gitelis S, Black J. Early sarcomatous degeneration near a cementless hip replacement. J Bone Joint Surg (Br) 1992: 74: 740–744

203. Goodfellow J. Malignancy and joint replacement (editorial). J Bone Joint Surg (Br) 1992: 74: 645

204. Vives P, Sevestre H, Grodet H, Marie F. Histiocytome fibreux malin du fémur après prothèse totale de hanche. Rev Chir Orthop 1987: 73: 407–409

205. Tait N P, Hacking P M, Malcom A J. Case reports: malignant fibrous histiocytoma occurring at the site of a previous total hip replacement. Br J Radiol 1988: 61: 73–76

206. Haag M, Adler C P. Malignant fibrous histiocytoma in association with hip replacement. J Bone Joint Surg (Br) 1989: 71: 701

207. Nelson J P, Phillips P H. Malignant fibrous histiocytoma associated with total hip replacement. Orthop Rev 1990: 19: 1078–1080

208. Troop J K, Mallory T H, Fisher D A, Vaughn B K. Malignant fibrous histiocytoma after total hip arthroplasty. Clin Orthop 1990: 253: 297–300

209. Solomon M I, Sekel R. Total hip replacement complicated by a malignant fibrous histiocytoma. J Arthroplasty 1992: 7: 549–550

210. Rock M G. Toxicity oncogenesis. In: Morrey B F, Ed. Biological, material and mechanical considerations of joint replacement. New York: Raven Press, 1993, pp 339–351

211. Aboulafia A J, Littelton K, Shmookler B, Malawer M M. Malignant fibrous histiocytoma at the site of hip replacement in association with chronic infection. Orthop Rev 1994: 23: 427–432

212. Iglesias M E, Vazquez Doval F J, Idoate F, Valenti J R, Quintanilla E. Malignant fibrous histiocytoma at the site of a total knee replacement. J Dermatol Surg Oncol 1994: 20: 848–849

213. Theegarten D, Sardisong F, Philippou S. Malignes fibroses Histiocytom im Bereich einer Totalendoprothese des Huftgelenkes. Chirurg 1995: 66: 158–161

214. Martin A, Bauer T W, Manley M T, Marks K E. Osteosarcoma at the site of total hip replacement. J Bone Joint Surg (Am) 1988: 70: 1561–1567

215. Brien W W, Salvati E A, Healy J, Bansal M, Betts F. Osteogenic sarcoma arising in the area of a total hip replacement. J Bone Joint Surg (Am) 1990: 72: 1097–1098

216. Van Der List J J, Van Horn J R, Slooff T J, Naudin Ten Cate L. Malignant epithelioid hemangioendothelioma at the site of a hip prosthesis. Acta Orthop Scand 1988: 59: 328–330

217. Himmer O, Lootvoot L, Deprez P, Monfor L, Ghosez J P. Angiosarcome après prothèse totale du genou. Rev Chir Orthop 1991: 77: 125–129

218. Eckstein F S, Vogel U, Mohr W. Fibrosarcoma in association with a total knee joint prosthesis. Virchows Archiv A Pathol Anat 1992: 421: 175–178

219. Weber P C. Epithelioid sarcoma in association with total knee replacement. J Bone Joint Surg (Br) 1986: 68: 824–826

220. Ryu R K, Bovill E G, Skinner H B et al. Soft tissue sarcoma associated with aluminium oxide ceramic total hip arthroplasty. Clin Orthop 1987: 216: 207–212

221. Lamovec J, Zidar A, Cucek-Plenicar M. Synovial sarcoma associated with total hip replacement. J Bone Joint Surg (Am) 1988: 70: 1558–1560

222. Gillespie W J, Frampton C M, Henderson R J, Ryan P M. The incidence of cancer following total hip replacement. J Bone Joint Surg (Br) 1988: 70: 539–542

223. Urist M R. Bone transplants and implants. In: Urist M R, Ed. Fundamental and clinical bone physiology. Philadelphia: J B Lippincott, 1980, pp 331–368

224. Burchardt H. The biology of bone graft repair. Clin Orthop 1983: 174: 28–42

225. Bassett C A. Clinical implications of cell function in bone grafting. Clin Orthop 1972: 87: 49–59

226. Elves M W, Pratt L M. The pattern of new bone formation in isografts of bone. Acta Orthop Scand 1975: 46: 549–560

227. Heiple K G, Goldberg V M, Powell A E, Bos G D, Zika J M. Biology of cancellous bone grafts. Orthop Clin North Am 1987: 18: 179–185

228. Goldberg V M, Stevenson S. Natural history of autografts and allografts. Clin Orthop 1987: 225: 7–16

229. Burchardt H. Biology of bone transplantation. Orthop Clin North Am 1987: 18: 187–196

230. Springfield D S. Massive autogenous bone grafts. Orthop Clin North Am 1987: 18: 249–256

231. Stevenson S, Horowitz M. The response to bone allografts. J Bone Joint Surg (Am) 1992: 74: 939–950

232. Kandel R A, Pritzker K P, Langer F, Gross A E. The pathologic features of massive osseous grafts. Hum Pathol 1984: 15: 141–146

233. Gross T P, Jinnah R H, Clarke H J, Cox Q G. The biology of bone grafting. Orthopedics 1991: 14: 563–568

234. Delloye C, De Nayer P, Allington N, Munting E, Coutelier L, Vincent A. Massive bone allografts in large skeletal defects after tumor surgery: a clinical and microradiographic evaluation. Arch Orthop Trauma Surg 1988: 107: 31–41

235. Enneking W F, Mindell E R. Observations on massive retrieved human allografts. J Bone Joint Surg (Am) 1991: 73: 1123–1142

236. Caldora P, Donati D, Capanna R et al. A histomorphologic study of explants of massive allografts: preliminary results. Chir Organi Mov 1995: 80: 191–205

237. Bucholz R W, Carlton A, Holmes R E. Hydroxyapatite and tricalcium phosphate bone graft substitutes. Orthop Clin North Am 1987: 18: 323–334

238. Ripamonti U. The morphogenesis of bone in replicas of porous hydroxyapatite obtained from conversion of calcium carbonate exoskeletons of coral. J Bone Joint Surg (Am) 1991: 73: 692–703

59

Chemotherapy of bone tumors

P. Pouillart   B. Laguerre   S. Scholl

OSTEOSARCOMA

The natural history of osteosarcomas (OS) of the extremities has been revolutionized by adjuvant chemotherapy, which was first advocated in the early 1970s. Two facts characterize this evolution: the substantial improvement of survival rates and the definite increase in limb preservation rates.

Prior to the adjuvant chemotherapy era, treatment consisted exclusively of radical surgery and metastatic progression occurred in 80–90% of patients at a median time interval to progression of 5–8 months.[1,2,3] Conventional adjuvant chemotherapy following surgery or, more recently, 2–4 courses of preoperative chemotherapy has substantially improved survival rates which are commonly quoted as being between 52% and 83%.[4,5,6,7,8] These encouraging results, mostly from pilot studies, have been confirmed by two randomized trials, thereby controlling for methodological flaws.[5,6]

Chemotherapeutic agents: principles of use and modes of delivery in OS

Phase II trials in patients with measurable disease led to the selection of the most potent cytotoxic agents. These are listed in Table 59.1. Three cytotoxic agents play a key role in the present treatment strategies: these are methotrexate given at high dose (HD.MTX), doxorubicin (DOX) and cis-platinum (CDDP).

The combination of these drugs is now considered as part of the standard treatment in OS, in both adjuvant and preoperative (neoadjuvant) treatment. Doses of HD.MTX vary between 8 and 12 g/m^2 according to the different protocols and the general tolerance of the patient. With these doses, concentrations of MTX are respectively 1.3 to 37 times greater than those of the surrounding healthy tissues. These results suggest a selective distribution as well as a specific action of MTX at this high dose.[9]

Table 59.1 Osteosarcoma. Chemotherapy: phase II studies

Drugs	Objective response rates
HD.MTX* q week	82%
HD.MTX* q 3 weeks	42%
Cyclophosphamide (CTX)	15%
Ifosfamide (IFM)	33%
Doxorubicin (DOX)	26%
Cis-platinum (CDDP)	33%
Actinomycin D (ACD)	15%
ACD + CTX + Bleo**	45%

* HD.MTX: High dose methotrexate + folinic acid rescue.
** Bleo: Bleomycin.

Doxorubicin is generally considered as the most active drug in metastatic OS, given at the minimal dose of 60 mg/m^2 per injection. With an objective tumor response level over 25% first reported in the early 1970s, DOX constituted, with HD.MTX, the basis of the first adjuvant trials. Subsequently, retrospective analysis has documented a positive correlation between dose intensity (mean dose administered in mg/m^2/week) and primary or secondary tumor response.[10,11,12]

Cis-platinum (CDDP) is also a major antitumor agent. With a 33% level of response, it plays a major role in adjuvant protocols in association with DOX.[13,14]

High-dose ifosfamide (IFM), administered at a dosage of 9–12 g/m^2 also appears to be an active agent although it provokes some hematological toxicity. The urinary complications of this drug are preventable.[15]

Finally, the association of cyclophosphamide (CPM), bleomycin (BLM) and actinomycin D (ACD), with a 45% response rate, was considered an effective combination of individually poorly active drugs and was proposed as an alternative treatment in the case of non-response to the preoperative chemotherapy.[16]

To summarize, the present strategies of cytotoxic treatment in OS are based on four drugs, HD.MTX, DOX, CDDP and IFM, generally considered as standard and present day limb-preserving strategies depend on an efficacious first-line preoperative chemotherapy

Therapeutic strategies: design and implication

Schematically, the treatment of OS has two aims: the regression of the primary tumor and control of clinically undetectable micrometastases.

With classic adjuvant treatments following radical surgery, disease-free survival rates between 35% and 55% are commonly obtained.[35,36,37] In this case, the objective of chemotherapy is the exclusive control of systemic micrometastatic disease. Preoperative chemotherapy regimes have now been in use over the last 15 years.

The theoretical advantages of this approach are threefold: the objective evaluation of tumor response to chemotherapy, the early start of systemic treatment and the reduction in tumor volume, allowing a more conservative surgical treatment. Furthermore, it appears that the risk of the occurrence of a spontaneous resistant clone is reduced, as well as the risk of dissemination during surgery.

The histological evaluation of tumor response to preoperative chemotherapy has been recognized as an essential parameter of prognosis: a poor response carries a high risk of metastatic recurrence, independent of the total duration of treatment with the same chemotherapy.[17] This correlation, first reported by clinicians from the Memorial Sloan Kettering Cancer Center, has since been confirmed by other centers.[19,20,21]

The evaluation of response according to standard clinical and radiological criteria (X-ray, CT scan, MRI, arteriography and dynamic scintigrams) contributes to the patient evaluation, but the only objective criterion of response is provided by the detailed histological assessment of the surgical specimen. The histological assessment as proposed by Huvos has remained the reference system according to which histological response is split into four categories, as shown in Table 59.2, whereby patients can be subdivided into favorable (grades 3 and 4) or unfavorable prognostic groups (grades 1 and 2).

Other studies have proposed less stringent criteria of evaluation. The COSS 80 study[23] suggested a high degree of tumor necrosis (>50%) to be a marker of good outcome. According to the MD Anderson evaluation scale,[24] three levels of response were designated as:

1. none or uncertain response (less than 40% tumor necrosis);
2. partial response (40–60% tumor necrosis);
3. objective response (60% tumor necrosis).

This seemingly straightforward evaluation system has the inconvenience of decreasing the differences in prognosis between subgroups and most investigators therefore prefer the Huvos system. This design uses the patient as their own control and allows separation into two groups: a first group which responds to chemotherapy with a favorable outcome and a second non-responsive group requiring an alternative treatment.

Initial results from the MSKCC appeared very promising, with 85–90% of initial poor responders remaining tumor free after an alternative regime (protocol T10).[7,8]

Table 59.2 Histological grading of response to preoperative chemotherapy in OS according to the histological scale of Huvos and Rosen[7]

Grade I	Little or no effect
Grade II	Area of acellular tumor osteoid and necrotic material related to the effect of preoperative chemotherapy associated with areas of histologically viable tumor
Grade III	Scattered foci of histologically viable tumor cells
Grade IV	No histological evidence of viable tumor cells

Two facts have since modified this early optimistic evaluation: the prolongation of follow-up beyond 3 years and the multiplicity of experiences from structured trials which did not confirm the first results.

Response rates and outcome

Objective response rates to first-line chemotherapy are in the order of 50% (range 30–85%). Higher response rates are achieved in younger patients (<20), due to higher dose intensities as well as a different modality of administration.[39]

Several cytotoxic agents have been assessed in intraarterial delivery: these were DOX, CDDP and 5-fluorouracil. These types of perfusions require precise technique and close surveillance to prevent the risks of extraarterial diffusion and necrosis of healthy peritumoral tissues.

Using intraarterial DOX and/or CDDP, very high local concentrations of the drugs can be achieved that are responsible for regression of the primary and an increase in the rates of conservative surgery.[25,27,30] Higher tumor response rates have been reported than following intravenous administration. However, disease-free and overall survival rates remain unchanged.[25–29]

The first multidisciplinary trials graded their patients according to their initial response to preoperative chemotherapy, with two objectives:

1. the evaluation of objective response rates and their correlation with the prognosis;
2. the evaluation of alternative regimens in patients with refractory tumors. Results of these principal trials are listed in Table 59.3.

Disease-free survival rates in these different trials are quite comparable. Overall, alternative therapeutic regimes did not modify the prognosis of patients whose tumors resisted first-line chemotherapy. In the absence of a really efficient, non-crossreacting second line of treatment, therefore, real progress can only be achieved by new drugs or by a better understanding of biological mechanisms that influence response.

Prediction of response

Despite major progress over the last two decades, all we

Table 59.3 Osteosarcoma. Disease-free survival (DFS) at 2 years in trials incorporating preoperative chemotherapy

Institutions	%DFS	Ref
Protocol T10	76	4
Mount Sinai	77	20
Rizzoli	58	31
M.D. Anderson	60	21
COSS 80	68	23
COSS 82	58	19

can offer today following failed first-line chemotherapy is the uncertainty of a second non-crossreacting regimen.

Fortunately, newer studies suggest that biological criteria may permit prediction of response, thereby allowing selection of potentially resistant tumors for more intensive treatments.

The loss of heterozygocity of the RB gene has been detected in 70% of a retrospective series of 47 patients.[32] It carries a poor prognosis and is associated with higher metastatic recurrence rates and earlier recurrences.

The evaluation of pleiotropic resistance mechanisms and in particular the P-glycoprotein (PGP) (170 kD protein) was originally thought to be the mainstay of drug resistance. PGP is expressed by the amplified mdr1 gene. Following a retrospective trial including 92 patients with high-grade OS, it appears that overexpression of PGP detected by immunohistochemical analysis may be an independent indicator of a poor outcome. In a multivariate analysis the PGP status (p=0.001) and the extent of postchemotherapy tumor necrosis (p=0.04) were independent predictors of clinical outcome. The overall risk of adverse events was 3.37-fold increased among patients with overexpression of PGP as compared with patients with normal levels of expression of PGP.[33,34] These advances will hopefully produce biological criteria to improve our design of therapeutic strategies in the near future.

EWING'S SARCOMA

Ewing's sarcoma is a rare tumor of young people with a peak incidence in adolescence. Originating from the bone tissue, it is characterized by a very high incidence of metastases in bone, bone marrow, viscera and the central nervous system.

A specific chromosome translocation t(11;22)(q24;q12) gives rise to the expression of a fusion protein (EWS/FLI-1) which is diagnostic of Ewing's sarcoma.[44–46] The detection of this fusion protein also allows screening for residual disease and thereby redefines the state of complete remission with a high degree of accuracy. The fine tuning of this enhanced detection of residual disease, together with the high chemosensitivity and the possibility of drug intensification, have been major advances in the treatment of Ewing's sarcoma.

Cytotoxic agents

The efficacy of the drugs was defined in metastatic patients and response rates are shown in Table 59.4. With a response rate of over 30%, doxorubicin, cyclophosphamide, vincristine and actinomycin D are considered as part of the standard treatment of Ewing's sarcoma. The combination of several drugs, DOX and CTX[48] or etoposide VP and ifosfamide (IFM),[47] gives high response rates of the order of 70–96%.

This combination is active in both primary and metastatic lesions.[48,49] Clinical factors found to influence response rates are tumor volume and, to a minor degree, the site of the primary, as well as the presence of visceral and lymph node metastases.

Therapeutic design

Objective responses in metastatic patients rapidly led to more complex strategies including adjuvant chemotherapy.

The results published by Rosen showed the advantage of multidisciplinary approaches combining preoperative and adjuvant chemotherapy with a local treatment which consisted of surgery and/or radiation therapy.[50] At a median follow-up time of 41 months, the reported survival rates of 70% are far superior to the previously reported 5% survival rates following exclusively local treatment.[51,52] Furthermore, these first experiences drew attention to the respective roles of surgery and radiation treatment for local control. Surgery is generally preferred as treatment of the primary but two goals guide the management of an individual lesion: the tumor control and the preservation of function.

A new era started with the use of chemotherapy as the first line of treatment. Multiple clinical trials focused on the determination of optimal dose and drug combinations. Following the documentation of combinations of vincristine, cyclophosphamide and actinomycin D (VAC) as active agents, a further breakthrough, with the addition of DOX to this combination (VACA), was documented by the increase in 5-year survival rates from 28% to 65%.[55] Other studies showed the combination of etoposide and ifosfamide (VI) to be very potent and response rates up to 96% have been reported.[47]

More recently, sequential regimes alternating VAC and VI have been suggested by investigators from MSKCC. The hematological toxicity could be decreased by the use of cytokines (GCSF) and disease-free survival rates in poor prognosis Ewing's sarcoma of up to 77% at 5 years have been reported.[56]

All these results stem from different clinical trials which are not totally comparable in their design and treat probably very heterogeneous patient populations. Beyond the gain in survival reported regularly by these trials, the role of preoperative chemotherapy, other than facilitating the local treatment, is above all in controlling systemic dissemination of the disease. Three factors that will influence prognosis are commonly reported: these are the tumor volume, the objective response to chemotherapy as evaluated on the surgical resection specimen and the dose intensity of cytotoxic drugs and in particular of DOX.[12,53–55]

While the overall results of treatments in Ewing's sarcoma are very encouraging, the treatment of some cases remains unsatisfactory. Very bulky tumors, in particular

Table 59.4 Ewing's sarcoma. Chemotherapy: phase II studies

Drugs	% Objective responses
Cyclophosphamide	51
Ifosfamide	32
Doxorubicin	40
Actinomycin D	30
Vincristine	30
Etoposide	30
Cis-platinum	7
BCNU	33
5-fluorouracil	33

of the pelvis, and metastatic tumors at diagnosis remain refractory to cure.

Chemotherapy intensification was a highly challenging goal in these highly proliferative tumors. Several trials, but all with small patient numbers, have been carried out since the early 1980s (Table 59.4). The results are encouraging but difficult to evaluate since none of these trials is controlled. However, the results of Burdach,[56–58] showing disease-free survival rates of 48% (in 17 patients), argue in favor of a large-scale prospective trial in the near future.

PERIPHERAL NEUROECTODERMAL TUMORS (PNET)

Peripheral neuroectodermal tumors are affiliated with Ewing's sarcoma and share the same chromosome translocation t(11:22)(q24:q12).

They are rare tumors and there are no prospective trials and no defined specific therapy. Some information has been gained from retrospective studies.[59,60]

Treatment strategies used in Ewing's sarcoma gave good chemosensitivity with a dose-response relation to cyclophosphamide. However, despite an improved outcome following surgical resection of the primary tumor, the 5-year survival rates remain very low at 20%.[59] An independent study from Germany,[60] albeit less pessimistic, confirms the poor prognosis of PNET in comparison to Ewing's sarcoma.

OTHER PRIMARY BONE TUMORS

These are rare tumors with quite dissimilar histological appearances but treated similarly to osteosarcomas. For each histological type, the clinical experience is limited and the specific therapeutic options ill defined.

Malignant fibrous histiocytoma (MFH) of long bones is among the commonest of these rare tumors. The natural history of MFH shows these tumors to be highly invasive locally and to present a high risk of local recurrence as well as a poor outcome, with survival rates close to those of osteosarcoma despite adequate local treatment. Results from the Rizzoli Institute,[40] as well as more recent results from Earl,[41] show these tumors to be chemosensitive to classic osteosarcoma-type protocols. In a limited series of 18 evaluable patients, preoperative chemotherapy was followed by an objective response in all patients and massive necrosis (>90%) was reported in 7/15 patients.[41] These results confirm the belief that this therapeutic strategy might be beneficial in these tumors.[42,43]

Objective responses have also been documented in a few cases of inoperable malignant giant cell tumors and poorly differentiated chondrosarcomas. The paucity of case reports means that it is impossible to validate or invalidate the use of osteosarcoma-type chemotherapy in these rare tumors.

REFERENCES

1. Marcove R C, Miké V, Hajek J V et al. Osteogenic sarcoma under the age of of twenty-one. J Bone Joint Surg (Am) 1970: 52: 411–423
2. Friedman M A, Carter S K. The therapy of osteogenic sarcoma: current status and thoughts for the future. J Surg Oncol 1972: 4: 482–510
3. Harvei S, Solheim O. The prognosis in osteosarcoma: Norwegian national data. Cancer 1981: 48: 1719–1723
4. Meyers P A, Heller G, Healey G et al. Chemotherapy for nonmetastatic osteogenic sarcoma: the Memorial Sloan-Kettering experience. J Clin Oncol 1992: 10: 5–15
5. Link M P, Goorin A M, Miser A W et al. The effect of adjuvant chemotherapy on relapse free survival in patients with osteosarcoma of the extremity. N Eng J Med 1986: 314: 1600–1606
6. Eilber F, Giuliano A, Eckardt J et al. Adjuvant chemotherapy for osteosarcoma: a randomized prospective trial. J Clin Oncol 1987: 5: 21–26
7. Rosen G, Marcove R C, Huvos A G et al. Primary osteogenic sarcoma: eight year experience with adjuvant chemotherapy. J Cancer Res Clin Oncol 1983: 106: 55–67
8. Rosen G, Marcove R C, Caparros B et al. Primary osteogenic sarcoma, the rationale for preoperative chemotherapy and delayed surgery. Cancer 1979: 43: 2163–2177
9. Grem J L, King S A, Wittes R E et al. The role of methotrexate in osteosarcoma. JNCI 1988: 80: 626–636
10. Hryniuk W M. Average relative dose-intensity and the impact on design of clinical trials. Sem Oncol 1987: 14: 65–74
11. Cortes E P, Holland J F, Glidewell O. Amputation and adriamycin in primary osteosarcoma: a 5-year report. Cancer Treat Rep 1978: 62: 271–277
12. Smith M A, Ungerleider R S, Horowitz M E, Simon R. Influence of doxorubicin dose-intensity on response and outcome for patients with osteogenic sarcoma and Ewing's sarcoma. JNCI 1991: 83: 1460–1470
13. Ettinger L J, Douglass H O, Mindell E R et al. Adjuvant adriamycin and cisplatin in newly diagnosed, nonmetastatic osteosarcoma of the extremity. J Clin Oncol 1986: 4: 353–362
14. Ochs J J, Freeman A L, Douglass H O et al. Cis-dichlorodiamine platinum (II) in advanced osteogenic sarcoma. Cancer Treat Rep 1978: 62: 239–245
15. Marti C, Kroner T, Remagen T et al. High dose ifosfamide in advanced osteosarcoma. Cancer Treat Rep 1985: 69: 115–117
16. Mosende C, Guttierrez M, Caparros M, Rosen G. Combination chemotherapy with bleomycin, cyclophosphamide and dactinomycin for the treatment of osteogenic sarcoma. Cancer 1977: 40: 2779–2786.
17. Rosen G, Caparros B, Huvos A G et al. Preoperative chemotherapy for osteogenic sarcoma: selection of postoperative adjuvant chemotherapy based on the response of the primary tumor to preoperative chemotherapy. Cancer 1982: 9: 1221–1230
18. Rosen G, Nirenberg A. Chemotherapy for osteogenic sarcoma: an investigative method, not a recipe. Cancer Treat Rep 1982: 66: 1687–1697
19. Winkler K, Berron G, Delling G et al. Neoadjuvant chemotherapy of osteosarcoma: results of randomized cooperative trial (COSS 82) with salvage chemotherapy based on histological tumor response. J Clin Oncol 1988: 6: 329–337
20. Weiner M, Harris M, Lewis M et al. Neoadjuvant high dose methotrexate, cisplatin and doxorubicin for the management of patients with non metastatic osteosarcoma. Cancer Treat Rep 1986: 70: 1431–1432
21. Hudson M, Jaffe M R, Jaffe N, Ayala A. Pediatric osteosarcoma. Therapeutic strategies, results and and prognostic factors derived from a 10-year experience. J Clin Oncol 1990: 8: 1988–1997
22. Goldie J H, Coldman A J. A mathematical model for relating the drug sensitivity of tumors to their spontaneous mutation rate. Cancer Treat Rep 1979: 63: 1727–1733
23. Salzer-Kuntschik M, Delling G, Beron G et al. Morphological grades of regression in osteosarcoma after polychemotherapy. Study COSS 80. Cancer Res Clin Oncol 1983: 106: 21–24
24. Jaffe N, Prudich J, Knapp J et al. Treatment of primary osteosarcoma with intra-arterial and intraveinous high-dose methotrexate. J Clin Oncol 1983: 1: 428–431
25. Eilber F R, Morton D L, Eckardt J et al. Limb salvage for skeletal and soft tissue sarcomas. Multidisciplinary preoperative therapy. Cancer 1984: 3: 2579–2584
26. Winkler K, Bielack S, Delling G et al. Effect of intraarterial versus intravenous cisplatin in addition to systemic doxorubicin, high dose methotrexate and ifosfamide on histologic tumor response in osteosarcoma (study COSS 86). Cancer 1990: 66: 1703–1710
27. Jaffe N, Robertson R, Ayala A et al. Comparison of intraarterial Cis-diamminodichloroplatinum II with high dose methotrexate and citrovorum factor rescue in the treatment of primary osteosarcoma. J Clin Oncol 1985: 3: 1101–1104
28. Benjamin R S, Chawla S P, Carrasco C H et al. Preoperative chemotherapy for osteosarcoma with intravenous adriamycin and intra-arterial cisplatinum. Ann Oncol 1992: 3 (suppl 2): 3–6
29. Lackman R D, Weiss A. Long term results of intra-arterial preoperative chemotherapy for osteosarcoma. ASCO 1996: abstr. 1697: 526
30. Malawer M M, Buch R, Reaman G et al. Impact of two cycles of preoperative chemotherapy with intra-arterial cisplatin and intravenous doxorubicin on the choice of surgical procedure for high grade bone sarcomas of the extremities. Clin Orthop Rel Res 1991: 270: 214–222.
31. Bacci G, Picci P, Ruggieri P et al. Primary chemotherapy and delayed surgery (neoadjuvant chemotherapy) for osteosarcoma of the extremities. The Istituto Rizzoli experience in 127 patients treated preoperatively with intravenous methotrexate (high versus moderate doses) and intraarterial cisplatin. Cancer 1990: 65: 2539–2553
32. Feugeas O, Guriec N, Babin-Boiletot A et al. Loss of heterezygosity of the RB gene is a poor prognostic factor in patients with osteosarcoma. J Clin Oncol 1996: 14: 467–472
33. Baldini N, Scotlandi K, Barbanti-Brodano G et al. Expression of P-glycoprotein in high grade osteosarcomas in relation to clinical outcome. N Engl J Med 1995: 333: 1380–1385
34. Rosier R N, Teot L A, Hicks D G et al. Multiple drug resistance in osteosarcoma. Iowa Orthop J 1995: 15: 66–73
35. Picci P. Osteosarcoma and the cancers of bone. Current Opin Oncol 1992: 4: 674–680
36. Jaffe N, Frei E, Traggis D et al. Adjuvant methotrexate and citrovorum factor treatment of osteogenic sarcoma. N Engl J Med 1974: 291: 994–997
37. Rosenberg S A, Chabner B A, Young R C et al. Treatment of osteogenic sarcoma. I Effect of high dose methotrexate after amputation. Cancer Treat Rep 1979: 63: 739–751
38. Sutow W W, Sullivan M P, Fernbach D J et al. Adjuvant chemotherapy in primary treatment of osteogenic sarcoma. A Southwest Oncology Group study. Cancer 1975: 36: 1595–1608
39. Smith M A, Ungerleider R S, Horowitz M E, Simon R. Influence of doxorubicin dose-intensity on response and outcome for patients

with osteogenic sarcoma and Ewing's sarcoma. JNCI 1991: 83: 1460–1470

40. Bacci G, Springfield D, Picci P et al. Adjuvant chemotherapy for malignant fibrous histiocytoma in the femur and the tibia. J Bone Joint Surg (Am) 1985: 67: 620–625

41. Earl H M, Pringle J, Kemp H et al. Chemotherapy of malignant fibrous histiocytoma of bone. Ann Oncol 1993: 4: 409–415

42. Urban C, Rosen G, Huvos A G et al. Chemotherapy of malignant fibrous histiocytoma of bone. A report of five cases. Cancer 1983: 51: 795–802

43. Weiner M, Sedlis M, Johnston A D et al. Adjuvant chemotherapy of malignant fibrous histiocytoma of bone. Cancer 1983: 51: 25–29

44. Delattre O, Zucman J, Plougastel B et al. Gene fusion with an ETS domain caused by chromosome translocation in human tumors. Nature 1992: 359: 162–165

45. Zucman J, Delattre O, Desmaze C et al. Cloning and characterization of the Ewing's sarcoma and peripheral neuroepithelioma t(11:2) translocation breakpoints. Genes Chromosomes Cancer 1992: 5: 271–277

46. Zucman J, Melot T, Desmaze C et al. Combinatorial generations of variable fusion proteins in the Ewing's family of tumors. EMBO J 1993: 12: 4481–4487

47. Meyer W H, Kun L, Marina L et al. Ifosfamide plus etoposide in newly diagnosed Ewing's sarcoma of bone. J Clin Oncol 1992: 10: 1737–1742

48. Hayes F A, Thompson E I, Hustu H O et al. The response of Ewing's sarcoma to sequential cyclophosphamide and adriamycin induction therapy. J Clin Oncol 1983: 1: 45–51

49. Hayes F A, Thompson E I, Meyer W H et al. Therapy for localized Ewing's sarcoma of bone. J Clin Oncol 1989: 7: 208–213

50. Rosen G, Caparros B, Nirenberg N et al. Ewing's sarcoma: ten years experience with adjuvant chemotherapy. Cancer, 1981: 47: 2204–2213

51. Bacci G, Picci P, Gitelis S et al. The treatment of localized Ewing's sarcoma. Cancer 1982: 49: 1561–1570

52. Bacci G, Toni A, Avella M et al. Long term results in 144 localized Ewing's sarcoma patients treated with combined therapy. Cancer 1982: 63: 1477–1486

53. Jürgens H, Exner U, Gadner H et al. Multidisciplinary treatment of primary Ewing's sarcoma of bone. A 6 year experience of a European cooperative trial. Cancer 1988: 61: 23–32

54. Kinsella T J, Miser J S, Waller B et al. Long-term follow up of Ewing's sarcoma of bone treated with combined modality therapy. Int J Rad Oncol Biol Phys 1991: 20: 389–395

55. Nesbit M E, Gehan E A, Burgert E O et al. Multimodality for the management of primary non metastatic Ewing's sarcoma of bone: a long term follow up of the first intergroup study. J Clin Oncol 1990: 8: 1664–1674

56. Kushner B H, Meyers P A, Gerald W L et al. Very high-dose short-term chemotherapy for poor-risk peripheral primitive neuroectodermal tumors including Ewing's sarcoma of bone. J Clin Oncol 1995: 13: 2796–2804

57. Burdach S, Jörgens H, Peters C et al. Myeloablative radiochemotherapy and hematopoietic stem-cell rescue in poor-prognosis Ewing's sarcoma. J Clin Oncol 1993: 11: 1482–1488

58. Horowitz M E, Kinsella T J, Wexler L H et al. Total body irradiation and autologous bone-marrow transplant in the treatment of high risk Ewing's sarcoma and rhabdomyosarcoma. J Clin Oncol 1993: 11: 1911–1918

59. Kushner B H, Hajdu S I, Gulati S C et al. Extra-cranial primitive neuro-ectodermal tumors: the Memorial Sloan Kettering Cancer Center experience. Cancer 1991: 68: 1825–1829

60. Schmidt D, Herremann C, Jürgens C et al. Malignant peripheral neuroectodermal tumor and its necessary distinction from Ewing's sarcoma. A report from the Kiel pediatric tumor registry. Cancer 1991: 68: 2251–2259

60

Radiotherapy of bone tumors

C. Alapetite   J. M. Cosset

CHAPTER CONTENTS

INTRODUCTION

The place of radiotherapy in bone tumor treatment has been profoundly modified during the last two decades with the introduction of efficient aggressive chemotherapy protocols and the progress in functional surgery. Improvement of definition of local disease extent with new imaging methods has also been of great benefit.

A better knowledge of both the efficiency and limitation of modern ionizing radiation treatments enables the clinician to select suitable indications for radiotherapy as a tool for achievement of local control.

LATE EFFECTS OF IRRADIATION ON NORMAL TISSUE

Growing bone

The effects of ionizing radiation on growing bones are of great concern when considering local treatment of bone tumors which arise predominantly during childhood. Indeed, radiation-related growth impairment as observed in the past has greatly influenced its application in the management of pediatric tumors. The use of tolerance doses in combination with other treatment modalities and careful radiation therapy technique can minimize the risk of serious late effects.

Our knowledge of the pathophysiology of ionizing radiation on growing long bone is incomplete but several rapidly proliferating cell populations of the epiphyseal plate, including the cells of the proliferative zone and the endothelial growth buds, may be important targets for radiation damage (for review see[1]).

Both clinical and laboratory research indicates a dose–effect relationship for reduction of the growth rate. This relationship is particularly steep between the doses of 15 and 30 Gy,[2,3] reaching a 'saturation dose' at about 40 Gy. This effect is strongly dependent on age at exposure or, more precisely, on the capacity for growth remaining at this time. Height impairment is most severe among prepubertal children, particularly when irradiated at under 6 years of age.[4,5]

The volume and site of irradiation are also of importance since proximal and distal growth plates do not participate to the same extent in long bone growth.

The fraction size is also of concern, as suggested by the α/β ratio for growing bone (a calculated end point which reflects the sensitivity to fractionation) of approximately 4.5 Gy in animal models.[6]

The effects of radiation on other locations of long bone have been described:[7] a metaphyseal irradiation results in reduced absorptive processes in calcified bone and cartilage and a diaphyseal irradiation alters periosteal activity.

Other treatment parameters which influence bone growth are the quality of radiation and beam energy. Indeed, energies predominantly absorbed through the photoelectric effect as kilovoltage beams should be proscribed since the dose to bone, related in this case to the atomic number, is several times higher than that delivered to soft tissues.

The influence of concomitant chemotherapy should also be considered.

Technical precautions as described below, based on these observations, should reduce not only severe growth impairment but also scoliosis, curvature deformities and slipped capital femoral epiphysis, which may occur when the femoral head of children less than 4 years of age receives doses exceeding 25 Gy.

Mature bone, muscle, soft tissue and peripheral nerves

Radiation injury to mature bone, mainly pathological fractures, has decreased in frequency with the use of megavoltage and the avoidance of large biopsies in osteolytic areas. Edema, fibrosis, atrophy or contraction stress the need to avoid doses higher than 55 Gy in large volumes.[8,9] Radiation doses greater then 60 Gy are associated with a risk of injury to peripheral nerves but their fractionation sensitivity is high.[10]

SECONDARY BONE SARCOMAS AFTER RADIOTHERAPY

As the success of the primary treatment of malignant neoplasms has increased in recent decades, so has the recognition of secondary cancers. Radiation risk is particularly high at young age and the study of pediatric cancer populations has provided important quantitative data.

Among them, a recent update of the Late Effects Study Group has studied 48 cases of bone cancer occurring among 9170 patients.[11] The absolute excess risk was 9.4 per 10 000 persons per year in the whole population and reached the highest rates in retinoblastoma (53.6 per 10^4 per year) and in Ewing's sarcoma (59.6 per 10^4 per year).

The risk increased significantly with diagnostic delay, from 0.6 per 10^4 per year when less than 5 years after the diagnosis to 36.1 per 10^4 per year when more than 20 years.

A high dose–effect relationship was found, with no cases before 10 Gy and a relative risk of six after 10–30 Gy and 21 after 40–60 Gy. In this series 69% of bone sarcomas were osteosarcomas, 17% chondrosarcomas, 5% Ewing's sarcomas, 3% fibrosarcomas, 3% unspecified sarcomas and 1.5% malignant mesenchymomas. This was in agreement with other series.[12]

These secondary sarcomas occur in the skull and mandible, in the axial skeleton and in the long bones, which is not the usual distribution at young age. These locations, where radical surgery is often impossible, may partly explain the difficulties in treating these secondary tumors.

Alkylating agents may potentiate the carcinogenic effects of radiotherapy in Ewing's sarcoma.[13]

The very high risk of bone sarcoma after treatment of Ewing's sarcoma suggests an association with a genetic predisposition, similar to retinoblastoma.

The risk of postirradiation sarcoma after benign bone tumors[14,15] and particularly after giant cell tumors, as reported in the 1960s, has not been confirmed in recent long-term follow-up studies of aggressive cases treated with megavoltage radiotherapy.[16]

RADIATION TECHNIQUE RECOMMENDATIONS

A careful radiation therapy technique is essential in order to deliver a sufficient dose of radiation to achieve maximal local tumor control while minimizing the treatment-related complications. Indeed, for both tumor and normal tissue, the dose–response curve is quite steep in the relevant range.

In order to obtain the required precision, the chain of treatment planning starts with the positioning of the patient, which has to be comfortable and reproducible. Immobilization devices are generally required, especially for children, and should be employed when possible for pretreatment imaging in order to adequately locate the target volume.

Computed tomography and magnetic resonance imaging best define the osseous and soft tissue tumor extent. Computer technology offers reconstruction of the relative tumor topography and critical normal tissue volumes, together with the individual conformation of the patient.

Physicist and dosimetrist together with the radiotherapist perform the optimization of beam planning using combinations of photons and electrons of megavoltage units. Wedges, beam weighting and compensators are often required.

For extremities, oblique opposed fields with wedges or conventional opposed anteroposterior fields may provide adequate dose distribution in the tumor and spare normal tissue (Fig. 60.1).

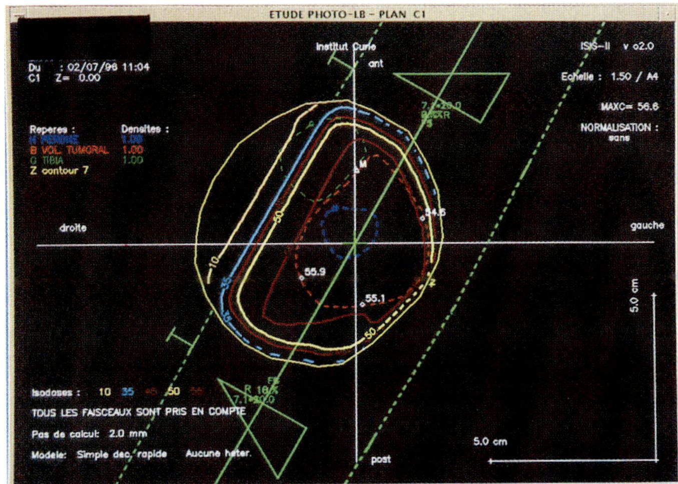

Fig. 60.1 Example of typical treatment planning for Ewing's sarcoma located in the fibula and associated with soft tissue extension. Note the sparing of a strip of normal tissue.

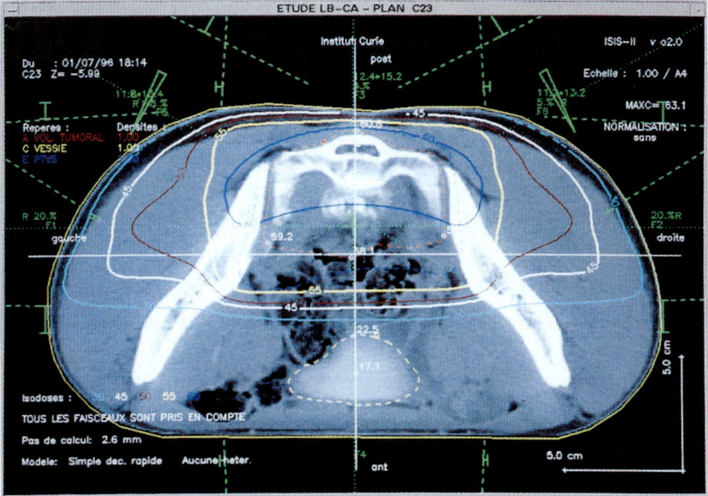

Fig. 60.2 Example of multifield treatment planning for Ewing's sarcoma of the sacrum offering the best protection of the bladder.

Multifield configurations are often required for pelvic lesions (Fig. 60.2) to protect the bladder.

Detailed explanations of the treatment process to the patient and the family are the best guarantee of the quality of the planned radiotherapy. Some recommendations are particularly important when considering radiation treatment of bones.

For lesions in the extremities, the actively growing epiphyseal cartilage should be excluded when possible without increasing the local tumor recurrence risk. If not possible, the entire growth plate should receive a homogeneous dose in order to avoid severe curvature deformities.

Vertebral bodies should also be completely covered by the radiation field without lateral or posterior-to-anterior dose gradients.

The capital femoral epiphysis should be shielded, especially in children under 4 in whom doses exceeding 25 Gy may result in slipped capital femoral epiphysis.

The joint should not be included in totality, particularly at the knee where irradiation of both epiphyses before fusion of the adjacent tibial and femoral growth plates may induce the most severe leg length discrepancies.

For extremities, sparing of a strip of linear soft tissue and avoidance of circumferential irradiation are vital to limit the risk of late fibrosis and functional limitation. The volume of irradiated soft tissue should be reduced after 55 Gy and the doses to peripheral nerves should not exceed 60 Gy. Fraction sizes equal or inferior to 1.8 Gy are recommended.

EWING'S SARCOMA

Although first described as a radioresponsive tumor by James Ewing,[17] the overall survival in early series with local irradiation alone averaged only 5–20% as a result of early distant recurrence.

The introduction of chemotherapy dramatically improved survival and permitted a local recurrence rate following radiotherapy of 15–20%.[18,19]

The relative roles of surgery and radiation therapy in local management are still under discussion.

A growing interest in the surgical approach is related both to the increased experience of limb salvage surgery or wide excisions for central tumors and the observation of second malignant tumors in long-term survivors after successful irradiation and effective adjuvant chemotherapy.[20,21]

At the present time, treatment at the primary site is either resection, resection and subsequent irradiation or irradiation alone. The decision requires coordinated discussions between orthopedic surgeons, radiotherapists, pathologists and chemotherapists.

The postchemotherapy surgical approach is considered in most cases where complete resection without tumor incision is compatible with preserving the patient's quality of life.

Postoperative irradiation takes into account the histologic response to chemotherapy and is indicated when microscopic or gross disease is documented at surgery.

A combined surgical and radiotherapeutic approach seems to be of particular value in locally advanced tumors where previous results after radiotherapy alone suggested some degree of radioresistance.[22,23,24] Radical irradiation remains essential when resection is not technically practicable.

Local control rates with multimodal therapies reported in recent updates are excellent, up to 95%.[23]

Radiotherapeutic technique for localized Ewing's sarcoma

Radiation technique is a prognostic factor for local control in Ewing's sarcoma as demonstrated by comparison of the CESS 81 and CESS 86 trials, where quality assurance in radiotherapy was part of the protocol with a central treatment planning program.[23]

Dose

The recommended doses for definitive irradiation are 45 Gy to the entire medullary cavity, often excluding the opposite epiphysis, and 55–60 Gy to the primary site. In postoperative situations, these doses are adapted to the histologic findings, from 45 Gy in good responders to 60 Gy for small volume boost when residual gross disease has been documented.

Conventionally fractionated irradiation delivers one daily fraction of 1.8–2 Gy 5 days per week. Reduced doses of 35 Gy in favorable cases (<8 cm in diameter and good response to preinduction chemotherapy) have been proposed in pediatric series[25] but should not be advised until further analysis confirms their effectiveness in local control.

Studies using altered fractionation schemes, such as hyperfractionated split course irradiation[23] (twice daily 1.6 Gy, break of 12 days after 22.4 Gy and 44.8 Gy total dose) or hyperfractionated irradiation[26] (twice daily 1.2 Gy to 36 Gy for initial volumes, 50.4 Gy total dose with complete regression of soft tissue mass, 55.2 Gy with partial response >50% and 60 Gy for bad responders), have demonstrated their usefulness. For pelvic, vertebral and rib lesions, technical modalities and total dose must take into account the tolerance doses of surrounding critical organs.

Volume

A precise estimate of the prechemotherapy intraosseous and adjacent soft tissue primary tumor extent is fundamental both in extremities and central locations. This is helped by computed tomography and magnetic resonance imaging.[23,27]

A traditional primary target volume includes the entire medullary cavity (exclusion of the opposite epiphysis appears to be safe) and a 3–5 cm margin beyond the soft tissue extension. However, sites of local recurrence are predominantly within the primary tumor volume and marginal failures occur infrequently.[28] This has led to proposals of diminished treatment volumes in tumors less than 8 cm in diameter in order to reduce adverse late effects.

Preliminary analysis confirms the efficacy of these 'tailored fields'.[25]

Radiation therapy for high-risk Ewing's sarcoma

Intensification protocols for high-risk localized or metastatic Ewing's sarcoma, including total body irradiation and autologous bone marrow transplant, have been used with variable results.[29,30]

A possible advantage of local irradiation to sites of metastatic disease at diagnosis (osseous and lung), if not completely surgically resected, has been reported.[31,32]

OSTEOSARCOMA

Before the era of chemotherapy, the 5-year survival rate after surgical ablation alone or exclusive radiotherapy did not exceed 20% because of early distant metastases. The treatment philosophy as defined by Cade was to spare unnecessary amputation in patients who will develop pulmonary metastasis. Delayed amputation was performed 6 months after primary radiation therapy in selected patients in whom there was no evidence of metastasis.[33,34,35]

At present, radiation treatment to the primary lesions is most often limited to surgically inaccessible sites: axial sites, frontal bones, base of skull, non-resectable pelvic bone sites and maxilla and mandible which demonstrate a high rate of local recurrences.

Preoperative radiotherapy has used doses up to 35 Gy after primary chemotherapy in order to increase limb salvage procedures.[36] An overall response rate of 81% has recently been reported[37] at sites irradiated with a hypofractionated accelerated radiotherapy protocol in patients with synchronous metastases or refusing amputation.

Because early studies indicated a relative resistance to irradiation of osteosarcomas with tumor sterilization at doses above 80–100 Gy[38] and persistence of tumor under 50 Gy, recommended doses in combination with chemotherapy should reach 60–75 Gy with conventional fractionation when normal tissue tolerance allows for it, with progressive shrinking of the treatment volume.

Three-dimensional computerized treatment planning and combination of proton and photon could offer technical possibilities of delivering higher doses to challenging locations.[39]

Radiotherapy provides a rapid and durable reduction of pain and should be considered for palliation of bone metastases. The benefit of whole lung irradiation to prevent the development of pulmonary metastases still has to be proven.[40,41]

CHONDROSARCOMA

Although considered as radioresistant, chondrosarcoma has been successfully controlled by irradiation which offers an alternative treatment when the lesion cannot be radically excised.[42,43]

Five-year actuarial survival rates of 48% are reported in well and moderately differentiated chondrosarcoma of the pelvic or shoulder girdle, axial skeleton, head and neck, rib or sternum. In unfavorable histology (mesenchymal, poorly or dedifferentiated) survival was 22%.[42]

The following indications are recommended: technically unresectable tumors without unacceptable morbidity, postoperative gross residual tumor or microscopically invaded margins and recurrence following local excision.[44]

Curative doses should reach 65–70 Gy with standard fractionation and effective palliation requires 50 Gy.

The postirradiation clinical regression is slow and takes many months. The affected bone never returns to a normal radiological aspect.

Aggressive mesenchymal chondrosarcomas are relatively radiosensitive, probably because of the round cell component.[45]

Due to their physical characteristics, the use of proton beams may optimize the dose distribution in critical locations such as base of skull and cervical spine where central nervous system structures limit both conventional radiation technique and surgical resection. An increment in dose of 15–35% is allowed and results of fractionated proton radiation therapy in combination with photons support the increase in control rate of these locally aggressive tumors.[46] Other charged particles have also provided promising results.[47]

MALIGNANT FIBROUS HISTIOCYTOMA AND FIBROSARCOMA OF BONE

Malignant fibrous histiocytoma (MFH) of bone is a rare high-grade bone tumor. The serious prognosis due to early dissemination suggests the need for adjuvant chemotherapy. The primary local treatment is a radical surgical resection. Control of the primary tumor is a critical problem and local recurrence occurs frequently.[48]

When adequate surgery cannot be achieved, radiotherapy should be considered, as also in palliative situations (metastatic disease, advanced age).

The primary local treatment of fibrosarcoma of bone with surgery and radiotherapy is limited to unresectable tumor and advanced metastatic disease.[49]

CHORDOMA

There has been little evidence of permanent local cure of chordomas with conventional megavoltage irradiation.

For this slow-growing tumor, long-term survival free of tumor regrowth over 10 years is rare although prolonged symptomatic relief was obtained with doses of 40–70 Gy.[50,51]

Location to critical sites such as sacrum and base of skull or adjacent to neurologic structures and a bone infiltration growth pattern make complete excision rarely feasible. The high rate of local recurrence and complications led to evaluation of postoperative charged particle irradiation for these locations[46,47,52] and the preliminary results of this optimized procedure are in favor of an increased local control.

GIANT CELL TUMOR OF BONE AND OTHER BENIGN BONE TUMORS

Although giant cell tumors demonstrate a high potential for local recurrence, radiation therapy has been reserved in the past for cases where complete resection was impossible, mostly in the spine. This followed the report that ionizing radiation increased the risk of malignant transformation of these tumors.[53]

Recent long-term follow-up studies of tumors irradiated because of inoperability or gross or microscopic postoperative residual disease did not report any case of radioinduced cancer among 21 patients. The most common megavoltage radiation regimen was 35 Gy in 15 fractions over 3 weeks.[16]

Before indicating radiation therapy for benign bone disease, one should consider the natural history of the lesion and the risk–benefit ratio of radiation treatment in comparison to other therapies. Indeed, irradiation should be limited to rare cases inaccessible to surgical treatment and with known radioresponsiveness, such as aneurysmal bone cyst,[54] vertebral hemangioma[55] or eosinophilic granuloma of bone.[56,57]

LYMPHOMAS OF BONE

Involvement of bone as a single extralymphatic site (stage IE) is rare and evaluation for dissemination has to be performed.

Treatment of stage IE non-Hodgkin's lymphoma of bone with favorable histology relies on radiotherapy of the entire involved bone up to 40 Gy with a boost of 10 Gy to the tumor area. In unfavorable histologies, radiotherapy is delivered after primary chemotherapy and includes regional lymph nodes.

An excellent local control is obtained for this radiosensitive tumor.[58] A recent report of four cases of Hodgkin's disease presenting as apparently solitary bone tumors demonstrated nodal involvement and potential for long-term survival could be obtained after aggressive combination treatment.[59]

Chemotherapy is considered according to the stage of the disease and for children responding to multiagent chemotherapy, the need for radiation therapy is questioned.[60]

SOLITARY PLASMACYTOMA OF BONE

Patients with plasma cell neoplasms rarely present with solitary bone lesions. Although it has been stated that most of them will develop systemic disease if followed over a sufficient period, long-term survival is significantly better than for multiple myeloma. Long-term local control of this radioresponsive tumor is obtained with doses of 40–50 Gy to the entire medullary cavity of the bone followed by a 10–15 Gy boost to the tumor site.[61,62]

BONE METASTASES

Radiotherapy is an essential tool for the treatment of bone metastases.

The mechanical threat due to destruction of the medullary structure and the cortical bone has to be considered first. Pathologic or impending fracture requires primary surgery to permit reliable stabilization of tumor defects and improve ambulation. Postoperative radiation therapy is always applied in order to limit the risk of local extension or recurrence. This attitude seems particularly important for lung and colorectal tumors and melanoma which tend not to heal.[63]

For limited osteolytic radioresponsive lesions such as secondary tumors of the breast, delayed bone reossification is obtained in more than 70% of cases.[64]

Around 80% of patients will have partial pain relief occurring as soon as 2 weeks after the completion of treatment. This rate increases until 3 months later.[65] Patients with prostate and breast primaries demonstrate a higher frequency of complete relief.

Various dose fractionation schedules have been proposed. Higher total radiation doses (2.7 Gy × 15 and 3 Gy × 10) appear to be associated with improved outcome when compared to short course programs (3 Gy × 5, 4 Gy × 5, 5 Gy × 5).[66]

Several factors have to be considered before determining the most appropriate radiation therapy strategy and technique: patient's performance status and symptoms, nature and prognosis of the disease, single or multiple sites of metastases, previous radiation treatment and distribution of bone marrow in the field with respect to myelosuppressive chemotherapy.

Hemibody irradiation has been used for widely disseminated bone metastases.[67]

The effectiveness of radiation therapy for metastatic spinal cord compression in combination with surgery or alone has recently been analyzed.[68] Early diagnosis, favorable histology and appropriate selection of patients are the most important factors governing the preservation of neurologic function.

Acknowledgments

We are most grateful to M.P. Marchand for her kind technical assistance and to L. Bonvalet for the dosimetry studies.

REFERENCES

1. Eifel P J, Donaldson S S, Thomas P R M. Response of growing bone to irradiation: a proposed late effects scoring system. Int J Radiat Oncol Biol Phys 1995: 31: 1301–1307
2. Gonzalez D G, Van Dijk J D P. Experimental studies on the response of growing bones to X ray and neutron irradiation. Int J Radiat Oncol Bio Phys 1983: 9: 671–677
3. Gonzalez D G, Breur K. Clinical data from irradiated growing long bones in children. Int Radiat Oncol Biol Phys 1983: 9: 841–846
4. Probert J C, Parker B R. The effects of radiation therapy on bone growth. Radiology 1975: 114: 155–162
5. Willman K Y, Cox R S, Donaldson S S. Radiation induced height impairment in pediatric Hodgkin's disease. Int J Radiat Oncol Biol Phys 1993: 28: 85–92
6. Eifel P J, Sampson C M, Tucker S L. Radiation fractionation sensitivity of epiphyseal cartilage in a weanling rat model. Int J Radiat Oncol Biol Phys 1990: 19: 661–664
7. Rubin P, Cassarett G W. Clinical radiation pathology, vols I and II. Philadelphia: WB Saunders, 1968
8. Stinson S F, Delaney T F, Greenberg J et al. Acute and long-term effects on limb function of combined modality limb sparing therapy for extremity soft tissue sarcoma. Int J Radiat Oncol Biol Phys 1991: 21: 1493–1499
9. Karasek K, Constine L S, Rosier R. Sarcoma therapy: functional outcome and relationship to treatment parameters. Int J Radiat Oncol Biol Phys 1992: 24: 651–656
10. Gillette E L, Mahler P A, Powers B E, Gillette S M, Vujaskovic Z. Late radiation injury to muscle and peripheral nerves. Int J Radiat Oncol Biol Phys 1995: 31: 1309–1318
11. Tucker M A, D'Angio G J, Boice J D et al. Bone sarcomas linked to radiotherapy and chemotherapy in children. N Engl J Med 1987: 317: 588–593
12. Newton W A, Meadows A T, Shimada H, Bunin G R, Vawter G F. Bone sarcomas as second malignant neoplasms following childhood cancer. Cancer 1991: 67: 193–201
13. Strong L C, Herson J, Osborne B M, Sutow W W. Risk of radiation: related subsequent malignant tumors in survivors of Ewing's sarcoma. J Natl Cancer Inst 1979: 62: 1401–1406
14. Steiner G C. Postradiation sarcoma of bone. Cancer 1965: 18: 603–612
15. Sim F H, Cupps R E, Dahlin D C, Ivins J C. Postradiation sarcoma of bone. J Bone Joint Surg (Am) 1972: 54: 1479–1489
16. Malone S, O'Sullivan B, Catton C, Bell R, Fornasier V, Davis A. Long-term follow-up of efficacy and safety of megavoltage radiotherapy in high-risk giant cell tumors of bone. Int J Radiat Oncol Biol Phys 1995: 33: 689–694
17. Ewing J. Diffuse endothelioma of bone. Proc N Y Pathol Soc 1921: 21: 17–24
18. Kinsella T J, Miser J S, Waller B et al. Long-term follow-up of Ewing's sarcoma of bone treated with combined modality therapy. Int J Radiat Oncol Biol Phys 1991: 20: 389–395
19. Nesbit M E, Gehan E A, Burgert O et al. Multimodal therapy for the management of primary, monometastatic Ewing's sarcoma of bone: a long-term follow-up of the first intergroup study. J Clin Oncol 1990: 8: 1664–1674
20. Kinsella T J, Lichter A S, Miser J, Gerber L, Glastein E. Local treatment of Ewing's sarcoma: radiation therapy versus surgery. Cancer Treat Rep 1984: 68: 695–701
21. Thomas P R M, Perez C A, Neff J R, Nesbit M E, Evans R G. The management of Ewing's sarcoma: role of radiotherapy in local tumor control. Cancer Treat Rep 1984: 68: 703–710
22. Jürgens H, Exner U, Gadner H et al. Multidisciplinary treatment of primary Ewing's sarcoma of bone. Cancer 1988: 61: 23–32
23. Dunst J, Jürgens H, Sauer R et al. Radiation therapy in Ewing's sarcoma: an update of the CESS 86 trial. Int J Radiat Oncol Biol Phys 1995: 32: 919–930
24. Jenkin R D. Ewing's sarcoma: radiation treatment at the primary site. Int J Radiat Oncol Biol Phys 1995; 32: 1253–1254. Comments about

Dunst J Hurgens H Saur R. Radiation therapy in Ewing's sarcoma: an update CESS trial. Int J Radiat Oncol Biol Phys 1995; 32: 919–930

25. Arai Y, Kun L E, Brooks M T et al. Ewing's sarcoma: local tumor control and patterns of failure following limited-volume radiation therapy. Int J Radiat Oncol Biol Phys 1991: 21: 1501–1508

26. Marcus R B, Cantor A, Heare T C, Graham-Pole J, Mendenhall N P, Million R R. Local control and function after twice-a-day radiotherapy for Ewing's sarcoma of bone. Int J Radiat Oncol Biol Phys 1991: 21: 1509–1515

27. Evans R G, Nesbit M E, Gehan E A et al. Multimodal therapy for the management of localized Ewing's sarcoma of pelvic and sacral bones: a report from the second intergroup study. J Clin Oncol 1991: 9: 1173–1180

28. Brown A P, Fixsen J A, Plowman P N. Local control of Ewing's sarcoma: an analysis of 67 patients. Br Radiol 1987: 60: 261–268

29. Marcus R B, Graham-Pole J R, Springfield D S et al. High-risk Ewing's sarcoma: end-intensification using autologous bone marrow transplantation. Int J Radiat Oncol Biol Phys 1988: 15: 53–59

30. Horowitz M E, Kinsella T J, Wexler L H et al. Total-body irradiation and autologus bone marrow transplant in the treatment of high-risk Ewing's sarcoma and rhabdomyosarcoma. J Clin Oncol 1993: 11: 1911–1918

31. Hayes F A, Thompson E I, Parvey L et al. Metastatic Ewing's sarcoma: remission induction and survival. J Clin Oncol 1987: 5: 1199–1204

32. Cangir A, Vietti T J, Gehan E A et al. Ewing's sarcoma metastatic at diagnosis. Cancer 1990: 66: 887–893

33. Stanley L E, Mackenzie D H. Osteosarcoma. A study of the value of preoperative megavoltage radiotherapy. Br J Surg 1964: 51: 252–274

34. Sweetnam R, Knowelden J, Seddon H. Bone sarcoma: treatment by irradiation, amputation, or a combination of the two. Br Med J 1971: 2: 363–367

35. Jenkin R D T, Allt W E, Fitzpatrick P J. Osteosarcoma. An assessment of management with particular reference to primary irradiation and selective delayed amputation. Cancer 1972: 30: 393–400

36. Eilber F R, Mirra J J, Grant T T, Weisenburger T, Morton D L. Is amputation necessary for sarcomas? A seven-year experience with limb salvage. Ann Surg 1980: 192: 431–438

37. Lombardi F, Gandola L, Fossati-Bellani F, Gianni M C, Rottoli L, Gasparini M. Hypofractionated accelerated radiotherapy in osteogenic sarcoma. Int J Radiat Oncol Biol Phys 1992: 24: 761–765

38. Gaintan-Yanguas M. A study of the response of osteogenic sarcoma and adjacent normal tissues to radiation. Int J Radiat Oncol Biol Phys 1981: 7: 593–595

39. Hug E, Fitzek M, Liebsch N, Munzenrider J E. Locally challenging osteo- and chondrogenic tumors of the axial skeleton: results of combined proton and photon radiation therapy using three-dimensional treatment planning. Int J Radiat Oncol Biol Phys 1995: 31: 467–476

40. Burgers J M V, Van Glabbeke M, Busson A et al. Osteosarcoma of the limbs. Cancer 1988: 61: 1024–1031

41. Marina N H, Pratt C B, Rao B N, Schema S J, Meyer W H. Improved prognosis of children with osteosarcoma metastatic to the lung at the time of diagnosis. Cancer 1992: 70: 2722–2727

42. Krochak R, Harwood A R, Cummings B J, Quirt I C. Results of radical radiation for chondrosarcoma of bone. Radiother Oncol 1983: 1: 109–115

43. McNaney D, Lindberg R D, Ayala A G, Barkley H T, Hussey D H. Fifteen year radiotherapy experience with chondrosarcoma of bone. Int J Radiat Oncol Biol Phys 1982: 8: 187–190

44. Harwood A R, Ivan Krajbich J I, Fornasier V L. Radiotherapy of chondrosarcoma of bone. Cancer 1980: 45: 2769–2777

45. Huvos A G, Rosen G, Dabska M, Marcove R C. Mesenchymal chondrosarcoma. Cancer 1983: 51: 1230–1236

46. Austin-Seymour M, Munzenrider J, Linggodd R et al. Fractionated proton radiation therapy of cranial and intracanial tumors. Am J Clin Oncol 1990: 13: 327–330

47. Castro J R, Linstadt D E, Bahary J P et al. Experience in charged particle irradiation of tumors of the skull base: 1977–1992. Int J Radiat Oncol Biol Phys 1994: 29: 647–655

48. Bacci G, Springfield D, Capanna R, Picci P, Bertoni F, Campaccini M. Adjuvant chemotherapy for malignant fibrous histiocytoma in the femur and tibia. J Bone Joint Surg (Am) 1985: 67: 620–625

49. Huvos A G, Higinbotham N L. Primary fibrosarcoma of bone. A clinicopathologic study of 130 patients. Cancer 1975: 35: 837–847

50. Cummings B J, Ian Hodson D, Bush R S. Chordoma: the results of megavoltage radiation therapy. Int J Radiat Oncol Biol Phys 1983: 9: 633–642

51. Fuller D B, Bloom J G. Radiotherapy for chordoma. Int J Radiat Oncol Biol Phys 1988: 15: 331–339

52. Schoenthaler R, Castrio J R, Petti P L, Baken-Brown K, Philipps T L. Charged particle irradiation of sacral chordomas. Int J Radiat Oncol Biol Phys 1993: 26: 291–298

53. Dahlin D C. Giant-cell tumor or vertebrae above the sacrum. Cancer 1977: 39: 1350–1356

54. Hay M C, Paterson D, Taylor T K. Aneurysmal bone cysts of the spine. J Bone Joint Surg (Br) 1978: 78: 406–411

55. Faria S L, Schlupp W R, Chimionazzo H. Radiotherapy in the treatment of vertebral hemangiomas. Int J Radiat Oncol Biol Phys 1985: 11: 387–390

56. Ochsner S F. Eosinophilic granuloma of bone. Experience with 20 cases. AJR 1966: 97: 719–726

57. Grennberger J S, Cassady J R, Jaffe N, Vawter G, Crocker A C. Radiation therapy in patients with histiocytosis: management of diabetes insipidus and bone lesions. Int J Radiat Oncol Biol Phys 1979: 5: 1749–1755

58. Mendenhall N P, Jones J J, Kramer B S et al. The management of primary lymphoma of bone. Radiother Oncol 1987: 9: 137–145

59. Ozdemirli M, Mankin H J, Aisenberg A C, Harris N L. Hodgkin's disease presenting as a solitary bone tumor. Cancer 1996: 77: 79–88

60. Loeffler J S, Tarbell N J, Kozakewich H, Cassady R, Weinstein H J. Primary lymphoma of bone in children: analysis of treatment results with adriamycin, prednisone, oncovin (APO), and local radiation therapy. J Clin Oncol 1986: 4: 496–501

61. Greenberg P, Parker R G, Fu Y S, Abemayor E. The treatment of solitary plasmacytoma of bone and extramedullary plasmacytoma. Am J Clin Oncol 1987: 10: 199–204

62. Mill W B, Griffith R. The role of radiation therapy in the management of plasma cell tumors. Cancer 1980: 45: 647–652

63. Gainor B J, Buchert P. Fracture healing in metastatic bone disease. Clin Orthop 1983: 178: 297–302

64. Garmatis C J, Chu F C H. The effectiveness of radiation therapy in the treatment of bone metastases from breast cancer. Radiology 1978: 126: 235

65. Tong D, Gillick L, Hendrickson F R. The palliation of symptomatic osseous metastases. Final results of the study by the radiation therapy oncology group. Cancer 1982: 50: 893–899

66. Blitzer P H. Reanalysis of the RTOG study of the palliation of symptomatic osseous metastasis. Cancer 1985: 55: 1468–1472

67. Salazar O M, Rubin P, Hendrickson F R et al. Single-dose half-body irradiation for palliation of multiple bone metastases from solid tumor. Cancer 1986: 58: 29–36

68. Maranzano E, Latini P. Effectiveness of radiation therapy without surgery in metastatic spinal cord compression: final results from a prospective trial. Int J Radiat Oncol Biol Phys 1995: 32: 959–967

A library for the pathologist

M. Forest

The classic and invaluable books around the microscope

Bullough P G. Bullough and Vigorita's orthopaedic pathology. 3rd ed. London: Mosby-Wolfe, 1997

Campanacci M. Bone and soft tissue tumors. Wien: Springer, 1990

Dorfman H D, Czerniak B. Bone tumors. St Louis: Mosby, 1997

Fechner R E, Mills S E. Tumors of the bones and joints. Atlas of tumor pathology, 3rd series, fasc 8. Washington: AFIP, 1993

Huvos A G. Bone tumors. 2nd ed. Philadelphia: W B Saunders, 1991

Milgram J W. Radiologic and histologic pathology of nontumorous diseases of bones and joints. South Lane Northbrook: Northbrook Publishing, 1990

Mirra J M. Bone tumors. Philadelphia: Lea & Febiger, 1989

Resnick D. Diagnosis of bone and joint disorders. 3rd ed. Philadelphia: W B Saunders, 1995

Schajowicz F. Tumors and tumorlike lesions of bone. 2nd ed. Berlin: Springer, 1994

Unni K K. Dahlin's bone tumors. 5th ed. Philadelphia: Lippincott-Raven, 1996

And more, for the passionate

Ackerman L V, Spjut H J, Abell M R, Eds. Bones and joints. Monographs in pathology no 17. Baltimore: Williams & Wilkins, 1976

Adler C P. Knochen-Krankheiten. Stuttgart: Georg Thieme, 1983

Adler C P, Kozlowski K. Primary bone tumors and tumorous conditions in children. London: Springer, 1993

Aegerter E, Kirkpatrick J A. Orthopedic diseases. 4th ed. Philadelphia: WB Saunders, 1975

Bartl R, Frish B. Biopsy of bone in internal medicine. Current histopathology vol 21. Dordrecht: Kluwer, 1993

Berry C L, Ed. Bone and joint disease. Curr topics in pathology vol 71. Berlin: Springer, 1982

Bogumill G P, Schwamm HA. Orthopedic pathology. Philadelphia: W B Saunders, 1984

Bonucci E, Motta P M, Eds. Ultrastructure of skeletal tissues. Boston: Kluwer, 1990

Bullough P G, Boachi-Adjei O. Atlas of spinal diseases. Philadelphia: J B Lippincott, 1988

Dominok G W, Knoch H G. Knochengeschwülste und geschwulstähnliche Knochenerkrankungen. 3rd ed. Stuttgart: Gustav Fisher, 1982

Fechner R E, Spjut H J, Haggitt R C. Diseases of bones and joints. Chicago: American Society of Clinical Pathology Press, 1986

Feldman F, Ed. Radiology, pathology, and immunology of bones and joints: a review of current concepts. New York: Appleton-Century-Crofts, 1978

Freyschmidt J, Ostertag H. Knochen-tumoren. Berlin: Springer, 1988

Greenfield G B, Arrington J A, Eds. Imaging of bone tumors. Philadelphia: J B Lippincott, 1995

Grundmann E, Ed. Malignant bone tumors. Recent results of cancer research vol 54. Berlin: Springer, 1976

Hajdu S I, Hajdu E O. Cytopathology of soft tissue and bone tumors. Monographs in clinical cytology vol 12. Basel: Karger, 1989

Hirohata K, Morimoto K, Kimura H. Ultrastructure of bone and joint diseases. 2nd ed. Tokyo: Igaku-Shoin, 1981

Hudson T M. Radiologic-pathologic correlation of musculoskeletal lesions. Baltimore: Williams & Wilkins, 1987

Jacobson S A. The comparative pathology of the tumors of bone. Springfield: Charles C Thomas, 1971

Jaffe H L. Tumors and tumorous conditions of the bones and joints. Philadelphia: Lea & Febiger, 1958

Jaffe H L. Metabolic, degenerative, and inflammatory diseases of bones and joints. Philadelphia: Lea & Febiger, 1972

Kricun M E. Imaging of bone tumors. Philadelphia: W B Saunders, 1993

Lichtenstein L. Diseases of bone and joints. 2nd ed. St Louis: C V Mosby, 1975

Lichtenstein L. Bone tumors. 5th ed. St Louis: C V Mosby, 1977

Lodwick G S. The bones & joints. Chicago: Year Book Medical Publishers, 1971

Marcove R C, Arlen M. Atlas of bone pathology. Philadelphia: J B Lippincott, 1992

McCarthy E F. Differential diagnosis in Pathology: Bone and Joint Disorders. New York: Igaku-Shoin, 1996

Mazabraud A. Anatomie pathologique osseuse tumorale. Paris: Springer, 1994

Moser R P. Cartilaginous tumors of the skeleton. AFIP atlas of radiologic-pathologic correlation. Fasc II. Philadelphia: Hanley & Belfus, 1990

Mulder J D, Schütte H E, Kroon H M, Taconis W K. Radiologic atlas of bone tumors. Amsterdam: Elsevier, 1993

Novak J F, McMaster J H, Eds. Frontiers of osteosarcoma research. Seattle: Hogrefe & Huber, 1993

Petterson H, Springfield D S, Enneking W F. Radiologic management of musculoskeletal tumors. New York: Springer, 1987

Price C H, Ross F G, Eds. Bone–certain aspects of neoplasia. London: Butterworth, 1973

Ranniger K, Ed. Bone tumors. Encyclopedia of medical radiology. Part 6 Diseases of the skeletal system vol V. Berlin: Springer, 1977

Revell P A. Pathology of bone. Berlin: Springer, 1986

Roessner A. Zur Zyto-und Histogenese der malignen und semimalignen Knochentumoren. Stuttgart: Gustav Fischer, 1984

Roessner A, Ed. Biological characterization of bone tumors. Current topics in pathology vol 80. Berlin: Springer, 1989

Rubens R D, Fogelman I, Eds. Bone metastases. London: Springer, 1991

Salisbury J R, Woods C G, Byers P D, Eds. Diseases of bones and joints. London: Chapman & Hall, 1994

Sandberg A A, Bridge J A. The cytogenetics of bone and soft tissue tumors. New York: Springer, 1995

Sanerkin N G, Jeffree G M. Cytology of bone tumours. Bristol: John Wright, 1980

Schajowicz F. Histological typing of bone tumours. WHO international histological classification of tumours. 2nd ed. Berlin: Springer, 1993

Schwamm H A, Millward C L. Histologic differential diagnosis of skeletal lesions. New York: Igaku-Shoin, 1995

Schulz A. Ultrastruktur-pathologie der Knochentumoren. Stuttgart: Gustav Fischer, 1980

Sissons H A, Murray R O, Kemp H B. Orthopaedic diagnosis. Berlin: Springer, 1984

Sundaresan N, Schmidek H H, Schiller A L, Rosenthal D I, Eds. Tumors of the spine. Philadelphia: W B Saunders, 1990

Uhthoff H K, Stahl E, Eds. Current concepts of diagnosis and treatment of bone and soft tissue tumors. Berlin: Springer, 1984

Unni K K, Ed. Bone tumors. Contemporary issues in surgical pathology vol 11. New York: Churchill Livingstone, 1988

Wilner D. Radiology of bone tumors and allied disorders. Philadelphia: W B Saunders, 1982

Wold L E, McLeod R A, Sim F H, Unni K K. Atlas of orthopedic pathology. Philadelphia: W B Saunders, 1990

Woods C G. Diagnostic orthopaedic pathology. Oxford: Blackwell, 1972

Index